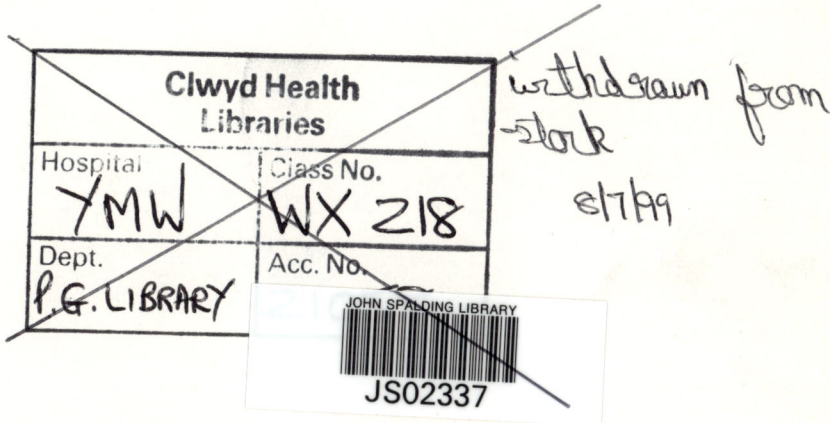
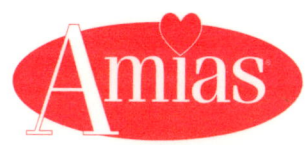

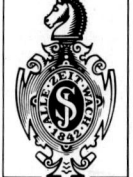

Care of the Critically Ill Patient

Edited by
Jack Tinker and Maurice Rapin

With 305 Figures

Springer-Verlag
Berlin Heidelberg New York 1983

Jack Tinker, BSc, FRCS, FRCP, DIC
Director, Intensive Therapy Unit
The Middlesex Hospital
London W1N 8AA, England

Maurice Rapin, MD
Chef du Service de Réanimation Médicale
Hôpital Henri Mondor
F-94010 Creteil, France

ISBN 3-540-11289-8 Springer-Verlag Berlin Heidelberg New York
ISBN 0-387-11289-8 Springer-Verlag New York Heidelberg Berlin

Library of Congress Cataloging in Publication Data
Main entry under title:
Care of the critically ill patient. Includes bibliographies and index. 1. Critical care medicine.
2. Critically ill. I. Tinker, Jack, 1936 — II. Rapin, Maurice. [DNLM: 1. Critical care. WX 218 C271]
RC86.7.C375 1982 616'. 028 82-5999
ISBN 0-387-11289-8 'U.S.) AACR2

Typeset by Polyglot Pte Ltd, 10 Dundee Road, Singapore 0314.
Printed and bound by William Clowes (Beccles) Ltd, Beccles, Suffolk.

2128/3916-543210

Preface

During the past decade there has been a considerable expansion in the understanding, assessment and treatment of critically ill patients. An attempt to portray our present knowledge of this diverse field in a comprehensive textbook is therefore a formidable and daunting undertaking. However, many colleagues in different disciplines and from different countries convinced us of the need for such a work and, greatly encouraged by their interest, we embarked upon the project.

Any single text, even a very long one, cannot cover every aspect of critical illness. Our first task was, therefore, to define those areas of the subject that had to be included. This we did on a systematic basis, and although the final emphasis of the book is very largely directed to clinical matters, we felt it pertinent to include in some detail accounts of relevant physiology and technology.

Care of the Critically Ill Patient is divided into twelve sections, each concerned with major facets of critical illness; each of the sixty-eight chapters includes a topical and often extensive bibliography. The many chosen contributors form an international group of specialists whose combined expertise embraces the topics that we have selected.

Editing presented certain conflicts and the final blend conveys our efforts to resolve these. Some material is intentionally repeated both for the convenience of the reader and also to place emphasis on certain issues. The aim has been to produce a comprehensive work of reference, and we hope that the book will provide a breadth of detailed and relevant information for the guidance of everyone who has to care for critically ill patients. For this we thank all who have contributed for their obvious professional expertise and for their collaboration during the many stages of preparation. It is difficult to make proper acknowledgement to the many people who, in smaller or larger measures, have helped to make the venture possible. It has been a particular pleasure to be associated with Springer-Verlag and we owe a special debt to Michael Jackson for his constant help, guidance and enthusiasm. Copy editing constituted a mammoth task which has been performed with outstanding skill, tact and considerable patience by Janet Dodsworth and Lindsay Toms. For putting all the pieces together so elegantly we thank Roger Dobbing and his staff.

For the editors nothing could have been achieved without the help of our secretaries Sonia Crossley and Helene Enjalbert. We owe a special debt of gratitude to Sonia Crossley for coordinating the recruitment and preparation of the manuscripts. By her patience and persistence she provided a tactful and effective liaison between authors, editors and publishers.

London and Paris
1982

Jack Tinker
Maurice Rapin

Acknowledgements

The following wish to acknowledge support for work published in this volume:

Warren M. Zapol, Robert L. Trelstad, Michael T. Snider, Henning Pontoppidan and François Lemaire (Chap. 18)—supported by NHLBI SCOR Grant HL 23591.

Richard D. Goodenough and John F. Burke (Chap. 38)— partially supported by USPH GM 21700–06 and GM 07035–05.

H. J. C. Swan and William Ganz (Chap. 57)—funded in part by NIH SCOR Grant #HL 17651.

Mary Ellen Leder Skalina, Richard J. Martin, and Avroy A. Fanaroff (Chap. 66)—supported in part by training grant 5–T32–HD07132–02.

Chapter 44 by Peter Safar was in part copied or adapted from some of the author's other publications on the subject (references [62–69] of that chapter).

Contents

Contributors

A. P. Adams,
Professor of Anaesthetics,
Guy's Hospital,
London, England

Maurice S. Albin,
Professor of Anesthesiology and Neurosurgery,
Director, Neuroanesthesia Service,
The University of Texas Health Center,
San Antonio, Texas, U.S.A.

Y. Aujard,
Maître de Conférence Agrégé,
Neonatal Unit,
Clinique de Pédiatrie de la Faculté Xavier Bichat,
Hôpital Bretonneau,
Paris, France

P. Babinet,
Service de Médecine,
Hôpital Delafontaine,
Saint–Denis, France

Maciej F. Babinski,
Associate Professor of Anesthesiology,
The University of Texas Health Science Center,
San Antonio,
Texas, U.S.A.

K. Balakumaran,
Thoraxcenter,
University Hospital "Dijkzigt",
Rotterdam, The Netherlands

Peter J. Barnes,
Physician,
Royal Postgraduate Medical School,
Hammersmith Hospital,
London, England

F. Beaufils,
Maître de Conférence Agrégé,
Medical Director,
Clinique de Pédiatrie de la Faculté Xavier Bichat,
Hôpital Bretonneau,
Paris, France

Arnold W. Berlin,
Assistant Professor of Surgery,
Albert Einstein College of Medicine;
North Central Bronx Hospital,
New York, U.S.A.

David J. Bihari,
Physician,
King's College Hospital,
London, England

Chantal Bismuth,
Associate Professor of Medicine,
Université de Paris VII;
Department of Toxicology,
Hôpital Fernand Widal,
Paris, France

Y. Bompard,
Maître de Conférence Agrégé,
Chef de Clinique Assistant,
Pediatric Intensive Care Unit,
Hôpital Bretonneau,
Paris, France

Jean–Louis Bourdain,
Centre Hospitalier Intercommunal Léon Touhladjian,
Poissy, France

Paul Bowden,
Consultant Psychiatrist,
Bethlem Royal and Maudsley Hospitals,
London, England

Marialuisa Bozza–Marrubini,
Professor of Neurology,
Servizio di Anestesia e Rianimazione I°,
Ente Ospedaliero Niguarda–Ca' Granda,
Milan, Italy

W. C. Brownlee,
Cardiologist,
The Royal Infirmary,
Manchester, England

Christian Brun-Buisson,
Centre Hospitalier Intercommunal Léon Touhladjian,
Poissy, France

John F. Burke,
Helen Andrus Benedict Professor of Surgery,
Chief of Trauma Services,
Massachusetts General Hospital and Harvard
Medical School,
Boston,
Massachusetts, U.S.A.

F. Cartier,
Professeur de Clinique des Maladies Infectieuses,
Service de Réanimation Médicale,
Hôpital Pontchaillou,
Rennes, France

J. H. Chamberlain,
Consultant Clinical Physiologist,
Guy's Hospital,
London, England

Antoine Chapman,
Professor and Head of Department of Internal Medicine,
Faculté de Médecine Paris–Ouest,
C. M. C. Foch,
Suresnes, France

J. Chastre,
Hôpital Boucicaut,
Paris, France

A. Cornil,
Chef, Service de Réanimation,
Hôpital Saint Pierre,
Brussels, Belgium

G. R. Cutfield,
Overseas Research Fellow, MRC (NZ),
Nuffield Department of Anaesthetics,
The Radcliffe Infirmary,
Oxford, England

Peter Daggett,
Physician,
The Middlesex Hospital,
London, England

A. De Coster,
Chef du Département des Voies Respiratories
Hôpital Universitaire Saint–Pierre,
Brussels, Belgium

J. De Groote,
Professor,
Academisch Ziekenhuis St–Raphael,
Leuven, Belgium

Harry M. Delany,
Professor of Surgery,
Albert Einstein College of Medicine;
North Central Bronx Hospital,
Bronx,
New York, U.S.A.

Leslie Donaldson,
Surgeon,
University Department of Surgery,
Glasgow Royal Infirmary,
Glasgow, Scotland

Robert M. Donaldson,
Cardiologist,
National Heart Hospital,
London, England

Najib Duedari,
Medical Director,
Val de Marne Blood Center,
Hôpital Henri Mondor,
Créteil, France

J. F. Duhamel,
Service de Gastroentérologie Pédiatrique et de Nutrition,
Hôpital des Enfants Malades,
Paris, France

D. Emslie–Smith,
Reader in Medicine,
Ninewells Hospital and Medical School,
Dundee, Scotland

P. L. Fagniez,
Professeur Agrégé,
Hôpital Henri Mondor,
Créteil, France

Avroy A. Fanaroff,
Professor of Pediatrics,
Rainbow Babies and Childrens Hospital,
Cleveland,
Ohio, U.S.A.

J. D. Fitzgerald,
Head of Research Department II,
ICI Limited,
Macclesfield,
Cheshire, England

D. C. Flenley,
Professor of Respiratory Medicine,
City Hospital,
Edinburgh, Scotland

William Ganz,
Professor of Medicine and Senior Research
Scientist—Cardiologist,
Cedars–Sinai Medical Center,
UCLA School of Medicine,
Los Angeles,
California, U.S.A.

Claude George,
Service de Réanimation Médicale,
Hôpital Henri Mondor,
Créteil, France

R. J. D. George,
Physician,
Central Middlesex Hospital,
London, England

Alan Gilston,
Consultant Anaesthetist,
National Heart Hospital,
London, England

Richard D. Goodenough,
Clinical and Research Fellow in Surgery,
Massachusetts General Hospital and Harvard
Medical School,
Boston,
Massachusetts, U.S.A.

M. Goulon,
Professor,
Clinique de Réanimation,
Service de Neurologie,
Hôpital Raymonde,
Garches, France

M. Haalebos,
Thoraxcenter,
University Hospital "Dijkzigt",
Rotterdam, The Netherlands

A. A. Habib,
Département de Neuro–Chirurgie,
Hôpital Lariboisière,
Paris, France

A. Harari,
Department of Anesthesiology,
Hôpital Cochin,
Paris, France

Charles E. Hartford,
Medical Director of the Burn Treatment Center,
Crozer-Chester Medical Center,
Upland,
Chester,
Pennsylvania, U.S.A.

G. B. Haycock,
Consultant Paediatric Nephrologist,
Guy's Hospital,
London, England

Edmund Hey,
Consultant Paediatric Physician,
The Princess Mary Maternity Hospital,
Newcastle upon Tyne, England

D. W. Hill,
Regional Scientific Officer,
North East Thames Regional Health Authority,
London, England

T. D. R. Hockaday,
Consultant Physician,
The Radcliffe Infirmary,
Oxford, England

P. G. Hugenholtz,
Professor of Cardiology,
Thoraxcenter,
University Hospital "Dijkzigt",
Rotterdam, The Netherlands

A. M. Joekes,
Consultant Nephrologist,
St Philip's Hospital,
London, England

Stephen N. Joffe,
Professor of Surgery,
University of Cincinnati Medical Center,
Cincinnati,
Ohio, U.S.A.

A. Kanfer,
Service de Néphrologie,
Hôpital Tenon,
Paris, France

O. Kourilsky,
Service de Néphrologie,
Hôpital Tenon,
Paris, France

J. Labrousse,
Professeur Agrégé,
Service de Réanimation et Médecine d'Urgence,
Hôpital Boucicaut,
Paris, France

C. A. Lawrence,
Research Fellow,
Institute of Urology,
London, England

William R. Lees,
Consultant Radiologist
The Middlesex Hospital,
London, England

J. R. Le Gall,
Professeur Agrégé,
Hôpital Henri Mondor,
Service de Réanimation Médicale,
Créteil, France

François Lemaire,
Professeur Agrégé,
Département de Réanimation,
Hôpital Henri Mondor,
Créteil, France

A. Levante,
Départment d'Anesthésie–Réanimation,
Hôpital Lariboisière,
Paris, France

Susan Lewis,
Former Assistant Superintendant and Senior
Intensive Care Physiotherapist,
The Middlesex Hospital,
London, England

François Lhoste,
Professeur Agrégé,
Département de Pharmacologie Clinique,
Hôpital Henri Mondor,
Créteil, France

I. Lightbody,
Lecturer in Therapeutics,
Ninewells Hospital,
Dundee, Scotland

Philippe Loirat,
Head of Intensive Care Unit,
C. M. C. Foch,
Suresnes, France

Samuel J. Machin,
Senior Lecturer
Department of Haematology,
The Middlesex Hospital,
London, England

D. Maclean,
Consultant Physician,
Ninewells Hospital,
Dundee, Scotland

P. Mannoni,
Canadian Red Cross—Blood Transfusion Service,
Edmonton,
Alberta, Canada

Richard J. Martin,
Assistant Professor of Pediatrics,
Rainbow Babies and Childrens Hospital,
Cleveland,
Ohio, U.S.A.

Jean Marty,
Interne des Hôpitaux de Paris,
Department of Anesthesiology and Intensive Care,
Hôpital Bichat,
Paris, France

Richard R. Mason,
Consultant Radiologist,
The Middlesex Hospital,
London, England

K. Messmer,
Professor of Surgery,
Klinikum der Universität Heidelberg,
Abteilung für experimentelle Chirurgie,
Heidelberg, West Germany

H. R. Michels,
Thoraxcenter,
University Hospital "Dijkzigt",
Rotterdam, The Netherlands

A. D. Milner,
Professor of Paediatric Respiratory Medicine,
University Hospital,
Queen's Medical Centre,
Nottingham, England

Jerome H. Modell,
Professor and Chairperson,
Department of Anesthesiology,
University of Florida College of Medicine,
J. Hillis Miller Health Center,
Gainesville,
Florida, U.S.A.

R. Naeije,
Service de Réanimation,
Hôpital Saint–Pierre,
Brussels, Belgium

François Nouailhat,
Consultation de Neurologie,
Centre Hospitalier Intercommunal Léon Touhladjian,
Poissy, France

Celia Oakley,
Consultant Cardiologist,
Hammersmith Hospital,
London, England

Henning Pontoppidan,
Medical Director of Respiratory/Surgical Unit,
Massachusetts General Hospital,
ARDS Specialized Center of Research,
Boston,
Massachusetts, U.S.A.

P. A. Poole–Wilson,
Reader in Cardiology and Honorary Consultant Physician,
Cardiothoracic Institute and National Heart Hospital,
London, England

David J. Price,
Consultant Neurosurgeon,
Pinderfields Hospital,
Wakefield, England

M. J. Purves,
Reader in Physiology,
University of Bristol,
Bristol, England

J. L. Ragguenea,
Département d'Anesthésie–Réanimation,
Hôpital Lariboisière,
Paris, France

Maurice Rapin,
Professor,
Service de Réanimation,
Hôpital Henri Mondor,
Créteil, France

B. Regnier
Professeur Agrégé,
Intensive Care Unit,
Hôpital Claude Bernard,
Paris, France

G. Richet,
Professor,
Service de Néphrologie,
Hôpital Tenon,
Paris, France

C. Ricour,
Professeur Agrégé,
Service de Gastroentérologie Pédiatrique et de Nutrition,
Hôpital des Enfants Malades,
Paris, France

Michael A. Rie,
Anaesthetist,
Massachusetts General Hospital,
Boston,
Massachusetts, U.S.A.

D. J. Rowlands,
Consultant Cardiologist,
Manchester Royal Infirmary,
Manchester, England

Michael Rudolf,
Consultant Physician and Honorary Senior Lecturer in Medicine
Royal Postgraduate Medical School,
Hammersmith Hospital,
London, England

W. J. Russell,
Director of Research and Development,
Royal Adelaide Hospital,
Adelaide, Australia

Peter Safar,
Distinguished Service Professor of Resuscitation Medicine,
University of Pittsburgh,
Pittsburgh,
Pennsylvania, U.S.A.

Kamran Samii,
Chef de Clinique Assistant,
Department of Anesthesiology and Intensive Care,
Hôpital Bicetre,
Le Kremlin Bicetre, France

P. W. Serruys,
Thoraxcenter,
University Hospital "Dijkzigt",
Rotterdam, The Netherlands

Harry M. Shizgal,
Professor of Surgery,
Royal Victoria Hospital,
Montreal,
Quebec, Canada

N. Simon,
Service de Réanimation,
Hôpital Léon Touhladjian,
Poissy, France

Mary Ellen Leder Skalina,
Clinical Assistant Professor of Pediatrics,
Rainbow Babies and Childrens Hospital,
Cleveland,
Ohio, U.S.A.

G. Smith,
Anaesthetist,
City Hospital,
Nottingham, England

Michael T. Snider,
Associate Professor of Anaesthesia,
University of Pennsylvania,
Hershey Medical Center,
Hershey, Pennsylvania, U.S.A.

J. D. Sraer,
Professeur Agrégé,
Service de Néphrologie,
Hôpital Tenon,
Paris, France

John M. Stevens,
Radiologist,
National Hospital for Nervous Diseases,
London, England

J. C. Stoddart,
Consultant in Charge,
Intensive Therapy Unit,
Royal Victoria Infirmary,
Newcastle Upon Tyne, England

Peter M. Suter,
Consultant in Charge,
Surgical Intensive Care Unit,
Hôpital Cantonal Universitaire,
Geneva, Switzerland

H. J. C. Swan,
Director of Cardiology,
Cedars–Sinai Medical Center,
UCLA School of Medicine,
Los Angeles,
California, U.S.A.

Barbara B. Tabeling,
Assistant Professor,
Department of Anesthesiology and Surgery,
J. Hillis Miller Health Center,
Gainesville,
Florida, U.S.A.

B. Teisseire,
Chef du Laboratoire des Echanges Gazeux
Hôpital Henri Mondor,
Créteil, France

A. Tenaillon,
Service de Réanimation,
Hôpital Boucicaut,
Paris, France

F. D. Thompson,
Consultant Nephrologist,
St Philip's Hospital,
London, England

C. Thurel,
Professeur Agrégé,
Département de Neuro–Chirurgie,
Hôpital Lariboisière,
Paris, France

Jack Tinker,
Director,
Intensive Therapy Unit,
The Middlesex Hospital,
London, England

John H. Tinker,
Chief, Cardiovascular Anesthesia Group,
Mayo Clinic and Mayo Medical School,
Rochester,
Minnesota, U.S.A.

Robert L. Trelstad,
Professor and Chairman,
Department of Pathology,
Rutgers Medical School,
Piscataway,
New Jersey, U.S.A.

F. Tremolières
Clinique de Réanimation Médicale,
Hôpital Claude–Bernard,
Paris, France

F. Vachon,
Professor,
Clinique de Réanimation Médicale,
Hôpital Claude Bernard,
Paris, France

J. A. M. White,
Senior Lecturer,
Department of Surgery,
University of Natal,
Durban, South Africa

Roger S. Wilson,
Assistant Professor of Anesthesia,
Associate Director, Respiratory Unit,
Department of Anesthesia,
Massachusetts General Hospital, Boston,
Massachusetts, U.S.A.

Warren M. Zapol,
Director of Specialized Center of Research,
Acute Respiratory Failure,
Massachusetts General Hospital,
Boston,
Massachusetts, U.S.A.

Section A
Applied Physiology

Chapter 1

Measurement and Control of Cardiac Output

P. A. Poole-Wilson

Cardiac output at rest and on exercise

In a normal person weighing 70 kg, the cardiac output at rest is approximately 6 litres/min (Table 1.1). The blood flow is sufficient to provide the body tissues with oxygen and substrate and to remove the products of metabolism, particularly carbon dioxide (CO_2) and heat.

Table 1.1. Cardiac volumes at rest and on severe exercise

	Rest	Severe exercise	Units
Heart weight	320	320	g
Cardiac output	6	25	litres/min
Heart rate	72	180	beats/min
Stroke volume	83	139	ml
End-diastolic volume	140	160	ml
End-systolic volume	57	21	ml
Ejection fraction	0.59	0.87	
Radius of heart in diastole	3.2	3.4	cm
Change in circumference	25	50	%
Systolic time per beat	300	200	ms
Diastolic time per beat	550	130	ms
Diastolic/systolic time	1.8	0.65	

Since the heart rate at rest is 72 beats/min, the amount of blood ejected from the heart with each beat, the stroke volume, is 83 ml. During exercise the requirements of the body for blood flow increase substantially. Cardiac output in trained athletes can be as high as 35 litres/min.

The energy for the movement of this large quantity of blood is provided not only by heart muscle but also from the pumping activity of skeletal muscle, the muscle pump. During severe exercise in an average person, cardiac output may increase five-fold to 25 litres/min. The increase is achieved by a doubling of the stroke volume and two and a half-fold rise in the heart rate (Tables 1.1–1.3). Stroke volume is increased partly by an increase in end-diastolic volume and partly by a decrease in end-systolic volume, that is, the heart is slightly enlarged and contracts to a smaller size. In mild exercise, end-diastolic volume is less than at rest. Although cardiac output can increase only five-fold on severe exercise, the oxygen (O_2) consumption of the body can increase ten-fold (Table 1.2).

Table 1.2. Body oxygen consumption at rest and on severe exercise

	Rest	Severe exercise	Units
Oxygen consumption	300	3000	ml/min
Cardiac output	6.0	25	litres/min
Arterial O_2 saturation	97	97	%
Arterial O_2 content	180	180	ml/litre
Venous O_2 saturation	71	33	%
Venous O_2 content	130	60	ml/litre
Arteriovenous difference	50	120	ml/litre
Haemoglobin concentration	14	14	g/100 ml

Table 1.3. Coronary flow and myocardial O_2 consumption

	Rest	Severe exercise	Units
Heart weight	320	320	g
Cardiac output	6	25	litres/min
Coronary flow	80	320	ml/min per 100g
Total coronary flow	264	1024	ml/min
Myocardial O_2 consumption	9	45	ml/min per 100g
Arterial O_2 content	180	180	ml/litre
Coronary venous O_2 content	68	39	ml/litre
Coronary venous O_2 saturation	37	21	%
Haemoglobin concentration	14	14	g/100 ml
Diastolic time	550	130	ms
Heart rate	72	180	beats/min
Time in diastole in 1 min	40	23	s
Mean perfusion pressure	100	120	mmHg
'Resistance'	1.25	0.375	units
'True resistance'	1.04	0.18	units

Chronic heart failure due to disease of heart muscle is termed myocardial failure. Unless failure is severe, the cardiac output and O_2 consumption at rest are normal, but on exercise cardiac output does not increase by the same amount as in healthy persons, and patients are limited in their exercise capacity either by fatigue or by shortness of breath. A similar limitation of cardiac function can occur after myocardial infarction, exacerbation of chronic heart failure, septicaemia, cardiac surgery, and rarer diseases of the heart. In these circumstances, management of patients is greatly aided by appropriate haemodynamic monitoring. The objective of treatment is to maximize tissue perfusion (increase of cardiac output) without causing pulmonary oedema by elevation of the left atrial pressure. Left atrial pressure can be estimated from the pulmonary artery end-diastolic pressure, or from the pulmonary capillary wedge pressure (PCWP), but the measurement of cardiac output is more difficult. Several books contain detailed descriptions of methods for the measurement of cardiac output [25, 34, 75, 82].

Direct Fick method

Adolph Fick enunciated his principle in 1870 [24], but the method was not applied to the heart until 1886 by Grehant and Quinquad [31]. It has since become a standard method for measurement of cardiac output (Fig. 1.1). The theory is impeccable and the method, used carefully, provides the standard by which other methods are judged.

If a substance, x, is added at a constant rate, dx/dt (dx is added in the small time dt), to a column of fluid flowing at a rate F, then the rate of entry of the substance equals the concentration of the substance before and after the exchange site multiplied by the rate of flow, that is:

$$\frac{dx}{dt} = F(C_2 - C_1)$$

or

$$F = \frac{dx/dt}{C_2 - C_1}.$$

The substance most frequently used is O_2, and the equation becomes

Cardiac output (litres/min)
$$= \frac{\text{Oxygen consumption (ml/min)}}{\text{Arterial } O_2 - \text{Venous } O_2 \text{ (ml/litre)}}.$$

In an average man at rest, the O_2 consumption is 300 ml/min, the arterial and venous O_2 contents being 180 and 130 (ml/litre), respectively.

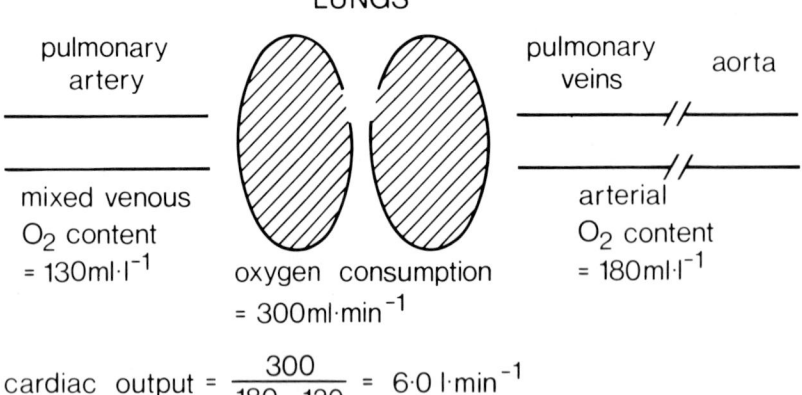

$$\text{cardiac output} = \frac{300}{180 - 130} = 6.0 \, l \cdot min^{-1}$$

Fig. 1.1 The Fick principle.

Hence

$$\text{Cardiac output (litres/min)} = \frac{300}{180 - 130}$$

$$= \frac{300}{50}$$

$$= 6.0 \text{ litres/min.}$$

The Fick principle can be applied to any column of fluid. There are, however, two absolute requirements. First, the measurements must be made in a steady state, and second, there must have been complete mixing of the added substance with the column of fluid when the concentration is measured both upstream and downstream to the exchange site.

In the circulation, the blood flow, O_2 consumption and venous O_2 content of body organs vary (Table 1.4) widely. Mixing occurs in the right atrium and ventricle. A sample of 'mixed venous blood' is usually obtained from the pulmonary artery through a cardiac catheter. A sample of arterial blood is obtained by direct puncture of an artery. Both techniques are invasive. The O_2 content of the samples can be measured by the Van Slyke technique [58], in which O_2 is displaced from the blood and its volume measured at a known temperature and pressure. The method is slow and requires considerable experience. More recently, polarographic apparatus has become available with which O_2 content can be measured directly (LEX–O_2–CON). The simplest and cheapest method, however, is to measure O_2 saturation with a spectrophotometric oximeter. The principle of this method is that light passed through blood is absorbed at different wavelengths, depending on whether or not haemoglobin is combined with O_2. The proportion of light absorbed at the two wavelengths gives the percentage saturation. One gram of haemoglobin can combine with 1.3 ml O_2, so that if the

haemoglobin concentration is 14 g/100 ml and the O_2 saturation of a sample of mixed venous blood is 71% then the O_2 content is 130 ml/litre (= 0.71 × 140 × 1.3).

The O_2 consumption of a person at rest can be obtained by reference to tables giving body weight and height. The cardiac output can be obtained by dividing by the measured difference in the arterial and mixed venous O_2 contents. This calculation is undertaken in catheter laboratories but the estimated cardiac output can be widely in error, since there is substantial variation in the assumed O_2 consumption at rest. Two methods are available for direct measurement of O_2 consumption. In the first, the subject breathes out into a Douglas bag over a timed period. A gas analyser is used to measure the concentration of O_2 in inspired air and in the bag containing expired air. The O_2 consumption is the concentration difference multiplied by the volume of gas expired into the bag. In the second method, the subject breathes through a mouth-piece connected to apparatus which records instantaneous air flow and O_2 concentration. If such apparatus is used to measure mixed venous O_2 content continuously at the same time as arterial O_2 remains constant, or if the arteriovenous O_2 content difference is measured continuously, then cardiac output can be recorded from moment to moment.

The accuracy of the method depends on several factors. Steady-state conditions are an absolute requirement and are not easy to ensure during exercise, when inevitably subjects become increasingly exhausted. Anxiety during the measurements may lead to real changes in cardiac output.

The O_2 content of mixed venous blood changes with respiration, so the sample should be withdrawn slowly over several breaths. If the subject is breathing a high concentration of O_2 rather than air, an error can arise from the amount of O_2 which is physically dissolved in

Table 1.4. Blood flow and oxygen consumption of body organs at rest

	Weight kg	Blood flow ml/min per 100g	% of cardiac output	O_2 consumption ml/min per 100g	% total O_2 consumption	A-VO_2 difference ml/litre	Venous O_2 content ml/litre	Venous O_2 saturation %
Heart	0.32	80	5	9	10	112	68	37
Kidneys	0.3	400	22	5	6	12.5	168	92
Liver and gastro-intestinal tract	4	50	23	3	30	60	120	66
Skin	2	10	4	0.2	2	20	160	88
Skeletal muscle	35	3	18	0.15	20	50	130	71
Brain	1.4	55	14	3	18	55	125	69
Remainder	27	3	14	0.15	14	50	130	71

blood but unattached to haemoglobin and which is not measured by photometric methods used to record O_2 saturation. The amount of dissolved O_2 in arterial blood is 3 ml/litre in a subject breathing air, and 20 ml/litre in a subject breathing O_2. The contribution of dissolved O_2 to the arteriovenous difference in a subject breathing O_2 is 19 ml/litre. This latter figure should be compared to an overall arteriovenous difference used to calculate cardiac output of 50 ml/litre (Tables 1.1 and 1.2). Large errors can arise from this source. Additional errors occur if the rate or depth of respiration changes. The volume of O_2 within the lung may alter and lead to an inaccurate measurement of O_2 consumption, particularly if the results are obtained over short periods of time.

Indicator-dilution method

A continuous infusion procedure was first used by Stewart in 1897 [71], and the single injection technique was validated by Hamilton and associates [25, 36]. This method (Fig. 1.2) is a variation of the Fick principle. Instead of a substance being added to the flow of blood, a single bolus of a substance is added and its appearance recorded distal to the injection site. The substance must mix with the total blood flow. The cardiac output equals the total

amount injected divided by the average concentration and the transit time determined at the recording site.

In practice, a dye, commonly indocyanine green (Cardiogreen), is injected into the pulmonary artery and the passage of the dye recorded in blood continuously removed from a peripheral artery. The blood is withdrawn past a photometer which records light absorbed at a particular wavelength. The amount of absorbed light is proportional to the concentration of the dye when the system has been calibrated. A curve such as that shown in Fig. 1.2 is obtained. A major problem with the method is that recirculation of the dye occurs and it is then not possible to determine the precise transit time. This problem is overcome by plotting the curve on a logarithmic scale and projecting the curve [34]. The assumption in this method is that the decrease in concentration of dye as the bolus passes the detection site is exponential, so that when plotted on a logarithmic scale, the curve becomes a straight line. Alternative and even more empirical methods have also been used.

For the method to be applicable, the indicator substance must be completely mixed and not lost from the circulation in the passage through the lungs. If the small volume of dye is injected into a peripheral vein or the right atrium and blood is sampled from the pulmonary artery,

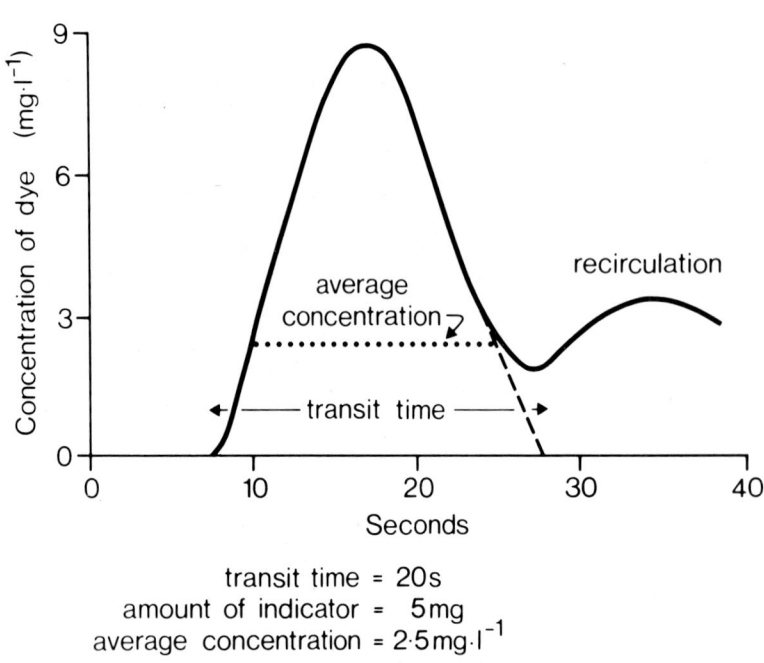

transit time = 20s
amount of indicator = 5 mg
average concentration = $2.5 \text{ mg} \cdot \text{l}^{-1}$

cardiac output = $\dfrac{5 \times 60}{2.5 \times 20}$

= $6.0 \text{ l} \cdot \text{min}^{-1}$

Fig. 1.2. Graphic representation of the dye dilution technique.

mixing is often inadequate. Repeated measurement cannot be made because dye accumulates in the circulation, increasing the background concentration. The accuracy of the method is least when the cardiac output is low, since the curve is flatter and more difficult to define. In addition, recirculation is more evident when the cardiac output is low and consequently the transit time is difficult to measure accurately. By contrast, the Fick method is more accurate when cardiac output is low since the arteriovenous difference increases, making small errors in the measurement of venous O_2 content less critical.

Thermodilution

The most widely used clinical method for measuring cardiac output is the thermodilution method [9, 26, 27, 79]. It is a variant on the indicator-dilution method, in which a bolus of heat in the form of cold fluid is used instead of dye. The advantages over the use of dye are that temperature can be recorded by thermistors and a bridge circuit with extreme ease and accuracy, and that recirculation is unimportant since heat is dissipated in passage of the cold bolus through the body organs.

The formula for calculation of cardiac output is:

$$\text{C.O.} = \frac{1.08 \times C_T \times 60 \times V_1 (T_B - T_1)}{T_B dt}$$

where C.O. = cardiac output, V_1 = volume of fluid injected, T_B = initial blood temperature, T_1 = initial injectate temperature, T_B = change of blood temperature, dt = increment of time, 1.08 = factor to account for difference in specific heat and density of injectate (5% dextrose) and blood, and C_T = factor to account for heat losses (see below).

In practice, a bolus of 5% dextrose (5 or 10 ml) is injected into the right atrium and temperature is recorded in the pulmonary artery. Special catheters are commercially available. These may be inserted from the neck (internal jugular vein or subclavian vein) or from the arm (brachial vein). The tip of the catheter is placed in a large pulmonary artery. Pulmonary artery pressure can be recorded from the tip and the thermistor is 1 or 2 cm from the tip. A second lumen in the catheter allows pressure to be measured in the right atrium and provides the entry site for the bolus of cold fluid. Measurements of cardiac output are repeated three times and a mean

taken. The difference between measurements is usually less than 10%. The commercially available catheters are for use with electronic equipment which gives an immediate digital readout of the cardiac output. The integral of the change in temperature in the pulmonary artery as the bolus of cold dextrose mixed with blood passes the thermistor is recorded electronically and the cardiac output calculated.

There are several important sources of error in the method. From the equation for deriving cardiac output, the entity $T_B - T_1$ appears in the numerator. Blood temperature is approximately 37°C. The injectate temperature may be either room temperature (25°C) or less if the injectate is stored in ice-cold fluid (0–4°C, measured accurately). Ice-cold injectate is preferable since any small error in the correct temperature of the injectate will have less effect on the value of $(T_B - T_1)$. However, if cold injectate is used its temperature should be known precisely and the syringe must not be handled excessively in the few moments prior to injection. Inevitably some dissipation of heat will occur between the proximal end of the catheter and the injection site in the right atrium. The dissipation of heat will be greater for catheters inserted into the brachial vein than for those inserted into the subclavian vein. For this reason, a correction factor (C_T) is used in the calculation of cardiac output. Values for C_T are provided by the manufacturers of commercially available catheters.

To achieve accurate and reproducible results, the cold bolus should be injected rapidly and smoothly. Special devices for automated injection are available, but their value is marginal. A more satisfactory procedure is to record on paper the temperature curve from the pulmonary artery thermistor. Results can then be repeated if the curve is not smooth, as occurs when the bolus is injected intermittently. It is also necessary to be certain that the volume injected is correct. In adults a volume of 10 ml rather than 5 ml has the advantages that any error in volume measurement will be proportionately less, that heat loss in the syringe and catheter will be less, and that mixing with the blood in the right atrium and ventricle is likely to be more thorough. The reproducibility of the method is less good in patients with atrial fibrillation and if the respiration rate is slow. Some users of the technique time the injection to a given part of the respiratory cycle. Despite these problems, the method is highly satisfactory in routine clinical practice and is the method of choice in most situations.

Electromagnetic flow probes

The principle of this method [67] is that a fluid flowing through an electromagnetic field generates a small electrical current. The magnetic field is created by an electrical coil. In most applications, the current generated is small and could not be measured accurately. The magnetic field is therefore switched on and off at a high frequency (sine wave or square wave) and the consequent small changes in current are detected. Such a device can be used to measure flow in an experimental circuit with great accuracy, since it is possible to design the probe to have a uniform magnetic field and the detectors of the electrical current across the column of fluid can be sited in optimal positions.

When flow is measured in blood vessels, several additional problems arise. Since the probe must be placed around the vessel externally it is difficult to ensure that the magnetic field is uniform. If it fits too snugly around the vessel the probe may distort the normal contour of the vessel. Detection of the electrical current is more difficult, since the electrical connection has to be made through the vessel wall. The position of the probe in relation to the vessel must remain fixed since rocking of the probe would appear as a change in flow.

Despite these problems, electromagnetic flow probes have been used to measure aortic and coronary blood flow at the time of cardiac surgery. Extractable probes have been developed, which can be inserted at the time of surgery around the aorta [80] or saphenous vein bypass grafts to the coronary artery [18]. Measurement can then be made in the recovery ward after the chest has been closed [48].

Impedance cardiography

In this method [41, 46], two pairs of electrical conductors are placed around the chest at a fixed distance apart. An oscillating electrical voltage is applied across one pair of conductors and the current measured across the other. The electrical impedance of the chest can then be determined. When the heart contracts, the volume of blood in the chest alters and the change in electrical impedance is recorded. Under some conditions, a good correlation is found between the change or rate of change of impedance and the cardiac output. The method is limited in application because many other factors alter impedance, e.g., sweating, respiration, lung volume, blood volume, and oedema.

Left ventricular angiography

For many years it has been possible to estimate ventricular volumes, ventricular muscle mass, and ejection fraction by radiographic methods. Early estimates of stroke volume were made from chest radiographs taken in systole and diastole. Left ventricular (LV) angiography is now routinely performed at cardiac catheterization to assess ventricular function [64]. A bolus of contrast material (30–50 ml) is injected in 2–3 s down a cardiac catheter sited in the left ventricle. Contraction of the ventricle is recorded on film. The film is usually taken with the patient in the right anterior oblique position, although some workers take pictures in two planes at right angles to assess the ventricular geometry more precisely. The film can subsequently be analysed frame by frame to obtain the contour of the left ventricle in systole and diastole. The method has been computerized [11, 62] so that areas of dyskinesis and wall thickness in different parts of the ventricle can be determined.

The calculation of cardiac output from stroke volume and heart rate by this method is not accurate. There are several reasons. The film is usually obtained in one plane only, and assumptions have to be made about the shape of the ventricle to calculate volumes. During contraction, the whole heart moves in the chest and some moving reference point such as the aortic valve has to be used to calculate the area in each frame of the film and the movement of one segment of the ventricular wall relative to another. Drawing the true contour of the left ventricle from the frames can be extraordinarily difficult in the region of the mitral valve, which may bulge in an irregular manner in the left ventricle. Injection of the dye into the left ventricle from the catheter frequently causes ventricular ectopic beats (VEBs). Finally, dye, when it enters the coronary arteries, strongly depresses ventricular contraction so that if a large quantity of dye is used to obtain clear pictures, ventricular function may already be reduced.

Echocardiography

In this technique a high-frequency sound is passed into the chest and the signal reflected from intrathoracic structures is recorded. With a single beam, the distance in the heart between two points on the anterior and posterior ventricular walls at a position in the ventricular chamber below the mitral valve can be measured with some accuracy. Changes in this distance (referred to as 'dimension') and the rate and timing of changes in dimension relate to reduced or incoordinate contraction of the left ventricle [29, 37]. Attempts have also been made to calculate stroke volume and hence cardiac output. This is unsatisfactory and has been largely discarded. Values were inaccurate and dependent on unjustified assumptions concerning the exact position of the single beam, the position of the beam in relation to the heart during contraction, and the shape of the left ventricle. Sources of error and the reproducibility and accuracy of echocardiography have been the subject of several recent papers [5, 14, 21, 23, 63]. More recently, with the use of multiple beams or a moving single beam, two-dimensional and soon maybe three-dimensional visualization of the heart may be possible. Computer analysis may eventually give reasonably accurate measurements of stroke volume.

Nuclear techniques

If a gamma-emitting isotope is injected into the circulation, then a signal can be recorded outside the body by a suitable nuclear detector. Cardiac output or stroke volume can be measured in three ways. First, an isotope such as technetium-99m can be tagged to a molecule such as albumin, which remains in the circulation. When the isotope is injected into a peripheral vein, the passage of the isotope through the heart is recorded [51]. From the wave, the cardiac output can be calculated with reference to the same principles as are at the basis of the indicator-dilution method (see above). Second, a gamma camera can be used to record the counts over the heart during systole and diastole. If the isotope is present only in the blood, the total counts are related to the ventricular volume and hence ejection fraction and stroke volume are estimated. Third, an isotope such as thallium-201 can be used to obtain an image of the ventricular muscle, since the isotope is taken up by the myocardium. The images can be analysed as for a LV angiogram.

Nuclear methods are relatively inaccurate and expensive. Although the methods are in one sense noninvasive, patients are exposed to radioactivity, which sets a limit on the number of times the procedure can be repeated. Several technical problems limit the accuracy, depending on which method is used. Resolution of gamma cameras is not less than 0.5 cm. Background counts have to be estimated and subtracted. Overlying structures, such as parts of the heart other than the left ventricle, have to be

discounted. For this reason, studies are often performed in the left anterior oblique position, which is an unsatisfactory view of the left ventricle for making measurements. Attenuation of the counts by the chest wall and lungs is a further source of error. Finally, it can often be difficult to define the location of the edge of the ventricle precisely. The edge may appear to move in systole because of shape changes of the ventricle during systole leading to a reduction in counts at a particular edge. Furthermore, as the position of the heart in the chest changes during systole, attenuation of counts at the edge may vary.

Velocity probes

An apparently simple method to determine cardiac output is the use of a catheter tip velocity catheter [45, 53]. If the blood velocity and the diameter of the aorta are known cardiac output can be estimated. Difficulties arise because the diameter of the aorta does change, if only slightly, with contraction of the heart, and the velocity of blood in the aorta is not uniform over the whole cross section. If the catheter is moving errors arise because velocity is greater in the centre of the aorta than at the edge.

Choice of method

Which method should be used to measure cardiac output? In human patients in whom the information is required for clinical reasons, the methods of choice are the direct Fick method and thermodilution. Nuclear techniques and echocardiography are not yet sufficiently accurate for routine application. For measurement of ventricular volumes, an LV angiogram with radiographic contrast material is invasive, but at present more accurate than nuclear techniques or echocardiography. For the assessment of LV function either by estimation of the ejection fraction or by detection of areas of dyskinetic myocardium, echocardiography (one- and two-dimensional) and nuclear techniques are probably as good as angiography.

Intrinsic properties of heart muscle

It has been customary since the time of Starling, in the early part of this century, to describe the properties of the heart as a pump in isolation, and then by consideration of the pressures which exist in the intact animal to make deductions about cardiac function and cardiac output in vivo. As discussed below, this approach underplays the important interactions which exist between the heart and the peripheral circulation. Nevertheless, I will first describe the intrinsic properties of the heart as a pump. More detailed descriptions can be obtained from books [8, 25, 56], or recent review articles [19, 32, 33, 40, 47, 55, 65, 77].

Effect of heart rate

Cardiac output is the product of heart rate and stroke volume. An increase in heart rate, if all other factors such as end-diastolic and systolic ventricular volumes and output impedance were held constant, would cause a proportional increase in cardiac output. This is rarely the situation in experimental models or in man.

In isolated strips of muscle, and in arterially perfused pieces of muscle, an increase of heart rate to a new steady state results in an increased strength of contraction [6, 7]. In an isometric preparation, where the muscle length is held constant, developed tension increases with heart rate. The increase occurs over the range 50–150 beats/min and the phenomenon is known as the 'Bowditch effect' [7] after its first description in 1873, or as 'a positive staircase'. At low heart rates (Woodworth effect) [81], at high heart rates, and under special experimental conditions the reverse is observed. That is, an increase in heart rate to a new steady state causes a reduction in the force of contraction. The Bowditch effect is observed in all species with the exception of the adult rat, which has an unusually short action potential. The effect is related to the availability and release of calcium from cellular stores to the myofibrils.

An increased contractility of the heart with increasing heart rate is more difficult to observe in whole animals or man. There are apparently contradictory results [15, 20, 38, 49, 52, 56, 61]. The discrepancies may arise partly because the increment in heart rate and the control heart rate are very different in these studies. Another problem is that an increase of heart rate may cause a transient increase of cardiac output, which then stimulates complex reflex changes. Baroreceptors may result in alteration of tone in the peripheral vessels and alteration of the stimulatory (sympathetic system) and inhibitory (parasympathetic system) reflexes to the myocardium. In addition, the diastolic filling pressure may fall, so that at the higher rate, the ventricle is contracting from a lower initial end-diastolic volume. Recent work suggests that in cats and dogs [20, 56] heart rate has only a small positive inotropic effect, but that the effect is greater in man, where the problem has been studied in patients with intact reflexes and in patients with transplanted (denervated) hearts [15, 52, 61].

Effect of preload

Starling's law of the heart [31, 70] states that the 'mechanical energy set free on passage from the resting to the contracted state depends . . . on the length of the muscle fibres'. Cardiac output was plotted against the venous pressure on the right side of the heart. The increase of cardiac output with increasing atrial pressure was shown to be similar to the increased developed tension observed in isometric twitches of isolated muscle when the initial length is increased. It is important to consider whether this comparison is valid.

Recent experiments in isolated muscle have related developed tension to the sarcomere length [42, 59, 69, 74]. The sarcomere is the basic contractile unit, made up of the interdigitating muscle proteins, actin and myosin. Shortening of the sarcomere causes muscle contraction. The natural length of cardiac muscle is that when the length of the sarcomere is approximately 1.6 μm. Above that length the muscle is stretched, and above 2.3 μm the muscle becomes increasingly stiff and is pulled apart (Fig. 1.3). Developed tension is small at a length of 1.4 μm, but increases to a maximum at approximately 2.3 μm. A vital piece of recent information is that in 'skinned muscles', developed tension is less dependent on initial length [22]. The increase in tension between lengths of 1.4 and 2.3 μm is only 40%. Skinned muscles have had the cell membrane removed by mechanical means or destroyed by chemical means. The results indicate, therefore, that much of the length-dependent increase of developed tension does not have a simple structural cause such as the degree of overlap of the muscle proteins, but is dependent on the integrity of the cell membrane. Other evidence which has recently been reviewed [40, 74] shows that alterations of muscle length change the amount of calcium which is available to the myofilaments to initiate contraction.

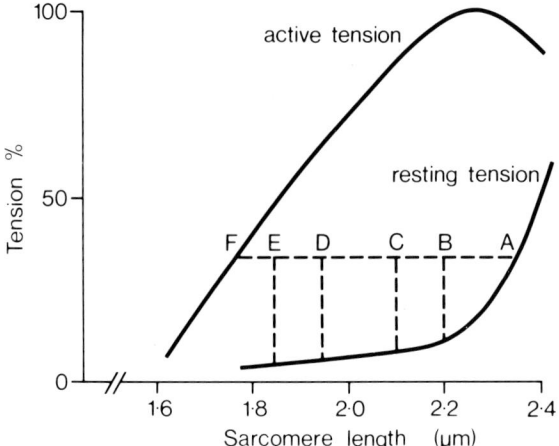

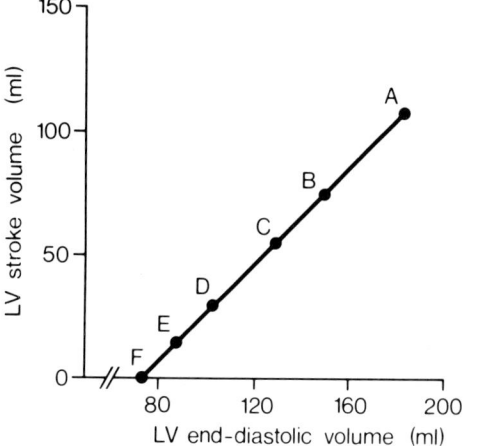

Fig. 1.3. *Top*: Tension plotted against sarcomere length in an isolated strip of myocardial muscle. The curve marked 'active tension' is obtained during isometric contractions. The curve marked 'resting tension' is obtained by passive stretch. In general the muscle contracts to point F regardless of the starting length A-E. The decline of tension above sarcomere lengths of 2.3 μm is due to physical dislocation of the muscle.

Bottom: Making simple geometrical assumptions the results in isolated muscle can be used to obtain a linear relation between stroke volume and left ventricular end-diastolic volume.

A second conclusion to be drawn from isolated muscle work is that there is no 'descending limb' of the curve relating tension to sarcomere length until sarcomere length is so great (2.4 μm) that resting tension is large and the muscle is effectively being pulled apart. In normal man at rest, the sarcomere length is 1.9 μm, so that the heart operates towards the top of the curve. In severe heart failure the sarcomere length rarely exceeds 2.1 μm [69]. Failure is, therefore, not due to a 'descending limb' of the tension–length curve at the level of the sarcomere, but to an abnormality of the mechanism of contraction.

A third important conclusion that can be drawn from Fig. 1.3 is that contraction of muscle, regardless of the initial length, proceeds until a point is reached on the curve relating developed tension to sarcomere length [74]. This statement is only an approximation if substantial shortening of the muscle occurs [12]. Similar results are obtained in cats [72] and dogs [50, 73], in which the ventricle contracts against varying afterloads. Ejection of blood from the heart ceases when a point is reached on the curve relating wall tension to LV volume obtained under isovolumetric conditions, i.e., without allowing volume to alter, equivalent to no blood passing through the aortic valve.

By making assumptions with regard to the shape of the ventricle, the sarcomere tension–length curve (Figs. 1.3 and 1.4) can be used to calculate the relation between LV pressure and volume. From the curves for tension in the sarcomere (Fig. 1.3), assuming that shortening continues until the point F (Fig. 1.3) is reached, it is apparent that if stroke volume is plotted against end-diastolic volume at a constant afterload, then the relationship must be linear (Fig. 1.3). The same argument applies to the whole heart as well as to strips of muscle (Fig. 1.4). Linear or almost linear curves have been obtained experimentally [34, 44, 65]. Curvature is almost certainly due to endocardial ischaemia, physical disruption of the sarcomeres, or other determinants of contraction. Usually in a clinical setting the so-called ventricular function curve is obtained by plotting stroke volume or cardiac output (on the *y*-axis) against LV end-diastolic pressure (on the *x*-axis) [8, 55, 65]. Because pressure is not linearly related to volume at end-diastole (Fig. 1.4) this relationship must inevitably be a curve, as depicted in Fig. 1.5. The curvature does not say anything about contractile function but is due to the nonlinear relation of pressure and volume and the constancy of end-systolic volume for a given afterload.

Contractility

A distinction has been made in the past between the effect of end-diastolic length or volume on developed tension or stroke volume and the effect of drugs which increase the force of contraction in the heart. The curves in Fig. 1.5, it has been argued, characterize cardiac function at a given afterload, and a change in the position of the curve represents an alteration in contractility. In that sense, the distinction is still true but it does not necessarily reflect

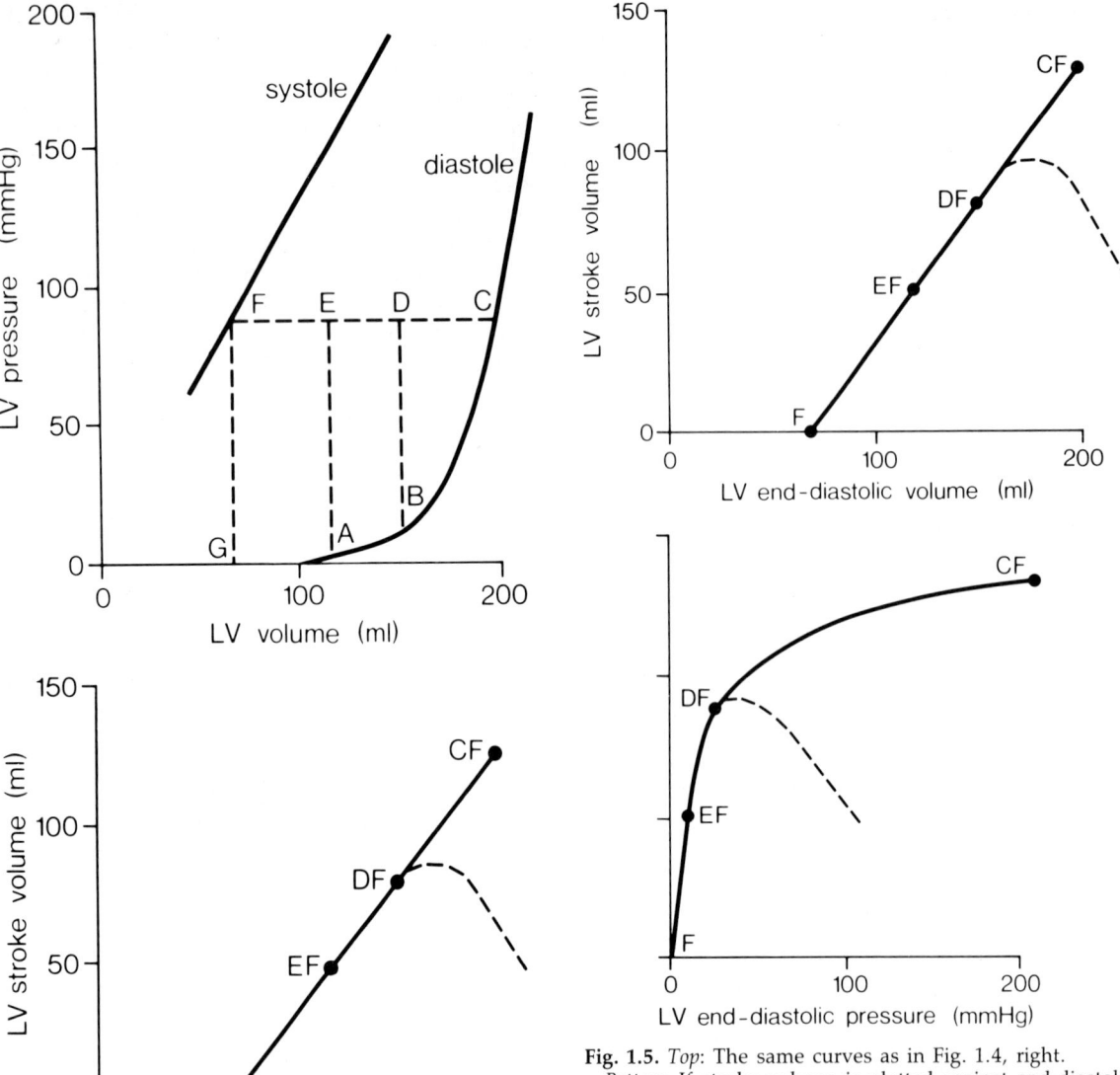

Fig. 1.4. *Top*: Left ventricular pressure plotted against left ventricular volume. The curves are similar to those obtained in isolated muscle in Fig. 1.3, left.

Bottom: The relation between stroke volume and end-diastolic volume is inevitably linear. In practice, stroke volume declines at high end-diastolic volumes and pressure because of endocardial ischaemia and other effects (*discontinuous line*).

Fig. 1.5. *Top*: The same curves as in Fig. 1.4, right.

Bottom: If stroke volume is plotted against end-diastolic pressure a curve is obtained because of the diastolic pressure–volume relation seen in Fig. 1.4, left. In practice, stroke volume declines at high end-diastolic volumes and pressure because of endocardial ischaemia and other effects (*discontinuous line*).

a fundamental biochemical difference. As described above, the shape of the function curve is determined by length-dependent changes in the activation of muscle. The release and availability of calcium to the myofilaments is altered. Exactly the same mechanism, a release of more calcium, is the cause of the inotropic effect of positive inotropic drugs such as the catecholamines. Thus changes in so-called contractility may not be fundamentally different, whether they arise from increase in end-diastolic volume or not.

Other factors

Many other factors determine the cardiac output in vivo [54]. Some become important in particular pathological conditions. The incompliant pericardium [39] and the splinting effect of the right ventricle can modify diastolic filling of the left ventricle. The pressure in the coronary arteries contributes to the shape of the ventricle in diastole and some of the recoil within the ventricle, because the arteries form an hydraulic lattice. Only on severe exercise does the sarcomere shorten to less than its natural length. In such circumstances there are restoring forces within the muscle, which in effect suck blood into the ventricle during early diastole.

Coronary blood flow

A normal cardiac output requires a normal coronary blood flow (Table 1.3). Probably the major cause for the apparent descending loop of the curve relating stroke volume to end-diastolic pressure in the ventricle (Fig. 1.5) is myocardial ischaemia. The subject is complex and the reader is referred to reviews of the subject [4, 30, 43, 78].

As much as 85% of the blood flow to the left ventricle occurs in diastole. Blood flow is required not only to supply oxygen and substrate but also to remove the products of metabolism, and in particular CO_2 and heat. Coronary sinus O_2 is low (Table 1.4) and substrate concentration relatively high, but it is not clear whether,

under limiting conditions, the availability of O_2 or the removal of CO_2 is more critical to normal myocardial function [60].

The fuel for contraction of muscle is adenosine triphosphate (ATP). The consumption of this fuel by the myocardium is determined principally by the heart rate, wall tension in the ventricle, and contractility [10, 66]. External work and other factors, such as energy for conduction of the electrical impulse across the heart, are relatively small. An estimate of O_2 consumption can be derived from the area under the LV pressure curve (Fig. 1.6), the tension–time index.

Coronary blood flow can be estimated from the pressure between the aortic pressure curve and the LV pressure curve in diastole. The ratio of the two areas has been regarded as an index of myocardial ischaemia [13]. Ischaemia exists when the consumption of ATP (related to O_2 consumption) exceeds the blood flow required to provide the substrates for the production of ATP and the removal of metabolites.

The presumption in this argument is that coronary blood flow is proportional to

$$\frac{\text{(Aortic diastolic pressure} - \text{Left ventricular diastolic pressure)}}{\text{Duration of diastole}}.$$

There are several possible errors. Because the coronary sinus drains into the right and not the

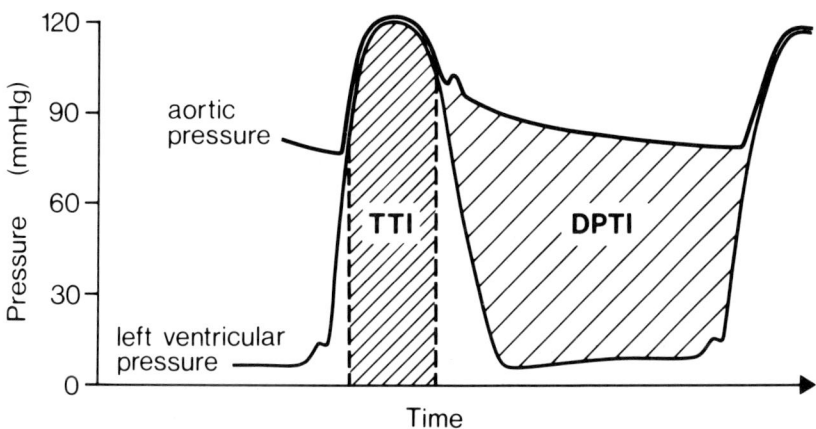

Energy consumed by heart ∝ tension-time index (TTI)
Coronary blood flow ∝ diastolic pressure-time index (DPTI)

Fig. 1.6. An estimate of the energy (ATP) consumed by the heart can be obtained from the area under the aortic pressure curve (tension time index = TTI) (77). Under normal conditions the ATP being utilized is related to oxygen consumption. It is probably more accurate but less practical to consider the area under the left ventricular pressure curve rather than the aortic curve.

Coronary flow occurs predominantly during diastole and is determined by the area marked DPTI (diastolic pressure time index). See text for discussion. The ratio of TTI to DPTI is approximately related to the development of myocardial ischaemia (77).

left atrium, and because tissue pressure may be appreciable, the subtraction of left ventricular diastolic pressure from the perfusion pressure may be incorrect. The relation between pressure and flow in the coronary circulation is non-linear and shows some degree of autoregulation, and a positive pressure still exists when flow is zero. That is, there is a critical closing pressure [68]. In addition, it should be noted that coronary blood flow depends on the duration of diastole (Table 1.3). During exercise the proportion of each minute spent in diastole is reduced. The definition of 'resistance' in the coronary circulation is therefore dependent not only on perfusion pressure and blood flow but also on the length of the diastole. It is also influenced by autoregulation at different pressures.

Assessment of the heart as a pump

Two methods have been advocated for the quantification of cardiac function. Traditionally, in the last two decades, stroke volume or cardiac output has been plotted against LV end-diastolic pressure [8, 65] (Fig. 1.7). The major criticism of this method [19] is that it does not convey any information on how the heart would alter its function with a change in afterload. A series of different curves are obtained for different afterloads. Any attempt in man to determine such a function curve by means of

vasoconstrictors, vasodilators, or removal of blood inevitably alters the curve as it is being determined.

An alternative proposal put forward by Elzinga and Westerhof [19] is to plot cardiac output against mean LV pressure (Fig. 1.8). These authors liken the function of the heart to a roller pump. An attractive feature of this proposal is that mean LV pressure is related to ATP and O_2 consumption [28, 76]. The disadvantage of this plot is that it cannot easily be determined in man and it takes no account of how the ventricle would respond to alterations of preload, which is held constant.

The most satisfactory representation of the heart as a pump seems to be a three-dimensional surface in which the axes are mean ventricular pressure, cardiac output, and LV end-diastolic volume [47].

Cardiac output during exercise and cardiac failure

What then determines the cardiac output in man? It is inconceivable that normal man was ordained to have a cardiac output of 6 litres/min at rest without powerful feedback mechanisms. The most detailed analysis of this problem has been made by Guyton [32–34]. The purpose of the heart and circulation is to provide the necessary blood flow to the body tissues. The body tissues have mechanisms whereby increased or reduced availability of substrates, particularly O_2, determines the resistance to blood flow in each tissue. The summation of the blood flow

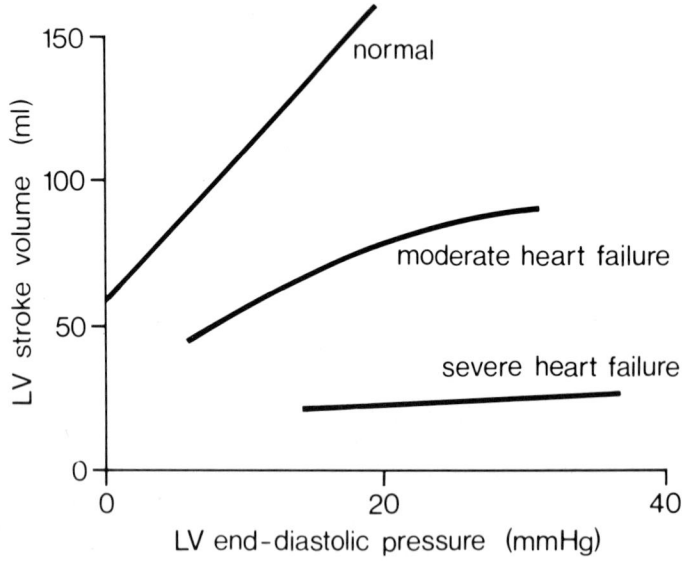

Fig. 1.7. Left ventricular function curves as measured in clinical situations. The curves are depressed in heart failure.

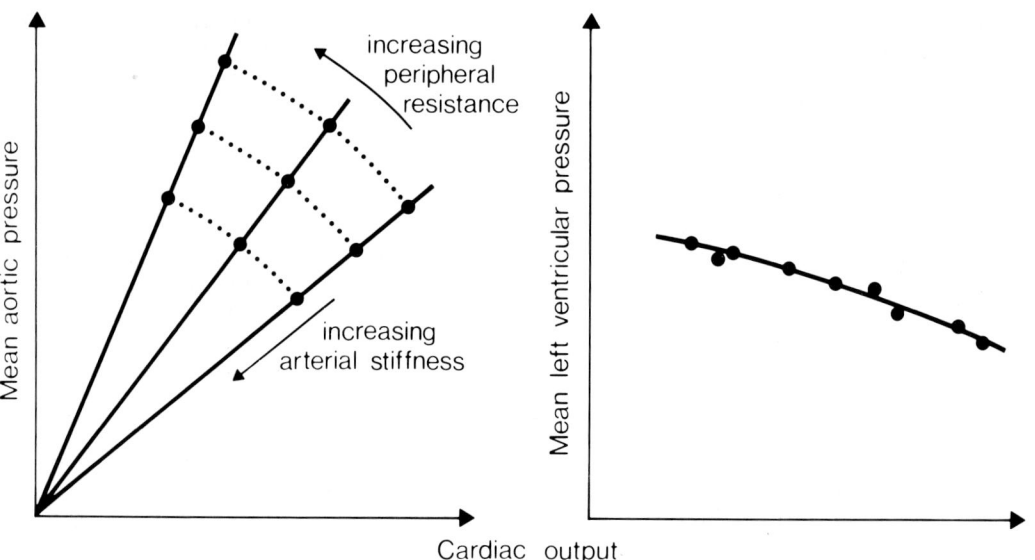

Fig. 1.8. *Left*: Plot of mean aortic pressure against cardiac output. The cardiac output is affected by changes in both arterial resistance and stiffness [41].

Right: A single relation is obtained if mean left ventricular pressure is plotted against cardiac output [41]. Mean left ventricular pressure is related in a simple manner to cardiac output.

needed by each tissue is the cardiac output, which is then provided by the heart. This idea is represented in Fig. 1.9. The cardiac function curve shows the relation between cardiac output as the pressure in the right atrium is increased. The curve is similar to ventricular function curves, but right and not left atrial pressure is used. The pressure in the right atrium, however, is also changed by alterations of blood flow round the circulation. Experimentally flow into the pulmonary artery can be altered and the venous pressure measured. The resultant curve

Fig. 1.9. Three curves show the increase of cardiac output as right atrial pressure increases ('cardiac function curve'). The three other curves show the increasing right atrial pressure as venous return is reduced, ('venous return curve'). The points where the curves intersect represent the equilibrium points, in normal conditions (N) and during exercise (E) and heart failure (F). See text and references [1], [37], and [38].

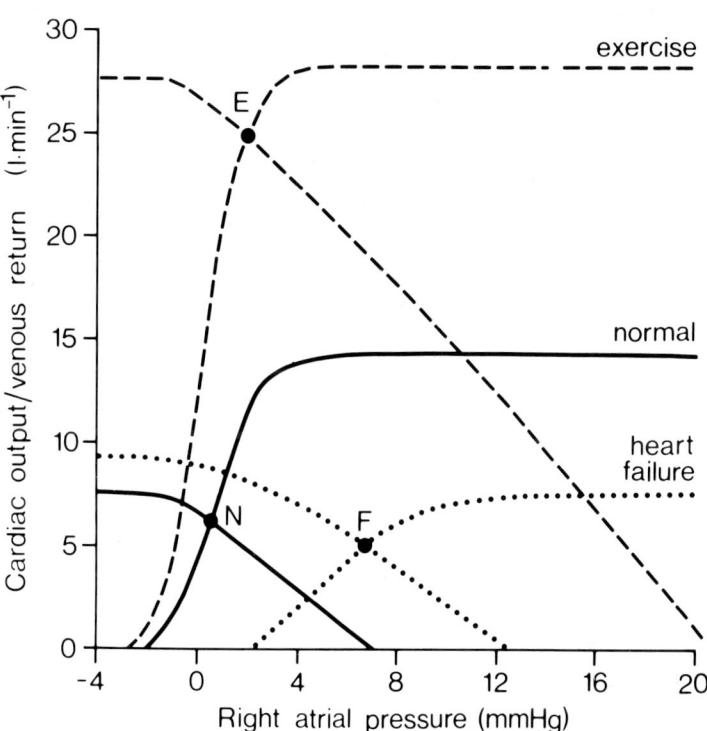

is called the 'venous return' curve. The two curves intersect at one point, which represents the cardiac output and filling pressure in the resting state.

During exercise, the increased sympathetic drive makes the cardiac function curve steeper. But the primary cause of an increased cardiac output is local vasodilatation of the skeletal muscles. The nervous system has little if any influence on vasodilatation [4, 46]. The vasodilatation causes a shift in the venous return curve. The equilibrium point moves from N to E (Fig. 1.9). In heart failure, the cardiac function curve is depressed but numerous factors such as sympathetic tone, increased renin and antidiuretic hormone, and sodium and water retention alter the venous return curve, so that in compensated heart failure cardiac output remains almost constant. The equilibrium point moves from N to F (Fig. 1.9). The main determinant of the cardiac output is the peripheral circulation. The heart is the means of providing the cardiac output required by the body organs (Table 1.4).

References

1. Anrep GV (1912) On the part played by suprarenals in the normal vascular reactions of the body. J Physiol (Lond) 45:307–317
2. Anrep GV (1936) Studies in cardiovascular regulation. Lane Medical Lectures, Stanford University Publications 3:199–312
3. Barcroft H, Dornhorst AC, McClatchey HM, Tanner RN (1952) On blood flow through rhythmically contracting muscle before and during release of sympathetic vasoconstrictor tone. J Physiol (Lond) 117:391–400
4. Belloni FL (1979) The local control of coronary blood flow. Cardiovasc Res 13:63–85
5. Bennett DH, Rowlands DJ (1976) Test of reliability of echographic estimation of left ventricular dimensions and volumes. Br Heart J 38:1133–1139
6. Blinks JR, Koch-Weser J (1961) Analysis of the effects of changes in rate and rhythm upon myocardial contractility. J Pharmacol Exp Ther 134:373–389
7. Bowditch HP (1871) Über die Eigenthümlichkeiten der Reizbarkeit, welche die Muskelfasern des Herzen zeigen. Ber Konigl Sachs Ges Wiss 23:652–689
8. Bradley RD (1977) Studies in acute heart failure. Arnold, London
9. Branthwaite MA, Bradley RD (1968) Measurement of cardiac output by thermal dilution in man. J Appl Physiol 24:434–438
10. Braunwald E (1971) Control of myocardial oxygen consumption. Physiologic and clinical considerations. Am J Cardiol 27:416–432
11. Brower RW, Meester GT (1976) Computer based methods for quantifying regional left ventricular wall motion from cineventriculograms. In: Computers in cardiology. IEEE Computer Society, Long Beach, pp 55–62
12. Brutsaert DL, DeClerck NM, Goethals MA, Housmans PR (1978) Relaxation of ventricular cardiac muscle. J Physiol (Lond) 283:469–480
13. Buckberg G, Fixler DE, Archie JP, Hoffman JIE (1972) Experimental subendocardial ischemia in dogs with normal coronary arteries. Circ Res 30:67–81
14. Crawford MH, Grant D, O'Rourke RA, Starling MR, Groves BM (1980) Accuracy and reproducibility of new M-mode echocardiographic recommendations for measuring left ventricular dimensions. Circulation 61:137–142
15. DeMaria AN, Neumann A, Schubart PJ, Lee G, Mason DT (1979) Systematic correlation of cardiac chamber size and ventricular performance determined with echocardiography and alterations in heart rate in normal persons. Am J Cardiol 43:1–9
16. Donald DE, Shepherd JT (1964) Initial cardiovascular adjustment to exercise in dogs with chronic denervation. Am J Physiol 207:1325–1329
17. Donald TC, Peterson DM, Walker AA, Hefner LL Afterload-induced homeometric autoregulation in isolated cardiac muscle. Am J Physiol 231:545–550
18. Donaldson R, Rickards AF, Wright JEC, Williams BJ, Russell D, Balcon R (1976) Effect of isoprenaline and nitroglycerine on pressure time indices and coronary graft blood flow in man. Cardiovasc Res 10:169–175
19. Elzinga G, Westerhof N (1979) Controversies in cardiovascular research: How to quantify function of the heart. The value of variables derived from measurements on isolated muscle. Circ Res 44:303–308
20. Elzinga G, Westerhof N (1980) Pump function of the feline left heart: Changes with heart rate and its bearing on the energy balance. Cardiovasc Res 14:81–92
21. Evans DH, McDicken WN, Robertson DAR (1976) The accuracy of cardiac function indices derived from ultrasonic time-position scans. Cardiovasc Res 10:65–73
22. Fabiato A, Fabiato F (1975) Dependence of the contractile actuation of skinned cardiac muscle cells on sarcomere length. Nature 256:54–56
23. Felner JM, Blumenstein BA, Schlant RC, Carter AD, Alimurung BN, Johnson MJ, Sherman SW, Klicpera MW, Kutner MH, Drucker LW (1980) Sources of variability in echocardiography measurements. Am J Cardiol 45:995–1004
24. Fick A (1870) Uber die Messung des Blutquantums in den Herzventrikeln. Sitz-Ber Physik-Med Ges Warzburg: 16
25. Folkow B, Neil E (1971) Circulation. Oxford University Press, Oxford
26. Ganz W (1971) A new technique for measurement of cardiac output by thermodilution in man. Am J Cardiol 27:392–396
27. Ganz W, Swan HJC (1972) Measurement of blood flow by thermodilution. Am J Cardiol 29:241–246
28. Gibbs CL, Gibson WR (1970) Effect of alterations in the stimulus rate upon energy output, tension development and tension time integral of cardiac muscle in rabbits. Circ Res 27:611–618
29. Gibson DG, Brown DJ (1976) Assessment of left ventricular systolic function in man from simultaneous echocardiographic and pressure measurements. Br Heart J 38:8–17
30. Gregg DE, Fisher LC (1963) Blood supply to the heart. In: Hamilton WF, Dow P (eds) Handbook of physiology. William and Wilkins, Baltimore, pp 1517–1584
31. Grehant H, Quinquad CE (1886) Recherches expérimentales sur la mesure du volume de sang qui traverse les poumons en un temps donné. CR Soc Biol (Paris) 30:159
32. Guyton AC (1967) Regulation of cardiac output. N Engl J Med 277:805–812

33. Guyton AC, Coleman TG, Granger HJ (1972) Circulation: Overall regulation. Annu Rev Physiol 34:13–41
34. Guyton AC, Jones CE, Coleman TG (1973) Circulatory physiology: Cardiac output and its regulation. Saunders, Philadelphia
35. Hamilton WF (1962) In: Hamilton WF and Dow P (eds) Handbook of physiology, sect 2 Circulation, vol 1. American Physiological Society, Washington, pp 551–584.
36. Hamilton WF, Moore JW, Kinsman JM, Spurling RG (1928) Simultaneous determination of the greater and lesser circulation times, of the mean velocity of blood flow through the heart and lungs, of the cardiac output and an approximation of the amount of blood actively circulating in the heart and lungs. Am J Physiol 85:377–378
37. Heikkilä J, Nieminen M (1975) Echoventriculographic detection, localization and quantification of left ventricular asynergy in acute myocardial infarction. A correlative echo and electrocardiographic study. Br Heart J 37:46–59
38. Higgins CB, Vatner SF, Franklin D, Braunwald E (1973) Extent of regulation of the heart's contractile state in the conscious dog by alteration in the frequency of contraction. J Clin Invest 52:1187–1194
39. Janicki JS, Weber KT (1980) The pericardium and ventricular interaction, distensibility and function. Am J Physiol Heart Circulat Physiol 7:H494–H503
40. Jewell BR (1977) A re-examination of the influence of muscle length on myocardial performance. Circ Res 40:221–230
41. Juett DA (1977) Impedance pneumography and plethysmography. Br J Clin Equipment 2:69–73
42. Julian FJ, Sollins MR, Moss RL (1976) Absence of a plateau in the length-tension relationship of rabbit papillary muscle when internal shortening is prevented. Nature 260:340–342
43. Kirk ES, Urschel CW, Sonnenblick EH (1974) Problems in cardiac performance: Regulation of coronary blood flow and the physiology of heart failure. In: Guyton AC, Jones CE (eds) Cardiovascular physiology. Physiology Series One, Vol 1. Butterworths, London, pp 299–334
44. Kissling G, Gallitelli MF (1977) Dynamics of the hypertrophied left ventricle in the rat. Effects of physical training and chronic pressure load. Basic Res Cardiol 72:178–183
45. Kolettis M, Jenkins BS, Webb-Peploe MM (1976) Assessment of left ventricular function by indices derived from aortic flow velocity. Br Heart J 38:18–31
46. Kubicek WG, Karnegis JN, Patterson RP, Witsoe DA, Mattson RH (1966) Development and evaluation of an impedance cardiac output system. Aerospace Med 37:1208–1212
47. Levy MN (1979) The cardiac and vascular factors that determine systemic blood flow. Circ Res 44:739–747
48. Lewis GR, Poole-Wilson PA, Angerpointer T, Coltart DJ, Williams BT (1978) Use of electromagnetic flow probes to assess myocardial performance in man. Eur J Cardiol 7/4:283–292
49. Mahler F, Yoran C, Ross J (Jr) (1974) Inotropic effect of tachycardia and poststimulation potentiation in the conscious dog. Am J Physiol 227:569–575
50. Mahler F, Covell JW, Ross J (Jr) (1975) Systolic pressure-diameter relations in the normal conscious dog. Cardiovasc Res 9:447–455
51. Maseri A (1972) The practice of dilution methods for the estimate of cardiac output, pulmonary and ventricular blood volume with radioisotopes. J Nucl Med Allied Sci 16:188–202
52. McLaughlin PR, Kleiman JH, Martin RP, Doherty PW, Reitz B, Stinson EB, Daughters GT, Ingels NB, Alderman EL (1978) The effect of exercise and atrial pacing on left ventricular volume and contractility in patients with innervated and denervated hearts. Circulation 58:476–483
53. Mills CJ, Shillingford JP (1967) A catheter tip electromagnetic velocity probe and its evaluation. Cardiovasc Res 1:263–273
54. Mirsky I, Rankin JS (1979) Special article: The effects of geometry, elasticity, and external pressures on the diastolic pressure-volume and stiffness-stress relations. How important is the pericardium? Circ Res 44:601–611
55. Noble MIM (1978) The Frank-Starling curve. Clin Sci 54:1–7
56. Noble MIM (1979) The cardiac cycle. Blackwell, Oxford
57. Patterson SW, Starling EH (1914) On the mechanical factors which determine the output of the ventricles. J Physiol (Lond) 48:357–379
58. Peters JP, Van Slyke DD (1932) Quantitative clinical chemistry, vol II, Methods. Williams & Wilkins, Baltimore
59. Pollack GH, Kreuger JW (1976) Sarcomere dynamics in intact cardiac muscle. Eur J Cardiol [Suppl] 4:53–65
60. Poole-Wilson PA (1975) Is early decline of cardiac function in ischaemia due to carbon-dioxide retention? Lancet II:1285–1287
61. Ricci DR, Orlick AE, Alderman EL, Ingels NB, Daughters GT, Kusnick CA, Reitz BA, Stinson EB (1979) Role of tachycardia as an inotropic stimulus in man. J Clin Invest 63:695–703
62. Rickards AF, Seabra-Gomes R, Thurston P (1977) The assessment of regional abnormalities of the left ventricle by angiography. Eur J Cardiol 5:167–182
63. Sahn DJ, DeMaria A, Kisslo J, Weyman A (1978) The Committee on M-mode standardisation of the American Society of Echocardiography. Recommendations regarding quantitation in M-mode echocardiography: Results of a survey of echocardiographic measurements. Circulation 58:1072–1082
64. Sandler M, Dodge HT (1968) The use of single plane angiograms for the calculation of left ventricular volume in man. Am Heart J 75:325–334
65. Sarnoff SJ, Mitchell JH (1962) The control of the function of the heart. In: Hamilton WF and Dow P (eds) Handbook of physiology, section 2 Circulation, vol 1. American Physiological Society, Washington, pp 489–532
66. Sarnoff SJ, Braunwald E, Welch GH, Case RB, Stainsby WN, Macruz R (1958) Haemodynamic determinants of oxygen consumption of the heart with special reference to the tension-time index. Am J Physiol 192:148–156
67. Shercliffe JA (1962) The theory of electromagnetic flow measurement. University Press, Cambridge
68. Sherman IA, Grayson J, Bayliss CE (1980) Critical closing and opening phenomena in the coronary vasculature of the dog. Am J Physiol Heart Circulat Physiol 7:H533–H538
69. Sonnenblick EH, Spotnitz HM, Spiro D (1964) Role of the sarcomere in ventricular function and the mechanism of heart failure. Circ Res 15/2:I170–I181
70. Starling EH (1918) The Linacre lecture on the law of the heart. Longmans, Green, London
71. Stewart GN (1897) Researches on the circulation time and on the influences which affect it, IV, The output of the heart. J Physiol (Lond) 22:159–173
72. Suga H, Yamakoshi K (1977) Effects of stroke volume and velocity of ejection on end-systolic pressure of canine left ventricle: End-systolic volume clamping. Circ Res 40:445–450
73. Taylor RR, Covell JW, Ross J (Jr) (1969) Volume-tension diagrams of ejecting and isovolumic contractions in left

ventricle. Am J Physiol 216:1097–1102

74. Ter Keurs HEDJ, Rijnsburger WH, Heningen R, Nagel-smit MJ (1980) Tension development and sarcomere length in rat cardiac trabeculae. Evidence of length-dependent activation. Circ Res 46:703–714

75. Wade OL, Bishop JM (1962) Cardiac output and regional blood flow. Blackwell, Oxford

76. Weber KT, Janicki JS (1977) Myocardial oxygen consumption: The role of wall force and shortening. Am J Physiol 233:H421–H430

77. Weber KT, Janicki JS (1979) The heart as a muscle-pump system and the concept of heart failure. Am Heart J 98:371–384

78. Weber KT, Janicki JS (1979) The metabolic demand and oxygen supply of the heart: Physiologic and clinical considerations. Am J Cardiol 44:722–729

79. Weisel RD, Berger RL, Hechtman HB (1975) Measurement of cardiac output by thermodilution. N Engl J Med 292:682–684

80. Williams BT, Sancho-Farnos S, Clarke DB, Abrams LD, Schenk WG (1972) The Williams-Barefoot flow probe: Design, transducer characteristics and clinical application in cardiac surgery. J Thorac Cardiovasc Surg 63:917–921

81. Woodworth RS (1902) Maximal contraction, "staircase contraction", refractory period and compensatory pause of the heart. Am J Physiol 8:213–249

82. Zierler KL (1962) Circulation times and the theory of indicator-dilution methods for determining blood flow and volume. In: Hamilton WF and Dow P (eds) Handbook of physiology, sect 2 Circulation, vol 1. American Physiological Society, Washington, pp 585–615

Chapter 2

The Systemic and Pulmonary Circulations

G. R. Cutfield

It is a fundamental physiological truism that the heart and circulation are servants to the oxygen and energy requirements of metabolically active tissues. In their classic work, 'Respiration', Haldane and Priestley [42] in explaining this relationship comment:

> The heart and vasomotor system are only the executive agents which carry out the bidding of the tissues, just as the lungs and nervous system do in the case of breathing.

This is a principle which is so easily overlooked by the student faced with the study of cardiovascular function, and yet crucial in the clinical care of patients, where many pathological states are manifestations of failure of this master-to-servant relationship. It follows therefore that we should begin this résumé by finding out what makes a good servant.

Functions of the circulation

The primary function of the circulation is the maintenance of a stable cellular environment, commensurate with our evolution from simple unicellular life-forms to multicellular organisms with specifically functioning organ systems. This requires the frugal provision of oxygen,

energy substrates and water to individual cells and the removal of carbon dioxide, excess water, heat and metabolites. Furthermore, the cardiovascular system must carry out this function in the face of changes in metabolic activity and substrate availability which may be sudden, marked and unpredictable. Obvious examples of such challenges are exercise, starvation, wound healing and external environmental stresses such as temperature change.

Other significant functions of the circulation include the transport of hormones from their sites of synthesis and release to their sites of action, and the provision of routes of access for the immune system in the defence of the body against foreign material.

Functional organization of the circulation

In the discussion which follows we shall study each of the anatomical entities illustrated in Fig. 2.1 in relation to function and its regulation.

In general terms the physiological functions of the circulation are subserved by the anatomical arrangement of two such circuits in

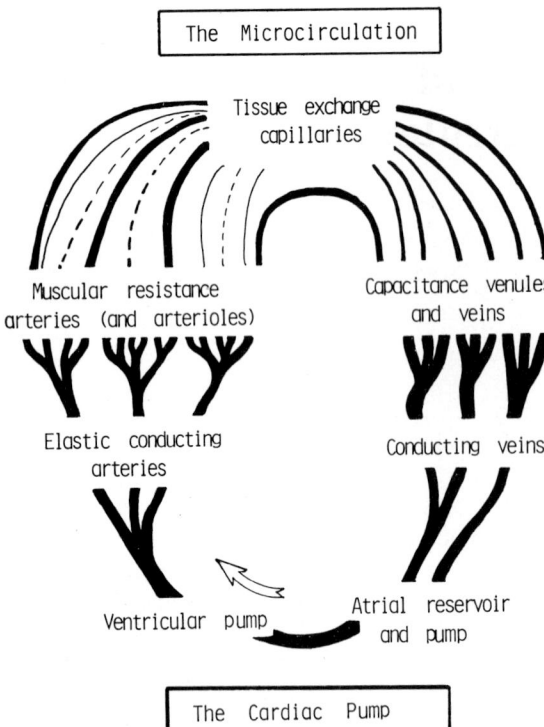

Fig. 2.1. Schematic diagram of the functional organization of the circulation, applicable to either the systemic or pulmonary circulations.

series. The *systemic* circuit provides suitably replenished arterial blood to the tissues and *vis a tergo* returns oxygen-depleted and carbon-dioxide-laden blood to the heart and the *pulmonary* circuit, in the exchange capillaries of which the surplus carbon dioxide is given up and the oxygen content restored. The basic anatomical elements are similar in each circuit and consist of a fixed-capacity *pressure* reservoir (the arterial system), supplied and energized by the cardiac pump, from which the exchange capillaries draw their flow in a selective manner, and a variable-capacity *volume* reservoir (the venous system), which collects and controls the return of blood to the cardiac pump. The functions and regulation of each circuit are different, however, and this justifies considering each separately.

The systemic circulation

While considering the systemic and pulmonary circulations in isolation, the reader must remember that this is purely for convenience and that, in vivo, the two are normally effectively integrated and interdependent.

The elastic conducting arteries

Anatomically this section of the arterial system comprises the aorta and its major branches. These are large-calibre vessels with a total cross-sectional area which is small in comparison with the distal peripheral vasculature (Table 2.1).

Histologically the wall structure is dominated by the internal elastic lamina, which may account for up to 60% of wall thickness [14, 43]. There are three main functions performed by the proximal arteries, fitting the physical properties conferred by their structure:

1) To act as *rapid transport* pathways between the ventricular pump and the distal arterial tree where the distribution of tissue blood flow is controlled.
2) To '*damp*' the large pressure fluctuations generated by the ventricular impulse to more constant pressures driving tissue perfusion.
3) To house the *sensor mechanisms* for the control of perfusion pressures.

The rapid transport function is characterized by high velocity blood flow at comparatively low energy cost. Resistance is low by virtue of the wide bore of the arteries, and high flow rates are achieved with very small pressure gradients, when measured, for example, between the aorta and the femoral artery.

The visco-elastic nature of the walls of the large arteries confers the ability to perform their damping function. Their compliance is 50 times that of the distal muscular arteries [95] and their elastance is significantly greater. Thus some of the kinetic energy of ventricular ejection is absorbed during systole, being stored as potential elastic energy with the rise in tension in the distended wall, thereby limiting the rise in systolic aortic pressure. As peak ventricular pressure declines, and in diastole, the stored elastic energy is transferred back to the contained blood, limiting the fall in diastolic pressure and maintaining the energy of forward blood flow. This property of large arteries has been the subject of intense interest, and more so since accurate methods have become available for the measurement, in conscious subjects, of internal vascular calibre [55], flow rates [100, 101], and intravascular pressures. Detailed discussion of arterial wall mechanics and pulsatile flow dynamics is available in reviews by McDonald [58], Patel and Vaishnav [70] and Caro et al. [11].

The high-pressure baroreceptors, located in the aortic arch and the carotid sinus, provide afferent information in the complex control of

Table 2.1. Calibre, numbers and total cross-sectional area of vessels in the systemic circulation in man [31, 32, 45, 58].

Vessel	Internal diameter (mm)	Number of vessels	Cross-sectional area (total) (cm^2)
Aorta	20.0	1	3.2
Large arteries	3.0	40	3.4
Main branches	2.0	600	3.4
Secondary branches	0.6	1800	4.0
Tertiary branches	0.2	76000	6.0
Terminal arteries	0.05	1×10^6	10.0
Terminal branches	0.03	13×10^6	16.0
Arterioles	0.02	4×10^7	30.0
Capillaries	0.008	1.2×10^9	80.0

tissue perfusion pressure. At first sight it would appear paradoxical that the only regulatory inputs are pressure derived, where the tissues would seem to require a regulated flow, and yet there are no known flow sensors as such in the circulation. This paradox is resolved when it is appreciated that local flow is controlled at tissue level, so that the main requirement from the proximal part of the systemic circulation is the provision of a stable head of driving pressure and a stable contained volume. The reflex control of these two variables will be discussed later.

Despite the great importance of the three functions just described, the proximal elastic arteries are subject to little regulation. Rather, the input to this section of the vasculature—ventricular performance—and the outlet from it—peripheral resistance—are subject to rigourous control. It has been demonstrated that autonomic stimulation and topical application of physiological concentrations of vaso-active agents exert only limited effects on large-vessel diameter [80]. This may serve to stiffen the vessel wall, so increasing wave velocity [57], but adds little to luminal pressure or resistance to flow [28, 71].

The muscular resistance arteries and arterioles

Eighty percent of the pressure reduction between the left ventricle and the right atrium occurs in this section of the arterial tree. Befitting the tree analogy, these vessels have multiple small branches, down to fourth-order divisions, which greatly increase the total cross-sectional area of this section. They have short courses and small calibre, ranging down to 20 μm. There is a predominance of vascular smooth muscle in the structure of the vessel

walls, which allows finely controlled alterations of calibre and hence the functions of the resistance vessels, which are:

1) The maintenance of a near *constant perfusion pressure* in the proximal vessels; the effector mechanism of baroreceptor reflex control.

2) The *regulation of blood flow*, at tissue level, in accordance with need.

3) The *adjustment of capillary hydrostatic pressure* in the regulation of capillary exchange and fluid volume control by the Starling mechanism [91, 93].

4) The *redistribution of blood flow* to vital organs in times of stress.

5) The feedback *control of stroke volume* of the left ventricle; total peripheral resistance makes up 90% of aortic input impedance, which represents the load resisting left ventricular stroke output.

The tone of the vascular smooth muscle, and hence the greater part of the resistance offered by these vessels, is capable of being altered by nervous, hormonal, chemical and physical means, and the interplay between these regulating factors is complex. In general, the nervous and hormonal stimuli are inputs from central control mechanisms, and the chemical and physical factors are local, reflecting tissue metabolism. As befits a circulation serving the demands of the tissues, local factors may override centrally mediated effects on vascular tone [76]. For example, local tissue hypoxia or hypercarbia will counter the vasoconstrictor effect of sympathetic stimulation in most regional vascular beds [21, 37, 53, 68]. Furthermore, there are regional variations in vascular responsiveness to these stimuli. This has been the subject of much recent research and is reviewed by Mellander and Johansson [64], Johansson [48, 50] and Blaustein [7]. As an example, the range of control of the arteriolar diameter by vascular smooth muscle in response to maximal sympathetic stimulation at given perfusion pressure in the coronary vessels is quite small, because resting tone is high. On the other hand, in the renal bed at the same perfusion pressure, maximum stimulation of vascular smooth muscle may lead to almost complete occlusion of arterioles [15]. The factors influencing overall vascular resistance and regional variation in reactivity of muscular arteries are summarized in Fig. 2.2.

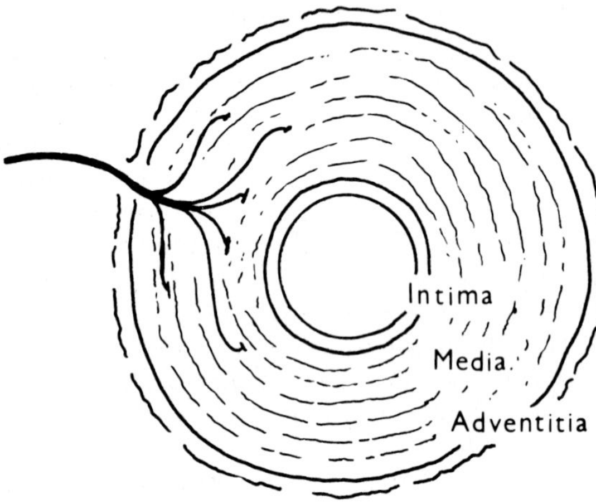

A detailed review of the mechanics of vascular smooth muscle contraction is beyond the scope of this chapter; however, because of its relevance to the control of the circulation, the aetiology of arterial hypertension and therapeutic implications which will be discussed in later sections, a simplified schema is presented in Fig. 2.3.

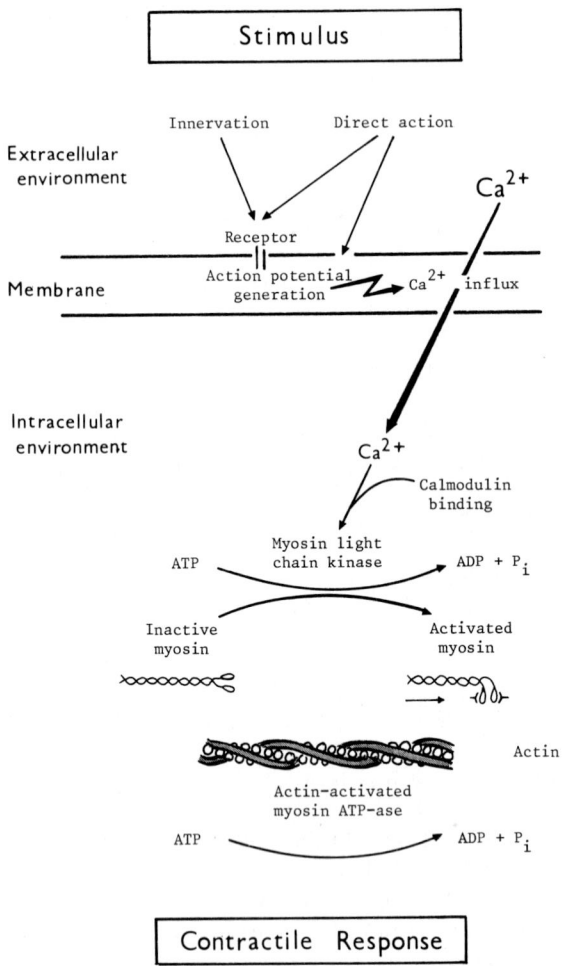

Fig. 2.3. Simplified schema of the current theories of the mechanism of vascular smooth muscle contraction [3, 50].

Active	Passive
1. Mass of vascular smooth muscle	1 Transmural pressure

2. Inherent contractility
   a) Resting tone
   b) Active tension
	2. Visco-elastic properties
	   a) Intima
	   b) Media
	      Muscle series elasticity
	      Collagen
	      Elastin

3. Contractile stimuli
   a) Type
   b) Intensity
   c) Interactions
	c) Adventitia

Fig. 2.2. Summary of factors influencing vascular resistance and regional variation in reactivity of muscular arteries.

It will be appreciated that this regional variation in responsiveness is important in times of stress when certain organ systems, such as brain and myocardium, deserve well-maintained perfusion. Sympathetic activity redistributes blood flow away from those regions where the sensitivity to alpha adrenergic stimulation is high and perfusion may be temporarily sacrificed (e.g. skin and gut) in favour of the vital regions. This is evident from the studies of the cerebral circulation [37, 54], which is not only poorly innervated by sympathetic nerves, but very much more responsive to perivascular carbon dioxide and oxygen tensions.

The interested reader is referred to the exhaustive and recent reviews of Casteels et al. [12] and Johansson [49]. There are several points worth noting in passing. Firstly, vascular smooth muscle contractility is ultimately controlled by intracellular calcium ion concentration and all factors affecting contractility will act either directly or indirectly on this final common pathway, from the extracellular environment to the contractile elements. Consider hypoxia as an example; low PO_2 appears to inhibit both the slow inward (calcium) current at the cell membrane, which is responsible for action potential generation, in turn preventing the influx of calcium ions upon stimulation, and also the calmodulin binding in the excitation-contraction coupling process. In contrast to the increased tone observed in skeletal muscle during hypoxia, the net result of these effects is an overriding relaxation of vascular smooth muscle which antagonizes other stimuli [3, 89]. On the other hand beta adrenergic stimulation promotes cyclic 3', 5' AMP accumulation, which is believed to stimulate removal of calcium ion from the cytoplasm and to inhibit (by increased phosphorylation) the myosin light chain kinase. Both mechanisms also result in relaxation of the muscle [3]. Secondly, measurement of vascular smooth muscle contractility is very difficult. What we may observe as a change in arteriolar calibre or resistance represents the net effect of the interaction of the contractile elements, passive elastic components of the entire vessel wall, and the rheology of the blood in small vessels. Less is known about the visco-elastic properties of the muscular resistance arteries compared with the large elastic arteries. Early work by Roach [78] and Burton [9] gave an analysis of the relative amounts of collagen and elastin supporting tissue which provided the explanation for the differing distensibility curves of arteries from differing regions. For instance, coronary arterioles are stiffer to passive inflation than other vessels and have little elastin in their media, most of the supporting tissue being collagen. More recently new techniques have been developed for dynamic studies of stress-strain relationships and these are described in a review by Intaglietta and Zweifach [46].

The tissue exchange capillaries

Having considered the resistance vessels (down to 20 μm diameter) above, this region of the circulation comprises the capillaries, together with their pre-capillary resistance sections. Structurally, the capillaries are ideally suited to their primary function of exchange between blood, interstitial fluid and tissue cells. The three processes known to be involved in this function are filtration and osmosis (generating the Starling capillary equilibrium [91, 93]), diffusion and active transport. The functional characteristics of the capillaries may be listed as follows:

1) Morphologically, they are minute vessels with a mean calibre of 8 μm, and they have a massive diffusional area relative to their contained blood volume, brought about by their profuse branching and huge numbers. Their abundance in tissues means that diffusion distances are very small, and exchange is further aided by the thin (1 μm or less) unicellular walls which are endowed with specialized intercellular junctions and specifically controlled pore-like fenestrations. At the same time, there is sufficient tensile strength in the walls to resist postural changes in venous hydrostatic pressures of 30–100 mmHg without rupture.

2) There are modest intra-luminal pressure gradients, sufficient only to maintain appropriate filtration pressures and forward blood flow. As a result, mean blood flow velocity is low at rest (0.7 mm/s), ensuring adequate red cell transit time and optimum oxygen unloading. In addition, there is a low intrinsic volume in the capillary circulation (less than 5% of the circulating blood volume), which prevents pooling and assists maximum exchange without stagnation.

3) The regulation of local tissue capillary blood flow and the exchange function of the capillaries is achieved by three means:
   Adjustment of *capillary perfusion pressure* by changes in pre- and post-capillary resistances;
   Adjustment of the number of 'open' capillaries and thus the *tissue capillary density*;
   Adjustment of *capillary membrane permeability*.
   Under these conditions flow will also be influenced by capillary length and diameter, rheology of flowing blood and the presence of shunts or anastomoses which bypass true exchange capillaries.

The overall regulation of capillary perfusion pressure is under autonomic nervous control, mediated through alpha adrenergic innervation, constricting and dilating the small resistance and capacitance vessels. However, this central control is modulated by local factors as described in the previous section.

Adjustment of the number of open capillaries is a function of the so-called pre-capillary sphincter. At the point of branching from the terminal arteriole, there is a region of capillary wall which appears to have the capacity to constrict or relax, although neither containing muscular elements nor receiving any direct innervation. It is believed therefore that the sphincter section is under the control of local factors and the likely contenders are: oxygen lack, carbon dioxide excess, potassium ion accumulation, adenosine and the prostaglandins.

The likely candidates and the criteria for meta-bolic controllers of local tissue blood flow have been extensively reviewed by Duling and Klitz-man [22], Rosell [81], Haddy and Scott [38] and Olsson [68]. These mechanisms most effectively couple the available oxygen and substrate sup-ply to tissue need, at the same time allowing a 'reserve' of closed capillaries which may be recruited when changes in metabolic activity occur. For example, considering skeletal muscle capillary density, the number of open capillaries per unit volume of tissue may be trebled in the transition from rest to maximum perfusion [52].

It is evident from recent research that there is normal variability in capillary permeability and that capillary endothelial pore numbers and dimensions are subject to physiological regula-tion. At present, information is sparse and based on indirect measurements such as *per-meability surface area product* for varying molecu-lar sizes [16], the *capillary isovolumetric pressure* when filtration and absorption are evenly ba-lanced [81], and the *capillary filtration coefficient* of Folkow et al. [77]. The current hypothesis is that local factors, such as histamine and kinins (which may be influenced also by central con-trol mechanisms), stimulate endothelial cellular contraction, so increasing pore dimensions. This is believed to occur particularly at the venular ends of the capillaries, where intercellu-lar junctions are relatively loose. The functional significance of changes in permeability in health has not been clearly identified, but a number of roles have been suggested. One example is that an increase in permeability would allow migra-tion of barrier-limited transport macromolecules (e.g. albumin in fatty acid transport) into the interstitial fluid and close to cellular mem-branes, thus facilitating the exchange of hydro-phobic species.

What is striking is that the control of the input to the microcirculation is so dominated by local factors, confirming the roles of the tissues as master and the circulation as servant.

The capacitance venules and veins

The applied physiology of the systemic venous system has been reviewed by Folkow and Mel-lander [25]. It is best understood in relation to its three interdependent functions:

1) The role of the venules in *post-capillary resist-ance* and the control of tissue fluid distri-bution by adjusting capillary hydrostatic pressure.

2) The *conduit* function; draining blood from the capillary beds and returning it to the heart with minimal resistance.

3) The *capacitance* function; acting as an adjust-able reservoir for blood volume, capable of adapting to sudden changes in distribution of circulating blood, thereby maintaining car-diac output.

The *fluid distribution* function highlights an inconsistency in regarding the venous system entirely as a collection of capacitance vessels, for in this regard the small post-capillary venules perform a highly significant *resistance* function. They contribute very little to overall circulatory flow resistance but are of prime importance in governing the movement of fluid between intravascular and interstitial compartments. The accepted terminology in this regard is the precapillary to post-capillary resistance ratio, changes in which will lead to variations in capillary hydrostatic pressure and thence, by the Starling equilibrium, to changes in filtration and reabsorption rates. For example, increases in the ratio, which are brought about by arterio-lar vasoconstriction and enhanced by post-capillary venular dilatation, will reduce capillary hydrostatic pressure, even below plasma onco-tic pressure, with the effect that net reabsorp-tion of interstitial fluid will occur until a new capillary equilibrium is established. In the ex-treme case of haemorrhagic hypovolaemia, this mechanism may reconstitute intravascular volume to the extent of 1000 ml per hour. As has been described in the previous section, pre-capillary resistance is set by neurohumoral vasomotor mechanisms, but greatly influenced by local factors. In contrast, the post-capillary resistance is little affected by local factors. The significance of this observation is that the role of the post-capillary resistance is crucial to the whole-body regulation of intravascular volume and the protection of the microcirculation against sudden alterations in venous pressure associated with postural changes. Both effects are mediated via the baroreceptor reflexes and control mechanisms of central origin, and will be discussed in the next section.

The *conduit* function is relatively straight-forward. The venules and veins are endowed with large calibre, changes in which lead to only small changes in resistance to flow, and there-fore allow brisk blood flow with small intra-luminal pressure gradients. The final pressure, right ventricular end-diastolic pressure, is slightly greater than zero—negative pressures lead to collapse of the conduit under the influence of extramural pressures and flow becomes fixed by the upstream driving pressure—and it is normally maintained within a narrow range by centrally controlled mechanisms affecting right heart function and venous capacitance (see below). Changes in posture alter the pressure gradients in veins very significantly and, if uncompensated, would severely embarrass venous return and cardiac output. Several counteracting mechanisms maintain homeostasis:

1) Changes in extramural pressure brought about by skeletal muscle tone in opposition to the effects of gravity, or by gravitational increases in interstitial fluid pressure (e.g. in the abdominal cavity).
2) The presence of valves in the limb veins which prevent backflow of blood and interrupt the continuous hydrostatic pressure head.
3) The *pumping* action of activity of adjacent skeletal muscle groups.
4) Active reflex venoconstriction, which limits dependent venous calibre and mobilizes blood from non-dependent regions of the venous system (see below).
5) Arteriolar vasoconstriction, which will reduce capillary blood flow and the tendency to filtration loss. As an example, on standing from supine rest there is a 70% reduction in the number of functionally open capillaries in the human foot [63].

The *capacitance* function, defined as the ability to accommodate changes in contained volume without major changes in intraluminal pressure, is inextricably linked with the two functions outlined above. It is in the venous system, and primarily in the venules and small veins with their wide bore and thin, distensible and lightly muscular walls, that 75% of the total blood volume at any given time is distributed. This capacitance represents a reservoir for the control of venous return and thus cardiac output. It is capable of being adapted to sudden changes in effective circulating blood volume, such as might result from changes in posture or intrathoracic pressure. The capacitance vessels have a compliance which is 20 times that of the arterial tree [66, 83] and, in health, can accomodate changes in enclosed volume of up to 7.5 ml/kg without significant changes in right heart filling pressures [88]. This is achieved by adrenergic control of smooth muscle tone, resulting in small changes of radius in large numbers of veins, predominantly in the splanchnic circulation [39, 40, 51].

Research in the field of regulation of venous capacitance, until this last decade, was less prolific than in other aspects of circulatory control, due no doubt to the difficulties in experimental design, particularly in intact subjects. The methods of study applied to date have been critically reviewed and evaluated by Hainsworth and Linden [41] and Robinson [79]. They fall into three main groups:

1) Isolated vein studies, measuring distensibility and responses to stimulation both in vitro and in vivo.
2) Regional circulatory studies, in which regions or limbs are isolated, with their inflow controlled, and capacitance measured in relation to outflow changes brought about by stimulation directly or indirectly from baroreceptor activation [40, 51].
3) Whole-body studies of *vascular capacity* [74, 85, 88], *total systemic compliance* [87] or *total systemic distensibility* [84].

These latter techniques require complex and highly invasive extracorporeal circuits which bypass heart and lungs, but allow assessment of changes in contained vascular volume at constant perfusion flow rates and pressures, in response to alterations in final 'venous' pressure, fluid infusion, or stimulation of baroreceptors or chemoreceptors.

Venous return is proportional to the pressure gradient between capillaries and the right heart, and the relationship is conveniently illustrated by venous return curves, popularized by Guyton et al. [34, 35, 36] (Fig. 2.4.). While the right atrial pressure is greater than zero (with respect to atmospheric pressure), venous return, $\dot{Q}$, is determined by the equation:

$$\dot{Q} = \frac{P_{ms} - P_{RA}}{R_{ven}}$$

where P_{ms} is the mean systemic pressure [92] that would be achieved at a given hydrostatic pressure level if the circulation is suddenly stopped, P_{RA} is the right atrial pressure, and R_{ven} is the resistance to venous return. Taking each term in turn:

P_{ms} may be measured experimentally in animals by the artificial means of fibrillating the heart, allowing 3–5 s for equilibration and defibrillating the heart. As reviewed by Green [33], P_{ms} is related to the 'stressed vascular volume' $(V - V_0)$, where V is the total blood volume or systemic vascular capacity and V_0 is the 'unstressed vascular volume' or that volume which would be accommodated in the vasculature before any rise in transmural pressure is induced. The other determinant of P_{ms} is the total systemic vascular compliance, C_{sys}, so that:

$$P_{ms} = \frac{V - V_0}{C_{sys}}$$

or graphically the relationship may be deduced from Fig. 2.5.

R_{ven}, or the resistance to venous return, normally accounts for 10% of the total resistance between the aorta and the right atrium. Most of this resistance is in the large veins and cavae and represents viscous flow resistance, the effect of extramural pressures, and the influence of adrenergic stimulation.

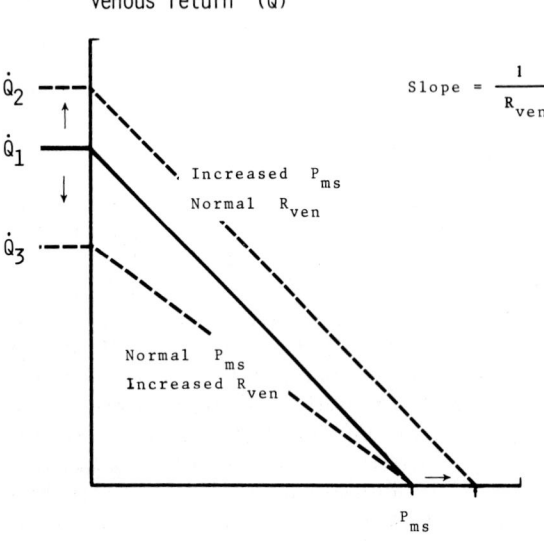

Fig. 2.4. The normal venous return curve and the effects of changing mean systemic pressure (P_{ms}) and venous resistance (R_{ven}), after Guyton et al. [35]. See text for discussion.

These two factors, P_{ms} and R_{ven}, are the prime extrathoracic determinants of venous return from the systemic circuit, as illustrated in Fig. 2.4. Changes in R_{ven} affect the slope of the venous return curve and changes in P_{ms} affect the pressure intercept, causing parallel shifts of the curve. Changes in P_{ms} may be brought about by altering V (e.g. by translocation of fluid between the interstitial and intravascular compartments), V_0 or C_{sys} (by variation of venomotor tone).

The regulation of venous capacitance is the product of four integrated factors [25]:

1) The functional characteristics of venous smooth muscle.
2) Superimposed neurohumoral control of venous smooth muscle.
3) Central and reflex integration of neurohumoral control.

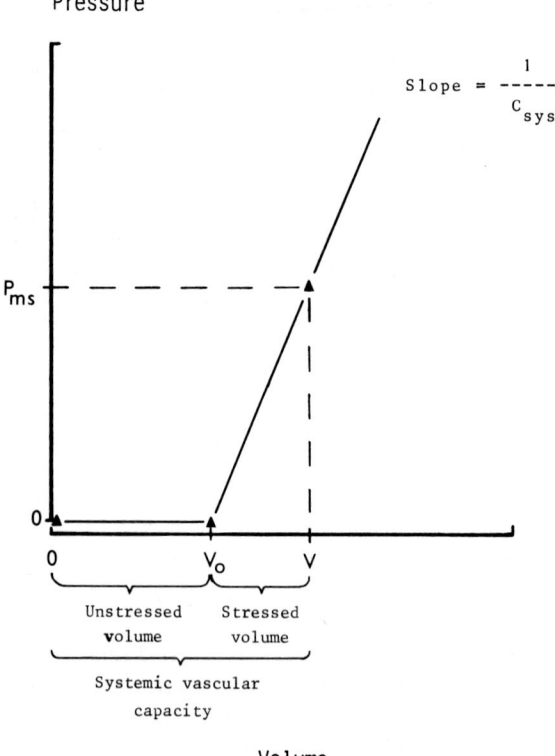

Fig. 2.5. Schematic representation of the static pressure–volume relationship for the systematic circulation. See text for discussion.

4) Interaction with local vasomotor influences.

Muscle content in venular walls is not uniform. Similarly basal tone in venular smooth muscle shows regional variation being generally higher in tissues where there is a greater difference in blood flow between rest and activity (e.g. skeletal muscle versus splanchnic venules). There is also considerably less inherent 'myogenic' activity than there is in arteriolar smooth muscle.

Venular smooth muscle is richly innervated, as befits its overall function in the regulation of whole-body venous return. The early work by Mellander et al. [62], substantiated by later studies [51], highlights a further differentiation between arteriolar and venular smooth muscles in terms of its responsiveness to sympathetic stimulation. At low frequencies of efferent nervous stimulation, capacitance vessels constrict more vigourously and more completely than arterioles. The significance of this observation is that as reflex sympathetic stimulation increases, venoconstriction precedes, and is more intense than, arteriolar constriction, so that tissue demand is still met by an adequate cardiac output.

As stimulation increases further, more venoconstriction is precluded but arteriolar constriction proceeds, particularly in less 'vital' tissues. Capillary hydrostatic pressure equilibrium is thus maintained or even displaced to favour reabsorption, thus further aiding venous return. The humoral activators differ slightly from those of arteriolar smooth muscle in that alpha and beta adrenergic stimulation appears to result in venoconstriction [84, 85] and angiotensin has a less pronounced effect on venular tone than it does on arterioles.

Central and reflex control will be discussed below, but in this respect it appears similar to the arterial system. There is a tonic sympathetic drive [5], the pattern of which may account for the apparently selective responses detailed above, modulated by inputs notably from the high-pressure baroreceptors. Reflex interactions from the cardiopulmonary mechanoreceptors and chemoreceptor activity appear to have less effect on venous capacitance [41].

Central and autonomic nervous system input to venous smooth muscle dominates completely, there being little evidence of interaction with metabolites known to have local vasoactive effects on arteriolar smooth muscle or pre-capillary resistance.

In summary, the venous system is of key importance in maintaining cardiac output and its control is a reflection of the whole-body reaction to alterations in regional perfusion. Although less responsible to the tissues per se, its relationship in the servant role of the circulation to tissue demands is evident. For example, as tissue demand increases, local arteriolar dilatation occurs with the consequence that:, (a) capillary flow and the upstream pressure driving venous return is increased, and (b) as peripheral resistance falls and *pari passu* arterial pressure diminishes, withdrawal of baroreceptor stimulation results in the adjustment of venous capacitance in tune with inotropic and chronotropic stimulation of the heart. The net response therefore is the protection of tissue perfusion by the maintenance of stable perfusion pressure, generated by increased venous return and increased flow from the heart into a reduced resistance.

Central control of the systemic circulation

As has been repeated throughout this chapter, the body tissues require of the systemic circulation a stable arterial perfusion pressure, from which (by local regulation of arteriolar and pre-capillary resistance) they may derive adequate nutrient blood flow. Consequently, the role of the central control of the circulation is to sense changes in tissue demands—by way of changes in perfusion pressure, blood volume and composition, tissue welfare and body temperature—and to integrate and effect appropriate cardiac, vascular and blood volume adjustments. Because of the extreme complexity of central circulatory control, the discussion which follows will concentrate on the three artificially separated aspects of *afferent input*, *central integration* and *efferent output*.

Afferent input

Table 2.2 summarizes the wide variety of sensory nerve endings, the central projections of which have been reported to influence cardiovascular control. The most significant afferent input in immediate control of arterial pressure in health is from the *arterial baroreceptors*. These are specialized stretch receptors which are juxtaposed with smooth muscle cells at the junction between the adventitia and the outer layers of the muscular media of the carotid sinus and the aortic arch [75]. They transduce variations in wall strain, induced by transmural pressure gradients, into variations in generator potential and spike output. The exact mechanism of this transformation is not known. There is also apparent differentiation of baroreceptor structure and function depending on whether they are served by myelinated (Aδ) or unmyelinated (C) axons [2, 8, 13, 18]. In the case of the carotid sinus the myelinated type predominate and their axons run in the glossopharyngeal and vagus nerves. These receptors provide a tonic discharge at normotension, with a smooth sigmoid curve of impulse frequency against pressure. By contrast, the unmyelinated baroreceptor endings which are more numerous in the aortic arch appear to be silent at normal pressures and respond only to sudden increases in pressure with an irregular discharge. Aortic arch baroreceptor axons run in the vagus nerve. The central projections of both inputs terminate in the nucleus of the solitary tract (NTS). From the NTS several connections have been identified, traffic in which has inhibitory effects on the sympathetic output from the brain, which is concerned with cardiovascular control.

Of the multiple *cardiopulmonary afferent receptors*, those with importance in normal circulatory control are the *low-pressure baroreceptors*.

Table 2.2. Sensory nerve endings with recognized or postulated roles in cardiovascular control [1, 8, 12, 18, 44, 60, 65].

Type	Site	Stimulus to discharge	Fibre type
Sensors of perfusion pressure			
High pressure baroreceptors	Carotid sinus / Aortic arch	Increased wall strain	Parasympathetic Aδ
Renal baroreceptors	Renal afferent arterioles	?	Parasympathetic Aδ,C
Sensors of blood volume and composition			
Low pressure baroreceptors	Atria and great veins	Increased wall strain	Parasympathetic Aδ,C
Peripheral chemoreceptors	Aortic bodies (Type 1) / Carotid bodies	Hypoxia (acidaemia, CO_2 ↑)	Parasympathetic C
Cardiopulmonary chemoreceptors Sympathetic Parasympathetic	Diffuse distribution in lungs and mediastinum	Hypoxia, lactate	Sympathetic Parasympathetic
Sensors of tissue welfare mechanoreceptors Cardiopulmonary Sympathetic Parasympathetic	Diffuse distribution in lungs and mediastinum	Light touch, myocardial tension and asynergy	Sympathetic Parasympathetic
Visceral nociceptors	Diffuse in viscera	Trauma and distension	Mixed Aδ,C
Somatic sensory receptors	Cutaneous, joint, muscle	Pain, temperature, movement	Somatic Aδ,C
(Pulmonary stretch receptors)	Lung parenchyma & pleura	Parenchymal deformation	Parasympathetic Aδ,C
(Diving reflex)	Facial skin	Cold water	Somatic (V) Aδ,C
Sensors of body temperature	Skin Anterior hypothalamus	Temperature change	Somatic Aδ,C

The other mechanoreceptors and chemoreceptors at these sites appear to have irregular activity in health but produce potent reflex effects during hypoxia, coronary arterial occlusion, epicardial tactile stimulation and other such disturbances. The precise location of the low-pressure baroreceptors and the mechanism of their impulse generation are not fully known, but they respond to strains in the walls of the atria, pulmonary arteries, and great veins in a fashion similar to the arterial baroreceptors, thus sensing and representing changes in left heart preload. They relay through unmyelinated fibres in the vagus nerve. As a generalization, sympathetic and somatic afferent stimulation results in enhanced sympathetic efferent output and attenuated vagal output from the brain, whereas parasympathetic afferent activity is manifest as reduced efferent sympathetic activity [13, 18].

Central integration

There are two important aspects of the central processing in cardiovascular control. These are the *source of the tonic sympathetic activity*, which appears to dominate circulatory efferent output and the *modulating effects of afferent input* on this tonic drive. Rather less is known for certain about the central origins of tonic cardiovascular controlling activity. In a recent review, Hilton and Spyer [44] counsel ignoring the traditional view of medullary 'depressor' and 'vasomotor' centres, on the grounds that evidence in support of their existence and prime co-ordinating activity is inadequate. Rather, these workers postulate that the major control is exercised by the dorsal hypothalamus, the autonomic output of which is related to inputs from the cortex, the stress/defence/arousal centres, and the peripheral baro- and chemoreceptors. This then is the tonic underlying output, and it is further modulated and differentiated by reflex interaction at brain stem and spinal cord level as illustrated in Fig. 2.6.

Such reflex interaction results in a high degree of selectivity and non-uniformity in the final response. Taking an illustrative example, withdrawal of carotid sinus baroreceptor input in man by the neck suction method results in tachycardia and more pronounced vasoconstriction in the splanchnic vascular bed, whereas

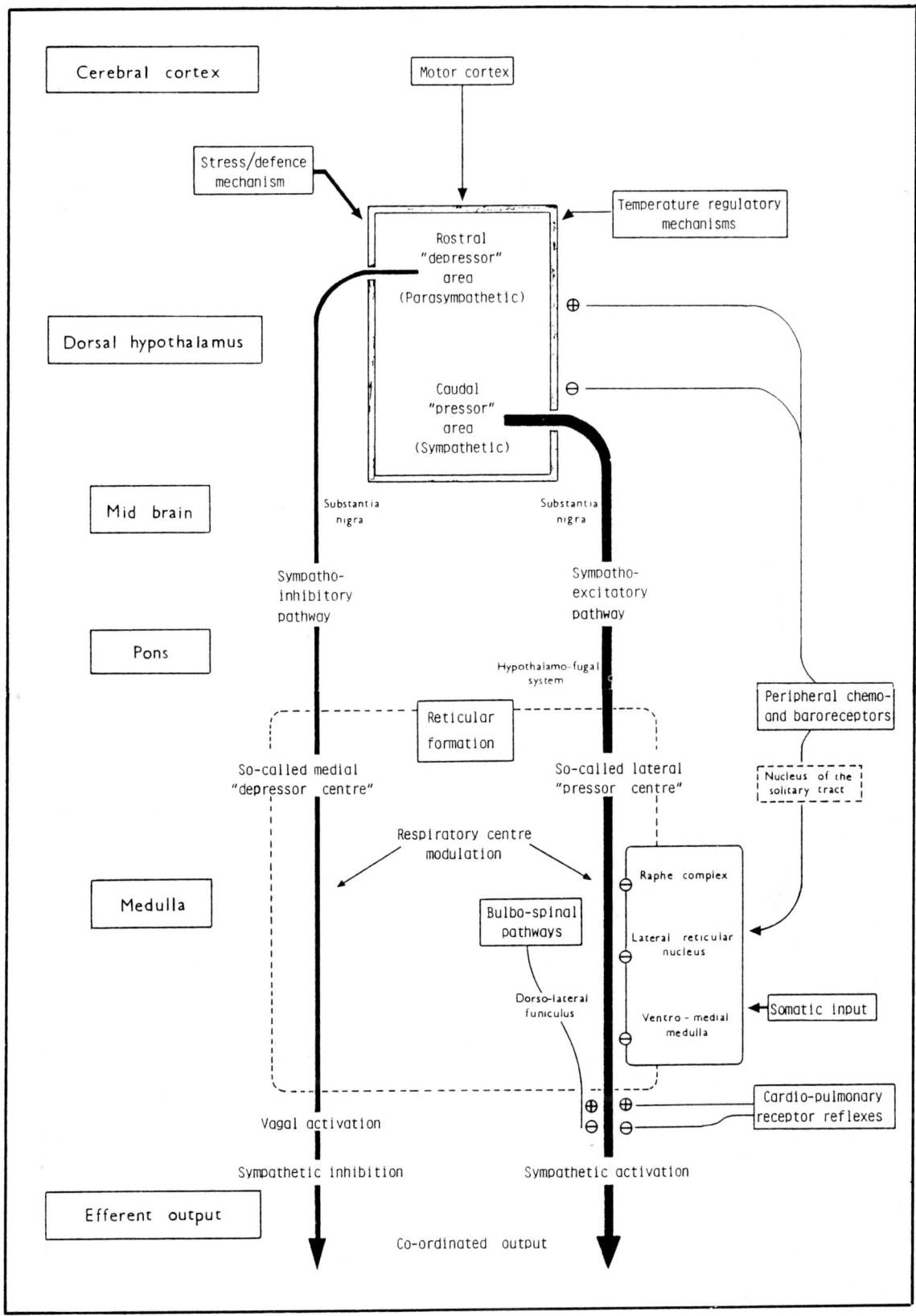

Fig. 2.6. Simplified schema of the central integration of cardiovascular control [44].

cardiopulmonary low-pressure baroreceptor activity results in greater changes in forearm vascular resistance and little change in heart rate. Thus the net response does not reflect the algebraic sum of the responses that would be expected if each reflex were to be elicited alone, but instead it represents a carefully co-ordinated set of appropriate 'commands' [1, 2].

Efferent output

The output of the central nervous system control of cardiovascular function is summarized in Fig. 2.7. It is generally recognized that in most species, including man, the sympathetic outflow dominates minute-by-minute circulatory adjustments in health and in stress [98], whereas the neurohumoral mechanisms (having greater latency) are more significant in long-term control of arterial pressure and blood volume. The final expressions of efferent stimulation are a reflection of a combination of factors, as already noted:

1) Functional characteristics of the effector, e.g. in the case of vascular smooth muscle these include the relative mass, intrinsic tone and inherent contractility.
2) The intensity of stimulation and the sensi-

tivity of the effector to neural or hormonal efferent activity.
3) Competition between central and local control mechanisms.

The pulmonary circulation

The pulmonary circulation is anatomically and functionally similar to the systemic circulation apart from some important distinctions, namely:

1) One organ system only (the lungs) is perfused with the entire cardiac output, whereas the systemic vasculature perfuses multiple parallel networks in various organ systems. Consequently, the rigorous external control of perfusion pressure and blood flow distribution appears to be less important in pulmonary perfusion, and there is no apparent regional differentiation as seen, for example, between the cutaneous and cerebral vessels.
2) All vessels are of larger calibre, with thinner walls than their systemic counterparts, so that functionally speaking this is a low-pressure, low-resistance circuit with short

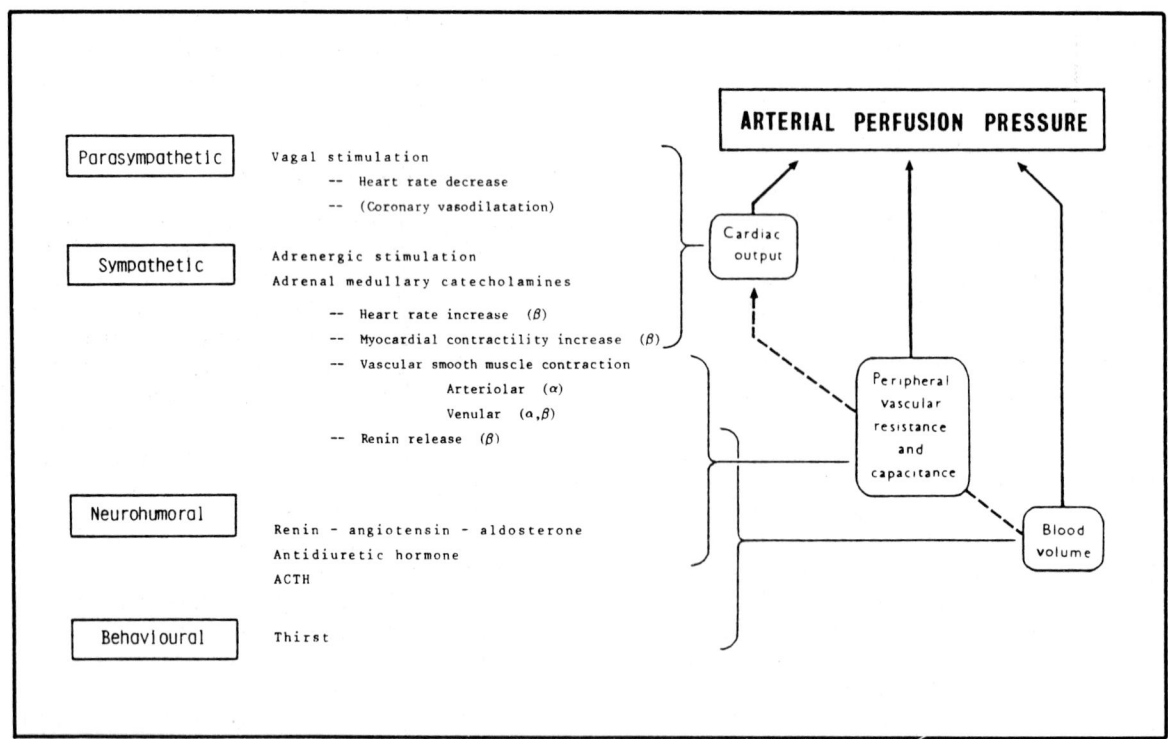

Fig. 2.7. Principal effector mechanisms in cardiovascular control [18, 86, 98].

hydrostatic columns. The mean pulmonary artery pressure is 15 mmHg and the mean gradient for blood flow is 6 mmHg. In health the pulmonary vessels will allow for changes in flow up to four-fold by matching changes in resistance, so that pulmonary vascular pressures change by only small increments. This is achieved by the two mechanisms of *distension* of open vessels and *recruitment* of vessels which are closed or subject to no flow at rest. The huge reserve capacity of recruitable vessels is amply demonstrated by the small changes in pulmonary artery pressures observed after unilateral pneumonectomy.

3) Although the lungs constitute only one organ system, the pulmonary circulation serves four major functions. These are:

a) *Gas exchange*: The functional analogue of the pulmonary microcirculation is a 0.2-μm membrane, 126 m^2 in area [27], onto which blood is pumped. The mean traverse time of red cells is 1 s. Diffusion of gases is normally rapid and complete unless diffusion barriers exist.

b) *A variable capacity reservoir of blood*: The normal intrapulmonary blood volume in man is about 500 ml, approximately equally shared between arterial, capillary and venous parts of the vasculature. Sjöstrand [90] demonstrated that increases in volume of about 600 ml could be accommodated with little change in pulmonary artery pressure when subjects changed from erect to supine posture, related to the distensibility and recruitment of vessels. On the other hand, rather less volume loss is tolerated, amounting to 25% of the resting pulmonary blood volume (i.e. 100 ml) on rising. The reservoir function allows for temporary adjustments in pulmonary blood volume associated with transient mismatching of left and right ventricular outputs, such as occur with changes of posture, the onset of severe exertion and abrupt changes in intrathoracic pressure.

c) *Filtration*: The pulmonary vasculature serves a useful 'sieve' function in the protection of the systemic circulation against embolism. That small venous emboli are arrested in the pulmonary vessels without serious parenchymal damage is a reflection of the efficacy of the reserve of function available, the fibrinolytic system activity, and the collateral flow available from the bronchial circulation. In the event, respiratory gas exchange continues relatively normally until recanalization occurs.

d) *Metabolic functions*: The pulmonary circulation aids in the support of normal cellular metabolism of pulmonary parenchymal cells. This is important for such functions as the regulation of capillary permeability, surfactant synthesis, and the biotransformation of hormones.

The pulmonary arteries

The mechanical properties and flow dynamics of the pulmonary arteries have been reviewed in detail by Caro et al. [11]. Research in this field has been hampered by the fact that access is difficult without causing profound disturbances in delicate interactions between extramural forces and vascular impedance. Morphologically, the main pulmonary artery is similar to the aorta, and is considered an elastic artery, as are its branches down to the tenth order. There is little smooth muscle or collagen in the walls of these vessels. From the tenth-order vessels, whose diameter averages 1 mm, there is a transition to muscular arteries. Here there is a striking contrast with the arrangement in the systemic circulation where this transition occurs much earlier, for example at the first-order divisions. The muscular pulmonary arteries are also thin walled and with peripheral progression the muscular component diminishes until at 30 μm diameter no vascular smooth muscle is discernible. Thus there is no equivalent to the muscular arterioles in the systemic arterial tree.

The pulmonary capillaries

The pulmonary capillary beds are profusely anastomotic and flow of blood resembles that in sheets of tissue rather than that in a reticular network [26, 29]. A further distinction is evident in that blood flow in the alveolar capillaries is pulsatile. The Starling equilibrium [91] in the capillaries is a function of the balance of hydrostatic pressure and osmotic pressure gradients between the capillary lumen and the alveolar interstitial space. Any excess of filtration over reabsorption is drained via pulmonary lymphatics, leaving a normal extravascular lung water volume of about 650 ml in a healthy man. Most of the pathological conditions encountered in which filtration is excessive are brought about by changes in either capillary permeability (allowing protein leakage into the interstitium and cancelling osmotic gradients favouring reabsorption), or by large elevations in capillary hydrostatic pressure. Detailed discussion of the pulmonary capillary fluid exchange and pulmonary oedema is given in recent reviews [69, 94].

The pulmonary veins

The pulmonary veins also differ functionally from their systemic counterparts in several respects; their walls are thinner, there are no valves present, and the smooth muscle is very sparse. As a consequence, they have a limited capacity to effect the post-capillary resistance and capacitance functions previously described.

The regulation of the pulmonary circulation

The factors affecting pulmonary blood flow and its distribution may be summarized as follows:

'Passive' factors:
  Cardiac output
  Lung volume
  Hydrostatic pressure gradients
'Active' factors:
  Tone in muscular arteries and the influences of;
    PO_2, PCO_2, and pH
    Sympathetic innervation
    Hormonal agents

Alterations in cardiac output will cause transient changes in pulmonary artery pressure and subsequent alterations in vascular distension and the numbers of recruited channels. As far as can be determined, these appear to be purely passive effects. This accounts for the reduction in overall pulmonary vascular impedance observed when venous return is augmented, thereby allowing increased flow for the same pressure gradient.

The effects of lung volume on pulmonary vascular resistance and therefore on pulmonary blood flow, are summarized in Fig. 2.8. The parabolic curve represents the sum of the resistance of the extra-alveolar vessels (precapillary arteries, arteries and veins) and the alveolar capillaries in relation to lung volume. It is evident that the total resistance is lowest at functional residual capacity. Expansion of the lung results in expansion of alveoli, with the result that the calibre of alveolar capillaries is reduced and their lengths are increased, thereby increasing resistance. At the same time there is a slight reduction in extra-alveolar vascular resistance, caused by their being pulled open by the action of elastic connective tissue

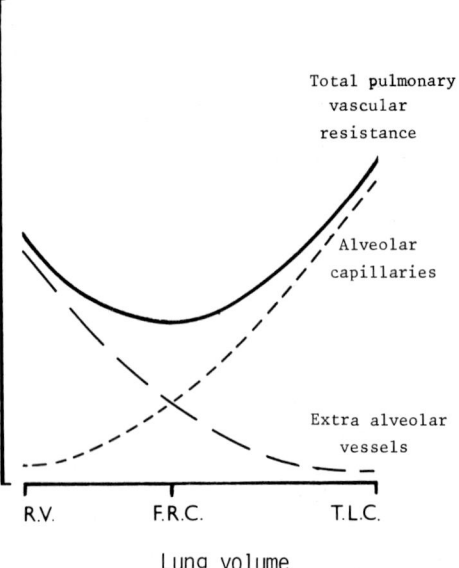

Pulmonary vascular resistance

Fig. 2.8. Diagrammatic representation of the relationship between lung volume and pulmonary vascular resistance [10, 17]. *RV*, residual volume; *FRC*, functional residual capacity; *TLC*, total lung capacity.

attachments along their course. Conversely, progression into the residual volume results in increases in extra-alveolar vascular resistance by the compressive effect of elastic recoil, but slight reductions in alveolar capillary resistance through regaining maximal calibre and shorter lengths [10, 17].

Hydrostatic pressure gradients are the most significant passive mechanical factors affecting pulmonary blood flow and its distribution, and this is a function of the combined effects of gravity and the alveolar capillaries acting as collapsible Starling resistors. The model of West et al. [97] affords a degree of simplicity to understanding the effects of gravity, intravascular pressure and alveolar pressure on blood flow distribution (Fig. 2.9).

Predictions from this model have been verified by the result of experiments in which regional pulmonary blood flow has been measured in intact subjects. Thus, in the least dependent regions of the lung, blood flow will be least because (a) the pulmonary artery pressure in these zones is opposed by the gravitational hydrostatic pressure head, (b) alveoli are held open by the most negative intrapleural pressure, so tending to collapse alveolar capillaries and (c) the alveolar capillaries are further collapsed by the zero or sub-atmospheric pressure in the pulmonary veins. Conversely,

Least dependent zone

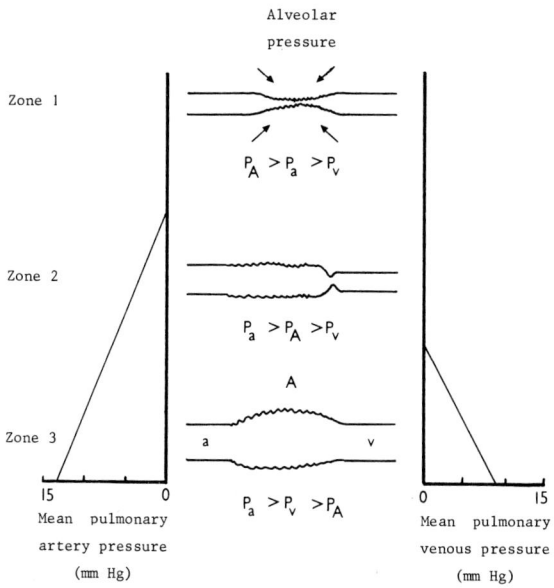

Zone 1

Zone 2

Zone 3

$P_A > P_a > P_v$

$P_a > P_A > P_v$

A

a   v

| 15 | 0 | | | 0 | 15 |
Mean pulmonary
artery pressure
(mm Hg)

$P_a > P_v > P_A$

Mean pulmonary
venous pressure
(mm Hg)

Most dependent zone

Fig. 2.9. The effects of gravity, vascular pressures and alveolar pressure on pulmonary blood flow distribution after West et al. [97].

in the most dependent zone of the lung, blood flow will be maximal because (a) pulmonary arterial pressure is not opposed by gravity, (b) intrapleural pressure is less negative and therefore alveoli are less distended, so that alveolar capillary resistance is reduced and (c), pulmonary venous pressure is positive, so preventing collapse of the alveolar capillaries, but there is sufficient gradient between arterial and venous pressures to maintain maximum flow.

Active tone in the vascular smooth muscle of the pulmonary arteries exerts some influence upon pulmonary blood flow distribution [24]. The pulmonary hypoxic vasoconstrictor response is a well-described phenomenon [4, 20, 67], whereby muscular pulmonary arteries constrict in response to *alveolar* hypoxia. The resultant effect is the redistribution of blood flow to attempt to maintain matching of alveolar perfusion to alveolar ventilation, optimizing blood gas exchange and systemic arterial oxygen content. This response is in direct contrast to the dilator effect of hypoxia on systemic vascular smooth muscle (q.v.) and the precise mechanism by which it occurs is not known. Humoral mediators have been implicated in the re-

sponse, which is also accentuated by hypercarbia and acidaemia [59, 82], and in the presence of high resting tone of vascular smooth muscle as seen in high altitude dwellers [24].

Resting tone is a composite of many factors, including muscle mass, the level of pulmonary arterial pressure, and the presence of neuro-humoral mediators.

Superimposed nervous stimulation of the richly innervated pulmonary arteries produces surprisingly little effect on the pulmonary blood flow [19, 99]. It does however result in stiffening of the large pulmonary arteries, so that although total pulmonary vascular resistance changes little, the added component of wave reflection to pulmonary impedance is increased. Hence in times of stress the afterload on the right ventricle is increased, which probably aids in the matching of left and right ventricular output, particularly when the inotropic state of each is similarly stimulated. Nevertheless the effects of the sympathetic stimulation of the adult pulmonary circulation are strikingly less pronounced than similar stimulation of the systemic vessels.

Hormonal agents exerting vaso-active effects on the pulmonary circulation include catecholamines (acting on alpha receptors), angiotensin, histamine, prostaglandins and the peptide neurotransmitters, all of which (depending on resting tone) cause vasoconstriction. Vasodilatation is stimulated by bradykinin and acetylcholine [6]. These agents have been thoroughly investigated as possible mediators of the pulmonary hypoxic vasoconstrictor response, but none alone entirely satisfies the criteria to be held responsible. Their actions in the normal subject are not well understood.

In summary, it might be tempting to regard the pulmonary circulation as a helpful but passive link in the continuity of the circulation; helpful because of its capacity to re-oxygenate, filter and 'recondition' arterial blood required by the tissues, but passive in that it appears to be regulated only to achieve optimum gas exchange, and perhaps to accommodate small changes of volume in times of stress to help keep the left and right sides of the heart in tune! That such a notion is absurd is plainly evident, not least in critical care medicine where almost all patients show the very significant effects of pathological disturbances of the physiology and control of the pulmonary circulation. Indeed, it is from this specialty that there is an increasing vogue for considering the heart and lungs together as a functionally integrated unit [56, 61, 96].

Implications of circulatory physiology in critical care

Understanding the applied physiology of the circulation should ideally be prerequisite to the care of critically ill patients for the reasons outlined below:

1) A significant proportion of patients are admitted to intensive care units with acute primary circulatory disorders. Examples of such cases are not difficult to find in any admission register and would include patients with hypovolaemic shock, acute left ventricular failure, massive pulmonary embolism or following open heart surgery.

2) Many patients present with acute illnesses superimposed on chronic cardiovascular disease, the existence and extent of which may not be known at the time of admission. In modern society coronary artery disease and essential hypertension, as two examples, are prevalent and may complicate care of seriously ill patients. The poorly controlled hypertensive patient, for example, will respond to stressful stimulation with markedly exaggerated pressor reactions, even under anaesthesia [73]. This arises because of the generally increased sympathetic tone due to poor buffering by baroreceptor input in these patients [72]. On the other hand the same patients tolerate hypovolaemia very poorly, partly because of their contracted circulations, and partly because of baroreceptor 'resetting' [102]. Reset baroreceptors in hypertensive patients have higher pressure thresholds for stimulation, and a reduced impulse frequency at resting blood pressures, hence reduced pressures are less well sensed, with the result that reflex responses to hypotension are obtunded. Both extremes will jeopardize myocardial oxygen supply to demand ratios in a seriously detrimental manner.

3) Most other medical emergencies will be associated with secondary circulatory effects, either because of or in compensation for the primary condition. A ready example is carbon monoxide poisoning which is typified by a hyperdynamic circulation. Because of tissue hypoxia, caused by the reduced oxygen availability following carboxyhaemoglobin complexing, peripheral vasodilatation occurs. In patients with diseased cerebral or coronary arteries, vasodilatation in these 'vital' beds is limited, so that tissue demand

may outstrip oxygen supply, resulting in fatal anoxia.

4) Therapeutic measures may affect circulatory physiology. Probably the most relevant example here is the response to techniques of artificial ventilation [23, 30, 47]. Very briefly, the elevation of mean intrathoracic pressure causes a chain of events which culminate in the depression of cardiac output. These events include initial impairment of venous return, increased pulmonary vascular impedance, the initiation of inhibitory cardiovascular reflexes by cardiopulmonary mechanoreceptors, and changes in left ventricular performance caused by alterations in diastolic compliance as a result of altered cardiac geometry. Right ventricular dilatation in response to increased loading contributes to leftward displacement of the septum and this, with the limitation imposed by intact pericardium, impairs left heart filling.

It is fitting that this chapter should close with the encouragement that a thorough knowledge of the underlying pathophysiology of patients' conditions, the likely compensatory mechanisms in action and the potential effects of therapy based on sound physiological principles will guide safe and effective management.

References

1. Abboud FM (1979) Integration of reflex responses in the control of blood pressure and vascular resistance. Am J Cardiol 44:903–911
2. Abboud FM, Eckberg DL, Johanssen VJ, Mark AL (1979) Carotid and cardiopulmonary baroreceptor control of splanchnic and forearm vascular resistance during venous pooling in man. J Physiol (Lond) 286:173–184
3. Adelstein RS, Hathaway DR (1979) Role of calcium and cyclic adenosine 3':5' monophosphate in regulating smooth muscle. Am J Cardiol 44:783–787
4. Barer GR, Howard P, Shaw JW (1970) Stimulus-response curves of the pulmonary vascular bed to hypoxia and hypercarbia. J Physiol (Lond) 211:139–155
5. Bassenge E, Holtz J, Kolin A (1978) Autonomic control of venous capacity and total vascular compliance in the conscious dog. J Physiol (Lond) 284: 105–106P
6. Bergofsky EH (1980) Humoral control of the pulmonary circulation. Ann Rev Physiol 42:221–233
7. Blaustein MP (1977) Sodium ions, calcium ions, blood pressure regulation and hypertension. A reassessment and a hypothesis. Am J Physiol 232:C165–173
8. Brown AM (1980) Receptors under pressure. An update on baroreceptors. Circ Res 46:1-10
9. Burton AC (1951) On the physical equilibrium of small blood vessels. Am J Physiol 164:319–329
10. Burton AC, Patel DJ (1958) Effect on pulmonary vascu-

lar resistance of inflation of the rabbit lung. J Appl
Physiol 12:239–246

11. Caro CG, Pedley TJ, Schroter RC, Seed WA (1978) The
    mechanics of the circulation. Oxford University Press,
    Oxford

12. Casteels R, Godfraind T, Rüegg JC (1977) Excitation-
    contraction coupling in smooth muscle. Elsevier/North
    Holland, Amsterdam

13. Coleridge HM, Coleridge JCG (1980) Cardiovascular
    afferents involved in regulation of peripheral vessels.
    Ann Rev Physiol 42:413–427

14. Cox RH (1978) Passive mechanics and connective tis-
    sue composition of canine arteries. Am J Physiol
    234:H533–541

15. Cox RH (1978) Regional variation of series elasticity in
    canine arterial smooth muscles. Am J Physiol
    234:H542–551

16. Crone C (1963) The permeability of capillaries in va-
    rious organs as determined by the use of the 'indicator
    diffusion' method. Acta Physiol Scand 58:292–305

17. Culver BH, Butler J (1980) Mechanical influences on the
    pulmonary microcirculation. Ann Rev Physiol 42:187–
    198

18. Donald DE, Shepherd JT (1980) Autonomic regulation
    of peripheral circulation. Ann Rev Physiol 42:429–439

19. Downing SE, Lee JC (1980) Nervous control of the
    pulmonary circulation. Ann Rev Physiol 42:199–210

20. Duke HN (1951) Pulmonary vasomotor responses of
    isolated perfused cat lung to anoxia and hypercapnia.
    Quart J Exp Physiol 36:75–88

21. Duling BR, Berne RM (1971) Oxygen and the local
    regulation of blood flow: possible significance of longi-
    tudinal gradients in arterial blood oxygen tension. Circ
    Res 28, 29 [Suppl I]:65–69

22. Duling BR, Klitzman B (1980) Local control of micro-
    vascular function—role in tissue oxygen supply. Ann
    Rev Physiol 42:373–382

23. Editorial (1981) Artificial ventilation and the heart. Br
    Med J 283:397–398

24. Fishman AP (1980) Vasomotor regulation of the pul-
    monary circulation. Ann Rev Physiol 42:211–220

25. Folkow B, Mellander S (1964) Veins and venous tone.
    Am Heart J 68:397–408

26. Fung YC, Sobin SS (1969) Theory of sheet flow in lung
    alveoli. J Appl Physiol 26:472–488

27. Gehr P, Bachofen M, Weibel ER (1978) The normal
    human lung: ultrastructure and morphometric estima-
    tion of diffusion capacity. Respir Physiol 32:121–140

28. Gerova M, Gero J (1967) Effector mechanisms induced
    by baroreceptor stimulation. In: Baroreceptors and
    hypertension. Pergamon, Oxford

29. Gil J (1980) Organisation of the microcirculation of the
    lung. Ann Rev Physiol 42:177–186

30. Goldberg HS, Rabson J (1981) Control of cardiac output
    by systemic vessels: circulatory adjustments to acute
    and chronic respiratory failure and the effect of thera-
    peutic interventions. Am J Cardiol 47:696–702

31. Green HD (1944) Circulation: physical principles. In:
    Glasser O (ed) Medical physics, vol I. Year Book
    Publishers, Chicago

32. Green HD (1950) Circulatory system: physical princi-
    ples. In: Glasser O (ed) Medical physics, vol II. Year
    Book Publishers, Chicago

33. Green JF (1979) Determinants of systemic blood flow.
    In: Guyton AC, Young DB (eds) Cardiovascular phy-
    siology III International review of physiology, vol 18.
    University Park Press, Baltimore

34. Guyton AC (1955) Determination of cardiac output by
    equating venous return curves with cardiac response
    curves. Physiol Rev 35:123–129

35. Guyton AC, Lindsey AW, Abernethy B, Richardson T
    (1957) Venous return at various right atrial pressures
    and the normal venous return curve. Am J Physiol
    189:609–615

36. Guyton AC (1963) Circulatory physiology: cardiac out-
    put and its regulation. Saunders, Philadelphia

37. Guyton AC, Ross JM Jr, Carrier O, Walker JR (1964)
    Evidence for tissue oxygen demand as the major factor
    causing autoregulation. Circ Res 15 [Suppl I] 60–68

38. Haddy FJ, Scott JB (1975) Metabolic factors in periph-
    eral circulatory regulation. Fed Proc 34:2006–2014

39. Hainsworth R, Karim F (1974) A method for measure-
    ment of changes in abdominal vascular resistance. J
    Physiol (Lond) 238:13–14P

40. Hainsworth R, Karim F (1976) Responses of abdominal
    vascular capacitance in the anaesthetised dog to
    changes in carotid sinus pressure. J Physiol (Lond)
    262:659–677

41. Hainsworth R, Linden RJ (1979) Reflex control of
    vascular capacitance. In: Guyton AC, Young DB (eds)
    Cardiovascular physiology III. International review of
    physiology, vol 18. University Park Press, Baltimore

42. Haldane JS, Priestley JG (1935) Respiration, 2nd edn.
    Oxford University Press, Oxford

43. Harkness MLR, Harkness RD, McDonald DA (1957)
    The collagen and elastin content of the arterial wall in
    the dog. Proc R Soc Lond [Biol] 146:541–551

44. Hilton SM, Spyer KM (1980) Central nervous regula-
    tion of vascular resistance. Ann Rev Physiol 42:399–
    411

45. Iberall AS (1967) Anatomy and steady flow characteris-
    tics of the arterial system with an introduction to its
    pulsatile characteristics. Math Biosci 1:375–395

46. Intaglietta M, Zweifach BW (1974) Microcirculatory
    basis of fluid exchange. Adv Biol Med Phys 15:111–119

47. Jardin F, Farcot J-C, Boisante L, Curien N, Margairaz
    A, Bourdarias J-P (1981) Influence of positive end-
    expiratory pressure on left ventricular performance. N
    Engl J Med 302:387–392

48. Johansson B (1974) Determinants of vascular reactivity.
    Fed Proc 33:121–126

49. Johansson B (1978) Vascular smooth muscle biophys-
    ics. In: Kaley G, Altura BM (eds) Microcirculation II.
    University Park Press, Baltimore

50. Johansson B (1981) Vascular smooth muscle reactiv-
    ity. Ann Rev Physiol 43:359–370

51. Karim F, Hainsworth R (1976) Responses of abdominal
    vascular capacitance to stimulation of splanchnic
    nerves. Am J Physiol 231:434–440

52. Kjellmer I (1964) The effect of exercise on the vascular
    bed of skeletal muscle. Acta Physiol Scand 62:18–30

53. Kjellmer I (1965) On the competition between meta-
    bolic vasodilatation and neurogenic vasoconstriction
    in skeletal muscle. Acta Physiol Scand 63:450–459

54. Kontos HA (1981) Regulation of the cerebral circula-
    tion. Ann Rev Physiol 43:397–407

55. Kolin A (1978) Methods of relative and absolute induc-
    tion angiometry for observation of changes in vascular
    compliance in conscious subjects. J Physiol (Lond)
    284:109P

56. Laver MB, Strauss HW, Pohost GM (1979) Right and
    left ventricular geometry: adjustments during acute
    respiratory failure. Crit Care Med 7:509–519

57. Lundholm L, Mohme-Lundholm E (1966) Length of
    inactivated contractile elements, length-tension dia-
    gram, active state and tone of vascular smooth muscle.
    Acta Physiol Scand 68:347–359

58. McDonald DA (1974) The elastic properties of the
    arterial wall. In: Blood flow in arteries, 2nd edn.
    Edward Arnold, London

59. Malik AB, Kidd BSL (1973) Independent effects of changes in H^+ and CO_2 concentrations on hypoxic pulmonary vasoconstriction. J Appl Phys 34:318–324
60. Mancia G, Ferrari A, Gregorini L, et al. (1979) Control of blood pressure by carotid baroreceptors in human beings. Am J Cardiol 44:895–902
61. Matthay RA, Wood LDH (1981) Cardiovascular function in respiratory failure. Introduction: The functionally integrated cardiovascular pulmonary unit. Am J Cardiol 47:683–685
62. Mellander S (1960) Comparative studies on the adrenergic neurohumoral control of resistance and capacitance blood vessels in the cat. Acta Physiol Scand 50 [Suppl 176] 1–86
63. Mellander S, Oberg B, Odelram H (1964) Vascular adjustments to increase transmural pressure in cat and man, with special reference to shift in capillary fluid transfer. Acta Physiol Scand 61:34–48
64. Mellander S, Johansson B (1968) Control of resistance, exchange and capacitance function in the peripheral circulation. Pharmacol Rev 20:117–196
65. Miller ED (1981) The role of the renin-angiotensin-aldosterone system in circulatory control and in hypertension. Br J Anaesth 53:711–718
66. Mintzner W, Goldberg HS (1975) Effects of epinephrine on resistive and compliant properties of the canine vasculature. J Appl Phys 39:272–280
67. Nisell O (1948) Effects of oxygen and carbon dioxide on the circulation of isolated and perfused lungs of the cat. Acta Physiol Scand 16:121–128
68. Olsson RA (1981) Local factors regulating cardiac and skeletal muscle blood flow. Ann Rev Physiol 43:385–395
69. Parker JC, Guyton AC, Taylor AE (1979) Pulmonary transcapillary exchange and pulmonary oedema. In: Guyton AC, Young DB (eds) Cardiovascular physiology III. International review of physiology, vol 18. University Park Press, Baltimore
70. Patel DJ, Vaishnav RN (1977) Mechanical properties of arteries. In: Hwang NHC, Norman NA (ed) Cardiovascular flow dynamics and measurements. University Park Press, Baltimore
71. Peterson LH, Jensen RE, Parnell J (1960) Mechanical properties of arteries in vivo. Circ Res 8:622–639
72. Philipp T, Distler A, Cordes V (1978) Sympathetic nervous system and blood pressure control in essential hypertension. Lancet 2:959–963
73. Prys-Roberts C, Green LT, Meloche R, Foëx P (1971) Studies of anaesthesia in relation to hypertension II: Haemodynamic consequences of induction and endotracheal intubation. Br J Anaesth 43:531–547
74. Rashkind WJ, Lewis DH, Henderson LB, Heiman DF, Dietrick RB (1953) Venous return as affected by cardiac output and total peripheral resistance. Am J Physiol 175:415–423
75. Rees PM, Sleight P, Robinson JL, Bonchek L, Doctor A (1978) Histology and ultrastructure of the carotid sinus in experimental hypertension. J Comp Neurol 181:245–252
76. Renken EM (1968) Neurogenic factors in microcirculatory low flow states. In: Shepro D, Fulton GP (eds) Microcirculation as related to shock. Academic, New York
77. Rippe B, Kamiya A, Folkow B (1978) Simultaneous measurements of capillary diffusion and filtration exchange during shifts in filtration-absorption and at graded alterations in the capillary permeability surface area products (PS). Acta Physiol Scand 104:318–336
78. Roach MR, Burton AC (1957) Reasons for the shape of the distensibility curves of arteries. Can J Biochem Physiol 681:35–47
79. Robinson BF (1980) Assessment of the effects of drugs on the venous system in man. In: Shanks RG (ed) Methods in clinical pharmacology I. Cardiovascular system. McMillan, London
80. Roddie IC, Wallace WFM (1980) Methods for the assessment of the effects of drugs on the arterial system in man. In: Shanks RG (ed) Methods in clinical pharmacology I. Cardiovascular system. McMillan, London.
81. Rosell S, Intaglietta M, Chisholm GM (1974) Adrenergic influence on isovolumetric capillary pressure in canine adipose tissue. Am J Physiol 227:692–696
82. Rudolph AM, Yuan S (1966) Response of the pulmonary vasculature to hypoxia and H^+ ion concentration changes. J Clin Invest 45:399–411
83. Rushmer RF (1970) Cardiovascular dynamics, 3rd edn. Saunders, Philadelphia
84. Rutlen DL, Supple EW, Powell WJ (1981) Adrenergic regulation of total systemic distensibility. Am J Cardiol 47:579–588
85. Rutlen DL, Supple EW, Powell WJ (1981) Beta adrenergic regulation of total systemic intravascular volume in the dog. Circ Res 48:112–120
86. Schmidt R, Kumada M, Sagawa K (1971) Cardiac output total peripheral resistance in the carotid sinus reflex. Am J Physiol 221:480–487
87. Shoukas AA, Sagawa K (1971) Total systemic vascular compliance measured as incremental volume-pressure ratio. Circ Res 28:277–289
88. Shoukas AA, Sagawa K (1973) Control of total systemic vascular capacity by the carotid sinus baroreceptor reflex. Circ Res 33:22–33
89. Sigurdsson SB, Orlov RS, Hellstrand P, Johansson B (1981) Response to ions and vasoconstrictor agents and changes of potassium fluxes in vascular smooth muscle during hypoxia. Acta Physiol Scand 112:455–462
90. Sjöstrand T (1953) Volume and distribution of blood and their significance in regulating the circulation. Physiol Rev 33:202–228
91. Starling EH (1896) On the absorption of fluids from connection tissue spaces. J Physiol (Lond) 19:312–326
92. Starling EH (1897) Some points in the pathology of heart disease. Lancet i:652–655
93. Starling EH (1909) The fluids of the body. WT Keener, Chicago
94. Staub NC (1974) Pulmonary oedema. Physiol Rev 54:678–811
95. Watt TB, Burrus CS (1976) Arterial pressure contour analysis for estimating human vascular properties. J Appl Phys 40:171–176
96. Weber KT, Janicki JS, Shroff S, Fishman AP (1981) Contractile mechanics and interactions of the right and left ventricles. Am J Cardiol 47:686–695
97. West JB, Dollery CT, Naimark A (1964) Distribution of blood flow in isolated lung: relation to vascular and alveolar pressures. J Appl Phys 19:713–724
98. Westfall T (1980) Neuroeffector mechanisms. Ann Rev Physiol 42:383–397
99. Widdicombe JG, Sterling GM (1970) The autonomic nervous system and breathing. Arch Intern Med 126:311–329
100. Wyatt DG (1968) The electromagnetic blood flowmeter. J Sci Instr (Series 2) 1:1146
101. Wyatt DG (1977) Theory, design, and use of electromagnetic flowmeters. In: Hwang NHC, Normann NA (eds) Cardiovascular flow dynamics and measurements. University Park Press, Baltimore
102. Zanchetti A (1979) An overview of cardiovascular reflexes in hypertension. Am J Cardiol 44:912–918

Chapter 3

Pulmonary Ventilation and Gas Exchange

Michael Rudolf

The prime function of the respiratory system is to ensure that there is effective gas exchange between air and blood. This means that the lungs must transfer sufficient O_2 from inspired air to arterial blood, so that ultimately tissue and cellular processes may proceed without interference, and at the same time metabolically produced CO_2 must be removed from venous blood into the expired air. The overall aim of pulmonary gas exchange is thus to keep the arterial and mixed venous O_2 and CO_2 tensions constant.

The physiological processes involved in ensuring that O_2 reaches the tissues in sufficient quantity can be broadly divided into four stages: (1) O_2 in inspired air must gain access to the alveoli of the lung where gas exchange takes place: this is the stage of ventilation; (2) O_2, now in the alveoli, must cross the blood–gas interface (the alveolar–capillary membrane): this is the stage of diffusion; (3) O_2, now in the pulmonary capillary blood, must be removed from the lung and gain access to the systemic circulation: this will depend on pulmonary blood flow; (4) O_2 must now be transported to the tissues where it will diffuse into tissue mitochondria so that cellular respiration may take place; this important aspect of respiratory physiology concerned with O_2 transport and consumption is dealt with in Chap. 4.

These four stages must also occur in reverse order for the successful elimination of CO_2 from the tissues, via the venous circulation, into expired air. It is the processes involved in stages (1), (2), and (3), namely ventilation, diffusion, and blood flow, and in particular the complex interactions of these processes, that are the elements of pulmonary gas exchange. It is therefore with these processes that this chapter will be concerned.

Anatomy

When vertebrates moved out of the sea onto dry land, the change in environment was accompanied by evolutionary changes in the respiratory system. The need to conserve water resulted in the development of an internal lung, in which blood is separated from the air by a tissue membrane. However, whereas the blood is brought to the lung by one system (pulmonary arterial) and removed by another (pulmonary venous), the airways are a complex system of branching tubes open to the atmosphere at one end only, and so have to subserve both inspiration and expiration. Thus, while blood flow in the lung is unidirectional and continuous, ventilation is intermittent and reciprocating. In each breath of tidal volume V_T there is a certain volume of air which is simply shunted in and out of the lung without ever taking part in gas exchange; this is the anatomical dead space V_D, and

$$V_T = V_D + V_A \qquad \text{[Eq. 3.1]}$$

where V_A (alveolar volume) is the amount of gas in each tidal breath that has actually reached the gas-exchanging part of the lung. The airways in the lung can therefore be divided into conducting airways (which make up the anatomical dead space) and the respiratory or gas-exchanging airways (where alveolar ventilation occurs).

Movement of air in the conducting airways is mainly by convective flow, but the mechanism by which gases in the respiratory airways become mixed is molecular diffusion [25]. This mechanism of molecular diffusion also occurs in the tissue phase across the alveolar–capillary membrane, and without it mammalian lungs would be unable to exchange O_2 and CO_2 between air and blood. Diffusion is a relatively slow process in tissues, but this is compensated for by the tissue membrane being extremely thin and having a very large surface area.

The structure and morphology of the airways are well adapted for efficient function with respect to the movement of gas; these correlations between structure and function have been well reviewed by Horsfield [24, 25].

Ventilation

Alveolar ventilation

Ventilation is concerned with how inspired air gets into the alveoli and how expired air is removed. Each expired tidal breath is made up of a dead space component V_D and an alveolar component V_A (Eq. [3.1]). If we now consider ventilation (i.e., volume per unit time) rather than volume, Eq. (3.1) becomes

$$\dot{V}_E = \dot{V}_D + \dot{V}_A \qquad \text{[Eq. 3.2]}$$

where $\dot{V}_E$ is expired minute volume, and $\dot{V}_D$ and $\dot{V}_A$ are the dead space and alveolar ventilation, respectively. As it is the alveolar (or gas-exchanging) ventilation that is of interest, we can rearrange this equation as

$$\dot{V}_A = \dot{V}_E - \dot{V}_D \qquad \text{[Eq. 3.3]}$$

Although $\dot{V}_A$ can be calculated by measuring $\dot{V}_E$ and assuming a value for dead space (or actually measuring it by Fowler's method [19]), another method of calculating $\dot{V}_A$ in normal subjects is to start from the concentration of CO_2 in alveolar gas. Since there is no gas exchange in the conducting airways and inspired air contains virtually no CO_2, all the expired CO_2 must come from alveolar gas, i.e.,

$$\dot{V}_{CO_2} = \dot{V}_A \times F_A CO_2 \qquad \text{[Eq. 3.4]}$$

where $\dot{V}_{CO_2}$ is the volume of CO_2 exhaled per unit time and $F_A CO_2$ is the fractional concentration of CO_2 in alveolar gas. Converting fractional concentration of gas to partial pressure, and rearranging,

$$\dot{V}_A = K \times \frac{\dot{V}_{CO_2}}{P_A CO_2} \qquad \text{[Eq. 3.5]}$$

where $P_A CO_2$ is now the partial pressure of CO_2 in alveolar gas and K is a constant. In traditional units (millimeters of mercury for pressure and millilitres STPD for gas uptake) K = 0.863, while in SI units (kilopascals for pressure and millimoles for gas uptake) K = 2.561. In either system of units, alveolar ventilation ($\dot{V}_A$) is in litres per minute BTPS, and the relationship between $\dot{V}_A$ and $P_A CO_2$ is shown graphically in Fig. 3.1.

In the steady state, the amount of CO_2 being eliminated by the lungs per minute ($\dot{V}_{CO_2}$) must be equal to the metabolic production of CO_2 by the tissues, and so Eq. (3.5) tells us that, if metabolic production of CO_2 remains constant, alveolar ventilation is inversely proportional to the alveolar PCO_2. Since in normal subjects the partial pressures of CO_2 in alveolar gas and arterial blood are virtually identical, $\dot{V}_A$ is inversely proportional to the arterial CO_2 tension $P_a CO_2$, i.e.,

$$\dot{V}_A \propto (P_a CO_2)^{-1} \qquad \text{[Eq. 3.6]}$$

Thus in clinical practice, changes in $P_a CO_2$ can often be interpreted as inverse changes in $\dot{V}_A$, assuming that CO_2 production remains unchanged.

Dead space

So far, dead space has been regarded as an anatomical concept, namely those parts of the lung (the conducting airways down to the level of the terminal bronchioles) where inspired air never comes into contact with the gas-exchanging part of the lung. But not all of the inspired air that does reach the alveoli is equally

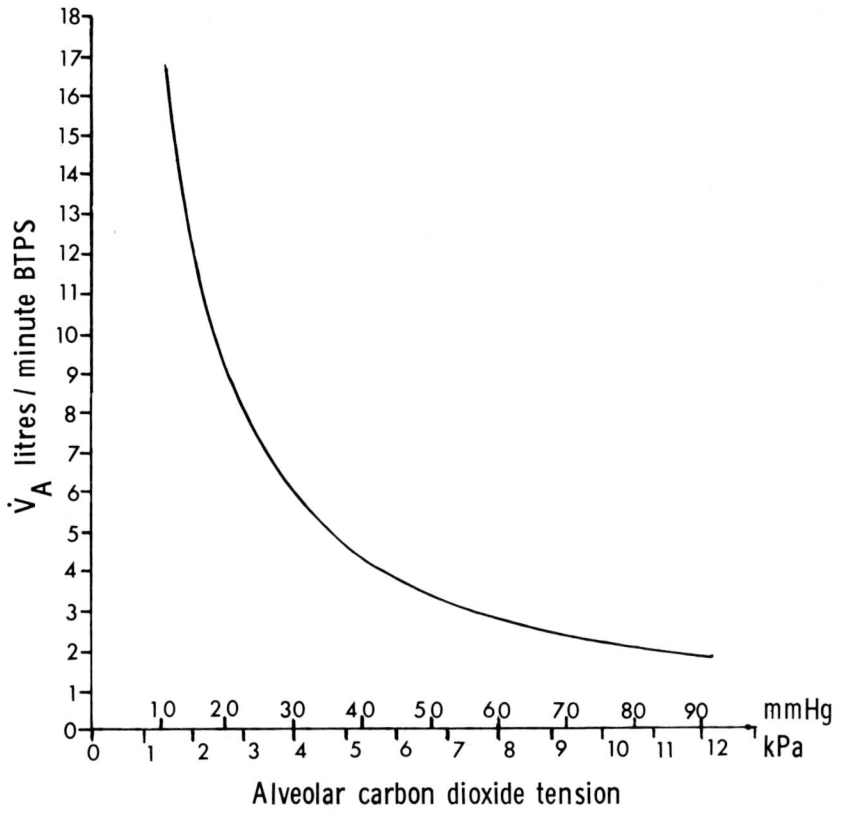

Fig. 3.1. The relationship between $\dot{V}_A$ and P_ACO_2 for $\dot{V}_{CO_2} = 200$ ml/min (9 mmol/min).

effective in arterializing mixed venous blood. Some alveoli, though ventilated, are not perfused at all with pulmonary capillary blood, and other alveoli, although both ventilated and perfused, are actually relatively overventilated and underperfused. In the same way that the anatomical dead space represents ventilation that is 'wasted' as regards gas exchange, so also the ventilation of such lung units which are either non-perfused or relatively underperfused represents 'wasted ventilation' and can be equated with an alveolar dead space [46].

As both the anatomical dead space and this alveolar dead space are unavailable for gas exchange, the sum of these two will give an overall 'effective' or physiological dead space, and this can now easily be calculated in terms of CO_2 elimination. The effective alveolar volume V_A is given by $V_A = V_E - V_D$, where V_D is now the overall physiological dead space and V_E is the volume of expired gas. It is still true that all the expired CO_2 must have come from gas-exchanging parts of the lung, and so $V_E \times F_E = V_A \times F_A$, where F_E and F_A are the fractional concentrations of CO_2 in mixed expired and alveolar gas, respectively. From these two equations, $V_E \times F_E = (V_E - V_D) \times F_A$,

and therefore

$$\frac{V_D}{V_E} = \frac{F_A - F_E}{F_A}.$$

Substituting partial pressures for fractional concentrations and P_aCO_2 for P_ACO_2, and equating V_E with the tidal volume V_T, we have the Bohr equation for physiological dead space:

$$\frac{V_D}{V_T} = \frac{P_aCO_2 - P_ECO_2}{P_aCO_2} \quad \text{[Eq. 3.7]}$$

In ideal lungs, there would be no alveolar dead space and the overall physiological dead space given by Eq. (3.7) would be identical with the anatomical dead space. In normal, as opposed to ideal, lungs the magnitude of the alveolar dead space (and hence the physiological dead space) depends on the distribution of pulmonary blood flow and the amount of wasted ventilation that occurs. It is minimal in the supine posture (in which position most of the alveoli are adequately perfused) and is increased in the upright posture, when there is relative underperfusion of apical alveoli.

The V_D/V_T ratio, which should normally be

less than 0.30, is a good indicator of inequality between ventilation and blood flow within the lung, and it is increased in a wide range of respiratory diseases. In the presence of a high physiological dead space, an increase in total pulmonary ventilation will be necessary to maintain CO_2 elimination and to keep P_aCO_2 normal. If limitations in lung mechanics preclude the increase in ventilation, alveolar PCO_2 will rise. This will enable the same amount of CO_2 to be eliminated by a lower alveolar ventilation (Fig. 3.1), but at the expense (and danger) of a raised alveolar, and hence arterial, CO_2 tension.

Distribution of ventilation

In the discussion on dead space, it was suggested that the distribution of pulmonary blood flow throughout the lung was not uniform, and that there were some alveoli which were either not perfused or relatively underperfused. The reasons for this distribution of blood flow will be discussed later. The distribution of ventilation throughout the lung is also not uniform, and studies with inhalation of radioactive xenon have shown that the lower regions of the lung ventilate more than the upper zones, i.e., regional ventilation decreases from base to apex in the upright posture [9]. This gradient in distribution of ventilation can be abolished when normal subjects lie supine, although in that posture the posterior (i.e., lowermost) lung has a greater ventilation than the anterior (uppermost) lung. In the lateral posture, ventilation is greatest in the dependent lung.

These experiments all suggest that regional differences in ventilation in the lung are largely due to gravity and the resulting gradient in pleural pressure [31], whereby, in the upright posture, the intrapleural pressure is more markedly negative at the apex than at the base. Thus basal regions of the lung are relatively compressed and will expand more on inspiration than the apical regions. The same reasoning explains the higher ventilation of dependent lung regions in the supine and lateral positions.

The distribution of ventilation depends not only on the pleural pressure gradient but also on the distributions of pleural pressure changes with tidal breathing, of resistance, of compliance, and of airway closure. The rate of inspiration and the lung volume from which inspiration commences are also important [3,20].

Alveolar gas tensions

Alveolar CO_2 tension

All the discussion on $\dot{V}_A$ has so far been concerned with the elimination of CO_2, and both Eq. (3.5) and Eq. (3.7) were obtained without paying any attention to O_2. Clearly ventilation is of prime importance in bringing O_2 into the alveoli so that gas exchange may occur, and we must now consider this in more detail. In calculating the alveolar O_2 tension (Eq. [3.10], below) it will again be necessary to assume that the alveolar and arterial tensions of CO_2 are equal. This assumption has already been made in deriving Eqs. (3.6) and (3.7), and it is now necessary to question this assumption and ask what exactly is meant by the term 'alveolar gas'

In deriving the relationship between $\dot{V}_A$ and alveolar PCO_2 (Eq. [3.5]), it was taken for granted that there is such an entity as a single value for P_ACO_2. But in real life, with lungs containing 300 million alveoli, all of which may have their own inequalities between ventilation and blood flow, the partial pressures of CO_2 in different parts of the lung may vary widely, and there is no single value for P_ACO_2. Nor is it possible to obtain a mean value for P_ACO_2 by analysing a sample of expired alveolar gas; first because different alveoli empty at different rates and so no spot sample of expired gas would be representative, and second because gas exchange is still taking place (and the alveolar gas tensions are altering) whilst such a sample is being collected [42].

It is for these reasons that we make the assumption that there is no significant difference between alveolar and arterial CO_2 tensions, and use the arterial PCO_2 as an estimate of the alveolar PCO_2. This represents a functional rather than a volumetric integration of the entire range of alveolar CO_2 tensions existing throughout the lung, although it will admittedly be weighted by the higher blood flow through the relatively well-perfused alveoli. Since P_aCO_2 is measured on a blood sample that has been collected through several ventilatory cycles, it will represent the mean effective PCO_2 at which the lung is working.

Alveolar O_2 tension

We can now move on to derive a formula for the alveolar tension of O_2 (P_AO_2). The amount of O_2 ($\dot{V}_{O_2}$) taken up by the lung per unit time and carried away by the pulmonary circulation must be equal to the difference between the amount of O_2 entering and leaving the alveoli, i.e.,

$$\dot{V}_{O_2} = (\dot{V}_A \times F_IO_2) - (\dot{V}_A \times F_AO_2) \quad \text{[Eq. 3.8]}$$

where F_IO_2 and F_AO_2 are the fractional concentrations of O_2 in inspired air and expired alveolar gas, respectively. This equation assumes that the inspired and expired alveolar gas volumes are identical. From Eq. (3.8),

$$F_AO_2 = F_IO_2 - \frac{\dot{V}_{O_2}}{\dot{V}_A}.$$

Substituting for $\dot{V}_A$ from Eq. (3.4),

$$F_AO_2 = F_IO_2 - \left(F_ACO_2 \times \frac{\dot{V}_{O_2}}{\dot{V}_{CO_2}}\right).$$

By definition, R (the respiratory exchange ratio) equals CO_2 output divided by O_2 uptake, i.e. $R = \dot{V}_{CO_2}/\dot{V}_{O_2}$. Therefore

$$F_AO_2 = F_IO_2 - \frac{F_ACO_2}{R}$$

and converting fractional concentrations of gases to partial pressures,

$$P_AO_2 = P_IO_2 - \frac{P_ACO_2}{R}. \quad \text{[Eq. 3.9]}$$

In fact, the inspired and expired alveolar gas volumes are not identical (because R is not equal to unity). The corrected form of Eq. (3.9) can be derived from the fact that the volumes of inspired and expired nitrogen are equal, and then, by simple but tedious algebra, it can be shown that

$$P_AO_2 = P_IO_2 - \frac{P_ACO_2}{R}$$
$$+ \left[\frac{P_ACO_2 \times F_IO_2 \times (1 - R)}{R}\right].$$

This correcting factor can usually be ignored, and, substituting P_aCO_2 for P_ACO_2, we have

$$P_AO_2 = P_IO_2 - \frac{P_aCO_2}{R} \quad \text{[Eq. 3.10]}$$

which is the alveolar air equation as usually used in clinical practice. By knowing the inspired O_2 tension P_IO_2, measuring P_aCO_2, and assuming a value of 0.8 for R, we can calculate P_AO_2. Note that this calculated P_AO_2 is the physiologically effective or 'ideal' alveolar O_2 tension that would be present throughout the alveoli of a perfectly homogeneous lung. In fact, just as with CO_2, the actual pressures of O_2 in

the alveoli may vary widely in different parts of the lung.

A more complicated analysis of the concept of ideal alveolar gas and the determination of alveolar gas tensions depends on equations which express the alveolar gas concentrations in terms of their relative alveolar ventilation and pulmonary blood flow [38, 40–43]. The simultaneous solution of these blood and gas respiratory exchange equations is most easily accomplished by a graphical method (the $O_2 - CO_2$ diagram [39]), which yields all the possible simultaneous alveolar PO_2 and PCO_2 values which could theoretically exist for any given mixed venous and inspired tensions of these gases. A full discussion of this topic is beyond the scope of this chapter.

Diffusion

Transfer of gas across the blood–gas interface (alveolar–capillary membrane) is by the process of molecular diffusion. This is a passive process and is governed by the usual physical laws: the rate of transfer of gas across the membrane is proportional to the pressure difference across the membrane and the area of the membrane, and inversely proportional to the membrane's thickness. The alveolar–capillary membrane in normal human lung has a total area of 50–100 m^2 and an average thickness of less than 1 μm, so that it is ideally suited for diffusion.

When a gas diffuses between a gaseous phase and a tissue phase, the rate of diffusion is also proportional to the solubility of the gas and inversely proportional to the square root of its molecular weight. Thus when comparing the rates of diffusion of O_2 and CO_2 (DO_2 and DCO_2), the ratio of

$$\frac{DO_2}{DCO_2} = \frac{\text{Solubility of } O_2}{\text{Solubility of } CO_2}$$
$$\times \frac{\sqrt{\text{Molecular weight } CO_2}}{\sqrt{\text{Molecular weight } O_2}},$$

which works out at about 0.05, so that CO_2 diffuses about 20 times more rapidly than O_2 through the alveolar–capillary membrane. It is therefore usually assumed that CO_2 elimination from the lung is not affected by any diffusion difficulties, and all further discussion on diffusion will be limited to its effect on O_2.

Oxygen

The overall diffusion pathway for an O_2 molecule from alveolar gas to the interior of a pulmonary capillary erythrocyte consists of the following [54]: (1) the surfactant layer lining alveoli; (2) the tissues of the alveolar wall (alveolar epithelium, interstitium, and capillary endothelium); (3) plasma in the capillary; (4) the red cell membrane. Once in the red cell, reaction kinetics with haemoglobin also have to be considered.

We have already seen that the structure of the alveolar–capillary membrane is ideally suited to diffusion, and it is now necessary to consider the pressure difference across the membrane and the time that is available for diffusion. The normal pressure gradient at the beginning of the pulmonary capillary is alveolar O_2 tension (100 mmHg or 13.3 kPa) on the gas side of the membrane, and mixed venous O_2 tension (40 mmHg or 5.3 kPa) on the blood side. The pressure difference is thus 60 mmHg (8 kPa), and this can be regarded as the 'driving pressure' for O_2 across the gas-blood interface. If there is alveolar hypoxia this driving pressure

will be decreased, and the experimental manipulation of alveolar hypoxia to differentiate between true diffusion defects and ventilation–perfusion inequality will be discussed later.

Pulmonary capillary transit time

The uptake of O_2 by blood as it traverses a pulmonary capillary [47] is represented schematically in Fig. 3.2. The PO_2 of a red cell entering the pulmonary capillary is 40 mmHg (5.3 kPa), i.e., mixed venous PO_2. On the other side of the membrane the PO_2 is 100 mmHg (13.3 kPa), and the PO_2 of the red cell will rapidly rise to very nearly reach this alveolar level within 0.25 s, which is well within the total time spent by an erythrocyte in a pulmonary capillary (usually about 0.75 s). Even when diffusion is abnormal due to pathological thickening of the membrane (Fig. 3.2B), the PO_2 of blood leaving the capillary will still be normal or only slightly reduced, so long as the red cells still have a full 0.75 s in which to become oxygenated. However, if the total time available for diffusion is reduced (Fig. 3.2A and B), then

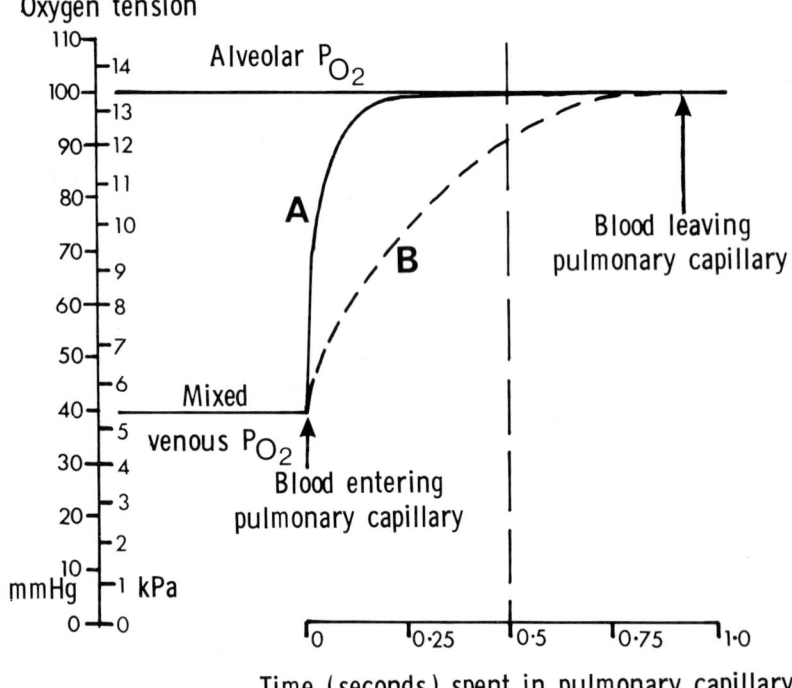

Fig. 3.2. *Continuous line*, **A**, shows time course of changes in PO_2 for red cells passing through pulmonary capillaries with normal diffusion properties; PO_2 rises from mixed venous to alveolar level within 0.25 s. With abnormal diffusion properties (*discontinuous line*, **B**), PO_2 still rises to almost reach alveolar level, but now takes 0.75 s. If time spent by erythrocytes in capillaries is reduced to 0.5 s (*vertical dashed line*), end-capillary PO_2 will be unchanged for red cells in normal capillaries (**A**), but will be decreased for blood in abnormal capillaries (**B**).

differences become apparent: with normal diffusion there is no appreciable change in the end-capillary PO_2, but with the abnormal diffusion time course the red cells no longer have sufficient time in which to become fully oxygenated and so there will be a measurable difference between alveolar and end-capillary O_2 tensions.

Such a situation may well arise on exercise where, due to the increase in cardiac output, there is a reduction in the amount of time that red cells spend in traversing the pulmonary capillary bed. This provides an explanation for the occurrence of hypoxaemia on exercise in patients with lung disease where diffusion is thought to be impaired. Exercise, with its resultant decrease in red cell pulmonary transit time, is an excellent method of stressing the diffusion properties of the lung.

Measurement of pulmonary diffusing capacity

To measure the pulmonary diffusing capacity for O_2, it is necessary to know the mean pressure gradient driving O_2 across the alveolar–capillary membrane. This can be determined by the Bohr integration procedure, but for routine clinical purposes it is much simpler to measure the diffusing capacity of the lung by means of a gas with physical properties which simplify the problem. Such a gas is carbon monoxide (CO) which, because it has such a high affinity for haemoglobin, has a negligibly low partial pressure in pulmonary capillary blood and so the pressure gradient across the membrane for CO is equal to its alveolar pressure.

Following inhalation of a small amount of CO and estimation of its alveolar concentration and how much has been taken up by the blood in a given time, the diffusing capacity of the lung for CO (D_LCO) can be calculated in $ml.min^{-1}.mmHg^{-1}$ (or $mmol.min^{-1}.kPa^{-1}$ in SI units). D_LCO is usually measured in the laboratory by a single-breath technique with 10 s breath-holding [34]. Recently, a bedside rebreathing technique has been described, which is ideally suited for critically ill patients [11].

The diffusing capacity measured in this way includes both a membrane component and a blood component:

$$\frac{1}{D_LCO} = \frac{1}{D_M} + \frac{1}{\theta.V_c} \quad \text{[Eq. 3.11]}$$

where D_M is the diffusing capacity of the alveolar–capillary membrane, θ is the reaction rate of CO with haemoglobin, and V_c is the blood

volume of the pulmonary capillary bed [44]. The value of θ will vary according to the prevailing O_2 tension and haemoglobin concentration, and changes in V_c occur with alterations in lung volume and posture, as well as in disease. Hence the overall D_LCO may well be affected by changes in θ and V_c that are not associated with any structural change in the membrane. When D_LCO is measured at different alveolar O_2 tensions (and therefore at different values of θ), Eq. (3.11) can be solved graphically for D_M and V_c, and it can be shown that both the membrane and blood components contribute approximately equally to the resistance to CO uptake by normal lungs [44].

Even static, extravascular red cells will take up CO, and there is a raised D_LCO in patients with pulmonary haemorrhage due to Goodpasture's syndrome [15]. Serial measurements of D_LCO can be used to monitor the progress of such patients [21].

The contribution—if any—of diffusion impairment to hypoxaemia in disease, and the relative importance of diffusion impairment against ventilation–perfusion inequality, will be discussed later.

Blood flow

Distribution of pulmonary blood flow

The pulmonary circulation is a low-resistance, low-pressure circulation. The pulmonary capillaries are unique in that they are virtually surrounded by gas. Although there is a layer of epithelial cells lining the alveoli, these provide little support for the capillaries, which consequently tend to become compressed or distended, depending on the prevailing intraluminal and transmural pressures [60]. Because of these factors, there is a large difference between the blood flow to the apex of the lung and that to the base in the upright posture.

In the same way that inhalation of radioactive xenon showed regional differences in ventilation, so the IV infusion of dissolved radioactive xenon can be used to demonstrate the distribution of blood flow throughout the lung [28]. Other radioactive gases, such as $C-^{15}O_2$ or, more recently ^{81m}Kr, can also be used [10, 59]. All these studies have shown that, in the upright posture, blood flow decreases almost linearly from base to apex.

There is thus a gravitational distribution of

pulmonary blood flow not dissimilar from that for ventilation. It is due to the hydrostatic pressure differences within the compressible and distensible pulmonary capillaries, and this was elucidated by West et al. in a series of elegant experiments on isolated dog lungs [60]. They found that the upright lung could be divided into three zones (Fig. 3.3):

Zone I. Arterial pressure is everywhere less than alveolar (atmospheric) pressure, so the capillaries collapse and there is no blood flow. Such a zone does not usually occur in man, but may do so if arterial pressure is reduced (e.g., low cardiac output) or if alveolar pressure is increased (e.g., during positive pressure ventilation [IPPV]).

Zone II. Due to hydrostatic effects, arterial pressure is higher and is now greater than alveolar pressure. Venous pressure is still less than alveolar, and under these conditions the capillary behaves as a Starling resistor; blood flow is determined by the arterial–alveolar pressure difference, and venous pressure has no influence. Since arterial pressure steadily rises down the zone while alveolar pressure remains constant, blood flow will steadily increase down zone II.

Zone III. Venous pressure is now greater than alveolar, so flow in the capillaries is determined by the arterial–venous pressure difference. Although this remains constant down the zone, the transmural pressure across the capillary wall steadily increases. This leads to distension of the capillaries, and so there is a steady increase in blood flow down zone III.

In addition to this overall gravitational pattern of pulmonary blood flow, there are also important local variations mediated by various mechanisms, the most important of which is hypoxic vasoconstriction.

Shunt

Not all the blood that enters the systemic arterial circulation has been in contact with alveolar gas and had a chance to become oxygenated. There is some true right-to-left shunting (via Thebesian and bronchial veins) in normal lungs, and there may of course be massive right-to-left shunting in patients with congenital cardiac defects or pulmonary arteriovenous malformations. Such factors will contribute to a real or anatomical shunt. In addition, due to ventilation–perfusion mismatch there will be some blood entering the arterial circulation which has come from alveoli that either are not ventilated at all or are underventilated relative to their blood flow. Such blood can be regarded as if a certain proportion of it had been shunted past the lungs without partaking in gas exchange, and this theoretical amount of shunt will obviously be increased in disease, where

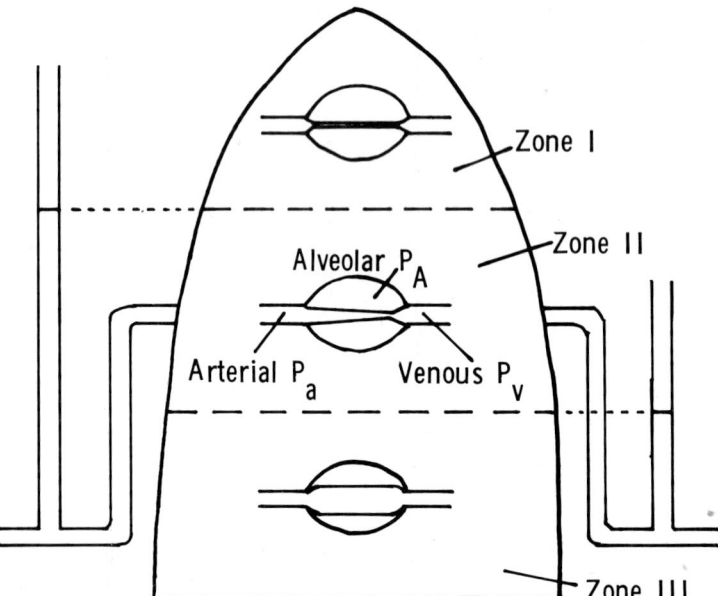

Fig. 3.3. Schematic representation of hydrostatic pressures within pulmonary capillaries and effect on distribution of blood flow. Alveolar pressure is everywhere atmospheric. In zone I, $P_A > P_a > P_v$, so capillaries collapse and there is no flow. In zone II, $P_a > P_A > P_v$, so capillaries behave as Starling resistors and flow is determined by $P_a - P_A$, which steadily increases down the zone. In zone III, $P_a > P_v > P_A$, and transmural pressure across the capillary wall increases down the zone, so there is progressive dilatation of vessels and increase in flow down the zone.

the inequality between ventilation and perfusion in the lungs is greater.

Thus in the same way as we developed the concept of an overall physiological dead space (made up of a true anatomical dead space plus an alveolar dead space, the latter due to unperfused or relatively underperfused alveoli), so too we can arrive at the concept of an overall physiological shunt, made up of a true anatomical shunt plus a theoretical shunt (called the venous admixture), the latter due to pulmonary blood flow that goes through unventilated or relatively underventilated alveoli.

Similarly, in the same way as it was possible to derive a formula (Eq. [3.7]) from which we could calculate the total physiological dead space as a fraction of the tidal volume, so too it is possible to derive an equation expressing the physiological shunt ($\dot{Q}_S$) as a fraction of the total cardiac output ($\dot{Q}_T$). The total blood flow entering the systemic circulation ($\dot{Q}_T$) is behaving as if some ($\dot{Q}_C$) has been through the pulmonary capillary bed and taken part in perfect (or ideal) gas exchange, and the remainder ($\dot{Q}_S$) has been effectively shunted past the pulmonary capillary bed and not taken part in any gas exchange. By definition,

$$\dot{Q}_T = \dot{Q}_C + \dot{Q}_S, \quad \text{or}$$
$$\dot{Q}_C = \dot{Q}_T - \dot{Q}_S.$$

$$[Eq. \ 3.12]$$

Now the total quantity of O_2 entering the circulation per minute must be equal to the amount being carried by the normally oxygenated blood plus the amount being carried by the shunted blood. Since the amount of O_2 being carried per minute for any particular blood flow $\dot{Q}$ is equal to $\dot{Q}$ multiplied by the content of O_2 in the blood, we can write

$\dot{Q}_T \times$ content of O_2 in arterial blood

$\quad = (\dot{Q}_C \times$ content of O_2 in normally oxygenated blood)

$\quad + (\dot{Q}_S \times$ content of O_2 in shunted blood).

If we assume that all the shunted blood has the composition of mixed venous blood, then

$$\dot{Q}_T \times C_aO_2 = (\dot{Q}_C \times C_{C'}O_2)$$
$$+ (\dot{Q}_S \times C_{\bar{v}}O_2) \quad [Eq. \ 3.13]$$

where C_aO_2, $C_{C'}O_2$, and $C_{\bar{v}}O_2$ are the O_2 contents of arterial, pulmonary end-capillary, and mixed venous blood, respectively. Substituting for $\dot{Q}_C$ from Eq. (3.12) into Eq. (3.13),

$$\dot{Q}_T \times C_aO_2 = ([\dot{Q}_T - \dot{Q}_S] \times C_{C'}O_2)$$
$$+ (\dot{Q}_S \times C_{\bar{v}}O_2),$$

whence

$$\frac{\dot{Q}_S}{\dot{Q}_T} = \frac{C_{C'}O_2 - C_aO_2}{C_{C'}O_2 - C_{\bar{v}}O_2}. \quad [Eq. \ 3.14]$$

C_aO_2 can either be measured directly on an arterial blood sample or calculated from the arterial PO_2, pH, and haemoglobin concentration, assuming a standard oxyhaemoglobin dissociation curve [45]. $C_{\bar{v}}O_2$ can similarly be measured or calculated from a mixed venous blood sample. If mixed venous blood is not available, it can be assumed that $C_{\bar{v}}O_2$ is 5 ml/100 ml (or 2.23 mmol/litre) less than C_aO_2 (i.e., that there is a constant arteriovenous O_2 content difference). $C_{C'}O_2$ is calculated as the content of blood with a PO_2 equal to the ideal alveolar O_2 tension (calculated from the alveolar air equation) and a pH equal to arterial pH.

The total physiological shunt can thus be calculated as a fraction of the cardiac output. To ascertain how much of this is due to true shunt and how much is due to ventilation–perfusion inequality, repeat measurements and calculations can be made after a period of breathing 100% O_2. This will effectively abolish any hypoxaemia due to ventilation–perfusion mismatch, and will yield a value for the true extrapulmonary shunt. This can then be subtracted from the first value, the difference representing the amount of shunt due to inequality of ventilation and perfusion within the lung. Note, however, that O_2 breathing can itself lead to the development of areas of atelectasis and the collapse of lung units with low ventilation–perfusion ratios [13], and so the calculated true shunt with 100% O_2 may be greater than that which actually exists when the patient is breathing air. In addition, even in normal subjects, breathing 100% O_2 does not always completely eliminate alveolar nitrogen, and this too can lead to an overestimation of the extrapulmonary true shunt.

Ventilation–perfusion relationships

Reference has already been made to the fact that the lung contains some 300 million alveoli, each of which will make its own contribution to gas exchange, depending on its ventilation and blood flow. For each individual alveolus or lung unit, the relationship between its ventilation $\dot{V}_A$ and its blood flow or perfusion $\dot{Q}$ can be described as its ventilation–perfusion ($\dot{V}_A/\dot{Q}$) ratio. The possible range of $\dot{V}_A/\dot{Q}$ ratios can extend from zero (alveoli that are perfused but completely unventilated) to infinity (alveoli that are ventilated but not perfused). For lung units with perfect matching between ventilation and blood flow, $\dot{V}_A/\dot{Q}$ will equal unity. Low $\dot{V}_A/\dot{Q}$ ratios (less than unity) describe alveoli that are relatively underventilated and overperfused, and conversely, high $\dot{V}_A/\dot{Q}$ ratios (greater than unity) describe alveoli that are relatively under-perfused and overventilated. In ideal lungs, both ventilation and blood flow would be per-fectly matched throughout ($\dot{V}_A/\dot{Q} = 1$), with local control mechanisms always ensuring that any change in the local distribution of ventila-tion was accompanied by an appropriate com-pensatory change in the distribution of blood flow, and vice versa.

Distribution of ventilation and blood flow

In normal, as opposed to ideal, lungs, we have seen that there are various factors (mainly gravi-tational) affecting the distributions of ventilation and of blood flow. In the upright posture, both ventilation and blood flow steadily increase from the apex down to the base, but blood flow increases more rapidly than ventilation (Fig. 3.4). Thus at the apex, where ventilation is greater than blood flow, there are lung units with $\dot{V}_A/\dot{Q}$ ratios greater than unity, whereas at the base, where blood flow is now greater than ventilation, $\dot{V}_A/\dot{Q}$ ratios will be less than unity. So even in normal lungs there is a scatter of $\dot{V}_A/\dot{Q}$ ratios, and, for healthy young subjects in the semirecumbent posture, the range of $\dot{V}_A/\dot{Q}$ ratios extends from 0.3 to 2.1 [49]. The disper-sion of this distribution of $\dot{V}_A/\dot{Q}$ ratios increases with age, and it becomes especially marked in the presence of disease, when maldistribution of ventilation and blood flow within the lung (or ventilation–perfusion inequality) becomes the single most important cause of inefficient gas exchange.

Three-compartment model

The effect on pulmonary gas exchange of mis-match between ventilation and blood flow within the lung (and especially within the dis-eased lung) has so far been analysed in terms of physiological dead space and shunt. This allows the total effect of $\dot{V}_A/\dot{Q}$ inequality on arterial and expired gas tensions to be represented as if a certain proportion of the ventilation failed to reach the alveoli (dead space) and as if a certain

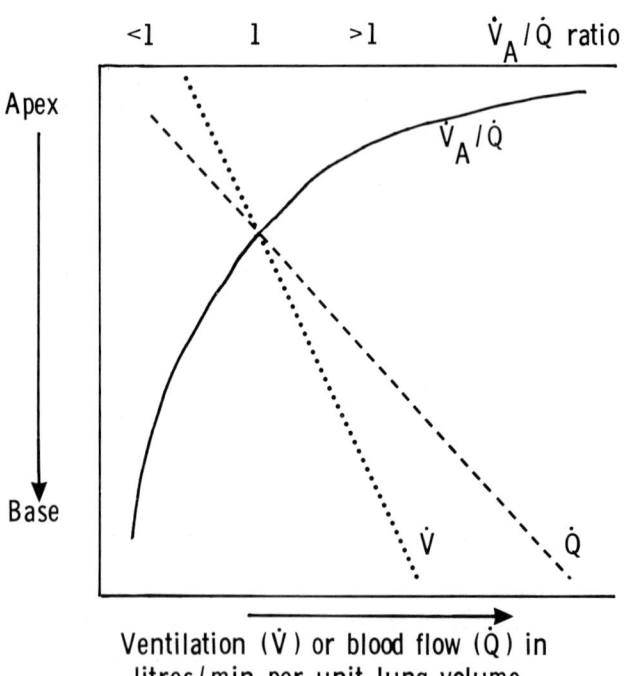

Fig. 3.4. Schematic representation of distribution of ventilation (-----), blood flow (– – –), and $\dot{V}_A:\dot{Q}$ ratios (———) in the normal upright lung. Both ventilation and blood flow increase from apex to base. At apex $\dot{V}_A/\dot{Q}$ ratios are >1, and at base $\dot{V}_A/\dot{Q}$ ratios are <1.

proportion of the pulmonary blood flow bypassed the lungs (venous admixture). In other words, the lung has been considered as a three-compartment model: one compartment acting as an ideal gas exchanger (with alveolar CO_2 tension equal to arterial CO_2 tension and alveolar O_2 tension being calculated from the ideal alveolar air equation), a second compartment acting as pure dead space ($\dot{V}_A/\dot{Q} = \infty$), and a third compartment acting as pure shunt ($\dot{V}_A/\dot{Q} = O$) [37]. Although such a three-compartment model is a useful concept, and calculation of the V_D/V_T and $\dot{Q}_S/\dot{Q}_T$ ratios allows the amounts of 'wasted' ventilation and pulmonary blood flow to be quantified, it is far more realistic to consider the continuous distribution of $\dot{V}_A/\dot{Q}$ ratios throughout the lung.

Computer techniques

One of the most important aids to our understanding of gas exchange and $\dot{V}_A/\dot{Q}$ ratios has been the development of appropriate computer techniques for dealing with the O_2 and CO_2 dissociation curves [30, 36], so that computer models could be constructed which allowed the behaviour of lungs with mismatched ventilation and blood flow to be studied [55]. In such models, ventilation, blood flow, and $\dot{V}_A/\dot{Q}$ ratios can be regarded as having a continuous logarithmic normal distribution throughout the lung, and the advantage of this is that the spread of each distribution can be described by a single parameter, the log standard deviation σ. Furthermore, the application of these computerized numerical techniques has allowed the development of experimental methods for determining the continuous distribution of $\dot{V}_A/\dot{Q}$ ratios in man, both in health and in disease. All these fundamental aspects of ventilation–perfusion relationships have been well reviewed in two key papers by West [55, 58].

Effect of ventilation–perfusion inequality on gas exchange

Oxygen

We are now in a position to consider how the uneven distribution of ventilation and blood flow can affect pulmonary gas exchange. The effect on O_2 uptake is comparatively easy to understand; indeed Haldane correctly described the effects of ventilation–perfusion mismatch on arterial oxygenation over 60 years ago [22]. He argued that if one area of the lung had its

normal share of blood flow but was relatively underventilated, then the pulmonary venous blood leaving that area would have a reduced O_2 content. If, to compensate for this, another area of lung had its normal share of blood flow but an increased amount of ventilation, this would not increase the oxygenation of pulmonary venous blood, since under normal circumstances this blood would already be almost fully saturated. Thus the overall result of this unequal distribution of ventilation relative to blood flow would be a fall in the arterial O_2 content.

Translating this into the modern terminology of gas exchange, we can say that blood coming from lung units with low $\dot{V}_A/\dot{Q}$ ratios will have a low O_2 tension and content, due to the shunt-like effect of these units. The resulting arterial desaturation cannot be compensated for by the presence of blood coming from lung units with high $\dot{V}_A/\dot{Q}$ ratios, for two reasons. First, alveoli with high $\dot{V}_A/\dot{Q}$ ratios usually have high ventilation and low blood flow, whereas alveoli with low $\dot{V}_A/\dot{Q}$ ratios often have a high blood flow. The major portion of arterial blood will therefore consist of blood coming from lung units where $\dot{V}_A/\dot{Q}$ is low. Second, although the blood coming from alveoli with high $\dot{V}_A/\dot{Q}$ does indeed have a higher O_2 tension than usual, because of the shape of the O_2 dissociation curve the O_2 saturation and hence content of this blood cannot be increased significantly above normal.

So a mixture of blood coming from both overventilated and underventilated alveoli will inevitably have an O_2 content and tension below normal. Even an increase in total alveolar ventilation will be ineffective in correcting this, due to the shape of the O_2 dissociation curve (cf. Section: *Carbon dioxide*, below). In a lung with no ventilation–perfusion inequality, the end-capillary O_2 tension (and hence the arterial O_2 tension P_aO_2) would be the same as the alveolar O_2 tension, P_AO_2, assuming that there were no diffusion defects or anatomical shunts. But the presence of inequality between ventilation and blood flow and the production of increasing numbers of alveoli with low $\dot{V}_A/\dot{Q}$ ratios will lead to the appearance of a gradient between P_AO_2 and P_aO_2, the alveolar-arterial O_2 difference was $D_{A-a}O_2$. The magnitude of this $D_{A-a}O_2$, although not linearly related to the degree of ventilation–perfusion mismatch (because of the non-linearity of the O_2 dissociation curve), does nevertheless provide a good rough guide to the severity of the impairment in O_2 uptake due to inequality between ventilation and blood flow.

Carbon dioxide

It is a common misconception that while, due to the reasons outlined above, ventilation–perfusion inequality interferes with O_2 uptake, it has no significant effect on CO_2 elimination. This is not true [56]. If, in a computer model of the lung within uniform ventilation and blood flow, a $\dot{V}_A/\dot{Q}$ in equality is imposed while everything else is held constant, both O_2 uptake and CO_2 output are impaired, i.e., the lung becomes less efficient as a gas exchanger for both O_2 and CO_2. As the extent of the inequality is made worse (by increasing the log standard deviation σ of the $\dot{V}_A/\dot{Q}$ distribution), so there is a steadily increasing interference with both O_2 and CO_2 transfer. When $\sigma = 2.0$ (representing a serious degree of ventilation–perfusion inequality), O_2 uptake is reduced to 45% of normal and CO_2 output is reduced to 55% of normal [55]. In this particular lung model all the lung units are assumed to be ventilated in parallel (Fig. 3.5A). But in disease, lung units may also be ventilated in series (Fig. 3.5B) and by collateral ventilation (Fig. 3.5C). Under these circumstances, where some lung units are receiving inspired gas from other lung units, CO_2 output may be impaired more than O_2 uptake [57].

So CO_2 elimination is certainly affected by ventilation–perfusion inequality. However, because the CO_2 dissociation curve, unlike the O_2 dissociation curve, is virtually linear in its physiological working range, it is often stated that any CO_2 retention caused by alveoli with low $\dot{V}_A/\dot{Q}$ can be compensated for by the increased amounts of CO_2 eliminated by alveoli with high $\dot{V}_A/\dot{Q}$. But this is not true either. First, and for the same reason as was put forward when the effect of $\dot{V}_A/\dot{Q}$ mismatch on O_2 uptake was considered, it is the alveoli with low $\dot{V}_A/\dot{Q}$ which contribute the major share of the arterial blood. Second, although the relationship between PCO_2 and CO_2 content is linear, the relationship between alveolar ventilation (and hence $\dot{V}_A/\dot{Q}$) and PCO_2 is hyperbolic (Fig. 3.1). This means that the increase in $\dot{V}_A$ needed to produce a given change in PCO_2 (and so to remove a given amount of CO_2) is greater when the PCO_2 is low than when it is high, i.e., overventilated (high $\dot{V}_A/\dot{Q}$) alveoli are less efficient than low $\dot{V}_A/\dot{Q}$ alveoli in terms of the volume of CO_2 eliminated per unit volume of ventilation. Therefore the overventilated lung units do not make up for the underventilated units, and the only way to eliminate CO_2 that would otherwise be retained is by increasing the total alveolar ventilation. This is in fact precisely what happens: the net end-result of $\dot{V}_A/\dot{Q}$ inequality is a low arterial O_2 tension (and a widened $D_{A-a}O_2$) and a normal arterial CO_2 tension, the latter obtained at the cost of an increase in ventilation. In patients who do not, or cannot, increase their ventilation (or do not increase it sufficiently), CO_2 retention results.

Measurement of ventilation–perfusion inequality

Arterial blood gases

Although abnormalities of the arterial blood gas tensions are the end-result of ventilation–perfusion mismatch, they do not allow the degree of $\dot{V}_A/\dot{Q}$ inequality to be assessed. The P_aCO_2 is virtually useless because it is so sensitive to the level of ventilation; a normal P_aCO_2 (attained at the expense of increased ventilation) can be present even when there is gross inequality of ventilation and blood flow. The P_aO_2 has as its main disadvantage the fact that its value is affected by other causes of hypoxaemia, such as anatomical shunt and true alveolar hypoventilation.

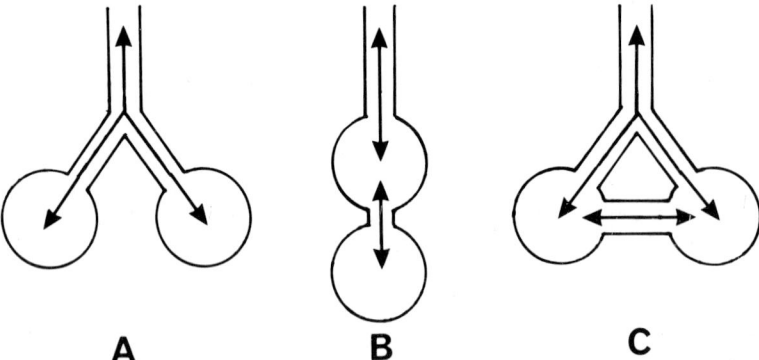

Fig. 3.5. Lung units ventilated in parallel (**A**), in series (**B**), and by collateral ventilation (**C**).

Alveolar–arterial O₂ difference

The $D_{A-a}O_2$ provides an extremely useful assessment of $\dot{V}_A/\dot{Q}$ inequality. It is derived from the measured P_aO_2 and the calculated ideal P_AO_2, and it is far less sensitive to alterations in the level of ventilation than the P_aO_2 alone. The normal $D_{A-a}O_2$ in young and middle-aged subjects is less than 15 mmHg (2 kPa), and is made up of true extrapulmonary shunt and the $\dot{V}_A/\dot{Q}$ inequalities that are present in normal lungs [23, 27, 33]; diffusion is not a limiting factor and does not contribute to the $D_{A-a}O_2$ at normal alveolar O_2 tensions [32, 47]. In routine clinical practice, calculation of the $D_{A-a}O_2$ from blood gas data (assuming a value for R) provides a good rough assessment of the efficiency of the lung as a gas exchanger.

Physiological dead space and shunt

Calculation of V_D/V_T and $\dot{Q}_S/\dot{Q}_T$ yields assessments of wasted ventilation and blood flow, respectively. These have already been fully discussed.

Inert gas elimination

Whilst blood gases, $D_{A-a}O_2$, V_D/V_T, and $\dot{Q}_S/\dot{Q}_T$ allow some quantification of the effect of ventilation–perfusion inequalities on gas exchange, they give us very little insight into the characteristics of the $\dot{V}_A/\dot{Q}$ distributions that actually exist.

It can be shown that when an inert gas, dissolved in saline, is infused into the venous circulation, the proportions of gas retained and excreted by a single lung unit depend on the blood–gas partition coefficient and the $\dot{V}_A/\dot{Q}$ ratio of that lung unit [16]. By using a mixture of six inert gases with a 10^5 range of solubilities (sulphur hexafluoride, ethane, cyclopropane, halothane, diethyl ether, and acetone) and measuring the retention and excretion patterns, it is possible to transform the data into distributions of ventilation and perfusion as a function of the $\dot{V}_A/\dot{Q}$ ratio for a 50-compartment model of the lung [50]. Possible limitations and inaccuracies in this technique will not be discussed here [29, 35], but there can be no doubt that the application of the inert gas method to clinical problems has been of great interest. With this technique, $\dot{V}_A/\dot{Q}$ distributions have been obtained for normal subjects (for whom the log standard deviation σ is of the order of 0.4) [49], patients with chronic obstructive pulmonary disease [52], asthmatics [53], and patients with interstitial lung disease [51].

Regulation of ventilation–perfusion ratios

The inequality of ventilation and blood flow within diseased lungs is mitigated to some extent by various mechanisms which tend to reduce the amount of ventilation–perfusion mismatch, and one of the most important of these factors controlling $\dot{V}_A/\dot{Q}$ ratios in disease is the relationship between alveolar O_2 tension and local pulmonary blood flow. Ever since the original observation by von Euler and Liljestrand that alveolar hypoxia increased the pulmonary artery pressure in the cat [48], there have been many demonstrations, both in experimental animals and in man, that pulmonary arterial vessels constrict in response to changes in local alveolar PO_2 [4, 26].

This compensatory hypoxic vasoconstriction is the main way in which reasonably constant $\dot{V}_A/\dot{Q}$ ratios are maintained in the presence of inequalities of ventilation, and accounts for the finding from inert gas elimination studies of surprisingly small amounts of blood flow to unventilated lung units in patients with chronic obstructive pulmonary disease and asthma [52, 53]. Relief of hypoxic vasoconstriction may be an important consideration when patients with these lung diseases are given O_2 to breathe, and it has been shown that O_2 treatment in a group of patients with chronic airways obstruction results in a diversion of blood flow away from well-ventilated to the more poorly ventilated areas [14]. The underlying mechanism of hypoxic pulmonary vasoconstriction remains to be elucidated [5, 6, 18, 26].

In addition to this compensatory reduction in blood flow to areas which are poorly ventilated, there is also a similar compensatory decrease in ventilation to alveoli which are poorly perfused, but this mechanism is probably only of minor importance in stabilizing local $\dot{V}_A/\dot{Q}$ ratios.

Ventilation–perfusion inequality versus diffusion defect

This chapter will now conclude with a brief account of one of the more controversial aspects of gas exchange, namely the question of whether or not impaired diffusion for O_2 actually contributes to hypoxaemia in clinical practice [7, 32].

The term 'alveolar–capillary block syndrome' was introduced in 1951 to explain the hypoxaemia in patients with fibrotic lung disease, where the thickened alveolar and capillary membranes were believed to act as a barrier to the diffusion of O_2 from alveoli into pulmonary capillary blood [2]. This concept was challenged by Finley et al. in 1962 [17], when they showed that in a group of 11 patients with a clinical diagnosis of alveolar–capillary block syndrome, the hypoxaemia at rest could be explained solely on the basis of unequal distribution of ventilation and perfusion and of venous admixture. Some simple calculations also showed that the observed degree of thickening of the membrane was unlikely to interfere seriously with O_2 diffusion without itself causing considerable inequality of ventilation and blood flow.

Briscoe and his colleagues, however, in a study on ten further patients with this syndrome, while agreeing that $\dot{V}_A/\dot{Q}$ inequalities were important in some patients, identified four patients with no ventilation–perfusion mismatch in whom the only disturbance of O_2 transfer was in the total diffusing capacity or in its distribution between different parts of the lungs. They therefore concluded that hypoxaemia in disease could be caused purely by reducing the diffusing capacity, especially if this change was distributed unevenly within the lung [1, 8].

More recently, when a series of patients with interstitial lung disease was studied by the inert gas wash-out technique, it was found that, at rest, the hypoxaemia of these patients could be accounted for by the pattern of ventilation–perfusion inequality alone [51]. But this was not so on exercise, when a component of their hypoxaemia had to be attributed to some other cause, presumably diffusion impairment secondary to the decrease in mean erythrocyte pulmonary transit time.

Exercise designed to stress the diffusion properties of the lung can also be utilized to investigate the relative contributions of diffusion block and of $\dot{V}_A/\dot{Q}$ inequality to the alveolar–arterial O_2 difference in normal lungs. In a series of ingenious experiments, equal degrees of alveolar hypoxia were produced either by breathing 14% O_2 at normal barometric pressure or by breathing pure O_2 at a low barometric pressure [12]. The alveolar–arterial O_2 difference was 9 mmHg (1.2 kPa) under the former conditions and zero under the latter, suggesting that the $D_{A-a}O_2$ of 9 mmHg was due to $\dot{V}_A/\dot{Q}$ inequality and not a diffusion defect. But exercise under the latter conditions increased the gradient to 13 mmHg(1.7 kPa), presumably due to diffusion impairment.

Clearly the terms 'alveolar–capillary block' and 'diffusion defect' are convenient, but misleading, oversimplifications. Figure 3.2, which depicts the changes in PO_2 as blood traverses a pulmonary capillary, shows that diffusion is not a fixed property of the alveolar–capillary membrane but is dependent on blood flow [47]. Diffusing capacity, D_L, will therefore vary in different alveoli according to their blood flow, and there will be a distribution of diffusing capacities throughout the lung. The contribution of each individual alveolus to O_2 transfer will depend on both its $\dot{V}_A/\dot{Q}$ and its $D_L/\dot{Q}$ ratios.

Nevertheless, the arguments about the relative roles of diffusion defects and $\dot{V}_A/\dot{Q}$ inequalities run on [7]. This at least ensures that the subject of pulmonary gas exchange continues to generate a good deal of physiological and clinical research.

References

1. Arndt H, King TKC, Briscoe WA (1970) Diffusing capacities and ventilation: perfusion ratios in patients with the clinical syndrome of alveolar capillary block. J Clin Invest 49:408–422
2. Austrian R, McClement JH, Renzetti AD, Donald KW, Riley RL, Cournand A (1951) Clinical and physiologic features of some types of pulmonary disease with impairment of alveolar-capillary diffusion. The syndrome of alveolar-capillary block. Am J Med 11:667–685
3. Bake B, Wood L, Murphy B, Macklem PT, Milic-Emili J (1974) Effects of inspiratory flow rate on regional distribution of inspired gas. J Appl Physiol 37:8–17
4. Barer GR, Howard P, Shaw JW (1970) Stimulus-response curves for the pulmonary vascular bed to hypoxia and hypercapnia. J Physiol (Lond) 211:139–155
5. Bergofsky EH (1974) Mechanisms underlying vasomotor regulation of regional pulmonary blood-flow in normal and disease states. Am J Med 57:378–394
6. Bohr DF (1977) The pulmonary hypoxic response. State of the field. Chest 71 [Supp]:244–246
7. Briscoe WA (1979) Does impaired diffusion for oxygen exist in diseased lungs? Bull Eur Physiopathol Respir 15:805–811
8. Briscoe WA, King TKC (1974) Analysis of the disturbance in oxygen transfer in hypoxic lung disease. Am J Med 57:349–360
9. Bryan AC, Bentivoglio LG, Beerel F, Macleish H, Zidulka A, Bates DV (1964) Factors affecting regional distribution of ventilation and perfusion in the lung. J Appl Physiol 19:395–402
10. Ciofetta G, Pratt TA, Hughes JMB (1978) Regional pulmonary perfusion assessed with continuous intravenous infusion of Kr-81m: A comparison with Tc-99m macroaggregates. J Nucl Med 19:1126–1130
11. Clark EH, Jones HA, Hughes JMB (1978) Bedside rebreathing technique for measuring carbon monoxide uptake by the lung. Lancet I:791–793
12. Cohen R, Overfield EM, Kylstra JA (1971) Diffusion component of alveolar-arterial oxygen pressure differ-

ence in man. J Appl Physiol 31:223–226

13. Dantzker DR, Wagner PD, West JB (1975) Instability of lung units with low $\dot{V}_A/\dot{Q}$ ratios during O_2 breathing. J Appl Physiol 38:886–895

14. Eiser NM, Jones HA, Hughes JMB (1977) Effect of 30% oxygen on local matching of perfusion and ventilation in chronic airways obstruction. Clin Sci 53:387–395

15. Ewan PW, Jones HA, Rhodes CG, Hughes JMB (1976) Detection of intra-pulmonary haemorrhage with carbon monoxide uptake. Application in Goodpasture's syndrome. N Engl J Med 295:1391–1396

16. Farhi LE (1967) Elimination of inert gas by the lung. Respir Physiol 3:1–11

17. Finley TN, Swenson EW, Comroe JH (1962) The cause of arterial hypoxaemia at rest in patients with 'alveolar-capillary block syndrome'. J Clin Invest 41:618–622

18. Fishman AP (1976) Hypoxia on the pulmonary circulation. How and where it acts. Circ Res 38:221–231

19. Fowler WS (1948) Lung function studies II. The respiratory dead space. Am J Physiol 154:405–416

20. Grant BJB, Jones HA, Hughes JMB (1974) Sequence of regional filling during a tidal breath in man. J Appl Physiol 37:158–165

21. Greening AP, Hughes JMB (1981) Serial estimations of carbon monoxide diffusing capacity in intrapulmonary haemorrhage. Clin Sci 60:507–512

22. Haldane JS, Meakins JC, Priestley JG (1919) The effects of shallow breathing. J Physiol (Lond) 52:433–453

23. Harris EA, Kenyon AM, Nisbet HD, Seelye ER, Whitlock RML (1974) The normal alveolar-arterial oxygen tension gradient in man. Clin Sci 46:89–104

24. Horsfield K (1974) The relation between structure and function in the airways of the lung. Br J Dis Chest 68:145–160

25. Horsfield K (1980) Gaseous diffusion in the lungs. Br J Dis Chest 74:99–120

26. Hughes JMB (1975) Lung gas tensions and active regulation of ventilation: perfusion ratios in health and disease. Br J Dis Chest 69:153–170

27. Hughes JMB (1980) Pulmonary gas exchange. Clin Sci 58:119–125

28. Hughes JMB, Glazier JB, Maloney JE, West JB (1968) Effect of lung volume on the distribution of pulmonary blood flow in man. Respir Physiol 4:58–72

29. Jaliwala SA, Mates RE, Klocke FJ (1975) An efficient optimization technique for recovering ventilation-perfusion distributions from inert gas data. J Clin Invest 55:188–192

30. Kelman GR (1968) Computer program for the production of O_2–CO_2 diagrams. Respir Physiol 4:260–269

31. Macklem PT, Murphy B (1974) The forces applied to the lung in health and disease. Am J Med 57:371–377

32. McHardy GJR (1972) Diffusing capacity and pulmonary gas exchange. Br J Dis Chest 66:1–20

33. Mellemgaard K (1966) The alveolar-arterial oxygen difference: Its size and components in normal man. Acta Physiol Scand 67:10–20

34. Ogilvie CM, Forster RE, Blakemore WS, Morton JW (1957) A standardized breath holding technique for the clinical measurement of the diffusing capacity of the lung for carbon monoxide. J Clin Invest 36:1–17

35. Olszowka AJ (1975) Can $V_A/\dot{Q}$ distributions in the lung be recovered from inert gas retention data? Respir Physiol 25:191–198

36. Olszowka AJ, Farhi LE (1968) A system of digital computer subroutines for blood gas calculations. Respir Physiol 4:270–280

37. Penman RWB (1967) Ventilation-perfusion inequality. Br J Dis Chest 61:12–24

38. Rahn H (1949) A concept of mean alveolar air and the ventilation-bloodflow relationships during pulmonary gas exchange. Am J Physiol 158:21–30

39. Rahn H, Fenn WO (1955) A graphical analysis of the respiratory gas exchange. The American Physiological Society, Washington DC

40. Riley RL, Cournand A (1949) Ideal alveolar air and the analysis of ventilation/perfusion relationships in the lungs. J Appl Physiol 1:825–847

41. Riley RL, Cournand A (1951) Analysis of factors affecting partial pressures of oxygen and carbon dioxide in gas and blood of lungs: Theory. J Appl Physiol 4:77–101

42. Riley RL, Lilienthal JL, Proemmel DD, Franke RE (1946) On the determination of the physiologically effective pressures of oxygen and carbon dioxide in alveolar air. Am J Physiol 147:191–198

43. Riley RL, Cournand A, Donald KW (1951) Analysis of factors affecting partial pressures of oxygen and carbon dioxide in gas and blood of lungs: Methods. J Appl Physiol 4:102–120

44. Roughton FJW, Forster RE (1957) Relative importance of diffusion and chemical reaction rates in determining rate of exchange of gases in the human lung, with special reference to true diffusing capacity of pulmonary membrane and volume of blood in the lung capillaries. J Appl Physiol 11:290–302

45. Severinghaus JW (1966) Blood gas calculator. J Appl Physiol 21:1108–1116

46. Severinghaus JW, Stupfel M (1957) Alveolar dead space as an index of distribution of blood flow in pulmonary capillaries. J Appl Physiol 10:335–348

47. Staub NC (1963) Alveolar-arterial oxygen tension gradient due to diffusion. J Appl Physiol 18:673–680

48. Von Euler US, Liljestrand G (1946) Observations on the pulmonary arterial blood pressure in the cat. Acta Physiol Scand 12:301–320

49. Wagner PD, Laravuso RB, Uhl RR, West JB (1974a) Continuous distributions of ventilation-perfusion ratios in normal subjects breathing air and 100% O_2. J Clin Invest 54:54–68

50. Wagner PD, Saltzman HA, West JB (1974b) Measurement of continuous distributions of ventilation-perfusion ratios: Theory. J Appl Physiol 36:588–599

51. Wagner PD, Dantzker DR, Dueck R, DePolo JL, Wasserman K, West JB (1976) Distribution of ventilation-perfusion ratios in patients with interstitial lung disease. Chest [Suppl] 69:256–257

52. Wagner PD, Dantzker DR, Dueck R, Clausen JL, West JB (1977) Ventilation-perfusion inequality in chronic obstructive pulmonary disease. J Clin Invest 59:203–216

53. Wagner PD, Dantzker DR, Iacovoni VE, Tomlin WC, West JB (1978) Ventilation-perfusion inequality in asymptomatic asthma. Am Rev Respir Dis 118:511–524

54. Weibel ER (1970) Morphometric estimation of pulmonary diffusion capacity. Model and method. Respir Physiol 11:54–75

55. West JB (1969) Ventilation-perfusion inequality and overall gas exchange in computer models of the lung. Respir Physiol 7:88–110

56. West JB (1971a) Causes of carbon dioxide retention in lung disease. N Eng J Med 284:1232–1236

57. West JB (1971b) Gas exchange when one lung region inspires from another. J Appl Physiol 30:479–487

58. West JB (1977) Ventilation-perfusion relationships. Am Rev Respir Dis 116:919–943

59. West JB, Dollery CT (1960) Distribution of blood flow and ventilation-perfusion ratio in the lung measured with radioactive CO_2. J Appl Physiol 15:405–410

60. West JB, Dollery CT, Naimark A (1964) Distribution of bloodflow in isolated lung: Relation to vascular and alveolar pressures. J Appl Physiol 19:713–724

Chapter 4

Oxygen Transport and Consumption

J. H. Chamberlain and A. P. Adams

The delivery of oxygen (O_2) to the tissues of the body depends on two main factors, the flow of blood and the amount of O_2 contained in that blood. The distribution of flow within a tissue is of importance, for although the overall total flow may be normal, some parts of the organ may be relatively underperfused i.e., an unevenness of distribution exists to a variable extent within the whole organ or tissue. The same is true of the distribution of the total cardiac output. The first section of this chapter concerns those factors affecting the amount of O_2 carried in the blood; the second section deals with total body O_2 consumption.

Carriage of oxygen in the blood

Quantitative aspects

Oxygen is carried in the blood in two forms, in physical solution and in chemical combination with haemoglobin (Hb).

Dissolved oxygen

The amount of O_2 carried in physical solution in the blood depends upon the partial pressure of O_2 and the solubility of O_2 in whole blood under given conditions. At 37°C, 0.000031 ml O_2 dissolves in each millilitre of blood for each millimetre of mercury O_2 pressure, so that in a subject whose PaO_2 is 100 mmHg, 0.31 ml O_2 is carried per 100 ml blood. In the absence of any pulmonary shunts, if the subject breathes 100% O_2 the PaO_2 will rise to approximately 670 mmHg (89 kPa) and the arterial blood will contain about 2.1 ml dissolved O_2 per 100 ml.

If the O_2 consumption were 250 ml/min and *complete* extraction of O_2 took place in the tissues, a cardiac output of approximately 80 litres/min would be required in a subject breathing air.

Combined oxygen

At STPD (standard temperature and pressure, dry) 1 g Hb combines with 1.34 ml O_2, so that in a subject with an Hb level of 15 g/100 ml blood, the total O_2 combined will be $15 \times 1.34 = 20.1$ ml if the blood is fully saturated. Thus the O_2 content of blood with a normal Hb concentration is increased about 60-fold because of the presence of Hb.

Again, if O_2 consumption were 250 ml/min and total O_2 extraction took place in the tissues the cardiac output would be only 1.25 litres/min. *Total* O_2 extraction would be difficult to achieve, and it appears undesirable physiologically. Normally only about 25% of the O_2 in the blood is used in the tissues as blood circulates around the body. This leaves the venous blood with 75% of its total possible amount (or 75% saturated). As only a quarter of the potential O_2 has been unloaded at the tissues the cardiac output is increased by a factor of about 3–4, which is the 'normal' cardiac output of 4–5 litres/min of resting man.

Oxygen affinity

The maximum possible quantity of O_2 that can be carried in the blood (O_2 capacity) depends very largely on the haemoglobin concentration. The *actual* amount carried (O_2 content) may be expressed in terms of the O_2 saturation:

O_2 saturation %

$$= \frac{(O_2 \text{ content} - \text{dissolved } O_2) \times 100}{O_2 \text{ capacity} - \text{dissolved } O_2}.$$

When blood is equilibrated with gases of widely differing O_2 partial pressures and the O_2 content is measured under each set of conditions, a curve relating content and PO_2 may be constructed. This is more usually shown as the relationship between saturation and PO_2 and is the familiar sigmoid O_2 dissociation or association curve.

Oxygen affinity is usually considered in terms of the PO_2 necessary to produce 50% saturation of Hb. This is called the P_{50} and is normally about 27 mmHg (3.6 kPa) (Fig. 4.1). If the P_{50} decreases (i.e., the dissociation curve shifts to the left) affinity increases and vice versa. There are numerous ways in which O_2 affinity can be changed. Some of these are physiological and others pathological (Table 4.1). Before these situations are discussed in detail, the under-

lying molecular mechanisms involved are explained, which allows an understanding of how these changes of affinity are effected.

Mechanism and physiology [64]

Haemoglobin is a fairly large and complicated molecule, achieving what is a relatively simple process—the reversible binding of oxygen— and it is reasonable to wonder why such a simple function needs to be wrapped in such complexity. The reason appears to arise from the fact that iron, the element to which O_2 is bound in the Hb, alters irreversibly from the ferrous to the ferric form when it is oxidized. Burying the iron, in the ferrous form, in the centre of the Hb molecule allows O_2 to combine with it in a loose way and prevents the formation of the stable but irreversible ferric form. The complex nature of the haemoglobin molecule also allows the strength of the chemical bond between O_2 and Hb to vary. In Fig. 4.2 a comparison is made between the O_2 dissociation curves for myoglobin and Hb. The relationship for myoglobin is that of a rectangular hyperbola, and the affinity for O_2 at all values of PO_2 is always higher than for Hb. This is of benefit in muscle, where myoglobin is an important O_2 carrier. Does the affinity of myoglobin for O_2 change with PO_2? It will be seen that it does not. This is best expressed by relating the PO_2 to the ratio of the number of oxymyoglobin molecules (Y) to reduced molecules $(1 - Y)$ and plotting both on a logarithmic scale. This is a graphical expression of the equilibrium between the free O_2 and the O_2 bound to myoglobin. As the slope of the line does not vary it is clear that the affinity of myoglobin for O_2 does not vary with the degree of its saturation. The intercept, where the myoglobin is half saturated (i.e., where $Y/[1 - Y] = 1$), gives the equilibrium constant, K_1, which is the PO_2 that is required to produce 50% saturation.

If the same process is followed for Hb a different result is obtained (Fig. 4.3) and a sigmoid curve results. At first, Hb is reluctant to bind O_2 but as the PO_2 increases the slope becomes steeper, until at near 100% saturation the slope decreases once more. A tangent drawn to the slope of this curve at the two extremities reveals the PO_2 at which the Hb would be 50% saturated under these two conditions, and it can be seen that the PO_2 at the lower end of the curve would require to be 100 times (30 vs 0.3 mmHg) that of the upper

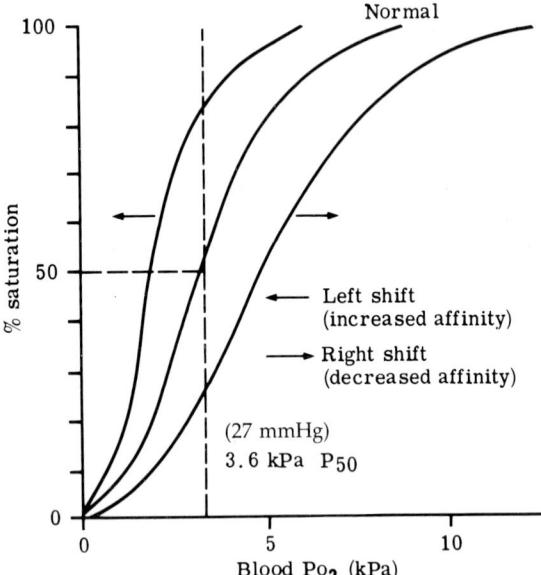

Fig. 4.1. ODC illustrating the effect of a change in affinity on the P_{50}.

Table 4.1. Changes in 2, 3-DPG and O_2 affinity for Hb in various disease states

Condition	Change[a] in		Mechanism[b]
	DPG	Oxygen affinity	
Hypoxaemia: Altitude	↑	↓	TO
Congenital heart disease R → L shunt	↑	↓	TO
acquired respiratory disease	↑ or ↓	↓ or ↑	TO,AB
Anaemia	↑	↓	TO
Defects of erythrocyte metabolism:			
Hexokinase deficiency	↓	↑	GR
Pyruvate kinase deficiency	↑	↓	GR
Polycythaemia (primary)	↓	↑	TO
Haemoglobinopathies	↑ or ↓	↓ or ↑	TO
Acid–base changes: Acidosis	↓	↓	AB
Alkalosis	↑	↑	AB
Low cardiac output	↑	↓	TO
Shock	↓	↓ or ↑	TO,AB,P
Blood storage (see text)	↓	↑	P,GR
Drugs: Propranolol	?	↓	?
Aluminium hydroxide	↓	↑	P
Anaesthetic agents	?	↓	?
Hormones: Thyroid excess	↑	↓	GR
Thyroid lack	↓	↑	GR
Cortisol and methyl prednisolone	↑	↓	?
Androgens	↑	↓	?
Pituitary deficiency	↓	↑	?
Diabetes	↑ or ↓	↓ or ↑	?
Cirrhosis	↑	↓	AB,TO,?
Angina	?	↓	?TO
Uraemia	↑ or ↓	↓ or ↑	P,AB,TO
IV Feeding	↓	↑	P
Exercise	↑	↓	?TO

[a]A fall of 2,3-DPG is associated with an increase in affinity and vice versa. In those instances where this reciprocal relationship does not occur there is a primary change in affinity which causes the secondary change in 2,3-DPG levels.
[b]TO, tissue oxygenation (e.g., poor flow, reduced O_2 content, etc.); P, change in phosphate supply; GR, Glycolytic rate; AB, acid-base change.

end to achieve the same results. In other words, when Hb is poorly saturated it becomes less able to combine with O_2, and when it is highly saturated it becomes very avid for O_2. Between these two extremes the affinity of Hb for O_2 is intermediate, and the slope of the straight line found here is expressed by Hill's constant n [41]. The normal value for n is 2.7, and it is

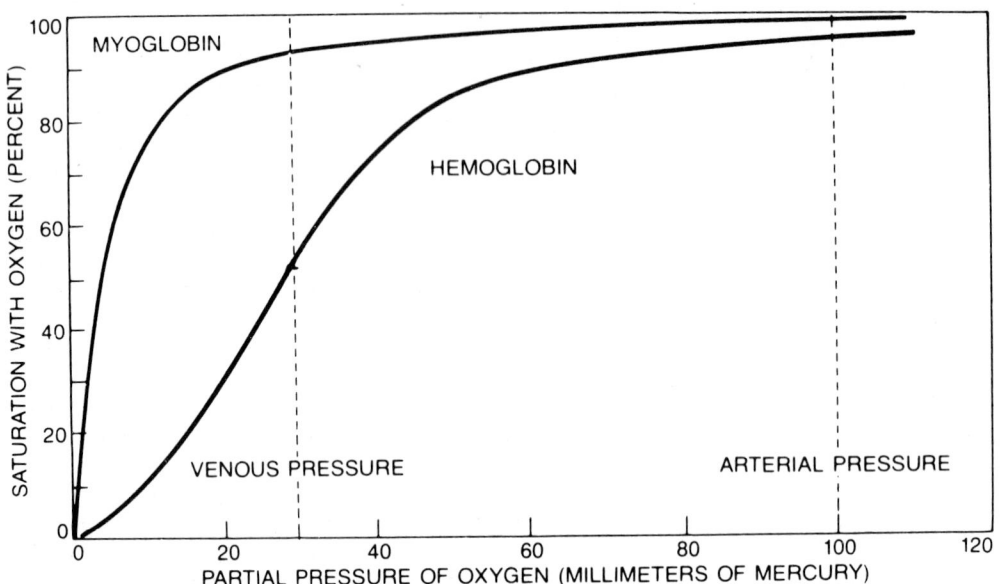

Fig. 4.2. ODCs for myoglobin and haemoglobin. From Perutz [64].

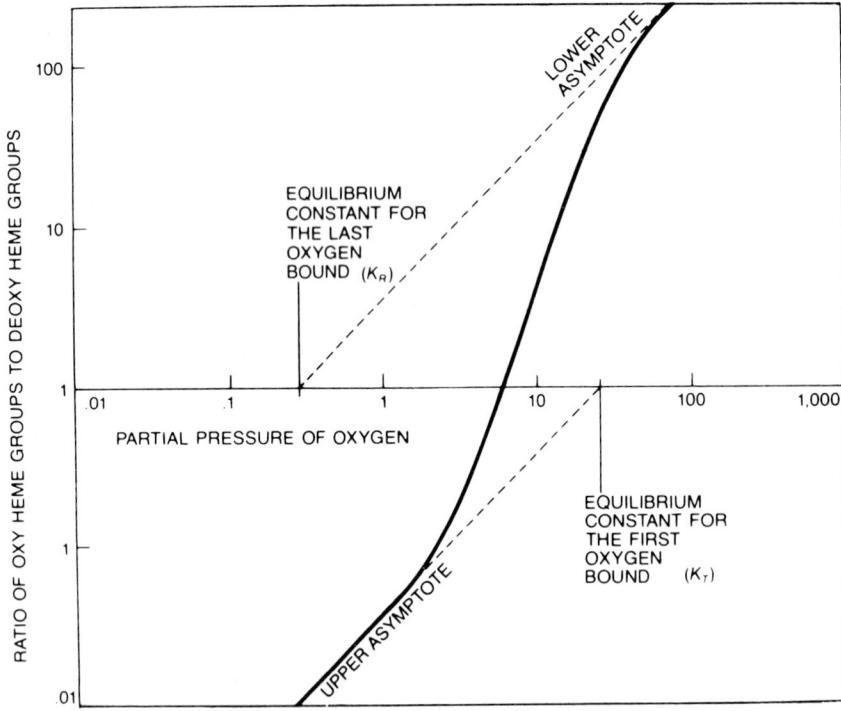

Fig. 4.3. Fractional saturation of HG plotted against the partial pressure of O_2, both on logarithmic scales. The equilibrium curve for myoglobin becomes a straight line on such a graph, showing that the affinity of myoglobin for O_2 does not change when the PO_2 alters. See text for explanation of haemoglobin curve. From Perutz [64].

increased in more sigmoid curves and decreased in more hyperbolic (less sigmoid) curves. Perutz has suggested a biblical parable to illustrate this phenomenon: "for unto everyone that has, shall be given, and he shall have abundance: but from him that hath not, shall be taken away even that which he hath." This curious effect is called haem–haem interaction because it results from the fact that the Hb molecule consists of four haem groups, each of which can combine with one molecule of O_2. These haem groups are not spatially fixed, relative to each other, and the combination of O_2 with one haem group subtly changes the spatial inter-relationships. In this process various structural and electrochemical changes occur which make those haem groups which lack O_2 more avid for it. Thus, by the time the third haem group in the molecule is oxygenated the last haem group is very avid indeed for O_2. This has the desirable physiological effect of increasing the O_2 content at values of high PO_2 which thus facilitates the on-loading of O_2 in the lungs and the off-loading of O_2 in the tissues where the PO_2 is low.

Furthermore, because of the difference between the rectangular hyperbola of the myoglobin dissociation curve and the sigmoid shape of the Hb dissociation curve, the latter is very much less saturated at a high PO_2 than is myoglobin. Tissue PO_2 does not need to fall to such low levels to accomplish the off-loading of O_2, and this protects the tissues from hypoxia and thus allows a much larger margin of error in the gradient for PO_2 between capillaries and tissues. Transport of O_2 within the muscle cell is facilitated by the fact that myoglobin will carry much larger amounts of O_2 at these low partial pressures than Hb. Because of the very steep slope at low PO_2 values the myoglobin is able to off-load very quickly as the PO_2 falls within the cell.

The two states of Hb, namely the saturated and unsaturated forms, are referred to as the relaxed (R) and tense (T) forms, respectively, reflecting the ease or difficulty with which O_2 is able to combine with the Hb molecule.

These extraordinary structural changes which Hb undergoes as it becomes saturated with O_2 are the basis of its changing affinity. In addition, there are other alterations of affinity, expressed in the form of a rightwards and leftwards shift in the whole dissociation curve (P_{50}), which are explained by other changes in the molecular structure of Hb. To understand these it is necessary to discuss the structure of Hb in more detail.

Haemoglobin consists of four subunits. Each subunit comprises a haem group enfolded within a polypeptide unit. The haem group (Fig. 4.4) is an iron complex of protoporphyrin, which is formed from four pyrolle rings. These rings are joined together by methane bridges and the iron atom occupies the centre position of the ring. There are two sequences of amino acids in the polypeptide chains attached to the haem units; these are the subunits alpha (α) and beta (β). The α chain consists of 141 amino acid residues and the β chain contains 146 residues; each chain is folded up in a similar way to form a three-dimensional structure. The whole is so arranged that the Hb molecule takes on the shape of an irregular tetrahedron. The haem groups lie buried in a pocket on the surface of

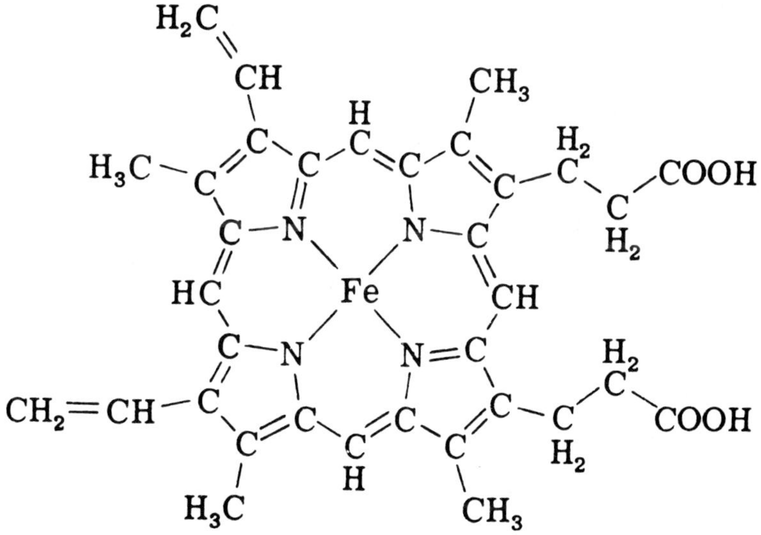

Fig. 4.4. Detailed structure of the haem group.

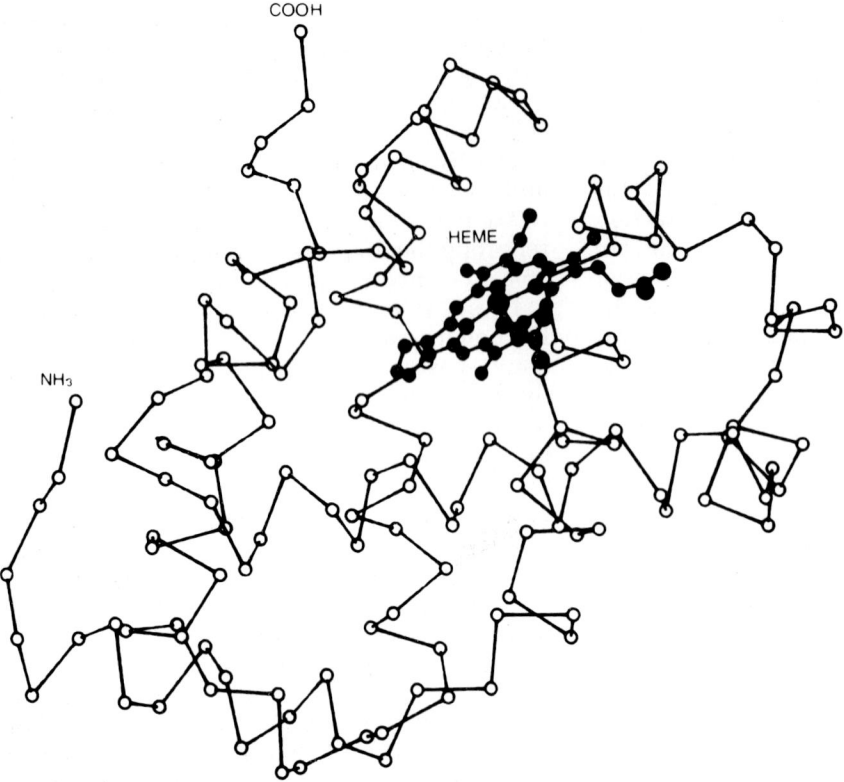

Fig. 4.5. The haem-group buried in a pocket of the enveloping polypeptide chain. From Perutz [64].

this structure at the four corners of the tetra-hedron (Fig. 4.5). In adult Hb there are two alpha (α_1 and α_2) and two beta (β_1 and β_2) units, which are bound together by various kinds of chemical bond. The contacts between α_1 and β_1 subunits, and those between the α_2 and β_2 subunits are effected through numerous hydro-gen bonds, and the spatial relationship *within* these pairs of dimers does not change when O_2 combines with haemoglobin. However, the con-tact *between* the two dimers is somewhat looser, and binding with O_2 results in considerable rotation of one pair of subunits with respect to the other (Fig. 4.6). It is this change of spatial relationship which is associated with the change from the R to the T form. There are many contacts between the two pairs of subunits, but these are not all as rigid as those bonds which hold the dimers themselves together. In addi-tion to hydrogen bonds, there are salt bridges, which are bonds between a positively charged nitrogen atom (N^+) and a negatively charged oxygen atom (O^-). It might be expected that in the T form the number of bonds formed be-tween the two pairs of subunits would be

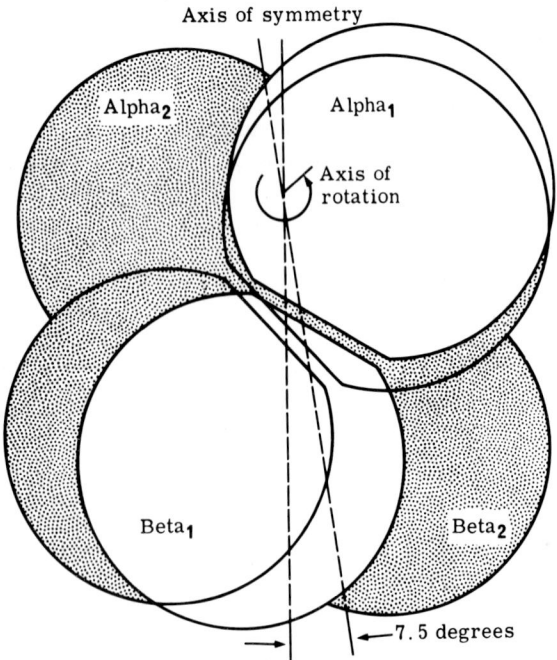

Fig. 4.6. Shows the way in which the two dimers change their spatial inter-relationship when Hb combines with O_2. From Perutz [64].

greater, making this form less susceptible to structural change and to combination with O_2. The extra salt bridges were found to fill this need. The components (N^+ and O^-) occur on the ends of the polypeptide chains (and elsewhere) and in the R state form no contact, whereas in the T state, because of the rotation of the subunit pairs, they make contact and form additional chemical bonds.

This behaviour also helps explain the well-known effect whereby a decrease in pH causes a reduction in O_2 affinity. The imidazole ring on the amino acid histidine (of which there are two in close association with the elemental iron) can be positively charged if both of its nitrogen atoms carry a hydrogen ion. This increases the likelihood of its forming a salt bridge with a negatively charged oxygen atom and changing the molecule from the R to the T form. In addition, this change also approximates other negatively charged oxygen atoms to uncharged nitrogen atoms on the histidine molecule, so that the amount of work required to render these nitrogen atoms positive is less and more protons are taken up from solution. It should be noted that the negatively charged oxygen atoms are part of the amino acid residues and have no connection with the O_2 which is reversibly combining with the Hb molecule.

The Bohr effect [10], whereby an increase of CO_2 produces a reduction in O_2 affinity of Hb, is also explained in a similar way. In this case the nitrogen atoms of the amino groups at the start of the polypeptide chains lose their protons in the presence of CO_2 and become negatively charged to form a carbamino group. These nitrogen atoms are attracted to positively charged groups of the protein globin and form the more stable T form. The opposite of this is called the Douglas Christiansen-Haldane (DCH) effect [15]. In this case, when the haemoglobin is oxygenated there is a decrease in CO_2 content.

When the Hb molecule changes from the R to the T form the gap between the two β chains becomes wider; lining the opening are a string of amino acids carrying positive charges. The 2,3-diphosphoglycerate (2,3-DPG) molecule exactly fits into this space and carries negative charges on its surface, which effectively neutralize the positive charges. The formation of these additional bonds stabilizes the Hb molecule in the T form and explains the loss of affinity which is related to an increase of 2,3-DPG concentration.

In summary, the Hb molecule can be likened to a switch which snaps between two states, the relaxed (R) state where its affinity for O_2 is high, and the tense (T) state where affinity is low. The change from one state to the other depends on a structural change in the molecule, which alters the relationship between certain key atoms in such a way that they are more (T) or less (R) firmly bound to each other. Certain physiological changes such as a fall in PO_2 and a rise in PCO_2, 2,3-DPG, and proton concentration favour the T structure and hence unloading of O_2. These changes are usually desirable in the sense that they favour off-loading (or on-loading) of O_2 at appropriate points of the circulation.

Quantitative aspects

The mechanism underlying the changes in affinity and their direction as PO_2, PCO_2, pH, and 2,3-DPG change have been discussed in the previous section. Here consideration is given to some quantitative aspects.

A few simple calculations performed on the Severinghaus blood gas calculator [72] allow an assessment of the effect of a change of pH on either the cardiac output or the mixed venous PO_2 ($P\bar{v}O_2$). In Table 4.2a it is assumed that the O_2 consumption is 250 ml/min, Hb 14.8 g/dl, and temperature 37°C, and that the $P\bar{a}O_2$ and $P\bar{v}O_2$ are held constant at 100 mmHg (13.3 kPa) and 40 mmHg (5.3 kPa), respectively. Varying the pH between 7.50 and 7.20 produces a change in P_{50} from 24 to 33 mmHg. So long as the $P\bar{v}O_2$ is constant the cardiac output required will vary from 3.6 litres/min at a pH of 7.2 to 6.9 litres/min at a pH of 7.50. If, on the other hand (Table 4.2b), the extraction of O_2 is held constant at 5.3 ml O_2/100 ml blood and the heart is assumed to be unable to alter its output in any way, the $P\bar{v}O_2$ will vary between 33 and 45 mmHg. Clearly life is not as simple as these calculations suggest, and the time scale and conditions at capillary level (to name but two factors) need to be considered. However, these considerations do suggest that changes in pH, which are commonplace in patients in ICUs, have considerable implications for the delivery of O_2.

Fetal haemoglobin and abnormal haemoglobins

Fetal haemoglobin (*HbF*) [61] has a greater affinity for O_2 than adult Hb (HbA) [2], which is of some advantage to the fetus who has to survive at a low PO_2. In the HbF molecule the β chains are replaced by Γ chains. The sequence of amino

Table 4.2. Effect of changing affinity by altering pH on cardiac output (**a**) and $P\bar{v}O_2$ (**b**)

| **a** | pH | % Saturation | | P_{50} (mmHg) | AV content (ml/100 ml) | Cardiac output (litres/min) |
		Venous	Arterial			
	7.35	71.5	97.2	28	5.3	4.7
	7.50	80.0	98.0	24	3.6	6.9
	7.20	61.5	95.8	33	7.0	3.6

b	pH	$P\bar{v}O_2$ (mmHg)	Content venous (ml/100 ml)	% Saturation, venous
	7.50	33	13.9	70.0
	7.20	45	13.71	69.9

All calculations have been made with a Severinghaus blood gas calculator [72].
Temperature = 37°C; Hb = 14.8 g/dl; PaO_2 = 100 mmHg; $\dot{V}O_2$ = 250 ml/min.
a $P\bar{v}O_2$ (= 40 mmHg) is held constant and cardiac output varies to satisfy the varying arteriovenous extraction.
b The cardiac output and hence extractions are held constant and the $P\bar{v}O_2$ varies.
Despite the slightly lower venous content and saturation at pH 7.2 than at pH 7.5, the $P\bar{v}O_2$ is much higher.

acids is different in only one position in the Γ chain: the 143-histidine of the β chain is replaced by serine. This uncharged residue prevents 2,3-DPG from sliding in and out of its pocket between the β chains. Hence the R form is favoured because the increased bonds present in the T form are not reinforced by the presence of 2,3-DPG [11].

Oxygen affinity changes after birth because HbF is replaced by HbA, and this process is complete in about 4–6 months post partum [61]. The influence that 2,3-DPG has on affinity under these circumstances is directly proportional to the amount of HbA present. Premature infants are born with high levels of HbF and low amounts of 2,3-DPG, and the normalization of affinity is much delayed [19]. Certain workers claim to have shown a favourable influence on survival as a result of exchange transfusion of premature infants with blood of a lower affinity [18, 31, 61].
Abnormal haemoglobins. Bellingham [6] has reviewed the numerous forms of Hb which are associated with altered O_2 affinity. Most of them are rare, the only exceptions being HbS in sickle cell disease and HbF in thalassaemia. In those haemoglobinopathies where the affinity is increased the red cell mass may be increased, and in states where the affinity is diminished the patients tend to be anaemic. However, because the red cell fragility is increased in many of these conditions, the Hb level does not always reflect only changes of affinity. Thalassaemia is associated with increased affinity. Sickle cell disease, on the other hand, is associated with

decreased affinity. Because a low PO_2 tends to exacerbate the sickling problem, exchange transfusion with normal blood may be appropriate under conditions such as surgery and anaesthesia, where the likelihood of sickling may be increased.

2,3-Diphosphoglycerate (2,3-DPG) metabolism

The importance of 2,3-DPG (and other phosphates, such as ATP) in affecting O_2 affinity was established in 1967 [9, 13]. We have already discussed how 2,3-DPG exerts its effect in the section: 'Mechanism and physiology'.

2,3-DPG is synthesized and broken down in the phosphoglycerate cycle of Rapoport and Luebering [67], a side-shuttle of the main Embden–Meyerof pathway (Fig. 4.7). There is approximately the same number of molecules of 2,3-DPG as of Hb in the red cell, but the actual amount is regulated by several factors:

1) The *concentration of 2,3-DPG* itself produces a negative feedback on 2,3-DPG mutase, the enzyme which facilitates its production from 1,3-DPG [69].
2) There is a reciprocal relationship between the *concentration of H^+ ion* and 2,3-DPG. Increasing the pH stimulates glycolysis and the formation of 2,3-DPG [70]. On the other hand, an increased concentration of 2,3-DPG in the cell leads (by an effect on the Donnan equilibrium) to a reduction in pH [21]. If sufficient time is allowed, usually 24 h or more, a change of pH is counter-balanced by a change in 2,3-DPG and

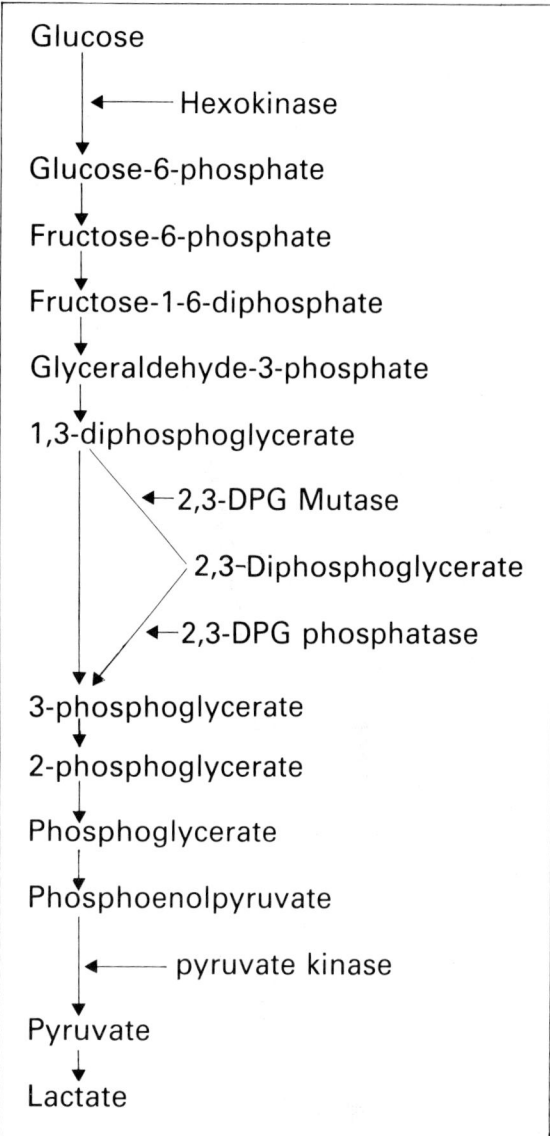

Fig. 4.7. The Embden-Meyerof pathway showing the side–shuttle of Rapoport and Luebering.

normal affinity is restored [1]. Thus, chronic disorders of acid–base balance are attended by an appropriate alteration in 2,3-DPG concentration, and a sudden restoration of the pH to normal will cause considerable shifts in the dissociation curve, which may not be advantageous to the patient. In acute situations such as cardiac arrest, insufficient time is available for 2,3-DPG levels to change, so that it may be more appropriate to correct any metabolic acidosis fully.

3) *Low inorganic phosphate concentrations* are associated with low 2,3-DPG levels [75, 81] and vice versa [49].

4) An *increase in glycolytic rate* occurs in thyrotoxicosis and may be responsible for an accumulation of 2,3-DPG [35, 54]. An enzyme deficiency above the level of the shuttle (hexokinase) causes a decrease in 2,3-DPG and one below the shuttle (pyruvate kinase), an increase [63].

Changes in affinity

The clinical conditions [35] in which alterations of O_2 affinity have been found are listed in Table 4.1. An attempt has been made to indicate the cause of the abnormality. Discussion follows of some of the more important conditions.

Hypoxaemia. In this context those conditions where arterial PO_2 is reduced are discussed, i.e., hypoxic hypoxaemia.

1) *Hypoxia of altitude*: Increased 2,3-DPG levels and reduced affinity have been found in those living at altitude and in persons taken to high altitude. The probable mechanism is a respiratory alkalosis which stimulates glycolysis, although there are some doubts as to whether this is the whole story. A rightward shift in the dissociation curve becomes a disadvantage above an altitude of 2500 m because the loading of O_2 in the lungs becomes less efficient [78].

2) *Congenital heart disease (R-to-L shunt)*: In most studies an increase in 2,3-DPG and in P_{50} has been found [23, 55, 62], although this has not always been paralleled by a similar increase of haematocrit [48].

3) *In chronic acquired respiratory disease* less consistent changes in affinity have been observed, and it is clear that these patients fall into a less homogeneous group than the previous two. Respiratory acidosis, the degree of polycythaemia, and the nature of the cardiovascular alterations present will all indirectly affect the need for changes in affinity [27, 62].

Anaemia. There have been many studies showing that in most types of chronic anaemia a rise in 2,3-DPG and P_{50} occurs [39, 80]. The potential advantages for O_2 delivery that this can confer are considerable. Figure 4.8 shows the interrelation between Hb concentration and P_{50}, at different values of cardiac output. This figure illustrates the fact that moderate changes in Hb concentration, say to 9 g/dl, may be readily compensated by a change in P_{50} (A−B) of 7.5 mmHg (1 kPa). Further reductions in Hb concentration require an increase in cardiac output to prevent a fall in mixed venous PO_2 (B−C). A case cited by Gillies is represented by the points D and E. D represents the cardiac output which would have been necessary had no shift in the ODC occurred. E was the measured point and the saving in cardiac output is considerable.

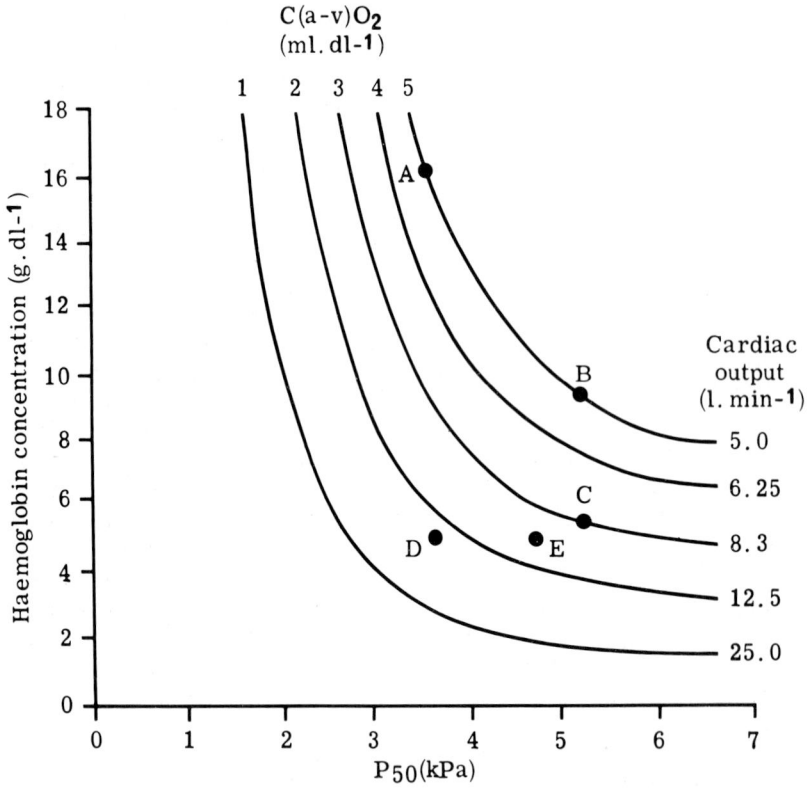

Fig. 4.8. Relationship between Hb concentration and O_2 affinity (P_{50}) at different levels of cardiac output. A → B illustrates how a rise in P_{50} can compensate for a drop in Hb and prevents any change in cardiac output from occurring. B → C illustrates that a further drop in Hb is not compensated for by an additional rise of P_{50} and an increase in cardiac output is required to maintain O_2 delivery. Points A–D represent an acute fall of Hb from 16 to 4.8 g.dl^{-1} and show the rise in cardiac output that would have been required to maintain O_2 delivery. E shows the actual measured point and illustrates how the rise in P_{50} reduces the increase of cardiac output required to maintain O_2 delivery. Modified from Gillies [30].

Shock. It might be supposed that in shock states where there is inadequate tissue oxygenation affinity would decrease, thereby facilitating O_2 delivery. However, this simple situation is complicated in these patients by a number of other factors, such as changes in pH, a low inorganic phosphate, and the transfusion of blood low in 2,3-DPG [52]. Suggestions [53, 77] that in endotoxic shock there is some other factor which shifts the ODC to the left inappropriately seem ill-founded [36, 37, 56, 84]. The available evidence indicates that alterations in pH probably override any stimulus from inadequate tissue oxygenation (and the precise nature of such a stimulus is still uncertain). In consequence, in vivo P_{50} may be more nearly normal than is desirable in O_2 delivery terms, due to the pH-induced alteration in 2,3-DPG concentration. Similar reasoning can be used to explain the effect of decreased phosphate concentration and the use of blood deficient in 2,3-DPG. The remedy is to correct the acid–base changes and the phosphate deficiency and to give blood which is rich in 2,3-DPG. Measures designed to deliberately decrease O_2 affinity have received insufficient support in the literature to recommend them [35, 52].

Low cardiac output. In the more stable situation of patients with chronic cardiac disease there is good evidence that in those whose cardiac output is low (NYHA grades III and IV), the 2,3-DPG level is increased and affinity decreased [94]. An unexplained observation by Shappell and co-workers is the increase in P_{50} of the blood from the coronary sinus immediately after pacing-induced angina [74].

Blood storage [82]. Blood stored at 4°C in acid citrate dextrose (ACD) will lose half its 2,3-DPG content in 4 days, and most of it in 7 days. Blood stored in citrate phosphate dextrose at 4°C also loses its 2,3-DPG content, but at about half this rate. If blood is frozen before any substantial decline in 2,3-DPG occurs (i.e., within the first 24 h in ACD and within 4 days in CPD) then normal levels will be maintained. On thawing, the erythrocytes have normal affinity. The addition of a solution containing pyruvate, inosine, glucose, phosphate, and adenine may increase 2,3-DPG levels above normal. If large amounts of blood deficient in 2,3-DPG are transfused, it takes several days for normal levels to be restored, and this may decrease P_{50} significantly. The rate of restoration will depend on such factors as pH and phosphate levels. Evidence that this is detrimental to the patient is difficult to evaluate because of the complex nature of the situation

attending massive transfusions [38, 86]. Despite this, it is clearly desirable that, in those conditions which limit O_2 delivery for other reasons, the transfusion of large quantities of old blood should be avoided whenever possible.

Uraemia. The interpretation of the changes of O_2 affinity found in uraemia is complex. It is probable that the underlying mechanisms involved include changes in pH and tissue oxygenation consequent upon anaemia. The end-result will depend on the balance of these factors and how they are modified by treatment (e.g., dialysis) [58]. There is no evidence of any unexplained factor peculiar to uraemia affecting the O_2 affinity [66].

Intravenous feeding. It is well recognized that prolonged IV feeding is associated with phosphate (PO_4) deficiency if adequate supplements are not given. Patients may also be PO_4-depleted as a result of their illness or an inadequate diet, and 2,3-DPG levels will be low in consequence. Restoration of normal levels will not be possible without a dietary supplement of PO_4 [76].

Carbon monoxide. Haemoglobin has an affinity for CO which is approximately 300 times the affinity for O_2. In addition, CO causes a leftward shift of the O_2 dissociation curve (ODC) [71]. Nunn [59] has shown that displacement of the ODC by 50% CO, when compared with anaemic blood of similar O_2 content, has only a small effect on the arterial blood, providing the PO_2 is greater than 60 mmHg (8 kPa), but will reduce the mixed venous blood PO_2 by about twice that of the anaemic blood.

Temperature. Temperature alters the affinity of oxygen for Hb. A rise in temperature decreases affinity and vice versa. The magnitude of this effect can be illustrated with the aid of a Severinghaus' blood gas calculator [72]. The conditions under consideration are the same as with the example used earlier for pH changes, viz. O_2 consumption 250 ml/min, PaO_2 100 mmHg (13.3 kPa), Hb 14.8 g/dl, and PvO_2 40 mmHg. If the temperature varies from 35°C to 39°C the mixed venous saturation varies between 77.5% and 61.5% at a pH of 7.35. To maintain the same O_2 delivery the cardiac output would vary between 6.4 litres/min at 35°C and 3.55 litres/min at 39°C.

Anaesthetic agents. The affinity of O_2 for normal adult Hb solutions is modified by the presence of increasing amounts of the anaesthetic halothane. P_{50} may increase by 25% with halothane at a partial pressure of 300 mmHg (40 kPa). The effect is not dependent upon pH or ionic strength. It is suggested that halothane–

Hb interactions may occur through hydrophobic linkage as occurs with short-chain diphatic hydrocarbons. However, the O_2-linked binding of halothane appears to be of minor importance in altering O_2 binding to Hb in vivo compared with other factors, such as chloride ion or 2,3-DPG [32]. Previous findings that halothane induced either no change or a decrease in O_2 binding may be explained now that it has been realized that the response of polarographic O_2 electrodes used in some of these experiments is altered by the presence of halothane.

Significance of changes in oxygen affinity

There is a considerable body of evidence showing that the affinity of Hb for O_2 varies widely in nature and does so in such a way as to facilitate O_2 delivery. Shappell and Lenfant [73] cite many intriguing examples from comparative physiology. The most obvious example in human physiology is the different affinity of HbF and HbA. We have discussed many other examples of both physiological (altitude) and pathological (anaemia) situations which have been associated with alterations of affinity. However, attempts to show that the prevention of such changes might have deleterious effects in the normal subject have not been completely successful [65, 83, 93]. Nonetheless, it seems likely that where one other factor in the delivery equation is also affected, such as coincident anaemia or a low cardiac output or poor local blood flow, then evidence of limitation of O_2 supply emerges. For example, the time to onset of pain in intermittent claudication was reduced in a group of patients who had their CO blood levels increased to 3%. In this instance the leftward shift of the ODC is superimposed on the flow limitation of the atherosclerosis, resulting in earlier ischaemia [3, 4].

The relevance of shifts in the ODC in critically ill patients is much more difficult to assess, because of the numerous simultaneous disturbances which occur in this group. Although claims have been made which imply benefit from deliberate manipulation of the P_{50} in such patients, these are difficult to substantiate. Despite this caveat, those responsible for the care of critically ill patients must always keep in mind the possible harmful effects of both leftward and rightward shifts in the ODC.

Cardiac output and oxygen content

The Fick equation relates to the cardiac output ($\dot{Q}t$), the total body O_2 consumption ($\dot{V}O_2$), and the arteriovenous O_2 content difference ($CaO_2 - C\bar{v}O_2$) in the following manner:

$$\dot{Q}t(Ca - C\bar{v}O_2) = \dot{V}O_2.$$

It is clear from this relationship that if O_2 consumption is held constant and the cardiac output falls, increased O_2 extraction occurs with a fall in mixed venous O_2 content ($C\bar{v}O_2$).

Some of the mixed venous blood will bypass the lungs through shunts of various kinds. The final arterial O_2 content (CaO_2) depends on the proportion of blood coming from the lungs which is fully oxygenated, and that bypassing the lungs through shunts. If each 100 ml arterial blood comprises a mixture of, say, 80 ml blood from the lungs, containing 20 ml O_2/100 ml, and 20 ml blood bypassing the lungs, containing 15 ml O_2/100 ml, the final arterial O_2 content will be

$$\frac{80 \times 20}{100} + \frac{20 \times 15}{100} = 19 \text{ ml } O_2/100 \text{ ml blood.}$$

Suppose that the cardiac output was halved at constant $\dot{V}O_2$: the CaO_2–$C\bar{v}O_2$ difference will be doubled and the mixed venous blood will now contain 10 ml O_2/100 ml blood. The resulting CaO_2 will be 18 ml O_2/100 ml. Notice that the percentage shunt (which in this example is 20%) is unchanged and that the only change which occurs is a reduction in cardiac output and the consequent fall in CvO_2.

Kelman et al. examined this problem in a theoretical manner, and in Fig. 4.9 and 4.10 the inter-relationship among $\dot{Q}t$, CaO_2, and PaO_2 is explored for different degrees of shunts [43]. It can be seen that substantial changes in arterial oxygenation can occur as a result simply of alteration of cardiac output.

Both Fairley et al. [26] and Kelman et al. [43] have demonstrated in theoretical models that the arterial PO_2 is depressed by both hypocapnia and hypercapnia in the presence of pulmonary venous admixture or shunt. The hypocapnic effect becomes evident at values of venous admixture greater than 14%. The effects are made worse by anaemia and reduction in cardiac output. These effects, together with those relating to a pharmacological depression of cardiac output due to hypocapnia [40], strongly suggest that maintenance of normocapnia or mild hypocapnia (i.e., $PaCO_2$ not less than 300 mmHg) is an important consideration in the maintenance of the delivery of O_2 by the blood from the lungs to the tissues.

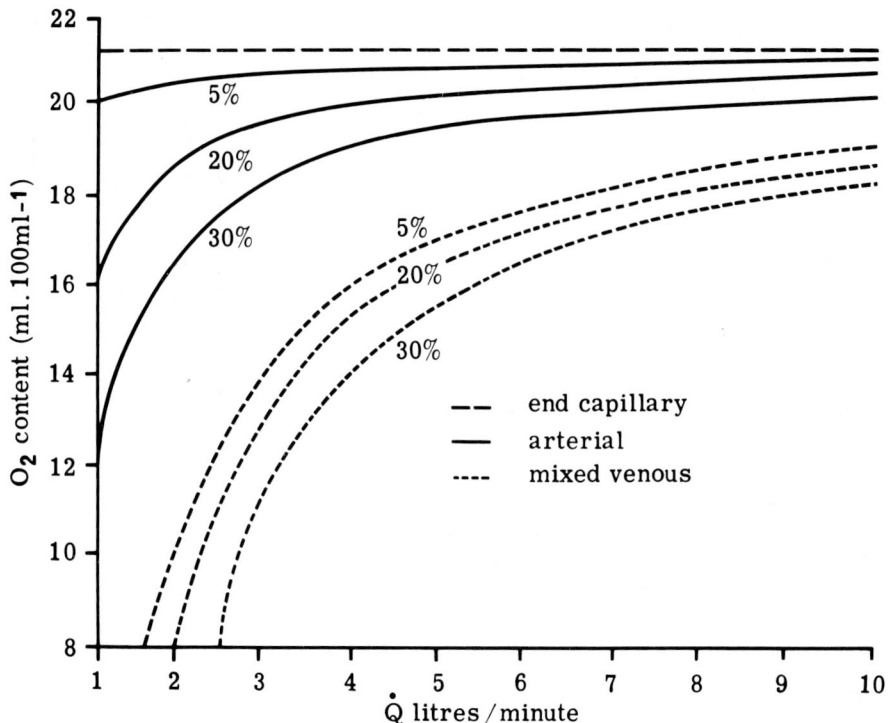

Fig. 4.9. Shows the effect of altering the cardiac output ($\dot{Q}$) on the O_2 content of end-capillary, arterial, and mixed venous blood for different degrees of right-to-left shunting. The percentage figures relate to the proportion of the cardiac output being shunted (i.e. Qs/Qt × 100). The alveolar PO_2 is held constant at 180 mmHg. Hb = 15 g.dl^{-1}. From Kelman et al. [43].

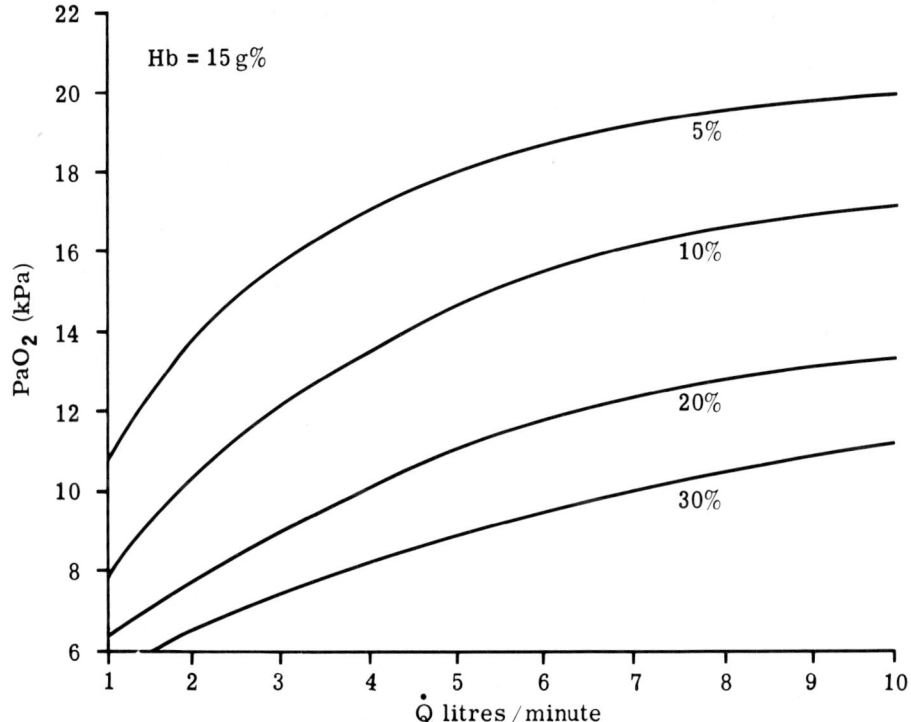

Fig. 4.10. Shows the effect of altering the cardiac output ($\dot{Q}$) on the arterial PO_2 for different levels of right-to-left shunting. The percentage figures relate to the proportion of the cardiac output being shunted. PAO_2 = 180 mmHg; Hb = 15 g.dl^{-1}. From Kelman et al. [43].

Oxygen stores

The O_2 stores of the body are meagre, and if replenishment ceases there is only sufficient O_2 to sustain life for a few minutes. In Table 4.3 the

Table 4.3. Oxygen stores

	While breathing air	While breathing 100% O_2
In the lungs (FRC)	450 ml	3000 ml
In the blood	850 ml	950 ml
Dissolved in tissue fluids	50 ml	100 ml
In combination with myoglobin	200 ml	200 ml
Total	1550 ml	4250 ml

principal stores are shown for a subject breathing air or pure O_2. During pure O_2 breathing the amount of O_2 stored in the lungs is considerably increased and extends the period of time before hypoxia develops to about 8 min. It is also interesting to note that if O_2 is supplied at the mouth during complete apnoea, adequate oxygenation may be continued for a very long time, albeit at the expense of a rising CO_2. This is because there is a diffusion gradient between the mouth, where the PO_2 is high, and the mixed venous blood, where it is low (40 mmHg). As the mixed venous CO_2 rises with continuing apnoea, the PO_2 falls by a similar amount. However, in contrast to air breathing, where the alveoli contain a high level of nitrogen and in consequence the PO_2 quickly falls to a low level, during O_2 breathing the PO_2 has further to fall and so remains at adequate levels for a longer time.

In addition to the small size of the O_2 stores, two other factors are worthy of mention. Firstly, because of the shape of the dissociation curve, loss of O_2 from the blood leads to an early and swift reduction of arterial PO_2 to levels associated with clinical evidence of hypoxia. Secondly, because the myoglobin dissociation curve is hyperbolic, release of O_2 from this source occurs only at very low PO_2 and so back-diffusion of O_2 from myoglobin into the blood is unlikely to occur as hypoxia supervenes.

After a period of hypocapnia, e.g., due to artificial ventilation of the lungs, body CO_2 stores are seriously depleted. Although resumption of spontaneous breathing following such a period of hypocapnia may occur at low levels of $PaCO_2$, little CO_2 is excreted through the lungs for periods of up to 1 h. In such circumstances CO_2 is then conserved by the body to replenish the stores. The consequence is that during this period the inevitable alveolar hypoventilation leads to dangerously low alveolar PO_2 levels during air breathing, and critically ill patients may be unable to respond to this added stress. Careful restoration of CO_2 stores before resumption of spontaneous breathing or the addition of O_2 to the inspired gas, or both, should be considered in such patients.

Oxygen consumption

Measurement

Theoretical and practical considerations

Calculations. The O_2 consumption ($\dot{V}_{O_2}$) is simply the difference between the quantity of O_2 in inspired and in expired gas, or

$$\dot{V}_{O_2} = \dot{V}_I.\, F_{I,O_2} - \dot{V}_E.\, F_{\bar{E},O_2}, \quad \text{[Eq. 4.1]}$$

where $\dot{V}_I$ and $\dot{V}_E$ are the inspired and expired minute volumes and F_{I,O_2} and F_{E,O_2} are the fractional concentration of O_2 in the inspired and expired gas. It is generally assumed that the volume of nitrogen in the inspired and expired gas is constant, since N_2 is neither taken up nor excreted by the lung, so that

$$\dot{V}_I.F_{I,N_2} = \dot{V}_E.F_{\bar{E},N_2} \quad \text{[Eq. 4.2]}$$

or

$$\dot{V}_I = \dot{V}_E.\frac{F_{\bar{E},N_2}}{F_{I,N_2}}. \quad \text{[Eq. 4.3]}$$

It is usual to measure the expired gas volume ($\dot{V}_E$) and, if air is being inspired, to assume that $F_{I,N_2} = 0.7904$. The expired N_2 concentration (F_{E,N_2}) is calculated by subtracting the mixed expired concentrations of O_2 and CO_2 which are measured:

$$F_{\bar{E},N_2} = 1 - F_{\bar{E},O_2} - F_{\bar{E},CO_2} \quad \text{[Eq. 4.4]}$$

Hence $\dot{V}_I$ may be calculated and the equation becomes

$$\dot{V}_{O_2} = \left(\frac{\dot{V}_E.F_{\bar{E},N_2}}{F_{I,N_2}}\right).\, F_{I,O_2} - \dot{V}_E.F_{\bar{E},O_2}.$$

$$\text{[Eq. 4.5]}$$

This is a general equation and may be used if the inspired O_2 concentration is different from air. However, it does assume a steady state in terms of O_2, CO_2, and N_2 stores and that only three gases, O_2, CO_2, and N_2 are involved. If

Eq. 4.4 is substituted in Eq. 4.5, further manipulation results in

$$\dot{V}_{O_2} = \dot{V}_E \left\{ \left[\frac{1 - F\bar{E},O_2 - F\bar{E}.CO_2}{1 - F_I,O_2} \right] . F_I,O_2 - F\bar{E},O_2 \right\}$$

[Eq. 4.6]

If the amount of CO_2 produced equals the amount of O_2 consumed ($RQ = 1$), then

$$F\bar{E},O_2 + F\bar{E},CO_2 = F_I,O_2 \qquad \text{[Eq. 4.7]}$$

and so the expression in the square brackets reduces to unity and $\dot{V}_{O_2}$ is simply the product of the O_2 extraction and the expired volume. The expression in the square brackets corrects for the small difference between the inspired and expired volumes. The error, if this correction is ignored, is fairly small (5%) if the inspired gas is air, although it increases somewhat as the RQ decreases. However, a much larger error is introduced if the subject breathes air which is enriched with O_2, so that ignoring the difference between the inspired and expired volumes under these circumstances is unacceptable.

Carbon dioxide production may be measured at the same time from the measurements already available:

$$\dot{V}_{CO_2} = \dot{V}_E . F\bar{E},CO_2. \qquad \text{[Eq. 4.8]}$$

Changes in steady state (Fig. 4.11) [14, 60]. It must be remembered that the time taken to reach a new steady state following, for example, a change in minute ventilation is quite different for O_2 and for CO_2. This is because the O_2 stores are so much smaller than the CO_2 stores. A new steady state occurs within 2 or 3 min for O_2, irrespective of direction of the change in ventilation. Because the CO_2 stores are large, a change in ventilation is attended by a very much slower achievement of the steady state. The direction of the ventilatory change is also important. An increase in ventilation leads to a new steady state within about 10 min, whereas a decrease in ventilation takes considerably longer, the *half*-time being about 16 min and completion taking up to 80 min. These facts must be borne in mind in the interpretation of respiratory exchange data from critically ill patients whose ventilatory pattern may be changing. It is also clear that the method of measurement should, as far as possible, avoid precipitating an unsteady state of this kind.

Conversion to indirect calorimetry. The importance of measuring the respiratory gas exchange is to calculate the energy requirements of the body. This process is termed indirect calorimetry, as against direct calorimetry, which measures the amount of heat produced by the subject directly by means of some form of

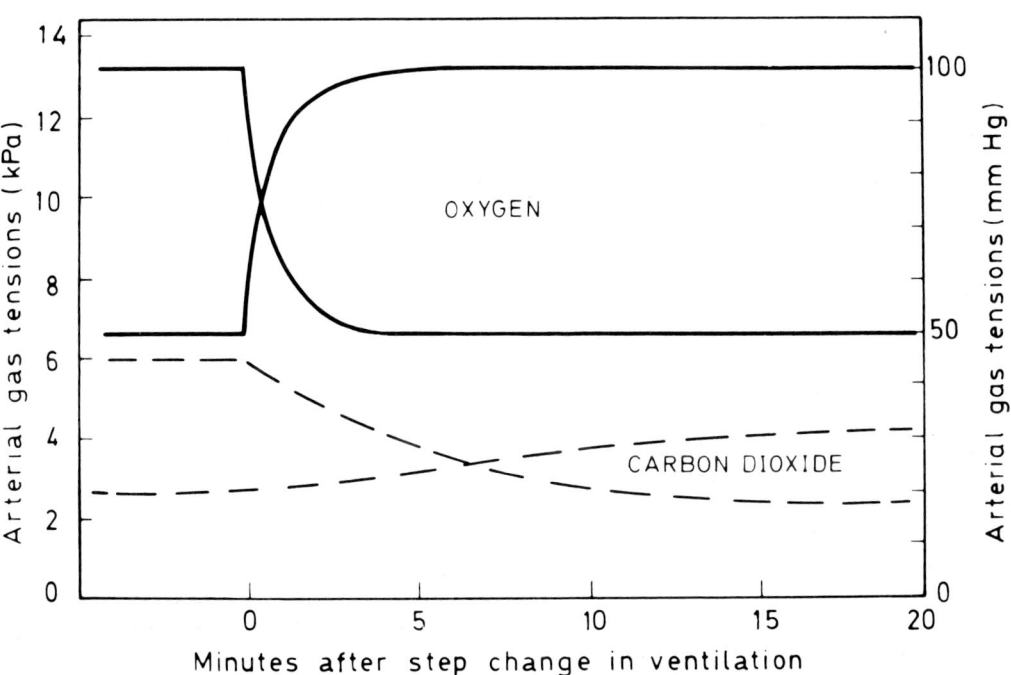

Fig. 4.11. Illustrates the effect of a step change in alveolar ventilation on the arterial PO_2 and PCO_2. A new steady state is far more quickly established for O_2 than for CO_2. From Nunn [59].

calorimeter. Discussion of direct calorimetry is beyond the scope of this chapter and the reader is referred to the work of Garrow [29].

Indirect calorimetry is based on a knowledge of the relationship between the quantity of O_2 consumed and CO_2 produced and the energy released when various reactions take place in the body. For example, the oxidation of glucose can be expressed as follows:

$$C_6H_{12}O_6 + 6O_2 = 6H_2O + 6CO_2 + 673 \text{ kcal.}$$

The quantity of gas involved is constant for any particular reaction, as is the heat produced. Previous workers have established how many calories are released for each gram of foodstuff oxidized (calorific value) and the relevant quantities of gas involved. In the above reaction the volume of O_2 consumed is the same as the volume of CO_2 produced, and the ratio of $\dot{V}O_2$ to $\dot{V}CO_2$, which is called the respiratory exchange ratio or respiratory quotient (RQ), is in this case unity. The calorific values and RQ for the different main foodstuffs are shown in Table 4.4. Normally the whole-body RQ will be between 0.7 and 1. It is possible, however, for the RQ to be greater than unity only if the administered carbohydrate is being converted to fat. An RQ outside the normal range probably reflects either an unsteady state or a fault in the measurement.

Table 4.4. The energy equivalents of body fuels

Food	Energy (kcal/g)		
	Bomb calorimeter	Human oxidation	Physiological value
Carbohydrate	4.1	4.1	4
Protein	5.4	4.2	4
Fat	9.3	9.3	9
Alcohol	7.1	7.1	7

The conversion of respiratory gas exchange into energy consumption (K) is represented by the following equation:

$$K \text{ k.cal} = 3.941 \, \dot{V}O_2 + 1.16 \, \dot{V}CO_2 - 2.17N,$$

where N = grams of nitrogen excreted in the urine in 24 h. The derivation of these formulae is to be found in Weir's paper [85].

Methods

Closed-circuit spirometry. The *spontaneous respiration method* [8] is illustrated in Fig. 4.12. The subject breathes in from a spirometer which is filled with 100% O_2. Expired gas is returned to the spirometer through the expiratory limb of the circuit via a CO_2 absorber. The descent of the spirometer bell indicates net gas exchange

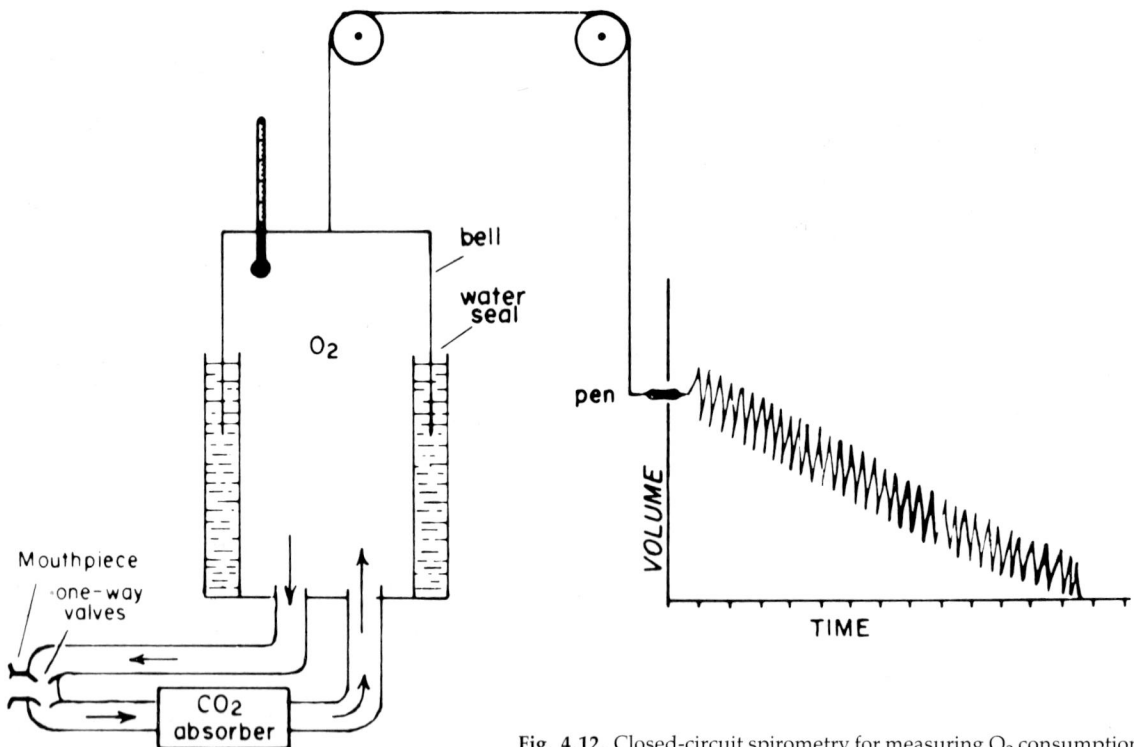

Fig. 4.12. Closed-circuit spirometry for measuring O_2 consumption.

minus CO_2 output, and providing the partial pressure of any inert gas (e.g., N_2) remains constant, this equals the O_2 consumption. Alternatively, the amount of O_2 required to keep the bell at a constant height may be measured. The co-operation of the subject is necessary to achieve a steady state and to avoid leaks. The accuracy is $\pm 7\%$.

In *artificial ventilation* [25, 47] the incorporation of a spirometer has been described, but it is clearly not a very simple technique.

Expired gas collection. In *spontaneous ventilation*, the collection of expired gas in a Douglas bag [20] or Tissot [79] spirometer is the classic open-circuit method for measuring respiratory gas exchange. Care needs to be taken to ensure a steady state during collection. A tight-fitting mask or mouthpiece, and a co-operative subject is essential. It is important to have leak-proof bags as CO_2 may diffuse out more rapidly than O_2 [70]. Ten-minute collection periods are usually required for accurate measurement of the expired gas volume. If the inspired gas is enriched with O_2 the F_{I,O_2} must be measured accurately and air entrainment avoided.

Expired gas collection is relatively simple in those *artificial ventilation* circuits which separate inspired and expired gases completely. If large minute volumes are being used the dilution of the expired gases will require careful measurement of the gas concentrations, as the inspired–expired concentration difference becomes quite small. Properly calibrated infrared (CO_2) [68] and paramagnetic (O_2) [24] gas analysers are fully capable of the required accuracy, as long as the output from these instruments is suitably amplified.

Open hood method. This method for use in *spontaneous ventilation* is illustrated in Fig. 4.13. The subject's head (or in the case of infants, possibly the whole body) is placed in a hood made of some clear plastic material such as Perspex. The hood is not air-tight. A large volume of air is sucked from the hood by a pump, creating a slightly negative pressure in the hood during all phases of ventilation. In this way all the expired

gas is also sucked out of the hood past the measuring system, and none escapes from the hood to the atmosphere. The air and expired gas are mixed in a chamber and the concentrations of O_2 and CO_2 measured together with the flow. The accuracy of measurement of the gas concentrations is crucial as considerable dilution of the expired gas occurs.

It has been suggested [42, 87] that the error involved in assuming a respiratory quotient of unity would be negligible and that the O_2 consumption could be calculated as follows:

$$\dot{V}_{O_2} = V \times (x - y)/100 \text{ litres/min},$$

where V = volume of expired gas and air and x and y are the percentage concentrations of O_2 in air and the mixture, respectively.

In fact this assumption is erroneous and the error is precisely the same as in the expired gas collection method if the RQ is assumed to be 1. This method is very convenient in the spontaneously ventilating subject in the ICU, as it does not require separation of inspired and expired gas and therefore does away with masks and mouthpieces, which are difficult to use in patients.

Neuhof and Wolf [57] indicate that they have used a similar system with an O_2-enriched atmosphere. They give no details of the potential or measured errors of their system, which can be quite considerable.

An adaptation of the open hood method for use in *ventilated subjects* has recently been described [68]. This is shown in Fig. 4.14. A portion of the inspired gas is shunted to mix with all the expired gas, and the mixture is sucked past the O_2 and CO_2 analysers and through a dry gas meter to measure volume. This system has the advantage of providing continuous estimates of O_2 consumption and CO_2 output. It can be used with those ventilators which mix inspired and expired gas at some other part of the circuit. It is possible to use it with high inspired O_2 concentrations and during PEEP, CPAP and IMV. It is not possible to use it with ventilators which require a pressure

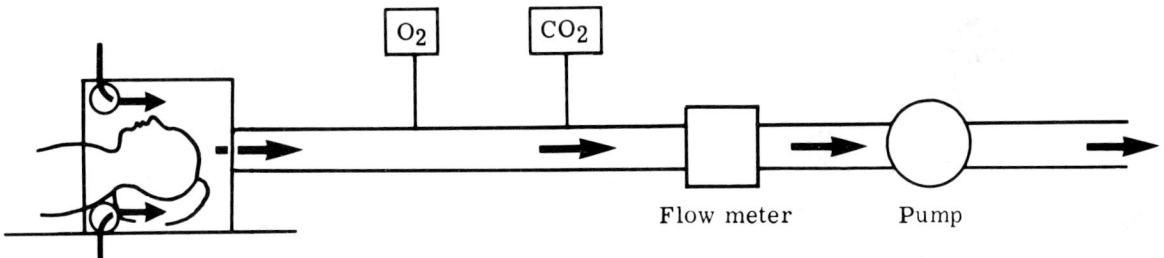

Fig. 4.13. Open hood method of measuring O_2 consumption.

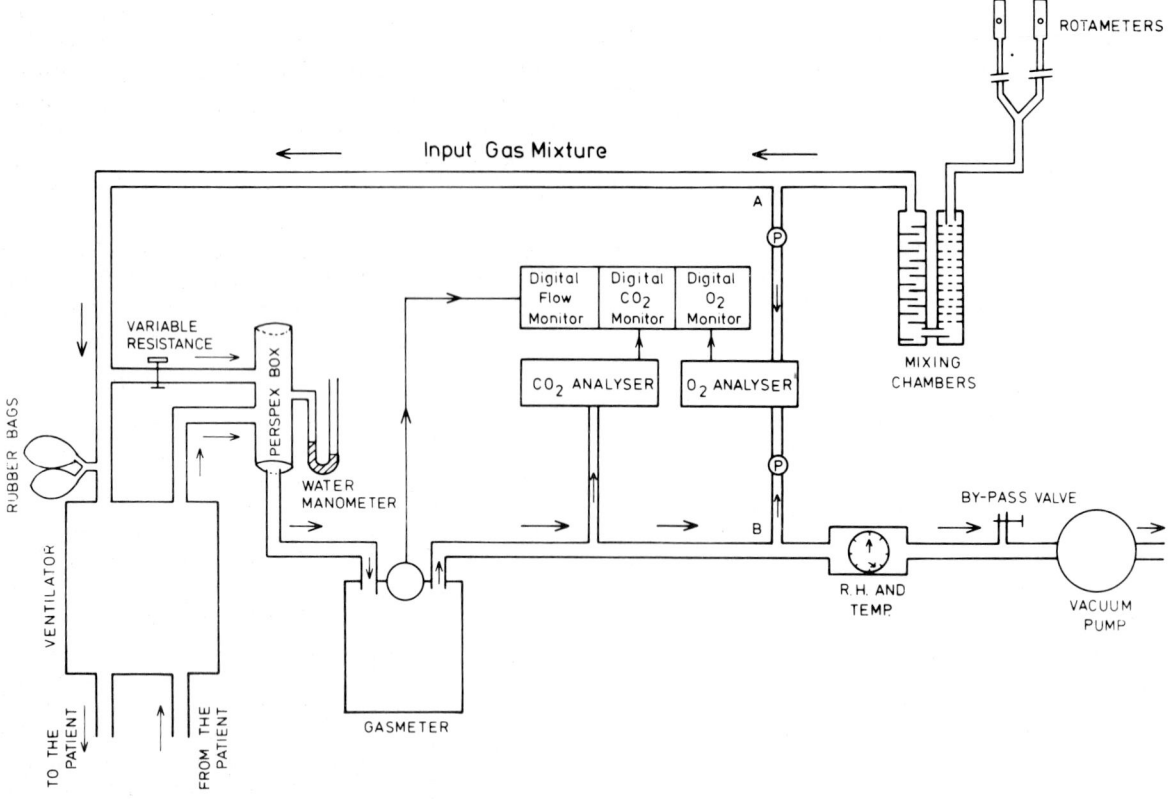

Fig. 4.14. Apparatus for continuous measurement of O_2 consumption and CO_2 production in ventilated subjects. From I. H. A. Rasool and J. H. Chamberlain, 1981, unpublished work.

source to drive them, but use with the Siemens servoventilator is possible when it is used in the anaesthetic mode.

Canopy method [45]. This is similar to the open hood method, but has the disadvantage that a gas-tight seal is necessary. The patient's head is placed in a hood or canopy as before, but an air-tight seal is placed around the neck. The inspired gas is either pumped in or sucked from the canopy, and the mixture of expired gas and inspired gas is analysed downstream. This system can be used with high inspired O_2, as described by Long et al. [51], but these workers give no details concerning accuracy. Except in this circumstance there does not seem to be any particular advantage in this system over the open hood method where leaks do not constitute a problem.

Changes in basal metabolic rate in critically ill patients

Standard tables

Various factors affect the basal metabolic rate (BMR) and need to be taken into account when calculating an individual's energy needs. These include body size, age, and sex. Table 4.5 provides the standard metabolic rates given by Fleisch [28] for different age groups and sex, corrected to body surface area.

Temperature

The ambient temperature is an important determinant of metabolic rate. A temperature of less than 23°C is associated in the normal patient with an increase in metabolic rate. If the ambient temperature rises above 37°C the body is incapable of getting rid of heat quickly enough and body temperature and metabolic rate increase [89]. Critically ill patients often have an elevated body temperature even in the absence of infection, and burned patients, when allowed to regulate their own environmental temperature, opt for a temperature of 30°C, almost 3 deg.C higher than controls. Wilmore [91], however, found that these patients continued to be hypermetabolic despite the elevated ambient temperatures, and could not confirm previous studies [5] which indicated a reduction in energy expenditure when patients

Table 4.5. Standard metabolic rates

Age in years	kcal/m² per h		kJ/m² per h	
	Men	Women	Men	Women
1	53.0	53.0	222	222
2	52.4	52.4	219	219
3	51.3	51.2	215	214
4	50.3	49.8	211	208
5	49.3	48.4	206	203
6	48.3	47.0	202	197
7	47.3	45.4	198	190
8	46.3	43.8	194	183
9	45.2	42.8	189	179
10	44.0	42.5	184	178
11	43.0	42.0	180	176
12	42.5	41.3	178	173
13	42.3	40.3	177	169
14	42.1	39.2	176	164
15	41.8	37.9	175	159
16	41.4	36.9	173	154
17	40.8	36.3	171	152
18	40.0	35.9	167	150
19	39.2	35.5	164	149
20	38.6	35.3	162	148
25	37.5	35.2	157	147
30	36.8	35.1	154	147
35	36.5	35.0	153	146
40	36.3	34.9	152	146
45	36.2	34.5	152	144
50	35.8	33.9	150	142
55	35.4	33.3	148	139
60	34.9	32.7	146	137
65	34.4	32.2	144	135
70	33.8	31.7	141	133
75 and over	33.2	31.3	139	131

were nursed in a warm environment. Zawacki et al. [95] also observed that preventing the evaporative loss by covering the burned area did not alter the metabolic rate.

Temperature was classically thought to have a consistent effect on energy expenditure. Nonetheless, the observation of Kinney and Roe [44] has shown this relationship in critically ill patients to be far from predictable. A high temperature is not uniformly associated with an increase in metabolism.

Physical activity

The level of physical activity will also affect energy requirements. In normal volunteers increases of up to 7% for sitting, 17% for standing, and over 100% for walking were reported by Kinney et al. [46, 50]. Increases of up to 25% when previously ventilated patients are allowed to respire spontaneously have been reported

[12]. However, it is not always certain from these reports what the pattern of respiratory activity is. It seems likely that if the transition from full artificial ventilation to spontaneous respiration is accomplished in a quiet and orderly fashion, and the patient is able to breathe without difficulty, then the O_2 cost is much less than 25%. 'Fighting' the ventilator, however, can be associated with considerable increases in O_2 consumption of up to 100%. Physiotherapy, both passive and active, will also increase energy demands (I. H. A. Rasool and J. H. Chamberlain, 1981, unpublished work).

Specific dynamic action

Administration of foods, particularly those containing nitrogen, either PO or IV, is associated with extra heat production. This is called the specific dynamic action. It is probably due to increased hepatic activity associated with the metabolism of the ingested foodstuffs. About 12% of the ingested protein is dissipated as heat in the subsequent 4 h. Fat (2%) and carbohydrate (6%) have a smaller effect and a mixed diet probably has an overall 6% loss. Wilmore [88] states that hypermetabolic patients exhibit even smaller increases in heat production following food. On the other hand, starvation is associated with a decrease in metabolic rate, at least in normal individuals. Benedict [7] showed that the basal metabolic requirements (BMR) had fallen on the 21st day of a fast to about 664 kcal/m² per day, from a starting level of 904 kcal/m² per day.

Change associated with illness

The foregoing discussion illustrates the multiplicity of factors which may affect the BMR of critically ill patients. In addition to these, studies on various categories of patients have indicated that the underlying condition itself is often associated with alterations in metabolic rate, which in some instances can be quite profound. The best-studied group is burned patients who usually have a considerable increase in metabolic rate, the degree of which is directly proportional to the percentage of the skin surface burned. The increase in BMR ranges from 25% for a 10% burn to 115% for a 70% burn [92]. At the other end of the spectrum, the routine uncomplicated surgical case does not usually exhibit any increased requirements above basal [22]. In between lie patients with fractures (20%–25%) [17], peritonitis

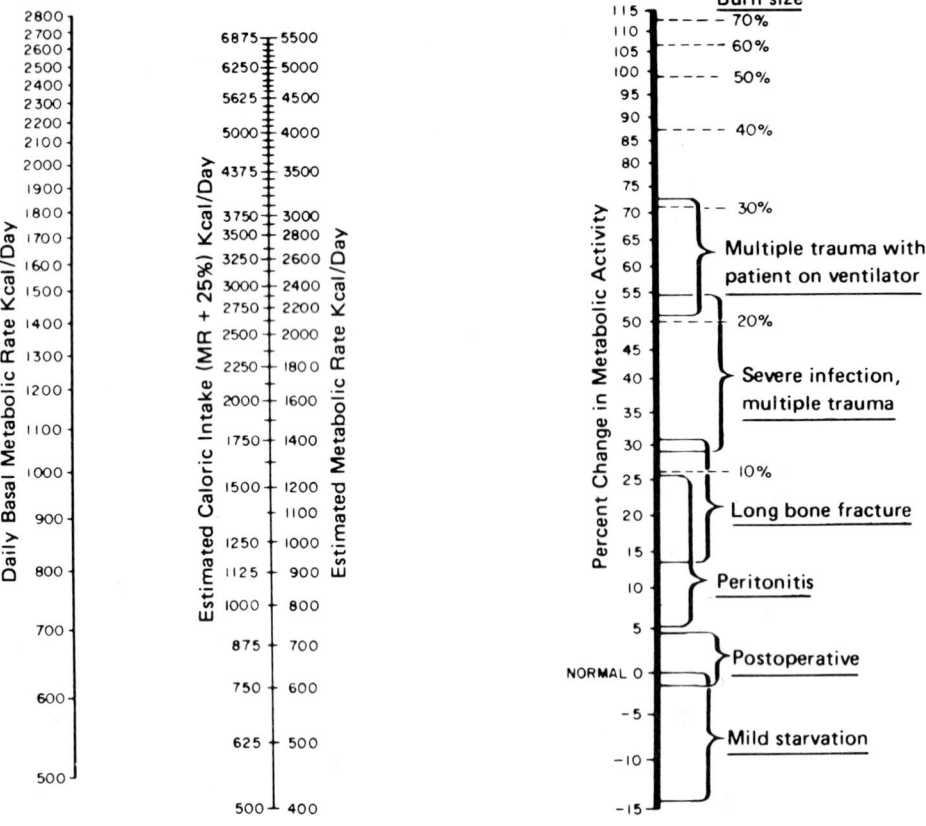

Fig. 4.15. Nomogram to calculate daily energy requirements on the basis of basal metabolic rate (taken from Table 4.5) and patient's clinical status. The estimated caloric requirement is given on the right-hand side of the *middle bar graph* and on the left-hand side an arbitrary 25% has been added to this to cover other possible sources of increased metabolic expenditure (see text for details). Taken from Wilmore [89].

(5%–25%) [22, 33], severe infection, and multiple trauma (30%–55%). The published reports are often short on data and long on discussion, and it is clear that the figures given above are only a rough and ready guide. Only one report [34] deals with ventilated patients, and this suggests that the metabolic rate of these patients, who were also septic, was even higher than that of septic patients who were breathing spontaneously. This was presumably a reflection of the seriousness of the underlying condition rather than the result of ventilation. The paucity of data reflects the difficulty of making meaningful measurements under these conditions, but such information is important if a rational approach to the nutritional support of these patients is to be forthcoming. Figure 4.15 gives a nomogram which enables the calculation of the energy requirements of a wide variety of patients. This should be used in conjunction with Table 4.5, which provides the estimation of BMR. An arbitrary 25% has been added to the estimated metabolic rate to cover those extraneous factors discussed above.

References

1. Alberti KGMM, Darley JJ, Emerson PM, Hockaday TDR (1972) 2,3-diphosphoglycerate and tissue oxygenation in uncontrolled diabetes mellitus. Lancet II: 391–395
2. Allen DW, Wyman T, Smith CA (1953) The oxygen equilibrium of foetal and adult human haemoglobin. J Biol Chem 203:84–87
3. Aronow WS, Isbell WW (1973) Carbon monoxide effect on exercise-induced angina pectoris. Ann Intern Med 79:392–395
4. Aronow WS, Stemmer EA, Isbell MW (1974) Effect of carbon monoxide exposure on intermittent claudication. Circulation 49:415–417
5. Barr PO, Broke G, Liljedahl SO, Plantin LO (1968) Oxygen consumption and water loss during treatment of burns with warm dry air. Lancet I: 164–168
6. Bellingham AJ (1976) Haemoglobins with altered oxygen affinity. Br Med Bull 32:234–238
7. Benedict FG (1915) A study of prolonged fasting. Carnegie Institute, Washington (Publication no 203)
8. Benedict FG (1918) A portable respiration apparatus for clinical use. Boston Medical and Surgical Journal 178:667–678
9. Benesch R, Benesch RE (1967) The effect of organic phosphates from the human erythrocyte on the allosteric properties of haemoglobin. Biochem Biophys Res Commun 26:162–167

10. Bohr C, Hasselbalch KA, Krogh A. (1904) Ueber einen in biologischer Beziehung wichtigen Einfluss, den die Kohlensaurespannung des Blutes auf dessen Sauerstoffbingung ubt. Acta Physiol Scand 16:402–412

11. Bunn HF, Briehl RW (1970) The interaction of 2,3-diphosphoglycerate with various haemoglobins. J Clin Invest 49:1088–1095

12. Bursztein S, Taitelman U, De Mythenacre S, Michelan M, Dahan E, Gepstein R, Edelman D, Melamed Y (1978) Reduced oxygen consumption in catabolic states with mechanical ventilation. Crit Care Med 6:162–164

13. Chanutin A, Curnish RR (1967) Effect of organic and inorganic phosphates on the oxygen equilibrium of human erythrocytes. Arch Biochem Biophys 121:96–102

14. Cheniak NS, Longobardo GS (1970) Oxygen and carbon dioxide gas stores of the body. Physiol Rev 50:196–243

15. Christiansen J, Douglas CG, Haldane JS (1914) The adsorption and dissociation of carbon dioxide by human blood. J Physiol (Lond) 48:244–271

16. Consolazio GF, Johnson RE, Percora LJ (1963) Physiological measurements of metabolic function in man. McGraw-Hill, New York, p 22

17. Cuthbertson DP (1932) Observations on disturbance of metabolism produced by injury to the limbs. Q J Med 25:233–246

18. Delivoria-Papadopoulos M, Miller M, Forster R (1976) Exchange transfusion in low birth weight infants. 1. Initial observations. J Pediatr 89:273–278

19. Delivoria-Papadopoulos M, Roncevic NP, Oski FA (1971) Postnatal changes in oxygen transport of term, premature and sick infants; the role of adult haemoglobin and red cell 2,3-diphosphoglycerate. Pediatr Res 5:235–245

20. Douglas CG (1911) A method for determining the total respiratory exchange. J Physiol (Lond) 42:17–18

21. Duhm J (1972) The effect of 2,3-DPG and other organic phosphates on the Donnan equilibrium and oxygen affinity of human blood. In Astrup P and Rorth M (eds) Oxygen affinity of haemoglobin and red cells acid base status. Munksgaard, Copenhagen, pp 583–594 (4th Alfred Benzon Symposium)

22. Duke JH, Jorgenson SB, Broell JR, Long CL, Kinney JM (1970) Contribution of protein to caloric expenditure following injury. Surgery 68:168–174

23. Edwards MJ, Novy MJ, Walters CL, Metcalfe J (1968) Improved oxygen release: An adaptation of mature red cells to hypoxia. J Clin Invest 47:1851–1857

24. Ellis FR, Nunn JF (1968) The measurement of gaseous oxygen tension utilising paramagnetism: An evaluation of the 'Servomex' OA 150 Analyser. Br J Anaesth 40:569–578

25. Engstrom CG, Herzoy P, Norlander O (1961) A method for the continuous measurement of oxygen consumption in the presence of inert gases during controlled ventilation. Acta Anaesthesiol Scand 5:115–128

26. Fairley HB (1967) The effect of hyperventilation on arterial oxygen tension. A theoretical analysis. Can Anaesth Soc J 14:87–93

27. Fairweather LJ, Walker J, Flenley DC (1974) 2,3-diphosphoglycerate concentrations and the dissociation of oxyhaemoglobin in ventilatory failure. Clin Sci 47:577–588

28. Fleisch A (1951) Le metabolisms basal standard et sa determination au moyen du 'Metobocalculator'. Helv Chir Acta 18:23–44

29. Garrow JS (1974) Energy balance and obesity in man. North Holland, Amsterdam, pp 57–61

30. Gillies IDS (1980) Anaemia in relation to anaesthesia. In: Prys-Roberts C (ed) The circulation in anaesthesia. Blackwell Scientific, Oxford, pp 351–372

31. Gottuso M, Williams M, Oski FA (1976) Exchange transfusion in low birth weight infants. II. Further observations. J Pediatr 89:279–285

32. Guesnon P, Bohn B, Bursaux E, Pyart C (1980) Oxygen linked binding of halothane to human adult haemoglobin. Br J Anaesth 52:1177–1181

33. Gump FE, Price JB, Kinney JM (1970) Whole body and splanchnic blood flow and oxygen consumption measurements in patients with intra-peritoneal infection. Ann Surg 171:321–328

34. Halmagyi DFJ, Kinney JM (1975) Metabolic rate in acute respiratory failure. Surgery 77:492–497

35. Harken AH (1977) The surgical significance of the oxyhaemoglobin dissociation curve. Surg Gynecol Obstet 144:935–955

36. Harken AH, Lillo R, Hufnager HV (1975) The direct influence of endotoxin on cellular respiration. Surg Gynecol Obstet 140:858–860

37. Harken AH, Woods M, Wright CB (1975) The influence of endotoxin on tissue respiration and oxygen dissociation in an isolated canine hind limb. Am Surg 41:704–709

38. Hechtman HB, Grindlinger GA, Vegas AM, Manny J, Valeri CR (1979) Importance of oxygen transport in clinical medicine. Crit Care Med 7:419–423

39. Hejm M (1969) The content of 2,3-diphosphoglycerate and some other phosphocompounds in human erythrocytes from healthy adults and subjects with different kinds of anaemia. Forsvars Medecin 5:219–226

40. Hewitt PB, Chamberlain JH, Seed RFL (1973) The effect of carbon dioxide on cardiac output in patients undergoing mechanical ventilation following open heart surgery. Br J Anaesth 45:1035–1042

41. Hill AV (1910) The possible effects of the aggregation of the molecules of haemoglobin on its dissociation curves. J Physiol (Lond) 40:iv

42. Kappagoda CT, Linden RJ (1972) A critical assessment of the open circuit technique for measuring oxygen consumption. Cardiovasc Res 6:589–598

43. Kelman GR, Nun JF, Prys-Roberts C, Greenbaum R (1967) The influence of cardiac output on arterial oxygenation: A theoretical study. Br J Anaesth 39:450–457

44. Kinney JM, Roe CF (1962) Caloric equivalent of fever. Ann Surg 156:610–620

45. Kinney JM, Morgan AP, Domigues FJ, Gildner KJ (1964) A method for continuous measurement of gas exchange and expired radioactivity in acutely ill patients. Metabolism 13:205–211

46. Kinney JM, Duke JH, Long CL, Gump FE (1970) Tissue salt and weight loss after injury. J Clin Pathol 23 [Suppl 4]:65–72

47. Lawler FG, White DC (1977) The measurement of oxygen uptake during anaesthesia. Br J Anaesth 49:5111–5112

48. Lenfant C, Way P, Ancutt C, Conz J (1969) Effect of chronic hypoxia on the oxygen Hb dissociation curve and respiratory gas transport in man. Respir Physiol 7:7–29

49. Lichtman MA, Miller DR, Cohen J, Waterhouse C (1971) Reduced red cells glycolysis, 2,3-diphosphoglycerate and adenosine triphosphate concentration and increased haemoglobin-oxygen affinity caused by hypophosphataemia. Ann Intern Med 74:562–568

50. Long CL, Kopp K, Kinney JM (1969) Energy demands during ambulation in surgical convalescence. Surg Forum 20:93–94

51. Long CL, Schaffel CN, Blakemore WS, Spencer JL, Broell JR (1979) A continuous analyser for monitoring respiratory gases and expired radioactivity in clinical studies. Metabolism 28:320–332

52. McConn R (1971) 2,3-DPG—What role in septic shock? In: Lillehie R and Stubbs S (ed) Shock in low and high flow states. Excerpta Medica, Amsterdam, pp 28–41 (International congress series, 247)

53. Miller LD, Oski FA, Diaco JF, Sugerman HJ, Gottlier AJ, Davidson D, Delivoria-Papadopoulos M (1970) The affinity of haemoglobin for oxygen: Its control and *in vivo* significance. Surgery 68:187–195

54. Miller WW, Delivoria-Papadopoulos M, Miller L, Oski F (1970) Oxygen-releasing factor in thyrotoxicosis. JAMA 211:1824–1826

55. Morse M, Cassels DE, Holder M (1950) The position of the oxygen dissociation curve of the blood in cyanotic congenital heart disease. J Clin Invest 29:1098–1103

56. Naylor BA, Welch MH, Shafer AW, Guenter CA (1972) Blood affinity for oxygen in haemmorhagic and endotoxic shock. J Appl Physiol 32:829–833

57. Neuhof H, Wolf H (1978) Method for continuously measured oxygen consumption and cardiac output for use in critically ill patients. Crit Care Med 6:155–161

58. Niness JR Kinsber RW, McDonald JW (1974) Erythrocyte 2,3-DPG, ATP and oxygen affinity in haemodialysis patients. Can Med Assoc J 5:661–667

59. Nunn JF (1977a) Applied respiratory physiology. Butterworths, London, pp 410–411

60. Nunn JF (1977b) Applied respiratory physiology. Butterworths, London, pp 354–358, 412–414

61. Oski FA (1979) Clinical implications of the oxyhaemoglobin dissociation curve in the neonatal period. Crit Care Med 7:412–418

62. Oski FA, Gottlier AJ, Delivoria-Papadopoulos M, Miller WW (1969) Red cell 2,3-diphosphoglycerate levels in subjects with chronic hypoxaemia. N Engl J Med 280:1165–1166

63. Oski FA, Marshall BE, Cohen PJ, Sugerman HJ, Miller LD (1971) Exercise with anaemia: The role of the left shifted or right shifted oxygen haemoglobin equilibrium curve. Ann Intern Med 74:44–54

64. Perutz MF (1978) Haemoglobin structure and respiratory transport. Sci Am 239:68–86

65. Pirnay F, Dajardin J, Deroanne R, Petit JM (1971) Muscular exercise during intoxication by carbon monoxide. J Appl Physiol 31:573–575

66. Raich PC, Rodriquez JM, Desai T, Korst DR, Shahidi NT (1971) Effect of haemodialysis on pH, inorganic phosphate and red cell 2,3-DPG in patients with uraemia. Clin Res 19:428

67. Rapaport S, Luebering J (1950) The formation of 2,3-diphosphoglycerate in rabbit erythrocytes: The existence of a diphosphoglycerate mutase. J Biol Chem 183:507–516

68. Rasool IHA, Chamberlain JH, Swan PC, Mitchell FT (1982) Measurement of respiratory gas exchange during artificial respiration. J Appl Physiol, to be published

69. Rose ZB (1968) The purification and properties of diphosphoglycerate mutase from human erythrocytes. J Biol Chem 243:4810–4820

70. Rose ZB (1970) Enzymes controlling 2,3-diphosphoglycerate in human erythrocytes. Fed Proc 29:1105–1111

71. Roughton FJW, Darling RC (1944) The effect of carbon monoxide on the dissociation curve. Am J Physiol 141:17–31

72. Severinghaus JW (1966) Blood gas calculator. J Appl Physiol 21:1108–1116

73. Shappell SD, Lenfant CJM (1975) Physiological role of the oxyhaemoglobin curve. In: Surgenor D McN (ed) The red blood cell, 2nd edn. Academic Press, New York, pp 842–871

74. Shappell SD, Murray JA, Nasser MG, Wills RE, Torrance JD, Lenfant C (1970) Acute change in haemoglobin affinity for oxygen during angina pectoris. N Engl J Med 282:1219–1224

75. Sheldon GF (1972) Hyperphosphataemia, hypophosphataemia and the oxygen dissociation curve. J Surg Res 14:367–372

76. Sheldon GF, Grzyb S (1975) Phosphate depletion and repletion: Relation to parenteral nutrition and oxygen transport. Ann Surg 182:683–689

77. Sugerman HJ, Miller LD, Oski FA, Diaco J, Delivoria-Papadopoulos M, Davidson D (1970) Decreased 2,3-diphosphoglycerate and reduced oxygen consumption in septic shock. Clin Res 18:418

78. Thomas HM, Lefrak SS, Irwin RS, Fritts HW, Caldwell PRB (1974) The oxyhaemoglobin dissociation curve in health and disease. Am J Med 57:331–348

79. Tissot J (1904) Nouvelle méthode de mesure et d'inscription du débit et des mouvements respiratoires de l'homme et des animaux. J Physiol (Paris) 6:688–700

80. Torrance JD, Jacobs P, Restrepo A, Eschbach J, Lenfant C, Finch CA (1970) Intraerythrocyte adaptation to anaemia. N Engl J Med 283:165–169

81. Travis SF, Sugerman HJ, Ruberg RL, Dudrick SJ, Delivoria-Papadopoulos M, Miller LD, Oski FA (1971) Alterations of red cell glycolytic intermediates and oxygen transport as a consequence of hypophosphataemia in patients receiving intravenous hyperalimentation. N Engl J Med 285:763–768

82. Valeri CR (1974) Oxygen transport function of preserved red cells. Clin Haematol 3:649–688

83. Vogel JA, Gleser MA, Wheeler RC, Whitten BK (1972) Carbon monoxide and physical work capacity. Arch Environ Health 24:198–203

84. Watkins GM, Rabelo A, Plzak LF, Sheldon GF (1974) The left shifted oxyhaemoglobin curve in sepsis. Ann Surg 180:213–220

85. Weir JB de V (1949) New method for calculating metabolic rate with special reference to protein metabolism. J Physiol (Lond) 109:1–9

86. Weisel RD, Dennis RC, Manny, Mannick JA, Valeri CR, Hechtman HB (1978) Adverse effects of transfusion therapy during abdominal aortic aneurysmectomy. Surgery 83:682–690

87. Wessel HU, Rorem D, Musters AS, Accuedo RE, Paul MH (1969) Continuous determination of oxygen uptake in sedated infants and children during cardiac catheterisation. Am J Cardiol 24:376–385

88. Wilmore DW (1977a) The metabolic management of the critically ill. Plenum, New York, pp 29–31

89. Wilmore DW (1977b) The metabolic management of the critically ill. Plenum, New York, pp 32–33

90. Wilmore DW (1977c) The metabolic management of the critically ill. Plenum, New York, p 36

91. Wilmore DW, Mason AD, Johnson DW, Pruitt BA (1975) Effect of ambient temperature on heat production and heat loss in burn patients. J Appl Physiol 38:593–597

92. Wilmore DW, Long JM, Mason AD, Skreen RW, Pruitt BA (1974) Catecholamines: Mediator of the hypermetabolic response to thermal injury. Ann Surg 180:653–669

93. Woodson RD, Wraune B, Detter JC (1973) Effect of increased blood oxygen affinity on work performance of rats. J Clin Invest 52:2717–2724

94. Woodson RD, Torrance JD, Shappell SD, Lenfant C (1970) The effect of cardiac disease on haemoglobin-oxygen binding. J Clin Invest 44:1349–1356

95. Zawacki BE, Spitzer KW, Mason AD, John LA (1970) Does increased evaporative water loss cause hypermetabolism in burned patients? Ann Surg 171:236–240

Chapter 5

Fluid and Electrolyte Balance

F. D. Thompson

The major function of the cardiorenal system is to maintain the fluid bathing the cells at a constant composition, for it is through this pericellular fluid that O_2 and nutrients are delivered and waste products of metabolism removed. The early marine vertebrates had an extracellular fluid similar to that of their salt water environment, but with evolution to fresh water and land there were various modifications, which included the development of an integument impermeable to water and modifications in renal function to allow the excretion or conservation of water and sodium according to the prevailing conditions. This chapter will outline the distribution of water and electrolytes throughout the body and the aspects of circulatory and renal physiology which are responsible for maintaining this steady state.

Distribution of body water

The total amount of water in the body is high and ranges between 50% and 60% of the body weight. The total water is measured by estimating the volume of distribution of a substance which will both pass freely throughout the body and enter the cells with ease. Such indicators are deuterium oxide and tritium oxide, and when these indicators are used averages of 500–600 ml/kg are obtained [17]. Fat contains little water, and when figures for the lean body mass are expressed the percentage of body water rises to 70. The total water is not evenly distributed, as well over half is found within the cells. The extracellular water is measured by the distribution of mannitol, sucrose, or inulin, and average figures of 180 ml/kg are obtained [7]. As the water in bone and dense connective tissue is not readily accessible, this figure may be low, and some workers suggest a more realistic estimate is 270 ml/kg. ^{121}I-albumin can be used to measure the circulating plasma volume, which is roughly 4.5% of the body weight. There is no indicator that will distribute itself solely within the cell, and so the intracellular fluid, which composes roughly 40% of the total body weight, is always a derived figure. Figure 5.1 illustrates the distribution of body water within the various body compartments.

The distribution of protein and electrolytes throughout the intra- and extracellular fluid is not equal. These differences in concentration can be conveniently expressed as histograms. This technique was introduced by Gamble in 1942 and allows a rapid visual assessment to be made of the major differencs (Fig. 5.2). It can be seen that for each compartment the anions and cations balance and that for extracellular fluid the major cation is sodium, with chloride being the major anion. The intracellular composition differs in that potassium is the major cation, whilst phosphate and sulphate maintain electrical neutrality [8]. A review of the mechanisms responsible for these major differences, which relates directly to the exchange between plasma

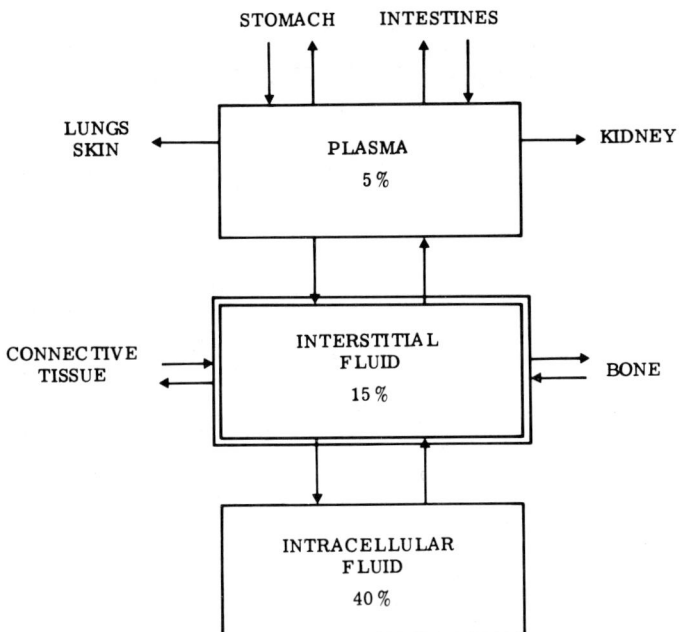

Fig. 5.1. Distribution of body water.

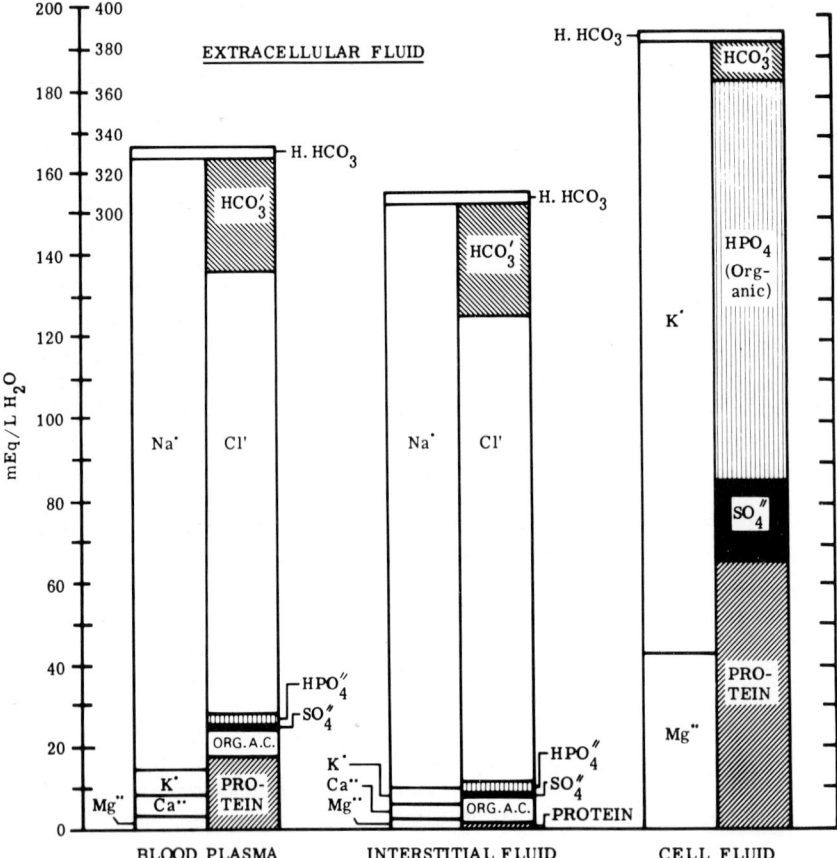

Fig. 5.2. Ion distribution in the fluid compartments of the body. J. L. Gamble: *Chemical Anatomy, Physiology and Pathology of Extracellular Fluid* (6th edn). Cambridge, Mass.: Harvard University Press. Copyright 1942, 1947, 1954, by the President and Fellows of Harvard College.

and interstitial fluid, and interstitial and intracellular fluid, will now be given.

Relationship between plasma and interstitial fluid

It is at capillary level that the interchange between the circulation and the interstitial fluid takes place. The large area of capillary endothelium permits an average production of 15 ml interstitial fluid/min and the reabsorption of 12 ml/min. The endothelial wall is one cell thick and is covered on its outer surface by a mucopolysaccharide basement membrane [3]. The forces which act across this thin cell wall are now well established [19] and are set out in Fig. 5.3. The major determinant of fluid movement is the hydrostatic pressure. At the arteriolar end of the capillary the hydrostatic pressure is 40–45 mm, falling along the capillary length until at the venous end the pressure is only 10–15 mmHg. The outward hydrostatic pressure is opposed mainly by the osmotic pressure of the plasma. This osmotic pressure is mainly due to the albumin fraction, this being the protein of the smallest molecular weight and highest concentration. The protein fraction exerts this osmotic influence, as the capillary wall is semipermeable to protein. However, it is freely permeable to the crystalloid component of plasma, and so this has no osmotic effect. It can be seen from Fig. 5.3 that the hydrostatic pressure is far greater than the osmotic pressure acting in the opposite direction at the arteriolar end of the capillary, and there is a net filtration of fluid in this high-pressure region. At the low-pressure venous end of the capillary the position is reversed, as the osmotic pressure is greater than the much reduced hydrostatic pressure, and here there is a net flux into the capillary. The turgor pressure of the tissues themselves opposes the outward passage of fluid, and this pressure depends on the volume of fluid present and the distensibility of the interstitial space. This can rise to pathological levels in cases of capillary damage when there is increased permeability of the capillary wall and in cases of lymphatic obstruction.

These forces acting on the capillaries are known as the Starling forces and it has been calculated that if these were the only factors responsible for fluid movement only 0.003 ml interstitial fluid/min would be produced. This level of production is clearly inadequate to provide adequate cell nutrition. A far greater volume of interstitial fluid is produced by simple diffusion. Whether this takes place throughout the cell membrane or only through discrete pores is uncertain. The rate of diffusion depends on the concentration gradient across the cell wall and the type of membrane involved.

The capillary beds of different organs have differing diffusion characteristics. The capillaries found in muscles, skin, heart, and lung are relatively impermeable to protein, whilst those found in the intestine and liver allow protein to pass freely. Even those capillary beds that are relatively impermeable to protein allow some to pass through into the interstitial fluid, and it may be that protein passes through large anatomical pores which are present in large numbers in capillary walls of the liver and gut. Another alternative mechanism to account for the passage of these large molecules is the formation of vesicles at the lumen surface which are released into the interstitial compartment, having migrated through the cell substance [16]. It has been estimated that even through the relatively impermeable capillaries of muscle, 1 mg protein per minute passes through for each 100 g tissue.

The rate of interstitial fluid production is governed by several factors. The muscular capillary sphincters are capable of alterations in tone,

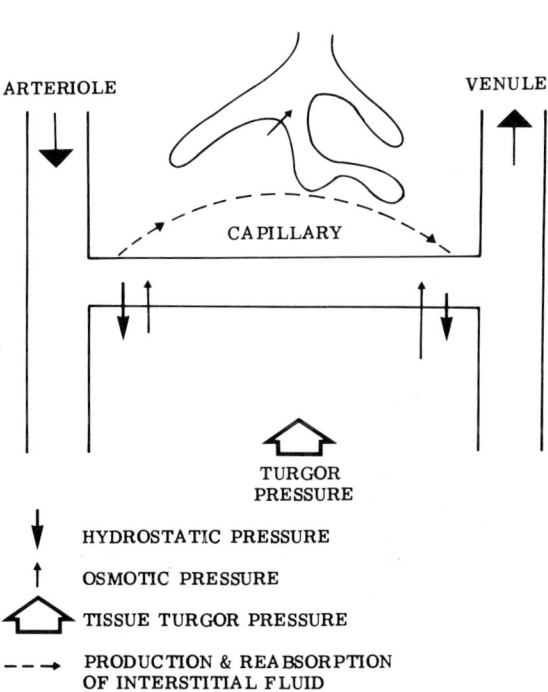

Fig. 5.3. Fluid exchange at a capillary level.

and with vasodilatation there is a greater production of fluid at the arteriolar end, the converse being true with vasoconstriction. A raised venous pressure will prevent the return of fluid at the venous end and so increase the amount of interstitial fluid, and in cases of dehydration and lowered venous pressure the interstitial compartment will be depleted at the expense of a circulating volume. In cases of hypoproteinaemia the reduced oncotic pressure permits greater interstitial fluid formation and subsequent oedema. These pathological processes will be dealt with in greater detail elsewhere.

It can be seen from Fig. 5.3 that not all the interstitial fluid produced at the arteriolar end of the capillary is reabsorbed at the venous end. The excess is carried away by the lymphatics. This lymphatic drainage is not insignificant as it accounts for at least 4 litres of fluid a day and it is this system that is responsible for returning the protein of the interstitial fluid back into the circulation [14].

Relationship of intracellular to extracellular interstitial fluid

The experimental evidence recorded in the histogram (Fig. 5.2) shows that the osmotic concentration within the cell and in the interstitial fluid is the same. However, there are major differences in the ionic composition, the major cations being potassium and magnesium, while the anions are represented by protein, sulphate, and phosphate. The physiological factors governing this unequal distribution of ions will now be considered. In general terms, cellular membranes are relatively impermeable to protein. There are notable exceptions, namely the absorption of macro-immunoglobulins from the intestine of the newborn and the secretion of pancreatic and salivary enzymes into the gastrointestinal tract. This process involves the incorporation of the protein molecule by the cell wall to form a vesicle which is transported through the body of the cell to be released at the opposite cell surface [6]. The mechanisms involved in the transport of ions and small molecules across cell membranes are an important and expanding subject. An outline of the more well-established mechanisms is given below.

Diffusion kinetics

The cell wall acts as a semipermeable mem-

brane, and ions and small molecules will diffuse across from high to low concentrations (Fig 5.4). It can be seen that with a simple diffusion process, higher concentrations mean greater net transport. The rate of solute diffusion of common biological substances such as sugars, amino acids, and ions do not follow this simple diffusion pattern, but exhibit a maximum rate of transfer (Fig. 5.5). With this mechanism a point is reached where increasing the concentration gradient does not increase the rate of diffusion, the system being saturated. This relationship is typical of a process involving a carrier which picks up the substance on the inside of the cell and transports it to the outer cell membrane [20]. In transport systems the carrier will be highly specific, which is why some amino acids are transported more readily than others. In other situations the various substrates will compete for the same carrier and in this complex situation the amount of substrate carried will depend upon its affinity for the carrier. Certain substances can move across a cell membrane by two distinct mechanisms; for example, sodium and potassium can move by simple diffusion in addition to their active transport across the cell membrane.

Sodium pump

An active transport mechanism for the extrusion of sodium from within the cell must exist, because without such a driving force the electrochemical gradient is such that sodium will freely enter the cell. To maintain electroneutrality there is a reciprocal exchange: as a sodium ion leaves the cell a potassium ion enters. Further support for an active process is given by the experimental facts that the efflux of ions across the cell membrane can be slowed by a reduction in temperature, that glucose is utilized during this process, and that the transport mechanism can be blocked by such substances as ouabain. The nature of this 'sodium pump', as it is now called, is the subject of much discussion, and Glynn and his co-workers have suggested that it is a linked carrier system with ATP as the carrier across the cell [10, 13].

Gibbs–Donnan equilibrium

The presence of protein on one side of a semipermeable membrane influences the ionic distribution across this membrane. This relationship of ions expressed by the Gibbs–Donnan relationship states that when equilibrium

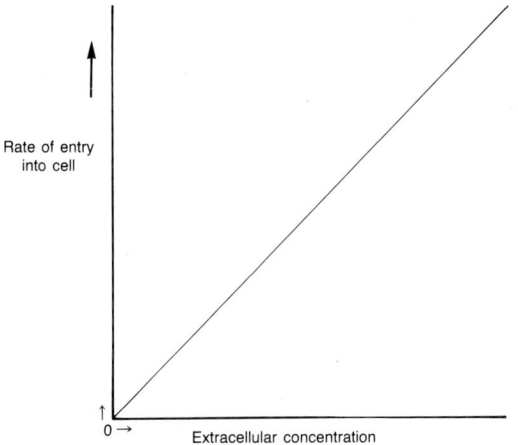

Fig. 5.4. Characteristics of simple diffusion.

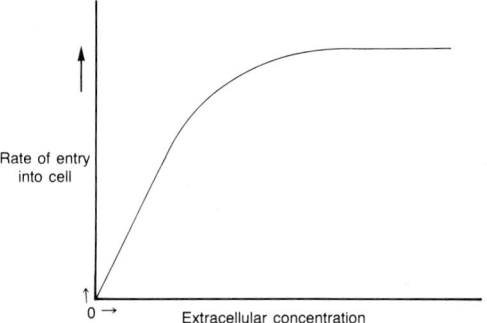

Fig. 5.5. Characteristics of carrier-mediated transport.

has been achieved, the concentration of the anions and cations which are freely diffusible is equal on each side of the membrane. If potassium and chloride are used as the diffusible ions to mimic the cellular situation, this can be presented as in Fig. 5.6. If the product of the potassium and chloride ions inside the cells is to be equal to the product of the potassium and chloride outside the cells, as these represent the freely diffusible ions, it will be seen that the negative charge on the intracellular protein which is not freely diffusible will exert an influence on the potassium and chloride concentration. To maintain electrical neutrality, extra potassium will remain within the cell to negate the effect of the negative charge on the protein. This will result at equilibrium in the intracellular chloride concentration being lower than that externally, whilst the potassium concentration intracellularly will be higher to satisfy the equation (Fig. 5.6).

This unequal distribution of ions generates an equilibrium potential across the membrane, E_m, which to some extent counteracts the effect of the chemical gradient [11]. This membrane potential can be expressed in general terms by the Nirnst equation:

$$E_m = 60 \log \frac{[K_1^+]}{[K_2^+]}.$$

These differences in intracellular and extracellular electrolyte composition are responsible for the cell wall's being polarized, being negative internally and positively charged on the external surface. This resting potential of 60–90 mV is the basis of nerve and muscle activity.

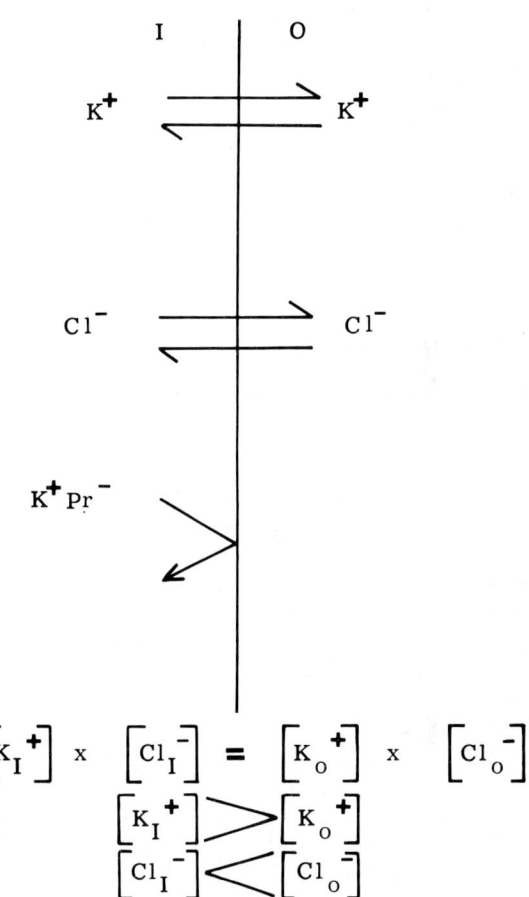

Fig. 5.6. The effect of non-diffusible protein molecules on freely diffusible ions. I, inside the cell; O, outside.

Movement of water between intra- and extracellular compartments

The majority of cell membranes are freely permeable to water, with the result that it is the relative osmotic pressures that govern the movement of water from one compartment to the other. If excess water is added to the extracellular compartment it will diffuse freely into the cells and the volume of both the intra- and extracellular fluid will increase at the expense of a reduction in osmolarity which is normally set at around 300 mosmol/litre. When the osmolarity of the extracellular fluid is increased by the addition of solute, water will move from out of the cell, expanding the extracellular compartment at the expense of the intracellular volume. If, on the other hand, an isotonic solution is added to the extracellular compartment there will be no shifts of water and only the extracellular compartment will expand. Loss of solute from the extracellular fluid will lower the osmolarity in that compartment, with the net result that the raised intracellular osmotic pressure will draw fluid into the cells, increasing their volume and water content [15].

Table 5.1 Normal daily volume, in an adult, of the various secretions into the alimentary tract

Source	Volume
Saliva	1500 cm^3
Gastric secretion	2500 cm^3
Bile	500 cm^3
Pancreatic juice	700 cm^3
Secretion of intestinal mucosa	3000 cm^3
Total	8200 cm^3
Normal plasma volume	3500 cm^3

Source: J.L. Gamble: *Chemical Anatomy*, Physiology and Pathology of Extracellular Fluid (6th edn). Cambridge, Mass.: Harvard University Press. Copyright 1942, 1947, 1954, by the President and Fellows of Harvard College.

Water and electrolyte balance

Water balance

The thirst mechanism which governs the intake of water is not clearly understood. The medial nuclei of the hypothalamus respond to changes in extracellular fluid osmolarity, and when the osmotic pressure rises the desire to drink is mediated by the central nuclei. Other factors, including a dry mouth, which promote the desire to drink may well by responsible. The intake of water is clearly balanced against the daily losses. From the skin and lungs alone the insensible loss due to vaporization can range between 800 ml and 1 litre/24 h, and this amount can be dramatically increased if sensible losses due to sweating are added, which may reach 2 litres/h in extremes of temperature.

Water and electrolytes are lost from the gastrointestinal tract, and on average the net loss of water ranges from 100 to 300 ml/24h. The secretions from the gastrointestinal tract may total 8 litres/24 h and in some pathological circumstances, which will be dealt with later, these secretions are lost from the body, producing an obvious deficit of water and electrolytes. A knowledge of the chemical composition of these secretions helps in clinical management, and the main constituents are listed in Fig. 5.7 and Table 5.1.

Urinary losses of water are variable, as the kidney is the main organ of water and electrolyte homeostasis. When losses of water far exceed the amounts ingested and dehydration occurs, the kidney will conserve water and, under maximal circumstances in man, a urine with an osmolarity of 1400 mosmol/litre can be produced in a volume of 500 ml/24 h. This hyperosmolar urine is the result of the antidiuretic hormone acting on the end of the distal tubule and collecting ducts, promoting the reabsorption of water, the drive to antidiuretic hormone production being a rise in extracellular fluid osmolarity in the region of the hypothalamic osmoreceptors [18]. Conversely, during periods of overhydration a large volume of urine, which may reach 20 litres in a 24-h period, is passed. The osmolarity of this urine is low and may well fall below 100 mosmol/litre. The factors governing the dilution of urine are not so clearly understood, but in the absence of the antidiuretic hormone the membranes of the distal tubule and collecting ducts are impermeable to water and the tubular contents remain hypotonic as a result of active extrusion of water along the ascending loop of Henle [12]. Many pathological states can alter the renal handling of water, e.g., when the solute load filtered at the glomeruli is high, the urine osmolarity is relatively low even during maximal antidiuretic hormone stimulation. This can occur in cases of advanced chronic renal failure.

Sodium balance

On average the body contains 60 mmol sodium per kilogram, 40% of which is bound to bone, 50% extracellular, and the remainder within the cell. Not all of this sodium is freely exchangeable. On average it is estimated that 42 mmol/kg is freely exchangeable, and this can be measured in man by the dilution technique involving ^{22}Na [2].

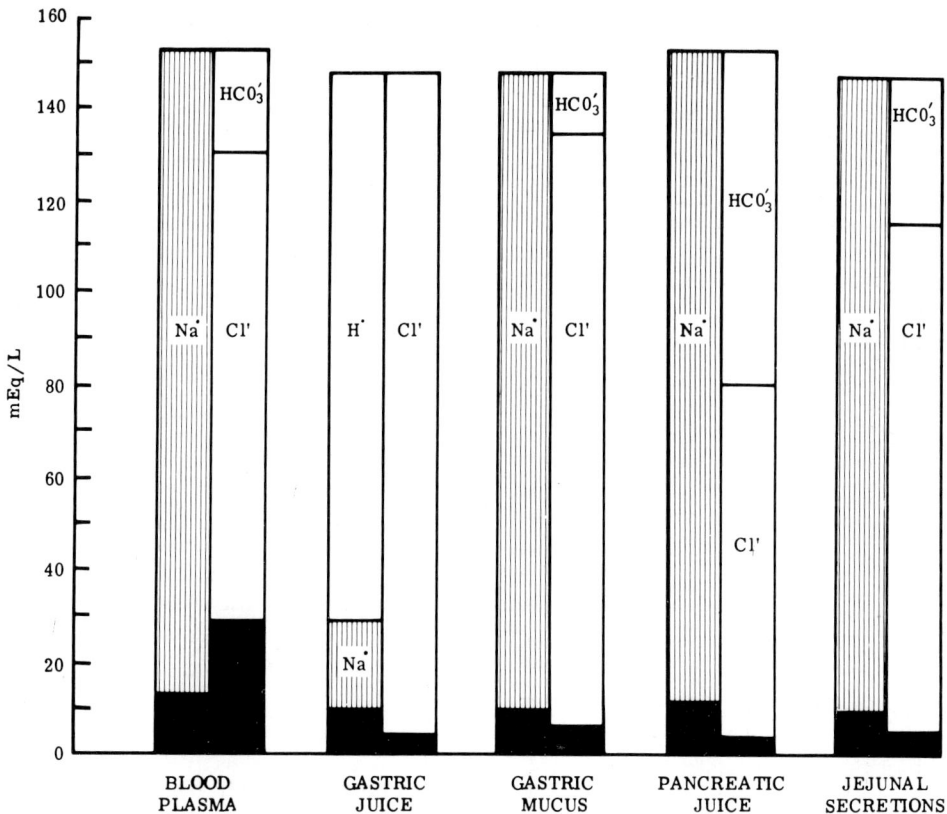

Fig. 5.7. The composition of the main alimentary secretions. Although differing in composition, they are all isotonic with plasma (expressed as mmol/litre fluid volume). J. L. Gamble: Chemical Anatomy, Physiology and Pathology of Extracellular Fluid (6th edn). Cambridge, Mass.: Harvard University Press. Copyright 1942, 1947, 1954, by the President and Fellows of Harvard College.

The intake of sodium clearly varies, but an average adult diet contains approximately 12 g sodium chloride per day. Again the kidney is the central organ for sodium homeostasis, and the urinary losses of sodium are governed by many interrelating factors. A detailed review of sodium homeostasis is beyond the scope of this chapter but many factors, such as the glomerular filtration rate, oncotic pressure of plasma, peritubular capillary pressure, and various hormonal factors (e.g., aldosterone, a possible third natriuretic factor) all play a part. The end result of these physiological processes is that in cases of sodium loss due to diarrhoea or excessive sweating, renal conservation is high and the urinary sodium concentration falls to extremely low levels; in some cases sodium may be completely absent. When sodium ingestion is excessive, however, renal compensation results in a high urinary sodium concentration [5].

Potassium

Total body potassium has been estimated at 42 mmol/kg and, as previously stated, the bulk of this ion is intracellular, only 2% of the body total being in the extracellular compartment. This unequal distribution is brought home when the numerical values for a standard 70-kg man are considered. In the extracellular fluid the total potassium would be approximately 60 mmol, whilst the intracellular total would reach 3400 mmol. For this reason the measurement of the plasma potassium is a very poor guide to overall potassium status, and several isotopic methods are available for the estimation of total body potassium. The commonly occurring isotope of potassium is ^{39}K but a small proportion of potassium is found as ^{40}K. The percentage of this rare isotope is constant, and so an estimate of the total body content of this isotope approximates to the total body stores. Not all potassium is freely exchangeable, and a dilution technique with ^{45}K can be used to estimate the exchangeable pool [2]. These values must be interpreted in the light of the clinical state of the patient; as potassium is found mainly in muscle, its value should be expressed in terms of lean body mass.

The dietary intake of potassium varies considerably, but the average adult's daily intake will be around 100 mmol. Again, the kidney is central in potassium homeostasis, and urinary concentrations vary considerably [5]. In cases of potassium depletion the urinary concentration may well fall to below 10 mmol/litre, whilst in the presence of normal function and a high intake, levels of up to 100 mmol/litre may be achieved. The physiological mechanisms associated with this variation of potassium excretion are complex. Only 5%–10% of the filtered potassium is found entering the distal tubule, and it appears that the major site of fine control is via tubular secretion in the distal tubule. The handling of potassium by the nephron is closely linked with that of sodium, hydrogen ion, and chloride, and is in part under the influence of aldosterone [9, 21].

Chloride

By and large, the intake of chloride is closely related to that of sodium and, apart from the active transport of chloride by the gastric mucosa and the loop of Henle in the kidney, its movements across cell membranes are generally thought to be passive. In cases of chloride loss due to vomiting or gastric suction, the anion gap is repleted by an increase in bicarbonate levels due to the interaction of sodium, hydroxyl and CO_2. The converse occurs in cases of chloride excess, when the plasma bicarbonate falls.

Calcium

Calcium present in low concentrations in plasma makes little contribution to the osmotic pressure and fluid regulation. However, as a cation it is extremely important in maintaining cell membrane integrity, is an active factor in blood coagulation, is an obvious component in bone, and plays a vital role in neuromuscular activity.

To some extent methodology governs the normal range of plasma calcium found in man. Whatever the method used, roughly 40% of the calcium is bound to protein and therefore does not diffuse through a semipermeable membrane. Of the remaining 60%, approximately 46% is free ionized calcium, and it is this fraction that plays a vital role in the above physiological mechanisms.

The calcium content in the normal diet varies considerably; the bulk of it is absorbed in the small intestine. Again, the mechanisms which govern the level of ionized calcium are complex and involve the interplay of parathyroid hormone, calcitonin, and vitamin D in both bone and the kidney. Parathyroid hormone promotes the release of calcium from bone and produces a phosphate diuresis in the kidney, and may promote gastrointestinal absorption of calcium. Calcitonin, on the other hand, tends to lower serum calcium concentration by inhibiting bone resorption and, with no dependence on parathyroid hormone, promotes the urinary loss of phosphate and calcium. Vitamin D promotes intestinal absorption of calcium, enhances the tubular reabsorption of phosphate by the kidney, and may act directly on the parathyroid glands, depressing hormone production [4]. This complex interplay of factors is clearly important when, at a later stage, patient management is considered, as the level of ionized calcium in plasma plays such a vital role in nerve and muscle activity.

Magnesium

Although magnesium is only the fourth cation in terms of concentration, it also plays a vital role, like calcium, in enzyme function and cellular metabolism. An average diet would contain approximately 25 mmol magnesium, roughly 40% of which is absorbed in the small intestine. The normal serum magnesium concentration ranges between 0.7 and 0.9 mmol/litre; 40% of this is protein-bound and the rest is complexed with citrate-phosphate. Sixty percent of magnesium is found in bone, but of this only 30% is freely exchangeable. Muscle is the other major pool of magnesium, as 20% of the total magnesium is found in this site. However, only 30% of the magnesium found in muscle is freely exchangeable, the rest being bound to lipo- and nuclear protein. In terms of renal handling of magnesium, the bulk of the filtered ion is reabsorbed in the proximal tubule and is closely associated with sodium and calcium reabsorption. There is some evidence to suggest that the tubular handling of magnesium is under the control of parathormone [1].

References

1. Alfrey AC (1976) Disorders of magnesium metabolism. In: Schrier RW (ed) Renal and electrolyte disorders. Little Brown, Boston, pp. 223–242
2. Belcher KH, Vetter H (1971) Radioisotopes in medical diagnosis. Butterworths, London
3. Bennett HS, Luft JH, Hampton JC (1959) Morphological characteristics of vertebrate blood capillaries. Am J Physiol 196:381–390
4. Borle AB (1974) Calcium and phosphate metabolism. Annu Rev Physiol 36:361–390
5. Brenner BM, Stein JH (1978) Sodium and water homeostasis. Churchill Livingstone, New York Edinburgh London
6. Christensen HN (1975) Biological transport, 2nd edn. Benjamin, London
7. Edelman IS, Liebman J (1959) Anatomy of body water and electrolytes. Am J Med 27:256–277
8. Gamble JL (1958) Clinical anatomy, physiology and pathology of extracellular fluid, 7th edn. Harvard University Press, Cambridge
9. Gennari FJ, Cohen JL (1975) Potassium homeostasis and acid base balance. Kidney Int 8:1
10. Glynn IM (1968) Membrane ATP-ase and cation transport. Br Med Bull 24:165–169
11. Hodgkin AL, Horowicz P (1959) The influence of potassium and chloride ions on the membrane potential of single muscle fibres. J Physiol (Lond) 148:127–160
12. Jamison RL, Maffly RH (1976) Osmotic concentration and dilution of urine. N Engl J Med 295:1059
13. Robinson JP, Flashner MS (1979) The $(Na^+ + K^+)$-activated ATPase enzymatic and transport properties. Biochimica et Biophysica Acta 549:145–176
14. Ruszynák I, Foldi M, Szabó G (1960) Lymphatics and lymph circulation. Elmsford, Pergamon, New York
15. Skelkurt EE (1976) Body water and electrolyte composition, Physiology, 4th edn. Little Brown, Boston
16. Stein WD (1967) The movement of molecules across cell membranes. Academic Press, New York
17. Strauss MB (1957) Body water in man. Little Brown, Boston
18. Verney EB (1947) Antidiuretic hormone and the factors which determine its release. Proc R Soc Lond [Biol] 135:25–106
19. Wiederhielm CA (1968) Dynamics of transcapillary fluid exchange. J Gen Physiol 52:29–63
20. Wilbrandt T, Rosenberg T (1961) The concept of carrier transport. Pharmacol Rev 13:109–183
21. Wright FS (1974) Potassium transport by the renal tubule, vol 6. University Park Press, Baltimore, (Physiology Series One. Kidney and urinary tract physiology) pp 79–105

Chapter 6

Acid–Base Balance

D. C. Flenley

Acids, bases and buffers

An acid is defined as a proton donor which in aqueous solution undergoes an ionic dissociation to form free protons, the chemical properties of these in solution being a function of the hydrogen ion activity $[H^+]$, which is related to the concentration of hydrogen ions by the activity coefficient; this can only be calculated theoretically for solutions of very low concentrations. In practice it appears that the biological properties of acids can all be related to the hydrogen ion activity, and also that it is this activity which is measured by the glass electrode, yielding the pH:

$$pH = \log \frac{1}{[H^+]}.$$

Thus in practice we shall refer only to hydrogen ion activity $[H^+]$ and not to concentration.

The pH scale stretches from 0 to 14, with neutrality, when proton acceptors exactly balance proton donors, at pH 7.0 when $[H^+]$ is 100 nmol/litre. In clinical practice arterial pH values outside the range 6.9–7.7 are very unlikely, and thus the arterial $[H^+]$ range compatible with life is from 126 nmol/litre to 18 nmol/litre, the normal values of arterial plasma pH in health being 7.38 to 7.42, or $[H^+]$ 42 to 38 nmol/litre.

Strong acids, such as hydrochloric or sulphuric acids, are fully dissociated in water, whereas weak acids, such as carbonic acid, acetic acid, and lactic acid, are only partially dissociated, to an extent defined by their dissociation constant (K). Salts of any acid are completely dissociated in solution, so that a solution of a weak acid will contain undissociated molecules [HA], anions from the salt $[B^+]$, acidic cations $[A^-]$ and $[H^+]$, activities of these components fitting the equation:

$$HA \rightleftharpoons H + A; \quad BA \rightarrow B + A;$$

$$\therefore [H^+] = K \frac{[HA]}{[BA]}.$$

Such a solution will resist or buffer a change in $[H^+]$, as an increase in $[H^+]$ will recombine to form undissociated HA. The buffer will be most effective at a range of pH values close to the pK of the acid. The concentration of the buffer salts will also determine the efficiency of the buffer in preventing a change of pH, so that in human plasma the most important physiological buffers are the bicarbonate system:-

$$H_2CO_3 \rightleftharpoons H^+ + HCO_3^-,$$

with a pK of 6.1; and the phosphate system:-

$$H_2PO_4^- \rightleftharpoons H^+ + HPO_4^{--},$$

with a pK of 6.8, along with the carboxyl and amino groups of plasma proteins. However, in whole blood the haemoglobin molecule forms an extremely important buffer, the imidazole groups of the histidine components of the globin chain contributing most of this effect. In addition, the buffering capacity of the haemoglobin molecule depends upon the oxygenation status of the haemoglobin (Bohr effect). The equation:

$$CO_2 \text{ (gas phase)} \rightleftharpoons CO_2 \text{ (in solution)}$$
$$+ H_2O \rightleftharpoons H_2CO_3 \rightleftharpoons H^+ + HCO_3^-$$

carbonic   ionic
anhydrase   dissociation

defines the acid–base status, as these components are all present in plasma, red cells, tissue fluids, CSF, and urine, and intracellularly. As the $[H^+]$ generated or lost in this equation is interchangeable with the $[H^+]$ in any other buffer system (the isohydric principle), a description of acid–base status based on this bicarbonate buffer system will also describe changes in $[H^+]$ which result from any other buffer system within that particular body compartment.

Application of the law of mass action to the dissociation of carbonic acid [13] yields:-

$$[H^+] = K_1'' \frac{S.PCO_2}{(HCO_3^-)}.$$

For human plasma at 38°C, $K_1'' = 7.94 \times 10^{-7}$, S (the solubility of CO_2 in plasma) being 0.03 mmol.litre^{-1}.mmHg^{-1}. In logarithmic notation this equation yields the Henderson–Hasselbalch equation for bicarbonic acid:-

$$pH = pK_1'' + \log \frac{(HCO_3^-)}{S.PCO_2}.$$

Changes which primarily affect the PCO_2 component of this equation are defined as respiratory acid–base disturbances, and those in which the HCO_3^- component (non-respiratory component) is primarily affected are defined as metabolic acid–base disturbances.

Clearly definition of any two components of this three-part system means that there can only be one unique value of the third. Terms used to describe the non-respiratory component are varied, the base excess being defined as the base required to titrate a blood sample to pH 7.40 at a PCO_2 of 40 mmHg (5.3 kPa) at 38°C [23]. Base excess has now replaced the older term standard bicarbonate, which was defined as the bicarbonate concentration of whole blood when this had been equilibrated with a gas phase of PCO_2 40 mmHg (5.3 kPa) at 38°C. The non-respira-

tory pH is an alternative way of expressing the same idea, this being the pH of a whole blood sample at a PCO_2 of 40 mmHg (5.3 kPa), again at body temperature. The old term buffer base was defined as the sum of the buffer salts which were capable of neutralizing strong acid in a biological solution, which in blood is the sum of the concentrations of bicarbonate and proteinate.

All the above measurements are independent of the PCO_2, and thus imply that this non-respiratory component will not change as the PCO_2 rises in the blood in life, within the body. In practice this is not true, as the extravascular fluids of the body are less well buffered than the blood, for they contain no red cells and thus no haemoglobin, but as the PCO_2 of body tissues rise hydrogen ions pass from the extravascular tissues into the blood. However, this cannot occur if CO_2 is added to the blood in vitro in a test tube, so that in this circumstance the non-respiratory measurements (base excess, standard bicarbonate, buffer base, non-respiratory pH) do remain constant. Nonetheless, this does not reflect the position which occurs in the body in vivo [2].

The equation derived by Henderson [13] can be used as a simple linear plot of $[H^+]$ against PCO_2. In one such a diagram (Fig. 6.1) lines of equal bicarbonate concentration radiate as a fan from the origin. Use of this linear notation (without the logarithmic pH scale) has some educational and conceptual advantages, at least for clinicians who are not experts in chemistry. Thus intuitively one expects more of a substance to be related to a larger numerical value,

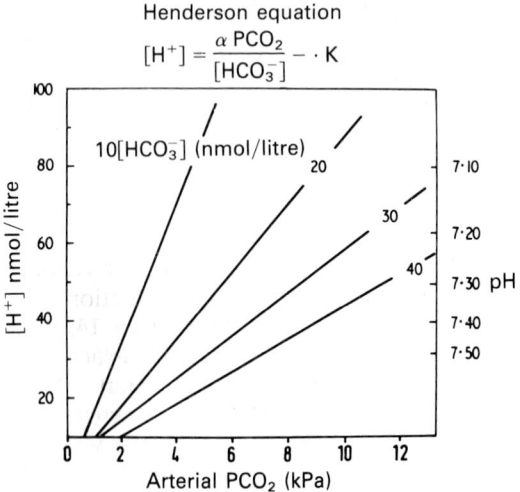

Henderson equation

$$[H^+] = \frac{\alpha PCO_2}{[HCO_3^-]} - \cdot K$$

Fig. 6.1. The Henderson (1908 [13]) equation, in the linear scales of $[H^+]$ plotted against PCO_2, with lines of equal bicarbonate concentration radiating from the origin, below the baseline.

not, as in the pH notation, to a smaller value, which gets smaller as a negative logarithm. On such a diagram one can plot the relationship between the $[H^+]$ or (pH) of the arterial blood in vivo against the PCO_2 of such a sample. When this is done in normal healthy subjects the normal range of these two variables is indicated by the shaded rectangle (Fig. 6.2). If such a normal healthy subject inspires gas with an increased CO_2 concentration in short-term experiment, his arterial PCO_2 will rise, and this is associated with a rise in $[H^+]$. The 95% confidence limits of this acute respiratory acidosis, as seen in the whole arterial blood in vivo, are defined by the band marked 'acute respiratory acidosis' in Fig. 6.2 [7].

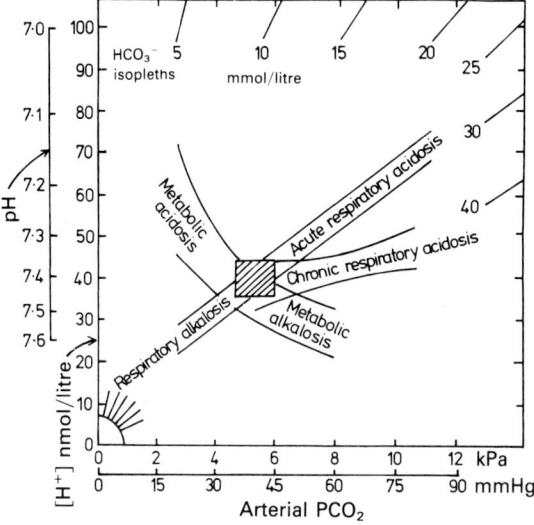

Fig. 6.2. The acid–base diagram, in $[H^+]$ PCO_2 plot, derived from Fig. 6.1, with significance bands of single disturbances as observed in human whole blood in vivo, the *shaded rectangle* ( ) defining the normal range. Flenley 1971 and 1978 [7, 8]. Reproduced, with permission, from the *British Journal of Hospital Medicine* and *The Lancet*.

If, however, this increased PCO_2 is maintained for some hours or days, an experiment which has never been carried out in man but has been attempted in dogs (who have similar mechanisms controlling their acid–base balance), it is empirically observed that the arterial $[H^+]$ is lower at any given level of PCO_2. This must be accompanied by an increase in plasma bicarbonate, as the physicochemical constraints require, and this is of course found in practice. Again, the observed empirical relationships between PCO_2 and $[H^+]$ in the arterial blood in vivo, in man, during such sustained chronic

hypercapnia resulting from disease are indicated by the 95% confidence limits (indicated in the chronic respiratory acidosis band in Fig. 6.2).

If a normal subject is asked to hyperventilate acutely, or, alternatively, moves to reside at high altitudes where hypoxia drives his ventilation, he will develop a relationship between arterial PCO_2 and $[H^+]$ like that indicated in the lower left-hand quadrant of Fig. 6.2, the acute respiratory alkalosis band. In practice it appears that data recorded in chronic respiratory alkalosis (as in people living at high altitudes) or in persistent hyperventilation lie in a relationship very similar to that in acute respiratory alkalosis. It is thus to be emphasized that primary disturbances in PCO_2, with either a lowering (hyperventilation) or an elevation (hypoventilation), indicating respiratory acid–base disturbances, lie in an oblique band across such diagrams from lower left to upper right.

In contrast, in a primary metabolic acidosis, where the initial abnormality in acid–base balance arises from excess of $[H^+]$, there is clearly an increase in the plasma $[H^+]$ activity (fall in pH). In man, in vivo, this is associated with an increase in ventilation as a result of acidic stimulation of the respiratory centres, although the PCO_2 falls. Again, the empirically observed relationships between PCO_2 and $[H^+]$ in the arterial blood in vivo in man during primary metabolic acidosis are shown as the 95% confidence limits, the curved band radiating slightly upwards and to the left from the rectangle of normal values in Fig. 6.2.

In primary metabolic alkalosis arterial $[H^+]$ is reduced (pH increased). In many subjects there is a tendency for the PCO_2 to rise a little. Thus relationships between $[H^+]$ and PCO_2, again in the arterial blood in vivo, lie within the 95% confidence limits shown in the lower right-hand part of Fig. 6.2. It is thus apparent that metabolic acid–base disturbances lie in a band more or less at right angles to that of respiratory acid–base disturbances, running from lower right to upper left in Fig. 6.2. All these significance bands are based upon actual measurements of human arterial blood in vivo during a single primary disturbance of acid–base balance, in the directions instanced.

Respiratory failure

Respiratory failure is conventionally defined as being present in a patient who, when at rest breathing air at sea level, has an arterial PO_2 lower than 60 mmHg (8.0 kPa) [3]. If this hypoxaemia is associated with a low or normal PCO_2 (below 50 mmHg; 6.6 kPa) it is referred to as type I respiratory failure; if, however, hypoxaemia is associated with CO_2 retention (PCO_2 above 50 mmHg; 6.6 kPa) this is defined as type II respiratory failure.

Type I

The commonest cause of hypoxaemia with a low or normal PCO_2 is maldistribution of ventilation ($\dot{V}$) to perfusion ($\dot{Q}$) in the lungs, so that some perfused alveoli receive a smaller amount of ventilation than normal ($\dot{V}/\dot{Q}$ ratio <0.8), thus tending to add poorly oxygenated blood to the arterial circulation, whereas in other areas well-ventilated alveoli receive a relatively inadequate perfusion. Such areas of high $\dot{V}/\dot{Q}$ ratio fail to correct the hypoxaemia in the arterial blood which results from low $\dot{V}/\dot{Q}$ ratios, although they do restore a normal PCO_2 level. This discrepancy between the PO_2 and PCO_2 in arterial blood results from the relative shape of their dissociation curves (Fig. 6.3). In practice such $\dot{V}/\dot{Q}$ imbalance is very common, often arising in pneumonia, acute pulmonary oedema, pulmonary thrombo-embolism, and bronchial asthma, and in many patients with chronic

bronchitis and emphysema which has not progressed to cor pulmonale [6]. Although it is tempting to attribute the low PCO_2 so often associated with the hypoxaemia in these conditions to hyperventilation resulting from hypoxic stimulation of peripheral chemoreceptors, two lines of evidence argue against such a mechanism. The first is recognition of the fact that correction of such hypoxaemia by oxygen therapy rarely restores PCO_2 values to normal; the second derives from the observation that in normal subjects made hypoxaemic to a similar degree, PCO_2 does not fall to the extent seen in disease, and indeed the hypoxic drive to breathing rarely becomes prominent in normal man unless the arterial PO_2 is reduced well below 60 mmHg (8.0 kPa).

Hypoxaemia without CO_2 retention (type I respiratory failure) is also common in patients with a right-to-left shunt, as in cyanotic congenital heart disease, or in the rare patients with arteriovenous anastamoses within the lungs. The alveolar capillary block syndrome, a term coined to indicate hypoxaemia with a low PCO_2, associated with a low transfer factor for carbon monoxide, shrunken and stiff lungs, was originally thought to result from thickening of the alveolar capillary membrane. This was thought to arise in such diseases as fibrosing alveolitis, widespread sarcoidosis, asbestosis, and other forms of pulmonary fibrosis, but it is now known that it usually results from mismatching of $\dot{V}/\dot{Q}$ ratios. The definition of respiratory failure excludes hypoxaemia due to a low inspired O_2 tension, such as that resulting from low O_2 concentrations at sea level, or to breathing air at a high altitude. In this context it is worth recalling that cabin pressure in commercial aircraft usually varies between 5000 and 8000 ft., when the inspired O_2 tension may be as low as 100 mmHg (13.3 kPa), as against the 150 mmHg (20 kPa) when air is breathed at sea level.

The treatment of type I respiratory failure is easy, for it consists of merely increasing the inspired O_2 concentration by giving the patient O_2 either by mask or by nasal prongs; even modest enrichment of the inspired O_2 concentration will raise the arterial O_2 tension towards normal values in patients with $\dot{V}/\dot{Q}$ imbalance. In a patient in whom a substantial fraction of the cardiac output is passing from the right to the left heart without exposure to ventilated alveoli (e.g., cyanotic congenital heart disease, or the profound intrapulmonary shunts of the adult respiratory distress syndrome), an increase in arterial O_2 tension is not readily obtained even

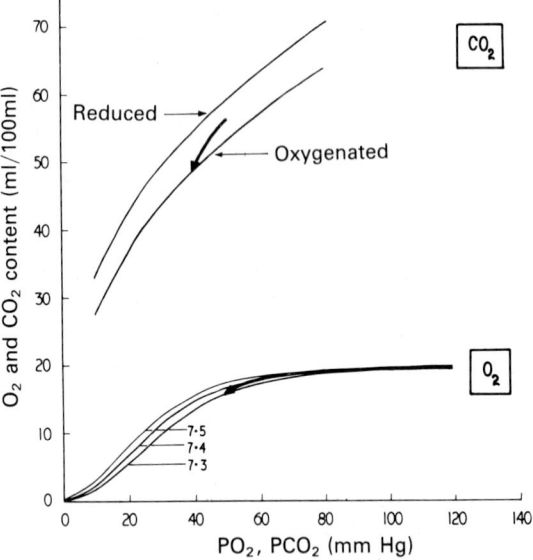

Fig. 6.3. O_2 and CO_2 dissociation curves of human blood, relating O_2 and CO_2 content (ml/100 ml) to PO_2 and PCO_2 (mmHg). Note the relatively linear slope of the CO_2 dissociation curve in the physiological range, contrasting with the markedly sigmoid shape of the O_2 curve over this range.

when high concentrations of inspired O_2 are breathed. This observation is the diagnostic hallmark of the presence of a right-to-left shunt as the cause of hypoxaemia. In patients with type I respiratory failure there is usually very little risk of provoking serious CO_2 retention by administration of high concentrations of O_2.

Type II

When CO_2 retention is combined with hypoxia it is clear that overall alveolar ventilation is depressed in relation to the metabolic demands of the patient for CO_2 excretion. By far the commonest cause of type II respiratory failure is an acute exacerbation of chronic bronchitis and emphysema, which most usually results from infection with *Haemophilus influenza* and *Streptococcus pneumoniae*, and can also arise from a drug overdosage with sedatives or from fractured ribs, or pneumothorax, in a patient with pre-existing chronic bronchitis and emphysema. In a patient with normal lungs, type II respiratory failure is rare, even in quite severe narcotic drug overdosage. Type II respiratory failure may also complicate the respiratory problems of patients with disorders of the chest wall arising either from abnormalities of the skeleton, as in scoliosis or ankylosing spondylitis, or as a late result of thoracoplasty; and in these conditions cough is usually preserved. In neuromuscular diseases involving the respiratory system, however (poliomyelitis, amyotrophic lateral sclerosis, muscular dystrophy, spinal cord injury, multiple sclerosis, myasthenia gravis, and peripheral neuropathy), muscular weakness usually impairs the cough reflex, so that recurrent aspiration pneumonia is a major problem.

Obese people are often also hypoxaemic, usually with type I respiratory failure with a relatively normal PCO_2, the hypoxaemia resulting from poor ventilation to perfused alveoli at the bases of the lungs. In contrast, some obese patients have the obesity hypoventilation syndrome (Pickwickian syndrome), with day-time somnolence in association with obstructive sleep apnoea, and in these patients hypoventilation causes hypoxaemia with CO_2 retention (type II respiratory failure) even when they are awake by day [11].

It has recently been recognized that failure of respiratory muscles may be a common but rarely recognized underlying problem in an acute exacerbation of chronic bronchitis and emphysema, as well as in other types of type II respiratory failure [5].

The treatment of type II respiratory failure depends on avoiding the dangers of severe CO_2 retention with the concomitant respiratory acidosis. In a recent retrospective analysis of 157 admissions of 135 patients suffering from an acute exacerbation of chronic bronchitis and emphysema causing hypoxaemia and CO_2 retention [28], the mainstay of treatment was controlled O_2 therapy. This aims to relieve hypoxaemia, yet without removing sufficient respiratory drive from hypoxia to cause a further exacerbation of CO_2 retention with worsening of respiratory acidosis. These patients had severe hypoxaemia when breathing air on admission to hospital (PO_2 23–50 mmHg; 3.1–6.6 kPa), and by definition had values of PCO_2 above 50 mmHg (6.6 kPa), ranging up to 97 mmHg (12.9 kPa). Acidosis was present in many patients, with $[H^+]$ values varying from 34 to 72 nmol/litre. Most patients had $[H^+]/PCO_2$ relationships within the chronic respiratory acidosis band on the acid–base diagram, but in a later series a considerable proportion tended to have an acute respiratory acidosis when breathing air on admission to hospital (Fig. 6.4).

During controlled O_2 therapy, which aimed to bring the arterial O_2 tension to over 50 mmHg (6.6 kPa) and in which the arterial PO_2 was never higher than 110 mmHg (14.6 kPa), the PCO_2 rose in most patients, with a concomitant rise in $[H^+]$. Analysis of the H^+/PCO_2 relationships at the time of the highest value of arterial $[H^+]$ during controlled O_2 therapy showed that death during an exacerbation was more likely if this $[H^+]$ value rose above 56 nmol/litre than in those cases where the arterial $[H^+]$ could be maintained below this level. The whole aim of controlled O_2 therapy in these patients is to steer between these twin dangers of severe hypoxaemia and severe respiratory acidosis. This study suggests that the empirical limits of obtaining a PO_2 above 50 mmHg (6.6 kPa) yet without causing $[H^+]$ in the arterial blood to rise above 56 nmol/litre may allow these aims to be successfully achieved. However, it should be recalled that the prognosis in these patients remains grave, and even following discharge from hospital only 30% or less of the patients survived for more than 6 years.

If these proposed limits of arterial blood gas tensions cannot be attained by controlled O_2 therapy alone, involving administration of the O_2 by nasal prongs at a flow rate of 1–3 litres/min, either respiratory stimulants or mechanical ventilation (MV) must be employed.

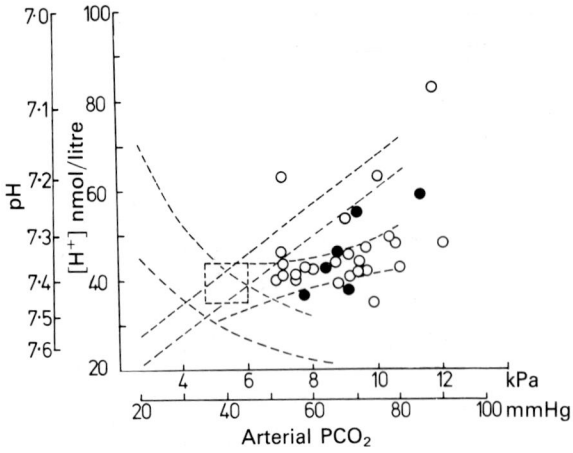

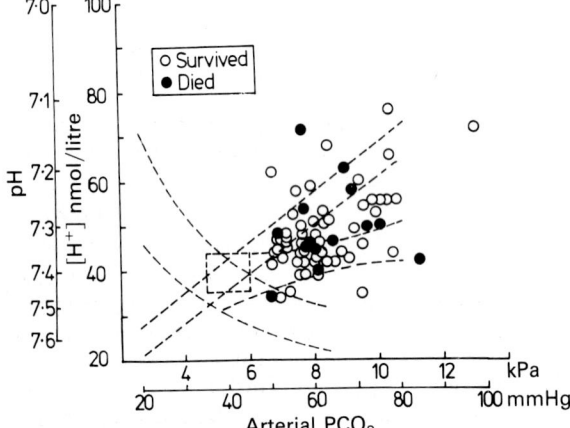

Fig. 6.4. Acid–base plots ($[H^+]/PCO_2$) in patients suffering from an acute exacerbation of type II respiratory failure, recorded while patients were breathing air on admission to hospital in the period 1961–1968 (above) or 1970–1976 (below). The patients in the later series more often had acute respiratory acidosis (values in *upper LH band*) and more of them died (*closed circles*).

The most potent respiratory stimulant at present available is doxapram, given by continuous IV infusion. Although this drug has many side-effects, including tachycardia, increased cardiac output, and tremor, it has been successful in lowering arterial PCO_2 and thus improving respiratory acidosis in many such patients during the critical period, so allowing control of the factors causing the acute exacerbation of their chronic respiratory failure [17]. MV is not often necessary in treating these patients in Britain, for controlled O_2 therapy, with or without respiratory stimulants such as doxapram, will suffice in most. There is also often some reluctance to use MV in these relatively elderly patients, who are suffering from a recurrent condition in which, even following correction of the acute excerbation, the long-term prognosis is extremely grave.

Bronchial asthma

Hypoxaemia is common in an acute attack of bronchial asthma, and is often poorly recognized due to the relative vasoconstriction which may result from the associated hypocapnia. This low PCO_2 results from alveolar hyperventilation, which may seem curious in a condition associated with an increased work of breathing, with severe airways obstruction. The mechanisms leading to this hyperventilation are not fully established, but it seems probable that they involve stimulation of irritant or other vagally innervated receptors in the lungs. In a typical attack a low PCO_2 is combined with hypoxaemia and respiratory alkalosis (Fig. 6.5). However, in the rare very severe case, the PCO_2 may rise due to alveolar hypoventilation, associated of course with respiratory acidosis. Early recognition of this complication of superimposed type II respiratory failure is very important in the asthmatic, for this is an acute respiratory acidosis and usually indicates a very serious outlook unless recognized and corrected early. This is in contrast with a similar level of PCO_2 in the chronic bronchitic, where as indicated above, CO_2 retention is usually chronic and an acute exacerbation merely causes a further rise in PCO_2 with an acute-on-chronic respiratory acidosis.

Clinical signs of CO_2 retention are highly variable, and the well-known triad of distended forearm veins, a rapid bounding pulse, and a coarse tremor of the outstretched hands correlates poorly with the actual level of PCO_2. In the asthmatic developing CO_2 retention this may be associated with an undue severity of acidosis, with $[H^+]/PCO_2$ values lying above the acute respiratory band. This 'extra' acid, over and above that due to the CO_2 retention itself, usually indicates a concomitant type A lactic acidosis due to a combination of arterial hypoxaemia with the low cardiac output which is so grave a feature of severe bronchial asthma. Reliance on controlled O_2 therapy alone in these cases is inappropriate, and large doses of bronchodilators, administered by positive pressure breathing (IPPB), combined with IV theophyllines and hydrocortisone are urgently required. If these measures do not prevent the PCO_2 from rising further endotracheal intubation and MV are urgently needed.

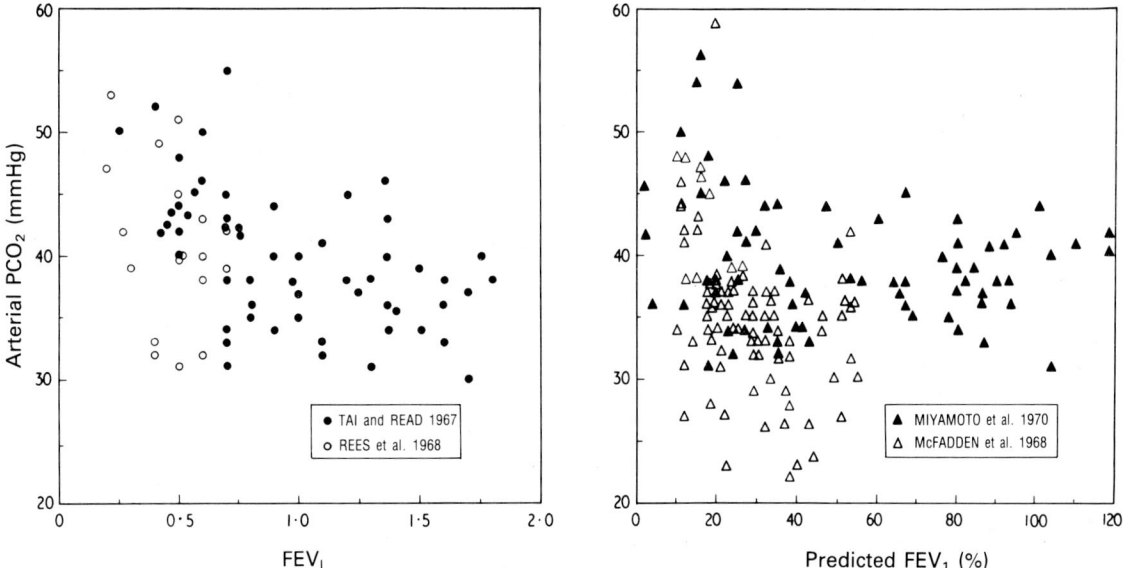

Fig. 6.5. Relationships between arterial PCO_2 and $FEV_{1.0}$ (absolute, *LH panel*, or as percentage of predicted normal value, *RH panel*) in patients with acute bronchial asthma. Note that as the $FEV_{1.0}$ falls with increasing severity of airways obstruction the PCO_2 tends to be lower, only rising in very severe attacks [15, 19, 20, 25].

Pulmonary oedema

Acute cardiogenic pulmonary oedema, like bronchial asthma, is also usually associated with hypoxaemia when breathing air, combined with alveolar hyperventilation resulting in a low PCO_2 in the arterial blood, with respiratory alkalosis. Also as in bronchial asthma, however, CO_2 retention may occur in pulmonary oedema and this may be associated with a greater rise in arterial $[H^+]$ than would be expected on the basis of acute CO_2 retention alone (Fig. 6.6). Once again a combination of type A lactic acidosis, due to hypoxaemia with a low cardiac output, is responsible for this extra acidity. As in bronchial asthma, when there is CO_2 retention MV may be urgently required, combined with infusion of bicarbonate to correct this additional metabolic component of the acid–base disturbance.

The clinical clue to CO_2 retention in acute pulmonary oedema can be clouding of consciousness, which is a very unusual feature in such patients, who are usually desperately breathless due to their acute pulmonary oedema. This combination of CO_2 retention with clouding of consciousness is characteristic of heroin-induced pulmonary oedema in drug abusers, and the clue again may be widespread pulmonary oedema, detected clinically and on the chest radiograph, coupled with pin-point pupils and impairment of conscious level. In other non-cardiogenic causes of pulmonary oedema (as in the adult respiratory distress syndrome) CO_2 retention and respiratory acidosis are usually not prominent, whereas hypoxaemia resistant to complete correction by administration of high concentrations of inspired O_2, is the characteristic feature [18, 24].

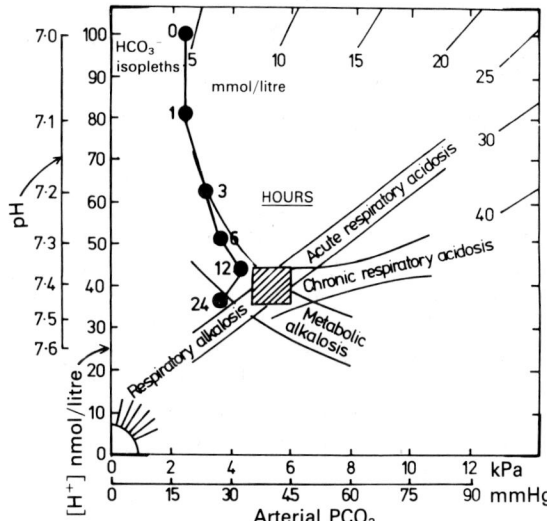

Fig. 6.6. Acid–base diagram ($[H^+]/PCO_2$ plot of sequential values at 0.2 and 4 h and on discharge $[D]$) in a patient with acute pulmonary oedema, with clouding of consciousness and CO_2 retention. Flenley 1978 [8]. Redrawn, with permission, from *British Journal of Hospital Medicine*.

Salicylate poisoning

In children salicylate poisoning causes an early transient respiratory alkalosis, reflecting the powerful ventilatory stimulant action of salicylate on the central nervous system (CNS). This is later complicated by a metabolic acidosis caused by the action of salicylate in uncoupling mitochondrial oxidative phosphorylation, with a resultant failure to generate ATP molecules, despite an active O_2 uptake. In the adult, however, controversy has surrounded the findings in acid–base disturbance following salicylate ingestion, some observers noting only metabolic acidosis, whereas others have claimed that respiratory alkalosis is virtually the only acid–base disorder. Recently Gabow et al. [10] have analysed their observations in 67 adult patients aged 16–77 years. One-third of their patients had also ingested another drug as well as the salicylate, and these other drugs usually included CNS depressants, which therefore formed an important component of the pattern of acid–base disturbance. Only 22% of their patients had simple respiratory alkalosis, whereas respiratory alkalosis with metabolic acidosis was found in over 50%, but there was no relationship between the initial salicylate level and the initial PCO_2 (Fig. 6.7). It should be noted, however, that in many of these patients PCO_2 values were very low, particularly in those who had only taken salicylate. The metabolic acidosis complicating salicylate intoxication was usually associated with ingestion of CNS-depressant drugs, but many

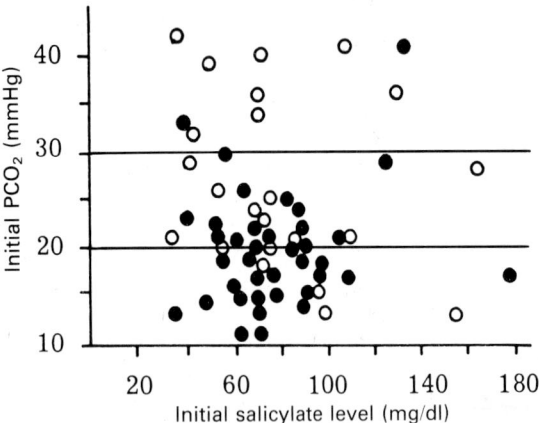

Fig. 6.7. Arterial PCO_2 and plasma salicylate level in adult patients with salicylate poisoning, with (●) and without (○) additional drugs. Note the low level of PCO_2 attained in many patients. Gabow et al. 1978 [10]. Reproduced, with permission, from *Archives of Internal Medicine*.

of the patients in this study had both a high anion gap (see section: Lactic acidosis) and ketonaemia, as well as increased lactic acid production.

Renal regulation of acid–base balance

A healthy adult eating a normal diet will require to excrete 40–80 mmol of $[H^+]$ in each 24 h. The ultrafiltrate of plasma which is formed in the renal glomerulus contains bicarbonate in a concentration equal to that of plasma, but 80%–90% of this bicarbonate is normally reabsorbed in the proximal renal tubule, as $NaHCO_3$, exchanging sodium for hydrogen, which is then excreted as water. Hydrogen ion $[H^+]$ is generated by the carbonic anhydrase present in the proximal tubular cell, the bicarbonate ion (HCO_3^-) then being reabsorbed into the peritubular blood, further bicarbonate reabsorption in the distal renal tubules reducing the urinary pH to about 6.0. Values of urinary pH lower than this mean that net acid excretion is occurring, particularly in the renal tubule segments distal to the ascending limb of Henle's loop. Net renal hydrogen ion excretion is thus measured by the sum of titratable acid (TA) excretion plus ammonium excretion (NH_4^+) minus bicarbonate excretion (HCO_3^-):

$$\text{Net acid excretion} = TA + (NH_4^+) - (HCO_3^-).$$

The major mechanisms controlling renal $[H^+]$ excretion thus consist of the absorption of bicarbonate, excretion of titratable acid, and excretion of ammonium [21].

Reabsorption of bicarbonate

The extracellular fluid volume is a major factor controlling bicarbonate reabsorption, so that when the extracellular volume is expanded (as in congestive heart failure, nephrotic syndrome, or following excess IV fluids, etc.) sodium reabsorption is inhibited, which then depresses bicarbonate reabsorption. Conversely, shrinkage of the extracellular space increases both sodium and bicarbonate reabsorption. In an extensive review of their experimental studies of renal acid–base balance, Schwartz and Cohen [22] conclude that the arterial $[H^+]$ is not a major determinant of the rate of acid excretion by the kidney, but that this depends largely upon the delivery of sodium to the distal tubular site, where it is exchanged for [H⁺]. If the extracellular fluid volume is contracted, the distal tubular cells will be stimulated to conserve sodium, and thus increase the excretion of hydrogen ion in the urine.

Other factors leading to an increase in bicarbonate reabsorption include potassium depletion, hypercapnia (as in chronic respiratory failure), hypoparathyroidism, and the hypercalcaemia of vitamin D overdosage. Nonetheless, extracellular fluid volume contraction is a major stimulus to increased bicarbonate reabsorption and so can completely overshadow these other effects, such as potassium loading.

Aldosterone plays an important role in the regulation of acid–base balance by the kidney, acting particularly on the collecting duct. Acid excretion increases in response to an excess of aldosterone, with resultant metabolic alkalosis, whereas deficiency of aldosterone is associated with metabolic acidosis.

Titratable acidity

Titratable acidity refers to the [H⁺] present in the urine as buffers, particularly as components of the phosphate buffer system (pK 6.8), creatinine and uric acid, but these last two only constitute a small proportion of the total titratable acid excreted. The lower the urinary pH the greater the amount of titratable acid present. However, in metabolic acidosis which does not result from a renal cause urinary pH is low, with an increase in titratable acid, but this increase is limited by the amount of buffer that can be excreted, as well as by the pK of that buffer.

Ammonium

Ammonia (NH₃) is formed in the distal tubular cells by complex chemical mechanisms, including the splitting of glutamine to form glutamate and ammonia. Ammonia is a small, noncharged molecule, which diffuses easily throughout the kidney and thus into the tubular fluid. In the acid urine of the distal tubular fluid, however:

$$NH_3 + [H^+] \rightleftharpoons NH_4^+$$

so that the ammonium ion NH_4^+ becomes trapped in the tubular fluid, as this epithelium does not allow the passage of a charged species, a process known as diffusion trapping. Chronic metabolic acidosis stimulates glutamine utilization, and thus increases NH₃ excretion [12].

It will be apparent from the above that metabolic acidosis which does not result from kidney disease will be associated with a low renal pH, increased NH₃ excretion, and high titratable acidity. Clearly, if the urinary pH is inappropriately high for the degree of arterial [H⁺] this must indicate that the metabolic acidosis is a result, in part at least, of a renal disorder.

Metabolic alkalosis

Metabolic alkalosis is a primary pathophysiological state associated with a gain in bicarbonate, or loss of non-volatile acid from the extracellular fluid. Extracellular fluid volume contraction and potassium depletion are both important physiological stimulants to metabolic alkalosis, and the importance of delivery of sodium to the distal tubular site, where it can be exchanged for [H⁺] in the tubular fluid, has been discussed above. The most frequently encountered causes of metabolic alkalosis include an excess loss of gastric fluid (as in vomiting), particularly in patients with hyperacidity and pyloric obstruction; and diuretic therapy, where potassium depletion and aldosterone excess combine with a shrunken extracellular fluid volume to cause the alkalosis. Less frequent causes include primary aldosteronism, the adrenogenital syndrome, renal artery stenosis, intrarenal vascular disease, and malignant hypertension, in all of which there may be increased production of mineralocorticoids.

Gastric juice normally contains sodium (10–30 mmol/litre) and potassium (5–40 mmol/litre), along with [H⁺] (65–150 mmol/litre) in a total volume of 400–5000 ml in 24 h. Thus in protracted vomiting, or following therapeutic aspiration of gastric contents, the plasma bicarbonate concentration is high and that of [H⁺] low, whereas urinary sodium chloride and bicarbonate are all low. Sodium bicarbonate is lost in the urine in large amounts early on in the vomiting, and the correction of gastric alkalosis depends upon the replacement of salt and water, and of the potassium deficit (which may be largely from intracellular sources), particularly in prolonged vomiting.

Excessive mineralocorticoid activity is also associated with metabolic alkalosis, as in Cushing's syndrome, adrenal adenoma, malignant hypertension, and the adrenogenital syndrome. However, in practice this type of metabolic alkalosis most commonly results from therapeutic administration of synthetic mineralocorticoids (fludrocortisone, DOCA, prednisolone, triamcinolone, etc.). All result to a greater or lesser degree in increased sodium re-absorption in the distal nephron, the increased extracellular volume depressing proximal sodium reabsorption, so that the increased distal delivery of sodium allows exchange for potassium and [H$^+$] at this site, these two ions (K$^+$ and [H$^+$]) thus being excreted.

In chronic hypercapnia the elevated PCO_2 results in an increased reabsorption of bicarbonate, as shown by the difference between the significance bands for the acute and chronic [H$^+$]/PCO_2 relationships in respiratory acidosis. If, however, the PCO_2 is rapidly returned to normal (e.g., by institution of a high level of ventilation by IPPV) the raised level of bicarbonate will persist, as bicarbonate excretion is slow, so that an alkalosis will develop at first. If such patients are treated with diuretics, however, bicarbonate reabsorption will remain high following the return of PCO_2 to normal, so that the post-hypercapnic metabolic alkalosis persists. The metabolic alkalosis following diuretic therapy is initially due to an increased acid excretion, associated with potassium depletion and secondary hyperaldosteronism, and is maintained by shrinkage of the extracellular fluid volume and by potassium depletion.

Severe metabolic alkalosis may be life-threatening, as the associated hypokalaemia may combine with the alkalosis to depress cardiac function. An arterial [H$^+$] below 30 mmol/litre (pH 7.52) is very uncommon, and even in these circumstances the arterial PCO_2 is still usually normal [26]. If alkalosis persists in spite of restoration of the extracellular fluid to normal, along with correction of potassium deficiency, the carbonic anhydrase inhibitor acetazolamide may be used to restore a normal acid–base balance. In cases where this has failed IV infusion of hydrochloric acid has been employed (Fig. 6.8) [30].

Metabolic acidosis

Metabolic acidosis is a pathophysiological state characterized by a gain of strong acid or a loss of bicarbonate from the extracellular fluid. Metabolic acidosis resulting from a loss of base is associated with a normal anion gap, whereas if the acidosis is due to a gain of acid there is an increase in the anion gap (see section: *Lactic acidosis*). Diabetic keto-acidosis is probably the commonest form of severe metabolic acidosis,

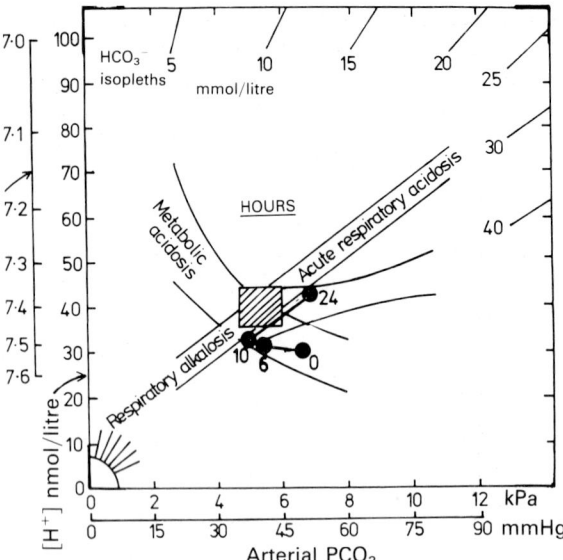

Fig. 6.8. Acid–base diagram ([H$^+$]/PCO_2 plot) in a 69-year-old man who developed severe metabolic alkalosis with ileus following resection of an aortic aneurysm, treated by infusion of HCl IV, values being shown of arterial [H$^+$] + PCO_2 at 0, 6, 10, and 24 h after infusion. Flenley 1978 [8]. Redrawn, with permission, from *British Journal of Hospital Medicine*.

but this may also result from chronic renal failure, and in both cases there will be a net gain in acid. Metabolic acidosis from loss of bicarbonate arises as a consequence of gastro-intestinal (GI) losses, e.g., in diarrhoea; following aspiration of pancreatic, biliary, or intestinal secretions; after ureterosigmoidostomy; and rarely following ingestion of calcium chloride, cholestyramine, or magnesium sulphate.

Renal causes of metabolic acidosis from bicarbonate loss include renal tubular acidosis, of either proximal or distal types. In the ammonium chloride loading test, which is used to confirm the diagnosis of renal tubular acidosis, ammonium chloride is given in capsules by mouth in a dose of 0.1 g/kg/day for 3 days, which should result in the urinary pH falling below 5.5 as a normal response. In the single-dose test [31] a single dose of ammonium chloride is given PO in a dose of 0.1 g/kg over 1 h, and the urinary pH should be below 5.5 some time between 2 and 8 h later. In the classic form of distal renal tubular acidosis, which may result either from drug toxicity or from systemic disease, the metabolic acidosis is associated with hypocalcaemia.

In renal acidosis from chronic renal failure, the glomerular filtration rate is usually less than 25% of normal, and in this form of metabolic acidosis the anion gap is increased. Although NH_3 excretion of each functional nephron is probably higher than normal, the acidosis results from overall failure of NH_3 excretion, due to reduction in the number of functional nephrons. Metabolic acidosis with a normal anion gap is a rare finding in renal failure, this form of hyperchloraemic acidosis being found in patients with either interstitial nephritis or salt-losing nephritis, and reduction in extracellular fluid volume appears to be invariable when this type of metabolic acidosis complicates renal failure.

Respiratory compensation

An increase in arterial $[H^+]$ stimulates ventilation, principally by acting directly on the respiratory centre, but may also potentiate any peripheral chemoreceptor drive from hypoxaemia, acting through the carotid bodies. The resultant hyperventilation lowers arterial PCO_2, and thus tends to reduce the arterial $[H^+]$, so serving as a compensatory mechanism. The limits of this compensation are clearly defined in man, and can be shown as the metabolic acidosis band on the $[H^+]/PCO_2$ plot (Fig. 6.9). It is clear that this band of the diagram crosses the bicarbonate isopleths almost at right angles. Thus if there is a clear clinical diagnosis of uncomplicated metabolic acidosis, as for example in diabetic ketoacidosis, the severity of the acidosis can be fairly precisely estimated by

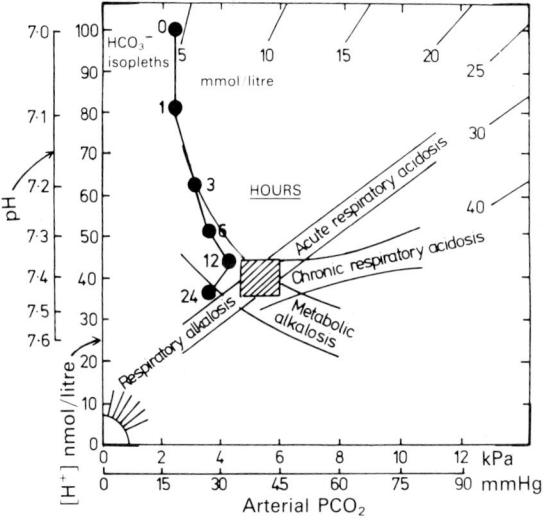

Fig. 6.9. Acid–base diagram ($[H^+]/PCO_2$ plot) showing sequential hourly values of arterial $[H^+]$ and PCO_2 in a 17-year-old girl with diabetic ketoacidosis, treated by insulin and IV NaCl. Note the changes across the bicarbonate bands on the diagram. Flenley 1978 [8]. Redrawn, with permission, from *British Journal of Hospital Medicine*.

measurement of the plasma bicarbonate level alone, for this will allow the probable arterial $[H^+]$ and PCO_2 values to be inferred from the intersection of that bicarbonate isopleth with the metabolic acidosis band on the $[H^+]/PCO_2$ plot. In contrast, in primary respiratory acid–base disturbances the plasma bicarbonate alone will give a very poor guide to the severity, or indeed the type of the acidosis, as the bicarbonate isopleths run more or less parallel to the bands of both acute respiratory acidosis and respiratory alkalosis on the $[H^+]/PCO_2$ plot.

Lactic acidosis

Metabolic acidosis associated with a high blood lactic level is defined as lactic acidosis. Lactic acid has a pK of 3.79 at 25°C, and is thus a relatively strong acid. Cohen and Woods [4] describe two types of lactic acidosis:-

Type A, which results from poor tissue perfusion as in shock and severe cardiac failure; and

Type B, which is due to diabetes, renal or liver failure, infections, toxic reactions to drugs and poisons (notably phenformin), and rare hereditary disorders such as glucose-6-phosphate deficiency.

In type A lactic acidosis the clinical picture is dominated by the causative shock state with hypotension, a pale clammy skin, and central cyanosis, associated with a hyperventilation from the acidic drive to breathing. Type B lactic acidosis usually develops rapidly over a few hours in patients who have received a drug (e.g., phenformin or a toxin which is known to cause the condition) and is heralded by hyperventilation, but may progress to drowsiness, vomiting, and eventually to coma. An increased anion gap, which is the biochemical clue to the probability of lactic acidosis, is only an apparent phenomenon, as clearly the anions in the plasma must be electrically balanced by the sum of the cations. Metabolic acidosis with a high anion gap can be due to renal failure; ketoacidosis; lactic acidosis (due to drugs and toxins such as phenformin directly causing lactic acidosis); or toluene, methanol, salicylate, paraldehyde, or ethylene-glycol, following poisoning from ingestion of anti-freeze [14].

In 114 patients hospitalized at the Bronx Municipal Hospital Center with chemically proven lactic acidosis or ketoacidosis [9] the highest values of serum lactate (18.3 ± 1.8 mmol/litre) were found in lactic acidosis due to phenformin, and in this group the mean blood pH was also very low at 6.79 ± 0.05, whereas in lactic acidosis not associated with phenformin the mean lactate levels were somewhat lower at 12.8 mmol/litre, with a pH on average of 7.17 ± 0.04. In diabetic ketoacidosis, although the mean pH in this group was 7.17 ± 0.02, the lactate level was only just above the normal range at 2.1 ± 0.1 mmol/litre, most of the acidosis arising from the dehydroxybrutrate, in a mean concentration of 10.8 ± 0.6 mmol/litre. In type A lactic acidosis, as for example in acute pulmonary oedema, the blood pH was much less depressed, at 7.29 ± 0.03, although the lactate levels were at least three times normal at 6.2 ± 1.3 mmol/litre.

It is clear that a rise in blood lactate must result from either an increase in the production or a failure of removal of the lactate; but the relative role of these two mechanisms in clinical lactic acidosis is not always clear. Lactate can be produced from skeletal muscle, erythrocytes, brain, and skin. In severe hypoxia the liver may produce, rather than consume, lactate, and this may also occur following fructose infusion. Lactate is removed by gluconeogenesis in the liver and kidney and also by oxidation in the heart and kidney. Lactate is produced by healthy contracting muscles, and the level will rise rapidly in the arterial blood during modest exercise in health, such as that producing an oxygen uptake of around 1 litre/min. The concentration achieves its peak at about 5 min from the start of exercise and then falls. If the exercise is more severe, however, the lactic concentration remains high throughout the exercise, and this is related to an increase in the respiratory exchange ratio (R) and a characteristic break in the linear relationship between oxygen uptake and minute ventilation (the anaerobic threshhold) [29].

Severe acidosis prevents the uptake of lactase in the isolated perfused rat liver, possibly due to inhibition of glycolytic enzymes. Although it is not yet certain whether this process occurs in man such a mechanism would explain the severe mortality from clinical lactic acidosis: obviously a self-perpetuating acidosis would then result as the major organ normally removing lactate, the liver, is prevented from doing so by the very acidosis which the lactate accumulation causes. Lactate metabolism also appears to depend upon a normal level of circulating glucose [16], as when hypoglycaemia complicates liver disease lactic acidosis can result, but this may be corrected following infusion of glucose. This has also been observed in the lactic acidosis complicated by phenformin treatment in diabetes.

Attempts to correct severe lactic acidosis by infusion of sodium bicarbonate have not always been successful, and the condition continues to carry a very grave outlook. Recently peritoneal dialysis with a bicarbonate-buffered fluid has been advocated for correction of the acidosis, and this was apparently achieved in four patients with lactic acidosis, one of whom had diabetes mellitus and three liver disease (two due to alcohol and one due to heroin overdose). The striking improvement in blood pH (from a mean of 7.05 before treatment to 7.39 after such dialysis) was associated with a fall in lactate levels from an average of 21.1 before treatment to 5.1 after dialysis [27].

In another new approach to treatment, particularly of type A lactic acidosis with shock, or diabetes with an anion gap of 39 mmol/litre attributed to lactate excess, successful resuscitation followed the infusion of nitroprusside, which was thought to improve tissue perfusion and so allow the correction of lactic acidosis [1].

References

1. Brezis M, Rowe M, Shalev O (1979) Reversal of lactic acidosis associated with heart failure by nitroprusside administration. Br Med J i:1399–1400
2. Bunker JP (1965) The great trans-Atlantic acid base debate. Anesthesiology 26:591–594
3. Campbell EJM (1965) Respiratory failure. Br Med J i:1451–1460
4. Cohen RB, Wood HF (1976) The clinical chemical and biochemical basis of lactic acidosis. Blackwell Scientific Publications, Oxford
5. Derenne JPH, Macklem PT, Roussos CH (1978) The respiratory muscles: Mechanics, control and pathophysiology. Am Rev Respir Dis, 118:119–133, 373–390, 581–601
6. Flenley DC (1970) Respiratory failure. Scott Med J 15:61–72
7. Flenley DC (1971) Another non-logarithmic acid-base diagram? Lancet I:961–965
8. Flenley DC (1978) Interpretation of blood-gas and acid-base data. Br J Hosp Med 20:384–394
9. Fulop M (1979) Serum potassium in lactic acidosis and ketoacidosis. N Engl J Med 300:1087–1089
10. Gabow PA, Anderson RJ, Potts DE, Schrier RW (1978) Acid-base disturbances in the salicylate-intoxicated adult. Arch Intern Med 138:1481–1484
11. Guilleminault C, Dement WC (eds) (1978) Sleep apnea syndromes. Alan R Liss, New York (Kroc foundation series, vol 11)
12. Hems DA (1975) Biochemical aspects of renal ammonia formation in metabolic acidosis. Enzyme 20:359–380
13. Henderson LJ (1908) The theory of neutrality regulation in the animal organism. Am J Physiol 21:427–448
14. Levinsky NG, Robert NJ (1979) Severe metabolic acidosis in a young man. N Engl J Med 301:650–657

15. Miyamoto T, Mizuno K, Furuya K (1970) Arterial blood gases in bronchial asthma. J Allergy Clin Immunol 56:248–254

16. Misbin RI (1977) Phenformin-associated lactic acidosis: Pathogenesis and ttreatment. Ann Intern Med 87:591–595

17. Moser KM, Luchsinger PC, Adamson JS, McMahon SM, Schleuter DP, Spivack M, Weg JG (1973) Respiratory stimulation with intravenous doxapram in respiratory failure. N Engl J Med 288:427–431

18. Murray JF (ed) (1977) Mechanisms of acute respiratory failure. Am Rev Respir Dis 115:1071–1078

19. McFadden ER, Lyons HA (1968) Arterial blood-gas tension in asthma. N Engl J Med 278:1027–1032

20. Rees HA, Millar JS, Donald KW (1968) A study of the clinical course and arterial blood gas tensions in patients in status asthmaticus. Q J Med 37:541–561

21. Sabatini S, Arruda JAL, Kurtzman NA (1978) Disorders of acid base balance. Med Clin North Am 62 6:1223–1255

22. Schwartz WB, Cohen JJ (1978) The nature of the renal response to chronic disorders of acid-base equilibrium. Am J Med 64:417–428

23. Siggaard-Andersen O (1964) The acid-base status of the blood, 2nd edn. Munksgaard, Copenhagen, p 26

24. Springer RR, Stevens PM (1979) The influence of PEEP on survival of patients in respiratory failure. Am J Med 66:196–200

25. Tai E, Read J (1967) Blood-gas tensions in bronchial asthma. Lancet I:644–646

26. Tuller MA, Mehdi F (1971) Compensatory hypoventilation and hypercapnia in primary metabolic alkalosis. Am J Med 50:281–290

27. Vaziri ND, Ness R, Wellikson L, Barton C, Greep N (1979) Bicarbonate-buffered peritoneal dialysis. An effective adjunct in the treatment of lactic acidosis. Am J Med 67:392–396

28. Warren PM, Flenley DC, Millar JS, Avery A (1980) Respiratory failure revisited: Acute exacerbations of chronic bronchitis between 1961–68 and 1970–76. Lancet I:467–471

29. Wasserman K, Whipp BJ, Koyal SN, Beaver WL (1973) Anaerobic threshold and respiratory gas exchange during exercise. J Appl Physiol 35:236–243

30. Worthley LIG (1977) The rational use of i.v. hydrochloric acid in the treatment of metabolic alkalosis. Br J Anaesth 49:811–817

31. Wrong O, Davies HEF (1959) The excretion of acid in renal disease. Q J Med 28:259–313

Chapter 7

Cerebral Blood Flow and Metabolism

M. J. Purves

The cerebral circulation has the same relation to the tissue which it perfuses as do blood vessels in other vascular beds. Oxygen and substrate must be supplied in proportion to metabolic rate, the chemical composition of extracellular fluid must be regulated to constancy, and temperature of tissue must be controlled with very narrow limits. There are, however, certain unique features about the brain and its circulation. First, brain has low O_2 stores and a limited capacity to respire anaerobically, so that the safety factor between O_2 supply and uptake is small. Vascular responses either to changes in metabolism or to systemic disturbances such as hypoxia, hypoglycaemia, and hypotension which threaten O_2 and substrate supply must therefore be very much more prompt than, for example, in voluntary muscle. Secondly, the rigid skull imposes a number of constraints. There cannot be significant changes in blood volume, or if there are, the associated changes in intracranial pressure (ICP) could well alter the resistance offered to blood flow by the small, thin-walled venules exposed to cerebrospinal fluid (CSF). Thirdly, it is almost certainly misleading to think of cerebral blood flow (CBF) and its regulation as homogeneous for, as will be discussed later, the levels of blood flow and metabolism in different parts of the brain may vary by up to an order of magnitude, while the difference in the speed of response of vessels to local changes in metabolism and to systemic disturbances suggests that quite different factors are involved. This chapter is concerned

mainly with mechanisms of control of cerebral blood vessels, and three topics are considered: the way in which cerebral blood vessels respond to the commoner systemic disturbances; cerebral metabolism and its regulation; and the way in which blood flow adjusts to metabolic need. This information, limited as it is, will provide the basis for a more complete understanding of how cerebral vascular control may be compromised in various disease states.

Cerebrovascular responses to systemic disturbances

The earliest experimental approach was simply to make a trephine hole and to measure the changes in the calibre of pial vessels in response to hypoxia, hypercapnia, and changes in arterial pressure. The results—which do not give quantitative estimates of changes in blood flow— were clear-cut. Hypoxia, hypercapnia, and hypotension cause pial vessel dilatation, and hypertension causes constriction [29, 112]. The responses were relatively sluggish and were not affected by section of the main afferent pathways from vasosensory receptors [29, 32]. On the other hand, it could be shown that electrical stimulation of these pathways affected the pial vessels. Stimulation of the cervical sympathetic nerve caused constriction [31], while stimulation of the sinus, vagus, and VII cranial nerves caused dilatation [3, 16, 31]. But the balance of opinion at the end of this phase of investigation in the 1940s was that the response of cerebral vessels to systemic disturbances involved intrinsic rather than reflex mechanisms.

After World War II, there were two important developments. There was first the application of electron microscopy to biological problems and the development of very much better histological and histochemical methods for determining the nature and projection of neural structures. Secondly, methods were developed for the measurement of CBF by means of clearance techniques based on the Fick principle. The first application of these methods was in man and nitrous oxide (N_2O) was used [57]; later modifications in which ^{133}Xe [67] and ^{85}Kr [65] were used followed by extensive investigation in experimental animals. Although the combination of these methods allowed quantitative description of the responses of cerebral blood vessels to physiological and pharmacological stimuli and much extended current knowledge of the neural pathways involved, there still remained great uncertainty about how these responses were brought about and, as in the 1930s, whether or how far neural pathways contributed.

The changes in blood flow are clear enough. If PaO_2 is altered in steps over the range of about 35–200 mmHg (4.7–26.7 kPa) the cerebrovascular response is hyperbolic and is potentiated by raising $PaCO_2$ [50, 72]. The response to step changes in $PaCO_2$ is sigmoid, being approximately linear over the physiological range but exhibiting reduced sensitivity at high and low CO_2 tensions [84]. The response to alterations in perfusion pressure, whether caused by changing arterial, venous, or intracranial pressures, is unusual. Blood flow is independent of pressure in the physiological range and some way above and below it: perfusion pressure has to be lowered to about half the control value before flow starts to fall, and flow starts to increase if pressure is raised to 50–60 mmHg above control values [66]. There are interactions between these variables. Thus, the vascular response to CO_2 is progressively reduced as perfusion pressure is reduced [44].

The strategy of these responses is also tolerably clear. If PaO_2 falls and metabolic rate remains unchanged, the increase in blood flow will diminish the arteriovenous (A-V) difference and so reduce the amount by which tissue PO_2 falls. The vulnerability of cells to hypoxia will also be reduced if, in addition, latent capillaries open and reduce the length of the diffusion pathway for O_2. This is known to occur as a long-term adaptation in acclimatization to hypoxia [105] and in infants with right-to-left shunts and significant haemoglobin (Hb) desaturation [20]. Outside physiological laboratories, pure hypoxia is almost as rare as pure hypercapnia; but in all the commoner forms of asphyxia, the potentiating effects of CO_2 will enhance the dilator response to hypoxia.

The independence of flow and perfusion pressure is similarly protective: it ensures, for example, that there is no significant change in CBF with everyday changes in pressure associated with changes in posture or intrathoracic pressure. Equally, it ensures that in acute hypertensive states associated, for example, with copulation or other violent forms of exercise or in pathological hypertensive states, within limits the blood–brain barrier is preserved.

How these changes are brought about is very much less clear. Broadly, there are two main hypotheses, which may not, however, be mutually exclusive. The first suggests that these vascular responses to systemic disturbances are wholly or in part determined by reflexes which involve (1) vasosensory or other receptors; (2) their afferent pathways; (3) a central and probably integrating group of vasomotor neurones in the reticular formation of the pons and medulla; and (4) efferent or motor fibres carried in the cervical sympathetic, VII and, possibly, other cranial nerves, which are distributed certainly to the carotid arteries, pial vessels, and to a very limited extent to intracerebral vessels. This reflex hypothesis has been supported by the results of series of experiments which have shown that stimulation of peripheral chemo- and baroreceptors cause substantial changes in CBF [82], responses which are abolished by section of the appropriate afferent nerves; that electrical stimulation of the VII cranial, sinus, and depressor nerves dilates cerebral vessels and increases blood flow [16, 90], and stimulation of sympathetic fibres constrict them; that discrete electrolytic lesions in the tegmentum of the reticular formation reduce or abolish the vascular response to CO_2 [92]; that the vascular response to CO_2 is reduced or abolished after section of the VII cranial nerve; that if the sympathetic nerves are cut in hypotension, the blood flow is higher than in the intact animal [28]; that if the sympathetic fibres are stimulated in hypertension, the upper limit of autoregulation is raised [8, 71]; and that electrical stimulation of the fastigial nucleus abolishes the characteristic flow/pressure relation [22], as does stimulation of the dorsal tegmentum after section of the sympathetic nerves [83].

Furthermore, it has now been quite clearly established that pial vessels at least possess noradrenergic [63] and cholinergic [64] receptors and that these are involved in vascular responses when the sympathetic and VII cranial nerves, respectively, are stimulated.

This impressive array of experimental results has been considerably eroded by a substantial number of essentially negative observations, namely, that stimulation of the vasomotor pathways results in only trivial changes in blood flow if any at all [48], and that as in the earlier experiments in the 1930s, vascular responses to systemic disturbances are not significantly affected by section of the afferent or efferent limbs of the reflex arcs [5, 48]. This divergence of results is so striking that if the technical competence of the various research workers can be assumed, it can only be explained by some important difference in the techniques used.

Broadly, and with some exceptions, those workers who have observed differences in CBF with section or stimulation of extrinsic nerves have used the indicator clearance technique, and mainly in primates, while those who have obtained negative results have used the indicator dilution technique with labelled microspheres, and mainly in dogs. The clearance technique involves the measurement of radioactivity with one or more externally placed counters and because of the limited penetration distance of gamma and, in particular, beta particles, such activity will tend to be in the more superficial layers of the cortex and subcortex, and will therefore presumably be heavily biased by the responses of pial vessels and their immediate branches. By contrast, the microsphere technique will more obviously measure rates of flow in intracerebral capillaries since the microspheres will be trapped in vessels 15 μm in size or smaller. The crucial question is then raised: do intracerebral capillaries respond to systemic disturbances, as do pial vessels, and could these two techniques in fact be measuring different functions of CBF? This question cannot be answered with certainty at present, since we have no independent method of separating pial and intracerebral vascular responses. Two pieces of information, however, suggest that this topic is worth pursuing. The first derives from experiments carried out to determine the contribution made by various parts of the vascular bed to overall cerebrovascular resistance [103]. The study was based on the view that the main conducting vessels, carotid and vertebral, the pial vessels and the 'downstream' intracerebral vessels effectively operate in series.

Under control conditions, these elements contribute to overall resistance in the ratio 39:21:40, respectively, but with an increase in arterial pressure, the ratio changes to 33:15:52. The reason for this disproportionate rise in the resistance offered by intracerebral vessels is unknown. It might be due to the existence of arterial 'cushions' at the origin of the intracerebral vessels [47, 75], which could be analogous to precapillary sphincters in other vascular beds. It could be due to an increase in postcapillary resistance as the thin-walled venules are compressed with the associated rise in ICP. Whatever the mechanism, these results suggest that intracerebral vessels may not be responding directly to the original disturbance but rather to the intermediate changes in flow/pressure in pial vessels in an attempt, for example, to maintain a constant head of pressure across the capillary bed. This type of compensatory response of intracerebral blood vessels could well also explain a second observation, namely, that if the sympathetic nerves are stimulated in rabbits, intracerebral blood flow, measured by heat clearance, at first falls but then rises to control levels as though stimulation is continued [93]. This observation also emphasizes how important the timing of responses is, something that is not possible with the discontinuous methods described above.

These observations have suggested to a number of workers (e.g. [45]) that the responses of the series components of the cerebral vascular bed are not homogeneous and to an unknown extent depend upon the responses of the vessels upstream. This view has a number of important implications. Thus cerebral blood flow will be more likely to be affected by the vulnerability of the main afferent vessels to go into spasm than in other vascular beds. Secondly, since the pial vessels appear to be central to the control system, relatively trivial or local effects upon pial vessels could profoundly affect intracerebral blood flow and cerebral function. One example of this could be the consequences of extravasation of blood in the subarachnoid space, which by paralysing pial vascular smooth muscle could well impair the compensatory ability of intracerebral vessels which were not directly affected. A further question might also then be asked: Whether or not it can be shown that intracerebral blood flow is dependent upon the responses of pial vessels, is there any evidence that intracerebral vessels are independently controlled? We briefly review two alternative mechanisms which have been proposed.

The first alternative is that the response of

cerebral vessels depends entirely upon intrinsic mechanisms. With respect to systemic hypoxia or hypercapnia, this would suggest that their action upon cerebral vessels is direct. There is at present no satisfactory evidence that hypoxia affects either pial or intracerebral vessels directly or indirectly. The possibility that hypoxia acts by causing the release of lactic acid, which then causes dilatation of vessels is unlikely, since blood flow increases before lactic acid is detectable [10] and even when the flow response to hypoxia is complete, the lactic acid concentration of 1.5 mM g^{-1} would be unlikely to cause a significant change in pH_{ECF}, especially since with hypoxia, Pco_2 falls [78]. There is some evidence that CO_2 dilates pial vessels by a direct action [94], but its action upon intracerebral vessels is unknown. CO_2 rarely if ever acts in molecular form; more commonly it alters extra- or intracellular pH. Although its action upon cells of cerebrovascular smooth muscle has not been analysed, it is reasonable that CO_2 should dilate since it is known to hyperpolarize and reduce spontaneous activity in smooth muscle elsewhere [38], and in general CO_2 inhibits excitable tissue [62, 101]. More directly, a low bicarbonate level has been shown to dilate pial vessels, though the suspicion arises from these experiments that the sensitivity of smooth muscle to external H^+ is rather low [110]. With respect to intracerebral vessels, it is probable that changes in pH_{ECF} are not of any significance in regulation, since with bicuculline seizures, amphetamine intoxication, hypoglycaemia, and hypoxia, pH_{ECF} does not obviously change, whereas local blood flow invariably increases [4].

To explain a direct action of pressure upon vascular smooth muscle, the 'myogenic' hypothesis coined by Bayliss [6], questioned by Anrep [2], and resuscitated by Folkow [30] has often been invoked. This mechanism, which supposes a change in the state of contraction of smooth muscle to oppose changes in intramural pressure, would if generally effective lead to positive feedback with infinitely constricted vessels and infinitely high blood pressure. Clearly this does not occur every time blood pressure rises, so if this mechanism exists it must be offset by mechanisms which dilate: together such mechanisms could determine the stability of blood vessel tone, but it is difficult to see how the myogenic mechanism by itself could account for the known dynamic and static responses of cerebrovascular smooth muscle to changes in perfusion pressure [114].

Proof that intrinsic factors exist or are impor-

tant will be obtained with difficulty, and then probably only by exclusion. An alternative possibility which could be more positively investigated is that blood vessels, and in particular those inside brain substance, are affected by the catecholaminergic pathways originating in pons and medulla, which project to most parts of the brain and which, through the liberation of noradrenaline and dopamine, profoundly affect the function of neuronal networks [9, 34, 35, 69, 109]. At present, we lack clear confirmation that fibres in these pathways genuinely innervate intracerebral blood vessels, though on two occasions at least, contact between some nerve fibres and small intracerebral vessels and even a capillary has been noted [19, 24, 46, 86]. But if no histological confirmation of such innervation exists, there is clear evidence that the responses of intracerebral vessels, particularly in the hypothalamus, are markedly affected if the pathway is destroyed [88] and that these vessels respond to endogenous noradrenaline [60] or acetylcholine [61]. These observations are of great interest and deserve to be extended, since they may provide a long-awaited basis for the integrated regulation of intracerebral blood vessels in response to systemic disturbances. If it can be established that these central aminergic pathways are of regulatory importance, it would then be crucial to know how these pathways are activated by, for example, hypoxia and hypercapnia.

In summary, we now know in some detail how CBF changes in response to alterations of PaO_2, $PaCO_2$, and perfusion pressure, and how these variables can interact. These descriptive results have been presented in terms of a strategy to maintain adequate O_2 and substrate supply when these are threatened. The experiments which have been designed to show how cerebral blood vessels respond to these stimuli have been far from decisive, in particular as to whether extrinsic neural pathways contribute. These discrepant results have, however, emphasized that the response of cerebral vessels is likely to be non-homogeneous and that in particular the responses of intracerebral and pial vessels may be different and differently controlled. This could account in turn for the discrepant measurements recorded with different techniques which, it is suggested, could be measuring different functions of CBF. A review of possible intrinsic factors suggests that these are unlikely to be of great importance. The possibility that central aminergic pathways regulate, in particular, intracerebral pathways holds considerable promise.

Cerebral metabolism

The first estimates of cerebral metabolic rate were derived from measurements of CBF based on the Fick principle and of the A-V O_2 difference [57]. The accuracy of the method depends upon satisfactory isolation of the venous drainage of the brain. This is practicable in primates, including man, but liable to error in most other experimental animals. In consequence, most of the earlier studies involved human subjects under control conditions and in various pathological states. The average value for cerebral O_2 consumption, 1.3–1.8 μmole.g^{-1}.min^{-1}, varies with age. In children, the value is significantly higher [53], and cerebral O_2 consumption falls progressively with age in parallel with cortical neurone density and CBF [55]. Cerebral O_2 consumption in man is unaffected by mental arithmetic [98]; it increases with epileptic seizures [41]; it is reduced with barbiturate anaesthesia [97] and in patients with diabetes, uraemia, and hepatic failure [99].

These values for average O_2 consumption are valuable, but a drawback is that they are likely to conceal not only regional or local differences but changes in them. A method which allows the measurement of such regional differences was developed by Ter-Pogossian et al. [13, 106, 107]. The injection of $^{15}O_2$-labelled water is used to measure CBF and $^{15}O_2$-labelled red cells to measure cerebral O_2 consumption. The technique is applicable to man, and values for these variables are similar to those obtained by N_2O wash-out [58]. The technique is limited of course to those who possess a cyclotron and by the number of external counters which can be applied.

An alternative approach has been adopted by Sokoloff et al. [100], who used ^{14}C-2-deoxyglucose and quantitative autoradiography to measure the distribution of glucose utilization in the brain. Deoxyglucose is transported across the blood–brain barrier and into cells as if it were glucose: both are phosphorylated by hexokinase but deoxyglucose-6-phosphate is not metabolized further and accumulates in the cell in proportion to the level of glucose uptake. If the relative concentrations of glucose and deoxyglucose in precursor pools and the kinetic constants of hexokinase with respect to these sugars are known, glucose utilization may be calculated from the concentration of ^{14}C-2-deoxyglucose in tissue. This in turn is calculated from the autoradiographic density of ^{14}C, with the aid of appropriate standards. The method depends critically upon a number of assumptions. In the first place, there must be minimal free deoxyglucose in the tissue and this requires 40–60 min equilibration before the termination of the experiment. Secondly, the method assumes that glucose is the principal substrate and if glucose utilization is thought of as an index of metabolic rate, that glucose is metabolized aerobically. This assumption is in general true: but there are important exceptions. Since glucose + $6O_2 \rightarrow 6CO_2 + 6H_2O$, the ratio A-V O_2 difference/A-V glucose difference will be equal to 6: or the glucose/oxygen index can be expressed as a percentage

100 A-V O_2 difference/6 A-V glucose difference.

This index has most commonly been found to be 100% or about 100% [18, 41, 56]. In absolute terms, glucose utilization in man has been found to be 0.29 μmole.g^{-1}.min^{-1} [41], but as Sokoloff et al. [100] have shown, this level varies very considerably between different parts of the brain. It must also be emphasized that under certain conditions, glucose utilization is not synonymous with metabolic rate. Thus, in hypoxia the glycolytic rate is enhanced; in hypercapnia it is inhibited.

It will be apparent from the descriptions above that all the methods at present available for estimation of cerebral metabolic rate have considerable drawbacks because they involve discontinuous measurements, because they involve potential inaccuracies in sampling arterial and, in particular, cerebral venous blood, because they yield average values for brain, or because values for glucose utilization require lengthy steady states and may not always and adequately define metabolic rate. There is one further difficulty. These measurements may describe changes in metabolic rate with various systemic disturbances, but they do not reveal how these disturbances affect cerebral tissue: nor do they reveal how tissue, as opposed to the vascular component, responds, if at all. These last points are essential for a complete understanding of how brain tissue may be vulnerable to the effects of, say, hypoxia or ischaemia. We therefore consider first how the effects of such disturbances are determined at tissue level and then consider briefly what is known about the vulnerability of the brain.

Cerebral metabolism and hypoxia

It is commonly known among clinicians and physiologists that PaO_2 may be raised or lowered by substantial amounts without significant change in integrative cerebral activity. If PaO_2 is reduced in stages, the following sequence of changes occur at the accompanying levels of hypoxia: at 85 mmHg (11.3 kPa) delayed dark adaptation; at 70 mmHg (9.3 kPa) impaired ability to learn a complex task; at 55 mmHg (7.3 kPa) impaired short-term memory; at 45 mmHg (6 kPa) loss of critical judgment; at 40 mmHg (5.3 kPa) an increase of CBF by 35%: at 35 mmHg (4.7 kPa) an increase of cerebral blood flow by 70%, and at 30 mmHg (4 kPa) loss of consciousness. These changes may occur at higher levels of PaO_2 if $PaCO_2$ falls to low levels with hyperventilation.

We might ask why in fact these changes in cerebral function occur, in particular those involving associative functions of the brain at the higher levels of PaO_2. The obvious answer would be that some cells or groups of cells become hypoxic, that mitochondrial respiration is impaired, and that in consequence insufficient ATP is formed. However, if this were the case, then there would be a clear fall in cerebral metabolic rate, since as is shown from the equation

$$dO_2/dt = K_{rate} \text{ (cytochrome } a_3^{2+})(O_2)$$

at the level of cytochrome a_3, which by accepting O_2 at the end of the respiratory chain, allows oxidative phosphorylation to occur and probably accounts for the overwhelming part of brain O_2 consumption, the rate of O_2 consumption (dO_2/dt) varies directly with PO_2. In fact, both in man [18] and in experimental animals [e.g., 7, 43, 52], no change in cerebral metabolic rate has been recorded even when PaO_2 has been lowered to 20–25 mmHg (2.7–3.3 kPa). This must imply that tissue PO_2, even at the lowest levels of PaO_2, is maintained above a critical PO_2 at which QO_2 starts to decrease. Strictly, such a critical PO_2 (defined for isolated mitochondria) is the PO_2 at which $\dot{Q}O_2$ is reduced by 50% (the apparent Michaelis constant [K_m]), and is considerably less than 0.1 mmHg [14, 15, 51]. Physiologically, it would be more important to know at what PO_2 a fall in QO_2 could be detected, and at present the evidence suggests that this is considerably below 5 mmHg (0.7 kPa) and probably less than 1 mmHg (0.13 kPa) [15, 102]. Confirmatory evidence that the cerebral energy state is not significantly affected until PaO_2 falls to very low levels has been provided [40, 91, 95]: all the results referred to have shown that no essential changes in the concentration of phosphocreatine, ATP, ADP, and AMP could be detected.

These somewhat paradoxical results raise two important questions: (1) what mechanism(s) maintain tissue PO_2 in all but the most severe levels of hypoxia above some critical level or threshold; and (2) why, if tissue PO_2 is so maintained, are there functional effects of hypoxia? The answer to the first question seems to be undoubtedly the vascular response discussed in a previous section, and this emphasizes the point that the vulnerability of the brain, and particularly those parts with initially high $\dot{Q}O_2$, will greatly increase with any form of impairment of vascular control. The answer to the second question is unknown: but one possibility may be proposed. In addition to the electron transfer oxidases such as cytochrome oxidase, there is a group of mixed function oxidases which catalyse the general reaction:

$$AH + 2e^- + O_2 \rightarrow AOH + O^{2-}(\rightarrow H_2O)$$

in which one O_2 atom is added to the reduced substrate (AH). It is of interest that the rate-limiting steps in the synthesis of the catecholamines dopamine and noradrenaline, and the indolamine serotonin, are catalysed by enzymes (tyrosine and tryptophane hydroxylase, respectively) which belong to this group. These enzymes have K_m values for O_2 of about 5–10 mmHg (0.7–1.3 kPa) [27, 33], which could provide a link between O_2 availability and function and, as discussed in a later section, act as sensors of O_2 concentration.

Cerebral metabolism and CO_2

As described in an earlier section, an increase in CO_2 causes an increase in CBF, and one effect of this is to raise the level of tissue PO_2. There is no evidence that this affects cerebral metabolic rate [25, 56, 77, 80]. The effect of hypocapnia has been studied in some detail since it has been shown that this impairs some aspects of mental function [61] and according to some anaesthetists [23, 42] hyperventilation reduces the required dosages of anaesthetics and relaxants and increases the pain threshold [17]. It is unclear whether these effects are due to hypoxia or to alkalosis. Hypocapnia causes a fall in cerebral blood flow and thus an increased extraction of O_2 and fall in tissue and venous PO_2. The alkalosis will cause a shift of the oxyhaemoglobin curve to the left which will further diminish venous PO_2.

In early studies, hypocapnia [$PaCO_2$ approx. 22 mmHg (2.9 kPa)] caused a reduction of about 40% in CBF in man [1, 58, 59, 111, 112], but in none of these studies did cerebral metabolic rate change. There did not therefore appear to be significant hypoxia. With more severe degrees of hypocapnia, e.g., $PaCO_2$ 9–10 mmHg (1.2–1.3 kPa) there was an increase in glucose consumption and lactate production, as was shown by a fall in the O_2/glucose index and a rise in the lactate/glucose index, suggesting some reduction in cellular oxygenation. Similar evidence showing a lack of any significant change in cerebral oxygen consumption with all but the severest degrees of hypocapnia has been found in experimental animals [12, 25, 39, 73].

Cerebral metabolism and ischaemia

Arrest of the circulation to the head in normal human subjects leads to fixation of the eyes in the midline in 5–6 s and loss of consciousness in 6–7 s. Large slow waves in the EEG appear at this time and the corneal reflex is lost after 10 s. Restoration of flow even after as long as 100 s interruption is followed by complete restoration of function, associated with the subject's being dazed, confused, and sometimes excited and euphoric [89]. Comparable results have been found in experimental animals [21, 49, 104]. The effects of ischaemia upon cerebral energy metabolism were first systematically studied by Lowry et al. and Goldberg et al. [37, 70]. These authors showed that in the absence of O_2 the tissue can only obtain energy by spending its energy-rich phosphate reserves (phosphocreatine [PCr], ATP, and by metabolizing its stores of glucose and glycogen to lactic acid. In 10 min, a total amount of 18 μmole ~P units/g was released. Of these, 14 were used in the first minute, and 16 in 2 min. Thus, after 2 min essentially no useful energy remained. All these observations indicate that whereas the brain can compensate satisfactorily for severe reductions in O_2, it cannot cope with a simultaneous reduction in substrate.

These changes with ischaemia can be modified in a number of ways. It was shown many years ago that hypothermia retarded the rate of fall of PCr and ATP concentrations and the rate of lactate increase with ischaemia [108]. This has been confirmed in subsequent studies [11, 74]. Anaesthetic agents also affect the rate of changes seen in ischaemia. Lowry et al. [70] and Gatfield et al. [36] showed that barbiturate anaesthesia retards the rate of change and similar results have been obtained with other anaesthetics [11]. Michenfelder and Theye [74] could not confirm this and it appears from later studies that these discrepant results relate to the time after institution of ischaemia when measurements are made. Thus Nilsson et al. [76]

and Nordstrom and Siesjo [79] showed that deep anaesthesia retards the rate of ~P use only in the initial period of ischaemia. In the first 5–10 s of ischaemia, ~P use in N_2O anaesthesia is approximately twice as high as with barbiturate anaesthesia: thereafter, with longer periods of ischaemia, any initial differences in the rate of energy use due to variations in the depth or type of anaesthesia disappear.

Metabolic regulation of CBF

The account in the previous sections on cerebral metabolic responses to various disturbances makes it clear that adequate cerebral function is dependent, as in other vascular beds, on an adequate O_2 and substrate supply, but it also indicates that the cerebral circulation can compensate, largely if not wholly, for all but the most severe degrees of hypoxia. Also, in an earlier section, it was pointed out that at present we are by no means certain how the cerebral vessels 'know' how severe the hypoxia is and by how much they have to increase blood flow to ensure such compensation. There is some doubt about the reflex component; we remain quite uncertain about a direct action of hypoxia upon vascular smooth muscle; it does not appear that the glycolytic production of lactic acid can account for the dilatation and increase in blood flow, and the operation of the intracerebral aminergic pathways, although provocative, has yet to be examined in detail. Similarly, we remain uncertain as to how a change in the metabolic rate of brain tissue brings about a compensatory increase in local blood flow. That it does is not in doubt. Leniger-Follert and Lübbers [68] and Silver [96] have shown quite clearly that if an area of cortex is activated, there is a highly localized increase in microflow within 1–2 s and a parallel increase in Po_2. This indicates that vascular response is very rapid and more than adequate in ensuring that O_2 supply is maintained. It also indicates that local hypoxia cannot be the trigger which induces the increase in flow. Leniger-Follert and Lübbers [68] also showed that with this type of cortical stimulation, local H^+ activity at first decreased and then increased after some seconds, whereas local K^+ activity increased very rapidly, within a few milliseconds.

These observations indicate that there is a very highly developed mechanism for the control of local CBF, but we remain ignorant about both the signal and the effector mechanism which increases or redistributes capillary flow. The subject of cellular O_2 tension sensors has been considered in detail by Reivich et al. [85], and we have described here some credible O_2 detectors. It is still not clear whether microflow is regulated by O_2 availability or by some dependent function, e.g., pH, ionic concentrations, or CO_2. The speed of response of arterioles suggests that they respond directly to hypoxia, but the slower capillary adjustments suggest a multifactorial mechanism. As to the effector mechanism, it is possible that (1) the capillary wall is contractile, and in favour of this view are the finding of contractile proteins in capillary walls [81] and recent electron microscope evidence that brain capillaries are innervated [86]; (2) the endothelial cells at the entrance to capillary branches may be able to swell and occlude the lumen; or (3) the elasticity of the endothelium may be altered by the environment or some neural mechanism. These questions have been dealt with in detail in a Ciba Foundation symposium [26].

The overall changes of cerebral metabolic rate and blood flow to the more important systemic disturbances such as hypoxia, hypercapnia, hypocapnia, and changes in perfusion pressure have now been recorded in detail in both man and experimental animals. The vascular responses are both prompt and, within limits, adequate to ensure that cerebral metabolism is largely unaffected. However, we remain largely ignorant as to how these vascular responses are brought about, that is, the effective signal and precisely which components of the vascular bed respond. Similarly, with respect to the vascular changes in response to local changes in metabolism, the prompt and more than adequate increase in O_2 supply has been documented but the coupling agent between metabolism and local flow eludes us. What this means for the clinician who has to manage a patient with a gross systemic disturbance is that the way in which the cerebral vasculature will attempt to respond should be tolerably clear, as will the way in which this response may be compromised if any component of the cerebral circulation is impaired. Since, however, our understanding of how the cerebral vessels sense and respond to these disturbances is very far from complete, there is little rational basis for intervention on the part of the clinician beyond the obvious course of minimizing the disturbance. It is perhaps fortunate for clinicians that many cerebrovascular disorders of this type are self-limiting.

References

1. Alexander SC, Cohen PJ, Wollman H, Smith TC, Reivich M, van der Molen RA (1965) Cerebal carbohydrate metabolism during hypocarbia in man. Studies during nitrous oxide anaesthesia. Anaesthesiology 26:624–632
2. Anrep GV (1912) On local vascular reactions and their interpretation. J Physiol (Lond) 45:318–327
3. Ask-Upmark E (1935) The carotid sinus and cerebral circulation. An anatomical, experimental and clinical investigation, including some observations on rete mirabile caroticum. Acta Psychiatr Scand [Suppl] 6:1–374
4. Astrup J, Heuser D, Lassen NA, Nilsson B, Norberg K, Siesjo BK (1976) Evidence against H^+ and K^+ as the main factors in the regulation of cerebral blood flow during epileptic discharges, acute hypoxemia, amphetamine intoxication and hypoglycemia. A microelectrode study. In: Betz E (ed) Ionic actions on vascular smooth muscle. Springer, Berlin, pp 110-115
5. Bates D, Sundt TM (1976) The relevance of peripheral baroreceptors and chemoreceptors to regulation of cerebral blood flow in the cat. Circ Res 38:488–493
6. Bayliss WM (1902) On the local reactions of the arterial wall to changes of internal pressure. J Physiol (Lond) 28:220–231
7. Berntman L, Carlsson C, Siesjö BK (1977) Cerebral oxygen utilization and blood flow in hypoxia: Influence of sympathoadrenal activation. Stroke 10/1:20–25
8. Bill A, Linder J (1976) Sympathetic control of cerebral blood flow in acute hypertension. Acta Physiol Scand 96:114–121
9. Bjorklund A, Lindvall O (1977) Anatomy of the catecholamine-containing projection systems of the brain stem reticular formation. In: Owman CH, Edvinsson L (eds) Neurogenic control of the brain circulation. Pergamon, Oxford, pp 409–428
10. Borgstrom L, Johansson H, Siesjö BK (1975) The relationship between arterial Po_2 and cerebral blood flow in hypoxic hypoxia. Acta Physiol Scand 93:423–432
11. Brunner EA, Passonneau JV, Molstad C (1971) The effect of volatile anaesthetics on levels of metabolites and on metabolic rate in brain. J Neurochem 18:2301–16
12. Cain SM (1963) An attempt to demonstrate cerebral anoxia hyperventilation of anaesthetized dogs. Am J Physiol 204:323–6
13. Carter CC, Eichling JO, Davis DO, Ter-Pogossian MM (1972) Correlation regional cerebral blood flow with regional oxygen uptake using ^{15}O method. Neurology 22:755–62
14. Chance B (1965) Reaction of oxygen with the respiratory chain in cells and tissues. J Gen Physiol 49:163–88
15. Chance B, Schoener B, Schindler F (1964) The intracellular oxidation-reduction state. In: Dickens F, Neil E (eds) Oxygen in the Animal Organism. Pergamon, Oxford, pp 367–92
16. Chorobki J, Penfield W (1932) Cerebral vasodilator nerves and their pathway from the medulla oblongata. Arch Neurol 28:1257–1289
17. Clutton-Brock J (1957) The cerebral effects of overventilation. Br J Anaesth 29:111–3
18. Cohen PJ, Alexander SC, Smith TC, Reivich M, Wollman H (1967) Effects of hypoxia and normocarbia on cerebral blood flow and metabolism in conscious man. J App Physiol 23:183–189
19. Csillik B, Jancso G, Toth L, Kozma M, Kalman G,

Karcsu S (1971) Adrenergic innervation of hypothalamic blood vessels. A contribution to the problem of central thermodetectors. Acta nat (Basel) 80:142–151

20. Diemer K (1968) Capillarisation and oxygen supply to the brain. In: Lubbers DW, Luft UC, Thews G, Witzleb E (eds) Oxygen transport in blood and tissue. Thieme, Stuttgart, pp 118–123

21. Dennis C, Kabat H (1939) Behaviour of dogs after complete temporary arrest of the cephalic circulation. Proc Soc Exp Biol Med 40:559–81

22. Doba N, Reis DJ (1972) Changes in regional blood flow and cardiodynamics evoked by electrical stimulation of the fastigial nucleus in the cat: Similarity to orthostatic reflexes. J Physiol (Lond) 227:729–748

23. Dundee JW (1952) Influence of controlled respiration on dosage of thiopentone and d-tubocurarine chloride required for abdominal surgery. Br Med J ii:893

24. Edvinsson L, Lindvall M, Nielsen KC, Owman CH (1973) Are brain vessels innervated also by central (non-sympathetic) adrenergic neuron? Brain Res 63:496–499

25. Eklof B, MacMillan V, Siesjö B (1973) The effect of hypercapnia acidosis upon the energy metabolism of the brain in arterial hypotension caused by bleeding. Acta Physiol Scand 87:1–14

26. Elliott K, O'Connor M (Eds) (1978) Cerebral Vascular Smooth Muscle and its Control. CIBA Foundation Symposium 56, Elsevier, Amsterdam

27. Fisher DB, Kaufman S (1972) The inhibition of phyenylalanine and tyrosine hydroxylases by high oxygen levels. J Neurochem 19:1359–65

28. Fitch W, MacKenzie ET, Harper AM (1975) Effects of decreasing arterial blood pressure on cerebral blood flow in the baboon. Circ Res 37:550–557

29. Fog M (1937) Cerebral Circulation. The reaction of the pial arteries to a fall in blood pressure. Arch Neurol 37:351–364

30. Folkow B (1964) Description of the myogenic hypothesis. Circ Res 14–15 (Supp 1) I:279–287

31. Forbes HS, Wolff HG (1928) Cerebral circulation. III. The vasomotor control of cerebral vessels. Arch Neurol 19:1057–1086

32. Forbes HS, Nason GI, Cobb S, Wortman RC (1937) Cerebral circulation. XLV. Vasodilation in pia following stimulation of the geniculate ganglion. Arch Neurol 37:776–781

33. Friedman PA, Kappelman AH, Kaufman S. (1972) Partial purification and characterization of tryptophane hydroxylase fom rabbit hind brain. J Biol Chem 247:4165–73

34. Fuxe K (1965) Evidence for the existence of monoamine neurons in the central nervous system. IV. Distribution of monoamine nerve terminals in the central nervous system. Acta Physiol Scand [Suppl] 64:37–85

35. Fuxe K, Hökfelt T, Ungerstedt U (1968) Localization of indolealkylamines in CNS. Adv Pharm Sci 6:235–251

36. Gatfield PD, Lowry OH, Schulz DW, Passonneau JV (1966) Regional energy reserves in mouse brain and changes with ischaemia and anaesthesia. J Neurochem 13:185–95

37. Goldberg ND, Passonneau JV, Lowry OH (1966) Effects of changes in brain metabolism on the levels of citric acid cycle intermediates. J Biol Chem 241:3997–4003

38. Golenhofen K (1970) Slow rhythms in smooth muscle (Minute rhythm) In: Bülbring E, Brading A, Jones A, Tomita T (eds) Smooth Muscle. Arnold, London

39. Gotoh F, Meyer JS, Takagi Y (1965) Cerebral effects of hyperventilation in man. Arch Neurol 12:410–23

40. Gottesfeld Z, Miller AT Jr (1969) Metabolic response of rat brain to acute hypoxia: Influence of polycythemia and hypercapnia. Am J Physiol 216:1374–9

41. Gottstein U, Bernsmeier A, Sedlmeyer I (1963) Der Kohlenhydratstoffwechsel des menschlichen Gehirns. I. Untersuchungen mit substratspezifischen enzymatischen Methoden bei normaler Hirndurchblutung. Klin Wochenschr 41:943–8

42. Gray TC, Rees GJ (1952) Role of apnoea in anaesthesia for major surgery Br Med J ii:891–2

43. Hägerdal M, Harp JR, Siesjö BK (1975) Influence of changes in arterial P_{CO_2} on cerebral blood flow and cerebral energy state during hypothermia in the rat. Acta Anaesthesiol Scand [Suppl] 57:25–33

44. Harper AM, Glass HI (1965) The effect of alterations in the arterial carbon dioxide tension on the blood flow through the cerebral cortex at normal and low arterial blood pressures. J Neurol Neurosurg Psychiatry 28:449–52

45. Harper Am, Desmukh VD, Rowan JO, Jennett WB (1972) Influence of sympathetic nervous activity on cerebral blood flow. Arch Neurol 27:1–6

46. Hartman BK, Zide D, Udenfriend S (1972) The use of dopamine β-hydroxylase as a marker for the central noradrenergic nervous system in rat brain. Proc Nat Acad Sci USA 69:2722–26

47. Hassler O. (1962) Physiological intima cushions in the large cerebral arteries of young individuals. Acta Pathol Microbiol Scand 55:19–26

48. Heistad DD, Marcus ML, Ehrhardt JC, Abboud FM (1976) Effect of stimulation of carotid chemoreceptors on total and regional cerebral blood flow. Circ Res 38:20–25

49. Hirsch H, Bolte A, Schaudig A, Tönnis D (1957) Uber die Wiederbelebung des Gehirns bei Hypothermie. Pflügers Arch 265:281–313

50. James IM, Millar RA, Purves MJ (1969) Observations on the extrinsic neural control of cerebral blood flow in the baboon. Circ Res 25:77–93

51. Jöbsis FF (1964) Basic processes in cellular respiration. In: Fenn WO, Rahn H (eds) Handbook of Physiology. Sect 3 Respiration, Vol 1. American Physiological Society, Washington, 63–124

52. Jóhannsson H, Siesjö BK (1975) Brain energy metabolism in anaesthetized rats in acute anaemia. Acta Physiol Scand 95:515–525

53. Kennedy C, Sokoloff L (1957) An adaptation of the nitrous oxide method to the study of the cerebral circulation in children: Normal values for cerebral blood flow and cerebral metabolic rate in childhood. J Clin Invest 36:1130–37

54. Kety SS (1956) Human cerebral blood flow and oxygen consumption as related to aging. J Chronic Dis 3:478–486

55. Kety SS (1957) The general metabolism of the brain in vivo. In: Richter D (ed) Metabolism of the Nervous System. Pergamon, New York, pp 221–236

56. Kety SS (1960) I, Blood-tissue exchange methods. Theory of blood-tissue exchange and its application to measurement of blood flow. In Bruner HD (ed) Methods in Medical Research, Vol 8. Year Book Publishers Inc, Chicago, pp 223–7

57. Kety SS, Schmidt CF (1945) The determination of cerebral blood flow in man by the use of nitrous oxide in low concentrations. Am J Physiol 143:53–66

58. Kety SS, Schmidt CF (1946) The effects of active and passive hyperventilation on cerebral blood flow, cerebral oxygen consumption, cardiac output, and blood pressure of normal young men. J Clin Invest 25:107–119

59. Kety SS, Schmidt CF (1948) The effects of altered arterial tensions of carbon dioxide and oxygen on

cerebral blood flow and cerebral oxygen consumption of normal young men. J Clin Invest 27:484–492

60. Klugman K, Mitchell G, Rosendorff C (1979) Evidence for an indirect cholinergic regulation of blood flow in the hypothalamus of conscious rabbits. Br J Pharmacol 66:217–221

61. Klugman KP, Mitchell G, Rosendorff (1980) Cholinergic regulation of intracerebral noradrenergic pathway-induced hypothalamic vasodilatation. Stroke (in press)

62. Krnjevic K, Randic M, Siesjö BK (1965) Cortical CO_2 tension and neuronal excitability. J Physiol (Lond) 176:105–122

63. Kuschinsky W, Wahl M (1976) The ability to influence the pial arterial tone by the sympathetic nervous system. In: Cervos-Navarro J (ed) The Cerebral Vessel Wall. Raven Press, New York

64. Kuschinsky W, Wahl M, Neiss A (1974) Evidence for cholinergic dilatatory receptors in pial arteries of cats. A microapplication study. Pflüegers Arch 347:199–208

65. Lassen NA, Munck O (1955) The cerebral blood flow in man determined by the use of radioactive Krypton. Acta Physiol Scand 33:30–49

66. Lassen NA (1959) Cerebral blood flow and oxygen consumption in man. Physiol Rev 39:183–238

67. Lassen NA, Høedt-Rasmussen K, Sorensen SC, Skinhoj E, Cronquist S, Bodforss B, Ingvar DH (1963) Regional cerebral blood flow in man determined by a radioactive inert gas (Krypton 85). Neurology (Minneap) 13:719–729

68. Leniger-Follert E, Lübbers DW (1976) Behaviour of microflow and local PO_2 of the brain cortex during and after direct electrical stimulation. Pflüegers Arch 366:38–44

69. Lindvall O, Bjorklund A (1974) The organization of the ascending catecholamine neuron systems in the rat brain as revealed by the glyoxylic acid fluorescence method. Acta Physiol Scand [Suppl] 412:1–48

70. Lowry OH, Passonneau JV, Hasselberger FX, Schultz DW (1964) Effect of ischaemia on known substrates and cofactors of the glycolytic pathway in brain. J Biol Chem 239:18–30

71. MacKenzie ET, McGeorge AP, Graham DI, Fitch W, Edvinsson L, Harper AM (1977) Breakthrough of cerebral autoregulation and the sympathetic nervous system. Acta Neurol Scand [Suppl] 64:(56) 58–49

72. McDowall, DG (1966) Interrelationships between blood oxygen tension and cerebral blood flow. In: Payne JP, Hill DW (eds) Oxygen measurements in blood and tissues. Churchill, London, 205–214

73. Michenfelder JD, Theye RA (1969) The effects of profound hypocapnia and dilutional anaemia on canine cerebral metabolism and blood flow. Anaesthesiology 31:449–57

74. Michenfelder JD, Theye RA (1970) The effects of anaesthesia and hypothermia on canine cerebral ATP and lactate during anoxia produced by decapitation. Anaesthesiology 33:430–9

75. Nelson E, Rennels M (1970) Innervation of intracranial arteries. Brain 93:475–490

76. Nilsson B, Siesjö BK (1976) A method for determining blood flow and oxygen consumption in the rat brain. Acta Physiol Scand 96:72–82

77. Nilsson B, Norberg K, Nordstrom C-H, Siesjö BK (1975) Influence of hypoxia and hypercapnia on CBF in rats. In: Harper M, Jennett B, Miller D, Rowan J (eds) Blood Flow and Metabolism in the Brain. Proc of Seventh Int Symposium, Aviemore. Churchill Livingstone, Edinburgh, pp 9, 19–9, 23

78. Norberg K, Siesjö BK (1975) Cerebral metabolism in hypoxic hypoxia. I. Pattern of activation of glycolysis, a re-evaluation. Brain Res 86:31–44

79. Nordström C-H, Siesjö BK (1978) Influence of phenobarbital on changes in the metabolites of the energy reserve of the cerebral cortex following complete ischaemia. Acta Physiol Scand 104:271–280

80. Novack P, Shenkin HA, Bortin L, Goluboff B, Soffe AM (1953) The effects of carbon dioxide inhalation upon the cerebral blood flow and cerebral oxygen consumption in vascular disease. J Clin Invest 32:696–702

81. Owman CH, Edvinsson L, Hardebo JE, Groschel-Stewart U, Unisicker K, Walles B (1977) Immunohistochemical demonstration of actin and myosin in brain capillaries. Acta Neurol Scand 56/Suppl 64:384–385

82. Ponte J, Purves MJ (1974) The role of the carotid body chemoreceptors and carotid sinus baroreceptors in the control of cerebral blood vessels. J Physiol (Lond) 237:115–340

83. Reis DJ, Dampney RAL, Doba NE, Kumada M (1977) Central control of blood pressure: A proposed localization of the 'tonic vasomotor center' of the medulla. In: Arterial Hypertension. ICS 410 Exercerpta Medica, Amsterdam, pp 6–8

84. Reivich M (1964) Arterial Pco_2 and cerebral hemodynamics. Am J Physiol 206:25–35

85. Reivich M, Coburn R, Lahiri S, Chance B (1977) Tissue Hypoxia and Ischaemia. Plenum Press, New York

86. Rennels ML, Nelson E (1975) Capillary innervation in the mammalian central nervous system: An electron microscopic demonstration. Am J Anat 144:233–241

87. Robinson JS, Gray TC (1961) Observations on the cerebral effects of passive hyperventilation. Br J Anaesth 33:62–8

88. Rosendorff C, Mitchell G, Scriven DRL, Shapiro C (1976) Evidence for a dual innervation affecting local blood flow in the hypothalamus of the conscious rabbit. Circ Res 38:140–145

89. Rossen R, Kabat H, Anderson JP (1943) Acute arrest of cerebral circulation in man. Arch Neurol 50:510–28

90. Salanga VD, Waltz AG (1973) Regional cerebral blood flow during stimulation of seventh cranial nerve. Stroke 4:213–217

91. Schmahl FW, Betz E, Dettinger E, Hohorst HJ (1966) Energiestoffweschel der Grosshirnrinde und Elektroencephalogramm bei Sauerstoffmangel. Pflüegers Arch 292:46–59

92. Scremin OU, Rubenstein EH, Sonnenschein RR (1977) Evidence for a cholinergic neurogenic component in the cerebral vasodilatation during hypercapnia in the rabbit. Fed Proc 36:568

93. Sercombe R, Aubineau P, Edvinsson L, Mamo H, Owman CH, Pinard E, Seylaz J (1975) Neurogenic influence on local cerebral blood flow. Neurology (Minneap) 25:954–963

94. Shalit MN, Shimojyo S, Reinmuth OM (1967) Carbon dioxide and cerebral circulatory control. I The extravascular effect. Arch Neurol 17:298–303

95. Siesjö BK, Johansson H, Ljunggren B, Norberg K (1974) Brain dysfunction in cerebral hypoxia and ischaemia. In: Plum F (ed) Brain Dysfunction in Metabolic disorders. Res Publ Assoc Res Nerv Ment Dis Vol 53 Raven Press, New York, pp 75–112

96. Silver IA (1978) Cellular microenvironment in relation to local blood flow. In: Elliott K, O'Connor M (eds) Cerebral vascular smooth muscle and its control, Ciba foundation symposium 56. Elsevier, Amsterdam, pp 49–67

97. Sokoloff L (1971) Neurophysiology and neurochemistry of coma. Exp Biol Med 4:15–33

98. Sokoloff L (1972) Circulation and energy metabolism of the brain. In: Albers RW, Siegel GJ, Katzman R, Agranoff BW (eds) Basic Neurochemistry. Little Brown, Boston, pp 299–325

99. Sokoloff L, Mangold R, Wechsler RL, Kennedy C, Kety SS (1955) The effect of mental arithmetic on cerebral circulation and metabolism. J Clin Invest 34:1101–1108

100. Sokoloff L, Reivich M, Kennedy C, Rosiers Des, Pettigrew KD, Sakurada O, Shinohara M (1977) The ^{14}C deoxyglucose method for the measurement of local cerebral glucose utilization: Theory, procedure and normal values in the conscious and anaesthetized albino rat. J Neurochem 28:897–916

101. Speckmann E-J, Caspers H (1969) Verschiebungen des corticalen Bestand-potentials bei Veranderungen der Ventilationsgrosse. Pflüegers Arch 310:235–250

102. Starlinger H, Lubbers DW (1973) Polarographic measurements of the oxygen pressure performed simultaneously with optical measurements of the redox state of the respiratory chain in suspensions of mitochondria under steady-state conditions of low oxygen tensions. Pflüegers Arch 341:15–22

103. Stromberg DD, Fox JR (1972) Pressures in the pial arterial microcirculation of the cat during changes in systemic arterial blood pressure. Circ Res 31:229–239

104. Sugar O, Gerard RW (1938) Anoxia and brain potentials. J Neurophysiol 1:558–70

105. Tenney SM, Ou LC (1970) Physiological evidence for increased tissue capillary in rats acclimatized to high altitude. Respir Physiol 8:137–150

106. Ter-Pogossian MM, Eichling JO, Davis DO, Welch MJ (1970) The measure *in vivo* of regional cerebral oxygen utilization by means of oxyhemoglobin labelled with radioactive oxygen-15. J Clin Invest 49:381–91

107. Ter-Pogossian, Davis MM, Eichling JO, Carter CC (1971) Regional cerebral oxygen metabolism and regional cerebral blood flow compartments measured by means of oxygen-15 in patients with cerebral abnormalities. In: Toole JT, Janeway R (eds) Seventh Conference on Cerebral Vascular Diseases. Grune and Stratton, New York, pp 103–8

108. Thorn W (1965) 'Der Phosphocreatingehalt des unbelasteten und des ischämischen Gehirns' Pflüegers Arch 285:331–4

109. Ungerstedt U (1971) Stereotaxic mapping of the monoamine pathways in the rat brain. Acta Physiol Scand [Suppl] 367:1–48

110. Wahl M, Deetjen P, Thurau K, Ingvar DH, Lassen NA (1970) Micropuncture evaluation of the importance of perivascular pH for the arteriolar diameter on the brain surface. Pflüegers Arch 316:152–163

111. Wasserman AJ, Patterson JL (1961) The cerebrovascular response to reduction in arterial carbon dioxide tension. J Clin Invest 40:1297–1303

112. Wolff HG, Lennox WG (1930) Cerebral circulation: Effect on pial vessels of variations in the O_2 and CO_2 content of blood. Arch Neurol 23:1097–1120

113. Wollman H, Alexander SC, Cohen PJ, Smith TC, Chase PE, Molen van der RA (1965) Cerebral circulation during general anaesthesia and hyperventilation in man. Anaesthesiology 26:329–34

114. Yoshida K, Meyer JS, Sakamoto K, Honda J (1966) Autoregulation of cerebral blood flow: Electromagnetic flow measurements during acute hypertension in the monkey. Circ Res 19:726–738

Chapter 8

Regulation of Body Temperature in Man

D. Emslie-Smith, I. Lightbody, and D. Maclean

Heat balance

Enzymes operate at optimal temperatures, and that is presumably the reason why the body temperature of homeotherms is kept within such narrow limits: a rise of 6°C seems always to lead to death [71]. If man is to remain in thermal equilibrium, the heat gained by his body must balance its losses (Table 8.1).

A simple heat balance equation for a man in thermal equilibrium would be:

$$M \pm R \pm C \pm K \pm E = 0,$$

where M is heat production from metabolism plus that from any work performed; R is the heat of radiation as either a gain or a loss from a heat source or to the surroundings; C is the heat of convection; K is that of conduction; and E is that of evaporation. To fulfil the first law of thermodynamics, or the second, applied physiologically, the summation of these terms must equal the energy stored as heat, but man stores heat only briefly after exercise or while lying in a hot bath and before mechanisms for dissipating heat become effective [75]: a man in thermal equilibrium stores no heat. Further accounts of the laws of heat flow to and from animals and man have been given by Monteith [61] and

Table 8.1. The heat balance of man

Heat gains	Heat losses
Metabolic	*Cutaneous vasodilatation*
Basal metabolism	Convection:
Specific dynamic action	Ambient temperature
(food)	Currents in air (and
Non-shivering thermogenesis	water during
Physical exercise	immersion)
Shivering	
Radiation	*Radiation* (long-wave)
Short-wave from sun	To surroundings and
Long-wave from	sky
surroundings	
	Conduction
	Immersion in cold
	water
Ingestion	*Evaporation*
Hot food and drink	Insensible water loss
Ventilation	Thermoregulatory
Hot climates	sweating
	Ventilation (panting)

Reduction of heat loss	Reduction of heat gain
Behaviour	*Behaviour*
Clothing	Reduction of clothing
Artificial heating	Increased radiative
	body surface
	Cooler environment
Vasoconstriction of skin	
(Pilo-erection)	

Colin et al. [17]. A recent general review of thermoregulation in man is that of Noak [68].

Mechanisms for heat gain

Man gains heat mostly from metabolic sources, at rest, during exercise and while shivering.

Metabolic mechanisms

The human body's daily energy production from ordinary metabolism amounts to about 13 MJ (3000 kcal). At least 95% of this is in the form of heat, which must be lost if the body temperature is not to rise. Much of this heat is produced in working skeletal muscles, but oxidative metabolism of the resting human body produces about 300 kJ (70 kcal) per hour. Apart from skeletal muscle, the tissues of the liver and other intra-abdominal organs and the brain are the most active sites of heat production. The brain is particularly important in the newborn, because of its relatively large size. Heat is steadily produced by resting man even in the fasting state (basal metabolism), and extra metabolic heat is produced after meals (diet-induced thermogenesis, DIT). The regulation of heat production at cellular level has been reviewed by Hochachka [44], Himms-Hagen [43], and Newsholme [67].

Non-shivering thermogenesis

If thermogenesis, or the metabolic rate, is plotted against the ambient temperature, a curve similar to those in Figs. 8.1 and 8.7 is obtained. At temperatures below the 'critical' temperature, where the metabolic rate rises and shivering may be induced, thermogenesis can be represented as in Fig. 8.1. Some non-shivering thermogenesis (NST) is obligatory, in the sense that it forms part of basal metabolism, but some is thermoregulatory. Usually the term 'non-shivering thermogenesis' is used to denote the thermoregulatory component, but NST, shivering, and voluntary skeletal muscle activity are additive in their contribution to total body heat production. The main mechanisms controlling NST as a response to a cold environment are shown in Fig. 8.2.

Brown adipose tissue

Brown adipose tissue (BAT) is histologically and functionally different from ordinary white adipose tissue. It is prominent and very important in newborn and young infants, in whom it is present in subcutaneous deposits between the scapulae, around the neck, and in the axillae, and in deep deposits behind the sternum and around the spine, the aorta, and the kidneys. These deposits are highly vascular and in infants the venous drainage of the interscapular sheet of BAT drains via vertebral plexuses to the azygos vein [49], in which the temperature of

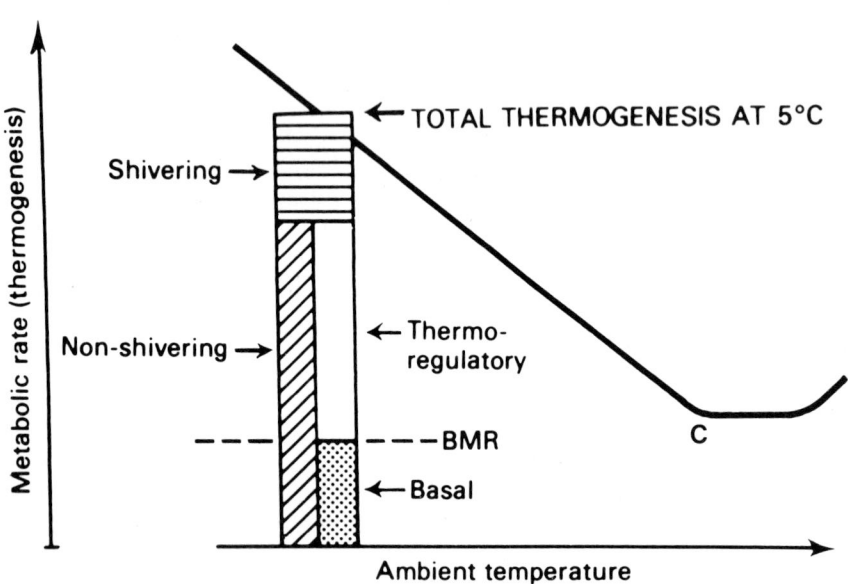

Fig. 8.1. Non-shivering thermogenesis. C, critical temperature. (Adapted from Hayward [35]) (*From Maclean and Emslie-Smith [57] by permission*)

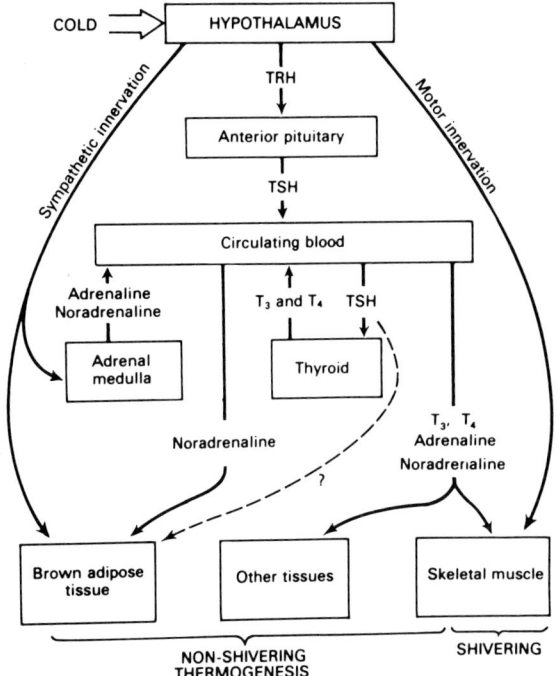

Fig. 8.2. Schema illustrating the main mechanisms of thermogenesis. (Modified from Hardy [34] and Doniach [26].) (*From Maclean and Emslie-Smith [57] by permission*)

blood may be 0.6°C higher than that in the vena cava [79]. Whereas white fat acts in thermoregulation like an insulating blanket, brown fat is actively thermogenic and may be regarded as like an electric blanket.

In the brown adipose cell many small vacuoles of fat are surrounded by many large mitochondria, so that the organelles of cellular oxidation lie close to the source of fuel. The overall system that controls the production of heat by BAT probably involves both nervous and humeral mechanisms. Cutaneous cold receptors send impulses to the hypothalamic temperature-regulating centres, which then relay impulses along sympathetic nerves whose endings release noradrenaline in the BAT. The noradrenaline stimulates the production of cAMP, which activates a lipase that splits triglyceride molecules into glycerol and free fatty acids. The BAT does not release from the cell the fatty acids produced by lipolysis. Most of them are re-synthesized to triglyceride or oxidized to CO_2 and H_2O inside the cell. The biochemical cycle turns the energy of chemical bonds into the energy of heat. The oxidative capacity of BAT may exceed that of heart muscle [25].

Brown adipose tissue plays an extremely important part in the thermal regulation of the newborn human infant, but until recently it was thought to play little part in later life in man. It may be depleted of lipid in hypothermic, malnourished children and old people [14, 36]. Recently, however, it has been suggested that BAT may still be important in the adult, possibly controlling NST and DIT and preventing the development of obesity [70].

Exercise

Skeletal muscle makes up about 50% of the body mass. At rest it contributes only about 20% of the heat production, but during activity it may increase its production of heat by ten times.

Shivering

When a resting man is exposed to cold, muscular tone increases in distal parts (thermal muscular tone or preshivering tone), which can increase the basal heat production by 50%–100%. When this increased muscle tone moves proximally, visible shivering develops and reaches its peak in 15–30 min. Shivering can increase metabolism by as much as 2–5 times [47], but the resulting increase in temperature is not maintained because of the heat loss by convection and the loss of insulation caused by the movements of the body. Heat produced by shivering and by exercise are not additive: shivering is inhibited by exercise [6] and the increase of blood flow in peripheral parts increases the rate of heat loss. There is some evidence that repeated exposure to cold can reduce the threshold of shivering in man [24].

Radiation

Man, like all objects containing heat, emits electromagnetic radiation in the infra-red range with wavelengths between 3.0 and 100 μm ('long wave' infra-red) and, irrespective of the colour of his skin, radiates heat to nearby solid objects rather than to the surrounding air, which is a comparatively poor heat absorber. Heat loss and heat gain by radiation are not uniform: some parts of the body can be warmed by absorbing radiant heat from the sun or a fire, while other parts may be cooled by the radiation of heat to a cold object, such as a window or the unclouded sky. The amount of heat lost is dependent upon the area of skin exposed. The naked body has an effective radiating surface of about 85% of its total surface area because surfaces such as the inner aspects of the thighs radiate to each other, rather than to the environment. Heat loss from radiation is greatest when the naked body is spreadeagled and least when it is huddled up in the fetal position.

Ingestion

The ingestion of physically hot food and drink leads to a temporary heat gain irrespective of the metabolic effect from any nutrient (DIT).

Mechanisms for reduction of heat loss

Behaviour

Man is really a tropical animal who, for various reasons, has often chosen to live in cold places. He maintains his heat balance chiefly by avoiding cold through intelligent behaviour, which includes the choice of local environment and appropriate clothing, by the use of artificially produced heat (fires, central heating), by taking exercise and, in the ultimate resort, by huddling up to reduce radiative and convective heat loss.

Cutaneous vasoconstriction

If, by his intelligence, man cannot manage to exist in a thermoneutral environment, he automatically protects his deep body temperature from change by first a fine, and then a coarse, mechanism. The fine mechanism is cutaneous vasoconstriction, which reduces the heat conductance of the body's 'shell' (see below). When vasoconstriction is complete, he produces heat by involuntary shivering [15]. Cutaneous vasoconstriction, and the reduction of blood velocity caused by increased viscosity induced by cold, both reduce the transfer of heat from deep tissues ('core') to the surface, thereby reducing the loss of heat by radiation and convection.

Mechanisms for heat loss

Cutaneous vasodilatation

The loss of heat from the skin by radiation, convection, conduction, and evaporation is greatly influenced by environmental conditions, such as the ambient temperature, relative humidity and air movements, being greatest, for example, when the weather is cool, dry and windy. It also depends on the heat conductance of the skin, which is controlled by the skin blood flow. Cutaneous vasodilatation can increase the superficial blood flow to as much as 100 times the minimum, thereby virtually abolishing the gradient between the deep tissues and the surface and allowing a greater loss of heat. Most of the heat produced by a man who is not sweating is lost by convection and radiation. Only during immersion in cold water is heat loss by conduction usually important. Alterations in skin conductance caused by cutaneous vasodilatation and vasoconstriction are considered below.

Evaporation

When the thermal conductance of the body reaches its maximum, with maximal cutaneous vasodilatation, and the ambient temperature still exceeds the body temperature, heat can no longer be lost passively by conduction, convection and radiation, but only through the evaporation of water. Powerful physiological mechanisms involving metabolic work then lead to cooling by evaporation [58]. At least 20% of man's total heat loss is the result of evaporation of water, about two-thirds from the surface of the skin and about one third from the respiratory tract. Respiratory loss is particularly important during MV for surgery under general anaesthesia [72]. In a thermoneutral environment man does not sweat, but water vapour diffuses continually through the skin without wetting it; this 'insensible perspiration' accounts for about 25% of the evaporated loss. This, together with the water loss from the respiratory tract, is called the 'insensible water loss' and amounts to about 30 g water every hour, of which every gram evaporated allows the loss of about 2.45 kJ (0.59 kcal).

There are two kinds of sweating. Emotional sweating develops all over the body, the amount of water lost being proportional only to the density of sweat glands in different areas of skin [1]. Conditions of stress or alertness cause emotional sweating, which can, of course, lower the body temperature but is not primarily thermoregulatory. Thermoregulatory sweating involves the evaporation of large amounts of water and is responsible for a major cooling effect on the body. Sympathetic neurones from the anterior hypothalamus synapse in the lateral horn of the first thoracic to second lumbar segments of the spinal cord and then run to the eccrine sweat glands. The post-ganglionic neurones release acetylcholine to these glands [69]. The water in sweat is derived from the blood, and rapid sweating demands a high skin blood flow. Sweat glands release a bradykinin-like polypeptide in the sweat, which in turn produces further vasodilatation. Thermoregulatory sweating begins on the dorsum of the foot and appears progressively up the legs, on the trunk, and lastly on the arms, hands, and brow.

When the ambient temperature is very high, the eccrine sweat glands are capable of producing over 4 litres dilute salt solution per hour. So long as the relative humidity and movement of the ambient air allow it, the water in sweat evaporates on the skin and reduces the skin temperature. Thermoregulatory sweating usually does not occur in man below an ambient temperature of about 29°C, but strenuous exercise in heavy clothing can cause profuse sweating. A circadian rhythm of sweating in man, different from that of core body temperature, has been suggested by Timbal et al. [76] and Wenger et al. [78], but the subject is compli-cated by the fact that sweating is reduced during REM (rapid eye movement) sleep [40 73].

Patients unable to produce and evaporate sweat, for example those with ectodermal dysplasia or quadriplegia are intolerant of heat [77].

Mechanisms for reduction of heat gain

Man reduces unnecessary heat gain by intelligent behaviour (reducing clothing and moving into the shade or an artificially cooled environment).

Some of these relationships between heat production and loss and the deep body temperature of a homeotherm are schematized in Fig. 8.3, which gives a good illustration of different zones and the relationships of various trends.

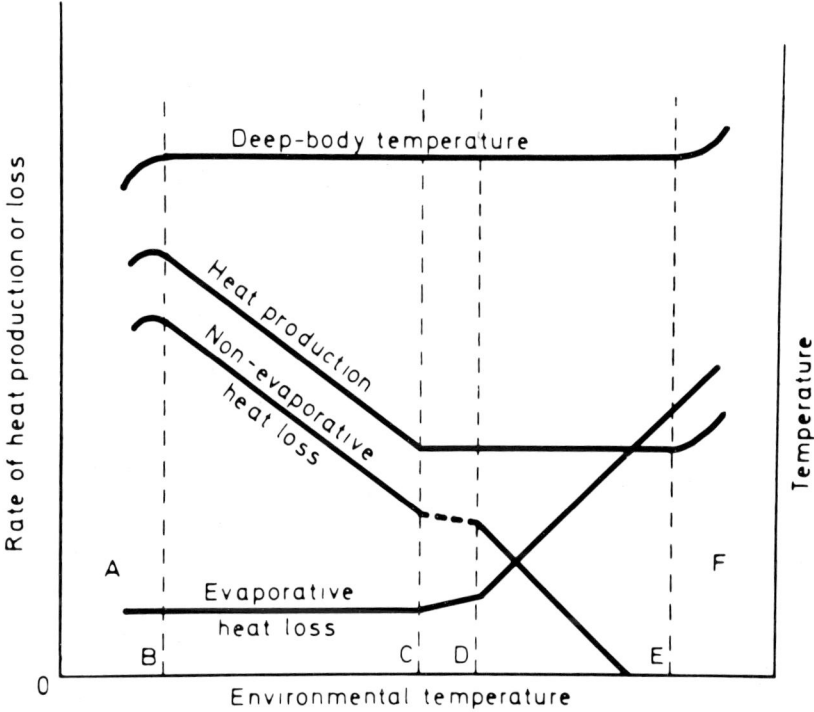

Fig. 8.3. Schematic representation of relationships between heat production, evaporative and non-evaporative heat loss and deep body temperature in a homeothermic animal, resting but free to move in a metabolic chamber where the air and mean radiant temperatures are equal to each other, convection is free and relative humidity is kept at 50%. (A) zone of hypothermia; (B) temperature of peak metabolism and incipient hypothermia; (C) critical temperature, ('lower critical temperature' in Fig. 8.7); (D) temperature of marked rise in evaporative heat loss; (E) temperature of incipient hyperthermal rise, ('upper critical temperature' in Fig. 7); (F) zone of hyperthermia; (CD) zone of least thermoregulatory effort; (CE) zone of minimal metabolism, ('thermoneutrality' in Fig. 8.7); (BE) thermoregulatory range. (From Mount [62]) (*From Maclean and Emslie-Smith* [57], *by permission*)

Co-ordination of heat gain and loss

Central regulation

A thermoregulating mechanism centrally based in the human nervous system is suggested by the great precision with which deep body temperature is kept about 37°C and also by the fact that both brain damage and drugs (such as psychotropic agents) that act centrally can modify or even abolish normal thermoregulation. Over the last 20 years thermal physiologists have been increasingly concerned with the construction of theoretical models involving the concepts of systems control. Essential features of a thermoregulatory control system are thermoreceptors that relay afferent signals to a central mechanism which somehow starts the efferent regulatory mechanisms that will keep the central body temperature as close as possible to the optimal. Any such control system would have to include two different afferent signals, changes in the temperature of arterial blood perfusing the brain and nervous impulses from the thermoreceptors. The first and simplest models involved the concept of a hypothalamic thermostat with an on–off control, which compared the temperature at the receptor sites with the central 'set-point' temperature. This concept of the set-point has now been called in question and alternative suggestions, such as servomechanisms, have been proposed [48]. The controversy has been well discussed by Bligh [13].

Many hypothetical 'circuit diagrams' of thermoregulation have been proposed, some comparatively simple, some exceedingly complicated with multiple feedbacks. The basic facts, however, are that in and around the hypothalamus at least three types of nerve cell have been identified. Some cells are specifically sensitive to temperature and act as sensors of the temperature of blood perfusing the hypothalamus: some cells fire when the temperature rises, others fire when the temperature falls. A second group of cells, when stimulated, sends impulses to the organs and tissues involved in the gain or loss of heat. Between these sensor and activator cells are cells of the third kind, which receive impulses from the sensors in the hypothalamus and elsewhere (mainly the skin) and in some way excite or inhibit the activators of the peripheral mechanisms for heat loss or gain [27].

A powerful proponent of the earlier, simpler concepts was Benzinger [8, 10, 11]. His conclusions were based on a great deal of experimental evidence recorded in man by the techniques of gradient layer calorimetry [10] and tympanic membrane thermometry [11]. Benzinger's concepts are not now fully accepted by many thermal physiologists, partly because of their 'uncompromising simplicity'. Fox [32] has provided a useful review of controversies about temperature regulation in man.

Whatever the mechanism, it does seem that hypothalamic thermoregulation is carried out *as if* there were a thermostat and set-point [46]; further, just because of the extreme simplicity of Benzinger's model, it may still prove the most practically useful one for clinicians.

Peripheral thermoreceptors are present in the skin all over the body and in the upper part of the gastrointestinal tract [42]. It is possible that two sets of receptors with similar response characteristics are connected with different effector systems. Both sorts send impulses to the afferent sensory nervous in-flow; one pathway carries impulses through the thalamo-cortical system to the cortex, producing a conscious sensation of cold, while the other runs to a group of cells in the posterior part of the hypothalamus. When this part of the hypothalamus is damaged experimentally, an animal cannot conserve heat when in the cold, but loses heat normally when it is in a warm environment. This area has been called the 'heat maintenance centre' or 'heat production and conservation centre'. In the pre-optic region of the anterior part of the hypothalamus (POAH) near the optic chiasma and internal carotid artery, there is another group of cells, the 'heat loss centre'. Experimental lesions of this area in an animal deprive it of its ability to lose heat in a hot environment, but leave intact its ability to maintain its normal temperature in a cold environment. Receptors sensitive to heat have been demonstrated in this site [37, 38]. Some receptor cells begin to fire at hypothalamic temperatures lower than the set-point, and Benzinger believes that their afferent pathway leads to the posterior centre, conveying inhibiting impulses from the anterior hypothalamic centre ('central warmth inhibition') (Fig. 8.4). Other cells in the anterior centre fire only at about the set-point temperature and give rise to pathways that initiate sweating.

Benzinger believes that the centre in the POAH acts as the 'temperature eye' of the body, the central sensory organ that ultimately controls all the thermoregulatory mechanisms, be they automatic or behavioural. He believes, too,

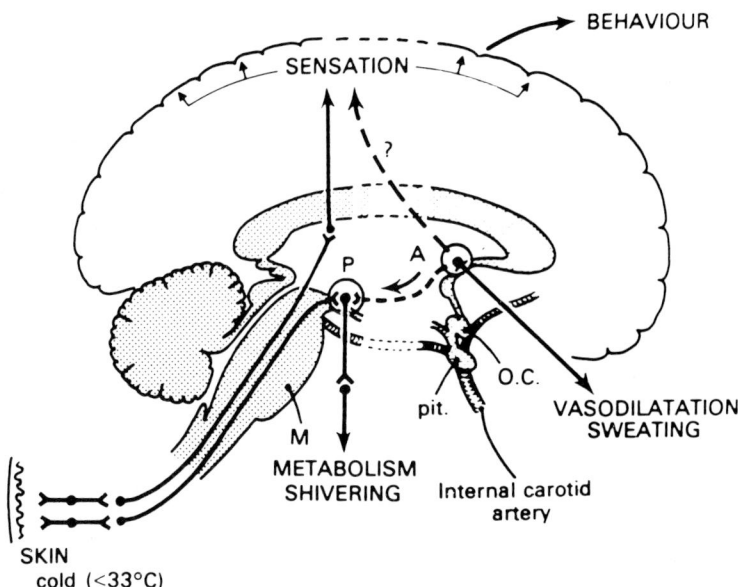

Fig. 8.4. Left-hand half of a sagittal section of human brain viewed from the mid-line, showing the medulla (*M*), the pituitary (*pit*), the optic chiasma (*O. C.*) and the internal carotid artery supplying the hypothalamus which is shown as split in the coronal plane for diagrammatic purposes. The two temperature regulating 'centres' are shown in the anterior (*A*) and posterior (*P*) hypothalamus, together with neural connections believed to be involved in thermoregulation. (Modified from Benzinger [9]). (*From Maclean and Emslie-Smith [57] by permission*)

that the posterior hypothalamic centre controls the mechanisms for metabolic heat production, including increases in metabolic thermogenesis and shivering, while the anterior centre sends afferent impulses via the sympathetic nervous system to control the mechanisms of heat loss—skin vasodilatation and sweating. He also thought that the anterior centre responded to warming by sending inhibitory impulses to the posterior centre when the temperature of the anterior centre reached a level of about 1°C below the temperature at which sweating was induced. The results of Benzinger's very elegant experiments on intact man [8] can well be interpreted as demonstrating something akin to a set-point in the human thermostat (Fig. 8.5). This set-point varies between different individuals and in the same individual at different times, at different ages, and in different states of physical well-being. It was estimated to average 36.7°C in the seven Mercury astronauts.

According to Benzinger's hypothesis, metabolic heat production in man is excited by the cold receptors of the skin and inhibited by the excitation of central warmth receptors stimulated by the temperature of blood in the perfusing internal carotid artery. When the intracranial temperature falls below the set-point, the metabolic response to cold is released. Metabolic thermogenesis is impaired when either the posterior centre is destroyed or the anterior

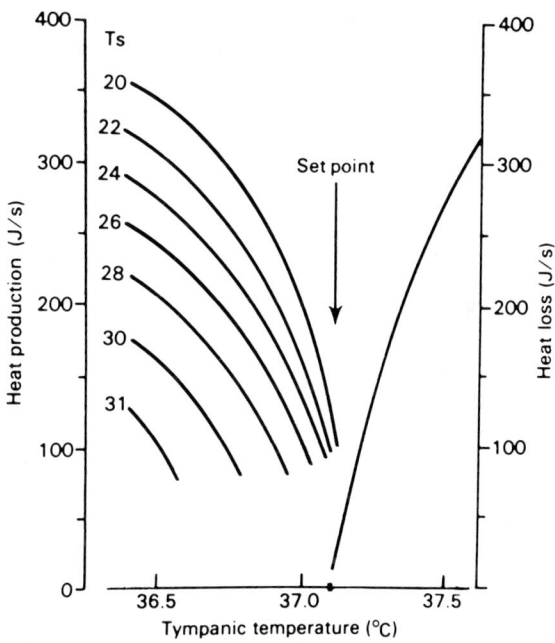

Fig. 8.5. Heat loss and heat production measured in the same subject. The central set-point is shown as 37.1°C. Above the set-point, at skin temperatures of 33 to 37.5°C. sweat loss rose to about 2 gallons per day; below the set-point, at skin temperatures (*Ts*) of 20 to 33°C metabolic heat production rose four-fold. (Adapted from Benzinger [8]) (*From Maclean and Emslie-Smith [57] by permission*)

centre is warmed beyond the set-point. Warmth impulses from the anterior centre then inhibit the reflex response to cold reception from skin at the posterior centre.

Although most interest has centred on the POAH as the principal site of central thermoregulation, some physiologists believe that the whole brain stem, from the POAH to the caudal hypothalamus, acts as sensor, integrator, and activator [80]. The rôle of the hippocampus and reticular formation was discussed by Horowitz et al. [46], while Simon [74] fully reviewed that of the spinal cord.

Endogenous chemical transmitters

Experiments in animals suggest that the set-point is controlled by various chemical substances [21]. There is a fairly high concentration of both noradrenaline and 5-hydroxytryptamine (5-HT) in the hypothalamus. The injection of these substances into the anterior hypothalamus causes rises and falls in body temperature, which vary in different species [36, 59]. Simple ions also seem to affect the set-point. In some animals a raised sodium ion concentration in the posterior hypothalamus raises the body temperature, whereas a raised calcium concentration produces a fall in body temperature or blocks the hyperthermia of exercise [59, 65, 66]. Sometimes the rise in body temperature produced by high sodium concentration is counteracted by the presence of calcium ions, the so-called calcium brake. Myers [63] has suggested that the balance between sodium and calcium ions determines the 'ionic set-point', but others, for example Hellon [39], consider that the present evidence for this idea is insufficient. Feldberg [29] found that the injection of prostaglandin E_1 into the third ventricles of the species that differ in their responses to 5-HT and monoamines causes a rise in temperature. He and others have suggested that this prostaglandin may be the common 'mediator' for raising temperature and may itself be released by pyrogens [30, 31, 39, 60]. In the cat, at least, its site of action seems to be the anterior hypothalamus. Hellon [39] considers that so far there is no evidence that the synthesis and release of prostaglandins play any part in normal temperature regulation in the absence of pyrogens. Leucocyte pyrogen causes fever when injected into the anterior hypothalamus, but not elsewhere [18]. Feldberg has suggested that it does so by removing the calcium brake, but it is uncertain whether or not the action of pyrogens causes a real change in the set-point [39].

Other substances such as dopamine, histamine, acetycholine, and thyrotrophin-releasing hormone (TRH) may also be implicated in the mediation of temperature regulation in animals [22, 56, 59, 64], but because of an almost total lack of understanding of neuronal circuitry and species-specificity, and of technical difficulties, there is a great deal of uncertainty about these ideas and their application to man is only conjectural [39].

The rise of temperature that accompanies ovulation may be the result of a raising of the set-point by progesterone acting through the anterior pituitary [41]. Figure 8.6 is based on one by Bligh [12], who has summarized various factors thought to influence the set-point and offered an explanation of the way in which thermoregulation is affected.

Central thermoregulatory responses and the circadian rhythm of temperature are disturbed in Wernicke's encephalopathy, but improve following successful treatment with thiamine [55]. The situation is less clear in anorexia nervosa, where loss of body fat seems to be a more important influence on thermoregulation than any loss of central control [23].

Effect of drugs

The narcotic analgesics have been shown consistently and in many species to influence body temperature profoundly [2]. Less well known is the fact that phenothiazines, apart from their better known effect of producing hypothermia, can, in hot environments, cause hyperthermia [28]. In rats, at least, beta-endorphin may act like morphine in affecting temperature regulation [45].

Peripheral regulation

Central thermoregulation in the brain initiates mechanisms that act peripherally, mainly through the autonomic nervous system, but also to some extent by way of the CNS, e.g., nerves supplying skeletal muscle. This peripheral thermoregulation is centred on the thermal conductivity of the skin, which is dependent on changes in cutaneous blood flow.

Thermal conductance

The thermal conductance of man is the rate of

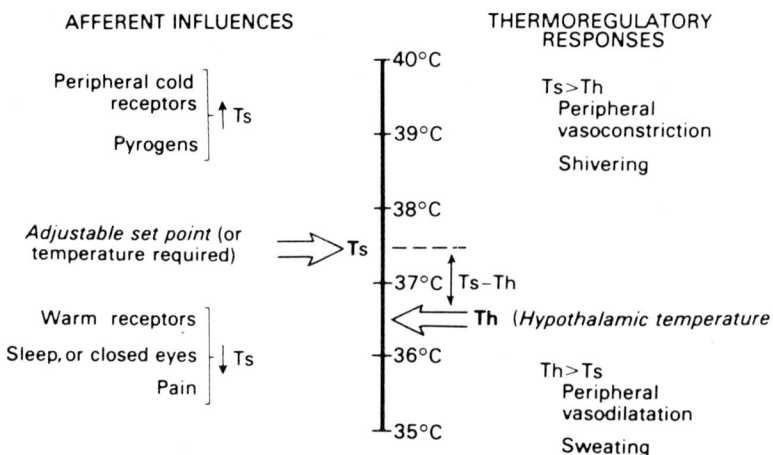

Fig. 8.6. Diagrammatic representation of the set-point theory of central thermoregulation based on the assumption that responses are controlled by and proportional to the difference between the set-point temperature (*Ts*) and the temperature of the hypothalamus (*Th*). (Adapted from Bligh [12]) (*From Maclean and Emslie-Smith [57] by permission*)

change of heat per centigrade degree difference in temperature between that of his body and his surroundings. It is very variable, being controlled by many thermoregulatory mechanisms, which are subject to continual short-term adjustments to allow him to remain in thermal balance. A homeotherm such as man can vary his thermal conductance rapidly by redistribution of blood flow without increasing his metabolic rate over a range of environmental temperatures, which is loosely regarded as his thermoneutral zone (TNZ). The lower temperature at which such metabolically inexpensive changes in thermal conductance can no longer maintain thermal equilibrium is known as his 'critical temperature', and below this he must increase his rate of thermogenesis. Most homeotherms increase their metabolism in a roughly linear manner, so that at about the critical temperature the thermal conductance is virtually minimal and constant. When faced with a rising ambient temperature, both body temperature and metabolic rate remain steady throughout the TNZ, so the thermal conductance must increase to reach its maximum just below the functional temperature of the body to allow heat to be lost to the environment. When the ambient temperature exceeds the body temperature, however, heat cannot any longer be passively lost by radiation, convection, and conduction, but only through the evaporation of water, such as sweating and panting. These activities involve metabolic work which is reflected in an increase in the rate of O_2 consumption (Fig. 8.7).

In man there are circadian rhythms in both the core-to-air conductance and the core-to-

skin conductance. In addition to this circadian rhythm of heat loss, different regions of the body behave in a different manner. For example, as the ambient temperature progressively

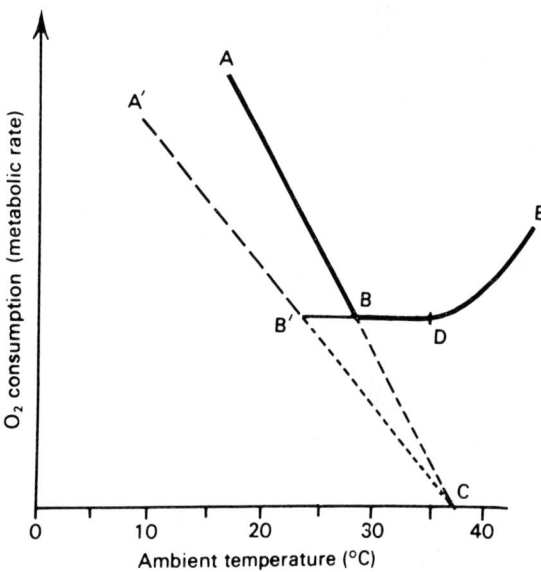

Fig. 8.7. Diagram to show the classical concept of thermoneutrality. (Compare with Fig. 8.3). Over the temperature range BD heat production remains constant and minimal (thermoneutral zone); below B (lower critical temperature) and above D (upper critical temperature) it rises: BA is linear, DE is not. The length of the zone of thermoneutrality (BD or B′D) is greater when body insulation is greater: below B (or B′) insulation can no longer conserve heat, so metabolism increases at a rate proportional to the gradient between the core body temperature and the ambient temperature. The line AB extrapolates to core temperature (C) at zero metabolism; the greater the insulation the flatter will be its slope (A′B′). E denotes evaporation. (*From Maclean and Emslie-Smith [57] by permission*)

falls, there seems to be no control over heat loss from the brow, but heat loss from the trunk, arms, and thighs steadily increases [5].

Cutaneous blood flow

Core and shell

A useful, simple concept suggests that in man the body contains a warm, central core within which the temperature remains almost constant, and a more peripheral shell through whose tissues there are various temperature gradients [3, 19]. The central core contains most of the vital organs and a variable amount of the deeper tissues of the limbs. Homeothermic animals like man normally maintain a core temperature higher than that of the ambient air, but heat is lost to the environment from the surface of the skin, which thus becomes cool, producing a temperature gradient between the core and skin surface which is varied by changes in the thermal conductance of the skin by alterations in blood flow. Figure 8.8 shows the effect of different ambient temperatures on the size of the core and the altered temperature gradients.

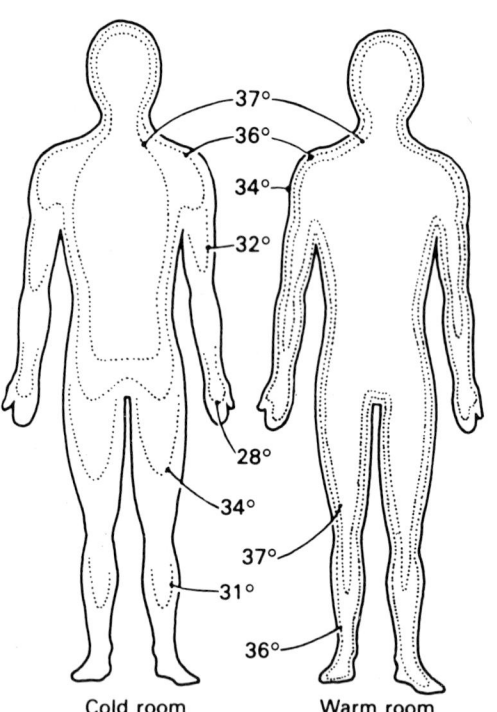

Fig. 8.8. Schematic representation of temperature gradients (°C) forming a 'core' and 'shell' in a man in a cold and warm environment. (Adapted from Aschoff and Wever [3]) (*From Maclean and Emslie-Smith* [57] *by permission*)

Vasoconstriction

The arteriolar and venous blood flow in skin can be so reduced that the thermal conductivity of the outside inch of the body becomes as low as that of cork. This lowered conductivity reduces the transfer of heat from the core to the surface so that the surface of the skin cools and less heat is lost by convection and radiation. Much of this vasoconstriction is mediated by sympathetic vasoconstrictor nerves that release noradrenaline in arteriolar smooth muscle. In addition, cold has a direct constrictor action on denervated arteries.

Vasodilatation

Relaxation of vasoconstrictor tone, and in some parts, e.g., the forearms, specific vasodilator impulses bring about cutaneous vasodilatation. The superficial blood flow may increase to as much as 100 times the minimum flow, virtually abolishing the gradient between the core and the surface and allowing a greater heat loss by convection and radiation from the skin because of its higher surface temperature.

Cold-induced vasodilatation

Cold-induced vasodilatation (CIVD) is a 'hunting' reaction in cutaneous vessels of fingers exposed to very cold water [54]. When the cold is severe enough to damage the skin the vasoconstriction induced by cold gives way to periodic episodes of vasodilatation with cyclical alterations in skin blood flow lasting about 20 min. The vasodilatation is greatest in the digits and serves to preserve fingers from cold injury. It is particularly noticeable in people who work in cold conditions, such as Eskimos, deep sea fishermen, and fish filleters [16]. However, during immersion of the body in cold water, CIVD may produce an adverse effect by increasing heat loss. Keatinge [52] has stated that even fat men, when immersed in water at 5°C, lose so much heat from CIVD that after 40 min they can no longer maintain their core temperature.

The mechanism of cold vasodilatation is still uncertain: cold-induced paralysis of the vascular smooth muscle may block neural and humoral vasoconstriction mechanisms [51]; there is also evidence to suggest that CIVD may be induced by bradykinin in a system involving the activation and inactivation of the enzyme, kininogenase, operating at a critical temperature of 15°C [50].

Temperature and energy exchange in man

Hardy et al. [33] studied the effects of ambient temperature on the energy exchange of resting unacclimatized nude male subjects. The graphs reproduced in Fig. 8.9 represent trend averages after 1 h exposure at each particular ambient temperature with the relative humidity between 40% and 60%. The measurements of 'metabolism' and 'evaporative loss' and of skin and internal body temperatures were all directly recorded. From these direct measurements the other relationships were derived.

Cold adaptation

The details of adaptation to chronic exposure to cold are beyond the scope of this review. Adaptation in animals occurs at cellular level and the endocrine system plays an important role in modulating these changes. The peripheral circulatory regulation of heat conservation and heat loss does change, as may central thermoregulatory mechanisms, but the applic-

ability of these observations to man remains largely untested [20].

Body temperatures

There is no single 'body temperature'. Temperatures recorded directly from the mouth and the axilla are too much influenced by the ambient temperature to be of great value in experimental work. The oesophageal temperature is technically harder to measure but it is likely to give a truer indication of the core temperature, and it reacts quickly to changes. The rectal temperature may be influenced by bacterial metabolism in the colon or by the temperature of blood returning from the legs, and its response to either cooling or heating of the body is slow compared with that of other 'deep' body temperatures. A fast response to such changes is shown by recordings made from the tympanic membrane [7]. It has been suggested that the tympanic membrane temperature is likely to be the nearest to that of the blood perfusing the hypothalamus, because both the tympanic membrane and the hypothalamus are supplied by branches from the internal carotid artery.

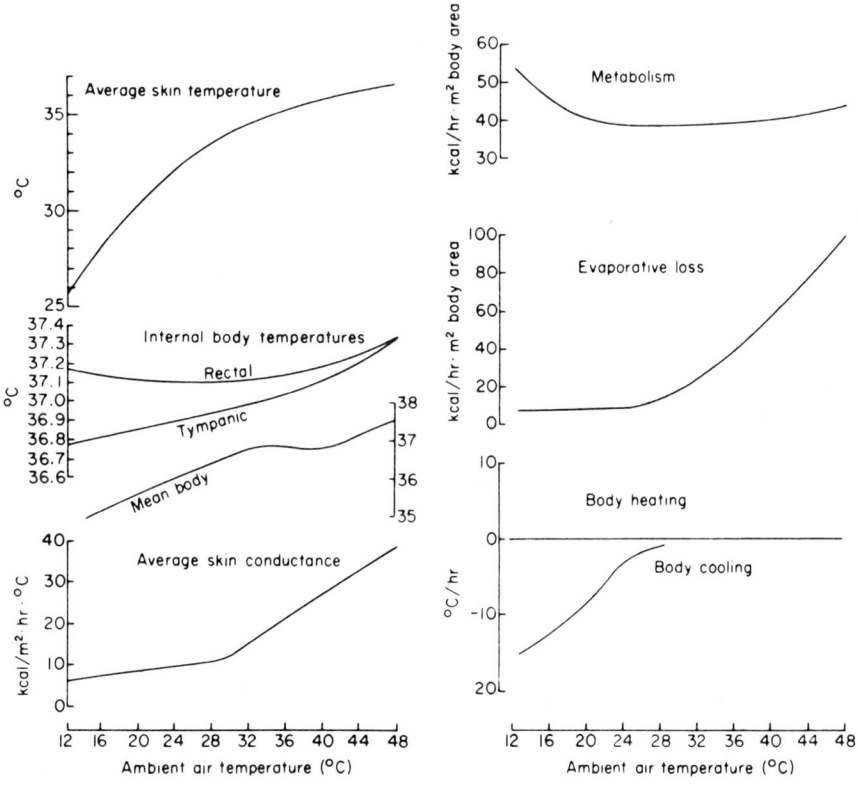

Fig. 8.9. Thermoregulatory responses of unclothed, quietly resting male subjects to ambient temperatures of 12 to 48°C, in still air, and at low relative humidity. (From Hardy et al. [33]). (*From Maclean and Emslie-Smith [57] by permission*)

Temperatures recorded from the external auditory meatus and not from the tympanic membrane itself are much less accurate, unless they are automatically and continuously corrected to eliminate the component derived from the temperature of the skin of the external auditory meatus [53].

There is a circadian rhythm in the core temperature of man: it is lowest at about 5 a.m. and highest at about 8 p.m., the range of variation being greatest in children and averaging about 1.5 deg C in men and 1.2 deg C in women. The rhythm is usually locked to daylight and darkness but men isolated from information about time and daylight develop a free-running periodic variation, usually varying between 24 and 26 h and unassociated with other rhythms such as sleep and activity [4].

The surface temperature of the body varies not only from place to place, but at different times of the day according to the skin blood flow. Various 'weightings' of skin temperatures have been suggested from which to estimate a 'mean skin temperature', but the very fact that different workers employ different formulae implies that none is generally regarded as satisfactory. The same is true of attempts to include the core temperature in such formulae to identify a so-called mean body temperature [71].

References

1. Allen JA, Armstrong JE, Roddie IC (1973) The regional distribution of emotional sweating in man. J Physiol (Lond) 235:749–759
2. Ary M, Lomax P (1979) Influence of narcotic agents on temperature regulation in neurochemical mechanisms of opiates and endorphins. In: Loh HH, Ross DH (eds) Advances in biochemistry and psychopharmacology, vol 20. Raven Press, New York
3. Aschoff J, Wever R (1958) Kern und Schale im Wärmehaushalt des Menschen. Naturwissenschaften 20:477–485
4. Aschoff J, Gerecke U, Wever R (1967) Desynchronization of human circadian rhythms. Jpn J Physiol 17:450–457
5. Aschoff J, Biebach H, Heise A, Schmidt T (1974) Day-night variation in heat balance. In: Monteith JL, Mount LE (eds) Heat loss from animals and man. Butterworths, London, pp 147–172
6. Bartholomew GA (1968) Body temperature and energy metabolism. In: Gordon MS, Bartholomew GA, Grinnell Jørgensen CB, White FN (eds) Animal function: Principles and adaptations. Macmillan, New York, pp 290–354
7. Benzinger TH (1959) On physical heat regulation and the sense of temperature in man. Proc Natl Acad Sci USA 45:645–659
8. Benzinger TH (1969) Heat regulation: homeostasis of central temperature in man. Physiol Rev 49:671–759
9. Benzinger TH (1970) Peripheral cold reception and central warm reception, sensory mechanisms of behavioural and autonomic thermostasis. In: Hardy JD, Gagge AP, Stolwijk JAJ (eds) Physiological and behavioral temperature regulation. Thomas, Springfield, pp 831–855
10. Benzinger TH, Kitzinger C (1963) Gradient layer calorimetry and human calorimetry. In: Herzfeld CM (ed) Temperature, its measurement and control in science and industry, 3, part 3: Biology and medicine. Reinhold, New York, pp 87–109
11. Benzinger TH, Taylor GW (1963) Cranial measurements of internal temperature in man. In: Herzfeld CM (ed) Temperature, its measurement and control in science and industry, 3, part 3: Biology and medicine. Reinhold, New York, pp 111–120
12. Bligh J (1966) The thermosensitivity of the hypothalamus and thermoregulation in mammals. Biol Rev 41:317–367
13. Bligh J (1975) Physiological responses to heat. In: Michaelson SM, Miller MW, Magin AR, Carstensen EL (eds) Fundamental and applied aspects of non-ionizing radiation. Plenum, New York, pp 143–164
14. Brooke OG, Harris M, Salvosa CB (1973) The response of malnourished babies to cold. J Physiol (Lond) 233:75–91
15. Cabanac M, Marsonet B (1977) Thermoregulatory responses as a function of core temperature in humans. J Physiol (Lond) 265:587–596
16. Carlson LD, Hsieh ACL (1965) Cold. In: Edholm OG, Bacharach AL (eds) The physiology of human survival. Academic Press, London, pp 15–51
17. Colin J, Timbal J, Boutelier C (1974) Les échanges thermiques dans le froid et les moyens d'évaluation d'une ambiance froide. Rev Med Liege 15:2621–2629
18. Cooper KE (1966) Temperature regulation and the hypothalamus. Br Med Bull 22:238–242
19. Cooper KE (1969) Regulation of body temperature. Br J Hosp Med 2:1064–1067
20. Cooper KE (1976) Mechanisms of human cold adaptation. In: Shephard RJ, Itoh S (eds) Circumpolar health. University of Toronto Press, Toronto
21. Cox B, Lomax P (1977) Pharmacologic control of temperature regulation. Annu Rev Pharmacol Toxicol 17:341–353
22. Cox B, Lomax P, Milton AS, Schönbaum E (eds) (1980) Thermoregulatory mechanisms and their therapeutic implications. Fourth International Symposium on the Pharmacology of Thermoregulation, Oxford, 1979. Karger, Basel
23. Davies CTM, Fohlin L, Thorén C (1977) Temperature regulation in anorexia nervosa. Proc Physiol Soc 268:8P–9P
24. Davis TRA (1974) Effects of cold on animals and man. Prog Biometeorol 1:215–227 and 633–634
25. Dawkins MJR, Hull D (1964) Brown adipose tissue and the response of new-born rabbits to cold. J Physiol (Lond) 172:216–238
26. Doniach D (1975) Possible stimulation of thermogenesis in brown adipose tissue by thyroid-stimulating hormone. Lancet II:160–161
27. Edholm OG (1978) Man—hot and cold. Arnold, London (Institute of Biology's Studies in Biology no 97)
28. Ellis F (1976) Heat wave deaths and drugs affecting temperature regulation. Br Med J ii:474
29. Feldberg W (1975) Body temperature and fever: Changes in our views during the last decade. Proc R Soc Lond [Biol] 191:199–229
30. Feldberg W, Saxena PN (1971a) Fever produced by prostaglandin E_1 J Physiol (Lond) 217:547–556

31. Feldberg W, Saxena PN (1971b) Further studies on prostaglandin E$_1$ fever in cats. J Physiol (Lond) 219:739–745
32. Fox RH (1974) Temperature regulation with special reference to man. In: Linden RJ (ed) Recent advances in physiology, vol 9. Churchill Livingstone, Edinburgh, pp 340–405
33. Hardy JD, Stolwijk JAJ, Gagge AP (1971) Man. In: Whittow GC (ed) Comparative physiology of thermoregulation: vol II Mammals. Academic Press, New York, pp 327–380
34. Hardy RN (1972) Temperature and animal life. Arnold, London
35. Hayward JS (1971) Discussion. In: Jansky L (ed) Nonshivering thermogenesis. Proceedings of a symposium. Academia, Prague, p 307 (Distributed by Swets and Zeitlinger, Amsterdam)
36. Heaton JM (1973) A study of brown adipose tissue in hypothermia. J Pathol 110:105–108
37. Hellon RF (1967) Thermal stimulation of hypothalamic neurones in unanaesthetized rabbits. J Physiol (Lond) 193:381–395
38. Hellon RF (1970) Hypothalamic neurons responding to changes in hypothalamic and ambient temperatures. In: Hardy JD, Gagge AP, Stolwijk JAJ (eds) Physiological and behavioural temperature regulation. Thomas, Springfield, p 463
39. Hellon RF (1975) Monoamines, pyrogens and cations: Their actions on central control of body temperature. Pharmacol Rev 26/4:289–321
40. Henane R, Buguet A, Roussil B, Bittel J (1977) Variations in evaporation and body temperatures during sleep in man. J Appl Physiol 42:50–55
41. Hensel H (1973) Neural processes in thermoregulation. Physiol Rev 53:948–1017
42. Hensel H, Brück K, Raths P (1973) Homeothermic organisms. In: Precht H, Christophersen J, Hensel H, Larcher W (eds) Temperature and life. Springer, Berlin, pp 503–761
43. Himms-Hagen J (1976) Cellular thermogenesis. Ann Rev Physiol 38:315–351
44. Hochachka PW (1974) Regulation of heat production at the cellular level. Fed Proc 33:2162–2169
45. Holaday JW, Loh HH, Hao Li C (1978) Unique behavioral effects of beta-endorphin and their relationship to thermoregulation and hypothalamic function. Life Sci 2217:1525–1526
46. Horowitz JM, Fuller CA, Horwitz BA (1976) Central neural pathways and the control of nonshivering thermogenesis. In: Jansky L, Musacchia XJ (eds) Regulation of depressed metabolism and thermogenesis. Thomas, Springfield, pp 3–25
47. Horvath SM, Howell CD (1964) Organ systems in adaptation: The cardiovascular system. In: Dill DB (ed) Handbook of physiology, Sect 4: Adaptation to the environment. American Physiological Society, Washington, pp 153–166
48. Houdas Y (1977) Development of a new concept on temperature regulation in man. Acta Physiol Pol 2814 [Suppl]
49. Hull D, (1973) Thermoregulation in young mammals. In: Whittow GC (ed) Comparative physiology of thermoregulation vol III. Academic Press, New York, pp 167–200
50. James PB (1975) A study of cold vasodilatation in human fingers. Ph D Thesis, University of Liverpool
51. Keatinge WR (1958) The effect of low temperatures on the responses of arteries to constrictor drugs. J Physiol (Lond) 142:395–405
52. Keatinge WR (1969) Survival in cold water: The physiology and treatment of immersion hypothermia and of drowning. Blackwell Scientific Publications, Oxford
53. Keatinge WR, Sloan REG (1975) Deep body temperature from aural canal with servo-controlled heating to outer ear. J Appl Physiol 38:919–921
54. Lewis T (1930) Observations upon reactions of vessels of human skin to cold. Hunting reaction. Heart 15:177–208
55. Lipton JM, Payne H, Garza HR, Rosenberg RN (1978) Thermolability in Wernicke's encephalopathy. Arch Neurol 35:750–753
56. Lomax P, Green MD (1975) Neurotransmitters and temperature regulation. Prog Brain Res 42:251–261
57. Maclean D, Emslie-Smith D (1977) Accidental hypothermia. Blackwell Scientific Publications, Oxford
58. McLean JA (1974) Loss of heat by evaporation. In: Monteith JL, Mount LE (ed) Heat loss from animals and man. Butterworths, London, pp 19–31
59. Metcalf G, Myers RD (1978) Precise location within the preoptic area where noradrenaline produces hypothermia. Eur J Pharmacol 51:47–53
60. Milton AS (1978) The role of prostaglandins in pyrexia. Biochem Soc Trans 6:727–731
61. Monteith JL (1974) Specification of the environment for thermal physiology. In: Monteith JL, Mount LE (eds) Heat loss from animals and man. Butterworths, London, pp 1–17
62. Mount LE (1974) The concept of thermal neutrality. In: Monteith JL, Mount LE (eds) Heat loss from animals and man. Butterworths, London, pp 426–439
63. Myers RD (1971) Hypothalamic mechanisms of pyrogen action in the cat and monkey. In: Wolstenholme GEW, Birch J (eds) Pyrogens and fever. Churchill Livingstone, Edinburgh, pp 131–146 (Ciba Symposium)
64. Myers RD, Waller MB (1975) 5-HT and norepinephrine-induced release of ACh from the thalamus and mesencephala of the monkey during thermoregulation. Brain Res 84:47–61
65. Myers RD, Gisolfi CV, Mora F (1977a) Calcium levels in the brain underlie temperature control during exercise in the primate. Nature 266:178–179
66. Myers RD, Gisolfi CV, Mora F (1977b) Role of brain Ca^{2+} in central control of body temperature during exercise in the monkey. J Appl Physiol 43:689–693
67. Newsholme EA (1978) Substrate cycles: Their metabolic, energetic and thermic consequences in man. Biochem Soc Symp 43:183–205
68. Noak R (1977) Regulation of body temperature. Prog Food Nutr Sci 2:473–481
69. Randall WC (1963) Sweating and its neural control. In: Herzfeld CM (ed) Temperature, its measurement and control in science and industry, 3, part 3: Hardy JD (ed) Biology and medicine. Reinhold, New York, pp 275–286
70. Rothwell NJ, Stock MJ (1979) A role for brown adipose tissue in diet-induced thermogenesis. Nature 281:31–35
71. Schmidt-Nielsen K (1979) Animal Physiology: Adaptation and environment, 2nd edn. University Press, Cambridge
72. Shanks CA (1975) Heat balance during surgery involving body cavities. Anaesth Intensive Care 3:114–117
73. Shapiro CM, Moore AT, Mitchell D, Yodaiken ML (1974) How well does man thermoregulate during sleep? Experientia 30:1279–1281
74. Simon E (1974) Temperature regulation: The spinal cord as a site of extrahypothalamic thermoregulatory functions. Rev Physiol Biochem Pharmacol 71:1–76
75. Snellen JW (1972) Set point and exercise. In: Bligh J, Moore RE (eds) Essays on temperature regulation. North-Holland, Amsterdam, pp 139–148
76. Timbal J, Colin J, Boutelier C (1975) Circadian variations in the sweating mechanism. J Appl Physiol 39:226–230

77. Totel GL (1974) Physiological responses to heat of resting man with impaired sweating capacity. J Appl Physiol 37:346–352
78. Wenger CB, Roberts MF, Stolwijk JAJ, Nadel ER (1976) Nocturnal lowering of thresholds for sweating and vasodilatation. J Appl Physiol 41:15–19
79. White FN (1968) Circulation. In: Gordon MS, Bartholomew GA, Grinnell Jørgensen CB, White FN (eds) Animal function: Principles and adaptation. Macmillan, New York, pp 152–229
80. Wünnenberg W (1976) Thermointegrative function of the hypothalamus. In: Jansky L, Musacchia XJ (eds) Regulation of depressed metabolism and thermogenesis. Thomas, Springfield, pp 26–41

Section B

Cardiovascular Disorders

Chapter 9

Cardiopulmonary Resuscitation (CPR)

Alan Gilston

With the exception of direct current counter-shock there have been few major advances in the techniques of cardiopulmonary resuscitation (CPR) since the combination of expired air resuscitation and external cardiac massage (chest compression) was introduced about 20 years ago. Even though the widespread adoption of these techniques, the development of coronary care ambulances and similar rescue services, and lay and paramedical training have unquestionably saved countless patients with 'hearts too good to die' [6], they are only a very small fraction of the potential survivors from cardiac arrest. Whilst there is no evidence that the long-term survival rate following CPR in suitable patients has improved in recent years, advances in management once spontaneous heart action has been restored have probably achieved this in patients treated in hospital, and the vital importance of postresuscitation care [51] as an integral part of the management of cardiac arrest is now widely recognized. It is difficult usefully to compare the results of CPR from different centres and at different periods because of wide differences in patient material, and such comparison even in well-defined conditions such as ischaemic heart disease must allow for many variables.

This chapter is not concerned with the prevention of cardiac arrest or with postresuscitation care; nor does it deal with the causes of cardiac arrest and their particular problems or the special field of neonatal resuscitation. It is largely an examination of selected topics in CPR, and in particular of our present understanding of the clinical pathophysiology of CPR and its influence on therapy. For obvious reasons, our knowledge in these areas is still extremely limited and this includes the two systems of paramount importance in this context, the cardiovascular system (CVS) and the CNS. Until we learn more about what is happening in these systems during CPR and during the often critical period which follows return of heart action, and until we can identify and monitor important changes and their response to therapy, treatment will remain, as now, largely empirical, in some ways probably valueless and perhaps even harmful. The pharmacology of the disease-arrested heart, for example, is largely a mystery, and present blunderbuss therapy during CPR compares unfavourably with modern therapy in other conditions. Experiments on healthy animals, including primates, valuable as they are, demand careful interpretation. Moreover, whilst there has always been a strong emphasis on the importance of brain protection, we now recognize that the heart too is highly vulnerable to ischaemic damage—witness the ravages of coronary artery disease—and its function may be permanently, even fatally depressed by delayed CPR, especially if there is already vascular insufficiency of the myocardium [2, 22, 39, 49, 87]. Moreover, protracted resuscitation itself may be harmful, and the sooner satisfactory spontaneous heart action is restored the better. From a pathophysiological viewpoint CPR is appropriately seen as a grave, unstable, and progressive metabolic lesion with especially deleterious effects on the heart and on its capacity to recover satisfactory function. Whilst slow recovery of normal brain function after successful but protracted resuscitation is acceptable, since it is not a threat to life if the patient is to survive, cardiac performance must swiftly return to a satisfactory level after CPR for proper perfusion of vital organs, including the heart itself, the kidneys, and if it is damaged, the brain.

Organization for CPR

Public education in the manual techniques of CPR is unquestionably worthwhile; even in hospital immediate resuscitation by professionals is not always instantly available. Unfortunately the results with resuscitation outside hospital, usually initiated by laymen of varying skill, are inferior to those inside. In particular, cardiac damage and cerebral damage are both more common [49, 115]. This may be partly related to the nature of the patient material, but it is more likely to reflect other factors, including delay in starting CPR [39, 74, 116], often from a natural hesitancy, lack of skill, and protracted interruptions. Delayed chest compression resulting from following the 'ABCD' sequence or from chest thumping may be additional factors. Resuscitation equipment (Appendix 2) must be available at strategic points throughout the hos-

pital, and the cardiac arrest alarm system swift and reliable. The equipment must be protected from casual depletion or theft and the electrical devices regularly tested. Ideally one physician, preferably an anaesthetist or intensive care specialist, should undertake the duties of Resuscitation Officer, with overall responsibility for organization [9, 46, 49, 66, 108, 121].

Definitions

Despite their importance, the terms 'cardiac arrest', 'circulatory arrest', 'failure of resuscitation', and 'death' do not have universally accepted meanings in the context of CPR. For the purposes of this chapter, these and other terms will be defined as follows.

Stages of CPR. There are three stages of CPR [51]: *Stage 1* is the restoration of the flow of oxygenated blood to vital organs, in particular the heart and brain. *Stage 2* is the restoration of spontaneous heart action. *Stage 3* is aftercare, which includes not only the management of the underlying condition, but the treatment of the complications of CPR and the prevention of further episodes of cardiac arrest.

Cardiac arrest. Classic definitions of cardiac arrest include such key words and phrases as 'sudden', 'unexpected', 'not expected to die', 'previously healthy (or apparently healthy) individual', and so on. Such definitions are nowadays obsolete and even inaccurate, because of our readiness to attempt CPR even in patients who are already gravely ill. Cardiac arrest is now most appropriately defined as 'the failure of the heart to pump sufficient blood completely to protect the brain from ischaemic damage'. In this sense any fatal condition is by definition preceded by cardiac arrest, and this is the logical implication of current practice in CPR, where the emphasis in hospital has changed from deciding when to initiate it to deciding when not to.

The onset of cardiac pump failure may be sudden, or it may be gradual, as in a steadily deteriorating low-cardiac-output state. There is no sharp margin between the different degrees of pump inadequacy, but a continuous spectrum from a normal cardiac output to complete loss of heart action, where no blood leaves the ventricle. However, even in a low-cardiac-output state cardiac arrest usually represents an abrupt deterioration in heart action, where the already inadequate tissue blood flow has now suddenly fallen to a level which threatens not merely depression of organ function but brain damage. Because heart action may not have ceased completely, the word 'arrest' is some-times inappropriate, but it is an accepted convention in this context.

Circulatory arrest. This term signifies complete cessation of blood flow to all organs and tissues. It may be due to cardiac arrest or to interruption of cardiac massage during CPR, as well as to deliberate use in certain types of surgery.

To avoid a confusion often present in the literature, the term 'cardiac arrest' will refer only to the state of the heart, and not to the circulatory state. Hence in this discussion the terms 'duration of cardiac arrest' and 'duration of circulatory arrest', for example, are not synonymous.

Heart action. In this discussion this term will imply spontaneous heart action, not cardiac massage.

Successful resuscitation. This term signifies that spontaneous heart action has been restored (stage 2 success).

Satisfactory CPR. This term indicates that CPR is effective in protecting the brain (stage 1 success).

Failure of cardiac resuscitation. This term is rarely used precisely, despite its importance. It has not one but two possible meanings [51]. Stage 1 failure is the failure to establish an artificial circulation with CPR sufficiently adequate to protect the brain. Stage 2 failure is the failure to restore a sufficient degree of spontaneous heart action to permit the cessation of cardiac massage, and this is its usual meaning. This distinction is most important when deciding about the abandonment of CPR.

Death. This term should be used only if CPR is not attempted, or is abandoned if attempted.

Survival of cardiac arrest

Some patients survive cardiac arrest only briefly, whilst others return to their previous physical and mental status and even a normal life. For practical purposes, and to clarify discussion, we can draw a distinction between 'initial survivors' and 'final' (or 'long-term') survivors. Initial survivors recover to a greater or lesser degree from the cardiac arrest and its ill-effects, but die from complications or from the underlying disease without leaving hospital. Final survivors leave hospital. This arbitrary distinction is not entirely satisfactory, and this is a problem hindering the comparison of results from different centres. A patient with a chronic illness, for example, may make a complete recovery from cardiac arrest and die in hospital

weeks or months later. Another may leave hospital, though handicapped by brain damage.

ABCD sequence

Whatever its supposed merits in the teaching of CPR to laymen, the widely propagated ABCD sequence [108] has little place in the skilled management of cardiac arrest except where this is clearly due to hypoxia. Whilst hypoxia or asphyxia from untreated respiratory problems are a common cause of death in hospital practice [15, 92], ischaemic heart disease is by far the commonest cause of unexpected cardiac arrest outside hospital [34]. There are many reasons for giving priority to cardiac massage over pulmonary ventilation in most cases of cardiac arrest and for teaching this approach to the public. They include the following [51]: the first aim in cardiac resuscitation is to protect the brain and heart from ischaemic damage by restoring their blood flow; the brain and heart tolerate even desaturated blood far better than ischaemia, and both organs have a limited capacity for anaerobic metabolism; artificial ventilation does not produce any significant artificial circulation; unless the patient was previously hypoxic there is still O_2 in the lungs at the moment of cardiac arrest; swift cardiac massage (or immediate countershock) may instantly restore spontaneous heart action whilst the myocardium is still well oxygenated; the respiratory centre may continue to function with the maintenance of cerebral blood flow, and hence the patient may continue to breathe satisfactorily; with a continuous supply of oxygen the patient may remain adequately oxygenated even though apnoeic; there is a natural aesthetic objection to expired-air resuscitation, which may delay CPR, and there is also a slight, but definite risk of the transfer of infection [1, 24, 26, 51]; if heart action returns immediately after chest compression is started, artificial ventilation may not be required; the risk of chest wall damage with chest compression is an acceptable price for successful resuscitation.

This question of whether cardiac massage or artificial ventilation should take priority may at first seem academic, since in skilled hands one swiftly follows the other. However, not only is artificial ventilation a more skilled manoeuvre than chest compression, which it may therefore delay, but current teaching emphasizes the importance of watching the patient for some moments to see whether his pulse returns, another delay, especially as even major pulses are not always as easy to detect as some experts suggest [49], especially in severe hypotension.

> Much emphasis has been placed on artificial respiration and on intravenous infusions, but the immediate decline in the functional state of the myocardium is caused not by hypoxia but by the accumulation of metabolites and potassium in the unperfused myocardium, a condition that can be partially corrected by massage even if the blood is not well-oxygenated. In the first attack therefore, priority should be given to massage and countershock, with absolute priority going to the earliest possible application of countershock [23].

Chest thumping

This manoeuvre is often recommended as the first step in CPR, chest compression being initiated only if thumping fails to restore heart action immediately. Since this manoeuvre is only rarely successful, and since it delays brain and heart protection if it fails it should only be used in ideal conditions, namely in hospital with full cardiovascular monitoring already established [49, 51]. Moreover, external cardiac massage itself may abolish a grave arrhythmia with the first few strokes.

Optimal chest compression

The grossly unphysiological technique of cardiac massage (internal or external) produces only a fraction of the normal cardiac output [51, 68]. There is also a fall in peripheral vascular resistance [19] which probably reflects vasoparalysis from intense tissue ischaemia and acidosis, and this aggravates the problem of maintaining an adequate cerebral and coronary blood flow, essential for the restoration of spontaneous heart action and brain protection. Recently described modifications of chest compression increase its effectiveness, whilst alpha-sympathetic agents antagonize vasodilatation, with consequent improvement of heart and brain perfusion.

For the best cardiac output the force and pattern of chest compression are more important than the rate [99, 113, 117, 118]. The systolic thrust [98] should not merely be a brief, albeit forceful, jerk, but a sustained squeeze, occupying about 60% of the compression cycle. Femoral, and presumably coronary and cerebral blood flow increase, though there is no evidence of improved brain protection or a reduction in metabolic acidosis. The cardiac output also depends on the degree of chest compression [5], and whilst there is a danger of excessive force in a small adult or child if the operator is unnecessarily vigorous, the possibly enhanced risk of

chest wall damage is an acceptable price for more effective resuscitation. Certainly there is often an improvement in signs of brain activity during CPR with more forceful chest compression.

Cerebral blood flow is also augmented by a change from alternate to simultaneous chest compression and lung inflation [16, 17, 99], but the need for endotracheal intubation to prevent gastric distension and regurgitation preclude its routine use. Whilst experimentally lung function is not impaired, it has yet to be shown that this method does not further aggravate the deterioration in the blood-gas state which commonly occurs during clinical CPR, unlike the experimental situation [70]. Experimentally abdominal compression also increases the effectiveness of chest compression, but the risk of liver laceration precludes its clinical use [54, 92].

Chest compression is eventually tiring, and manual compression devices such as the Rentsch Press (US Medical Controls Inc., P.O. Box 364, East Hartford, Connecticut, USA) are useful in protracted resuscitation, in recurrent cardiac arrest, and when the patient is moved, though they are powerful devices and must be applied with care. Complex artificially powered devices cannot be justified since their introduction can dangerously interrupt chest compression. In addition, they do not improve the survival rate [112a]. One of the operators can use the heel of his foot if the patient is on the floor [11].

Effects on the CNS

Clinical experience suggests that prompt and efficient CPR usually protects the brain against permanent damage, though protracted resuscitation is often followed by a period of unsatisfactory brain function before full recovery. If brain damage does occur despite swift resuscitation it suggests a failure of technique or an organic cause which reduces the effectiveness of CPR [51]. The higher incidence of cerebral damage in patients resuscitated outside hospital is due to delay in initiating skilled CPR [74, 115, 116]. The blood flow required for normal brain function far exceeds the minimum flow needed for the prevention of ischaemic brain damage, which is about one-seventh of normal [51], and this is provided by efficient CPR. The brain also receives relatively more blood than other organs during cardiac massage

[112]. However, the brain is exquisitely sensitive to interruption or fluctuations in its blood flow during CPR. [124], probably because this is already at a critical level, with the associated physiological consequences, and the margin between ischaemic depression of brain function and ischaemic damage is extremely narrow, being only a matter of a few millilitres of blood flow per minute [77].

There is no clinical way of monitoring the adequacy of cerebral blood flow with certainty during CPR, or of assessing cerebral integrity; this is one of the greatest practical problems. Whilst certain signs of brain activity [51] (Appendix 1, Table 9.A.3) do suggest that the brain is adequately protected, their absence or their disappearance, common during protracted CPR, does not necessarily mean it is in jeopardy or permanently damaged [51]. Even the electroencephalogram (EEG) is an uncertain guide, since cerebral electrical activity disappears before cerebral blood flow reaches the critical level for damage [77]. This uncertainty about the state of the brain during CPR, and especially during protracted CPR, prohibits the abandonment of resuscitation on the grounds of supposed irreversible brain damage (stage 1 failure). Unfortunately, even if cerebral protection is correctly judged inadequate, if the situation has lasted some minutes it may be too late to save the brain, for example by opening the chest, because of its susceptibility to ischaemic damage, though promising recent work on its therapy justifies continued resuscitation even in this situation.

The central localization of the signs of brain activity during CPR is not clear, though for example struggling, frowning, head shaking, and an eyelash reflex suggest cortical activity is satisfactory, and hence cerebral protection is adequate, since the cortex is highly susceptible to ischaemic and hypoxic damage because of its high metabolic rate and high blood flow [14, 84]. Full consciousness and speech are rare and soon disappear, no doubt because of the gross impairment of cerebral blood flow and the dependence of intellectual function on normal brain metabolism. If any sign of brain activity persists it usually indicates there will be complete recovery of brain function once satisfactory heart activity returns, and the recovery will be swift if cardiac arrest lasts for only a few minutes.

The gradual deterioration in brain activity with protracted resuscitation may be due to various factors [51]. They include gradual deterioration of the artificial circulation, and

increasing cerebral functional depression, resulting not only from ischaemia and hypoxaemia, but from the secondary cerebral lactic acidosis which is inaccessible to alkali correction because of the blood-brain barrier [51, 67]. This lactic acidosis, which develops in the brain [41, 51, 67] as in other tissues, has important functional consequences during and after CPR. It antagonizes and eventually abolishes cerebral autoregulation, and it probably also depresses brain function [64]. The loss of autoregulation critically affects cerebral blood flow, since this now changes from an active, physiological, regulatory mechanism which normally maintains a constant flow, despite changes in perfusion pressure, by varying the calibre of the vascular bed, to a passive, hydrostatic mechanism where cerebral blood flow is completely dependent on the perfusion pressure. Respiratory acidosis too inhibits autoregulation, and it is commonly present in CPR. The duration, degree and distribution of the loss of autoregulation after heart action returns probably depends on many factors, especially the severity of cerebral insult [125], and this is influenced by the duration of CPR and its effectiveness. It probably lasts some hours, and perhaps even days, after protracted resuscitation, especially if there is brain damage [21, 51, 89, 125], since lactic acid disappears far more slowly in the brain than in the systemic circulation because of the relative impermeability of the blood brain barrier to hydrogen and lactate ions. Moreover the mean perfusion pressure during CPR is commonly below 50 mmHg, i.e., below the lower limit of autoregulation in normotensive persons, a limit raised in hypertensive and often much older patients who may already have impairment of autoregulation and reduction of cerebral blood flow resulting from cerebrovascular disease and other factors [7, 59, 78]. It is clear that alpha-sympathetic agents can help to protect the brain by raising the perfusion pressure both during and after CPR. Marked depression of cerebral metabolic rate might conceivably enhance cerebral protection during CPR, but unfortunately the dose of barbiturate required would probably also depress the heart. Whilst there may be an intracranial pressure (ICP) wave with each chest compression stroke [97] its effect on cerebral perfusion is uncertain. There is no evidence to support the idea [80] that the high venous pressure which can develop during CPR leads to cerebral oedema.

There is good reason to believe that the apparent marked susceptibility of the brain to ischaemic damage is largely due to the additional insult of inadequate perfusion once heart action is restored, and the brain can recover from about 20 min of complete ischaemia at normal temperature, (and experimentally for much longer, though here some brain damage does occur) if this is followed immediately by normal cerebral blood flow from circulatory support [48, 51]. This may well reflect the critical effect of the loss of autoregulation on cerebral haemodynamics, since a neurone which has been insulted by delayed or inadequate CPR is additionally injured and even permanently damaged by a low cardiac output and hypotension afterwards. Similarly, the risk of cerebral damage from cardiac arrest is enhanced by pre-existing brain ischaemia [53]. The benefit of circulatory support after CPR may therefore lie in its increasing the salvage rate of potentially recoverable neurones. Inadequate heart action and hypotension, which are common after CPR, must be swiftly and vigorously treated, especially whilst the patient is unconscious and presumably still has impaired autoregulation. Respiratory acidosis is an indication for mechanical ventilation combined with volume expansion to combat its circulatory ill-effects, though PEEP (positive end-expiratory pressure) is probably best avoided if there is any possibility of cerebral damage [47]. There are interesting temporal links between the functional manifestations of complete cerebral ischaemia and its pathophysiological effects. For example, sudden and complete cerebral ischaemia leads to complete loss of consciousness and cessation of cerebral electrical activity within a few seconds, and this corresponds in time with the depletion of the very limited oxygen stores of the brain [58]. Irreversible brain damage resulting from more than 3–4 min total ischaemia at normal temperature corresponds with the time for exhaustion of the energy-rich phosphate stores [103]. Recovery of neuronal function is possible even after 15–20 min of complete ischaemia if the circulatory state which follows is good, and this period corresponds with complete exhaustion of the glucose stores of the brain from anaerobic metabolism [58]. Clearly this is not a simple relationship, however, for whilst hypoglycaemia aggravates the effect of cerebral hypoxia [79], experimentally, glucose loading before cardiac arrest also increases the susceptibility of the brain to ischaemic damage [64], possibly by increasing lactic acid formation [81]; and haemorrhage, which removes one source of glucose, possibly reduces it [48].

Full neurological recovery within the first 12 h of cardiac arrest probably signifies almost complete absence of neuronal damage, rather than masked damage, and the complete reversal of functional derangement [20, 83]. Even if there is damage, and this is likely to be present with even transient abnormalities [12], such as amnesia and nightmares [27, 36, 100], recovery may reflect reversal of neuronal injury as well as masking by normal neurones [110]. There is probably no sharp margin between the various degrees of transient functional depression of neuronal function and fully reversible neuronal damage. This is a question of semantics, and complete and rapid recovery from post-CPR coma, for example, may be regarded as either.

Our knowledge of the pathophysiological events in the brain soon after successful CPR is sparse. Experimental findings in non-primates, such as the 'no-reflow phenomenon' may not be relevant to man [48]. Few centres can measure various important parameters, such as cardiac output, cerebral blood flow, the state of autoregulation, and cerebral metabolic rate, or their global and regional changes with therapy. The study of such changes has only recently been initiated in a few centres, and the few reports presently available are mostly unsatisfactory since they do not describe the highly relevant circulatory state of the patients, most of whom have brain damage [48]. Compared with the management of other organ failure, current special therapy for post-cardiac arrest brain damage is largely empirical and often worthless. Such therapy includes steroids in conventional or massive doses, and diuretic therapy for cerebral oedema, though this may not even be present [13, 88], certainly not immediately and its importance is still in doubt [52], hyperventilation and hypothermia. Massive barbiturate therapy (Chap. 44) may prove of value, though presently there seems to be no benefit of this medication in head injury (W. B. Jennett, personal communication). One of our problems is that head injury, and strokes, about which we know a great deal, are often regarded as clinical models for the treatment of global ischaemic brain damage, and whilst this is to some degree justified the conditions are not identical.

Failure to regain consciousness after CPR may be related to several factors. These include brain damage, especially as a result of delayed or unskilled resuscitation, intracerebral acidosis, osmolar changes resulting from sodium bicarbonate therapy, and reduced cerebral blood flow due to a low cardiac output. Unless there are immediate focal signs, it is very difficult to determine the likely outcome soon after heart action returns, and even dilated pupils do not necessarily indicate cerebral damage. However, protracted coma has a bad prognosis.

Effectiveness of CPR

Whilst the presence of brain activity is a sure sign that CPR is producing a satisfactory artificial circulation, its absence or its disappearance do not mean CPR is ineffective, especially in prolonged resuscitation. The compression pulse is of less value and its presence does not necessarily mean there is a cardiac output, though the patient is unlikely to survive if it cannot be detected [9], particularly if there is no sign of brain activity and the pupils are large (diameter $\geq$ 8mm). In such cases resuscitation may reasonably be judged unsatisfactory, though more forceful chest compression and vasoconstrictor therapy may improve the pulse and the neurological state, an indication of the difficulty of reliably judging the effectiveness of CPR and the integrity of the brain.

Pulmonary function

Lung function may deteriorate markedly during CPR [42, 51, 75], and it may already have been compromised beforehand from other causes, including surgery, cardiac lesions, circulatory problems, pulmonary disease, and terminal inhalation of secretions and vomit. In spite of apparently adequate or even vigorous artificial ventilation respiratory acidosis is common and the $PaCO_2$ may rise to 60 mmHg (8 kPa) or more, especially with sodium bicarbonate therapy, which releases carbon dioxide as it neutralizes lactic acid [10]. Arterial desaturation from a marked fall in PaO_2 despite ventilation with pure oxygen is also common. These changes may be due to various cardiorespiratory abnormalities [51]. Possibly the most important is the combination of airway closure and atelectasis from chest compression with greatly reduced lung perfusion from the very low cardiac output. This leads to ventilation–perfusion mismatch, a rise in physiological dead space, and an increase in venous admixture including a high physiological shunt. The physiological shunt effect on the PaO_2 is exaggerated by the low mixed venous O_2 tension associated with the low cardiac output [45, 96]. Other possible factors in these functional changes include in-

adequate coordination between chest compression and artificial ventilation, inhalation of secretions and vomit, pulmonary oedema and diaphragmatic displacement from gastric distension. These abnormalities in lung function improve after heart action returns, especially with mechanical ventilation. A PEEP valve for use with a self-inflating bag is now available, but it has little or no place in CPR because of the danger of a further reduction in cardiac output and hence cerebral blood flow [47], though this may not be a valid objection to its use if the cardiac output from chest compression is indeed due to a generalized rise in intrathoracic pressure [73a].

Respiratory acidosis is probably not as harmful as metabolic acidosis because of its stimulant effect on the sympathetic nervous system, though it can depress heart action if severe [10]. It also impairs cerebral autoregulation and the patient must be artificially ventilated if he remains unconscious once heart action returns.

Drug therapy

Whilst drug therapy is invaluable in CPR which lasts more than a few minutes, with the possible exception of sodium bicarbonate there is, at the moment, no 'correct' list of drugs, no ideal dosage, no proper combination, and no established sequence of administration. The sick, arrested heart behaves quite differently from the normal heart. At the moment drug therapy during CPR is based on a combination of empiricism, clinical experience, and experimental evidence, though it has improved in recent years with the introduction of some new and potent agents and the abandonment of others which are less effective or more toxic. This unsatisfactory situation is due not only to the obvious difficulties of investigating human cardiac arrest, but to the enormous variation in material and patient response. One thing is clear: the gross impairment of the circulatory state during CPR leads to equally severe derangement of organ function and tissue metabolism and their response to stimulant drugs. At the moment we do not know whether drug therapy eventually does not do as much harm as good and finally even perpetuate cardiac arrest.

Inotropic agents

Sympathomimetic agents are invaluable during

CPR, despite their stimulation of myocardial oxygen consumption in a situation where this is already in jeopardy from the greatly reduced coronary perfusion and maybe from ischaemic heart disease [61]. We use three agents in particular: isoprenaline, adrenaline, and noradrenaline (Appendix 1). More recently introduced sympathomimetic agents have yet to show an advantage in CPR.

Experimentally the results of CPR are not only greatly improved by the use of powerful alpha-sympathetic agents such as adrenaline and noradrenaline or pure vasoconstrictors such as phenylephrine, but recent experimental work suggests that the beta-sympathetic effect is far less important in this context [86, 93, 123]. However, experience during open-heart surgery constantly demonstrates the value of beta-sympathetic stimulation in restoring and improving satisfactory heart action, and the value of this pharmacological effect is well established in heart failure. Beta-sympathetic stimulation is not entirely beneficial for the heart, since it disproportionately increases myocardial oxygen consumption in a situation where this is already severely restricted and may have been impaired by ischaemic heart disease even before arrest [37, 82]. On the other hand, ventricular fibrillation also greatly increases myocardial oxygen consumption [49, 56], and this factor, together with the ill-effects of prolonged CPR, justifies the swift use of agents which promote the restoration of heart action.

Alpha-sympathetic stimulation raises the blood pressure and so improves cerebral blood flow and coronary blood flow. These benefits follow a rise in peripheral vascular resistance, which may fall during CPR, probably as a result of tissue acidosis and ischaemia [51], and also, perhaps, calcium therapy [109]. This acidosis not only paralyses the cerebrovascular bed and abolishes autoregulation, making cerebral blood flow pressure-dependent, but it may also account for the need for and tolerance of huge doses of sympathomimetic agents during CPR, though these agents are still effective even at low pH levels [93]. Little is known about the mechanics of coronary blood flow during CPR, though the diastolic pressure is probably the most important, as in the normal state [66], and this is raised by vasoconstrictors [93].

The ECG (electrocardiogram) is a poor guide to the correct inotropic agent or its dose during CPR, but poor-quality (slow, low voltage) ventricular fibrillation may improve with any of the sympathomimetics, in particular isoprenaline,

and with calcium therapy. Inotropic support must be continued as an infusion after spontaneous heart action returns if it is inadequate, and this is especially important if there is cerebral damage. The choice of agent largely depends on the views of the operator, though we choose adrenaline and isoprenaline as the initial drugs [47].

Despite its intense alpha-sympathetic properties, we have found noradrenaline a beneficial drug in cardiac resuscitation, and experimentally it has major benefits [51]. We have also found it invaluable when used early, and without hesitation, in severe heart failure, especially in patients resistant to other agents because of beta-adrenergic blockade therapy [47]. Physiologically, both adrenaline and noradrenaline play an essential role in cardiovascular homeostasis, regulating the action of the heart and the peripheral distribution of blood. Significantly, too, the cardiac store of noradrenaline is depleted in heart failure. Clearly the current obsession with alpha- and beta-sympathetic activities, and the unfavourable view of alpha effects is not always justified, especially in severe heart failure and cardiac resuscitation.

Calcium chloride is another valuable drug during CPR, and indeed the sympathetic agents act on the heart through the calcium ion. Here too the proper dose is unknown, though the gluconate salt must not be used since it releases calcium ions through metabolism in the liver, whose blood flow is now greatly reduced. Calcium also antagonizes the ill-effects of hyperkalaemia, a common problem in CPR, especially after extensive tissue damage or major surgery. There are complex relationships between calcium ionization, PCO_2, and lactic acid concentration [102], which may be important during CPR.

Myocardial depressants

Abolition of resistant or recurrent ventricular fibrillation, ventricular tachycardia, or ventricular tachyarrhythmia is generally not possible without pharmacological depression of ventricular excitability. Lignocaine is one of the best drugs in this context, since it only slightly depresses myocardial contractility [51] though its value in preventing arrhythmias in ischaemic heart disease is less certain [38]. A more potent drug is required if it fails, more specifically a short-acting beta blocker, such as practolol. In some centres bretylium tosylate has been found to be effective [72, 101]. It is very difficult to compare powerful drugs of this type in clinical ventricular fibrillation because of the gravity of the situation, their probable equal effectiveness in the initial stages of CPR, and the increasing unlikelihood of success with protracted cardiac arrest, where pharmacological depression of myocardial contractility may itself become a factor in failure. However, sometimes one drug succeeds where another has failed.

Metabolic acidosis

In health and at rest there is little lactate in the circulation even though the red cells themselves are a major source, lacking mitochondria to oxidize it [95]. Normally excess lactate is swiftly metabolized, especially by the liver [18], its half-life in the plasma being only 10–15 min [32]. Even if lactate production rises markedly, as in exercise or in severe heart failure, there is little or no rise in its serum level, since consumption matches production, though there can be a temporary marked rise in extreme exertion in athletes, with a pH fall below 7 [104]. However, as the cardiac output falls markedly not only does the production of lactate exceed the capacity of the liver to metabolize it but this capacity steadily falls as hepatic blood supply falls, and eventually the liver itself contributes to lactate formation [31]. This situation occurs in a low-cardiac-output state, of which CPR is an extreme example. The cardiac output during CPR is difficult to measure with accuracy, since it is probably close to the limit of experimental error [69], but present evidence suggests it is only a fraction of the normal resting level, as little as one-sixth or less, and at most one half [51, 68]. The gross tissue hypoxia from this marked reduction in O_2 transport, frequently aggravated by coexisting hypoxaemia, inevitably leads to a severe and progressive metabolic acidosis, far worse than in the most advanced shock, and recurring despite repeated correction with alkali [42, 94].

Whilst there is a wide variation in the rate of accumulation of lactate [94] it is probably closely related to the degree of tissue hypoxia [3], and it can therefore be diminished by O_2 therapy during CPR [94]. The acidosis needs about 0.5 mmol sodium bicarbonate per litre of extracellular fluid per minute of CPR for neutralization [42, 94].

Despite its well-recognized ill-effects and the importance of correcting lactic acidosis, there is no justification for administering a large dose of sodium bicarbonate immediately after the initiation of CPR, and no evidence this step is beneficial, though it has been authoritatively recommended [108]. The only exception is when the patient has a known or suspected metabolic acidosis before cardiac arrest, for example as a result of cardiogenic shock or other low-cardiac-output state. If spontaneous heart action returns swiftly there will be little or no acidosis but the patient will have received an unnecessary dose of alkali. Not only are the ill-effects of metabolic acidosis significant only when it is severe (pH ≤ 7.2, base deficit ≥ 13 mmol/litre, standard bicarbonate ≤ 15 mmol/litre) but sympathetic agents are still effective in this situation [92]. Most important, unnecessary alkali therapy itself has significant disadvantages. They include hypernatraemia due to the sodium load (8.4% sodium bicarbonate solution contains seven times as much sodium as physiological saline), which is especially undesirable in a patient with a cardiac lesion; an increase in serum osmolality, which can lead to neurological derangement and even damage [20, 76]; and metabolic alkalosis, which can lead to hypokalaemia and shifts the oxyhaemoglobin dissociation curve to the left, so impairing tissue oxygenation [29]. In one series metabolic alkalosis was far more common than acidosis in unsuccessfully resuscitated patients [19]. Not only is sodium lactate formed from the neutralization of lactic acid metabolized to bicarbonate once the circulatory state recovers [40, 94], with an added risk of alkalosis, but residual lactic acid too is converted to bicarbonate within a few hours [40]. Finally, gravely ill patients frequently develop a metabolic alkalosis from several causes, and this situation carries a high mortality [18, 20]. It is clear that the amount of alkali administered during and after CPR should be strictly limited and used only to correct *severe* acidosis.

If the degree of acidosis is known it can be corrected according to formula A in Table 9.A.5 [71]. This is more accurate than the popular Astrup formula. We correct acidosis only when the base deficit reaches 10 mmol/litre. If the degree of acidosis during CPR is not known, it can be corrected according to formula B in Appendix 1, which is based on clinical data and on the rate of formation of lactic acid [42, 94].

A constant infusion of bicarbonate is preferable to repeated large boluses. This not only prevents surges in osmolality, but avoids the dangers of sudden release of large volumes of CO_2 in a situation where pulmonary ventilation is already impaired, with the risk of neurological depression as the CO_2 diffuses into the brain [8]. An uncontrolled infusion is also undesirable, though it is a common fault during CPR. The rate should be adjusted to about 7–8 ml 8.4% sodium bicarbonate solution per minute in an adult, or about 100 drops per minute from a standard infusion set.

Electrolyte disturbances

There are few reports on the electrolyte changes accompanying and following CPR, even experimentally, despite their probable importance. As might be expected with sodium bicarbonate therapy, the serum sodium is frequently high [75]. Hyperkalaemia too is common, especially after extensive trauma such as open-heart surgery, where damaged tissue readily leaks potassium into the circulation (A. Gilston and E. Lockey, 1979, unpublished work), and this is probably aggravated by acidosis. We have found that whilst glucose and insulin therapy during CPR can temporarily reduce the serum potassium level, this gradually rises during protracted resuscitation and may reach a toxic level. Sometimes hyperkalaemia leads to a coarse writhing type of ventricular fibrillation, seen during internal cardiac massage, when calcium chloride therapy may be beneficial. Whilst it is uncertain whether diuretic therapy can protect the kidney against the ill-effects of ischaemia, it is justified after CPR to encourage sodium loss. If the circulatory state recovers the serum potassium level gradually falls. We are unable to explain the common significant difference between the arterial and venous potassium level during CPR, and its direction is not consistent, (A. Gilston and E. Lockey, 1979, unpublished work).

Routes of drug administration

Intravenous administration of drugs is satisfactory during CPR despite the greatly prolonged circulation time. Because of its dangers [51], intracardiac injection is justified only when IV injection fails, and a recent favourable report was hardly justified by the results it described [25]. Intratracheal administration has also been reported, but like others we have found it too uncertain for CPR and the solution often splashes back during ventilation.

Cannulation of vessels

A reliable route for the IV administration of drugs during CPR is essential if heart action does not return swiftly, though its establishment must not interrupt resuscitation. A good peripheral vein is satisfactory for the initial stages of resuscitation, but often none can be found. Of the major veins, the subclavian is excellent in experienced hands, though it carries a definite risk of complications, including pneumothorax. We prefer the safer internal jugular route, though this is more difficult because of the jerking during chest compression. The femoral vein is also convenient [50] but it is not always easy to determine whether the cannula is in the femoral vein or the femoral artery, since the blood may be desaturated, its escape pulsatile, and the pressure high at both sites during chest compression. However, the simultaneous cannulation of both vessels will usually show which is artery and which vein. It is best to administer powerful vasoconstrictors through a large vein to avoid skin damage; hence the value of a major vessel. Sodium bicarbonate too can cause extensive skin damage if it escapes into the tissues. Calcium chloride and sodium bicarbonate must not be infused together as this leads to precipitation of insoluble calcium carbonate. Sympathomimetic agents are also inactivated by alkalis. If no separate line is available it is best to flush bicarbonate from the infusion tubing before administering other drugs.

Arterial cannulation has great advantages during CPR. It not only allows frequent blood gas analysis, but even if a transducer is not available an air bubble trapped in the manometer line will oscillate with each chest compression and then spontaneously when heart action returns [47]. This oscillation is a far better monitor of heart action than the ECG, which is quite unreliable in this context, and may even show sinus rhythm when heart action has ceased, a clear demonstration of the importance of distinguishing between electrical and contractile activity.

Fluid expansion

As in severe shock [107], intense tissue acidosis resulting from tissue ischaemia leads to vasoparalysis in the brain and other tissues during CPR, with a marked fall in peripheral vascular resistance. However, although there may also be a leakage of intravascular fluid through the capillaries in severe shock [107], perhaps this is not a significant feature of CPR, where the blood volume may even rise slightly [19], though this finding may be the result of the hyperosmolar effect of sodium bicarbonate therapy [122]. Experimentally transfusion is of no benefit during CPR [54, 60], unless of course there is blood or fluid loss. Whilst haemodilution may improve tissue flow by reducing blood viscosity, at the moment it seems that with vasoconstrictors and sodium bicarbonate therapy volume expansion during CPR is of limited value.

Defibrillation

Successful electrical abolition of ventricular fibrillation, ventricular tachyarrhythmia, or ventricular tachycardia is most likely when the countershock is so rapidly applied that there is no time for the development of myocardial hypoxia or acidosis [2, 62, 63]. In other words, the sooner the shock is applied the better, and if instantly available it should take precedence over chest compression. Since ventricular fibrillation is the commonest arrhythmia in adults, and has a far better prognosis than asystole, 'blind' defibrillation is mandatory when the ECG has not yet been connected. The correct energy level does not depend on body or heart weight [62, 73], and 200 joules is usually adequate [73, 105]. Excessive (>300 j) or repeated high energy countershock can eventually damage the heart [28, 51, 111].

Artificial pacemaking

Asystole only very rarely responds to an artificial pacemaker during CPR, and this device has no place in the routine management of cardiac arrest, nor is it an essential item of resuscitation equipment. Asystole during CPR usually represents not a simple failure of atrioventricular conduction or of the intrinsic ventricular pacemaker, but 'power failure' with grave, and if it persists irreversible, depression of both the contractile and the electrical activity of the heart. It commonly follows delayed CPR [2, 49], an indication of the vulnerability of the heart to ischaemia. Attempted pacemaking in this situation, a common mistake with the unskilled physician, unnecessarily interrupts chest compression and it is an unacceptable brain insult. Like thumping, it is justified only in ideal hospital conditions or if the patient has known complete heart block before cardiac arrest.

Abandoning CPR

It is impossible to diagnose the onset of brain death during CPR with certainty, and resuscitation cannot justifiably be abandoned because there are no signs of brain activity, even if the pupils are widely dilated (diameter $\geqslant 8$ mm). It should be abandoned only when spontaneous heart action cannot be restored (stage 2 failure), and then only after a full review of therapy, including drugs, countershock, O_2 therapy, correction of severe acidosis, and treatment of hyperkalaemia. Once initiated it is proper to continue CPR for at least 1 h and in certain circumstances, e.g., hypothermia and cold-immersion near-drowning, for very much longer, until the patient has been rewarmed [51, 114].

Internal cardiac massage is justified nowadays only where there is a specific reason for not using or for abandoning chest compression [51]. Such reasons include cardiac tamponade or laceration, major thoracic trauma, and in specialized units massive pulmonary embolism or cardiac lesions amenable to surgery. The risks of serious cardiac damage with internal cardiac massage, except when performed by a skilled operator, alone restrict its use.

Complications of chest compression

In view of its nature, it is hardly surprising that mechanical complications of chest compression are common [4, 51]. Some, e.g., damage to abdominal viscera, are probably avoidable with a careful technique, but others, especially chest wall and cardiac damage, are not. There is presently no way of judging the degree of chest compression in an individual patient to produce the least damage and the best cardiac output, and the two aims may be incompatible [5].

Chest compression may also be partially responsible for the serious deterioration in lung function during CPR [51]. If breathing is clinically and functionally unsatisfactory afterwards, mechanical ventilation must be used without hesitation, especially if either the neurological or the cardiovascular state is also unsatisfactory [43, 44]. An endotracheal tube inserted during CPR is always best left in place until the patient's respiratory state is satisfactory and until his protective reflexes at least have returned.

Outcome of CPR

Two factors in particular favour a successful outcome of CPR, namely a relatively healthy heart and swift and efficient resuscitation. One common, favourable situation is appropriately described as 'electrical failure' [55]. In these circumstances, heart function is satisfactory before cardiac arrest is precipitated by a sudden grave rhythm disturbance such as 'primary ventricular fibrillation' [85] following an acute coronary attack which is accompanied by little or no myocardial damage. In this situation ventricular fibrillation can very often be immediately abolished and satisfactory spontaneous heart action restored within seconds by countershock, without any need even to initiate the manual techniques of CPR. Such an approach is now a standard feature of intensive and coronary care units. At the other extreme the outlook is bad and the patient is unlikely to survive if cardiac arrest is due to power failure [55], because of extensive myocardial damage [33] or depression. Power failure may be due to ischaemic heart disease, delayed resuscitation, or gross deterioration of heart function from disease, drugs, anoxia and asphyxia, and other fatal conditions. In this situation asystole is often dominant, since the damaged heart cannot even generate an electrical signal. This type of cardiac arrest is seen in the gravely ill and here CPR is rarely successful and often cannot be justified, 'death with dignity' [57] being an appropriate concept in this situation.

Other factors besides myocardial integrity and the swiftness of CPR can influence the outcome and decide whether the patient is a long-term survivor with unimpaired cerebral function, the only worthwhile criterion of success, or at most an initial survivor. Such factors include the duration of cardiac arrest, its frequency, the skill of the operators, the facilities at their disposal, and the aftercare of the patient. His management after spontaneous heart action is restored can frequently influence the chances of further arrest, depending on the underlying condition, as well as the rate and degree of recovery from the complications of CPR.

Whilst the relatively short duration of cardiac arrest in most longterm survivors, 15 min or less [51], is probably related to the potential of a 'good' heart for recovery, rather than to the efficiency of CPR, it is at least possible that more patients could be saved if the duration of CPR, and hence its ill-effects on the heart, could be reduced by better use of available techniques. Such ill-effects include myocardial ischaemia from the very poor coronary blood flow, aggravated by hypoxaemia from lung dysfunction, increased myocardial oxygen consumption from ventricular fibrillation [49, 56] and sympathetic stimulants, myocardial trauma from chest compression [4, 51, 91], acidosis, alkalosis, electrolyte disturbances, and continued poor coronary flow from poor heart action after resuscitation.

Repeated cardiac arrest is common with very sick hearts, and it has a bad prognosis unless the chief problem is heart block. Certain arrhythmias also carry a bad prognosis if they persist. They include bradycardia, nodal rhythm, and idioventricular rhythm [35]. Possibly they reflect hypoxic myocardial damage [20].

Long-term survival rate after CPR depends on many factors, not least the patient material and the site of resuscitation [49, 90]. Approximately 60% of the patients with ischaemic heart disease leave hospital, of whom about a quarter die within the first year [119]. Only half may regain their previous degree of activity, either because of cardiac impairment or, and this applies in particular to those resuscitated outside hospital, because of neurological impairment [106, 119].

Appendix 1

Summary of CPR

Stage 1: Protect the brain
Stage 2: Restore heart action
Stage 3: Aftercare

Stage 1

Diagnosis of cardiac arrest

Sudden deep unconsciousness
No pulse (radial artery unless an expert)
Pupils may dilate (unreliable)
Apnoea (unreliable)
Cyanosis (daylight)
Fit (occasionally)
The ECG may show a lethal arrhythmia, but it cannot exclude cardiac arrest, whatever rhythm it
  shows

Management (Table 9.A.1)

Note the time
External cardiac massage
Clear airway
Artificial ventilation (1 inflation/5 compressions alternately), with extra oxygen if possible
Tracheal intubation (Table 9.A.2)
Large stomach tube if recent meal

Table 9.A.1. Actions to be avoided

DO NOT
Wait for ECG for diagnosis
Wait for ECG for countershock
Confuse the electrical with the mechanical activity of the heart
Thump the chest
Hesitate in doubt
Transfer the patient from his bed to the floor
Interrupt chest compression for more than 10 s for tracheal intubation or countershock
Start CPR if cardiac arrest has not been witnessed
          if there is not the slightest chance of success
          if the patient has a chronic lethal and distressing illness

---

Table 9.A.2. Indications for tracheal intubation in CPR

Vomiting and regurgitation
Epistaxis
Unsatisfactory artificial ventilation
Prolonged resuscitation
Internal cardiac massage
Stage 3 management (neurological/respiratory problems)

If jaw is clenched use muscle relaxant or anaesthetic agent

Signs of effective resuscitation

Neurological signs (Table 9.A.3)
Compression pulse

Signs of ineffective resuscitation

(Stage 1 failure)
None certain but very likely if:
  No neurological signs from beginning of swift CPR
  Pupils remain large (≥8 mm) or become so
  No compression pulse
Increase force of chest compression; use alpha-sympathomimetic agents

Stage 2

Management

Immediate countershock, if available, for ventricular fibrillation, or use blindly
Start IV infusion
Give drugs (Tables 9.A.4 and 9.A.5)
ECG
Arterial cannulation, if possible

Table 9.A.3. Neurological signs indicating satisfactory protection of the brain

Pupils become smaller
Eyelash reflex
Struggling
Stiffly held limbs
Frowning/swallowing
Tight jaw
Strong respiratory efforts

Table 9.A.4. Important drugs in CPR

Drug	Dose	Frequency
Adrenaline[a]	2–4 mg (2–4 mg 1% solution)	3–4 min intervals
Noradrenaline[a]	2–4 mg	5–10 min intervals
Isoprenaline[a]	2–4 mg	3–4 min intervals
Calcium chloride[a]	50–100 mg (5–0 ml 1% solution)	5–10 min intervals
Lignocaine	100 mg (10 ml 1% solution)	5–10 min intervals in ventricular fibrillation
Practolol	2–5 mg	5–10 min intervals in intractable ventricular fibrillation

[a]Can be used blind before ECG trace is available.

Table 9.A.5. Sodium bicarbonate therapy in CPR

A. Acidosis known

$$\text{Dose (mmol)} = \frac{\text{base deficit} \times \text{estimated weight (kg)}}{5}$$

B. Acidosis unknown

$$\text{Dose (mmol)} = \frac{\text{duration arrest (min)} \times \text{estimated weight (kg)}}{10}$$

  or 70 mmol/10 min arrest (adults)
  or 100 drops/min (standard infusion set)
  (of 8.4% sodium bicarbonate solution)

Return of spontaneous heart action

Spontaneous pulse (best sign)
Neurological state improves (if brief cardiac arrest may recover consciousness immediately)
Pupils do not enlarge
Eyes stay central
ECG shows acceptable rhythm
IMPORTANT: Monitor the pulse and ECG for at least 5 min in case arrest recurs

Absence of spontaneous heart action

(Interrupt chest compression for only a few seconds at most)
No spontaneous pulse
Neurological deterioration
Pupils may enlarge
Eyes drift sideways
IMPORTANT: Resume chest compression immediately whatever the ECG shows

Persistent cardiac arrest

(Stage 2 failure)
Check CPR technique, including drug therapy
Check blood-gas state
Check acid-base state
Check serum potassium level
Consider internal cardiac massage (selected cases only)

Abandoning CPR

Stage 1 failure: Impossible to be certain brain is irreversibly damaged: continue resuscitation
    (Table 9.A.6)
Stage 2 failure: continue resuscitation for at least 1 h if previously satisfactory cardiac status or if
    hypothermic
Review previous medical status
Continue CPR till rewarmed if hypothermic
Continue CPR for not less than 1 h

Table 9.A.6 Possible causes of
failure of CPR in stages 1 and 2

Delayed CPR
Inefficient CPR
Airway/ventilation problems
Organic causes

Favourable factors in CPR

Swift resuscitation
Relatively healthy heart
Duration of cardiac massage not more than 15 min
Only one episode
Dominant rhythm during CPR is not asystole

Stage 3

Record details of cardiac arrest

Maintain clear airway till conscious
Oxygen therapy
Continue mechanical ventilation if breathing unsatisfactory, especially if still unconsciousness, regardless of blood-gas state
Blood-gas and acid-base analysis
Management of brain damage: general and special measures
Support poor circulatory state
Continue monitoring till cardiovascular state satisfactory and stable
Chest radiograph if prolonged resuscitation

Appendix 2

Equipment for cardiac resuscitation [42, 47]

Table 9.A.7. Essential airway and ventilation equipment

Airways
Artery forceps
Bandage or tape
Endotracheal catheter mount
Endotracheal tubes (assorted, with connections, and ready for use)
Introducer
Laryngoscope (adult and child blades, with spare batteries and bulbs)
Magill forceps
Oxygen cylinder, flowmeter, and line
Plastic bag for false teeth
Portable sucker and tubing
Scissors
Self-inflating bag and masks
Stomach tube (large)
Suction catheters
Swabs (gauze)
Syringe (labelled 'cuff')
Yankauer sucker

Table 9.A.8 Disposables

Adhesive tape (especially highly effective type)
Ampoule files
Infusion set
Intravenous cannulas (various)
Manometer lines
Microinfusion set
Mixing quills
Needles
Scalpel
Scalpel blades (size 11 for skin puncture)
Self-adhesive labels (for labelling syringes)
Skin sutures (straight needle for anchoring cannulas)
Spirit swabs
Sterile gloves
Sterile swabs
Syringe caps for blood-gas samples
Syringes (plenty and a wide variety of sizes)
Taps

Table 9.A.9. Electrical equipment

DC defibrillator (maximum 400 J) with adult and child paddles and electrode jelly
ECG
Pacemaker?
Torch (large, with spare bulbs and batteries)

Table 9.A.10 Other items

Board or tea-tray
Clip-board with paper
Pen
Sphygmomanometer
Stopwatch
Thoracotomy set (optional)
Tourniquet (self-releasing)
Towels (two skin towels)[a]

[a]For removal of electrode jelly
between countershocks

Table 9.A.11. Essential drugs

Drug	Presentation
Adrenaline	5-ml (0.1% solution) ampoules
Atropine	1-mg ampoules
Calcium chloride	10-ml (1% solution) ampoules
Dextrose	500 ml 5% solution
Heparin	5-ml (1000 units/ml) ampoules
Isoprenaline	2-mg ampoules
Lignocaine	100-mg ampoules
Methohexitone	100-mg ampoules
Diazepam	10-mg ampoules
Noradrenaline	4-mg ampoules
Pavulon	4-mg ampoules
Practolol	5-mg ampoules
Saline	10 ml ampoules
	500 ml pack
Sodium bicarbonate	50-ml (8.4%) ampoules
	200-ml (8.4%) packs
Succinylcholine	100-mg ampoules

References

1. Achong MR (1979) Hazards of mouth-to-mouth resuscitation (letter). Lancet II:1025.
2. Adgey AA, Nelson PG et al (1969) Management of ventricular fibrillation outside hospital. Lancet I:1169
3. Alpert NR (1970) Regulation of lactate metabolism. Helv Chir Acta 35:335
4. Atcheson SG, Fred HL (1975) Complications of cardiac resuscitation. Am Heart J 89:263
5. Babbs CF, Voorhees WD et al (1979) Dependence of cardiac output on the amplitude of chest compression during CPR in dogs (abstract). Crit Care Med 7:127–130
6. Beck CS, Leighninger DS (1960) Hearts too good to die—our problem. Ohio State Med J 56:1221
7. Bentsen N, Larsen B, Strandgaard S (1975) Chronic impairment of CBF autoregulation in man. Observations in hypertensive and diabetic patients (abstract). In: Cerebral blood flow and metabolism. CBF Congress VII, Aviemore, Scotland, p 48
8. Berenyi KJ, Wolk M, Killip T (1975) Cerebrospinal fluid acidosis complicating therapy of experimental cardiopulmonary arrest. Circulation 52:319
9. Bernhard WN, Turndorff H, et al (1979) Impact of CPR training on resuscitation Crit Care Med 7:257
10. Bishop RL, Weisfeldt ML (1976) Sodium bicarbonate administration during cardiac arrest: Effect on arterial pH, PCO_2 and osmolality. JAMA 235:506
11. Bilifield LH, Regula GAA (1978) New technique for external heart compression. JAMA 239:2468
12. Blackbrough AE, Brierley JB, Nicholson AN (1973) Behavioural and neurological disturbances associated with hypoxic brain damage. J Neurol Sci 18:475
13. Brierley JB (1972) The neuropathology of brain hypoxia. In: Critchley M, O'Leary JL, Jennet B (eds) Scientific foundations of neurology. Heinemann Medical Books, London, p 243
14. Brierley JB, Adams JH, et al (1971) Neocortical death after cardiac arrest: 2 cases. Lancet II:560
15. Camarata SJ, Weil MH et al (1971) Cardiac arrest in the critically ill: A study of predisposing causes in 132 patients. Circulation 44:688
16. Chandra N, Rudikoff M, et al (1979) Augmentation of carotid blood flow during cardiopulmonary resuscitation (CPR) in the dog by simultaneous compression and ventilation with high airway pressure (abstract). Am J Cardiol 43:422
17. Chandra N, Rudikoff M, Weisfeldt ML (1980) Simultaneous chest compression and ventilation at high airway pressure during cardiopulmonary resuscitation. Lancet I:175–178
18. Cohen RD, Simpson R (1975) Lactate metabolism. Anesthesiology 43:661
19. Cohn JD, Del Guercio LRM (1966) Cardiorespiratory analysis of cardiac arrest and resuscitation. Surg Gynecol Obstet 123:1066
20. Caronna JJ (1979) Diagnosis, prognosis and treatment of hypoxic coma. Adv Neurol 26:21
21. Cold GE, Jensen FT (1978) Cerebral autoregulation in unconscious patients with brain injury. Acta Anaesthesiol Scand 22:270
22. Copley DP, Mantle JA, et al (1976) Reduction of morbidity and mortality with early cardiorespiratory resuscitation by bystanders (abstract). Circulation 54 [Suppl] 2:225
23. Cranefield PF (1973) Ventricular fibrillation. N Engl J Med 289:732
24. Davies JNP (1979) Operator risk in mouth-to-mouth resuscitation. Lancet II:593
25. Davison R, Barresi V, et al (1979) Intracardiac injections during cardiopulmonary resuscitation, a low risk procedure (abstract). Crit Care Med 7:126

26. Deetz TR (1979) Operator risk in mouth-to-mouth resuscitation. Lancet II:912

27. Dobson M, Tattersfield AE, et al (1971) Attitudes and long-term adjustment of patients surviving cardiac arrest. Br Med J iii:207

28. Doherty PW, McLaughlin PR, et al (1979) Cardiac damage produced by direct current countershock applied to the heart. Am J Cardiol 43:225

29. Douglas ME, Downs JB Mantini EL (1979) Alteration of oxygen tension and oxyhaemoglobin saturation: A hazard of sodium bicarbonate administration. Arch Surg 114:326

30. Downing SE, Talner NS, Gardner TH (1965) Cardiovascular responses to metabolic acidosis. Am J Physiol 208:237

31. Editorial (1978) Lactic acidosis and a possible new treatment. N Engl J Med 298:564

32. Editorial (1970) Lactic acidosis. Br Med J iv:258

33. Editorial (1971) Myocardial infarction and shock. N Engl J Med 285:174

34. Editorial (1972) Cardiorespiratory resuscitation: Status report. N Engl J Med 286:1000

35. Editorial (1974) Pre-hospital ventricular defibrillation. Lancet II:1361

36. Editorial (1978) The experience of dying. Lancet I:1347

37. Editorial (1979) Treatment for heart failure: Stimulation or unloading? Lancet II:777

38. Editorial (1979) Antidysrhythmic treatment in acute myocardial infarction. Lancet I:193

39. Editorial (1979) Ventricular fibrillation outside hospital. Lancet II:508

40. Emmet M, Narins RG (1977) Clinical use of the anion gap. Medicine 56:38

41. Feldman RA, Yashon D, et al (1971) Lactate accumulation in primate spinal cord during circulatory arrest. J Neurosurg 34:618

42. Gilston A (1965) Clinical and biochemical aspects of cardiac resuscitation. Lancet II:1039

43. Gilston A (1976a) A clinical scoring system for adult respiratory distress. Anaesthesia 31:448

44. Gilston A (1976b) Facial signs of respiratory distress after cardiac surgery. Anaesthesia 31:385

45. Gilston A (1977) The effects of PEEP on arterial oxygenation. An examination of some possible mechanisms. Intensive Care Med 3:267

46. Gilston A (1979a) Equipment for a cardiac resuscitation service in hospital. Br J Clin Equip 4:236

47. Gilston A (1979b) Techniques and complications in cardiac surgery. In: Hewer CL, Atkinson RS (eds) Recent advances in anaesthesia and analgesia, 13th edn. Churchill Livingstone, Edinburgh London New York p 57–94

48. Gilston A (1979c) Complete circulatory recovery after prolonged circulatory arrest. Intensive Care Med 5:193

49. Gilston A (1979d) Cardiac resuscitation services. Principles and practice. Intensive Care Med 5:49

50. Gilston A (1976) Cannulation of femoral vessels. Br J Anaesth 48:500

51. Gilston A, Resnekov L (1971) Cardio-respiratory resuscitation. Heinemann Medical Books, London

52. Ginsberg MD (1979) Delayed neurological deterioration following hypoxia. Adv Neurol 26:21

53. Graham DI (1977) Pathology of hypoxic brain damage in man. J Clin Pathol 30 [Suppl]:170

54. Harris LC, Kirimli B, Safar P (1967) Augmentation of artificial circulation during cardiopulmonary resuscitation. Anesthesiology 28:73

55. Hellerstein HK, Turell DJ (1964) The mode of death in coronary artery disease. An electrocardiographic and clinicopathological correlation. In: Surawicz B, Pelleg-rino ED (eds) Sudden cardiac death. Grune & Stratton, New York, Chap 3

56. Hottenrot C, Maloney JV, Buckberg G (1974) Studies of the effects of ventricular fibrillation on the adequacy of regional myocardial blood flow. J Thorac Cardiovasc Surg 68:515

57. Jackson DL, Youngner S (1979) Patient autonomy and 'death with dignity'. N Engl J Med 301:404

58. Jennett WB (1967) The central nervous system. In: Wells C, Kyle J (eds) Scientific foundations of surgery, Heinemann Medical Books, London, p 365

59. Jones JV, Strandgaard S (1975) Autoregulation of cerebral blood flow in chronic hypertension. In: Harper AM, Jennett WB, Miller JD, Rowan JO (eds) Blood flow and metabolism in the brain. Churchill Livingstone, Edinburgh, London, New York, p 5, 10

60. Jude JR, Neumaster T, Kfoury E (1968) Vasopressor-cardiotonic drugs during cardiac resuscitation. Acta Anaesthesiol Scand [Suppl] 29:147

61. Katz A (1978) A new inotropic agent: Its promise and a caution. N Engl J Med 299:1409

62. Kerber R, Sarnit W (1977) Influence of body weight and heart weight on the success of defibrillation (abstract). Circulation 56 Suppl III:97

63. Kerber RE, Sarnat W (1979) Factors influencing the success of ventricular defibrillation in man. Circulation 60:226

64. Kaltzo I (1979) Cerebral oedema and ischaemia. In: Smith WT, Cavanagh JB (ed) Recent advances in neuropathology. Churchill Livingstone, Edinburgh London New York, p 27

65. Klocke F, Ellis AK, Orlick AE (1980) Sympathetic influences on coronary perfusion and evolving concepts of driving pressure, resistance and transmural flow regulation. Anesthesiology 52:1–5

66. Kortilla K, Vertio H, Savolainen K (1979) Importance of using proper techniques to teach cardiopulmonary resuscitation to laymen. Acta Anaesthesiol Scand 23:235

67. Lassen NA, Christensen MS (1976) Physiology of cerebral blood flow. Br J Anaesth 48:719

68. Letac B, Pascal JY (1970) Etude hémodynamique du massage cardiac externe. Presse Med 78:1735

69. Levett JM, Replogle RL (1979) Thermodilution cardiac output. Review of the literature. J Surg Res 27:392

70. Lee WR, Bailue HD et al (1971) An experimental comparison in dogs of expired air and oxygen ventilation during external cardiac massage. Br J Anaesth 43:38

71. Li WK, Holder BS (1969) Sodium bicarbonate for correction of metabolic acidosis in open heart surgery. Anesth Analg (Cleve) 48:381

72. Lie KI, Liem KL, Durrer D (1978) Management in hospital of ventricular fibrillation complicating acute myocardial infarction. Br J Hosp Med 40 [Suppl 78]

73. Lown B, Crampton RS, et al (1978) The energy for ventricular defibrillation—too little or too much? N Engl J Med 298:1252

73a. Luce JM, Cary JM, Ross BK, et al (1980) New developments in cardiopulmonary resuscitation. JAMA 244: 1366

74. Lund I, Skulberg A (1976) Cardiopulmonary resuscitation by lay people. Lancet II:702

75. Martinez LR, Holland S, et al (1979) pH homeostasis during cardiopulmonary resuscitation in critically ill patients. Resuscitation 7:109

76. Mattar JA, Weil MH, et al (1974) Cardiac arrest in the critically ill. II hypersosmolal states following cardiac arrest. Am J Med 56:162

77. McDowall DG (1980) Clover lecture. Royal College of Surgeons.

78. Melamed E, Lavy S, et al (1980) Reduction in regional cerebral blood flow during normal aging in man. Stroke 11:31–35

79. Meldrum BS, Horton RW, Brierley JB (1971) Insulin-induced hypoglycaemia in the primate. Relationship between physiological changes and neuropathy. In: Brierley JB, Meldrum BS (eds) Brain hypoxia. (Clinics in developmental medicine no 39140). Heinemann, London, p 207

80. Messert B, Quagleri CE (1976) Cardiopulmonary resuscitation. Lancet II:410

81. Myers RE (1979) A unitary theory of causation of anoxic and hypoxic brain injury. Adv Neurol 26:195

82. Mueller H, Ayres SM, Grace WJ (1973) Principle defects which account for shock following acute myocardial infarction in man. Implications for treatment. Crit Care Med 1:27

83. Negovsky VA (1979) General problems of the post-resuscitation pathology of the brain. Resuscitation 7:73

84. Nemoto EM (1978) Pathogenesis of cerebral ischemia-anoxia. Crit Care Med 6:203

85. Oliver MF, Julian DG, Donald KW (1967) Problems in evaluating coronary care units. Am J Cardiol 20:465

86. Otto CW, Yakaitis RW, Blitt CD (1979) Mechanism of action of epinephrine during resuscitation. Anesthesiology 51, S:152

87. Pantridge JF (1979) Ventricular fibrillation outside hospital (letter). Lancet II:702

88. Pappius HM (1976) Pathophysiology of cerebral edema. The search for an ideal therapeutic agent. In: Morley TP (ed) Current controversies in neurosurgery. Saunders, Philadelphia, London, Toronto, p 587

89. Paulsen GW, Locke GE, Yashon D (1971) Cerebral spinal fluid lactic acid following circulatory arrest. Stroke 2:565

90. Peatfield RC, Sillett RW et al (1977) Survival after cardiac arrest in hospital. Lancet II:1223

91. Pomerantz M, Delgado F, Eiseman B (1971) Unsuspected depressed cardiac output following blunt thoracic or abdominal trauma. Surgery 70:865

92. Redding JS (1979) Cardiopulmonary resuscitation: An algorithm and some common pitfalls. Am Heart J 98:788

93. Redding JS (1971) Abdominal compression cardiopulmonary resuscitation. Anesth Analg (Cleve) 50:668

94. Rackwitz VR, Jahrmarker H, et al (1975) Pathogenese und therapie der azidose bei reanimation. Intensivmedizin 12:1

95. Relman AS (1978) Lactic acidosis. In: Brenner BM, Stein JH (ed) Acid Base and Potassium Homeostasis. Churchill Livingstone, Edinburgh, London, New York, p 65

96. Rocha AGDL, Edmonds JF et al (1978) Importance of mixed venous oxygen saturation in the care of critically ill patients, Can J Surg 21:227

97. Rogers MC, Nugent SK Stidham GL (1979) Effect of closed-chest cardiac massage on intracranial pressure. Crit Care Med 7:454

98. Rudikoff MT, Tucker M, et al (1976) Importance of compression rate during closed chest cardiac massage in man (abstract). Circulation 54 [Suppl]:225

99. Rudikoff MT, Freund P, Weisfeldt ML (1977) Mechanisms of blood flow during cardiopulmonary resuscitation (abstract). Circulation 56 [Suppl]:97

100. Sabom MB, Kreutziger S (1977) Near death experiences. N Engl J Med 297:1071

101. Sanna G, Arcidiacono R (1973) Chemical ventricular defibrillation of the human heart with bretylium tosylate. Am J Cardiol 32:982

102. Schaer H (1976) Effects on ionized calcium of a correc-tion of acidosis with alkalinizing agents. Br J Anaesth 48:327

103. Siesjo BK, Nordstrom CH, Rehncrona S (1977) Metabolic aspects of cerebral hypoxia-ischemia. Adv Exp Med Biol 78:261

104. Sigaard-Anderson O (1974) The acid-base status of the blood, 4th edn. Munksgaard, Copenhagen

105. Sipes JN, Sascho JA et al (1977) First shock cross ventricular defibrillation in coronary disease (abstract). Circulation 56 [Suppl 3]:115

106. Snyder BD, Lowenstein RB, et al (1980) Neurologic prognosis after cardiopulmonary arrest II. Level of consciousness. Neurology 30:52–58

107. Stalker AL (1970) The microcirculation in shock. J Clin Path 23 [Suppl 4]:10

108. Standards for Cardiorespiratory Resuscitation (CPR) and Emergency Cardiovascular Care (ECC) (1974) JAMA 227 [Suppl]

109. Stanley TH, Amaral JI, et al (1976) Peripheral vascular versus direct cardiac effects of calcium. Anesthesiology 45:46

110. Symon L, Branston NH et al (1977) The concept of thresholds of ischaemia in relation to brain structure and function. J Clin Path 30 [Suppl 11]:149

111. Tacker WA, Ewy GA (1979) Emergency defibrillation dose: Recommendations and rationale. Circulation 60:223

112. Tacker WA, Babbs CF, Woorhees WD (1979) Blood flow to vital organs during cardiopulmonary resuscitation (abstract). Crit Care Med 7:126

112a. Taylor GJ, Rubin R, et al (1979) External cardiac compression. A randomized comparison of mechanical and manual techniques. JAMA 240:644

113. Taylor GJ, Tucker WM, et al (1977) Prolonged compression during cardiopulmonary resuscitation in man. N Engl J Med 296:1515

114. Theilade D (1977) The danger of fatal misjudgement in hypothermia after immersion. Anaesthesia 32:889

115. Thomassen A, Wernberg M (1979) Prevalence and prognostic significance of coma after cardiac arrest outside intensive care and coronary care units. Acta Anaesthesiol Scand 23:143

116. Thompson RG, Hallstrom AP, Cobb LA (1977) Beneficial effect of bystander-initiated CPR in out-of-hospital ventricular defibrillation (abstract). Circulation 55 [Suppl III]:436

117. Vaagenes P (1979) Reply to Gilston A Crit Care Med 7:255

118. Vaagenes P, Lund I, et al (1978) On the technique of external cardiac compression. Crit Care Med 6:176

119. Wernberg M, Thomassen A (1979) Long-and short-term mortality rates in patients who primarily survive cardiac arrest compared with a normal population. Acta Anaesthesiol Scand 23:211

120. Wilson RF, Gibson D, et al (1972) Severe alkalosis in critically ill surgical patients. Arch Surg 105:197

121. Woollam CHM (1979) Teaching aids in resuscitation. Br J Clin Equipment 4:182

122. Worthley LIG (1976) Sodium bicarbonate in cardiac arrest (letter). Lancet II:903

123. Yakaitis RW, Otto CW, Blitt CD (1979) Relative importance of alpha and beta adrenergic receptors during resuscitation. Crit Care Med 7:293

124. Yashon D, Wagner FC, White RJ (1969) Pressure and electrical correlates indicating cerebral viability during cardiac arrest and resuscitation. Trans Am Neurol Assoc 94:350

125. Zimmer R, Lang R, Oberdorster G (1971) Post-ischaemic reactive hyperemia of the isolated perfused brain of the dog. Pfluegers Arch 328:332

Chapter 10

Cardiac Arrhythmias and Their Treatment

W. C. Brownlee and D. J. Rowlands

The clinician involved in the care of the critically ill patient may be concerned with the management of cardiac arrhythmias in any or all of three main areas. These are coronary care, post-cardiac surgery intensive care, and more general intensive or respiratory care, often given in units reserved for patients requiring ventilatory support. Although the management of cardiac arrhythmias may take on a different emphasis among these three groups, the principles of diagnosis, the criteria for treatment, and the management are common to all three. In this chapter, therefore, these groups of patients will not be considered separately, except where it is felt that the management or the aetiology of the arrhythmia differs between one group and another.

It is now widely appreciated that arrhythmias are extremely common following myocardial infarction and that arrhythmias occurring in the early hours after infarction can lead to death [10, 24, 43]. As a result, management decisions regarding arrhythmias probably most frequently become necessary in coronary care units (CCUs). The realization that such arrhythmias could be treated with drugs and electrical DC countershock was the stimulus that led to the development of CCUs with continuous monitoring of the ECG. Only con-tinuous monitoring reveals the extremely high incidence of arrhythmias after acute myocardial infarction (AMI). For example, Grace and Chadbourne [19], with intermittent rhythm strips taken in a coronary ambulance, detected ventricular ectopic beats (VEBs) in 10% of patients, whereas Pantridge et al. [41], using continuous oscilloscope monitoring, found VEBs in 58% in the first hour and in 93% in the first 4 h following AMI. Reliable computer monitoring techniques demonstrate an even higher incidence of arrhythmias, reaching 100% in one series [35].

Although a casual look at patients seemingly comfortably nursed in a quiet CCU might not lead one to suppose that they are critically ill patients, various estimates show that about 40% of patients diagnosed as having AMI will die within the first 4 weeks. Possibly between 30% and 50% of these deaths occur in the first hour, many instantaneously from ventricular fibrillation [9]. Because of delays in obtaining medical assistance these patients do not usually arrive in CCUs. Despite this preselection the in-patient mortality remains at about 15% following AMI. In the first few hours a significant proportion of the deaths are still due to arrhythmia, mainly ventricular fibrillation, but later most deaths are from cardiac failure consequent upon myocardial necrosis. Since some disturbance of rhythm is almost invariable after infarction and since some arrhythmias are associated with a significant mortality in these patients, the problem of how to handle these arrhythmias is clearly of the highest importance.

In many respects, the patient returning to intensive care after open heart surgery is potentially similarly at risk from acute cardiac arrhythmias. Despite coronary perfusion or cold cardioplegia the heart will have undergone relative ischaemia. There will also, almost inevitably, be a ventricular incision giving a small area of ventricular necrosis. Many of the patients will have had rhythm disturbances (such as atrial fibrillation) pre-operatively and in addition will have impaired ventricular function as a result of long-standing valvular disease or ischaemic disease. Corrective surgery for congenital abnormalities may have compromised the conduction tissue, thus predisposing to significant incidents of both acute and chronic heart block after such operations. Most centres reporting their series with reference to the results of coronary artery bypass grafting (CABG) for ischaemic heart disease show that there is a significant peri-operative infarction rate, in the region of 10%, and it is likely that these patients are subject to the same arrhythmias as patients with AMI.

In the general intensive care unit (ICU) or respiratory care unit an appreciation of the role of cardiac arrhythmias in the overall context of the patient's illness is of paramount importance. Many of the patients have multiple pathologies, and the haemodynamic consequences of cardiac arrhythmias may assume major importance as a determinant of overall tissue perfusion. The management of arrhythmias in this area is often difficult. The arrhythmias may be due to pre-existing heart disease or secondary hormonal or metabolic abnormalities (such as catecholamine excess or electrolyte or acid–base abnormalities), hypoxia, inflammatory conditions, poisoning, or direct trauma to the heart.

It is clear that decisions regarding the management of arrhythmias in each of these three areas may be critical to patient survival.

The cardiac rhythm

The rhythm of the heart is the ordered sequence of depolarization of the myocardium [48]. The term 'cardiac rhythm' encompasses within its meaning:

1) The site of origin of the depolarization process
2) The temporal and spatial sequence of the spread of that depolarization throughout the myocardium
3) The temporal relationship of that depolarization to those that precede and follow it [48].

It is important to realize that although the rhythm of the heart (normal or abnormal) is dictated by the performance of the specialized pacemaker and conduction tissue, the rhythm is recognized by the subsequent electrical activity of myocardial cells, for it is the activity of these cells which gives rise to the surface ECG.

The normal cardiac rhythm is sinus rhythm, with a regular rate of 60–100 beats/min. An arrhythmia is any cardiac rhythm which deviates from this definition. In clinical usage the term sinus rhythm indicates not only that depolarization arises from the pacemaker cells within the sinus node, but also that the depolarization then spreads through the atrial myocardium, through the atrioventricular (AV) node (with appropriate delay) and is distributed to the ventricular myocardium via the His–Purkinje system within the normal time limits. Thus we consider that disturbances of conduction and of initiation of the impulse may be considered to be cardiac arrhythmias. The definition of sinus rhythm that we have given also means there are three possible forms of deviation beyond the limits of the definition, which are deviations only in degree. Thus sinus tachycardia and sinus bradycardia differ from the normal rhythm only in falling outside the arbitrary rate limits. Sinus arrhythmia (which is an irregular sinus rhythm in which the cycle length varies by more than 10% [38a]) differs only in being irregular.

Classification of arrhythmias

The foregoing definition of arrhythmia permits the following functional classification without implying any assumptions regarding the mechanisms or aetiology:

1) Variations of impulse formation at the sino-atrial node
2) Ectopic impulse formation
3) Disturbances of conduction
4) Combinations of the above

Table 10.1. Classification of arrhythmias

Group 1 Variations of impulse formation at the sino-atrial node

Sinus arrhythmia
Sinus tachycardia
Sinus bradycardia
Sinus arrest

Group 2 Ectopic[a] impulse formation

Atrial premature[a] beats
Atrial tachycardia
Atrial flutter
Atrial fibrillation
Wandering atrial pacemaker
Nodal (junctional) escape beats
Nodal (junctional) premature[a] beats
Nodal (junctional) rhythm
Nodal (junctional) tachycardia
Ventricular premature[a] beats
Ventricular tachycardia
Ventricular fibrillation
Idioventricular rhythm (slow ventricular tachycardia)

Group 3 Disturbances of conduction

Sino-atrial block
Intra-atrial block
Atrio-ventricular dissociation
Interference dissociation
Fusion beats
AV block
  First-degree
  Second-degree (Mobitz types I and II)
  Third-degree
Left anterior hemiblock (Left superior intraventricular block)
Left posterior hemiblock (Left inferior intraventricular block)
Left bundle-branch block
Right bundle-branch block
Ventricular pre-excitation

Combinations of arrhythmias

Combinations from the above three groups

[a]An 'ectopic' impulse is one that arises at any site other than the sino-atrial node. A 'premature' impulse is one that arises earlier than one would anticipate from observation of preceding beats. Whilst, very rarely, a premature impulse may arise at the sino-atrial node and, also rarely, an ectopic impulse may not be premature, in the majority of cases ectopic impulses are premature and vice versa.

Table 10.1 shows a list of the common arrhythmias classified in this way.

Mechanisms

Groups 1 and 3

Histological examination of the sinus node of patients who suffer from chronic sino-atrial disorder (sick sinus syndrome) has shown that many of the specialized pacemaker cells seem to have been replaced with fibrous tissue out of all proportion to the age of the patient [14]. In other cases the sinus node is seen to be very small or vestigial, and virtual isolation of the node by adipose tissue has been recorded in several instances. In chronic AV block similar degenerative processes are seen in the conduction tissue, involving the bundle branches or the His bundle and AV node. It is not unreasonable to suppose that this degeneration of the specialized pacemaker and conduction tissue gives rise to many of the variations of impulse formation at the sinus node and to the disturbances of conduction. It is also reasonable to suppose that functional disturbances within these structures can easily be caused by interruption of their blood supply, and in AMI relative or absolute deprivation of blood supply to these areas is an obvious arrhythmic mechanism.

Group 2

The mechanisms involved in ectopic impulse formation appear much more complex. Some of the rhythms can be understood in terms of escape rhythms if we assume that areas of the specialized conduction tissue have pacemaker activity: thus non-paroxysmal nodal rhythms and nodal escape beats appear to arise from the automatic focus normally present at the AV junction, and usually coincide with depressed sinus node activity. Similary the slower idioventricular rhythms seen in complete AV block may be explained as a slower, lower focus, taking over where there is nodal and His bundle disease.

To explain other ectopic-impulse arrhythmias two further mechanisms have to be considered, that of the focal tachycardia and that of reciprocating tachycardia involving re-entry pathways. This latter type of mechanism typically occurs in the Wolff–Parkinson–White syndrome, where an anatomically separate AV pathway may complete an electrical circuit involving the AV node and sustain a tachycardia. Intracardiac electrophysiological studies (particularly premature stimulation techniques) have demonstrated that many atrial and nodal tachycardias, particularly of the paroxysmal type, are related to re-entry pathways in and around the AV node. From the clinical point of view, distinction between the focal and the re-entry mechanism is usually not possible with the surface ECG.

The ventricular arrhythmias, particularly ventricular fibrillation, are most commonly associated with ischaemic heart disease. In most other disorders of the heart, the frequency of ventricular arrhythmias tends to correlate with the severity of ventricular damage and, in the case of valvular disease, with the degree of ventricular failure; and on the whole the arrhythmias do not have a serious prognosis unless they are induced by digitalis and associated with hypokalaemia. However, in acute ischaemia, clinical observation and animal experiments suggest that many different mechanisms may be responsible for ventricular arrhythmias. Ventricular fibrillation occurring soon after the onset of infarction seems to be due to re-entry within the myocardium. However, the onset of infarction is also associated with an increase in the automatism of ischaemic but non-necrotic Purkinje fibres. The infarct border seems to be important in the generation of metabolic and electrophysiological differences between normal and ischaemic tissue. Acute potassium loss is involved in reduction of resting cell membrane potential and decreased velocity of the fast response of depolarization. There is shortening of action potential duration and an increase in tissue cyclic adenosine monophosphate (cAMP). All these factors appear to be important in the production of these ventricular arrhythmias [40]. Finally, when the acute event has subsided ventricular arrhythmias may be due to re-entry phenomena around the border zone of an electrically inactive area, such as a ventricular aneurysm.

Consequences

The range of haemodynamic disturbance caused by cardiac arrhythmias can extend from the negligible (unnoticed by the patient, and only found in the so-called normal population by ambulatory monitoring) to the catastrophic haemodynamic consequences of ventricular fibrillation.

An arrhythmia may give rise to its haemodynamic consequences as the result of the following possible changes:

1) Change in heart rate
2) Loss of atrial transport
3) Increase in myocardial oxygen requirements
4) Decrease in myocardial blood flow
5) Loss of synchronicity of ventricular contraction
6) Any combination of the foregoing.

Heart rate changes

In the normal resting adult in sinus rhythm wide variations in heart rate from approximately 40–160 beats/min produce very little change in cardiac output [46]. However, in patients with significant valvular disease or with impaired LV function the range over which the heart rate can be compensated by changes in stroke volume is much narrower. Increases in heart rate are mainly produced by reduction in the duration of diastole and at high rates ventricular filling time is much reduced and may become critical. The presence of AV valve narrowing or decreased ventricular compliance (as in ventricular hypertrophy) greatly exacerbates the haemodynamic consequence of ventricular filling time reduction produced by tachycardia. In extreme bradycardia cardiac output can only be maintained by an appropriate increase in stroke volume. This can be achieved by increasing the ejection fraction of the ventricle, its end-diastolic volume, or both. The margin of effective compensation is limited, and at heart rates below 40 beats/min ventricular volume limitations preclude total compensation even in the normal heart. This limitation is again more apparent in patients with myocardial disease, and cardiac output may become critically low or heart failure supervene even though the ventricular rate is maintained above 40 beats/min. In addition, the duration of the bradycardia has a bearing on the haemodynamic response. Thus, in chronic heart block cardiac output may be reasonably maintained at rates which cause appreciable cardiac embarrassment in acute heart block.

Atrial transport function

In an otherwise healthy heart the loss of atrial transport appears to be of little haemodynamic consequence except at a very fast rate or during exercise [4]. In the diseased heart (e.g., following AMI) atrial transport may become extremely important in maintaining the cardiac output [8]. Similarly, atrial transport may prove to be very important in the long-term treatment of some patients with chronic complete heart block or sino-atrial disease [54].

Myocardial oxygen requirements and supply

Heart rate is one of the most important determinants of myocardial O_2 requirements. Tachycardia consistently increases the O_2 need of the myocardium per unit of time. Coronary flow, particularly to the LV myocardium, occurs predominantly during diastole, and since the total duration of diastole is rate-dependent and is reudced during tachycardia, myocardial blood flow falls. Tachycardia thus both increases myocardial O_2 requirements and decreases myocardial O_2 supply. This effect will obviously be aggravated by the presence of significant coronary artery disease.

Synchronicity of ventricular contraction

Effective ventricular function depends upon the organized, nearly synchronous contraction of the left ventricle. In the presence of an intraventricular conduction disturbance ventricular myocardial depolarization is less synchronous. The resulting contraction is also less synchronous and is marginally less effective. This effect is not noticeable in an otherwise normal heart functioning at a normal rate. But in the presence of a diseased ventricle or at high rates such as are recorded in ventricular tachycardia there may be a significant effect. The total loss of ventricular function associated with ventricular fibrillation is, of course, related to the total disorganization of ventricular contraction in this arrhythmia.

Thus the haemodynamic consequences of any arrhythmia are extremely variable, but are always likely to be more pronounced in the presence of valvular, coronary artery, or myocardial disease.

Indications for treatment

Before any attempt is made to treat a cardiac arrhythmia it is important to have in mind a definite indication, for the mere deviation of the rhythm from normal is not, in itself, an adequate reason for interference. Ambulatory monitoring has demonstrated the frequency of asymptomatic ventricular arrhythmias in the normal population, particularly in those in middle age [21]. Similarly unsuspected and asymptomatic sino-atrial dysfunction is frequently found by such monitoring [34]. The temptation to treat such grave-looking ventricular arrhythmias and pauses is great, but there is ample evidence that in the absence of any other signs of heart disease such ventricular arrhythmias are benign. However, ventricular

arrhythmias may be the first manifestation of ischaemic heart disease or cardiomyopathy. Therefore, when frequent ectopic beats, multiform beats, or R-on-T phenomena are seen in apparently normal individuals further investigation may be warranted, and if exercise testing, echocardiography, or coronary arteriography defines significant disease, treatment of the arrhythmias may be indicated in an attempt to improve the prognosis. Follow-up of patients with sino-atrial disease has shown that the overall survival of patients with established and potential dysfunction was apparently indistinguishable from that of the normal population. Pacemaker implantation had little discernible effect on mortality [50], suggesting that asymptomatic sino-atrial disorder should not be treated prophylactically. Arrhythmia which does not degrade cardiac function, is not likely to give rise to any more serious arrhythmia, and does not cause the patient any symptoms therefore does not require treatment.

Conversely, the indications for treatment of a cardiac arrhythmia may be considered to be the following:

1) Where the arrhythmia produces immediate deterioration in cardiac performance (as is always the case with ventricular fibrillation, is usually the case with ventricular tachycardia, and is sometimes the case with atrial fibrillation)
   or
2) When the arrhythmia gives no immediate deterioration in cardiac function but its persistence may be expected to give rise to such a deterioration (e.g., atrial tachycardia)
   or
3) When in a given clinical context the arrhythmia carries a risk of giving rise to subsequent arrhythmias, which could in turn depress overall cardiac performance (e.g., R-on-T ectopic beats or frequent and multifocal ectopic beats in the postinfarction situation)
   or
4) When the arrhythmia, though apparently doing no harm and carrying little risk, is causing the patient distressing symptoms (e.g., multiple atrial premature beats)
   or
5) In the absence of demonstrable haemodynamic disturbance treatment has been shown to improve survival (e.g., in chronic complete heart block).

In each case, the indication for treatment should be seen within the clinical context; for example, if the patient develops complete heart block following acute inferior myocardial infarction, has an adequate blood pressure, satisfactory urine output, and no impairment of consciousness, artificial pacing may be unnecessary. Further, any arrhythmia should only be treated if some method of treatment is available which has a reasonable chance of success and is reasonably safe. These are simple, commonsense guidelines, but they are frequently neglected in the haste to apply treatment once an arrhythmia has been detected.

Management

The management of arrhythmias will be discussed with particular reference to AMI, as this model seems to hold good in the treatment of critically ill patients in other areas, as explained in the introductory section of this chapter.

Treatment of haemodynamically significant cardiac arrhythmias usually has two objectives, the first being to restore sinus rhythm and the second to prevent relapse. The first objective may not always be possible or necessary, for instance if a patient has valvular disease and is in chronic atrial fibrillation. In the acute situation where haemodynamic deterioration is secondary to cardiac arrhythmias, if drugs are to be given they should almost always be administered IV as absorption following intramuscular (IM) injection can be slow and variable in patients who have impaired cardiac function, and absorption following oral administration too slow. In prevention of relapses, however, the oral route is always to be preferred. Once the decision either to treat or to prevent a cardiac arrhythmia has been made, it is important to review the patient as a whole. The important points to look for are pain, fear, hypoxia, electrolyte imbalance, fluid, and acid–base imbalance. All these should be treated and corrected as far as possible in association with the appropriate treatment for the cardiac arrhythmia.

Variations in impulse formation at the sino-atrial node

Sinus arrhythmia

This requires no treatment. It is only technically an arrhythmia and has no deleterious haemodynamic effects.

Sinus bradycardia

This frequently follows inferior myocardial infarction [17]. Between 8% and 38% of patients seen within 4 h after the onset of symptoms of AMI have sinus bradycardia [41, 52]. Sinus bradycardia in association with AMI is usually benign, resolves spontaneously within hours, and is of little haemodynamic consequence [1]. However, if there is a detectable haemodynamic consequence (such as hypotension, reduced cerebral, or renal profusion) the arrhythmia should be treated. There has been some suggestion that sinus bradycardia in association with hypotension in the prehospital phase of AMI is associated with a higher mortality if left untreated. This increase in mortality is thought to be related to the effect of the bradycardia in giving rise to (1) haemodynamic deterioration; (2) electrical instability; (3) enlargement of the zone of infarction; or any (4) combination of the foregoing.

The bradycardia may respond to the simple manoeuvre of elevating the legs. Failing this, IV atropine is the drug of choice. We give between 0.5 mg and 1.5 mg in 0.5 mg increments every 3 min. A single treatment is usually effective but sometimes the effect is short-lived and repeated doses may be necessary. On the rare occasions when this treatment fails, temporary pacing may be justifiable [36]. Where there is no disturbance of AV conduction atrial pacing is the method of choice. It is our practice, however, if inserting a temporary atrial electrode to insert a temporary ventricular electrode at the same time in case of instability in the atrial pacing system or development of AV conduction disturbances. Occasionally pacing will be instituted because of electrical instability; usually this is seen as multifocal VEBs, short runs of ventricular tachycardia, or more prolonged attacks of atypical ventricular tachycardia, often now called 'torsade de pointes' [28]. Again, where there is no disturbance in AV conduction atrial pacing is the treatment of choice. However, where there is no associated hypotension right ventricular pacing is usually satisfactory, and once this is established antiarrhythmic drugs are not usually necessary in addition. Conversely, it is dangerous to attempt to treat such ventricular arrhythmias in the presence of marked sinus bradycardia with antiarrhythmics without the presence of a temporary pacemaker. It is certainly not established that bradycardia in the absence of hypotension or electrical instability requires treatment. Experimental evidence in the dog shows that increases in the heart rate by atropine or ventricular pacing can increase infarct size and the incidence of ventricular arrhythmias [22, 58] and it should be noted that the in-patient mortality of patients with sinus bradycardia but without hypotension is lower than the mortality of all patients with AMI [6]. Chronic sinus bradycardia not associated with recent myocardial infarction or cardio-active drug treatment is often the dominant rhythm of patients with sino-atrial disorder [13]. Where the patient has symptoms related to this bradycardia or has symptomatic longer pauses due to either sinus arrest or sino-atrial exit block or requires drug suppressant therapy for associated tachyarrhythmias, permanent pacing is the treatment of choice. Conventional ventricular pacing is usually satisfactory in these patients, although long-term transvenous atrial pacing in the absence of AV conduction disease confers the advantages of increased cardiac performance and probable freedom from systemic thromboembolism and advances in pacemaker technology mean that a second ventricular lead can be inserted at the time of implantation, in case the patient has unexpected AV nodal disease and will later require ventricular pacing [23].

Sinus tachycardia

After AMI, sinus tachycardia usually indicates the occurrence of appreciable myocardial damage and may be indicative of a degree of LV failure, although it is important to appreciate that both anxiety and pain may contribute to the tachycardia. The in-patient mortality for patients with sinus tachycardia in AMI is significantly higher than that for all patients with AMI [6]. The fact that these excess deaths are usually due to ventricular failure emphasizes the relationship of sinus tachycardia to the extent of myocardial damage. The arrhythmia has no significant haemodynamic consequences and is a response of the heart, to attempt to maintain cardiac output in the presence of ventricular damage. In this setting it does not require treatment, as reducing the heart rate will lower the cardiac output and aggravate the situation as far as perfusion of the body is concerned. However, a rapid heart rate has been shown experimentally to be one of the factors favouring the extension of infarction, particularly when the rapid rate is associated with sympathetic overactivity [51]. This is one reason for considering the use of beta blockers in AMI, particularly for patients with sinus tachycardia

[37]. However, a randomized trial comparing propranolol, atenolol, and placebo has shown that there was no significant difference between the three groups with respect to mortality at 1 year [57]. Chronic sinus tachycardia is always the response to some underlying disorder, and it is underlying disorder, rather than the tachycardia, that should be treated.

Atrial ectopic arrhythmias

In general, atrial arrhythmias are relatively benign. In the absence of an accessory pathway the refractory period of the AV node imposes an upper limit on the ventricular rate (this constraint does not operate in the case of ventricular arrhythmias). In addition, intraventricular conduction is often normal and thus two of the mechanisms by which arrhythmias can give rise to marked haemodynamic deterioration are attenuated or eliminated. Further, the arrhythmia is often short-lived and frequently stops spontaneously. It may pass unnoticed by the patient and may not require treatment. Arrhythmias giving rise to sustained high ventricular rates which are symptomatic and which give rise to haemodynamic deterioration do justify treatment, both in association with AMI and in the long term.

Atrial premature beats

Of no haemodynamic significance in themselves, atrial premature beats may supply the premature stimulation required to trigger a re-entry arrhythmia. Generally no treatment is required except in the situation where supraventricular tachycardia is known to be induced by these premature beats and it becomes desirable to suppress them to prevent recurrence. In such a situation, after AMI, short-term suppressive therapy may be indicated. Drugs used on a long-term basis in an attempt to suppress paroxysmal tachyarrhythmias may, in part, act to reduce the number of attacks by reducing the incidence of premature beats. Where treatment is required it should be given as described in the section: *Atrial tachycardia.*

Atrial tachycardia

In patients with normal LV function atrial tachycardia may be tolerated for many hours without marked haemodynamic deterioration. However, in the patient who has just sustained a myocardial infarction or has impaired ventricular function for other reasons, the increase in heart rate together with the reduction in or loss of atrial transport usually has important haemodynamic consequences, and unless the rhythm resolves spontaneously within a few minutes of its onset this arrhythmia requires treatment.

It is always worthwhile trying carotid sinus massage in the first instance. The ECG should always be monitored during this manoeuvre and it is a convenient time to produce a tracing for the patient's records. Carotid sinus massage may do one of three things. It may (1) terminate the arrhythmia, restoring sinus rhythm; (2) increase the degree of AV block, allowing the distinction to be made between an atrial tachycardia, junctional tachycardia, and atrial flutter with a lesser degree of AV block; or (3) have no apparent effect whatever.

If carotid massage does not terminate the arrhythmia and the arrhythmia is not associated with immediate profound haemodynamic deterioration, drug therapy is indicated. Verapamil IV is the drug of choice for termination of this arrhythmia. It should be used with caution in the acute phase after AMI, because of its depressant effect on muscle contractility. However, if the patient's haemodynamics are not unduly disturbed by the tachycardia it is safe to give verapamil even after AMI: 5 mg is given over 5 min and the dose may be repeated every 5 min until conversion occurs or the dose totals 20 mg. Verapamil may be continued orally after successful conversion, in doses of 40 or 80 mg three or four times a day. If there is concern about LV function IV administration of a digitalis preparation is indicated to convert the rhythm. Digitalis is contraindicated, however, if the patient is already digitalized or there is any suggestion that the arrhythmia was induced by digitalis. It is also contra-indicated if there is hypokalaemia. The preparation of choice is ouabain 0.5 mg given IV. The onset of action is within 5–10 min, the peak effect at about 30–120 min after injection, and the plasma half-life about 21 h [18]. Alternatively, digoxin can be given IV up to a dose of 1 mg in divided doses. If this first attempt at conversion with either verapamil or a digitalis preparation has failed, the choices for converting the arrhythmia are other drugs, synchronized DC cardioversion, and overdrive pacing. Against the setting of AMI it is our practice to proceed to DC cardioversion if the first choice has failed, as inevitably further I.V. therapy involves the use of drugs which additionally depress myocardial contractility. However, the drugs which may be useful include practolol 5–20 mg, disopyramide in a dose of 2 mg/kg, phenytoin 50–100 mg at 5-min intervals until therapeutic or toxic effect is observed up to a total dose of 1 g (all doses for IV use). Verapamil and any beta blocker should never be given together, because of their profound depressant activity on both myocardial and conduction tissues. Severe myocardial depression and profound bradycardia may ensue, with catastrophic consequences. The effect on the conduction tissue is particularly dangerous if the patient has already been given digoxin. If there is any possibility that the atrial tachyarrhythmia is related to chronic digitalis treatment, withdrawal of the digitalis is essential. Under these circumstances, and particularly if there is any evidence of hypokalaemia, IV potassium therapy 25–100 mmol potassium chloride with 500 ml 5% dextrose given over 4–6 h is helpful and phenytoin is particularly effective in suppressing digitalis-induced arrhythmias.

If the chosen drug therapy has failed to control the arrhythmia within 20–30 min, DC countershock is indicated. DC countershock is indicated as first-line therapy without any prior trial of drugs if the onset of arrhythmia is associated with immediate appreciable haemodynamic deterioration. DC countershock is almost universally successful in these arrhythmias, except where a digitalis preparation is implicated in the causation; under these circumstances DC countershock is relatively contra-indicated. If DC countershock is resorted to, drug treatment is indicated to try to prevent a recurrence of the tachyarrhythmia. As already stated, verapamil is useful, as is digoxin, quinidine (in the form of 250-mg Durules), disopyramide, or a beta blocker. The individual dose regimen needs to be tailored to the particular situation but typical doses would be: for digoxin 0.25 mg twice daily; for quinidine (Kinidin) 250 mg (Durules) three times daily; for disopyramide 100–200 mg three times daily; for propranolol (Inderal LA) 160 mg daily. In the case of digoxin it is particularly important to take account of the patient's age, physical size, renal state, and thyroid function when deciding on the long-term oral dose.

In rare cases the arrhythmia may fail to respond to any of the drugs listed and also to DC countershock, or the countershock may be successful for only a short time, with the arrhythmia recurring. Such cases can be extremely difficult to handle, as repeated DC countershock is undesirable. Under these circumstances combinations of drugs may be required, but if such multiple-drug treatment is to be undertaken the approach can be made safer by the prior insertion of a temporary ventricular pacing system; at the same time an atrial electrode may be inserted, as atrial overdrive or atrial burst pacing may well be effective, particularly in re-entry arrhythmias, and is certainly preferable to repeated DC cardioversion.

We have already made reference on several occasions to digitalis-induced arrhythmias. Digitalis-induced atrial tachycardia is particularly likely to be associated with some degree of AV block, and if the patient is taking digitalis in any form the safest rule is to assume that the atrial tachycardia has been induced by digitalis despite the absence of other signs of digitalis intoxication. This is a particularly wise assumption when the tachycardia is associated with AV block. It should be remembered also that many patients receiving digitalis are also taking diuretics and may have a degree of hypokalaemia. It is imperative to check for this and correct any hypokalaemia.

Chronic forms of paroxysmal supraventricular tachycardia are not usually associated with marked haemodynamic deterioration in the patient unless there is existing ventricular disease. Most patients can be successfully managed on a drug treatment regimen such as that outlined in this section. However, some patients who have repeated frequent symptomatic tachycardias may be best managed by permanent pacing systems which are triggered by the tachycardia and outpace the arrhythmia or interrupt the circulation of the tachycardia by introduction of timed premature beats. Often e.g., in the Wolff–Parkinson–White syndrome, the arrhythmia is associated with an aberrant pathway, and where the arrhythmia has defied pharmacological and pacemaker control (and particularly if the aberrant pathway has the ability to conduct fast atrial rates and if atrial flutter or fibrillation has been demonstrated) it may be necessary to consider a surgical solution. At operation the aberrant pathway can be localized (with difficulty) by recording ECGs from the surface of the heart, and the aberrant pathway can be incised or ablated [16]. Undoubtedly the most effective anti-arrhythmic drug for the control of such chronic tachycardias is amiodarone. Since use of this preparation was started in the present authors' patients, none has had to be referred for surgical ablation of aberrant pathways.

Nodal AV junctional tachycardia

As already explained, this is often indistin-

guishable in practical terms from atrial tachycardia, and is managed in the same way.

Atrial flutter

When atrial flutter is seen in conjunction with AMI it can be approached in a similar manner to atrial tachycardia so long as two important points are borne in mind: (1) atrial flutter is never terminated by carotid sinus massage, which more usually transiently increases, the degree of AV block, making the rhythm more obvious on the surface ECG; and (2) atrial flutter responds well to low-energy DC shock, and it is common practice to proceed to DC shock at an early stage in the management of atrial flutter, particularly when associated with AMI. The treatment of choice for atrial flutter beginning de novo is cardioversion. Atrial flutter generally responds badly to antiarrhythmics, requiring often almost toxic doses of digoxin to produce an increase in AV block. Similarly, IV verapamil can bring about an acute increase in the degree of AV block and may make the ventricular rate more manageable, but is usually of little use in chronic treatment. Acutely atrial flutter can often be managed by atrial overdrive pacing, either via a transvenously placed endocardial electrode or with an oesophageal electrode, and this can sometimes be used as an alternative to cardioversion, particularly when the arrhythmia keeps recurring.

Chronic atrial flutter appears to be an unstable arrhythmia, usually degenerating to atrial fibrillation or reverting to sinus rhythm, and it is usually managed with chronic digoxin therapy.

Digoxin alone or in combination with quinidine *or* verapamil *or* beta blockers (in the doses outlined above in the section: *Atrial tachycardia*) may be used to suppress the recurrence of atrial flutter, though the success of this treatment is uncertain.

Atrial fibrillation

Atrial fibrillation is a much commoner arrhythmia than atrial flutter, both in AMI [6] and in the chronic condition. When associated with AMI, both arrhythmias are often transient, 90% resolving to sinus rhythm within 24 h [15]. Left ventricular failure is the most common haemodynamic abnormality associated with these attacks of atrial flutter or fibrillation. Whether the rhythm disturbance is secondary to or precipitates LV failure has not been established [6], but in a series of 16 patients with atrial fibrillation after AMI it was noted that 12 were in congestive cardiac failure, but in only one instance did the arrhythmia seem to be responsible for the failure [53]. The immediate treatment for atrial fibrillation when associated with haemodynamic deterioration is digitalization, preferably with IV ouabain 0.5 mg. (If sinus rhythm returns or if the ventricular rate is satisfactorily controlled maintenance treatment with digoxin is indicated and should probably be continued for at least a week because of the possibility of recurrence with the return of a rapid ventricular response.) If a rapid ventricular response to the atrial fibrillation persists despite this dose of ouabain, or if there is immediate substantial haemodynamic deterioration, DC cardioversion is indicated. The acute prior administration of a digitalis preparation is not a contra-indication for such cardioversion, although low energies in the order of 25–50 J should be tried first because of the risk of inducing ventricular tachyarrhythmias [25].

Chronic atrial fibrillation is found mainly with a rheumatic valvular heart disease or ischaemic heart disease and it may complicate heart failure from any cause. It may be associated with thyrotoxicosis, and in all these situations the age of the patient appears to be a major factor determining the onset of atrial fibrillation, it being unusual in patients under 40 years of age with mitral disease or thyrotoxicosis but common in those over 45.

When atrial fibrillation is not related to any known cardiac abnormality or systemic disease it is often termed 'lone atrial fibrillation', although it is apparent that some of the patients so affected have sinus node disease; they cannot be restored to sinus rhythm for any length of time. Similarly paroxysmal atrial fibrillation may develop with sino-atrial disease and may occur in bursts for years before, as a rule, becoming established. Whatever the cause of chronic atrial fibrillation it can usually be managed with oral digoxin to control the ventricular rate, in the doses indicated in the section: *Atrial tachycardia*. Cardioversion to sinus rhythm under these circumstances is usually not indicated unless some intervention has occurred (such as treatment of thyrotoxicosis or mitral valvotomy for mitral stenosis) which will increase the chance of the patient remaining in sinus rhythm for some considerable time after cardioversion. Whenever atrial fibrillation occurs, whether of acute or chronic onset, consideration should be given to anticoagulation to reduce the risk of systemic

embolization. When the development of chronic atrial fibrillation seems inevitable (as in the patient with severe mitral stenosis) it is prudent to start permanent anticoagulant therapy while the patient is still in sinus rhythm.

Wandering atrial pacemaker and nodal (AV junctional) premature beats

Beats of this kind are never of any great haemodynamic significance and do not require treatment.

Ventricular ectopic arrhythmias

Ventricular ectopic beats

Ventricular arrhythmias are particularly associated with ischaemic heart disease and the incidence of VEBs following AMI is variously reported as 34% to 100% but is probably nearly 100% if continuous automated observations are made [6, 55]. Both CCU and in-hospital mortality from myocardial infarction have been correlated with the frequency of paired, multiform, and R-on-T VEBs but one cannot with confidence assume a cause-and-effect relationship, since large infarcts are generally associated with a higher frequency of VEBs [53]. Infrequent VEBs are not generally associated with significant haemodynamic deterioration. However, as they become more frequent, and particularly when bigeminal rhythm supervenes, they may give rise to a haemodynamic deterioration due to the relative bradycardia induced, and this arrhythmia may require treatment in its own right. More often, VEBs are treated because of the fear that they may anticipate the development of ventricular tachycardia or fibrillation. In 1967 Lown et al. [33] suggested that VEBs of frequency greater than 5 min, of R-on-T type, of multiform appearance, of runs of two or more, and of bigeminal type commonly predispose to ventricular fibrillation. These arrhythmias were termed 'warning' arrhythmias. However, more recently many workers have questioned these principles, and perusal of several more recent papers [5, 11, 12, 29, 31, 42, 44] reveals the following points: Many episodes of ventricular fibrillation are not preceded by warning arrhythmias. Where warning arrhythmias are detected they do not necessarily lead on to ventricular tachycardia or fibrillation. Furthermore, as we have already seen, detection of such arrhythmias is related more to the technique used for monitoring than to their presence or absence. These observations cast considerable doubt on the value of initiating antidysrhythmic treatment on the detection of such 'warning' arrhythmias, and to date there has been no large controlled trial evaluating the effect of suppressing VEBs on the incidence of ventricular fibrillation within the first few hours of the onset of AMI. Trials with prophylactic administration of lignocaine, propranolol, procainamide, quinidine, and diphenylhydantoin have all been undertaken, but there is no unanimous view on the roll of routine antiarrhythmic therapy in AMI. In some units antiarrhythmic therapy is prescribed following the recognition of warning arrhythmias as described by Lown, while in others antiarrhythmic prophylaxis for 48 h after the onset of the symptoms of AMI is recommended. Antiarrhythmic therapy is usually given for some time after a recurrence of ventricular tachycardia or fibrillation.

Controlled trials have shown that prophylactic drug therapy by various agents will reduce the incidence of ventricular ectopic rhythms, but as already stated the more important question of whether these drugs will prevent primary ventricular fibrillation or decrease the mortality has not been answered. Bloomfield et al. [7] showed that quinidine reduced the incidence of ventricular arrhythmias after AMI. Propranolol was tried by Balcon et al. [3], and more recently Wilcox et al. [57] have compared propranolol, atenolol, and placebo, confirming no reduction in the mortality at 1 year in the treated groups. Koch-Weser et al. [26] conducted a controlled double-blind trial of procainamide in AMI and showed a statistically significant reduction in the incidence of VEBs together with a reduction in the incidence of primary ventricular fibrillation, though the latter did not reach statistical significance. Lie et al. [30] used continuous infusions of lignocaine 3 mg/min for 48 h after AMI, and showed a statistically significant decrease in the incidence of warning arrhythmias, ventricular tachycardia, and ventricular fibrillation in the treated group, though the mortality rates were similar in both the treated and the control groups and it should be noted that all deaths but one were accounted for by causes other than cardiac arrhythmia (such as cardiogenic shock, cardiac rupture, or pulmonary oedema).

Taking all this into account, our policy is to treat with antiarrhythmic drugs those patients who have haemodynamically significant ventricular ectopic arrhythmias; those in whom we have detected the R-on-T phenomenon; those in whom episodes of ventricular tachycardia have either been detected or treated by cardioversion; or those who have experienced any episode of primary ventricular fibrillation. Whatever policy is adopted concerning these antiarrhythmic drugs after infarction or after cardiac surgery, current evidence suggests that lignocaine is the most suitable drug to use. Various dosage regimens are described. We use 1 mg/kg IV over 1–2 min, followed by continuous infusion of 2–3 mg/min. A second bolus dose of half the amount in the first bolus can conveniently be given 10 min after the start of the infusion. Occasionally infusion rates of up to 4 mg/min may be required to control the ectopic rhythms which were the indication for treatment. Lignocaine is excreted mainly by hepatic metabolism, and if there is any evidence of liver impairment or markedly reduced cardiac output these doses should be halved. Side-effects commonly encountered involve the CNS and consist in dizziness, drowsiness, speech disturbances, tremor or, rarely, agitation. Occasionally cardiac side-effects are noted, such as hypotension or sudden increases in conduction disturbances. All these side-effects are indications to reduce the dose. Should such a regimen fail to suppress the arrhythmia despite the development of toxic side-effects, alternative treatment should be substituted. Disopyramide can be used with a loading dose of 2 mg/kg IV followed by maintenance, administered either IV or orally, with up to 1 g/day, although atropine-like effects and cardiac depression tend to be more of a problem when this preparation is given IV than is commonly observed with lignocaine. Mexiletine is pharmacologically very similar to lignocaine, but has the advantage that oral preparations can be used. It is more toxic than lignocaine when given IV but is very useful orally. Treatment should start with a loading dose of 400 mg, followed by 200–250 mg three or four times a day. Quinidine may also be used orally in doses of 250 and 500 mg twice a day in the sustained-release preparation (Kinidin Durules), and propranolol in doses of 160 mg a day or higher (as Inderal LA, 160 mg) can be used. Procainamide by mouth is useful, but hypotension often restricts its use by the IV route. It is our practice to institute some oral antiarrhythmic therapy 12 h or so after initiation of IV therapy, halving the IV therapy dose and terminating it entirely at 24 h while continuing the oral regimen for at least a week during mobilization.

Ventricular tachycardia

Ventricular tachycardia has been defined by the New York Heart Association as being present "whenever three or more ventricular premature contractions occur in sequence, having approximately the same contour and separated by a fixed interval". The rate "is usually from 140 to 200 beats a minute but may be somewhat slower or faster". The rate "is regular but 0.01 to 0.02 seconds variations in cycle time are seen" [38b]. There is usually AV dissociation but this is not always easily seen on surface ECGs and thus supraventricular tachycardias associated with bundle-branch block may cause some diagnostic problems. The haemodynamic consequences of the shortest and slowest ventricular tachycardia are negligible, but sustained tachycardias or those with a rate over about 140 beats/min tend to be associated with profound haemodynamic disturbance. Ventricular tachycardia after AMI demands immediate treatment as it is likely to lead to ventricular failure or ventricular fibrillation. If the patient has no profound haemodynamic disturbance treatment can be instituted with IV lignocaine given as described above for VEBs. If this fails or if the arrhythmia is associated with profound and immediate haemodynamic disturbance DC cardioversion is advisable. If the arrhythmia occurs repeatedly (even if in short runs and self-terminating) drug treatment is indicated and, as already stated, after DC cardioversion drug therapy is instigated in the hope that this will reduce the likelihood of recurrence. We favour the use of IV lignocaine together with the oral administration of mexiletine, IV lignocaine providing cover until the oral mexiletine can be expected to be effective. However, as both drugs have CNS side-effects a significant incidence is noted with this regimen, but any such side-effects are a reliable indication that the lignocaine should be given in smaller doses or discontinued. With care during the 'overlap' period between the effects of IV lignocaine and oral mexiletine the incidence of side-effects is kept acceptably low.

Idioventricular rhythm (slow ventricular tachycardia)

Sinus slowing, intermittent sinus arrest or sino-atrial block may lead to the appearance of a ventricular rhythm at or near to normal rates caused by the release of a lower ventricular focus accelerated by the effect of the infarction above the usual rate of between 40 and 60 beats/min. In some cases the QRS complexes are narrow, indicating an AV junctional focus rather than a lower ventricular focus. On the whole it causes little haemodynamic disturbance, as the only consequence is the loss of atrial transport and a minor degree of asynchronicity in ventricular contraction. The phenomenon is generally benign and does not usually require treatment. If, however, there is any haemodynamic deterioration it can usually be returned to sinus rhythm, as it is not usually associated with any AV conduction disturbance, by speeding up the sinus node with atropine.

Ventricular fibrillation

The only management is immediate defibrillation with all associated aspects of management [47]. Of course, the object of antiarrhythmic therapy in AMI is to attempt to prevent primary ventricular fibrillation. Although ventricular fibrillation is most likely to occur in the first few hours after infarction it is also quite likely to occur during the convalescent phase of myocardial infarction a week or more after the onset of the acute event, when it is sometimes termed 'late ventricular fibrillation'. It seems possible to make some prediction as to whether this phenomenon will occur. The patients involved have usually had an initial stormy passage with acute pulmonary oedema, a fairly persistent third heart sound, cardiomegaly, and prolonged, persistent ST segment elevation; and it seems reasonable to keep such patients under more prolonged supervision than is the current practice for uncomplicated infarction [32], perhaps keeping these patients in hospital for 2–3 weeks. It must be said, however, that as yet there has been no study to show that antiarrhythmic therapy for such patients is beneficial. It has been known for many years that the risk of sudden death after myocardial infarction diminishes fairly progressively over the first 6 months and then remains at a relatively low level. There is a strong association between LV dysfunction and death [20], and several reports have shown that there is a relationship between ventricular arrhythmias and subsequent sudden death, whether the arrhythmias were detected on routine ECGs, on exercise testing, or on 24 h tape monitoring [20, 27, 49, 56]. It may be that these arrhythmias are simply a measure of ventricular dysfunction rather than involving any great risk in themselves, and this may explain why so far the several trials on chronic antiarrhythmic drug therapy seem to have been relatively ineffective. Long-term prophylaxis with quinidine, procainamide, diphenylhydantoin, mexiletine, alprenolol, practolol, propranolol, and atenolol have all been tried, most showing small but not statistically significant benefits. Many of these trials are reviewed by Bigger et al. [6]. The most hopeful results have been obtained with the long-term use of beta blockers. A case can be made out for the permanent use of beta blockers (provided no contra-indication exists) after myocardial infarction or for the use of mexiletine for 3–6 months after infarction if life-threatening arrhythmias develop at any stage after infarction, but there is certainly no conclusive evidence that this course of action is helpful. Further large trials with mexiletine, disopyramide, and beta blockers are under way in an attempt to resolve these problems.

Disturbances of conduction

First-degree AV block

A not-infrequent arrhythmia which is most often associated with inferior infarction, first-degree AV block rarely causes significant haemodynamic deterioration, and if it progresses to second-degree block it usually gives rise to the Wenckeback phenomenon (Mobitz type I block) and so is unlikely to progress to asystole. However, observation should be more careful if there is associated bundle-branch block, as this suggests problems of conduction in the His–Purkinje system, and if there is a progression to a higher grade of block there is more likelihood of a bradycardia or asystole. Treatment for first-degree AV block is not usually required.

Second-degree heart block of Mobitz type 1 (Wenckeback phenomenon)

In the acute situation this is almost always a benign arrhythmia and when associated with inferior infarction, as it commonly is, it almost always yields eventually to sinus rhythm. When it is associated with narrow QRS complexes and an adequate ventricular rate, treatment is hardly ever indicated either in the short or in the long term, unless it can be proved that the rhythm is unstable and symptoms are due to the instability in the rhythm.

Second-degree heart block of Mobitz type II

The rhythm in Mobitz type II heart block (i.e., with no progressive increase in the P–R interval preceding the failure to conduct) is associated with damage to the conduction tissue in the low AV node and the His system. When it is seen in association with AMI it often progresses to complete heart block [39], and in view of this some clinicians recommend the insertion of a prophylactic temporary transvenous pacing system. This policy is not universally accepted; some do not insert a pacemaker unless there is recognizable haemodynamic deterioration. If ventricular demand pacing is decided upon it should be appreciated that atrial transport will be lost and it may be better to leave such a system set at a slow on-demand rate which allows atrial transport but protects the patient from asystole.

Third-degree (complete) heart block

When complete heart block develops simultaneously with AMI and is associated with haemodynamic deterioration, or with the development of ventricular instability such as multiple VEBs, temporary transvenous on-demand pacing is indicated. In the majority of cases where complete heart block develops in association with inferior myocardial infarction, the conduction disturbance is temporary and usually resolves within a week of the AMI. The temporary transvenous pacing system can be removed after it has been shown that conduction has been adequate for about 48 h. Where complete heart block develops suddenly in association with anterior myocardial infarction the prognosis is extremely poor, as the development of block in this situation implies extensive coronary disease and a large infarction. The majority of such patients usually succumb from cardiogenic shock or other complications of large infarctions.

It can thus be seen that it is unusual to have to convert a temporary pacing system put in after acute infarction into a permanent pacing system, but this should always be considered where complete heart block persists after AMI.

Fascicular blocks

It is now well recognized that the left bundle-branch system has electrophysiologically two discrete divisions [45], the posterior (inferior) fascicle having a dual blood supply from both the right and the left coronary arteries. The development of left posterior fascicular block (left posterior hemiblock, left inferior intraventricular block) usually implies more extensive cardiac damage that when there is left anterior fascicular block (left anterior hemiblock, left superior intraventricular block).

Furthermore, the combination of right bundle-branch block and left posterior hemiblock appears more likely to precede complete heart block than that of right bundle-branch block and left anterior hemiblock, and some authors recommend insertion of temporary pacing systems whenever such a combination of conduction disturbances complicates AMI (as a prophylaxis against very slow ventricular rates or asystole if the block progresses to a higher grade). Some physicians make similar recommendations even for the less ominous combination of right bundle-branch block and left anterior hemiblock when this complicates an acute infarct [2]. If bifascicular block is associated with a prolonged PR interval this suggests that there is disease in all three fascicles and probably warrants prophylactic pacemaker insertion. Where fascicular blocks are seen that are not associated with proven episodes of infarction, and where they are associated with an unstable cardiac rhythm, or proven symptoms, permanent pacing is indicated. The mere presence of fascicular block without any symptoms attributable to high grades of block or any ECG evidence of higher grades of block does not in itself constitute an indication for permanent pacing.

Temporary second-degree and third-degree heart block not uncommonly complicate cardiac surgery, particularly reconstructive surgery of congenital abnormality where suture lines or cardiotomies occur close to the AV node and His system. It has become a routine in most centres to insert temporary epicardial pacing leads onto the ventricle during closure of a thoracotomy in such patients, and many centres practise this as a routine for all such patients and indeed all valve replacement patients, routinely attaching a demand pacemaker set at a comparatively slow standby rate in case of bradycardia. There is no doubt that this adds a certain element of safety and confidence to the acute post-operative management of such patients. As a general rule we do not recommend the insertion of a permanent pacing system at the time of cardiac surgery even if a known pre-existing conduction disturbance requiring permanent pacing has been diagnosed. We manage these patients on temporary pacing systems, converting to a permanent transvenous system when the wound from cardiac surgery has soundly healed.

The term 'cardiac arrhythmia' encompasses an extremely heterogeneous group of rhythms, ranging from the totally innocent (e.g., sinus arrhythmia) to the immediately catastrophic (ventricular fibrillation). There clearly cannot be any uniform management policy. Furthermore, the same arrhythmia may have very different consequences, depending on (1) the clinical context in which it occurs and (2) the presence and severity of myocardial or valvular disease. The sensible approach to the management of arrhythmias demands an understanding of the mechanisms and consequences of the rhythm disturbance and on the possibilities of safe, effective intervention. Arrhythmias only require treatment when they are associated with current or potential haemodynamic impairment and when relatively safe, effective treatment is available.

References

1. Aber C (1973) Coronary care. Churchill Livingstone, Edinburgh London, pp 34–113
2. Atkins JM, Leshin SJ, Blomqvist G, Mullins, CB (1973) Ventricular conduction blocks and sudden death in acute myocardial infarction. Potential indications for pacing. N Engl J Med 288:281
3. Balcon R, Jewitt DE, Davis JPH (1961) A controlled trial of propranolol in acute myocardial infarction. Lancet II:917
4. Benchimol A, Ellis JG, Diamond EG (1965) Haemodynamic consequences of atrial and ventricular pacing in patients with normal and abnormal hearts. Effects of exercise at a fixed atrial and ventricular rate. Am J Med 39:911
5. Bennett MA, Pentacost BL (1972) Warning of cardiac arrest due to ventricular fibrillation and tachycardia. Lancet I:1351
6. Bigger JT, Dresdale RJ, Heissenbuttel RH, Weld FM, Wit AL (1977) Ventricular arrhythmias in ischaemic heart disease: Mechanisms, prevalence, significance and management. Prog Cardiovasc Dis 19:255
7. Bloomfield SS, Romhilt DW, Chou T (1971) Quinidine for prophylaxis of arrhythmias in acute myocardial infarction. N Engl J Med 285:979
8. Chamberlain DA, Leinback RC, Vassaux CE, Kastor JA, De Sanctis RW, Sanders CA, (1970) Sequential atrio-ventricular pacing in heart block complicating acute myocardial infarction. N Engl J Med 282:577
9. Cobb LA, Baum RS, Alvarez H, Schaffer WA (1975) Resuscitation from out-of-hospital ventricular fibrillation. Four years follow-up. Circulation 51/52 [Suppl III]:223
10. Day HW, (1963) An intensive coronary care area. Diseases of the Chest 44:423
11. Dhurandhar RW, MacMillan RL, Brown KWG, (1971) Primary ventricular fibrillation complicating acute myocardial infarction. Am J Cardiol 27:347
12. El-Sherif N, Myerbury RJ, Scherlag BJ, Befeler B, Aranda JM, Castellanos A, Lazzara R (1976) Electrocardiographic antecedents of primary ventricular fibrillation: Value of the R-on-T phenomenon in myocardial infarction. Br Heart J 38:415
13. Eraut D, Shaw DB (1971) Sinus bradycardia. Br Heart J 33:742
14. Evans R, Shaw DB, (1977) Pathological studies in sino-atrial disorder (sick sinus syndrome). Br Heart J 39:778

15. Fluck DC, Olsen E, Pentecost BL, Thomas M, Fillmore SJ, Shillingford JP, Mounsey JPD (1967) Natural history and clinical significance of arrhythmias after acute cardiac infarction. Br Heart J 29:170

16. Gallagher JJ, Gilbert M, Svenson RH, Sealy WC, Kasell J, Wallace AG (1975) Wolff–Parkinson–White syndrome. The problem, evaluation, and surgical correction. Circulation 51:767

17. George M, Greenwood TW (1967) Relation between bradycardia and the site of myocardial infarction. Lancet II:739

18. Goodman LS, Gillman A (1975) The pharmacological basis of therapeutics, 5th edn. Macmillan, London, p 673

19. Grace WJ, Chadbourne JA (1970) The first hour in acute myocardial infarction (AMI): Observations in 80 patients. Circulation 41/42 [Suppl III]:160

20. Greene HL, Reid PR, Schaeffer AH (1978) In: Sandoe E, Julian DG, Bell JW (eds) Management of ventricular tachycardia. Excerpta Medica, Amsterdam

21. Hinkle LE, Carver ST, Stevens M (1969) The frequency of asymptomatic disturbances of cardiac rhythm and conduction in middle-aged men. Am J Cardiol 24:629

22. Hon J (1973) Atropine and acute myocardial infarction. Circulation 47:429

23. Joseph SP, White J (1979) Long-term atrial pacing for sinus node disease with output terminal programmable pacemakers. J Thorac Cardiovasc Surg 78:292

24. Julian DG, Valentine PA, Miller GG (1964) Disturbances of rate, rhythm and conduction in acute myocardial infarction. Am J Med 37:915

25. Kleiger R, Lown B (1966) Cardioversion and digitalis. Circulation 33:878

26. Koch-Weser J, Klein SW, Foo-Cantor LL, Kastor JA, De Sanctis RW (1969) Antiarrhythmic prophylaxis with procaineamide in acute myocardial infarction. N Engl J Med 281:1253

27. Kotler MN, Tabatruk B, Mower MM, Tominaga S (1973) Prognostic significance of ventricular ectopic beats with respect to sudden death in the late post-infarction period. Circulation 47:959

28. Krikler DM, Curry PVL (1976) Torsade de pointes, an atypical ventricular tachycardia. Br Heart J 38:117

29. Lawrie DM, Higgins MR, Godman MJ, Oliver MI, Julian DG, Donald KW (1968) Ventricular fibrillation complicating acute myocardial infarction. Lancet II:523

30. Lie KL, Wellens HJ, VanCapelle FJ, Durrer D (1974) Lidocaine in the primary prevention of ventricular fibrillation N Engl J Med 291:1324

31. Lie KL, Wellins HJJ, Downar E, Durrer, D (1975) Observations on patients with primary ventricular fibrillation complicating acute myocardial infarction. Circulation 52:755

32. Lie KL, Liem KL, Durrer D (1978) Management in hospital of ventricular fibrillation complicating acute myocardial infarction. Br Heart J [Suppl] 40:78

33. Lown B, Fakhro AM, Hood WB, Thorn, GW, (1967) The coronary care unit: New perspectives and directions. JAMA 199:188

34. Macleod AA, Jewitt DE (1978) Role of 24-hour ambulatory electrocardiography monitoring in a general hospital. Br Med J i:1197

35. Mogensen L (1971) A controlled trial of lignocaine prophylaxis in the prevention of ventricular tachyarrhythmias in acute myocardial infarction. Acta Med Scand 513:1

36. Morris A, Bluestone R (1966) Treatment of slow heart rates following acute myocardial infarction. Br Heart J 28:631

37. Mueller HS, Ayres SM (1977) The role of propranolol in the treatment of acute myocardial infarction. Prog Cardiovasc Dis 19:405

38. New York Heart Association, Criteria Committee (1973) Nomenclature and criteria for diagnosis of diseases of the heart and great vessels, 7th edn. Little Brown, New York, p 196 (a); p 219 (b)

39. Norris RM (1970) In: Sandoe E, Flenstead-Jensen E, Olesen KH (eds). Symposium on cardiac arrhythmias. Astra Elsinore

40. Opie LH, Nathan D, Lubbe WF, (1979) Biochemical aspects of arrhythmogenesis and ventricular fibrillation. Am J Cardiol 43:131

41. Pantridge JF, Adgey AAJ, Geddes JS, Webb SW (1975) The acute coronary attack. Grune & Stratton, New York, pp 27–42

42. Raferty EB, Rehman MF, Banks DC, Oram S (1969) Incidence and management of ventricular arrhythmias after acute myocardial infarction. Br Heart J 31:273

43. Robinson, JS, Sloman JG, McRae C (1964) Continuous electrocardiographic monitoring in the early stages after acute myocardial infarction. Med J Aust 1:427

44. Romhilt DW, Bloomfield SS, Chou TC, Fowler NO (1973) Unreliability of conventional electrocardiographic monitoring for arrhythmia detection in coronary care units. Am J Cardiol 31:457

45. Rosenbaum M (1970) In: Sandoe E, Flenstead-Jensen E, Olesen, KH (eds). Symposium on cardiac arrhythmias. Astra Elsinore

46. Ross J, Linhart JW, Braunwald E (1965) Effects of changing heart rate by electrical stimulation of the right atrium in man: Studies at rest, during muscular exercise and with isoproterenol. Circulation 32:549

47. Rowlands DJ (1976) Cardiac arrest. Br J Hosp Med 16:310

48. Rowlands DJ (1978) The management of arrhythmias following an acute myocardial infarction. Intensive Care Med 4:13

49. Ruberman W, Weinblatt E, Goldberg JD, Frank CF, Shapiro S (1977) Ventricular premature beats and mortality after myocardial infarction. N Engl J Med 297:750

50. Shaw DB, Holman RR, Gowers JI (1980) Survival in sino-atrial disorder (sick sinus syndrome). Br Med J i:139

51. Shell WE, Sobel BE (1973) Deleterious effects of increased heart rate on infarct size in the conscious dog. Am J Cardiol 31:474

52. Skjaeggestad O, Berstad S (1974) Arrhythmias in the earliest phase of acute myocardial infarction. Acta Med Scand 196:271

53. Sobel BE, Roberts R, Ambos HD (1974) The influence of infarct size on ventricular dysrhythmia. Circulation 49/50 [Suppl III]:110

54. Sutton R, Citron P (1979) Electrophysiological and haemodynamic basis for application of new pacemaker technology in sick sinus syndrome and atrioventricular block. Br Heart J 41:600

55. Vetter NJ, Julian DG (1975) Comparison of arrhythmia computer and conventional monitoring in a coronary care unit. Lancet I:1151

56. Vismara LA, Amsterdam EA, Mason DT (1975) Relation of ventricular arrhythmias in the late hospital phase of acute myocardial infarction to sudden death after hospital discharge. Am J Med 59:6

57. Wilcox RG, Roland JM, Banks DC, Hampton JR, Mitchell JRA (1980) Randomised trial comparing propranolol with atenolol in immediate treatment of suspected myocardial infarction. Br Med J i:885

58. Zipes DP, Knoeble SB (1972) Rapid rate dependent ventricular ectopics. Adverse responses to atropine induced rate increase. Chest 62:255

Chapter 11

The Pathophysiology of Shock

R. J. D. George and Jack Tinker

Inadequate or inappropriate tissue perfusion sufficient to cause cellular hypoxia and the accumulation of toxic metabolites results in abnormal cellular metabolism and is the final common path in all causes of shock. Viewed in these terms, the complex reactions and countereactions of the body to the diverse causes of shock are all attempts towards restoring the normal 'milieu intérieur'.

This unified concept of shock as an inseparable breakdown of cellular metabolism and microcirculatory homeostasis leading to irreversible cardiovascular collapse has led us in this chapter to consider its pathophysiology in these terms.

Traditionally, shock is considered in three broad categories:

1) In *cardiogenic shock*, the cardiac output fails to meet the body's needs despite an adequate filling pressure. Acute myocardial infarction is the most important cause. Shock usually follows infarction of more than 45% of the left ventricular myocardium [20, 108], when mortality may be as high as 90% [124].

2) *Hypovolaemic shock* is due to a reduction in actual circulating blood volume from haemorrhage, indirectly by electrolyte losses, or from loss of plasma, e.g., in burns. A reduction of up to 25% may be accommodated by regional vaso-constriction in healthy subjects [167]. Early fluid replacement rapidly reverses these changes with a good prognosis. This is the most common cause of shock [85].

3) *Septic shock* may occur in any infection associated with the release of foreign polysaccharides or proteins [159]. The initiation of shock due to sepsis occurs in the microcirculation (Fig. 11.4), when alterations in nutrient capillary flow, permeability and disseminated intravascular coagulation (DIC) disrupt tissue oxygenation sufficiently to compromise intermediary metabolism and organ function. Cellular oxygen consumption and energy production is also reduced at an early stage. Initially the systemic circulation is spared and cardiac output may, in fact, increase in what is termed warm or hyperdynamic shock [145, 159, 161, 168]. The ability to maintain a normal or elevated cardiac output and respond to a fluid load are important prognostic markers [97, 143, 161]. A mortality of 25% in warm hypotension rises to greater than 60% in those with low cardiac output [159]. The importance of sepsis in hospital practice is well known: it occurs in 1% of the hospital population (100 000–300 000 patients) in the United States [170]. In the United Kingdom septic shock most commonly follows gastro-intestinal surgery [84].

The evolution of shock (Fig. 11.1)

In the early stages of shock, the changes observed are directly related to the initial pathology. But as the microcirculation, and particularly the cell, become increasingly disrupted, metabolites are liberated into the circulation in significant quantities. These changes are independent of the primary aetiology and herald the establishment of shock proper. These vasoactive byproducts may alter capillary permeability, dilate arterioles and propagate DIC to exacerbate regional ischaemia and cellular damage still further. The paralysed microcirculation ultimately expands and fluid leaks into the extracellular space causing tissue oedema. Thus hypovolaemia, myocardial oedema, and nonspecific toxic metabolites all continue to impair cardiac output further. In addition, sustained ischaemia in the gut increases its permeability and allows systemic invasion by the gut flora.

In the late stages, therefore, distinction between the three types of shock is lost and, more important, the patient develops features of hypovolaemia, myocardial failure, and septicaemia as momentum gathers and death ultimately supervenes.

In terms of diagnosis and management, shock is most conveniently considered from the viewpoint of the systemic circulation, as objective measurement and therapy are expressed initially in these terms. However, pathophysiologically it is more logical and less repetitive to begin at the final common abnormality, cellular hypoxia, and piece together the changes that give irreversible shock its momentum.

The cell

Normal cellular respiration

All cells must oxidize substrates to provide fuel for exergonic (energy-utilizing) functions. The currency is the high-energy phosphate bond, and the commonest compound is adenosine triphosphate (ATP). Synthesis and transport of specialized cellular products, neuromuscular function, and maintenance of transmembrane potentials are all exergonic.

High-energy phosphate bonds are generated by glycolysis of glucose-6-phosphate (G6P) to pyruvate, an anaerobic process yielding two ATP molecules. Kreb's citric acid cycle provides the final common path for the major oxidative

energy-yielding reactions. Both fatty acids and pyruvate enter via acetyl-coenzyme A to produce CO_2 and NADH. NADH then passes down the electron transport chain of cytochromes to form water and NAD. This last step is termed oxidative phosphorylation and probably occurs on the inner mitochondrial membrane [1]. Aerobic metabolism of one glucose molecule yields a total of 38 ATP molecules.

In the absence of oxygen, energy is only available from anaerobic glycolysis. The essential regeneration of NAD under these circumstances is achieved by reduction of pyruvate to lactate and this is one of the causes of acidosis in hypoxia. Breakdown of ATP is possibly a major cause of acidosis in the myocardium, but this is a subject of much controversy.

Hypoxia

Transient hypoxia is a normal event in certain tissue, notably exercising muscles and certain metabolic organs. Several mechanisms therefore exist to circumvent this temporary lack of oxygen. In general, resistance to hypoxia depends upon blood supply and tissue glycogen content. For example, astrocytes have only enough reserves for 15 s, but the liver may continue functioning anaerobically for several hours [173]. Skeletal muscle is the only organ capable of storing oxygen in significant quantities, which it does as myoglobin. Additional substrate and high-energy phosphate bonds are stored as glycogen and creatine phosphate. In cardiac muscle an oxygen debt may not be incurred and the only source of high energy bonds is anaerobic glycolysis [108]. Skeletal muscle can be anoxic for up to 30 min [1]. Local acidosis is considerable. During hypoxia cell permeability to glucose rises, as does catecholamine-induced glycogenolysis, to provide sufficient substrate for anaerobic glycolysis [18, 121]. The increased glycolysis under hypoxic conditions is known as the 'Pasteur effect'.

Under normal circumstances cardiac output rises and local metabolites increase regional flow to accommodate the need for additional

Fig. 11.1. Summary of the interrelationships between cardio ▷ vascular, microcirculatory, and cellular changes in the evolution of shock. The complexity of this flow diagram emphasizes the plethora of positive feedback loops at all levels in shock and integrates Figs. 11.2, 11.4, and 11.5. ———, cardiovascular changes; −−−−, microcirculatory changes; −·−·−·−, cellular changes. The line coding shown is common to all the flow diagrams in this chapter.

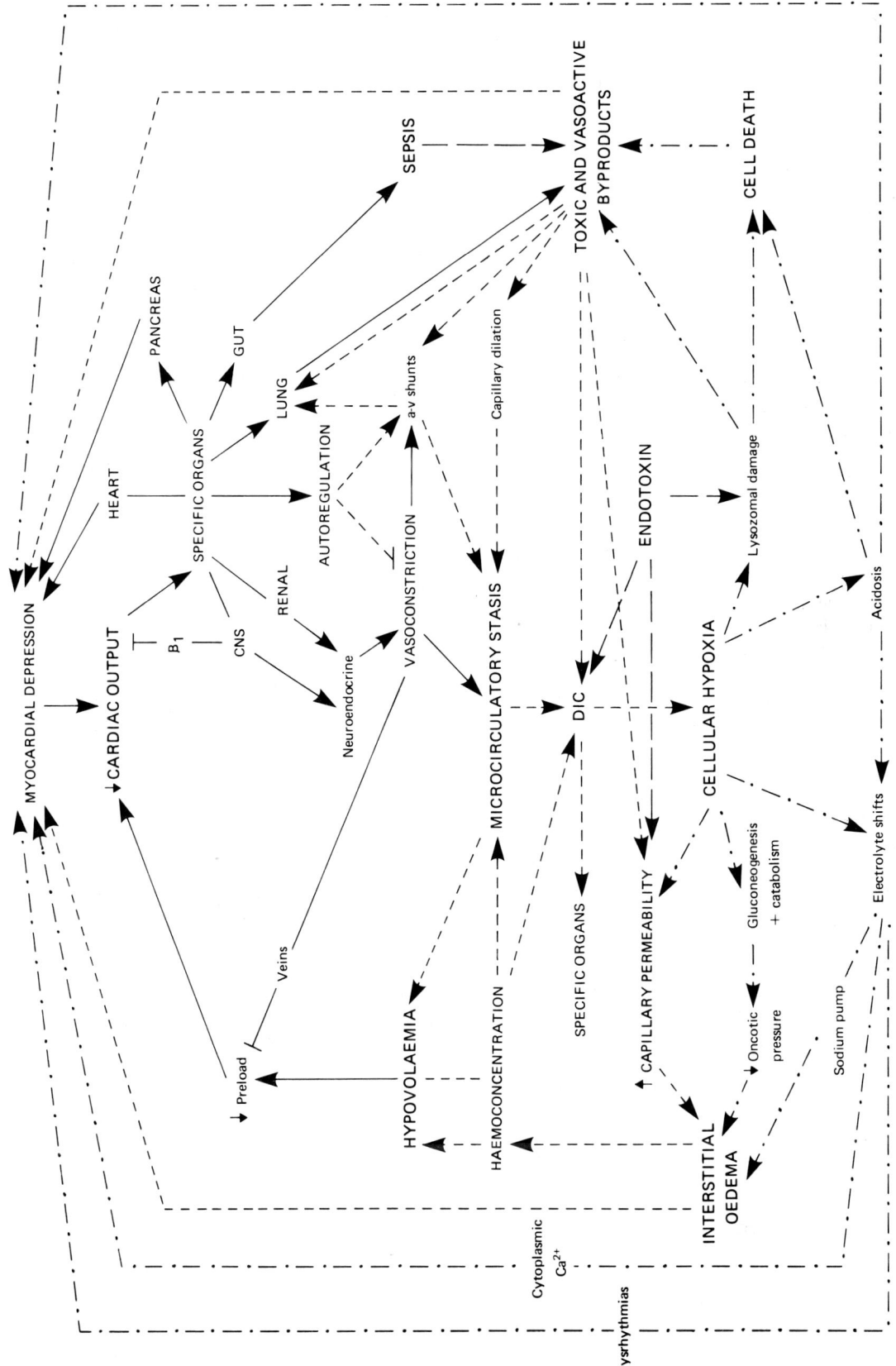

oxygen. Respiration and tissue oxygen extraction also rise [69].

Consequences of sustained hypoxia: The sick cell (Fig. 11.2)

The most obvious consequence of sustained hypoxia is a precipitous drop in ATP concentration, so that exergonic reactions eventually cease. The importance of this is highlighted by the fact that survival of experimental animals in the recovery phase of shock is dependent upon the rate of rise of cellular ATP [68] and in shock models in which 100% mortality is expected this may be reduced to 27% by infusion of ATP–$MgCl_2$ solution [21].

The exergonic function vital to all cells is the sodium pump. As this fails, transmembrane potentials are lost and ultimately sodium and water enter the cell and potassium leaves it. The resulting cellular oedema affects all intracellular organelles, and the mitochondria and lysozomes in particular [36, 134]. In addition to cellular respiration the mitochondria are responsible for major intracellular stores of calcium. As intracellular phosphate rises (due to dissociation of ATP to ADP + PO_4), calcium leaves the organelle. This is facilitated by the increased permeability of both the mitochondrial and cellular membranes [60]. The net effect is a sustained rise in intracellular calcium ([Ca]i); and there is positive feedback as [Ca]i inhibits ATP translocase and impairs ATP release by the mitochondrion [75].

The central role played in the myocardium by calcium is well documented. It is responsible for both the plateau phase of the cardiac action potential (CAP) and excitation–contraction (e–c) coupling [126]. It is the flux of calcium via slow Ca^{2+} channels in the sarcolemma that produces the characteristic CAP and couples activation with optimum contraction. Persistence of a high [Ca]i will result in failure of muscular relaxation and arrest in systole [172]. Cyclic AMP and ATP contribute to the propogation of these fluxes by phosphorylation of a membrane-bound gating protein which allows passage of Ca^{2+} to and fro [126, 151].

Cyclic AMP (cAMP) is probably also of particular significance as the common path in the regulation of [Ca]i. Sperelakis and Schneider [151] proposed that a control over exergonic activities in the myocardial cell (i.e., excitation and contraction) was achieved via ATP, the concentration of which would determine the number of Ca^{2+} channels open, and therefore the cells' contractility and energy expenditure.

They also suggested that [Ca]i itself could be a sensor. Subsequently, work in turkey red cells [154] and glioma cells [15], both good sources of adrenergic-adenylcyclase receptor complexes, has implied that adenylcyclase is, in fact, Ca^{2+}-sensitive via allosteric binding and has a biphasic response. At low [Ca]i, there is a 40% increase in activity up to 1 μmol, and then at levels of 10–100 μmol, progressive inhibition. One may speculate that a similar arrangement is present in the myocardial cell, where this ingenious feedback system would allow a [Ca]i of 10 μmol to be reached rapidly and produce optimum e–c coupling [151]. Any wasteful excess Ca^{2+} shift would be abbreviated by the feedback inhibition and energy expenditure kept to a premium. This model may explain several observations.

1) The fall of intracellular cAMP and loss of sensitivity to beta-adrenergic stimuli with sustained hypoxia in both the myocardium and peripheral vasculature;
2) The disruptive effect of acidosis; Regional myocardial ischaemia is sufficient to cause pH to fall below 6.8, and complete Ca^{2+} slow channel inactivation will occur at pH 6.4 [151]. This inactivation is, in part, due to competitive inhibition of calcium-dependent reactions by hydrogen ions.
3) The negative inotropism and peripheral vasodilatation of certain endotoxins (via smooth muscle dilatation), as endotoxins significantly impair ATPase dependent Ca^{2+} uptake by the sarcoplasmic reticulum [130, 150, 172];
4) The positive inotropism of (a) Ca^{2+} infusions and (b) dexamethasone via increased Ca^{2+}/ATP movement in the mitochondrion [75] and the effects of $ATPMgCl_2$ infusions on survival [20].

Aside from the particular changes in the myocardial cell, the important repercussions of cellular hypoxia which influence the organism as a whole are the release of toxic by-products. These amplify local changes through the microcirculation and ultimately lead to systemic vascular collapse (see section: *The microcirculation*).

In sepsis, apart from the effects of hypoxia, there is a primary abnormality of cellular metabolic processes such that amino acid, fat, and glucose handling is significantly altered. The mechanism is unclear, but is evident through a

Fig. 11.2. The intracellular consequences of sustained hypoxia. (See text for commentary.) $\triangleright$

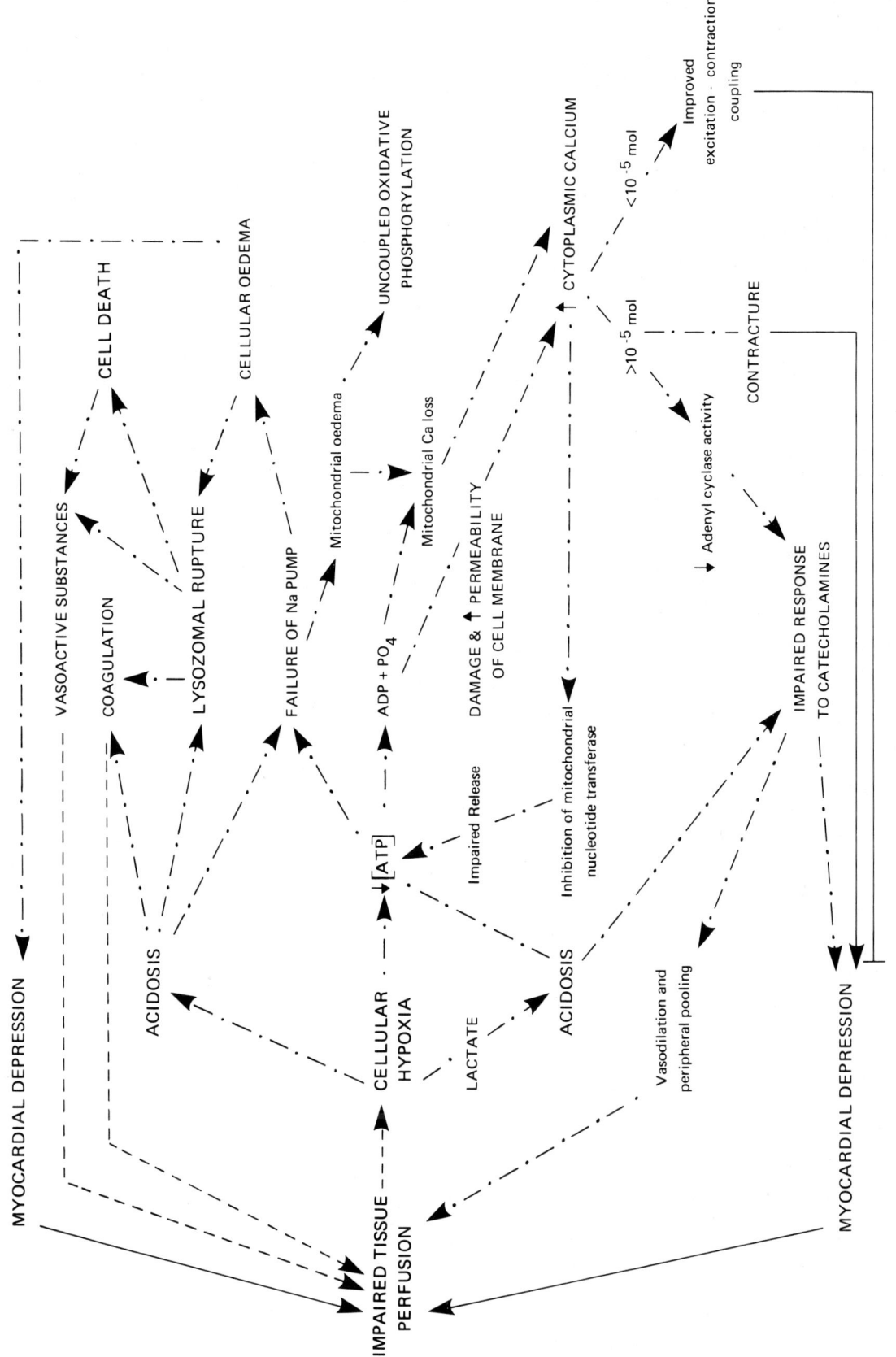

rise in pyruvate concentration. This is suggested by the multiple regression equations developed by Siegel [145] to characterize the changes seen in the metabolism of the septic cell. It seems that particular patterns of cellular and haemodynamic abnormalities occur together, which is strong evidence in favour of a cellular or metabolic concept of shock.

The microcirculation

Anatomy

The microcirculation is the delivery and exchange network of the cardiovascular system. Its function is to modify regional flow according to need by integrating central and peripheral control mechanisms. For simplicity, it may be considered as a unit comprising the terminal arteriole and precapillary sphincter, the capillary exchange bed and the postcapillary venule. Both the arterioles and venules contain smooth muscle capable of altering vessel calibre, and the arteriole is the site of maximum peripheral resistance. It appears that the hallowed precapillary sphincter is not muscular, but may be an aggregation of cells capable of swelling and shrinking according to ambient conditions [146]. Some authorities believe that it responds only to regional humoral changes [72].

Theoretical considerations

Rheology

The physics of a non-Newtonian fluid such as blood flowing in a pulsatile fashion through distensible tubes makes any succinct discussion of rheology impossible. Nonetheless, isolated statements may be made and the reader referred to specialist texts [14, 26, 73].

1) In general terms at a microcirculatory level, Poiseuille's Law still applies:

$$\text{Flow} = \frac{\pi r^4 \Delta P}{8l \, \eta},$$

where r = radius, ΔP = pressure drop along tube, l = length of tube, η = viscosity of fluid.

2) The viscosity of blood is inversely proportional to flow rate for two reasons: the plasma is both a colloid of proteins and a suspension of red cells. At high flow rates the red cells deform to become elliptical, and this lowers viscosity. At low flow rates, therefore, there is a significant rise in viscosity and, in addition, reversible aggregation of red cells and platelets. Though not contributing significantly to the overall changes of viscosity, the plasma proteins, in particular fibrinogen, maintain red cell flexibility [7, 30].

3) The haematocrit is thus the most important determinant of viscosity at high and low flow rates. In vitro, viscosity remains effectively constant to a PCV of 40%, above which it rises rapidly. An optimum of 30% to accommodate both adequate O_2 carrying capacity and flow is suggested by Hanson (53). In sepsis, where oxygen demand is high, there is no significant haemodynamic upset to 15 mg% Hb [167].

4) Plasma skimming, a phenomenon in which the red cells congregate centrally in the vessels, goes some way to reduce viscosity.

Practically, therefore, the physician should aim for vessel patency, an adequate head of pressure, and blood with optimum O_2-carrying capacity and viscosity, which is achieved at a haematocrit between 30% and 40%.

Physiology

The capillary endothelium provides a selectively permeable membrane between the blood and the extracellular space, across which there is exchange of nutrients and metabolites. The balance of fluid between these two compartments, and therefore the integrity of the circulating blood volume, depends upon three factors; plasma colloid oncotic pressure (COP), capillary hydrostatic pressure and capillary permeability. The COP depends almost entirely upon the serum albumin concentration, (COP = [albumin] × 0.57) [119], as the endothelium is virtually impermeable to molecules of this size. Any albumin entering the extravascular fluid space is either membrane bound and metabolised or cleared by the lymphatics [139]. Capillary hydrostatic pressure, usually in the region of 15 mmHg, depends upon the relative arteriolar and venular tone, factors of enormous importance in acute hypovolaemia.

The relationship of COP, hydrostatic pressure and fluid shifts was first described by Ernest Starling in 1896 [152], at which time capillaries were considered impermeable to proteins. The equation has since been modified to accommodate capillary permeability [44]:

$$JV = Kfc \, [Pc-Pt - \sigma(\pi c - \pi t)],$$

where JV = fluid exchange; Kfc = capillary filtration coefficient; P = hydrostatic pressure;

π = oncotic pressure; σ = capillary membrane reflections coefficient; c = capillary; t = tissue. σ = 1 for solute exclusively confined to the capillary, σ = 0 for water, σ = 0.9 for protein.

Under normal circumstances, there is a net imbalance in favour of fluid egress into the interstitium of about 1 mmHg. Lymphatic flow copes with this and maintains a tissue oncotic pressure approximately two-thirds that of plasma [44]. Similarly, in the face of a falling oncotic pressure, the increased transcapillary flow is accommodated by a rise in lymphatic drainage, but the susceptibility to oedema is increased. Changes in capillary permeability are of greater importance. (General application to the capillary bed will be made below. The particular case of the lung is dealt with elsewhere.)

Normal microcirculation

Tissue blood flow and autoregulation

The relative importance of rheology and physiology varies from tissue to tissue according to blood flow and this in turn is an integration of central nervous (principally sympathetic) and regional control. However, 'Whenever conflict arises, local metabolic control predominates' [123]. This is particularly in evidence in the vital organs; brain, heart, kidney and, to a lesser extent, skeletal muscle, where the effect of local myogenic and humoral mechanisms maintain tissue blood flow at a near constant level over a wide pressure range (Fig. 11.3). This 'autoregulation' therefore assures adequate oxygen delivery over all but extremes of pressure. Two mechanisms exist for autoregulation.

1) The *myogenic response* (Bayliss effect) is an inherent sensitivity of the precapillary arterioles to intravascular pressure, and was first suggested by Bayliss [5]. A rise in either arteriolar or venous pressure (transmitted retrogradely) will result in vasoconstriction so that the important capillary hydrostatic pressure gradient is preserved [72]. This response is very rapid, taking about 3 s.

2) In the *humoral response*, the metabolic changes seen in hypoxic cells release a plethora of vaso-active substances. However, the conceptual difficulty of a distal metabolite affecting the precapillary sphincter is obvious. Microscopic observation of capillaries has shown that under normal circumstances the direction of flow down a capillary is frequently reversed and that isolated venular constriction results in extensive changes in flow patterns within the capillary bed [14]. This may allow metabolites to reach a more uniform concentration in the capillary bed as a whole and thus exert some influence upon the anatomically proximal sphincter region. Furthermore, experimental observation on rat mesentery shows that distal capillary stimulation causes the endothelial cells in the region of the precapillary sphincter (itself cellular) to swell [146].

Many mediators have been implicated in autoregulation, and indeed these may vary between organs [146]. Adenosine, PO_4 and 5^1-nucleotidase are potent coronary vasodilators [108], whereas PCO_2 (via pH) and csf HCO_3 concentrations are probably of greater significance in cerebral blood flow [81]. Other important possible vasodilators are K^+ and lactate.

As the essential role of autoregulation is preservation of an adequate oxygen supply, hypoxia must be the sensor determining local flow, appropriately set for each organ. A direct effect on capillary wall PO_2 is unlikely, as this

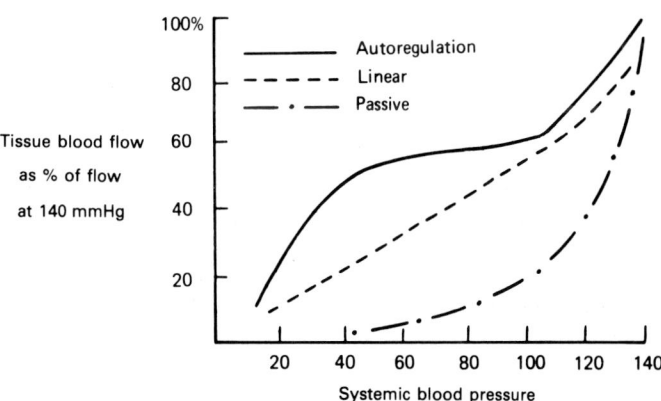

Fig. 11.3. The pressure-flow relationships that may occur in arterioles (adapted with kind permission from Ledingham I McA (ed) *Shock—Clinical and Experimental Aspects.* Excerpta Medica, Amsterdam 1976, p 3).

Autoregulation flow is characteristic of privileged organs, where flow is maintained constant over a wide pressure range; linear flow is characteristic of rigid tubes, e.g., atheromatous vessels; passive flow is characteristic of distensible vessels, namely normal arterioles without autoregulation, e.g., skin and all ischaemic tissue with toxic arteriolar paralysis.

must be very low. The respiratory enzymes or ATP/adenosine ratios are also candidates, but no firmly accepted mechanism exists [146].

Particular characteristics of regional auto-regulation clearly will depend upon the requirements of the organ in question. The effectiveness of myogenic control lies in its rapidity, which may be of especial advantage in muscle. The brisk response to changes observed by Silver in 1977 [146] in the brain may also be myogenic, as other workers stress this component of cerebral autoregulation [81]. The integration of central function may also be relevant here, as for example, cholinergic dilator, low-resistance channels are seen in skeletal muscle, whose function may be to modify flow during exercise [123].

The effects of the sympathetic nervous system are highlighted in the cerebral circulation where a rise in the noradrenaline concentration shifts the autoregulation curve in Fig. 11.3 to the right, presumably as protection against potential arterial hypertension. This also occurs in other tissues [72].

The abnormal microcirculation

Failure of autoregulation

The effectiveness of autoregulation is entirely dependent upon sphincter and smooth muscle sensitivity to appropriate metabolites and the physical ability of vessels to dilate under these circumstances. In the early phases of cardiogenic and hypovolaemic shock, where sympathetic tone is high, the autoregulation curve shifts to the right. As ischaemia persists, the local by-products exert an increasing influence on arteriolar tone until they dominate, and the capillary beds re-open [12]. The flow characteristics then become passive and pressure-dependent (Fig. 11.3).

Vessel distensibility is frequently compromised by atherosclerosis. In addition to the adoption of a linear pressure–flow curve, regional perfusion pressures are disproportionately reduced by large atheromatous plaques. Autoregulation is therefore active at an earlier stage, and so toxic arteriolar paralysis is also an earlier event. Autoregulation in surrounding, healthy tissue will produce a relatively larger calibre change than the atheromatous neighbour, resistance will be lower, and blood will therefore divert preferentially to these less needy areas. The result is that healthy tissue will be assured of survival, but critically ischaemic tissue may infarct.

The cerebral circulation is particularly susceptible, and pressures that would easily sustain a youthful cortex may cause signs of ischaemia in elderly patients [171]. The critical effect of ischaemia on brain stem function is obvious. The diseased myocardium is also at risk, as collateral vessels, essential in maintaining flow to ischaemic areas, are less distensible than the preferred anatomical routes [108]. Infarction may therefore complicate a potentially reversible hypovolaemia with cardiogenic shock. The renal circulation is of particular interest, as autoregulation is over-ridden in acute hypotension [8]. (See section on the kidney under *Effect of shock on specific organs*.)

Evolution of irreversible shock and microcirculatory collapse (Fig. 11.4)

In the early and reversible stages of shock where, for example, volume expansion will restore the circulation, the compensatory mechanisms (sympathetic discharge and autoregulation) have provided an alternating, obligatory, and intermittent flow to non-vital areas sufficient to ensure survival and a sustained supply to essential organs. Established and irreversible shock supervenes when the previously restricted beds open and venous return is lost by peripheral pooling [111]. These changes are almost exclusively due to the interactions of vasoactive substances and the development of DIC. They are summarized in Fig. 11.4.

The progression of ischaemia to stagnant hypoxia was first suggested by Lillehei [92] in an elegant analysis. The initial sympathetic vasoconstriction in response to hypotension affects the precapillary arterioles more than the postcapillary venules. The resultant fall in hydrostatic pressure in the capillary exchange bed allows the blood volume to be augmented by interstitial fluid. Should ischaemia persist, however, anaerobic respiration leads to the changes detailed in the section: *The cell*. Acidosis, often as low as pH 6.9 [59, 146], antagonizes catecholamines directly, and lysozomal rupture promotes the formation of vasoactive and toxic metabolites. In addition to the loss of sympathetic control and disruption of controlled autoregulation, these humours influence capillary permeability and myocardial contractility, and they precipitate intravascular coagulation. The

Fig. 11.4. Summary of the changes that form the basis of ▷ irreversibility in shock. The omnipotence of both vaso-active by-products and endotoxin is emphasized.

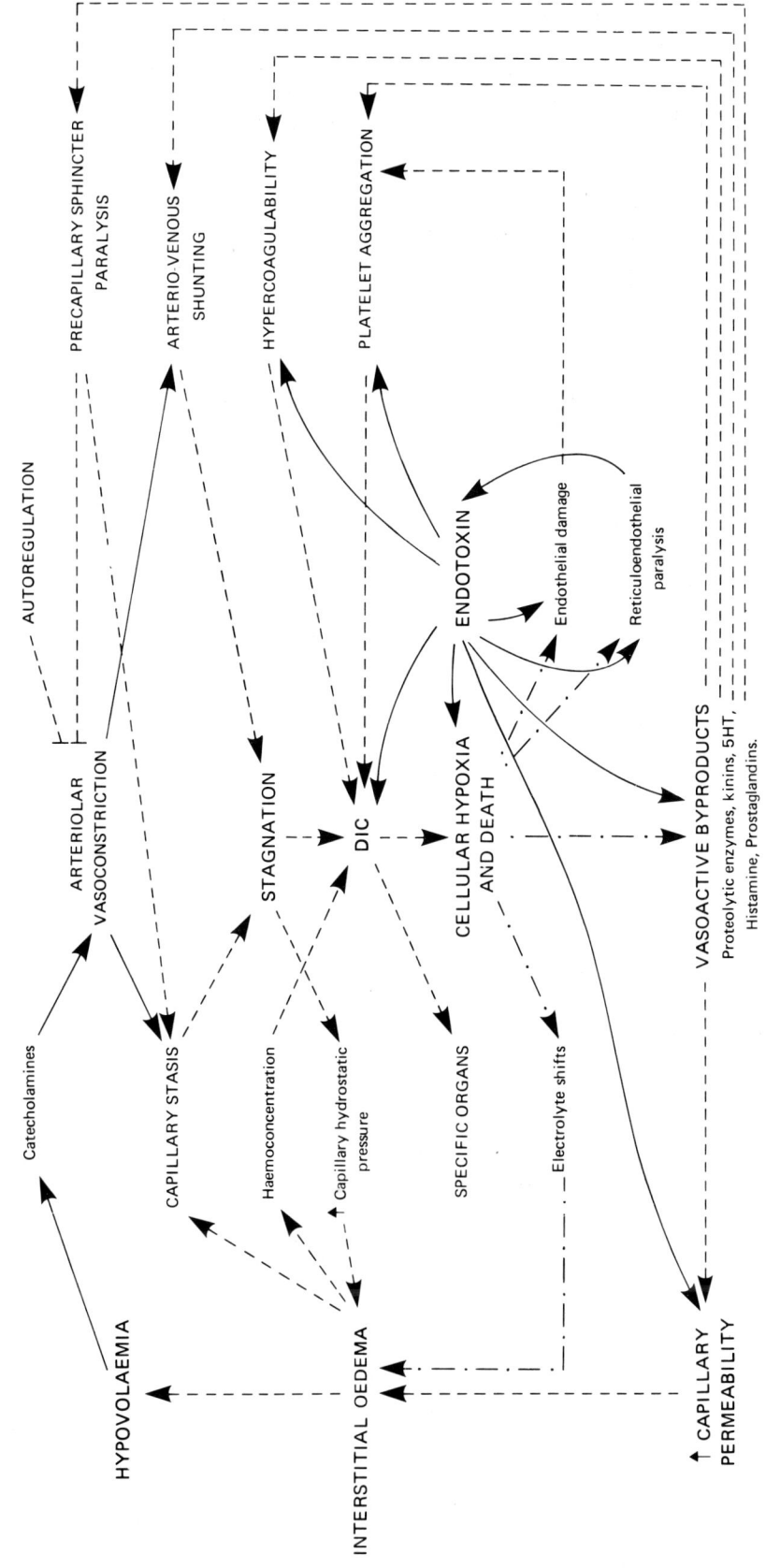

main contenders have recently been reviewed in detail by Nagler and McCohn [111]. In the flow diagrams these are grouped under vaso-active substances (Figs. 11.1 and 11.4).

The net effect of these changes is precapillary sphincter paralysis, arteriolar dilatation, and peripheral pooling in the previously closed capillary beds. Venular smooth muscle is more resistant to vasodilators [123], so that there is capillary stagnation, a rise in hydrostatic pressure, and reversal of the early compensatory interstitial fluid recruitment. Fluid therefore leaves the vascular space aided by the increased vascular permeability. Local haematocrit and viscosity must rise and susceptibility to coagulation becomes inevitable. The interstitial oedema completes the cycle by mechanically occluding the capillaries.

Vaso-active substances

Lysozomal enzymes and kinins

Lysozomal enzymes are in abundance in liver, kidney, spleen and polymorphs [111]. The stimuli to release, other than cell death, are hypoxia, ischaemia, sepsis and acidosis [70, 148, 163]. Their role is significant, as (a) the concentrations measured in blood are related to the duration of shock [41]; (b) their effect in sepsis may be blocked by aprotinin to reduce pneumonitis in the isolated, perfused lung [23]; and (c) pretreatment with steroids interferes with lysozomal release to good effect [166]. Apart from direct cytotoxicity, myocardial depression, and coronary vasoconstriction [47], lysozomal enzymes digest endogenous protein, and α_2 globulin in particular with the release of kinins from kininogen [107].

There are many kinins, the archetype being bradykinin. The group has four main actions; profound vasodilatation, increased capillary permeability [111], myocardial depression [142], and a close interrelationship with Hageman factor and the activation of coagulation [155]. Kinins are considered to be especially prominent in the mediation of endotoxic shock [122], when the principal source is the gut [77]. Most endotoxins have no direct circulatory effect. The lung may also be involved in kinin activity in shock as it is known to be capable of both their production and inactivation [33, 46, 51]. Nagler and McCohn suggest that a number of as yet unidentified kinins may be responsible for shock.

Induced histamine

The suggestion of histamine as an initiating humour was reintroduced by Schayer [133] when he found a significant rise in histidine decarboxylase activity accompanying the early hypotensive phase of septic shock. The arguments are only persuasive for endotoxaemia, however. It must be stressed that this 'induced histamine' is independent of the endogenous mast cell histamine and is not blocked by antihistamines [167].

Prostaglandins

This heterogeneous group of carboxylic acids is in the middle of a renaissance following recent interest in the latest additions, prostacyclin (PGI_2) and thromboxane (PGA_2). The omnipotence of the group as a whole upon the vascular endothelium and aggregation properties of platelets is almost certainly of significance in the pathophysiology of shock [38].

Table 11.1. Vascular actions of prostaglandins

	PGA₂	PGD₂	PGE₁	PGE₂	PGF₂α	PGI₂
Vasdilation				√		√
Vasoconstriction	√				√	
↑ Permeability		√		√		
Platelet aggregation	√			√		
Aggregation inhibition		√	√			√

Table 11.1 summarizes the main prostaglandins contributing to changes in the microvasculature. Group E and F have directly opposing vasomotor effects, to the extent that their relative concentrations are of most significance. Both are metabolized by the lung and ordinarily are present in arterial blood in very low concentrations [35]. In experimental endotoxic and haemorrhagic shock, the levels rise. However, the relative increase of $PGF_{2\alpha}$ in haemorrhagic shock implies that these levels are regulated in some way rather than being consequent upon passive changes [37]. $PGF_{2\alpha}$ may also play a part in the early pulmonary hypertension of endotoxic shock.

The roles of prostacyclin and thromboxane are discussed in the section on DIC.

Endotoxins

The ubiquity of this group of toxins is self-evident (Figs. 11.1 and 11.4). However, the brunt of the attack is born by the microcirculation. Distinction between gram-positive and gram-negative infections in pathophysiological terms [78, 98, 161, 165] is now obsolete [167]. Both groups produce toxins, e.g., staphylococci, in addition to a local coagulase, liberate an α toxin which vasoconstricts, causes endothelial damage and platelet aggregation, increases membrane permeability, and uncouples oxidative phosphorylation [159]. The classic endotoxin released by dead gram-negative bacteria is lipid A, which is a concealed membrane fragment with low antigenicity. The effects of endotoxin are legion, but may be grouped broadly.

Vascular effects. The reduction of peripheral resistance and mean circulating time in all septic shock [143] strongly implicates arterio-venous shunting through the resistance bypass channels. This is probably not a direct effect but the result of increased catecholamines, released by endotoxin, closing the capillary beds [82]. In sepsis the arterio-venous shunts appear to escape intrinsic control and are either open or closed according to the ambient pressure. The major evidence in favour of this concept is the small change in oxygen consumption relative to flow [98]. However, these changes are probably only half the story, as recent work suggests that capillary flow through muscles in shock is unchanged [174] and that defective oxygen utilisation and abnormal cellular respiration is an early event in sepsis [145]. Defective uptake of oxygen may therefore account significantly for this paradox.

Tissue damage. Endotoxin is itself cytotoxic. Both the cellular and mitochondrial membranes may be modified by interpolation of lipid A. In the latter, this is probably the mechanism by which oxidative phosphorylation is uncoupled [159]. (See section: *The cell.*) Endothelium and other exposed tissue is destroyed and the reticulo-endothelial system disrupted with the release of neutrophil procoagulant [159] and impaired phagocytosis of thrombogenic fibrinogen complexes [86]. The role of complement seems to vary with the type of lipid A and activation may occur via both classic and alternate pathways to amplify toxicity. C_3 levels have been used as prognostic markers [91].

Disseminated intravascular coagulation

DIC may be defined as an acute, widespread but transient clotting of blood in the microcirculation [55]. DIC is widely accepted as a major factor in irreversible shock [55, 59, 116, 120], and its role in certain organs, especially the lungs, is a subject of much debate [24, 29].

In the classic triad of Virchov changes in blood flow, the vessel wall and the blood components are necessary for coagulation. From rheological studies, we see that the sluggish capillary flow in shock is sufficient for long rouleaux of red cells and clumps of platelets to accumulate. This occurs with a four-fold reduction in flow rate. These aggregates are reversible, but highly susceptible to the most trivial additional stimulus for coagulation, e.g., hypoxia, acidosis, toxins, etc. [14]. As stagnation of blood continues, coagulation is inevitable. It appears not only that the integrity of the endothelium is important to prevent exposure of the highly thrombogenic collagen, but that the cells also actively prevent irreversible platelet aggregation by the production of prostacyclin (PGI_2). This recently discovered prostaglandin is not only a potent inhibitor of platelet aggregation [104] but also causes vasodilatation [103] (Table 11.1).

Changes in the blood per se are legion. Hypovolaemia itself is sufficient to cause hypercoagulability [56] but the metabolic changes of cellular hypoxia [148], acidosis [58], endotoxins, either directly via procoagulants (106) or indirectly via the reticulo-endothelial system [114, 120], platelet damage and the kinins [155, 159] are all known precipitants of intravascular coagulation.

In summary, therefore, microthrombi may form via vessel damage and the extrinsic cascade, or via Hageman factor and the intrinsic cascade in a highly susceptible, viscous, and sluggish circulation. Ischaemia lasting in excess of 1 h is sufficient to cause cell death [55].

Aside from the individual cellular consequences, consumption of the clotting factors over a sustained period will lead to a secondary bleeding diathesis, and specific changes in various organs. (See section: *The effect of shock on specific organs.*)

The most significant end-products of microcirculatory failure are profound hypovolaemia, both in real terms with a loss of fluid through leaky capillaries at a rate as high as 200 ml/h, and functionally with capillary stasis. Together with myocardial depression systemic vascular collapse becomes irreversible and other organs fail; arterial hypoxia develops, acute renal failure further disrupts fluid balance, consciousness is clouded, and there may be haemorrhagic enterocolitis. (See section: *The effect of shock on specific organs.*)

The systemic circulation

Physiology

The function of the heart is to pump blood, and its output is the product of stroke volume and heart rate.

Stroke volume is the objective result of myocardial fibre shortening, dependent upon the intrinsic myocardial contractility, end-diastolic fibre length (preload), and the resistance to ejection (afterload). Anything that modifies cardiovascular function must act through one or other of these 'intrinsic' physiological variables. Figure 11.5 shows the interrelationships of the intrinsic variables and the ways in which extrinsic factors may exert their influence.

Intrinsic factors

Myocardial contractility

This is the ability of cardiac muscle to develop tension from a given end-diastolic fibre length. It is dependent upon the sarcomere length, the optimum being 22 μm when actin/myosin overlap is maximum [74]. Myocardial contraction may then proceed provided there is adequate intracellular ATP and Ca^{2+} for excitation/contraction coupling [151]. This forms the mechanical basis for Starling's law of the heart [153]. Extrinsic factors may influence myocardial contractility by changing ATP availability or calcium handling by the cell, or by disordered patterns of myocardial contraction.

Preload: The Frank–Starling relationship

Otto Frank, using the isolated frog heart [40], and later Ernest Starling, using the dog heart–

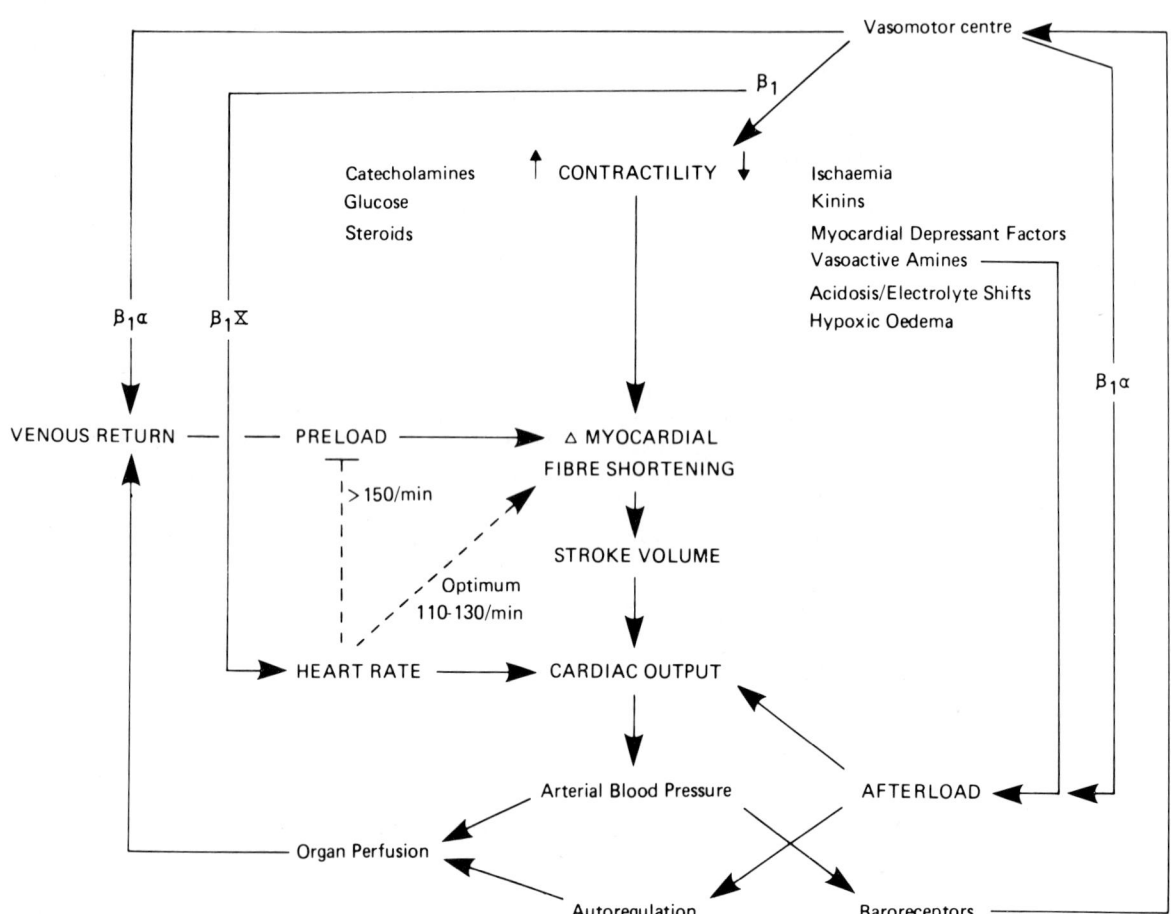

Fig. 11.5. Interrelationships of intrinsic variables in the systemic circulation and ways in which extrinsic factors may exert their influence.

lung preparation [153] discovered the dependence of myocardial contractility upon initial fibre length: 'The law of the heart is thus the same as the law of muscular tissue generally, that the energy of contraction, however measured, is a function of the length of the muscle fibre' [153]. In the presence of a constant afterload this may be extrapolated to relate ventricular end-diastolic pressure (VEDP) to stroke volume or cardiac output [132]; these are variables easily measured in man.

Heart rate

In the normal heart, the VEDP depends upon atrial emptying and, therefore, the duration of diastole, such that a rise in heart rate is accompanied by a fall in stroke volume and cardiac output remains constant [149]. However, contractility may, in fact, rise with heart rates between about 50 and 150 beats/min above which stroke volume and cardiac output fall disproportionately [127, 167]. Oxygen consumption at rates above 100 is considerable.

Afterload

This is the resistance against which each ventricle pumps. In the case of the left heart, it represents total systemic vascular resistance. A rise in afterload leads to a rise in ventricular and aortic pressure.

This peripheral resistance is predominantly generated by the arterioles. The vascular tone is the resultant of vasoconstricting alpha-adrenergic stimulation and the predominantly local vasodilating metabolites. Beta-adrenergic and cholinergic vasodilator fibres do exist

regionally as well. Organ flow is therefore regulated physiologically by the extent of alpha-adrenergic innervation and the existence of regional autoregulation [147]. (See section: *The normal microcirculation*.)

The relationship of right and left heart

The heart is usually considered in the singular; but the realization that it is two pumps in series is germane to any physiological discussion [13]. As a generalization the right heart is a low-pressure circuit, where pulmonary vascular resistance is low. The principal intrinsic denominator of stroke volume is therefore the preload (venous return). Conversely, the left heart is a high-pressure system and stroke volume is therefore more dependent upon afterload (systemic vascular resistance). The left ventricle is necessarily more muscular and less compliant, so that for a given end-diastolic volume its preload must be proportionately greater, and so therefore must the pulmonary capillary hydrostatic pressure. Under normal circumstances, the Starling curves for right and left ventricles are essentially parallel. In univentricular failure this no longer applies and each ventricle must then be considered separately (Fig. 11.6). This is of particular importance in left ventricular failure if capillary permeability and colloid oncotic pressure are abnormal, as pulmonary oedema may develop at a lower pulmonary capillary pressure [160]. (See section: *Theoretical considerations* under *The microcirculation*.)

As the left heart is responsible for systemic perfusion, and impaired systemic tissue perfusion is the basic defect underlying shock, the

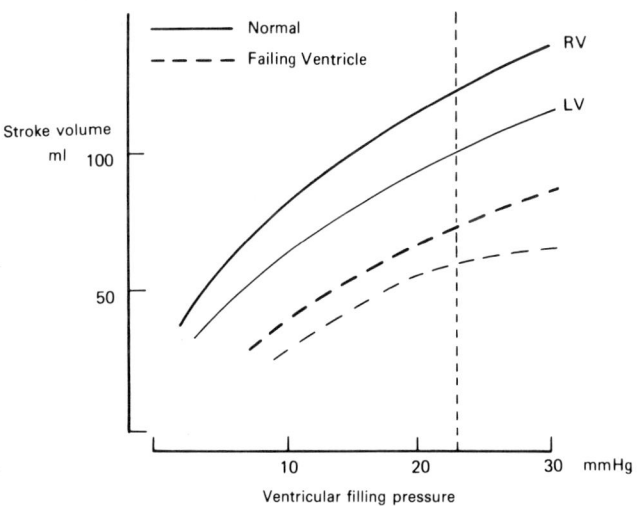

Fig. 11.6. Relationship of right and left ventricles in the normal and the failing heart.

clinician's attention must focus primarily upon the performance of the left ventricle. For effective control, therefore, an accurate index of preload must be available. Left atrial pressure is not easily and safely accessible, but pulmonary capillary pressure closely equates with left ventricular end diastolic pressure providing mitral valve function is normal [156]. This may be measured with a wedged pulmonary artery catheter. The same catheter can be used to measure cardiac output by thermodilution (see Chap. 57). With this monitoring at the bedside, the extrinsic influences upon the heart may be assessed accurately.

Extrinsic factors

Sympathetic nervous system

Central integration of neural cardiovascular control occurs in the medullary vasomotor centre (VMC). The major peripheral stimulus is a change in blood pressure sensed by stretch receptors in the aortic arch, carotid body, and major arteries [62]. The firing pattern at a given pressure is greater when the pressure is rising rather than falling, which makes the response rapid and accurate [79]. Other afferent information comes via the hypothalamus. The chemoreceptors may also modify VMC responses to changes in PO_2 and PCO_2 [80].

Alpha receptors are responsible for increases in vascular tone both in the arteriolar resistance vessels and venous capacitance vessels. Beta receptors increase myocardial contractility and heart rate, and peripherally act as vasodilators [82]. The parasympathetic supply to the heart is vagal and slows heart rate. Within the autonomic control of vascular tone, the overall change in tone depends upon the ratio of alpha to beta receptors [147]. Where alpha receptors predominate, such as skin, gut and, to a lesser extent, kidney, there is dramatic vasoconstriction. The cerebral and coronary flows are virtually uninfluenced, except that the autoregulatory pressure flow curves are shifted to a higher pressure [50].

Humoral factors

Aside from the humoral mechanisms discussed in the microcirculatory section, a large proportion of the peripheral metabolites have a direct effect upon myocardial function as well as afterload. Myocardial failure is therefore a major factor in the later stages of shock of any aetiology.

Positive inotropes

Catecholamines released by the autonomic nervous system, the adrenal medulla, and therapeutically by the physician are all positively inotropic. They increase intracellular cAMP and myocardial permeability to Ca^{2+} thereby facilitating e–c coupling (section: *The normal microcirculation*). Glycogen breakdown also increases the concentration of glucose, which is the only energy substrate that may be metabolized anaerobically. Heart rate is variably affected and the rise in preload obviously influences myocardial performance via the Frank–Starling relationship. With the increasing acidosis of sustained shock, the effect of catecholamines on the myocardium is gradually lost [22].

The direct actions of corticosteroids on myocardial performance are debatable. Some workers have found them to be positive inotropes (66), although the effect was inconstant, whilst others have failed [87]. This may be due to different experimental models (dogs and cats, respectively). However, an increase in coronary blood flow is an accepted finding [66, 158] and dexamethasone is known to influence ATP and Ca^{2+} handling by myocardial mitochondria [60].

Negative inotropes

The heterogeneous population of vasoactive substances released by hypoxic tissue include a number of myocardial depressants. These originate largely from the pancreas and splanchnic region and are cellular proteins fragmented by released proteolytic lysozomal and zymogen enzymes [52, 88]. At present, some nine substances, small polypeptides of between 250 and 1000 mol. wt, have been isolated by a number of workers and found to be negatively inotropic on both intact animal hearts and isolated papillary muscle preparations. This action is independent of pH, Na^+, and K^+ concentrations, coronary blood flow or preload [128]. The archetype of this group, myocardial depressant factor (MDF), probably interferes with the calcium and the e–c coupling process, as very high calcium concentrations (7.5 mmol) will reverse its effect upon muscle strips [89]. In addition to its effect upon the myocardium, MDF provides two positive feedback mechanisms: further splanchnic vasoconstriction and impaired macrophage phagocytosis, which ensure that the level of these toxic peptides remains high within the blood [88].

Although the bulk of the cardiotoxic peptides are splanchnic in origin, the reticulo-endothelial system is the source of a high molecular weight (16 000) aggregated γ globulin with the cumbersome name passive transferable lethal factor (PTLF) [110]. It is present in shocked patients and post-cardiopulmonary bypass in concentrations proportional to the clinical state. Again the negative inotropism is independent of coronary blood flow [88, 111, 128].

The apparent ubiquity of these toxins (detection has been reported in haemorrhagic, endotoxic, and cardiogenic shock and in shock following splanchnic ischaemia, pancreatitis, and burns [27, 93, 129]) has led recently to the reappraisal of steroids, and in particular of aprotinin, in the preventive management of potentially susceptible patients [48, 68].

In addition to their production of toxic proteolytic fragments, lysozomal enzymes are direct negative inotropes and coronary vasoconstrictors [47].

The myocardial depression of sepsis is not due to endotoxin, which alone has no cardiotoxicity [65]. Only with the release of the abovementioned toxins is there any tangible effect on the cardiovascular system [28]. The effects of myocardial oedema, etc., are discussed in the next section.

The systemic circulation in shock

Hypovolaemic and cardiogenic shock are both primarily failure of the intrinsic cardiovascular variables. Septic shock affects both afterload and the myocardium. Late in all forms of shock, peripheral vascular paralysis, interstitial fluid loss, and toxic myocardial depression invariably coexist.

Hypovolaemia

Following loss of volume in a closed system, there are two avenues of compensation: an increased turnover, with the product of stroke volume and heart rate returning cardiac output to normal, or a shrinkage of the effective volume to be perfused. In addition to these, the circulation may recruit fluid from the interstitial space.

Acute hypovolaemia such as follows haemorrhage leads to an initial fall in venous return. Stroke volume, cardiac output, blood pressure, and baroreceptor discharge all therefore fall, and the vasomotor centre (VMC) responds by increasing adrenergic discharge:

(a) Heart rate and myocardial contractility rise due to beta stimulation; (b) Volume deficit is compensated by preserving only essential organ perfusion. Heart, brain, hepatic and diaphragmatic flow is essentially unaffected and the percentage cardiac output in these organs rises [147]; (c) Venous constriction reduces venous capacitance and augments the reduced preload via alpha and possibly beta receptors. (d) Interstitial fluid supplements blood volume, as discussed in the section: *The microcirculation*. The vasoconstriction in the arterioles exceeds that of the veins, so that hydrostatic pressure within the capillaries falls and fluid will enter the vascular space until the balance is redressed. In the acute phase, this flow may approach 1 litre/h, with falls of as much as 27% in plasma protein [19]. Falls in cardiac output of 50% and in volume of 35% can be accommodated briefly, and volume replacement will reverse all the changes. As 'physiological' ischaemia continues, the likelihood of irreversible microcirculatory damage rises dramatically.

These compensatory mechanisms are extremely effective in the acute stage of shock from any cause, to the extent that hypovolaemia may pass unnoticed until local ischaemia unmasks its presence. Clinically, it is important to realise that in an otherwise healthy individual, a 25% reduction in plasma volume may occur without hypotension [57]. The need to ensure that the plasma volume and preload are adequate at all times cannot be overemphasized.

Changes in afterload and endotoxic shock

The secondary rise in afterload in response to a falling cardiac output has been discussed. Primary changes in the peripheral vasculature and therefore in afterload and preload are associated with septic shock, and the effects on the systemic circulation are manifest in this way. Myocardial depression, though probably a relatively early change, is initially obscured by the inotropic effect of endogenous catecholamine release. As sensitivity to adrenaline and noradrenaline is lost, myocardial failure per se is more obvious [63].

The single common feature of septic shock due to either gram-positive or gram-negative bacteria is a fall in peripheral resistance [63, 137, 143, 161, 162, 168, 169], and clinically the two are indistinguishable [159]. The fall in peripheral resistance is due to dilatation of the low-resistance AV shunts that bypass the capillary networks, with the result that the tissues remain hypoxic.

The evidence for shunting with continuing precapillary vasoconstriction may be summarized as follows [143]:

(a) Narrow A-V O_2 difference confirms impaired O_2 extraction. This may be as low as 10%–15% [167]. (However, the contribution of impaired O_2 extraction has been mentioned in this context.) (b) Higher flow rates, often 2–3 times normal, are necessary for a given O_2 consumption [98]. (c) O_2 consumption in ventilated patients is directly related to myocardial work, which implies a constant, reduced body O_2 consumption. (d) Mean transit time is low.

In spite of continuing closure of the capillary beds, peripheral pooling and extravasation of fluid may be sufficient to reduce the preload. This apparent hypovolaemia and its effect on cardiac output is not uncommon [63, 168] and a feature of septic shock is the dramatic response to plasma expansion [162, 174]. An adequate preload is essential and the ability to respond a good prognostic sign [98, 161].

The overall effect of a reduced afterload, a variable preload and progressively increasing myocardial depression (see below) is that the cardiac index [cardiac output per unit surface area (CI)] may be several times normal or only a fraction of that required for adequate perfusion [2, 98, 143]. It may also fluctuate [143]. Opinions vary as to the significance of the CI on survival [115, 143, 157], but the consensus of opinion is that a high output is a good prognostic sign [161]. In an appraisal of several series it was found that a CI > 3.1 litres/min per m^2 at the onset of shock correlated well with survival ($r = 0.86$). McLean [98] found that in a series of 28 patients with early sepsis an ability to increase CI by 1 litre/min per m^2 in response to a fluid load was the best predictor of survival.

In summary, an elegant model of the initial compensations in sepsis is the adaptation of the circulation to an acute, major AV fistula, e.g., VSD [140] or a central AV fistula [112]. The sudden evolution of a shunt leads to hypotension as the afterload falls dramatically. The baroreceptors and sympathetic axis release catecholamines in an attempt to restore systemic blood pressure with arteriolar vasoconstriction and an increase in heart rate, myocardial contractility, and venular tone (maintaining a CVP). The capillary beds are therefore rendered ischaemic. However, the metarteriolar shunts in sepsis have no adrenergic innervation and represent the VSD, which stays open passively as the preferrred path of least resistance. The peripheries remain warm and apparently well perfused. With the late onset of myocardial failure, cardiac output falls, the passive shunts close, and the patient becomes cold and clammy. Ultimately, the capillary beds re-open

and there is stagnant peripheral pooling and hypovolaemia.

Changes in the myocardium

The initial sympathetic and evoked endocrine responses to hypotension all continue to improve myocardial performance via beta receptors, mobilization of glucose, and release of steroids from the adrenal cortex. The point at which myocardial performance itself is of importance depends upon the aetiology of the shock.

Oxygen availability and coronary blood flow

As coupling of energy supply and demand is essential in the myocardium, where an O_2 debt may not be incurred, inotropism, in the absence of depressants, depends upon O_2 availability. This is met by increased blood flow as O_2 extraction is very high, normally 65%, and a rise to 75%–80% is a sign of significant myocardial hypoxia [108]. In essence, therefore O_2 supply is determined by Aortic pressure/Coronary vascular resistance (modified Poisseuille). The privilege of autoregulation normally preserves flow down to pressures of approximately 50 mmHg. Owing to the high intraventricular pressures, the subendocardium is the least well-supplied area, and so autoregulates at higher pressures. This increases its susceptibility to hypoxia and lactic acid gradients [131]. Heart rate and ventricular end-diastolic volume are also important in this context.

The predilection of atheroma for the coronary arteries means that autoregulation is frequently disrupted, and the pressure: flow relationship becomes linear (Fig. 11.3). This may put a significant area of myocardium at risk, and is of great importance in uncomplicated myocardial infarction, or shock with complicating ischaemic heart disease. Under these circumstances an adequate perfusion pressure is mandatory, but inevitably this requires the expenditure of more energy and an increase O_2 requirement. The development of ischaemia in sepsis is a grave prognostic sign [162]. An interesting study in dogs showed that myocardial infarction is well tolerated before exposure to shock and myocardial depressants, but if this insult succeeds toxaemia, ventricular fibrillation is universal and only adequately treated by lignocaine [128]. A reasonable compromise is to maintain a systolic pressure of 80 mmHg [61].

Myocardial hypoxia

From the section: *The cell* we see that hypoxia at a cellular level in an organ so dependent upon ionic fluxes as the heart may lead to aberrations of contraction and excitation before cellular damage is irreversible. In the myocardium, hyperkalaemia, acidosis, and changes in ionized calcium all impair performance, either by the development of dysrhythmias or by interfering with e–c coupling. As myocardial oedema develops, it reduces capillary flow further (especially in the subendocardium where the intramyocardial pressure is already high), impairs O_2 diffusion and reduces myocardial compliance. Contractility therefore suffers [63, 162]. Vaso-active, hypoxic by-products compound capillary permeability, and some are selective coronary vasoconstrictors.

Limitation of myocardial hypoxia is a balance between generating pressure to provide adequate coronary perfusion and, at the same time, reducing myocardial work. This unique combination is, in fact, provided by intra-aortic counterpulsation [108, 125]. Pharmacological agents such as beta blockers, vasodilators, and inotropes, provide only one or the other [3, 61, 108]. This is discussed in detail in Chapter 12.

The effect of shock on specific organs

Brain and neuro-endocrine axis (Fig. 11.7)

The brain stem is the integrator of minute-to-minute cardiovascular control (see section: *The systemic circulation*). However, the influence of neural mechanisms stretches beyond this, in that survival, in spite of adequate coronary flow, depends ultimately upon the brain [49].

The central role of the brain at all stages in shock probably depends upon the neuro-endocrine axis, which coordinates the sympathetic nervous system, the hypothalamus, and the pituitary. In the early phase of hypotension, compensation is neural and the sympathetic discharge is dependent upon the medullary vasomotor centre in the brain stem, though the denervated heart will respond slowly to changes in haemodynamics according to Starling's law [31]. In addition to volume sensors, pH, PCO_2, osmolality, hypoxia, sepsis and so on, all evoke central responses. The nucleus of this neuro-endocrine axis is probably the hypothalamus, whence the medullary reticular formation and autonomic outflow provide the prime neural efferents, and the hypothalamus and pituitary the endocrine axis [32]. Responses may be divided simply into

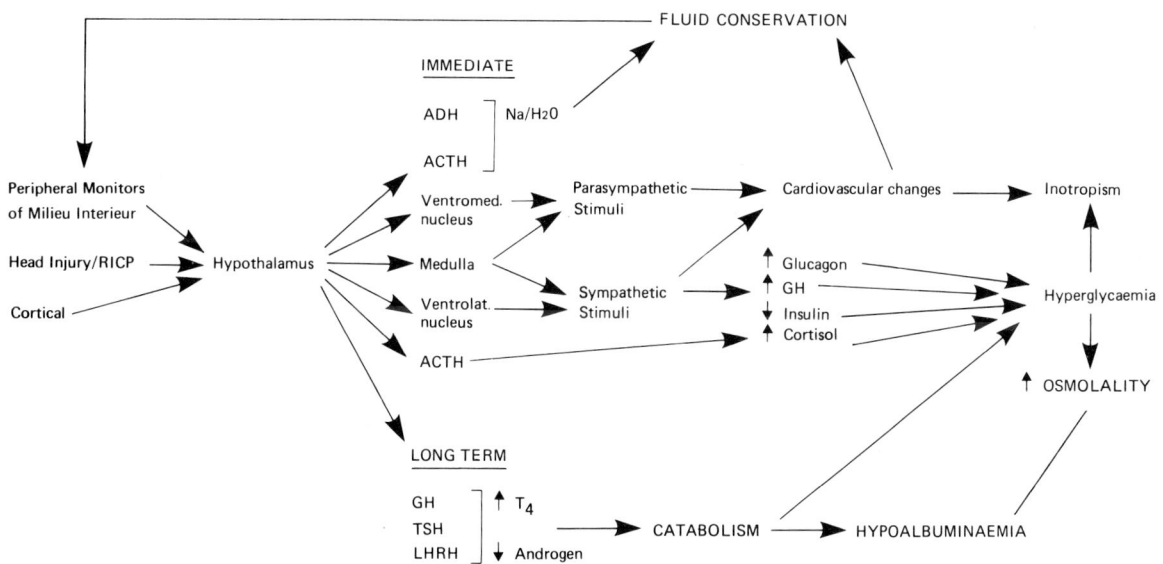

Fig. 11.7. The neuro-endocrine axis in shock.

those of immediate benefit and long-term compensation. They are detailed in Fig. 11.7.

Immediate benefit. Haemodynamics are adjusted by catecholamine release from the adrenals and sympathetic nerves (see section: *The systemic circulation*). ADH, aldosterone and cortisol are released by both renal and central osmolar changes to conserve sodium and water and maintain plasma volume.

Impaired O_2 delivery increases the need for glucose as the only anaerobic energy source (see section: *The cell*). Hyperglycaemia is promoted by catecholamines, glucagon, cortisol and growth hormone release, with inhibition of insulin secretion. This is hypothalamic in origin [42]. As insulin is essential for transmembrane glucose transport, the efficacy of glucose–insulin–potassium cocktails has been a source of much research. The acute catabolic response is unhindered [16, 17] but haemodynamics and myocardial carbohydrate metabolism both improve [118, 164].

Long-term compensation. Thyroxine secretion and antagonism of androgens by catecholamines help provide a sustained catabolic response as a source of glucose [32]. However, this is ultimately deleterious, as plasma albumin falls to exacerbate tissue oedema, immunoparesis develops and healing may be delayed.

Shock due to primary cerebral pathology

Shock associated with raised intracranial pressure is due to stimulation of adrenoreceptors, as pulmonary oedema may be blocked by alpha blockade or cord section [9, 117]. Myocardial necrosis, possibly adrenergically mediated, also occurs in subarachnoid haemorrhage, and this is presumably due to brain stem compression [113].

Pulmonary oedema in head injury is considered to be due to venular constriction in the pulmonary bed [117].

Kidney

The pathophysiology of acute renal failure is discussed in Chapter 24. In the face of impaired organ perfusion, the kidney contributes principally by conserving blood volume. It may also aid in peripheral vasoconstriction.

Consequences of falling renal blood flow (Fig. 11.8)

The responses to acute haemorrhage and slow sustained hypotension are different. In the latter, autoregulation is unimpaired and so the glomerular filtration rate (GFR) is preserved down to systemic pressures of approximately 70 mmHg [6]. However, in acute hypotension, renal blood flow (RBF) is sacrificed early by the relatively rich sympathetic supply, which initially overrules local factors. Alpha blockade will abolish this effect [8].

The pattern of RBF has been a subject of debate mainly due to methodology, but it is now accepted that flow in deep cortical nephrons is maintained selectively. The mechanism is very complex and varies with the cause of hypotension. Prostaglandins, renin, and sympathetic nerves all interact to produce selective juxtamedullary flow [105]. Deep cortical

RENAL COMPENSATION IN SHOCK

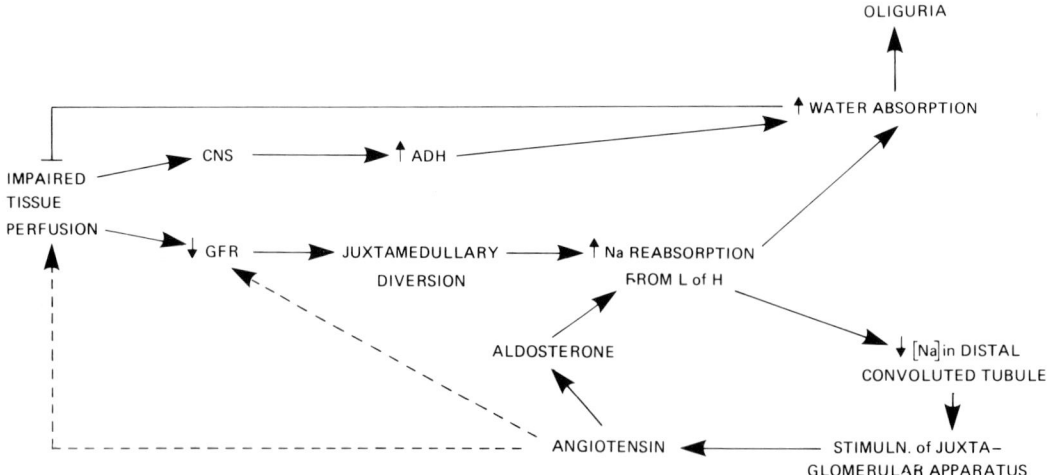

Fig. 11.8. Renal compensation in shock.

nephrons are those with predominantly long loops of Henle, and this redistribution therefore allows maximum sodium reabsorption and preservation of the countercurrent medullary concentration gradient. The superficial cortical nephrons are also said to secrete more renins [67]. The mode of redistribution is probably afferent vasoconstriction modulated by angiotensin and prostaglandins [76, 105].

The combined fall in GFR and Na^+ concentration in the distal convoluted tubule prompts renin secretion and conversion of angiotensinogen to angiotensin I and II and aldosterone. Whether angiotensin confines its vasoconstriction to the afferent renal arteriole is not known, but it does increase Na^+ reabsorption further and helps preserve intravascular volume. A fall in urinary Na^+ to less than 10 mmol is a useful sign of intensive renal compensation in hypovolaemia.

The precise mechanism is unknown, but sepsis frequently causes inappropriate polyuria with hypovolaemia. In the absence of renal failure, this may give a clinical suspicion of sepsis [94].

Lung

Preservation of the pulmonary circulation and adequate gas exchange is vital. Changes that may compromise most organs mildly are devastating to the enormous area of exchange membranes in the lung, as the juxtaposition of alveolar epithelium and capillary endothelium is directly responsible for gas exchange (especially O_2) and essential for efficient oxygenation. The additional function of the lung as a metabolic organ must not be dismissed.

The adult respiratory distress syndrome (ARDS) is discussed in detail in Chapter 18. In summary, the pattern of pulmonary changes in shock begins with hyperventilation, alkalosis, and mild hypoxia, followed by increasingly impaired oxygenation and metabolic acidosis as lactate from anaerobic respiration spills into the systemic circulation. Microvascular changes of irreversible shock: increased capillary permeability, pulmonary hypertension resulting from vaso-active metabolites, and DIC herald overt pulmonary failure [24].

Septic shock is associated with respiratory failure in the majority of cases. In one survey [25], 91% of patients with respiratory failure and intermittent positive pressure ventilation (IPPV) showed evidence of sepsis and sepsis was associated with respiratory problems in 42% of

cases. Pure hypovolaemia was complicated by respiratory problems in only 7% of patients in another survey [43].

Alkalosis, which accompanies both hypovolaemic shock and sepsis, is neurogenically mediated via pulmonary J receptors in response to congestion, humoral agents (possibly the main mechanism in sepsis), and lung mechanics, e.g., falling compliance [29, 71]. The reflex is abolished by vagotomy, and is probably the origin of pulmonary complications in head injury [117].

Pulmonary hypertension, best assessed as a PAEDP greater than 4 mmHg above PCWP, is again a universal finding, though the aetiology is multifactorial [10, 25, 175]; but this is another field of research which is dogged by the problems of animal models and species variation. Venular constriction may be either centrally mediated, secondary to the vaso-active amines (histamine and 5HT) liberated by damaged platelets, a side-effect of fibrinolytic fragment D (which is a by-product of DIC) [96], or due to the mechanical effect of pulmonary oedema [4, 11, 23, 25, 71, 120, 141].

Systemic hypoxia is due to ventilation/perfusion mismatch, caused by both micro-atelectasis and the AV shunts that develop parri passu with microcirculatory damage. This is especially prominent in the hyperdynamic septic patient, where an increased cardiac output is required for the same O_2 capacity. In terminal stages, the rising capillary permeability leads to pulmonary oedema.

The metabolic functions of the lung have been emphasized in shock as the normal pulmonary circulation inactivates NA/5HT/histamine and prostaglandins [100]. Latterly, it has also been suggested as an amplifier in DIC [120].

Splanchnic circulation

The importance of the splanchnic circulation in established shock in dogs is clearly shown by the fact that removal of the abdominal viscera prior to induction of shock delays its onset [111]. Once mucosal integrity is lost, endotoxin enters the circulation and vaso-active products are produced in abundance. Lysozomal enzymes, induced histamine, myocardial depressant factor, angiotensin and unspecified kinins not only produce systemic effects (see sections: *The microcirculation* and *The systemic circulation*), but intensify local vasoconstriction and permeability as a positive feedback [47, 52, 100, 111].

Gut

The adrenergic innervation of the alimentary tract is rich, and the fall in circulation following acute hypotension is accordingly high. The gut is relatively resistant to this ischaemia, but once a critical level is passed irreversible damage almost always ensues. The most susceptible area of gut is the villus. Normally a countercurrent arrangement, analogous to the nephron, allows transfer of substances between afferent and efferent loops of the capillaries. However, at low flow rates, O_2 tends to shunt across the base and the tip of each villus becomes ischaemic. Oedema, haemorrhage, and bacterial invasion result in the sloughing of a pseudomembrane [102]. Subsequent free access of endotoxin to the circulation ultimately complicates all forms of shock.

In addition to the humoral contribution, activation of histidine decarboxylase releases histamine with pooling of blood in the splanchnic and portal beds [64]. Plasma is then lost through leaky capillaries and significant hypovolaemia occurs. Superior mesenteric artery occlusion in an otherwise healthy experimental model will cause a mean fall of 54% in plasma volume [101].

Liver

There is relatively little close scrutiny of the liver considering its function as a toxic filter and metabolic organ. It is well protected from all but extreme ischaemia, when irreversible damage occurs in 24 h [136]; it has autoregulation and a dual blood supply. However, normal liver function is of great importance, particularly in sepsis. The cardiovascular abnormalities in cirrhosis are very similar to those in sepsis, with shunting and a high cardiac output [109, 115, 144]. Shock complicated by chronic liver disease or jaundice carries a poor prognosis [85]. The detoxifying effects of the liver (via Kuppfer cells) was shown by the significant increase in myocardial depression due to lysozomes when the liver and reticulo-endothelial system were bypassed [47].

The metabolic abnormalities are very complex, but an impaired ability to metabolize amino acids and proteolytic products and to produce urea are prominent sequelae of prolonged ischaemia. In the early phases, the liver is an important source of glycogen.

Pancreas

It seems that the pancreas suffers particularly marked oligaemia in acute haemorrhage, flow falling to 15%–20% of its normal level, and this ischaemia persists after re-infusion of shed blood [147]. In addition, pancreatic lysozomes are especially sensitive to hypoxia and readily release proteolytic enzymes into the cell [90]. As the pancreas is a tissue designed to produce enzymes capable of digesting dietary substrate, their intracellular release is grave. The actions of these toxic factors have been discussed in detail in the section: *The systemic circulation*.

Haemodynamic and clinical correlations in shock

The complexity of shock in physiological terms makes management both challenging and difficult. Central to an adequate therapeutic approach is reproducible and objective information on haemodynamics, and the clinically accessible indices, namely systemic blood pressure, heart rate, urine output, and jugular venous pressure, fall short. Haemodynamics from bedside invasive techniques, especially the Swan–Ganz catheter [45] in combination with arterial and mixed venous blood gas analysis allow measurement of left ventricular filling pressure indirectly, cardiac output by thermodilution, and derivation of a whole gamut of variables, e.g., stroke work and peripheral shunts [135]. From these, haemodynamic subsets may guide the therapy of acute myocardial infarction [39] or predict categories of shock in terms of therapy and survival [138]. Similar analysis is now being effectively applied to correlate physiology and abnormal cellular metabolism in sepsis [145].

Arterial blood pressure

The variable influence of stroke volume, arterial compliance, and afterload upon blood pressure makes absolute interpretation unhelpful. However, as a generalization, diastolic pressure depends upon the peripheral resistance and systolic pressure upon stroke volume. The best guide to changes in blood flow is therefore the pulse pressure and volume [167]. Arterial pressure is most accurately measured by an intra-arterial cannula, when the waveform is also of diagnostic use [74, 119]. This is essential in severely hypotensive patients [167].

Systolic pressure is of particular importance in the use of vasodilators to assure that pressures do not fall below 70 mmHg when coronary blood flow is threatened [61, 119].

Cardiac output

The prognostic value of cardiac output measurement in sepsis has been discussed. With the feasibility of bedside monitoring this is accessible to all acute services [45, 54] and, when it is considered in combination with intra-arterial blood pressure and ventricular filling pressure, myocardial performance may be assessed effectively [119].

Ventricular filling pressure

Clinically the jugular venous pulse reflects right-sided filling pressures, and a central venous catheter will quantify this. As we have seen however, (section: *The systemic circulation*), faced with abnormal Starling curves (Fig. 11.6), filling of the left ventricle may no longer be inferred from measurement of right atrial pressure or CVP. As therapy in shock is directed primarily at the systemic circulation, and left-sided filling influences the pulmonary exchange bed, and therefore oxygenation, measurement of left ventricular end-diastolic pressure is important. Pulmonary capillary wedge pressure equates sufficiently well to be used widely. Differences seldom exceed 4 mmHg [119] even in circumstances of mitral valve disease, severe heart failure, atrial fibrillation, or chronic lung disease [34, 39, 95].

For optimum fluid balance, left ventricular end-diastolic pressure must be balanced with the fluid shifts in the pulmonary capillary circulation (Fig. 11.6). In the face of a normal oncotic pressure, pulmonary oedema occurs at about 26 mmHg [99]. Nonetheless, as colloid oncotic pressure is 0.57 the albumin concentration, halving albumin, as may well occur in the postoperative, catabolic patient with sepsis, reduces this critical pulmonary capillary pressure to 13 mmHg. With the increased capillary permeability of sepsis this may drop to zero [78]. Presented with a radiograph of pulmonary oedema, diagnosis and management of the dominant problem may only be continued with such haemodynamic measurements. Furthermore, cardiogenic pulmonary oedema may take up to forty-eight hours to resolve after return to

a normal left ventricular end-diastolic pressure and this phase lag must again be considered [99].

Prospects for the future

The realization that shock is a cellular problem from which all the multisystematic problems stem has led to rapid and rational conclusions as to the mechanisms that render circulatory changes irreversible. The paramount role of humoral mechanisms at a regional level are accepted, and exciting work is being done to clarify the role of the new prostaglandins and protein fragments that have such potent vasoactivity. The cell may be manipulated crudely with glucose–insulin–potassium cocktails, and ATP/Mg^{2+} improves the chances of survival in many experiments. Future research must continue to deepen our understanding and improve our manipulation of these basic mechanisms.

References

1. Alberti KGMM (1977) Biochemical consequences of hypoxia. J Clin Pathol 30 [Suppl II]:14–20
2. Albrecht M, Clowes GHA (1964) Increased circulatory requirements in the presence of inflammation. Surgery 56:150–171
3. Apps MCP, Tinker J (1978) The measurement and control of myocardial infarct size. Int Care Med 4:21–27
4. Bayley T, Clements JA, Osbahr AJ (1967) Pulmonary and circulatory effects of fibrinopeptides. Circ Res 21:469–485
5. Bayliss WM (1902) On the local reactions of the arterial wall to changes of internal pressure. J Physiol (Lond) 28:220–231
6. Beeuwkes R III, Brenner BM (1978) The kidney. In: Johnson PC (ed) Peripheral circulation. Wiley Medical, New York, pp 167–192
7. Begg TB, Hearns JB (1966) The relative contribution of haematocrit, plasma fibrinogen and other proteins to plasma viscosity. Clin Sci 31:87–93
8. Bell G (1971) Renal blood flow during haemorrhagic shock. In: Ledingham I McA, McAllister IA (eds) Conference on shock. Kimpton, London, pp 20–26
9. Berman R, Moseley RV, Doty DB, Gutierrez VS (1971) Post-traumatic alka-losis in young men with combat injuries. Surg Gynaecol Obstet 133:11–15
10. Beyer A (1979) Shock lung. Br J Hosp Med 23:248–258
11. B G, Hognestad J (1971) Thrombocytes and pulmonary vascular resistance during haemorrhagic hypotension. Acta Physiol Scand 82:218–228

12. Bond RF, Manley ES, Green HD (1967) Gutaneous and skeletal muscle vascular responses to haemorrhage and irreversible shock. Am J Physiol 212:488–497

13. Bradley R (1976) Studies in acute heart failure. Arnold, London pp 1–7

14. Branemark PI (1968) Rheological aspects of low flow states. In: Shepro D, Fulton GP (eds) Microcirculation as related to shock. Academic Press, London, pp 161–180

15. Bronstrom MA, Bronstrom CO, Breckenbridge BM, Wolff DJ (1979) Regulation of adenylate cyclase from glial tumour cells by calcium and calcium binding protein. J Biol Chem 254:7548–7557

16. Cahill GF Jr (1970) Starvation in man. N Engl J Med 282:668–675

17. Cahill GF (1971) Physiology of insulin in man. Diabetes 20:785–799

18. Cain SM (1969) Diminution of lactate rise during hypoxia, PCO_2 and β blockade. Am J Physiol 217:110–116

19. Carey LC, Lowery BD, Cloutier CT (1971) Haemorrhagic shock. Curr Prob Surg pp 1–48 (Monograph)

20. Cauldfield JB, Dunkman WB, Leinbach RC (1972) Cardiogenic shock. Myocardial morphology with and without artificial left ventricular counterpulsation. Arch Pathol 93:532–536

21. Chaudry IH, Sayeed MM, Baue AE (1974) The effect of adenosine tri-phosphate–magnesium chloride administration in shock. Surgery 72:220–227

22. Christy JH (1971) Pathophysiology of gram-negative shock. Am Heart J 81:694–701

23. Clowes GHA (1973) The pulmonary response to circulating agents post-traumatic and septic states. In: Haberland GL, Lewis DH (eds) New aspects of trasyslol therapy: The lung in shock. Schattauer, Stuttgart, p 71

24. Clowes GHA, Farrington GH, Zuschmeid W, Cossette GR, Saravis C (1970) Circulating factors in the aetiology of pulmonary insufficiency and right heart failure accompanying severe sepsis. Ann Surg 17:663–678

25. Clowes GHA, Hirsch MFE, Williams L, Kwashik E, O'Donnell TF, Cuevas P, Saini VK, Moradi I, Farizan M, Saravis C, Stone M, Kuffler J (1975) Septic lung and shock lung in man. Arch Surg 181:681–692

26. Cokelet GR (1978) Haemodynamics. In: Johnson PC (ed) Peripheral circulation. Wiley Medical, New York, pp 81–110

27. Crampton RS, Wangensteen SL, Glenn TM, Lefer AM (1971) Presence of a myocardial depressant factor in patients with circulatory shock. Surgery 70:223–231

28. Cuevas P, Fine J (1973) Production of fatal endotoxin shock by vasoactive substances. Gastroent erology 64:285–291

29. Douglas ME, Downs JB, Dannemiller FJ, Hodges MR (1976) Acute respiratory failure and intravascular coagulation. Surg Gynaecol Obstet 143:555–560

30. Editorial: (1965) Hyperglycaemia and diabetes after burns. Lancet I:225

31. Editorial: (1980) Function of the transplanted heart. Br Med J ii:529

32. Egdahl RH, Meguid MM, Aun F (1977) The importance of the endocrine and metabolic responses to shock and trauma. Crit Care Med 5:257–263

33. Erdos EG (1971) Enzymes that inactivate vasoactive peptides. Concepts in biochemical pharmacology Pt 2. Springer, Berlin Heidelberg New York, p 620

34. Falicov RE, Resnekov L (1970) Relationship of the pulmonary artery end diastolic pressure to the left ventricular end-diastolic and mean filling pressures in patients with and without left ventricular dys-function.

Circulation 42:65–73

35. Ferriera SH, Vane JR (1967) Prostaglandins: Their disappearance from and release into the circulation. Nature 216:868–873

36. Flear CT, Singh CM (1973) Hyponatraemia and sick cells. Br J Anaesth 45:976–994

37. Fletcher JR, Ramwell PW (1979) Modulation of prostaglandins E and F by the lungs in baboon haemorrhagic shock. J Surg Res 26:465–472

38. Fletcher JR, Ramwell PW (1980) The effects of prostacyclin on endotoxin shock and endotoxin induced platelet aggregation in dogs. Circ Shock 7:299–308

39. Forrester JS, Diamond G, Chatterjee K, Swan HJC (1976) Medical therapy of acute myocardial infarction by application of haemodynamic subsets. N Engl J Med 295:1356–1413

40. Frank O (1895) Zur Dynamik des Herzmuskels. Z Biol 32:370

41. Fredlund PE, Ockerman PA, Vang JO (1972) Plasma activities of acid hydrolases in experimental oligaemic shock in the pig. Am J Surg 124:300–306

42. Frohman LA, Bernadis LL (1971) The effect of hypothalamic stimulation on plasma glucose, insulin and glucagon levels. Am J Physiol 221:1596–1603

43. Fulton RL, Jones CE (1975) The aetiology of post-traumatic pulmonary insufficiency in man. Rev Surg 32:84–85

44. Gabel JC, Drake RE (1979) Pulmonary capillary pressure and permeability. Crit Care Med 7:92–97

45. George RJD (1980) How to insert a flotation catheter. Br J Hosp Med 24:296–301

46. Gillis CN (1973) Metabolism of vasoactive hormones by the lung. Anaesthesiology 39:626–632

47. Glenn TM, Lefer AM, Beardsley AC, Fergusson WW, Lopez-Razi AM, Serate TS, Morris JR, Wangensteen SL (1972) Circulatory responses to splanchnic lysozomal hydrolases in the dog. Ann Surg 176:120–127

48. Glenn TM, Tauber PF, Miller AG, Goldfarb RD, Mustafa SJ (1976) Alteration of haemodynamic and biochemical sequelae associated with acute coronary artery ligation by aprotinin. In: Cantin M, Haberland GL, Schnells G, Seyle H (eds) New aspects of trasylol therapy. Schattauer, Stuttgart, vol 8 p. 329–336

49. Golden PF, Jane JA (1973) Experimental study of irreversible shock and the brain. J Neurosurg 39:434–441

50. Green HD, Kepchar J (1959) Control of peripheral resistance in major systemic vascular beds. Physiol Rev 39:617–686

51. Greenbaum LM, Freer R, Chang J. Semente E, Yamafuji K (1969) Poly-morphonuclear leucocyte kinin and kinin metabolising enzymes in normal and malignant leucocytes. Br J Pharmacol 36:623–634

52. Haglund U, Lundgren O (1978) Intestinal ischaemia and shock factors. Fed Proc 37:2734–2740

53. Hanson GC (1978) Pathophysiology of shock. In: Hanson GC, Wright PL (eds) Medical management of the critically ill. Academic Press, London, pp 293–300

54. Hanson GC, Bennett ED (1978) Monitoring in shock. In: Hanson GC, Wright PL (eds) Medical management of the critically ill. Academic Press, London, pp 301–332

55. Hardaway RM (1965) Microcoagulation in shock. AM J Surg 110:298–301

56. Hardaway RM (1967) Disseminated intravascular coagulation in experimental clinical shock. Am J Cardiol 20:161–173

57. Hardaway RM (1979) Monitoring of the patient in a state of shock. Surg Gynaecol Obstet 148:339–345

58. Hardaway RM, Elovitz MJ, Brewster WR, Houchin DN (1964) The clotting time of heparinised blood—

influence of acidosis. Arch Surg 89:701–705

59. Hardaway RM, James PM, Anderson RW, Bredenberg CE, West RL (1967) Intensive study and therapy of shock. JAMA 199:779–790

60. Haugaard N, Haugaard ES, Lee NH, Horn RS (1969) Possible role of mitochondria in the regulation of cardiac contractility. Fed Proc 28:1657–1662

61. Herbert P, Tinker J (1980) Inotropic drugs in acute circulatory failure Intensive Care Med 6:101–11

62. Heymans C, Neil E (1958) Reflexogenic areas of the cardiovascular system. Churchill, London

63. Hinshaw LB (1974) Role of the heart in the pathogenesis of endotoxin shock. J Surg Res 17:134–145

64. Hinshaw LB, Emerson TE, Iampietro PF, Brake CM (1962) A comparative study of the haemodynamic actions of histamine and endotoxin. Am J Physiol 203:600–606

65. Hinshaw LB, Archer LT, Black MR, Elkins RC, Brown PB (1974a) Myocardial function in shock. Am J Physiol 226:357–366

66. Hinshaw LB, Archer LT, Black NR, Greenfield LJ (1974b) Effects of methylprednisolone sodium succinate on myocardial performance, haemodynamics and metabolism in normal and failing hearts. In: Glenn TM (ed) Steroids and shock. University Park Press, Baltimore, pp 253–273

67. Horiuchi K, Tanaka H, Yamamoto K, Neda J (1971) Distribution of renin in the dog kidney. Life Sci 10:727–734

68. Horpacsy G, Schnells G (1980) Energy metabolism and lysozomal events in haemorrhagic shock after aprotinin. Circ Shock 7:49–58

69. Intaglietta M, Johnson PC (1978) Principles of capillary exchange. In: Johnson PC (ed) Peripheral Perfusion. Wiley Medical, New York, pp 141–166

70. Janoff A, Weissmann G, Zwelfach BW, Thomas L (1962) Pathogenesis of experimental shock: 'in vitro' studies of lysozomal enzymes in normal and tolerant animals subjected to lethal trauma and endotoxaemia. J Exp Med 116:451–466

71. Jastrzebski J, Hilgaro P, Henry K, Sykes MK (1975) Early cardio-respiratory effects of endotoxin shock in dogs. Effects of pre-treatment with EACA. Cited in: Ledingham I McA (ed) Shock: Treatment and experimental aspects. Excerpta Medica, Amsterdam, pp 21–42

72. Johnson PC (1978) Principles of peripheral circulatory control. In Peripheral Circulation, ed. Johnson PC, Wiley Medical, New York, pp 111–139

73. Kelman GR (1977a) Physical principles in applied cardiovascular physiology, 2nd edn. Butterworths, London, pp 1–20

74. Kelman GR (1977b) The heart in applied cardiovascular physiology, 2nd edn. Butterworths, London, pp 22–66

75. Kimura S, Rasmussen H (1977) Adrenal glucocorticoids, adenine nucleo-tide translocation and mitochondrial calcium accumulation. J Biol Chem 252:1217–1225

76. Kleinecht D (1980) Pathogenesis of acute reversible intrinsic renal failure (acute tubular necrosis). In: Chapman A (ed) Acute renal failure. Churchill Livingstone, London, pp 5–18

77. Kobald EE, Lovell R, Katz W, Thal AP (1964) Chemical mediators released by endotoxin. Surg Gynaecol Obstet 118:807–813

78. Kwaan HM, Weil MH (1969) Mechanisms of shock caused by bacterial infections. Surg Gynaecol Obstet 128:37–45

79. Landgren S (1952) On the excitation mechanisms of the carotid baroreceptors. Acta Physiol Scand 26:1–34

80. Landgren S, Neil E (1951) The contribution of carotid chemoreceptor mechanisms to the rise of blood pressure caused by carotid occlusion. Acta Physiol Scand 23:152–157

81. Lassen NA (1978) Brain. In: Johnson PC (ed) Peripheral circulation. Wiley Medical, New York, pp 337–358

82. Ledingham I McA (1976) Pathophysiology of shock. In: Ledingham I McA (ed) Shock, clinical and experimental aspects, Excerpta Medica, Amsterdam, p 3

83. Ledingham I McA (1979) Pathophysiology of shock. Br J Hosp Med 23:472–482

84. Ledingham I McA, McArdle CS (1978) Prospective study of the therapy of septic shock. Lancet I: 1194–1197

85. Ledingham I McA, McArdle CS, Fisher WD, Maddern M (1974) The incidence of the shock syndrome in a general hospital. Postgrad Med J 50:420–424

86. Lee L (1962) Reticuloendothelial clearance of circulating fibrin in the pathogenesis of the generalised Schwartzmann reaction. J Exp Med 115:1065–82

87. Lefer AM (1974) Myocardial action of steroids. In: Glenn TM (ed) Shock. University Park Press, Baltimore, pp 253–273

88. Lefer AM (1978) Properties of cardioinhibitory factors produced in shock. Fed Proc 37:2734–2740

89. Lefer AM, Revotto MJ (1970) Influence of a myocardial depressant factor on the physiological properties of heart muscle. Proc Soc Exp Biol Med 134:269–73

90. Lefer AM, Spath JA (1974) Pancreatic hypoperfusion and the production of a myocardial depressant factor in haemorrhagic shock. Ann Surg 179:868–876

91. Levin J, Poore TE, Young NS (1972) Gram-negative sepsis: detection of endotoxaemia with the limulus test. With studies of associated changes in blood coagulation, serum lipids and complement. Ann Intern Med 76:1–7

92. Lillehei RC, Longerbeam JK, Block JH, Manax WG (1964) The nature of irreversible shock: experimental and clinical observations. Ann Surg 160:682–710

93. Lovett WL, Wangensteen SL, Glenn TM, Lefer AM (1971) Presence of a myocardial depressant factor in patients in circulatory shock. Surgery 70:223–31

94. Lucas CE, Rector FE, Werner M, Rosenberg IK (1973) Altered renal homeostasis with acute sepsis. Arch Surg 106:444–449

95. Luchsinger RC, Seipp HW, Patel DJ (1962) Relationship of pulmonary artery wedge pressure to left atrial pressure in man. Circ Res 11:315–318

96. Luterman A, Manwaring D, Curreri PW (1977) The role of fibrinogen degradation products in the pathogenesis of the adult respiratory distress syndrome. Surgery 82:703–709

97. Maclean LD, Mulligan GN, Mclean APH, Duff JA (1967a) Alkalosis and septic shock. Surgery 62:655–662

98. Maclean LD, Mulligan GN, Mclean APH, Duff JH (1967b) Patterns of septic shock in man. A detailed study of fifty-six patients. Ann Surg 166:543–562

99. McHugh TJ, Forrester JS, Adler L, Zion D, Swan HJC (1972) Pulmonary vascular congestion in acute myocardial infarction, haemodynamic and radiological correlations. Ann Intern Med 76:29–33

100. McNeil JR (1971) Role of vasopressin and angiotensin in response of splanchnic resistance vessels to haemorrhage. Adv Exp Med Biol 23:127–144

101. Marston A (1962) The bowel in shock. Lancet II:365–370

102. Marston A (1977) Responses of the splanchnic circulation to ischaemia. J Clin Pathol 30 [Suppl II]:59–67

103. Moncada S, Vane JR (1978) Unstable metabolites of arachidonic acid and their role in haemostasis and thrombosis. Br Med Bull 34:129–135

104. Moncada S, Gryglewski R, Bunting S, Vane JR (1976) An enzyme isolated from arteries transforms prostaglandin endoperoxidases to an unstable substance that inhibits platelet aggregation. Nature 263:663–665

105. Montgomery SB, Jose PH, Slotkoff LM, Lilienfield LS, Eisner GM (1980) The regulation of intrarenal blood flow in the dog during ischaemia Circ Shock 7: 71–82

106. Morrison DC, Cochrane CG (1974) Direct evidence for Hageman factor (Factor XII) activation by bacterial lipopolysaccharides (endotoxins) J Exp Med 14:797: 811

107. Movat HZ, Steinberg SG, Habal FM, Ramadive NS (1973) Demonstration of a kinin-generating enzyme in the lysozomes of human polymorphs. Lab Invest 29:699–784

108. Mueller HS (1977) The heart and oxygen transport. In: Thompson WL (ed) The organ in shock. Upjohn Co. Kalamazoo, pp 38–49

109. Murray JT, Dawson AM, Sherlock S (1958) Circulatory changes in chronic liver disease. Am J Med 24:358–367

110. Nagler AL, Levenson SM (1975) The nature of the toxic material in the blood of rats subjected to irreversible haemorrhagic shock. Circ Shock 1:252–264

111. Nagler AL, McConn R (1976) The role of humoral factors in shock. In: Ledingham I McA (ed) Shock: Clinical and experimental aspects. Excerpta Medica, Amsterdam, pp 79–109

112. Nakano J, Fisher RD (1965) Effects of an arterio-pulmonary artery shunt on cardiovascular haemodynamics. Cardiologia 47:1–13

113. Neil-Dwyer G, Walter P, Cruickshank JM, Doshi B, O'Gorman R (1978) Effects of propranolol and phentolamine on myocardial necrosis after subarachnoid haemorrhage. Br Med J ii:990–992

114. Niemetz J, Herbert V (1971) The role of protein synthesis on the generation of tissue factor activity by leucocytes. Proc Soc Exp Biol Med 139:1276–1279

115. Nishijima H, Weil MH, Shubin H, Cavailles J (1973) Haemodynamic and metabolic studies on shock associated with gram-negative bacteria. Medicine (Baltimore) 52:287–294

116. Olsson P, Radegran K, Taylor GA (1970) Haemodynamic changes resulting from thrombin-induced intravascular coagulation. Cardiovasc Res 4:443–451

117. Paintal AS (1973) Vagal sensory receptors and their reflex effects. Physiol Rev 53:159–227

118. Pindyck F, Drucker MR, Brown RS, Shoemaker WC (1974) Cardiorespiratory effects of hypertonic glucose in the critically ill patient. Surgery 75:11–19

119. Poole-Wilson PA (1978) Interpretation of haemodynamic measurements. Br J Hosp Med 23:371–382

120. Preston FE (1979) Haematological problems associated with shock. Br J Hosp Med 24:232–245

121. Randle PJ, Smith GH (1958) Regulation of glucose uptake by muscle. Biochem J 70:490–508

122. Reichgott JJ, Forsyth RP, Melmon KL (1971) Effects of bradykinins and autonomic nervous system inhibition of systemic and regional haemodynamics in unanaesthetised Rhesus monkeys. Circ Res 29:367–374

123. Renkin EM (1968) Neurogenic factors in microcirculatory low flow states. In: Shepro D, Fulton GP (eds) Microcirculation as related to shock. Academic Press, New York, pp 139–148

124. Resnekov L (1973) Circulatory assistance for the failing heart. Br Heart J 35:1265–70

125. Resnekov L (1978) Cardiogenic shock. Br J Hosp Med 23:232–241

126. Reuter H, Scholz H (1977) A study of ion selectivity and the kinetic properties of the calcium dependent slow inward current in mammalian cardiac muscle. J Physiol (Lond) 264:17–47

127. Ricci DR, Oruck AE, Alderman RL, Ingels NB, Daughters GT, Kusnick CA, Reitz BA, Stinson EB (1979) Role of tachycardia as an inotropic stimulus in man. J Clin Invest 63:693–703

128. Rogel S, Hilewitz H (1978) Cardiac impairment and shock factors. Fed Proc 37:2718–2723

129. Rosenthal SL, Hawley PL, Hakim AA (1972) Purified burn toxic factor and its competition. Surgery 71:527–536

130. Rubanji G, Korovách AGB, Koltay E, Nagy-Dora T, Bologh I, Somogyi E (1980) The effect of haemorrhagic shock on the performance, oxygen consumption and ultrastructure of isolated rat hearts. Circ Shock 7:59–70

131. Rubio R, Berne RM (1978) Myocardium. In: Johnson PC (ed) Peripheral circulation. Wiley Medical, New York, pp 231–253

132. Sarnoff SJ, Berglund (1954) Starling's law of the heart studied by means of simultaneous right and left ventricular function curves in the dog. Circulation 9:706–718

133. Schayer RW (1962) Evidence that induced histamine is an intrinsic regulator of the microcirculatory system. Am J Physiol 202:66–72

134. Schumer W, Sperling R (1968) Shock and its effect on the cell. JAMA 205:75–79

135. Shabot MM, Shoemaker WC, State D (1977) Rapid bedside computation of cardiorespiratory variables with a programmable calculator. Crit Care Med 5:105–111

136. Sherlock S (1975) Diseases of the liver and biliary system, 5th edn. Blackwell Scientific, Oxford, p 90

137. Shoemaker WC (1971) Cardiorespiratory patterns in complicated and uncomplicated septic shock. Ann Surg 174:119–125

138. Shoemaker WC (1977) Pathophysiology and therapy of shock states. Use of haemodynamic and oxygen transport variables to predict survival and to guide therapy. In: Thompson LW (ed) The organ in shock. Upjohn, Kalamazoo, pp 75–87

139. Shoemaker WC, Hauser CJ (1979) Critique of crystalloid versus colloid therapy in shock and shock lung. Crit Care Med 7:117–124

140. Siegel JH (1961) A study of the mechanisms of cardiovascular adaptation to an acute ventricular septal defect. J Thorac Cardiovasc Surg 14:523

141. Siegel JH (1979) Ventilation perfusion maldistribution secondary to the hyperdynamic cardiovascular state as the major cause of increased pulmonary shunting in human sepsis. J Trauma 19:432–460

142. Siegel JH, Sonnenblick EH, Judge RD, Wilson WS (1965) Occult myocardial failure and vasopressors in shock. Cardiologia 47:353–379

143. Siegel JH, Greenspan M, Del Guercio LRM (1967) Abnormal vascular tone, defective oxygen transport and myocardial failure in human septic shock. Surgery 62:655–662

144. Siegel JH, Greenspan M, Cohn JD, Del Guercio LRM (1968) Prognostic implications of altered physiology in operations for portal hypertension. Surg Gynaecol Obstet 126:249–262

145. Siegel JH, Cerra FB, Coleman B, Giovannini I, Shetye M, Border JR, McMenamy RH (1979) Physiological and metabolic correlations in human sepsis. Surgery 86:163–193

146. Silver IA (1977) Local factors in tissue oxygenation. J Clin Pathol [Suppl II]:7–13
147. Slater GI, Vladeck BC, Bassin R, Kark AE, Shoemaker WC (1973) Sequential changes in distribution of cardiac output in haemorrhagic shock. Surgery 73:714–722
148. Slater TF (1969) Lysozomes in experimentally induced tissue injury. In: Pringle JT, Fell HR (eds) Lysozomes in biology and pathology. Elsevier, Amsterdam, p 469
149. Sleight P (1978) In: Sleight P (ed) The control of the cardiovascular system. ICI Pharmaceuticals, Alderley Park, Macclesfield, Cheshire, Chap I, pp 3–12
150. Soulsby ME, Bennett CL, Hess ML (1980) Canine arterial calcium transport during endotoxin shock. Circ Shock 7:139–148
151. Sperelakis N, Schneider JA (1976) A metabolic control mechanism for calcium ion influx that may protect the ventricular myocardial cell. Am J Cardiol 37:1079–1085
152. Starling EH (1895/6) On the absorption of fluids from the connective tissue spaces. J Physiol (Lond) 19:312–326
153. Starling EH (1918) The Linacre lecture on the law of the heart (Cambridge 1915). Longman Green, London
154. Steer ML, Atlas D, Levitzki A (1975) Inter-relations between β-adrenergic receptors, adenylate cyclase and calcium. N Engl J Med 292:409–414
155. Stormorken H (1977) Activation and interaction of sub-defence systems Churchill Livingston, London, (Recent advances in blood coagulation, no. 2, pp 46–58)
156. Swan HJC, Ganz W, Forrester J, Marsuc H, Diamond G, Chonette D (1970) Catheterisation of the heart in man with use of a flow-directed balloon-tipped catheter. NEJM 283:447–451
157. Udhoji VN, Weil MH, Sambhi MP, Rossoff I (1963) Haemodynamic studies in clinical shock associated with infection. Am J Med 34:461–469
158. Vyder JK, Nagasawa K, Corday E, Parmley WW, Swan HJC (1974) Haemodynamic aspects of corticosteroid administration in the treatment of acute myocardial infarction. In: Glenn TM (ed) Steroids in shock. University Park Press, Baltimore, pp 211–232
159. Wardle N (1979) Bacteraemic and endotoxin shock. Br J Hosp Med 23:223–231
160. Weil MH, Henning RJ (1979) New concepts in the diagnosis and fluid treatment of circulatory shock. Anesth Analg (Cleve) 58:124–132
161. Weil MH, Nishijima H (1978) Cardiac output in bacteraemic shock. Am J Med 64:920–922
162. Weisel RD, Vito L, Dennis RC, Valeri CR, Hechtman HS (1977) Myocardial depression during sepsis. Am J Surg 133:512–521
163. Weissman G, Thomas L (1962) Studies in lysozomes D. J Exp Med 116:433–450
164. Weisul JP, O'Donnell TF Jr, Stone MA, Clowes GHA Jr (1975) Myocardial performance in clinical septic shock: effects of isoprpterenol and glucose–potassium–insulin. J Surg Res 18:357–363
165. Wiles JB (1980) The systemic septic response. Does the organism matter? Crit Care Med 8:55–59
166. Wilson JW (1974) Cellular localisation of 3H-labelled corticosteroids by electron-microscopic autoradiography after haemorrhagic shock. In: Glenn TM (ed) Steroids and shock. University Park Press, Baltimore, pp 275–299
167. Wilson RF (1980) The pathophysiology of shock. Intensive Care Med 6:89–100
168. Wilson RF, Sarver EJ, Leblanc PL (1971) Factors affecting haemodynamics in clinical shock with sepsis. Ann Surg 174:939–943
169. Winslow EJ, Loeb HS, Rahimtoola SH, Kamath S, Gunner RM (1973) Haemodynamic studies and results of therapy in fifty patients with bacteraemic shock. Am J Med 54:421–432
170. Wolff SM, Bennett JV (1974) Gram negative rod bacteraemia. N Engl J Med 291:733–734
171. Wollner L, McCarthy ST, Soper NDW, Macy DJ (1979) Failure of cerebral autoregulation as a cause of brain dysfunction in the elderly. Br Med J i:1117–1118
172. Woo P, Carpenter MA, Trunkey D (1979) The effect of septic shock on ionised calcium in the human. J Surg Res 26:605–610
173. Woods HF, Krebs HA (1971) Lactate production in the perfused rat liver. Biochem J 125:129–139
174. Wright CJ, Duff JH, Mclean APH, Maclean LD (1971) Regional capillary blood flow oxygen uptake in sepsis. Surg Gynaecol Obstet 132:637–644
175. Zapol WM, Snider MT (1977) Pulmonary hypertension in severe, acute respiratory failure. N Engl J Med 296:476–480

Chapter 12

The Management of Shock

David J. Bihari and Jack Tinker

The veins unfill'd, our blood is cold, and then
We pout upon the morning, are unapt
To give or to forgive; but when we have stuff'd
These pipes and these conveyances of our blood,
With wine and feeding, we have suppler souls
Than in our priest-like fasts.

Coriolanus V, i, line 51

A sound heart is the life of the flesh.

Proverbs Chap. 14, v. 30

In the previous chapter, shock has been examined in terms of its final common pathway—the development of inadequate or inappropriate tissue perfusion, sufficient to cause cellular hypoxia, with accumulation of toxic metabolities. Restoration of a normal *milieu interieur* is attempted by homeostatic physiological mechanisms, and the aims of management include manipulations to maintain blood flow, and hence oxygen delivery, to vital organs, whilst at the same time treating the underlying cause of shock.

The state of shock constitutes a syndrome which is but one cause of acute circulatory collapse, and in this chapter attention will centre on the three conventional categories of shock: hypovolaemic, cardiogenic, and septic.

The shock syndrome is a dynamic process in which the measurable haemodynamic and metabolic variables are continually changing, and this betrays the simplistic nature of a formal classification. Myocardial function, distribution of cardiac output and the magnitude of the circulating blood volume are major haemodynamic considerations, and the manipulation of these is the basis of management. Immediate end-points of therapy remain the same whatever the cause, or category, and depend upon the maintenance of an adequate delivery of substrate to respiring tissues, with the prevention or reversal of anaerobic respiration.

The fundamental pathogenesis of the syndrome is either a reduction in cardiac output, due to an acute reduction in circulating blood volume or an acute deterioration in myocardial function, or a maldistribution of blood flow, which commonly occurs with a normal or raised cardiac output. It is usual for the high-cardiac-output, maldistributive type of shock to evolve into a more severe state with a low cardiac output; hypovolaemia, absolute or relative, is common in all forms.

Irreversible shock

The development of irreversible, refractory shock has been reviewed in the previous chapter, and the role of the microcirculation and subsequent changes at cellular and subcellular levels emphasized. Prolonged shock, of any cause, results in impaired myocardial function, and some authors [82] consider this to be of prime importance. Animal studies have demonstrated the direct relationship between myocardial oxygen availability and ventricular performance in haemorrhagic shock [83]. The balance between myocardial oxygen demand and delivery is an extremely important consideration in the management of all forms of shock, as most forms of medical therapy have substantial effects on myocardial oxygen demand. It has a special relevance in shock following acute myocardial infarction where limitation of infarct size, with preservation of jeopardized myocardial tissue, forms a part of treatment. Four major factors effect myocardial oxygen consumption: preload, afterload, contractility, and heart rate and a knowledge of the effect of an intervention on both cardiac metabolism and function is critical to therapeutic decision making, as was emphasized by Forrester [50].

Effects on other organs

The shock syndrome has profound effects on the function of other organs, and prevention of 'multisystem failure' is yet another aspect of management. Shock has a domino effect, triggering problems in other systems—acute respiratory failure, acute renal failure, and hypoxic cerebral damage being the most common. To prevent the development of these complications, various therapeutic regimens have been designed, such as early mechanical ventilation with PEEP, the use of mannitol, frusemide and low-dose dopamine 'barbiturate coma'; but the most effective form of prevention remains the prompt treatment of the initiating cause of shock, so minimizing the haemodynamic disturbance. Of prime importance in this respect is rapid diagnosis and accurate assessment of the degree of circulatory and metabolic derangement.

The diagnosis of shock

This is a two-stage process which depends upon recognition of the critical nature of the illness and the definition of the underlying cause. Clinical assessment aims to classify the shock syndrome into one of the two broad categories described: 'pump failure', or 'maldistribution of flow'. Although extremely important in the initial approach to therapy, clinical assessment is limited and can only be an impression. There are a number of ways in which it can mislead about the state of cardiac function [50]. The correlation between clinical signs of pulmonary oedema and haemodynamic data is poor, and a 'phase lag' of as much as 48 h between haemodynamic stabilization and the resolution of abnormal physical and radiological signs has been described [94]. Pulmonary capillary pressure may be raised in chronic heart failure, with no signs of pulmonary congestion, due to substantial thickening of the pulmonary vascular wall. Chronic obstructive airways disease may present with pulmonary clinical features similar to those of pulmonary oedema, but is distinguished by a normal pulmonary capillary pressure.

Perhaps the most significant problem in the management of the shock syndrome is assessment of the adequacy of cardiac output. A clinical impression of this is gained from the patient's temperature, the state of the peripheral vasculature, the mean arterial pressure, and the urine output. However, the high cardiac output of maldistributive shock may not be recognized when it is associated with cutaneous and renal vasoconstriction, and arteriovenous shunting. The failure to recognize a high cardiac output might result in the inappropriate use of inotropes.

Intimately related to the estimation of cardiac output is the question of oxygen transport and the diagnosis of hypoxia. Arterial hypoxaemia per se is not diagnostic of cellular hypoxia and must be related to total oxygen transport, consumption, and extraction. The concentration of haemoglobin and its saturation are critical in oxygen transport, and cardiac output is the third factor determining oxygen delivery. Hypoxia can only be safely diagnosed following an 'oxygen flux test'. Oxygen delivery, consumption, and extraction rate must be measured and then delivery increased. If there is no change in oxygen consumption, and extraction rate, no conclusion can be drawn concerning oxygen utilization. However, if oxygen consumption increases, then one can assume that the patient was previously hypoxic, with an oxygen debt which had to be paid off. An increase in consumption, following an increase in oxygen delivery, is a good prognostic sign in all forms of shock, whereas the onset of irreversible shock in animals correlates well with an accumulated oxygen debt of more than 20 ml/kg [96]. The importance of the oxygen flux test is in situations where oxygen delivery is seemingly adequate, i.e. Hb. $\geq$ 10 g%, with an arterial saturation of more than 90%, cardiac index $\geq$ 2.2 litre/min. Nevertheless in a group of patients with maldistributive shock, this delivery may not be adequate, and hence there is an oxygen debt, with the development of cellular hypoxia. This hypoxia can only be recognized by increasing the oxygen delivery (best done by increasing the cardiac output) and noting an increase in oxygen consumption. Despite this form of systemic appraisal, regional hypoxia may still go unnoticed.

Clinical assessment

The limitations of clinical assessment have been mentioned, but most patients will be allocated to their diagnostic category by the context of their presentation. Hypovolaemia following surgery or trauma is usually obvious as a cause of circulatory collapse, and a history of some underlying disease process is helpful in determining the likelihood of pump failure or maldistribution of flow.

The aim of physical examination is to obtain some estimate of organ blood flow and tissue perfusion with reference to the blood volume of the patient. In the absence of cerebral pathology the level of consciousness is an indication of brain perfusion and its adequacy. Specific neurological signs are rare, but when present suggest a neurological cause of circulatory collapse. Skin perfusion is readily judged by colour, temperature and the state of the peripheral vessels; capillary filling can be assessed in the nail bed. Signs suggesting the cause of circulatory collapse may be present, e.g. new cardiac murmurs following myocardial infarction, and there may be other signs suggesting the onset of the complications of shock, e.g. the development of respiratory distress. A source of sepsis must be sought and pre-existing disease excluded.

Haemodynamic assessment

Haemodynamic monitoring is discussed in detail in Chap. 11; suffice it to say that the measurement of the pulmonary capillary pressure (PCP) using a flotation catheter has been described as a 'quantum leap' in critical care [139]. Swan estimates that between one and two million flow-directed catheters have been inserted since 1970 [156]. The PCP, measured in this way, in the presence of normal mitral valve function, corresponds to the left ventricular end-diastolic pressure. However, in critically ill patients Calvin et al. [22] have described a poor correlation between PCP and left ventricular preload as measured by left ventricular end-diastolic volume using radionuclide angiography. They suggest that changes in left ventricular compliance account for the poor correlation. Despite this finding, in the absence of facilities for carrying out radionuclide angiography, PCP remains the best guide to left ventricular filling. Its value is influenced by changes in circulating blood volume and left ventricular function, and it is a major factor in the genesis of pulmonary oedema when related to plasma oncotic pressure and capillary permeability.

Central venous pressure (CVP) is not a reliable guide to left ventricular filling because of the wide disparity that can exist between left and right ventricular function in seriously ill patients [49]. Systemic venous tone is an important determinant of CVP, and a normal CVP may be seen in patients with reduced blood volumes, because of increased venous constriction. Right ventricular infarction is another cause of disparity between CVP and PCP. Such considerations justify the use of flotation catheters in patients presenting with shock. A further advantage of using thermistor-tipped flotation catheters is the direct measurement of cardiac output by thermodilution. Patients can then be immediately classified into the two groups— those with a high cardiac output, and a maldistribution of flow, and those with a low cardiac output suffering from hypovolaemia or pump failure. Therapy can then be rational, and the effects of intervention appropriately assessed.

Continuous monitoring of right atrial oxygen tension using a catheter incorporating a Clark-type oxygen sensor at its tip has been suggested as an alternative to intermittent determinations of the cardiac output [108]. This technique lends itself equally well to pulmonary artery oxygen tension monitoring, but access to this position is more difficult, as the catheter is not flow directed. In patients who have had a proven myocardial infarct, a fall in oxygen tension is associated with the clinical features of a low cardiac output. A comparison of published data suggests that at venous oxygen saturations below 60% [tensions of 30 mmHg (4 kPa)] there is a high incidence of complications and death.

Lactic acidaemia is present at these levels [78], suggesting anaerobic respiration secondary to poor tissue perfusion. The major defect in this monitoring system is that it does not take into account the arteriovenous shunting that occurs in prolonged shock. A normal or raised venous oxygen saturation may be seen in patients with shock associated with maldistribution of flow, and/or cellular hypoxia. However, it remains a useful guide to tissue perfusion in patients suffering from pump failure.

Measurement of the core-peripheral temperature deficit has been widely used for assessing peripheral blood flow [130], but the notable shortcomings of this method are the mode of heat lost and the fact that skin temperature and cutaneous blood flow may vary independently. Rithalia et al. [126] reported a study of 28 critically ill patients in which the peripheral temperature and the core–peripheral temperature deficit made no contribution to patient management. In the same study, the advantages of the relatively non-invasive, continuous method of monitoring blood gases using transcutaneous PO_2 and pH electrodes were emphasized. In those circumstances, where cardiovascular collapse had occurred, hypotension, tachycardia, and oliguria were preceded by a fall in transcutaneous pH and PO_2. It was also noted that a sustained low transcutaneous pH, even in the presence of normal arterial blood gases, was a universally poor prognostic sign. These results suggest that transcutaneous monitoring of blood gases may be a useful index of tissue blood flow, but the problem remains as to the clinical relevance of measurements of skin perfusion in situations where blood flow to the brain, heart, and kidneys is all-important.

Assessment of oxygenation

Hypoxia in the shock syndrome may occur at four different levels, and an approach to therapy depends upon accurate diagnosis. Pulmonary hypoxia resulting in arterial hypoxaemia is the form most readily identified. Pulmonary dysfunction as a result of ventilation–perfusion mismatching (pulmonary shunting) is a common occurrence in the shocked patient. It may be the result of pulmonary oedema (left ventricular failure, low-pressure pulmonary oedema of the ARDS), pulmonary infection or a functional disturbance of the pulmonary circulation secondary to vasoactive factors. It is recognized by the measurement of the arterial PO_2 and haemoglobin saturation. Arterial oxygen content may be measured directly or calculated from the formula:

$$(Hb) \times \% \text{ saturation} \times 1.34 = \text{vol. } O_2 \text{ in } 100 \text{ ml blood}$$

A PO_2 of less than 60 mmHg (8 kPa) or a saturation of less than 90% is unacceptable and requires some form of intervention.

Arterial oxygen content depends upon the quantity of haemoglobin available to take up and carry oxygen to the tissues, and 'anaemic' hypoxia may occur during and after blood loss. Shifts in the oxygen–haemoglobin dissociation curve may contribute to anaemic hypoxia. In haemorrhagic shock, the curve is shifted somewhat to the right, providing delivery of more oxygen to the tissues at any given arterial oxygen tension. It appears that the shape of the curve, and the red cell 2, 3 DPG content are not disturbed, but paradoxically the red cell ATP increases [81]. Similar increases in the P_{50} value have been reported in cardiogenic shock [1], and are considered to be a protective response. Anaemic hypoxia becomes a problem when the patient's haemoglobin concentration drops below 10 g%, and this deficiency is corrected with stored blood. In the acute situation, oxygen transport is not increased because the red cell content of 2, 3 DPG in stored blood is very low, resulting in a shift of the dissociation curve to the left. Desaturation of haemoglobin occurs only at low oxygen tensions, so that there is a relative reduction in oxygen delivery to the tissues. Transfused red blood cell 2, 3 DPG returns to normal levels over a 24–48 h period, but this is an important consideration in fluid therapy.

Two other major determinants of the position of the oxygen–haemoglobin dissociation curve are pH and temperature. An acidosis shifts the curve to the right, and injudicious bicarbonate therapy reverses this protective effect, the resulting alkalosis producing a decrease in oxygen delivery to the tissues. Hypothermia has two effects on oxygen metabolism. Although the dissociation curve is shifted to the left, resulting in reduced delivery, oxygen consumption falls, so that requirements are reduced. The fall in consumption is much more marked than the reduction in delivery, and hypothermia has been used as a form of therapy to protect organs from ischaemic damage. Hyperthermia is dangerous for this reason—the increase in oxygen consumption—and should be treated aggressively with physical cooling and antipyretic agents. In general, to avoid anaemic hypoxia the haemoglobin concentration should be maintained above 10 g%, preferably using fresh blood, and the arterial pH should be maintained between 7.26 and 7.36.

The third form of hypoxia is that associated with a low cardiac output. Despite a high arterial oxygen tension and an adequate concentration of haemoglobin, hypoxia may result secondary to pump failure. Oxygen delivery is derived from the formula:

oxygen delivery (ml O_2 per min) = arterial oxygen content (ml O_2 per 100 ml blood $\times$ cardiac output (litres/min) $\times$ 10

From this formula it can be seen that the cardiac output is a major determinant of oxygen delivery, and a small reduction in its value has important consequences for tissue metabolism.

The final form of hypoxia in the shock syndrome is termed 'cellular hypoxia'. Oxygen consumption is reduced secondary to cellular poisoning due to circulating 'toxins'. The nature of these toxins is obscure, and the diagnosis is presumptive, following the lack of response to an oxygen flux test. It is difficult to distinguish this form of hypoxia from a reduced oxygen consumption secondary to arteriovenous shunting. Measurement of the pulmonary shunt is helpful as a large shunt correlates well with low lactate levels, and suggests peripheral arteriovenous shunting as the cause of a low oxygen consumption. Careful monitoring of the pH, base excess, and lactate levels will give some clue to whether one is dealing with cellular poisoning or shunting. Both of these phenomena occur in the late stages of shock, are difficult to manage, and have a poor prognosis.

In conclusion, it is not possible to diagnose hypoxia using blood gas measurements alone, unless the problem is that of pulmonary hypoxia. The three other forms of hypoxia must be borne in mind, and oxygen delivery and extraction studies are essential. The practical implications of this discussion are that the physician must aim to maintain the haemoglobin concentration above 10 g%, the arterial oxygen tension above 60 mmHg (8kPa), the haemoglobin saturation above 90%, and the cardiac output above 3 litres/min. The detection and treatment of cellular hypoxia and arterio-venous shunting are difficult (see Figs. 12.1, 12.2).

Blood viscosity

The rheological aspects of blood flow in shock are discussed in the preceding chapter, but it is important to emphasize that the major determinant of blood viscosity is the haematocrit. Certain forms of shock, such as that induced by thermal injury, are associated with intravascular aggregation of red cells, white cells, and platelets. These aggregates cause an increase in blood viscosity. Another source of aggregates is stored blood, and large amounts of bank blood should be avoided [43]. The role of these aggregates in the pathogenesis of ARDS following resuscitation with large volumes of unfiltered bank blood remains controversial [129], but it would seem prudent to use effective blood micropore filters to avoid increasing the risk of development of acute respiratory failure [71].

The optimum haematocrit for maximum oxygen transport is 25% for the coronary circulation and approximately 45% for the systemic circulation in dogs with haemorrhagic hypotension. Oxygen consumption of the myocardium increases with haemodilution to a peak at 25%, but total body oxygen consumption is constant over a wide range of haematocrit, between 25% and 45% [72].

Therefore, the aim should be to maintain optimum O_2-carrying capacity with a low viscosity, at a haematocrit between 30% and 40%.

Oncotic pressure

The plasma colloid oncotic pressure (COP) is one factor in the balance of fluid between the blood and the extracellular space, as first described by Starling [150]. The plasma COP has been used to predict excess lung water, with low values appearing to correlate with an increase in respiratory problems [123]. There is a uniform mortality once the plasma COP has fallen below 12.5 mmHg (1.7 kPa) [131].

The clinical use of the plasma COP in conjunction with measured PCP may be a more reliable basis for guiding fluid therapy and diagnosing non-cardiogenic pulmonary oedema. The oncotic–hydrostatic gradient (COP–PCP) is a more sensitive index for separating patients with or without cardiogenic pulmonary oedema than capillary pressure alone [167]. Normal COP [21 $\pm$ 3 mmHg (2.8 $\pm$ 0.4 kPa)] generates a gradient of more than 8 mmHg (1.1 kPa), protecting the lungs from the formation of pulmonary oedema. This gradient is reversed if the hydrostatic pressure exceeds the COP and the result is pulmonary oedema. Plasma COP may be measured directly, or can be calculated from the serum albumin.

However, most of the studies validating these measurements have been in cardiac patients

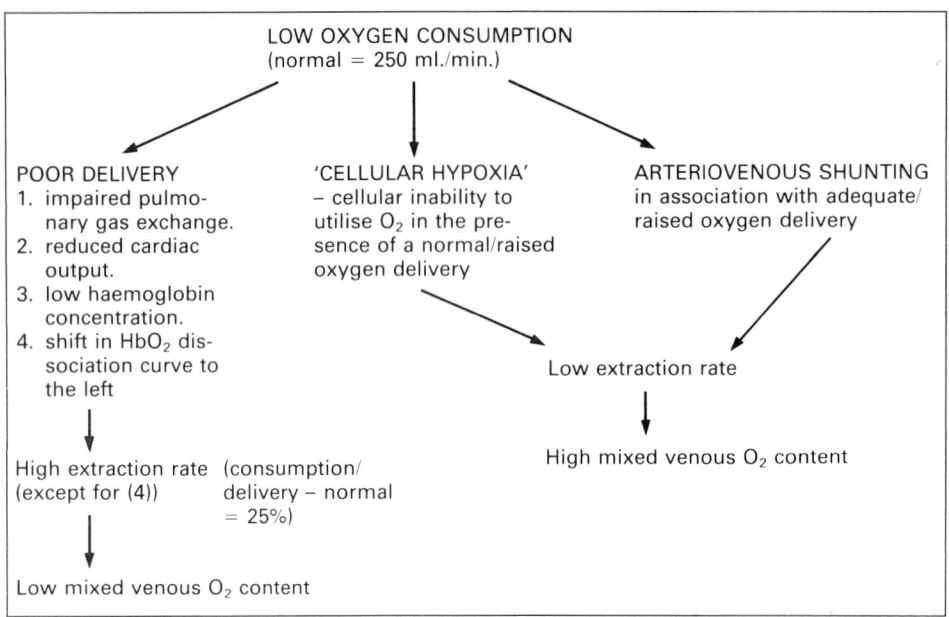

Fig. 12.1. Low oxygen consumption.

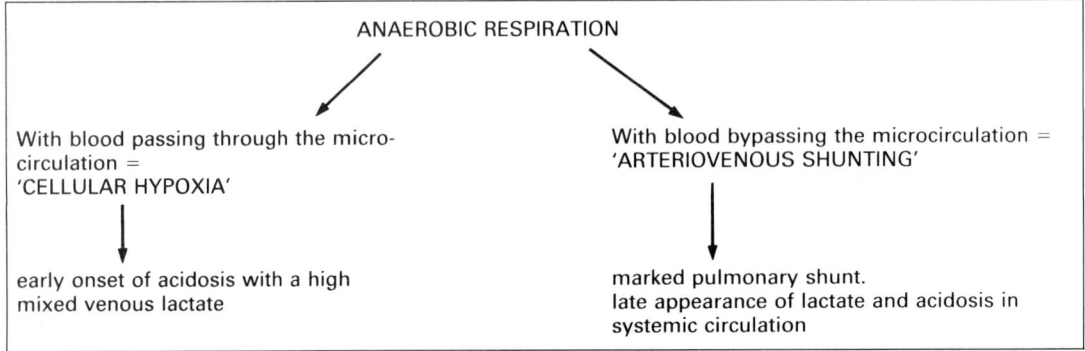

Fig. 12.2. Low oxygen consumption with low oxygen extraction rate, despite adequate delivery.

where the capillary membrane was intact and the primary problem was an increase in hydrostatic pressure. Another important gradient to be considered in the formation of pulmonary oedema is the plasma–interstitial COP gradient. Alteration in membrane permeability will greatly modify this value. Staub has demonstrated that interstitial COP varies with changes in filtration rate [151]. The plasma oncotic-hydrostatic gradient does not take into account changes in the interstitial COP. Experiments in the chronic lung lymph fistula sheep model of pulmonary oedema suggest that falls in the plasma COP are well compensated for by falls in the interstitial COP, and that the filtration rate correlates poorly with the plasma COP–PCP gradient because of the large changes in interstitial COP. When E. coli endotoxin is used to disrupt membrane permeability, large increases in fluid filtration are seen, with essentially no change in the balance of Starling forces [36].

These observations limit the usefulness of measuring plasma COP as a guide to fluid therapy.

Plasma volume

Accurate assessment of plasma volume in critically ill patients is a difficult but crucial judgement. Shoemaker [80] has described a group of patients in whom cardiac output, CVP, PCP and other vital signs were normal, who nevertheless were hypovolaemic when plasma volume was measured directly with I^{131}-labelled albumin. He emphasizes that reliance on routine vital signs may give a false sense of security. Other studies [140] have shown that a high percentage of patients returning from operative procedures after their fluid deficit had been replaced according to conventional clinical criteria have significantly reduced plasma volumes. Other workers [7] have not found the measurement of plasma volume useful in the management of shock as the required plasma volume may be much greater than the predicted 'normal'. In general, measurement of cardiac filling pressures is an adequate and convenient guide to plasma volume, but their limitations must be remembered.

Metabolic derangement

The problems of assessment of adequate oxygenation have been emphasized, and the complexity of the necessary measurements add to the clinical problem. The acid–base status is a more convenient parameter which can be monitored closely.

The form of acid–base disorder depends upon the severity and the stage of development of the shock syndrome. In a study of patients in Vietnam, one-third presented with an acidosis, but the other two-thirds had either normal or alkalotic pH because of respiratory compensation [106]. A transient respiratory alkalosis is common in the early phase of septicaemia [41] in association with hyperventilation. Respiratory alkalosis is rapidly supplanted by a metabolic acidosis, due to the accumulation of lactic acid as anaerobic metabolism becomes predominant. The severity of the metabolic acidosis (lactate concentration) correlates well with prognosis in shock [31]. Recent work has indicated that endotoxaemia interferes with the production of new glucose from alanine, glycerol, and lactic acid. Apparently this is caused by depression of the rate-limiting enzymes (specifically phosphoenolpyruvate kinase and fructose diphosphatase) as well as an energy deficit, since ATP is necessary for converting these precursors into glucose. Depressed gluconeogenesis may also contribute to the increase in lactic acid since it is not taken up by the liver for new glucose formation. There have been reports of a positive correlation between serum endotoxin and lactate in septic shock, and a negative correlation between blood glucose and endotoxin in animals. The glucose:lactate ratio may be a useful prognostic and therapeutic pointer in the management of shock [135].

Blood glucose may be high (reflecting catecholamine-mediated glycogen breakdown), normal, or low. Hypoglycaemia secondary to the inhibition of gluconeogenesis requires an exogenous source of glucose, and in this situation the use of glucose insulin and potassium solutions has some therapeutic value. Glucose

homeostasis, avoiding hyper- and hypoglycaemia, is an important aim in management.

The correction of the metabolic acidosis eventually depends upon an improvement in tissue perfusion, but a serum pH of less than 7.25 may cause myocardial depression and reduce the effectiveness of endogenous/exogenous catecholamines on myocardial function [114]. Correction of the severe forms of metabolic acidosis is therefore indicated, but the dangers of bicarbonate therapy make the routine use of sodium bicarbonate hazardous. Left shifts of the oxygen–haemoglobin dissociation curve with a reduction in tissue delivery of oxygen have been mentioned, and sodium overload is another consideration, especially in the presence of poor renal function.

Coagulation status

Consumption coagulopathy (DIC) plays an important role in the development of refractory unresponsive shock, especially in association with sepsis. Its cardinal manifestation is the onset of severe, sudden abnormal bleeding which may appear from incisional margins of surgical wounds, or venepuncture sites. Haematuria, bleeding from the nose and gums, and ecchymoses are not uncommon, in association with a general reduction in organ function. Tests of coagulation are essential for accurate diagnosis, but no single test is diagnostic. An attempt to evaluate the activity of the fibrinolytic system should be made, because the degree to which fibrinolysis has been activated can affect the course of the syndrome.

Other organ function

Renal and pulmonary function may alter significantly. Serial measurements of serum electrolytes are essential, and special attention should be paid to the serum potassium concentration in order to avoid cardiac instability.

Hourly urine output, urinary electrolytes, and urine:plasma osmolality ratios are important indices of renal function. Serum level of creatinine, in relation to urinary excretion of creatinine (creatinine clearance) is the most commonly used measure of glomerular filtration; the blood urea is another useful measure but has more limitations.

Mechanical ventilatory assistance is often required in the management of these patients, and therefore monitoring must include the alveolar–arterial gradient, respiratory rate, tidal volume, vital capacity, effective compliance, arterial O_2 tension, and arterial CO_2 tension.

The principles of therapy
(Fig. 12.3)

The principles of haemodynamic management depend upon a classification of patients into two groups: those with an inadequate cardiac output and impaired tissue perfusion, and those with an adequate or high cardiac output, and impaired tissue perfusion due to maldistribution of flow. Recognition of these two groups can only be made once hypovolaemia as a cause of shock has been treated, with the establishment of an adequate preload.

---

1. Maintain adequate cardiac filling pressures.
   CVP 8–12 mm.Hg., PCP 12–18 mm.Hg.

2. Maintain adequate oxygenation.
   Arterial PO_2. 60 mm.Hg., saturation 90%, haemoglobin 10 gm.%.

3. Maintain the optimum viscosity of blood.
   PCV = 30–35%.

4. Correct the acidosis.
   Maintain pH between 7.25 and 7.35.

5. Maintain normal levels of electrolytes.

6. Maintain normoglycaemia.

7. Maintain sinus rhythm.
   Treat arrhythmias.

Measurement of the cardiac output

Low cardiac output = pump failure

High cardiac output = maldistribution of flow

Fig. 12.3. An approach to the diagnosis and management of shock.

Volume replacement therapy— optimization of preload

The objectives of IV fluid administration are two-fold: to replace body fluid, and to increase preload and increase cardiac output.

The need for fluid replacement is obvious in frank haemorrhagic shock, and in shock associated with reduction in extravascular salt and water. Rapid and appropriate intervention will

reverse this form of shock rapidly and completely and haemorrhagic shock has a good prognosis, provided bleeding is controlled and the complications of transfusion are avoided. The haemodynamic hallmarks of a reduction in effective vascular volume include: tachycardia, hypotension, arteriolar constriction, reduced systemic venous pressure, reduced ventricular filling pressures, and the concomitant reduction in cardiac output. Prompt fluid replacement will reverse these changes, but a delay in treatment may lead to a form of 'irreversible' shock with hypotension persisting in the face of restitution of blood volume. In such cases the shock syndrome proper has developed, with a reduction in pump function, and/or maldistribution of blood flow.

The form of fluid that is given should be selected in accordance with the pattern of fluid depletion, and so may be blood, colloid, or crystalloid. In the case of water loss, with hypernatraemia and haemoconcentration, hypotonic sodium crystalloid replacement is indicated; shock due to sodium depletion requires repletion with normal saline. Haemorrhage requires blood replacement, but if necessary colloid and crystalloid can be used as stopgap measures.

The colloid vs crystalloid controversy

This debate is ancient and remains unresolved. Several authors [23, 109] have proposed the use of sodium-rich fluids in shock and trauma to correct hypovolaemia and to expand extracellular fluid, whereas others [161] advocate colloidal fluid therapy on the assumption that decreased blood volume, rather than extracellular fluid deficit, is the primary problem. Experimentally, large volumes of crystalloid, amounts equivalent to three times the blood loss, are not sufficient to reverse hypovolaemia. Such excessive volumes of crystalloid reduce plasma COP and decrease the oncotic–hydrostatic pressure gradient. Studies in rats made hypotensive by exteriorisation of the intestine [33] suggest that five times the volume of crystalloid vs colloid must be given to maintain haematocrit values at pre-shock levels. Animals infused with crystalloid show a 50% weight gain, with no improvement in survival. This is in contrast to those animals receiving colloid, who show only a 10% weight gain with high survival rates. Fluid loading in sheep with chronic lung lymph fistulae [35] suggests that crystalloid resuscitation following haemorrhagic shock leads to an increase in pulmonary vascular pressures and an increase in lung lymph flow. Conversely, albumin resuscitation of hypovolaemic shocked patients has been reported to impair pulmonary function, with increases in the alveolar–arterial PO_2 gradient and pulmonary shunt [91], and to impair salt and water excretion [90]. In a definitive study of oxygen transport responses to colloid and crystalloid infusions in critically ill patients, Shoemaker's group demonstrated greater and more prolonged increases in plasma volume, cardiac index, arterial pressure, and oxygen delivery and consumption in those hypovolaemic patients treated with colloid [64]. Plasma expansion with lactated Ringer's solution produced only a short-lived expansion of the plasma volume, with a fall in oxygen consumption and pulmonary oxygen transport. There was no evidence of capillary leakage of albumin in these patients.

Because of the absence of a consensus view, it is not possible to be dogmatic about fluid replacement. The hazards of colloid are obvious in the presence of a capillary leak, their action being to increase interstitial colloidal pressure and so add to the tendency of oedema formation. In such a situation, all fluid therapy is hazardous, and the patient must be maintained with the lowest possible PCP compatible with an adequate cardiac output.

When neither clotting factors nor red cells are required, albumin preparations containing over 98% albumin are the colloids of choice. However, their cost is high and hence their availability is limited to those patients who are hypoproteinaemic, e.g. in acute hepatic failure or the nephrotic syndrome. Purified protein fraction contains 90% albumin and is free from contaminants such as Australia antigen (HBsAg). It is an excellent solution for volume expansion but again, use has to be restricted because of its short supply. Various plasma substitutes are available for use, but all have disadvantages. An ideal plasma substitute should have an oncotic pressure similar to plasma, remain in the circulation long enough to exert its effect, and then be disposed of by metabolic degradation or excretion. Gelatins, dextrans, and hydroxyethyl starches are all available and have been used with success (see Chap. 32). However, these agents have no oxygen carrying capacity and can only act through volume expansion.

Fluorocarbons

Much interest has been aroused by the development of fluorocarbons, in particular Fluosol-DA, and the possibility of its role in oxygen transport in shock. The properties of fluorocarbons were first exploited in the development of 'liquid respiration'. J. A. Kylstra (State University of New York, Buffalo) presented a paper at the American Society of Artificial Organs in 1962 entitled 'Of mice as fish', and demonstrated that mammals could respire within oxygen-rich liquids. Others followed up this fascinating demonstration and fluorocarbons were found to dissolve as much as 60% oxygen by volume. A major problem was the development of an emulsion, because these compounds were immiscible with blood. Using bovine albumin or a family of surfactants, 'Pluronics', H. A. Sloviter at the University of Pennsylvania developed such an emulsion, and since then the majority of research has centred on the use of the most appropriate fluorocarbon. The initial compounds were unsuitable because they tended to concentrate in the liver and spleen of injected animals, and cause capillary blockage.

L. C. Clark, at the University of Cincinnati, made a major breakthrough when he found that perfluorodecalin was completely eliminated by expiration, or by transpiration through the skin. This compound still had a tendency to agglomerate and block capillaries, and subsequently Ryoichi Naito, of the Green Cross Corporation, tried mixing perfluorodecalin with a small amount of perfluorotripropylamine to obtain a stable emulsion. This compound emulsion is stable and forms the main constituent of Fluosol-DA, but it has an extremely long half-life, in the region of 50 days. The first clinical test of Fluosol-DA took place when Naito infused himself and some of his colleagues at Green Cross with the emulsion. These investigators survived and now Fluosol-DA has been used in other clinical situations. Fluosol also contains hydroxyethyl starch and a mixture of electrolytes to maintain plasma iso-osmolality. It has been used in decerebrate subjects with no adverse effects, and at present the Food and Drug Administration approves the use of Fluosol on a named case basis. It has been used with success in the resuscitation of Jehovah's Witnesses, and Shoemaker reported the oxygen-carrying characteristics of the emulsion at the third World Congress of Critical Care [164]. He monitored the haemodynamic and oxygen transport characteristics of three severely anaemic Jehovah's Witnesses following a pre-operative infusion of 20 ml/kg body wt. Fluosol. He reported that at normal alveolar oxygen tension levels, Fluosol acts as a plasma expander, and only becomes a significant part of the oxygen delivery system at alveolar oxygen tensions of more than 200 mmHg (26.7 kPa). At the same meeting, Nishimura reported results in 185 patients given 6–25 ml/kg body wt. Fluosol [111]. Increased arterial oxygen content, increased oxygen consumption, and acid–base normalization were noted when inspired oxygen concentrations were greater than 50%. Further research in this field of oxygen transport continues, and fluorocarbon investigation centres on the search for a non-toxic, rapidly excreted compound.

Other crystalloids

Refractory hypovolaemic shock which has not responded to vigorous fluid replacement has been treated with hyperosmotic sodium chloride with some success [34]. The use of hyperosmotic crystalloid solutions—glucose, mannitol, and sodium chloride—is not new, and investigations in dogs suggest that no appreciable plasma volume expansion occurs initially, indicating that fluid shift into the vascular bed plays no essential role in this response [166]. While these solutions may reduce myocardial oedema and subendocardial ischaemia, an important factor in the pump failure associated with irreversible shock, there is no good evidence that hyperosmotic solutions, including dextrose–potassium–insulin solutions, are more effective than more conventional fluid replacement.

Level of preload

Optimum filling pressures in the heart will ensure a maximum cardiac output for a given state of the myocardium, and the values of these are increased in the shock syndrome because of changes in compliance of the left and right ventricles [148]. Following myocardial infarction, there is a decrease in ventricular compliance [38], and various levels of CVP and PCP have been recommended in therapy. In the presence of a normal COP and intact capillaries, filling pressures should be maintained at higher than normal levels: CVP 10–15 mmHg, and PCP 12–18 mmHg. These levels ensure that preload is adequate and that hypovolaemia is not a factor in the circulatory collapse. The danger of fluid overload is obvious, and pulmonary oedema may occur at these levels if oncotic pressure falls, or if there is a disruption of the capillary membrane.

There is no clinical indication for a reduction of preload other than pulmonary oedema with impaired gas exchange, and a reduced preload will almost always lead to a reduction in cardiac output. The shape of the cardiac function curve will determine the magnitude of this fall, which may be small if the curve is flat, but large if the curve is steep. The reduction of preload using venesection, diuretics, and venodilators is contraindicated in the management of shock, unless pulmonary oedema is a major contributing factor to systemic hypoxia. A well-known maxim, 'No-one ever died from swollen ankles,' is particularly apt, and drugs which reduce preload should, in general, be avoided. However, it must be noted that there is a role for the reduction of preload in the control of myocardial infarct size. Preload is a major determinant of myocardial oxygen consumption and, in the presence of an adequate cardiac output following myocardial infarction, it is reasonable to reduce preload in order to reduce myocardial oxygen demands. Nitroglycerin, sublingual, cutaneous, or IV, is fashionable for this reason, and has been found to be effective in the control of persistent angina [32], and to reduce infarct size [44]. After coronary occlusion in the experimental animal, nitroglycerin has been shown to reduce ST segment elevation, improve ventricular function, raise ventricular fibrillation threshold, and enhance the electrical stability of the heart by decreasing differences in refractory periods between ischaemic and non-ischaemic areas [66]. Similar effects have been observed in patients with acute myocardial infarction [46]. Patients with severe left ventricular impairment respond best, but in patients with normal or reduced left ventricular filling pressures, nitroglycerin produces a fall in cardiac output with an associated reflex tachycardia [47]. Further ST segment elevation in this group of patients has been reported [13]. These observations underline the importance of maintaining optimum preload, and the complications of nitroglycerin—hypotension, pulmonary shunting, methaemoglobinaemia, and headache—should also be remembered. Haemodynamic monitoring is essential, and the superiority of IV nitroglycerin over more traditional therapeutic modalities, e.g. diuretics, has not been proved.

In conclusion, optimization of preload is the first principle of the management of all shock, and the importance of volume replacement cannot be overemphasized. The form of fluid used to maintain preload, in the absence of blood loss, is open to question, but in the presence of normal capillary permeability, colloid is indicated.

The pharmacological management of pump failure

Pump failure as a primary cause of circulatory collapse, or as an end-point in the progression of shock, demands active intervention.

Primary causes of pump failure are numerous, and include progressive chronic cardiomyopathies, mechanical factors such as valvar obstruction and regurgitation, intracardiac septal defects, and pericardial tamponade. Pump failure following cardiopulmonary bypass is an important cause of a low cardiac output, but the most common cause of defective pump function is myocardial ischaemia. 'Cardiogenic shock' is the global term often given to these conditions and this defines a diseased heart as the source of the haemodynamic catastrophe. 'Pump failure' is a less specific term and indicates that circulatory collapse in association with failure of the heart to pump adequately may occur in individuals with previously healthy hearts. It is an obvious truism to say that most people die with an inadequate cardiac output.

Pump failure accompanying acute myocardial infarction is the paradigm of this form of shock, and has been extensively reviewed. Most patients exhibit triple vessel coronary disease with extensive involvement of the left anterior descending coronary artery [168]. The underlying infarction usually involves the majority of the left ventricle but there is a variant of pump failure secondary to acute myocardial infarction in which the right ventricle is the predominant area of damage. In this form of shock, right ventricular dysfunction (a low cardiac output with a raised right ventricular filling pressure, and a reduced left ventricular filling pressure) is the cause of systemic hypoperfusion. An increase in left ventricular preload by volume loading is essential in management, and the general prognosis is better than that form of shock associated with left ventricular infarction [11].

The clinical features of pump failure secondary to acute myocardial infarction occur in 10%–15% of patients who survive sufficiently long to reach hospital [59]. Systemic hypoperfusion with reflex sympathetic cutaneous vasoconstriction and diaphoresis is marked, and arterial hypoxaemia secondary to pulmonary oedema may form a major component of the general hypoxic state. Cardiac signs may be minimal, but a gallop rhythm, a pericardial rub, or signs of acute mitral incompetence or ventricular septal rupture occasionally are found. Diminished urine output is characteristic, and

acute tubular necrosis may develop, especially with the injudicious use of diuretics in the presence of absolute or relative hypovolaemia. A full 12-lead electrocardiogram is essential.

All therapeutic interventions are geared to increasing cardiac output by manipulating the two major determinants of pump function: the heart rate and the stroke volume. The management of complicating arrhythmias is dealt with in Chap. 10. Optimization of preload has been discussed, and it remains to consider myocardial contractility and the reduction of afterload.

Myocardial contractility and the control of infarct size

A low cardiac output, secondary to myocardial dysfunction and pump failure, is the terminal event of all irreversible forms of the shock syndrome. The exact mechanisms which result in these profound functional changes in a healthy heart are unknown, but compromised coronary perfusion, increased metabolic requirements of the heart in shock, a decline in the ratio of subendocardium to subepicardium perfused, and myocardial interstitial oedema all play some role [147]. One part of the management is the care of the stressed myocardium, healthy or diseased, with special attention following acute myocardial infarction to the limitation of infarct size.

Numerous studies have identified the extent of myocardial damage as an important prognostic factor in both the early and late mortality following acute myocardial infarction. Measurement of infarct size is difficult, and although studies of creatine kinase release, electrocardiographic mapping techniques, and isotopic localization have all been used with certain degrees of success, they are time consuming, and give results only in retrospect. A functional classification of myocardial performance by the application of haemodynamic subsets, as suggested by Forrester et al. [50], is probably more useful in the patient with pump failure. However, more recently, two additional concepts have been suggested to be of prognostic importance: incomplete myocardial infarction, that is, areas of viable myocardium remaining in the distribution of the artery responsible for infarction; and the presence of viable but potentially jeopardized myocardium, that is myocardium with preserved function but supplied by a severely narrowed coronary artery [119]. It is with regard to these considerations that a number of therapeutic manoeuvres have been practised in the management of pump failure associated with acute myocardial infarction.

O_2 therapy alone has been shown to reduce infarct size in animals, and many patients with acute myocardial infarction are hypoxic secondary to pulmonary oedema and/or a low cardiac output, and may benefit from O_2 therapy [97]. Glucose–insulin–potassium cocktails have been used in animals to improve myocardial function and reduce the extent of myocardial necrosis following experimental coronary occlusion, but there is no controlled evidence of an effect in man. It is very difficult to separate any direct effect of such cocktails from volume loading per se. Hyaluronidase, given by infusion, and mannitol have been used to increase collateral blood flow to jeopardized myocardium, and have both been shown to reduce infarct size in animals. Their role in patient management is as yet undefined.

There was a vogue for the administration of corticosteroids in acute myocardial infarction, but this has not been sustained. Although animal studies suggested a role in the limitation of infarct size, some studies in man suggested a higher mortality in groups treated with steroids [127]. One major risk of their use is that healing may be affected and that cardiac rupture or a ventricular aneurysm may develop.

It is possible to reduce the size of myocardial infarction in animals and man by reducing the amount of work done by the heart. Beta blockade in this context has undergone extensive investigation, but is not appropriate for the patient with pump failure. In the shock syndrome secondary to pump failure, there are only two methods of reducing myocardial work, and hence myocardial oxygen consumption: the control of inappropriate and disruptive tachyarrhythmias, and the reduction of afterload. Therapeutic reduction of afterload must be undertaken with considerable caution since too-vigorous administration of peripheral vasodilators may result in a substantial fall in aortic diastolic pressure, in which case the decrease in myocardial perfusion and reflex increase in heart rate may exceed the reduction in oxygen demand. Nitroprusside is the agent of choice since this has only a small effect on preload.

The effects of the various inotropes on the imbalance between myocardial oxygen supply and demand are somewhat variable. Any increase in cardiac output achieved through increasing myocardial contractility must be associated with an increase in myocardial oxygen consumption. Isoprenaline consistently increases heart rate, produces arrhythmias, lowers aortic diastolic pressure, and further impairs myocardial metabolism, as evidenced by increases in coronary sinus lactate concentrations [110]. Noradrenaline increases myocardial oxygen demand but this increase may be equalled by an increase in delivery secondary to an increase in aortic diastolic pressure, particularly if profound hypotension exists [110].

Dopamine, perhaps the most popular inotrope in use at the present time, has a variety of effects depending upon the infusion rate. At low doses it acts only on dopaminergic receptors, causing an increase in renal and splanchnic blood flow. This effect is similar to reducing afterload, and may be accompanied by a fall in mean arterial pressure, with a variable effect on cardiac output. As the infusion rate is increased, the drug has a positive inotropic effect by stimulating the myocardium directly, and also indirectly through release of noradrenaline stores. It has less chronotropic effects than isoprenaline, but in higher doses alpha vasoconstriction and the generation of arrhythmias become more prominent [55]. It is difficult to predict its effects on the balance between myocardial oxygen demand and supply, but comparison with dobutamine suggests that the latter is superior in this respect.

Dobutamine is the result of systematic modification of the chemical structure of isoprenaline and is now recommended by some as the inotrope of choice following myocardial infarction [149]. It acts directly on the beta-1 receptors in the myocardium to produce an increase in contractility. It has only a weak chronotropic effect, and peripheral vasoconstriction is unusual even at maximal doses. A comparison of dobutamine and dopamine in patients with low output cardiac failure demonstrated that for the same increases in cardiac output and heart rate, dobutamine decreased mean arterial and pulmonary capillary pressures, whereas dopamine did not change arterial pressure, and increased pulmonary capillary pressure [88]. Similar findings were demonstrated in a crossover study of dopamine and dobutamine, in patients with congestive cardiomyopathy and heart failure. Dobutamine produced a progressive rise in the cardiac output by increasing stroke volume, while simultaneously decreasing systemic and pulmonary vascular resistances and filling pressures. There was no increment in heart rate or premature ventricular contractions. As arterial pressure rose with increased doses of dopamine, pulmonary capillary pressure also rose, and the incidence of ventricular extrasystoles increased. The product of heart rate (HR) times systolic blood pressure (SBP) increased with the administration of both drugs, but the rise was more dramatic with dopamine. At the same HR × SBP product, dopamine increased the cardiac index by 0.60 litre/min whereas dobutamine increased it by 1.31 litre/min. During the 24-h infusion, only dobutamine produced a sustained increase in stroke volume, cardiac output, urine flow, urine sodium concentration, creatinine clearance, and peripheral blood flow. Renal and hepatic blood flow was not significantly altered by either drug [85]. In patients following cardiopulmonary bypass, dobutamine is a potent inotropic agent, and produces an increase in cardiac output with few arrhythmias, and a less prominent tachycardia compared with isoprenaline [162]. The effect of dobutamine on coronary blood flow depends upon the pressure gradient generated between aortic diastolic pressure and the filling pressure of the left ventricle. The data above suggest that the net effect of dobutamine is to increase coronary blood flow, and animal studies have confirmed an increase in myocardial blood flow to all areas of the heart in models of acute myocardial infarction [175]. Its use in patients with acute myocardial infarction has not been associated with an increase in infarct size, or an increase in ventricular arrhythmias [54]. Dobutamine would seem to be the inotrope of first choice following myocardial infarction.

Digoxin is another agent which can increase cardiac output, myocardial oxygen consumption, and myocardial infarct size in animals [99]. In man, there is no evidence concerning digoxin's effect on infarct size, and in cases where the drug produces a reduction in preload, or in heart rate, oxygen demand is reduced [28]. It seems likely that inotropes seldom improve the imbalance between myocardial oxygen supply and demand, and frequently aggravate it, emphasizing the role of mechanical support of the circulation in the post-infarct situation.

Recently it has been shown that intracoronary infusion of streptokinase can restore patency of an obstructed coronary artery during the early hours of myocardial infarction [52]. Reperfusion may actually promote injury under some circumstances [17], but Braunwald's group have demonstrated a substantial increase in nutrient flow resulting in salvage of jeopardized myocardium following intracoronary streptokinase infusion [98]. The use of intracoronary prostacyclin as a means of restoring blood flow is also being explored [6].

Limitation of infarct size, and the effect of pharmacological intervention on the balance between myocardial oxygen supply and demand, are important considerations in the management of patients with pump failure, whether the aetiology of the pump failure is ischaemic or not, because in all forms of shock myocardial function must be protected.

Inotropic agents have this reputation of 'thrashing the myocardium to death', but are invariably required in pump failure states. In the setting of severe hypotension and low cardiac output a choice of agents has to be made (see Chap. 16). Suffice it to say that there are no magic potions available and all such agents have their disadvantages. There is sometimes value in combining two inotropes in the management of the critically ill patient, and a low-dose dopamine infusion to protect renal perfusion is often of value in combination with another catecholamine, such as dobutamine, or noradrenaline which provides full inotropic support. Glucagon is another agent which has been used with some success, especially in heart failure associated with beta blockade. However, clinical trials of this agent have produced equivocal results in the treatment of pump failure, and the beneficial effects are only marginal [105]. Prenalterol is a new beta-1 stimulant with little effect on the peripheral circulation. Although clinical experience is limited, increases in cardiac index have been reported in such varying states as pump failure secondary to myocardial infarction, septic shock, and following cardiopulmonary bypass. There is no evidence of its superiority over any of the other drugs mentioned, and there is a suggestion that it is only a partial agonist of the beta-1 receptor, and at high doses may cause beta-1 blockade, preventing a full response to adrenaline or noradrenaline. The toxicity of digoxin makes it an unsuitable drug for use in critically ill patients, especially when there are many other more effective inotropes available [65].

It remains to be restated that the ideal inotropic agent would increase vital organ perfusion by increasing cardiac output without excessively increasing myocardial oxygen consumption. It should have a minimal chronotropic effect because rapid heart rates reduce coronary blood flow. The data at present are confusing and contradictory, but it would seem that dobutamine and dopamine are currently the inotropes of choice. Noradrenaline has a role in profound hypotension, and following cardiopulmonary bypass to maintain coronary perfusion, but can only be used for short periods. The choice may end as a personal matter depending upon the physician's familiarity with the different inotropes available, but of great importance is the ability to monitor responses to therapy. Earlier introduction of mechanical support, before the myocardium is thrashed to death, is recommended.

Reduction of afterload—vasodilator therapy in pump failure

If after attempts to optimize preload and improve myocardial contractility the haemodynamic state remains unsatisfactory, then reducing ventricular afterload may be helpful. Such vasodilator therapy has been described by Braunwald as a 'physiological approach to heart failure' [14]. Myocardial systolic tension is a major determinant of myocardial fibre shortening and oxygen consumption, and a reduced afterload permits greater ventricular muscle shortening with an increase in ejection fraction and cardiac output. This improvement in pump performance is generally accomplished with a reduction in myocardial oxygen consumption due to the reduction in systolic tension generated, and the reduction in heart size. When the left ventricle is normal, a reduction in afterload achieved by reducing aortic impedance does not greatly augment left ventricular stroke volume, and the arterial pressure may fall. Reflex tachycardia may compensate for the fall in peripheral resistance by increasing cardiac output and maintaining arterial pressure. The more abnormal the function of the left ventricle, however, the greater the stroke volume will rise as afterload is reduced, and thus a smaller fall in arterial pressure is observed [26]. A venodilator may lower afterload by reducing ventricular volume without altering systemic vascular resistance.

The three main indications for the reduction of afterload are: evidence of vasoconstriction and oliguria in the presence of a systolic pressure of 90 mmHg; pulmonary oedema with a low cardiac output; and pulmonary oedema in association with acute mitral incompetence, or a ruptured interventricular septum [161]. It can only be considered if the systolic pressure is maintained at 90 mmHg, for severe hypotension, with concomitant decreases in coronary, cerebral, and renal blood flow, is a major hazard. Preload may also fall precipitously as nearly all vasodilator drugs cause some venodilatation, and this must be countered with volume expansion. Careful haemodynamic monitoring is essential as the response to such drugs as nitroprusside and nitroglycerine is sometimes unpredictable. A high filling pressure is essential at the start of therapy in order to minimize the drop in preload. Reflex tachycardia is a possible sign of inadequate preload and must also be avoided in order to minimize myocardial oxygen consumption. One question that remains to be resolved concerns the distribution of the increase in cardiac output that occurs in this situation. There is little information regarding the regional vascular effects of many of these drugs, and only dopamine, in low doses, is used specifically to dilate the renal vascular bed. There is some suggestion that the increase in cardiac output following afterload reduction using vasodilators is mainly distributed to the splanchnic bed, and this may not constitute a useful increase in vital organ perfusion.

The ideal vasodilator for the treatment of acute pump failure should have a rapid onset and brief duration of action when administered by IV infusion. The drug should be non-toxic. The available vasodilators vary in their haemodynamic effects, depending on their major locus of action—arteriolar dilatation or venodilatation (Fig. 12.4). The selection of a specific agent depends upon the pathophysiological state of the patient. The major controversy in therapy at the present time revolves around the advantages and disadvantages of nitroprusside and nitroglycerine.

Nitroprusside remains the more suitable agent for acute afterload reduction because it has a lesser effect on the venules, and produces a more rapid and predictable response, which is easily terminated. It has been suggested that increases in subendocardial blood flow are more profound with nitroglycerine but there is no good evidence of this in man. The controversy is, in fact, a non-issue, as nitroglycerine has an important role in the management of patients with a low output state and pulmonary oedema. In this situation, reduction of preload and afterload is indicated and is achieved best with this drug (Fig. 12.5).

Alpha adrenergic blocking drugs, in particular phentolamine and phenoxybenzamine, have been used successfully in the past but are probably obsolete. Beta-2 agonists such as salbutamol have been used following myocardial infarction [160] and cardiac surgery [120], but the relevance of increasing flow to the skeletal muscle and splanchnic beds is highly doubtful.

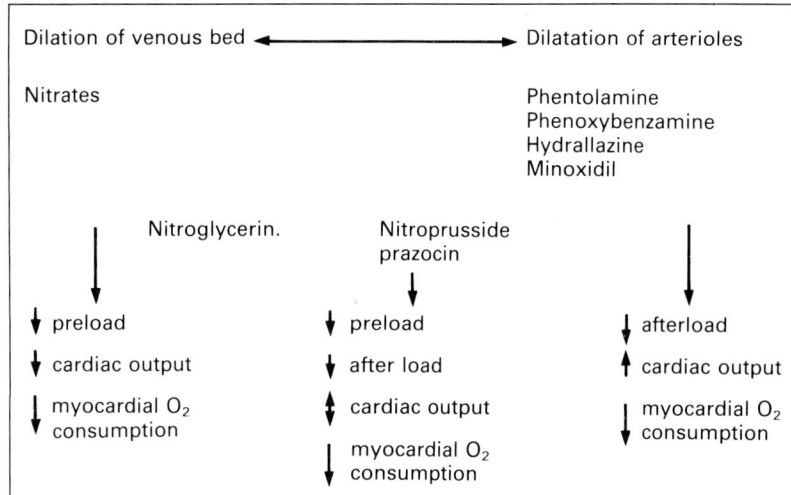

Fig. 12.4. Vasodilator spectrum of activity.

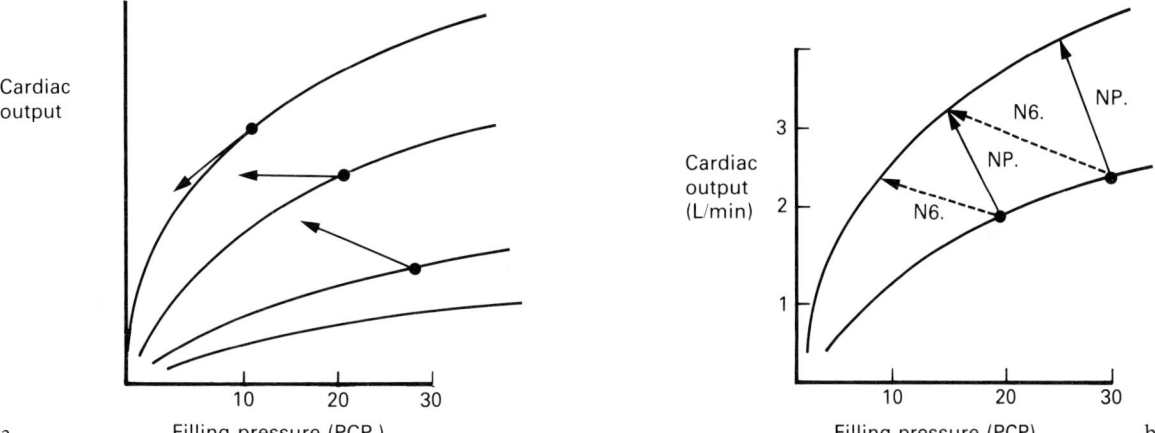

Fig. 12.5. a Haemodynamic changes reported with nitroprusside and nitroglycerin at different filling pressures in pump failure—the lack of controversy. **b** The varying effects of nitroglycerin on cardiac output according to filling pressure, and myocardial contractile state.

The pharmacological balloon pump

Inotropes and vasodilators used in combination in severely shocked patients have been reported as being more effective than when used singly [113]. Combinations such as dobutamine/dopamine and nitroprusside/nitroglycerin have become commonplace in the CCU and in the management of the critically ill, but their use begs the question concerning early and appropriate application of the mechanical balloon pump, with special reference to the preservation of jeopardized myocardium.

Other drugs

A number of other drugs have recently been used in the management of pump failure, and include captopril, a converting enzyme inhibitor, and naloxone.

Captopril. Evidence that the renin–angiotensin–aldosterone system may be activated in patients with severe decompensated cardiac failure has raised the possibility that angiotensin may be responsible for the increase in peripheral resistance seen in pump failure. This has been reported in animal models of experimental heart failure [170], and multiple lines of evidence suggest that the kidney may have a central role in the pathogenesis of congestive heart failure. Plasma renin is often, but not always, raised [19], and converting enzyme inhibition not only improves renal perfusion but also increases the glomerular filtration rate, with a naturesis [67]. Excessive intrarenal angiotensin-2 may cause afferent arteriole constriction and accelerate the decline in renal function associated with pump failure [19]. A converting enzyme inhibitor could well correct these functional changes in the kidney, and also act advantageously by reducing the total peripheral resistance (after-load), and venous tone (preload).

There have been several reports of a good response to teprotide (an intravenous convert-ing enzyme inhibitor), and captopril in patients with chronic congestive heart failure, but data in the acute situation are scant. Hollenberg's group have reported spectacular results using captopril in patients with severe pump failure [42]. Eight patients were studied, and all had severe pump failure resistant to maximal con-ventional therapy, including vasodilators. Five patients were previously receiving nitroprus-side, and three of these also required dopamine in order to maintain an adequate systemic perfusion pressure. Captopril resulted in a dramatic improvement, with significant in-creases in cardiac index and creatinine and p-aminohippurate clearances, and with a fall in levels of serum creatinine, and blood urea ni-trogen. Improvement was sustained over a mean follow-up period of 7 months, and the time each patient spent in hospital was reduced markedly. This study was not controlled and randomized, but it suggests an important area of investiga-tion.

Naloxone. Since the demonstration of opiate re-ceptors in the central nervous system in 1973 [118], infusion of beta endorphin has been shown to be a potent hypotensive stimulus. Furthermore, stressful stimuli have been dem-onstrated to increase endogenous beta endor-phin concentration in the blood.

There has been much speculation about the role of beta endorphin in the generation of the shock syndrome, and there is some evidence that naloxone, a specific opiate-competitive antagonist, may be helpful in the management of shock. Both exogenous and endogenous opiates depress myocardial function, and Faden and Holaday have reported that in rats sub-jected to haemorrhagic shock, specific opiate receptor blockade with naloxone dramatically improved the mean arterial pressure and pulse pressure, and prolonged survival [45]. Further studies in mongrel dogs subjected to haemor-rhagic shock have confirmed the protective effects of naloxone [58]. Naloxone produced a dose-dependent increase in mean arterial pres-sure, cardiac output, stroke volume, and left ventricular contractility. Survival at 72 h was related to the dose of naloxone given at the time of onset of shock, and no dog survived the experiment without receiving naloxone. Other animal experiments using haemorrhaged cats have demonstrated an inhibition of proteolysis, a stabilization of lysosomal membranes, and a

reduction in circulating myocardial depressant factor [30]. A modest positive inotropic effect on isolated cat papillary muscle was also observed.

Studies in critically ill patients have been limited to a few case reports. In the few patients reported, naloxone has had a beneficial effect in what appeared to be irreversible cardiogenic and septic shock [40, 159]. The dose of naloxone seems to be critical, and although 0.1 mg/kg body wt. has been reported to be effective in shock in man, 8 mg/kg body wt. per hour has been used in animals. Patients with chronic liver disease who develop septic shock with a high cardiac output have responded to nalox-one, with an increase in cardiac output of up to 30%.

In conclusion, naloxone may be indicated in unresponsive shock and may buy time to insti-tute other, more permanent, measures such as mechanical support of the circulation.

The mechanical support of the circulation

Despite intensive pharmacological support and volume replacement therapy, pump failure associated with acute myocardial infarction con-tinues to be a lethal syndrome. Fifteen percent of all myocardial infarction patients develop shock associated with pump failure, and when the diagnosis is strict it is associated with a reported mortality of 85% [133]. The develop-ment of temporary mechanical methods of circulatory assistance has been an important priority in cardiovascular research, and the assist device that has proved to be the most practical, and with which the most clinical ex-perience has been gained, is the intra-aortic balloon counter-pulsation device (IABCP).

The concept of augmentation of the arterial diastolic pressure, and hence coronary blood flow, was first explored by Kantrowitz and Kantrowitz [75] in 1953, and they demonstrated that retardation of the systolic pressure pulse could increase coronary blood flow by 22%–53%. Further studies of diastolic augmentation were achieved by wrapping the left hemi-diaphragm around the thoracic aorta and syn-chronously stimulating the intact left phrenic nerve during diastole [76]. At the third World Congress of Cardiology in Brussels in 1958, Claus et al. introduced the concept of diastolic assistance for the failing heart, and coined the term 'counterpulsation'. Their first counter-pulsation device withdrew blood from bilateral femoral arterial catheters during systole, and reinfused it during diastole. Using this device, these workers were able to show a decrease in the ventricular tension time index, myocardial oxygen consumption, and an increase in sur-vival of animals following coronary occlusion [24]. The two concepts of diastolic augmentation and counterpulsation were combined by Moulo-poulos in 1962, who devised the first IABCP device [107]. The principle was simple: a cath-eter with a sausage-shaped balloon was passed into the descending thoracic aorta, and was rapidly inflated in diastole, thus raising the pressure with which the coronary arteries were perfused and so increasing coronary blood flow. Sudden deflation immediately before systole in order to reduce left ventricular afterload would lead to an increase in stroke volume and ejec-tion fraction, and decrease the tension in the myocardial wall and myocardial oxygen con-sumption. The first clinical application of IABCP was carried out by Kantrowitz in 1967 [77] in two patients with left ventricular pump failure, one of whom survived to be discharged from hospital. Since these pioneering studies, there has been extensive world-wide experience in the use of the IABCP for the support of the circulation, and it has been shown to improve haemodynamic performance in a wide variety of clinical situations.

A number of balloon variables have been described that may directly affect the magnitude and duration of diastolic augmentation, and the decrease in left ventricular work [171]. The position of the balloon in the thoracic aorta, its volume of displacement, the balloon configura-tion and occlusivity, and inflation–deflation timing, are all important in determining the ultimate effect of IABCP. Arrhythmias are a relative contra-indication to the use of IABCP because they may not trigger the balloon pump appropriately. Studies in animals to examine changes in coronary blood flow induced by IABCP have produced variable results depend-ing upon the initial state of the animals' circu-lation. In general, coronary blood flow is significantly increased using IABCP in hypo-tensive animals with pre-existing reductions in coronary blood flow [22]. If, however, coro-nary blood flow is normal, IABCP is unlikely to effect an increase. Counterpulsation in com-bination with mannitol or propranolol has been shown to increase collateral blood flow to ischaemic myocardium over and above changes effected by a single intervention [73]. Studies

in humans with left ventricular pump failure suggest average increases in coronary blood flow of 23 ml/min per 100 g left ventricle, and correlates with changes in arterial perfusion pressure [86]. Reductions in afterload [110] and in preload [171] have been described in associa-tion with IABCP resulting in decreased left ventricular work. Therefore, IABCP may pro-duce a decrease in myocardial oxygen consump-tion by reducing ventricular work, while at the same time increasing coronary blood flow and oxygen delivery. Studies on acute myocardial ischaemia models in dogs have found IABCP to be effective in reducing the size of ischaemic damage, measured using ST segment mapping [100], and it has also been shown to improve lactate levels in ischaemic myocardium, increase ATP levels, and improve the histochemical and electron microscopic appearance of the is-chaemic myocardium [45].

Unfortunately, in the past, the practice of IABCP in the clinical situation was not simple. The standard catheter was inserted through a dacron sidearm sewn into the femoral artery, and required the expertise of a vascular sur-geon. Complications were common, and in-cluded dissection of the aorta, perforation of a major artery, thrombosis, embolism, and infec-tion [69]. Most of the complications seemed to occur at the time of the insertion of the catheter, but this situation has changed with the introduction of percutaneous IABCP. A single chamber percutaneous balloon catheter, constructed around a central guidewire, may be inserted using a 12F sheath into the common femoral artery with the conventional Seldinger technique. Several reports of experience with this catheter have appeared in the literature [15, 16, 154a], and it seems that insertion is rapid—5 min to the onset of IABCP—and the complica-tion rate is low. This method of balloon inser-tion may justify earlier intervention with IABCP in the future.

The best defined indication for the use of IABCP is after cardiac surgery in cases when it proves difficult to take the patient off cardiopul-monary bypass, and when a limited period of pumping may allow the myocardium to recover from the ischaemic damage caused by the operation. In an extensive series reported from the Texas Heart Institute [154], 419 patients with postoperative low output syndrome were supported with IABCP. Overall, 226 patients (54%) were successfully weaned from pump-ing support and 188 (45%) were subsequently discharged from hospital. Survival was di-rectly related to haemodynamic status, with a mortality rate of 46.3% in those patients with a cardiac index between 1.2 and 2.1 litre/min per square metre and a peripheral resistance less than 2100 dyn. $s^{-1}.cm^{-5}$. In those patients with a cardiac index less than 1.2 litre/min per square metre and a systemic vascular resistance of more than 2100 dyn. $s^{-1}.cm^{-5}$ the mortality rate was 96.6%. Patients with balloons of 40 and 30 ml had significantly better survival rates than those with 20 ml balloons. An effect of IABCP on the right side of the circulation was also noted, with reductions in right atrial pressure, pulmonary artery pressure, and pulmonary vascular resistance. This extensive report demonstrates that in this group of post-cardiac-surgery patients, IABCP produces immediate and predictable haemodynamic effects, and the accruing clinical results show increasing survival and hospital discharge rates.

The role of pre-operative IABCP is less well defined, but may also be useful to maintain the patient and his heart in the best possible condition while preparations for surgery are being made [57]. Pump failure secondary to acute mitral regurgitation or ventricular septal defect following myocardial infarction is an indication for IABCP support. Emergency surgery following acute myocardial infarction is difficult because of the problems of operating on tissue that is undergoing active necrosis, and if haemodynamic stabilization can be achieved for 1 week or more, the results of surgery are generally improved [21]. Full investigation and diagnosis of the cardiac lesion by cardiac catheterization using the haemodynamic support of IABCP may be carried out, and patients who would benefit from surgery may be identified. The time course of the sequence of IABCP—cardiac catheterization—surgery is controversial, and there have been reports of increased myocardial necrosis with temporal delay [29], and subtle haemodynamic deterioration may occur within a few hours after stabilization with IABCP [39]. Nevertheless, in cases of emergency surgery for mechanical causes of cardiogenic shock, long-term patient survival may exceed 40% [103]. Survival following mitral valve replacement is more common than survival following surgery for a ruptured intraventricular septum [25].

The use of IABCP in pump failure secondary to acute myocardial infarction with no correctable mechanical lesion, has been disappointing. Despite the theoretical advantages of mechanical support—improved myocardial oxygen delivery, reduction of myocardial oxygen consumption, protection of ischaemic myocardium,

facilitation of removal of toxic metabolites accumulating in the myocardium—the majority of patients treated in this way become balloon dependent, and definitive long-term survival has not been demonstrated [51]. The incidence of sudden death among short-term survivors is very high [87], and the quality of life of the long-term survivors has been poor. One problem in the assessment of this form of therapy is the time delay between presentation and the initiation of IABCP. By the time mechanical support is instituted, most patients have been in shock for more than 6 h, and have received conventional pharmacological support which may increase infarct size. Clinicopathological correlations have demonstrated that in patients who die of pump failure following myocardial infarction, more than 40% of the left ventricle is infarcted by either new or old infarction. Therefore, it has been suggested that if pump failure ensues following acute myocardial infarction and the process is not rapidly reversed, a much larger area of myocardium will be enveloped by the infarction process [115]. IABCP in combination with pharmacological intervention may be able to prevent further myocardial damage.

A recent paper from Rotterdam has described experience of early IABCP in 181 patients, 71 of whom were diagnosed as suffering from cardiogenic shock. Although these patients had already been treated by conventional means, and were expected to have a high mortality, about half of them survived more than 3 months. Forty-two further patients with angina at rest, unresponsive to medical treatment, in danger of full infarction, were treated with the balloon pump, and in 41 relief of pain was rapid, and surgery was performed later with a low complication rate [102]. Other studies have demonstrated abolition of pain, reversal of ST segment changes, and improvement in haemodynamic status in patients with 'pre-infarction' or 'crescendo' angina [172]. Similarly, in post-infarction angina where extension of the infarct is threatened, pain and ECG changes may be ameliorated by IABCP. IABCP has been used in the management or right ventricular infarction with a low output state [68] with some success, and Shumway's group have carried out counterpulsation with a pulmonary artery balloon for acute right ventricular failure following cardiac surgery [104]. Others have demonstrated experimentally the beneficial effects of aortic counterpulsation on right heart haemodynamics [171], and have suggested a role for IABCP in the management of shock associated with pulmonary embolism.

IABCP may have a role in the management of septic shock, especially in the late stages where myocardial depression is the prominent feature. Coexisting coronary artery disease and myocardial ischaemia is an important element in this form of myocardial depression, particularly in the elderly patient, and the maintenance of coronary blood flow is a fundamental consideration. Berger employed IABCP in two patients in advanced septic shock, reversing the shock state with survival of both patients [5].

In conclusion, the available evidence suggests that IABCP should be used earlier than it currently is, because it is clear that not many lives are saved in the reasonably long term once the shock syndrome has developed. There is no satisfactory clinical trial establishing a higher survival rate in patients with left ventricular failure, without shock, following acute myocardial infarction, treated with balloon support, than in similar patients receiving rigorous medical therapy, although there is an attractive rationale for its use. However, the balloon is of considerable value in the stabilization of patients with cardiogenic shock, particularly if there is a surgically correctable cause of shock such as acute mitral regurgitation, or ventricular septal rupture. Criteria for surgical intervention in the balloon-dependent group who do not have these mechanical causes of pump failure, are not precise, but are determined by the adequacy of the function of the left ventricle, the presence of a discrete aneurysm, and perhaps bypassable coronary arterial obstruction.

In order to reduce mortality by treating patients with lesser degrees of circulatory and pump failure following acute myocardial infarction, a non-invasive method that is simpler to apply, and that would result in fewer complications, has been sought. External pressure circulatory assistance has been investigated for several years [116]. It can produce effective diastolic augmentation of the arterial pressure, but studies on coronary blood flow have given varied results [143, 155]. It has been shown to be less effective than IABCP in reducing the afterload of the left ventricle and some studies have reported persistence of the excess lactate production by the myocardium [18]. A recent study in 23 patients suggested improvements in regional wall motion abnormalities following acute myocardial infarction, but there was no reduction in post-infarction angina. Also, pulmonary oedema developed in one patient 15 min after the initiation of treatment [132]. A co-operative clinical trial studied a total of 258 patients in 25 institutions and reported a significant reduction in mortality in patients less than 46 years of age, who received external circulatory support for at least 3 h in the first 24 h of hospitalization. There was a reduction in mortality of the whole group who received external support for at least 4 h in the first 24 h [3]. This study had all the problems of collaborative trials with poor definition of the initial clinical status of the patients, unequal numbers of patients from the various institutions, and an absence of haemodynamic measures. The conclusions of the study—that further application and investigation of external circulatory assistance in myocardial infarction are needed—cannot be doubted, but no more than that can be said. The complications of the technique are minimal, with patients complaining of leg cramps, a distressing feeling of confinement, and skin irritation. There is no evidence that the procedure causes injury or trauma, and in particular deep venous thrombosis and pulmonary embolism have not been associated with this form of support.

'Paracorporeal left ventricular support' is a blanket term used to describe a variety of mechanical support measures which have been employed in desperation, usually in order to take a patient off cardiopulmonary bypass. These methods are designed to unload the traumatized left ventricle totally while also maintaining adequate levels of systemic blood flow. The return of left ventricular contractile function in such patients requiring mechanical support may be detected utilizing radio-isotope gated cardiac blood pool imaging [157]. Left ventricular ejection fraction will show a significant improvement in the first 72 h of this form of support, if any significant recovery of cardiac function is going to take place at all, and one may infer that continued support of the circulation after 6 days, with no improvement in left ventricular ejection fraction, is not indicated. This is not always the rule, however, and there is a report of a patient who required 3 weeks of mechanical circulatory support until his cardiac performance had improved sufficiently to allow separation from the mechanical device [79]. More recently, Pierce et al. have reported their experience of ventricular assist pumping in patients with cardiogenic shock after cardiac operations [118a]. The ventricular assist pump was used to support the circulation in eight patients who could not be separated from cardiopulmonary bypass after open heart surgery. Three patients with left ventricular failure survived after 7 days of pumping, and one patient with right ventricular failure, in whom the pump was used to convey blood from the right atrium into the pulmonary artery, also survived. These results provide further evidence that in patients who cannot be weaned off cardiopulmonary bypass, the myocardial derangement is often reversible. The implications of successful paracorporeal support are extensive [51a], but the application of this form of therapy awaits further investigation and technological advance.

The management of high cardiac output 'distributive' shock

Physiologically inappropriate regional vasodilatation with systemic hypotension and a reduced peripheral resistance is central to this alternative form of the shock syndrome (Fig. 12.6). Although this clinical entity usually occurs in association with sepsis, it is also seen as a sequel to a neurological insult, or in association with toxic, metabolic, and endocrine depression of vasomotor tone; anaphylaxis is another important cause. The major problem consequent on the systemic hypotension is compromised perfusion of vital organs because of impaired perfusion pressure. Although flow has been recently emphasized as the essential determinant of oxygen delivery and substrate supply to tissues, it is vital to remember that below a certain mean arterial pressure, auto-

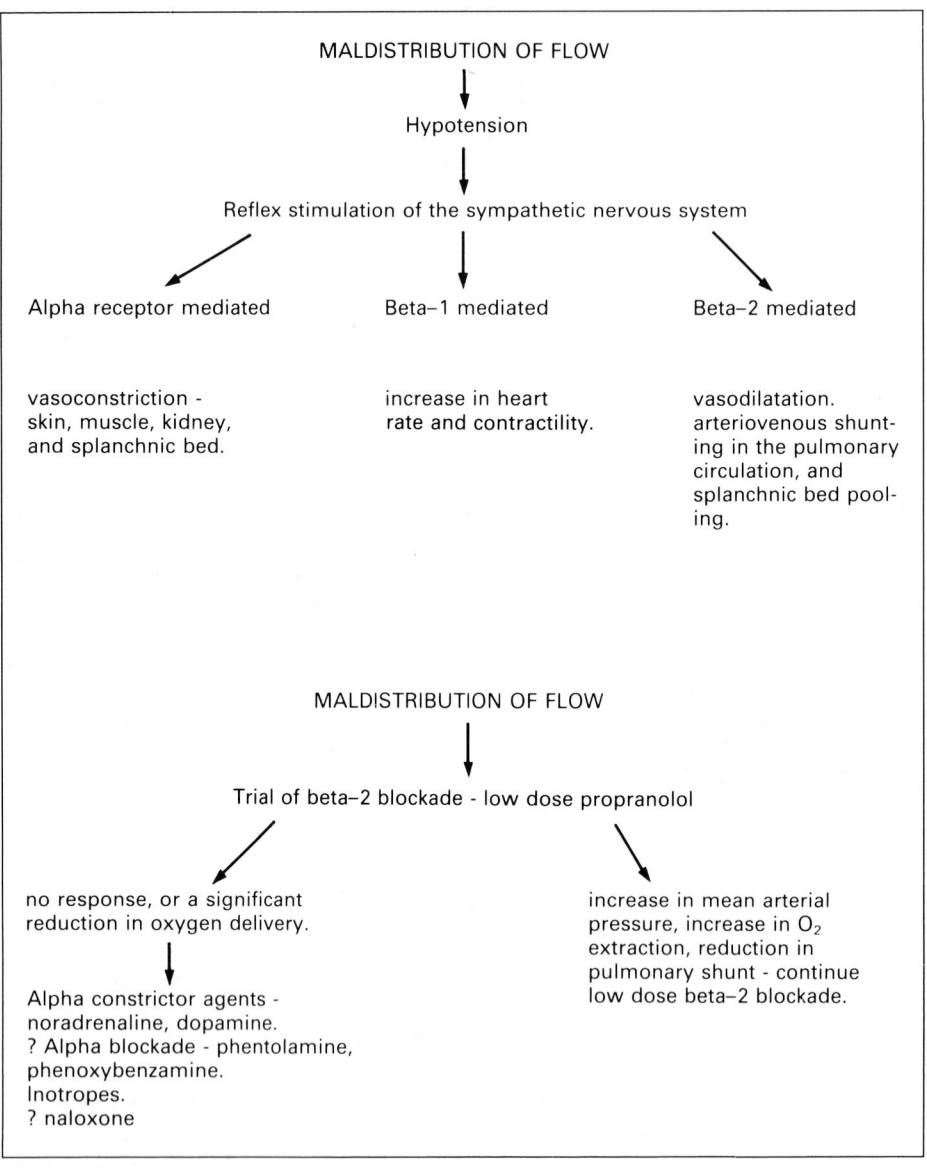

Fig. 12.6. Consequences and treatment of the maldistribution of blood flow.

regulation of blood flow to the cerebrum, the kidneys, and within the coronary circulation, does not take place. At these low levels of arterial pressure, flow is dependent entirely on pressure, so that pressure must be maintained. Reduction of systemic arterial pressure below 60 mmHg is accompanied by a marked decline in cerebral blood flow [63]. Therefore, in order to maintain perfusion of these vital organs, therapy must be aimed at the redistribution of blood flow with maintenance of systemic arterial pressure.

The initial lowering of arterial pressure and marked reduction in oxygen consumption, with a normal or raised cardiac output, is not explained exclusively by a decline in total peripheral vascular resistance and perfusion pressure of vital organs. There is evidence of regional arteriovenous shunting which may impair nutrient blood flow [177], and it is likely that there is direct inhibition of mitochondrial function [101]. Furthermore, myocardial dysfunction becomes prominent in the later stages of this form of shock, leading to irreversibility. Although it is widely held that high cardiac output shock changes to pump failure shock as the shock becomes prolonged, one study has demonstrated a 60% mortality in high cardiac output septic shock, as against 25% in those with a low cardiac output [62]. This study emphasized the role of hypovolaemia in those with a low cardiac output, and once hypovolaemia was corrected, cardiac output improved. Inappropriate vasodilatation results in a greatly expanded vascular tree, and a normal blood volume is not sufficient to fill this extensive vascular space. Careful monitoring of CVP and PCP is essential in the management of this form of shock, as hypovolaemia may occur at any time—at presentation, or later, with the development of a capillary leak. Enough fluid must be given to fill newly opened capillaries and venules, and produce an adequate venous return to the heart. Hardaway emphasizes the strong element of hypovolaemia in low output, high peripheral resistance septic shock which responds well to intravenous fluids [60]. Optimization of preload is again fundamental.

The role of vasoactive drugs

Once preload has been assessed and deemed to be sufficient, attention must turn to pharmacological methods of manipulating organ blood flow in order to maintain cerebral, coronary, and renal blood flow. General supportive measures should not be forgotten, i.e. maintenance of arterial oxygen content, correction of a severe metabolic acidosis, optimization of the haematocrit, correction of electrolyte and blood sugar abnormalities, and attention to clotting abnormalities. This will ensure the best possible circumstances in which pharmacological intervention may act. If systemic hypotension persists despite these measures, in combination with adequate fluid replacement, there are a number of possible approaches.

Inotropes. These drugs are commonly administered in high cardiac output shock, but have no role in rational therapy. All such agents increase myocardial oxygen consumption, and in the setting of an already raised cardiac output, can only jeopardize the myocardium and may hasten the onset of pump failure.

Vasodilators. The rationale for the use of these drugs (alpha blockers: phentolamine, phenoxybenzamine, chlorpromazine; beta stimulants: isoprenaline, salbutamol; dopaminergic: dopamine; direct action on smooth muscle: nitroprusside, hydrallazine) rests on the accepted theoretical consideration that the observed systemic hypotension is partly induced by arteriolar vasoconstriction with the opening up of many low-resistance arteriovenous shunts. It is suggested that vasodilators will improve actual tissue perfusion and correct this form of circulatory abnormality. The essential prerequisite for the use of vasodilators is normovolaemia, with adequate preload, otherwise profound hypotension will ensue. Beta-2 stimulants have undesirable affects on heart rate and rhythm and are therefore contra-indicated. They also lower diastolic blood pressure and impair coronary perfusion. A low-dose dopamine infusion to maintain renal blood flow is a useful therapeutic manoeuvre, especially in combination with other efforts to raise systemic arterial pressure, but by itself is inadequate in the treatment of severe shock. It increases splanchnic blood flow, which may further exaggerate splanchnic blood pooling and hypotension.

Successful use of phenoxybenzamine in septic shock, in the presence of an adequate blood volume, has been reported by Hardaway [61], but the majority of his patients seemed to have low cardiac indices, and so a reduction in afterload was probably appropriate. Chlorpromazine may be used as a weak alpha blocking agent but is unlikely to make much impression on the clinical picture. It is difficult to justify vasodilatation in profoundly hypotensive patients with a high cardiac output and a low peripheral resistance, and although some argue that flow to vital tissues is improved, perfusion of vital organs may be compromised. Production of severe irreversible hypotension is a major hazard, and a more appropriate aim should be the generation of a systemic perfusion pressure of 90 mmHg.

Vasoconstrictors. There is no doubt that arterial pressure can be restored to satisfactory levels using alpha agonists (methoxamine, noradrenaline, high-dose dopamine, metaraminol). Although most authorities insist that the generalized vasoconstriction produced results in further compromise of vital organ perfusion, noradrenaline may produce increases in myocardial blood flow, but its effect on cerebral blood flow is unpredictable, depending upon the state of the blood–brain barrier [5]. Renal vasoconstriction may be prevented by a simultaneous infusion of low-dose dopamine. In the face of profound, persistent hypotension, the judicious administration of noradrenaline is justifiable, but again, it must be emphasized that continuous monitoring of oxygen delivery and extraction is essential in order to assess this hazardous pharmacological intervention. The complications of vasoconstrictor therapy, with the development of ischaemic digits and the sloughing of skin, must be considered, and this management can only be temporary, buying time so that the primary cause of shock is eliminated.

Propranolol. A less aggressive approach to vasoconstriction is the institution of beta-2 blockade, at present using propranolol. The use of propranolol in maldistributive shock depends upon a theory of shock propagated by Berk [8]. The theory states that the release of catecholamines in shock is compensatory in the main part, i.e. the resulting alpha-mediated vasoconstriction and the beta-1-mediated increase in heart rate and contractility produce an increase in cardiac output, and an increase in perfusion pressure of vital organs—the brain, the heart, and the kidneys. However, the high levels of circulating adrenaline also cause beta-2 activation, which may be considered to be a decompensatory effect, resulting in a propagation of the maldistribution of flow.

Berk hypothesizes that the splanchnic bed pooling and the pulmonary shunting so characteristic of this form of shock is a result of beta-2 stimulation in these regions. His conclusion is that a major therapeutic aim in the management of the problem is beta-2 blockade. This can be achieved with small doses of propranolol, 2–4 mg IV bolus, which at this dosage preferentially blocks the beta-2 receptor.

Other investigators [125] have demonstrated

the importance of the beta-2 receptor in the control of hepatic blood flow. Berk himself [9] has shown that an infusion of adrenaline in healthy mongrel dogs caused in increased pulmonary shunt, with an increase in the pulmonary vascular resistance. These changes could be prevented by pretreatment with propranolol, and in addition could be reversed with the beta blocker after the adrenaline infusion had been started. Further studies in critically ill patients [10] confirmed the results of these animal experiments, and an increase in mean arterial pressure with a fall in pulmonary shunt occurred in shocked patients treated with propranolol.

There is an additional reason for using beta blockade in the treatment of shock, in so far as animal experiments suggest that beta blockade may protect the kidneys against the development of acute tubular necrosis. Renin release may well be a beta-2 mediated effect and this hormone is thought to play a part in the development of acute tubular necrosis.

The problem of using a non-specific beta blocker in this situation is only too obvious; not only does it disguise an important clinical sign of bleeding (i.e. rise in pulse rate) but a fall in cardiac output may also occur secondary to the reduction in heart rate, or as a result of the direct negative inotropic effect of the drug. Haemodynamic monitoring is obligatory, but the beneficial effect of the drug can only be judged by direct measurement of the pulmonary shunt and oxygen consumption.

Oxygen transport studies in patients with acute liver failure and maldistributive shock suggest that although oxygen delivery may fall following the administration of propranolol, primarily through a reduction in cardiac output, oxygen consumption is significantly increased. Mean arterial blood pressure also increases in this clinical situation. These data suggest that propranolol acts either to reduce the peripheral arteriovenous shunting or, by splanchnic bed constriction, to increase the effective circulating blood volume. Beta blockade has another side effect detrimental to the therapy of shock, that is the potentiation of hypoglycaemia.

A trial of beta-2 blockade is therefore justified in patients with acute circulatory failure who have been shown to have a high cardiac output with a low peripheral resistance and a large pulmonary shunt. Small doses of propranolol should be administered with great care in order to avoid the beta-1 blockade, which will result in cardiac depression. Oxygen transport and extraction studies should be performed to monitor the effect of treatment, and the pulmonary shunt must be measured. If there is no improvement in these parameters, or if the mean arterial pressure remains low, alpha vasoconstrictors should be used to maintain perfusion of vital organs.

In conclusion, the management of the patient with profound hypotension and a normal or raised cardiac output is extremely difficult (Fig. 12.7). If severe vasoconstriction is present,

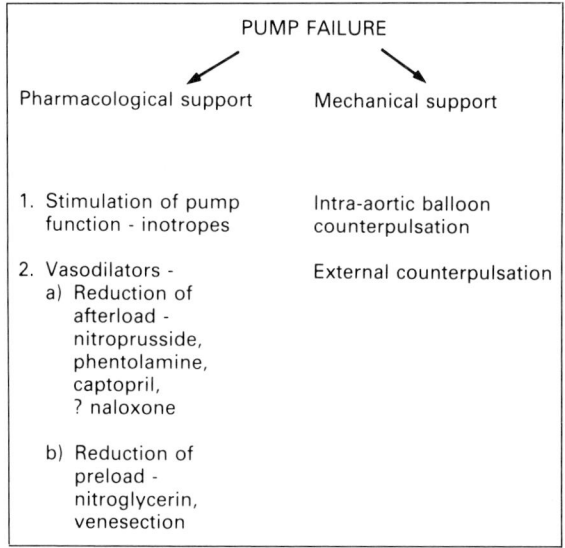

Fig. 12.7. Possible means of treating pump failure.

and an adequate arterial pressure maintained, vasodilatation in association with fluid replacement is the treatment of choice. Frequently, however, arterial pressure is too low to contemplate a further reduction in peripheral resistance, and vasoconstriction is indicated. Beta-2 blockade will increase peripheral resistance and is usually associated with an increase in mean arterial pressure, a reduction in pulmonary shunting, and an increase in oxygen consumption. Finally, and perhaps desperately, alpha agonists can be used and, when administered with due care, produce good results.

The diagnosis and management of sepsis

Sepsis continues to be a major cause of death in critically ill patients despite the use of specific antibiotics, aggressive surgical intervention, and intravenous/enteral hyperalimentation. The incidence of septic shock has increased almost 20-fold over the last 25 years [92]. A few years ago, there were approximately 71 000 documented cases of gram-negative sepsis in the United States, to which 18 000 deaths were directly attributable [176]. The increased use of immunosuppressive agents and corticosteroids enhance susceptibility to infection, and patients with an increased risk of infection—severely injured patients, the transplant recipient, diabetics, patients with cancer, the elderly patient—are living longer. The use of devices such as indwelling intravenous catheters (especially those used for parenteral nutrition) and bladder catheters increases the risk of sepsis developing in the critically ill. Frequent instrumentation, the widespread practice of extensive abdominal and pelvic surgery with the universal use of broad-spectrum antibiotics, have all contributed to the increasing incidence of septic shock.

Any micro-organism capable of infecting the human host ultimately may produce an overwhelming septicaemia that evolves into septic shock. Fungal organisms, viruses, rickettsiae, gram-positive aerobic bacteria, and gram-negative anaerobic bacteria have all been incriminated in causing this form of circulatory collapse, but the organisms of major importance are the gram-negative aerobic rods, which produce endotoxin. In several large series, the most commonly isolated pathogen was *E. coli*, followed by *Klebsiella pneumoniae*, *Proteus sp.*, and *Pseudomonas aureginosa* [4]. *Staphylococcus aureus* and *Streptococcus pneumoniae* are the most frequent gram-positive causes of septic shock. Anaerobes, particularly *Bacteroides*, are responsible for about 10% of cases following abdominal surgery. One discrete entity that has recently emerged is that known as the 'toxic shock' syndrome [163]. It has been described in young menstruating women in association with tampon use, but the disease may also occur in men and young children. It is strongly associated with a focal staphylococcal infection, and is probably caused by some staphylococcal extracellular product or products [136]. The vast majority of such patients (presenting with such innocuous signs as conjunctivitis, pharyngitis and strawberry tongue) do not have a bacteraemia, but develop widespread organ damage.

The role of endotoxin, a lipoprotein–carbohydrate complex found in the cell wall of all gram-negative organisms, in the pathogenesis of septic shock remains a highly controversial subject. Endotoxin can damage capillary and post-capillary venular endothelium, and the lipid-A of endotoxin is recognized as one cause of vasospasm and intravascular coagulation. Animal models using injections of endotoxin do not produce the clinical picture of septic shock seen in man, and recent clinical studies have failed to demonstrate significant blood elevations of endotoxin in the majority of patients who have documented gram-negative sepsis [153]. Even when endotoxin is identified, its level is quite low, far below the levels necessary to produce endotoxic shock in animals [121]. Some authorities have emphasized that sepsis and endotoxin shock are separate entities [169], so that extreme caution must be exercised in using the experimental findings with endotoxin models as the basis for pharmacological therapy in septic patients.

Although the clinical picture of septic shock depends in part upon the nature of the causative organism, it frequently entails chills and rigors, in association with a pyrexia, which rapidly evolves over a few hours into the full-blown hypotensive syndrome of septic shock. Hyperpyrexia may occur and cerebral function is commonly impaired. Vasodilatation with a warm and dry skin may be prominent during the initial phase but later, as shock progresses and becomes refractory, vasoconstriction occurs, and there is a decline in cardiac output. Oliguria is also noted at this stage, but polyuria may occur in association with the vasodilatation, and go on to high urine output renal failure. Hyper- and hypocoagulability occur with these clinical manifestations. The disorders of glucose metabolism have already been described.

The microbial investigation of such patients depends upon immediate culture of blood, urine, sputum, cerebrospinal fluid (in those with signs of meningism), and where present, wound exudates. Blood cultures remain the most important investigation, and blood-culture-negative septic shock has a worse prognosis than that in which the pathogen is identified, and its sensitivity to antimicrobial agents documented [152]. Anaerobic and aerobic media should be used, and a gram stain of a turbid broth often gives valuable information about the likely microbial diagnosis. As most bacteria can be isolated from the blood culture broth after only 1 day's incubation, a routine 24 h sub-culture is recommended. Gas liquid chromatography may help the more rapid detection of anaerobes in blood cultures [137]. Clinical findings often indicate the source of infection, and stress must be placed upon a thorough examination of all systems, including a pelvic examination. The detection of circula-tion antigens can be attempted by counter-current immunoelectrophoresis, but this is applicable to only a few bacterial species, e.g. *S. pneumoniae* and *Klebsiella aerogenes* [144]. The Limulus assay for the detection of endotox-aemia has been used in the diagnosis of septic shock, but has given variable results [153] and is not recommended. Rapid assays for C5a and endorphins may have a role in the future of the early diagnosis of septic shock, but at the moment remain a research tool.

Certain radiographic studies are indicated in the evaluation of the patient with septic shock. A conventional chest x-ray will provide evidence of a primary pulmonary infection; it may demonstrate the presence of septic pulmonary emboli, and give some indication concerning the development of ARDS. Plain x-ray films of the abdomen may reveal evidence of mechanical bowel obstruction, intestinal perforation, or a soft tissue density with gas, suggesting a localized abscess. An ultrasonic examination of the abdomen may reveal intra-abdominal or pelvic cystic collections, or demonstrate obstruction of the biliary tree, or a pyonephrosis. Although gallium-67 citrate and indium^{111}-labelled white cells may localize inflammatory foci, they do not differentiate sterile from septic collections, or provide anatomical information enabling safe percutaneous needle aspiration. In this respect, ultrasonography and CT scanning are superior [53].

The primary therapy of septic shock—administration of antimicrobial drugs

In the absence of specific antimicrobial therapy, mortality is almost inevitable within 48 h, and survival may be enhanced as much as three-fold using appropriate and vigorous antimicrobial agents [141]. Therapy is by necessity situational and empirical; that is, at the time of prescription, the organism is unknown, and information on its sensitivity to antimicrobials is unavailable. Surgical intervention for the drainage of localized septic foci must be considered a first priority, and occasionally, septic shock responds only to the drainage of pus. Resuscitation, in order to make the patient fit for general anaesthesia and the surgical procedure, requires control of the haemodynamic and clotting abnormalities, but courageous surgical intervention in overwhelming sepsis may still be required.

The choice of antimicrobial agents depends upon a number of considerations. Of great importance is the setting of the infection, i.e. was the infection acquired in hospital, or in the community, and has the patient been on antibiotics? The second question relates to the anatomical site of infection, if one can be detected. Infections that develop below the xiphoid are caused by gram-negative organisms, either alone or in concert with anaerobic organisms. Anaerobic infection is common in two situations: spillage of bowel contents into the peritoneal cavity, and female pelvic infections. In these instances, and in the case of septic shock associated with pulmonary aspiration, broadening antimicrobial coverage to include anaerobes is justifiable [74].

Community-acquired infections occuring above the xiphoid are usually caused by gram-positive organisms, and are sensitive to penicillin. The child with meningitis deserves special consideration as *Haemophilus influenzae* must be covered using Chloramphenicol. Pneumonia in the alcoholic or in the elderly debilitated patient may be caused by gram-negative organisms, and so requires broader spectrum cover. A gram stain examination of sputum is useful in detecting gram-negative rods. A third consideration is the increasing recognition of pneumonia caused by *Legionella pneumophilia*. If this organism is suspected (the clinical suggestions include an epidemic in the geographical region; pneumonia in the middle-aged; recent history of travel, especially to a 'convention or Spain'; diarrhoea; encephalopathy; relative bradycardia in association with a pyrexia; leucocytosis; hyponatraemia; hypertransaminasaemia; and renal failure), high dose erythromycin or rifampicin is indicated [27].

If the history includes recent hospitalization, or prolonged antibiotic administration, as is most commonly seen in cases of septic shock, gram-negative organisms are involved in almost all nosocomial infections, regardless of site. The only gram-positive organism regularly causing infection in hospitalized patients is the penicillin-resistant *Staphylococcus*. Infection due to *Staphylococcus* may be controlled by an aminoglycoside, but in the case of septic shock, specific anti-staphylococcal therapy with two anti-microbial agents is indicated, using high doses of cloxacillin/flucloxacillin, or vancomycin with fucidin. *Pseudomonas* is an important pathogen in the critically ill and must also be covered. Carbenicillin, or one of the new semi-synthetic penicillins (ticarcillin, azlocillin), which contain less sodium, should be used.

The above considerations apply to the immunologically compromised host, but such patients demonstrate exceptional susceptibility to certain organisms, related to their specific immunological defect. Those patients with defective humoral immunity or recently splenectomized are unusually susceptible to encapsulated organisms, such as *S. pneumoniae*, and *H. influenzae*. Patients with defective immunity, including the transplant population, are unusually susceptible to Cytomegalovirus, and *Pneumocystis carinii*, and so may require cotrimoxazole.

The previous discussion renders impossible a recommendation concerning the exact antimicrobials to use in septic shock, and many ICUs have their own antimicrobial policy. Suffice it to say that gentamicin remains the mainstay of treatment of gram-negative septicaemia. Its complications are well known, and blood levels are readily available. In combination with ampicillin and metronidazole, if anaerobic infection is suspected, most organisms are covered. Staphylococcal infection would require the introduction of a beta-lactamase stable penicillin and fucidin. The third generation cephalosporins are in ascendence, since they have not been reported to cause renal impairment. Cefuroxime (covering *Staphylococcus*, gram negatives but not *Pseudomonas* or the anaerobes) and cefoxitin are alternatives, but remain extremely expensive.

The haemodynamic management of septic shock is discussed in the sections: *High cardiac output maldistributive shock* and *Pump failure*.

Secondary therapy in septic shock

Many other measures such as the administration of glucose–potassium–insulin cocktails [173], the use of anti-histamines to antagonize histamine-mediated vasodilatation [89], and the administration of inhibitors of prostaglandin synthesis [48] have been explored in the experimental and clinical situation, but their clinical efficacy has not been established. General supportive measures, with the prevention of multi-organ failure, remain central to management.

The role of steroids in the management of shock

The role of steroids in the therapy of shock has been a widely promulgated, but still controversial topic for years. Blalock [12] in 1940 recognized the need for 'adrenal extract' in the circulatory collapse associated with Addison's disease, but was sceptical concerning its use in other situations of shock. Proponents of the use of steroids have noted an increase in cardiac output [165], peripheral vasodilatation, restoration of phagocytic function of the reticuloendothelial system [2], stabilization of lysosomal enzyme levels [158], with a reduction in formation of platelet aggregates, protection of the lung, and prevention of ARDS [146], and favourable effects on the oxygen affinity of haemoglobin, with enhanced oxygen delivery to the tissues [20]. The problem has been assessed most frequently in the treatment of septic shock. There have been reports of increased clearance of endotoxaemia [124], an event known to occur in septic shock, the relevance of which is open to doubt but may have a role in the development of final irreversible shock. However, it is important to note that the Food and Drug Administration recently reviewed the indications for the use of steroids in septic shock, focusing on the package insert for Solu-Medrone (methyl prednisolone succinate, Upjohn). The decision was made to remove septic shock from the insert as an indication for the use of high-dose methyl prednisolone.

There have been few clinical trials of satisfactory design established to investigate the actions of steroids, and the major report of a favourable effect in septic shock remains Schumer's trial published in 1976 [134]. He carried out a prospective and retrospective study of 500 patients, diagnosed as having septic shock, in order to determine mortality rate and complication rate in steroid-treated and control groups. The prospective study was randomized and double blind. There was no significant difference between the study groups compared for age, severity of shock, presence of underlying disease, and the use of other therapeutic regimens. Overall mortality was significantly reduced in the steroid treated groups: 10.4% vs 38.4% in saline-treated controls in the prospective study; 14% vs 42.5% of untreated controls in the retrospective study; and the prevalence of complications associated with steroid administration was 6%. The major problem of this study is the definition of death

due to sepsis. Many patients survive the initial hypotensive episode associated with septic shock, but go on to die later of multiple organ failure. Although Schumer states that the longest period between an original onset of shock and a death attributable to the shock was 4 weeks, there is no further information concerning the time course or the ultimate cause of death.

There have been other clinical studies showing a favourable effect of massive doses of corticosteroids on morbidity in septic shock, but many have not [174]. Therefore, despite the substantial amount of data accumulated in the animal laboratory suggesting that early therapy with corticosteroids will prevent the manifestations of septic shock, clear-cut benefits have been difficult to demonstrate in human beings. In an excellent review of the problem, Sheagreen suggests that because in all previous clinical trials, the full-blown syndrome of septic shock had to be present before steroids were given, they were given too late to effect the course of the syndrome [138].

The mechanism by which corticosteroids could influence the development of the septic shock syndrome probably resides in their ability to inhibit complement-mediated activation of the polymorphonucleocytes. Corticosteroids can inhibit granulocyte production of superoxide [56], and the approximate plasma level of methylprednisolone (1 mg/ml) after the infusion of 30 mg/kg almost completely prevents granulocyte aggregation in vitro in response to activated C5a [70]. In all the in vitro models of complement-granulocyte interaction, corticosteroids prevent aggregate formation more effectively when they are introduced before, rather than after, complement activation [112]. Higher concentrations of corticosteroid are required to disaggregate polymorphonuclear leucocytes (PMNs) than to prevent their aggregation in the first place. Complement activation (primarily by endotoxin in gram-negative bacteraemia, and by techoic acid in gram-positive bacteraemia) is a central feature of septic shock, and is the prime cause of the development of the capillary leak. Sibbald [142] has recently reported that most patients with sepsis have a prompt decrease in pulmonary capillary leakage after a massive dose of corticosteroid. The patients who did not respond were found, in retrospect, to have had leakier capillaries than the responders. This observation, with the in vitro studies, suggests that the earlier the dose of corticosteroid is administered, the more effective it will be in stopping the capillary leak. Clinically, if adequate predictors of deterioration could be found, the use of steroids might prove more rewarding in a prophylactic setting, rather than in their present therapeutic role, administered after the damage has been done. A further action of corticosteroids in shock may be the inhibition of beta lipotrophin secretion from the pituitary, since this stress hormone originates from the same molecule of ACTH. Since massive doses of corticosteroid inhibit the secretion of ACTH, the release of beta lipotrophin—the precursor of beta endorphin—is probably also suppressed by the early administration of steroids. The role of beta endorphin in shock has been discussed.

A major consideration concerning the administration of steroids in shock, is the safety of their action. The mechanism by which corticosteroids probably work in the intravascular space to inhibit complement activation of PMNs could lead to an increased likelihood of more extensive infection outside the vascular system because of impaired migration and function of the PMNs. The other unwanted effects of steroids are well known, and gastrointestinal bleeding and glucose intolerance are common problems in the critically ill even in the absence of steroids. Clearly, the controversy has not been resolved, despite dogmatic statements on both sides, and a large prospective double blind trial of the use of steroids in early bacteraemia is required.

The management of the capillary leak syndrome

A major problem that develops in many cases of shock, where the patient survives the initial haemodynamic insult, is the development of generalized oedema. Septic shock is the major cause of this fluid distribution problem, and usually the disorder becomes apparent through the development of acute respiratory failure. There is no single causal factor and oedema formation relates more to a number of variables—a decline in COP, shrinking of the vascular tree following resuscitation, the use of excessive volumes of fluid in resuscitation, afferent arteriole dilatation with venular constriction, and increases in capillary permeability.

Alveolar capillary damage is a consistent finding in ARDS, and it seems that following shock two forms of respiratory failure may develop. The first form, 'wet lungs', has a good prognosis and responds to diuretics, dialysis, or fluid restriction. It is associated with a normal pulmonary capillary pressure, but pulmonary hypertension and right ventricular dysfunction do not develop. A Swan–Ganz pulmonary angiogram will demonstrate patent arterioles and emphasizes the interstitial nature of the disorder (Fig. 12.8). The second form of respiratory failure following shock is more severe, and is associated with a poor prognosis. Pulmonary hypertension and right ventricular dysfunction are features of this condition, and a Swan–Ganz pulmonary angiogram will demonstrate pruning and beading of the arterioles, suggesting the formation of fibrin microemboli (Fig. 12.9). Respiratory failure is rapid and commonly irreversible, despite active intervention with heparin, streptokinase infusions, and extracorporeal membrane oxygenation.

Once resuscitation has been achieved and the haemodynamic state of the patient stabilized, fluid therapy must be given with care to avoid generating oedema formation, and post-resuscitative hypertension. The prophylactic role of steroids has been mentioned, and the problems of colloidal resuscitation have been discussed. In this aftermath of shock, large-molecular-weight compounds administered intravenously have been shown to appear rapidly in the intra-alveolar fluid [128], and there is no reason to believe that there is not leakage from other capillaries taking place. Resolution of oedema in such patients may be slowed by the administration of colloid. Therefore the use of albumin and other colloids should generally be avoided, other than in hypo-albuminaemia, or where capillary permeability remains unimpaired.

Water retention in patients ventilated mechanically, especially where PEEP is also used, is a recognized problem [117]. Attention to fluid balance is essential, and one aims to maintain fluid balance in a negative state, in order to avoid the accumulation of peripheral oedema. The minimum PCP for an adequate cardiac output and systemic blood pressure is the ideal for such patients with 'leaky' capillaries, and the judicious use of diuretics is advised. Management on a weigh bed is advantageous, as oedema accumulation is rapidly detected. There is no point in 'chasing' a CVP/PCP in this situation as all fluid, crystalloid or colloid, rapidly leaves the circulation to form oedema in the interstitial space.

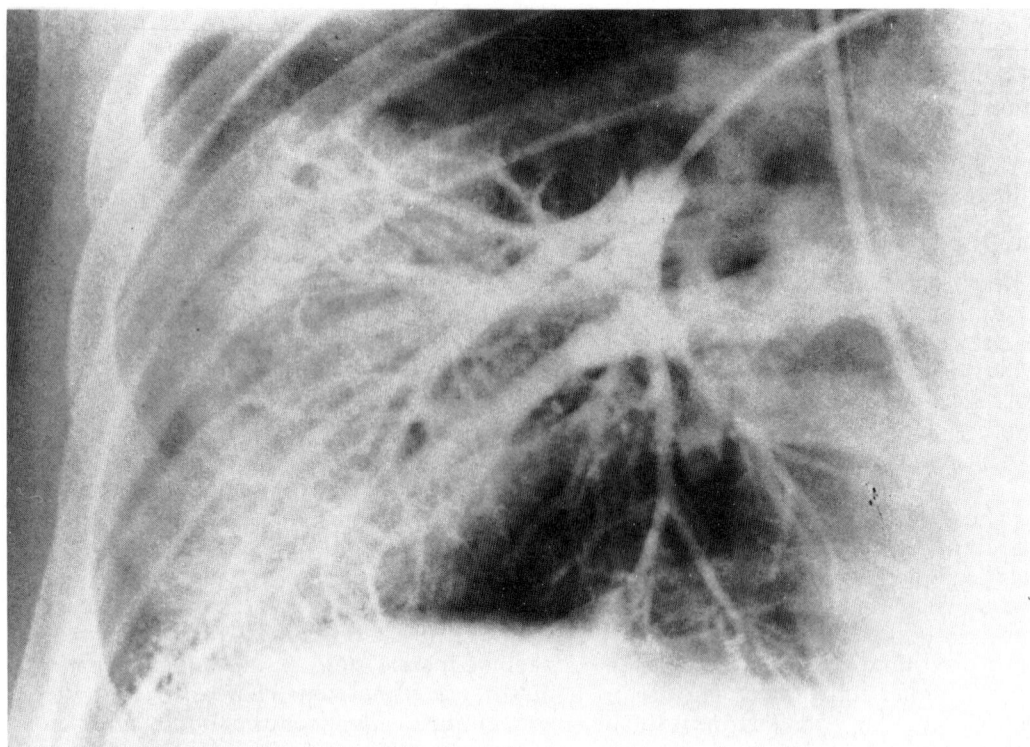

Fig. 12.8. Pulmonary angiogram showing patent pulmonary arterioles.

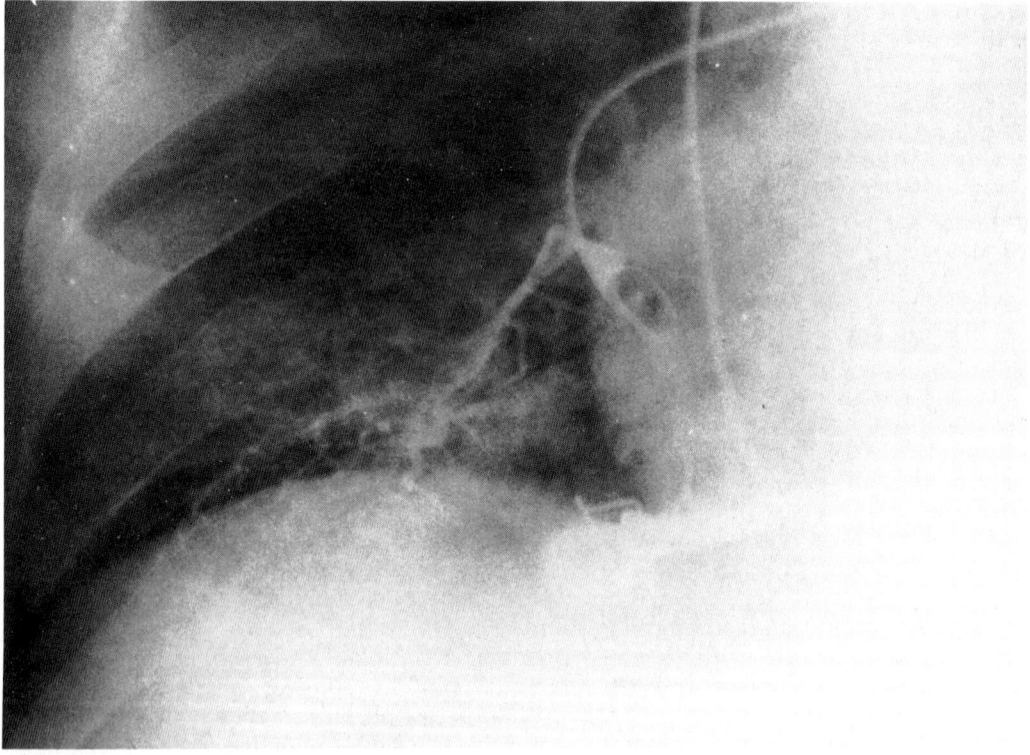

Fig. 12.9. Pulmonary angiogram in a patient with the adult respiratory distress syndrome in pulmonary hypertension. Pruning of the arteriolar tree is seen.

Arachidonic acid metabolites

There has been much interest in the use of prostaglandin compounds and prostacyclin in the therapy of shock. Prostaglandin E_1 in a standard haemorrhagic shock model in beagles has been shown to increase the cardiac output and decrease peripheral resistance [93]. Animals treated with prostaglandin E_1 showed significantly longer survival times compared to controls.

Prostacyclin infusions in animals have been found to be beneficial in diminishing the systemic injury produced by trauma [84], and in man following cardiopulmonary bypass. Other animal studies have demonstrated a reduction in mortality from experimentally induced haemorrhagic shock. Observations using the chronic lung lymph fistula preparation in adult sheep suggest that there is an increase in lymph prostacyclin and PGF_{2a} in response to injected *E. coli* endotoxin, early on in the course of septic shock [37]. These workers propose that the cause of pulmonary hypertension in this form of lung injury is the vasoconstrictor PGF_{2a}, and prostacyclin is released as a protective response. Prostacyclin infusions in this situation reduce the pulmonary hypertension and the lung lymph flow response. There appears to be a direct membrane stabilizing effect apart from the effect on the filtration pressure. Interestingly, none of the four sheep infused first with endotoxin plus prostacyclin died of systemic shock, whereas there were three fatalities in the untreated group from severe hypotension. The relevance of these observations to the syndrome of septic shock in man is unknown, but they open up a new approach to the treatment of ARDS.

In summary, an approach to the management of shock has been outlined which focuses on cellular metabolic derangement, and its correction as an ultimate goal.

The diagnosis of shock is not simply a haemodynamic set of measurements, but requires careful assessment of the oxygen metabolism of the patient. The difficulties of making a diagnosis of 'hypoxia' have been emphasized, and the importance of eliminating an 'oxygen debt' with concomitant anaerobic respiration and lactic acidosis forms a central theme in therapy.

The dynamic process of the shock syndrome, with the ever-present possibility of hypovolaemia, makes classic categories of description simplistic, and obscures the fundamental principles of treatment. Tissue oxygen and other vital substrate delivery must be maintained in terms of improving cardiovascular performance. The underlying cause of shock must be treated. Myocardial oxygen consumption, especially in the setting of an ischaemic pump, requires careful consideration determining further therapeutic intervention.

Optimization of preload, improving myocardial contractility, with the reduction of afterload where appropriate, constitute the basis of the approach to the problem of a low cardiac output. Redistribution of blood flow is essential where cardiac output is apparently adequate but arteriovenous shunting exists, exaggerating tissue hypoxia. At present, oxygen consumption is the important measure of successful intervention in both situations, but in the future, one hopes that more direct measures of cerebral, cardiac and renal function will be available to govern the use of vasoactive drugs.

The prevention of multisystem failure is another fundamental aim in the management of shock, but when organ failure supervenes, prognosis deteriorates. In particular, capillary leak is a difficult problem to overcome, and requires careful fluid management to prevent massive oedema formation.

Shock is a common problem and is often fatal. Improved survival depends upon adherence to a number of physiological principles, with the application of appropriate haemodynamic and metabolic monitoring. Critical interpretation of measured and derived data is essential in the assessment of the shocked patient, and governs the various therapeutic interventions, However, despite the many advances in the understanding of the pathogenesis, and the management of shock, this clinical syndrome remains difficult to treat, and sometimes impossible to reverse.

Most forms of shock are potentially reversible and demand early, aggressive treatment (with optimistic enthusiasm).

References

1. Agostoni A, Lotto A, Stabilini R et al. (1975) Haemoglobin oxygen affinity in patients with low output heart failure and cardiogenic shock following acute myocardial infarction. Eur J Cardiol 3:53–58
2. Altura BM, Altura BT, (1974) Peripheral vascular actions of glucocorticoids and their relationship to protection in circulatory shock. J Pharmacol Exp Ther 190:300–315

3. Amsterdam EA, Banas J, Criley JM et al. (1980) Clinical assessment of external pressure circulatory assistance in acute myocardial infarction, a report of a cooperative clinical trial. Am J Cardiol 45:349–356

4. Barnett JA, Sandford JP (1969) Bacterial shock. JAMA 209:1514–1517

5. Berger RL, Saini VK, Long W, Hechtman H, Hood W (1973) The use of diastolic augmentation with the intraaortic balloon in human septic shock with associated coronary artery disease. Surgery 74:601–606

6. Bergman G, Daly K, Atkinson L et al. (1981) Prostacyclin: haemodynamic and metabolic effects in patients with coronary artery disease. Lancet 1:569–572

7. Berk JL (1975a) Monitoring the patient in shock. Surg Clin NA 55:713–720

8. Berk JL (1975b) Use of vasoactive drugs in the treatment of shock. Surg Clin North Am 55:721–728

9. Berk JL, Hagen JF, Koo R (1968) Pulmonary insufficiency caused by adrenaline. Ann Surg 178:423–435

10. Berk JL, Hagen JF, Mary G, Koo R (1972) The treatment of shock with B adrenergic blockade. Arch Surg 104:46–51

11. Bihari DJ (1982) Right ventricular infarction, a diagnosis not to miss. Br J Hosp Med 27:287–289

12. Blalock A IN: Principles of surgical care, Shock and other problems. Kimpton (London) p 165

13. Borer JS, Redwood DR, Levitt B (1975) Reduction in myocardial ischaemia with nitroglycerin or nitroglycerin plus phenylephrine administered during acute myocardial infarction. N Engl J Med 293:1008–1012

14. Braunwald E (1977) Vasodilator therapy, a physiological approach to the treatment of heart failure. N Engl J Med 297:331–333

15. Bregman D, Casarella WJ (1980) Percutaneous intraaortic balloon pumping, initial clinical experience. Ann Thorac Surg 29:153–155

16. Bregman D, Nichols AB, Weiss MB et al. (1980) Percutaneous intraaortic balloon insertion. Am J Cardiol 46:261–264

17. Bresnaham GF, Roberts R, Shell WE, Ross J, Sobel BE (1974) Deleterious effects due to haemorrhage after myocardial reperfusion. Am J Cardiol 33:82–86

18. Broder MI (1975) External counterpulsation in low cardiac output states. Surg Clin North Am 55:561–572

19. Brown JJ, Davies DL, Johnson VW, Lever AF, Robertson JIS (1970) Renin relationships in congestive cardiac failure, treated and untreated. Am Heart J 80:329–342

20. Bryan-Brown CW (1975) Tissue blood flow and oxygen transport in critically ill patients. Crit Care Med 3:103–108

21. Buckley MJ, Mundth ED, Dagget WM et al. (1971) Surgical therapy for early complications of myocardial infarction. Surgery 70:814–820

22. Calvin JE, Driedger AA, Sibbald WJ (1981) Does the capillary wedge pressure predict left ventricular preload in critically ill patients? Crit Care Med 9:437–443

23. Carrico CJ, Canizarro PC, Shires GT (1976) Fluid resuscitation following injury, rationale for the use of balanced salt solutions. Crit Care Med 4:46–54

24. Claus RH, Birtwell WC, Albertal G et al. (1961) Assisted circulation, the arterial counterpulsator. J Thorac Cardiovasc Surg 41:447–465

25. Cohn LH (1975) Intraaortic balloon counterpulsation in low cardiac output states. Surg Clin North Am 55:545–559

26. Cohn JN, Franciosa JA Vasodilator therapy of heart failure. N Engl J Med 297:27–31, 254–258

27. Cordes LG, Fraser DW (1980) Legionellosis, Legionaire's disease, and Pontiac fever. Med Clin North Am 64:395–416

28. Covell JW, Braunwald E, Ross J (1966) Studies on digitalis. XVI. Effects on myocardial oxygen consumption. J Clin Invest 45:1535–1542

29. Cox JL, McLaughlin VW, Flowers NC, Horan LG (1968) The ischaemic zone surrounding acute myocardial infarction. Its morphology as detected by dehydrogenase staining. Am Heart J 76:650–659

30. Curtis MT, Lefer AM (1980) Protective actions of naloxone in haemorrhagic shock. Am J Physiol 239:H416–H421

31. Daniel AM, Pierce CH, MacLean LD (1976) Lactate metabolism in the dog during shock from haemorrhage, cardiac tamponade, and endotoxin. Surg Gynaecol Obstet 143:581–586

32. Dauwe F, Affaki G, Waters DD, Theroux P, Mizgala HF (1979) Intravenous nitroglycerin in refractory unstable angina (abstract). Am J Cardiol 43:416

33. Dawidson I, Gelin L, Hedman L, Soderburg R (1981) Haemodilution and recovery from experimental intestinal shock in rats. Crit Care Med 9:42–46

34. De Felippe J, Timouer J, Velasco IT, Lopes OH, Rocha-e-Silva M (1980) Treatment of refractory hypovolaemic shock by 7.5% sodium chloride injections. Lancet II 1002–1004

35. Demling RH, Mareher M, Will JA (1980a) Response of the pulmonary microcirculation to fluid loading after haemorrhagic shock and resuscitation. Surgery 87:552–559

36. Demling RH, Duy N, Manohar M, Proctor R (1980b) Comparison between lung fluid filtration rate and measured Starling forces after haemorrhagic and endotoxic shock. J Trauma 2:856–860

37. Demling RH, Smith M, Gunther R, Gee M, Flynn J (1981) The effect of prostacyclin infusion on endotoxin-induced lung injury. Surgery 89:257–263

38. Diamond G, Forrester JS (1972) Effects of coronary artery disease and acute myocardial infarction on the left ventricular compliance in man. Circulation 45:11–19

39. Dilley RB, Ross J, Bernstein EF (1972) Serial haemodynamics during intraaortic balloon counterpulsation for cardiogenic shock (Abstract). Circulation 45 [Suppl. II]:76

40. Dirksen R, Otten MH, Wood GJ et al. (1980) Naloxone in shock (letter). Lancet II 1360–1361

41. Duff P (1980) Pathophysiology and management of septic shock J Reprod Med 24:109–117

42. Dzam VJ, Colucci WS, Williams GH et al. (1980) Sustained effectiveness of converting enzyme inhibition in patients with severe congestive heart failure. N Engl J Med 302:1373–1379

43. Eirich FR (1967) The adsorption of solvated macromolecules and its relation to the viscosity and stability of dispersion. In: Copely AL (ed) Haemorheology. Oxford, Pergamon, p 67

44. Epstein SE, Kent KM, Goldstein RE, Borer JS, Redwood DR (1975) Reduction of ischaemic injury by nitroglycerin during acute myocardial infarction. N Engl J Med 292:29–35

45. Faden AJ, Holaday JW (1979) Opiate antagonists—a role in the treatment of hypovolaemic shock. Science 205:317–318

46. Flaherty JT, Reid PR, Kelly DT et al. (1975) Intravenous nitroglycerin in acute myocardial infarction. Circulation 51:132–139

47. Flaherty JT, Corne PC, Baird MG (1976) Effects of intravenous nitroglycerin on left ventricular function and ST segments in acute myocardial infarction. Br Heart J 38:612–621

48. Fletcher JR, Herman CM, Ranwell PW (1976) Im-

proved survival in endotoxaemia with aspirin and indomethacin in pretreatment. Surg Forum 27:11–12

49. Forrester JS, Diamond G, McHugh TG, Swan HJC (1971) Filling pressures in the right and left side of the heart in acute myocardial infarction. A reappraisal of CVP monitoring. N Engl J Med 285:190–193

50. Forrester JS, Diamond G, Chatterjee K, Swan HJC (1976) Medical therapy of acute myocardial infarction by application of haemodynamic subsets. N Engl J Med 295:1356–1362, 1404–1413

51. Forssell G, Nordlander R, Nyquist O, Schenck-Gustavsson K (1979) Intraaortic balloon pumping in the treatment of cardiogenic shock complicating acute myocardial infarction. Acta Med Scand 206:189–192

51a. Frommer PL (1981) Ventricular assist pumping. N Engl J Med 305:1645–1646

52. Ganz W, Buchbinder N, Marcus H (1981) Intracoronary thrombolysis in evolving myocardial infarction. Am Heart J 101:4–13

53. Gerzof SE, Robbins AH, Johnson WC, Birkett DH, Nasbeth DC (1981) Percutaneous catheter drainage of abdominal abscess, a five year experience. N Engl J Med 305:653–657

54. Gillespie TA, Dieter-Ambos H, Sobel BE, Roberts R (1977) Effects of dobutamine in patients with acute myocardial infarction. Am J Cardiol 39:588–594

55. Golberg LI, Hsieh Y-y, Resnekov L (1977) Newer catecholamines for the treatment of heart failure and shock: an update on dopamine and a first look at dobutamine. Prog Cardiovasc Dis 19:327–340

56. Goldstein IM, Roos D, Weissman G, Kaplan HB (1976) Influence of corticosteroids on human polymorpholeucocyte function in vitro, reduction of lysosomal enzyme release and superoxide production. Inflammation 1:305–315

57. Gunstein J, Goldman BS, Scully HE, Huckell VF, Adelman AG (1976) Evolving indications for preoperative intraaortic balloon pump assistance. Ann Thor Surg 22:535–543

58. Gurll NJ, Vargish T, Reynolds DG, Lechner RB (1980) Opiate receptors and endorphins in the pathophysiology of haemorrhagic shock. Surgery 89:364–369

59. Haddy FJ (1970) Pathophysiology and therapy of shock of myocardial infarction. Ann Intern Med 73:809–827

60. Hardaway RM (1980a) Endotoxaemic shock. Dis Colon Rectum 23:597–604

61. Hardaway RM (1980b) Treatment of severe shock with with phenoxybenzamine. Surg Gynaecol Obstet 151:725–734

62. Hardaway RM, James PM, Anderson RW, Bredenburg CE, West RL (1967) Intensive study and treatment of shock in man. JAMA 199:779–790

63. Harper AM (1966) Autoregulation of cerebral blood flow; influence of arterial blood pressure on the blood flow through the cerebral cortex. J Neurol Neurosurg Psychiatry 29:398–403

64. Hauser CJ, Shoemaker WC, Turpin I, Goldberg SJ (1980) Oxygen transport responses to colloids and crystalloids in critically ill surgical patients. Surg Gynaecol Obstet 150:811–816

65. Herbert P, Tinker J (1980) Inotropic drugs in acute circulatory failure. Intensive Care Med 6:101–111

66. Hill NS, Antman EM, Green LH, Alpert JS (1981) Intravenous nitroglycerin, a review of the pharmacology, therapeutic effects and complications. Chest 79:69–76

67. Hollenburg NK, Swart SL, Passan DR, Williams GH (1979) Increased glomerular filtration rate after converting enzyme inhibition in essential hypertension. N Engl J Med 301:9–12

68. Iqbal M, Liebson PR (1981) Counterpulsation and dobutamine, their use in the treatment of cardiogenic shock due to right ventricular infarction. Arch Intern Med 141:247–249

69. Isner JM, Cohen SR, Virmani R, Lawrinson W, Roberts WC (1980) Complications of the intraaortic ballon counterpulsation device; clinical and morphological observations in 45 necropsy patients. Am J Cardiol 45:260–268

70. Jacob HS, Craddock PR, Hammerschmidt D, Moldow CF (1980) Complement induced granulocyte aggregation, an unsuspected mechanism of disease. N Engl J Med 302:700–704

71. James OF (1976) The occurrence and significance of microaggregates in stored blood. Intensive Care Med 2:163–166

72. Jan KM, Heldman J, Chien S (1981) Coronary haemodynamics and oxygen utilisation after haematocrit variations in haemorrhage. Am J Physiol 40:H326–H332

73. Jett GK, Dengle SK, Barnett PA et al. (1981) Intraaortic balloon counterpulsation, its influence alone and in combination with various pharmacological agents on regional myocardial blood flow during experimental acute coronary occlusion. Ann Thorac Surg 31:144–154

74. Johanson WG, Harris GD (1980) Aspiration pneumonia, anaerobic infections and lung abscess. Med Clin North Am 64:385–394

75. Kantrowitz A, Kantrowitz A (1953) Experimental augmentation of coronary flow by retardation of the arterial pressure pulse. Surgery 34:678–687

76. Kantrowitz A, McKinnon WMP (1958) Experimental use of the diaphragm as auxillary myocardium. Surg Forum 9:266–268

77. Kantrowitz A, Tjonneland S, Freed PS et al. (1968) Initial clinical experience with intra aortic balloon pumping in cardiogenic shock. JAMA 203:113–118

78. Kasnitz P, Druger GL, Yorra F, Simmons DH (1976) Mixed venous oxygen tension, hyperlactaemia and survival in severe cardiopulmonary disease. JAMA 236:570–574

79. Koffsky RM, Litwak RS, Mitchell BL (1976) A simple left heart device for use after open intracardiac surgery: development, deployment, and clinical experience. J Artificial Organs 2:257–262

80. Lazrone S, Waxman K, Shippy C, Shoemaker WC (1980) Haemodynamic, blood volume and oxygen transport responses to albumin and hydroxyethyl starch infusions in critically ill postoperative patients. Crit Care Med 8:302–306

81. Lecompte F, Aberkane H, Azonlay E, Mouffat-Joly M, Pocidalo JJ (1975) Blood affinity for oxygen in experimental haemorrhagic shock with metabolic acidosis. Pfluegers Arch 359:147–152

82. Ledingham I McA, Heimbach DM, Hutton I (1971) Cardiac function in haemorrhagic shock. BJ Surg 58:868–869

83. Lee JC, Downing SE (1976) Myocardial oxygen availability and cardiac failure in haemorrhagic shock. Am Heart J 92:201–209

84. Lefer AM, Sollot M, Galvin MJ (1979) Beneficial actions of prostacyclin in traumatic shock. Prostaglandins 17:761–767

85. Leier CV, Heban PT, Huss P, Bush CA, Lewis RP (1978) Comparative systemic and regional haemodynamic effects of dopamine and dobutamine in patients with cardiomyopathic heart failure. Circulation 58:466–475

86. Leinbach RC, Buckley MJ, Austen WG et al. (1971) Effects of intraaortic balloon pumping on coronary flow

and metabolism in man. Circulation [Suppl.] 43:1–77

87. Limet R, Demoulin JC, Fourny J (1980) Five year experience with intraaortic balloon pumping. Acta Cardiol (Brux) 35:121–130

88. Loeb HS, Bredakis J, Gunnat RM (1976) Superiority of dobutamine over dopamine for augmentation of cardiac output in patients with chronic low output cardiac failure. Circ Shock 3:55–63

89. Lowry P, Blanco T, Santiago-Delphin EA (1977) Histamine and sympathetic blockade in septic shock. Am Surg 43:12–19

90. Lucas CE, Ledgerwood AM, Higgins RF (1979) Impaired salt and water excretion after albumin resuscitation from hypovolaemic shock. Surgery 86:544–549

91. Lucas CE, Ledgerwood AM, Higgins RF, Weaver DW (1980) Impaired pulmonary function after albumin resuscitation from shock. J Trauma 20:446–451

92. McCabe WR (1974) Gram negative bacteraemia. Adv Intern Med 19:135–158

93. Machiedo GW, Rush BF (1979) Comparison of corticosteroids and prostaglandins in the treatment of haemorrhagic shock. Ann Surg 190:735–739

94. McHugh TJ, Forrester JS, Adler L (1972) Pulmonary vascular congestion in acute myocardial infarction, haemodynamic and radiological correlations. Ann Intern Med 76:29–33

95. McKenzie ET, McCulloch J, O'Keane M, Pickard JD, Harper AM (1976) Cerebral circulation and noradrenaline, the relevance of the blood brain barrier. Am J Physiol 231:483–488

96. McNay JL, Abe Y (1970) Pressure dependent heterogeneity of renal blood flow in dogs. Circ Res 27:571–587

97. Madias JE, Madias NE, Hood WB (1975) Precordial ST segment mapping. 2. The effects of oxygen inhalation on ischaemic injury in patients with acute myocardial infarction. Circulation 53:411–417

98. Markis JE, Malagold M, Parker JA et al. (1981) Myocardial salvage after intracoronary thrombolysis with streptokinase in acute myocardial infarction. N Engl J Med 305:777–782

99. Maroko PR, Kjekshus JK, Sobel BE (1971) Factors influencing infarct size following experimental coronary occlusion. Circulation 43:67–82

100. Maroko PR, Bernstein EF, Libby P et al. (1972) Effects of intraaortic balloon counterpulsation on the severity of myocardial ischaemic injury following acute coronary occlusion. Counterpulsation and myocardial injury. Circulation 45:1150–1159

101. Mela L, Bacalzo LV, Miller LD (1971) Defective oxidative metabolism of rat liver mitochondria in haemorrhagic and endotoxic shock. Am J Physiol 220:571–577

102. Michels R, Haalebos M, Kint PP (1980) Intraaortic balloon pumping in myocardial infarction and unstable angina. Europ Heart J 1:31–43

103. Miller MG, Weintraub RM, Hedley-White J, Restall DS, Alexander M (1974) Surgery for cardiogenic shock. Lancet ii:1342–1345

104. Miller CD, Moreno-Cabral RJ, Stinson EB, Shinn JA, Shumway NE (1980) Pulmonary artery balloon counterpulsation for acute right ventricular failure. J Thorac Cardiovasc Surg 80:760–763

105. Modlin IM, Jaffe BM (1980) Clinical usefulness of glucagon. Surgery 87:470–472

106. Moss GS, Saletta JD (1974) Traumatic shock in man. N Engl J Med 290:724–726

107. Moulopoulos SD, Topaz S, Kolff WJ (1962) Diastolic balloon pumping in the aorta. A mechanical assistance for the failing circulation. Am Heart J 63:669–675

108. Moxham J, Armstrong RF (1981) Continuous monitoring of right atrial oxygen tension in patients with myocardial infarction. Intensive Care Med 7:1–8

109. Moyer CA (1954) Fluid balance. Year Book Medical Publishers, Chicago

110. Mueller H, Ayres SM, Gianelli S (1972) Effect of isoprenaline, noradrenaline and intraaortic counterpulsation on haemodynamics and myocardial metabolism in shock following acute myocardial infarction. Circulation 45:335–351

111. Nishimura N (1981) Cardiovascular changes with 'Fluosol DA' in man (abstract). Crit Care Med 9:167

112. O'Flaherty JT, Craddock PR, Jacob HS (1977) Mechanism of anticomplementary activity of corticosteroids in vivo. Possible relevance in endotoxin shock. Proc Soc Exper Biol Med 154:206–209

113. Oliver LE, Horowitz JD, Dyron MK et al. (1980) Use of dopamine and prazocin combined in the treatment of cardiogenic shock. Med J Austr [Suppl.] July 42–45

114. Opie LH (1965) Effect of extracellular pH on the function and metabolism of isolated perfused rat heart. Am J Physiol 209:1075–1080

115. Page DL, Caulfield JB, Kastor JA, De Sanctis RW (1971) Myocardial changes associated with cardiogenic shock. N Engl J Med 285:133–137

116. Parmley WW, Chatterjee K, Charnzi Y, Swan HJC (1974) Haemodynamic effects of noninvasive systolic unloading (nitroprusside), and diastolic augmentation (external counterpulsation), in patients with acute myocardial infarction. Am J Cardiol 33:819–825

117. Permutt S (1979) Mechanical influences on water accumulation in the lungs. In: Fishman AP, Renkin EM (eds) Pulmonary oedema. American Physiology Society, Bethesda, p 175

118. Pert CB, Snyder SH (1973) Opiate receptor—demonstration in nervous tissue. Science 179:1011–1014

118a. Pierce WS, Parr GVS, Myers JL et al. (1981) Ventricular assist pumping in patients with cardiogenic shock after cardiac operations. N Engl J Med 305:1606–1610

119. Pitt (1981) Prognosis after acute myocardial infarction (Editorial). N Engl J Med 305:1147–1148

120. Poole-Wilson PA, Lewis G, Angerpointer T et al. (1977) Haemodynamic effects of salbutamol and nitroprusside after cardiac surgery. Br Heart J 39:721–725

121. Postel J, Schloerb PR, Furtado D (1975) Pathophysiological alterations during bacterial infusions for the study of bacteraemic shock. Surg Gynaecol Obstet 141:683–692

122. Powell WJ, Daggett WM, Margro AE et al. (1970) Effects of intraaortic balloon counterpulsation on cardiac performance, oxygen consumption, and coronary blood flow in dogs. Circ Res 26:753–764

123. Rackow EC, Fein IA, Leppo J (1977) Colloid osmotic pressure as a prognostic indicator of pulmonary oedema and mortality in the critically ill. Chest 72:709–713

124. Raflo GT, Jones RCW, Wangansteen SL (1975) Inadequacy of steroids in the treatment of severe haemorrhagic shock. Am J Surg 130:321–327

125. Richardson PDI, Withrington PG (1977) The role of beta adrenoreceptors in the responses of hepatic arterial vascular bed of the dog to phenylephrine, isoprenaline, noradrenaline and adrenaline. Br J Pharmacol 60:239–249

126. Rithalia S, George R, Tinker J (1981) Continuous tissue pH and transcutaneous pO_2 measurement as an index of tissue perfusion in the critically ill. Resuscitation 9:61–74

127. Roberts R, Dernello V, Sobel BE (1976) Deleterious effects of methylprednisolone in patients with myocardial infarction. Circulation (Suppl.) 53.1:204–206

128. Robin ED, Cary LC, Grenvik A, Glauser F, Gaudio R (1972) Capillary leak syndrome with pulmonary oedema. Arch Intern Med 130:66–71

129. Rosen AJ (1975) Shock lung, fact or fancy? Surg Clin North Am 55:613–626

130. Ross BA, Brock L, Aynsley-Green A (1969) Observations on central and peripheral temperature in the understanding and management of shock. Br J Surg 56:877–882

131. Rozkovec A, De Leon S, Tinker J (1978) Pulmonary oedema and capillary permeability. Intensive Care Med 4:115–118

132. Sawin H, Morganroth J, Chen C (1980) The effect of external counterpulsation on regional wall motion abnormalities during acute myocardial infarction (abstr.). Clin Res 28:209

133. Scheidt S, Arscheim R Killip T (1970) Shock after myocardial infarction, a clinical and haemodynamic profile. Am J Cardiol 26:556–564

134. Schumer W (1976) Steroids in the treatment of clinical septic shock. Ann Surg 184:339–341

135. Schumer W (1979) Septic shock. JAMA 242:1906–1907

136. Shands KN, Dan BB, Schmid GP (1981) Toxic shock syndrome, the emerging picture. Ann Intern Med 94:264–266

137. Shanson DC (1978) Blood culture techniques. In: Williams JD (ed) Modern topics of infection. Heineman, London

138. Sheagreen JN (1981) Septic shock and steroids. N Engl J Med 305:456–458

139. Shoemaker WC (1981) Diagnosis and management of shock. In: Shoemaker WC, Leigh Thompson W (eds) Society of Critical Care Medicine handbook, 'The state of the art' Vol. 1 Society of Critical Care Medicine, USA

140. Shoemaker WC, Bryon-Brown CW, Quigley L (1973) Body fluid-shifts in depletion and poststress states and their correction and adequate nutrition. Surg Gynaecol Obstet 136:371–374

141. Shubin H, Weil MH (1976) Bacterial shock. JAMA 235:421–424

142. Sibbald WJ, Anderson RR, Reid B, Holliday RL, Driedger AA (1981) Alveo-capillary permeability in human septic Adult Respiratory Distress Syndrome. Chest 79:133–142

143. Silverstein DM, Hamilton GW, Hammermeister KE (1974) The effect of external pressure diastolic augmentation on the perfusion of the acutely ischaemic myocardium (abst.). Circulation 49–50 [Suppl. 11]: 111–140

144. Simpson RC, Speller DCE (1977) Detection of bacteraemia by countercurrent immuno-electrophoresis (letter). Lancet I:206

145. Siska K, Ziegelhoffer A, Fedelesora M et al. (1974) Effect of intraaortic balloon counterpulsation on experimental myocardial injury following acute coronary occlusion. Biochemical ultrastructure, and physiological aspects. Cardiovasc Res 8:404–416

146. Sladen A (1976) Methylprednisolone—pharmacological doses in shock lung syndrome. J Thorac Cardiovasc Surg 71:800–806

147. Sobel BE (1980) Cardiac and noncardiac forms of acute circulatory collapse (shock). In: Braunwald E (ed) Heart disease, a textbook of cardiovascular medicine. Saunders, Philadelphia

148. Sonnenblick EH, Siegel JH, Sarnoff SJ (1963) Ventricular distensibility and pressure–volume curves during sympathetic stimulation. Am J Physiol 204:1–4

149. Sonnenblick EH, Frishman WH, LeJemkel TH (1979) Dobutamine, a new synthetic cardioactive sympathetic amine. N Engl J Med 300:17–22

150. Starling EH (1895) On the absorption of fluids from the connective tissue spaces. J Physiol 19:312–326

151. Staub NC (1974) Pulmonary oedema. Physiol Rev 54: 678–681

152. Stokes EJ (1974) Blood culture technique. Association of Clinical Pathologists, Broadsheet No. 81.

153. Stumacher RJ, Kovnat MJ, McCabe WR (1973) Limitations in the usefulness of the limulus assay for endotoxin. N Engl J Med 288:1261–1264

154. Sturm JT, McGee MG, Fuhrman TM et al. (1980) Treatment of postoperative low output syndrome with intraaortic balloon pumping, experience with 419 patients. Am J Cardiol 45:1033–1036

154a. Subramanian VA, Goldstein JE, Sos TA, McCabe JC, Hoover EA, Gay WA (1980) Preliminary clinical experience with percutaneous balloon pumping. Circulation 62 [1]:123–129

155. Sugg WL, Watson JT, Platt MR, Willerson JT (1974) Similarities between external counterpulsation and intraaortic ballon pumping. Influence on collateral coronary blood flow in ischaemic myocardium (Abstract). Circulation 49–50 [Suppl] III: 69

156. Swan HJC, Ganz W (1979) Complications of flow directed balloon tipped catheters (letter). Ann Intern Med 91:494

157. Sweet SE, Sussman HA, Ryan TJ, Bernhard WF, Berger RL (1980) Sequential imaging during paracorporeal left ventricular support. Chest 78:423–428

158. Tanaka K, Iizuka Y (1968) Suppression of enzyme released from isolated rat liver lysosomes by nonsteroidal noninflammatory drugs. Biochem Pharmacol 17:2023–2032

159. Tiengo M (1980) Naloxone in irreversible shock (letter). Lancet i:690

160. Timmis AD, Fowler MB, Chamberlain DA (1981) Comparison of haemodynamic responses to dopamine and salbutamol in severe cardiogenic shock complicating acute myocardial infarction. Br Med J 282:7–9

161. Tinker J (1979) Shock, a pharmacological approach to the treatment of shock. Br J Hosp Med 261–268

162. Tinker JH, Tarhan S, White RD (1976) Dobutamine for inotropic support during emergence from cardiopulmonary bypass. Anesthesiology 44:281–286

163. Todd J, Fishant M, Kapral F, Welch T (1978) Toxic shock syndrome associated with phage 1 staphylococcus. Lancet ii: 1116–1118

164. Tremper KK, Shoemaker WC (1981) Oxygen transport effects of 'Fluosol', a perfluorochemical blood substitute (Abstract). Crit Care Med 9:167

165. Vargish T, Shircliffe A, James PM (1974) Effects of steroids on cardiac function. Ann Surg 40:688–696

166. Velasco IT, Pontieri V, Silva RE, Lopes ON (1980) Hyperosmotic sodium chloride and severe haemorrhagic shock. Am J Physiol 239:H664–673

167. Vij D, Babcock R, Magilligan D (1981) A simplified concept of complete physiological monitoring of the critically ill patient. Heart Lung 10:75–82

168. Wackers FJ, Lie KI, Becker AE, Durrer D, Wellens HJJ (1976) Coronary artery disease in patients dying from cardiogenic shock or congestive heart failure in the setting of acute myocardial infarction. Br Heart J 38:906–910

169. Waisbren BA (1964) Gram negative shock and endotoxic shock. Am J Med 36:819–824

170. Watkins L, Burton JA, Haber E et al. (1976) The renin angiotensin aldosterone system in congestive heart failure in conscious dogs. J Clin Invest 57:1606–1617

171. Weber KT, Janick JS (1974) Intraaortic balloon counterpulsation. A review of the physiological principles,

clinical results and device safety. Ann Thorac Surg 17:602–620

172. Weintraub RM, Vonkydis PC, Araesy JM (1974) Treatment of preinfarction angina with intraaortic balloon counterpulsation and surgery. Am J Cardiol 34:809–814

173. Weisul JP, O'Donnell TF, Stone MA, Clowes GHA (1975) Myocardial performance in clinical septic shock, effects of isoprenaline and glucose/potassium/insulin. J Surg Res 18:357–363

174. Weitzman S, Berger S (1975) Clinical trial design in studies of corticosteroid for bacterial infections. Ann Intern Med 81:36–42

175. Willerson JT, Hutton I, Watson JT (1976) Influence of dobutamine on regional myocardial blood flow and ventricular performance during acute and chronic myocardial ischaemia in dogs. Circulation 53:828–833

176. Wolff SM, Bennet JV (1974) Gram negative rod bacteraemia. N Engl J Med 291:733–734

177. Wright CJ, McLean APH, MacLean LD (1971) Regional capillary blood flow and oxygen uptake in severe sepsis. Surg Gynaecol Obstet 132:637–644

Chapter 13

The Diagnosis and Management of Pulmonary Embolism

Celia Oakley

Incidence and prevention

The incidence of fatal pulmonary embolism is unknown. In a previously healthy population pulmonary embolism has probably been over-diagnosed [25] but in a hospital population acute pulmonary embolism has been the most common cause of sudden unexpected death in some series and has been estimated to occur in up to 1% of all postoperative patients [10, 22].

At a French surgical congress held in 1974 and devoted to pulmonary embolism it was estimated that pulmonary embolism was responsible for 20 000 deaths a year in France and for 1200–18 000 deaths in postoperative patients [13]. No doubt many of these deaths could have been prevented or successfully treated by medical means if the event had happened where the facilities were available, although many of the deaths may have been a merciful last event in terminal malignancy. Nonetheless, the large number of postoperative deaths was surprising in view of world-wide surgical interest and progress in preventing this. Surgical concentration upon prevention by the use of heparin SC, head-down tilt during anaesthesia, anti-embolism stockings, and seemingly also simply by taking an interest, has greatly reduced the incidence of this unnecessary com-plication. In our own hospital over the past 10 years there have been only three fatal cases of postoperative pulmonary embolism in non-malignant disease.

The risk of venous thrombo-embolism in cardiac patients has only been greatly reduced by the more intensive use of anticoagulants in chronic heart failure and by the ability of cardiac surgeons (seemingly unlike most other surgeons) to operate on patients despite warfarin treatment and while the thrombotest (or PTT) is in the therapeutic range.

The fact that heparinization of the blood is necessary in cardiopulmonary bypass undoubtedly accounts for the rarity of postoperative pulmonary embolism in such cases, most of whom were routinely given warfarin postoperatively. Over the last few years patients have tended to leave hospital even more quickly after major cardiac surgery. It is now common for patients to be discharged 10 days after coronary artery bypass, so that there is hardly time to establish warfarin medication, and many surgeons now do not use postoperative anticoagulants, relying on stockings, physiotherapy, and 'antiplatelet' drugs. Of all these measures the increasing use of early mobilization has probably contributed most to the prevention of pulmonary embolism in high-risk groups.

The data on the effectiveness of SC heparin in the prevention of venous thrombosis and pulmonary embolism in high-risk grroups are quite persuasive. The dose is 5000 u SC every 12 h. Postoperative blood loss is statistically slightly increased by this regimen but serious bleeding is not usually a problem. Prophylactic heparin does not seem to work in patients undergoing hip replacement or prostatectomy.

Aetiology

Virchow's classic triad of vascular stasis, damage to the vessel wall, and changes in the coagulability of the blood are still regarded as the usual predisposing conditions to venous thrombosis. Stasis is by far the most important of these and accounts for thrombosis occurring in the chronically sick, in postoperative patients, and occasionally in the healthy who have been sitting for many hours in the economy seats of crowded jumbo jets.

The least well understood predisposing cause is a hypercoagulable state, although this may contribute to thrombo-embolism associated with pregnancy and parturition. A congenital deficiency of antithrombin III is the only abnormality of the clotting mechanism which has been demonstrated to be related to heightened risk of thrombosis, although patients who have undergone splenectomy are also predisposed [27].

The most common source of pulmonary emboli is the deep veins of the legs [5, 29, 30]. Although such thrombi can be found in nearly 100% of fatal cases of pulmonary embolism, clinically evident deep venous thrombosis is often absent in pulmonary embolism. Sevitt showed that nearly all patients who die after surviving more than a few days after severe burns or road traffic accidents have thrombosis in leg and pelvic veins but that routine use of oral anticoagulants in such cases can prevent this [28].

Rarely, venous thrombosis may occur in other veins such as axillary or renal veins and give rise to pulmonary emboli [9]. Recurrent pulmonary embolism may occur from the renal veins in the nephrotic syndrome and give rise to a distinct clinical syndrome with breathlessness and pulmonary infiltrates on x-ray [23].

Tumour embolism may occur in chorionepithelioma and renal carcinoma, even mimicking major or recurrent pulmonary embolism [35].

Fat embolism may follow fracture [8]; bone marrow may be released during severe traumatic injury [26]; amniotic fluid may embolize during protracted or assisted labour or following caesarean section [21]; and air embolism may complicate wounds of the great veins in the neck or careless cannulation technique [7].

Pathophysiology

Pulmonary embolism may be massive and almost immediately lethal [2, 3, 4, 17, 19, 22]. Minor embolism usually precedes major and the recognition of minor embolism may permit prevention of a major episode. Minor pulmonary embolism may be recurrent and lead to progressive thrombo-embolic pulmonary hypertension. Recurrent thrombo-embolism and thromboembolic pulmonary hypertension are outside the scope of this chapter, although it is important to mention now that the apparently acute major pulmonary embolism may be superimposed upon chronic recurrent pulmonary embolism and thrombo-embolic pulmonary hypertension.

Generous reserves of pulmonary vascular capacity together with the extraordinarily efficient fibrinolytic activity of the pulmonary arterial endothelium account for the clinical silence of many pulmonary emboli. Peripheral embolism only results in clinical symptoms if it causes infarction of a segment of lung or is associated with clinically discernible venous thrombosis. Pulmonary infarction only complicates peripheral embolism if the embolus happens to fit and to clog the pulmonary artery branch in which it lodges, so that blood-borne fibrinolysins cannot reach the thrombus and stasis may lead to rapid propagation of thrombosis. More surprisingly, even a large mass of embolic material may be silent for it only causes major circulatory obstruction if the embolus fails to move onwards from the central pulmonary arteries into the periphery. Although most major pulmonary emboli come from the ileofemoral veins any accompanying signs of ileofemoral thrombosis or even minor calf thrombosis are relatively uncommon. The reason is that the thrombus which becomes an embolus was never adherent or occlusive. That is why it became detached altogether from the vein wall or anchoring thrombus. If there was an anchoring thrombus which was occlusive then there may be persisting signs of venous obstruction. The thrombus which becomes an embolus may have been in the vein for some days and is already partially autolysed, so it readily breaks up when it reaches the pulmonary vascular tree. This means that a pulmonary embolus, if not immediately lethal, tends to clear extremely rapidly, so that the patient who at one moment may be close to death may be apparently recovered within the space of a few hours. The hazard then is the possibility of further embolism before resolution of the embolic material by natural or augmented fibrinolysis.

Major pulmonary embolism occurs often but not exclusively in postoperative, postpartum, medically sick, or bed-ridden patients, particularly those with terminal malignant disease. Unfortunately it sometimes occurs quite unexpectedly in otherwise fit people. They may have been sitting in cramped conditions, as during a long plane journey in a crowded plane, or they may have suffered a leg injury in a rugby tackle or they may have a still hidden adenocarcinoma; but equally they may have no discernible precipitating factors at all. In this last category of patients the diagnosis is not only much more often missed, but the catastrophic episode is also more likely to be fatal because by its nature it occurs outside hospital. Sudden obstruction to RV emptying is responsible for the circulatory collapse caused by acute massive pulmonary embolism, but arguments have been brought to suggest that there may also be neurohumoral factors which add vasoconstriction to the mechanical burden.

Experiments nearly half a century ago showed that occlusion of more than two-thirds of the pulmonary artery cross-sectional area is required to cause right ventricular failure [12]. McIntyre and Sasahara showed a linear relationship between the extent of pulmonary vascular obstruction as measured by angiography and the mean pulmonary artery pressure in patients without previous heart or lung disease, suggesting that vasoconstrictive factors played no part in the mechanism of development of pulmonary hypertension [14]. In clinical massive or major pulmonary embolism the pulmonary artery systolic pressure rarely exceeds 60 mmHg as more severe obstruction produces RV failure, a further fall in output and even a fall in pulmonary artery pressure; in the most severe cases therefore the pulmonary artery pressure may be hardly abnormal but the RV diastolic pressure and right atrial pressure will be very high, 15–25 mmHg, and equal to the diastolic pressure in the pulmonary artery. No relationship exists between the angiographically determined amount of pulmonary vascular obstruction and the pulmonary artery pressure in patients with pre-existing heart or lung disease [14], in whom RV hypertrophy and pulmonary vasoconstrictive reflexes may combine to cause marked and transient rises in pressure.

There does seem to be a difference between experimental occlusion of the left or right main pulmonary artery which causes no change in RV pressure or output [31] and pulmonary embolism when this amount of obstruction to the pulmonary circulation is usually associated with a rise in PAP and in calculated PVR. In addition, mechanical factors alone cannot fully explain the abnormalities in pulmonary gas exchange that occur in pulmonary embolism, so it seems that reflex or humoral factors must contribute to the clinical picture [3, 15, 17].

Naturally occurring thrombo-emboli encourage platelet aggregation on their surfaces and initiation of the platelet release phenomenon with liberation of prostaglandins as well as histamine and serotonin may be responsible for constriction of pulmonary vascular and bronchial smooth muscle [4]. Plasmin activated through local fibrinolytic channels can augment these reactions through stimulating tissue mast cells to release their vaso-active substances.

Bronchoconstriction occurs in airways up to 3 mm in diameter following experimental micro-embolization [6]. Bronchoconstriction and closure of distal lung units both in embolized and in normal areas can cause wheezing and increase dyspnoea. The invariable hypoxaemia occurring after pulmonary embolism is also explained by these ventilation-perfusion imbalances. Hyperpnoea and tachypnoea stem from anxiety, low cardiac output, vagal stimulation of lung afferent pathways, and from hypoxaemia itself [33]. These reactions are likely to be intense but short-lived and this fits in with the rapidly evolving time course of clinical pulmonary embolism.

Clinical manifestations of massive and major pulmonary embolism

The pathophysiology of massive pulmonary embolism has only recently been described with precision, since very seriously sick or moribund patients have been investigated before performance of pulmonary embolectomy or institution of fibrinolytic therapy.

Massive pulmonary embolism is a cause of sudden death. While clinical death may be instantaneous, electromechanical dissociation is

common, with no circulation but regular electrical activity on the ECG. In such patients immediate cardiac massage, aided by lifting the
legs in the air for autotransfusion, may cause
the central occluding material to break up and
pass on into the first- and second-order pulmonary artery branches, where the cross-
sectional area is much greater. Consciousness
may then be regained and the circulation rapidly restored although a low cardiac output due
to persisting central obstruction is likely to pre-
vail. The clinical signs and prognosis then become those of major pulmonary embolism.

When an embolus lodges in the main pulmonary artery or T junction the right ventricle
suddenly becomes unable to empty its contents
or to transport blood to the left ventricle. The
right ventricle distends and its filling pressure
abruptly rises. The forward output fails and the
starved left ventricle discharges a much diminished stroke volume. Reflex catecholamine sup-

port causes systemic vasoconstriction and
tachycardia. Syncope may occur but in the
supine position intense vasoconstriction may
preserve the blood pressure despite a low stroke
volume. The pulses are jerky and ill-sustained,
but a near-normal blood pressure can lead to
grave underestimation of the seriousness of the
situation (Fig. 13.1). The blood pressure may be
only tenuously maintained, and if the patient is
raised to examine the venous pulse the arterial
pressure may well disappear. the venous pressure is high but may be difficult to see because of
exaggerated respiratory effort. Tachypnoea and
hyperpnoea are striking and help to differentiate major pulmonary embolism from other conditions such as acute myocardial infarction
which may be thought of in differential diagnosis. Auscultation invariably reveals a loud triple
rhythm, though this may only be audible at
the xiphisternum because augmented breath
sounds tend to obscure the heart sounds in

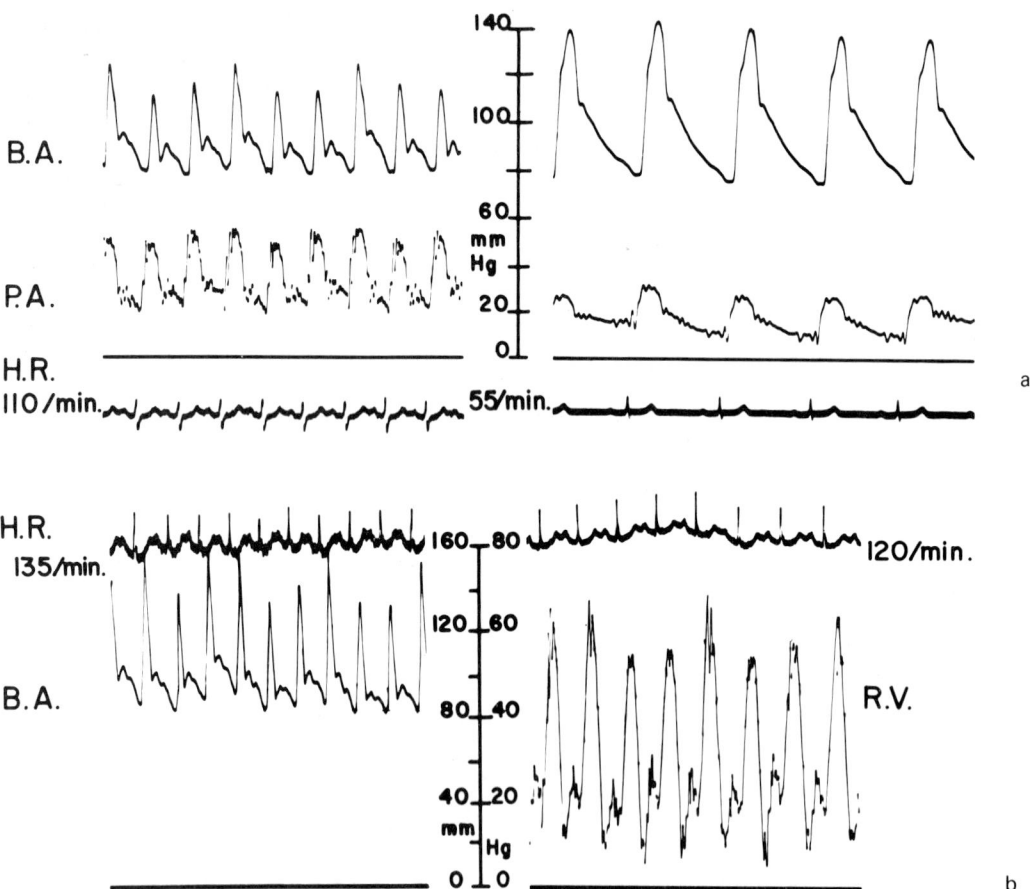

Fig. 13.1. a Massive pulmonary embolism. The brachial artery (*BA*) side trace shows the tachycardia and narrow, ill-sustained
arterial pulse with pulsus paradoxus. The pulmonary artery (*PA*) pressure is raised to 50 mmHg and also shows paradox. On
the *right*, 1 month later the same patient shows normal BA and PA pressures.
 b In same patient as in Fig. 1a, the RV diastolic pressure is greatly raised and equals the PA pressure of 25 mmHg.

other areas. Pulmonary closure is usually inaudible because of the failing right ventricle, whose diastolic pressure usually has risen to equal the diastolic pressure in the pulmonary artery. If pulmonary valve closure can be heard or is loud this usually indicates pre-existing pulmonary hypertension.

No single symptom or combination of symptoms is diagnostic of pulmonary embolism. In large series of patients such as the 327 cases of thrombo-embolism published by Bell [3], chest pain occurred in 88%, shortness of breath in 84%, apprehension in 59%, cough in 53%, haemoptysis in 30%, sweating in 27%, and syncope in 13%. Massive embolism, not surprisingly, was more often associated with syncope and apprehension and minor embolism with cough, chest pain, and haemoptysis. The plebeian symptoms of cough and chest pain were often felt by the patient several days before the diagnosis of pulmonary embolism was made. Apprehension, sweating, and syncope were acute, often presaging collapse or death.

In the same series tachypnoea was the most common sign. Lung crackles, tachycardia, and fever were next. Gallop rhythm, sweating, and phlebitis were found in a third and oedema and cyanosis in a quarter. It should be emphasized that this large series included patients with pulmonary emboli of varying size and acuteness of onset.

The lungs are overventilated by a vagally induced increased drive to breathe, which results in alveolar hyperventilation despite the increase in physiological dead space caused by the areas of non-perfused lung. Arterial PO_2 is usually very low, even though only about a quarter of adults have a patent foramen ovale through which to shunt when the right atrial pressure rises. When 25% or less of the pulmonary vascular bed is obstructed arterial hypoxaemia may be the only sign, so it is of great clinical value. The PCO_2 is also low except in patients on the verge of circulatory arrest. Sinus rhythm is nearly always maintained and the rate is fast, but bradycardia may herald circulatory arrest.

Although a metabolic acidosis rapidly builds up because of the inadequate cardiac output pulmonary hyperventilation may result in a misleadingly normal pH.

The chest radiograph is an anteroposterior portable film and usually of low quality (Fig. 13.2a). It may look misleadingly normal but is useful in diagnosis if it shows a previous herald infarct (previous peripheral emboli will otherwise be invisible). Its other use is for the exclusion of lung collapse, tension pneumo-

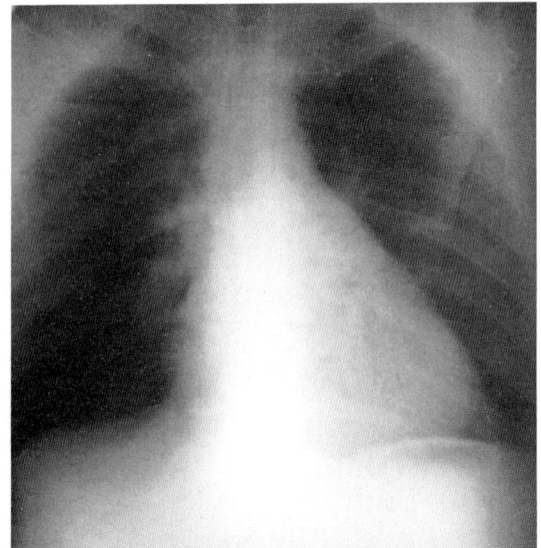

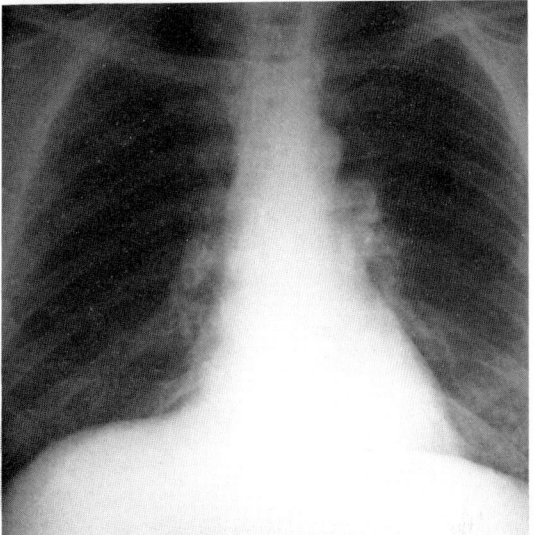

Fig. 13.2. Massive pulmonary embolism (same patient as in Fig. 13.1). The portable anteroposterior chest radiograph (a) shows no definite abnormality and is mainly useful for excluding overt lung pathology and pre-existing heart disease. b PA radiograph after recovery.

thorax, or pericardial tamponade, which may superficially mimic major pulmonary embolism.

Soon after massive or major pulmonary embolism the ECG may appear normal (Fig. 13.3a), though comparison with pre-existing or later ECGs may reveal that an axis shift to the right and posteriorly has been caused by dilatation of the right atrium and right ventricle and true anatomical clockwise rotation of the heart. Hyperventilation may be

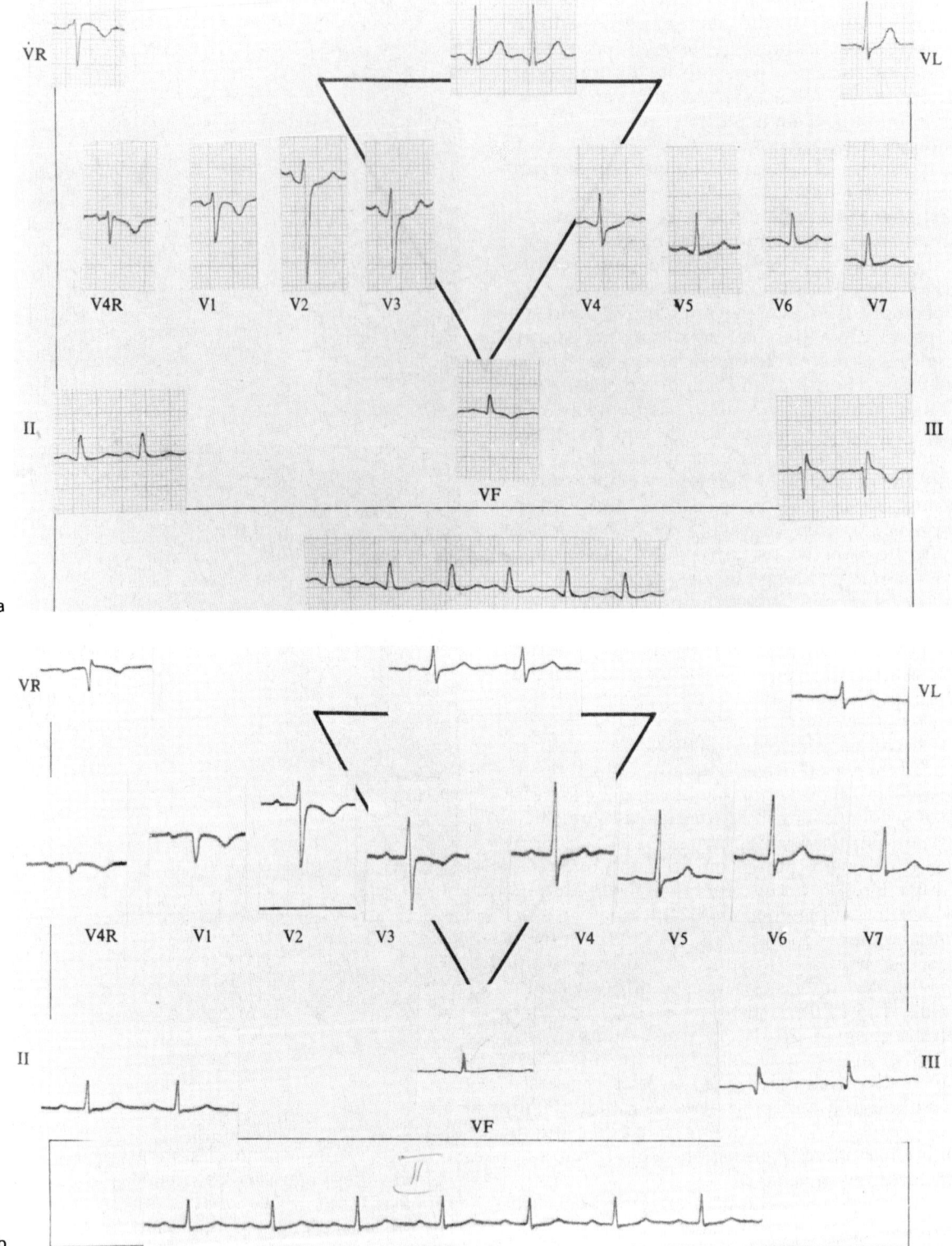

Fig. 13.3. Massive pulmonary embolism. The immediate ECG (**a**) shows sinus tachycardia and no very definite abnormality, although 'classical' changes are seen in leads III and VF. Lead III shows an r Sr with T wave inversion and VF a q with T wave inversion, which are points of difference from the record (**b**) of a few hours after the episode, when the heart rate has already slowed but T wave inversion has appeared in leads V_1 to V_3 and there is a small late r wave in VR, with axis shift to the right indicative of RV dilatation.

associated with T wave inversion in the right-sided V leads but this change may be both delayed and transient (Fig. 13.3b). Dilatation of the right ventricle may be associated with the development of a late terminal R wave in AVR or low RSR in V_1 and S in V_6. A spikey right atrial P wave is rarely seen. If major pulmonary embolism complicates recent AMI then these features may be obscured.

When the picture of major pulmonary embolism is typical the diagnosis should leave not a moments doubt. The anguish giving way to extreme restlessness with catecholamine-induced widened palpable fissures and proptosis, distended veins, exaggerated respiratory efforts with normal lung sounds, third heart sound gallop and close to normal ECG and chest x-ray with hypoxaemia, hypocapnoea and normal pH in the arterial blood can leave no room for doubt.

Special tests

Pulmonary angiography

Pulmonary angiography and lung scans are appropriate and provide specific information (Figs. 13.4 and 13.5). In suspected pulmonary embolism it is illogical to carry out special tests

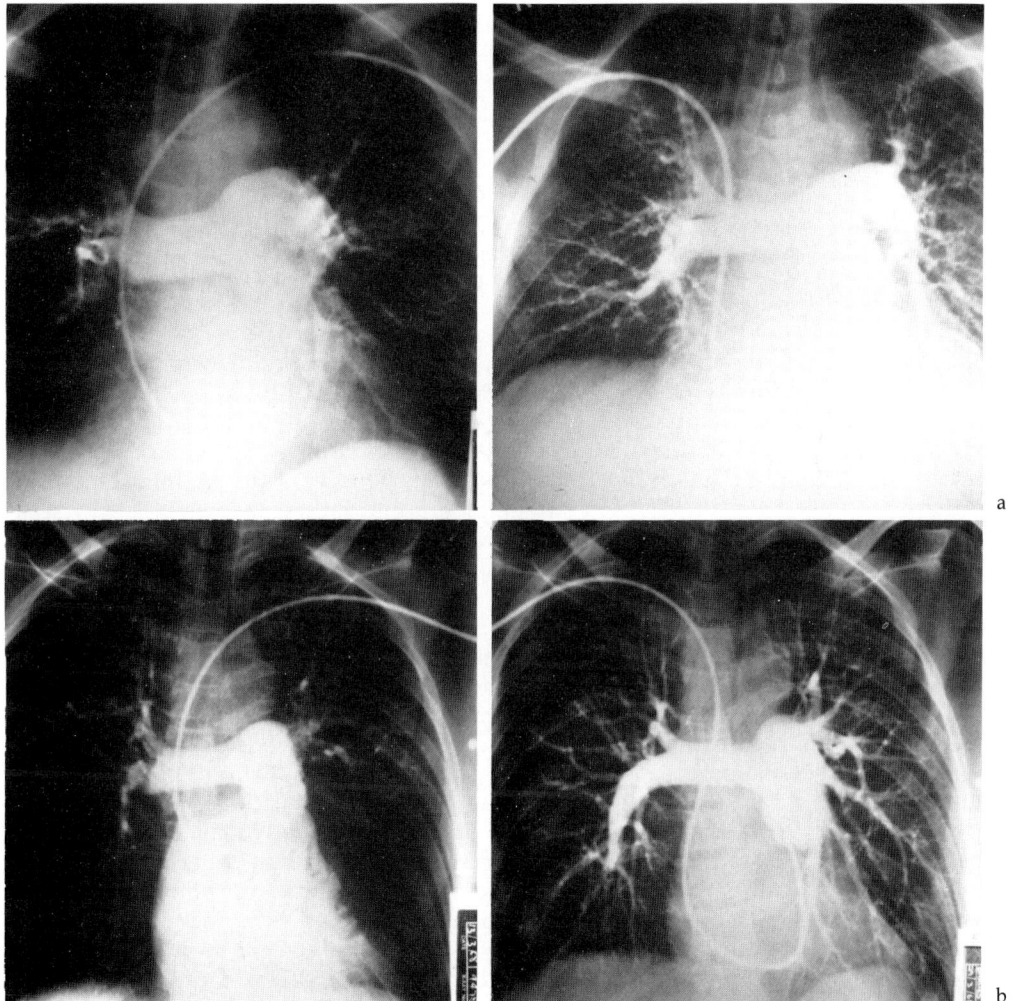

Fig. 13.4. a Massive pulmonary embolism. On the *left* is the angiogram recorded 2 h after the episode and immediately after the chest radiograph shown in Fig. 13.2a. The main PA is considerably dilated. Emboli are seen obstructing the orifices of almost all the main branches of the left and right PA. On the *right* is the serial pulmonary angiogram recorded 1 month later.
b Massive pulmonary embolism. Another case, showing limited circulation only to a few upper lobe PA segments and on the *right* a normal pulmonary angiogram recorded 3 weeks later.

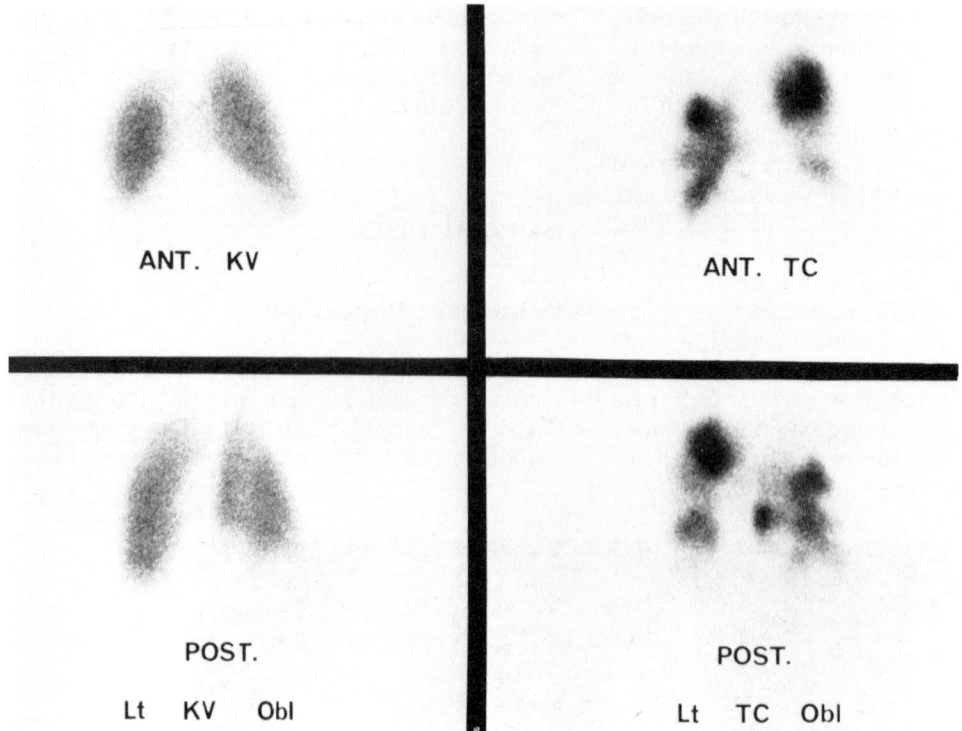

Fig. 13.5. Krypton ventilation (*KV*) and technetium perfusion (*TC*) lung scan from a patient who had sustained major pulmonary embolism 3 days earlier on a background of multiple emboli for the previous month since abdominal surgery. The ventilation scan is normal. The perfusion scan shows multiple avascular areas in both lungs due to emboli. It was $2\frac{1}{2}$ months before the perfusion scans became normal.

on the legs to diagnose mischief in the thorax, and in any case peripheral venography may be normal after major pulmonary embolism although it can occasionally reveal a floating ileofemoral thrombus threatening the life of the patient a second time.

Pulmonary angiography provides both a definitive diagnosis and precise localization and quantitation of the site and severity of pulmonary arterial obstruction. It provides a basis from which to recognize the occasional patient in whom rapid resolution fails to occur. For the equally rare patient who fails to recover rapidly or who has a second embolus before the first has resolved and who needs emergency surgery, the pulmonary angiogram gives the surgeon guidance in knowing in which part of the lungs the obstructions are situated.

In most patients with circulatory collapse from pulmonary embolism who previously had no cardiac or pulmonary fault the flow is usually found to have been cut off to more than the equivalent of one lung. In patients with previous chronic respiratory or cardiac disease less than this may cause severe distress. In patients with previous chronic thrombo-embolic disease the superimposition of any further pulmonary

emboli may cause a critical decline in condition.

Pulmonary angiography is usually well sustained even in seemingly moribund patients. It can be carried out quickly by using the brachial or subclavian venous route for introduction of the angiographic catheter, since it is unwise to enter via the femoral route with the risk of propelling dormant ileal femoral thrombus into the central vascular compartment. The injection of 0.6 mg atropine down the catheter at the beginning of the procedure and of 0.3 mg phenylephrine before injecting contrast will overcome the potentially hazardous complications of vagally induced bradycardia or of contrast-induced vasodilatation. Because the circulation is hypokinetic the dilution volume is reduced and invariably a small amount of contrast provides for first class opacification of the pulmonary artery. AP cut films are usually preferable to cine, as a 9-in. image intensifier as usually available will only allow inclusion of one lung field at a time. The catheter should be placed in the central pulmonary artery, however; there should be no fear then of entering the clot, because the catheter can only do good by breaking it up and encouraging it to move onwards into branches where the total cross-sectional area of the lung is greater to accommodate the broken-up clot.

Injection of 0.5 ml 76% urografin or equivalent per kg body wt. through a no. 8 angio- or pigtail catheter at a rate of 25 ml/s will provide excellent pictures.

The appearances of the pulmonary angiogram vary according to the length of time which has elapsed since the impact of the embolus in the main pulmonary artery. If the angiogram is done immediately after resuscitation or the development of symptoms of collapse the embolus may be seen trapped in the T junction or the pulmonary artery bifurcation and barely extending to the first branches. An hour or two later, particularly after cardiac massage has been done, the thrombus may have already left or partially left the main pulmonary artery, be broken up, and be seen hung up on bifurcations of the first and second branches. Because emboli are not adherent to the arterial wall contrast is often seen seeping around the occlusive material, providing very characteristic pictures.

The catheter may be left in situ when desired so that serial pictures can be taken to monitor progress and to facilitate the infusion of streptokinase, although it should be emphasized that streptokinase need not be infused centrally as it exerts the same effect whether infused centrally or peripherally, and progress can be monitored almost as well by serial perfusion scans, particularly once the initial pulmonary angiogram has been done.

Ventilation–perfusion scans

In the extremely sick patient lung scans are more time-consuming and require positioning of the patient, so they are more arduous as well as providing less specific information than pulmonary angiography. For patients who are less ill and can co-operate perfusion lung scanning provides very good information on the extent and the location of pulmonary emboli (Fig. 13.5), and moreover can be followed serially to gauge progress. Particularly in patients with pre-existing lung disease simultaneous ventilation scans are invaluable. This is because chronic lung disease causes static defects in ventilation and perfusion which are largely matched and do not change. In pulmonary embolism the ventilation scan is normal and in pulmonary embolism complicating chronic lung disease unmatched pulmonary perfusion defects are seen in areas with normal ventilation; moreover the perfusion defects change and diminish rapidly when serial scans are done.

A characteristic of pulmonary embolism is the rapidity with which defects in perfusion diminish. Sometimes, however, after major pulmonary embolism one sector or even one lung may show a very slow evolution. Usually this clears up eventually and becomes normal, rarely requiring surgical interference.

Peripheral venography

The patient with massive pulmonary embolism is very ill and there is in general no place for peripheral venography, certainly not in the emergency situation. Whether there is a place for venography in a patient who is less ill or after recovery from the crisis can be argued. Venography certainly has no place in the diagnosis of major pulmonary embolism and the argument centres on whether or not it has a place in its management. Recognition of persisting thrombotic material in peripheral veins, particularly in the ileofemoral system after major pulmonary embolism, is potentially valuable, as trailing thrombus may represent a further threat to life if it becomes dislodged. Unfortunately this cannot be prevented by anticoagulant or fibrinolytic treatment. If venography is done and 'floating' thrombus is seen then the question of either an inferior vena cava umbrella or a local ileofemoral thrombectomy should be considered. Unless a vascular surgeon who is expert in venous procedures is available locally there seems to be no reason to visualize the peripheral veins.

Blood tests

The triad of raised LDH and bilirubin and normal SGOT (aspartate transaminase; AST) has been regarded as diagnostically specific and useful in differentiation from myocardial infarction and pneumonia [34]. In practice it is neither specific nor useful; not useful because the results are not immediate and not specific because the enzyme results are highly variable, depending on the time lapse since the onset of pulmonary embolism.

An arterial blood sample for blood gases provides immediate useful and nearly specific information. The combination of hypoxaemia, hypocapnoea, and a normal or low pH is most helpful, although admittedly a normal arterial PO_2 does not exclude the diagnosis and a normal or even a raised PCO_2 may be found in patients with previous chronic lung disease (in such patients the observation of a drop in PCO_2 has value).

Recent interest has focussed on the detection of fibrin split products [24]. This test may be over-sensitive and its specificity awaits further determination.

Management of massive and major pulmonary embolism

Management is determined by the severity of the circulatory compromise. In massive embolism cardiac massage, elevation of the legs and O_2 are the first emergency measures. Intense vasoconstriction is needed, but usually this is achieved reflexly and exogenous vasoconstriction probably achieves nothing extra. Vasodilators must be avoided at all costs and there is no place for IV digoxin, dobutamine, or dopamine in most instances. Ten thousand units of heparin should be injected IV immediately as a bolus.

It is important to appreciate that the vast majority of patients who do not die within 30 min of massive pulmonary embolism recover completely with no aftermath. The aims of treatment are therefore to support life and to prevent recurrence. The few patients who die at a greater interval from the onset of the crisis die because of a second major embolus.

Intravenous heparin should be continued in a dose sufficient to prevent platelet-thrombus interaction. This is usually 5000–7500 u 4-hourly, but occasionally can be very much more and laboratory control is essential. It has been shown that continuous IV infusion of heparin is significantly less likely to be associated with bleeding complications than 4-hourly dosage. One thousand units per hour by constant infusion pump is the usual requirement. The partial thromboplastin time is usually preferred to the whole-blood clotting time. Heparin should be continued until the patient's circulatory state has stabilized and until warfarin has been introduced and shown to have achieved therapeutic thrombotest or prothrombin levels.

Oral anticoagulants should be continued for 3 months in most cases, the duration being determined by the presence or absence of associated clinical venous thrombosis or of a continuing predisposing cause. Deep vein thrombosis resolves clinically by the development of collateral channels and not by recanalization of the blocked main veins, and an arbitrary 3 months may be allowed for this to be accomplished to an optimal extent, warfarin meanwhile being continued to reduce the risk of recurrent thrombosis. If pulmonary embolism follows a predisposing cause such as operation or illness which is transient, anticoagulants need not be continued longer than about 6 weeks, but if the pulmonary embolism occurred without warning and without any determinable or removable predisposing causes then it is logical to continue oral anticoagulants on a very long-term or indefinite basis—usually until there is some reason to stop. The same is true if there has been previous recurrent thrombo-embolism.

Heparin is not thrombolytic. Two thrombolytic agents, streptokinase and urokinase, have been extensively investigated over the past 10 years. Urokinase has the disadvantage over streptokinase of being exceedingly expensive, but has other major advantages since it is neither antigenic nor pyrogenic and its dosage does not have to be rigidly controlled. In a national randomized trial in the United States heparin and urokinase (followed by heparin) were compared in 160 patients with acute pulmonary embolism proven both by pulmonary angiography and perfusion lung scans [18]. The group receiving urokinase progressed faster in the first 24 h, with more rapid resolution of the haemodynamic, pulmonary angiographic, and lung scan abnormalities than the group receiving heparin.

The differences were most marked in the patients with massive embolism (who would have been most at risk from the consequences of further emboli occurring during this vulnerable early period). After the first 24 h the differences between the lung scans of the two groups gradually became less noticeable, until by the end of a week there was no difference. There was no significant difference in mortality later and no difference between the groups when lung scans were repeated at 3, 6, and 12 months.

This important study from the United States suggested that urokinase is only useful for patients with massive pulmonary embolism in shock (and who might previously have been candidates for pulmonary embolectomy in some institutions). In Britain only streptokinase is generally available and this is vastly inferior to urokinase, being antigenic and pyrogenic, needing careful laboratory control of dosage, and being more likely to cause haemorrhage. In addition, a patient who has had a recent streptococcal infection may be resistant to its action.

Despite these drawbacks the use of streptokinase has been growing, which may be due to some unwise usage in patients who would probably have been better treated with heparin. A further disadvantage of streptokinase is the need to achieve a smooth transfer back onto adequate anticoagulation without any gap, since otherwise rebound thrombosis seems to occur. The recommended dosage schedule for streptokinase is 1 000 000 U IV followed by 250 000 u hourly for 24 h. Administration for longer than this is probably unnecessary and the patient should of course be given IV heparin before and after the streptokinase infusion. There is no advantage in giving the streptokinase directly into the pulmonary artery, unless for convenience when serial pulmonary angiography is planned. Serial perfusion lung scans have really made repeated angiography superfluous; the first lung scan can be compared with the angiogram and resolution thereafter followed on the scan. Further angiography would then only be needed if a major lung scan abnormality persisted or there was doubt about the resolution of pulmonary hypertension.

The place for emergency pulmonary embolectomy is small. For a patient who has died in hospital and who cannot be resuscitated by cardiac massage a modern modification of the old Trendelenburg operation may be life-saving. A modern operation can be done through a right thoracotomy with venous occlusion by means of snares round the superior and inferior vena cavae and an incision in the right pulmonary artery through which a Fogarty catheter can be inserted and most of the thrombus extracted with a sucker. There is no need to try and clear it all, because this is unnecessary and involves time and too much lung handling. Provided a pathway is restored the right ventricle will remuster and the patient himself will utilize fibrinolytic forces to remove any embolic material which remains.

A patient who is fit to be transferred into hospital from home or work or from a small hospital to a regional centre indicates by his very survival that pulmonary embolectomy is not going to be required. Only sudden deterioration resulting from a further major embolus or failure of resolution due to persisting obstruction of a major pulmonary artery may bring a need for pulmonary embolectomy.

The diagnosis may be obvious but is not always so, especially when circulatory arrest is virtually instantaneous and pulmonary angiography is usually obligatory if operation on a mistaken diagnosis is to be avoided.

A heavily modified Trendelenberg operation or embolectomy via sternal split on cardiopulmonary bypass can be undertaken. Cardiopulmonary bypass can only be contemplated where the procedure can be mounted with minimal delay. Femoro-femoral bypass under local anaesthesia may prove life-saving when the blood pressure is extremely low during the induction of anaesthesia.

Many surgeons routinely clip the inferior vena cava or place an umbrella in it before completion of the operation [11], but others emphasize the rarity of embolism following pulmonary embolectomy and stress both the morbidity and the failure of inferior vena cava interference to prevent future pulmonary emboli.

Massive haematemesis is a not uncommon complication of acute pulmonary embolism and results from acute gastric erosion akin to the Curling's ulcer after burns. This bleeding may preclude effective use of either thrombolytic agents or anticoagulants until it has ceased, and cimetidine has a limited usefulness in the treatment of gastric erosion as distinct from duodenal ulceration. From among such patients may come a rare indication for operation on the inferior vena cava because of the inability to treat by other means [11]. It should be remembered, however, that pulmonary embolism gets better without the aid of either external thrombolytic agents or anticoagulants provided the patient does not have recurrent emboli so that it may be judged preferable to avoid operation if the haemodynamic status is reasonably satisfactory rather than to expose the patient to the further stress of major surgery.

Operations on the inferior vena cava

Surgical interference with the inferior vena cava has never been as popular in Britain as in the mainland of Europe and the United States. The idea is to interrupt the inferior vena cava or to so partition it that large, potentially fatal, emboli cannot pass up it. The very many different ways of tackling the problem testify to the still unsatisfactory results. They vary from ligation, partial ligation, partition with sutures, staples, staples or clips, through filters and sieves to the Mobin–Udin umbrella [11]. The last method is now the most popular as the umbrella can be passed venously without the need for laparotomy and the umbrella opened in the chosen position just above the renal veins. All the various partitioning devices and the umbrella are apt to be followed by total thrombotic occlusion of the cava. None of the procedures is free from risk to life or from complications and there is an incidence of recurring, even lethal, pulmonary embolism. Total occlusion of the cava may lead to proximal propagation of thrombus and embolization or to retrograde thrombosis involving the renal veins. The development of wide collaterals may themselves convey fatal emboli while poor collateralization may be followed by disability from oedema and the likelihood of further venous thrombosis. Anticoagulants are still needed.

Inferior vena caval interruption should be considered when anticoagulants cannot be given, such as when massive haematemesis has occurred or further major surgery is contemplated. The risk inherent in laparotomy is highest in those patients who might gain most from such an operation, so that the umbrella has gained in popularity. Its disadvantage is the danger of incorrect placement or dislodgement.

Prognosis

Seventy-five percent of all deaths from pulmonary emboli occur within 60 min of the onset of symptoms and the remainder within the next 48 h [1, 2]. This most important fact means that the vast majority of those who survive long enough to be diagnosed and treated get better.

Natural fibrinolysis begins within hours of embolism (but is slower in humans than it is in experimental dogs) but early recovery is mostly attributable to fragmentation and onward movement of embolized material. That is why clinical improvement precedes lung scan improvement (though it has to be followed on daily pulmonary angiograms). Nowadays serial lung scans show that complete resolution takes between 8 days and 1 month, a very few patients taking even longer [32]. In the United States Natural Cooperation trial of urokinase, lung scans had improved by 50% at 14 days, but 16% still showed some residual abnormality at the end of a year.

The vast majority of patients return to their normal state of health and have no residual disability of massive or major pulmonary embolism, and unresolved embolism is uncommon except in patients with pre-existing heart disease. The risk of chronic thrombo-embolic pulmonary hypertension or recurrent embolism in the series was less than 1% [20]. In fact very few patients with chronic thrombo-embolic pulmonary hypertension have a history of major embolism.

The long-term prognosis in previously well patients who have had a major pulmonary embolus is therefore very good.

References

1. Alpert JS, Smith RE, Ockene IS, Askenazi J, Dexter L, Dalen JE (1975) Treatment of massive pulmonary embolism: The role of pulmonary embolectomy. Am Heart J 89:413
2. Alpert JS, Smith R, Carlson J, Ockene IS, Dexter L, Dalen JE (1976) Mortality in patients treated for pulmonary embolism. JAMA 236:1477
3. Bell WR, Simon TL, Demets DL (1977) The clinical features of submassive and massive pulmonary emboli. Am J Med 62:355
4. Bo G, Hognestad J (1972) Effects on the pulmonary circulation of suddenly induced intravascular aggregation of blood platelets. Acta Physiol Scand 85:523
5. Byrne JJ, O'Neil EE (1952) Fatal pulmonary emboli. A study of 130 autopsy proven fatal emboli. Am J Surg 83:47
6. Clarke SW, Graf PD, Nadel JA (1970) In vivo visualization in cats and dogs. J Appl Physiol 29:646
7. Deal CW, Fielden BP, Monk I (1971) Haemodynamic effects of pulmonary air embolism. J Surg Res 11:533
8. Dines DD, Linscheid RL, Didier EP (1972) Fat embolism syndrome. Mayo Clin Proc 47:237
9. Falicov RE, Resnekov L, Peyasnick J (1970) Progressive pulmonary vascular obstruction and cor pulmonale ducts repeated embolism for axillary vein thrombosis. Ann Intern Med 73:429
10. Freiman DG, Suyemoto J, Wessler S (1965) Frequency of pulmonary thromboembolism in man. N Engl J Med 272:1278
11. Gardiner AMN (1978) Inferior vena cava interruption in the prevention of fatal pulmonary embolism. Am Heart J 95:679
12. Haggart GE, Walker AM (1923) The physiology of pulmonary embolism as disclosed by quantitative occlusion of the pulmonary artery. Arch Surg 6:764
13. Marion P, Bient JP (1974) Embolies pulmonaires. In: Rapport du 76e Congrès Français de Chirurgie. Paris, Masson
14. McIntyre KM, Sasahara AA (1971) Haemodynamic response to pulmonary embolism in patients free of prior cardiopulmonary disease. Am J Cardiol 28:228
15. McDonald IG, Hirsh J, Hale GS, O'Sullivan EF (1972a) Major pulmonary embolism: a correlation of clinical findings, haemodynamics, pulmonary angiography and pathological physiology. Br Heart J 34:356
16. McIntyre KM, Sasahara AA, Sharma GV (1972b) Pulmonary thromboembolism: Current concepts. Adv Intern Med 18:199
17. Miller GAH, Sutton GL (1970) Acute massive pulmonary embolism. Clinical and haemodynamic findings in 23 patients studied by cardiac catheterisation and pulmonary arteriography. Br Heart J 32:518
18. National Cooperative Study (1973) The urokinase–pulmonary embolism trial. Circulation 47:[Suppl II] 1
19. Oakley CM (1970) Diagnosis of pulmonary embolism. Br Med J ii:773

20. Paraskos JA, Aldestein SJ, Smith RE, Rickman FD, Grossman W, Dexter L, Dalen J (1973) Late prognosis of acute pulmonary embolism. N Engl J Med 289:55

21. Peterson EP, Taylor HB (1970) Amniotic fluid embolism: An analysis of 40 cases. Obstet Gynaecol 35:787

22. Poe ND, Dore EK, Swanson LA, Taplin GU (1969) Fatal pulmonary embolism. J Nucl Med 10:28

23. Pollak VE, Kark PM, Pirani CL, Shafter HA, Muehrcke RC (1956) Renal vein thrombosis and the nephrotic syndrome. Am J Med 21:496

24. Rickman FD, Handin R, Howe JP, Alpert J, Dexter L, Dalen JE (1973) Fibrin split products in acute pulmonary embolism. Ann Intern Med 79:664

25. Robin ED (1977) Overdiagnosis and overtreatment of pulmonary embolism: the Emperor may have no clothes. Ann Intern Med 87:775

26. Rogel S, Rosenmann E, Rachmilewitz EA (1965) Multiple pulmonary infarctions caused by bone marrow emboli. N Engl J Med 272:732

27. Rosenburg RD (1976) Hypercoagulability and methods for monitoring anticoagulant therapy. US Department of Health Education and Welfare, Washington. (USDHEW publication no. 76, p 866)

28. Sevitt S (1962) Deep venous thrombosis and pulmonary embolism. Am J Med 33:703

29. Sevitt S, Gallagher N (1961) Venous thrombosis and pulmonary embolism. Clinico-pathological study in injured and burned patients. Br J Surg 48:475

30. Sharma GURK, O'Connell DC, Wheeler HB, Belko JS, Sasahara AA (1974) Deep venous thrombosis as a diagnostic clue to pulmonary embolism. Am J Cardiol 33:170

31. Swenson EW, Fuley TN, Guzman SV (1961) Unilateral hypoventilation in man during temporary occlusion of one pulmonary artery. J Clin Invest 40:828

32. Tow DE, Wagner HN Jr (1967) Recovery of pulmonary arterial blood flow in patients with pulmonary embolism. N Engl J Med 276:1053

33. Vaage J (1976) Vagal reflexes in the bronchoconstriction occurring after induced intravascular platelet aggregation. Acta Physiol Scand 97:94

34. Walker WE, Rosenthal M, Snodgrass PJ, Amador E (1961) A triad for the diagnosis of pulmonary embolism and infarction. JAMA 178:8

35. Winterbauer RH, Elfenbein IB, Ball WC Jr (1968) Incidence and clinical significance of tumour embolization to the lungs. Am J Med 45:271

Chapter 14

Hypertensive Crises

John H. Tinker

Critically ill patients can become severely hypertensive—often to their detriment. In this chapter, we are not particularly concerned with the precise causes of these hypertensive crises, but rather with their acute therapy. Here, perhaps contrary to the best principles of general medicine, we are interested in getting the blood pressure under control rapidly and safely. The pharmacology (and toxicology) of various acutely-used vasodilator drugs will be discussed with emphasis on sodium nitroprusside (SNP) because it is widely used and is immediately effective but not clinically easy to use, and because of the possible problems of cyanide (CN) toxicity [60]. Although other drugs, such as nitroglycerine and phentolamine, may possess theoretical advantages over SNP in certain circumstances, in fact they are not as widely employed in critical care situations, probably because they are less effective in achieving the immediate objective, namely taking and keeping control of a severely elevated blood pressure.

Whether 'controlling' a severely elevated arterial pressure makes sense is another matter. If, for example, a severely elevated intracranial pressure has driven up the arterial pressure (Cushing reflex), obviously therapy must then be directed at the cause. If, on the other hand, a severely vasoconstricted patient with a relatively low cardiac output is hypertensive, the restoration of normal vascular tension may immediately result in better vital organ perfusion.

A common hypertensive crisis in critically ill patients occurs following cardiac surgery during the period of emergence from anesthesia. As the anesthetic agent 'wears off,' even if the patient is sedated with analgesic and hypnotic agents, arterial pressure can increase to alarming levels. This situation is most likely after aortic valve replacement. Perhaps the thickened ventricle, which pumped so valiantly against a stenotic valve so recently in the past, is now 'feeling its oats.' A more rational explanation is that aortic pressure receptors have been disrupted by the surgery, and are not permitting the brain as accurate a 'picture' of arterial pressure as in normal circumstances. This is illustrative of a hypertensive crisis in which the etiology is clouded. In any event, this patient, often with a systolic blood pressure >200 mmHg, is truly in crisis, for the aortic suture line may become compromised. Coronary artery bypass surgery is also often associated with severe postoperative hypertensive crises. Again the root area of the aorta has been operated upon, and again, tenuous suture lines are at risk. In this patient, the greatly increased O_2 demand is also deleterious, for the heart cannot be expected to have been entirely 'revascularized' by this procedure.

These postoperative hypertensive crises may be accompanied by tachycardia, but if this is not present during the hypertension, acute lowering of the blood pressure can result in a reflex tachycardia. Loeb et al. [33] have clearly shown in patients with coronary artery disease that tachycardia is considerably more dangerous than hypertension with respect to the conversion of a potentially to an actually ischemic myocardial area. The ever-increasing number of coronary artery bypass operations has now made this form of hypertensive crisis probably the most common seen in critical care units, at least in the United States. These patients do need their pressures controlled, but their heart rates must also be carefully controlled, as will be discussed.

Other hypertensive crises, such as malignant hypertension, thyroid storm, eclampsia, and the like, are now rare, because of improved antihypertensive medication, renal angiography, subsequent renal artery reconstruction surgery, and better understanding of thyrotoxicosis and eclampsia.

Sodium nitroprusside

Historical aspects

Sodium nitroprusside (SNP) (Fig. 14.1) was probably known to Claude Bernard, and was studied in animals as early as 1886 [22]. Charles Johnson [24] injected the substance, also known as sodium nitroferricyanide, into three humans in 1929. One of these was a hypertensive patient, and Johnson reported that relief of the hypertension lasted approximately 2 h. Irvine

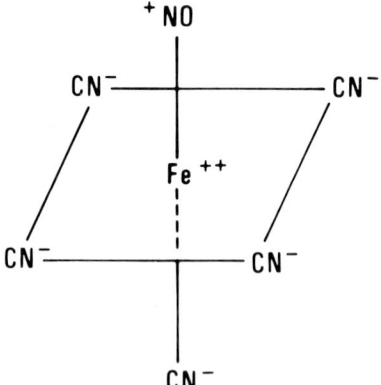

Fig. 14.1. The iron coordination complex of sodium nitroprusside. From Tinker JH, Michenfelder JD: *Anesthesiology* 45:341, 1976, by permission.

Page and his associates conducted the first clinical trials of SNP in the early 1950s [46, 47]. They tried it as an oral medication with no success, but also gave it IV, and reported excellent success in controlling malignant hypertension unmanageable by conventional means. By 1959, SNP was a recognized, if 'last ditch' therapy for severe hypertensive crises [18]. The drug was first used to produce deliberate hypotension during surgery in 1962 [40] and first tried as an 'afterload reducer' to treat congestive heart failure in 1972 [19]. In the United States, Federal Food and Drug Administration approval of this substance for any human usage did not come until 1974, and then only for hypertensive crises. Cyanide toxicity was reported by the earliest investigators [22, 24], who noted that the livers of the animals smelt of 'bitter almond.'

Pharmacology and mechanism of action

Few would dispute that SNP is a generalized vasodilator, roughly equally effective on the arterial and venous circulations [54]. This sharply contrasts with the propensity of nitroglycerin (TNG) to dilate the venous capacitance vessels, and explains why many clinicians use SNP when severe arterial hypertension is present. Nitroglycerin reduces arterial pressure, in part at least, by a 'back door' method, namely venous capacitance vessel dilatation leading to a decrease in right and then left ventricular preload, in the hope that decreased LV output will result. Clinicians who have tried both usually resort to SNP when the immediate objective is to decrease rapidly a severely elevated arterial pressure.

Needleman et al. [42] have extensively studied SNP's mechanism of action, along with that of a number of other vasodilators. SNP's cell membrane receptor is separate from that for TNG or isoproterenol, and contains SH groups. Apparently, although there are different cell surface receptors, there is a common intermediary vasodilator mechanism. How this works to induce vascular smooth muscle relaxation is unknown.

Tachyphylaxis is of importance with respect to these vasodilator drugs not only because in critical care relatively long-term usage is required, but also because, in the case of SNP, tachyphylaxis leads to dosage levels that can be associated with CN toxicity. Some earlier reports suggested that SNP never involves problems of tachyphylaxis. It is true that, compared with the effect of the ganglionic blocker trimethaphan, for example, SNP tachyphylaxis develops slowly. Nonetheless, as the hours, even days, go by, SNP dosage requirements often increase to the point where the likelihood of CN toxicity precludes further usage of the drug. Of all the currently used IV vasodilators, it is probable that the slowest development of tachyphylaxis is seen with SNP.

Metabolism and CN toxicity

Hermann, in 1886, observed the odor of bitter almond in livers of animals treated with SNP and concluded that they had died of CN toxicity [22]. Johnson, in 1929, was certain that SNP would not lead to CN toxicity if used judiciously [24]. Page et al. [47] were also convinced of the safety of the drug with regard to CN toxicity. Davies et al., in 1975, reported on three patients in whom SNP was employed for deliberate intraoperative hypotension [9, 10]. Very large (5–10 mg/kg) doses were required over relatively short time periods (1–5 h), presumably due to initial resistance to SNP rather than tachyphylaxis. When SNP was discontinued, the blood pressure did not rapidly return to normal, and severe metabolic acidosis was noted. Cardiac arrest without successful resus-

citation occurred in one patient [9]. The impossibility of resuscitating such a patient was, in retrospect, a hallmark of CN toxicity.

Figure 14.2 depicts the concept of SNP metabolism of Smith and Kruszyna [57]: oxyhemoglobin donates an electron to SNP without enzyme catalysis, producing an unstable nitroprusside radical that dissociates into five free CN^- ions. The fate of the iron-nitroso (^-NO) group is unknown. One of the free CN^- ions joins the methemoglobin produced via the above electron donation, to become cyanmethemoglobin. The remaining four CN^- groups are eventually detoxified into thiocyanate (SCN). This reaction requires a liver (and kidney?) enzyme, a sulfuryl transferase termed rhodanese, and a sulfur donor, often thiosulfate (SSO_4^-) [31]. There is ample evidence that rhodanese is present in abundance, and that sulfur donor availability limits the rate of CN detoxification [36, 37].

The resultant compound, SCN, is much less, and differently, toxic than CN. It enters the chloride pool and is thus distributed in both extra- and intravascular water and is *not* rapidly excreted, having a half-life of approximately 12 days [56]. SCN was tried as an oral antihypertensive agent in the early 1950s [46, 47], and SCN toxicity (a neurotoxic syndrome)

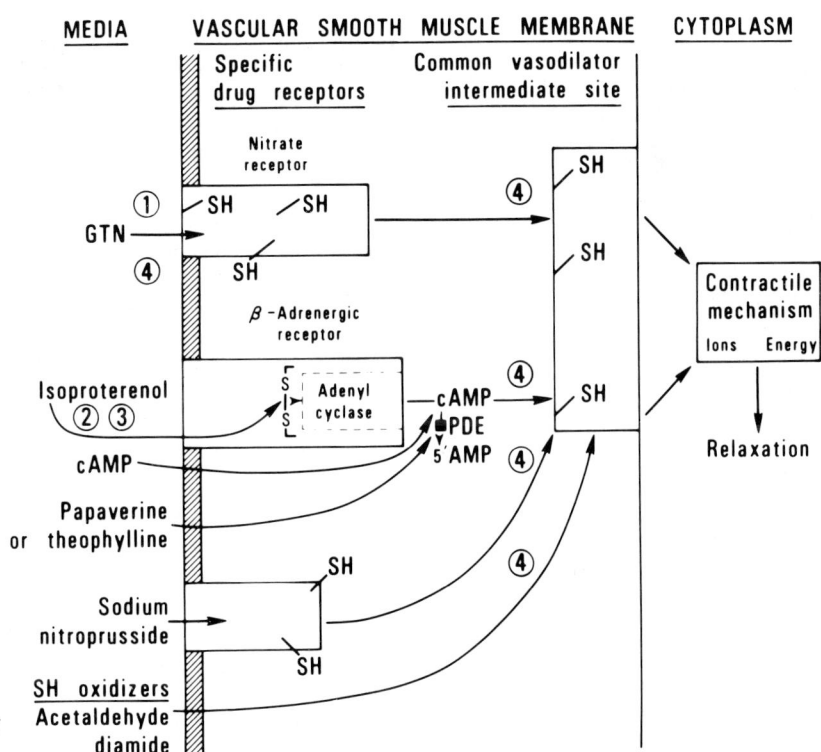

Fig. 14.2. The concept of nitroprusside breakdown of Smith and Kruszyna [57]. From Tinker JH, Michenfelder JD: *Anesthesiology* 45:345, 1976, by permission.

apparently occurred when serum SCN levels reached 10 mg/dl [19]. This serum level somehow found its way into the nitroprusside literature and it is commonly believed that SCN levels (easy to measure) can be used to monitor chronic SNP usage, to warn against impending CN toxicity. In fact, when CN is the generator of SCN, in the absence of exogenously administered sulfur donor, CN toxicity due to cytochrome oxidase blockage by CN supervenes long before SCN levels reach 10 mg/dl [36, 37, 63–65]. This is the situation during SNP administration. It is now quite clear that SCN blood levels reflect not only blood CN levels, but also the availability of sulfur donor, and are thus not adequate monitors of CN toxicity.

We have conducted 48-h intensive care studies of SNP-induced CN toxicity in dogs [37, 62]. When SNP was given at 0.5 mg.kg^{-1}.h^{-1} (~8 μg.kg^{-1}.min^{-1}), blood CN levels increased modestly and then leveled off; all dogs survived 48 h. At SNP doses of 0.75 and 1.0 mg.kg^{-1}.h^{-1} all dogs died at 30–36 h, with near-linear increases in blood CN, metabolic acidosis, and increases in mixed venous PO$_2$. If exogenous sulfur donor (thiosulfate: 6 mg.kg^{-1}.h^{-1}) was given along with SNP at the previously toxic dose of 1.0 mg.kg^{-1}.h^{-1}, the dogs could be protected against CN toxicity. SCN levels were highest in these animals, despite survival, indicating that monitoring SCN levels is not adequate protection against CN toxicity. The development of metabolic acidosis seemed the best early warning of CN toxicity. These dosage 'limits' of 0.5 mg.kg^{-1}.h^{-1} [37] are supported by other studies [64, 65] and by the development of CN toxicity in a patient receiving SNP chronically, who developed tachyphylaxis after 8 days of therapy. CN toxicity did not develop until the SNP dose had increased above 0.5 mg.kg^{-1}.h^{-1} [37].

Patients receiving SNP infusions can be protected against CN toxicity very simply by first never permitting a dose of over 0.5 mg.kg^{-1}.h^{-1}. Secondly, if the dose has increased to near these levels, careful acid-base status determinations must be made frequently. The development of a metabolic acidosis in a patient receiving SNP at or near 0.5 mg.kg^{-1}.h^{-1} is CN toxicity until proven otherwise, and the drug should probably be stopped. Lowering the dosage may suffice if, for example, propranolol can be added. However, CN toxicity to the point of metabolic acidosis is a serious, late manifestation—cytochrome oxidase may be largely inactivated. Of course the critically ill patient receiving SNP may well develop metabolic aci-

dosis for any of numerous other reasons, but the SNP must be first considered the culprit.

Often, patients are given SNP in situations where cardiac output is low and peripheral resistance low; oliguria or anuria may be present or supervene. What should be done about the dose of SNP that will presumably be required to produce the desired vasodilation? We have recently studied this question in anuric dogs [62], and found them to be surprisingly more resistant to SNP-induced CN toxicity, presumably due to increased sulfur donor availability due to excretory failure. We believe that the SNP dose does not need to be arbitrarily decreased just because a patient has become oliguric or anuric [62].

Many patients with cardiac lesions are given SNP. Because the heart extracts such a high percentage of delivered O$_2$, we were concerned that that organ might be especially sensitive to SNP-induced CN toxicity [61]. In fact, EEG isoelectricity indicative of cerebral CN toxicity occurred at blood CN levels significantly lower than those associated with the first decrease in overall myocardial O$_2$ consumption. We do not believe that CN derived from SNP is a special problem with respect to the myocardium [61].

The vitamin B$_{12}$–nitroprusside controversy

Vitamin B$_{12}$ is cyanocobalamine, and an analog of this compound, hydroxycobalamine, can exchange its hydroxy group for a CN group. The cyan derivative is less protein-bound and thus more easily excreted. Hydroxycobalamine has thus been advocated as an antidote for CN toxicity and as an adjunct to prevent CN toxicity during SNP administration [41, 52, 63]. The compound is expensive, turns sclerae of experimental animals pink [52] and is not widely available. In addition, mole-for-mole amounts are required, making large doses (in milligrams) necessary. Thiosulfate, on the other hand, is inexpensive, generally available in hospital pharmacies, and quite nontoxic. It does result in an osmotic diuresis when given in excess. A. Ivankovich (personal communication) has tested hydroxycobalamine, thiosulfate, sodium nitrite plus thiosulfate, and cysteine as antidotes for CN poisoning, and found thiosulfate alone to be superior in a dog model.

CN poisoning and its treatment

Assuming that the SNP dose has strayed above 0.5 mg.kg^{-1}.h^{-1}, and that a metabolic acidosis is present, the SNP should be stopped. If hemodynamics are adequate, thiosulfate 150 mg/kg should be administered IV. This can be repeated in 10–15 min. Reversal of metabolic acidosis indicates treatment efficacy, and is obscured by administration of bicarbonate. Nonetheless, we would simultaneously give appropriate bicarbonate.

If CN toxicity has progressed to severe metabolic acidosis (base deficit > -15 mmol/liter), cardiac arrest is possible and resuscitation will be difficult. In this case, 5 mg sodium nitrite/kg IV or an ampule of amyl nitrite can be administered before the thiosulfate to convert some hemoglobin into methemoglobin, which will then attract CN to form cyanmethemoglobin. The nitrites are *not* benign hemodynamically and must be slowly (over 5 min) administered. It must be emphasized that CN toxicity during chronic SNP use, while an ever-present possibility, is very unlikely in any event, and has not been reported at all when SNP dosages have not exceeded 0.5 mg.kg^{-1}.h^{-1} [19, 61].

Resistance and tachyphylaxis

Nitroprusside is less likely than trimethaphan to be associated with early tachyphylaxis, but this is most certainly possible, especially after many days of antihypertensive therapy. In one case [37], the dose required to keep arterial pressure between narrow limits remained virtually unchanged for 7 days. On the 8th day, the SNP dosage requirement increased in an exponential fashion, rapidly achieving levels greater than 0.5 mg.kg^{-1}.h^{-1}, with CN toxicity and death shortly thereafter. Mechanisms of tachyphylaxis are rarely understood for any drug, and SNP is no exception. Grayling et al. [20] have suggested that build-up of CN may render vascular smooth muscle less sensitive to SNP vasodilation; however, this study was performed in vitro, with relatively high concentrations of CN.

Some patients, often younger individuals, demonstrate initial resistance to SNP [9, 10, 37]. These are obviously at earliest risk for CN toxicity. The dog often requires relatively high dosages of SNP to produce a given degree of vasodilation and thus appears resistant in human terms [36]. This makes the dog a reasonable model to study SNP CN toxicity, because CN release from SNP, which does not require enzymatic catalysis [57] proceeds apace in that species [36]. There are two human conditions, namely Leber's optic atrophy and tobacco amblyopia, which are associated with abnormally high blood CN levels [67]. This indicates that CN metabolism can be abnormal in some individuals (CN is a dietary residue), but offers little explanation for resistance or tachyphylaxis to SNP. These two conditions are often listed as contraindications for SNP use, despite the absence of reports of SNP having been used in those situations.

Contraindications

SNP releases CN which is detoxified by the liver. From this, some workers have concluded that SNP is contraindicated in hepatic failure [21]. There is no evidence that this is true; indeed, rhodanese is not likely to be the limiting factor in CN detoxification. There is one report [44] that suggested that chronic SNP might lead to hypothyroidism. Vitamin B$_{12}$ levels do decrease during SNP therapy, leading to the speculation that relatively chronic SNP therapy might seriously deplete B$_{12}$ stores [15]. Still, the drug is not likely to be employed over long enough periods for the implied threat of pernicious anemia to be serious. As noted above, anuria seems, if anything, to enhance CN metabolism into SCN, although this might eventually result in excessive SCN build-up and the syndrome of SCN neurotoxicity [62].

Clinical use

The potency and efficacy of this vasodilator make the use of a calibrated drug infusion device mandatory. The drug is usually administered in a solution containing 200 mg/1000 ml. The solution has to be protected against breakdown by light. This breakdown of SNP does *not* involve the release of CN [48, 60]. In many ICUs SNP solutions are changed every 4 h, for the above reason; this practice is probably overcautious.

Often, control of blood pressure can be achieved with <1.5 μg SNP/kg^{-1}.min^{-1}, which is well below the toxic range. With SNP, especially initially, 'roller coaster' blood pressure is possible until experience is gained in SNP usage. If blood pressure decreases too far, it is best merely to turn the SNP down, or off, and wait. A pressor agent should not be given, since it would arrive at about the same time as SNP's effect is diminishing, resulting in a large overshoot.

A good method of achieving initial control is to start with a relatively large SNP dose, about 3 μg. kg^{-1}. min^{-1}. This dose should be continued until the very first tendency for the arterial pressure to decrease is noted. When the SNP dose should be reduced very markedly to about 0.25 μg. kg^{-1}. min^{-1}. The pressure will continue to fall for a few minutes and, just as it begins an upward tendency again, the SNP dose should be increased to almost but not quite the same level as previously, to about 2.7 μg. kg^{-1}. min^{-1}. If this 'bracketing the target' method of wide initial swings in the dosage administered by the drug pump is used, the resultant blood pressure tracing will record a smooth steady decline. If, on the other hand, the therapist opts for more sedate initial adjustments in SNP dose, the familiar roller coaster blood pressure will result. In either case, the dose required to keep the arterial pressure at the desired level should be achievable within 30 min or less of starting the drug.

Tachycardia may develop in response to acutely decreasing arterial pressure with any agent. This is especially undesirable in patients with coronary artery disease [33] because tachycardia increases myocardial O_2 demand while decreasing diastolic coronary perfusion time. Whether or not tachycardia will develop depends on the degree of sedation/anesthesia and extent of cardiac illness. Patients in severe congestive failure are not necessarily capable of increasing their heart rates in response to afterload reduction therapy [6].

The development of tachycardia may also oppose the antihypertensive therapy, and may increase gradually over several hours or days, necessitating gradual increases in vasodilator dose, with possible CN toxicity. We would treat this tachycardia with beta-adrenergic blockade if possible, rather than by increasing the dosage of SNP to merely treat the increasing hypertension. Heavy sedation of such a critically ill patient is often much less satisfactory than beta blockade in terms of treating this tachycardia. Often the postoperative aortic valve replacement patient is in this category. We see no reason why intermittent IV boluses of propranolol cannot be administered by nurses whenever heart rates increase to undesirable levels while the patient is also receiving SNP. These boluses might need to be as small as 0.5 mg propranolol at least initially, until a response tendency is noted. The addition of beta blockade to SNP-induced generalized vasodilatation has one further very significant benefit in addition to controlling tachycardia; namely it

allows the continuation of small SNP doses and the postponement of the time when SNP will need to be discontinued due to tachyphylaxis.

Nitroglycerine vs nitroprusside

Nitroglycerine (TNG) obviously does not release CN, and has been widely used as an IV vasodilator. In the United States, Food and Drug Administration approval has not yet been issued, and thus lack of a commercial preparation hinders its widespread adoption. TNG is a volatile substance, which would rather adhere to many types of glass and plastic surfaces than remain dissolved in aqueous solutions. Thus care must be taken in its pharmaceutical preparation, to ensure that the drug is in fact being administered.

TNG is more a venodilator than a generalized vasodilator, differing substantially from SNP in this regard. If the immediate objective is to decrease arterial blood pressure, to do so with a capacitance vessel dilator may prove difficult. Dilating capacitance vessels decreases preload, resulting in reductions of first right and then left ventricular outputs. This may be rapidly followed by reflex attempts at vasoconstriction, and those arterial side effects may not be effectively blocked by TNG. Translating this into practical terms, there is commonly a clinical impression that TNG is not as effective as SNP when the objective is rapid control of severely hypertensive arterial pressure. Conversely, TNG may be preferable if LV preload reduction is desired, e.g., during acute failure secondary to myocardial infarction. There is some controversy as to whether these two agents have similar or disparate effects on the coronary circulation, especially during acute myocardial ischemia. Chiariello et al. [7], in 1976, compared TNG with SNP in patients with AMI, and in dogs following coronary ligation. Administration of each drug until similar reductions were obtained in both mean arterial and pulmonary capillary wedge pressure resulted in significant improvement of myocardial ST segment 'maps' with TNG (i.e., reduction of potential infarct size), whereas these same ST segments worsened considerably with SNP. Chiariello et al. concluded that somehow SNP directed coronary flow away from the ischemic myocardial zone, whilst TNG had the opposite effect. This report and others [34] gave rise to concern over the use of SNP for the treatment of postoperative hypertensive crises in patients with coronary artery disease, and over the use of SNP to treat LV failure in patients with AMI.

By contrast, Kerber et al. [26] have more recently reported no differences between TNG and SNP in several regional perfusion and functional parameters in dogs during acute myocardial ischemia. Their studies demonstrated no differences between TNG and SNP, when they were used to decrease mean arterial pressure by either 7% or 15% in regional ventricular wall systolic: diastolic thickness ratios, regional wall stress reductions, or regional myocardial perfusion [27]. Their studies also did not show any promising benefit of afterload reduction in the 'treatment' of acute myocardial ischemia. Use of vasodilators to reduce preload when myocardial ischemia is so severe as to have resulted in congestive failure *is* efficacious, however. In this case, TNG seems theoretically superior to nitroprusside. Nonetheless SNP is a mainstay drug in many CCUs.

Other agents for treatment of hypertensive crises

There are many other short-acting antihypertensive agents that can be employed during hypertensive crises. The ganglionic blocking agents are a large class of agents, lately reduced by attrition to trimethaphan. This agent can dramatically reduce arterial pressure in a crisis, and possesses no specific toxicity other than the side-effects expected from ganglionic blockade. It is a problematic drug, however, in that tachyphylaxis often rapidly supervenes. Trimethaphan is the agent to which many would turn if nitroprusside became unsuitable due to the threat of CN toxicity. The ganglionic blocking agents have been recently reviewed [27, 38, 55].

Diazoxide [49, 59] is largely an arteriolar dilator, having a direct action. Its mechanism of action, although possibly related to calcium antagonism, is not known. A bolus injection of 5 mg/kg IV will often rapidly alleviate an hypertensive crisis situation, but reflex tachycardia will cause a return toward the former problems in 20–30 min. A second dose often lasts somewhat longer. As usual, propranolol potentiates activity and can be used to prevent the reflex tachycardia. The problem with diazoxide is that it cannot be administered in a continuous infusion, and the intermittent bolus technique may not result in as smooth control of arterial pressure as desired.

There are many alpha-adrenergic blocking agents, but the one of interest in a discussion of hypertensive crises is phentolamine. The degree of vasodilatation obtained with phentolamine in any particular vascular bed is dependent on the prior regional degree of vasoconstriction; thus the drug is somewhat less predictable in its actions than is nitroprusside. Phentolamine also apparently has some beta-stimulating capacity, so that the tachycardia resulting may be worse than would be expected from reflexes alone. Logically, phentolamine plus propranolol should be ideally suited for the pre- and intraoperative therapy of hypertensive crises associated with pheochromocytoma. Actually nitroprusside may be easier to use intraoperatively as a continuous infusion. Alpha-adrenergic blocking agents have been recently reviewed by El-Etr and Glisson [14].

Hydralazine is a direct arteriolar vasodilator, the mechanism of action of which is again unknown. In contrast to nitroprusside and TNG, hydralazine has little effect on capacitance vessels. Circulatory reflexes are entirely unimpaired; hence tachycardia and compensatory increases in venous return are likely. Concurrent propranolol administration can make the drug a valuable addition to a critical care armamentarium. As is true with other antihypertensives, renin activity increases during the use of hydralazine, gradually opposing its effects. Intravenous hydralazine takes effect in 15 min, and may be effective for 3–4 hours, especially if propranolol is used to control the tachycardia. Once again, hydralazine is not our first-choice drug in a severe hypertensive crisis, but after several days of nitroprusside therapy, if the causative factors for the hypertensive crisis are still present, alternative therapy must be sought [1, 53].

Newer agents such as the direct vasodilating agents prazosin [4, 13, 16, 23, 29, 58] and minoxidil [2, 8, 39, 45]; alternative beta-adrenergic blocking agents such as timolol [3, 25] and labetalol [11, 35, 50]; anti-renin agents such as saralasin [12]; centrally acting antihypertensive drugs like clonidine [32, 43, 66]; calcium antagonists such as nifedipine [5, 30, 51] are outside the scope of this chapter and are not yet in general usage for IV therapy of hypertensive crises in critically ill patients. The interested reader is referred to the recent references listed for each of these agents.

References

1. Albrecht RF, Toyooka ET, Polk SLH, et al (1978) Hydralazine therapy for hypertension during the anesthetic and postanesthesia periods. Little Brown, Boston, pp 299–312 (Int Anesth Clin 16/2)
2. Andersson O, Sivertsson R (1979) Minoxidil in refractory hypertension. Acta Med Scand 205:213–219
3. Aronow WS, Van Herick R, Greenfield R, et al (1978) Effect of timolol plus hydrochloro-thiazide plus hydralazine on essential hypertension. Circulation 57:1017–1021
4. Aronow WS, Lurie M, Turbow M, et al (1979) Effect of prazocin vs. placebo on chronic left ventricular heart failure. Circulation 59:344–350
5. Bartorelli C, Magrini F, Moruzzi P, et al (1978) Hemodynamic effects of a calcium antagonistic agent (nifedipine) in hypertension. Clin Sci Mol Med [Suppl] 55:291s–292s
6. Chatterjee K, Parmley WW, Ganz W, et al (1973) Hemodynamic and metabolic responses to vasodilator therapy in acute myocardial infarction. Circulation 48:1183–1193
7. Chiariello M, Gold HK, Leinback RC, et al (1976) Comparison between the effects of nitroprusside and nitroglycerin on ischemic injury during acute myocardial infarction. Circulation 53:766
8. Compese JM, Stein D, DeQuattro V (1979) Treatment of severe hypertension with minoxidil: Advantages and limitations. J Clin Pharmacol 19:231–241
9. Davies DW, Kadar D, Steward DJ, et al (1975) A sudden death associated with the use of sodium nitroprusside for induction of hypotension during anesthesia. Can Anaesth Soc J 22:547–552
10. Davies DW, Greiss L, Steward DJ, et al (1975b) Sodium nitroprusside in children: Observations on metabolism during normal and abnormal responses. Can Anaesth Soc J 22:553–560
11. Dawson A, Johnson BF, Smith IK, et al (1979) A comparison of the effects of labetalol, bendrofluazide and their combination in hypertension. Br J Clin Pharmacol 8:149–154
12. Delaney TJ, Miller ED (1979) Blood flow alteration induced by saralasin on SNP. Anesthesiology [Suppl] 51:S73
13. Desch CE, Magorien RD, Triffon DW, et al (1979) Development of pharmacodynamic tolerance to prazocin in congestive heart failure. Am J Cardiol 44:1178–1182
14. El-Etr A, Glisson SN (1978) Alpha-adrenergic blocking agents. Little Brown, Boston, pp 239–259 (Int Anesth Clin, vol 16/2)
15. Fahmy NH (1980) Vitamin B_{12} levels decrease during sodium nitroprusside administration. Proc Cong Int Anesth Res Soc
16. Fauchald P, Helgeland A (1979) Treatment of hypertension with prazocin. An open study in general practice. Acta Med Scand [Suppl] pp 141–142
17. Franciosa JA, Guiha NH, Limas CJ, et al (1972) Improved left ventricular function during nitroprusside infusion in acute myocardial infarction. Lancet I:650–654
18. Gifford RW (1959) Current practices in general medicine. 7. Treatment of hypertensive emergencies including use of sodium nitroprusside. Proc Mayo Clin 34:387–394
19. Goodman LS, Gilman A (1975) The pharmacological basis of therapeutics, 5th edn. MacMillan, New York, pp 715–717
20. Grayling GW, Miller ED, Peach MJ (1978) Sodium cyanide antagonism of the vasodilator action of sodium nitroprusside in the isolated rabbit aortic strip. Anesthesiology 49:21–24
21. Greiss L, Tremblay NAG, Davies DW (1976) The toxicity of sodium nitroprusside. Can Anaesth Soc J 23:480–486
22. Hermann L (1886) Ueber die Wirkung des Nitroprussidnatriums. Arch Ges Physiol 39:419–424
23. Hua AS, Myers JB, Kincaid-Smith P (1978) Studies with prazosin—a new effective antihyypertensive agent. Med J Aust 1:45–48
24. Johnson CC (1929) The actions and toxicity of sodium nitroprusside. Arch Int Pharmacodyn Ther 35:489–496
25. Karatzas NB, Papazchos G, Clouva P, et al (1979) Timolol and bendroflumethiazide in the treatment of hypertension. J Int Med Res 7:215–220
26. Kerber RE, Martins JB, Marcus ML (1979) Effect of acute ischemia, nitroglycerin and nitroprusside on regional myocardial thickening, stress and perfusion. Circulation 60:121
27. Klowden AJ, Ivankovich AD, Miletich DJ (1978) Ganglionic blocking drugs, general considerations and metabolism. Little Brown, Boston, pp 113–150 (Int Anesth Clin, vol 16/2)
28. Koch-Weser J, Graham RM, Pettinger WA (1979) Drug therapy, Prazocin. N Engl J Med 300:232–236
29. Kuokkanen K, Mattila MJ (1979) Antihypertensive effect of prazocin in combination with methyldopa, chlonidine, or propranolol. Ann Clin Res 11:18–24
30. Kuwajima I, Ueda K, Kamata C, et al (1978) A study of the effects of nifedipine in hypertensive crises and severe hypertension. Jpn Heart J 19:455–467
31. Lang K (1933) Die Rhodanbildung im Tierkörper. Biochem Z 259:243–256
32. Lilja M, Jounela AJ, Juustila H, et al (1979) Antihypertensive effects of clonidine. Clin Pharmacol Ther 25:864–869
33. Loeb HS Sandje A, Croke RP, et al (1978) Effects of pharmacologically-induced hypertension on myocardial ischemia and coronary hemodynamics in patients with fixed coronary obstruction. Circulation 57:41–46
34. Mann T, Cohn PF, Holman LB, et al (1978) Effect of nitroprusside on regional myocardial blood flow in coronary artery disease. Results in 25 patients and comparison with nitroglycerin. Circulation 57:732–738
35. McGrath BP, Matthews PG, Walter NM, et al (1978) Emergency treatment of severe hypertension with intravenous labetalol. Med J Aust 2:410–411
36. Michenfelder JD (1977) Cyanide release from sodium nitroprusside in the dog. Anesthesiology 46:196–201
37. Michenfelder JD, Tinker JH (1977) Cyanide toxicity and thiosulfate protection during chronic administration of sodium nitroprusside in the dog: Correlation with human case. Anesthesiology 47:411–448
38. Miletich DJ, Ivankovich AD (1978) Cardiovascular effects of ganglionic blocking drugs. Little Brown, Boston, pp 151–170 (Int Anesth Clin, vol 16/2)
39. Mitchell HC, Pettinger WA (1978) Long-term treatment of refractory hypertensive patients with minoxidil. JAMA 239:2131–2138
40. Moraca PP, Bitte EM, Hale DE, et al (1962) Clinical evaluation of sodium nitroprusside as a hypotensive agent. Anesthesiology 23:193–199
41. Mushett CW, Kelley KL, Boxer GE, et al (1952) Antidotal efficacy of vitamin B_{12a} (Hydroxocobalamine) in experimental cyanide poisoning. Proc Soc Exp Biol Med 81:234–237
42. Needleman P, Jakschik B, Johnson EM (1973) Sulfhydryl requirement for relaxation of vascular smooth muscle. J Pharmacol Exp Ther 187:324–331

43. Niarchos AP (1978) Evaluation of intravenous clonidine for hypertensive emergencies. J Clin Pharmacol 18:220–228

44. Nourok DS, Glassock RJ, Solomon DH, et al (1964) Hypothyroidism following prolonged sodium nitroprusside therapy. Am J Med Sci 248:129–138

45. Onesti G, Fernandes J (1978) Recent acquisitions in antihypertensive therapy, clonidine, minoxidil, and prazocin. Cardiovasc Clin 9:273–289

46. Page IH (1951) Treatment of essential and malignant hypertension. JAMA 147:1311–1318

47. Page IH, Corcoran AC, Dustan HP, et al (1955) Cardiovascular actions of sodium nitroprusside in animals and hypertensive patients. Circulation 11:188–198

48. Palmer RF, Lasseter KD (1975) Sodium nitroprusside. N Engl J Med 293:294–297

49. Paulissian R (1978) Diazoxide. Little Brown, Boston, pp 201–231 (Int Anesth Clin, vol 16/2)

50. Pearson RM, Havard CW (1978) Intravenous labetalol in hypertensive patients given by fast and slow injection. Br J Clin Pharmacol 5:401–405

51. Pederson OL, Mikkelson E, Christensen NJ, et al (1979) Effect of nifedipine on plasma renin, aldosterone and catecholamines in arterial hypertension. Eur J Clin Pharmacol 15:235–240

52. Posner MA, Tobey RA, McElroy H (1976) Hydroxocobalamine therapy of cyanide intoxication in guinea pigs. Anesthesiology 44:157–160

53. Ram CV, Kaplan NM (1979) Alpha receptor blocking drugs in the treatment of hypertension. Curr Probl Cardiol 3:1–53

54. Rowe GG, Henderson RH (1974) Systemic and coronary hemodynamic effects of sodium nitroprusside. Am Heart J 87:83–87

55. Salem MR (1978) Therapeutic uses of ganglionic blocking drugs. Little Brown, Boston, pp 171–200 (Int Anesth Clinics, vol 16/2)

56. Smith RP (1973) Cyanate and thiocyanate: Acute toxicity. Proc Soc Exp Biol Med 142:1041–1044

57. Smith RP, Kruszyna H (1974) Nitroprusside produces cyanide poisoning via a reaction with hemoglobin. J Pharmacol Exp Ther 191:557–563

58. Stokes GS, Frost GW, Graham RM, et al (1979) Indoramin and prazocin as adjuncts to beta adrenoceptor blockade in hypertension. Clin Pharmacol Ther 25:783–789

59. Thien TA, Huysmans FT, Gerlag PG, et al (1979) Diazoxide infusion in severe hypertension and hypertensive crisis. Clin Pharmacol Ther 25:795–799

60. Tinker JH, Michenfelder JD (1976) Sodium nitroprusside: Pharmacology, toxicology, and therapeutics. Anesthesiology 45:340–354

61. Tinker JH, Michenfelder JD (1978) Cardiac cyanide toxicity induced by nitroprusside in the dog: Potential for reversal. Anesthesiology 49:109–116

62. Tinker JH, Michenfelder JD (1980) Increased resistance to nitroprusside-induced cyanide toxicity in anuric dogs. Anesthesiology 52:40–47

63. Vesey CJ, Cole PV, Linnell JC, et al (1974) Some metabolic effects of sodium nitroprusside in man. Br Med J ii:140–142

64. Vesey CJ, Cole PV, Simpson PJ (1976) Cyanide and thiocyanate concentrations following sodium nitroprusside infusion in man. Br J Anaesth 48:651–654

65. Vesey CJ, Cole PV, Simpson PJ (1977) Nitroprusside and cyanide (correspondence). Br J Anaesth 49:395

66. Whitsett TL, Chrysant SG, Dillard BL, et al (1978) Abrupt cessation of clonidine administration. Am J Cardiol 41:1285–1290

67. Wilson L (1965) Leber's optic atrophy: A possible defect of cyanide metabolism. Clin Sci 29:505–515

Chapter 15

The Management of Unstable Angina Pectoris

P. G. Hugenholtz, H. R. Michels, K. Balakumaran,
M. Haalebos, and P. W. Serruys

Of all the acute coronary events seen in the ICU, such as arrhythmias, myocardial infarction, and cardiogenic shock, the patient with unstable angina progressing to myocardial infarction has entered more and more into the limelight, particularly now that newer drugs (e.g., beta blockers and Ca antagonists) and surgical procedures (such as balloon pump support and early revascularization) have become available to modify the course of events.

Mortality and prognosis in ischaemic heart disease

Unstable angina pectoris is conceptually midway between stable angina pectoris and acute myocardial infarction (AMI). At the ends of this spectrum are asymptomatic myocardial ischaemia and sudden ischaemic cardiac death. When the condition is viewed as a continuum, one can readily accept that the prognosis for survival in ischaemic heart disease deteriorates as one moves from asymptomatic disease towards sudden death. Thus, although it is increasingly clear that the syndrome of sudden ischaemic cardiac 'death' can be reversed [3, 32] the chance of survival, even with prompt and trained assistance, is still only in the order of

14%–18%, with a 1-year mortality rate, in survivors, of 30% [32, 49]. Acute myocardial infarction has a somewhat better prognosis, 50%–60% [7, 40] surviving the acute attack, with a further 6%–10% death rate in the first year thereafter [29, 36, 40].

In angina pectoris, early studies [8, 52, 60] have revealed a yearly mortality ranging from 2.5% [60] to around 12% [52]. The Framingham study showed an annual mortality rate of 5% after 1 to 10-year follow-up [30]. Subsequent studies [12, 13, 44, 53] in patients with proven coronary sclerosis yielded an annual mortality varying between 5.5% [12] and 15% [13], depending on the degree of coronary artery disease and the extent of left ventricular (LV) dysfunction.

The most puzzling aspect in this context is the phenomenon of unstable angina pectoris and impending, often unrecognized, myocardial infarction [36]. Follow-up studies in unstable angina pectoris have yielded a wide spread of mortality rates. Bertolasi et al. [6] recorded a 20% mortality in 40 patients at 8 months, which rose to 35% in a high-risk group. Conti et al. [16] recorded 5 deaths within 6 months in 73 medically treated patients, and Duncan [19] published similar findings. Gazes et al. [22], in a study of 140 patients, found an 18% mortality at 1 year and were able to define a high-risk group of 54 patients with a 43% mortality at the end of the first year. It is in this area where reduction of death rates appears to be the big current challenge to the ICU.

When these results are viewed as a whole, however, it has to be concluded that the criterion of mortality in the first year after recognition does not distinguish clearly between unstable angina pectoris and stable angina pectoris. This is perhaps partly attributable to the fact that unselected angina pectoris patients include a proportion of cases with the unstable form, thus mixing the groups. The only proper way to clarify this matter would be to compare the prognosis in an untreated cohort of patients with well-defined stable angina pectoris with that in one of patients with well-defined unstable angina pectoris. Such a study has never been done and can no longer be expected. Yet one intuitively feels that within unstable angina pectoris, there must be a subset of patients at high risk of myocardial infarction and sudden death [6, 22]. The identification of this high-risk group is of singular importance, for there is increasing evidence that intensive medical therapy can help to 'cool' this emergency and improve its prognosis [29, 38]. Furthermore, while urgent coronary artery bypass surgery is perhaps an attractive alternative therapeutic approach directed at modification of the sombre immediate prognosis, the central issue here is whether these patients are identifiable as a group or groups.

Unstable angina pectoris

Patients with crescendo angina, or repeated attacks of severe angina at rest, ending in infarction or sudden death, make a vivid impression. But there are other cases with equally dramatic 'prodromata', which subsequently 'cool off' without infarction or death and so tend to be forgotten. Yet they dilute the high-risk group and blur the progression through the spectrum of impending infarction to established infarction and/or sudden death. The most useful distinguishing feature between stable and unstable angina pectoris is the predictability of the former in relation to its occurrence, duration, induction, presentation, and severity. Attacks of unstable angina pectoris, by contrast, are unexpected in one or more of these features: they occur in circumstances that are unusual for the particular patient affected or are excessively prolonged (but not excessively curtailed), or they arise unprovoked by effort, emotion, cold, meals, or arrhythmias, or are unusually severe (but not unusually mild); angina which, although provoked, arises from milder degrees of provocation than usual would also be included in this concept. Furthermore, recent-onset angina and the early return of angina after infarction must be similarly classified, because in these circumstances newness makes for unpredictability. The characteristics of unstable angina are thus a rather mixed bag, related only by their unpredictability. In all cases there may also be the clinical impression that something is amiss with the patient under observation.

The attacks are usually simultaneous with or preceded by transient ST or T wave changes in the ECG. These include T wave inversion (partial or complete), ST depression or ST elevation, and they may mimic the early stages of AMI. It is said that T wave inversion and ST depression reflect subendocardial ischaemia while ST elevation indicates a more severe form of transmural ischaemia. The latter is more often associated with haemodynamic disturbances and ventricular arrhythmias, although this is not always the case since arrhythmias can arise via re-entry phenomena even with small focal areas of ischaemia.

Pathophysiology

In general, O_2 delivery to the myocardium varies with coronary blood flow, the latter being determined by the perfusion pressure, i.e., the aortic diastolic pressure, and coronary vascular resistance. Coronary blood flow is capable of autoregulation, rising in situations with increasing O_2 demand and falling with lower O_2 demand (Fig. 15.1). This adjustment is achieved by means of appropriate alterations in coronary vascular resistance via various, mainly humoral, factors. Further, as the major part of coronary flow occurs during diastole, tachycardia that encroaches upon diastole tends to reduce coronary flow, as does increased LV diastolic pressure, for the perfusion pressure proper in the distal coronary circulation is the difference between the aortic pressure and the LV diastolic pressure. Myocardial ischaemia is essentially a regional phenomenon. If blood flow becomes inadequate with respect to the O_2 demand, as it does in coronary artery disease during exercise, emotion or tachycardia, or O_2 delivery

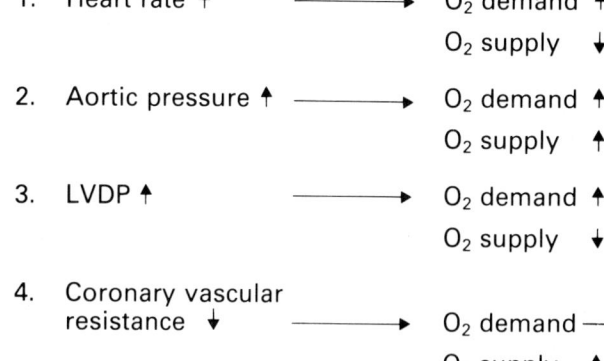

Fig. 15.1. Myocardial ischaemia: haemodynamic consequences and secondary effects. The usual haemodynamic changes due to myocardial ischaemia on the left, are enumerated with the influence of these changes on myocardial O_2 demand and O_2 supply on the right.

decreases primarily through coronary spasm [25, 34, 45], myocardial ischaemia will occur and the contractile function of ischaemic cells is rapidly lost [56]. A state resembling that of regional cardiac failure may ensue [10, 11]. It is often observed at catheterization that such ischaemia leads to immediate, yet reversible, regional abnormalities, such as dyskinesia or even akinesia. If the area is extensive, LV end-diastolic pressure (LVED) rises rapidly and the ventricular wall becomes stiffer, thus reducing diastolic capillary blood flow even further. If pain ensues, sympathetic stimulation will lead to further tachycardia and perhaps even to raised blood pressure, thus further augmenting O_2 demand [27]. Although autoregulation of the coronary blood flow may compensate the shortfall initially, this is often insufficient during longer episodes of myocardial ischaemia [5]. Friesinger [21], in a review of the literature on this subject, concluded that a raised LVED pressure was usual, and a raised blood pressure and tachycardia were frequent, in both spontaneous and provoked angina. Grossman and Mann [24], as well as our group in Rotterdam [38], have found by direct measurements during pacing-induced angina that despite increased coronary flow, there may be a rise in LVED pressure and a moderate rise in blood pressure. These changes would of themselves tend to produce direct or indirect alterations in myocardial O_2 demand and delivery. In any case, increased LVED pressure and raised blood pressure, i.e., increased preload and afterload, will increase ventricular wall stress and hence O_2 demand for the ventricle as a whole. This stiffer ventricle has the additional effect of increasing coronary vascular resistance, reducing coronary flow further, and worsening the discrepancy between supply and demand.

The various options open to correction (or further disbalance) of the regulatory system are

given in Figs. 15.2 and 15.3. These schemes show that while the onset of myocardial ischaemia tends to generate a mounting spiral of increasing ischaemia, the onset of recovery from ischaemia may set in motion a spreading wave of recovery. In other words, both the tendency to deterioration and that to recovery are subject to multiplier, or cascade, effects. Hence, one might expect every attack of myocardial ischaemia to find its equilibrium through the interplay of these two tendencies. If the equilibrium is reached with all regions non-ischaemic, the attack will be one of angina pectoris. If the equilibrium is achieved later, the pain is likely to have been prolonged and the

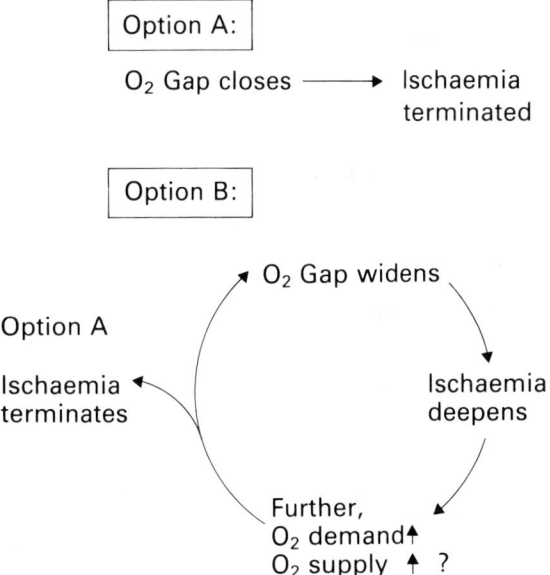

Fig. 15.2. The first minutes after myocardial ischaemia, which itself alters both demand and supply of myocardial O_2 (Fig. 15.1). This would have repercussions on the O_2 demand-supply gap. Two possible developments are schematized here: Option A, where the gap closes with termination of ischaemia, and option B, where the gap widens with deepening ischaemia.

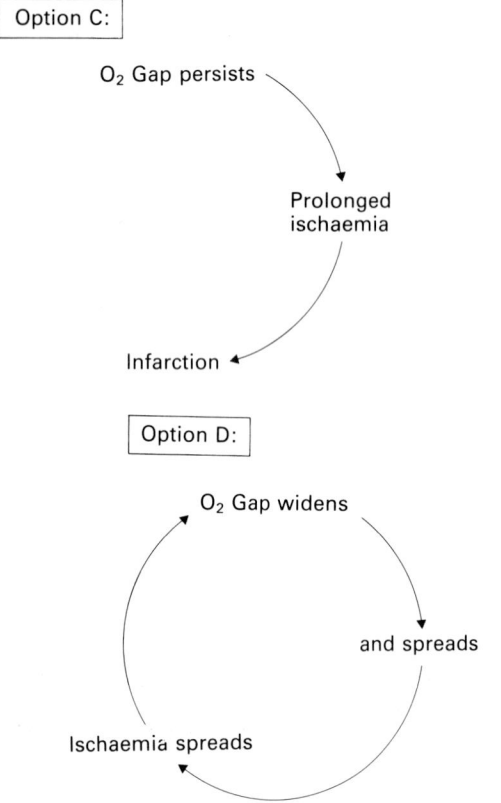

Fig. 15.3. Schematic representation of two more possible developments of a myocardial O_2 demand-supply gap just after myocardial ischaemia: Option C, where persistence of the gap leads to infarction, and option D, where the gap spreads to non-ischaemic regions of the myocardium leading to extensive ischaemia: the domino effect.

attack will be described as acute coronary insufficiency. When equilibrium is reached still later, with a region or regions of persisting ischaemia, a myocardial infarction may result. If equilibrium is not reached until extensive loss of ventricular function has taken place cardiogenic shock, and even sudden death, may follow [47]. Thus, serious events can evolve from relatively trivial initiating causes. The necessary condition is that the initiating event should generate a situation within which lies the possibility of further aggravation. The magnification of these effects by a multiplier or cascade mechanism is of special significance in attempts to assess and grasp a clinical situation where no sufficient cause is evident at first glance. Since unstable angina pectoris is inherently unpredictable (because no sufficient cause directly antedates the attack, among other reasons), mechanisms with some form of multiplier effect must be comprehended completely to be treated correctly. It is in this situation that the physician in intensive

care medicine meets the greatest challenge and may experience his or her 'finest hour'.

It is now necessary to ask whether one can detect any direct evidence for such a multiplier mechanism early in angina pectoris. The first event and the early rounds of the multiplier seem too subtle to be detectable. Most reported observations are indeed of the prefinal events and the more advanced complications. Maseri et al. [35], however, were able to make detailed ECG, haemodynamic, and clinical recordings of attacks of 'spontaneous' angina pectoris. The sequence they invariably found was: electrical ischaemia → mechanical dysfunction → haemodynamic changes → symptoms → further haemodynamic changes. This was often spontaneously followed by a subsidence in the reverse order. A multiplier of aggravation interacting with or cancelling a multiplier of improvement would seem an eminently suitable model to explain this sequence. Furthermore, if the multiplier mechanism were of importance in angina pectoris one would expect a greater preponderance of subclinical ischaemic episodes over clinical attacks; continuous ECG monitoring of ST segment changes [50] has indeed shown that this is the case. The logical conclusion is therefore that continuous (preferably computer-assisted to detect the majority of ischaemic events) monitoring of electrical and haemodynamic functions is essential.

What, then, are the underlying anatomical disturbances? Until recently, spasm and fixed coronary artery stenosis have been regarded as two separate, and mutually exclusive, causes of ischaemia and infarction. The current concept of the pathophysiology suggests, however, that spasm, or more accurately coronary vascular motility, and fixed stenosis are interrelated (Fig. 15.4). Actually both may act in combination, i.e., spasm of a major vessel around a fixed obstruction may lead to a critical reduction in flow, which in turn leads to ischaemia. In fact, in the past few years publications by several authors such as Maseri et al. [35], Hillis and Braunwald [26], Yasue et al. [59], Muller and Gunther [39], Van Ekelen and Robles de Medina [55], and Curry et al. [15] have brought about this shift in attitude towards the pathophysiological derangements underlying myocardial infarction. Instead of requiring fixed coronary artery obstruction only, it is now accepted that temporary obliteration of coronary flow by spasm in the vascular wall of the longer arteries, even in the absence of a fixed stenosis, can lead to unstable angina and, if lasting long enough,

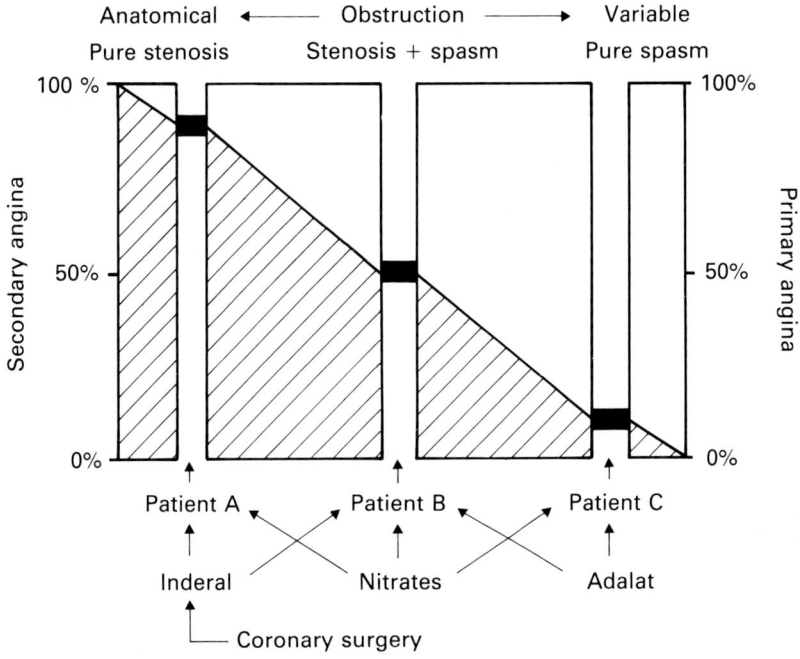

Fig. 15.4. Causes of angina pectoris: The stenosis–spasm axis. The initiation of angina pectoris depends on coronary stenosis, coronary spasm, or a varying combination of the two. Increased O_2 demand plays a prominent role in the angina of stenosis, and decrease in O_2 supply in the angina of spasm. Protection in the former consists in holding down O_2 demand with beta blockers and in the latter, in maintaining O_2 supply with Ca blockers. Nitrates affecting both supply and demand are useful over the whole range.

to myocardial infarction. Most probably, spasm and fixed stenosis will always act in combination; that is, spasm of a major vessel around a fixed obstruction causes the critical reduction in flow which leads to irreversible ischaemia. In addition, thrombocyte aggregates may form, and these in conjunction with altered choles-terol levels may worsen the functional obstruction. It has been postulated that prostaglandin metabolism may be disturbed and that excessive levels of thromboxane A2 will lead to further spasm, thus setting up the vicious circle shown in Fig. 15.5. The process may also abort, when vascular obstruction and ischaemia subside and

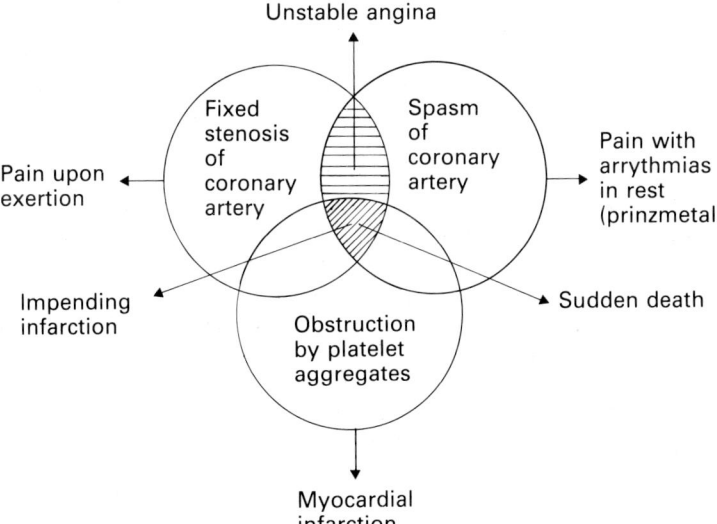

Fig. 15.5. The interplay of causes of angina pectoris, arrhythmias, myocardial infarction, and sudden death.

ECG changes disappear. In these instances myocardial cell death has been avoided and enzyme levels will vary little from control. These concepts open new avenues for treatment, for if coronary spasms could be recognized in time, its timely relief should completely reverse the process of impending infarction. Our studies over the past 5 years relate to a number of experiences which may provide a partial answer to the potential efficacy of various approaches in this concept of events.

Treatment

Beta blockade and Ca agonists

First of all the principle of vasodilator therapy, in particular the action of calcium channel blockers such as nifedipine, and of beta blockers such as propanolol need to be considered. Nifedipine's powerful action leads to strong vessel dilation, the efficacy of which has been proven without doubt in classic cases of Prinzmetal's angina, where spasm is known to be the main causative mechanism. In our laboratory direct intracoronary injection of nifedipine has been observed to lead to prompt restoration of the normal calibre of a completely blocked vessel [28]. There are other actions of nifedipine, however, which may make this drug equally attractive for the treatment of patients with unstable angina pectoris. Measurements of LV function, both in the pig and in man, have shown that local mechanical contraction ceases for up to 5 min when nifedipine is injected into the coronary artery supplying that section of cardiac muscle. This suppression of O_2 consumption in patients with unstable angina might be the best protective action for ischaemic cells provided that coronary flow can be increased at the same time, while electrical activation continues normally. With these and other observations in mind, a group of patients was studied who had been admitted to the coronary care unit with angina pectoris occurring at rest and with transient ST or T wave changes, but without any proof of AMI such as excessive enzyme release. Usually this high-risk group of patients with unstable angina pectoris is managed with bedrest, O_2, sedatives, long-acting nitrates and beta blockers in a sufficient dosage to reduce the heart rate to 50–60 beats/min. The objective of this treatment is to bring these patients with signs of myocardial

ischaemia back into a stable and asymptomatic state (option A in Fig. 15.2), thereby hopefully preventing the occurrence of an infarction.

Detailed data were collected in 720 patients with various symptoms of coronary artery disease who had been admitted to the coronary care unit in a 9-month period [28]. Forty-seven of these 720 had precordial pain at rest typical of angina pectoris, which persisted or worsened despite treatment with nitrates and beta blockers and thus met our definition. Over the same period, 370 of the 720 patients proved to have a myocardial infarction. In all 47 patients transient ST–T changes but no new Q wave formation were documented during angina at rest while in the coronary care unit. The haemodynamic characteristics of these patients are given in Table 15.1.

All patients were semi-isolated in private rooms, although they remained directly accessible to the nursing staff. Haemodynamic monitoring was initiated immediately by means of a Swan–Ganz thermodilution catheter, which was inserted through the subclavian vein, the right jugular vein, or an arm vein into the pulmonary artery. Also, if either hypotension or hypertension was present initially, an arterial line was inserted in the left radial artery under local anaesthesia. All patients were lightly heparinized through the IV line (< 30 000 units IV/24 h). A semi-automated monitoring system facilitated the continuous recording of heart rate and cardiac rhythm, while pressures and cardiac output were determined at regular intervals. During and following every attack of pain a 12-lead ECG was recorded, and if pain persisted the ECG was repeated at 15-min intervals. Upon admission and 6 h after each attack of pain, CPK, CPK-MB, and α-HBDH cardiac enzymes were measured. After initial sedation, usually with oral diazepam (5–10 mg t.i.d.), isosorbide dinitrate was given sublingually in a dose of 5 mg every 2 h, or if necessary, IV. In addition, propranolol was administered IV at dosages varying from 1 to 10 mg/kg until a heart rate of 60 beats/min was reached. Thereafter, propanolol was given PO at dosages ranging from 400 to 800 mg/24 h. When propanolol was contraindicated, as in the presence of lung disease, a cardioselective beta blocker was chosen, such as metoprolol.

Of the 47 patients so selected, 37 were male and 10 female. Their ages ranged from 29 to 77 years, with a mean of 58. Three subgroups of patients could be identified: 12 had no history whatsoever of previous coronary artery disease (group I); 25 had long-standing histories of

Table 15.1. Results following addition of nifedipine (N) to treatment regimen when standard therapy with beta-blockers and long-acting nitrates had failed in 12 patients for whom pretreatment haemodynamic values were available[a].

hr	Heart rate (beats/min)			MAP (mmHg)			PAPS (mmHg)			PAPD (mmHg)			PCWP (mmHg)		
	Median	Range	n	Median	Range	n	Median	Range	n	Median	Range	n	Median	Range	n
0	69	46–74	12	97	75–136	12	24	16–30	12	6.5	3–11	12	6	2–10	12
1	75	46–81	12*	94.5	75–115	12	23	16–37	12	7.5	4–13	12	7	3–11	12
4	68	43–84	12	92.5	76–116	12	24	16–37	12	7.5	2–13	12	8.5	2–11	12
8	71	49–85	11	92	78–120	11	25	16–28	11	8	4–13	11	7	3–13	11
24	70	54–86	11	90	80–105	11	23	20–31	9	6	3–12	9	5	3–9	9

N →

Table 15.1. (continued)

hr	CO (litres/min)		
	Median	Range	n
0	4.6	3.4–7.3	10
1	5.0	3.6–7	10
4	5.2	3.6–6.3	5
8	5.0	3.7–5.5	5
24	4.8	3.2–5.5	5

[a]After 1 h a small but significant (*, $P < 0.05$) rise in heart rate was recorded; MAP decreased gradually; there were no demonstrable changes in pulmonary pressures or CO.

coronary artery disease (group II); and the remaining 10 had noted a return of angina at rest within 2 weeks after discharge from the hospital, where they had been admitted for an AMI (group III). Two patients in group II and one in group III had previously undergone coronary artery bypass grafting (CABG). Most were submitted to cardiac catheterization as soon as their condition made this possible; of the three groups, group III showed the worst prognosis.

Of these patients with unstable angina who were treated for at least 3 and up to 8 h with propranolol or other beta blockers, nitrates, etc., 16 became asymptomatic within this set period. The 31 remaining patients were then all given nifedipine PO in addition, in doses of 10 mg six times a day, and, 27 of them became asymptomatic within 30 min on average and remained so for the rest of their hospital stay. Four patients from group II or III failed to respond to nifedipine. Two of these sustained a myocardial infarction within 24 h, and one died. Because of persistent pain, two other patients received intra-aortic balloon pumping, with immediate relief of their symptoms. Both underwent CABG and both are alive. Coronary arteriography showed that three of these four patients had more than 75% obstruction in three vessels, while one of the four patients, a 73-year-old male, had 90% left main coronary

artery obstruction and suffered a fatal myocardial infarction shortly after the coronary arteriogram. Elective coronary angiography and left-heart catheterization had been planned, while they returned to some physical activity in the intermediate care unit, for 20 of the 27 patients who experienced initial relief of symptoms with the addition of nifedipine to their therapeutic regimen. However, one patient with postinfarction angina sustained a fatal myocardial infarction prior to catheterization and within 7 days of initiation of nifedipine treatment. Of the 19 patients catheterized, left main coronary artery obstruction greater than 90% was found in one individual, three-vessel obstruction greater than 75% in nine, two-vessel disease with more than 75% obstruction in three patients, and single-vessel obstruction of a similar degree in six patients.

Apart from the patient with fatal infarction, four more patients suffered a non-fatal infarction within 2 weeks, after the initial relief of their symptoms. In two patients this was related to angiography; both had severe pain, with ST–T changes but without new Q wave formation, and a slight rise of cardiac enzymes. Two other patients suffered a non-fatal infarction; in one of these, no CABG was planned. In the remaining patient, coronary artery spasm was documented during angiography. In this individual administration of nifedipine into the coronary artery involved led to immediate relief.

Thus, of the total group of 27 patients whose condition could be managed with nifedipine and who had not responded to adequate beta blockade, five sustained an infarction within 2 weeks following initial stabilization. During further follow-up (3–5 months) no other myocardial infarction was noted. So far 15 of the 19 have undergone elective CABG. In these, the indication for surgery was their past history of unstable angina and an advanced degree of coronary artery stenosis, plus the feasibility of bypass grafting. All of them are alive and well. The other 11 patients have remained asymptomatic and have been maintained with nifedipine therapy.

Intra-aortic balloon pumping

Earlier experience in our coronary care unit, before nifedipine became available, had led us to institute intra-aortic balloon pumping (IABP) in these patients when the response to beta blockade was unsatisfactory and the anginal attacks persisted [38]. The effect of IABP is twofold. The abrupt presystolic balloon *defla*tion decreases afterload, while the diastolic balloon *inflation* enhances coronary perfusion pressure. The latter is the major determinant of coronary blood flow in the presence of critical stenosis, and therefore a most significant mode of support. In addition, the reduction of afterload increases stroke volume and the ejection fraction without increased effort by the heart. As the heart empties better, wall tension and preload, and thus O_2 consumption are decreased. It has been suggested that counterpulsation may open dormant collateral channels and that IABP increases flow to the subendocardium by augmenting existing collateral circulation. While afterload reduction reduces O_2 demand, diastolic augmentation increases O_2 availability. The ratio of the diastolic pressure time index (DPTI) representing myocardial blood flow to the systolic tension time index (TTI), which is related to myocardial O_2 consumption, is termed the endocardial viability ratio (EVR). While only a conceptual term, EVR can be regarded as a reflection of the balance between availability and consumption of O_2.

The clinical use of IABP was originally advocated for cardiogenic shock following CSMI and severe LV failure after acute infarction. Angina pectoris at rest refractory to medical therapy has more recently been accepted as an indication for IABP. In 1979, Weintraub et al. [57] published their results in 82 patients seen between 1972 and 1978. Of the 80 with angina, 60 underwent IABP and most received CABG. There was prompt relief of symptoms with only two deaths, whilst 77% of the survivors were considered employable. Our own experience [38] extends to 59 patients seen from 1975 to early 1979. Forty-two had angina at rest, either of new onset or superimposed on previously stable angina, while 17 had angina at rest within 2 weeks after infarction.

Pain relief after the institution of IABP was prompt in 41 of 42 (98%) patients. Their ages (range 35–65 years, mean 62 years) and most characteristics were similar to those of the 47 patients described earlier. In one patient, a 65-year-old male, with long-standing three-vessel CAD, symptoms worsened. This patient developed a non-fatal AMI and was no longer a candidate for CABG. The other 41 were all catheterized. Left main coronary artery obstruction was found in one patient (3%), three-vessel obstruction in 19 (46%), two-vessel obstruction in 14 (34%), and single-vessel obstruction (all proximal obstruction of the left anterior descending artery) in eight patients (19%). Forty-one patients underwent CABG. Two patients (4%) had an AMI during surgery and in one of these the infarction (and subsequent death) may have been attributable to trapping of gas in a kinked balloon.

The myocardial infarction rate for the whole group was 11% (5/42): one patient had an AMI despite IABP, two patients had an AMI during CABG, and in two patients who died within 24 h an AMI could not be excluded. The total mortality rate was 7% (3/42): one patient died during the surgical procedure, two high-risk patients with three-vessel disease, poor LV function and severe associated disease, (diabetes mellitus) died within 24 h. Of the 38 patients who survived CABG, one had an AMI within 3 months, four had mild stable angina pectoris (New York Heart Association NYHA class II), and none died (follow-up ranged from 3 months to 5 years).

Our results indicate a relatively high perioperative mortality in patients with refractory angina pectoris treated with IABP. The series is small (42 patients), however, and it should be noted that death was attributable to intractable diabetes in two patients. One of these was also at high risk because of severe three-vessel obstructive disease and poor LV function. In a third patient the IABP may have contributed to death. It should be stressed that no surgical mortality could de demonstrated in the 12 patients undergoing CABG for post-infarct angina at rest. When considering the whole group, surgical mortality is 6% (3/53). While this is definitely higher than the mortality for patients undergoing CABG under stable conditions (around 1% in our institution) the 6% surgical mortality is similar to that described by others.

It should be emphasized that the patients selected for IABP were completely refractory to any form of medical therapy and had rapid progression of their symptoms. They thus constitute a special high-risk group. We now do not recommend the use of IABP, which may be unnecessarily hazardous, unless all pharmacological efforts have failed. The experience with nitrates, beta blockade, and above all Ca antagonists as a first priority has made it very evident that balloon pumping, while efficient, should only be used as a last resort. In fact, our current management is conducted along the scheme shown in Fig. 15.6.

Discussion

This chapter contains an attempt to explain why unstable angina threatening to proceed myocar-

dial infarction provides intensive cardiac care units with a major challenge today. New pharmacological and surgical interventions carry the promise of a major advance in therapy, provided the underlying pathophysiologic disturbances are properly recognized and altered in time.

From experience with the traditional approach depicted in the upper half of Fig. 15.7, in which bed rest, O_2, sedatives, nitrates, and beta blockade all play their role, it has become clear that not all patients respond as expected. The multiplier effect and even the domino theory provide a ready explanation why other factors must be considered in the events that predate the onset of infarction. In fact, the role of excessive platelet aggregation and its attendant biochemical changes has not so far been sufficiently well understood to be included in the overall strategy as it appears in Fig. 15.7. Even so, it is our firm conviction that a number of recommendations regarding management can be given now.

From the entire set of observations, which indicate primary O_2 sparing and spasm-relieving effect of nifedipine, the application of this drug in this type of patients with unstable angina and impending infarction has become essential. Indeed, the hypothesis has been put forward that the subset of patients where coronary artery spasm is suspected as a primary

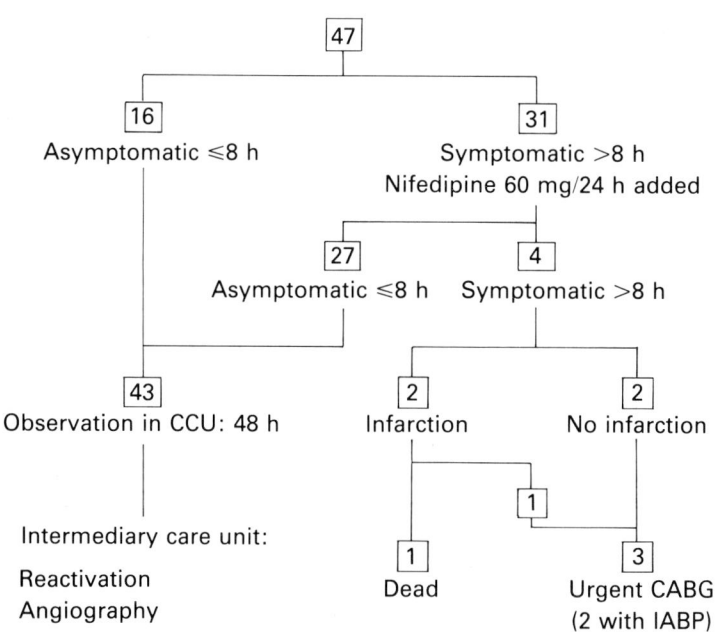

Fig. 15.6. Sequence of events in 47 patients with unstable angina, admitted to the coronary care unit with suspected impending infarction. All had angina at rest, ST/T wave changes, and no Q formation or enzyme ↑ (impending infarction). All were treated with ≤8 h bed rest, beta blockade, and nitrates.

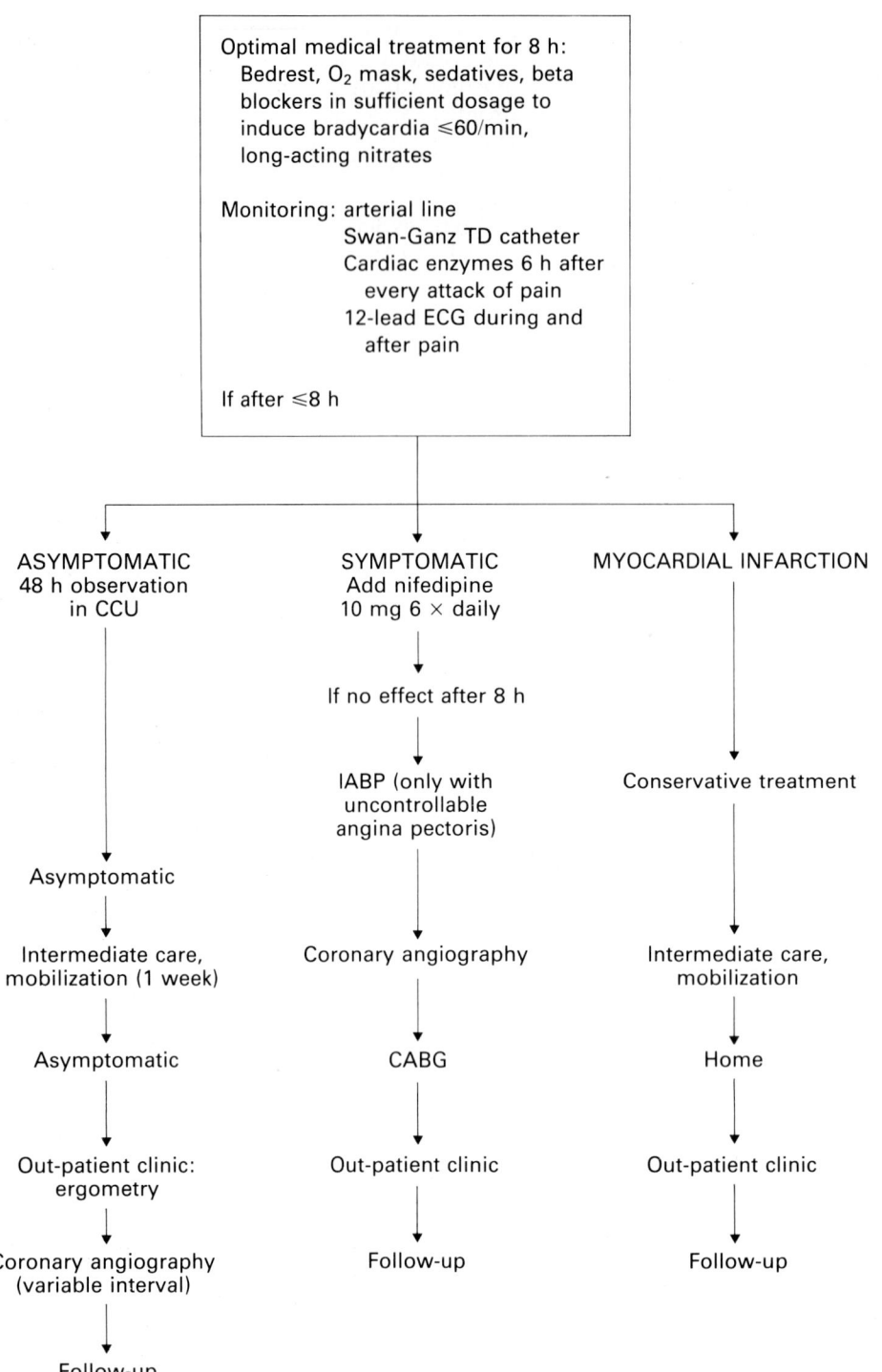

Fig. 15.7. Approach to treatment in angina at rest.

or secondary factor may not benefit from beta adrenergic blockade at all. In fact, Yasue [56] has specifically argued against its use in this group of patients. Then as there are other reports of the inconclusive efficacy of beta block-ade, which has failed to relieve symptoms within the first hours despite reduction of heart rate and blocking of adrenergic impulses, the addition of nifedipine, or perhaps the use of nifedipine alone, may be the more logical approach.

To sort out the best solution a multicentre trial is currently under way in the Netherlands to establish the most effective use of the various drugs in cases where surgery (CABG) does not have a primary role.

In any case with a view to reversing the multiplier effect, the inhibition of transmembrane calcium influx into cardiac muscle fibres may be the quickest way to reduce phosphate-bound energy being transformed into mechanical work by calcium-dependent myofibrillar adenosine triphosphate (ATP). This in turn leads to an immediate decrease in cardiac oxidative metabolism. In recent experiments de Jong et al. [18] showed that even in brief periods of ischaemia promptly followed by reperfusion, massive release of nucleosides, indicating breakdown of high-energy phosphates, followed. Thus an attempt at reducing O_2 need is vital. In addition, the reduction of the calcium-dependent contractile tone of the larger epicardial coronary arteries—and perhaps to some extent the capillaries as well (dramatically illustrated by the sudden collapse of the ventricular wall thickness after intracoronary drug admission) leads to increased flow, which in turn will promote the rapid restoration of the regional O_2 supply. Finally, the dilatation of large systemic arteries and arterioles will diminish afterload, which may result in a further, albeit indirect, decrease of cardiac O_2 demand. All three mechanisms may vary in significance, but they are essential.

Data provided by Clark and Henry [14], as well as by other workers, have also indicated that even when an area around an infarct is already ischaemic, a reduction in the amount of ischaemic cells can be achieved. The response to nifedipine, in some patients unresponsive for hours to beta blockade was so dramatic and so rapid that one was struck by the similarity to the response to IABP. Although the study was non-randomized and in many other aspects lacked the requirements for a stringent clinical trial, the reduction in symptoms was so impressive that we have become convinced that a spastic component plays a major role in this subgroup. Twenty-seven of the 31 patients in whom the drug was added became asymptomatic within a very short period and remained so in nearly all instances. Given the brittle nature of these patients, and the fact that all other supportive therapy had failed, there is little doubt that nifedipine was the sole agent tipping the dominoes in their favour. In contrast, in those patients in whom nifedipine did not evoke a similarly favourable response, the extent of organic fixed stenosis, as demonstrated by arteriography, was such that the lack of response to the drug was hardly surprising. Their subsequent response to IABP and emergency bypass surgery proved that the organic stenotic element in these individuals was the prevailing component. Viewing these data and the literature as a whole, our group has arrived at the following recommendations for management. These views correspond to a considerable degree with those put forward by Neill and co-workers [42] recently.

Bed rest and reduction of anxiety are important supportive measurements which should be provided at the onset.

Anticoagulation. None of the earlier trials that indicate the efficacy of anticoagulation [4, 43, 54, 58] meet the statistical criteria currently mandatory for such studies [58]. As coronary thrombosis, rather than preceding myocardial infarction may well be the consequence of infarction [9, 48], widespread nihilism with these drugs for this diagnosis has occurred. It is our belief that to date no well-designed studies are available to support the use of anticoagulants in unstable angina. On the other hand, heparin appears to be well accepted. Since vaso-active substances that may induce vasospasm are released during platelet aggregation, platelet aggregation inhibitors may come to play a major role, yet the usefulness of these drugs in unstable angina has not been established. As a consequence, short-term anticoagulants are advocated in all patients with prolonged bedrest, to avoid deep vein thrombosis and pulmonary artery thrombosis in patients being monitored with intravascular catheters. Heparin 30 000 units/24 h IV is still the ideal choice under subsequent laboratory control.

Nitrates. Nitroglycerine tablets sublingually relieve most anginal attacks. The direct vasodilating effect on the venous system lowers preload and wall stress in the left ventricle. An additional dilating effect on the larger arteries will lower afterload and may increase coronary flow. Recently Shafer et al. [51] have also indicated that nitrates may have an anti-aggregation action, thus augmenting their efficacy. But unwanted side-effects do occur [13]. Hypotension and bradyarrhythmias can be managed by raising the legs to improve venous return, and if not effective, atropine, 0.25–1.1 mg IV and plasma infusions can be used. While nitroglycerine sublingually acts within minutes, the duration of action is equally short. Nitroglycerine ointment for topical application has a prolonged effect, as has isosorbide dinitrate, and is especially effective to prevent angina attacks at night. The 5-mg tablets of isosorbide nitrate for sublingual use are effective within minutes, and their action extends from 1 to 3 h. The 20-mg tablets for oral administration provide a longer-lasting effect. When they are administered PO there is a quick first-pass effect through the liver, where isosorbide dinitrate is transferred by luthation-S transferase into two metabolites, isosorbide 2-, and isosorbide 5- mononitrate. These two metabolites were found to persist in the dog for over 4 h after IV administration. A sustained effect on exercise performance in patients with angina pectoris has been demonstrated both for the IV administered monoitrates, and for orally administered isosorbide dinitrate. Even so these drugs are not always effective and beta-blockade has been employed more and more.

Beta blockers, Ca antagonists, balloon pumping, surgery. There is a vast literature on this subject, and the interested reader is likely to be partisan to one or more approaches. He is also referred to various articles on this subject. It is our current policy always to include beta blockers, unless they are specifically contraindicated. It is also a policy that when they are not beneficial within hours nifedipine should be added (Fig. 15.6). Finally, if all these measures fail, we have recourse to IABP within 24 h after admission for persisting angina.

In all cases, cardiac catheterization is carried out as soon as the situation has stabilized. During the drug regimen that has proven effective, elective CABG is planned for those individuals in whom the anatomical situation of the coronaty arteries requires surgical corrections. In keeping with recommendations made by other authors, surgical intervention is withheld when symptoms subside during pharmacological therapy and when the anatomical situation does not dictate CABG.

The most recent developments with intra–coronary streptokinase treatment to dissolve obstructing platelet aggregates, provide yet another possible approach to therapy in this category of critically ill patients (P.G. Hugenholtz, to be published).

References

1. Abrams J (1980) Current concepts: Nitroglycerin and long-acting nitrates. N Engl J Med 302:1234
2. Antman E, Muller J, Goldberg S, et al (1980) Nifedipine therapy for coronary-artery spasm: experience in 127 patients. N Engl J Med 302:1269
3. Baum RS, Alaverez H, Cobb LA (1974) Survival after resuscitation from out-of-hospital ventricular fibrillation. Circulation 50:1231
4. Beamish RE, Storrie VM (1960) Impending myocardial infarction. Recognition and management. Circulation 21:1107
5. Berne RM (1963) Cardiac nucleotides in hypoxia: possible role in regulation of coronary blood flow. Am J Physiol 204:317
6. Bertolasi CA, Trongé JE, Carreno CA, et al (1974) Unstable angina—prospective and randomized study of its evolution with and without surgery. Am J Cardiol 33:201
7. Blackburn H (1974) Progress in the epidemiology and prevention of coronary heart disease. In: Yu PN, Goodwin JF (eds) Progress in cardiology vol, 3 Lea & Febiger, Philadelphia, pp 1–36
8. Block WJ Jr, Crumpacker EL, Dry TJ, Gage RP (1952) Prognosis of angina pectoris. Observations in 6 882 cases. JAMA 150:259
9. Branwood AW, Montgomery GL (1956) Observations on the morbid anatomy of coronary disease. Scott Med J 1:367
10. Braunwald E (1971) Control of myocardial oxygen consumption. Am J Cardiol 27:416
11. Braunwald E, Sonnenblick EH, Ross JR (1976) Mechanisms of contraction of the normal and failing heart, 2nd edn. Little, Brown, Boston
12. Bruggraf GW, Parker JO (1975) Prognosis in coronary artery disease. Circulation 52:146
13. Bruschke AVG, Proudfit WL, Sones FM (1973) Progress study of 590 consecutive nonsurgical cases of coronary disease followed 5–9 years. Circulation 47:1147
14. Clark RE, Henry PD (1978) Protection of ischemic myocardium by nifedipine. In: Lichtlen PR, Kimura E, Taira N (eds) International Adalat Panel discussion. Excerpta Medica, Amsterdam, Oxford, Princeton, pp 24–29
15. Come PC, Pitt B (1976) Nitroglycerin-induced severe hypotension and bradycardia in patients with acute myocardial infarction. Circulation 54 [suppl 4]:624
16. Conti R, Gilbert JB, Hodges M, et al (1975) Unstable angina pectoris: Randomized study of surgical vs medical therapy. (Abstract) Am J Cardiol 35:129
17. Curry CR Jr, Pepine CJ, Sabom MB, Conti CR (1979) Similarities of ergonovine-induced and spontaneous attacks of variant angina. Circulation 59:307
18. De Jong JW, Harmsen E, Keijzer E (1980) Release of purine metabolites from the isolated ischemic working rat heart. (Abstract) VIII European Congress of Cardiology, Paris
19. Duncan B, Fulton M, Morrison SL, et al (1976) Prognosis of new and worsening angina pectoris. Br Med J i:981
20. Engel HJ, Wolf R, Hundeshagen H, Lichtlen R (1980) Regional myocardial blood flow at rest and during angina induced by atrial pacing before and after nitroglycerin. In: Kreuzer H, Parmley WW, Rentrop P, Reiss HW (eds) Quantification of myocardial ischaemia. Witzstock, New York, pp 327–341
21. Friesinger GC (1977) Haemodynamics. In: Julian DG (ed) Angina pectoris. Churchill Livingstone, Edinburgh
22. Gazes PC, Mobley Jr EM, Faris HM Jr et al (1973) Pre-infarctional (unstable) angina—a prospective study. Ten year follow-up. Circulation 48:331–337
23. Gifford RH, Feinstein AR (1969) A critique of methodology in studies of anticoagulant therapy for acute myocardial infarction. N Engl J Med 280:351
24. Grossman J, Mann JT (1978) Evidence for impaired left ventricular relaxation during acute ischaemia in man.

Eur J Cardiol 7 [Suppl]:239

25. Hellstrom HR (1979) Coronary artery vasospasm: The likely immediate cause of acute myocardial infarction. Br Heart J 41:426

26. Hillis LD, Braunwald E (1978) Coronary-artery spasm. N Engl J Med 299:695

27. Hood WB Jr (1971) Pathophysiology of ischaemic heart disease. Prog Cardiovasc Dis 14:297

28. Hugenholtz PC, Michels HR, Serruys PW, Brower RW (1981) Nifedipine in the treatment of unstable angina, coronary spasm and myocardial ischaemia. Am J Cardiol 47:163–173

29. Juergens JL, Edwards JE, Achor RWP, Burchell HB (1960) Prognosis of patients surviving first clinically diagnosed myocardial infarction. Arch Intern Med 105:134

30. Kannel WB, Feinleib M (1972) Natural history of angina pectoris in the Framingham study. Am J Cardiol 29:154

31. Krauss KR, Hutter AM Jr, De Sanctis RW (1972) Acute coronary insufficiency. Course and follow-up. Circulation 45 [Suppl I]:I–66

32. Liberthson RR, Nagel EL, Hirschman JC, Nussenfeld SR (1974) Pre-hospital ventricular fibrillation. Prognosis and follow-up course. N Engl J Med 291:317

33. Maseri A, Mimmo R, Chirchia S, et al (1975) Coronary artery spasm as a cause of acute myocardial ischaemia in man. Chest 68:625

34. Maseri A, L'Abbate A, Pesola A, et al (1977) Coronary vasospasm in angina pectoris. Lancet I:713

35. Maseri A, L'Abbate A, Baroldi G, et al (1978) Coronary vasospasm as a possible cause of myocardial infarction. N Engl J Med 299:1271

36. Medalie JH, Goldbourt U (1976) Unrecognized myocardial infarction: Five-year incidence, mortality and risk factors. Ann Intern Med 84:526

37. Meester GT (1980) Computer analysis of cardiac catheterization data. Doctor of Medicine thesis, Erasmus University, Rotterdam, The Netherlands

38. Michels R, Haalebos M, Hagemeyer F, Balakumaran K, Brand M.v/d, Serruys PW, Hugenholtz PG (1980) Intraaortic balloon pumping in myocardial infarction and unstable angina. Eur Heart J 1:31

39. Muller JE, Gunther SJ (1978) Nifedipine therapy for Prinzmetal's angina. Circulation 57:137

40. Myocardial Infarction Community Registers (1976) WHO, Copenhagen

41. National Cooperative Study Group (1978) Unstable angina pectoris. In-hospital experience and initial follow-up. Am J Cardiol 42:839

42. Neill WA, Wharton TP Jr, Fluri-Lundeen J, Cohen IS (1980) Acute coronary insufficiency—coronary occlusion after intermittent ischaemic attacks. N Engl J Med 302:1157

43. Nichol ES, Phillips WC, Gasten GG (1959) Virtue of prompt anticoagulant therapy in impending myocardial infarction. Experience with 318 patients during a 10-year period. Ann Intern Med 50:1158

44. Oberman A, Jones WB, Riley CP, et al (1972) Natural history of coronary artery disease. Bull NY Acad Med 48:1109

45. Oliva PB, Breckinridge JC (1977) Arteriographic evidence of coronary arterial spasm in acute myocardial infarction. Circulation 56:366

46. Opie LH (1980) Drugs and the heart. Lancet I:693, 750, 806, 861, 912, 966, 1011

47. Raizes G, Wagner GS, Hackel DB (1977) Instantaneous non-arrhythmic cardiac death in acute myocardial infarction. Am J Cardiol 39:1

48. Roberts WC, Buja LC (1972) The frequency and significance of coronary arterial thrombi and other observations in fatal acute myocardial infarction. Am J Med 52:423

49. Schaffer WA, Cobb LA (1975) Recurrent ventricular fibrillation and modes of death in survivors of out-of-hospital ventricular fibrillation. N Engl J Med 293:259

50. Schang SJ, Pepine CJ (1977) Transient asymptomatic ST segment depression during daily activity. Am J Cardiol 39:396

51. Shafer AI, Alexander RW, Handson RI (1980) Inhibition of platelet function by organic nitrate vasodilators. Blood 55:649

52. Sigler LH (1951) Prognosis of angina pectoris and coronary occlusion. Follow up of 17,000 cases. JAMA 146:998

53. Slagel RC (1972) Natural history of angiographically documented coronary artery disease. (Abstract) Circulation 45 [Suppl II]:II–60

54. Vakil RJ (1964) Preinfarction syndrome—management and follow-up. Am J Cardiol 14:55–66

55. Van Ekelen WAJJ, Robles de Medina EO (1978) Variant forms of angina pectoris. Eur J Cardiol 8/3:305

56. Verdouw PD, Ten Cate FJ, Hugenholtz PG (1980) Effect of nifedipine on segmental myocardial function in the anesthetized pig. Eur J Pharmacol 63:209

57. Weintraub RM, Aroesty JM, Paulin S, et al (1979) Medically refractory unstable angina pectoris. I. Long-term follow-up of patients undergoing intraaortic balloon counterpulsation and operation. Am J Cardiol 43:877

58. Wood P (1961) Acute and subacute coronary insufficiency. Br Med J i:1779

59. Yasue H, Touayama M, Shimamoto M, et al (1978) Role of autonomic nervous system in the pathogenesis of Prinzmetal's variant of angina. Circulation 50:137

60. Zuckel WJ, Cohen BM, Mattingly TW and Hrubec Z (1969) Survival following first diagnosis of coronary heart disease. Am Heart J 78:159

Chapter 16

Cardiovascular Pharmacology

J. D. Fitzgerald

Disturbances of cardiovascular function are amongst the most commonly encountered events in the critically ill patient. The aim of therapy is to maintain adequate tissue perfusion by normalization of blood volume, pH, and gas tension. Drug therapy is frequently needed if this normalization has not achieved the desired effect. In this chapter, drugs which act primarily on the cardiovascular system will be divided on the basis of their pharmacological classification and described in terms of: (1) therapeutic application and pharmacological classification; (2) mode of action; (3) pharmacokinetics; (4) unwanted effects. It is hoped that the information will be sufficient to permit the rational selection and safe use of cardiovascular agents.

Clinical pharmacokinetics

In order to be effective, specific therapeutic agents should be present at the site of action, in the correct concentration, for the required period of time. Dosing recommendations have usually been based upon data relating drug administration to therapeutic effect. Additional data has become available over the past 25 years, relating dose to both drug concentration in blood and biological effect. In most instances, it is not possible to measure the concentration of drug at the effector site, but knowledge of the change in concentration of the drug in accessible fluids such as blood and urine has improved the design of therapeutic regimens. For many drugs, there is a minimal effective plasma concentration and a higher concentration associated with unwanted effects. Plasma concentrations lying between these two extremes are regarded as being in the therapeutic range. Knowledge of how a drug behaves in the body should lead to the more frequent achievement of therapeutic plasma levels and hence a reduction in drug toxicity. It may also help to explain the basis of certain drug interactions and failure of drug therapy.

Pharmacokinetics may be defined as the study of the rates of transfer of drug between various parts of the body and therefore includes the kinetics of drug absorption, distribution, metabolism and excretion. The object of studying these processes is to obtain indirect data on the drug concentration at the site of action.

Compartmental analysis

The technique of compartmental analysis has

been introduced to describe the various phases of a drug in the body, from the time of administration to its final disappearance. A compartment may be regarded as a kinetically homogeneous pool, and such a compartment may not necessarily have an anatomical equivalent. Many different compartmental schemes have been proposed as a means of describing the change in drug concentration in fluids and tissue over time, but a generally accepted scheme comprises the following components:

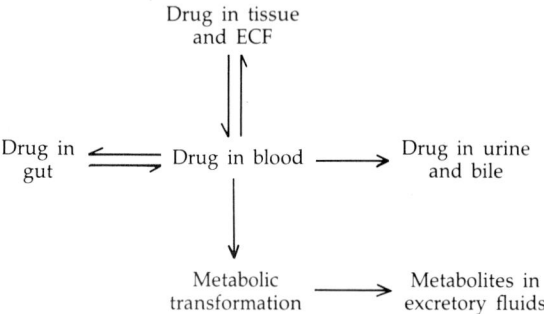

Kinetic analysis is based on compartmental schemes ranging from the simplest single-compartment open model to a multi-compartment model, though the model of choice is the one that contains the fewest compartments but is adequate to explain the observed changes in drug concentration. A two-compartment open model can accommodate most drug kinetic analyses and this will be used to introduce the various concepts of pharmacokinetics. A two-compartment open system may be depicted as

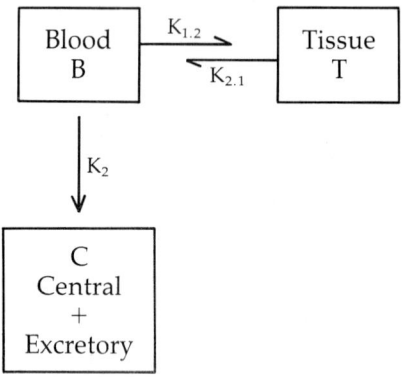

The letters B, T, and C refer to drug concentrations in the relevant compartments. The drug passes reversibly between blood and tissues and therefore the model is described as open, because drug loss at C will affect drug concentration in both B and T. In such a system the ratio between the drug concentration in blood and in tissues may not reach equilibrium. The term $K_{1.2}$ refers to the first-order rate constant for transfer of drug from blood (compartment one) to tissues (compartment two), while $K_{2.1}$ is the rate constant for transfer from compartment two to compartment one. Elimination from the blood compartment is described by the rate constant K_2.

Rate constants

The essence of pharmacokinetics is the determination of the rate at which drugs are transferred from one compartment to another and also of the amount of drug transferred. The rate of transport from, for example, blood to tissue can be expressed as $-dC/dt = KC^n$, where C represents the concentration of drug in blood, the power, n, represents the order of the reaction, and K represents the proportionality constant of transfer between B and T. From this equation it may be concluded that the rate of decrease of transferable drug C with time is the product of the constant K and the transferable concentration C.

These concepts can be exemplified by examining the change in drug concentration in plasma following IV administration of a drug. In Fig. 16.1 it can be seen that the concentration of drug in the blood initially falls very rapidly and then more slowly. The alterations in plasma concentration over time are due to transport of the drug from the blood compartment to the tissue compartment, or to drug elimination. As described above, the transfer process for a drug from one compartment to another is associated with a rate constant.

In most instances the transfer process will be first-order, which means that the rate of transfer is dependent only upon the drug concentration. In some uncommon instances drugs may transfer from one compartment to another at a rate which is constant over time and *independent* of the drug concentration. Such a transfer rate is defined as a zero-order process and the rate equation above ($dC/dt = -KC^n$) becomes $dC/dt = K_0$. If the factors t and C are integrated then the equation $C_t = C_0 - K_0 t$ is obtained, and this equation is used to determine the zero-order rate constant K_0.

Distribution and elimination phases

The one-compartment model illustrated in Fig. 16.1 shows an early rapid decline in plasma

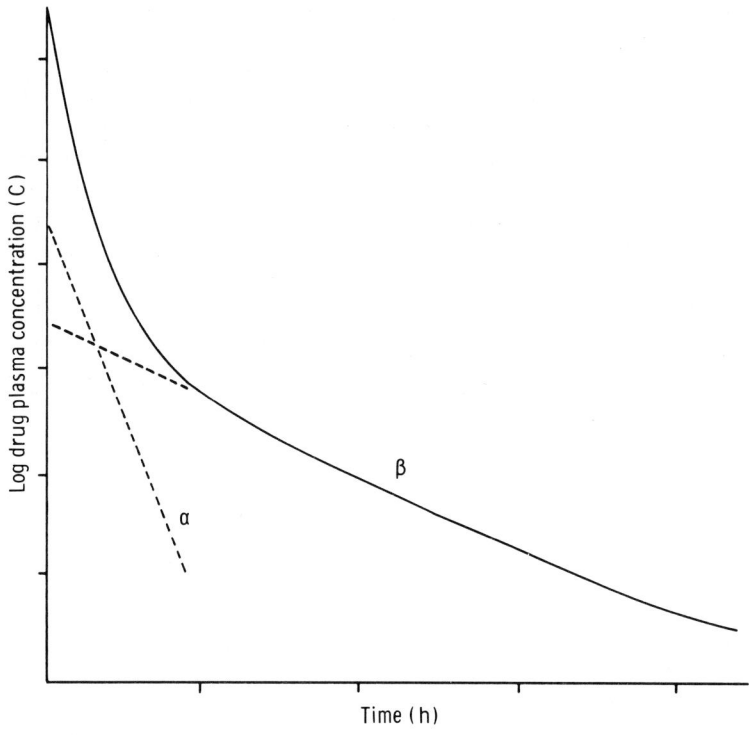

Fig. 16.1. Alteration in drug plasma concentration over time following IV administration. The curve comprises an initial rapid (alpha) phase, representing drug distribution, and a slower later (beta) phase, representing drug elimination. The *dotted lines* represent the slopes for the alpha and beta phases.

levels, followed by a more gradual decline. The rapidly declining phase is attributed to that period following administration when the drug is diffusing into the various compartments from the plasma. This portion of the curve is referred to as the distributive or alpha phase, whilst the more gradual slope represents drug elimination and is referred to as the beta phase. The curve representing alterations in plasma concentration of the drug with respect to time can be described by the equation:

$P = Ae^{\alpha t} + Be^{-\beta t}$, where P is concentration of drug in plasma; and A and B are the concentrations of drug in the α and β phases, respectively, at time zero.

The constants alpha and beta are derived as complex functions from the previously described rate constants $K_{1.2}$, $K_{2.1}$ and K_2.

If an accurate bi-exponential curve is to be constructed a large number of plasma level determinations should be obtained early in the phase following injection and also carried out over a long period of time [96].

The practical purpose of mathematical analysis of compartmental modelling is to obtain pharmacokinetic parameters which are of clinical value. An effective dosing regimen depends upon the knowledge of rate of transfer of the

drug from the gut (depot), determination of how long the drug persists in the body, and knowledge of the distribution, as well as routes and rates of elimination. An accurate plot of the log concentration of a drug in plasma versus time can provide the valuable information itemized below.

Drug half-life

The half-life of a drug ($t\frac{1}{2}$) is the time required for the drug concentration (C) to become equal to half the initial drug concentration. This definition applies to a first-order process. The derived equation for calculating the half-life is $t\frac{1}{2} = 0.693/K_1$, where K_1 is the first-order rate constant. Since the rates of disappearance of drug from the blood compartment are mostly first-order processes the $t\frac{1}{2}$ is independent of the initial plasma concentration and is uniform throughout the entire process. The half-life is usually obtained by measuring blood concentration data, but it may also be obtained by observing the rate of decline of a biological response. The relationship between plasma half-life and biological half-life is not always directly proportional. If the biological half-life is defined by means of blood concentration data then it may be defined as the time required for the body to *eliminate* half the drug that is in the body.

The biological half-life is calculated from the equation $t\frac{1}{2} = 0.693/\beta$. The term β was defined previously and this represents the rate constant of elimination of the drug from the body. It is obtained by measuring the slope of the first-order plot based on the elimination phase. The $t\frac{1}{2}$ may be altered by factors such as age, renal failure, or alterations in metabolic disposition, which will all modify the elimination phase.

Area under the curve

An important concept illustrated in Fig. 16.2 is that of the area under the curve (AUC). When kinetics are first-order, the AUC plotted from zero to infinity is a linear function of the dose of drug. Determination of the area under the curve following IV and PO administration of a drug can be used to compare differing forms of drug dosage. It can also give a measure of systemic bioavailability of the drug, and furthermore can be used to determine its volume of distribution.

Apparent volume of distribution

The term 'volume of distribution' (VD) is a conceptual one, defined as the volume of body water which would be required to contain the amount of drug in the body if it were uniformly present in the same concentration as it is in the blood. The term 'apparent' is used since drugs are not uniformly distributed throughout all body compartments. It is used to determine the amount of drug present in the body by measuring the concentration of drug in the blood and it can be calculated from the equation $VD = D/AUC \times \beta$, where D is the dose at time zero. Several other approximations can be used to determine the VD, depending on the information available.

Drug clearance

This term is used to express the rate constant for the loss of drug from the body. It refers mostly to clearance by the kidney, since determination of drug levels can be most easily performed in

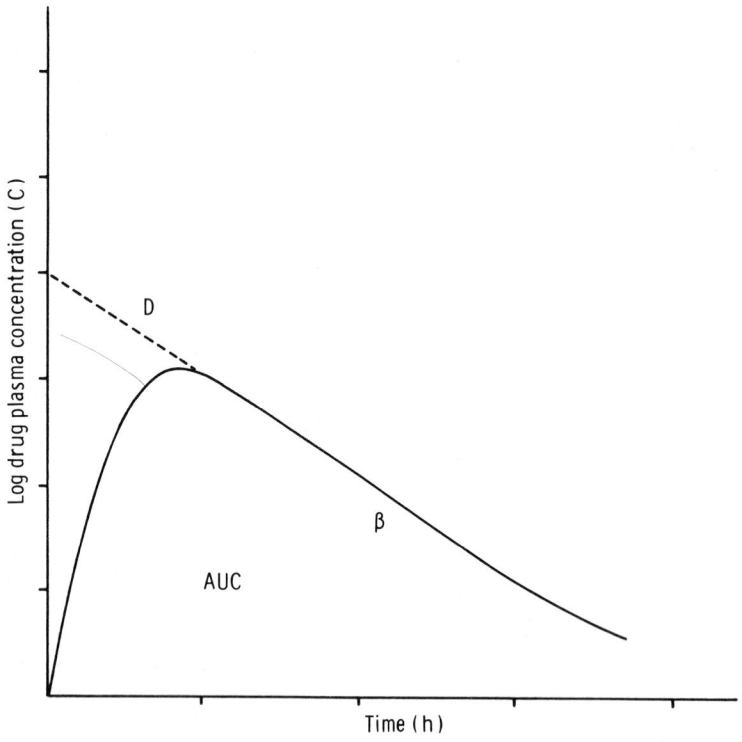

Fig. 16.2. The alteration of plasma concentration of a drug over time after oral drug administration. The *slope* of the declining curve (beta) represents drug elimination and the term AUC refers to the area under the curve. The *dotted line* D represents extrapolation of the β phase to obtain the plasma concentration at time zero (C_0) as used to determine the volume of distribution $V_0 = dose/C_0$.

the urine. Whole-body clearance should also include determination of the loss by metabolism and non-renal excretion. The clearance of the drug may be expressed as C_t/χ where C_t is the amount eliminated per unit time (t) and χ is the concentration of drug in the blood at that time. The concept of total-body clearance is clearly analogous to the concepts developed by physiologists in determining renal clearance. Renal clearance (Cr) may be defined as that volume of plasma which is cleared of the substance by the kidneys in 1 min and is calculated from the equation $Cr = UV/P$, where U is the concentration in the urine, V is the volume of urine excreted during 1 min, and P is the concentration in the plasma. In other words the term 'clearance' relates to the amount excreted in the urine in 1 min divided by the amount contained in 1 ml plasma.

In summary, combined analysis of the blood level curves in Figs. 16.1 and 16.2 may provide information on the rate of drug distribution (alpha phase), the rate of drug elimination (beta phase), and its apparent volume of distribution, as well as its biological half-life and the rate of clearance from the body.

Achieving therapeutic blood levels

Therapy usually involves repeated drug administration, with the aim of maintaining an effective concentration at the receptor site during the period of therapy, and therefore the pharmacokinetic profile described in Fig. 16.2 has to be re-evaluated to include an understanding of how sustained therapeutic blood levels are achieved. The concentration/time profile of a drug is determined by the dose and frequency of its administration. In addition, it is determined by the rate constants between the compartments, as shown:

$$\text{Depot} \xrightarrow{K_1} \text{Blood} \underset{K_{2.1}}{\overset{K_{1.2}}{\rightleftharpoons}} \text{Tissue}$$

$$\text{Blood} \xrightarrow{K_2} \text{Excretion}$$

Variation in the rate constants (K_1, $K_{1.2}$, $K_{2.1}$, K_2), which are associated with absorption, metabolism, and excretion respectively, are important determinants of the plasma drug concentration curve. The theoretically desirable features of the concentration curve are shown in Fig. 16.3 and the aim of therapy is to maintain plasma levels between the minimal and maxi-

mum points of the therapeutic range. Since the rate constants for an individual do not normally vary greatly, the major determinants of the shape of the drug concentration curve for long-term administration are the dose and frequency of drug administration. In multidose regimens, plasma steady-state concentration (P_{ss}) is equal to the AUC divided by the fixed time interval of dosing (r):

$$P_{ss} = \frac{AUC}{r}$$

Steady-rate plasma levels are achieved when the rate of supply equals the rate of drug elimination and the latter is reflected in the $t\frac{1}{2}$. If a steady state is to be maintained, then an amount of drug that is equal to the dose administered must be eliminated from the body during the fixed interval r. It is important in devising long-term dose regimens to understand therefore the determinants of both drug supply and drug elimination.

Drug absorption (supply)

The absorption of a drug from the gut depends upon a variety of related factors. Absorption occurs by a process of passive diffusion across a lipid/protein cell membrane. The drug must first be in solution not only for absorption to take place, but also for it to exert its pharmacological action. Therefore, drug absorption is determined firstly by the rate at which the drug enters solution (i.e., dissolution rate) and secondly by the diffusion rate across the gastro-intestinal membrane. Solid dosage forms should disintegrate rapidly. Disintegration rate depends on the excipients in the formulation, the type of coating and the degree of compression used in preparation. If the disintegration rate is rapid, then the dissolution rate depends upon the solubility of the agent and its surface area, in that a finely powdered drug presenting a large surface area enters solution more rapidly.

The important factors that determine drug absorption once it is in solution are its lipid solubility and the extent to which it is ionized. Absorbability of a drug from the gastro-intestinal tract can be correlated with its oil/water partition coefficient, i.e. the ratio of concentration in non-aqueous to aqueous solution. Increasing rates of absorption are associated with increased partition coefficients. Many drugs are either weak acids or weak bases which dissociate in solution depending upon

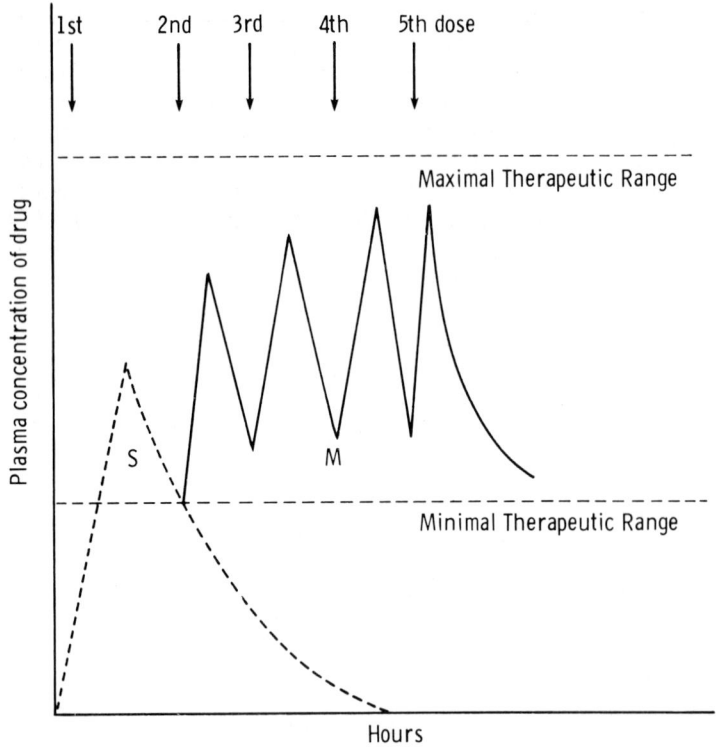

Fig. 16.3. Alteration in drug plasma concentration over time after repeated oral dosing. The *dotted line* represents the pattern following a single dose (*S*) and the *solid line*, the pattern after multiple dosing (*M*). The maximal and minimum therapeutic plasma concentrations represent the range of drug concentration associated with a therapeutic response and minimal unwanted effects. The frequency of dosing depends on the elimination half-life.

the pH. The undissociated neutral species diffuses into lipid membranes more easily and therefore absorption of a drug is influenced by the pH of the environment. For example, a weak organic acid in an alkaline solution will lose H^+ ions (protons) and become negatively charged. This results in reduced lipid solubility and hence reduced absorption. In essence, the factors which influence drug absorption are the concentration of drug in solution, its lipid solubility, and its molecular size. Environmental factors such as pH, regional intestinal motility, and the presence of other agents may also modify the pattern of absorption.

Once a drug is absorbed, it is dissolved in the aqueous phase of the body fluids. Within the vascular compartment, drugs can be bound to red cells, lipoproteins, or plasma proteins. Plasma albumin can reversibly bind drugs, especially those which are acidic. A drug may bind not only to specific sites on albumin, but also to secondary and tertiary sites. The extent of binding depends on the affinity of the albumin-binding site, as well as the concentration of albumin, the pH, and the ionic composition of the solution. The practical importance of protein binding is that drug action, distribution, and excretion depends on the concentration of free drug in solution and alterations in albumin binding modify free drug concentration. Thus, if a drug with high affinity for albumin is administered in the presence of a previously administered drug which has a lower affinity for albumin, the latter compound will be displaced and its free concentration will rise. This may result in enhanced concentration at its site of action or enhanced excretion.

Drug elimination

Drugs are removed from the body by excretion in bile and urine, but small amounts may also occur in sweat, saliva, and milk. Lipid soluble drugs require biotransformation to render them more water-soluble prior to excretion. Recently, the concept of clearance has been applied to the entire process of metabolism and excretion, because it permits a fuller description of the removal of drug from its site of action. Total systemic clearance (CL_{ss}) of a drug is defined as the sum of all the clearances carried out by various organs. It may be determined by giving a drug IV (I) and measuring the area under the curve (i.e., $CI_S = D_I/AUC_I$, when D is the total dose of drug). The primary clearance organs are the liver and the kidney. The former clears the drug by metabolism as well as by biliary excretion. Hepatic clearance depends on liver blood flow and the activity of drug-metabolizing enzymes [117, 136].

Drug metabolism commonly involves an oxidative step in which a hydroxyl group is inserted into the molecule (phase I metabolism). Thereafter, the molecule may be conjugated with glucuronic or acetic acid, resulting in the formation of water-soluble metabolites (Phase II metabolism). These soluble metabolites may then undergo renal excretion. Drug-metabolizing enzymes are situated in the smooth endoplasmic reticulum of the hepatic parenchymal cell. The activity of these enzymes is modified by genetic variation, age, exposure to other chemicals, and hepatic disease.

Certain drugs such as propranolol and lidocaine are avidly cleared by the liver. When such a drug is given PO a large proportion is cleared as it enters the liver from the gut via the portal circulation. The oral drug clearance can be determined by dividing the total oral dose by the area under the curve D (oral)/AUC (oral). Such a calculation gives a measure of the drug's systemic bioavailability and extensive hepatic clearance following oral dosing is termed the 'first-pass effect'.

The renal excretion of drugs occurs by either glomerular filtration or tubular secretion, or by both. Glomerular filtration depends upon the extent of protein binding of the drug and its molecular size. It also depends upon the hydrostatic pressure gradient across the membrane of Bowman's capsule. In contrast, tubular secretion is an energy-dependent process with organic acids and bases, including drugs being secreted by this process.

Summary

In this section certain pharmacokinetic concepts of clinical relevance have been described. Drug administration is followed by its distribution throughout the body and this process may be described by the technique of compartmental analysis. The rate of transfer of a drug determines the concentration of the drug within any compartment at time t. The aim of dosing regimens is to obtain the concentration of drug at the effector site which will achieve the desired therapeutic effect, without causing unwanted effects. An indirect guide to drug concentration at the effector site is given by measurement of plasma drug levels, which depend upon the rates of supply, distribution, and clearance of the drug. Measurement of plasma and urine drug concentration over time, and application of these data to compartmental analysis provide data on the rate of absorption, persistence within the body, and elimination half-life of a drug, which forms the basis for the recommendations on dose and frequency of drug administration. In addition, the effect of age, race, sex, and disease on drug kinetics can be ascertained by studying the appropriate population [75, 80, 123].

Drug kinetics in critical care

Cardiac failure and shock frequently modify the normal pattern of drug disposition. In this aspect, drug kinetics has been studied mostly in various forms of heart failure, and the principles extrapolated to the shock state. Cardiac failure is associated with fluid and salt retention, resulting in expanded blood volume. There is increased autonomic activity, which is associated with changes in blood distribution to favour the heart and brain, while flow to the liver, kidneys and voluntary muscles is reduced. These abnormalities may affect drug absorption, distribution, and elimination. Thus, intestinal absorption may be reduced because of altered motility and blood flow, together with oedema of the intestinal tissue. Drug distribution may be modified because of the increased blood volume and reduced cardiac output, associated with increased flow to brain and heart and reduced flow elsewhere. Hepatic blood flow and metabolism are altered in heart failure, and drug clearance may be reduced as a consequence. Specific examples of the effect of heart failure on drug disposition will be described in the appropriate sections [4, 58, 107].

Drugs modifying autonomic function

The autonomic system

The heart and blood vessels are innervated by the autonomic system and many drugs exert their cardiovascular effects by modifying autonomic function.

The autonomic system comprises (1) the thoracolumbar sympathetic efferent outflow extending from the first thoracic to the second lumbar segments of the spinal cord; and (2) the craniosacral parasympathetic efferent outflow arising from the pons and medulla as well as the 2nd to 4th sacral segments of the spinal cord.

The sympathetic medullated nerves arise in the intermediospinal portion of the cord passing out anteriorly to join the sympathetic ganglia lying on either side of the spinal column. These preganglionic medullated fibres terminate at different levels in the sympathetic chain or in sympathetic ganglia such as the coeliac and mesenteric ganglia. Their terminal axons release the neurotransmitter acetylcholine. Postganglionic sympathetic nerves are non-medullated and innervate smooth muscle and glands, releasing the neurotransmitter noradrenaline.

The preganglionic fibres of the cranial parasympathetic nerve run in the IIIrd cranial nerve to the pupil; VIIth and IXth cranial nerves to the lacrymal and salivary glands; the Xth and XIth nerves to the thoracic and abdominal viscera. The cell bodies of the preganglionic fibres are found in the accessory nucleus of the mid brain for the IIIrd nerve; the superior salivatory nucleus of the ponto medullary junction of the VIIth nerve; the inferior salivary nucleus of the XIth, and the dorsal vagal nucleus in the medulla for the vagus nerve.

The sacral parasympathetic nerves arise in the grey matter of the spinal cord at the level of the first lumbar vertebra and pass out in the IInd, IIIrd, and IVth sacral nerves to the inferior hypogastric plexus. They supply the lower portion of the colon and the urogenital system. The preganglionic parasympathetic nerves, which are medullated and much longer than the preganglionic sympathetic nerves, terminate in ganglia close to the organ which they innervate. Acetylcholine is the neurotransmitter released at both the preganglionic and postganglionic parasympathetic nerve endings.

The discharge pattern of the efferent autonomic system is determined by the level of afferent nerve input especially from the baroreceptor and chemoreceptor areas, and also by the activity of the centres in the medulla, hypothalamus, and cortex. These higher centres determine the integrated response of the cardiovascular system to environmental change and influence the relative distribution of blood flow, blood pressure and cardiac output, for the express purpose of maintaining appropriate tissue perfusion [38].

Neurotransmitters

Noradrenaline is formed from L-tyrosine in the cell bodies or terminal varicosities of postganglionic sympathetic nerves. It is stored in the nerve varicosities in electron-dense, large- and small-core vesicles, the contents being released into the synaptic cleft by the action potential. Released noradrenaline can (1) interact with the postsynaptic adrenoceptor; (2) be taken up into extraneuronal tissues, such as glands and cardiac and smooth muscle, by a separate uptake mechanism (uptake 2); (3) interact with the presynaptic adrenoceptor on the nerve ending; (4) be taken up into the sympathetic nerve by a stereospecific energy-dependent mechanism (uptake 1); (5) be degraded by catechol-O-methyltransferase (COMT) and monoamine oxidase (MAO), giving rise to numerous biologically inactive metabolites (Fig. 16.4). Drugs may specifically modify this series of events by (1) reducing noradrenaline release (adrenergic neurone blockers); (2) antagonizing adrenoceptors (alpha and beta blockers); (3) reducing noradrenaline uptake (uptake 1 blockers, e.g., desipramine); and (4) reducing enzymatic breakdown (MAO inhibitors) [132].

Acetylcholine is the neurotransmitter released not only from post-ganglionic parasympathetic nerves, but also from all preganglionic autonomic nerves, from motor nerves to voluntary muscle and at numerous synapses within the CNS. This neurotransmitter is formed within the nerve ending from choline and acetyl coenzyme A, and released into the synapse where it exerts its effect by binding to cholinoreceptors. Its action is terminated by the enzyme cholinesterase situated near the receptor, or by diffusion from the synaptic cleft.

Dopamine is a catecholamine formed from L-tyrosine by decarboxylation of the intermediate dihydroxyphenylalanine (DOPA). Its major physiological function is as a neurotransmitter within the CNS, where it is present in the basal ganglia, medulla oblongata, and hypothalamus. It is also present in peripheral sympathetic nerves. Dopamine differs from adrenaline and noradrenaline in that it binds not only to alpha and beta adrenoceptors, but also to specific dopaminergic receptors in renal, splanchnic, coronary, and collateral blood vessels. Its agonist action at dopaminergic receptors is prevented by pimozide and metoclopramide. In addition, dopamine causes release of noradrenaline from nerve endings so it has a modest indirect sympathomimetic action [130].

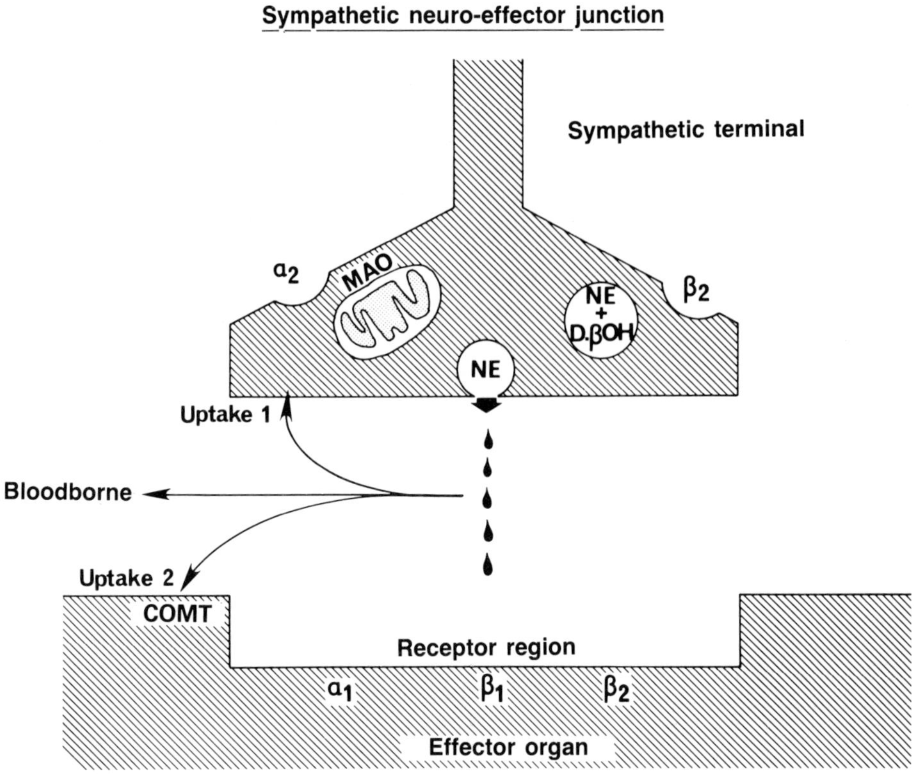

Sympathetic neuro-effector junction

Fig. 16.4. Diagrammatic representation of the fate of neuronally released noradrenaline. Uptake 1 is a stereospecific energy-dependent mechanism. *MAO*, monoamine oxidase; *DβOH*, dopamine β-hydroxylase; *NE*, noradrenaline; *COMT*, catechol-O-methyl transferase. α_2-Adrenoceptor activation inhibits noradrenaline release and β-adrenoceptor activation facilitates release.

Classification of autonomic receptors

A receptor may be defined as that molecular component of a cell which interacts with a specific ligand to elicit a biological response. The receptors are classified on the basis of their interaction with chemically defined agonists and antagonists, and this classification is therefore purely operational. Thus cholinoreceptors are subdivided into muscarinic and nicotinic. The term 'muscarinic' is derived from the original observation that the plant alkaloid muscarine, when administered to animals, induces changes similar to electrical stimulation of the vagus nerve. Muscarinic receptors are activated by acetylcholine or the synthetic agonists methacholine or carbachol, and the specific antagonist is atropine. Nicotinic receptors are so designated because nicotine initially stimulates and then antagonizes them. They are activated by acetylcholine or by synthetic agonists such as urocanylcholine (ganglionic cholinoreceptors) or suxemethonium (neuromuscular cholinoreceptors). The specific antagonists are mecamylamine, or hexamethonium at auto-

nomic ganglia, and gallamine or (+) tubo-curarine at neuromuscular junctions.

Adrenotropic receptors are subdivided into alpha and beta receptors. The alpha adrenoceptors respond preferentially to noradrenaline and the synthetic agonist phenylephrine, their effects being specifically antagonized by phentolamine and phenoxybenzamine. These receptors are further subdivided into α_1, situated on the postsynaptic membrane, and α_2, present on the presynaptic neuronal membrane. Appropriate agonists and antagonists of α_1 and α_2 receptors are shown in Table 16.1. The beta receptors respond preferentially to

Table 16.1. Drugs used to characterize adrenoceptor responses

	Alpha receptor	Beta receptor
Agonist	Norepinephrine	Isoproterenol
Antagonist	Phentolamine	Propranolol
Response	Excitatory	Inhibitory (except heart)

isoprenaline and are specifically antagonized by propranolol. They are subdivided into β_1 and β_2, both of which are postsynaptic. These receptors are also found on the presynaptic neuronal membrane, but their categorization and physiological function require further definition [76].

Adrenoceptors are present in most tissues. In general, alpha activation results in excitatory or contractile responses, e.g., in vascular smooth muscle, whereas beta activation is inhibitory, with the important exceptions of cardiac beta adrenoceptors and those mediating lipolytic responses.

Nicotinic receptor antagonists

Agents which specifically antagonize the action of acetylcholine at nicotinic receptors on sympathetic ganglia may be used to induce controlled hypotension during anaesthesia or for the medical management of dissecting aortic aneurism. Their use is limited and the preferred agents are mecamylamine and trimethaphan.

Pharmacological effects. Ganglion blockade impairs the function of both the sympathetic and the parasympathetic portions of the postganglionic autonomic system. The cardiovascular effects are dependent on posture and are minimal in the horizontal position. In the upright position, blood pressure is markedly decreased due to reduced arteriolar and venous tone. Cardiac output falls and there is a reduction in renal and splanchnic blood flow. Ganglion blockade results in atony of the gastrointestinal and genito-urinary smooth muscle, causing paralytic ileus and urinary retention, respectively.

Trimethaphan camsylate (Arfonad). This is a short-acting ganglion-blocking agent used primarily to control blood pressure in hypotensive anaesthesia, in dissecting aortic aneurism, and in the management of hypertensive crisis. It is administered IV in a saline or dextrose solution by dissolving 250 mg in 250 ml. There is no data on its pharmacokinetics. Unwanted effects arise from its pharmacological action, namely hypotension, gut and bladder dysfunction, and failure of ocular accommodation.

Agents acting at muscarinic receptors

Atropine. Atropine is the only widely used muscarinic antagonist for the management of sinus bradycardia and AV block, especially when associated with acute myocardial infarction

(AMI). It acts by reversing the hyperpolarization of the spontaneously depolarizing tissue in the sinus and AV nodes, which is caused by the action of acetylcholine on cardiac muscarinic receptors. Atropine has less effect on inter-atrial conduction and no effect on the His–Purkinje system [2].

Atropine can be given PO, SC, or IV. In critical care, it is given IV in an initial dose of 0.3 mg, increasing by 0.3 mg at 15-min intervals to a maximum of 2 mg. In AMI it may reduce bradycardia and improve impaired AV conduction, resulting in a reduction in ventricular ectopic beats (VEBs) and increased ventricular rate. Atropine, when given IV, is cleared rapidly by the kidney, and 90% of a single dose is removed within 24 h. It undergoes some hepatic metabolism, but 30% of a dose appears unchanged in the urine.

Atropine will antagonize all muscarinic receptors, resulting in dry mouth, visual disturbances, and bladder and bowel dysfunction. Large doses cause marked CNS manifestations, such as hallucinations and hyperpyrexia, leading to coma. The action of atropine can be overcome by giving an anticholinesterase such as physostigmine (1–2 mg IV), which reduces the breakdown of acetylcholine.

Adrenoceptor agonists

Drugs that stimulate adrenotropic receptors are termed sympathomimetics. Naturally occurring stimulants are the catecholamines, dopamine, noradrenaline, and adrenaline, though there are numerous synthetic analogues, including the alpha agonists phenylephrine and methoxamine and the beta agonists isoprenaline, salbutamol, and dobutamine. Since these agents act on the heart and blood vessels they are widely used in the management of cardiogenic and septic shock, and occasionally for the short-term management of heart block. The choice of agent for a particular type and severity of shock is dealt with elsewhere. This section will discuss only the pharmacological actions of these agents.

Pharmacological effects. Sympathomimetic agents differ from each other both in potency and in the ratio of alpha- to beta-adrenergic stimulation. They will activate those adrenoceptors for which they have a specific affinity causing alterations in cardiovascular, metabolic, and respiratory function.

Cardiovascular effects. Catecholamines are used in critical care to restore tissue perfusion. This may be achieved by increasing cardiac function (beta stimulation), raising blood pressure (alpha vasoconstriction), or reducing vascular tone (beta stimulation). The haemodynamic effects of catecholamines will depend on the affinity of the agonist for alpha and beta receptors. Noradrenaline binds predominantly to alpha and β_1 adrenoceptors, adrenaline to both alpha and β_2 receptors, and isoprenaline solely to β_1 and β_2 receptors. In addition, the net haemodynamic effects will be influenced by the cardiovascular reflexes activated by the primary haemodynamic effects of the catecholamines. Prediction of the net haemodynamic effect of catecholamine administration provides a valuable exercise in applied pharmacology.

Noradrenaline causes generalized vasoconstriction of blood vessels supplying renal, splanchnic, muscular, and cerebral beds, resulting in a fall in blood flow. The haemodynamic effects of an infusion of noradrenaline (5–15 μg/min) are a sharp rise in systolic and diastolic pressures and a reflexly mediated cardiac slowing. Cardiac output will alter according to the net effect of the acute rise in afterload and preload, as well as direct stimulation of ventricular beta adrenoceptors. Usually cardiac output is slightly reduced, but cardiac work is increased by these effects and hence myocardial blood flow increases despite the direct constrictor action of noradrenaline on coronary vessels.

Adrenaline, having significant β_2- and alpha-agonist actions, causes a different spectrum of cardiovascular responses. Vessels in the renal, hepatic, and cutaneous beds are constricted, but vessels in the splanchnic and voluntary muscle beds are relaxed. There is a significant increase in blood flow in mesenteric and splanchnic veins, but a reduction in renal blood flow. Adrenaline (0.1–0.2 μg/kg/min) causes a rise in systolic blood pressure due to the direct inotropic and chronotropic cardiac actions, whilst diastolic pressure falls due to β_2-mediated vasodilation. Heart rate rises due to the chronotropic β_1 action but because the blood pressure rise is much less than with equivalent doses of noradrenaline there is a diminished degree of reflex vagal inhibition. Cardiac output rises, as does cardiac work and coronary flow. Adrenaline enhances the rate of depolarization in the sinus node and Purkinje tissue and the rate of AV conduction, while shortening the refractory period of atrial and ventricular muscle. These cardiac electrophysiological actions account for the arrhythmogenic actions of adrenaline [45].

Isoprenaline, which activates only β_1 and β_2 adrenoceptors, dilates splanchnic and skeletal muscle vessels, but has little effect on renal, cutaneous, and hepatic blood vessels. It increases heart rate, cardiac contractility, and left ventricular (LV) work, but decreases ventricular volume. Thus when an infusion of isoprenaline is given at doses equal to adrenaline, it causes a greater and more prolonged tachycardia, an enhanced fall in diastolic blood pressure and an increase in cardiac output. The fact that an isoprenaline infusion (2–10 μg/min) causes an improvement in cardiac output and tissue perfusion has led to its use in shock states, especially cardiogenic shock. Recently detailed haemodynamic studies [49, 93] show that whilst an isoprenaline infusion may double cardiac output in shocked subjects, this is accompanied by a disproportionately greater increase in myocardial metabolism, especially lactate production. Thus, isoprenaline does not appear to have the appropriate balance of pharmacological effects for routine use in cardiogenic shock.

Salbutamol has predominantly β_2-agonist actions, and is used primarily for its bronchodilator actions in the management of asthma. Gibson and Coltart [42] have studied its haemodynamic effects and shown that in doses of 0.4–2.0 μg/kg/min IV it causes a marked fall in peripheral resistance accompanied by an increase in heart rate and cardiac output. The chronotropic response was secondary to the fall in diastolic blood pressure and was prevented by atropine administration, indicating that only the vascular selective β_2 actions of salbutamol were present at those doses. In cardiogenic shock and also low-output states after cardiac surgery, salbutamol causes an increase in cardiac output and clinical improvement [140]. It has also been shown to improve patients with congestive cardiomyopathy since it causes a fall in LV end-diastolic pressure without significant alteration in blood pressure and heart rate. Such observations emphasize the significance of vascular tone rather than cardiac stimulation in restoring cardiac function.

Dopamine, administered systemically, acts primarily on the cardiovascular system, though it also causes stimulation of the exocrine pancreas and inhibits release of growth hormone and prolactin. In low doses, it causes vasodilatation of renal and splanchnic vessels due to specific activation of dopaminergic receptors, and an increase in heart rate and contractility due to beta-adrenoceptor activation. These latter effects are due both to a direct action and to enhanced release of neuronal noradrenaline.

In higher doses, dopamine causes an alpha-receptor-mediated vasoconstriction and a direct dopamine receptor-mediated increase in renal excretion of sodium.

Thus the overall haemodynamic consequences of dopamine infusion depend upon the proportion of differing receptors activated. Infusions in the range 2–10 μg/kg/min cause an increase in cardiac output in normal subjects accompanied by a fall in vascular resistance with little change in heart rate and blood pressure. Doses in excess of 30 μg/kg/min cause generalized alpha-mediated vasoconstriction and an increase in blood pressure. The effect on blood pressure is complex in that low doses can cause hypotension which can be of both direct and neurogenic origin [44, 46]. Similarly, its effects on cardiac function and metabolism are complex and dose-dependent. In general there is a rise in myocardial O_2 consumption and coronary flow due to its inotropic actions, but infusion rates can be achieved that improve cardiac output and reduce vascular resistance without increasing myocardial O_2 consumption [81].

Dobutamine is a sympathomimetic amine possessing a novel combination of adrenotropic actions. It differs significantly from the natural catecholamines and isoprenaline in that its major action is on cardiac β_1 adrenoceptors with minor β_2- and alpha-adrenergic actions. Unlike dopamine, it does not act on dopaminergic receptors, nor does it cause release of noradrenaline. In conscious dogs, it was observed that dobutamine had an impressive inotropic action accompanied by little alteration in heart rate and blood pressure [55]. Under similar experimental conditions, noradrenaline caused a marked rise in blood pressure, whereas dopamine induced a rise in heart rate and fall in blood pressure. Dobutamine appears to have a biphasic effect on peripheral blood vessels in that low doses (5 μg/kg/min) cause some increase in tone whilst higher doses (30 μg/kg/min) induce muscular relaxation. These observations indicate that dobutamine has a distinctly different profile of cardiovascular actions to isoprenaline and dopamine. Its ability to improve ventricular contractility without markedly increasing heart rate or dilating resistance vessels suggests that dobutamine may have value in shock states associated with depressed cardiac function.

In normal subjects, dobutamine (2.5, 5, and 10 μg/kg/min) caused a dose-dependent increase in contractility with minimal increase in heart rate [30]. In patients with depressed cardiac function due to aortic stenosis [62] or chronic congestive cardiac failure [6, 81], dobutamine (2–10 μg/kg/min) caused a dose-dependent increase in stroke volume and LV dp/dt, and a reduction in LV end-diastolic pressure, accompanied by a rise in cardiac output with little change in heart rate or blood pressure. When administered to patients with myocardial infarction, dobutamine caused a greater reduction in LV end-diastolic pressure than dopamine, with little rise in heart rate and blood pressure for an equivalent increase in cardiac output. At equivalent inotropic doses, isoprenaline causes a much greater rise in heart rate and cardiac output, accompanied by a fall in diastolic blood pressure. The optimal indications for the use of dobutamine in cardiogenic shock and congestive heart failure require careful evaluation. The net haemodynamic response depends very much on the clinical setting and the main reason for caution is the extent of co-existing coronary artery disease. Dobutamine increases cardiac work and myocardial O_2 consumption, but in general this increase is less than that caused by dopamine and particularly isoprenaline. In the presence of adequate coronary perfusion, dobutamine is probably the inotropic agent of choice. In the peri-infarction period and following coronary artery bypass surgery (CABS), caution is required since some studies suggest that in this setting it may cause a disproportionate increase in myocardial O_2 consumption. Thus Myer et al. [94] observe an increased inhomogeneity of flow due to dobutamine, in patients with severe coronary artery disease and its net effect in this setting is difficult to predict, since studies by Schell et al. [120] were not able to show an increase in infarct size when dobutamine was given to patients with AMI. In shocked patients with severe hypotension, *dopamine* may be the preferred agent because of its greater alpha vasoconstrictor action combined with the dopaminergically mediated increase in renal and splanchnic perfusion.

Prenalterol (H133/22) is a new selective β_1-adrenoceptor agonist used for the management of acute cardiac failure and the cardiovascular effects of shock. It is a directly acting sympathomimetic agent which differs from the classic agents in that it causes a significant increase in myocardial contractile force, whilst having little effect on heart rate or blood pressure [14]. Prenalterol is available for clinical study, as either a parenteral formulation or a slow-release tablet. For parenteral use the recommended dose is 0.5–20.0 μg/kg/min according to the haemodynamic and clinical response. In normal subjects, prenalterol causes a dose-dependent increase in heart rate and systolic blood pressure, and a variable reduction in diastolic pressure. There is a correlation between biological effect and plasma level in the range of 15–50 mmol/litre. The indirect indices of cardiac function derived from measurement of systolic time intervals, i.e., pre-ejection periods, LV ejection time and total electromechanical systole are all shortened [63]. The cardiovascular effects persist for about 1 h after the infusion is stopped.

In patients suffering from AMI or septic shock, infusion of prenalterol (2.5–15 μg/kg/min) causes an increase of about 30% in cardiac contractility, accompanied by a small increase in heart rate [49]. Cardiac output may increase by 10–20% depending upon the initial level of output. Myocardial O_2 consumption rises, as does lactate extraction [108]. Prenalterol also causes a modest rise in plasma levels of free fatty acids and insulin.

Following IV injection, prenalterol is rapidly distributed throughout the body, the alpha phase lasting about 8 min. The beta elimination phase is about 2 h [111]. After administration PO, haemodynamic effects can be observed within 30 min and persist for 45 h. It is well tolerated and the reported effects of tachycardia, palpitations, and feeling of tension are due to its beta-stimulant actions.

Other actions of adrenoceptor agonists. Adrenaline relaxes bronchial smooth muscle and causes respiratory stimulation, by both a central and a peripheral action. In therapeutic doses, it is a mild CNS stimulant causing apprehension, anxiety, and tremor. It has marked metabolic effects causing a rise in plasma free fatty acids (FFA), glucose, lactate, and potassium, accompanied by a reduction in plasma insulin levels. These metabolic effects are associated with a rise in total-body O_2 consumption, possibly due to an increased metabolism in brown adipose tissue.

Noradrenaline does not have as great an effect as adrenaline in these systems, and causes only a mild hyperglycaemia.

Isoprenaline causes similar beta-adrenoceptor effects to adrenaline resulting in a rise in FFA, but insulin levels also rise because of the beta stimulant effects on the islet cells in the pancreas. Its calorigenic actions are equivalent to those of adrenaline.

Salbutamol also causes a rise in plasma insulin, free fatty acids and lactate.

Pharmacokinetics. The naturally occurring catecholamines, noradrenaline and adrenaline, undergo rapid and extensive metabolism and excretion when given parenterally. They are rapidly removed from the circulation by the uptake I and uptake II mechanism resulting in a plasma half-life of only 3–5 min. Thereafter, they are metabolized by monoamine oxidase and catechol-O-methyl transferase enzymes, (COMT) giving rise to a wide range of free and conjugated metabolites. The major metabolites are 4-hydroxy, 3-methoxy mandelic acid (VMA) and metanephrine sulphate [72]. Both catecholamines are rapidly destroyed by enzymes in the gut and liver.

Isoprenaline sulphate is absorbed from the gut or sublingually. An effect is observed within 30 min and persists for 60–90 min. Isoprenaline is extensively metabolized in the gut and liver, giving rise to inactive conjugates which are excreted in the urine. A small amount of isoprenaline is excreted unchanged and one metabolite, 3-methoxyisoprenaline, has weak antagonist activity. When isoprenaline is given by infusion, plasma levels fall rapidly on termination of the infusion, with a half-life of 5 min. A secondary additional decline takes place over 2 h.

Salbutamol is rapidly absorbed from the gut and its pharmacological effects last 3–5 h. Peak plasma levels are observed 3 h after a dose of 4–8 mg PO. It is not degraded by COMT and sulphatases, which may explain its more persistent effects. About 80% of a single dose is excreted in the urine within 24 h, and half the excreted dose is in the form of a conjugated metabolite. Similar patterns of metabolism are observed after inhalation of the aerosol formulation [134].

Dopamine is inactive when given PO, and when given parenterally it undergoes rapid metabolism to noradrenaline by dopamine beta-hydroxylase. The plasma half-life of dopamine is 5 min.

Dobutamine is not active when given PO. The usual infusion of 10 μg/kg/min gives plasma levels of 150–250 ng/ml. The average clearance rate is 3.5 litre/min with an elimination half-life of 3 min. The volume of distribution (VD) varies considerably and this may account for the wide range of plasma levels for a given infusion rate [66].

Unwanted effects of adrenoceptor agonists. These are due primarily to the specific pharmacological actions of the agents and an appreciation of the differing spectrum of properties explains the differing effects. Thus adrenaline is a powerful arrhythmagenic agent and will also cause tremor, anxiety and hyperventilation.

Noradrenaline causes marked vasoconstriction and the major concern is hypertension and regional ischaemia in patients with arterial disease. Dopamine is less arrhythmagenic than noradrenaline, but it can also cause gangrene in limbs, due to excess vasoconstriction in shocked patients [126]. Dobutamine appears to be the least arrhythmagenic of these sympathomimetic amines, but it may also cause tremor and tachycardia in high doses.

Adrenoceptor antagonists

Drugs are available which will specifically antagonize the various subdivisions of both alpha and beta adrenoceptors. The main application of antagonists is in the management of hypertension, cardiac arrhythmias, and coronary artery disease. Alpha antagonists have not been widely used in the past, but the specific α_1 antagonist, prazosin, is now commonly used to manage essential hypertension because it appears to cause less postural hypotension and reflex tachycardia than the non-selective antagonists. The majority of patients receiving these drugs are not critically ill and this section will be confined to the consideration of those adrenotropic antagonists which may be of value in managing the critically ill patient. Additional comment will be made on the influence of these agents on patients taking drugs chronically, who may subsequently become critically ill.

Alpha adrenergic antagonists may be used to lower blood pressure in hypertensive crises especially those associated with phaeochromocytoma and also to reduce afterload in acute ventricular failure.

Phenoxybenzamine (POB) is the reference alpha antagonist, though it has several drawbacks in that its onset of action is slow because it is not a competitive antagonist. Furthermore, it antagonizes histaminic, serotinergic, and muscarinic receptors. When given IV to the supine subject there is a widening of pulse pressure, due to blockade of vascular alpha adrenoceptors and a secondary reflex increase in heart rate. Rapid injection causes a sharp fall in blood pressure as a result of its non-specific actions. Blood flow in the renal, splanchnic, and skin regions increases, with little effect on coronary and cerebral blood flow. Cardiac output increases slightly depending on the height of the afterload, prior to administration. In addition, phenoxybenzamine blocks the metabolic effects of alpha-mediated catecholamine stimulation.

For the pre-operative management of phaeochromocytoma, POB is given IV in a daily dose of 1 mg/kg for 3 days prior to operation. The blood volume thus expands slowly and if there is a disproportionate fall in blood pressure, blood transfusion should be given. On the day of operation, an additional dose of 50 mg phenoxybenzamine is given IV. Propranolol is also given for 2 days pre-operatively (240 mg daily) [25].

More recently POB has also been used to lower afterload in patients with cardiogenic shock. In these situations it is given in a dose of 1 mg/kg in 200 ml saline, and careful monitoring of pulmonary wedge pressure (PWP) is essential, since excessive reduction of venous return may cause clinical deterioration [19].

Phenoxybenzamine is available in 2-ml ampoules (50 mg/ml). The oral dose is 30–90 mg daily, but the drug is irregularly and incompletely absorbed from the gut. About 80% appears in the bile and urine within 24 h, but total body clearance may take more than a week.

Phenoxybenzamine causes numerous side-effects such as dizziness, tachycardia, failure of ejaculation, and nasal stuffiness, which are all associated with its alpha-adrenoceptor action.

Phentolamine is a short-acting competitive non-selective alpha-adrenoceptor antagonist, which has also been used in the management of phaeochromocytoma, hypertensive crisis, acute ventricular failure, and accidental catecholamine overdosage. To obtain a controlled fall in systemic blood pressure, it is administered by infusion at a dose of 0.1–2.0 mg/min. If there is depressed cardiac output associated with high aortic impedance and abnormally elevated end-diastolic pressure (>18 mmHg) administration of phentolamine will decrease end-diastolic pressure, and this will be accompanied by a small reduction in systolic blood pressure, an increase in heart rate and a marked increase in cardiac output. Myocardial O_2 consumption is relatively unaffected. In contrast, when end-diastolic pressure is normal there may be a reduction in cardiac output and an unwanted reflex tachycardia, due to an inappropriate reduction in systolic pressure [90].

Phentolamine is rapidly metabolized, particularly in the liver, and excreted in the urine. The unwanted effects are similar to those encountered with other non-selective alpha antagonists.

Thymoxamine is a relatively specific alpha blocker which has a very short duration of action when given IV, causing a fall in blood pressure and a small rise in cardiac output. Its oral absorption is uncertain and it appears to be of limited value.

Indoramin is a competitive alpha blocker used primarily in the treatment of hypertension. Like phenoxybenzamine, it has several other pharmacological properties such as local anaesthesia, antihistamine, and antiserotonin effects. It is a moderately effective antihypertensive agent.

Prazosin has recently been introduced for the management of hypertension and differs from other alpha-adrenoceptor antagonists in that it is highly selective for the α_1 adrenoceptor which is found on the postsynaptic membrane, mediating the vasoconstrictor response [12]. The α_2 receptor is situated on the presynaptic membrane and stimulation by noradrenaline inhibits further noradrenaline release, i.e., a negative feedback loop. This negative feedback loop is therefore preserved in the presence of prazosin, thus preventing the reflex tachycardia which normally follows the fall in blood pressure. Given IV to hypertensive patients, prazosin (0.1 mg) causes a fall in blood pressure within 30 min, which is accompanied by little change in heart rate or cardiac output unless the supine subject is tilted. In follow-up of long-term prazosin therapy it has been observed that there is a reduction in blood pressure and total peripheral resistance, with no alteration in the heart rate, cardiac output, and stroke volume responses to exercise [82]. Prazosin has approximately an 80-fold greater affinity for alpha receptors of veins than of arteries, and its spectrum of vascular activity is more closely related to glyceryltrinitrate than to classic arterial dilators such as hydrallazine.

The recommended oral dose for prazosin is 1–7.5 mg daily, but the initial dose should be low and the patient must be warned of the possibility of transient syncope and dizziness. The oral dose can be increased every 3 or 4 days to a maximum of 7.5 mg daily. After a single dose of 2–5 mg PO, peak plasma levels range between 23 and 40 ng/ml, but there is a wide individual variation. The plasma half-life is between 2 and 4 h and prazosin is highly bound to plasma proteins with a VD of between 75 and 120 litres. It undergoes extensive first-pass metabolism in the liver, with 90% of the drug being excreted in the faeces within 24 h and the remainder in the urine. Thus most of the drug is excreted by the biliary system in the form of dealkylated and conjugated metabolites.

Prazosin is well tolerated and the commonest side-effects are postural dizziness, palpitations, dyspnoea, fatigue, and nasal congestion. The most important side-effect is the 'first dose phenomenon' which is characterized by palpitations, faintness, and dizziness on receiving the initial dose of the drug. The symptoms resemble those of postural hypotension and may be due to the greater effect of prazosin on the venous capacitance vessels, causing a sudden decrease in the venous return.

Beta antagonists were introduced 20 years ago, initially for the management of angina pectoris and cardiac arrhythmias, but subsequently for numerous clinical indications (Table 16.2). In critically ill patients, beta antagonists may be used to control arrhythmias unresponsive to the first-line therapy of lidocaine and procainamide.

Table 16.2. Clinical indications for propranolol

Cardiovascular	Endocrine	Other
Angina pectoris	Thyrotoxicosis	Certain anxiety reactions
Arrhythmias	Phaeochromocytoma	Essential tremor
Essential hypertension		
Hypertrophic obstructive cardiomyopathy		
Migraine		
Tetralogy of Fallot		

They may be of particular value in the management of inappropriate tachycardia which can cause heart failure rather than arising as a result of ventricular failure. Propranolol is also used in the management of thyroid crisis, phaeochromocytoma and the cardiovascular manifestations of tetanus and acute prophyria. Although there are numerous beta antagonists available, relatively few have been appropriately evaluated for use in critical care. This section will therefore describe the general pharmacology of beta antagonists, but only propranolol will be discussed in detail.

Beta adrenoceptors are widely distributed throughout the body, although the clinically important ones are found in the heart, where they mediate positive inotropic, chronotropic, and dromotropic responses (β_1 effects) and in vascular and bronchial smooth muscle, where receptor activation causes relaxation (β_2 effects). In addition beta-adrenoceptor stimulation increases lipolysis (β_1), muscle glycogenolysis (β_2), and release of the hormones, insulin, and renin.

Propranolol. Propranolol was introduced in 1964 and is the reference agent. It is a potent specific antagonist of beta adrenoceptors, having five times greater affinity for β_2 than for β_1 receptors [36]. Atenolol and metoprolol differ from propranolol in acting primarily at β_1 adrenoceptors, but there is no clinically available β_2-selective analogue. In high concentrations, propranolol has local anaesthetic or quinidine-like actions which are not thought to contribute to its clinical actions [41]. Other beta antagonists, such as oxprenolol and pindolol, differ from propranolol in that they not only antagonize catecholamine effects at the adrenoceptor, but also mildly stimulate the adrenoceptor. This dual action is called partial agonism and the degree of partial agonism will determine the haemodynamic profile of the beta antagonist.

There are various *cardiovascular effects:* In the exercising healthy subject, propranolol (0.1 mg/kg IV) reduces heart rate, cardiac output, LV work, and systolic blood pressure by 15%–20%, with the degree of reduction depending on the extent of prior beta receptor activation. The fall in cardiac output is due both to the reduction in heart rate and ventricular function [127]. In patients with cardiac disease, the haemodynamic effect of propranolol depends on the nature and extent of the disease. In the hypertensive subject with good LV function, propranolol will reduce heart rate and cardiac output. In a patient with LV failure it may worsen failure and cause pulmonary oedema and hypotension, because the activation of cardiac adrenoceptors is necessary to maintain ventricular function. Propranolol increases ventricular volume and in patients with coronary artery disease can cause abnormalities of ventricular wall motion, leading to incoordinate contraction and reduced ejection fraction. Propranolol reduces myocardial O_2 consumption by reducing cardiac work and this is the basis for its use in angina pectoris. It alters the utilization of myocardial energy substrates by reducing FFA extraction and increasing glucose utilization, so that the latter contributes up to 60% of cardiac energy requirements. This action favours preservation of glycogen stores and conservation of O_2 supply. The reduction in myocardial work and O_2 demand thus reduces coronary flow by 15%–20%. In peripheral blood vessels, there is a reflex increase in vasoconstriction resulting from the fall in cardiac output.

Propranolol lowers circulating levels of FFAs and lactate produced by exercise and catecholamine stimulation, but has no effect on blood glucose. In the presence of hypoglycaemia, it will antagonize the homeostatic responses designed to reverse the hypoglycaemia and will also mask the cardiovascular accompaniments.

There are some *rare indications for propranolol in critical care:*

1) *Thyroid storm* or *crisis* is a medical emergency characterized by fever, tachcardia, CNS disturbances, and vomiting. The aim of therapy is to reduce the production and secretion of thyroid hormones and to lessen their metabolic effects. Fever is controlled by cooling, and thyroid secretion by methimazole (80 mg) or propylthiouracil (800 mg). In addition, 1 g saturated solution of potassium iodide is given. The symptoms of exaggerated sympathetic activity such as tachycardia, nervousness, tremor, and diarrhoea are reduced by beta blockade with propranolol. To achieve an immediate effect, propranolol is given IV (1–10 mg) over 10 min. Thereafter, it is given orally, 40 mg, four times daily. Propranolol helps to reduce fever and total body O_2 consumption and improves nitrogen balance [83, 116]. It does not reduce circulating levels of thyroid hormone.

2) *Acute intermittent porphyria* (AIP) is an inborn error of metabolism characterized by cardiovascular, gastro-intestinal (GI), and neuropsychiatric disturbances. The cardiovascular manifestations are tachycardia and hypertension, which may progress to acute LV failure. Increased plasma and urine levels of catecholamines are found during an attack of AIP and there is evidence of increased release of neuronal noradrenaline. Propranolol (80–160 mg daily) reduces the tachycardia and hypertension over 4–7 days, and long-term therapy appears to control cardiovascular symptoms [88]. Atsmon [31] has reported control of a very severe case of AIP by giving propranolol 280 mg IV over a period of 24 h.

3) The *symptomatic management of tetanus* requires the use of large doses of sedatives (e.g., diazepam 10–20 mg IM) and occasionally muscle relaxants and artificial ventilation. In severe cases of tetanus, the heart rate and blood pressure increase. Propranolol may be given (2–10 mg IV) over 10 min and repeated at intervals, to maintain a heart rate below 110 beats/min and a systolic pressure below 150 mmHg [114]. *Pharmacokinetics.* The initial therapeutic dose of propranolol is 40 or 80 mg, and this may be increased up to 420 mg daily. The paediatric dose is initially 30 mg per day increasing to effect. Propranolol should always be given PO unless a rapid effect is essential. Great care is required when it is given IV and the dose is

3–5 mg given over a period of 10 min and not more rapidly than 1 mg/min. Heart rate and blood pressure should be monitored during the injection in case there is an inappropriate bradycardia due to unopposed vagal activity. If it is necessary to infuse propranolol it is suggested that a loading dose of 8 mg is given slowly, followed by 0.02 mg/min to maintain therapeutic plasma levels.

Propanolol is rapidly and completely absorbed from the gut, but undergoes extensive metabolism by the liver (first-pass effect). The metabolites are excreted in the urine with less than 10% in the faeces. Over 90% of propranolol is excreted in the form of metabolites of which a major metabolite is 4-hydroxypropranolol which also has beta-antagonist activity. Variations in hepatic metabolism account partly for the 20-fold variation in plasma level for a given dose of propranolol and therefore it must be titrated for effect. Effective blockade is associated with plasma levels of 50–100 ng/ml. Propranolol is widely distributed amongst tissues, with the highest concentrations in brain, lung, and kidney. In man, there is a 30-fold higher concentration in brain than blood. The volume of distribution is 3 litres/kg and the plasma half-life is 2–4 h after an IV dose, and 3–6 h after long-term oral dosing. In the presence of renal disease the half-life is decreased because alterations in hepatic metabolism lead to an increase in faecal excretion and there is evidence of retention of propranolol metabolites. In severe hepatic disease, the half-life is increased as is the volume of distribution because of reduced binding of propranolol to plasma protein [118].

Unwanted effects. Propranolol should be given with care in situations where beta-adrenoceptor activation is maintaining function. Thus, in the presence of heart block or bradycardia, blockade of endogenous sympathetic activity may cause severe bradycardia, which should be reversed by giving atropine. In the presence of cardiac enlargement or a history of congestive heart failure, propranolol must be given with care and a diuretic is probably indicated initially. Patients with a history of bronchospasm should not receive propranolol unless it is deemed essential, and they should be carefully observed since severe status asthmaticus can be induced rarely. Patients suffering from hypoglycaemia should not be given propranolol since it reduces the availability of alternative energy substrates. In addition, patients with hypertension due to phaeochromocytoma should not receive a beta blocker unless alpha-adrenoceptor blockade has already been established since beta blockade alone will potentiate alpha-mediated vasoconstriction and enhance the hypertension.

Sudden cessation of propranolol therapy may result in rebound effects characterized by a rise in heart rate and blood pressure. In patients with coronary artery disease it may result in a syndrome of increasing chest pain, cardiac arrhythmias, and myocardial infarction. In the latter setting, deaths have been reported but the incidence of this 'withdrawal syndrome' is less than 5%. The onset may occur 1–14 days after therapy is stopped and is more likely to be seen in those who remain active during this time. The mechanism underlying the withdrawal syndrome is not understood. Some studies indicate that there is an increased responsiveness to beta agonists within the 5-day period after stopping propranolol and this enhanced responsiveness may be due to an increase in beta receptor population [119]. Other investigators have not been able to confirm enhanced responsiveness during the acute phase of withdrawal, but prudence suggests that in certain situations this may occur and therefore the dose should be reduced gradually over 10–14 days.

In the critical care situation, patients may be admitted who are receiving long-term beta blockade for hypertension or coronary artery disease. Considerable judgement needs to be exercised in deciding whether to stop therapy because, firstly, in the stress of acute illness inappropriate cardiovascular responses to the situation will be reduced by beta blockade. Secondly, acute cessation of therapy at this point may precipitate a withdrawal syndrome. Therefore the potential benefits of stopping therapy must be very carefully assessed.

The commonest non-specific side-effects associated with propranolol therapy are fatigue and GI disturbances. Central nervous effects include vivid dreams, visual disturbances, hallucinations, and sleep disorders. The important cardiovascular effects are bradycardia and hypotension, as well as cold extremities and Raynaud's phenomena, although the incidence of the latter is about 5%.

If patients are to undergo general anaesthesia the anaesthetic of choice is halothane, since other anaesthetic agents, such as ether, chloroform and trichlorethylene, will cause excessive cardiac depression in the presence of beta blockade. The normal clinical signs of hypovolaemia and shock during anaesthesia will be reduced by beta blockade.

Many *new beta antagonists* have been introduced clinically over the last 10 years. For the clinician, the important question is whether they offer any advantage in safety and efficacy. The differences of practical importance are (1) pharmacokinetic profile; (2) degree of partial agonist activity; (3) selectivity for cardiac beta adrenoceptors. Opinions differ concerning the importance and relevance of such differences and the interested reader should consult the relevant literature [133].

In the critical care situation, practical advice is required as to the choice of beta antagonist and to the management of acutely ill patients who may be admitted, receiving one of eight or ten different beta antagonists. The clinician who is unfamilar with the specific beta antagonists may be reassured that they all have qualitatively the same type of pharmacological profile as propranolol and their differing properties do not require any modification of the general principles outlined in the section on propranolol.

If it becomes necessary to withdraw a patient from their beta-blocking regimen the effect will be lost within 48 h. Alprenolol and oxprenolol have the shortest half-lives (2–3 h) and sotalol and timolol the longest (10–12 h).

Practolol is without doubt, the beta antagonist of choice for IV administration in the urgent control of cardiac arrhythmias in critically ill patients. It causes much less haemodynamic alteration than propranolol for an equivalent therapeutic effect, and there has been considerable experience of its use in this context. The haemodynamic difference is attributed to the type and degree of partial agonist activity observed with practolol [41]. Practolol is no longer available for long-term oral administration because it can induce the unique oculomucocutaneous syndrome [139], but it is acceptable for acute IV use and is still available in Europe for this purpose.

Pindolol is a potent non-selective beta antagonist with high partial agonist activity. Recent studies indicate that it causes less reduction in cardiac function in normal subjects and in patients with coronary artery disease [39]. Further evaluation is required to determine if it is a suitable alternative to practolol for the control of arrhythmias in the critically ill patient.

Labetalol is dealt with separately from other beta antagonists, because it possesses both alpha and beta adrenoceptor blocking activity, although it is five times more potent a beta antagonist than an alpha antagonist. It resembles propranolol in having membrane-stabilizing activity and no partial agonist properties, but it has only one quarter the potency of propranolol.

The cardiovascular effects resemble a combination of alpha- and beta-blocking actions. It reduces heart rate, LV dp/dt, cardiac output, and total cardiac work, by antagonizing cardiac beta adrenoceptors. When given IV to hypertensive subjects (50 mg) it causes a rapid fall in blood pressure, which persists for 6–18 h. In the supine position, the fall in pressure is accompanied by little change in heart rate and cardiac output, but in the erect position both these parameters are significantly reduced, particularly during exercise, when it causes a dose-dependent reduction in exercise tachycardia. Following long-term oral administration to hypertensive patients, the heart rate and blood pressure are reduced, but cardiac output is normal. Thus, labetalol differs from propranolol in that it reduces total peripheral resistance with minimal effects on cardiac output, whereas propranolol reduces cardiac output and increases peripheral resistance.

The initial dose of labetalol is 100 mg, three times daily and an effect on blood pressure is seen within 2 h. It is rapidly absorbed from the gut, with peak plasma levels obtained at $1–1\frac{1}{2}$. It undergoes extensive hepatic metabolism and about 60% of the dose is recovered in the urine, mainly in the form of metabolites, the remainder being excreted in the gut, via the biliary system. One of the conjugated metabolites is hydroxy-labetalol, which has significant pharmacological activity. Labetalol is minimally bound to plasma proteins and has an elimination half-life of $3\frac{1}{2}–5$ h.

Labetalol can be given by IV infusion for the rapid control of elevated blood pressure and it may have an advantage over such agents as diazoxide, because it reduces renin secretion and is not bound to plasma proteins. It may also be of value in the acute management of phaeochromocytoma and clonidine withdrawal crisis.

The commonest side-effect of labetalol is postural hypotension related to its alpha-blocking properties and this is more likely to be observed during the initial phase of treatment or if the dosage is increased too rapidly. Other effects are sedation, dry mouth, vivid dreams, headache, bowel disturbance, and occasional difficulty in urination [109]. Since it is a beta antagonist it is contra-indicated in patients with AV block, and care is also required in patients prone to bronchospasm. Similarly it should not be given to patients with heart failure unless they have received diuretics and, if necessary, digitalis.

Vasodilator agents

Vasodilator drugs may be used in a range of indications including hypertension, angina pectoris, cardiac failure, AMI, and peripheral vascular disease. Classifying these agents in a single group is unsatisfactory in that no one agent is of clinical value in all these indications and furthermore they differ widely both in their mechanism of action and site of optimal effect within the vascular tree. Thus the clinical indication is primarily dependent upon whether the major site of action is on arteriolar (resistance) vessels or venous (capacitance) vessels. Robinson [22] has proposed that vasodilator agents can be classified into (1) non-selective, e.g., diazoxide; (2) relatively venous selective, e.g., glyceryl trinitrate, sodium nitroprusside and prazosin; (3) relatively arterio-selective, e.g., hydrallazine.

These differences in vascular responses to vasodilator drugs may be explained on the basis of Golenhofer's observations that vascular smooth muscle is activated by two mechanisms [47]. One mechanism, the phasic or P-type, is associated with spike discharges, particularly in arteriolar resistance vessels, in man and is dependent on the extracellular calcium concentration. It is specifically inhibited by the calcium antagonists, verapamil, and nifedipine. The second mechanism is the tonic or T-type, and is not associated with spike discharges, being minimally dependent upon extracellular calcium concentrations. This contractile mechanism is found in venous smooth muscle in man, and is specifically inhibited by nitroprusside and nitrites. The practical significance of these differences is that the net haemodynamic responses to these vasodilators differ markedly and can be accounted for by the selective actions on veins or arteries.

Relatively venoselective vasodilators

Sodium nitroprusside (nipride)

This agent was first used to reduce blood pressure in 1919, but only in the last 10 years has its full potential been realized. When given by continuous IV infusion it can be of value in the management of hypertensive crises, aortic dissection, some forms of congestive cardiac failure, and certain forms of AMI.

Nitroprusside relaxes arterial and venous smooth muscle and has no effect on uterine, GI, or myocardial muscle. It acts by interfering in the sequence of excitation/contraction at a point beyond the mechanism responsible for the depolarization of the cell membrane. Though it has been shown to inhibit ^{45}Ca uptake in rabbit aorta, its action is not solely dependent upon antagonism of calcium uptake, because it blocks the rapid phase of contraction to noradrenaline which is mediated by release of intracellular stores of calcium.

The haemodynamic response to infusion of nitroprusside comprises a reduction in systemic and pulmonary vascular resistance and a decrease in arterial pressure and LV filling pressure. In normal subjects it causes little change or even a reduction in cardiac output, which is accompanied by a reflex increase in heart rate. In the presence of elevated LV filling pressure and heart failure it causes an increase in cardiac output, which is accompanied by an increase in stroke work index and therefore a reduction in LV filling pressure. Thus it causes a reduction in both preload and afterload. The effect on cardiac output depends on the LV end-diastolic pressure, prior to administration. When this is more than 12 mmHg, end-diastolic pressure is reduced and there is a significant increase in cardiac output. When the end-diastolic pressure is below 10 mmHg, the pressure will fall further and this will be accompanied by a reduction in cardiac output, which can be reversed by volume expansion. Therefore, to obtain an optimal effect it is necessary to ensure that the preload is maintained in the range of 10–13 mmHg [90]. Used in this manner, nitroprusside is valuable in the short-term management of cardiac failure associated with cardiomyopathy, mitral and aortic valve incompetence, myocarditis, ventricular septal defects, and certain forms of AMI. Its use in the latter should be confined to those patients who are hypertensive and have chest pain, with some degree of LV failure. It should not be used in normotensive patients with adequate ventricular function.

Pharmacokinetics. Nitroprusside is available in 50-mg ampoules and should always be made up freshly and protected from light and alkaline solution. It should not be mixed with other agents. Therapy is commenced with an infusion rate of 3 μg/kg/min and the rate increased until an optimal hypotensive response is obtained, though the recommended maximal dose is 10 μg/kg/min. Frequent monitoring of blood pressure is essential, and in patients with AMI or complex cardiac dysfunction, monitoring of pulmonary artery wedge pressure is desirable. Nitroprusside has a very short half-life in the body, being rapidly converted to cyanide and then to thiocyanate. The incidence of side-effects is related to the rate of formation of cyanide and its disposal. Poisoning is a possibility, but rarely occurs unless there is liver disease, or a high dose is given for a prolonged period. Infusion rates of less than 5 μg/kg/min for less than 3 days are regarded as safe. The earliest sign of cyanide toxicity is metabolic acidosis. Thiocyanate accumulation causes CNS disturbances such as stupor, aphasia, and weakness. These signs are associated with a thiocyanate plasma level in excess of 10 mg/100 ml. A satisfactory antidote is the infusion of hydroxycobalmin (25 mg/h), which combines with cyanide to form cyanocobalamin.

Nitrates and nitrites

These agents are primarily used in the management of angina pectoris, but their marked venodilating properties have favoured their use in the management of certain forms of cardiac failure because they unload the left ventricle. The reference nitrate is nitroglycerine. Its brevity of action is a major disadvantage and attempts have been made to prolong its effect, either by combining it in a nitroglycerine ointment or by modifying either its formulation or its chemical structure to prevent degradation.

Nitrates relax smooth muscle, but the mechanism is not fully understood. They appear to act at a specific cellular site, since they do not interfere with the response of smooth muscle to other stimulants, such as noradrenaline, or inhibitors, such as histamine and acetylcholine. Furthermore, when tachyphylaxis in response to the relaxing action of nitrates is induced it does not alter the relaxation effects of other agonists. It has been speculated that they act either by causing a rise in intracellular cyclic GMP or by inhibiting the synthesis of the prostagladin, thromboxane A_2, which has potent vasoconstricting actions. Nitrates relax smooth muscle not only in the vasculature, but also in the gut, genito-urinary tract, and respiratory system, and therefore differ from nitroprusside.

The cardiovascular effects of nitroglycerine result from its primary effect on the venous bed. It causes a fall in ventricular filling pressure and stroke volume and hence a fall in cardiac output in the upright position, though this may be offset to some extent by the reflex tachycardia. Blood pressure is reduced as a result of the reduction both in cardiac output and peripheral resistance. In the presence of an attack of angina pectoris, which is accompanied by elevation of LV filling pressure and an increase in end-diastolic volume, the venodilating effect of nitroglycerine reduces ventricular dimensions and intramyocardial tension, resulting in reduced myocardial O_2 consumption and improved coronary flow. Controversy continues over the effect of nitrates on coronary blood flow. Nitroglycerine relaxes coronary arterial muscle and increases blood flow in the isolated canine heart. In the presence of obstruction to coronary flow it may cause a reduction in flow in the segment distal to the obstruction. Hence it has been argued that nitrates act predominantly by a peripheral effect in reducing venous return rather than by primarily increasing coronary flow. However, it is now thought that nitrates will relax large coronary vessels and have little effect on small vessels and hence both the peripheral and cardiac effects contribute to its overall anti-anginal action [21]. It also causes relaxation of pulmonary blood vessels and this too may contribute to the unloading of the left ventricle.

Pharmacokinetics. Nitroglycerine is available in the form of tablets in the following strengths: 150, 300, 400, and 600 μg. Tablets should be protected from light, high temperatures, and contact with cotton wool. Nitroglycerine is rapidly absorbed from skin and mucous membrane, and a dose of 0.5 mg gives detectable plasma levels of about 3 ng/ml within 4 min, with a plasma half-life of 1–3 min. It is metabolized primarily in the liver by means of a glutathione-dependent organo-nitrate reductase, leading to the formation of inorganic nitrite and 1,3- and then 1,2-dinitroglycerine. These products may either be excreted in the urine or further degraded to glycerin mono-nitrate, which is conjugated and excreted as the glucuronide in urine [95].

The long-acting nitrates include isosorbid dinitrate, penta-erythritol tetranitrate, and erythrityl tetranitrate. Isosorbid is the only one likely to be used in the critical care situation, where it may be of value in certain forms of cardiac failure associated with AMI, cardiomyopathy, or valvular heart disease. Isosorbid dinitrate (ISDN) causes a reduction in mean systemic arterial pressure and vascular resistance, resulting in a sustained reduction in LV filling pressure. The effect on heart rate and cardiac output depends on the initial filling pressure and if this is high, cardiac output will rise as ventricular pressure falls, whilst heart rate will vary according to the degree of systemic hypotension.

The duration of haemodynamic effect depends on the dose and route of administration. A dose of 10–20 mg PO can reduce ventricular filling pressure for up to 5 h [137]. Isosorbid is available in 5- or 10-mg scored tablets and can be taken sublingually or swallowed. Absorption is rapid and complete, but isosorbid undergoes rapid denitration to the 2- and 5-isosorbid mononitrates as well as to isosorbid itself. There is also a chewable form of isosorbid dinitrate and when the drug is given in this form or sublingually the extent of hepatic metabolism is reduced. About 80% of isosorbid is excreted in urine within 24 h, the majority in the form of the metabolite 5-isosorbid mononitrate and lesser amounts as 2-isosorbid mononitrate and free isosorbid itself. These metabolites are also present as glucuronide conjugates. Isosorbid dinitrate is cleared very rapidly from the blood and cannot be detected 30 min after an oral dose, though the metabolites have a half-life of 3 h.

Unwanted effects. The unwanted effects of nitrates are due primarily to their vasodilating properties. Thus headache, dizziness, and postural hypotension are not uncommon, and in the elderly cerebral ischaemia can be precipitated. Therefore, they should not be given to patients with cerebral injury, haemorrhage, or severe anaemia. The commonest side-effect is vascular headache, which can be reduced by introducing the drug initially in a low dose. Nitrates may also cause a rise in intra-ocular pressure. Prolonged exposure to nitrates can lead to the development of tolerance and a reduced vasodilator effectiveness, though this has not been shown in patients who are taking nitrates for angina pectoris and further studies on this aspect are still needed. Prolonged exposure to the manufacture of nitrates can lead to nitrate dependence in the factory workers. Thus, when they are not exposed every day, symptoms of headache and flushing, going on to chest pain and peripheral arterial spasm have been reported. Therefore the possible problems of tolerance and dependence should be kept in mind when treating patients for prolonged periods on nitrates. High doses can cause haemoglobinaemia, hypotension, vomiting and CNS stimulation.

Arterioselective vasodilators

Hydrallazine

Hydrallazine is the best-known example of this type of agent, and acts primarily on the resistance vessels in the arterial tree, causing an increase in blood flow to most vascular beds, except skin and muscle. As a consequence, both diastolic and systolic blood pressure are reduced and this is accompanied by a reflexly mediated rise in heart rate, cardiac contractility and cardiac output. Since it has much less effect on the venous system, postural hypotension is unusual. In exercising subjects, hydrallazine causes a greater increase in cardiac output and a reduction in systemic vascular resistance, in comparison with control conditions. Prolonged administration of hydrallazine causes an increase in both blood and plasma volume, which reduces its hypotensive effectiveness. Since its primary effect is to reduce afterload, its value in the management of severe mitral and aortic regurgitation has been studied. Both Chatterjee [20] and Fitchitt [35] have shown that a dosage of 75 mg three times a day reduces elevated ventricular filling pressure and improves cardiac function. It is thought that hydrallazine acts by interfering with calcium influx at the arteriolar cell membrane, causing a reduction in the phasic calcium dependent tone of this tissue.

Pharmacokinetics. Hydrallazine is available in tablets (10, 25, 50, 100 mg) and ampoules (20 mg/ml). Oral therapy should be commenced with a dose of 10 mg four times a day, and increased according to the cardiovascular response. Doses in excess of 200 mg daily may lead to the development of a systemic lupus syndrome. If it is to be used for rapid reduction of afterload in hypertensive emergencies or acute LV failure, hydrallazine is rapidly and completely absorbed from the gut, but undergoes extensive first-pass hepatic metabolism, so that its systemic bioavailability is about 30%. In liver, it undergoes *n*-acetylation by the action of hepatic acetyltransferase. There is a wide individual difference in acetyltransferase activity, which is genetically determined, so that subjects who are slow acetylators may have a 30% higher blood level for a given dose of hydrallazine, than those who are fast acetylators. Hydrallazine is 90–95% bound to plasma proteins and has a volume of distribution of 2 litres/kg. About 90% of absorbed hydrallazine is excreted in the urine, the remainder appearing as triazole derivatives and hydrazines, either free or as glucuronide conjugates.

Unwanted effects. The commonest unwanted effects of hydrallazine are headache, tachycardia, palpitation, and postural hypotension. These are due to its pharmacological action on arteriolar smooth muscle. Non-specific effects such as sleep disturbances, diarrhoea, and sedation have also been reported. The most important unwanted effects are acute and delayed rheumatoid-like conditions. There is an acute syndrome consisting of fever, myalgia, arthralgia, and lymphadenopathy, which can be observed within 3 weeks of starting therapy. Following prolonged hydrallazine therapy, a toxicity syndrome closely resembling systemic lupus erythematosis has been reported, particularly in patients taking doses in excess of 400 mg daily. The syndrome presents as arthritis, with various skin lesions, and antinuclear antibodies can be detected [102].

Minoxidil

This is a specific arteriolar vasodilator resembling hydrallazine, but with prolonged dose-dependent hypotensive effect. Its clinical use is restricted to cases of severe refractory hypertension and certain cases of pulmonary hypertension. It is therefore unlikely to be used in the critical care situation. It causes a marked fall in systemic vascular resistance with a reflex rise in heart rate, cardiac contractility, and cardiac output. Since it is so potent, chronic administration can lead to a high cardiac output syndrome. It causes marked retention of sodium and an increase in blood volume, so that it is always used in combination with a diuretic and beta antagonist. It is available in 5-mg tablets and the daily dose is 20–40 mg. Its potent vasodilator action leads to fluid retention, weight gain, tachycardia and possible hypertension. It may also cause hypertrichosis.

Non-selective vasodilators

Diazoxide

Diazoxide is a benzothiazine derivative related to the thiazide diuretics, but without significant diuretic activity. It exerts equal vasodilating actions on both the resistance and capacitance vessels and causes an increase in blood flow in the cerebral, coronary, and renal vascular beds. Arteriolar dilatation is accompanied by a reflex rise in heart rate, cardiac output, and renin release, while despite the increase in renal blood flow there is a reduction in glomerular filtration rate and renal plasma flow, resulting in fluid and sodium retention.

Unlike other vasodilators, diazoxide has a significant additional pharmacological action in that it inhibits insulin release from the pancreatic beta cell and raises plasma catecholamine levels.

Diazoxide is primarily used to achieve a rapid reduction of blood pressure in patients with hypertensive crisis. It is available in ampoules containing 300 mg/ml and the initial IV dose is 150–300 mg given as a bolus over 30–120 s. The optimal speed and dose of administration are controversial, but the usual response to such a regime is 25% reduction in blood pressure within an hour. Diazoxide is extensively bound to plasma proteins and its plasma half-life is greater than 24 h, though the hypotensive effect may last for 12–16 h. It is metabolized in the liver to give hydroxymethyl and carboxymethyl derivatives, which are excreted in the urine along with the unchanged drug. The important unwanted effects of diazoxide are salt and water retention, hyperglycaemia, hyperuricaemia, and occasionally extrapyramidal symptoms. They do not limit its usefulness in the acute reduction of blood pressure, but do so when the drug is used for long-term management of hypertension. Care is required in administering the drug to patients with atherosclerotic, cardiac, and cerebral vascular disease, because of the dangers due to excessive reduction in blood pressure. For example, myocardial ischaemia can be precipitated by rapid reduction in blood pressure following diazoxide. The hypotensive effects of other vasodilator drugs and beta antagonists are potentiated by diazoxide. Anticoagulants, which are also albumin-bound, may be displaced by it and their effects enhanced.

Calcium antagonists

This group of drugs share the common effect of interfering with the flux of calcium ions through the slow channel in the plasma membrane of cardiac and vascular tissue. They are used in the management of angina pectoris, hypertension, and cardiac arrhythmias. The reference calcium antagonist is verapamil. Other examples are nifedipine, prenylamine, and perhexilene, although the last two agents are rarely used in the critical care situation. There are important pharmacological differences between these various agents in that they differ particularly in the ratio of specific to non-specific pharmacological effects. Calcium antagonists act primarily on the cardiovascular system and have pronounced negative inotropic, chronotropic and vasodilator actions [37].

Verapamil

In experimental studies in dogs, verapamil (0.5 mg/kg IV) causes a reduction in heart rate, cardiac contractility, and myocardial O_2 consumption, which is accompanied by an increase in coronary blood flow. It also prolongs AV conduction, reduces LV dp/dt max and elevates LV end-diastolic pressure. It reduces both systolic and diastolic blood pressure, but in general the extent and alteration in cardiovascular function is modest in the doses used clinically. Verapamil causes a reduction in heart rate, which is not reversed by atropine and is thought to be dependent on its calcium antagonist action. It has a more dramatic effect in prolonging conduction through the AV node, so that the PR interval is lengthened, but there is no change in the QRS or Q-TC.

Verapamil is available in 40-mg tablets, and the daily dose is 40–100 mg three times daily. When the preparation is used parenterally, the dose is 1–10 mg given at a rate of 1 mg/min with monitoring of the blood pressure and ECG. It is used IV, primarily in the management of supra-ventricular tachycardia, because of its marked effect in reducing conduction through the AV node. Verapamil is rapidly absorbed from the gut, plasma levels peaking at about 45 min, but it undergoes extensive first-pass hepatic metabolism. The plasma half-life of verapamil is about 3 h but its metabolites persist for up to 24 h in the body. The extensive first-pass metabolism of verapamil explains its low systemic bioavailability and the tenfold difference between the PO and IV dose [116]. Verapamil is excreted in the urine and about 80% of ^{14}C-labelled verapamil can be recovered from urine over 5 days. The nature and kinetics of verapamil metabolites have not been described.

Nifedipine

This is a more recently introduced calcium antagonist, which is more specific than verapamil and has a slightly different spectrum of action. In experimental studies, nifedipine (30 μg/kg IV) causes an increase in heart rate and a marked increase in coronary blood flow accompanied by a reduction in LV end-diastolic pressure, but little change in the indices of contractility, while intra-arterial pressure is significantly reduced. Nifedipine acts on both arteriolar resistance vessels, to reduce afterload and venous capacitance vessels to reduce preload. It causes a lesser rise in myocardial O_2 consumption than nitroglycerine, for a given fall in afterload, because its calcium antagonistic actions reduce the discharge rate of the sinus node. In man, nifedipine (10–20 mg PO) reduces blood pressure by reducing total peripheral resistance. This is accompanied by a reduction in LV systolic and end-diastolic pressures, with a modest increase in cardiac output and heart rate. Blood flow is increased in the coronary and splanchnic beds. Nifedipine has a strikingly less pronounced effect on cardiac conduction than does verapamil, so that little change in the PR or QRS complex is observed in the dose range that causes significant haemodynamic change.

Nifedipine is administered in a dose of 30–90 mg daily and is well absorbed from the gut. Blood levels peak at 1–2 h and a single dose of 10 mg is associated with plasma levels of 15–20 ng/ml. It is significantly bound to plasma proteins and undergoes extensive metabolism to inactive derivatives. Studies with ^{14}C-labelled material suggest a half-life of 3–4 days, with 80% of the material excreted in the urine and 15% in the faeces.

Unwanted effects. The unwanted effects of calcium antagonists relate primarily to their known pharmacological actions. Verapamil has a much greater effect on myocardial calcium kinetics than nifedipine, and therefore verapamil should be used cautiously in patients with heart failure and is contra-indicated in the presence of depressed sinus node and AV function. Verapamil may interact with beta antagonists to produce cardiac standstill, but nifedipine can be used in their presence. Both agents will potentiate the effect of other hypotensive drugs. Non-specific side-effects reported are nausea, flushing, headache, and tremor. Overdose due to calcium antagonists causes hypotension and severe cardiac depression. This can reversed by either adrenoceptor agonists, such as adrenaline or dobutamine, or calcium gluconate, which has been shown to be useful for the management of verapamil overdosage [101].

Cardiac stimulants

This section will deal with those drugs (cardiac glycosides and xanthines) that have a direct stimulant effect on ventricular muscle. Sympathomimetic agents, whilst having a marked cardiac stimulant effect, have been discussed in the section on autonomic drugs. Theoretically, inotropic agents are used where depressed ventricular function is suspected, in diseases such as cardio-myopathy, coronary artery disease, valvular heart disease, and 'toxic shock'. During the last 10 years there has been a marked change in attitude towards the role of inotropic agents, so that in practice their use is mainly confined to the management of the acutely failing heart in normal sinus rhythm. Their contribution to the management of chronic heart failure appears to be more limited. Specifically, there are now considerable reservations as to the value of cardiac glycosides in the treatment of chronic heart failure with normal rhythm and the modification of preload and afterload is thought by many to be of more value [86].

Cardiac glycosides

It is estimated that at any one time 300 000 patients are receiving digoxin in the United Kingdom, whilst in the United States about 27 million prescriptions for glycosides were issued in 1978. An understanding of the practical usage is therefore essential, but the literature on the subject is so extensive that only a summary can be given here. The most commonly available glycosides are digoxin, digitoxin, lanatoside C, and ouabain. The majority of patients are treated with digoxin and in the discussion that follows the term 'digoxin' is used instead of digitalis or glycoside.

The purpose of digoxin administration is to attain a concentration of glycoside at the cardiac membrane which either causes a significant inotropic response or a marked reduction in ventricular rate. Digoxin remains the drug of choice for slowing ventricular rate in atrial fibrillation. But its role in the long-term management of heart failure with normal rhythm is currently undergoing re-evaluation. Evidence of a sustained benefit for patients in sinus rhythm is so small, compared with the possible risks, that digoxin administration should be used only after diuretic therapy has failed to achieve an optimal effect [50]. This, possibly controversial, view has a direct bearing on the recommendations for dose regimens.
Cardiovascular effects. The primary action of digoxin is upon the heart and blood vessels, but

it also has effects on the CNS and the autonomic system as well as the kidney and GI tract. The therapeutically desirable actions of digoxin are depression of conduction through the AV node and an increase in the force of cardiac contraction. Cardiac function can be described by the relationship between the cardiac performance and ventricular end-diastolic volume (Frank–Starling mechanism) (Fig. 16.5). When cardiac performance is increased by physical activity there is initially an increase in the contractile state of the muscle. At higher performance levels, end-diastolic volume also increases, so that enhanced cardiac performance is achieved by an increase in both diastolic fibre length and contractile state. This force velocity relationship is depressed in cardiac failure which represents an inability of the heart to pump blood at a rate sufficient to achieve adequate tissue perfusion. Thus, heart failure is associated with a reduction in intrinsic velocity of shortening (V max) and, as it progresses, there is an additional depression in maximal isometric force [9, 124]. Digoxin acts on the heart to move the ventricular function curve upwards and to the left so that more stroke work is derived at any given end-diastolic fibre length (Fig. 16.5). It therefore increases the velocity of shortening and the maximal tension generated in muscle fibres.

The haemodynamic effects of digoxin depend on the initial state of the circulation. In the absence of cardiac failure, digoxin increases cardiac contractility but the cardiac output is unchanged. This occurs because there is a rise in peripheral vascular resistance, due to the direct contractile response of arteriolar and venous smooth muscle to digoxin and an indirect increase in sympathetic vasoconstrictor tone. These peripheral actions can reduce venous return, and hence cardiac output may be unaltered despite the increase in cardiac contractile force. Established heart failure is associated with elevated end-diastolic filling pressure, increased muscle mass, and a reflex increase in autonomic tone. In this setting, digoxin causes a marked increase in cardiac contractility resulting in a fall in end-diastolic pressure and heart rate with an increase in cardiac output and subsequent clinical improvement. The inotropic and negative dromotropic actions of digoxin are dose-dependent, but the upper dose is limited by the development of cardiac arrhythmias. When cardiac function improves, arteriolar and venous tone are reduced as a consequence of reduced autonomic tone, though in certain forms of heart failure peripheral resistance may remain high.

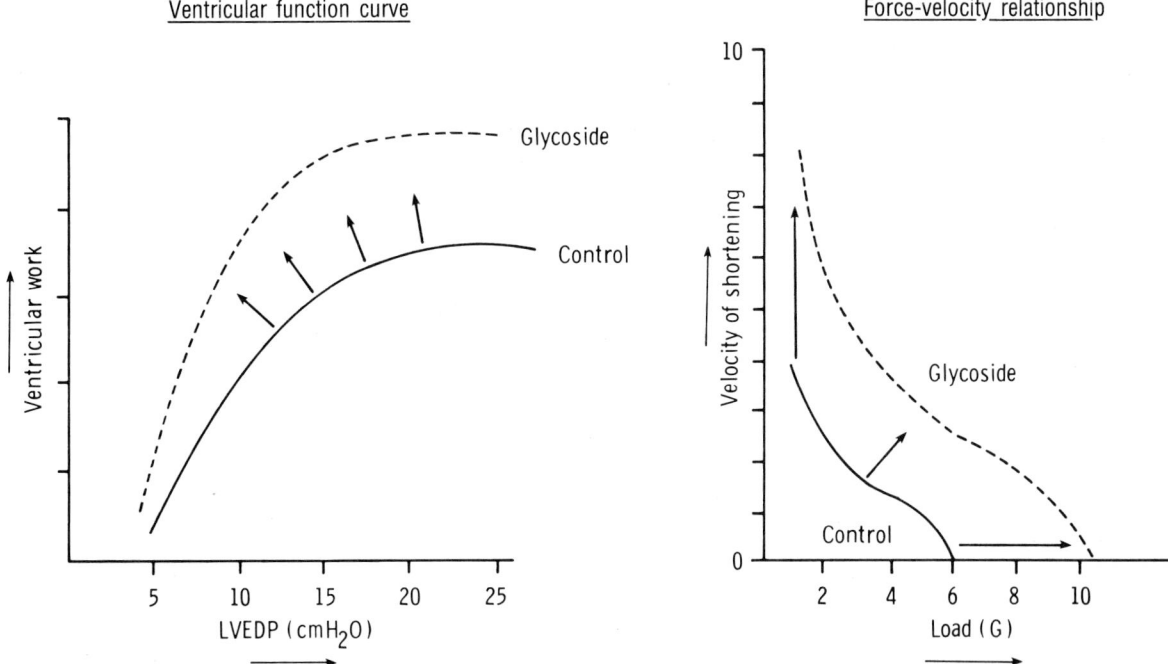

Fig. 16.5. Schematic representation of the effect of glycosides on two parameters of cardiac muscle function. The ventricular function curve relates ventricular work to end-diastolic pressure and glycosides permit more work for a given end-diastolic pressure. The force velocity curve depicts the relationship between resting tension (load) and velocity of muscle contraction. Glycosides increase both the velocity of contraction and the maximal force of contraction [125].

The electrophysiological effects of digoxin arise from its direct action on cardiac tissue and also its indirect effect in modifying autonomic tone. In therapeutic doses it prolongs the PR intervals of the ECG, shortens the rate corrected QT interval and reduces T wave amplitude. The ST segment becomes downward sloping and the T wave flattened or inverted. In toxic doses, it enhances spontaneous depolarization of Purkinje tissue, leading to the development of arrhythmias. In addition, digoxin enhances vagal activity by increasing afferent, central and efferent autonomic activity [91]. In therapeutic doses, it acts synergistically with acetylcholine to induce depression of AV conduction. Catecholamines potentiate the arrhythmagenic effect of digoxin both at the cardiac level and indirectly by increasing central sympathetic neural discharge [89].

The mode of action of digoxin at a molecular level is not completely understood, but it exerts its inotropic effect by modifying the transmembrane flux of calcium. Cardiac glycosides bind specifically to sarcolemmal Na^+/K^+ ATPase, causing a dose-dependent inhibition of the enzyme. This inhibition is thought to result in an increase in the transient flux of sodium, leading to a secondary increase in flux of calcium, whilst sodium is subsequently removed from the cell in the early phase of each cardiac cycle. The increase in intracellular calcium makes more calcium available for binding to the troponin–tropomyosin complex resulting in disinhibition of the actin–myosin contractile binding sites [1].

Digoxin causes a significant diuresis in patients with congestive heart failure. Congestive failure results in sodium and fluid retention due to a reduction in effective arterial blood volume. Homeostatic responses in this situation include increase retention of salt and water, which can lead to oedema associated with a reduced renal filtration fraction. Improvement in cardiac function by digoxin reverses these effects, leading secondarily to a natriuresis and hence the diuretic effect of digoxin is due to the improvement in cardiac function.

Pharmacokinetics. Digoxin is available in the following formulations: Tables 125 and 250 μg; P.G. tablets 62.5 μg; P.G. elixir 50 μg/ml; ampoules 250 μg/ml. Digoxin is rapidly but incompletely absorbed from the gut. Peak plasma levels are attained at about 1 h and the plasma half-life is 36 h, in subjects with normal renal function [57].

The intestinal absorption of digoxin is markedly influenced by the formulation and manufacturing process. Variations in systemic bioavailability are due to differences in tablet dissolution rates. In addition, drugs which reduce intestinal transit, such as metoclopramide, reduce systemic absorption. Furthermore, agents such as cholestyramine, kaopectate, magnesium trisilicate, neomycin, and activated charcoal bind digoxin in the gut and reduce its systemic bioavailability. Digoxin is widely distributed throughout the tissues of the body and is concentrated in the heart, kidneys, liver, and skeletal muscle. Approximately 80% of a given dose of digoxin appears unchanged in the urine over 7 days, so that only a small amount of digoxin is converted to metabolites. Excretion is by glomerular filtration and when renal function is normal about 30% of the body load of digoxin is excreted daily. There is a close correlation between digoxin clearance and creatinine clearance so that age and renal disease, which reduce renal function, prolong the elimination half-life of digoxin [129].

Dosing regimens. Selecting the appropriate dosing regimen of digoxin requires a knowledge of digoxin pharmacokinetics which has then to be applied to the individual patients, since factors such as renal function, age, electrolyte disturbance, and changes in thyroid function can modify the individual response. In addition, the ease with which the clinical response can be measured will influence the dose regimen. For example, the effect of digoxin intervention is easily assessed in patients with atrial fibrillation. On the other hand, if the assessment has to be made in a patient with congestive cardiac failure with normal rhythm, then the relationship between the therapeutic and toxic dose is very difficult to assess. The therapeutic plasma level of digoxin is between 0.8 and 2.5 ng/ml. Chamberlain has demonstrated a relationship between plasma level and ventricular slowing in patients with atrial fibrillation, and plasma levels have also been correlated with inotropic effect in healthy subjects [18].

It is customary to separate the dosing of digoxin into the loading phase and the maintenance phase. The total loading dose should lie between 10 and 20 μg/kg body unless electrolyte imbalance or depressed renal function is suspected. This total dose is divided into three or four dose intervals separated by 5 or 6 h. Before receiving the next dose the patient is assessed for evidence of response. If rapid digitalization is desired for a patient with severe cardiac failure or rapid fibrillation the total loading dose can be given as a single dose, but there will be an enhanced risk of digitalis toxicity.

Rapid digitalization can be achieved by IV administration. In this situation the dose should be one-third of that used by the oral route. The digoxin solution (0.25 ng/ml) should be given slowly over 3 min. In the presence of renal failure the loading dose should be reduced by 50%.

The daily maintenance dose is that required to replace the daily loss of digoxin, which in the presence of normal renal function is about 34%. Thus, the daily maintenance dose can be calculated by multiplying the loading dose by the percentage eliminated. An alternative approach, when rapid digitalization is not necessary, is to give the calculated maintenance dose daily. Adequate therapeutic levels should then be reached at about five times the elimination half-life, i.e., 7–8 days. The patient should always be monitored during the digitalization procedure, and therefore if this cannot be done it is better to give a loading dose followed by a maintenance dose. In the presence of potassium depletion, i.e., a plasma level below 3 mmol/litre, the dose of digoxin should be reduced by a third. The dose should also be reduced by about half in patients with clinical myxoedema and in patients above the age of 65 years.

Digoxin is the glycoside of choice for paediatric use. It is available in tablet strengths of 62.5 μg and also as an elixir (50 μg/ml). There are no significant differences between adults and infants in the pharmacokinetic profile, except that it is more rapidly absorbed. Children in the 4 weeks to 2 years age group need relatively higher plasma levels to attain an optimal effect. A satisfactory regimen is 50 μg/kg per 24 h (80 μg/kg for 4 weeks to 2 years) in two divided doses.

Others

Digitoxin is a potent glycoside and is administered in a loading dose of 1.5 mg divided into six equal doses. The average maintenance dose is 100 μg daily with a range of 50–200 μg. It is rapidly and completely absorbed in the gut and has a plasma half-life of 4–8 days. The therapeutic plasma concentration is 15–25 ng/ml and digitoxin is extensively bound to plasma protein. It can thus be displaced from albumin-binding sites by such drugs as phenylbutazone, warfarin, tolbutamide, and clofibrate. It undergoes extensive hepatic metabolism and about 60% of the daily dose is excreted in the urine and 30% in the faeces. About 10% undergoes enterohepatic circulation.

Lanatoside C is given in a daily dose of 1–1.5 mg. Approximately 75% is absorbed from the gut but is not significantly bound to plasma proteins. The plasma half-life is 2–3 h and it undergoes extensive metabolism. Of any given dose, 90% is excreted in the urine, mainly in the form of digoxin.

Oubain is very poorly absorbed from the gut and is only used IV. The dose by this route is 0.25–0.7 mg IV. Its half-life is 14–21 h and it is excreted by the kidney (70%) and the liver (30%).

Unwanted effects. There is a narrow margin between therapeutic and toxic doses of cardiac glycosides and the incidence of digitalis toxicity has been variously reported as between 10% and 30% of patients treated. Estimating the true incidence of toxicity is difficult because firstly there are no completely unequivocal signs of digitalis toxicity and furthermore, many extrinsic and intrinsic factors modify the individual sensitivity to glycosides. The commonest manifestations of digitalis toxicity are disturbances of cardiac rhythm, GI symptoms, CNS disturbances.

Glycoside excess can induce a range of rhythm disturbances, the commonest being VEBs or prolonged PR interval with Wenckebach phenomenon. Excess digitalis can also induce cardiac failure.

The commonest GI side-effects are nausea, vomiting, and anorexia, which has been correlated with elevated digoxin levels. In elderly patients cardiac glycosides can precipitate intestinal ischaemia by causing vasoconstriction.

The CNS manifestations of toxicity are fatigue, weakness and mental disturbance. Thus, in elderly patients digitalis can cause confusion, hallucinations, delirium, and seizures. Disturbances of vision are also common including photophobia, and changes in colour perception.

Since cardiac glycosides are so widely prescribed, excessive overdosage for suicidal purposes is not uncommon. In healthy subjects overdose will present as depression of cardiac automaticity and conduction, but in patients with previous cardiac disease cardiac arrhythmias are more likely to develop.

There are several drug interactions of importance. Firstly, drugs that modify absorption can lead to irregularity in dosing or underdosing. Thus, morphine, anticholinergics, metoclopramide, antacids, and ion exchange resins will modify the systemic bioavailability of glycosides. Diuretics and infusions of electrolyte solutions will modify the response to glycosides. Recently it has been shown that quinidine has an important interaction with glycosides in that it will increase the plasma digoxin levels by upto 50% and induce digitalis toxicity [7].

Management. If digitalis toxicity is suspected, glycosides should be withdrawn and the serum electrolytes measured. If the patient's condition is stable no further action may be required. If there are cardiac disturbances leading to deterioration of the clinical condition additional therapy is called for. Sinus bradycardia or notable AV block can be improved by atropine (0.5 mg) given by slow IV injection. Ventricular ectopic arrhythmias may be controlled by potassium chloride or by diphenylhydantoin. This is given IV in a dose of 100 mg every 5–10 min under careful ECG and blood pressure monitoring. Lidocaine may be given in a dose of 15–50 μg/kg IV. If propranolol is used there is a significant risk of inducing AV block and sinus bradycardia, but it is effective in controlling ectopic beats.

The most satisfactory approach to the management of digitalis toxicity is prevention. Before administering a glycoside to a patient it is important to consider whether the renal function is normal or has been modified by disease or age and whether the patient has any significant deviation of lean body mass (LBM) from the predicted norm. Consideration must be given to factors that might sensitize the patient to the normal dose of glycoside, and these factors are low serum potassium levels and concomitant cardiac disease.

Suicidal overdose with cardiac glycosides can be treated by gastric lavage if ingestion has been recent. Activated charcoal should then be given, although there is no clear evidence as to its efficacy. Severe cardiac slowing can be managed with ventricular pacing and ectopic arrhythmias by diphenylhydantoin or lidocaine. There may be an associated hyperkalaemia and an attempt should be made to reduce potassium levels.

Xanthines (theophylline)

Theopylline stimulates cardiac muscle and relaxes vascular and bronchial smooth muscle, as well as increasing urine flow. It also has central stimulant properties. Theophylline is a competitive inhibitor of cyclic nucleotide phosphodiesterase and therefore prevents inactivation of the second messenger cAMP. Thus many of the pharmacological effects of theophylline are due to raised intracellular levels of cAMP. It also causes an alteration in calcium ion flux in skeletal and myocardial muscle, and inhibits adenosine activation of specific receptors found in the CNS and on platelets.

Pharmacological actions. Theophylline dilates veins and arteries, and has both direct and indirect chronotropic and inotropic effects. In healthy subjects it causes a dose-dependent increase in forearm blood flow and venous distensibility with an accompanying increase in heart rate and shortening of systolic time intervals [99]. In patients with cardiac failure, IV theophylline causes an increase in cardiac output and a reduction in filling pressure and pulmonary vascular resistance. The haemodynamic changes are due to a variety of actions, including relaxation of vascular smooth muscle, direct stimulation of the heart, and secondary alterations in autonomic tone, as well as to the release of adrenaline.

Theophylline inhibits the tone of bronchial smooth muscle and has a direct effect on renal tubules, which increases the excretion of sodium and chloride ions.

Pharmacokinetics. Theophylline is usually formulated as the double salt of theophylline ethylenediamine (aminophylline) and is available in a variety of tablets and capsules as well as in ampoules containing 25 mg/ml.

Following oral administration theophylline is rapidly and completely absorbed, peak plasma levels being observed at 1–2 h. The therapeutic plasma level is 10–20 μg/ml, but unwanted effects occur with plasma levels greater than 25 μg/ml. The plasma half-life of theophylline is variable, ranging from 30 h in premature infants to 6 h in healthy adults. It is eliminated by hepatic biotransformation and urinary excretion. About 12% of a dose of theophylline appears unchanged in the urine, and its elimination is decreased by cardiac, pulmonary, and hepatic disease. In general the initial dose of theophylline is 5.6 mg/kg as a loading dose and a maintenance dose of 24 mg/kg per 24 h for children or 13 mg/kg for adults [98].

Unwanted effects. The common side-effects of theophylline are anxiety, nervousness, and tremor, which are due to its central stimulant actions. It may also cause nausea, vomiting, and abdominal pain. When plasma levels exceed 40 μg/kg, convulsions, cardiac arrhythmias, and cardiorespiratory arrest can occur. Toxicity is particularly likely to occur in children, because they may receive an adult dose by mistake.

Diuretics

Diuretic agents are effective in the management of cardiac, renal, and hepatic oedema, though their commonest use is as antihypertensive agents and they can be of value in the management of hypercalcaemia, hypercalsuria, and diabetes insipidus. Their desired pharmacological effect is to increase the secretion of water and urinary electrolytes. There are a wide variety of diuretic agents and they can be classified according to their saluretic potency.

Mode of action

The class I diuretics include the high ceiling diuretics, which cause a greater than 20% excretion of the filtered sodium load. Examples of diuretics in class I are frusemide, bumetanide, ethacrynic acid, and the organo-mercurials. The major site of action of frusemide is in the medullary portion of the ascending limb of the loop of Henle. It causes a concentration-dependent reduction in sodium reabsorption in this thick segment, resulting in a marked increase in the filtered sodium load. Frusemide also increases urinary calcium excretion, possibly by inhibiting the shared calcium–sodium transport mechanism in the ascending limb. In addition, it reduces uric acid secretion and has a mild inhibitory effect on carbonic anhydrase. The mode of action of frusemide at the cellular level is not clear, but it has been suggested that it inhibits the membrane sodium–potassium ATPase of the tubular cell, resulting in a depression of sodium transport and its retention within the lumen.

Class II diuretics are the benzothiadiazines and related agents which have a lesser saluretic potency than the class I agents, causing between 5% and 15% excretion of the filtered sodium load, following a maximal dose of the drug. These agents differ widely in their duration of diuretic action. They act primarily on the cortical portion of the loop of Henle to inhibit sodium reabsorption at that point. Thus, thiazides reduce free water clearance, which would suggest that their primary effect is on the early portion of the distal tubule, found in the cortical region of the kidney. Thiazides also reduce uric acid secretion in the distal tubule and cause an increased potassium loss because the excess of sodium in the distal tubule promotes sodium–potassium exchange.

The class III diuretics are the potassium-sparing agents, spironolactone, triamterene, and amiloride. These agents act on the distal tubule, but in differing ways. Amiloride and triamterene act on the luminal surface of the tubular cell membrane, blocking the sodium–potassium or hydrogen ion exchange in the distal tubule. As a result, sodium reabsorption is depressed in the distal segment causing a saluresis, which is not accompanied by increased loss of potassium and hydrogen ions. In contrast, spironolactone acts by antagonizing the effect of the hormone aldosterone, which stimulates sodium–potassium ATPase. This stimulation normally promotes the removal of sodium from the distal tubule cell and increases potassium entry. Spironolactone acts to block this action and secondarily increases sodium loss.

Several other agents have diuretic effects. For example, mannitol and isosorbide undergo glomerular filtration and increase fluid loss because of their osmotic effects. On the other hand, theophylline acts directly on the renal tubule to cause diuresis. A recently introduced agent, ticrynafin, has a potency similar to that of class II benzothiadiazines but in addition causes an increase uric acid secretion. This agent has recently been withdrawn from use in man because of unexpected hepatic toxicity. The detailed pharmacology of diuretics has recently been reviewed [77, 128].

Extrarenal pharmacological effects of diuretics

Cardiovascular actions. Diuretics cause a modest fall in blood pressure, which averages about 20/12 mmHg in hypertensive subjects, though this depends on the initial blood pressure. The immediate haemodynamic effect is a reduction in cardiac output and a small rise in peripheral resistance accompanying the fall in blood pressure. The reduction in cardiac output is attributed to alterations in plasma and extracellular fluid volume, secondary to loss of water and sodium. Class I diuretics such as frusemide cause the most dramatic fall in blood pressure, but because of its short duration of action frusemide has lesser effect, for a given saluretic dose, than milder thiazides which act for a prolonged period of time. In patients with elevated left atrial or pulmonary wedge pressure, frusemide causes a dramatic decrease, which is observed before the onset of natriuresis [29]. This fall is attributed to peripheral venous dilatation, resulting in a reduction in pulmonary blood volume. Cardiac output and blood pressure do not change much during this acute phase. However, in chronic heart failure frusemide causes a reduction in blood volume, secondary to the saluresis, resulting in a reduction in intraventricular volumes and pressures [104].

In contrast, prolonged thiazide therapy in hypertensive patients who are not in heart failure results in a sustained reduction in blood pressure, which is due to a fall in peripheral vascular resistance and is not accompanied by an alteration in cardiac output. Effective blood pressure reduction depends on the duration of action of the diuretic rather than on its saluretic potency, and thus long-acting agents such as chlorthalidone are more effective than the short-acting ones, such as frusemide. The cause of the reduction in peripheral vascular resistance brought about by diuretic administration is not understood. It is not due to a direct effect of the drug on vascular smooth muscle, since the hypotensive effective persists for several days after withdrawal of the diuretic, which is not observed with agents that are direct vasodilators. It is likely that the changes are secondary to reduced extracellular volume and electrolyte distribution. The reduction in extracellular volume activates the renin–angiotensin system, so that the final effect of the diuretic is dependent upon the individual homeostatic response. In general, there is a reduction in extracellular fluid volume and plasma volume with an accompanying elevation of angiotensin II levels [24].

Metabolic effects. Chronic administration of diuretic agents may cause electrolyte depletion characterized by sodium loss and hypokalaemia, possibly accompanied by alkalosis and hyperuricaemia. Thiazides may also cause glucose intolerance, which is often referred to as the diabetagenic effect, though there is no evidence that permanent diabetes is induced by thiazide administration. The mechanism is not understood but is possibly due to enhanced hepatic glycogenolysis due to either a direct effect on the liver or secondary to increased catecholamine release, associated with blood volume depletion.

Pharmacokinetics

Class I diuretics. Frusemide is available in 40 and 80 mg tablets and also in ampoules containing 10 mg/ml. The usual IV dose is 20–40 mg and the initial oral dose is 40–80 mg once daily. Frusemide is rapidly absorbed from the gut and has a systemic bioavailability of about 50%.

Peak plasma levels are observed within 1 h and this coincides with the peak saluretic effect. The plasma half-life is about 80 min and frusemide is bound to plasma proteins and does not undergo significant biotransformation. Its biological effect is usually complete within 8 h following a single dose. About 70% of a parenteral dose appears in the urine within 4 h and renal excretion is by both glomerular filtration and proximal tubular secretion. In the presence of severe renal failure frusemide is excreted by the biliary tract [68].

Bumetanide is available in tablets of 1 and 5 mg and ampoules containing 250 µg/ml. It is about 40 times more potent than frusemide, and is rapidly and completely absorbed from the gut. There is a correlation between the saluretic response and plasma levels and hence the onset of effect is rapid. It is highly bound to plasma proteins and has a volume of distribution of 12 litres. The diuretic effect is observed for about 6 h following a single dose. Bumetanide does not undergo biotransformation and is excreted in the urine [53].

Class II diuretics. Thiazide diuretics make up a large group of agents, which differ from each other in chemical structure and duration of saluretic effect. Thiazides are well absorbed from the gut, with the exception of chlorthalidone, which has a systemic bioavailability of less than 40%. Most are only modestly bound to plasma proteins, but polythiazide is 85% bound. The plasma half-lives of thiazides vary greatly from the very short-acting, such as hydrochlorothiazide, which has a half-life of 3–6 h to cyclothiazide and chlorthalidone, which have half-lives of 36–48 h. Thiazides are concentrated in the kidney, particularly in the proximal tubular cells, and the extent of cellular accumulation has been correlated with both potency and liposolubility. Thiazides are also concentrated in the liver, but with the exception of mefruside they do not undergo extensive hepatic metabolism or excretion. They are generally excreted in the urine and are cleared by both glomerular filtration and tubular secretion [103].

Class III diuretics. *Spironolactone* is available in tablets of 25 and 200 mg, and the initial dose is 400 mg daily in divided doses. Data on the pharmacokinetics of spironolactone are incomplete because of the difficulties with assay methods. Its systemic bioavailability depends markedly on the tablet formulation; hence systemic bioavailability varies between 50% and 90%. The plasma half-life is 48–72 h and is reduced during prolonged administration. Spironolactone undergoes extensive hepatic bio-

transformation giving rise to the active metabolites canrenoic acid and canrenone, which are more active than spironolactone as aldosterone antagonists and have elimination half-lives of 20–40 h. Several other metabolites and glucuronide conjugates have also been detected. Spironolactone metabolites are excreted by the kidney, undergoing both glomerular filtration and proximal tubular secretion, in addition to biliary excretion [65].

Amiloride (5 mg tablets) is given in a daily dose of 5–20 mg. It is incompletely absorbed and peak plasma levels are observed at 4 h. A diuretic effect is observed 2 h after administration and it may persist for 12 h. The half-life of amiloride is 6 h and it does not undergo significant metabolism or protein binding. Amiloride is excreted through the kidney and 50% of a given dose appears in the urine within 24 h.

Triamterene is available in 10- and 100-mg capsules and therapy commences with 50 mg twice daily. It is irregularly absorbed from the gut and peak plasma levels are observed within 3 h. Its plasma half-life is about 2 h and it is extensively bound to plasma proteins. Its modest diuretic effect commences 2 h after administration and lasts 12 h. Triamterene undergoes extensive hepatic biotransformation to an inactive metabolite, hydroxyphenylpteridine. Triamterene and its metabolites are excreted through the kidney and cleared within 12 h.

Unwanted effects. The commonest unwanted effects of thiazides are due to their pharmacological effects on the kidney. The most prominent are depletion of sodium and potassium, accompanied by alkalosis and hyperuricaemia.

Sodium depletion. A rapid loss of sodium from the body can result in hypotension and impaired renal function, characterized by a raised blood urea and serum creatinine. It can be accompanied by serious haemodynamic disturbances, especially in seriously ill or elderly patients. The syndrome is more likely to occur with class I diuretics when the atrial pressure is normal, or when cardiac output is dependent on a higher-than-normal filling pressure, as seen in mitral stenosis and constrictive pericarditis. Similarly, in patients with hepatic cirrhosis too rapid a diuresis can result in hypokalaemia and uricaemia, and hepatic coma may be precipitated. Chronic sodium depletion is characterized by lethargy, hypotension, and decreased skin turgor. In some patients who have oedema there may be a hyponatraemia, and diuretics given in this situation will worsen the clinical situation. Chronic dilutional hyponatraemia should be managed by osmotic diuretics and IV theophylline [34].

Hypokalaemia. Prolonged administration of class I and class II diuretics may result in depletion of the body stores of potassium and in hypokalaemia. The clinical symptoms are muscle weakness and lassitude. If the patient is also receiving cardiac glycosides the first indication of hypokalaemia may be cardiac arrhythmias. Potassium depletion is due to the enhanced delivery of sodium to the distal renal tubule. In the distal tubule there is a sodium–potassium exchange mechanism, and the extent of the potassium loss depends on local conditions at this point, such as the tubular cellular potassium concentration, the ambient aldosterone level, and the urine flow within the tubule. If the serum potassium is above 3.5 mmol/litre potassium depletion is not likely, whilst levels below 3.2 mmol/litre usually indicate hypokalaemia. Serum potassium levels do not directly reflect the intracellular level of potassium, and potassium depletion is unlikely to be a problem in the younger hypertensive patient who is receiving a normal diet and has no other disease. On the other hand, hypokalaemia can cause clinical problems in disease states, such as diabetes and hepatic cirrhosis, as well as in patients above 65 years of age. Particular care is required in patients who are receiving steroids, carbenoxelone therapy and cardiac glycosides.

Potassium depletion can be managed either by modifying the diet, giving a potassium supplement, or using a potassium-sparing diuretic. Such measures are called for once the plasma potassium falls below 3.1 mmol/litre. The daily replacement needs are about 30 mmol potassium per day, and this can be achieved by giving either slow-release tablets which contain 8–12 mmol potassium or certain diuretic–potassium combinations which usually contain 6–8 mmol potassium per tablet [92].

Prolonged diuretic therapy may be accompanied not only by potassium loss, but also by an extracellular alkalosis due to loss of potassium, hydrogen, and chloride ions and extracellular volume depletion. This can be largely corrected by the administration of potassium chloride.

Carbohydrate intolerance. Diuretics can impair glucose homeostasis in non-insulin-dependent diabetics. In older patients they may induce hyperosmolar non-ketotic diabetic coma accompanied by hyperglycaemia [78]. In such a situation the diuretic must be withdrawn.

Other unwanted effects. A wide range of non-specific side-effects can be associated with diuretic administration. The commonest are GI disturbances such as nausea, flatulence, and skin rashes. Frusemide may cause blood dyscrasia. It may also cause tinnitus, headache and some loss of auditory activity. This latter is usually associated with high doses of a diuretic and is reversible.

Spironolactone administration may cause GI disturbances such as nausea, abdominal pain, and diarrhoea. In addition, it may cause gynaecomastia in the male and menstrual disorders and breast enlargement in females. Particular care is required with the use of class III diuretics in the presence of renal and hepatic failure. These agents are potassium-sparing and in the presence of renal failure abnormally high potassium levels may result. Class III diuretics may also cause CNS disturbances and can induce hepatic coma in cases of hepatic cirrhosis.

Drug interactions. Diuretics will potentiate the hypotensive effect of other antihypertensive agents. The class I and class II diuretics also potentiate the effects of cardiac glycosides, due to the reduction in plasma potassium levels. Diuretics may impair diabetic control and increased doses of insulin and oral hypoglycaemics may be needed. In this situation any hypokalaemia should be corrected. Furthermore, since diuretics also cause uric acid retention in patients with gout, the dose of uricosuric agent may need to be increased.

In the intensive care situation it is particularly important to note that class I diuretics may potentiate the toxicity due to aminoglycosides, such as gentamicin. This is more likely to occur if there is concomitant renal failure.

Pharmacokinetic characteristics of anti-arrhythmic drugs

The management of cardiac arrhythmias is described in Chapter 10, in which the major emphasis is upon diagnosis and overall approaches to therapy. The indications for anti-arrhythmic agents are clearly delineated but no details are given concerning pharmacological aspects of these agents. This section, therefore, will describe the clinical pharmacokinetics of the available anti-arrhythmic drugs with the aim of providing safer and more specific therapy. Whilst the major emphasis is upon pharmacokinetic characteristics, some general comments on the classification and mode of action of these agents are appropriate because there is currently some controversy in the literature on this subject.

Cardiac arrhythmias result from disturbances of normal automaticity and/or conduction in cardiac cells. The initiation and propagation of the cardiac impulse can be related to phasic changes in the electrical activity of the heart. If a micro-electrode is inserted into a myocardial fibre, a resting potential of −90 to −95 mV is observed with respect to the outside of the cell. The arrival of a propagated action potential results in a rapid depolarization followed by a slower phase of repolarization, and the recorded changes in potential have been subdivided into (Fig. 16.6) (1) phase 0, which is the rapid depolarization associated with the movement of sodium ions, into the cell; (2) phases 1 and 2, representing the early slow repolarization period during which calcium is entering the cell (slow current) and sodium ions are being removed; (3) phase 3, the rapid repolarization phase; and (4) phase 4, the resting diastolic potential.

In pacemaker tissue and Purkinje fibres, phase 4 is not a stable negative potential but shows a tendency to spontaneous depolarization. When the negative potential declines from −90 to about −65 mV the cell undergoes spontaneous depolarization.

Disturbances of automaticity arise from an alteration in the slope of the resting diastolic potential (phase 4) or the appearance of spontaneous depolarization in abnormal sites. Alteration at the resting potential or the maximal rate of depolarization (phase 0), results in changes in conduction velocity and an imbalance between conduction velocity and the refractoriness of cardiac tissue may result in re-entrant arrhythmias.

The classification of anti-arrhythmic drugs is based upon their observed effects on the conformation of a normal cardiac action potential, and is summarized here because it is frequently described in detailed reviews on these agents. It is useful, in that the ordering of any large group of agents into categories is an aid to understanding and communication. However it is of limited value in describing which agent to use for a specific arrhythmia, because each agent has more than one electrophysiological effect depending upon both the dose and the presence of additional pharmacological properties. For example disopyramide has both quinidine-like (class 1A) actions and antimuscarinic effects. Furthermore, the quantitative and temporal relationships of the ionic disturbances associated with cardiac arrhythmias are not known. Bearing these limitations in mind, the following classification based upon the studies of Vaughan-Williams [131], Singh [121], and Hoffman and Bigger [54] is of practical value (Table 16.3).

Classification

Class Ia

Drugs in this group all depress the rate of rise and over-shoot of phase 0 of the action potential without changing the resting potential. The classic example is quinidine, and this group also includes disopyramide, procainamide, ajmaline, and the more recently developed agents lorcainide and encainide. In addition, all these agents prolong phase 3 of the action potential.

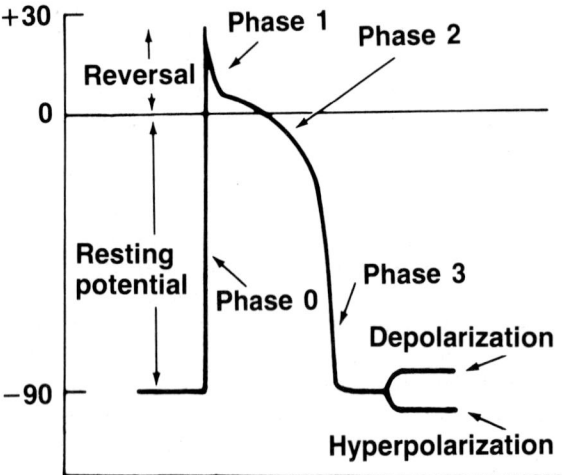

Fig. 16.6. Diagram of an action potential recorded from a Purkinje fibre. The resting potential is −90 mV. A stimulus causing depolarization leads to a rapid reversal of the potential to +30 mV. The repolarization phase is divided into three components, phases 1 and 3 being rapid and phase 2 slow repolarization. Phase 4 is the resting potential, which is flat in Purkinje tissue but sloping upwards in pacemaker tissue leading to spontaneous discharge at about −60 mV. Reproduced from Cranefield PF (1976) The conduction of the cardiac impulse. With permission of the Futura Publishing Company, New York.

Table 16.3. Classification of anti-arrhythmic drugs according to electrophysiological effect

Class	Drugs	Primary electrophysiological action
Ia. Quinidine-like	Quinidine, disopyramide, procainamide, lorcainide, encainide	Depress rate of rise of action potential (AP) without altering resting potential. Inhibition of fast Na^+ channel
Ib. Lignocaine-like	Lignocaine, phenytoin, mexilitine, tocainide (aprindine)	As above but selectively less effect on atrial and AV tissues
II. Beta-adrenoceptor antagonists	Propranolol and numerous congeners	1. Antagonize effects of catecholamines on spontaneous depolarization (phase 4) of pacemakers 2. Prevent effects of catecholamines on slow channel (? Ca) 3. No effects on rate of rise of AP
III.	Amiodarone	Prolongs duration of repolarization without affecting resting potential or rate of rise of AP
IV. Calcium slow channel inhibitors	Verapamil (Lidoflazine diltiazam)	Inhibition of slow Ca^{2+} current causing reduction in action potentials of SA and AV nodes and ectopic foci

Class Ib

This group differs from class Ia only in that these drugs shorten rather than lengthen phase 3. They include lignocaine, phenytoin, mexiletine, and tocainide.

Class II: Adrenoceptor antagonists

Stimulation of cardiac beta adrenoceptors causes an increase in spontaneous depolarization and spread of conduction through the AV node and myocardial tissue. The beta antagonists propranolol, oxprenolol, metoprolol, atenolol, etc. block these cardiac effects of catecholamines and hence cause slowing of heart rate and conduction velocity insofar as these are dependent upon catecholamine activity.

Class III

Agents in this group prolong the duration of the action potential and is represented by amiodarone and bretylium.

Class IV: Calcium channel inhibitors

Conduction through the AV node relies on a slow inward calcium current, and a similar current is associated with certain ectopic discharges. Specific antagonism of the calcium channel will prolong conduction and reduce ectopic discharge. The calcium antagonist verapamil is the best-studied example in this class.
Pharmacokinetics of class I drugs. Quinidine is used in the management of supraventricular and ventricular arrhythmias. It is available as quinidine sulphate, gluconate, bisulphate, or polygalacturonate. The commonest formulation is quinidine sulphate (tablets or capsules, containing 100, 200, or 300 mg). A longer-acting preparation is also available (Kinidin durules, 250 mg). Prior to initiation of quinidine therapy, it is good practice to administer a test dose of 200 mg in case the patient exhibits an idiosyncratic response. Subsequently, doses of 200–400 mg are given every 2–4 h, to a total of 3 g daily. The cardiac response should be checked prior to each subsequent dose. The normal maintenance dose is 100–200 mg, three to six times daily.

Quinidine sulphate is rapidly absorbed from the gut, achieving peak plasma concentrations in 2–3 h. Absorption varies and is depressed in patients with cardiac failure. The systemic bioavailability is 40%–80%. It is widely distributed throughout the body, the VD being 2.6 litres/kg. The plasma half-life is approximately 6 h and 80% of quinidine is bound to plasma albumin. Quinidine undergoes extensive hepatic metabolism, the metabolites being eliminated in the urine and approximately 10%–30% of quinidine is recovered unchanged in the urine within 24 h. The major pathways of quinidine elimination are hydroxylation to monohydroxy-quinidine and dihydroxy-quinidine.

The plasma level of quinidine associated with therapeutic benefit lies in the range of 0.3–5.0 μg/ml when a specific assay method is used. Toxicity is associated with plasma levels greater than 9.0 μg/ml [97]. In the presence of cardiac failure, the rate and extent of intestinal absorption of quinidine is reduced and a decreased volume of distribution is observed. This latter effect causes a reduction in the amount of quinidine appearing in urine per 24 h and an elevation in the plasma levels, for any given dose.

Unwanted effects. Quinidine is poorly tolerated in about 30% of patients. The commonest symptoms are GI disturbances such as anorexia, nausea, vomiting, and diarrhoea. More importantly, quinidine can induce syncope by precipitating cardiac arrhythmias such as ventricular flutter, ventricular tachycardia, and asystole. Such changes have been observed in the presence of therapeutic plasma levels and may be associated with either sudden alterations in the dose regimen or changes in serum potassium levels. Occasionally patients may exhibit a hypersensitivity response consisting of tinnitus, vertigo, skin eruptions, GI pain, and fever. This can be accompanied by hypotension, cyanosis, and collapse. More rarely quinidine can cause blood dyscrasias manifest as thrombocytopenia, haemolytic anaemia, or agranulocytosis.

Overdose of quinidine can result in cinchonism, which is a syndrome comprising headache, abdominal pain, skin rashes, and visual disturbances. In this situation quinidine elimination can be enhanced by either dialysis or by urinary acidification.

Quinidine is contraindicated in the presence of heart block, severe hypotension, and known drug hypersensitivity. Caution is needed in the digitalized patient and in untreated congestive heart failure. Drug interactions of clinical significance are as follows:

1) Potentiation of the anti-coagulant effect of coumarin drugs
2) Enhancement of the action of hypotensive agents and the cardiac actions of beta blockers
3) Potentiation of muscle relaxants
4) Reduced anti-arrhythmic effects in patients taking phenobarbitone.

Quinidine causes a 30%–50% increase in free digoxin levels and therefore administration of quinidine to a patient receiving digoxin may precipitate digitalis toxicity. The increase in serum digoxin concentrations has been attributed to reduced renal clearance of digoxin accompanied by a reduced volume of distribution [7].

Disopyramide was shown to be an antiarrhythmic agent of the quinidine type in 1962, and became available for general clinical use in 1974. Its electrophysiological and ECG characteristics closely resemble those of quinidine and

procainamide. It is effective in the management of atrial fibrillation, ventricular premature beats, and tachycardia. It is available in capsules of disopyramide phosphate containing 100 and 150 mg or as disopyramide base containing 100 mg. Normally an initial loading dose of 300 mg is given, followed by 100–150 mg disopyramide base every 6 h. This dosing regimen should be reduced in the presence of renal or hepatic insufficiency or a history of cardiac failure. If a rapid effect is required, disopyramide may be given IV in a bolus injection of 2 mg/kg administered over 10 min, but this total dose should not exceed 150 mg. Following oral administration, disopyramide is rapidly absorbed and has a systemic bioavailability varying from 60% to 85% [51]. It is rapidly distributed throughout the body and the volume of distribution is 40–80 litres in healthy volunteers, but this is reduced by a half to two-thirds in patients with myocardial infarction or severe renal failure. Disopyramide is bound to plasma proteins, the extent of binding being concentration-dependent, and only about 30% is bound in the therapeutic range of 5–6 μg/ml. Peak plasma levels following oral administration are observed after 2 h but this may be depressed in patients with AMI. Prolonged dosing at 150 mg every 6 h results in therapeutic plasma levels of between 2 and 3 μg/ml.

Disopyramide is metabolized in the liver to form the *n*-monode-alkylated metabolite, but approximately two-thirds of disopyramide is excreted unchanged. Urinary excretion accounts for about 80% of an administered dose, the remainder appearing in the faeces. The elimination half-life in healthy subjects is 4–8 h but this is increased to 11 h in patients with recent myocardial infarction and two to three times this figure in patients with severe renal failure. Disopyramide is also excreted in breast milk and significant amounts appear in fetal tissue.

Unwanted effects. Disopyramide has similar therapeutic indications to quinidine and it may be regarded as a satisfactory replacement for quinidine in that it has a lower incidence of adverse reactions. The commonest unwanted effect, due to its anticholinergic properties, are dryness of the mouth and difficulty in urination in 10%–40% of patients. Urinary retention has also been reported. It should therefore be used with care in patients with prostatic hypertrophy and also in elderly patients with glaucoma. Disopyramide depresses both cardiac conduction and contraction and should not be used in patients with second- or third-degree heart block. Its negative inotropic actions are greater than were first appreciated and considerable care is required in administering the drug to patients with cardiomegaly or with a history of heart failure. A recent report suggests that if there is a history of congestive heart failure disopyramide may precipitate a recurrence in up to 50% of such cases [105].

Rare adverse reactions have also been reported, such as intrahepatic cholestasis, peripheral neuropathy and CNS depression. Important drug interactions have not been reported, but care is clearly required in administering disopyramide in the presence of beta blockers or procainamide since there is likely to be an additive negative inotropic effect.

The electrophysiological actions of *procainamide* closely resemble those of quinidine, but it has lesser effects on AV conduction. It is effective in the management of atrial, junctional, and ventricular arrhythmias. Procainamide hydrochloride is available in capsules (250, 375, and 500 mg) and in a sustained release formulation (procainamide durules, 500 mg). The daily dose is 50 mg/kg given in divided 4-hourly doses, except in cases of renal failure when the dose should be reduced. To achieve rapid effects, procainamide can be slowly given IV in a dose of 50 mg/min, to a maximum of 1 g. Ampoules of procainamide for parenteral use contain 100 and 500 mg/ml.

Following oral administration, it is rapidly absorbed and peak blood levels are achieved at 60–90 min. Procainamide is widely distributed (VD = 0.11/kg) and less than 20% is bound to plasma protein. The plasma half-life is 2–4 h and about 60% of unchanged drug is excreted in the urine. It undergoes both hydrolysis and acetylation in the liver to form paraminobenzoic acid and *n*-acetyl derivates of both the parent compound and the hydrolysis product. The degree of acetylation depends on the genetically determined acetylator status and, interestingly, *n*-acetyl procainamide (NAPA) has valuable anti-arrhythmic properties. The therapeutic blood level for anti-arrhythmic effect lies between 4 and 10 μg/ml, whilst side-effects are associated with levels of 12–16 μg/ml. The short plasma half-life means that close attention must be paid to the dosing schedule. Sustained-release preparations have recently become available, which give lower peak plasma levels, which are, however, more prolonged, so that doses of 1–1.5 g 8-hourly are satisfactory [70].

The kinetics of procainamide are modified in cardiac and renal failure. Absorption is depressed following AMI and chronic heart failure. The elimination half-life can be markedly prolonged in renal failure, since excretion is by renal tubular secretion and there is an inverse correlation between drug administration and the renal excretion of procainamide and its metabolites. In particular, NAPA levels tend to accumulate and can be detected for 3–4 days after therapy is stopped. Hydrolysis of procainamide is reduced in chronic heart failure and in respiratory failure, but acetylation rates are not altered [32].

Unwanted effects. Procainamide causes nausea, vomiting, and rashes in a significant number of patients. Prolonged administration can cause a syndrome resembling lupus erythematosis in up to 20% of subjects. This comprises fever, rash, musculoskeletal pain, pleurisy and pericarditis. Antinuclear antibodies can be detected in the majority of patients, but less than a quarter develop the lupus syndrome.

Intravenous dosing is associated with hypotension due to a direct relaxing effect on vascular smooth muscle. Bradycardia and prolongation of conduction may also occur. Hypotension responds to sympathomimetic agents such as phenylephrine. Procainamide will enhance the effects of many hypotensive agents and also the action of beta blockers and some muscle relaxants.

Lorcainide, a new anti-arrhythmic drug, acts predominantly on the fast Na^+ channel to cause a depression in the maximal rate of depolarization. It slows conduction and reduces pacemaker activity in the sinus node and Purkinje tissue [15]. It can be given PO in doses between 190 and 300 mg or IV in doses of 1–2 mg/kg. It is well absorbed but undergoes extensive first-pass hepatic metabolism. Its systemic bioavailability is low but becomes much higher during prolonged therapy due to saturation of the hepatic extraction mechanism. It is widely distributed and the elimination half-life is 6–8 h. It is excreted in the urine and less than 2% appears as unchanged drug [59].

Pharmacokinetics of class Ib drugs

Lidocaine is the reference anti-arrhythmic agent in this group. It causes a concentration-dependent reduction in the rate of rise of depolarization (Vmax) and therefore depresses membrane responsiveness. Unlike the class Ia drugs, it shortens the action potential duration and the refractory period of Purkinje fibres. Lidocaine is effective in controlling VEBs of any origin and raises the cardiac fibrillation threshold. Its bioavailability following administration PO is less than 35% because of extensive first-pass hepatic extraction and metabolism [5]. Therapeutic blood levels can be obtained if high doses are administered PO, but these are accompanied by severe GI and CNS side-effects, possibily due to the formation of metabolites by the liver. It is therefore only used parenterally. Following a bolus injection, the kinetics of lidocaine are best described by a three-compartmental model. The initial alpha distribution phase lasts about 6–10 min, and during this period lidocaine is being distributed preferentially to the lungs, heart, brain, and kidney. Subsequently there is a secondary redistribution phase lasting about 42 min, representing uptake into muscle and adipose tissue. The third and longest phase, lasting 2–3 h, represents hepatic metabolism and possibly distribution to relatively avascular tissues. The steady-state volume of distribution, following infusion, varies from 80 to 150 litres and is much reduced in cardiac failure. Because of these pharmacokinetic characteristics, a steady-state myocardial concentration can best be maintained by giving an infusion, because after a single IV dose, peak levels may be transiently attained in the myocardium, but then rapidly fall due to the secondary redistribution phase.

Lidocaine is about 70% bound to plasma proteins, and is extensively metabolised by microsomal enzymes in the liver. The major metabolites are monoethyl glycinexylidide (MEGX) and glycinexylidide (GX) and these tend to accumulate during prolonged intravenous infusion. The former metabolite is as potent an anti-arrhythmic and anticonvulsant agent as lidocaine itself, and the GX metabolite is about one-third as potent. Lidocaine and its metabolites are excreted in urine.

The effective therapeutic blood level for the suppression of ventricular arrhythmias lies between 1 and 5 μg/ml. These therapeutic blood levels can be attained by administering an initial bolus of 1–2 mg/kg body followed immediately by an infusion of 2 mg/min rising to 4 mg/min according to the response. If an infusion cannot be given, an IM dose of 4–5 mg/kg, given into the deltoid muscle, is recommended.

Certain disease states have marked effects on lidocaine kinetics. In patients with myocardial infarction there is a tendency for lidocaine concentrations to increase during prolonged infusion. For example, Le Lorier observed a fourfold increase in lidocaine concentrations during a constant infusion lasting 12 h [79]. This progressive rise is attributed to non-linear clearance resulting from saturation of hepatic metabolism or from the accumulation of lidocaine metabo-

lites. The clearance of lidocaine depends primarily on hepatic blood flow, and if this is depressed the lidocaine half-life is increased. On the other hand, renal impairment does not affect the pharmacokinetics of lidocaine [23].

Unwanted effects. The most prominent unwanted effects of lidocaine are upon the CNS and consists of an initial phase of excitation manifested by restlessness, excitement, dizziness, vomiting, and convulsions. This may be followed by depression of the CNS resulting in drowsiness, respiratory failure, and coma. These may be accompanied by bradycardia and some degree of heart block together with hypotension. In the seriously ill patient it may be difficult to decide whether lethargy, hypotension, and confusion are due to the primary cardiac condition or to excess lidocaine. A recently described rapid serum lidocaine determination can be useful in clarifying such a problem [28]. There are no reports of significant drug interactions, though clearly, agents that affect cardiac output and hepatic blood flow may be expected to alter the normal pharmacokinetic profile of lidocaine.

Phenytoin (diphenylhydantoin) is used primarily as an anticonvulsant drug, but is also effective in the management of digitalis-induced arrhythmias, particularly paroxysmal atrial tachycardia. In the absence of digitalis toxicity, it is used in the management of lidocaine-resistant ventricular arrhythmias. The electrophysiological effects of phenytoin have been the subject of controversy. It clearly depresses the rate of rise and overshoot of the action potential and is regarded as a quinidine-like drug.

It shortens the duration of the action potential in ventricular and Purkinje fibres and has minimal effects on AV conduction time; it is therefore considered more like lidocaine than quinidine.

Phenytoin is available in capsules containing 30, 50, or 100 mg/kg. The oral dose is 50–100 mg/kg three times daily, increasing to 200 mg three times daily according to the response. It is also available in ampoules containing 100 or 250 mg for IV use if rapid control of the arrhythmia is essential. The parenteral solution is alkaline and very irritant so a central IV catheter is recommended. The solution should not be mixed with other agents. Varying dose schedules are recommended for achieving rapid control by parenteral administration, and a favoured one is 50–100 mg IV every 5 min until control is achieved or toxicity supervenes, but the total dose should not exceed 1 g [8]. Alternatively 5 mg/kg can be given IV, followed by 1 mg/kg commencing 15 min after the initial dose.

Phenytoin is well absorbed from the gut but peak plasma concentrations may not be achieved for 8–12 h and it may be several days before stable plasma levels are attained following oral therapy. Phenytoin is taken up and concentrated in many tissues, especially in the liver and is over 90% bound to plasma proteins. It crosses most membranes and is found in the brain, milk, and fetus.

The therapeutic plasma concentration lies between 10 and 20 μg/ml and most responsive ventricular arrhythmias are controlled with plasma levels below 18 μg/ml [74]. The plasma half-life of phenytoin is dose-dependent but the therapeutic plasma levels have a half-life of approximately 22 h.

Phenytoin undergoes extensive hepatic metabolism and the major metabolite is 5-phenylparahydroxyphenylhydantoin. Following hydroxylation, the metabolites are conjugated and excreted in bile with subsequent reabsorption and excretion in the urine, less than 5% appearing as phenytoin. There are wide individual variations in the plasma level and half-life of phenytoin and the variability is attributed to differences in the rate and extent of hepatic metabolism. Reduced hepatic metabolism can lead to drug accumulation and toxicity. *Unwanted effects.* The most common unwanted effects are those of the CNS and they are related to plasma level. Plasma levels in the range 20–25 μg/ml are associated with nystagmus, ataxia, and dizziness, whilst lethargy, mental confusion, and hallucinations are observed at plasma levels of 35–40 μg/ml [106]. During long-term therapy unwanted effects such as blood dyscrasias, including megaloblastic anaemia and thrombocytopenia, are described. Lymphadenopathy and gum hyperplasia are specifically associated with long-term phenytoin therapy. Parenteral phenytoin may cause hypertension, tachycardia, and asystole, which can be avoided by careful monitoring of the blood pressure and ECG during administration.

Mexiletine is a recently introduced antiarrhythmic agent, which is a primary amine analogue of lidocaine and has similar electrophysiological properties in that it reduces action potential duration in Purkinje fibres. In normal subjects it has little effect on ventricular conduction time, but conduction time may be lengthened in patients with defects of the His–Purkinje system [64, 85, 112]. Mexiletine is used primarily in the management of ventricular

arrhythmias and offers advantages over lidocaine in that it is active following administration PO, with a much longer duration of effect. It is available as capsules (50 and 200 mg) and injection (25 mg/ml). The oral dose is 400–600 mg initially, followed by 0.6–1.6 g daily at 8–hourly intervals. The recommended regimen for IV use is 100–200 mg (1–3 mg/kg) given slowly over 10 min. Subsequently 250 mg is given by infusion over 1 h, followed by 250 mg over 2 h. Thereafter an infusion of 0.5–1.0 mg/min should give plasma levels in the therapeutic range [13].

Mexiletine is rapidly and completely absorbed from the gut and peak plasma levels are observed between 2–4 h. Therapeutic plasma levels vary from 0.5 and 2.0 μg/ml, but unwanted effects may occur with plasma levels in the range 1.5–3.0 μg/ml. It is widely distributed (VD = 5.0 litres/kg) and about 70% is bound to plasma proteins. It undergoes hepatic metabolism and both mexiletine and its metabolites are excreted in the urine. This excretion is markedly influenced by urinary pH, in that at pH 5 the terminal plasma half-life may be reduced from 10 to 3 h. This could influence the use of mexiletine in the acute situation, since therapy being given at the same time to combat acidosis would increase the urinary pH and hence reduce mexiletine excretion which could cause drug accumulation [69].

Unwanted effects. Originally it was considered that mexiletine had a wide therapeutic margin, but it is now being realized that CNS effects may occur with low plasma levels. These effects are tremor, dizziness, drowsiness, diplopia, ataxia, paraesthesia, and hallucinations. Most of these can be avoided by careful attention to the dosing regimen and thereafter the only significant effects may be nausea and tremor. After parenteral administration, hypotension, bradycardia, and conduction defects may be observed if the rate of injection is not appropriately controlled.

Tocainide is also a primary amine analogue of lidocaine with similar electrophysiological properties, but like mexiletine it is active following PO administration and has a long duration of action. The clinical indications are similar to those for lidocaine. The usual oral dose is 600–800 mg daily, and the IV dose is 0.5–0.75 mg/kg given over 15 min. Tocainide is rapidly and completely absorbed and its VD is about 1.6 litres/kg, with about 50% bound to plasma proteins. The plasma half-life is 12–14 h and about 40% of the drug is excreted unchanged in the urine. Therapeutic levels are in the 4–10 μg/ml range [87]. Unwanted effects resemble those of lidocaine and mexiletine, and include tremor, dizziness, paraesthesia, and convulsions [26].

Encainide is currently undergoing clinical evaluation. Its electrophysiological effects resemble those of lidocaine and are both time and concentration-dependent. It shortens action potential duration and lengthens the effective refractory period. In high concentrations it depresses the V_{max} of the action potential without changing the resting potential.

Encainide hydrochloride is available for study in 25-mg tablets. It is rapidly absorbed but has a variable systemic bioavailability and there is a non-linear relationship between dose and steady-state plasma concentration. The elimination half-life is 2–3 h and the therapeutic plasma concentration is in the range 1–56 μg/ml with side-effects being observed at levels above 150 μg/ml. These side-effects are ataxia and diplopia [110].

Pharmacokinetics of class II agents. These are the beta-adrenoceptor antagonists, and their kinetic properties are described on pp. 276–277.

Pharmacokinetics of class III agents. Amiodarone is the reference drug in this group, which also includes bretylium and possibly the beta-blocker sotolol [92, 93]. The characteristic electrophysiological features are a prolongation of the action potential duration with little change in the rate of deplorization (phase 0). Amiodarone prolongs the refractory period in the atrium, the AV node, and the ventricle. It is effective in controlling arrhythmias associated with the Wolff–Parkinson–White syndrome. Amiodarone may control both atrial and ventricular arrhythmias resistant to other forms of therapy. Unlike class I and class II agents it does not depress ventricular function in clinical doses [122, 135].

The daily oral dose of amiodarone is 300–600 mg. It is slowly absorbed from the gut and widely distributed throughout the body, high levels being found in the thyroid, adipose tissue, and muscle. The plasma level associated with control of arrhythmias is not known. It is excreted very slowly and the terminal half-life is 25–30 days [10]. Furthermore, the onset of action is very slow and it may be 3–5 days before an optimal effect is observed. Thus amiodarone is of limited value in the acute management of arrhythmias. It is mostly excreted unchanged from the urine and a small amount is dehalogenated so that about 9 mg iodine/day may be found in the urine following a standard oral dose of 300 mg amiodarone.

Unwanted effects. In general, amiodarone is well tolerated, but on prolonged therapy microdeposits appear in the cornea, though they do not impair vision. Skin rashes and photodermatitis have also been reported. Circulating levels of thyroxine are elevated, and consequently T_3 levels are decreased. Thus cases of disturbance of thyroid function have been reported [106].

Pharmacokinetics of class IV (calcium slow channel inhibitors). Verapamil is the reference example in this group of anti-arrhythmic agents. It differs from drugs in class Ia and Ib in that it has no effect on the resting membrane potential or on the rapid upstroke (phase 0) of the action potential. Furthermore it does not alter the overall rate of repolarization. Recent electrophysiological studies have shown that the process of depolarization in normal tissue can be divided into two separate components: (1) a fast sodium-dependent channel, and (2) a slow mixed sodium/calcium-dependent channel. Verapamil acts on the calcium component of the slow channel. This calcium-dependent slow channel potential can be demonstrated in the normal sinoatrial node, in the AV node, and in mitral valve leaflets [67]. Verapamil, by reducing the calcium current in these sites, decreases both automaticity and speed of conduction. Calcium-dependent slow response potentials induced by catecholamines or ischaemia in atrial, ventricular, or Purjinke tissue are abolished by verapamil [113]. This effect may explain its value in controlling many atrial and junctional arrhythmias. Its lesser effectiveness in the majority of ventricular arrhythmias suggests that the slow calcium response may be less important in the genesis of these latter arrhythmias.

Verapamil is available in 40-mg tablets and the oral dose is 40–100 mg three times daily. Ampoules containing 2.5 mg/ml are available for parenteral use and the recommended dose is 1–10 mg given over 10 min. The pharmacokinetics of verapamil are described on p. 283.

Unwanted effects. In general, verapamil is well tolerated and the majority of its side-effects are due to its pharmacological action upon the cardiovascular system. Blockade of the slow calcium channel by verapamil causes not only alterations in cardiac conduction, but also a reduction in cardiac contractility and vasodilatation. These combined cardiovascular effects result in a fall in systemic blood pressure, which is more likely to be encountered during parenteral administration. It follows therefore that verapamil should not be given to patients with established heart block, bradycardia, hypotension, or heart failure. In particular, there is a danger of an interaction with both digitalis and beta blockers, resulting in severe bradycardia, heart block, or asystole [73].

Drugs affecting blood coagulation

The transportation of blood can only be maintained if it is in a state of appropriate fluidity. However, a breach of a blood vessel may lead to a serious loss of circulating fluid and such an event is combated rapidly by local clotting of blood. Normal blood fluidity is maintained by an interplay between factors leading to clotting and factors which either solubilize clots (fibrinolysis) or inhibit the clotting process. This section will deal with the pharmacology of agents that interfere with this balance. The agents that act as anti-coagulants are the coumarins (warfarin), indanediones (phenindione), heparin, and drugs modifying platelet function. The agents enhancing clot removal (fibrinolysis) are streptokinase and urokinase.

The coagulation system

Clot formation

The process leading to haemostasis following injury to a blood vessel involves the interaction of platelets, endothelial factors, and circulating coagulation factors. Effective haemostasis depends finally on the formation of a stable clot composed of fibrin and platelets. The formation of fibrin is preceded by a complex series of biochemical interactions between coagulation factors in the blood and factors released from the damaged endothelium and from activated platelets [138]. The 'clotting cascade' leading to blood coagulation can be divided into three phases and is more easily understood if the process is described in the reverse order. The elements comprising the cascade are, by convention, described by Roman numerals (Fig. 16.7). The final phase in the clotting process (phase 3) comprises the action of the protease enzyme, thrombin, on fibrinogen. Thrombin acts on fibrinogen to release fibrin monomers which polymerize to form an insoluble fibrin clot which is further stablized by the action of a circulating factor (factor XIII).

Thrombin activity is initiated by the action of factor X on prothrombin (factor II) in the presence of calcium. This is phase 2 of the cascade. Phase 1 comprises the events leading to factor X formation. The initiating trigger is contact of the blood with a 'foreign' surface such as collagen, which leads to activation of factor XIII to form factor XIIIA. The suffix A is used to describe the activated form of the enzyme.

Once factor XIIIA is formed, a series of other enzymes (factors XI, IX, VIII, and X) is activated in sequence. The process requires the presence of calcium ions and certain co-factors. Furthermore, the process can be limited by the presence of inhibitors such as anti-thrombin (AT III) and inhibitors of factors XI and XII. With the exception of factors XIII and VIII, the plasma protein-clotting factors are formed in the liver.

The fibrinolytic system

Plasma contains a beta globulin called plasminogen, which on activation forms plasmin. Plasmin is a protease that acts on established fibrin polymers to form soluble degradation products, and its action results in clot lysis. Plasmin also inactivates fibrinogen, prothrombin, and factors V and VIII. Clearly plasmin can prevent the normal coagulation process and also resolve fibrin clots. The inactive form, plasminogen, is activated by a plasminogen activator, which in turn is stimulated by factor XII. Thus, tissue damage initiates not only the coagulation cascade but also the fibrinolytic system. Plasminogen activators may be found in many secretions, including human urine (urokinase).

Haemostasis

Injury to a blood vessel evokes a series of events leading to haemostasis. The initial event is activation of circulating platelets leading to their aggregation and the subsequent formation of a platelet–fibrin plug. Exposure of platelets to damaged endothelium leads to their aggregation, possibly by the local release of adenosine diphosphate (ADP) and by thromboxane A_2 and thrombin. Aggregated platelets undergo viscous metamorphosis resulting in the release of coagulation factors. Subsequently, fibrin is laid down to form a red thrombus. The platelet therefore plays a key role in haemostasis and reduction in circulating platelets leads to a haemorrhagic state.

Phase 1   Phase 2   Phase 3

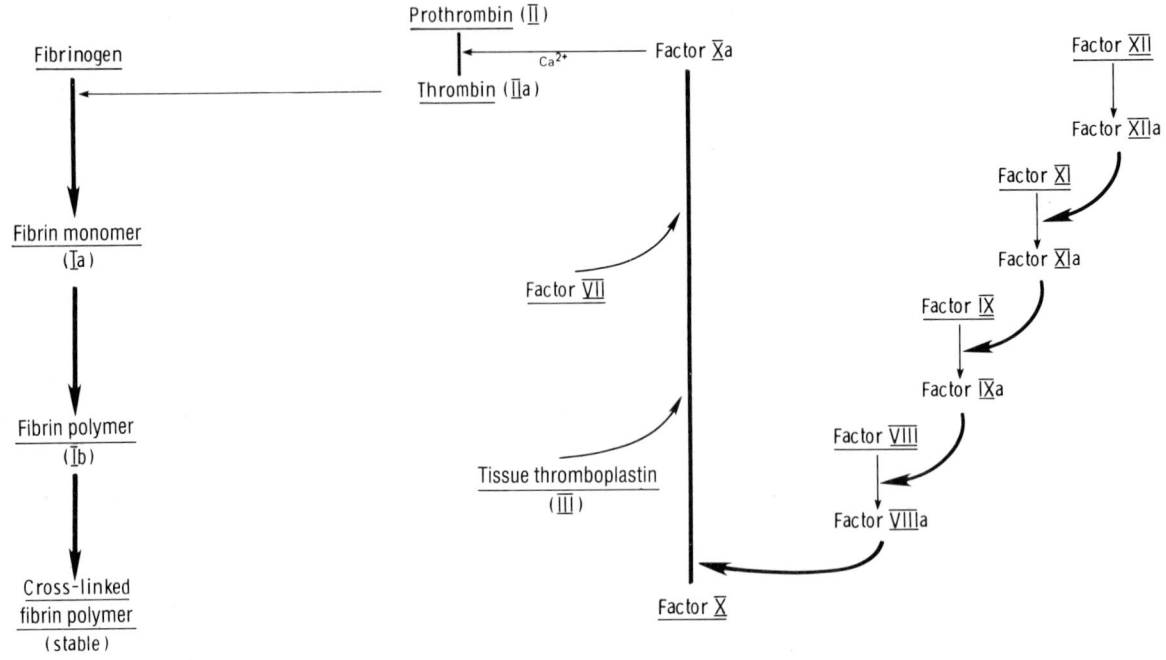

Fig. 16.7. Scheme of biochemical events leading to fibrin clot formation. Phase 3 is the series of initiating steps of enzymatic activation leading to factor VIIIa formation. Phase 2 leads to thrombin activation (factor IIa) and phase 1 is the formation of stable fibrin from fibrinogen.

Drugs modifying prothrombin formation

Vitamin K

The formation of prothrombin and factors VIII, IX, and X depends upon the availability of vitamin K. Vitamin K_1 is a fat-soluble phytoquinone present in liver and some plants. It should be distinguished from vitamin k_2 (menaquinone), which is of bacterial origin. The sole pharmacological action of vitamin K is to promote the formation of coagulation factors, and this effect can only be shown when body stores of vitamin K are depleted. Administration of vitamin K_1 to deficient animals leads to restoration of depressed levels of prothrombin and factors VII, IX, and X. Its mode of action is not precisely known, but has been attributed either to facilitation of glycoprotein attachment during the synthesis of coagulation factors or to its action as a co-factor in gamma carboxylation of glutamic acid residues in the proteins involved in coagulation [125].

Vitamin K_1 (phytomenadione) is used to treat hypoprothrombin states in neonatal haemorrhage or as an antidote to anticoagulant over-dose. It is available as a tablet (5 mg) or injection (2 and 10 mg/ml). The dose for infants is 0.5–1 mg and for adults 5–20 mg PO or by slow IV injection. Phytomenadione is rapidly absorbed from the gut and accumulates in the liver, but is not stored elsewhere in the body. Following IV administration, phytomenadione can cause tachycardia and hypotension as well as sweating, bronchospasm, and facial flushing. An IV injection should, therefore, be given very slowly.

Vitamin K antagonists (oral anticoagulants)

These agents are derivatives of either coumarin or indanedione. Warfarin (sodium) is the reference anticoagulant and is one of the coumarin derivatives, others being dicoumarol, acinocoumarol, and phenprocoumon. The indanedione group comprises phenindione, anisindione, and diphenadione. All anticoagulants are used in the management of venous thrombosis and pulmonary embolism as well as in established rheumatic heart disease and certain cases of AMI. They act by interfering with the action of vitamin K on the hepatic synthesis of the clotting factors.

Their precise mode of action is not clearly understood, since the role of vitamin K in forming the clotting factors is not agreed. Presumably by interfering with either glycoprotein formation or gamma carboxylation of glutamic acid, they reduce the hepatic synthesis of coagulation factors and hence decrease circulating levels of factors II (prothrombin), VII, IX, and X. The rate of decline in plasma levels is determined by the half-life of these factors, so that factor VII falls most rapidly, and factor II reduction is slowest. The effect of these agents can be reversed by large doses of vitamin K.

Pharmacokinetics. Warfarin (sodium), the reference anticoagulant, is available in a variety of tablet strengths, ranging from 1 to 25 mg, and also in an injectable form (50–75 mg/ampoule). It is rapidly and completely absorbed from the gut, becoming extensively bound to plasma proteins, and is metabolized in the liver to form 7-hydroxywarfarin, 6-hydroxywarfarin, and also alcohols of warfarin. It is widely distributed throughout the body and accumulates in the liver, lungs, kidney, and red cells. Warfarin may also be excreted in the milk and can cross the placenta, thus affecting the neonatal coagulation system. The plasma half-life is 48 h, with a range of 14–55 h, but the biological effect persists for 4–6 days, following cessation of therapy [52]. The therapeutic dose of warfarin varies greatly between individuals and is dependent upon the rate of metabolism and availability of vitamin K. The response is also altered by numerous factors including alteration in hepatic function, pregnancy, concomitant drug therapy, and extent of protein binding. Though maximum warfarin plasma levels are observed within 6 h of dosing, there is a delay of 1–3 days before the maximal effect is observed [3]. Therapeutic effect is determined by monitoring the prothrombin conversion time, which is sensitive to factors II, VII, and X. The normal range of prothrombin time is 11–13 s and the aim of therapy is to increase the time by 1.25–1.75 of the normal value or 15–30% of normal prothrombin activity. Previously a time of 2–2.5 times the normal prothrombin time was recommended, but this can lead to an increase in the incidence of haemorrhage. Dosing commences with 10–15 mg warfarin daily and the subsequent doses are modified according to the prothrombin time results.

Drug interactions. Numerous drug interactions with anti-coagulants have been described and warfarin has been the agent most commonly implicated. The classes of drug most commonly involved are listed in Table 16.4. Only those agents for which there is clinical evidence of an interaction are included. Experimental studies in vitro or in animals have implicated numerous additional drugs but the interaction has not been confirmed clinically. As a general principle, meticulous attention should be paid to concomitant drug therapy before treatment with oral anticoagulants is initiated. If there is any doubt a reference book on drug interaction should be consulted. No attempt is made in this text to explain the mechanism of the drug interactions listed, since many of the explanations are not well proven. In general, the concomitant drugs interfere with either protein binding of the anticoagulant or its hepatic binding and metabolism [71, 100].

Unwanted effects. The commonest unwanted effect is haemorrhage, which occurs mostly from the GI tract but may be found in the

Table 16.4. Drug interactions with oral anticoagulants

Drug class	Effect on response to anticoagulant
1. Alcohol	Reduce plasma $T\frac{1}{2}$
2. Analgesics	
Mephanemic acid	Potentiation[a]
Salicylates, sulphinpyrazone Phenylbutazone	Potentiates. Additional bleeding tendency due to GI damage and platelet inhibition
3. Antibiotics	
Chloramphenicol, neomycin, rifampicin	Potentiation
Griseofulvin	Inhibition[b]
4. Anticonvulsants	
Phenytoin	Dicoumarol prolongs $T\frac{1}{2}$ of phenytoin
5. Antidepressants	
Tricyclics	Potentiation
6. Hypolipidaemics	
Clofibrate	Marked potentiation
Dextrothyroxine	Potentiation
Cholestyramine	Reduces both vitamin K and anticoagulant absorption. (Combination probably contraindicated)
7. Oral hypoglycaemics	Complex effects on both protein binding and hepatic metabolism. Doses of both types of agent require adjustment
8. Sedative hypnotics	
Barbiturates	Inhibition
Glutethimide	Inhibition
Chloral hydrate	Initially potentiates and returns to normal after 10–14 days

[a]Increased anticoagulant activity and bleeding tendency.
[b]Reduced anticoagulant activity.

kidney, brain, skin, or uterus. Haemorrhage is due to the known pharmacological action of this group of agents and should not be regarded as a toxic effect. Treatment consists of stopping the drug administration and if bleeding is severe, giving phytomenadione (vitamin K_1), 5–10 mg IV over 10 min. Whole fresh blood should also be available.

Non-specific side-effects, such as anorexia, vomiting, and diarrhoea can occur. Rarely alopecia and urticaria have been reported. Warfarin and other anticoagulants should not be given (1) in acute cerebral haemorrhage; (2) after recent haemorrhage of any sort; (3) in severe hypertension; (4) during or after traumatic surgery; (5) in ulcerative conditions of the gut; (6) during pregnancy (first 3 months or after the 37th week); or (7) during breast feeding.

Other anticoagulants

These differ from warfarin in their potency, duration of action, and incidence of side-effects. With the exception of diphenadione, the indanedione anticoagulants are less frequently used because of increased incidence of toxicity.

Dicoumarol is available in 25, 50, and 100 mg tablets or capsules. It is irregularly absorbed from the gut and greatly bound to plasma proteins. It is extensively metabolized in the liver, producing metabolites which are excreted in the urine. The plasma half-life varies greatly between 36–72 h and the biological effect persists for 5–6 days after therapy is stopped.

Diphenadione This anticoagulant has a prolonged duration of effect for up to 20 days after stopping therapy. It is available in 5-mg tablets and the initial dose is 20–30 mg on the first day, followed by 2.5–5 mg daily, according to the prothrombin time response. The unwanted effects and contraindications are similar to those given for warfarin.

Heparin is a unique anticoagulant of natural origin, which can be extracted from beef lung and pork intestinal mucosa. It is a mucopolysaccharide consisting of a series of polymers formed from sulphated d-glucosamine and d-glucuronic acid. The chain length of the polymers varies ten fold and the molecular weight ranges from 7 600–19 700. Recent studies on the chemistry and biology of heparin suggest that it has many properties other than acting as an anticoagulant. It is a highly negatively charged (acidic) molecule and is one of a group of linear anionic polyelectrolytes which are highly reactive with cations, forming complexes with enzymes and other proteins. Thus, heparin appears to have many additional biological properties other than acting as an anticoagulant though it is remarkably well tolerated. At present only its anticoagulant actions are used for therapeutic purposes [16].

Mode of action. The primary therapeutic use of heparin is to prevent or reduce thrombus formation in veins and arteries, particularly following surgery and myocardial infarction. It also reduces thrombus formation in indwelling catheters and during extracorporeal circulation. These effects are achieved by activating the endogenous prothrombin inhibitor (AT III), which is a protease present in the α_2 globulin fraction of serum. Activation of AT III by heparin inhibits the actions of factors IXA, XA, X1A and XIIA, resulting in decreased thrombin formation (Fig. 16.7); and it is likely that the key action of heparin is to prevent the action of factor XA. Activated AT III also combines with thrombin to prevent fibrin formation but higher concentrations are required than those which neutralize factor XA [141]. Furthermore, higher concentrations of AT III plus heparin also inhibit thrombin-induced platelet aggregation. It is probable that heparin also reduces thrombosis by binding to endothelial cells lining blood vessels to enhance the electronegative potential of these cells and hence reduce thrombus deposition. Intravenous heparin in doses not affecting coagulation also causes the release of lipoprotein lipase from the vascular endothelial cells. This causes hydrolysis of circulating triglycerides and subsequent elevation of FFA levels. The physiological relevance of this is not known.

Pharmacokinetics. Heparin is inactive when given PO and must be administered parenterally. It is well absorbed from subcutaneous and muscular tissue. After IV injection, heparin is rapidly removed from the blood and the half-life ranges from 50 to 150 min, depending upon the dose. It is taken up by endothelial cells, macrophages, and cells of the reticulo-endothelial system. It is also degraded by a heparinase found in liver and kidney. Heparin is excreted in urine partly as desulphated uroheparin. The complexities of heparin dosage and kinetics have recently been reviewed [33].

Dosage of heparin is determined by the whole blood clotting time which should be kept to 2–2.5 times the control value (5–10 min). A more convenient and accurate test is the thrombin time, and this should be increased to three to four times normal. The initial dose of heparin required to achieve a rapid anticoagulant effect is 10 000–12 500 USP units IV followed by 6000–12 000 units, four to six times daily. If given by continuous infusion, 20 000–30 000 units of heparin are added to 1 litre of 5% dextrose in 0.9% saline solution and given at a rate of 15–30 units/min. Since the anticoagulant effect following such an infusion may take 2–3 h to develop, an initial bolus of 5000 units should be given. The dose for children is 50 units/kg per 24 h. It must be noted that heparin is incompatible with certain antibiotics, and should not be mixed with streptomycin, erythromycin, gentamicin and tetracycline.

The SC dose of heparin is 10 000–20 000 units initially followed by 8000–10 000 units three times a day. The IM route is not recommended because of haematoma formation. Recently 'low dose' heparin has been recommended for the prevention of deep vein thrombosis (DVT) and pulmonary embolism associated with abdominal and orthopaedic surgery. The precise dose schedule varies slightly but excellent results have been obtained by giving 5000 units SC 2 h prior to surgery and then 8-hourly for 7 days. Such doses of heparin do not alter the normal clotting test and it is postulated that low doses can prevent factor XA activation without changing the normal coagulation tests [142].

Unwanted effects. Heparin is remarkably well tolerated, but occasionally febrile or allergic responses are encountered. In subjects with a history of allergy, it is customary to give a test dose of 1000 units of heparin prior to initiating therapy. Rarely alopecia, diarrhoea, osteoporosis, and spontaneous fractures may occur after prolonged heparin administration. Heparin overdose is manifest as epistaxis, haematuria, and ecchymosis. If necessary the effects of heparin overdose can be rapidly reversed by giving protamine sulphate IV, which acts by neutralizing the negative charges on the surface of heparin. The dose required is not easy to predict, but a useful guide is to give 1 mg protamine sulphate per 100 units of heparin administered, without giving more than 50 mg protamine in any 15-min period [60]. Heparin should not be given to patients receiving ethacrynic acid since this appears to potentiate its anticoagulant activity. Similarly, care is required if a patient is also receiving aspirin, since the combined effects on AT III and inhibition of platelet adhesiveness may cause haemorrhage.

Thrombolytic agents

The resolution of a recently formed thrombus can be accelerated by activation of the endogenous fibrinolytic system. The plasminogen activators, urokinase and streptokinase, are used to promote plasmin formation which will solubilize fibrin. The specific role of these agents in therapy remains controversial, but it has been established that they have a beneficial effect in severe pulmonary embolism [11, 115].

Urokinase is the plasminogen activator isolated from human urine, which is available in powder form in ampoules containing 5000, 25 000, or 100 000 plough units (equivalent to 7500, 37 500, or 150 000 IU). The following regimen is recommended: urokinase 2000 units/lb body wt is infused IV over 10 min followed by 2000 units/lb/h for 12 h. Thereafter heparin is given IV in the normal dose range. Overdose with urokinase can be reversed by giving aprotonin 50 000–100 000 units/h IV until haemorrhage is controlled. The principal side-effect with urokinase is haemorrhage, but occasionally fever has been reported.

Streptokinase is a large-molecular-weight protein obtained from cultures of haemolytic streptococci. It is used to resolve thrombi in pulmonary embolism and arterial and venous thrombosis, and though some of the indications for its use remain controversial its major indication is established in the management of major pulmonary embolism. It is available in sterile ampoules (100 000; 250 000 and 600 000 IU). Streptokinase is administered by IV infusion and the recommended initial dose is 300 000–600 000 units given over the first hour followed by a 100 000 units hourly for 1–3 days according to the clinical response. Following parenteral administration, peak fibrinolytic activity is observed within 20 min. Highest concentrations are found in the liver and about 6% of a single dose can be recovered in the urine within 4 h. Antibodies to streptococci occur commonly in man and can inactivate streptokinase, but this problem can be overcome by using large initial doses (250 000–600 000 units) [11]. Allergic responses are therefore common and hydrocortisone (100 mg) should always be given at the beginning of treatment. A response to therapy can be measured by determining the plasma thrombin time, which should be increased two to threefold. Frequent monitoring is not necessary. The effectiveness of streptokinase depends upon the availability of circulating plasminogen, and as levels of plasminogen fall increasing the dose of streptokinase becomes less effective. When the infusion has been stopped heparin should be given within 4 h to prevent rebound thrombosis.

Unwanted effects. The antigenic and anticoagulant effects of streptokinase account for its unwanted effects. Allergic responses take the form of fever, rash, hypotension, and bronchospasm. The incidence is reduced by the concomitant administration of steroids. Bleeding can be controlled by stopping therapy and if necessary giving a blood transfusion. Since stretopkinase is rapidly cleared from the body it is not often necessary to reverse its action with aprotonin. Streptokinase should not be used in cases of recent trauma or surgery and the usual contraindications to anticoagulant therapy also apply.

Antiplatelet agents

Since platelets are intimately involved in thrombus formation, drugs which prevent platelet function have been evaluated in thrombo-embolic disease. The current status of antiplatelet agents has recently been reviewed [40]. The agents of clinical significance are aspirin, sulphinpyrazone, and dipyramidole. Clinical syndromes in which these agents have been shown to be effective are given in Tables 16.5 and 16.6, and it must be emphasized that the effectiveness of these agents, as assessed by controlled trials, varies considerably according to the thrombo-embolic indication.

Aspirin (acetyl salicylic acid) acts by prolonging platelet survival and reducing platelet aggregation by inhibition of the enzyme platelet cyclo-oxygenase, which causes a reduction in thromboxane A_2 formation. This effect is achieved by irreversible inhibition of the cyclo-oxygenase enzyme in the platelet, which leads to a reduction in the formation of thromboxane A_2; this in turn is responsible for platelet aggregation.

The usual dose of aspirin is 300–1500 mg daily in four divided doses. It is rapidly and completely absorbed and plasma levels of about 50 μg/ml are observed after a single dose of 1 g. Six doses of 1 g each at hourly intervals, however, give much higher levels of about 180 μg/ml. Aspirin is rapidly hydrolysed in the intestine and plasma to form salicylic acid. Both aspirin

Table 16.5 Summary of results[a] of clinical trials of antiplatelet agents

Indication		Foreign surface interaction			Cerebral ischaemia	Myocardial infarction	Venous thrombosis
	Drug	Arterial surgery	Prosthetic valves	A/V shunt			
Aspirin		+	+[b]	?	+[c]	−[d]	+[f]
Dipyridamole		?	+[b]	?	?		+[g]
Sulphinpyrazone		−	−	+	−	+[e]	−

[a] +, benefit; −, no benefit; ?, not evaluated.
[b] Only when combined with oral anticoagulants.
[c] Only in male subjects.
[d] Four large studies show a positive trend.
[e] Apparently reduced sudden death but not infarction rate.
[f] Effective in reducing thrombosis after hip surgery but not after general surgery.
[g] Aspirin and dipyridamole may be effective after general surgery but heparin is preferable.

Table 16.6. Clinical indications[a] for antiplatelet drugs

Drug dose Indications	Aspirin	Dipyridamole	Sulphinpyrazone
Prosthetic valves	500 mg + oral anticoagulant	100 mg q.i.d. oral anticoagulant	−
A/V shunt	−	−	200 mg t.i.d.
Arterial surgery	1.5 g/daily	−	No effect
Venous thrombosis (hip surgery	1.5 g/daily	−	−
Cerebral ischaemia (males only)	325 mg q.i.d.	No effect	No effect
Myocardial ischaemia	Possibly effective but not fully proven	Possibly effective with aspirin	Results controversial

[a] Where dose is given the indication is established; −, not tested.

and salicylic acid are widely distributed and salicylic acid is highly protein bound. The plasma half-life is about 4 h and this is markedly prolonged at higher doses. Salicylic acid is metabolized in the liver to at least four metabolites, the major one being salicyluric acid. Aspirin and its metabolites are cleared by the kidney and the rate of renal excretion is pH-dependent [27, 43].

Unwanted effects. These are numerous and well recognized. The important adverse effects are: (1) gastric ulceration and GI distress; (2) a bleeding tendency due to depression of platelet function and to possible reduction of plasma prothrombin; (3) renal damage as evidenced by albuminuria and casts. Hypersensitivity reactions to aspirin occur in about 1 in 500 subjects and are seen as rashes, urticaria, and occasionally bronchospasm [17].

Dipyridamole reduces platelet adhesion as well as inhibiting platelet release and aggregation. It inhibits platelet phosphodiesterase, causing a rise in intracellular cAMP and hence inhibition of platelet function. It also inhibits adenosine deaminase and this may facilitate its platelet-inhibitory action.

Dipyridamole is available in tablets (25 and 100 mg) and ampoules (5 mg/ml). It is rapidly and completely absorbed and subsequently found in high concentrations in the liver. The plasma half-life is 2–3 h and since its antiplatelet action is concentration-dependent it should be given in a dose of 100 mg four times daily. It is excreted mostly in the bile and there is a small amount of intestinal reabsorption.

Unwanted effects. These are GI disturbances, skin rashes, headache, and flushing. Administration of dipyridamole IV can cause hypotension.

Sulphinpyrazone was originally introduced as a uricosuric agent. It was subsequently shown to prolong platelet survival and reduce platelet turnover. It appears to act in a similar manner to aspirin in that it inhibits platelet cyclooxygenase and thus reduces the formation of thromboxane A_2, but differs from aspirin in not causing irreversible inhibition. Sulphinpyrazone is available in tablets (100 mg) and capsules (200 mg) and the recommended dose is 200 mg every 6 h. It is rapidly and completely absorbed and plasma levels of 20 μg/ml are observed after a single dose of 200 mg. The volume of distribution is about 6 ml/kg body wt and more than 90% of sulphinpyrazone is bound to plasma proteins. The plasma half-life is 2.5–3 h and it is metabolized in the liver to hydroxylated metabolites. It has recently been

suggested that a thioether metabolite has a much longer half-life and is a potent inhibitor of platelet aggregation, thus accounting for the observed inhibition of collagen-induced platelet aggregation when plasma concentrations of sulphinpyrazone are no longer detectable [86]. Excretion of both sulphinpyrazone and its metabolites occurs via the urine.

Unwanted effects. Sulphinpyrazone causes nausea, vomiting, and abdominal pain. It may exacerbate peptic ulcer and gout. Occasionally blood dyscrasias have been observed and it is recommended that blood cell counts are made at regular intervals if prolonged therapy is used.

References

1. Akera T (1977) Membrane adenosinetriphosphatase: A digitalis receptor? Science 198:569–574
2. Averill KH, Lamb LE (1959) Less commonly recognised action of atropine on cardiac rhythm. Am J Med Sci 237:304–307
3. Bachmann K, Shapiro R (1977) Protein binding of coumarin anticoagulants in disease states. Clin Pharmacokinet 2:110–126
4. Benet LZ (ed) (1976) The effect of disease states on drug pharmacokinetics. American Pharmaceutical Association, Washington
5. Benowitz NL, Meister W (1978) Clinical pharmacokinetics of lignocaine. Clin Pharmacokinet 3:177–201
6. Berkowitz C, McKeever L, Croke RP, Jacobs WR, Loeb HS, Gunner RM (1977) Comparative responses to dobutamine and nitroprusside in patients with chronic low-output cardiac failure. Circulation 56:918–924
7. Bigger JT (1979) Quinidine–digoxin interaction: What do we know about it? N Engl J Med 301:779–781
8. Bigger JT, Schmidt PH, Kutt H (1965) Relationship between the plasma level of diphenylhydantoin sodium and its cardiac antiarrhythmic effects. Circulation 38:363–374
9. Braunwald E, Bloodwell RD, Goldberg LI, Morrow AG (1961) Studies on digitalis. Observations in man on the effects of digitalis preparations on the contractility of the non-failing heart and on total vascular resistance. J Clin Invest 40:52–59
10. Broekhuysen J, Laruel R, Sion R (1969) Etude comparée du transit et du metabolisme de l'amiodarone chez diverses especes animales et chez l'homme. Arch Int Pharmacodyn 177:340–359
11. Brogden RM, Speight TM, Avery GS (1973) Streptokinase: A review of its clinical pharmacology, mechanism of action and theraputic uses. Drugs 5:357–445
12. Cambridge D, Davy MJ, Massingham R (1977) Prazosin. Selective antagonist of post-synaptic alpha adrenoceptors. Br J Pharmacol 59:514P–515P
13. Campbell NPS, Kelly SG, Adgey AAJ, Shanks RG (1978) The clinical pharmacology of mexiletine. Br J Clin Pharmacol 6:103–108
14. Carlsson E, Dahlof C-G, Hedberg A, Persson H, Tangstrand B (1977) Differentiation of cardiac chronotropic and inotropic effects of beta-adrenoceptor agonists. Naunyn Schmiedebergs Arch Pharmacol 300:101–105

15. Carmeliet E, Janssen PJ, Marsboom R, Van Neuten JM Xhonneux R (1978) Antiarrhythmic, electrophysiologic and haemodynamic effects of lorcainide. Arch Int Pharmacodyn 231:104–130

16. Carter JN, Eastman CJ, Kilham HA, Lazarus L (1975) Rational therapy for thyroid storm. Aust NZ J Med 5:458–461

17. Chafee RH, Settipane GA (1974) Aspirin intolerance. J Allergy Clin Immunol 53:193–204

18. Chamberlain DA, White RJ, Howard IR, Smith TW (1970) Plasma digoxin concentration in patients with atrial fibrillation. Br Med J iii:429–431

19. Chatterjee K, Parmley WW (1977) The role of vasodilator therapy in heart failure. Prog Cardiovasc Dis 19:301–325

20. Chatterjee K, Parmley WW, Massie B, Greenberg B, Werner J, Klausner S, Norman A (1976) Oral hydralazine therapy for chronic refractory heart failure. Circulation 54:879–883

21. Cohen MV, Kirk ES (1973) Differential response of large and small coronary arteries to nitroglycerin and angiotensin. Circ Res 33:445–453

22. Collier JG, Lorge RE, Robinson BF (1978) Comparison of effects of tolmesoxide (RX 71107), diazoxide, hydrallazine, prazosin, glyceryltrinitrate and sodium nitroprusside of forearm arteries and dorsal hand veins of man. Br J Clin Pharmacol 5:36–47

23. Collinsworth KA, Strong JM, Atkinson AJ, Winkle RA, Perlroth F, Harrison DC (1975) Pharmacokinetics and metabolism of lignocaine in patients with renal failure. Clin Pharmacol Ther 18:59–64

24. Conway J (1977) Anti-hypertensive effect of diuretics. In: Gross F (Ed) Anti-hypertensive agents. Springer, Berlin (Hdb Exp Pharm, vol 39, pp 477–494)

25. Crout JR, Brown BR (1969) Anaesthetic management of phaeochromocytoma: The value of phenoxybenzamine and methoxyflurane. Anaesthesiology 30:29–35

26. Danilo P (1979) Tocainide. Am Heart J 97:259–262

27. Davison C (1971) Salicylate metabolism in man. Ann NY Acad Sci 179:249–268

28. Deglin SM, Deglin JM, Wurtzbacher J, Litton M, Rolfe C, McIntire C (1980) Rapid serum lignocaine determination in the coronary care unit. JAMA 244:571–573

29. Dikshit K, Vyden JK, Forrester JS, Chatterjee K, Prakash R, Swan HJJ (1973) Renal and extra-renal haemodynamic effects of furosemide in congestive heart failure after acute myocardial infarction. N Engl J Med 288:1087–1090

30. Dollery CT, Follath F, Lewis GRJ (1975) Cardiovascular effects of dobutamine. Br J Clin Pharmacol 2:182P

31. Douer D, Weinberger A, Pinkhas J, Atsmon A (1978) Treatment of acute intermittent porphyria with large doses of propranalol. JAMA 240:766–768

32. Du Souich P, Erill S (1978) Metabolism of procainamide in patients with chronic heart failure, chronic respiratory failure and chronic renal failure. Eur J Clin Pharmacol 14:21–27

33. Estes JW (1980) Clinical pharmacokinetics of heparin. Clin Pharmacokinet 5:204–220

34. Fichman MP, Vorherr H, Kleeman CR, Telfer M (1971) Diuretic-induced hyponatraemia. Ann Intern Med 75:853–857

35. Fitchett DH, Nato JAM, Oakley CM, Goodwin JR (1978) Oral hydrallazine in management of congestive cardiomyopathy. Br Heart J 40:454–461

36. Fitzgerald JD, O'Donnell SR (1978) The antagonism by propranolol and alpha-methyl propranolol (ICI 77602) of vascular and cardiac responses to isoprenaline in anaesthetised dogs. Clin Exp Pharmacol Physiol 5:579–586

37. Fleckenstein A (1977) Specific pharmacology of calcium in myocardium, cardiac pacemakers and vascular smooth muscle. Annu Rev Pharmacol Toxicol 17:149–166

38. Folkow B, Neil E (1971) Circulation. Oxford University Press, London, pp 307–363

39. Frishman W, Davies R, Strom J, Elkyam U, Stampfer M, Ribner H, Weinstein J, Sonnenblick E (1979) Clinical pharmacology of the new beta-adrenergic blocking drugs. 5. Pindolol (LB46) therapy for supraventricular arrhythmia: A viable alternative to propranolol in patients with broncho spasm. Am Heart J 98:393–398

40. Gallus AS (1979) Anti-platelet drugs: Clinical pharmacology and theraputic use. Drugs 18:439–477

41. Gibson DG (1977) Pharmacodynamic properties of beta-adrenoceptor blocking drugs in man. In: Avery GS (ed) Cardiovascular drugs: vol 2, Beta-adrenoceptor blocking drugs. Addis Press Australasia, New York, pp 1–39

42. Gibson DG, Coltart DJ (1971) Haemodynamic effects of intravenous salbutamol in patients with mitral valve disease: Comparison with isoprenaline and atropine. Postgrad Med J 47 [Suppl]:40–46

43. Gibson T (1975) The kinetics of salicylate metabolism. Br J Clin Pharmacol 2:233–241

44. Goldberg LI (1972) Cardiovascular and renal actions of dopamine. Potential clinical applications. Pharmacol Rev 24:1–37

45. Goldberg LI, Tally RC (1971) Current therapy of shock. Adv Intern Med 17:363–372

46. Goldberg LI, Hsieh YY, Resnekov L (1977) Newer catecholamines for treatment of heart failure and shock. An update on dopamine and a first look at dobutamine. Prog Cardiovasc Dis 19:327–336

47. Golenhoffer K (1976) Theory of P and T systems for calcium activation in smooth muscle. In: Bulbring E, Suba MF (eds) Physiology of smooth muscle. Raven Press, New York, pp 111–126

48. Gunnar RN, Loeb HS, Pietras RJ, Tobin JR Jr (1967) Ineffectiveness of isoproterenol in shock due to acute myocardial infarction. JAMA 202:1124–1127

49. Hatton I, Murray RG, Boyes RN, Rae AP, Hillis WS (1980) Haemodynamic effects of prenalterol in patients with coronary heart disease. Br Heart J 43:134–137

50. Haywood R, Hamer J (1979) Digitalis. In: Hamer J (ed) Drugs for heart disease. Chapman & Hall, London, pp 244–317

51. Heel RC, Brogden RN, Speight TM, Avery GS (1978) Disopyramide: A review of its pharmacological properties and therapeutic uses in treating cardiac arrhythmias. Drugs 15:331–368

52. Hewick DS, McEwen J (1973) Plasma half-lives, plasma metabolites and anticoagulant efficacies of the enantiomers of warfarin in man. J Pharm Pharmacol 25:458–465

53. Hoffbrand BI, Jones G (eds) (1975) Bumetanide. Postgrad Med J 51 [Suppl 6]

54. Hoffman BF, Bigger JT Jr (1971) Anti-arrhythmic drugs. In: DiPalma JR (ed) Drill: Pharmacology in medicine. McGraw-Hill, New York, pp 824–852

55. Holloway GA, Fredrickson AL (1974) Dobutamine, a new beta-agonist. Anaesthesia 53:616–621

56. Hoobler SW, Kashima T (1977) Central nervous system actions of clonidine in hypertension. Mayo Clin Proc 52:395–402

57. Iisalo E (1977) Clinical pharmacokinetics of digoxin. Clin Pharmacokinet 2:1–16

58. James IN (1974) Diseases affecting drug response. Br J Hosp Med 12:823–834

59. Janchen E, Bechtold H, Kasper W, Kersting R, Just H,

Heykants J, Meinertz T (1979) Lorcainide: Saturable presystemic elimination. Clin Pharmacol Ther 26:187–195

60. Jaques LB (1973) Protamine: Antagonist to heparin. Can Med Assoc J 108:1291–1297

61. Jaques LB (1979) Heparins: Anionic polyelectrolyte drugs. Pharmacol Rev 31:99–167

62. Jewitt D Birkhead J, Mitchell A, Dollery CT (1974) Clinical cardiovascular pharmacology of dobutamine: A selective inotropic catecholamine. Lancet II:363–365

63. Johnsson G, Jordo L, Lundborg P, Ronn O, Wegelin-Fogelberg I, Wikstrand (1978) Haemodynamic and tolerance studies in man of a new orally active selective beta-1 adrenoceptor agonist H80/62. Eur J Clin Pharmacol 13:163–170

64. Joseph SD, Kelly B, Holt D, White J (1978) Mexiletine: Effective therapy in Wolff–Parkinson–White syndrome. Br Heart J 40:458P–459P

65. Karim A (1978) Spironolactone: disposition, metabolism, pharmacodynamics and bioavailability. Drug Metab Rev 8:151–188

66. Kates RE, Leier CB (1978) Dobutamine pharmacokinetics in severe heart failure. Clin Pharmacol Ther 24:537–541

67. Kawai C, Konishi T, Matsuyama E, Okazaki H (1977) Effects of calcium antagonists on the sinoatrial and atrioventricular nodes. J Mol Cell Cardiol 9 [Suppl]: 19

68. Kelly MR, Cutler RE, Forrey AW, Kimpel BM (1974) Pharmacokinetics of orally administered furosemide. Clin Pharmacol Ther 15:178–183

69. Kiddie MA, Kaye CM, Turner P, Shaw TRT (1974) The influence of urinary pH on elimination of mexiletine. Br J Clin Pharmacol 1:229–234

70. Koch-Weser J (1971) Pharmacokinetics of procainamide in man. Ann NY Acad Sci 179:370–382

71. Koch-Weser J, Sellers EM (1971) Drug inter-actions with coumarin anticoagulants. N Engl J Med 285:487–490, 547–551

72. Kopin IJ (1972) Metabolic degradation of catecholamines. The relative importance of different pathways under physiological conditions and after administration of drugs. In: Blaschko H, Muscholl E (eds) Catecholamines. Springer, Berlin (Hdb Exp Pharm, vol 33, pp 270–282)

73. Krikler DM, Spurrell RA (1974) Verapamil in the treatment of paroxysmal supraventricular tachycardia. Postgrad Med J 50:447–453

74. Kutt H (1971) Biochemical and genetic factors regulating dilantin metabolism in man. Ann NY Acad Sci 179:704–712

75. La Du DN, Mandel HG, Way EL (eds) (1971) Fundamentals of drug metabolism and disposition. Williams & Wilkins, Baltimore

76. Langer SZ (1974) Presynaptic regulation of catecholamine release. Biochem Pharmacol 23:1793–1796

77. Lant AF, Wilson GM (1972) Diuretics In: Black DAK (ed) Renal disease. Blackwell Scientific, Oxford, pp 655–671

78. Lavender S, McGill RJ (1974) Non-ketotic hyperosmolar coma and furosemide therapy. Diabetes 23: 247–248

79. LeLorier J, Grenon D, Latour Y, Caille G, Dumont G, Brosseau A, Solignac A (1977) Pharmacokinetics of lignocaine after prolonged intravenous infusions in uncomplicated myocardial infarction. Ann Intern Med 87:700–702

80. Levy G, Gibaldi M (1975) Pharmacokinetics. In: Gillett JR, Mitchell JR (eds) Concepts in biochemical pharmacology. Springer, Berlin (Hdb Exp Pharm, vol 28/3, pp 11–34)

81. Loeb HS, Bredakis J, Gunner RM (1977) Superiority of dobutamine over dopamine for augmentation of cardiac output in patients with chronic low output cardiac failure. Circulation 55:375–379

82. Lund-Johansen P (1974) Haemodynamic changes at rest and during exercise in long-term prazosin therapy of essential hypertension. In: Cotton C (ed) Prazosin—Evaluation of a new antihypertensive agent. Exerpta Medica, Amsterdam, pp 43–53

83. Mackin JF, Canary JJ, Pittman CS (1974) Thyroid storm and its management. N Engl J Med 291:1396–1398

84. Margulies EH, White AM, Sherry S (1980), Sulfinpyrazone: A review of its pharmacological properties and theraputic use. Drugs 20:179–197

85. McComish M, Robinson C, Kitson D, Jewitt DE (1977) Clinical electrophysiological effects of mexiletine. Postgrad Med J 53 [Suppl 1]:85–91

86. McHaffie DJ, Purcell H, Mitchell-Higgs D, Guz A (1977) Are digitalis glycosides of benefit to the patient in sinus rhythm with cardiac failure due to myocardial disease? QJ Med 184:587–598

87. Meffin PJ, Winkle RA, Blaschke TF, Fitzgerald JW, Harrison DC (1977) Response optimisation of drug dosage, antiarrhythmic studies with tocainide. Clin Pharmacol Ther 22:42–57

88. Menawat AS, Kochar DK, Panwar RB, Joshi CK (1979) Propranolol in acute intermittent porphyria. Postgrad Med J 55:546–547

89. Mendez R, Mendez C (1953) The action of cardiac glycosides on the refractory period of heart tissue J Pharmacol Exp Ther 107:24–31

90. Miller RR, Vismara LA, Williams DO, Amsterdam EA, Dearia AN, Mason DT (1977) The concept of afterload reduction therapy in congestive heart failure. Clinical applications and spectrum of peripheral vasodilator drugs. In: Mason DT (ed) Advances in heart disease. Grune & Stratton, New York, pp 25–44

91. Moe GK, Han J (1969) Digitalis and the autonomic nervous system. In: Fisch C, Surawicz B (eds) Digitalis. Grune & Stratton, New York, pp 110–117

92. Morgan TO (1973) Clinical use of potassium supplements and potassium-sparing diuretics. Drugs 6:222–229

93. Muller H, Ayres SM, Gregory JJ, Gianelli S, Grace J (1970) Haemodynamics coronary blood flow and myocardial metabolism in coronary shock. Response to L-norepinephrine and isoproterenol. J Clin Invest 49:1185–1889

94. Myer SL, Curry GC, Donsky M, Zwieg D, Parkey R, Willerson JD (1976) The influence of dobutamine on haemodynamics and coronary flow in patients with and without coronary artery disease. Am J Cardiol 38:103–109

95. Needleman P (1976) Organic nitrate metabolism. Ann Rev Pharmacol 17:81–102

96. Notari RE (1980) Biopharmaceutics and clinical pharmacokinetics: An introduction, 3rd edn. Marcel Dekker, New York, pp 46–106

97. Ochs HR Greenblatt DJ, Woo E (1980) Clinical pharmacokinetics of quinidine. Clin Pharmacokinet 5:150–168

98. Ogilvie RI (1978) Clinical pharmacokinetics of theophylline. Clin Pharmacokinet 3:257–272

99. Ogilvie RI, Fernandez PG Winsberg F (1977) Cardiovascular response to increasing theophylline plasma concentrations. Eur J Clin Pharmacol 12:409–414

100. O'Malley K, Stevenson IH Ward CA, Wood AJT, Crooks J (1977) Determinants of anticoagulant control in patients receiving warfarin. Br J Clin Pharmacol 4:309–318

101. Perkins CM (1978) Serious verapamil poisoning: Treat-

ment with intravenous calcium gluconate. Am J Cardiol 41:770–772

102. Perry HM (1973) Late toxicity to hydrallazine resembling systemic lupus erythematosis or rheumatoid arthritis. Am J Med 54:58–72

103. Peters G, Roch-Ramel F (1969) Diuretics. In: Herken H (ed) Handbook of experimental pharmacology, vol 24. Heffter & Heubner, Berlin, pp 257–385

104. Plumb VJ, James TN (1978) Clinical hazards of powerful diuretics furosemide and ethacrynic acid. Mod Concepts Cardiovasc Dis 47:91–94

105. Podrid PJ, Schoeneberger A, Lown B (1980) Congestive heart failure caused by oral disopyramide. N Engl J Med 302:614–617

106. Pritchard DA, Singh BN, Hurley PJ (1975) Effects of amiodarone on thyroid function in patients with ischaemic heart disease. Br Heart J 87:856–860

107. Reidenberg NM (1974) Kidney disease and drug metabolism. Med Clin North Am 58:1059–1068

108. Reiz S, Friedman A (1980) Haemodynamic and cardiometabolic effects of prenalterol in patients with Gramnegative septic shock. Acta Anaesthesiol Scand 24:5–10

109. Richards DA, Turner P (eds) (1976) Labetalol. Br J Clin Pharmacol 3:[Suppl 3]

110. Roden DM Reele SB, Higgins SB, Magal RF, Gammans RE, Oates JA, Woosley RE (1980) Total suppression of ventricular arrhythmia by encainide. N Engl J Med 302:877–882

111. Ronn O, Fellenius E, Graffner C, Johnsson G, Lundborg P, Svensson L (1980) Metabolic and haemodynamic effects and some pharmacokinetics of a new selective β-1 adrenoceptor agonist prenalterol in man. Eur J Clin Pharmacol 17:81–86

112. Roos JC, Paalman DCA, Duning AJ (1976) Electrophysiological effects of mexiletine in man. Br Heart J 38:1262–1269

113. Rosen MR, Wit AL, Hoffman BF (1975) Electrophysiology and pharmacology of cardiac arrhythmias. VI. Cardiac effects of verapamil. Am Heart J 89:665–673

114. Saady A, Zorda TA (1973) Tetanus: Principles of management and review of thirty-seven cases. Anaesth Intensive Care 1:226–231

115. Sasahara AA, Hyers TM Cole CM, Edever H, Murray JA, Wenger NK, Sherry S, Stengle JM (1973) The urokinase pulmonary embolism trial. A national cooperative study. XI. Morbidity and mortality. Circulation 47 [Suppl 2]:66

116. Schomeius M, Spiegelhalden B, Stieren B, Eichelbaum M (1976) Physiological disposition of verapamil in man. Cardiovas Res 10:605–609

117. Shand D, Turner P (1978) Clinical pharmacokinetics in recent advances in clinical pharmacology, no 1. Churchill Livingstone, London, pp 1–16

118. Shand DG (1976) Pharmacokinetics of propranalol: A review. Postgrad Med J 52 [Suppl 4]:22–29

119. Shand DG Wood AJJ (1978) Propranalol withdrawal syndrome, Why? Circulation 58:202–203

120. Shell WE, Sobell BE (1974) Protection of jeopardized ischaemic myocardium by reduction of ventricular afterload. N Engl J Med 291:481–483

121. Singh BN, Hauswirth O (1974) Comparative mechanisms of action of antiarrhythmic drugs. Am Heart J 87:367–374

122. Singh BN Jewitt DE Downey JM, Kirk ES, Sonnenblick EH (1976) Effects of a amiodarone and L8040, novel anti-anginal and antiarrhythmic drugs on cardiac and coronary haemodynamics and cardiac intracellular potentials. Clin Exp Pharmacol Physiol 3:427–442

123. Smith SE, Rawlins ND (1973) Variability in human drug response. Butterworths, London

124. Sonnenblick EH, Williams JR, Glick G, Mason DT, Braunwald E (1966) Studies on digitalis, XV. Effect of cardiacglycosides on myocardial force velocity relations in the non-failing human heart. Circulation 34:532–541

125. Stenflow J, Suttie JW (1977) Vitamin K-dependent formation of gamma carboxyglutamic acid. Annu Rev Biochem 46:157–172

126. Stetson JP, Reading GP (1977) Avoidance of vascular complications associated with the use of dopamine. J Can Anaesth Sox 24:727–728

127. Stone HL, Bishop VS, Dong E (1967) Ventricular function in cardiac denervated and cardiac sympathectomized conscious dogs. Circ Res 20:587–592

128. Suki UM, Eknoyan G, Martinez-Maldonado M (1975) Tubular sites and mechanisms of diuretic action. Ann Rev Pharmacol 13:91–106

129. Taggart AS, McDevitt DG (1980) Digitalis: its place in modern therapy. Drugs 20:398–404

130. Thorner NO (1975) Dopamine is an important neurotransmitter in the autonomic nervous system. Lancet I:662–664

131. Vaughan Williams EM (1974) Electro-physiological basis for a rational approach to antidysrhythmic drug therapy. In: Harper NJ, Simmonds AB (eds) Advances in drug research. Academic Press, London, pp 69–97

132. Von Euler US (1972) Synthesis, uptake and storage of catecholamines in adrenergic nerves. The effects of drugs. In: Blaschko H, Muscholl E (eds) Catecholamines. Springer, Berlin, pp 186–221

133. Waal-Manning HJ (1976) Experience with beta-adrenoceptor blockers in hypertension. Drugs 11 [Suppl 1]:164–171

134. Walker SR Evans ME, Richards AJ, Patterson JW (1972) The clinical pharmacology of oral and inhaled salbutamol. Clin Pharmacol Ther 13:861–867

135. Wheeler PJ, Puritz R, Ingram DP, Chamberlain DA, (1979) Aminodarone in the treatment of refractory supraventricular and ventricular arrhythmias. Postgrad Med J 55:1–9

136. Wilkinson CR, Shand DG (1975) The physiological approach to hepatic drug clearance. Clin Pharmacol Ther 18:377–390

137. Williams DO, Bonner WJ, Miller RR, Amsterdam EA, Mason DT (1977) Haemodynamic assessment of peripheral vasodilator therapy in congestive heart failure: Prolonged effectiveness of isosorbid dinitrate. Am J Cardial 39:84–89

138. Williams WJ (1978) Sequence of coagulation reactions. In: Williams WJ (ed) Haematology, 2nd edn. McGraw-Hill, New York, pp 108–132

139. Wright P (1975) Untoward effects associated with practalol administration: Oculomucocutaneous syndrome. Br Med J i:595–597

140. Yacoub NH, Bayland E (1973) Cardiovascular effects of intravenous salbutamol after open heart operation. Lancet I:1260–1262

141. Yin ET Wessler S, Stoll PJ (1971) Biological properties of the naturally occurring plasma inhibitor to activated factor X. J Biochem 246:3703–3711

Section C

Respiratory Disorders

Chapter 17

Acute Respiratory Failure

Michael A. Rie and Roger S. Wilson

Respiration is an integrated sequence of events that produces gas exchange—the uptake of O_2 and the elimination of CO_2 between an organism and its environment. 'Respiratory failure' defines a condition which makes this process less efficient.

The intensive care physician often cares for such patients and provides treatment without benefit of a full medical history and diagnosis. In this chapter we overview the physiologic approach to diagnosis and therapy of respiratory failure. No attempt will be made to deal with specific disease states, but rather we consider physiologic features common to the broad categories of respiratory failure. When appropriate, problems inherent in the diagnosis, prevention, and correction of gas exchange abnormalities in the critically ill patient are illustrated by use of selective clinical cases.

Physiologic classification of respiratory failure

Respiration is dependent on central and peripheral nervous system function, mechanical properties of the lungs and chest wall, the exchange of gases in the pulmonary parenchyma, and circulatory transport and distribution of O_2 and CO_2 to meet the metabolic needs of the body tissues. For a more complete discussion of normal respiratory physiology, the reader is referred to Chapters 4 and 5 and contemporary texts [21, 43, 77]. Understanding of the benefits and limitations of respiratory care requires the realization that ventilatory therapy is physiologically supportive and not etiologically therapeutic. As such, the goals of treatment are restoration or maintenance of lung structure and function during acute physiologic insults to the organism. Fundamental to the success of such therapy is the capacity of the host organism to regain functional autonomy through removal of the offending pathogenic factor. Our ability to maintain gas exchange without biologic cure of the chronic and acute 'respiratory failures' creates major medical, social, and ethical problems for society.

Although classic teachings have defined respiratory failure by abnormalities in the arterial blood gases beyond the predicted normal ranges, we have found it therapeutically helpful to categorize the 'respiratory failures' by the state of the resting (end-expiratory) communicating intrathoracic gas volume or functional residual capacity (FRC), as detailed in Table 17.1. Therapeutic interventions follow different goals and guidelines in the supernormal and subnormal lung volume states. Furthermore, patients with supernormal lung volume may develop respiratory failure due to those conditions in the subnormal FRC category requiring individual alterations in therapy (see Case II).

The intensive care physician is often required to deliver emergency life support to patients when gas exchange abnormalities are far advanced and the medical history is incomplete.

In such circumstances clinical and physiologic data will usually elucidate the broad category of respiratory pathology in question while empiric supportive care is instituted. Table 17.2 provides one such approach. With diffuse parenchymal injury, as in the adult respiratory distress syndrome (ARDS), etiology is multifactorial, especially with the passage of time

and the evolution of superimposed iatrogenic risks. Case I illustrates the therapeutic utility of the classification system.

Case I. A 22-year-old, 80-kg man was injured in an automobile accident sustaining multiple right sided rib fractures and a right pulmonary contusion evident on x-ray (see Fig. 17.1). He was taken to a local hospital and found to be unconscious without skull fracture. A left cerebral contusion was noted on computerized tomograms of brain. Fluid restriction, corticosteroids, nasotracheal intubation, and MV were begun. With 40% inspired O_2 arterial blood gases were $PaO_2 = 104$ mmHg (13.9 kPa), $PaCO_2 = 36$ mmHg (4.8 kPa), pH = 7.39. Over the next 48 h progressive hypoxemia developed with PaO_2 falling to 50 mmHg (6.7 kPa) with $F_{IO_2} = 1.0$ and 5 cmH_2O PEEP. Severe ARDS was suspected and transfer to a regional ICU requested. Examination at this time revealed a pharmacologically paralyzed (pancuronium) patient with small pupils. Vital signs were: temperature 37.5°C, blood pressure 130/70 mmHg, heart rate 150/min, respiration 14/min on a volume-cycled ventilator with tidal volume of 900 ml and peak inspiratory airway pressure of 40 cmH_2O with 5 cmH_2O PEEP. Platelet count was 150 000/mm³. Pulmonary artery catheterization revealed a pulmonary artery pressure of 40/15 mmHg (mean pressure 30 mmHg) and cardiac output of 6 litres/min. Mixed venous O_2 tension was 37 mmHg (4.9 kPa). The ICP was unknown. A chest x-ray (Fig. 17.2) was obtained, thiopentone sodium was administered [39], and chest physiotherapy was begun, yielding moderate mucoid secretions with white cells and no organ-

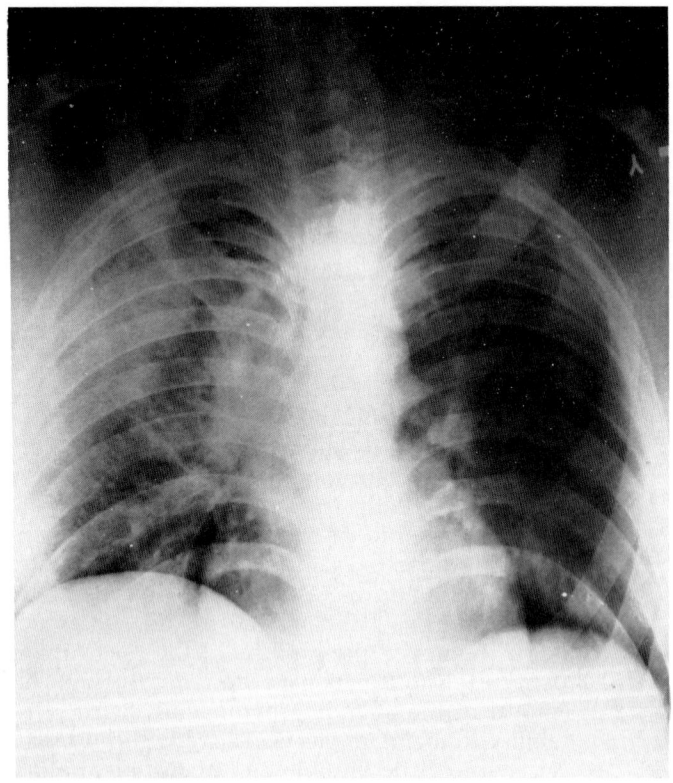

Fig. 17.1. Case I shortly (30 min) after trauma, showing multiple rib fractures and right-sided pulmonary contusion without hemopneumothorax.

Table 17.1. Classification of acute respiratory failure

A. SUPERNORMAL LUNG VOLUME STATES
    1. Acute exacerbation of chronic obstructive pulmonary disorders (COPD, cystic fibrosis)
    2. Status asthmaticus and other acute and chronic bronchoconstrictive states
B. NORMAL OR SUBNORMAL LUNG VOLUME STATES
    1. Acute decrease of FRC without major pulmonary vascular dysfunction
        a. Neuromuscular diseases (e.g., myasthenia gravis, polyneuritis, cervical spinal cord transection)
        b. Acute postoperative atelectasis and retention of secretions
        c. Localized pneumonitides
        d. Inadequate neural sensation and stimulation (brain injury, drug overdose, anesthesia, and neuromuscular relaxants)
    2. Acute decrease of FRC with major vascular dysfunction
        a. Pulmonary venous hypertension with normal vascular resistance
            I. LV failure
            II. Decreased LV compliance
            III. Fluid overload states
            IV. Pulmonary veno-occlusive diseases
        b. Pulmonary arterial hypertension with elevated vascular resistance
            I. Chronic restrictive lung disease with exacerbation (interstitial fibrosis, mitral stenosis, idiopathic pulmonary hypertension, etc.)
            II. Adult respiratory distress syndromes
            III. Neurogenic pulmonary edema

Table 17.2. Clinical diagnosis of respiratory failure

	Supernormal FRC (COPD)	Retention of secretions and lobar syndromes	ARDS	Hydrostatic pulmonary edema
D(A-a) O_2	Normal at $F_{I_{O_2}} = 1.0$ ↑ at $F_{I_{O_2}} = 0.21$	↑	↑↑	↑↑
V_D/V_T	↑↑	NORMAL	↑ (with progression)	↓
Ventilatory requirement	↑	NORMAL	Normal initially but ↑ with progression	↓
Effective dynamic compliance	Normal or ↑	NORMAL	↓↓	NORMAL
Response to chest physiotherapy	+	+++	NONE (early)	NONE (early)
Pulmonary vascular resistance	Normal or ↑ with cor pulmonale	NORMAL	↑	↓
Platelet count	NORMAL	NORMAL	Sequential ↓ often present over hours/days	NORMAL
Response to PEEP	Nil or hemodynamic deterioration	No Response	+	++
Chest radiographic opacities	Nil or patchy	Nil or patchy	Diffuse with slow clearing	Diffuse and rapidly resolving

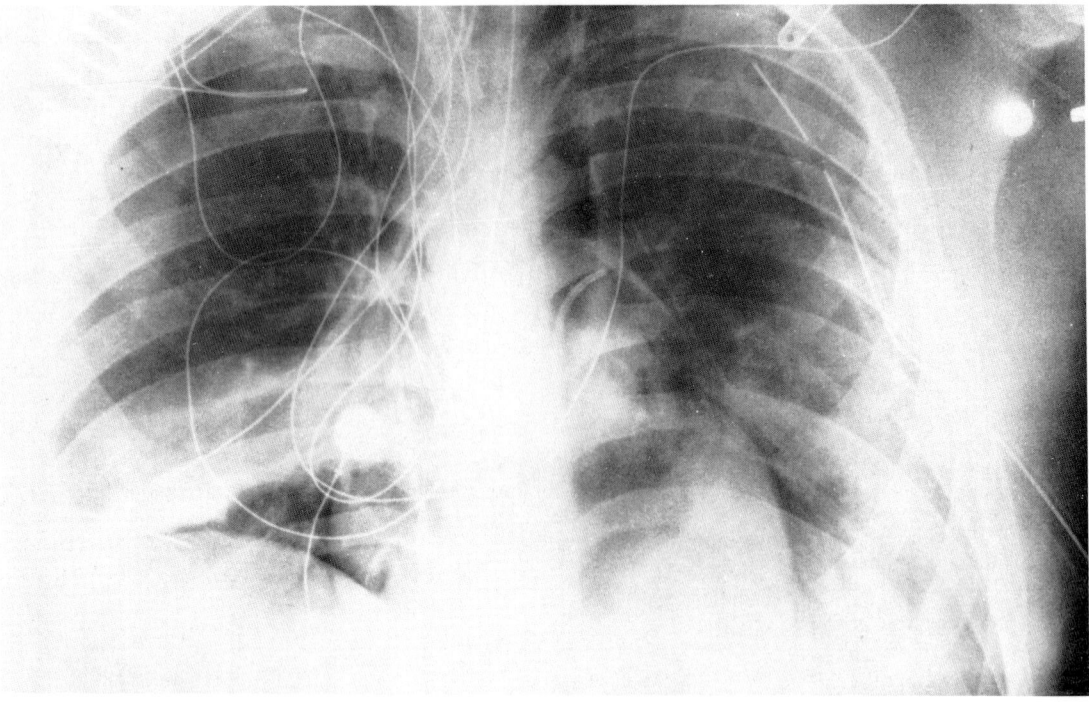

Fig. 17.2 Case I, 2 days after trauma, when hypoxemia first presented. Note regional opacity in right chest consistent with right middle lobe atelectasis.

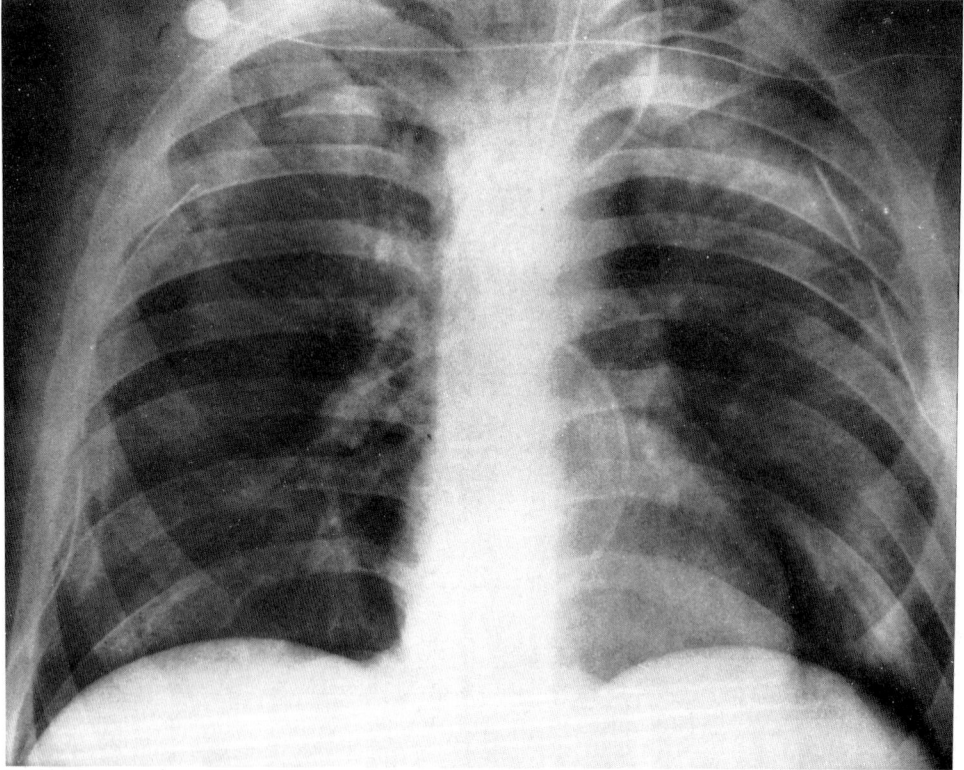

Fig. 17.3 Case I, 1 h after chest physiotherapy led to correction of severe shunting. Lung field is now clear.

isms on Gram stain. Within 6 h (Fig. 17.3) the chest radiograph was clear and PaO_2 had increased to 385 mmHg (51.3 kPa) with an F_{Io_2} of 1.0. F_{Io_2} was reduced to 0.4. Heart rate was 80/min with mean pulmonary artery pressure (PAP) of 20 mmHg and normal pulmonary vascular resistance (PVR). Three days later the patient remained comatose with a temperature of 40°C. Blood cultures revealed *Acinetobacter calcoaceticus*. *A. calcoaceticus* sinusitis was diagnosed. A tracheostomy was performed and antibiotics were administered. Oxygenation deteriorated over the next 12 h, with the thrombocyte count falling to 30 000/mm³ while PVR tripled and mean PAP rose to 30 mmHg. Serial x-rays over the next week showed progressive right middle and lower lobe consolidation progressing to necrosis with bronchopleural fistula and diffuse bilateral infiltration (Fig. 17.4)

Comments:

1) The initial hypoxemic episode was thought to be ARDS because of the prior lung contusion; yet the dramatic changes of PaO_2 and chest x-ray with physiotherapy clearly pointed to lobar shunting due to atelectasis.

2) The second hypoxemic episode originated from a nonpulmonary septic focus. The physiologic profile was consistent with ARDS prior to conventional confirmatory findings of lung infection (x-ray and sputum cultures).

3) Prolonged atelectasis in the right middle lobe, though successfully treated, left that area of lung susceptible to bacterial invasion and destruction many days later.

4) Head trauma and corticosteroid therapy imply potentially fatal risks of nasotracheal intubation not evident with oral intubation.

Hypercapnea

Arterial PCO_2 may be elevated acutely or chronically above the normal range [40 ± 4 mmHg (5.3 ± 0.5 kPa)]. Hypercapnea and respiratory acidosis are characteristic of chronic ventilatory failure and status asthmaticus. By contrast, progressive hypocapnea [$PaCO_2$ < 36 mmHg (4.8 kPa)] is the common physiologic response associated with mild asthma and low-FRC states (crushed chest, postoperative atelectasis, ARDS and hydrostatic pulmonary edema) in the absence of large airway obstruction or CNS depression. Progressive reduction of FRC results in tachypnea with decreased tidal volume thought to be secondary to neural activation of 'J' receptors within the lung. Hypoxemia ensues secondary to airways closure and impaired clearance of secretions. Hypoxemia further augments the minute ventilation [76], leading to a further decrease in $PaCO_2$. A return to normal values generally heralds impending pulmonary or cardiopulmonary arrest.

Hypoxemia

In chronic hypercapnic respiratory failure (CRF) hypoxemia is common during air breathing. PaO_2 may be elevated by a small increase of

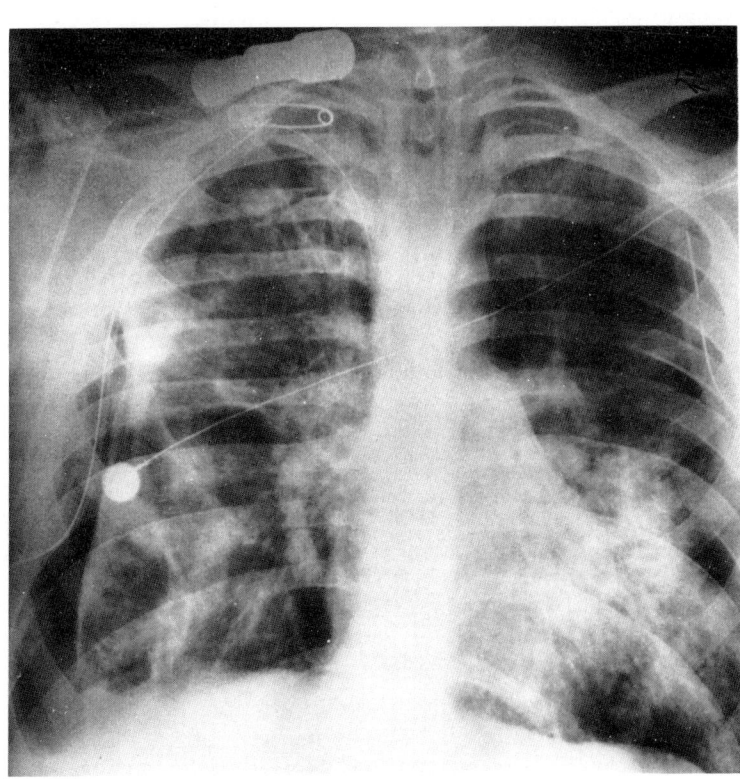

Fig. 17.4. Case I, 1 week after radiograph in Fig. 17.3. Pneumonitis in right middle and lower lobes has necrotized, producing empyema, bronchopleural fistula, and spread of infection to left lung. Emergency right middle and lower lobectomies successfully treated the bronchopleural fistula. Patient died 1 week later with progressive ARDS.

F_{Io_2} (≤ 0.4). In CRF the common causes of hypoxemia are: (1) ventilation–perfusion (VA/Q) inequalities due to regional differences in airways resistance and (2) decreased alveolar PO_2 at $F_{Io_2} = 0.21$ due to increased alveolar PCO_2. In acute respiratory failure (ARF) with decreased FRC, hypoxemia requires therapy directed at increasing the FRC.

While a rise or fall in PaO_2 at constant F_{Io_2} may signify improvement or deterioration in lung function, circulatory and metabolic determinants of the PaO_2 (see Table 17.3) may

Table 17.3. Determinants of the arterial O_2 tension

A. VENTILATORY
1. F_{Io_2}
2. $PaCO_2$ (via hemoglobin dissociation curve)
3. FRC

B. CIRCULATORY
1. Cardiac output (see Chaps. 5 and 18)
2. $C\bar{v}O_2$
3. Regional distribution of the pulmonary vascular resistance
4. Left atrial pressure (recruitment)

C. METABOLIC
1. O_2 consumption
2. pH (via hemoglobin dissociation curve)

obscure the interpretation of this value in critically ill patients. Therapeutic interventions that change circulatory and metabolic determinants of the PaO_2 may result in a striking increase in PaO_2 and decrease of F_{Io_2}. Measurement of $\dot{Q}_S/\dot{Q}_T$ may be necessary for more accurate appraisal of the intrapulmonary gas exchange and its response to ventilatory interventions. In summary: (1) PaO_2 may vary widely with no change in lung function; (2) sudden changes of PaO_2 are usually circulatory or metabolic in origin if gross ventilatory changes have been excluded (pneumothorax, bronchial intubation, change in F_{Io_2}, ventilator malfunction, etc.); and (3) elevated PaO_2 (even with low F_{Io_2}) may be present with progressive parenchymal lung disease when compliance is low and physiologic dead space is elevated.

Clinical diagnostic methods for ARF

It is well recognized that clinical symptoms are a late manifestation of CRF [54]. The majority of ARF syndromes also develop in a slow insidious fashion, with a time course of hours to days [47]. Progressive decrease of lung volume, abnormalities of gas exchange, and mortality can be reduced if physiologic derangements are detected and reversed early by simple prophylactic measures. It is now widely accepted that elective or 'prophylactic' ventilatory support is rational therapy in selected patients following anesthesia and surgery and other stresses (see Tables 17.4 and 17.5). In situations requiring prophylactic MV the rationale for support dictates that a period of stability exist and that the patient 'prove his respiratory apparatus is unlikely to fail' prior to the discontinuation of support. For example, a patient coming to surgery with fecal contamination of the peritoneum is at risk of developing sepsis with diffuse pulmonary injury in the immediate postoperative period despite surgical drainage and appropriate antibiotics. In such cases (even in young, previously healthy individuals) it is prudent to keep the endotracheal tube in place postoperatively for some hours, until progressive lung injury and hypoxemia are ruled in or out. A clear chest x-ray in the recovery room is no guarantee of healthy lungs and will change more slowly than intrapulmonary gas exchange and lung–thorax compliance.

Table 17.4. Therapeutic indications for MV

A. Resuscitation from total or impending cardiopulmonary collapse

B. Hypoventilation and apnea [definition: $PaCO_2 > 50$ mmHg (6.7 kPa) during spontaneous ventilation except in the case of COPD]
1. Anesthesia
2. Drug overdose
3. Need for muscle paralysis (status epilepticus, tetanus)
4. CNS dysfunction
5. Peripheral neuromuscular failure (polyneuritis, myasthenia gravis)

C. Hypoxemia [$PaO_2 < 70$ mmHg (9.3 kPa) on O_2 mask except in the case of COPD]
1. Adult respiratory distress syndrome
2. Hydrostatic pulmonary edema inadequately responsive to conservative therapy
3. Acute lobar syndromes (pulmonary embolism, lobar and bronchopneumonia, lobar or regional atelectasis)

D. Loss of mechanical integrity of the respiratory apparatus (crushed chest with flail, lacerated diaphragm, sternal instability post-sternotomy, etc.)

E. Discoordination syndrome

F. Nonspecific weakness—inability to meet demands of increased respiratory work

Table 17.5. Prophylactic indications for MV

A. Prolonged shock of any cause

B. Postoperatively
   1. With extreme obesity (especially in abdominal procedures)
   2. Where likelihood of massive sepsis is high (e.g., bowel content soilage of the peritoneal cavity)
   3. In the patient with COPD undergoing major abdominal surgery
   4. Debilitation and marked electrolyte imbalance
   5. With left lung contusion following thoracic aneurysm repair

C. Situations in which reduced O_2 consumption and work of breathing will remove additional stress on the cardiovascular system
   1. Following open-heart surgery—especially in the case of mitral stenosis with severe pulmonary hypertension
   2. Shivering during postoperative rewarming in the patient with coronary artery disease (sedate, ventilate, and curarize if necessary)

D. Acid aspiration syndrome

E. Cachexia—debilitation with major superimposed physiologic insult

Bedside assessment and the clinical decision to employ MV

Isolated measurements cannot adequately assess the respiratory reserve or likelihood of total respiratory failure in any given patient. For example, pneumococcal pneumonia would probably require ventilatory support in an obese octogenarian with congestive heart failure, but would present trivial physiologic stress to an asthenic 30-year-old patient. Therefore, it is necessary to use sequential measurements to evaluate patient performance trends; some test of ventilation, respiratory mechanics, and oxy-genation should be done in each patient. The frequency of determinations depends on the pace with which respiratory dysfunction is developing. Those parameters that we and others have found to be of value are summarized in Table 17.6.

Numerical parameters are broad guidelines that should be applied in the clinical context of the particular case; a vital capacity below 15 ml/kg body weight may be adequate if the patient is cooperative and can cough effectively, provided that hypoxemia is not progressive. Conservative management may on occasion produce surprising improvement and obviate the need for, and inherent iatrogenic risk of, invasive therapy. In other instances, especially where multiorgan failure exists, marginal numerical performance may be entirely insufficient to avoid respiratory assistance if the patient is incapable of defending his natural airway from aspiration of secretions or if sepsis and increased metabolic rate are present. A program of conservative care is unlikely to succeed with insufficient monitoring, nursing, and chest physiotherapy services. It is often poorly appreciated that vastly greater time and effort needs to be expended to care effectively for the nonintubated patient; preoccupation with invasive circulatory monitoring may result in a prolonged supine position and secondary atelectasis.

Airway management

A patent airway is the first priority of cardiopulmonary resuscitation and the first question to

Table 17.6. Sequential measurements to evaluate the efficiency of pulmonary mechanics, oxygenation and ventilation

	Normal range	Tracheal intubation and ventilation indicated
Mechanics		
Respiratory rate	12 to 20	>35
Vital capacity (ml/kg of body weight[a])	65 to 75	<15
FEV_{1S} (ml/kg of body weight[a])	50 to 60	<10
Inspiratory force (cmH$_2$O)	−75 to −100	<−25
Oxygenation		
$\dot{Q}_S/\dot{Q}_T$ (%)	5 to 9	>20
PaO_2 (mmHg)	75 to 100 (air)	<70 (on mask O_2)
Ventilation		
$PaCO_2$ (mmHg)	35 to 45	>55[b]
V_D/V_T	0.25 to 0.40	>0.60

[a]'Ideal' weight is used if weight appears grossly abnormal.
[b]Except in patients with chronic hypercapnia.

consider when assessing a patient with 'difficult breathing.'

Flaring of the alae nasae and intercostal muscle retraction may be due to a diffuse pulmonary disorder. However, when these are seen in conjunction with a 'tracheal tug' (suprasternal notch retraction of airway and soft tissue), obstruction of the upper airway should be suspected. Auscultation over the mouth or neck will confirm the diagnosis. The old dicta that 'noisy breathing = obstructed breathing' and that 'inspiratory stridor and wheezing occur in large airway obstruction (mouth down to subsegmental bronchi) while expiratory wheezing arises in the small airways' remain unchallenged. Failure to diagnose upper airway obstruction makes other resuscitative measures ineffective and is a common cause of unsuccessful resuscitation following cardiac arrest. Patients with upper airway obstruction show agitation, tachycardia, hypertension, tachypnea, and diaphoresis. Sedatives, narcotics, and neuromuscular relaxing drugs should not be administered until it is clear that mechanical airway obstruction is not present and that an artificial airway can be safely secured. A complete discussion of lesions causing upper airway obstruction is beyond the scope of this chapter [24, 36, 47]. The most common problems confronting the critical care physician are outlined in Table 17.7

Table 17.7. Common causes of upper airway obstruction in critical care units

A. ACUTE
  1. Trauma—oropharyngeal, maxillofacial and laryngotracheal
  2. Foreign body aspiration
  3. Inhalation injury with edema
  4. Complications of artificial airways
     a. Postextubation glottic edema and stenosis
     b. Tracheomalacia
     c. Tracheal stenosis
  5. Cervicomediastinal external tracheal compression due to traumatic, postsurgical, and invasive vascular catheterization hematomas
  6. CNS depression
     a. Postanesthetic depression
     b. Drug overdose
     c. Brain stem lesions and cranial nerve dysfunction
B. CHRONIC
  1. Sleep apnea syndromes
  2. Lesions of the pharynx, larynx, trachea, mediastinum, great vessels (e.g., tumors, cysts, strictures, palsies, tuberculosis, other chronic infections, sarcoidosis, aneurysms)
  3. Congenital lesions of pharynx, larynx and trachea

Management of common causes of large airway obstruction

Postanesthetic airway obstruction

This is common in the recovery room. The best treatment is to position the patient on his side so that the tongue will fall away from the posterior pharyngeal wall; if necessary an oropharyngeal or nasopharyngeal airway may be inserted. Excessive pharyngeal secretions should be ruled out by gently suctioning the pharynx. Humidified O_2 by face mask (not nasal cannula) should be given until consciousness is regained. If signs of airway obstruction persist, then postextubation edema of the vocal cords should be considered. Although uncommon in adults, it follows difficult traumatic intubation and is seen in patients undergoing laryngoscopy and bronchoscopy with pre-operative glottic inflammation or lesions. Post extubation, glottic edema may clinically present from the moment of extubation for up to 48 h. If this is detected early, a trial of conservative therapy is indicated and is usually successful. Such therapy might include the following:

1) Upright posture (sitting) when awake
2) Cool humidified mist inhalation
3) Racemic epinephrine 0.25-0.50 ml 1:200 solution in 3 ml saline, administered by nebulized face mask every 3–4 h
4) Dexamethasone inhaler every 4 h
5) Short course (less than 72 h) of pharmacologic doses of corticosteroid (e.g., dexamethasone 4 mg every 4–6 h)
6) Fluid restriction and diuretic drugs rarely produce immediate benefit.

External compression of the cervicomediastinal trachea

This complication is occasionally seen after head and neck surgery; it develops rapidly and is fatal if not promptly treated. Hematoma accumulation following thyroid surgery is usually detectable by inspection and palpation of the neck. This problem is usually solved by prompt opening of the wound to permit decompression of the hematoma. Hematoma formation following an anterior approach to the cervical spine may develop behind the trachea adjacent to the membranous wall, develop in a more insidious manner, be less obvious, and not be relieved by wound opening. Oral intubation is often difficult or impossible because of displacement of the larynx and emergency surgical re-exploration and cricothyrotomy or tracheostomy may be life-saving. A rapid tracheal cannulation method employing a large-bore intravenous polyethylene cannula and pediatric endotracheal tube adapter has been described [4] and has been successful in securing airway access and ventilation in our experience.

Tracheal injury secondary to prolonged intubation and tracheostomy

This has become a significant and well-recognized problem, since large numbers of patients are now surviving treatment for ARF. Tracheal stenosis may rarely occur following brief periods of intubation (24 h), though the majority of patients have had an artificial airway for longer intervals. Stomal lesions now occur far less frequently with proper tracheostomy care and swivel adapters. The lesion may be evident at extubation or remain undetected for months to years while being confused with asthma or chronic obstructive disease of the lower airways. Differentiation of tracheal stenosis or malacia from lower airways disease is made by the medical history, careful examination for narrowing of the tracheal air column on routine radiographs of the chest, lateral oblique and tomographic films of the cervicomediastinal trachea, auscultation of inspiratory wheezing over the mouth and neck, and rarely by the distinct 'amputation and flattening' of the expiratory and/or inspiratory flow volume loop at pulmonary function testing [34].

Specific treatment for the patient with tracheal stenosis requires sound judgment to avoid further iatrogenic complications. Superimposed upper respiratory infection may exacerbate the obstruction, with edema converting a stable chronic problem into an emergency situation. A program as outlined for vocal cord edema with addition of chest physiotherapy may often improve the situation. If an artificial airway is required, a small-bore rigid endotracheal tube should be cautiously placed after a period of denitrogenation with spontaneous ventilation and $F_{Io_2} = 1.0$. If time permits, anesthesia may be induced with an inhalation agent (usually halothane) in preparation for rigid bronchoscopy. This is of value to confirm the diagnosis, evacuate secretions and attempt via direct visualization to determine the extent of the lesion and dilate the obstructed area. In cases of airway emergency a rigid pediatric bronchoscope may be advanced under direct vision at the bedside. This procedure is hazardous but may be the only way to pass the

obstruction and establish an airway. Once an airway is established from above, a new tracheostomy may be electively created through the previous incision and the diseased portion of trachea, and not over other healthy cartilaginous tracheal rings. This will spare further loss of healthy trachea, which will simplify the ultimate resection and reconstruction that will be required [24, 25]. Such operations are elective and await the time when the patient has stable cardiopulmonary function and postoperative MV support, high F_{Io_2}, and airway protection are no longer required.

Artificial airways

The indications for endotracheal intubations are:

1) The establishment of a secure airway in patients with neurologic dysfunction who cannot be adequately treated by pharyngeal airway
2) Institution of positive pressure ventilation
3) Prevention of aspiration
4) Removal of tracheobronchial secretions by catheters or fiberoptic bronchoscopy.

The relative safety of moderately prolonged (less than 14 days) intubation by either the nasal or the oral route is well established [66]. Although many patients have been treated with intubation for periods of weeks to months, it remains unclear that long-term laryngeal lesions and dysfunction are not greater in this group. There are clearly certain types of patients in whom tracheostomy carries such a great risk of complication (e.g., airway and neck burns) as to make the risks of prolonged intubation preferable. However, with the widespread practice of very prolonged intubation (greater than 3 weeks) we perceive [25] an increasing number of patients referred from other hospitals with cuff stenosis of the trachea with associated laryngeal injuries. Surgical results for uncomplicated tracheal cuff stenosis are excellent [24, 25]. By contrast, long-term laryngeal dysfunction is observed with greater frequency following laryngeal injury, [41] with or without repair. We have therefore tended to take a cautious view in the debate of how long to keep the adult patient intubated. We maintain endotracheal tubes in situ for 7–14 days before converting to tracheostomy. However, if it is likely that prolonged airway access will be required, we will perform a tracheostomy within 7–14 days of intubation. It is noteworthy that prospective studies of the airway following intubation and tracheostomy [2, 66] show a very high incidence (>50%) of laryngeal lesions at the time of extubation and at later follow-up. Although stomal malacia and airway narrowing at that site are common compared with postintubation cases, surgical reconstruction is not commonly necessary. Stauffer's series used larged-bore tracheostomy tubes (8 and 9 mm internal diameter), which required larger surgical opening of the trachea than the 7 mm tube that is our largest standard tube for adult tracheostomy. The role of surgical technique in the performance of tracheostomy needs to be considered in light of Stauffer's series, for which a very high (36%) incidence of stomal hemorrhage was reported. It is surprising to note the diversity of surgical techniques used to perform tracheostomy and the paucity of surgical data relating operative techniques to late-outcome results at the stoma.

The choice between nasal and oral intubation is largely dependent on technical considerations summarized in Table 17.8. The introduction of large volume, highly compliant cuffs and improvements in the biocompatibility of materials from which endotracheal tubes are fabricated have increased the margin of safety for use of these devices. The large cuffs have considerable length (4–5 cm), which is approximately 50% of the average length of the adult human trachea from the cricoid cartilage to the carina. x-Rays demonstrate the proximal end of these cuffs in or just below the larynx. This location is neces-

sary (especially when the trachea is short) to maintain the appropriate position of the distal end of the tube. Laryngeal position is often detected by inability to seal the cuffed tube with the usual volume of air required. Sudden increases in cuff air volume should immediately raise this possibility, which is often the precursor of unintended extubation. Endotracheal or tracheostomy tube cuffs should be periodically deflated (after pharyngeal suction) and reinflated to the volume where audible air leakage disappears. The volume and pressure required to reach this point should be recorded daily. Progressive increases of cuff air requirement over days to weeks may signal the development of tracheomalacia. In this circumstance we have chosen to change from air-filled cuffs to foam-filled cuffs until positive pressure ventilation is no longer required [31]. In conclusion, routine meticulous care of the artificial airway is essential to minimize the short-term complications of airway obstruction and inadvertent extubation as well as the longer-term laryngotracheal injuries [16].

For patients who have had prolonged ventilatory support and are slowly regaining neurologic and cardiorespiratory function, it is common to progress to tracheostomy removal in a gradual fashion. When the patient can breathe spontaneously with the tracheostomy cuff deflated, a stomal stent is usually inserted. This historically included plugged fenestrated tracheostomy tubes [8] or stomal button prosth-

Table 17.8. Clinical considerations in the choice of nasal and oral intubation

Nasal intubation	Oral intubation
Advantages	
1. Easily held in place	1. Large bore and shorter length make suctioning easier
2. Better tolerated by patients	2. More easily inserted by inexperienced personnel
3. May be inserted blindly without laryngoscopy when neck motion or visualization is limited	
4. Allows surgical and nursing access to oral cavity if required	
Disadvantages	
1. Choanal size limits diameter of tube that can be inserted	1. Easily dislodged and may be occluded if precautions are not taken to prevent patient from biting the tube
2. Occasional difficulty in passing suction catheter	2. May be poorly tolerated by some patients
3. Relative contraindications:	
a. Risk of epistaxis in anticoagulated patient or patients with bleeding tendency	
b. Inability to drain paranasal sinuses. Longer-term use associated occasionally with septicemia secondary to sinusitis (especially immunocompromised host)	
c. Maxillary and facial fractures	
4. Gastric rupture (if patient has cuff airleak, pharyngeal obstruction, and no gastric drainage tube)	

esis [32]. Both of these involve the risk of airway obstruction. More recently the Olympic Tracheostomy Button (Olympic Medical Corporation, Seattle) has been employed with the prospect of increased safety, airway access, and versatility. Long et al. [37] recently reported a prospective series employing the Olympic Button in 168 mixed, medical, surgical, and neurologic cases at the Massachusetts General Hospital and have employed the button in out-patients for up to 1 year without major problems. The advantages of this device are (see Figs. 17.5 and 17.6) its ease of insertion, the

ability to custom-fit the appliance to a given patient, and the ease with which the plug may be removed and the IPPB adapter inserted if suctioning or resumption of positive pressure breathing are required. As noted by Long et al., the latter is particularly advantageous considering that 10% of patients required reinsertion of standard tracheostomy tubes because of clinical deterioration of the underlying cardiorespiratory pathology.

For patients with severe laryngotracheal stenosis or malacia at the time of decannulation, the Montgomery silastic silicone T-tube pros-

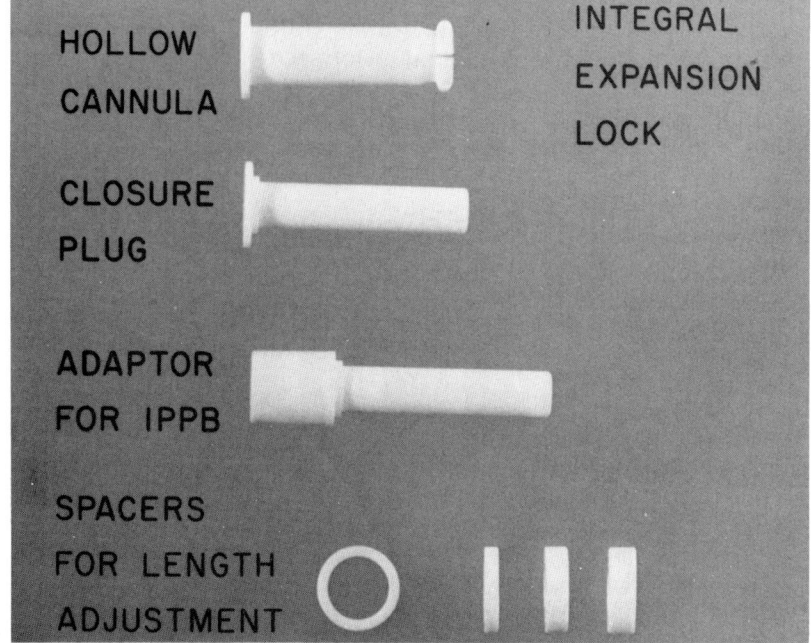

Fig. 17.5. Olympic Tracheostomy Button with associated appliances. Expansion lock in closed position.

HOLLOW CANNULA

CLOSURE PLUG

ADAPTOR FOR IPPB

SPACERS FOR LENGTH ADJUSTMENT

INTEGRAL EXPANSION LOCK

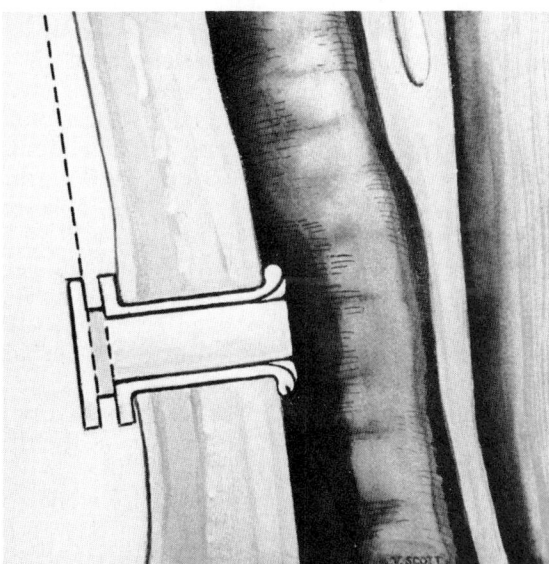

Fig. 17.6. Schematic view of the Olympic Tracheostomy Button in situ. When closure plug is in place the expansion lock holds tube securely in place at the anterior tracheal wall.

thesis [42] offers atraumatic stenting until the patient is ready for elective surgical repair of the airway. This tube is well tolerated for months to years in patients who are not surgically curable.

Postoperative pulmonary complications

Perhaps the greatest incidence of acute ventilatory failure in general hospitals is to be found in those patients recovering from anesthesia and surgery. It is well recognized that the classic postoperative pulmonary complications (PPC) (exacerbation of bronchitis, retention of secretions, atelectasis and progressive respiratory failure) occur with greatest frequency in patients with pre-existing pulmonary abnormalities [72]. Patients with normal pre-operative vital capacity and expiratory flow rates have a 3% incidence of PPC, while those with a diminished vital capacity have a 70% incidence [67, 68]. In addition, 95% of all PPC occur in patients with abnormal pre-operative vital capacity and expiratory flow rates. The therapeutic and financial implications of this are enormous, particularly when expensive technology and manpower are expended for post-operative preventive respiratory care in patients at low risk of PPC [49]. While there is general agreement on the indications for pre-operative pulmonary function testing, there are few systematic data on the potential benefit of conservative measures applied in prophylactic fashion to the nonintubated postoperative patient [49]. However, certain basic physiologic principles govern the diagnostic and therapeutic approach in this situation. The principal effects of anesthesia and surgery upon the respiratory system are (1) a decrease in the FRC and forced vital capacity (particularly following upper abdominal surgery); (2) a decreased lung-thorax compliance secondary to airways closure, ablation of sighing, and muscle splinting, with (3) a consequent decrease in PaO_2 at the ambient F_{IO_2}; and (4) reduced lung defenses (decreased cough, decreased macrophage function, and possibly bacterial colonization of the lower airways).

When these effects are superimposed upon pre-existent disease of the airways, the increased incidence of PPC requires therapeutic efforts addressed at increasing the frequency of sighing (deep breaths), clearing the airway of secretions by promotion of coughing and re-

storation of the upright posture (removing the weight of the abdominal contents from the diaphragm), and breathing exercises designed to improve function of the diaphragm and muscles required for lateral costal expansion. In considering the overall respiratory care needs of the surgical population, guidelines for pre-operative pulmonary function testing and treatment are proposed in Tables 17.9–17.13.

Surgery should be delayed and conservative therapy given to patients with cor pulmonale with polycythemia, bronchiectasis, and uncontrolled bronchitis and those with chronic pulmonary disease with superimposed upper respiratory infections or pneumonia. There is little benefit from pre-operative treatment in

Table 17.9. Indications for preoperative lung function tests (without and with bronchodilator)

A. Prior history of pulmonary disease
B. History of restrictive pulmonary factors
   1. Obesity (>20% above ideal weight)
   2. Kyphoscoliosis
   3. Neural or musculoskeletal disease affecting the trunk
C. Surgery that significantly induces pulmonary restriction
   1. Ventral herniorrhaphy
   2. All forms of intrathoracic and chest wall surgery
   3. All patients >50 years of age having upper abdominal surgery
D. Smokers and heavy ex-smokers (>20 pack years)
E. Recent (<30 days) history of upper respiratory infection
F. All patients >60 years of age

Table 17.10. Preoperative treatments to reduce postoperative complications[a]

1. Stop smoking (>1 week)
2. Expectorants and antibiotics as indicated by bronchitis and sputum cultures and sensitivities
3. Bronchodilators if indicated by pulmonary function tests (flow volume loop)
4. Aerosol humidification
5. Chest physiotherapy, postural drainage, and preoperative instruction in breathing and coughing exercises by a trained chest physiotherapist

[a]Therapy as recommended by Stein and Cassara [67] demonstrating a prospective two-thirds reduction in PPC. Note the absence of intermittent positive pressure breathing devices and other expensive machinery.

Table 17.11. Indications for pre-operative regional studies of lung ventilation and perfusion in patients undergoing pulmonary resection

1. $FEV_{1S} < 1.5$ liters (lobectomy)
2. $FEV_{1S} < 2.0$ liters (pneumonectomy)
3. $FEV_{1S} < 50\%$ of predicted
4. $MBC < 50\%$ of predicted

Table 17.12. Pre-operative pulmonary contraindications to elective lung resection

ABSOLUTE	RELATIVE
1. Predicted postoperative $FEV_{1S} < 800$ ml (if ideal weight > 50 kg)	1. $D_{L_{CO_{SB}}} < 50\%$
2. $PaCO_2 > 44$ mmHg (resting blood gas by indwelling cannula)	2. $PaO_2 < 50$ mmHg ($F_{I_{O_2}} = 0.21$)

Table 17.13. Pharmacologic preoperative preparation for patients with chronic lung disease

1. Complete therapy for airway infection and congestive heart failure
2. Replace potassium losses, especially for patients with chronic CO_2 retention receiving steroids and diuretics (consider NH_4CL therapy for those with normokalemia and base excess $> +5$ mmol/liter)
3. Schedule patients for surgery in late morning after pre-anesthesia chest physiotherapy if indicated (bronchiectasis, cystic fibrosis, lung abscess)
4. Bronchodilators to be given on call to surgery for those receiving them
5. For patients receiving aminophylline:
   a. Measure blood level 1 day preoperatively to assure therapeutic range
   b. Avoid bolus therapy intraoperatively for wheezing; maintenance IV drip to begin prior to anesthesia induction
6. Consider maintenance IV fluids beginning the night prior to surgery to avoid urgent intravascular volume expansion with induction of anesthesia and secondary circulatory preload depression from positive pressure breathing

hospital for those patients who have been intensively treated as out-patients and are functioning at their best basal performance, in those patients with pure emphysema without secretions and unresponsive to bronchodilators, and in those patients with severe chronic lung disease who become acutely immobilized (e.g., fractured hip with traction). In such situations it is usually necessary to plan for prophylactic postoperative ventilatory support. Skillfully managed this should require less than 1 week in the majority of cases. When major elective abdominal surgery is planned for a patient with severe obstructive lung disease and chronic hypercarbia, the prognosis of the lung disease is often as poor as the risk of no surgery [52] and this should be discussed with the patient. In our experience, many surgeons and their patients are not aware of these data.

Case II. A 68-year-old man is scheduled for a right thoracotomy for removal of a right upper lobe squamous carcinoma. Two years ago he underwent left upper lobectomy for excision of bullae and a squamous carcinoma. Spontaneous pneumothorax occurred 1 year prior to admission, and was treated by excision of right middle and lower lobe blebs. Postoperative artial fibrillation required digitalis therapy. He can climb one flight of stairs without difficulty and is ambulatory in the home. A productive morning cough is present. Physical examination reveals markedly diminished breath sounds in the left chest with poor motion of the left hemidiaphragm. The vital capacity is 3.50 liters and the FEV_{1S} is 2.0 liters without improvement from bronchodilators. Chest radiographs and pre-operative lung scans are depicted in Figs. 17.7–17.9. Pre-operative arterial blood gases while the patient is breathing room air are $PaO_2 = 61$ mmHg (8.1 kPa), $PaCO_2 = 45$ mmHg (6 kPa), and pH = 7.40

Anesthesia was performed with a left-sided Robertshaw double-lumen tube; there was 'difficulty' in seating the tube in the left main bronchus, and several attempts at placement were required. Surgery was uneventful and the patient was extubated at the end of the procedure. Atelectasis developed in the left lower lobe 24 h after surgery and failed to clear with chest physiotherapy. Two fiberoptic bronchoscopies evacuated copious purulent mucous from the left main bronchus but the bronchoscope could not enter the distal remaining lower lobe bronchus because of mucosal edema and marked constriction secondary to upward displacement of the bronchus. Persistent atelectasis of the left lower lobe resulted in fever (40°C), hypotension, and atrial fibrillation. Intubation and MV, chest physiotherapy, aerosol therapy, antibiotics, and digitalis were administered but failed to expand the left lower lobe. Two rigid bronchoscopies provided evacuation of secretions and dilatation of the left lower lobe bronchus with transient distal aeration. Persistent aeration of the left lower lobe was achieved with addition of 12 cmH_2O PEEP to the ventilatory pattern. Hypercapnea and recurrent atrial fibrillation developed with the appearance of pneumonia in the right lower lobe. Although spontaneous ventilation, normocarbia, and normal sinus rhythm returned with clearing of right lower lobe infiltrate, continuous positive airway pressure (CPAP) for several weeks was required because of repeated left lower lobe collapse when it was removed. The patient was successfully extubated 6 weeks after surgery when the left bronchial edema subsided. Two years later he is asymptomatic, with markedly diminished left-sided breath sounds.
Comments:
1) A minimally functional left lower lobe became a life-endangering source of infection when endobronchial intubation produced edema superimposed on an already diseased bronchus.
2) Detailed knowledge of regional lung function pre-operatively suggested that the patient could physiologically tolerate a right upper lobectomy and that he would be dependent on the functional integrity of his right lower lung in the immediate postoperative period. When that area was compromised, hypercarbic respiratory failure ensued.
3) Despite the evident bullous disease and obstructive physiology with supernormal lung volume, PEEP and subsequently CPAP therapy were of major therapeutic benefit in maintaining the patency of the large airways during prolonged weaning.
4) Torsion of lobar bronchi is not infrequently seen following lobectomy in patients with chronic obstructive lung disease.

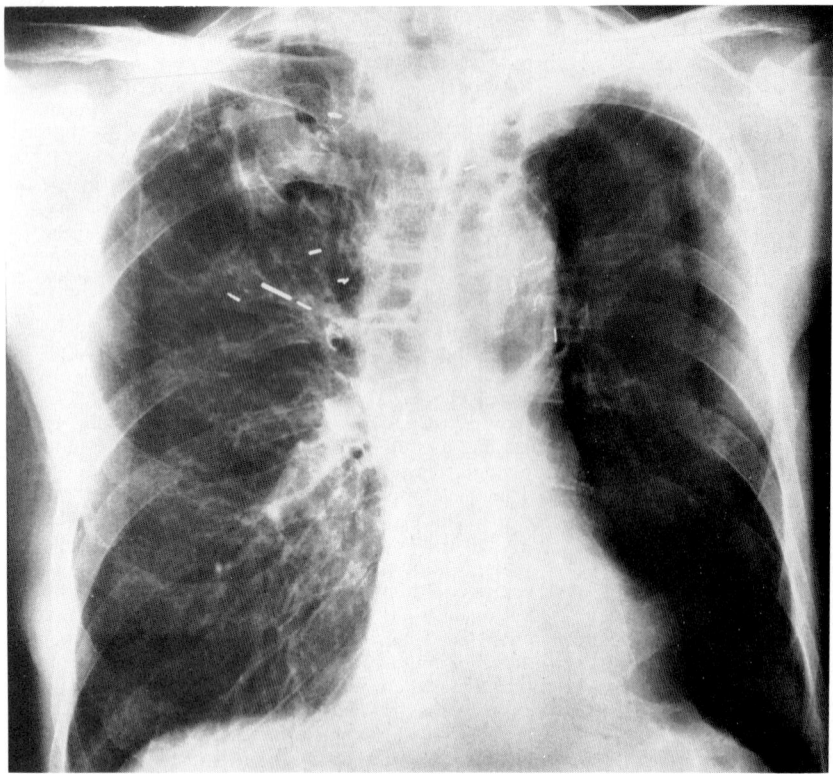

Fig. 17.7. Pre-operative chest x-ray in Case II. Note diminished vascular markings in the left chest with upward displacement of left bronchus.

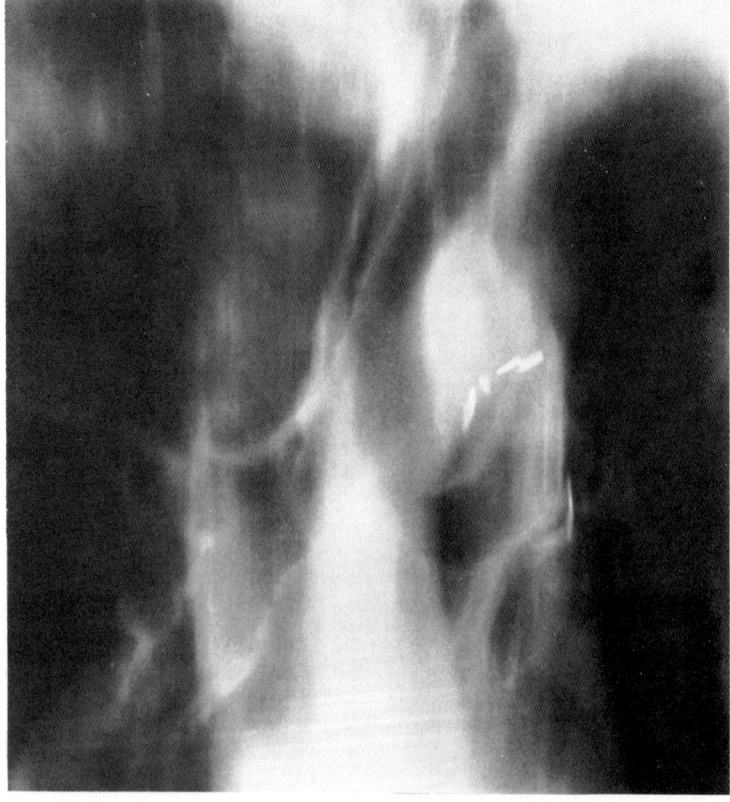

Fig. 17.8. Pre-operative tomogram of Case II. Note the area of left bronchostenosis below the surgical clips placed 2 years prior.

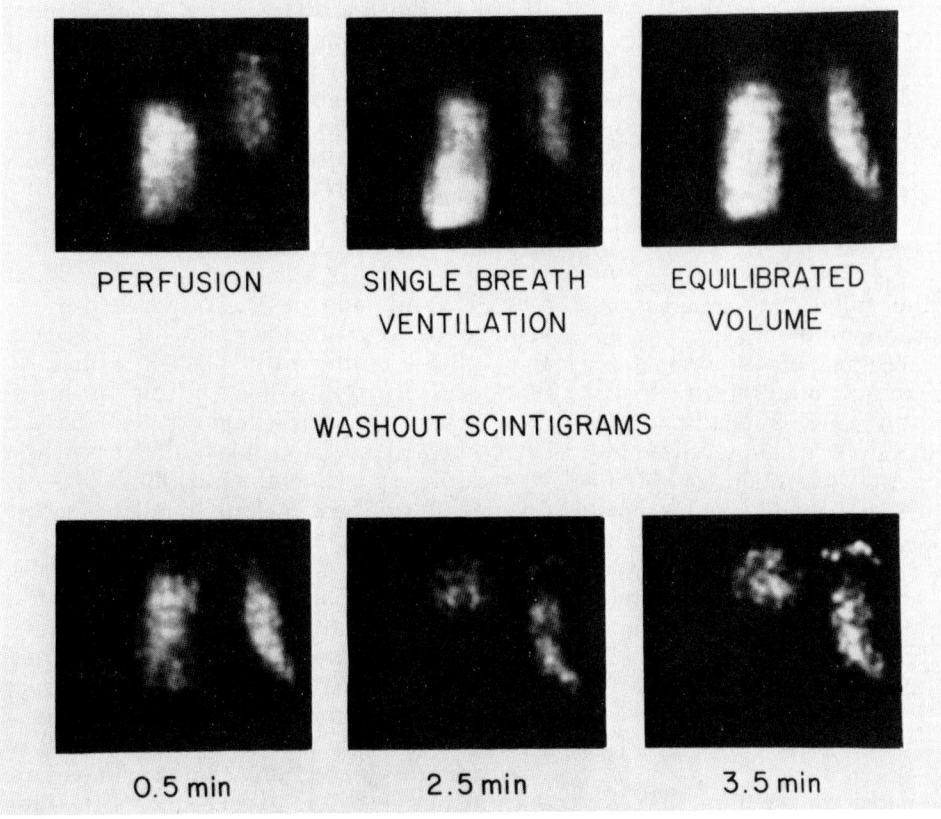

Fig. 17.9. Pre-operative N^{13} perfusion and ventilation scans obtained in Case II. 60% of perfusion goes to right lower lung field, while the right upper lung field is neither perfused or ventilated. Note marked decrease in left lung perfusion and the marked delay of left lower lung field washout at 3.5 min.

Mechanical aids to lung expansion in the nonintubated postoperative patient have been reviewed by Pontoppidan [49]. Maneuvers to promote maximal sustained inspiratory lung volume such as the incentive spirometer [6] and by face mask CPAP [1] are recent promising additions to clinical therapy, though full evaluation is not at hand. There is little or no evidence that IPPV by mask or mouthpiece provides as effective therapy as does the 'stir-up' regimen combined with chest physiotherapy or maximal inspiratory maneuvers.

Monitoring

Clinical laboratory

Bacteriology

Patients with suspected acute pulmonary infections commonly present at ICUs before the need for an artificial airway and ventilatory support exists. Traditional diagnostic approaches have involved the acquisition of spontaneous or induced expectorated sputum with examination by Gram staining and appropriate culture techniques. Many patients will demonstrate colonization of the respiratory tract with a variety of Gram-negative and Gram-positive organisms influenced by the duration of prior hospital stay, the severity of underlying illnesses and injuries, and extent of immunocompromise [28]. In recent years the fiberoptic bronchoscope has gained widespread popularity as a means of obtaining lower airway specimens for more specific regional bacteriologic diagnoses [55]. Recent studies [5] suggest that cultures obtained by pharyngeal passage of the bronchoscope are contaminated by upper and large airway organisms and may give misleading results for selection of antibiotic therapy. These authors [80] have described a double-sheathed brush catheter with distal polyethylene glycol plug that may be passed at the time of either rigid or fiberoptic bronchoscopy to obtain lobar or segmental samples uncontaminated by upper airways organisms. This approach appears rational and promising as preliminary experience in ICUs is gained. Aseptic technique and prompt processing of samples is essential. We have been impressed in evaluation of this technique by the realization that specific organisms and density of growth from equivocal regions in the chest radiograph may occasionally provide early and more reliable diagnostic material than tracheal or bronchoscopic aspirates.

Hematology

Patients with ARDS or diffuse and progressive acute pulmonary processes should be periodically screened for coagulation abnormalities with thrombocyte count, prothrombin time, partial thromboplastin time, and fibrinogen levels. Thrombocytopenia usually precedes evidence of coagulopathy (elevation of fibrin degradation products and rarely lung hemorrhage) in our experience. A progressive fall in thrombocyte count is an important correlate of severe ARDS, as discussed in Chapter 18, while hypoxemic respiratory failure with normal levels suggests other potentially reversible etiologies (Table 17.2).

Chemistry

Frequent measurements of sodium, potassium, chloride, and osmolality of blood and urine are helpful in patients receiving prolonged MV. Mechanically ventilated nonseptic patients are unable to excrete excess free water loads in association with inappropriate antidiuretic hormone (ADH) secretion and alterations in systemic hemodynamics [28]. Progressive hyponatremia is particularly common in patients receiving large volumes of hypertonic glucose for parenteral nutrition. Prolonged parenteral nutrition requires periodic measurements and adjustments of the serum phosphate as hypophasphatemia is an important cause of muscle weakness that may impair ventilator weaning. Patients with progressive ARDS and pulmonary hypertension commonly develop right-sided cardiac dysfunction with hepatomegaly, jaundice; peripheral edema, and diminishing urine output in the face of adequate systemic blood flow and pressure. Extensive blood sampling for a variety of chemical values is frequently over-used in this setting and should be carefully controlled to avoid additional blood transfusions.

Respiratory function

Monitoring of respiratory function is essential to (1) define the severity of injury; (2) assess change in functional status, i.e., improvement or worsening of injury; (3) assess effectiveness of therapy and (4) predict appropriateness of withdrawing (weaning) ventilatory support. As previously indicated (Table 17.6) assessment of function must consider oxygenation, ventilation, and mechanical properties.

Decreased efficiency of oxygenation, expressed as the alveolar to arterial O_2 tension difference (A-aDO_2), right-to-left shunt ($\dot{Q}_S/\dot{Q}_T$), and ratio of arterial O_2 tension to inspired O_2 concentration (PaO_2/$F_{I_{O_2}}$) are valuable indices in the early stages of disease. Efficiency of oxygenation is the principal measurement to assess potential benefit derived from therapeutic modalities such as chest physical therapy, diuresis, and PEEP. It is not uncommon for these measurements to reach a steady state or plateau following initial improvement during the first few hours or days, then only to become less 'sensitive' and less reliable indices of the overall condition of lung function as time progresses. Although numerous publications have stressed the importance of measuring intrapulmonary shunt fraction or (A-aDO_2) at $F_{I_{O_2}} = 1.0$, we no longer do this. The bases for discontinuing this technique are documented in several recent studies showing increase in $\dot{Q}_S/\dot{Q}_T$ with short-term administration of 100% O_2. Suter et al. [70] demonstrated a significant increase in $\dot{Q}_S/\dot{Q}_T$ when the $F_{I_{O_2}}$ was increased from maintenance levels of 0.3–0.6 to 1.0 for measurement of $\dot{Q}_S/\dot{Q}_T$. In addition to increase in $\dot{Q}_S/\dot{Q}_T$, Suter demonstrated a decrease in FRC (6% ± 6%) and total compliance (10% ± 6%). Since $\dot{Q}_S/\dot{Q}_T$ is increased with 100% O_2 breathing during MV and may produce functional loss of lung volume and compliance, presumably due to absorption atelectasis, there is no justification for performing this test. A measured increase in PaCO_2, although of primary importance in conditions such as CNS depression and failure of peripheral motor function, is uncommon in the early stages of parenchymal disease and thus is of limited value. Measurement of the efficiency of CO_2 elimination (V_D/V_T), although often not abnormal in the early stages, will reflect progression of disease when persistently elevated over several days. In our experience a V_D/V_T of 0.50 or greater frequently correlates with major $\dot{V}_A/\dot{Q}$ mismatch associated with obstructive pulmonary vascular hypertension, pulmonary fibrosis, and other forms of serious pulmonary injury. In general, sustained elevation of V_D/V_T in the absence of pre-existing chronic pulmonary disease is associated with a poor prognosis for recovery. A V_D/V_T greater than 0.55–0.60 is usually not compatible with the patient's ability to wean fully from MV.

The most difficult aspect of assessment, albeit the most important, is the area of mechanical function. The ability to sustain spontaneous respiration is a function of demand and the ability to meet the demand. With reference to the respiratory system, demand is the amount of 'work' the individual must perform to provide a given amount of ventilation. Work is expressed as a function of pressure required to produce a given volume change per unit time [78]. During spontaneous ventilation (and during MV) work must be done to overcome elastic, resistive, and inertial properties of the system. Since inertia is of minor importance, focus is directed at the elastic and resistive components. Elastic work is determined by the compliance characteristics of the lung and the chest wall and the magnitude of the tidal volume. Resistive work is determined by airways resistance and flow rate. Thus, factors which decrease chest wall or pulmonary compliance (volume change per unit pressure change) and increase airways resistance will increase the amount of work necessary for a given volume change. Inability to meet this increase in demand for work will result in respiratory failure.

Description of the detailed methods of measurements have been reviewed in several recent publications [22, 45, 46, 78]. Bedside measurements of mechanical function (Table 17.6) include respiratory rate, vital capacity, inspiratory force, and occasionally measurement of flow, i.e., FEV_{1s}. Although these measurements have proven to be reliable for guidelines concerning intubation, weaning, and extubation, they do not reflect overall pulmonary function during acute disease requiring MV.

Respiratory system compliance, easily measured in the intubated and ventilated patient, provides useful information to guide therapy and when measured serially is of prognostic significance [47, 78, 79]. Compliance (Δ volume/Δ pressure) is strictly defined by the methods and site of pressure measurement. Transrespiratory pressure (airway pressure relative to atmosphere) defines the characteristics of lung and chest wall. If pleural pressure (e.g., esophageal, chest tube, etc.) is used, transpulmonary (airway–pleural) pressure change during volume change will define compliance characteristics of the lung alone. A true measurement of elastic recoil requires that airway resistance (i.e., flow) be eliminated. Static compliance measured in the paralyzed patient with a 1-liter calibrated plexiglass syringe is optimal, since airway pressure reaches true equilibrium when downstream intrapulmonary gas distribution is complete following each 200–250 ml volume increase. Dynamic compliance (peak inspiratory pressure — atmosphere or EEP), measured when gas flow ceases in the upper airway, does not allow time for intrapulmonary gas distribution. Dynamic compliance includes a component of airways resistance and will yield a compliance figure lower than that obtained simultaneously with the static technique. Plateau or effective compliance, measured with end-inspiratory hold (approx. 0.5 s) or with an inspiratory time exceeding 2 s, approximates the static technique, is easy to perform, does not require muscle paralysis, and is suitable for clinical use.

Suter et al. used maximal total respiratory system compliance to define the best or optimal level of PEEP in patients with acute lung injury [69]. Serial measurement, i.e., on a daily basis, is perhaps the most sensitive index of change in overall respiratory system function. In our experience, progressive decrease in compliance, in the presence of a stable chest x-ray and unchanged oxygenation, is a prognostically unfavorable sign. The ultimate amount of information is provided when total mechanical function including airways resistance, elastic and flow-resistive inspiratory work, compliance and inspiratory, expiratory, and peak pressures are measured. This requires simultaneous flow and pressure measurements during several respiratory cycles and on-line analysis done with the aid of a digital computer [57, 78]. As described by Peters et al. [45, 46], measurements of airways resistance, resistive work, compliance, or elastic work will define the physiological abnormality, will give indication for use of specific therapy, e.g., bronchodilators, provide documentation of effect, and provide information for evaluation of the ability to wean.

Respiratory work is of prime importance in weaning. It is recognized [22] that total work per minute or breath may be altered by a change in the level of end-expiratory pressure. PEEP, well recognized for its effect on oxygenation, provides additional benefit in improving compliance probably secondary to airspace recruitment until the level of PEEP is reached at which overdistention becomes prominent. CPAP, if administered in appropriate settings, may not only improve oxygenation but may, through improvement in mechanical function, obviate the need for MV.

Radiology

Portable anteroposterior chest radiographs are an essential part of monitoring during respiratory failure. As in other thoracic radiology applications, comparison of sequential films and their response to therapy is essential, and this is facilitated by having all chest radiographs kept in the ICU. This permits prompt answers to clinical management issues. It is helpful in interpreting ICU chest x-rays to obtain the radiographs with consistent technique. We obtain full inspiration radiographs on the ventilator or with manual breathing bags to facilitate comparison. In our experience, daily review with a radiologist in the ICU increases diagnostic yield. As a rule, physiologic changes (deterioration or improvement) precede radiographic changes.

Cardiovascular

Patients with mechanical ventilatory failure only (e.g., myasthenia gravis) can usually be monitored by a well-alarmed ECG heart rate monitor, frequent (every 1–2 h) blood pressure measurements, and periodic measurements of urine output. An indwelling arterial cannula

may facilitate blood gas analysis but is not essential for blood pressure monitoring. Conscious ventilator-dependent patients can usually sense dyspnea due to inadequate ventilation, airway secretions, etc., before vital signs and blood gases show change; thus it is important for ICU staff to develop some means of communicating with the patient. The ECG monitor should be maintained in all ventilator-dependent patients, irrespective of their cardiovascular stability, because it is an additional monitor of respiratory inadequacy when ventilator alarms malfunction or are 'turned off' (Fig. 17.10).

Arterial pressure, central venous pressure, and urine output are usually sufficient to assess bronchopneumonia, postoperative pulmonary complications, and volemic status in acute MV failure. When ischemic heart disease, chronic LV failure or LV dysfunction are suspected, then balloon-tipped flow-directed pulmonary artery catheterization may be of value. There are no absolute indications or contra-indications for the use of this device. Insertion of pulmonary artery catheters in respiratory failure should be considered when (1) the contribution of left atrial hypertension to pulmonary edema is in

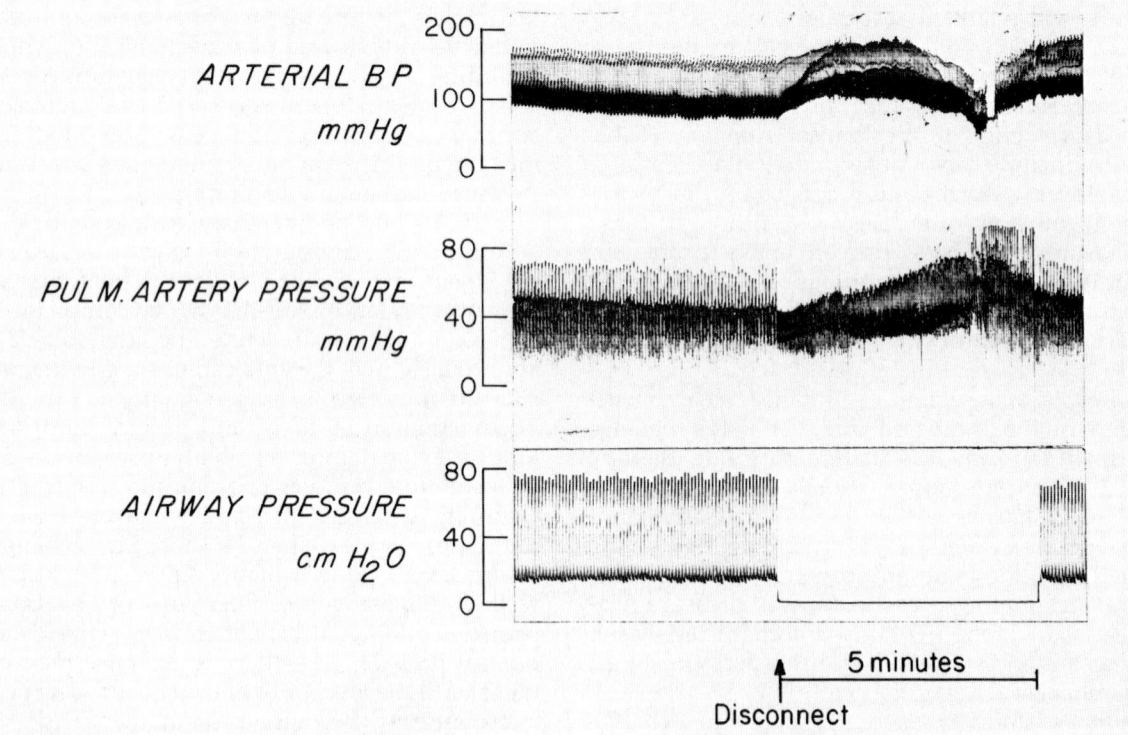

Fig. 17.10. Paper chart recording of airway disconnection from MV in a curarized 20-year-old man with ARDS. Ventilator alarms malfunctioned and the situation was diagnosed when ECG rate monitor detected bradycardia. Exact time interval was known from recorder speed. Note hypertension and tachycardia (*upper panel*) followed by hypotension and bradycardia. Pulmonary artery pressure increase is probably secondary to associated vasoconstriction and hypoxemia.

question; (2) large volume losses and requirements exist in a patient with acute parenchymal lung disease; (3) there is a prior history of acute right heart dysfunction in a patient with a new pulmonary process, and (4) assessment and management of ARDS is needed. The use of pulmonary artery catheter monitoring facilitates acquisition of cardiac output via thermodilution, mixed venous O_2 tension, or content, and permits computation of $\dot{Q}_S/\dot{Q}_T$ and pulmonary vascular resistance, both of which are sophisticated diagnostic parameters (Table 17.2) when the etiology of hypoxemia is in doubt or major unexplained changes in PaO_2 are occurring. Thermodilution technology is not adequate if an intracardiac shunt is suspected. In such situations dye dilution cardiac output (e.g. indocyanine green) is recommended [27], usually revealing the characteristic double-peaked curve of early recirculation.

The interpretation of cardiovascular variables during positive pressure breathing with acute or chronic lung injury [35, 48] is often confusing and difficult. The major effects of respiration on the cardiovascular system are summarized in Tables 17.14 and 17.15. Acute lung injury and pulmonary hypertension are other factors affecting the cardiovascular function and its monitoring (Chap. 18). For the patient with ARF the goal of cardiovascular monitoring is to define and maintain adequate systemic blood flow to meet metabolic demands without deleterious effects to the patient. In this regard we offer three simple principles of hemodynamic monitoring during ARF.

Principle I. Artifacts of pressure measurement are universally present in the critically ill patient. In classic cardiac catheterization the spontaneously breathing patient is asked to exhale and relax so as to bring the intrathoracic pleural pressure toward zero and thus permit transducers (which are calibrated to atmospheric pressure)

Table 17.14. Effects of negative (spontaneous) pressure breathing upon the cardiovascular system

A. Increased right heart preload [35, 48, 53]
   1. Increased RV end-diastolic volume (RVEDV)
   2. Increased RV end-diastolic transmural pressure (RVEDP)
   3. Increased RV stroke volume (RVSV) and pulmonary blood flow
B. Increased LV afterload [13, 53]
   1. Decreased LV stroke volume (LVSV)
   2. Decreased LV ejection fraction (LVEF)
   3. Unchanged or increased LV end-diastolic transmural pressure (LVEDP)
C. Increased pulmonary blood volume

Table 17.15. Effects of positive pressure breathing upon the cardiovascular system

A. Cardiac output, biventricular stroke volumes, and blood pressure usually decrease secondary to decreased venous return (but exceptions exist)
B. Right ventricular afterload rises if PVR rises secondary to pulmonary over-distention
   1. Postulated increase in RVEDV
   2. Postulated decrease in RVEF
C. Decreased LV volumes (systolic and diastolic) are associated with leftward displacement of the interventricular septum [29, 35, 48]
   1. Increased LVEF
D. Decreased transmural LVEDP (initially but may rise at higher levels of mean airway pressure)
   1. Postulated decrease in LV compliance secondary to ventricular interdependence [35]
   2. Postulated localized pleuro-pericardial pressure compression of left ventricle [15]
E. Increased venous pressure to organs outside the thorax and redistribution of systemic blood flow [28]

to record values approaching the transmural pressure. In the ICU this is rarely possible, as steady-state end-expiratory transmural filling pressures are not attainable without esophageal or pleural catheters. If the patient has compliant lungs, positive-pressure breathing will usually generate higher levels of pleural pressure and intrathoracic pressure readings than with the ventilatory system disconnected [50]. Thus, absolute transducer-generated values must be correlated with other indices of patient performance [blood pressure, cardiac output, $\dot{Q}_S/\dot{Q}_T$, urine output (without diuretic)] if the data are to have clinical value.

Principle II. All observers of cardiovascular monitors must record data by similar methods if the data are to detect patient performance. We recommend measurement of CVP, PAP, PCWP, and LAP at end-expiration on the ventilator, as this is the physiologic state that the patient must tolerate. Airway disconnection ('popoff') may show an incremental drop of filling pressures but is a 'preload surge' stress test and is therefore poorly representative of the circulatory state during MV. Furthermore, the correlated cardiac output measurement is also taken during MV, though the timing of indicator injection during the respiratory cycle is usually not standardized. Measurements of the vascular pressures should be taken from calibrated electronic screen or paper recorders. Digital displays on present-generation ICU monitors are notoriously inaccurate during respiratory activity because their preamplifiers summate data over several seconds at different points in the respiratory cycle.

Principle III. With positive pressure ventilation and ARF the conventional Frank–Starling relationship may be radically altered by a host of interrelated factors. Weber et al. [74] and Laver et al. [35] have summarized the concept of the 'cardiopulmonary unit.' Cardiac ventricles are separated by the interventricular septum and reside within a rigid pericardium which in turn is located in an enclosed thoracic cage with distensible lungs. For these reasons elevation of CVP or PCWP may not always be indicative of hypervolemia or ventricular failure or be attributable to transmitted pleural pressures. Elevated PCWP or LVEDP with normal cardiac output can occur because of the effects of MV (Table 17.15) or acute and chronic lung injury [48]. Interpretation of 'state of the art' monitoring must remain clouded because the clinician lacks bedside monitors of biventricular ejection fractions and volumes during systole and diastole. Even when such measurements are brought to the bedside [13, 29, 62] the interreactive relationship of variables confuses the analysis [15]. We believe that biventricular transmural end-diastolic pressures, volumes and ejection fractions may change dynamically throughout the respiratory cycle and that such measurements, when clinically available, will have to be acquired instantaneously at the same point in the respiratory cycle for reproducible sequential monitoring.

In summary, the critical care physician must correlate invasive cardiovascular monitoring data with other vital life functions (urine output, cardiac output, blood pressure) and accept the imprecision of artifactual data. Trend changes in response to therapeutic challenges provide the most useful information about benefit and dosage of treatment.

Sedatives and neuromuscular relaxants

Before narcotics or sedatives are given to depress respiratory efforts of the patient, the ventilatory pattern being provided must be checked for adequacy. Disconnect the ventilator and try to over-ride the patient's urge to inspire by using manual ventilation with a self-inflating bag and delivering frequent deep breaths; if this fails to bring the patient 'in phase,' then blood gases should be obtained and examination of the chest performed to rule out hypoxemia or other unforeseen problems. In similar fashion, blood pressure and hemodynamic performance should be thoroughly scrutinized as agitation and dyspnea are typical of the hypovolemic or shock patient. When these maneuvers are performed and $PaCO_2$ is slightly depressed (35–40 mmHg) most patients will be content and often fall asleep on the ventilator. Circumstances where this is not the case include (1) severe pain or discomfort that the patient is unable to communicate (e.g., distended urinary bladder); (2) severe ARDS, particularly where FRC has been reduced 50% or more below predicted normal; (3) florid systemic sepsis with or without shock, (4) irritation from orotracheal tubes in certain individuals (especially the young); (5) shivering and increased metabolic rate in hypothermic patient who are being rewarmed; (6) central neurologic dysfunction or injury, and (7) metabolic acidosis of whatever cause.

In the first five situations narcotics and sedatives are indicated. Small frequent doses of IV narcotic to titrate against the patient's needs are useful. Young, previously healthy individuals may require large doses of narcotic (e.g., morphine, 20–30 mg IV every 1–3 h). These drugs should be dispensed as needed in each case and frequent blood gas analysis should be done to prove that ventilation and oxygenation are adequate. We have found that painful or irritating procedures (wound dressings or bronchoscopies) can be carried out with the ultra-short-acting thiobarbiturates. The redistribution of the drug allows for rapid awakening and resumption of lower rate IMV or weaning. In preparation for bronchoscopy one may thus avoid topical anesthesia, which is bacteriostatic and will interfere with bacterial culture results.

An occasional patient in one of the first five situations mentioned above may require neuromuscular relaxants as well. In the case of neurologic dysfunction, sedatives and narcotics should be avoided and neuromuscular relaxants used to facilitate control of ventilation. For patients with elevated ICP, barbiturate therapy may be used to prevent further ICP elevation during periods of chest physiotherapy and airway suctioning [39]. The effects of nondepolarizing neuromuscular relaxant drugs may be electively reversed with cholinesterase-inhibiting drugs, permitting periodic assessment of neurologic function. The following practical pharmacologic facts about the nondepolarizing (long-acting) neuromuscular relaxants may be helpful to those physicians infrequently employing these drugs.

d-Tubocurarine (curare or DTC) is the oldest natural compound of this drug class in clinical use. It blocks acetylcholine receptors at postsynaptic neuromuscular junctional membranes to inhibit impulse transmission. It has no sedative or depressant effect on the CNS. This drug causes release of histamine and if it is given rapidly may induce transient hypotension. It has no effect on impulse formation and transmission in the heart, and it is ideal for patients with heart disease and tachyarrhythmias. It should be given slowly in 1–3 mg (1 ml = 3 mg) increments to an initial dose of approximately 0.3–0.5 mg/kg (60-kg adults usually require 25–30 mg). Thereafter, 6–9 mg every 30–60 min is usually required to maintain the desired neuromuscular relaxation. An alternative method for long-term use in the ICU is to administer a continuous infusion (e.g., 200 mg DTC in a total volume of 100 ml with 5% dextrose in water, and initially infuse 15–20 mg over 20 min, thereafter controlling the drip rate at 5–15 mg/h as necessary via a controlled infusion pump). This method obviates undesirable hypotensive effects from sudden bolus administration of drug and is more easily employed by nursing personnel in a well-staffed ICU. Dosages should be periodically reassessed by terminating the drip to assure that large stores of the drug are not accumulating in the patient. This drug is partly metabolized in the liver and excreted in the urine and bile. It may be used in patients with acute renal failure in reduced dosage.

Metocurine (formerly dimethyltubocurarine) is the trimethylated derivative of d-tubocurarine, being 1.8 times as potent as the parent compound but without ganglionic depression [58]. It has a weak histamine-releasing effect and is without effect on heart rate. These pharmacologic properties translate clinically into an agent that has minimal effects on cardiovascular function and this agent is undergoing increasing clinical use in anesthesia for patients with cardiac disease. The usual clinical dosage is 0.2–0.3 mg/kg initial IV dose in increments (12–18 mg for 60-kg adult). This may be supplemented with doses of 0.02–0.03 mg/kg at 40–60 min intervals as necessary. This high-molecular-weight compound is excreted almost entirely via the kidney and is very poorly dialyzable. Prolonged paralysis (days to weeks) may result in patients with serious renal dysfunction and it may not be recommended in renal failure.

Pancaronium bromide (Pavulon) is a synthetic drug of the same class as DTC and with approximately the same duration of action. It has no clinically significant ganglionic-blocking effect, and therefore hypotension is not a side-effect. It generally increases the intrinsic sinus rate of the heart due to blockade of cardiac muscarinic receptors and may produce supraventricular and nodal tachycardias in susceptible patients. It may aggravate or precipitate fatal ventricular arrhythmias in patients with unstable ischemic heart disease, and should be used with extreme caution in these patients. The usual initial dosage for neuromuscular blockade approximates 0.06–0.10 mg/kg given in IV increments (4–6 mg in a 60-kg adult). This may then be supplemented with 0.01–0.02 mg/kg (1–2 mg) every 40–60 min as necessary. The route of excretion is via the kidneys; it cannot be recommended for use in acute renal failure.

Practical application of ventilatory support systems and PEEP

Several objectives must be met when MV is applied. The first is to provide adequate gas exchange without harmful consequences to the respiratory or other organ systems; the second, to create an optimal condition for potential healing of the primary pulmonary injury; and the third, to initiate resumption of spontaneous ventilation as early as possible in the course of recovery.

The optimal approach to ventilatory management of acute pulmonary injury and respiratory failure is still in dispute. Patients vary so widely in pathophysiologic and clinical manifestations that individualized management is necessary. Numerous studies have demonstrated that the most efficient respiratory pattern during MV is one utilizing a large (12–15 ml/kg) tidal volume and a slow (10–12 breaths/min) respiratory rate for adequate CO_2 elimination. Events that influence the inspiratory pressure wave form, such as slow flow, accelerating or decelerating flow patterns, and inspiratory hold, have been shown to be of no clinical importance in improving the efficiency of gas exchange. The manipulation of the expiratory phase, namely use of PEEP, is of major importance. Regional reduction in lung volume with secondary airways closure, atelectasis, $\dot{V}_A/\dot{Q}$ inequality, and increased shunting are the most common pulmonary complications in hospitalized patients with acute lung injury. Restoration of functional residual capacity toward normal values is achieved with PEEP or CPAP. Therapy is usually directed toward improving arterial oxygenation, since the measurement of intrathoracic gas volume and/or demonstration of airways closure are not easily performed. PEEP influences the distribution of both ventilation and pulmonary blood flow and most probably has other effects on such factors as the quantity and distribution of extravascular lung water, pulmonary and systemic lymphatic drainage, reduction of RV preload, and large airways stabilization (see Case II). In most patients there is a direct relationship between increase in arterial oxygenation and increase in FRC as PEEP increases. The improvement in FRC is directly related to the level of PEEP and total respiratory system compliance. Although there is a linear increase in arterial PO_2 with an increase in FRC, increasing levels of PEEP are associated with other, less favorable changes,, including increases in mean intrathoracic pressure and pulmonary vascular resistance, potential for increased afterload to the right ventricle with RV dysfunction, and the risk of pulmonary barotrauma. Since the use of PEEP must balance both benefits and complications of therapy, there is no agreement on what level of PEEP is optimal and what criteria are to be used in any given clinical setting.

Suter et al. have proposed that the optimal or 'best PEEP' is that level of PEEP associated with maximal O_2 transport (the product of cardiac output and arterial O_2 content) [69]. In a study of 15 patients with acute respiratory failure, the best PEEP coincided with maximal total respiratory system compliance as measured by the ratio of delivered tidal volume to plateau inspiratory minus end-expiratory pressure. The 'best PEEP' levels varied widely among patients, ranging from zero to 15 cmH_2O. Patients who had abnormally low FRC at zero PEEP required higher levels of PEEP to reach this optimal point than did patients with initially normal or high levels of FRC. Improvement in arterial O_2 tension was related in a linear fashion to increase in PEEP as previously discussed. One practical difficulty in the clinical application of the 'best PEEP' concept is that the magnitude of cardiac output decrease (the limiting factor in O_2 transport) is dependent on the pre-existing cardiovascular state (preload, contractility, afterload) and the ability to restore the O_2 transport with volemic replacement or inotropic support. It is clear that while compliance will reflect the optimal PEEP level at any given 'state of circulation,' one can modify the circula-

tory conditions to increase O_2 transport at higher levels of PEEP where total compliance is beyond its maximum and falling.

Although Suter et al. used a large (12 ml/kg) tidal volume in the above studies, they have recently demonstrated the feasibility of reducing the size of the tidal volume, reducing peak and mean airway pressure, as a level of end-expiratory pressure is increased [71]. In a series of 12 patients requiring therapy with MV for acute respiratory failure, they were able to show that when a small tidal volume (i.e., 5 ml/kg) was used compliance was initially low and at the upper limit of PEEP (15 cmH_2O) had not improved to the levels reached when larger tidal volumes (7, 10, 12, 15, 20 ml/kg) were used at incremental levels of PEEP. As tidal volume was increased and PEEP applied in incremental steps, peak compliance was reached earlier at the largest tidal volumes (i.e., at lower levels of PEEP) than with lower tidal volume. Thus, varying tidal volume altered the position of the tidal ventilation on the pressure volume curve, resulting in an increase in compliance both with increasing tidal volume and with PEEP up to a point. As in their previous study, when overdistention becomes a critical factor then compliance will decrease. Since FRC is the primary determinant of improvement in arterial oxygenation, one can utilize these findings in a clinical setting by increasing PEEP and reducing the undesirable effects of higher levels of PEEP by reducing tidal volume, thus reducing both mean and peak airway pressures.

Thus, when MV is applied together with PEEP, one must consider (1) the efficiency of arterial oxygenation; (2) the prior state of the systemic and pulmonary circulation; (3) the initial level of PEEP and tidal volume; and (4) the effect of the ventilatory pattern upon compliance in mediating increases in PaO_2 with incremental increases in PEEP.

Weaning from ventilatory support

There are several available techniques to wean patients from MV. The 'conventional' technique employs periodic disconnection from the ventilator with use of a T-piece or CPAP for increasing intervals as tolerated by the patient [19]. The use of intermittent mandatory ventilation (IMV) with or without CPAP is now the most commonly employed technique [17, 20]. Weaning is accomplished with a gradual decrease in the ventilator frequency to rates as low as one or fewer breaths/min. High frequency ventilation (HFV) has been considered as an alternative under special physiologic conditions [14]. Regardless of the technique employed, certain criteria must be met before successful weaning can be considered possible [48, 56]. These include a stable clinical condition, adequate circulation with a cardiac index of greater than 2 liters per minute/m^2, the absence of sepsis, and a normal metabolic state. Given these conditions, the predictability for successful weaning is evaluated by assessing mechanical function of the respiratory system and gas exchange. Work of breathing affords the most useful information, although technical difficulties of measurement limit its clinical utility. Mechanical function may be assessed by vital capacity, inspiratory force, and (when IMV weaning is employed) the spontaneous respiratory rate. The latter should not exceed 30 breaths/min as this commonly results in fatigue, CO$_2$ retention, and respiratory acidosis. Rates greater than 30 breaths/min indicate a need to reduce weaning time (or frequency) with conventional techniques or increase the mandatory frequency with IMV. Arterial P$_{CO_2}$ in itself is difficult to interpret as it is influenced by previous metabolic and respiratory status. Hence pH appears to be a more reliable index of ventilatory adequacy. Several authors have cited the ability to maintain pHa > 7.35 during spontaneous breathing (either conventional or IMV weaning) as the desirable level. The failure to wean from MV presents a difficult and serious clinical problem having no simple solution. Inability to wean or 'weaning failures' can be traced to difficulties associated with the patient, the ventilator system, or the airway.

Patient factors

When considering the patient-related problems there are five factors that can cause inadequate spontaneous ventilation. These include (1) intrinsic pulmonary and airways disease, (2) deranged chest wall mechanics, (3) low cardiac output, (4) sepsis, and (5) hypermetabolic states. Intrinsic pulmonary disease can produce weaning difficulties either by way of decreased recruitable airspace or by an increase in airways resistance. In the case of decreased recruitable airspace, the common causes are extensive atelectasis, consolidation, edema, and occasionally fibrosis. The manifestations of these conditions are a decreased FRC at low or zero PEEP and a decreased compliance which is not improved with PEEP. Application of PEEP results in a marked increase in the work of breathing, associated with an elevated V$_D$/V$_T$. Therapy under such circumstances is directed toward continued MV or IMV support with levels of PEEP sufficient to produce optimal gas exchange and mechanical function and treatment of the primary lung pathology. This includes attention to fluid balance, identification of infectious pathogens, and intensified chest physical therapy. Increase in airways resistance secondary to pre-existing chronic and/or reversible airways disease manifests itself by wheezing, and often by an increase in FRC and an increase in V$_D$/V$_T$. These changes will result in increased resistive work of breathing, tachypnea, and ultimately CO$_2$ retention. Successful therapy must include continued use of low-rate IMV or standard MV and PEEP and a diligent search to determine a reversible cause of increased airways resistance. Such patients may only wean if hypercarbia [PaCO$_2$ = 55–60 mmHg (8 kPa)] is accepted during the convalescent stage.

A second factor to consider is derangement of chest wall function. Specific entities include direct chest wall trauma, gross abdominal distention with or without obesity, CNS disease, muscle weakness, phrenic palsy, and respiratory muscle discoordination. The physiologic basis for weaning difficulties when one or more of these problems exists relates to the need for a coordinated and well-integrated function between the chest wall (rib cage) and the diaphragm during spontaneous breathing. A detailed description of the complex interrelationship between chest wall, diaphragm, and abdominal muscles is not here possible and the reader is referred to appropriate references [23, 38, 40, 59]. Abnormal chest wall function is characterized by a discoordinate or rocking respiratory motion where chest wall and abdomen appear to be dysrhythmic during spontaneous breathing, especially during a vital capacity maneuver. This results in less gas movement than would be expected from the measurement of inspiratory force. These patients appear to be working much harder than would be thought necessary from the clinical setting, moving less air, and being unable to meet the demand for respiratory work. Therapy of discoordinate breathing is continued use of ventilatory and nutritional support. Specific diagnostic tests such as fluoroscopy of the diaphragm, strain gauge or magnetometer studies to demonstrate chest wall and abdominal activity, and a search for central or periheral neuromuscular pathologies are helpful in detecting the cause of weaning difficulties but do not facilitate specific therapy.

Abnormal cardiac function also limits weaning. It is well recognized that the intravascular blood volume requires expansion during positive pressure ventilation to maintain appropriate systemic blood flow. Where intrinsic limitation of cardiac function exists, as in ischemic or valvular heart disease, relative fluid overload may be produced when mean intrathoracic and airway pressures are abruptly reduced during the weaning process, leading to congestive hear failure [7]. A high index of suspicion confirmed by appropriate circulatory monitoring is essential, and diuresis and/or inotropic support may be necessary to facilitate weaning.

Hypermetabolic states limit the ability to wean. Common causes of hypermetabolism include sepsis, burns, and fever. Hypermetabolism is manifested physiologically by increases in O_2 consumption, CO_2 production, and minute ventilation requirement which may exceed the patient's capacity to meet the demand. Another recently described cause of hypermetabolism in nonseptic patients is an elevated respiratory quotient and CO_2 production secondary to parenteral nutrition with large glucose loads [3].

Here therapy is reduction of glucose intake and addition of protein and fat to the diet (see 'Fluid balance').

Ventilatory system factors

Ventilator design and PEEP devices are a major source of weaning problems. As shown in Fig. 17.11, there are three types of IMV–PEEP ventilatory systems for weaning. An increase in respiratory work may be produced by the ventilator system due to additional work required to activate valves and/or inability to supply peak flow upon patient demand. This produces an increase in the work of breathing with progressive tachypnea, dyspnea, and wide fluctuations in airway pressure during the respiratory cycle. This in turn leads to an increased loading of the respiratory system and a potential for decrease in compliance; activation of stretch receptors may in turn lead to further tachypnea and ultimately a subsequent increase in the work of breathing. Systems that incorporate a demand valve may be inadequately responsive in terms of time cycling and/or demand flow when spontaneous ventilatory rates reach 30 breaths/ min or greater. Meticulous attention must be paid to the appropriate settings of flow and

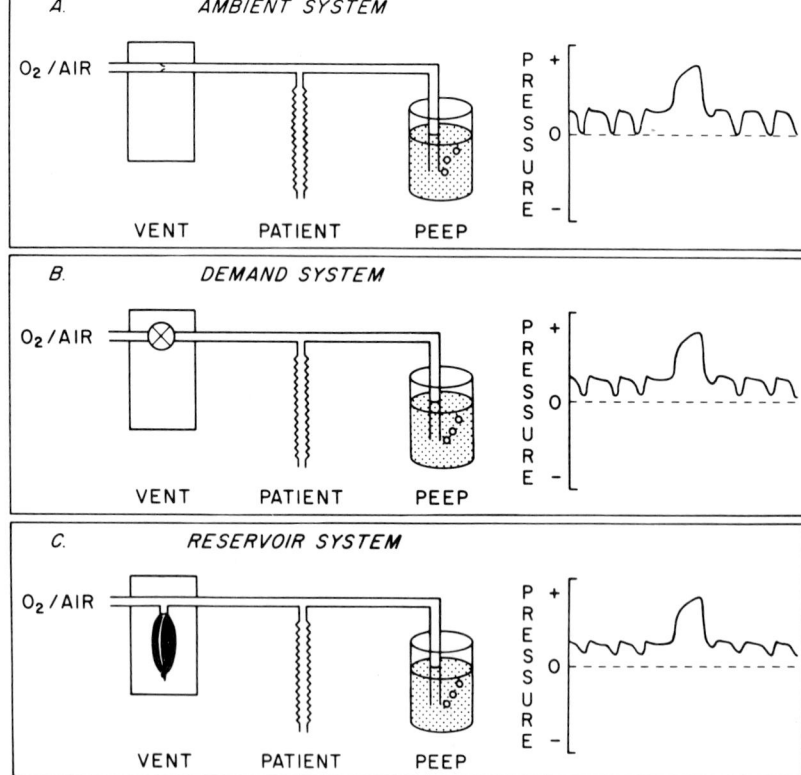

Fig. 17.11. Ambient system (A) provides continuous gas flow through the ventilator circuit during spontaneous breaths; airway pressure during inspiration falls to ambient or subambient levels. (B) Demand valve and (C) reservoir systems provide a sufficient volume of gas to meet inspired demand during peak inspiratory flow periods resulting in smaller pressure fluctuations during spontaneous breathing. See text for discussion.

sensitivity when IMV is used at rates approaching this threshold. CPAP should be produced with a system that provides a minimum of external work for the patient. As shown in Fig. 17.12, a simple system may be produced to maintain adequacy of flow during the respiratory cycle and eliminate fluctuations in airway pressure greater than ±2–3 cm H_2O above and below the level of PEEP.

Airway factors

The artificial airway may also produce weaning problems. It is recognized that small internal diameter endotracheal tubes require increased patient effort during spontaneous ventilation. The use of the nasotracheal approach with soft plastic tubes often produces major limitations of the internal diameter in the nasopharynx and in the posterior pharynx, as these tubes accomodate to the natural angulation of the airway. These restrictions may produce a major increase in resistive work of breathing. Tube obstruction is often overlooked as a source of sudden and marked change in weaning ability. Obstruction may be produced by inspissation of secretions, blood, foreign bodies such as granulation tissue, and malposition of the tracheostomy tube with ball-valving effect against the tracheal wall.

Fluid and electrolyte therapy

Fluid therapy for volemic maintenance and metabolic needs during acute respiratory failure remains controversial. Despite extensive past and recent researches into the pathogenesis of pulmonary edema states [63, 64] and better understanding of the effects of MV and PEEP on the liver and kidney [28], there are no easy, reliable, and clinically applicable methods to study extravascular lung water content (pulmonary edema) in man [65]. Although the double-indicator dilution method is promising in normal lungs, perfusion inequality and marked regional reductions of lung perfusion in ARDS pathologies (see Chap. 18) lead to inaccurate measurements compared with gravimetric methods. Chest radiographs and blood gas analyses are late indicators of hydrostatic pulmonary edema. The underlying principles of transcapillary fluid exchange (Starling's equation) remain unchallenged and are:

$$Qf = K_f[(Pmv - Ppmv) - \delta(\pi\, mv - \pi\, pmv)]$$

where:

Qf = net transvascular fluid flow
Pmv and π mv = microvascular hydrostatic and protein osmotic pressures

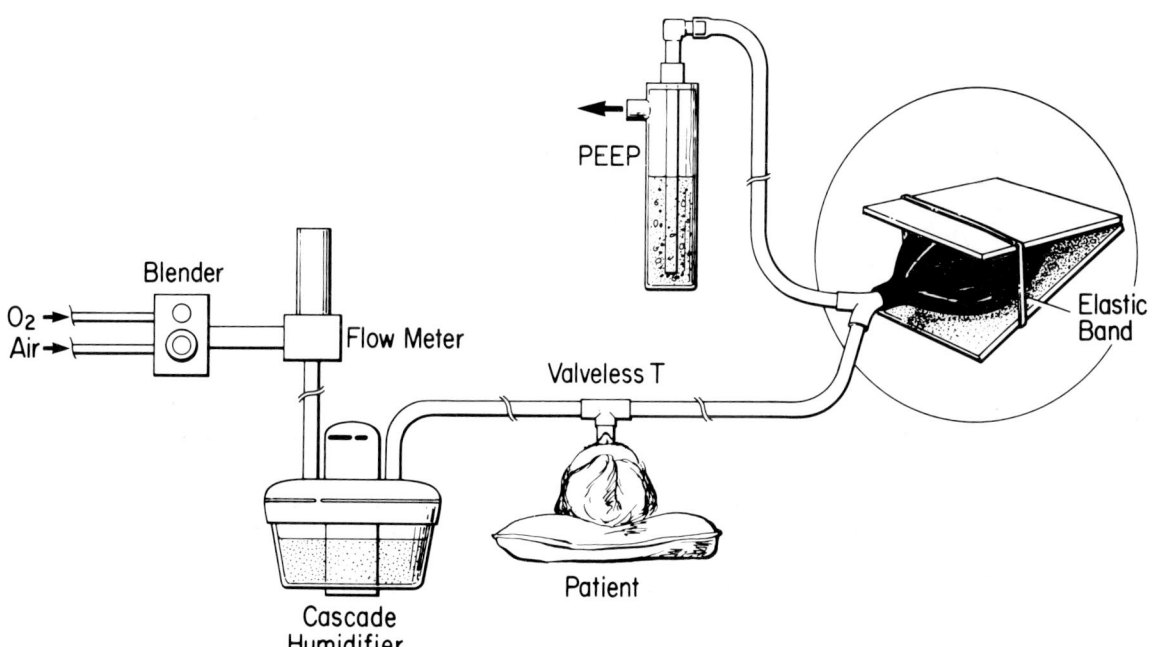

Fig. 17.12. Valveless CPAP system. Flow should be sufficient to avoid rebreathing and maintain pressure. Bag-in-board with elastic loading serves as a capacitance to maintain pressure with inspiratory and expiratory volume changes.

Ppmv and π pmv = perimicrovascular (interstitial) hydrostatic and colloid osmotic pressures

Kf = apparent fluid filtration coefficient of the filtering membrane

δ = apparent reflection coefficient of the membrane for protein.

While it is evident that we can directly measure pulmonary or systemic arterial colloid osmotic pressure (COP), the assumption that the PCWP (or even left atrial pressure) represents Pmv may be incorrect, particularly in the critically ill patient. Although aliquots of the pulmonary lymphatic effluent can be obtained in sheep, the precise anatomical vessels from which this emanates and their relative proportions during stress remain unknown. Staub [63] computes Pmv as

$[P_{(left\ atrium)} + 0.4\ P_{(pulmonary\ artery)}]$ where 0.4 expresses the ratio

$$\frac{Venous\ resistance}{(Arterial + venous)\ resistances}.$$

This factor of 0.4 derives from measurements of upstream and downstream resistances in healthy animals and assumes a capillary resistance of zero. Thus, with an extensively branched, autonomically innervated pulmonary circulation with series and parallel elements, it is possible that major changes of the vascular resistance will alter regional Pmv and regional transcapillary fluid exchange, particularly in the face of pulmonary arterial hypertension. Alveolar hypoxia in animals and man induces vasoconstriction resulting in pulmonary arteriolar hypertension. In newborn lambs [10] (but not adult sheep) this is accompanied by increased lymphatic effluent with low left atrial pressure. Reversing the pulmonary arterial pressure with alpha blockers (but not the hypoxic stimulus) returns lymphatic production to basal levels. Vasoconstriction has been documented in adult ARDS (see Chap. 18), suggesting that Pmv may be variable despite a steady measure of PCWP via balloon-occluded catheters. While attention of clinicians to fluid balance in ventilatory failure and acute lung injury has focused on the obvious findings of radiographic opacities, hypoxemia, and increases in pulmonary extravascular water at lung biopsy or autopsy, the relevance or irrelevance of the choice of fluid in the natural history of the disease is rarely addressed. One school of thought [51, 75] tries to use the (COP–PCWP) gradient as an indicator of pulmonary edema risk. There can be little argument that hypo-oncotic animals or humans will be more likely to develop hydrostatic pulmonary edema when left atrial pressure and Pmv are elevated [26]. Others [73] point out that patients with normal lungs maintained at normal levels of left atrial pressure may undergo extensive crystalloid volemic fluid resuscitation with hypo-oncotic blood and low (COP–PCWP) gradient without developing pulmonary edema or hypoxemia. Animal data [44, 81] demonstrate the predilection of crystalloids for the soft connective tissues (skin) and the ability of the lung to reduce Ppmv in proportion to a falling Pmv. It is not known whether such principles are applicable with sepsis, multiple vital organ dysfunctions over time, and alteration of the pulmonary vascular resistance.

It is classically argued [11, 63, 64] that the toxic pulmonary edemas (capillary permeability defect) show higher protein concentrations in the pulmonary lymphatic effluent than does hydrostatic edema, while small elevations in left atrial pressure result in large increases in transvascular fluid flux. Although these findings of augmented lung lymph flux were originally demonstrated in animals with elevated PAP and PVR, it is evident that toxic pulmonary edema may exist when gross pulmonary hemodynamics are normal [18]. This has been interpreted by most observers to indicate that it is advantageous to keep the left atrial and Pmv pressures as low as possible to minimize pulmonary edema. Such theory demands caution when treating patients with ARDS, because of the substantial risks of inducing inadequate systemic and renal perfusion during MV with PEEP. The NHLBI ECMO additional data collection study (see Chap. 18) showed a striking increase in mortality to 85% when renal failure supervened during hypoxemic respiratory failure, as against a 40% mortality when hypoxemic respiratory failure alone was present. The practice of keeping patients 'slightly hypovolemic' is fraught with the substantial risk of renal hypoperfusion and acute renal failure in our experience. Since we have abandoned the practice of extreme dehydration (serum osmolality > 320 mosmol/liter) and primarily directed our therapy at the maintenance of adequate systemic blood flow, the incidence of acute renal failure in our ARDS patients has decreased. Although many physicians continue to give concentrated protein solutions and diuretics in attempts to achieve the 'hyperoncotic state,' there are no data to show that these manipulations either decrease transvascular fluid exchange at normal or elevated Pmv or reverse toxic pulmonary edema and progressive respiratory failure. Although transient improvements in gas exchange clearly occur in fluid overloaded ARDS patients, we are not aware of reports of prolonged systematic elevation of COP being effective in improving gas exchange, pulmonary edema or lung pathology during experimental or human ARDS. Figure 17.13 demonstrates the futility of protein and diuretic therapy in one prospectively studied case of severe ARDS. We believe that only reversal of the primary etiology will reverse the clinical course while excessive dehydration or hypervolemia will transiently be deleterious.

Parenteral nutrition during acute respiratory failure

While it is well known that glucose and fat are aerobically metabolized with respiratory quotients of 1.0 and 0.7, respectively, it was only recently noted that total parenteral nutrition (TPN) with glucose as the principal caloric macronutrient may produce increases in CO_2 production resulting in augmented ventilatory requirements [3]. This has prompted increased use of IV lipid infusions in attempts to balance the percentage of total calories administered as glucose, protein, and fat. Whereas previous work suggested a decrease in the CO-diffusing capacity of lungs during such infusions, Jarnberg and co-workers [30] have presented evidence that these effects may be minor in critically ill patients. Whether augmented fat nutrition can decrease CO_2 production in chronic hypercapnic respiratory failure and improve exercise tolerance is unknown. Also unknown is the contribution of arachidonic acid infusion to prostaglandin metabolism and turnover in ARDS. These endogenous compounds are thought possibly to be related to ARDS pathogenesis.

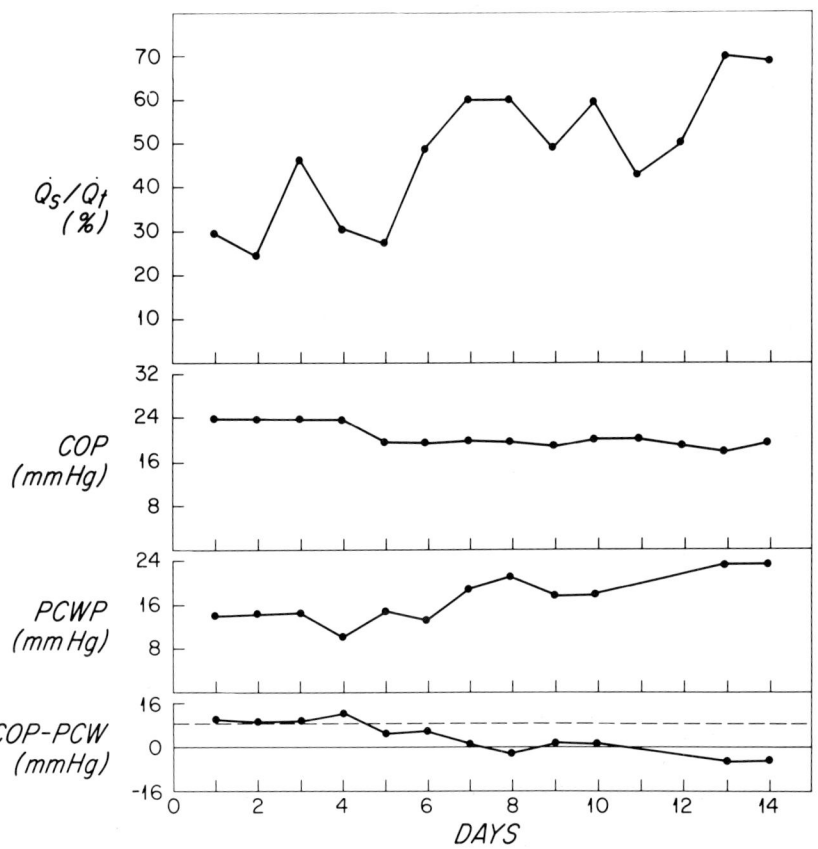

Fig. 17.13. A well-nourished 18-year-old man entered hospital with a 1-day history of staphylococcal pneumonia following influenza-like illness. Note independence of $\dot{Q}_S/\dot{Q}_T$ from COP, which was maintained at normal levels by infusions of fresh plasma and diuresis. *Dashed line* signifies (COP–PCWP) gradient of 9 mmHg [51] said to be associated with pulmonary edema. PCWP was measured while 30 cmH$_2$O PEEP was applied. Elevation of PCWP after day 6 was associated with RV dysfunction, elevated cardiac index and LVEF = 0.7 (Tc^{99m} gated cardiac blood pool scan). At autopsy the lungs weighed 2000 g with edema and hemorrhage.

High-frequency ventilation

For the last 30 years positive pressure ventilation has remained the primary means of providing gas exchange during acute and chronic respiratory failure. Recently, high-frequency ventilation (HFV) has been proposed as an alternative technique of potential therapeutic value. A number of investigators have demonstrated adequate ventilation with high frequencies and small tidal volumes approaching the estimated anatomic dead space in animal models, normal subjects, and patients.

High-frequency ventilation incorporates the following characteristics: (1) Rate exceeds 60 breaths/min or 1 Hz; (2) tidal volume approaches or is less than the anatomic dead space; (3) system compression volume and apparatus compliance must be minimal; and (4) low airway pressure and subambient extrapleural pressures exist throughout the respiratory cycle. High-frequency ventilation may be subdivided into three categories based on technique and rate. Low-frequency rates range between 60 and 100 breaths/min and gas exchange is produced by means of a jet technique with substantial air entrainment. The second category employs a high frequency of 100–200 breaths/min and is generally produced by similar jet techniques or with a variety of airway oscillators. A third method consists of oscillation at rates of 900–3000 breaths/min (15–50 Hz) produced by sine wave generators including loudspeaker systems and piston pumps. A vast amount of experience has been summarized in several reviews concerning the use of low-frequency ventilation to provide gas exchange during anesthesia for bronchoscopy and laryngoscopy [60, 61]. Limited data have been published concerning the use of this technique in acute lung injury. Jet ventilation at rates of 100–200 breaths/min has been successfully utilized in acute lung injury, particularly in patients with bronchopleural fistula [14]. Oscillation techniques at frequencies of 5–30 Hz have been demonstrated to produce adequate gas exchange in laboratory animals, neonates, and selected patients with chronic and acute respiratory disease.

A limiting factor in the successful application of HFV is the question of how these techniques provide gas exchange [9, 33]. Ventilation in the normal lung is produced by a combination of convective flow to the most distal portion of the airway, where diffusion becomes the important process. Although low-rate HFV relies in great part on convective flow, enhanced diffusion must be considered when the tidal volume approaches the volume of the anatomical dead space. At oscillatory frequencies in the range of 15–50Hz where bulk flow in the airway is negligible, diffusion of gases must be considered to be of prime importance. The lack of understanding of the relative importance of convection versus enhanced diffusion limits the true scientific and clinical application at present. Nevertheless, several potential benefits are obvious in the use of HFV. The ability to produce gas exchange at low mean airway pressure with subatmospheric pleural pressure would be advantageous in providing greater cardiovascular stability and perhaps less barotrauma than with conventional MV. In addition, improved or enhanced diffusion may provide better $\dot{V}_A/\dot{Q}$ distribution and hence better gas exchange in patients with chronic obstructive pulmonary disease where regional differences in airways resistance exist. HFV may conceivably enhance mucociliary clearance mechanisms and function as 'endogenous chest physiotherapy.' Finally, HFV has potential application both during anesthesia and during acute and chronic respiratory failure.

The future application of HFV in clinical medicine will depend on further definition of its physiologic and structural effects upon the lung. Widespread application will require evidence that it offers advantages not presently available with conventional techniques and as yet unknown risks that are preferable to those of MV.

References

1. Andersen JB, Olesen KP, Eikard B, Qvist J (1980) Periodic continuous positive airway pressure, CPAP, by mask in the treatment of atelectasis: A sequential analysis. Eur J Respir Dis 61:20–25
2. Arola MK, Puhakka H, Makela P (1980) Healing of lesions caused by cuffed tracheostomy tubes and their late sequelae: A follow-up study. Acta Anaesthesiol Scand 24:169–177
3. Askanazi J, Rosenbaum SH, Hyman AL, Silverberg PA, Milic-Emili J, Kinney JM (1980) Respiratory changes induced by the large glucose loads of total parenteral nutrition. JAMA 243:1444–1447
4. Attia RR, Battit GE, Murphy JD (1975) Transtracheal ventilation. JAMA 234:1152–1153
5. Bartlett JG, Alexander J, Mayhew J, Sullivan-Sigler N, Gorbach SL (1976) Should fiberoptic bronchoscopy aspirates be cultured? Am Rev Respir Dis 114:73–78
6. Bartlett RH, Brennon ML, Gazzaniga AB, Hanson EL (1973) Studies on the pathogenesis and prevention of

post operative pulmonary complications. Surg Gynecol Obstet 137:925–933

7. Beach T, Millen E, Grenvik A (1973) Hemodynamic response to discontinuance of mechanical ventilation. Crit Care Med 1:85–89

8. Bendixen HH, Egbert LD, Hedley-Whyte J, Laver MB, Pontoppidan H (1965) Respiratory care. Mosby, St. Louis

9. Bohn DJ, Miyasaka K, Marchak BE, Thompson WK, Froese AB, Bryan AC (1980) Ventilation by high frequency oscillation. J Appl Physiol 48:710–716

10. Bressack MA, Bland RD (1981) Intravenous infusion of tolazoline reduces pulmonary vascular resistance and net fluid filtration in the lungs of awake hypoxic newborn lambs. Am Rev Respir Dis 123:217–221

11. Brigham KL, Wolverton WC, Blake LH, Staub NC (1975) Increased sheep lung permeability caused by pseudomonas bacteremia. J Clin Invest 54:792–804

12. Browne AGR, Pontoppidan H, Chiang H, Geffin B, Wilson R, (1972) Physiological criteria for weaning patients from prolonged artificial ventilation. Abstracts of scientific papers, Annual Meeting of the American Society of Anesthesiologists, pp 69–70

13. Buda AJ, Pinsky MR, Ingels NB, Daughters GT, Stinson EB, Alderman EL (1979) Effect of intrathoracic pressure on left ventricular performance. N Engl J Med 301:453–459

14. Carlon GC, Kahn RC, Howland WS, Ray C Jr, Turnbull AD (1981) Clinical experience with high frequency jet ventilation. Crit Care Med 9:1–6

15. Cassidy SS, Gaffney FA, Johnson RL (1981) A perspective on PEEP. N Engl J Med 304:421–422

16. Department of Nursing (1980) Massachusetts General Hospital Manual of Nursing Procedures. Little, Brown, Boston

17. Downs JB, Klein EF Jr, Desautels D (1973) Intermittent mandatory ventilation: A new approach to weaning patients from mechanical ventilators. Chest 64:331–335

18. Erdmann AJ, Zapol WM (1980) 100% Oxygen breathing increases lung permeability and lung water in awake sheep. Am Rev Respir Dis 121:460(S)

19. Feeley TW, Hedley-Whyte J (1975) Weaning from controlled ventilation and supplemental oxygen. N Engl J Med 292:903–906

20. Feeley TW, Saumarez R, Klick JM, McNabb TG, Skillman JJ (1975) Positive end-expiratory pressure in weaning patients from controlled ventilation; a prospective randomized trial. Lancet II:725–729

21. Fishman AP (1980) Pulmonary diseases and disorders. McGraw-Hill, New York

22. Gherini S, Peters RM, Virgilio RW (1979) Mechanical work on the lungs and work of breathing with positive end-expiratory pressure and continuous positive airway pressure. Chest 76:251–256

23. Goldman MD, Mead J (1973) Mechanical interaction between the diaphragm and rib cage. J Appl Physiol 35:197–204

24. Grillo HC (1976) Congenital lesions neoplasms and injuries of the trachea. In: Sabiston DC, Spencer FC (eds) Gibbon's surgery of the chest. Saunders, Philadelphia, pp 256–293

25. Grillo HC (1979) Surgical treatment of post intubation injuries. J Thorac Cardiovasc Surg 78:860–875

26. Guyton AC, Lindsey AW (1959) Effect of elevated left atrial pressure and decreased plasma protein concentration on the development of pulmonary edema. Circ Res 7:649–657

27. Guyton AC, Jones CE, Coleman TG (1973) Circulatory physiology: Cardiac output and its regulation. Saunders, Philadelphia

28. Hedley-Whyte J, Burgess GE, Feeley TW, Miller MG (1976) Applied physiology of respiratory care. Little, Brown, Boston

29. Jardin F, Farcot JC, Boisante L, Curien N, Margairaz A, Bourdarias JP (1981) Influence of positive end expiratory pressure on left ventricular performance. N Engl J Med 304:387–392

30. Jarnberg PO, Lindholm M, Eklund J (1981) Lipid infusion in critically ill patients: Acute effects on hemodynamics and pulmonary gas exchange. Crit Care Med 9:27–31

31. Kamen JM, Wilkinson CJ (1971) A new low pressure cuff for endotracheal tubes. Anesthesiology 34:482–485

32. Kistner RL, Hanlon CR (1960) A new tracheostomy tube in treatment of retained bronchial secretions. Arch Surg 81:259–262

33. Klain M, Smith RB (1977) High-frequency percutaneous transtracheal jet ventilation. Crit Care Med 5:280–287

34. Kryger M, Bode F, Antic R, Anthonisen N (1976) Diagnosis of obstruction of the upper and central airways. Am J Med 61:85–93

35. Laver MB, Strauss HW, Pohost GM (1979) Right and left ventricular geometry: Adjustments during acute respiratory failure. (Herbert Shubin Memorial Lecture) Crit Care Med 7:507–519

36. Lindholm CE (1969) Prolonged endotracheal intubation. Acta Anaesthesiol Scand 33:1–130(S)

37. Long J, West G (1980) Evaluation of the Olympic trach-button as a precursor to tracheostomy tube removal. (Abstract) Respiratory Care 25:1242

38. Macklem PT (1980) Respiratory muscles: The vital pump. Chest 78:753–758

39. Marsh ML, Marshall F, Shapiro HM (1977) Neurosurgical intensive care. Anesthesiology 47:149–163

40. Mead J, Peterson N, Grimby G, Mead J (1967) Pulmonary ventilation measured from body surface movements. Science 156:1383–1384

41. Montgomery WW (1973) Surgery of the upper respiratory system, vol II. Lea & Febiger, Philadelphia

42. Montgomery WW (1974) Silicone tracheal T-tube. Ann Otol Rhinol Laryngol 83:1–5

43. Murray JF (1976) The normal lung: The basis of diagnosis and treatment of pulmonary disease. Saunders, Philadelphia

44. Pappova E, Bachmeier W, Crevoisier JL, Kollar J, Kollar M, Tobler P, Zahler HW, Zaugg D, Lundsgaard-Hansen P (1977) Acute hypoproteinemic fluid overload: Its determinants, distribution and treatment with concentrated albumin and diuretics. Vox Sang 33:307–317

45. Peters RM, Hilberman M (1971) Respiratory insufficiency: diagnosis and control of therapy. Surgery 70:280–287

46. Peters RM, Hilberman M, Hogan JS (1972) Objective indications for respirator therapy in post-trauma and post-operative patients. Am J Surg 124:262–269

47. Pontoppidan H, Geffin B, Lowenstein E (1973) Acute respiratory failure in the adult. Little, Brown, Boston

48. Pontoppidan HP, Wilson RS, Rie MA, Schneider RC (1977) Respiratory intensive care. Anesthesiology 47:96–116

49. Proceedings of the Conference on the Scientific Basis of In-hospital Respiratory Therapy (1980) Am Rev Respir Dis 122:1–146(S)

50. Qvist J, Pontoppidan H, Wilson RS, Lowenstein E, Laver MB (1975) Hemodynamic responses to mechanical ventilation with PEEP: The effect of hypervolemia. Anesthesiology 42:45–55

51. Rackow EC, Fein IA, Leppo J (1977) Colloid osmotic pressure as a prognostic indicator of pulmonary edema

and mortality in the critically ill. Chest 72:709–713

52. Renzetti AD, McClement JH, Litt BD (1966) The veterans administration cooperative study of pulmonary function. Am J Med 41:115–129

53. Robotham JL, Lixfeld W, Holland L, MacGregor D, Bryan AC, Rabson J (1978) Effects of respiration on cardiac performance. J Appl Physiol 44:703–709

54. Rodman T, Sterling FH (1969) Pulmonary emphysema and related lung diseases. Mosby, St. Louis

55. Sackner MA (1975) Bronchofiberoscopy. Am Rev Respir Dis 111:62–88

56. Sahn SA, Lakshminarayan S (1973) Bedside criteria for discontinuation of mechanical ventilation. Chest 63:1002–1005

57. Saklad M, Paliotta J, Weyerhaeuser R (1973) On-line monitoring of ventilatory parameters. In: Dornette WHL (ed) Clinical anesthesia, vol 9. F.A. Davis, Philadelphia, nos. 2 and 3

58. Savarese JJ, Ali HH, Antonio PR (1977) The clinical pharmacology of metocurine: Dimethyltubocurarine revisited. Anesthesiology 47:277–284

59. Sharp JT, Goldberg NB, Druz WS, Fishman HC, Danon J (1977) Thoracoabdominal motion in chronic obstructive pulmonary disease. Am Rev Respir Dis 115:47–56

60. Sjöstrand U (1977) Review of the physiological rationale for the development of high-frequency positive pressure ventilation—HFPPV. Acta Anaesthesiol Scand 64:7–27(S)

61. Sjöstrand U (1980) High-frequency positive pressure ventilation (HFPPV): A review. Crit Care Med 8:345–364

62. Snider MT, Rie MA, Bingham JB, Lauer J, Urbina A, Strauss HW (1980) Right ventricular performance in ARDS: Radionuclide scintiscan and thermal dilution studies. (Abstract) Am Rev Respir Dis 121:192

63. Staub NC (1974) Pulmonary edema. Physiol Rev 54:678–811

64. Staub NC (1978) The forces regulating fluid filtration in the lung. Microvasc Res 15:45–55

65. Staub NC, Hogg JC (1981) Conference report of a workshop on the measurement of lung water. Crit Care Med 8:752–759

66. Stauffer JL, Olson DE, Petty TL (1981) Complications and consequences of endotracheal intubation and tracheostomy: A prospective study of 150 critically ill adults. Am J Med 70:65–76

67. Stein M, Casara EL (1970) Preoperative pulmonary evaluation and therapy. JAMA 211:787–790

68. Stein M, Koota GM, Simon M, Frank HA (1962) Pulmonary evaluation of surgical patients. JAMA 181:765–770

69. Suter PM, Fairley HB, Isenberg MD (1975a) Optimum end-expiratory airway pressure in patients with acute pulmonary failure. N Engl J Med 292:284–289

70. Suter PM, Fairley HB, Schlobohm RM (1975b) Shunt, lung volume and perfusion during short periods of ventilation with oxygen. Anesthesiology 43:617–627

71. Suter PM, Fairley HB, Isenberg MD (1978) Effect of tidal volume and positive end-expiratory pressure on compliance during mechanical ventilation. Chest 73:158–162

72. Tisi GM (1979) Pre-operative evaluation of pulmonary function. Am Rev Respir Dis 119:293–310

73. Virgilio RW, Rice CL, Smith DE, James DR, Zarins CK, Hobelmann CF, Peters RM (1979) Crystalloid versus colloid resuscitation: Is one better? Surgery 85:129–139

74. Weber KT, Janicki JS, Sharoff S, Fishman AP (1981) Contractile mechanics and interaction of the right and left ventricles. Am J Cardiol 47:686–695

75. Weil MH, Henning RJ, Morissette M, Michaels S (1978) Relationship between colloid osmotic pressure and pulmonary artery wedge pressure in patients with acute cardiopulmonary failure. Am J Med 64:643–650

76. Weil JV, Byrne-Quinn E, Sodal IE, Friesen WO, Underhill B, Filley GF, Grover RJ (1970) Hypoxic ventilatory drive in normal man. J Clin Invest 49:1061–1072

77. West JB (1977) Pulmonary pathophysiology: The essentials. Williams & Wilkins, Baltimore

78. Wilson RS (1976) Monitoring the lung: Mechanics and volume. Anesthesiology 45:135–145

79. Wilson RS, Rie MA (1975) Management of mechanical ventilation. Surg Clin North Am 55:591–602

80. Wimberly N, Faling LJ, Bartlett JG (1979) A fiberoptic bronchoscopy technique to obtain uncontaminated lower airway secretions for bacterial culture. Am Rev Respir Dis 119:337–343

81. Zarins CK, Rice CL, Peters RM, Virgilio RW (1978) Lymph and pulmonary response to isobaric reduction in plasma oncotic pressure in baboons. Circ Res 43:925–930

Chapter 18

Pathophysiologic Pathways of the Adult Respiratory Distress Syndrome

Warren M. Zapol, Robert L. Trelstad,
Michael T. Snider, Henning Pontoppidan,
and François Lemaire

To achieve a better understanding of the pathogenesis of acute lung injury and effective prevention and therapy, the intensive care physician must recognize that most hospitalized patients with acute lung disease fall into two broad categories:

1) A large group has 'classic' pulmonary complications. These often develop after surgery and are due to small airway closure, atelectasis, and/or pulmonary edema resulting from an elevated left atrial pressure without abnormally increased microcirculatory permeability. This type of acute respiratory failure (ARF) is characterized by preservation of basic pulmonary architecture, and as a rule it is preventable and reversible provided effective treatment is instituted early [43].

2) A smaller population in which diffuse alveolar capillary membrane injury is commonly diagnosed as the adult respiratory distress syndrome (ARDS) [23, 40, 41]. Table 18.1 lists some of the diverse conditions which can produce this type of severe lung injury; each injury is characterized by an increased permeability to plasma proteins by the alveolar capillary membrane. Table 18.2 suggests possible pathophysiologic mechanisms leading to the acute lung injury.

The precise causes and mechanisms of ARDS are poorly understood in man, and despite supportive treatment with mechanical ventilation (MV) and diuretics, more than one-half of ARDS patients die [39]. The mortality of both types of ARF was found to be far higher than

had been generally realized [41] in a recent collaborative study sponsored by the U.S. National Heart, Lung, and Blood Institute [40]. In this 18-month-long study, in nine medical centers 686 patients over the age of 12 years were studied, who required: (1) intubation and MV for 24 h or more, and (2) an inspired O_2 concentration of 50% or more. Detailed data were collected from 5 days before tracheal intubation and for 15 days thereafter (Fig. 18.1).

The mortality rate of a subgroup of 490 patients (aged 12–65 years) having isolated respiratory failure was 41%, while the death rate rose to 68% for patients over 65 years of age. When additional acute injury to other organ

Table 18.1. Some injuries causing ARDS

Severe trauma (thoracic or extrathoracic)
Fat embolization
Bacteremia
Aspiration of gastrointestinal contents
Smoke or toxic gas inhalation (including O_2)
Surface burns
Hydrocarbon ingestion
Toxic drugs (heroin, paraquat)
Neurogenic pulmonary edema
Viral, mycoplasma, bacterial pneumonia
Legionnaire's disease, Pittsburgh agent
Acute vasculitis
Goodpasture's syndrome
Anaphylactic reaction to drugs and blood
Radiation of thorax
Immunosuppression and infection (pneumocystis)
Thrombus, amniotic fluid, or tumor embolism to the lung

Table 18.2. Possible mechanisms of acute lung injury

Mechanisms	Comments
Lung trauma	Direct injury to lung cells, intrapulmonary hemorrhage
Infection	
Bacterial/viral pneumonia	Inflammatory edema secondary to direct alveolar and/or pulmonary capillary cell injury
Endotoxin	Thromboxane A_2 release and pulmonary hypertension [12]
	Animal studies and clinical reports of increased capillary permeability and pulmonary edema: may also be mediated via other mechanisms listed below, e.g., DIC
Toxins	
Inhaled oxidants	Altered permeability with inhaled toxin [14]; O_2, phosgene, ozone, oxides of nitrogen, etc.
Circulating	Picture of diffuse vasculitis and endothelial injury; alloxan and oleic acid animal studies? Similar to endotoxin in man
Vasoactive substances	Injury produced secondary to liberation of histamine, serotonin, and thromboxanes. Vasoactive substances may play a major role in inflammatory, immunologic, endotoxin and hemorrhagic shock injury
Microembolization	Diffuse endothelial damage of pulmonary capillaries—many etiologies are possible including embolization, endotoxemia, tissue trauma. Major role in ARDS? Fibrino-peptides increase vascular permeability [3]. Role of inhibited fibrinolysis [49]?
Fat embolism	Most often associated with trauma (skeletal and/or tissue burns). Pathophysiology is uncertain; mechanisms include alveolocapillary damage from free fatty acids? Vasoactive substances and ? intravascular coagulation
Massive transfusions	Pulmonary vascular obstruction by platelet–leukocyte aggregates, with marked degenerative cellular changes in interalveolar septum. Cardiopulmonary bypass in man may show similar pathology; probably preventable with fine-pore filters
Immunologic reactions	Etiologies include: drug hypersensitivity, idiosyncratic reactions, anaphylaxis (e.g., heroin, antibiotics), allergic alveolitis. Injury appears to result from release of chemical mediators
Shock	Pulmonary insufficiency associated with extrathoracic trauma and low cardiac output: additional factors, e.g., myocardial failure, overhydration and mechanisms listed above may play essential roles
Loss of surfactant	Decreased surfactant from O_2, toxins, and dilution with plasma may cause atelectasis and increased shunt

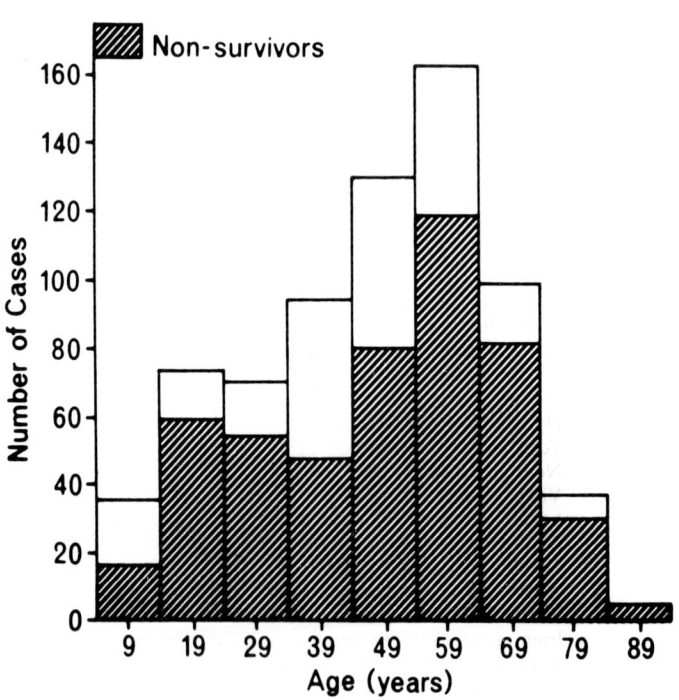

Fig. 18.1. NHLBI additional data collection from nine University hospitals: Incidence and mortality of the 686 patients in ARF by age [40]. *Open boxes* depict survivors, *shaded boxes* non-survivors.

systems was present on admission or developed during the study period (85% of 686 patients) the chances of surviving were greatly reduced (Fig. 18.2). For example, only 40% of patients aged 12–65 years with ARF and another organ system failure survived.

With such high mortality rates, it is essential that intensive care physicians, nurses, and respiratory therapists be cognizant of the factors that can cause pulmonary complications or primary lung injury. Unnecessary delay in treating acute lung injury may add to lung damage, increasing the need for high inspired O_2 concentrations, large tidal volumes, and the high airway pressures necessary to achieve adequate gas exchange.

Supportive therapy for ARDS is notably unsuccessful without removal of the primary cause. If standard methods do not reveal a definite etiologic agent open lung biopsy should be performed. Hill et al. [22] and Nellems et al. [42] have reported on large groups of ARDS patients who underwent biopsy. Although the salvage rate remained low, diagnostic information on infection and the pathologic status of the lung was useful in optimizing therapy. Open lung biopsy by a skilled surgeon infrequently causes the complications of bronchopleural fistula or bleeding.

The pathophysiological manifestations of acute lung injury as characterized by bedside pulmonary function and hemodynamic studies are similar in the many diseases causing acute lung injury listed in Table 18.1. The common

hallmarks are bilateral chest radiograph infiltrates, a marked decrease in end-expiratory communicating intrathoracic gas volume (FRC), with a reduction to 50% of normal or less; reduced dynamic and static compliance with a marked decrease in the slope of the static pressure–volume curve; and a rising alveolar–arterial O_2 tension difference ($AaDO_2$), right-to-left intrapulmonary shunt (Q_S/Q_T), dead space-to-tidal volume ratio (V_D/V_T), and decreased diffusion capacity (D_{LCO}) [43].

In patients with the more common 'classic' lung complications and in those in the early stages of ARDS, the V_D/V_T is only moderately elevated (usually below 0.4), and the pulmonary vascular resistance is near normal [44]. However, in all patients with severe ARDS, pronounced reductions of FRC and compliance with impaired O_2 and CO_2 exchange are accompanied by an increase in the pulmonary vascular resistance [58].

We will now examine the alterations seen in severe ARDS as they evolve in separate lung compartments, within the pulmonary circulation, the alveoli, and small airways, at the alveolar–capillary membrane, and in the interstitial space. This general morphologic classification is employed for didactic reasons and is based on the concept that lung injury patterns are common to the syndrome and independent of the specific causes listed in Table 18.1. Our information is based upon biopsy and autopsy pathology studies and clinical studies of hemodynamics and gas exchange.

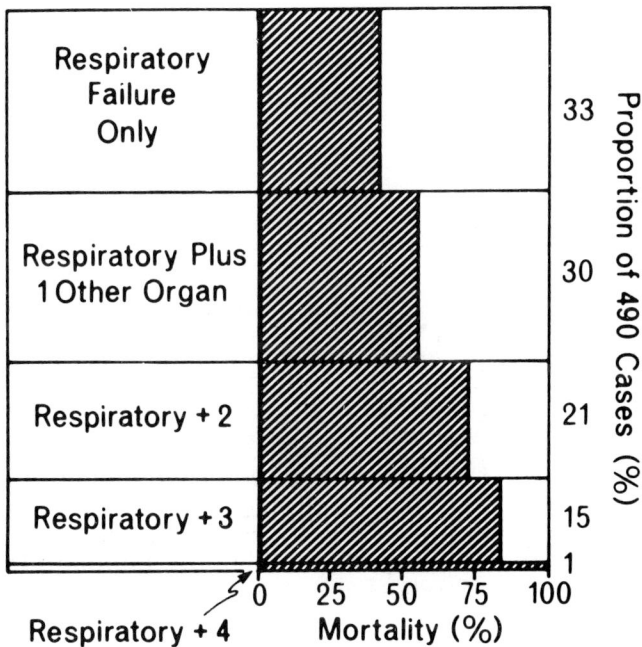

Fig. 18.2. NHLBI additional data collection: Incidence and mortality of organs system failure in the 495 ARF patients aged 12–65. Organs or systems considered for failure were: kidneys, liver, brain, heart, immune (sepsis) and coagulation (DIC) [40].

For a review of normal pulmonary structure, function and pathophysiology, two recent monographs are recommended [38, 57].

Lung alterations in early ARDS (hours to days)

Vasculature

A characteristic feature is pulmonary venous and capillary congestion, often accompanied by endothelial cell swelling and necrosis (Fig. 18.3). Recent studies of pulmonary hemodynamics in early and mild ARDS have not demonstrated a markedly elevated pulmonary vascular resistance within 24 h of injury (with notable exceptions in certain types of severe ARDS) [60]. Within a few days most patients develop pulmonary artery hypertension (PAH), defined as a mean pulmonary artery pressure (PAP) exceeding 20 mmHg (Fig. 18.4), and the pulmonary vascular resistance (PVR) eventually rises to two or three times the normal value (Fig. 18.5). PVR is calculated as the difference between mean PAP and pulmonary capillary wedge pressure (PCWP) divided by cardiac output. The normal value in adults is below 1.0 mmHg/min/litre [2]. In each patient there is an inverse relationship between the PVR and the cardiac index (CI) (Fig. 18.6a); therefore, sequential measurements of PVR should be referred to a specific CI; that is, a

PVR–CI curve should be constructed before changes of PVR are interpreted as changes in the status of the pulmonary vessels.

We do not know precisely what determines

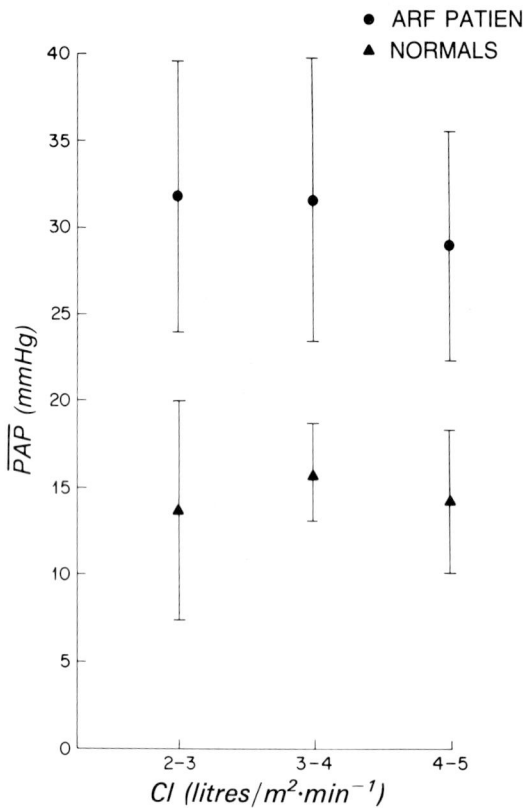

Fig. 18.4. Mean PAP as a function of CI for 30 patients in ARF and for normal controls [58].

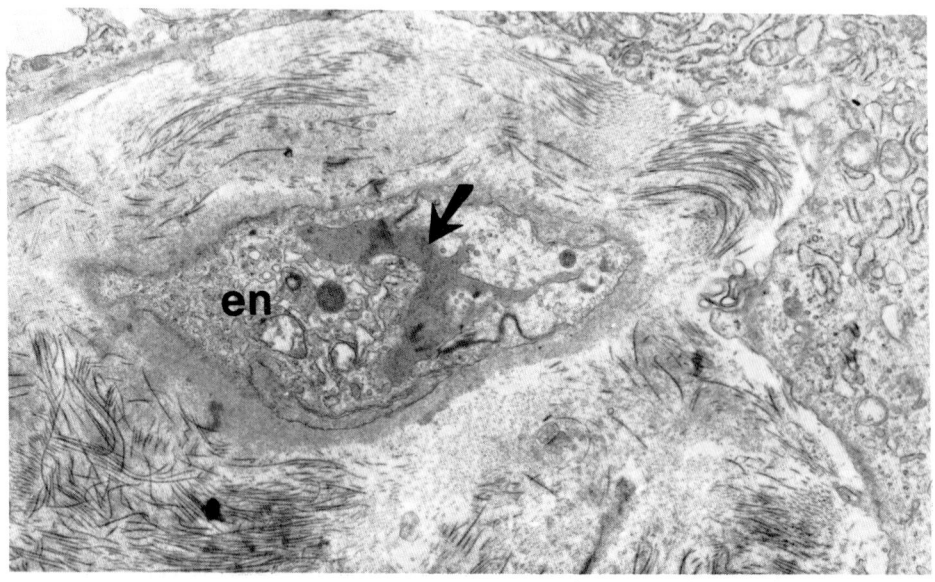

Fig. 18.3. Alveolar capillary with swollen endothelial cells (*en*) nearly occluding the lumen (*arrow*). (×6000)

the shape of the PVR–CI curve. It is our belief that in ARDS a markedly increased lung interstitial pressure raises the 'opening pressure' of the pulmonary vessels from 5–10 mmHg to 20–30 mmHg and thus increases the PAP. In early ARDS, the interstitium fills with plasma exudate and reversible vascular compression may occur (Fig. 18.6b). Figure 18.7 illustrates serial measurements of PAP and CI in a patient recovering from acute post-traumatic ARDS. With intensive therapy lung function improved, the patient progressed from moderate to mild ARDS, radiographic infiltrates cleared, and the opening pressure decreased.

In early ARDS after lung vessels are 'opened' there does not appear to be an increased resistance to flow. Figure 18.8a shows the effects on pulmonary artery pressure of increasing pulmonary blood flow by isoprenaline infusion. Early in ARDS doubling of cardiac output (CO) from 3.5 to 7 litres/min increases mean PAP by only 3 mmHg (from 44 to 47 mmHg). However, 3 days later, in more severe ARDS, the PAP had increased to 55 mmHg. We were unable to increase CO over 4 litres/min despite infusing inotropic drugs. In addition to physical obstruction [5] a large number of endogenous and exogenous mediators are capable of increasing pulmonary vascular tone [7]. Interstitial and vascular wall edema, reactive vasoconstriction secondary to hypoxia and acidosis, or mediator-induced constriction may be implicated in the

early PAH. Special attention is now being devoted to the vasodilator and vasoconstrictor roles of some arachidonic acid metabolites (thromboxane A_2, endoperoxides, and prostacyclin) [27, 37]. These potent vasoactive agents are short-lived and difficult to measure. At present their metabolites, thromboxane B_2

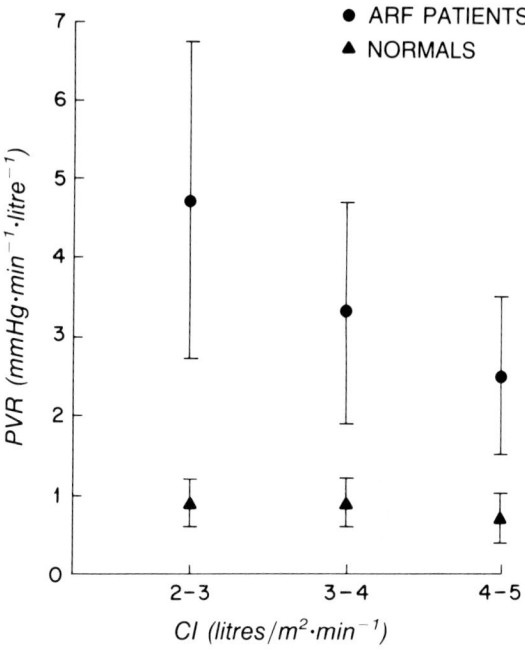

Fig. 18.5. PVR as a function of CI for 30 patients in ARF and for normal controls [58].

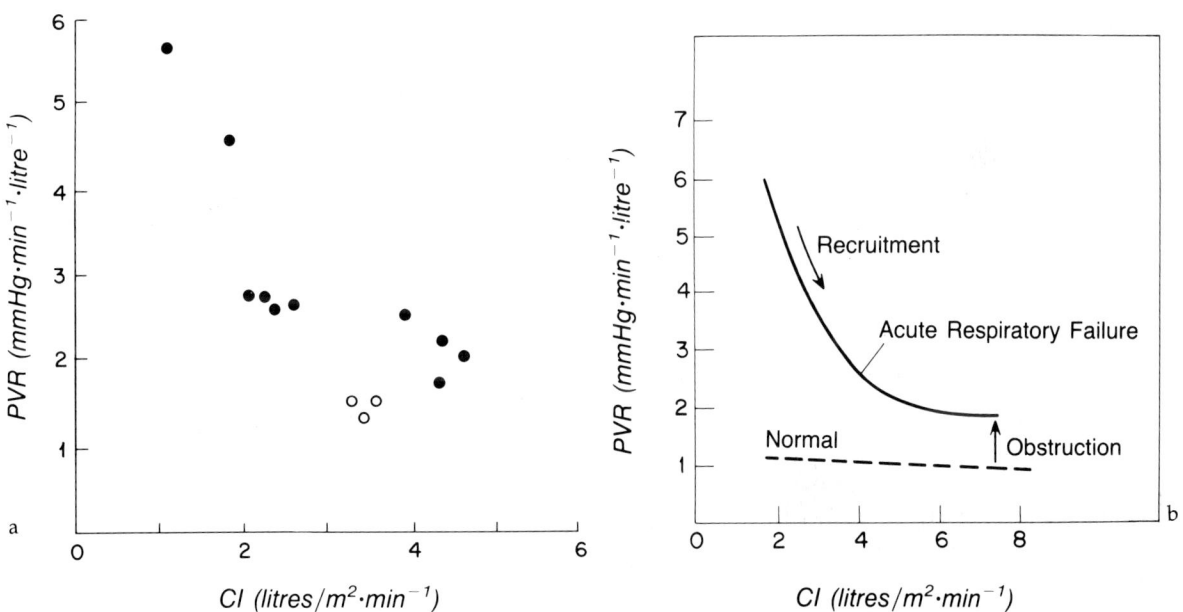

Fig. 18.6. a Variation in CI resulting from a change in bypass blood flow rate during severe varicella pneumonia (*closed circles*) and 6 months after recovery (*open circles*) [58].
b. Schema of possible events influencing the relationship of PVR with the CI.

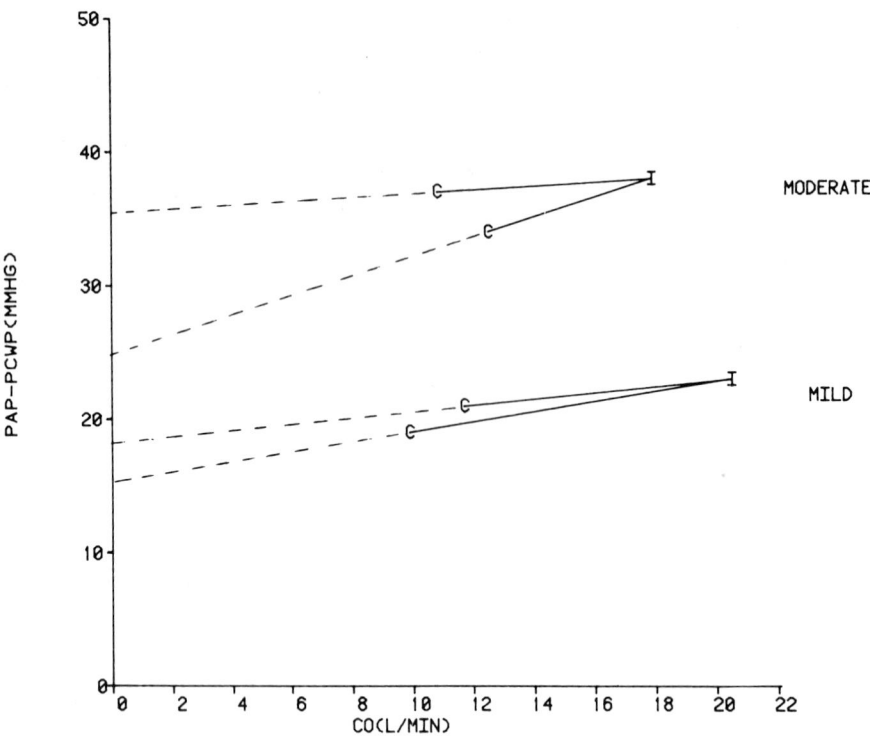

Fig. 18.7. PAP minus PCWP plotted against cardiac output in post-traumatic ARF. *C* indicates control, *I* indicates isoprenaline infusion. Linear intercepts to zero cardiac output (*CO*) may provide an indication of interstitial lung pressure. The intercept pressure rises in severe ARF.

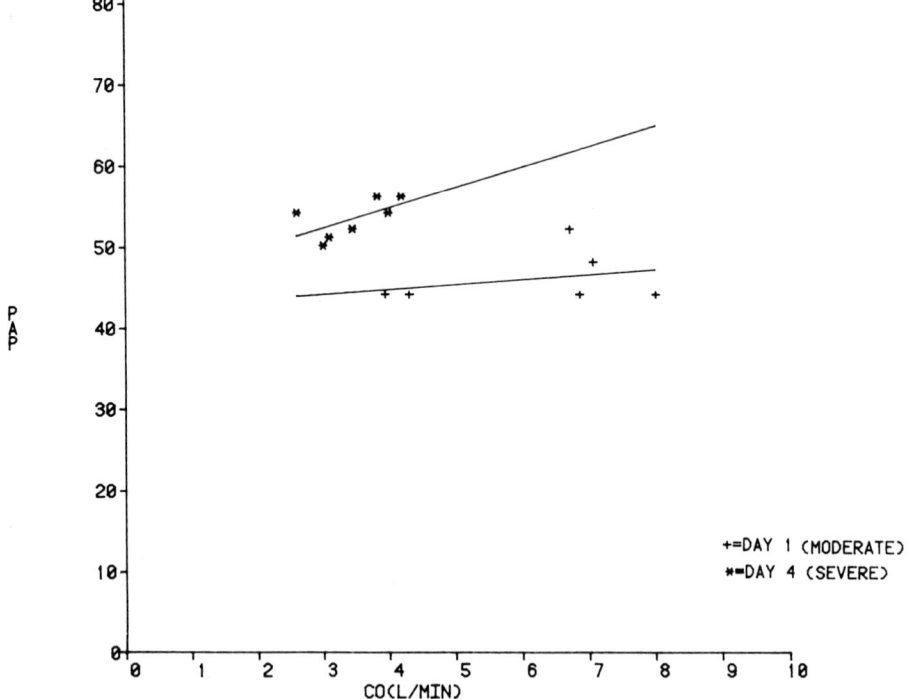

Fig. 18.8. a Mean PAP for one patient plotted against cardiac output during moderate (+) and severe (*) respiratory failure.

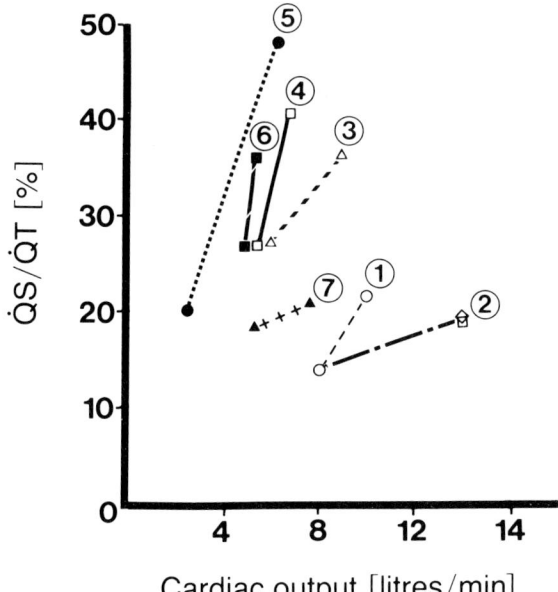

Fig. 18.8. b Cardiac output plotted against shunt ($\dot{Q}_S/\dot{Q}_T$) in ARF of differing severity: 1, mild ARF; cardiac output changes induced by nitroprusside infusion; 2, mild ARF; isoproterenol infusion; 3, moderate ARF: nitroprusside infusion [53]; 4, moderate ARF in shock patients; dopamine infusion [46]; 5, severe ARF; treated by venoarterial partial bypass [31]; 6, moderate ARF in septic shock patients; treated by plasma volume expansion [26]; 7, mild ARF in shock patients; dobutamine infusion [47].

and 6 keto-$PGF_{1\alpha}$ are measured by radioimmunoassay. Complement activation of leukocytes with subsequent vasoconstriction may be another factor producing pulmonary hypertension and transvascular leakage [13]. Recent studies suggest leucocyte occlusion of pulmonary vessels is not the cause of PAH [18, 63].

Snider et al. have reported [51] that intravenous infusion of nitroprusside during early ARDS of varied etiology reduces the PVR as well as the PAP and PCWP. The patients concerned were not hypoxemic. This provides evidence that diffuse pulmonary vascular constriction or spasm is present in ARDS. Prostacyclin, a vasodilator, and ibuprofen (an inhibitor of cyclooxygenase) are presently under clinical investigation as means of lowering PAP [56].

Vasculature–airway interaction in early ARDS: Factors determining and modifying the extent of hypoxemia

Airway pressure and alveolar recruitment

Increased alveolar–capillary permeability is the common feature of ARDS, with alveolar flooding by edema, followed by distal airway collapse producing arterial hypoxemia by an increased right-to-left shunt. A direct correlation may exist between the radiological pattern and the severity of hypoxemia.

Increasing the level of end-expiratory pressure markedly reduces $\dot{Q}_S/\dot{Q}_T$, presumably by recruiting and opening closed airway units, as evidenced by an increased FRC [16]. Gas exchange during acute pulmonary disease may be completely modified by varying the balance of alveolar edema and collapse with alveolar recruitment, the latter determined primarily by the level of end-expiratory pressure. In the short term, the severity and extent of lung damage is not altered by PEEP, i.e., extravascular lung water is not decreased [24]. After increasing airway pressure the same quantity of alveolar edema is simply spread over an increased alveolar surface area [34].

For some ARDS patients $\dot{V}/\dot{Q}$ inhomogeneity is a prominent factor in gas exchange and the PaO_2 improves markedly after an increase of the inspired O_2 concentration (FIO_2). In other ARDS patients, increasing the FIO_2 to 100% does not improve hypoxemia, their shunt is 'fixed', and only an increase in PEEP can reduce it [17, 28].

Pulmonary capillary pressure

Sustained elevation of lung hydrostatic pressure markedly increases the efflux of lymph [8]; extravascular lung water increases [25] and results in alveolar edema. Such phenomena occur in ARDS at a considerably lower hydrostatic pressure than in cardiogenic pulmonary edema [48]. The long-term deleterious effect on gas exchange of an elevated vascular hydrostatic pressure must be clearly separated from the short-term effect of increased pulmonary artery pressure on vascular recruitment (see below).

Mixed venous oxygenation

At constant shunt, PaO_2 decreases when $P\bar{v}O_2$ decreases (e.g., due to a low cardiac output or increased $\dot{V}O_2$). Increasing cardiac output by vasoactive drug infusion (dopamine, isoprenaline, or dobutamine) reduces the $P(A-a)O_2$ difference, raises $P\bar{v}O_2$, and minimizes the increase of $\dot{Q}_S/\dot{Q}_T$. In addition, an increased $P\bar{v}O_2$ may suppress hypoxic pulmonary vasoconstriction, thereby increasing $\dot{Q}_S/\dot{Q}_T$. Such an effect, as well as denitrogenation atelectasis, may explain the often reported increase of $\dot{Q}_S/\dot{Q}_T$ during pure O_2 ventilation [55].

Vascular recruitment

Factors influencing pulmonary vascular recruitment have been studied for over 30 years. Some major factors are: pulmonary blood flow, transmural pulmonary artery and capillary pressure, left atrial pressure, alveolar pressure, and lung volume. Few of these factors have been studied in clinical ARDS. Hypoxic vasoconstriction may play a major role in diverting blood from low $\dot{V}/\dot{Q}$ units towards better-ventilated ones [4]. This protective constriction could reduce $\dot{Q}_S/\dot{Q}_T$ and improve PaO_2, but may increase the PAP and PVR. The extent to which this phenomenon occurs in the absence of a decreased $P\bar{v}O_2$ is poorly understood [11]. Pulmonary vasodilatation following nitroprusside infusion without concomitant alteration of the $P\bar{v}O_2$ has provided evidence for normoxic vasoconstriction in ARDS [53]. Pulmonary and systemic vasodilation due to nitroprusside infusion increases the cardiac output and decreases PAP and PVR while increasing $\dot{Q}_S/\dot{Q}_T$ and decreasing the PaO_2 [53].

A linear correlation has been measured between cardiac output and Q_S/Q_T in ARDS (Fig. 18.8b) [30] and animal studies [33].

Decreasing cardiac output with partial venoarterial bypass [29] or augmenting cardiac output with dopamine [46] induces simultaneous changes in $\dot{Q}_S/\dot{Q}_T$ and PaO_2. These changes are more marked when cardiac output variations are accompanied by concomitant alterations of PAP and PCWP. Increased shunting as cardiac output increases is less obvious in the final stages of acute lung disease [53] and at high levels of PEEP [21, 32, 51].

Pulmonary vascular occlusion

Open lung biopsies from pneumonia patients within 1 week following intubation frequently reveal thrombi or emboli in small vessels [22]. Following trauma there may be embolization of marrow elements to lung vessels. Thrombotic vascular obstruction is the anatomic basis for the filling defects observed in lung arteries over 0.5 mm diameter by segmental balloon occlusion ('wedge') angiograms (Fig. 18.9). Pulmonary artery filling defects were reported by Greene et al. in 19 of the 40 ARDS patients

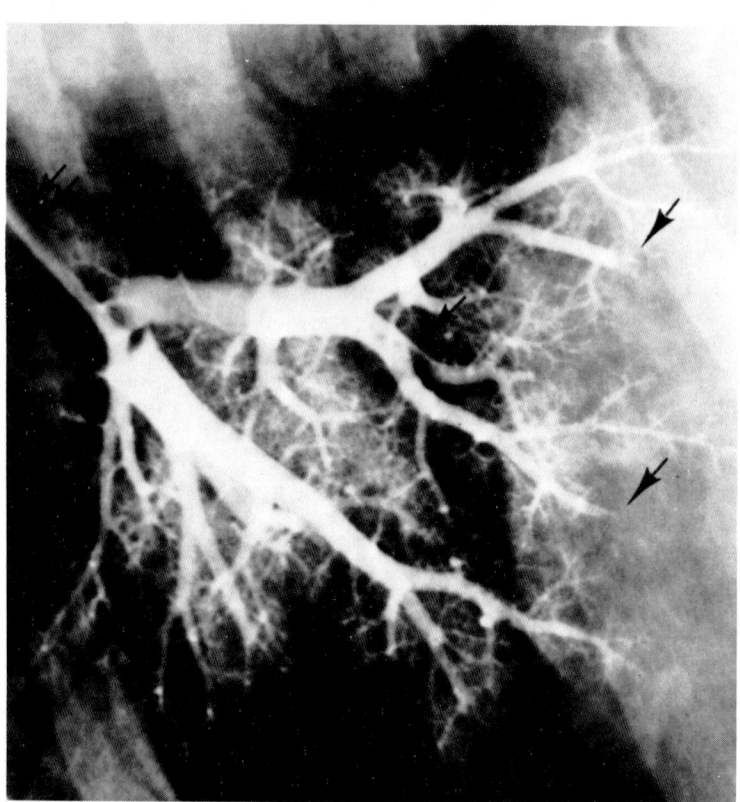

Fig. 18.9. Balloon occlusion wedge arteriogram after severe extra-thoracic trauma. *Single arrows* indicate vascular occlusion, subsequently proven at open lung biopsy to represent bone marrow emboli. *Double arrow* points to Swan–Ganz catheter. Arteriogram courtesy of Dr Reginald Greene.

he studied [20]. Pulmonary vascular occlusion correlated with both an elevated PVR (> 2.5 mmHg/min/litre) and the presence of disseminated intravascular coagulation.

It remains to be learned in man whether microthromboembolism constitutes a common primary embolic pathologic event in ARDS [49] or is a secondary phenomenon due to intravascular thrombosis within severely damaged lung parenchyma. Microthromboemboli were uncommon in lung ultrastructural morphometric studies of nine patients dying of septicemia [1] and in 40 patients examined in a collaborative study of bypass in ARDS [45]. However, both studies were based on small tissue samples. Eeles and Sevitt, using standard pathologic techniques in trauma patients, found frequent evidence of large pulmonary artery occlusion [15]. Recently, careful lung vascular injection studies by Zapol et al. [61] and Snow et al. [54] indicated widespread microvascular occlusion in ARDS.

Coagulopathies are common in severe ARDS. Thrombocytopenia due to a shortened platelet lifespan [50] is common. Platelet lifespan can be short despite the absence of lung infection, septicemia or DIC [evidenced by an elevated fibrinogen degradation product (FDP) concentration]. Saldeen has reported impaired fibrin clearance from the injured lung [49]. However, Carvalho has measured high plasma concentrations of FDP and soluble fibrin complexes, suggesting active fibrinolysis in the majority of ARDS patients [50]. Grant et al. [19] and Carvalho et al. [10] have measured markedly elevated levels of an abnormal factor VIII antigen produced by endothelial cells in the plasma of ARDS patients despite normal levels of coagulant factor VIII.

The role of heparin anticoagulation or fibrinolytic agents in ARDS is controversial. No prospective and randomized studies have been reported.

Alveolar lining and alveolar space

Hyaline membranes form within the first few days of injury and are a common histologic finding within 3–4 days (Fig. 18.10a). They consist of necrotic type I alveolar lining cells and coagulated intra-alveolar proteins derived from the exudate that floods the airspace following increased vascular permeability and loss of alveolar integrity. The thin type I cells, which cover 90% of the gas exchange surface, are highly vulnerable to injury and incapable of reproduction (Fig. 18.10b and c). The denuded

alveolar surface left behind by the sloughed type I cells becomes covered through vigorous hyperplasia and lateral extension of the type II epithelial cell (the granular pneumocyte). Moreover, the progenitors of the type I cells are these proliferative type II cells.

Interstitium

Swelling and edema of the interstitial space and interlobar septae are universal early features. The extracellular matrix, rich in collagen, elastin, and some proteoglycans, becomes a highly hydrated gel, leading to possible vascular compression and reduced compliance. Perivascular and peribronchial edema and interstitial hemorrhage imply major interruptions of the vascular channels.

By the end of the first week following lung injury, fibroblasts throughout the lung's interstitium reveal cytologic features consistent with an activated state in that the volume of the cell cytoplasm increases, as does that of many organelles such as the endoplasmic reticulum (Fig. 18.11). Although the cytologic features of the interstitial cells suggest accelerated biosynthetic activity there is also a substantial increase in matrix degradation. The manner of matrix breakdown is poorly understood, but probably involves hydrolases both released by local cells and present in phagocytic vacuoles. Leukocyte infiltrates are not a prominent feature in most cases of early ARDS, and macrophages are normally present in the alveolar space. Whether the leukocytes and macrophages are the major source of the catabolic activity is not clear, since many of the hydrolases which affect the matrix can also be produced by the interstitial fibroblasts.

Pulmonary edema, microvascular hydrostatic pressure (MHP) and colloid osmotic pressure (COP)

Pulmonary interstitial edema figures prominently in acute lung injury. The role of COP and the COP–MHP gradient is currently disputed and is reviewed to emphasize that in ARDS the integrity of the walls of the pulmonary capillary and small extra-alveolar vessels are compromised and the egress of plasma facilitated. There are no useful tools to measure either the metabolic function of the pulmonary vascular wall or its permeability to plasma proteins and cells. Clinical measurements of extravascular lung water, by either double indicator dilution or

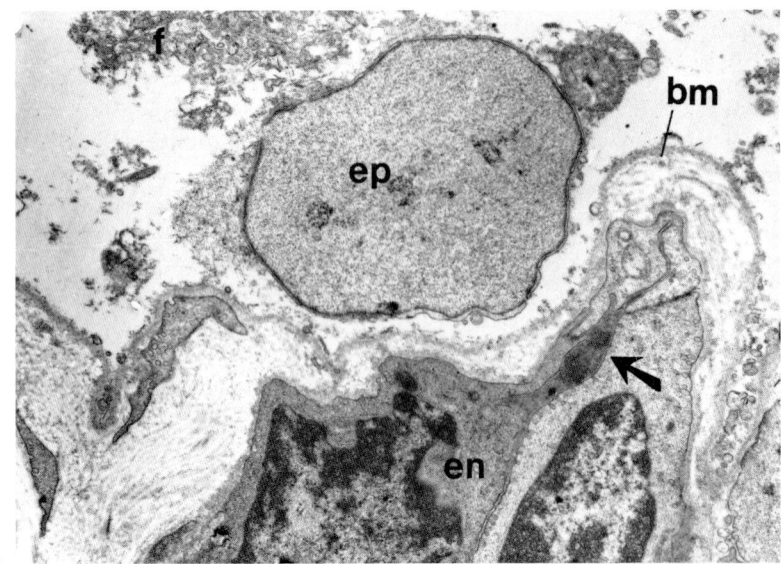

Fig. 18.10. a A round swollen epithelial cell (*ep*): debris, fibrin (*f*), and amorphous material are present in the alveolar space. The basement membrane (*bm*) is denuded. Swollen endothelial cells (*en*) nearly occlude the capillary lumen (*arrow*). (×6000)

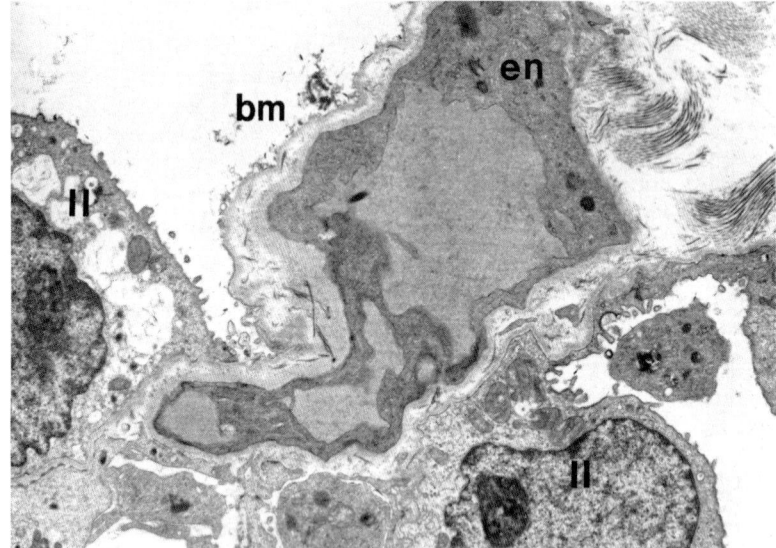

b Hyperplastic type II pneumocytes line both surfaces of the alveolar septum. The remnants of a type I pneumocyte are present on an otherwise denuded basement membrane (*bm*). The alveolar capillary endothelium (*en*) appears intact. (×6000)

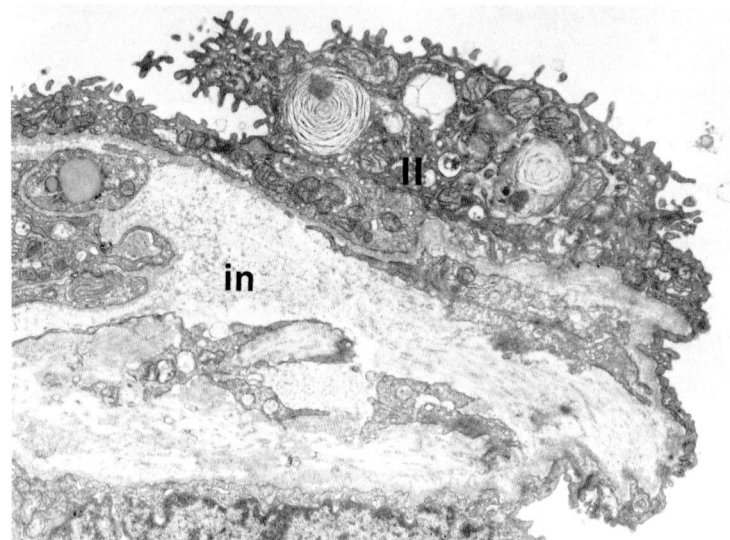

c Hyperplastic type II pneumocyte. There is moderate swelling in the interstitium (*in*). (×6000)

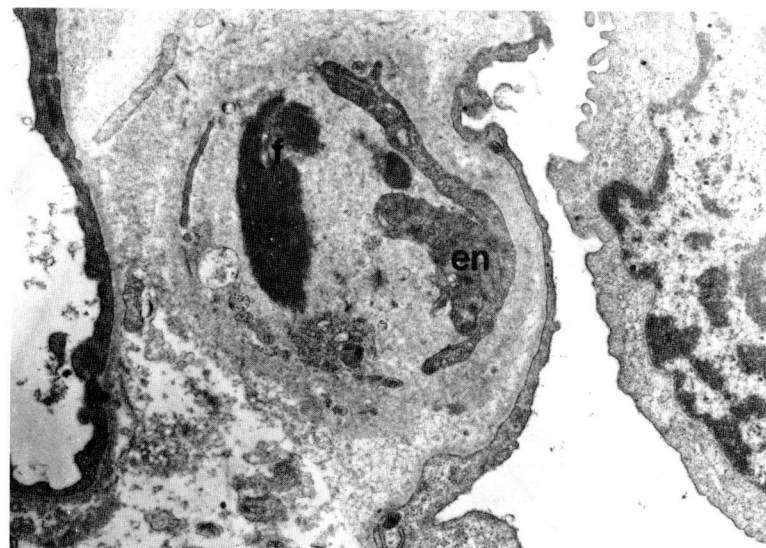

Fig. 18.11. a Remnants of an alveolar capillary. The endothelial cells (*en*) have condensed and exhibit retracted cytoplasmic processes. Fibrin is present in the ablated lumen. (×6000)

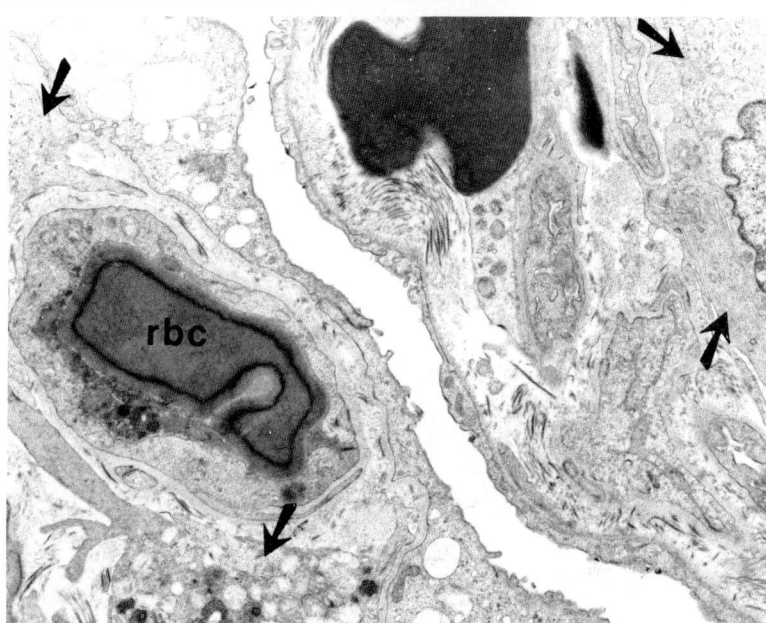

b Occluded capillary containing a crenated red blood cell (*rbc*) and fibrin. Another red cell is present in the extravascular space. The interstitial cells (*arrow*) have more highly developed cytoplasmic organelles than normal. (×6000)

permeability surface area product, underestimate pulmonary edema (probably because edematous regions are unperfused) [9, 36]. Inhaled gas techniques to assess the extent of pulmonary edema also underestimate edema, probably due to closure of airways leading to injured alveoli.

MHP is usually estimated as mean left atrial pressure plus 0.4 times the difference between mean pulmonary artery and left atrial pressure [6]. In ARDS there is often pulmonary artery vasoconstriction and thrombotic pulmonary vascular obstruction of both arteries and veins, and any MHP estimate is clearly imprecise.

However, if MHP is 15–25 mmHg any distinction between high-pressure pulmonary edema and that resulting from vascular wall injury is rarely clear-cut. The safest course of action is to suppose abnormal vascular wall permeability is widespread. Once plasma enters the interstitial space, the transvascular wall COP difference disappears and MHP and lymphatic drainage rate become the major determinants of extravascular plasma content. In ARDS there are no data concerning the role of COP in altering pulmonary edema formation. Practically, the MHP and PCWP should be maintained at the lowest levels consistent with allowing sufficient cardiac output to provide adequate perfusion of critical organs (usually urine output and composition are used to assess the adequacy of perfusion).

In summary, the major changes occurring during the first few days of acute lung injury are intra-alveolar and interstitial edema of high protein content, hemorrhage, hyaline membrane formation, necrosis of alveolar lining epithelium and endothelial cells, and activation of type II and interstitial cells, with appearance of microthrombi in small pulmonary arteries (Fig. 18.11). The changes at this time do not suggest substantial alterations in the underlying architecture of the lung, although these may have begun. A basically normal pattern of alveolar space and interstitial matrix is retained. Recruitable airspace and vasculature appears to be present in most cases. Reversibility of the morphologic changes in early stages would seem likely were effective primary therapeutic measures available for clinical application.

Late alterations in severe ARF (days to weeks)

Vasculature

Thrombi in small and medium-sized pulmonary arteries are identifiable by balloon occlusion angiography (Fig. 18.9). Intact megakaryocytes

may be present in small vessels. Endothelial cell necrosis (Fig. 18.11a) is commonly observed but neovascularization is not detectable. Postmortem lung vascular perfusion with low-viscosity silicone rubber infused at 75 mmHg has shown extensive loss of microvascular units in the respiratory regions of the lung [61]. However, the precise cause of vessel loss, such as thrombosis, embolism, or resorption, was not identified.

At this stage PAH is more pronounced, with mean PAP frequently exceeding 30–40 mmHg due to a PVR elevated more than threefold. Evidence for right ventricular (RV) dysfunction during ARF has been obtained. A decreased RV ejection fraction (25% or less) and an increased RV end-diastolic volume has been observed in 15 patients with severe ARF examined by both thermal washout techniques and gated pool scanning [52]. This may be due in part to the increased RV afterload or myocardial injury. Dilatation of the right ventricle is common, and leads to a marked increase of the RV wall tension necessary for systolic ejection (Fig. 18.12) [35]. At this time, no therapy has been proved consistently effective in reducing the pulmonary vascular resistance or improving cardiac function in severe ARF.

Alveolar lining and alveolar spaces

The alveolar lining now features a cuboidal epithelium representing vigorous hyperplasia of type II epithelial cells, and presumably

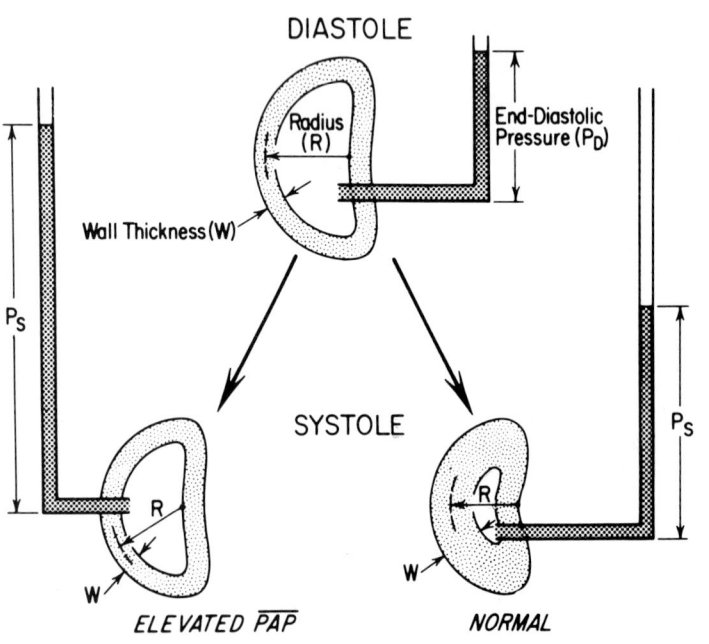

$$\text{WALL STRESS (S) =} \frac{P \times R}{W} \ (\text{dynes} \cdot \text{cm}^{-2})$$

Fig. 18.12. The Laplace relationship states that an increased RV end-systolic volume due to a decreased stroke volume or marked increase in RV end-diastolic volume will result in a higher peak systolic wall stress. If enlargement of the cavity is accompanied by a reduced wall thickness then RV wall stress will further increase. S, wall stress; P, intravascular pressure; R, internal radius; W, wall thickness. Taken from Martyn, et al. [35].

reflects regenerative efforts (Fig. 18.10c). The taller, thicker alveolar lining provided by the type II cells in conjunction with residual intra-alveolar hyaline membranes causes marked interference with the normal ventilation perfusion relationships, gas diffusion, and blood gas exchange; $\dot{Q}_S/\dot{Q}_T$ often exceeds 0.4. Bachofen and Weibel have measured a marked increase of gas diffusion distance in ARDS lungs studied by morphometric methods [1]. V_D/V_T often exceeds 0.6, causing progressive difficulty with CO_2 elimination.

Discontinuities of the alveolar basement membranes (Fig. 18.13) allow activated interstitial cells to enter the alveolar air space and are a key step in the initiation of intra-alveolar fibrosis. This is further aggravated as the lung disease process advances and diffuse intra-alveolar fibrosis with production of an obliterative matrix becomes widespread.

Interstitium

Light and electron microscopy show a substantial increase in connective tissue matrix, particularly fibrillar collagen (Fig. 18.14a). These fibrotic changes have been confirmed by biochemical analysis of total lung collagen content, which in severe ARDS increases two- to threefold in 3 weeks (Fig. 18.14b) [62]. There is a concomitant increase of total dry lung mass due to hemorrhage, plasma and cellular infiltration reducing the apparent collagen concentration. In addition to extensive interstitial fibrosis there appears to be a change in the character of the interstitial matrix, with diminished elastic tissue

detected by staining and light microscopy. A schematic diagram of the destructive and proliferative alterations which occur in the alveolar wall is shown in Fig. 18.15. Destruction of alveolar wall architecture with obliteration of the vasculature of the lung contributes to the increasing PVR. The overall alveolar architecture is severely disrupted; increased turnover or degradation of matrix components occurs simultaneously with substantial deposition of new matrix. The rapid matrix turnover destroys the architecture of gas-exchanging units, and such changes are probably irreversible. Mechanical ventilation at elevated airway pressures to maintain gas exchange often results in overdistension of terminal airways and alveolar spaces, with the resultant formation of large cavities and cystic spaces (Fig. 18.16) [28].

Distribution of lesions

Although pulmonary morphologic changes are frequently described as 'diffuse,' they often are not global but consist of diseased areas interspaced with 'spared' areas of relatively well-preserved normal lung. The focal but diffuse nature of pulmonary vascular and alveolar injury may drastically alter the distribution of ventilation, perfusion, and diffusion. Pulmonary hypertension in ARDS may remove or reduce zones 1 and 2 described by West [57]. Numerous 'mini-zones' of unknown geographical distribution may characterize the deranged ventilation and flow relationships throughout the lungs. Subpleural areas appear especially involved in ischemic necrosis

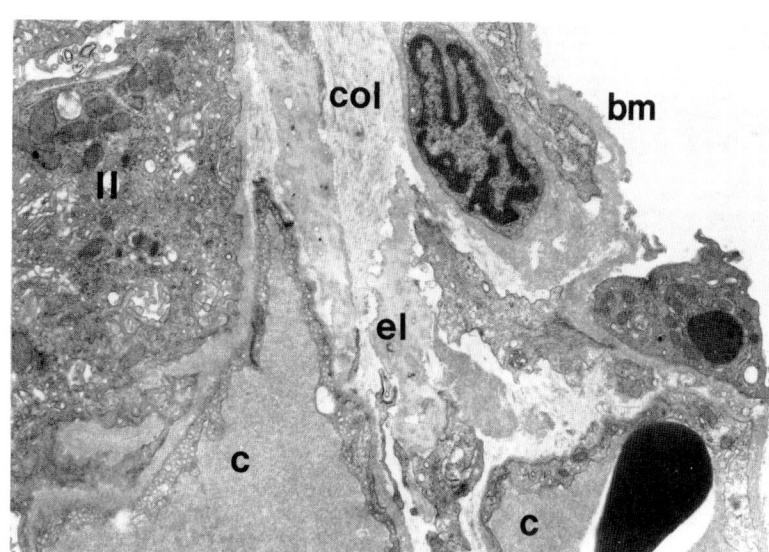

Fig. 18.13. The alveolar surface is partly denuded, with exposed basement membrane (*bm*), Interstitial cell processes are near the basal surface of the basement membrane and closely appose elastin (*el*) fragments. Collagenous (*col*) bundles in the interstitium are increased. Two intact capillaries (*c*) and hyperplastic type II pneumocytes are present.

(Fig. 18.16) and undergo autolysis. As these areas are well ventilated, rupture of their pleural surface gives rise to a tension pneumothorax and bronchopleural fistula. As lung disease advances a functional separation of airspace and vasculature becomes apparent and the normal circulatory response to large changes of airway pressure is blunted or entirely ablated [58]. Figure 18.17 shows no change of PAP in a patient with severe ARDS, despite increasing PEEP from 0 to 30 cmH_2O. This implies that airway pressure is no longer transmitted to the pulmonary vascular bed and large amounts of unventilated and shunting lung vasculature are available for perfusion.

A histologic feature of patients surviving severe ARDS is a greater proportion of spared regions of 'normal' lung. In contrast, dying patients show diffuse progression of disease within the entire lung.

The optimal therapy for late-stage ARDS with its profound derangement of oxygenation, CO_2 elimination, and pulmonary mechanics is disputed. The role of conventional, controlled MV with moderate (e.g., 15 cmH_2O) end-expiratory pressure, as against the use of intermittent mandatory ventilation with extremely high levels of end-expiratory pressure, high-frequency positive pressure ventilation, or extracorporeal membrane oxygenation for selected acute lung diseases still needs definition [59].

We believe it is unlikely that manipulation of MV patterns or temporary membrane lung perfusion will reverse the inexorable progression of lung disease and prevent death. It is our opinion that new therapies must be developed, to be administered in the earliest stages of acute lung disease to block the acute phase reactions, especially those that involve subsequent destruction of lung architecture. Improving our understanding of the basic pathophysiology of ARDS will point the way to such therapies, and possibly increase the survival rate of ARDS patients.

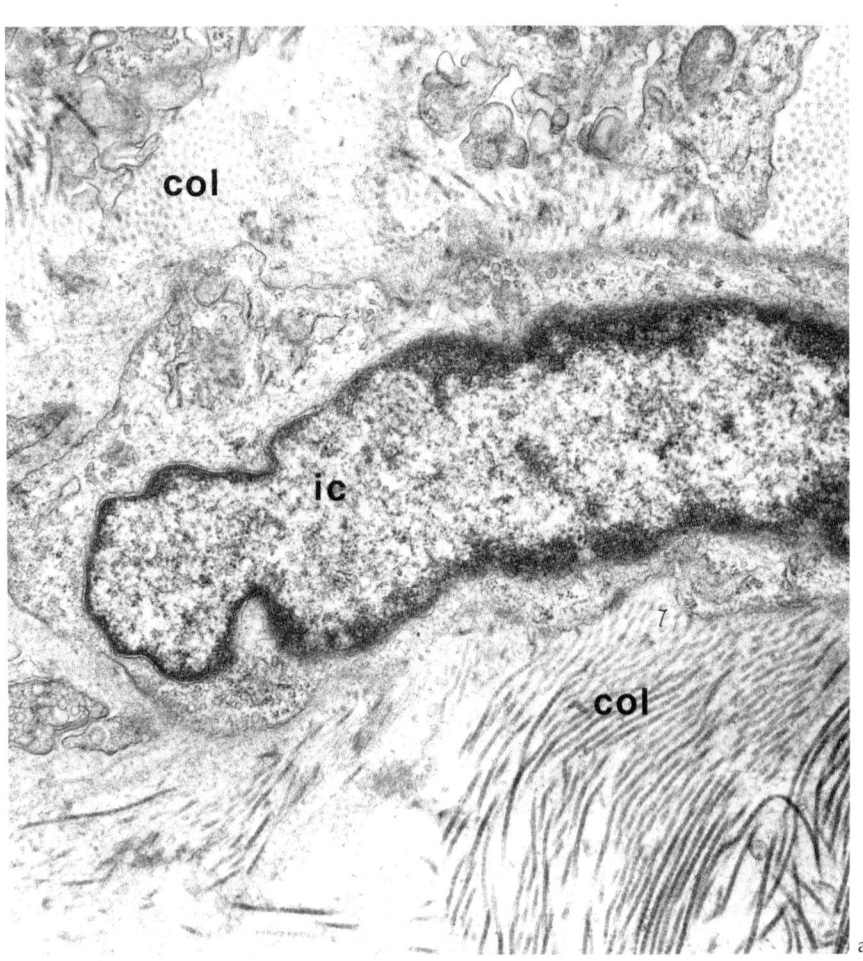

Fig. 18.14. a Interstitial cells (*ic*) with bundles of collagen (*col*) in longitudinal and cross section. ($\times$ 16 800)

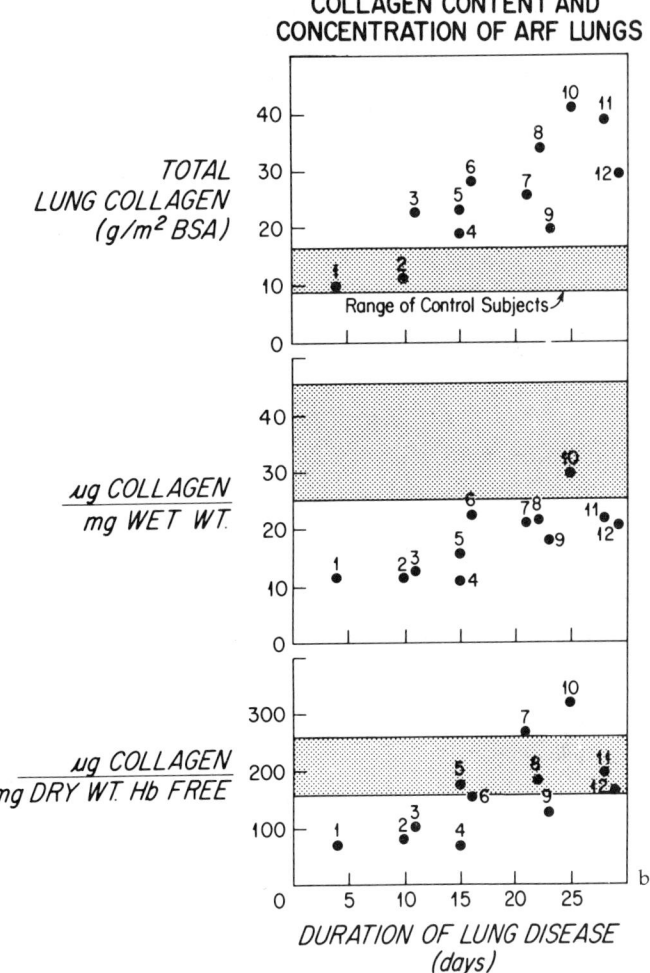

COLLAGEN CONTENT AND CONCENTRATION OF ARF LUNGS

TOTAL LUNG COLLAGEN (g/m² BSA)

µg COLLAGEN / mg WET WT.

µg COLLAGEN / mg DRY WT. Hb FREE

DURATION OF LUNG DISEASE (days)

Range of Control Subjects

Fig. 18.14. b Total collagen (g/m² body surface area [*BSA*], and collagen concentration in the lungs of patients at various times after the onset of ARF. Each point is the mean for a large number of post-mortem lung samples. The *shaded areas* encompass the mean values for nine normal lungs, whereas the numbers associated with the *closed circles* identify patients with ARF. *Hb*, hemoglobin [63].

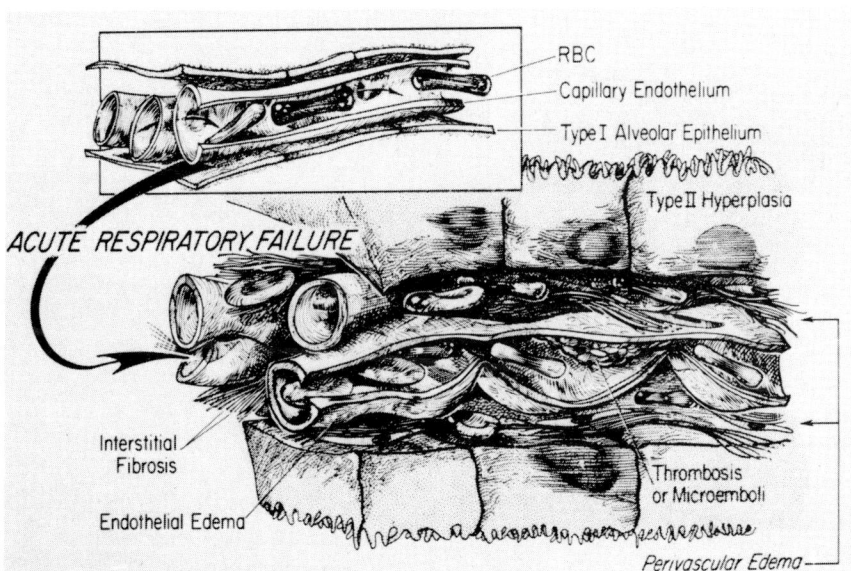

RBC
Capillary Endothelium
Type I Alveolar Epithelium
Type II Hyperplasia
ACUTE RESPIRATORY FAILURE
Interstitial Fibrosis
Endothelial Edema
Thrombosis or Microemboli
Perivascular Edema

Fig. 18.15. Pathologic alterations of lung structure in severe ARF with normal structure. Vascular occlusion by endothelial and interstitial edema, thrombosis, and microembolism is shown. Type II cell hyperplasia is prominent and increases the diffusion distance for respiratory gas exchange.

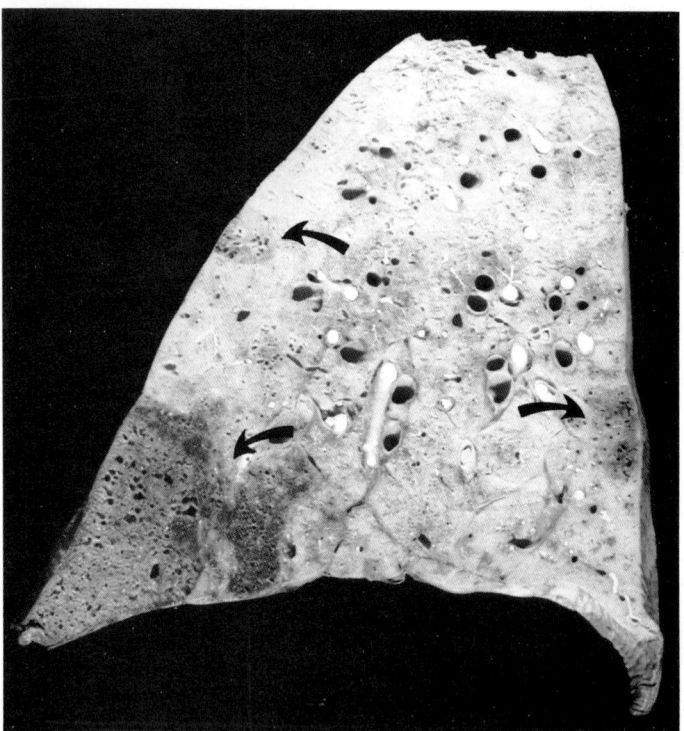

Fig. 18.16. Fixed post-mortem lung slice following 3 weeks of intensive care after amniotic fluid embolism. Vessels are filled by white silicone polymer. Regions of subpleural ischemic necrosis (*arrows*) are becoming cystic. Pleura at lower left ruptured, causing a bronchopleural fistula. Photograph courtesy of Dr. K. Kobayashi.

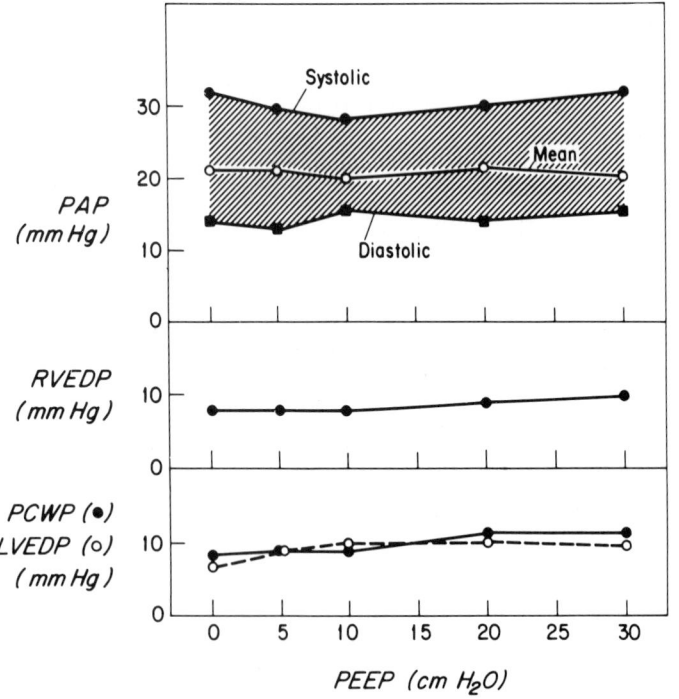

Fig. 18.17. PAP and PCWP, RV end-diastolic pressure (*RVEDP*) and LV end-diastolic pressure (*LVEDP*) as a function of PEEP during severe viral pneumonia. $\hat{C}_T$, total thoracic compliance [58]. Pulmonary and ventricular pressures are independent of PEEP; C_T, = 13 ml/cmH$_2$O.

References

1. Bachofen M, Weibel ER (1977) Alterations of the gas exchange apparatus in adult respiratory insufficiency associated with septicemia. Am Rev Respir Dis 116:589–61

2. Barratt-Boyes BG, Wood EH (1958) Cardiac output and related measurements and pressure values in the right heart and associated vessels, together with an analysis of the hemodynamic response to the inhalation of high oxygen mixtures in healthy subjects. J Lab Clin Med 51:72-90

3. Bayley T, Clements JA, Osbahr AJ (1967) Pulmonary and circulatory effects of fibrinopeptides. Circ Res 21:469–485

4. Benumof J (1979) Hypoxic vasoconstriction and infusion of sodium nitroprusside. Anesthesiology 50:481–483

5. Blaisdell FW, Lewis FR Jr (1977) Respiratory distress syndrome of shock and trauma, Vol XXI in the series Major problems in clinical surgery. Saunders, Philadelphia

6. Blake LH (1978) Mathematical modeling of steady state fluid and protein exchange in lung. In: Lung water and solute exchange. Marcel Dekker, New York, p 118

7. Bowers RE, Ellis EF, Brigham KL, Oates J (1979) Effects of prostaglandin cyclic endoperoxides on the lung circulation of unanesthetized sheep. J Clin Invest 63:131–137

8. Brigham KL, Woolverton WC, Blake LH, Staub NC (1974) Increased sheep lung vascular permeability caused by pseudomonas bacteremia. J Clin Invest 54:792-804

9. Brigham KL, Snell JD, Harris TR, Marshall S, Haynes J, Bowers RE, Perry J (1979) Indicator dilution lung water and vascular permeability in humans. Circ Res 44:523–530

10. Carvalho AC, Bellman S, Saullo J, Lauer J (1981) Factor VIII in adult respiratory distress syndrome. Am Rev Respir Dis 123:98

11. Colley PS, Cheney FW, Hlastala MP (1979) Ventilation-perfusion and gas exchange effects of sodium nitroprusside in dogs with normal and edematous lung. Anesthesiology 50:489–495

12. Cook JA, Wise WC, Halushka PV (1980) Elevated thromboxane levels in the rat during endotoxic shock. J Clin Invest 65:227–230

13. Craddock PR, Fehr J, Brigham KL, Kronenberg RS, Jacob HS (1977) Complement and leukocyte-mediated pulmonary dysfunction in hemodialysis. N Engl J Med 296:769–774

14. Deneke SM, Fanburg BL (1980) Normobaric oxygen toxicity of the lung. N Engl J Med 303:76–86

15. Eeles GH, Sevitt S (1967) Microthrombosis in injured and burned patients. J Pathol Bacteriol 93:275–293

16. Falke KJ, Pontoppidan H, Kumar A, Leith DE, Geffin B, Laver MB (1972) Ventilation with end expiratory pressure in acute lung disease. J Clin Invest 51:2315–2323

17. Fallat RJ, Lamy M, Koeninger E, Hill JD (1976) Use of physiologic and pathologic correlations in evaluating adult respiratory distress syndrome. In: Zapol WM, Qvist J (eds) Artificial lungs for acute respiratory failure. Academic Press, New York, pp 391–404

18. Fountain SW, Martin BA, Musclow CE, Cooper JD (1980) Pulmonary leukostasis and its relationship to pulmonary dysfunction in sheep and rabbits. Circ Res 46:175–180

19. Grant K, Rodvien R, Mielke CH (1978) Altered factor VIII complexes in patients with acute respiratory insufficiency. Thromb Haemost 40:326–334

20. Greene R, Zapol WM, Snider MT, Reid LM, Snow R, O'Connell R, Novelline RA (1981) Early bedside angiographic diagnosis of pulmonary vascular occlusion during acute respiratory failure. Am Rev Resp Dis (in press)

21. Hemmer M, Suter PM (1979) Treatment of cardiac and renal effects of PEEP with dopamine in patients with acute respiratory failure. Anesthesiology 50:399–403

22. Hill JD, Ratliff JL, Parrott JCW, Lamy M, Fallat RJ, Koeniger E, Yaeger EM, Whitmer G (1976) Pulmonary pathology in acute respiratory insufficiency: Lung biopsy as a diagnostic tool. J Thorac Cardiovasc Surg 71:64–71

23. Hill JD, Rodvien R, Snider MT, Bartlett RH (1978) State of the Art Address: Clinical extracorporeal membrane oxygenation for acute respiratory insufficiency. Trans Am Soc Artif Intern Organs 24:753–763

24. Hopewell PC, Murray JF (1976) Effects of continuous positive-pressure ventilation in experimental pulmonary edema. J Appl Physiol 40:568–574

25. Huchon GJ, Hopewell PC, Murray JF (1980) Interaction between increased permeability and increased hydrostatic pressure on water and blood contents in dog lungs. Am Rev Respir Dis 121:435

26. Jardin F, Eveleigh MC, Gurdjian F, Delille F, Margairaz A (1979) Venous admixture in human septic shock: Comparative effects of blood volume expansion, dopamine infusion and is isoproterenol infusion on mismatching of ventilation and pulmonary blood flow in peritonitis. Circulation 60:155-159

27. Kadowitz PJ, Capnick BM, Feigen LP, Hyman AL, Nelson PK, Spannhake EW (1978) Pulmonary and systemic vasodilator effects of the newly discovered prostaglandin PGI_2. J Appl Physiol 45:408–413

28. Lamy M, Fallat RJ, Koeniger E, Dietrich H-P, Ratliff JL, Eberhart RC, Tucker HJ, Hill JD (1976) Pathologic features and mechanisms of hypoxemia in adult respiratory distress syndrome. Am Rev Respir Dis 114:267–284

29. Lemaire F, Harari A, Rapin M, Jardin F, Teisseire B, Laurent D (1976) Assessment of gas exchange during venoarterial bypass using the membrane lung. In: Zapol WM, Qvist J (eds) Artificial lungs for acute respiratory failure. Academic Press, New York, pp 421–433

30. Lemaire F, Gastinne H, Regnier B, Teisseire B, Rapin M (1978a) Perfusion changes modify intrapulmonary shunt Q_S/Q_T in patients with ARDS. Am Rev Respir Dis 117:144

31. Lemaire F, Jardin F, Regnier B, Loisance D, Goudot B, Lange F, Eveleigh MC, Teisseire B, Laurent D, Rapin M (1978b) Pulmonary gas exchange during venoarterial bypass with a membrane lung for acute respiratory failure. J Thorac Cardiovasc Surg 75:839–846

32. Lemaire F, Regnier B, Simoneau G, Harf A (1980) PEEP suppresses the increase of shunting caused by dopamine infusion. Anesthesiology 52:376–377

33. Lynch JP, Mhyre JG, Dantzker DR (1979) The influence of cardiac output on intrapulmonary shunt. J Appl Physiol 46:315–321

34. Malo J, Ali J, Duke K, Gallagher W, Wood LDH (1980) How does PEEP reduce $\dot{Q}_S/\dot{Q}_T$ in pulmonary edema. Fed Proc 39:280

35. Martyn JAJ, Snider MT, Szyfelbein SK, Burke JF, Laver MB (1980) Right ventricular dysfunction following acute thermal injury. Ann Surg 191:330–335

36. Meignan M, George C, Lemaire F (1978) Extravascular lung water during acute respiratory distress syndrome in adults. Bull Eur Physiopathol Respir 14:617–628

37. Moncada S, Vane JR (1979) Arachidonic acid metabolites and the interactions between platelets and blood-vessel walls. N Engl J Med 300:1142–1147

38. Murray JF (1976) The normal lung: The basis for diagnosis and treatment of pulmonary disease. Saunders, Philadelphia

39. Murray JF (1977) Conference report: Mechanisms of acute respiratory failure. (National Heart, Lung, and Blood Institute) Am Rev Respir Dis 115:1071–1078

40. National Heart, Lung, and Blood Institute, Division of Lung Diseases (1979) Extracorporeal support for respiratory insufficiency: A collaborative study. National Institutes of Health, Bethesda

41. National Heart and Lung Institute, Lung Program (1972) Respiratory diseases task force report on problems, research, approaches and needs. National Institutes of Health, Bethesda (DHEW publication no. 73–432)

42. Nellems JM, Cooper JD, Henderson RD, Peng T, Phillips MJ (1976) Emergency open lung biopsy. Ann Thorac Surg 22:260–264

43. Pontoppidan H, Geffin B, Lowenstein E (1973) Acute respiratory failure in the adult. Little Brown, Boston

44. Pontoppidan H, Wilson RS, Rie MA, Schneider RC (1977) Respiratory intensive care. Anesthesiology 47:96–116

45. Pratt PC, Vollmer RT, Shelburne JD, Crapo JB (1979) Pulmonary morphology in a multihospital collaborative extracorporeal membrane oxygenation project. I. light microscopy. Am J Pathol 95:191–214

46. Regnier B, Rapin M, Gory G, Lemaire F, Teisseire B, Harari A (1977) Hemodynamic effects of dopamine in septic shock. Intensive Care Med 3:47–53

47. Regnier B, Safran D, Carlet J, Teisseire B (1979) Comparative haemodynamic effects of dopamine and dobutamine in septic shock. Intensive Care Med 5:115–120

48. Robin E, Thomas ED (1954) Some relations between pulmonary edema and pulmonary inflammation. Arch Intern Med 93:713–724

49. Saldeen T (1979) The microembolism syndrome, a review. In: Saldeen T (ed) The microembolism syndrome. Almqvist Wiksell International, Stockholm, pp 7–44

50. Schneider R, Zapol WM, Carvalho A (1980) Platelet consumption and sequestration in severe acute respiratory failure. Am Rev Respir Dis 122:445-451

51. Snider MT, Zapol WM (1976) Assessment of pulmonary oxygenation during venoarterial bypass with aortic root returns. In: Zapol WM, Qvist J (eds) Artificial lungs for acute respiratory failure. Academic Press, New York, pp 251–274

52. Snider MT, Rie MA, Bingham JB, Lauer J, Urbina A, Strauss HW (1980a) Right ventricular performance in ARDS: Radionuclide scintiscan and thermal dilution studies. Am Rev Respir Dis 121:192

53. Snider MT, Rie MA, Lauer J, Zapol WM (1980b) Normoxic pulmonary vasoconstriction in ARDS: Detection by sodium nitroprusside and isoproterenol infusions. Am Rev Respir Dis 121:191

54. Snow RL, Zapol WM, Reid LM (1980) Morphology of the pulmonary circulation in adult respiratory distress syndrome. Am Rev Respir Dis 121:192

55. Suter PM, Fairley HB, Schlobohm RM (1975) Shunt, lung volume and perfusion during short periods of ventilation with oxygen. Anesthesiology 43:617–627

56. Watkins WD, Peterson MB, Crone RK, Shannon DC, Levine L (1980) Prostacyclin and prostaglandin E_1 for severe idiopathic pulmonary artery hypertension. Letter to the Editor. Lancet I:1083

57. West J (1977) Pulmonary pathophysiology: The essentials. Williams & Wilkins, Baltimore

58. Zapol WM, Snider MT (1977) Pulmonary hypertension in severe acute respiratory failure. N Engl J Med 296:476–480

59. Zapol WM, Snider MT (1980) Membrane lungs for acute respiratory failure: Current status. Editorial/Am Rev Respir Dis 121:907–909

60. Zapol WM, Snider MT, Schneider RC, Rie MA (1976) Pulmonary hypertension in severe acute respiratory failure. In: Zapol WM, Qvist J (eds) Artificial lungs for acute respiratory failure: Theory and practice. Academic Press, New York, pp 435–454

61. Zapol WM, Kobayashi K, Snider MT, Greene R, Laver MB (1977) Vascular obstruction causes pulmonary hypertension in severe acute respiratory failure. Chest 71 [S]:306S–307S

62. Zapol WM, Trelstad RL, Coffey JW, Tsai I, Salvador RA (1979) Pulmonary fibrosis in severe acute respiratory failure. Am Rev Respir Dis 119:547–554

63. Zapol WM, Peterson MB, Wonders T, Kong D, Watkins WD (1980) Plasma thromboxane and prostaglandin metabolites in sheep partial cardiopulmonary bypass. Trans Am Soc Artif Intern Organs 26:556–559

Chapter 19

Severe Asthma

A. De Coster, R. Naeije, and A. Cornil

The pathophysiology of respiratory failure has been widely investigated for many years and the therapeutic procedures related to intensive care in respiratory failure are well known. Consequently there is a great deal of information and results of MV in many patients with both acute and chronic respiratory failure are available. By contrast much less is known of the pathophysiology of severe asthma and its treatment.

Definition and classification

Asthma may be defined as an acute attack of shortness of breath, induced by a variety of agents or by exercise, and accompanied by clinical signs of bronchial obstruction which are totally or partially reversible. It corresponds with a sudden increase of airways resistance of immunological or non-immunological origin [54b].

Severe asthma is more difficult to define and the term 'status asthmaticus' is frequently used [28]. This has been defined by the American Thoracic Society as 'an acute asthmatic attack in which the degree of bronchial obstruction is either severe from the beginning or increases in severity and is not relieved by the usual treatment such as epinephrine or aminophylline' [9]. Several workers have attempted to quantify the degree of severity. Bellamy [4] uses the severity

of the airflow obstruction and its failure to respond to bronchodilator treatment; the refractoriness to some of the commonly used drugs is also highlighted by Hugh-Jones [28]. Whilst resistance to therapy is found in many cases it is not common to all, for refractoriness to treatment and severe asthma are not always associated. Other authors [32, 48] have used descriptive clinical terms such as 'an asthmatic attack', 'patient too dyspnoeic to speak', or 'patient confined to chair or bed by dyspnoea'. However, even in such circumstances, bronchospasm may disappear with adequate treatment, so that intensive therapy is not necessary. This is also true for those patients who are unable to perform a forced expiratory manoeuvre to test the severity, as proposed by Franklin [19].

The intensity of dyspnoea, because it is difficult to evaluate, is not a good test. It is also unpredictable: a severe attack may last for several days but then respond perfectly well to another drug, or even stop only when the patient is admitted to hospital.

We feel that patients with severe asthma can be classified into three groups.

1) *Group I*: Patients who are in coma
2) *Group II*: Patients who are disorientated, drowsy, or agitated because of hypoxia and perhaps hypercapnia
3) *Group III*: Patients who remain conscious but who are completely exhausted by their attack and have not responded to treatment for several days.

Criteria for diagnosis

Clinical features

History

The diagnosis of acute respiratory failure in relation to hypoxia and hypercapnia is usually easy, although it must always be confirmed by arterial blood gas analysis. It is also important to obtain details of any relevant past history (allergies; results of previous skin tests or RAST [radio-allergo-solvent test]) to identify the presence of any recent bacterial or viral respiratory infection, and to know which drugs have been used, especially the type and dose of sympathomimetic agents used in the previous days or hours.

The onset of bronchial obstruction may sometimes be very sudden in an atopic subject exposed to a high concentration of antigen.

Physical findings

In addition to the mental disturbances previously mentioned, the patients may have signs of hypercapnia: profuse sweating, peripheral vasodilatation, arterial hypertension, or sometimes hypotension. Tachycardia is a constant feature and heart rates of 140–160 beats/min are not unusual. In patients who are exhausted, dyspnoea is usually extreme and they are unable to speak, sleep, eat, or even drink. The combination of sweating and reduced fluid intake may lead to significant hypovolaemia. Wheezing is usually obvious and breath sounds are diminished over both lungs, so that sometimes a pneumothorax may be misdiagnosed or, if present, not recognized. There is also an excessive use of the accessory respiratory muscles with indrawing of the lower ribs, in relation to the low position of the diaphragm.

Pulsus paradoxus has been proposed as an indicator of severity, but it is not easy to measure and is only present if there are variations of more than 10 mmHg in systolic pressure [11, 35]. It will be present in 70% of the patients in whom the peak expiratory flow is less than 30% and in all patients in whom the FEV_1 is less than 20% of the theoretical values [54]. However, pulsus paradoxus may also be influenced by the inspiratory flow rate; for the same tidal volume the systolic variations of arterial pressure are greater when the inspiratory time is shorter. It may also occur in severe emphysema, so that it is not necessarily related to the severity of asthma and it is therefore not always a reliable guide.

Radiology

In acute asthma, signs of overinflation of the lungs are frequent (hyperlucency of the parenchyma, horizontal ribs, and flat diaphragm). Indeed, in extreme cases it may be difficult to differentiate the features from those of bilateral pneumothorax without a shift of the mediastinum.

Biochemistry

Hypovolaemia may be suspected if there is an increase in plasma protein content and haematocrit [68]. Hypokalaemia, if present, may be a consequence of previous corticosteroid treatment.

The most important features, however, are changes in the PaO_2 and acid–base balance. It is well known that in asthma hypoxaemia, slight or severe, is usually present because of pulmonary ventilation–perfusion imbalance. In some series [43, 54], hypoxaemia was present in 90–100% of cases, and in our series of 33 patients the values for PaO_2 were between 32 and 75 mmHg (4.3–10 kPa). In moribund patients they are usually very low, in the order of 30–40 mmHg (4.0–5.3 kPa).

It is generally considered that in asthma there is a low $PaCO_2$ and a respiratory alkalosis. However, in severe cases there is an increase of $PaCO_2$, often marked, and in our experience only in exhausted patients does the $PaCO_2$ actually remain normal.

It is widely agreed that an increased $PaCO_2$ developing during an asthmatic attack indicates a poor prognosis [7, 46, 49, 61], the mortality being very high in such patients [7, 48, 49, 54]. The acid–base balance of some of our patients is shown in a diagram published by Davenport (Fig. 19.1), and it is apparent that in most cases the acidosis has both respiratory and metabolic components. The reported frequency of metabolic acidosis, which is usually a lactic acidosis [17, 39] varies in different series: 50% in the series of Jardin [31], 14% in that of Roncoroni [57]. It has been reported by others, but only in a few cases [34, 55, 64]. Its mechanism remains obscure. Hypoxaemia is probably not responsible, in patients with chronic respiratory insufficiency when breathing low O_2 mixtures there is no significant increase in lactate and, on the other hand, breathing pure O_2 does not de-

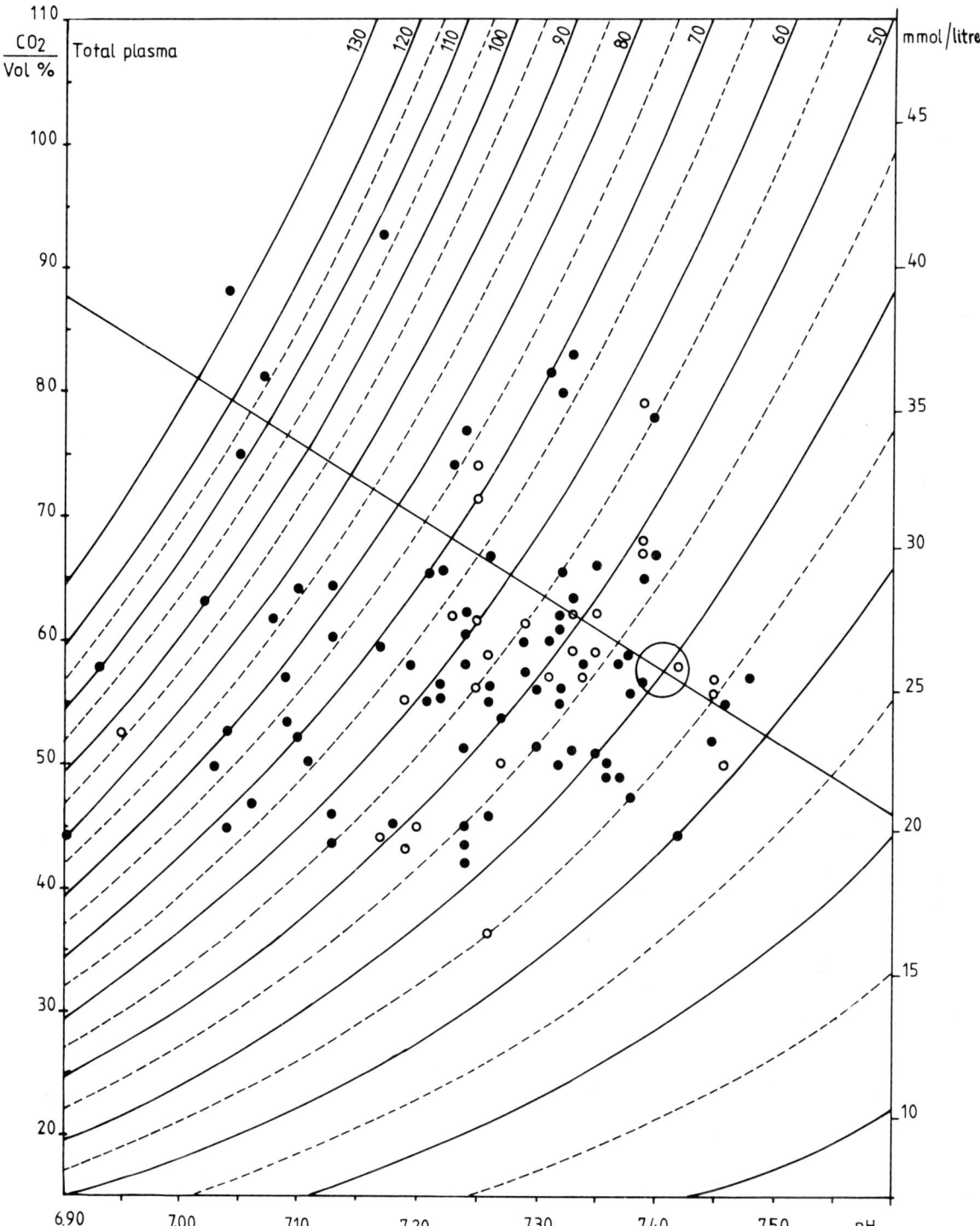

Fig. 19.1. Acid–base balance in severe asthma.

crease the slightly elevated levels of lactate in such patients [17]. Starvation can also be excluded because ketosis is not frequent and when present, disappears rapidly with glucose infusions without parallel correction of the acidosis. Other factors that might be incriminated are a decreased lactate uptake by the liver, peripheral circulatory failure and the presence of increased levels of circulating catecholamines.

Electrocardiogram

Sinus tachycardia is a very frequent finding and ST-T wave changes are common. P pulmonale may appear in leads II or III and there may be right axis deviation [1, 62].

In a number of patients atrial and ventricular ectopic beats, and occasionally more severe arrhythmias, may occur. Usually these abnormalities disappear as the asthmatic attack improves.

Precipitating factors

It is difficult to analyse and define the factors which are really responsible for the sudden onset of an asthmatic crisis or for the progressive deterioration of an episode of bronchospasm.

In about 50% of patients a viral or bacterial infection of the upper respiratory tract or bronchi may be found [4]. Alterations in treatment, such as the sudden interruption, or reduction, of corticosteroids, overdosage of sedatives, and abuse of bronchodilators, may all be responsible for a worsening clinical situation, and it must be remembered that some therapeutic procedures are not without danger. A severe attack may follow desensitization procedures, skin testing, or provocation tests with grass pollen. In some cases, the induction of anaesthesia with certain drugs may induce an acute episode of bronchial obstruction [72]. As in many other conditions it is always difficult to appreciate the role of psychological factors in the onset of a severe asthmatic attack. Table 19.1 summarizes some factors that might be involved [4, 7, 76].

Table 19.1 Precipitating factors in 127 patients with severe asthma

Factor	No. of cases
Upper respiratory tract infection	41
Excessive use of sympathomimetic aerosols	20
Psychological factors	8
Desensitizing vaccine	5
Interruption of corticosteroid therapy	3
Skin test	2
Beta-blocking drugs	2
Dust	2
Provocative test	1
Printing ink	1
Hair lotion or dye	1
Bronchography	1
Sedative overdosage (diazepam)	1
Unknown	39

Pathophysiology

Airway resistance

The primary factor in asthma is an increase of airways resistance; this is due to three main factors that vary in importance from one case to another:

Oedema of the bronchial mucosa, which may be accompanied by interstitial oedema, is secondary to liberation of histamine from the mast cells. In severe cases, degranulated mast cells can be seen in the alveoli; the basement membranes may be thickened and an increase of capillary permeability may be suspected [18].

Increase in tone of the bronchial muscles, which may also be hypertrophied. These muscles, together with their sympathetic innervation, play a dominant role in the onset of bronchial obstruction.

Mucous plugs both in the bronchi and in the small airways are also important These plugs are thick, inspissated, and tenacious, and are very difficult to remove even at autopsy. When they are wide-spread gas exchange is severely affected and asphyxia occurs.

The increase in airways resistance has important effects on both the mechanical aspects of respiration and gas exchange.

Respiratory mechanics

During an attack of asthma, the airway obstruction is manifest in a marked decrease of forced expiratory flow and a large increase in airway resistance. There are also modifications of lung volumes with a pronounced decrease in vital capacity, an increase of functional residual capacity, and sometimes an enormous increase of total lung capacity (up to 200% of the predicted value in a few cases) [27, 80]; a finding that is in agreement with the radiological appearances. These changes all relate to a modification of the elastic properties of the lungs; the pressure–volume curve is shifted upwards and to the left [40, 51, 80] and the maximal static intrapleural pressure is markedly decreased [80]. The cause of these modifications of the elastic properties of the lungs is still a matter of discussion [40, 51, 80].

During an asthmatic attack the patient breathes at a high lung volume, and whilst this increases the work of breathing, it also serves to keep the airways open. A very high negative intrapleural pressure may develop during inspiration with a positive pressure at the end of expiration. There are therefore wide swings of intrapleural pressure with a mean negative pressure [2, 73].

Disturbances in ventilation and perfusion

Because the airway obstruction is not uniform, some regions of the lungs are better ventilated than others and perfusion is not exactly adapted to the ventilation. Studies with inhaled and injected isotopes have clearly demonstrated a $\dot{V}/\dot{Q}$ imbalance, which may explain the shunt effects responsible for moderate to severe hypoxaemia [28, 75]. Airway closure at low lung volume may enhance the shunt effect.

Finally, if the obstruction becomes severe and widespread throughout both lungs alveolar hypoventilation occurs, leading to hypoxaemia and hypercapnia.

Pulmonary haemodynamics

In the few studies available on pulmonary haemodynamics in acute asthma, a normal cardiac output and a normal or only slightly increased PAP have been reported [22, 23, 25, 26, 74, 81]. This was at first somewhat unexpected in view of the frequent ECG changes that suggested right heart strain. It was especially puzzling to find patients with a P pulmonale and normal PVR. Recent investigations on the interrelationships between the mechanics of breathing and pulmonary haemodynamics have, however, clarified these observations. In the interpretation of cardiac catheterization measurements, it has to be remembered that the heart and intrathoracic vessels are exposed to the intrathoracic pressure rather than to the atmospheric pressure, which is taken as the zero reference level. During an acute asthmatic attack, markedly negative intrapleural pressures with large lung volumes have to be developed to overcome the tendency to small airway closure [73]. Since the mean intrapleural pressure remains markedly negative [66], the transmural pressures across the heart and intrathoracic vessels are increased. Moreover, because of air trapping during expiration, the alveolar and airway pressures become higher than the pleural pressure, necessitating a still higher PAP to propel blood through the lungs. The net result of these forces is an increased PVR, marked strain on both right and left ventricles, and pulsus paradoxus [66, 73].

Treatment

All patients with the features of severe asthma, as previously defined, must be admitted immediately to an ICU.

General measures

Oxygen therapy

Since many of these patients are hypoxaemic and hypercapnic, O_2 must always be given; because of the hypercapnia it may be necessary to administer it at a low flow rate.

Fluid and electrolyte balance

Decrease of fluid intake, sweating, and hyperventilation lead to a marked water deficit, which will be further increased by the work of breathing and the presence of fever, possibly due to a respiratory infection (56). Adequate water and electrolyte replacement are essential and proper hydration may also decrease the viscosity of the mucous plugs. When hypovolaemia leads to circulatory failure plasma expanders will be required [79] (Chap. 32).

Correction of a metabolic acidosis

In cases where the metabolic component of acidosis is judged to be important, infusion of sodium bicarbonate has been proposed [7, 8, 45], but it is important to recognize that the CO_2 resulting from the combination of sodium bicarbonate with an acid has to be eliminated via the lungs, which is difficult in patients with severe respiratory failure [45]. We feel that sodium bicarbonate, or other buffers, are hardly ever indicated in severe asthma, except in the aftermath of a cardiac arrest. Correction of metabolic acidosis has been described in adults, but is more frequent in children.

Specific measures

The three main factors responsible for hypoxaemia and hypercapnia, namely contraction of the bronchial muscles, oedema of the bronchial mucosa and the presence of mucous plugs, are the objects of specific therapeutic measures.

Pharmacological treatment

This whole problem has been comprehensively discussed recently by Paterson and co-workers

[50]. Both adrenergic and cholinergic mechanisms are involved in the control of bronchial muscle tone. The role of the cholinergic system is well known to be stimulation of the vagus nerve inducing bronchoconstriction and, in practice, atropine and its derivatives have been used for many years to block the effect. The adrenergic regulatory mechanism is more complex. The role of the alpha receptors in man is questionable, whereas the beta receptors play an important role and research efforts are directed at the development of drugs with a selective beta-2 action on bronchial smooth muscle.

At the cellular level, an increase of cAMP is accompanied by bronchodilatation and the role of different drugs to produce this is well known [73].

Bronchodilators may be administered by aerosol (wet or dry), by mouth, or by a parenteral route. In the critically ill patient, a very rapid effect is needed and the IV route is preferred for the rapid relief of the bronchospasm, although it is associated with side-effects. Aerosols are completely ineffective because the very sick patient is unable to use them correctly. In severe cases, the use of IPPV has been advocated for administration of an aerosol, but the results are not convincing [77].

Adrenaline has been widely used in the past but when given IV it produces side-effects related to its sympathetic stimulation. However, it is a rapid and powerful bronchodilator which may sometimes relieve otherwise intractable bronchospasm. The usual dosage is 0.3–0.5 mg IM or SC in aqueous solution. Labrousse et al. [37] administer it IV in a dosage of 0.05–0.3 mg over 1 min, followed by an infusion at 4–8 μg/min for 1 or 2 days.

Isoprenaline was used until fairly recently, mostly in children. Parry [49], in a well-documented study, treated 34 children with severe asthma, isoprenaline being infused at a constant rate of 0.1 μg/kg/min. The infusion was maintained for several hours and produced a favourable response in 27 cases. However, this drug causes a tachycardia that is much more pronounced than that caused by more selective drugs, such as salbutamol [65]. Simpson [65] regards the use of isoprenaline as the last effort before MV is considered.

'Selective' beta-2 agonists. A selective bronchial beta-2 agonist does not yet exist, but there are a number of drugs that are more 'effective' on bronchial muscle although they do have effects on beta-2 receptors elsewhere. The bronchodilator effect of these drugs is well established and their use in critically ill patients can be recommended; the cardiac effects occur at doses some three to six times higher than those at which bronchodilatation occurs, so that their adverse cardiovascular effects are much lower than those of adrenaline or isoprenaline [77].

Salbutamol can be given by IV administration at a dose of 200 μg over 10 min; it causes tachycardia but this is less pronounced than that caused by isoprenaline [77].

Alpha-adrenergic blocking drugs. The role of alpha receptors in the human bronchial tree is not very important, and adrenergic antagonists such as phentolamine have only a small bronchodilator effect though they may potentiate the effect of beta-2 stimulants. For this reason, the use of phentolamine aerosols in cases of severe asthma has been proposed by Marcelle [41], but has not gained acceptance.

Theophylline is an alkaloid in the family of xanthines, and also acts on the nervous system, the kidney, and the heart. It inhibits phosphodiesterase, increasing the level of cAMP and relaxing smooth muscle tone, the desired effect in patients with bronchial asthma. However, the optimal use of theophylline may be difficult and it is worth noting, initially, that different preparations of theophylline contain different amounts of the active drug. Recent studies have also focused attention on a number of conditions that may interfere with its metabolism [36, 44]. Smoking increases the metabolism of the drug, whilst hepatic cirrhosis, heart failure, and severe airways obstruction decrease its elimination [52]. Side-effects may be severe, and include nausea, vomiting, insomnia, and seizures. Cardiovascular effects such as tachycardia and arrhythmias may also occur [5, 10]. The optimal therapeutic level of theophylline is between 10 and 20 μg/ml [70], which is not far removed from its toxic level.

Measurements of plasma theophylline levels are regarded as essential by some workers to control its administration [36]. Powell [52] recommends that the first measurement should be made approximately 24 h after the start of treatment. Unfortunately, however, the measurements are not easy and only a few laboratories are able to do them on a routine basis. For that reason, empirical schemes have been established. The nomogram of Jusko [33] is based on body weight, cardiac and hepatic function, and any previous administration of theophylline; it is claimed that this enables an optimal therapeutic level of the drug to be attained in 72% of cases.

From a practical point of view, in severe asthma, it is appropriate to give an initial loading dose of theophylline of 6 mg/kg, infused over 20 min. This is followed by a continuous infusion of 0.9 mg/kg/h. Good results may also be obtained by the intermittent administration of 4 mg/kg over 20 min every 4 h.

If these guidelines are followed, theophylline has a very good bronchodilator effect. Increases in heart rate may be observed, and a paradoxical decrease of PaO_2 due to an increase of ventilation/perfusion disturbances [47] has frequently been reported. Therefore, it must always be given together with O_2 therapy.

Combination of theophylline and beta-2 agonists has been recently reviewed by Paterson [50]. From a clinical point of view the problem is very difficult, because asthma is never a stable disease and it is extremely difficult to appreciate the properties of different beta-2 agonists in clinical trials, let alone demonstrate additive or synergistic effects. Also in severe asthma, when only IV agents are used the clinician often makes his choice on the basis of past treatment.

Corticosteroids have been used for many years in the treatment of asthma, but even now we are ignorant of their mechanisms of action [13]. Hydrocortisone increases the level of cAMP in leucocytes and lymphocytes of normal as well as asthmatic subjects. Corticosteroids have no effect on type I IgE-mediated reactions, but the delayed response is suppressed. This means that the time needed to obtain a beneficial effect is in the order of several hours. They also have well known anti-inflammatory properties and enhance cellular sensitivity to catecholamines, so that a single injection of corticosteroids will restore the responsiveness of the bronchial tree to isoprenaline [60]. It has also been demonstrated that the dosage of corticosteroids required to produce a beneficial effect is independent of the pre-existing level of cortisol, which may be low in patients who have previously been treated for a long time.

The best route for administration is IV, in a dose of 4 mg hydrocortisone/kg body wt. given every 4–6 h [13], the total dosage being approximately 1 g/24. As previously mentioned, the maximum effect is obtained after 6–8 h, with bronchodilatation starting after 2–3 h. This implies that hydrocortisone is never a drug of 'primary emergency,' but must be considered more as a drug to counteract 'the steady-state period of airways obstruction'.

Intravenous prednisolone or methylprednisolone may be preferred to hydrocortisone, because of their less potent salt-retaining activity.

Resistance to bronchodilating drugs. The 'paradoxical' effect of adrenaline has been recognized for a long time, and earlier clinicians observed in cases of severe asthma that repeated administration of adrenaline, the only drug then available, could induce bronchoconstriction instead of decreasng airways resistance. More recently, an increase in the number of deaths in asthmatic patients was observed in the United Kingdom but not in the United States; it was attributed to the sale of aerosols containing high doses of isoprenaline [67].

On the other hand, the regular use of beta-2 bronchodilators in 'physiological doses' is not accompanied by a decrease of efficacy; studies have shown that there is the same response to salbutamol before and after 1 month of its regular use [24]. There is no doubt that some patients may inhale an enormous amount of beta-2 agonist (one bottle of salbutamol in 1 day), well above physiological doses, without any improvement of bronchial obstruction but, on the contrary, with a progressive worsening of the bronchospasm. Rebound of bronchoconstriction may also be seen after injection of isoprenaline [50].

Clinically, therefore, resistance does exist but its mechanism has not been established. It has been postulated that acidosis decreases the response to adrenaline, but this is certainly not always the case, and infusions of sodium bicarbonate to restore a more physiological pH do not always improve the efficacy of beta-2 stimulants [64]. Release of other mediators which overcome the bronchodilator effect of adrenaline has been postulated but not demonstrated [20]. The most widely accepted hypothesis is a progressive decrease in the number of beta-receptor sites on the cell membranes [69]. This has been demonstrated by the studies on white blood cells of both normal and asthmatic subjects; there is also a decrease in the production of cAMP after incubation of the cells with isoprenaline or salbutamol [21]. Increasing tolerance leads to increased dosages of beta-2 stimulants, and eventually any benefit is overshadowed by their side-effects. At this stage the drugs must be completely stopped and replaced with corticosteroids.

Bronchial lavage

Mucous plugs impair alveolar ventilation, and Ramirez et al. [53] have proposed the sophisticated technique of bronchial lavage, derived from that used with success for alveolar proteinosis. After general anaesthesia, the patient was intubated with a Carlens tube and one lung ventilated with pure O_2 whilst the other was successively filled with saline and emptied. During the procedure, hypoxaemia was aggravated and $PaCO_2$ rose. However, no deleterious cardiovascular effects were reported.

Removal of plugs through a rigid or flexible bronchoscope may also be attempted, and different lavage fluids have been proposed [6, 53, 61]. Such procedures are not without danger, however; they regularly aggravate hypoxaemia, may produce acid–base disturbances, and necessitate a general or local anaesthetic, which may induce severe bronchospasm. Certain of the drugs used in the lavage fluid, such as acetylcysteine, may irritate the bronchial mucosa when administered topically, and it is not always easy to remove the total quantity of liquid that is injected. It is also fair to say that the procedure has been declared successful by some authors who have used it in patients who were not always seriously ill [6, 53]. It is therefore our opinion that bronchial lavage should not be used in severe asthma.

Physiotherapy

Active physiotherapy (Chap. 22) is required as soon as possible. Relaxation of muscles, quiet diaphragmatic breathing, and clapping to free bronchial casts, followed by coughing, are all essential and must be repeated several times a day.

Mechanical ventilation

Intubation and MV (IPPV) are seldom required in severe asthma. It was necessary in only 0.3% of all admissions for asthma in a general hospital [76]. However, it can be a life-saving procedure in patients who are in extremis on admission, or whose condition is deteriorating in spite of optimal medical treatment [2, 76].

Youth, a long history of asthma, previous admissions for status asthmaticus, and attacks that have lasted for more than 24 h (up to weeks) at the time of hospitalization are characteristics shared by patients who will need IPPV or who otherwise will die from asthma [30, 42, 76]. The clinical identification of high-risk patients is certainly difficult, and in patients admitted to hospital the assessment of severity is commonly inadequate, even when made by experienced physicians [37a].

Accepted indications for IPPV are: respiratory arrest, exhaustion, deterioration in mental status, and increased $PaCO_2$ to values above 60–70 mmHg (8–9.3 kPa). When IPPV has to be instituted, the largest possible endotracheal tube should be used. Small tubes (less than 8 mm in diameter) increase airways resistance, make suction more difficult, and may easily become plugged with thick mucus. The nasotracheal route is preferred if possible, because of positional stability and comfort. Sedation will often be required because of intense agitation and maladaptation to the respirator. Histamine-releasing drugs such as morphine and meperidine are best avoided; a suitable regimen is diazepam in combination, if necessary, with pancuronium bromide [58].

A volume-cycled ventilator must be used to ensure a constant tidal volume. With the advent of modern techniques of respiratory monitoring, it has recently been recognized that IPPV in the presence of increased airways resistance may considerably increase the end-expiratory lung volume [38, 71]. This aggravates the overdistension of the lungs, with unfavourable haemodynamic effects and an augmented risk of alveolar rupture [38]. During IPPV, expiration is a passive phenomenon, and in asthmatic patients airways resistance rises to the extent that the time needed for expiration is greatly prolonged. Therefore, slow respiratory rates must be used, sometimes as low as 10/min [58, 71], when it becomes difficult to maintain an acceptable alveolar ventilation. However, in our experience, a moderate degree of hypercapnia can be tolerated if arterial oxygenation is maintained at levels that permit normal O_2 transport to the tissues.

It is recommended that IPPV settings are adjusted to the functional requirements of the patients, with constant monitoring of pulmonary mechanics, expired CO_2, and arterial blood gases [71]. Respiratory rate will be reduced and expiration time prolonged so as to obtain optimal dynamic compliance and VD/VT ratios, a moderate hypercapnia can be tolerated (up to 60 mmHg) and arterial O_2 saturation should be maintained above 90%.

IPPV has resulted in the salvage of many asthmatic patients who would otherwise have died. However, the procedure may be associated with a high rate of morbidity and mortality [58], and complications associated with ventilation are not infrequent.

The mortality rate reported from intensive care units with experience in the treatment of asthma are shown in Table 19.2. The results are variable [26], with the mortality expressed as percentages of the number of episodes of

Table 19.2 Reported mortality rates in severe asthma

Authors	Number of patients	Number of episodes	Number of deaths	Percentage of deaths
Iisato et al. [29]	26	29	4	14
Weiztman and Wilson [75]	39	42	4	9.5
Wood et al. [79]	22	30	1	3.3
Scoggins et al. [58]	19	21	8	38
Darioli et al. [15]	13	18	0	
Sheehy et al. [59]	22		2	9
Ambiavagar [3]	22		4	18
Williams [78]	18		2	11

Table 19.3 Patients with severe asthma treated in our ICU from 1964 to 1979

	Coma	Drowsiness, mental confusion	Exhaustion	Total
Number of patients	58	39	30	127
Treated with MV	46 (3 deaths)	21 (4 deaths)	12	79 (7 deaths)
Treated without MV	12	18	18	48

asthma treated, ranging form 0% to 38%. In our series seven patients out of seventy-nine needing artificial ventilation died (Table 19.3); deaths outside the hospital are probably also frequent [12, 14].

For the future it is hoped that recent advances in ventilator technology and respiratory monitoring will improve the prognosis of those asthmatic patients who require IPPV.

Some important practical points

It is vital to distinguish between patients with a recent and sudden onset of an asthmatic attack and those who have suffered from acute bronchospasm for several days and will probably have used, correctly or incorrectly, a number of bronchodilator drugs.

ACTH is contra-indicated because the adrenals may be unable to respond.

Sedatives or morphine derivatives must not be used unless ventilation is planned.

Cough sedatives should not be used, since they can abolish the cough reflex and encourage the retention of inspissated mucus.

Respiratory stimulants are contra-indicated.

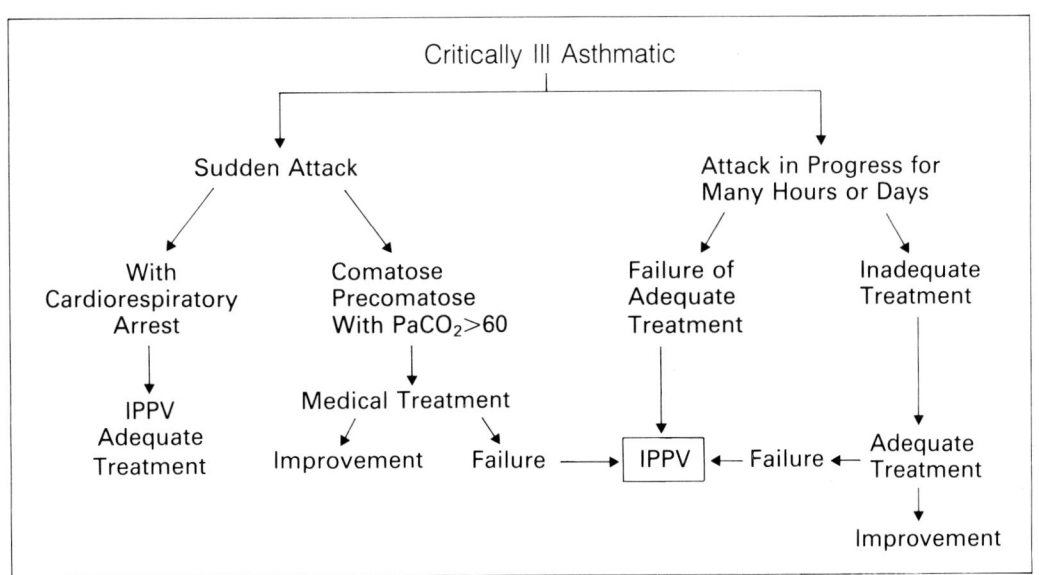

Fig. 19.2. Management of patients with severe asthma.

Beta-blocking drugs are absolutely contra-indicated. In our series two patients became asphyxic and had cardiac arrests after taking these drugs.

On the basis of our personal experience, our approach to the management of the patient with severe asthma is summarized in Fig. 19.2.

References

1. Ahonen A (1979) Analysis of the ECG changes in status asthmaticus. Respiration 37:85–90
2. Ambiavagar M, Sherwood-Jones E (1967) Resuscitation of the muribond asthmatic. Use of intermittent positive pressure ventilation, bronchial lavage and intravenous infusions. Anaesthesia 22:375–391
3. Ambiavagar M, Sherwood-Jones E, Roberts DV (1967) Intermittent positive pressure ventilation in severe asthma. Mechanical effects on the circulation. Anaesthesia 22:134–139
4. Bellamy D, Collins JV (1979) 'Acute' asthma in adults. Thorax 34:36–39
5. Beswick K, Davies J, Davey AJ (1975) A comparison of intravenous aminophylline and salbutamol in the treatment of severe bronchospasm. Practitioner 214:561–566
6. Birley DM, Rochford J (1968) Bronchial lavage. Proc R Soc Med 61:1159–1161
7. Bocles JS (1970) Status asthmaticus. Med Clin North Am 54:493–509
8. Bocles JS (1969) L'asthme grave. Etude de 80 observations d'asthme mortel. Ann Med Interne (Paris) 120:97–107
9. Busey JF, Fenger Epk, Hepper NG, Kent DC, Kilburn KH, Mathews LN, Simpson DG, Grzybowski S (1968) Management of status asthmaticus: A statement by the committee on therapy. Am Rev Respir Dis 97:735–736
10. Camarata JS, Weil MH, Hanashiro PK, Shubin H (1971) Cardiac arrest in the critically ill. A study of predisposing causes in 132 patients. Circulation 44:688–695
11. Chang Shim, Williams MH Jr (1978) Pulsus paradoxus in asthma. Lancet I:530–531
12. Cochrane GM, Clark TJH (1975) A survey of asthma mortality in patients between ages 35 and 64 in the Greater London Hospitals in 1971. Thorax 30:300–305
13. Collins JV, Jones D (1977) Corticosteroids in the treatment of severe acute asthma. Acta Tuberc Pneumol Belg 68:63–73
14. Crompton GK, Grant IWB (1975) Edinburgh emergency asthma admission service. Br Med J iv:680–682
15. Darioli R, Domenighetti G, Perret C (1979) Mechanical ventilation for severe respiratory failure in status asthmaticus. Paper presented at the International Congress on Respiratory Diseases, Basel, Switzerland, 10–13 October
16. De Coster A, Cornil A, De Troyer A, Thys JP, Degaute JP, Ectors M (1978) Treatment of severe attacks of asthma in intensive care units: 12 years experience. Thorax 33:533 [abst]
17. De Coster A, Messin R, Degre S (1980) Lactate and pulmunary pathology. In: Moret PR, Weber J Haissly JC, Denolin H (eds) Lactate, physiologic, methodologic and pathologic approach. Springer, Berlin Heidelberg New York, pp 145–152
18. Dugué P, Ohresser P, Orehek J, Charpin J (1978) Physiopathologie de l'état de mal asthmatique. Bull Eur Physiopathol Respir 14:347–366
19. Franklin W (1974) Treatment of severe asthma. N Engl J Med 290:1469–1472
20. Friedlaender S (1970) Newer concepts of managing asthmatic patients. Postgrad Med J 47:94–95
21. Galant SP, Duriseti L, Underwood S, Insel PA (1978) Decreased beta-adrenergic receptor on polymorphonuclear leucocytes after adrenergic therapy. N Engl J Med 299:933
22. Gelb AF, Lyons HA, Fairshter RD, Glauser FL, Morrissey R, Chetty K, Schiffman P (1979) P pulmonale in status asthmaticus. J Allergy Clin Immunol 64:18–22
23. Gunstone RF (1971) Right heart pressures in bronchial asthma. Thorax 26:39–45
24. Harvey JE, Tattersfield AE (1979) Beta-adrenergic responsiveness in asthmatic and atopic non-asthmatic subjects. Thorax 34:416 [abst]
25. Helander E, Lindell SE, Soderholm B, Westling H (1962) Observations on the pulmonary circulation during induced bronchial asthma. Acta Allergol 17:112
26. Hetzel MR, Clark TJH, Branthwaite MA (1977) Asthma: Analysis of sudden deaths and ventilatory arrests in hospital. Br Med J i:808–811
27. Holmes PW, Campbell AH, Barter CE (1978) Acute changes of lung volumes and lung mechanics in asthma and in normal subjects. Thorax 33:394–400
28. Hugh-Jones P (1978) Status asthmaticus. Bull Eur Physiopathol Respir 14:233–236
29. Iisato El, Iisato EU, Tala ES (1969) Death from asthma with special reference to the last drug regimen. Acta Med Scand 185:45–50
30. Iisato EU, Iisato EI, Vapaovuori MJ (1969) Prolonged artificial ventilation in severe status asthmaticus. Acta Med Scand 185:51–55
31. Jardin F, Barthelemy M (1977) Fréquence de l'acidose métabolique au cours de l'état de mal asthmatique de l'adulte. Nouv Presse Med 6:329–332
32. Jones ES (1971) The intensive therapy of asthma. Proc R Soc Med 64:1152
33. Jusko WJ, Koup JR, Vance W, Schentag JJ, Kuritzky P (1977) Intravenous theophylline therapy: Nomogram guidelines. Ann Intern Med 86:400–404
34. Karetzky MS (1975) Blood studies in untreated patients with acute asthma. Am Rev Respir Dis 112:607–613
35. Kelsen SG, Kelsen DP, Fleeger BF, Jones RC, Rodman T (1978) Emergency room assessment and treatment of patients with acute asthma. Am J Med 64:622–628
36. Kordash TR, Van Dellen GR, McCall JT (1977) Theophylline concentrations in asthmatic patients after administration of aminophylline. JAMA 238:139–141
37. Labrousse J, Bousser JP, Tenaillon A, Lissac J (1977) Artificial ventilation in status asthmaticus. Intensive Care Med 3:114
37a. Leading article (1979) Fatal asthma. Lancet II:337–338
38. Lemaire F (1979) Ventilation mécanique et hypoventilation alvéolaire des bronchopneumopathies chroniques. Bull Eur Physiopathol Respir 15:[suppl] 280–289
39. Lissac J, Labrousse J, Tenaillon A, Bousser JP, Labrousse F, Jacquot C (1975) Les désordres acidobasiques dans l'état de mal asthmatique. Bull Physiopathol Respir 11:745–756
40. Mansell A, Dubrawsky C, Levison H, Bryan AC, Langer H, Collins-Williams C, Orange RP (1974) Lung mechanics in antigen-induced asthma. J Appl Physiol 37:297–301
41. Marcelle R (1969) Traitement de l'état de mal asthmatique par la phentolamine. Allergy 24:432–446

42. McDonald JB, McDonald ET, Seaton A, Williams DA (1976) Asthma deaths in Cardiff 1963–74: 53 deaths in hospital. Br Med J ii:721–723
43. McFadden ER, Lyons HA (1968) Arterial blood gas tension in asthma. N Engl J Med 278:1027
44. Mitenko PA, Ogilvie RI (1973) Rational intravenous doses of theophylline. N Engl J Med 89:600–603
45. Mithoefer JC, Runser RH, Karetzki MS (1965) The use of sodium bicarbonate in the treatment of acute bronchial asthma. N Engl J Med 272:1200–1203
46. Ostrea EM, Odell GB (1972) The influence of bicarbonate administration on blood pH in a closed system. Clinical implications. J Pediatr 80:671–680
47. Pain MCF, Charlton GC, Read J (1967) Effect of intravenous aminophylline on distribution of pulmonary blood flow in obstructive lung disease. Am Rev Respir Dis 95:1005–1014
48. Palmer KNV (1969) Progress in asthma. Postgrad Med J 45:336–347
49. Parry CWH, Martorano F, Cotton ER (1976) Management of life threatening asthma with intravenous isoproterenol infusions AM J Dis Child 130:39–42
50. Paterson JW, Woolcock AJ, Shenfield GM (1979) Bronchodilator drugs. Am Rev Respir Dis 120:1149–1188
51. Peress L, Sybrecht G, Macklem PT (1976) The mechanism of increase in total lung capacity during acute asthma. Am J Med 61:165–169
52. Powell JR, Vozeh S, Hopewell P, Costello J, Sheiner LB Riegelman S (1978) Theophylline disposition in acutely ill hospitalized patients. Am Rev Respir Dis 118:229–238
53. Ramirez SR, Obenour WH (1971) Bronchopulmonary lavage in asthma and chronic bronchitis: Clinical and physiologic observations. Chest 59:146–152
54. Rebuck AS, Read J (1971) Assessment and management of severe asthma. Am J Med 51:788–798
54a. Regional Office for Europe of WHO/Executive Committee and the European Society of Clinical Respiratory Physiology (1978) Nomenclature and definitions in respiratory physiology and clinical aspects of chronic lung diseases. Bull Physiopathol Respir 11:937–959
55. Rees KA, Miller JS, Donald KW (1968) A study of the clinical course and arterial blood gas tensions of patients in status asthmaticus. QJ Med 37:541–561
56. Richards W, Siegel SC, Strauss JS, Leich DM (1967) Status asthmaticus in children. JAMA 201:75–81
57. Roncoroni AJ, Adrogue HJA, De Obrutsky CW, Marchisio ML, Herrera MR (1976) Metabolic acidosis in status asthmaticus. Respiration 33:85–94
58. Scoggins CH, Sahn SA, Petty TL (1977) Status asthmaticus: Nine-year experience. JAMA 238:1158–1162
59. Sheehy AF, Di Benedetto R, Lefrak S, Lyons HA (1972) Treatment of status asthmaticus. Arch Intern Med 130:37–42
60. Shenfield GM, Hodson ME, Clarke SW, Paterson JW (1975) Interaction of corticosteroids and cathecholamines in the treatment of asthma. Thorax 30:430–435
61. Sherwood E Jones (1971) The intensive therapy of asthma. Proc R Soc Med 64:1152
62. Siegler D (1977) Reversible ECG changes in severe acute asthma. Thorax 32:328–332
63. Simons FER, Pierson WE, Bierman CW (1977) Respiratory failure in childhood status asthmaticus. Am J Dis Child 131:1097–1101
64. Simpson H, Forfar JO, Grubb DJ (1968) Arterial blood gas tension and pH in acute asthma in childhood. Br Med J iii:460–464
65. Simpson H, Mitchell I, Inglis JM, Grubb DJ (1978) Severe ventilatory failure in asthma in children; Experience of 13 episodes over six years. Arch Dis Child 53:714–724
66. Stalcup SA, Mellins RB (1977) Mechanical forces producing pulmonary edema in acute asthma. N Engl J Med 297:592–596
67. Stolley PD (1972) Asthma mortality. Am Rev Respir Dis 105:883–890
68. Straub EW, Buhlmann AA, Rossler PI (1969) Hypovolemia in status asthmaticus. Lancet I:923–926
69. Svedmyr NLV, Larson SA, Thiringer GK (1976) Development of "resistance" in beta-adrenergic receptors of asthmatic patients. Chest 69:479–483
70. Svedmyr K, Mellstrand J, Svedmyr N (1977) A comparison between effects of aminophylline, proxyphylline and terbutaline in asthmatics. Scand J Respir Dis [Suppl] 101:109–146
71. Thomas L, Robert D, Perrin F (1978) Exploration fonctionnelle sous ventilation artificielle. Application au choix des réglages. Nouv Presse Med 7:719–724
72. Webb AK, Bilton AH, Hanson GC (1979) Severe bronchial asthma requiring ventilation. A review of twenty cases and advice on management. Postgrad Med J 55:161–175
73. Weiss EB, Summer WR (1978) Physiological changes in the acute asthmatic attack. In: Status asthmaticus. University Park Press, Baltimore, pp 81–99
74. Weitzenblum E, Pauli G, Roeslin N, Vandevenne A, Bohner C, Oudet P (1971) Les donnes hémodynamiques pulmonaries au cours de la crise d'asthme: Incidence des conditions mécaniques endothoraciques. J Fr Med Chir Thor 25:487–509
75. Weiztman RH, Wilson AF (1974) Diffusing capacity and overall ventilation/perfusion in asthma. Am J Med 57:767–774
76. Westerman DE, Benatar SR, Potgieter PD, Ferguson AD (1979) Identification of high-risk asthmatic patient. Experience with 39 patients undergoing ventilation for status asthmaticus. Am J Med 66:565–572
77. Williams S, Seaton A (1977) Intravenuous or inhaled salbutamol in severe acute asthma. Thorax 32:555–558
78. Williams NE (1968) Bronchial lavage in status asthmaticus Proc R Soc Med 61:1161
79. Wood DN, Downes JJ, Lecks HI (1968) The management of respiratory failure in childhood status asthmaticus. Experience with 30 episodes and evolution of a technique. Allergy 42:261–267
80. Woolcock AJ, Read J (1968) The static elastic properties of the lungs in asthma. Am Rev Respir Dis 98:788–794
81. Zimmerman HA (1951) A study of the pulmonary circulation in man. Chest 20:46

Chapter 20

Intermittent and Continuous Positive Pressure Ventilation

Peter M. Suter

Mechanical ventilation with intermittent or continuous application of positive pressure (IPPV or CPPV) on the airways has become an essential tool in the management of acute respiratory problems. This treatment is efficient for the prevention and the treatment of severe respiratory failure after major surgical interventions or trauma. The judicious application of the techniques of ventilatory support improves the prognosis substantially in many medical diseases complicated by an impairment of pulmonary gas exchange, such as neuromuscular diseases, severe pulmonary edema, sepsis or pneumonia.

The purpose of this chapter is to review briefly the pathophysiology of acute respiratory failure treated by MV, to provide some guidelines for the patterns of ventilatory support producing an appropriate gas exchange and to discuss the overall effects of this treatment on the different systems and organs of the body.

Pathophysiology of acute respiratory failure and positive pressure ventilation

It is important to recognize some important morphologic, physiologic, and functional changes occurring in the respiratory system in order to understand the implications of MV on lung function. Ventilatory insufficiency, i.e., alveolar hypoventilation is discussed separately from pulmonary parenchymal failure to simplify the analysis and distinguish two different therapeutic approaches.

Ventilatory insufficiency

The inability of a patient to produce a sufficient pulmonary ventilation can be defined by an inadequate CO_2 elimination. This situation is characterized by an alveolar hypoventilation and an increase in the partial pressure of CO_2 in the arterial blood ($PaCO_2$), associated with a respiratory acidosis. Some frequent causes of ventilatory failure are listed in Table 20.1. The lung parenchyma can be normal; if it is not, the comments in the next section may apply.

The treatment of pure ventilatory insufficiency is easy and does not require sophisticated respiratory equipment. Intermittent positive pressure ventilation (IPPV) is employed with the usual tidal volume of 12–15 ml/kg body weight. The respiratory frequency is adjusted to produce adequate CO_2 elimination resulting in a normal $PaCO_2$, except in the case of chronic obstructive pulmonary disease (COPD) with CO_2 retention, where values of $PaCO_2$ existing before the acute illness should be obtained.

Table 20.1. Frequent causes of ventilatory insufficiency (alveolar hypoventilation) defined by an acute rise in $PaCO_2$ and respiratory acidosis

Respiratory center dysfunction
Drug overdose
Anesthesia
Peripheral neuromuscular disease
   Polyneuritis
   Myasthenia
   Cervical spinal cord injury
Therapeutic muscle paralysis
   Postoperative phase in selected cases
   Tetanus
   Status epilepticus and some other CNS diseases
Loss of chest wall integrity and function
   Flail chest
   Ruptured diaphragm
Severe respiratory movement discoordination
Inability to eliminate CO_2 adequately for other reasons
   Hypermetabolic state (severe burns, sepsis) associated
      with weakness, marked obesity, or debilitation

When prolonged MV, e.g., for more than 24 h, is necessary, one or several of the following techniques should be applied to prevent atelectasis and the retention of secretions: position changes; periodic manual hyperinflation by nurses or respiratory therapists; endotracheal suction when bronchial secretions accumulate in the airway. The addition of a positive end-expiratory pressure (PEEP), i.e., 5 cmH$_2$O, can also help to restore resting lung volume to normal or near-normal and to prevent airway closure and alveolar collapse.

Pulmonary parenchymal failure and pulmonary edema

The majority of patients requiring prolonged MV have some form of acute pulmonary parenchymal disease. The factor most frequently responsible for insufficient gas exchange is pulmonary edema (PE). Because fluid filtration from the microvasculature of the lung is frequently altered in these patients and positive pressure ventilation interferes with some factors that determine PE formation, this topic will be briefly discussed here.

Depending on body position and activity a certain leakage of fluid occurs continuously from the pulmonary capillaries and probably from the arterioles. The lymphatic system is capable of draining this fluid, however, and can increase the removal rate to up to ten times the normal rate [118]. A number of other 'safety factors' exist against interstitial PE [116], and the

alveolar epithelium represents a second barrier (Table 20.2). In so-called high-pressure PE, also named *hydrostatic or cardiogenic PE*, the micro-

Table 20.2. Safety factors against PE [116]

Interstitial edema
   Microvascular barrier
      Low fluid and small molecule conductance
      Very low protein conductance
   Perimicrovascular fluid pressure
   Plasma protein concentration
   Lymphatic system
Alveolar flooding
   Alveolar barrier
      Very low fluid and small molecule conductance
      Ultra-low protein conductance
   Low interstitial fluid pressure [96]
   Lymphatic system
   Alveolar gas pressure and surface tension

vascular pressure is increased. In this situation the extent of fluid extravasation and accumulation in the pulmonary interstitium depends upon this hydrostatic pressure and thus on the function of the left side of the heart. In addition, the plasma osmotic pressure and the intrathoracic pressure influence lymphatic flow, as does the pressure in the superior vena cava, which is a function of body position, intravascular volume, and right heart function. The filtration also depends on the interstitial compliance and the reflection coefficient for proteins of the endothelial and epithelial layers of the lung [3, 16, 19, 56, 57].

Positive pressure ventilation may decrease fluid filtration from the microvasculature [18] or have no effect on the lung fluid balance [132]. The increased intrathoracic pressure can impede lymphatic flow. It can also impair RV function and increase central venous pressure [86]. These factors tend to aggravate interstitial PE during positive pressure ventilation. The 'alveolar barrier', separating the air spaces from interstitial tissue and capillaries, affords nearly complete protection against leakage of fluid into the alveolar lumen, even when the lung has accumulated substantial amounts of edema fluid [116]. When alveolar flooding occurs, i.e., when edema fluid enters the air spaces, the alveolar barrier appears to undergo a transformation and become freely permeable to fluid and protein [116]. Ventilation with intermittent or continuous positive pressure improves pulmonary gas exchange in PE, possibly by changing the distribution of the ventilation and edema fluid within the gas exchange units and the lung [92, 119, 126]. It is unlikely that the intercellular junctions of the alveolar epithelium are pulled open by stretch due to high intra-alveolar pressures or that this occurs only at very high lung volumes [43]. However, substantial bulk flow of fluid and protein across the alveolar barrier can also be observed at relatively low lung volumes [54].

In contrast to high-pressure PE, *increased permeability PE* is characterized by an increased filtration coefficient of the endothelial barrier, whereas its reflection coefficient is decreased, indicating a change in the integrity of the microvascular wall [115]. This type of PE is typical of the early phases of the adult respiratory distress syndrome (ARDS: cf. Chap. 17), and it can be observed in a variety of acute diseases resulting in pulmonary parenchymal insufficiency, such as hypersensitivity reactions, multiple emboli, oxygenator and dialyser membrane injury, shock, septic and endotoxin injury, and some bacterial and viral pneumonias. The major and probably sole significant sites of transvascular fluid and protein exchange are the intercellular junctions of the lung endothelium, which are more important than the transport by pinocytotic vesicles in these cells [116]. There is no correlation between microvascular, interstitial hydrostatic, and oncotic pressure in 'permeability PE' [38].

In this type of PE, positive pressure continuously applied to the airways and the alveoli decreases alveolar and bronchial fluid egression, but it does not decrease the total water content of the lung [71]. As in high-pressure PE, positive pressure ventilation improves pulmonary gas exchange by improving regional or general ventilation/perfusion mismatching. Therefore the mechanisms of recruitment and maintenance of ventilation to perfused areas, by reversing and preventing alveolar collapse and airway closure, play a major role, whereas perfusion and edema are probably not directly influenced by MV [24, 130].

A third type of PE is probably due to *high vascular distending pressure*. This can be seen in severe left atrial hypertension, in increased linear velocity of pulmonary blood flow in pulmonary embolism, following extensive pulmonary resection, in neurogenic PE, and in high-altitude PE [116]. For its ventilatory support by positive pressure ventilation, considerations and effects are similar to those applicable in the two other forms of PE.

Guidelines for ventilatory support

In this section a number of practical considerations are outlined for the setting and regulation of MV. It must be emphasized that there is no unique ventilatory pattern for good oxygenation in all patients; the modalities of this treatment must be adapted to each individual situation and modified according to the patient's response in terms of pulmonary gas exchange and the function of other vital systems and organs. The aim of the guidelines described below is to establish an adequate lung ventilation; the secondary effects of MV on the respiratory system and others organs will be discussed in the section: *Secondary effects and complications of positive pressure ventilation*. A schematic representation of the ventilatory patterns described here is given in Fig. 20.1.

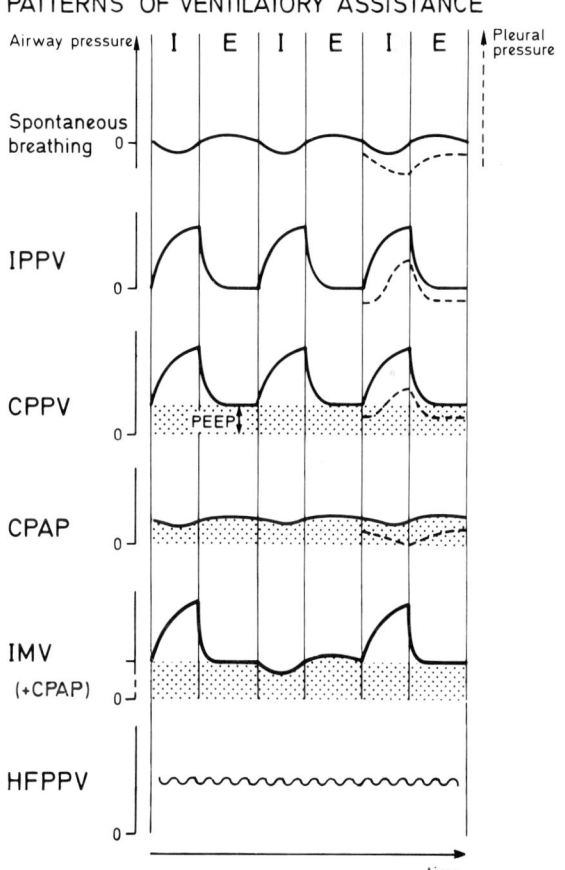

Fig. 20.1. Airway pressure – time diagrams of the types of MV most frequently used. Airway pressure is indicated by the *full line*, estimated pleural pressure by the *dashed line* on the right border of the figure. *I*, inspiration; *E*, expiration. For other abbreviations, see text.

Intermittent positive pressure ventilation

IPPV is defined as an intermittent application of a certain positive pressure (i.e., higher than atmospheric) to the airways, thereby producing insufflation of a tidal volume into the lungs. During expiration, the airway pressure falls to zero or atmospheric pressure. IPPV can be performed with pressure-preset ventilators (e.g., Bird mark VII or Bennett PR–2), which deliver a variable tidal volume, depending on changes in the compliance and the resistance of the patient's respiratory system. These devices are inexpensive, but their use is restricted to the ventilation of relatively normal lungs and respiratory therapy, because of the low peak pressure that they attain and the variability of the tidal volume. By contrast, the volume-preset ventilators deliver a constant tidal volume in almost all respiratory conditions and are used preferentially for the treatment of acute pulmonary failure.

The optimal pattern for MV varies from patient to patient, but Table 20.3 gives some practical guidelines for the initial settings. The

Table 20.3. IPPV: Ventilatory modes used preferentially and safety devices

a) Initial settings

Tidal volume	12–15 ml/kg ideal body wt.
Respiratory frequency	8–15/min, to achieve normal $PaCO_2$ and pH
Mode	Assisted/controlled
Time ratio I:E	1:4–1:1 (–4:1, see section: *Other types of ventilatory support*)
Inspiratory time	1.5 s (1–2 s)
Inspiratory pause	0–0.6 s
Inspired O_2 fraction (F_IO_2)	0.4–1.0, to achieve adequate PaO_2

b) Safety devices
   Inspiratory (high-pressure) relief valve with alarm
   Disconnect (low-pressure) alarm
   Fail to cycle alarm

c) Modes without proven value:
   Periodic mechanical hyperinflations (sigh)
   Differential inspiratory flow patterns

tidal volume of 12–15 ml/kg ideal body wt results in adequate gas exchange and patient comfort. When lower tidal volumes are employed the patients frequently complain of dyspnea and of inadequate chest wall expansion, whereas lung function deteriorates progressively secondary to small airway closure and an increase in intrapulmonary shunt [87, 100]. These complications can be avoided by the application of PEEP or by periodic hyper-

inflation of the lungs ('sigh'). The use of the mechanical sigh given by the ventilator is not recommended, because it has no advantage when appropriate tidal volumes are employed; in addition it is unpleasant for the patient and potentially harmful for the lung tissue due to the high intrapulmonary pressure produced. Tidal volumes above 15 ml/kg ideal body wt are rarely indicated and may be dangerous, because of their effect on peak intrapulmonary pressure and function of surfactant [46]. The form of the inspiratory flow pattern is of lesser importance than the duration of inspiration and consequently than the inspiration: expiration time ratio (I:E). The inspiratory time is normally adapted to between 1 and 2 s, and the expiratory time and I:E ratio will vary depending on respiratory frequency. An inspiratory pause or hold applied at the end of the mechanical insufflation allows the determination of 'quasi-static' or 'effective' compliance and decreases the dead space-to-tidal volume ratio (V_D/V_T), but does not improve arterial oxygenation [52, 123]. The inspired fraction of O_2 (F_IO_2) is adjusted to as high a level as is necessary to achieve adequate tissue oxygenation and is lowered as soon as possible to avoid the potential hazards of O_2 toxicity, resorption atelectasis, and increased $\dot{Q}_S/\dot{Q}_T$ [39, 121].

Continuous positive pressure ventilation

CPPV consists in the intermittent insufflation of a tidal volume in the inspiratory phase, associated with the maintenance of a positive airway pressure during the expiratory phase (IPPV with PEEP). The advantage of CPPV over IPPV is an improved pulmonary gas exchange in those cases where alveolar collapse, a decreased functional residual capacity (FRC), and closure of small airways are central events in the pathophysiology of respiratory failure (Fig. 20.2). Accordingly, CPPV is frequently used in postoperative and posttraumatic respiratory failure, ARDS, severe cardiogenic PE, diffuse viral or bacterial pneumonia, and permeability PE. In these conditions the addition of PEEP to IPPV causes a marked improvement in pulmonary gas exchange, an increase in FRC and a decrease in $\dot{Q}_S/\dot{Q}_T$ [7, 8, 44, 81, 84, 99]. In most instances, but not in all, PEEP increases the compliance of the respiratory system [45, 100, 122, 124], depending on the initial compliance, the duration of the pulmonary disease, the closing volume [88, 105, 111, 126] and the level of PEEP applied. Cardiovascular performance and O_2 transport are also affected by PEEP [36, 77, 91, 120, 122].

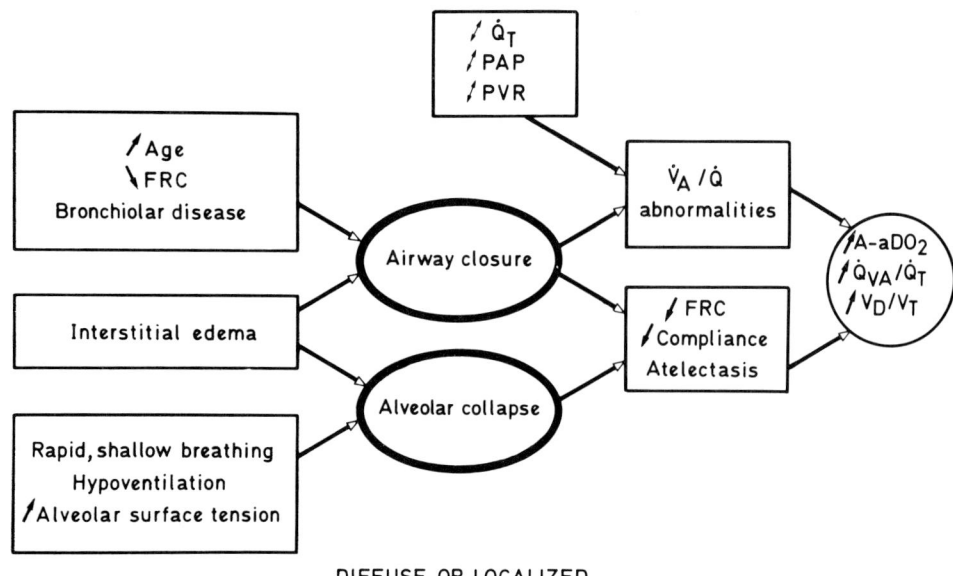

Fig. 20.2. Schematic representation of some etiologic factors, central events, and resulting lung function changes in acute pulmonary failure. In the acute phase, interstitial edema is the most important factor leading to airspace collapse. Ventilation perfusion ($\dot{V}_A/\dot{Q}$) abnormalities are a consequence of these elements combined with changes in cardiac output ($\dot{Q}_T$), PAP, and PVR. All these factors lead to an impaired gas exchange, increased alveolar–arterial O_2 tension difference (A-aDO_2), venous admixture ($\dot{Q}_{VA}/\dot{Q}_T$) and dead space fraction (V_D/V_T).

The direction and importance of the changes produced depend on the intravascular volume and cardiac filling pressures [104, 125], the level of PEEP applied [41, 63, 100, 101], and the precise effect of PEEP on intracardiac pressures, volumes, and geometry [20, 21, 25, 27, 28, 31, 33, 49, 86] as well as cardiac performance [58] and pre-existing cardiac and pulmonary disease [106–108, 114, 127]. These interactions of MV in general, and PEEP in particular, with other organ functions will be presented in more detail in the section: *Secondary effects and complications of positive pressure ventilation.*

For the inspiratory phase, the considerations and rules that apply for CPPV are similar to those discussed for IPPV. PEEP can be produced by a spring- or pressure-loaded valve, or by an underwater seal. The levels employed vary widely and depend on personal experience, the goals to be achieved with CPPV, the patient population, the type and importance of pulmonary parenchymal disease, associated organ dysfunction, cardiovascular filling and function, and the use of vasoactive drugs. Where as 10 years ago PaO_2 was the most important variable determining the efficiency of ventilatory support, more recently interest has focused more on other systemic effects.

Of the measurements used to regulate the level of PEEP, the following are the most frequently used: PaO_2, mixed venous O_2 tension

($P_{\bar{v}}O_2$), total static compliance of the respiratory system, O_2 transport, cardiac output, and the function of other systems and organs. The advantages and shortcomings of these values are listed in Table 20.4. The effects of PEEP on the respiratory function can best be evaluated by separate examination of its influences on lung function and cardiac output, the two main factors determining O_2 availability and CO_2 elimination at the cellular and tissue level.

The changes in lung function produced by PEEP are: (1) an increase in FRC, determined by the applied level of PEEP, the compliance of the respiratory system, and the volume of lung tissue recruited; (2) an increase in compliance at low lung volumes and in the presence of collapsed or closed lung regions which can be opened and kept open by PEEP while there is no change or decrease in compliance at high lung volumes (emphysema, overdistension) or in the late stages of pulmonary failure, which are characterized by parenchymal consolidation and interstitial fibrosis; (3) an improvement in the exchange of O_2 and CO_2, which is most marked for CO_2 at low levels of PEEP and V_D/V_T, while high levels of PEEP frequently produce an increase in V_D/V_T; PaO_2 increases progressively and continuously with increasing levels of PEEP [45, 81, 101, 122]. These changes in lung function with progressive distension can best be explained by the phenomenon of

Table 20.4. CPPV: Variables used to regulate the level of PEEP

	Advantages	Disadvantages
Gas exchange		
PaO_2	Important determinant of cellular and organ function	Depends not only on pulmonary gas exchange, but also on $P_{\bar{v}}O_2$
	Easy to measure	Does not correlate with $\dot{Q}_T$
$P_{\bar{v}}O_2$	Reflects pulmonary gas exchange, $\dot{Q}_T$, and systemic oxygen reserve	Sample difficult to obtain
		Difficult to interpret in situations with metabolic disturbances
Lung mechanics		
FRC	Correlates with gas exchange surface area	Normal or optimal values are difficult to define
Compliance	Correlates with:	Does not correlate with PaO_2
	Recruitment and	Does not correlate with O_2 transport in chronic stages, in patients with very low compliance
	Overdistension of gas exchange areas	
	Oxygen transport in most cases in the acute phase of pulmonary failure	Dependent on tidal volume
V_D/V_T	Estimates effective alveolar gas exchange area	Interpretation of changes difficult because of the addition of three different variables: anatomic, alveolar, shunt-dependent dead space
	Correlates with pulmonary vascular involvement	Dependent on tidal volume
Oxygen transport	Best estimate of overall systemic effects and benefits	Dependent on pulmonary gas exchange, cardiac output, hemoglobin
		O_2 consumption varies with O_2 transport in ARDS [35]
Other organ functions		
CNS	Almost always determine the final outcome	Function depends on previous state and 'reserves'
Cardiac output	Easy to 'estimate'	
Renal function	Determined by and also influence the respiratory function	Difficult to 'measure' precisely
Hepatic function		Changes in performance depend on several factors, namely oxygenation, organ perfusion, metabolic state

alveolar collapse, airway closure or opening and a decrease in the compliance of the lung tissue with overdistension (Fig. 20.3).

The effects of the increased intrathoracic pressure and PEEP on cardiac output are secondary to the following mechanisms (Fig. 20.4):

1) The *venous return and the cardiac filling pressures* are influenced by PEEP: this results in a decrease of $\dot{Q}_T$ in hypovolemic and normovolemic patients at moderate or high pressure levels [81, 104, 122, 125], whereas $\dot{Q}_T$ does not change or improves with PEEP in the presence of hypervolemia [104, 125, 131].

2) The *pulmonary vascular resistance* decreases between residual lung capacity and FRC, and with the application of small amounts of PEEP in acute respiratory failure [25]; at high distending pressures this vascular resistance increases, probably due to the transmission of alveolar pressure to the capillaries (Fig. 20.5) [13].

3) The *ensuing right heart distension* alters right and left heart geometry, volumes, and end-diastolic pressures [74, 75, 86, 98, 103, 108, 131], resulting in decreased systolic volume and $\dot{Q}_T$ despite a normal ejection fraction.

4) A *compression of the heart and the coronary* circulation by the increased intrathoracic pressure has been proposed, but Pepine has shown that the decrease in coronary blood flow is secondary to decreased myocardial demands [97].

5) *Humoral or reflex mechanisms originating in the lung* may also contribute to a decrease in cardiac output by impairing myocardial contractility [42, 61].

The individual response of O_2 transport to PEEP is very variable, depending among other factors on transmission of airway pressure to the pleural space, which is decreased when significant consolidation of lung parenchyma is present [31, 41, 44], and on the state of myocardial contractility and the pulmonary vascular bed [133].

Intermittent mandatory ventilation

IMV is a combination of mechanical (mandatory) insufflations with unassisted spontaneous breathing between the tidal volumes delivered by the machine. This technique was initially

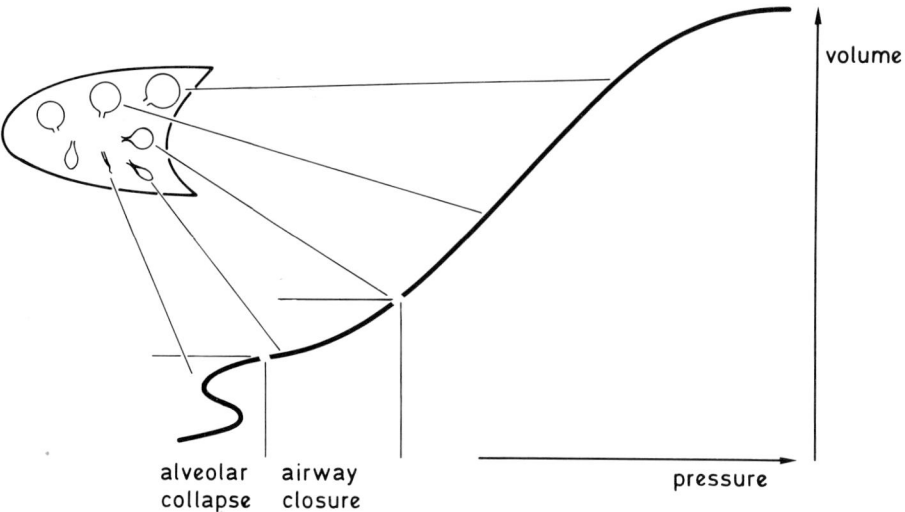

Fig. 20.3. Pressure–volume diagram with the corresponding alveolar structures of the lung in the supine patient. This figure depicts schematically lung regions and mechanics for alveolar collapse [118], airway closure [37, 73, 88], normal distension by ventilation, and overdistension at high airway pressures. In the healthy upright adult, tidal volume coincides with the steepest part of the pressure–volume curve. During positive pressure ventilation, a similar condition for pulmonary mechanics and gas exchange can be obtained by the addition of PEEP, thereby avoiding airway closure and alveolar collapse during expiration. Application of high levels of airway pressure or PEEP will result in overdistension of lung tissue, a fall in compliance, and an increase in dead space ventilation.

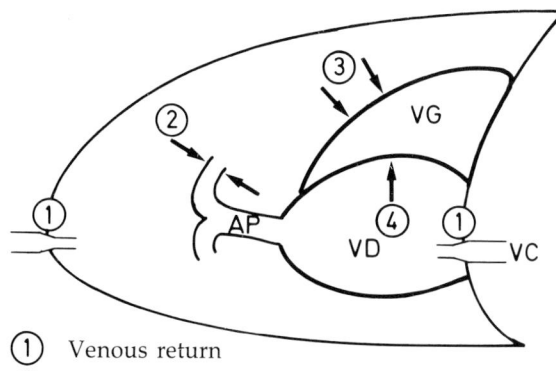

①　Venous return
②　Pulmonary vascular resistance
③　'Tamponade'
④　Deviation of septum
⑤　Humoral factors

Fig. 20.4. Etiologic factors involved in cardiovascular depression by increased intrathoracic pressure during IPPV and CPPV.

introduced to facilitate weaning from MV [40]. It has, however, become an established pattern that is used from the beginning to the end of the therapy of acute respiratory failure by ventilatory asistance. IMV differs from conventional MV in that synchronization of the mandatory inspiration with the spontaneous breathing movements does not appear to be important [68]. IMV seems to facilitate the transition from MV to spontaneous breathing after prolonged

ventilator treatment, but weaning is no more easily or rapidly achieved with this technique in good-risk patients who require postoperative ventilatory support for only a few hours [64, 90]. The regulation of IMV is shown schematically in Fig. 20.6. The greatest advantages of this technique over the conventional pattern of transition from MV to a T-piece are the decreased need for close monitoring in the weaning phase and the smoother changes in cardiac filling volumes and pressures in patients with cardiocirculatory instability. Better tolerance of high levels of PEEP (above 25 cmH$_2$O) than during conventional CPPV has been reported with IMV [78].

Continuous positive airway pressure

Continuous positive airway pressure during spontaneous breathing (CPAP) is frequently applied in the treatment of the idiopathic respiratory distress syndrome of the newborn [60] and also in adult patients with postoperative or posttraumatic pulmonary parenchymal failure [58, 95, 109]. As a preventive measure, CPAP decreases the postoperative pulmonary morbidity and mortality in high-risk patients [109] and improves arterial oxygenation during weaning from MV [47, 48]. It is clear that this technique can only be used in patients who have a normally functioning respiratory center and who

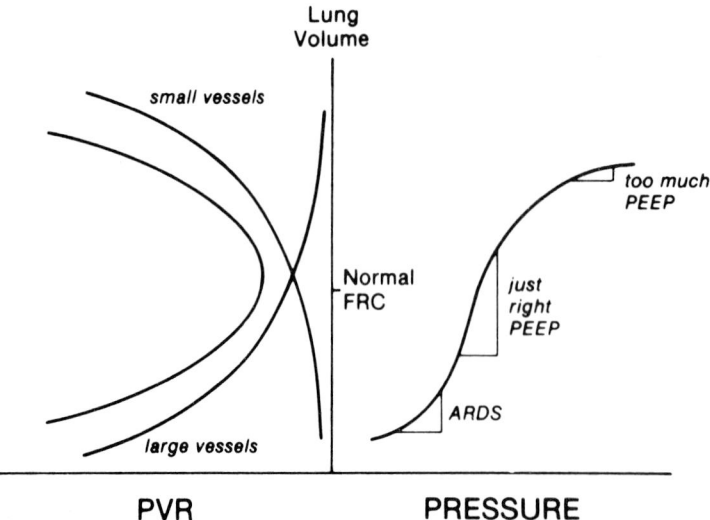

Fig. 20.5. Relationship between lung volume (*vertical axis*), distending pressure (*right half* of the figure, representing a pressure-volume curve, pressure increases from left to right), and PVR (*left* part of the figure, decreasing from left to right). In ARDS, increasing lung volume toward normal FRC by PEEP results in a decrease in PVR due to changes in the large vessels. When the lung volume is increased to high volumes and distending pressures, PVR increases secondary to the resistance in small vessels. Benumof [13], reproduced with permission.

are able to perform the work of ventilation. CPAP increases FRC, decreases or increases ventilatory work, depending on lung volume and compliance, increases PaO_2 with a decrease in $\dot{Q}_S/\dot{Q}_T$, and decreases respiratory frequency in association with an increase in tidal volume [55, 128]. The changes in the functioning of other organs are similar to those observed with PEEP, but being a consequence of the increased intrathoracic pressure, they are dependent on the level of CPAP applied and are often less important than those encountered in CPPV.

One important advantage of CPAP over IPPV and CPPV is that it can be a applied via a tightly fitting face mask, thereby avoiding endotracheal

intubation [59]. This form of treatment can only be given intermittently, but is efficient in preventing alveolar collapse, airway closure, and arterial hypoxemia in many forms of pulmonary parenchymal disease, such as hydrostatic or permeability PE, fat embolism, and postoperative atelectasis [59, 95, 109, 128].

The level of CPAP must be increased until the desired effect is obtained, but without exhaustion of the patient due to increased work of ventilation. An adequate positive pressure must be maintained during the expiratory *and* the inspiratory phase to keep the respiratory effort low and also to obtain an increase in FRC. The levels of CPAP required to achieve this vary between 5 and 15 cmH_2O when applied by a

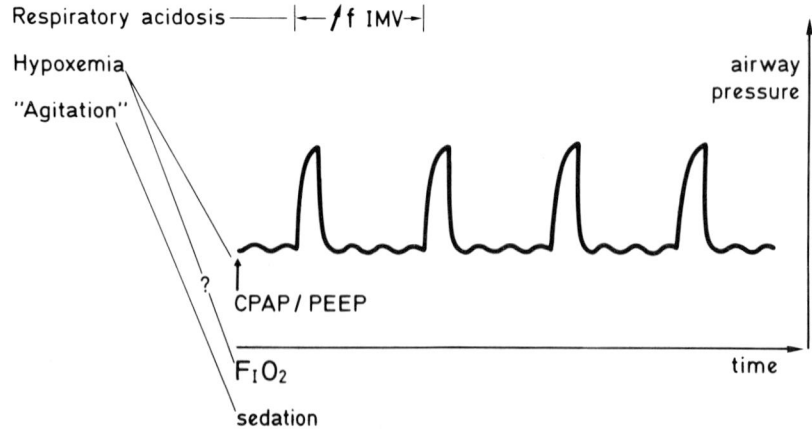

Fig. 20.6. Airway pressure-time diagram of IMV. Indicated are the regulation possibilities for respiratory acidosis (increase frequency of IMV), hypoxemia (increase first CPAP/PEEP, increase F_IO_2 only when first step inefficient), and inadequate patient adaptation to IMV (give appropriate sedation).

face mask; in the intubated patient levels between 5 and 25 cmH$_2$O are needed.

Other types of ventilatory support

High-frequency positive pressure ventilation

A different form of MV with high frequencies (60–3000/min) and low tidal volumes (5–100 ml) has been under investigation for more than 10 years in animal models and also in man. This type of ventilatory support is called high-frequency positive pressure ventilation (HFPPV) or high-frequency ventilation (HFV) for frequencies between 60 and 200/min, and high-frequency oscillation (HFO) between 200 and 3000/min. Most of the clinical investigations have been carried out during bronchoscopy or laryngeal surgery [80, 112, 113]. Recently the first experiences with HFPPV in ARF in infants [17] and adults [11, 23] have been reported. These data appear promising, but further clinical application and controlled studies are required to evaluate the long-term effects of this ventilatory mode on the respiratory system and other organs. At this time the best results are obtained in patients who have developed bronchopleural fistula during conventional MV [26, 79]. The physiopathology of pulmonary gas exchange during HFPPV is not fully understood, but it is suggested that there is an improvement of convective flow, alveolar mixing and diffusion. More investigation is necessary before this form of therapy can be fully understood [51, 79, 107, 114].

Low-frequency positive pressure ventilation with extracorporeal CO$_2$ removal

After the disappointing results of treating severe acute pulmonary failure with extracorporeal membrane oxygenation [134], only a few centers continued to investigate and develop this technique. Gattinoni et al. have worked on the concept of extracorporeal CO$_2$ removal by a membrane lung associated with the supply of O$_2$ in the patient's lung, ventilated two or three times per minute by a conventional ventilator and by a continuous endotracheal flow, which maintains a certain level of PEEP [53]. The results obtained so far with LFPPV-ECCO$_2$R are encouraging, but the problems it involves include bleeding and lack of a generally accepted index of severity of pulmonary failure for its institution—a common problem in evaluation of all modes of ventilatory support in man.

Inversed ratio ventilation

IRV is defined as a ventilatory pattern allowing a longer time for the inspiratory phase than for expiration, thereby producing an I:E ratio greater than 1:1 [12]. Depending on the expiratory time and the time constant of the passive expiration, this technique can result in a substantial level of PEEP and gas trapping in the lungs. Pulmonary gas exchange is usually improved by IRV, but cardiovascular depression can be significant and the patient has to be heavily sedated or curarized to tolerate the ventilatory pattern.

Differential lung ventilation

Selective application of a ventilatory pattern to the left and the right lung has been used for the treatment of marked unilateral lung disease [29, 102, 129]. This technique consists in the administration of different tidal volumes, F$_I$O$_2$, and PEEP to each lung by one or two ventilators through a double-lumen endotracheal tube. In this way differences in the time constants of the distribution of ventilation and in the mechanical properties and the perfusion of the two lungs can be compensated for, enabling a substantial improvement of gas exchange. The main disadvantages of differential lung ventilation are the complicated tubing circuit, the problem of synchronization of the two ventilators, and the amount of monitoring equipment that is required. In a number of patients with unilateral lung disease, an improvement in lung function can be achieved by adequate positioning and frequent posture changes alone [105].

Chest physical therapy during MV

Chest physical therapy must be applied whenever necessary. Postural changes achieved by turning the patient from the right to the left side or vice versa regularly every 1–2 h around the clock can be of value in the prevention of both atelectasis and skin breakdown. The prescription of fixed time intervals for percussion and endotracheal suction for all patients is inappropriate, because it can cause significant impairment of arterial oxygenation [32]. The schedules for manual hyperinflation and clearing of the airway by gentle suction and instillation of a few milliliters of isotonic saline must be adapted to each individual patient. The greatest benefit of these maneuvers is seen in patients with increased sputum production [32]. Before and during chest physiotherapy adequate oxygenation must be assured.

The endotracheal tube must always be handled with strict aseptic techniques in intubated patients, to decrease the danger of exogenous superinfection. Adequate humidification of the inspired gas is also essential for the function of physiological clearing mechanisms of the airways and avoids drying of the mucus [30, 50].

Secondary effects and complications of positive pressure ventilation

MV is an efficient but potentially harmful therapy. Therefore all patients receiving this treatment must be monitored carefully, for many of the 'accidents' in ICUs that are due to human error or equipment malfunction are related to respiratory equipment [1].

Most or all the side-effects of MV are due to the increased intrathoracic pressure. The mechanisms involved include a direct mechanical interference of the positive pressure with intrathoracic structures or neural receptors [61, 72, 103, 104, 106], changes in the perfusion of extrathoracic organs secondary to alterations in arterial or venous pressure [67, 94, 110], and reflex or humoral responses originating from intrathoracic or other organs [61, 70, 83].

Respiratory system

During IPPV and CPPV, the distribution of ventilation is different from that during spontaneous breathing: nondependent lung regions presenting with a high ventilation/perfusion ratio ($\dot{V}_A/\dot{Q}$) receive a greater part of the tidal volume, and dependent areas (low $\dot{V}A/\dot{Q}$) receive less. With PEEP, ventilation is probably more evenly distributed [65, 66]. Lung blood flow is also redistributed during IPPV in favor of dependent, less ventilated areas. During CPPV total pulmonary perfusion can decrease, the vertical gradient of blood flow increases, and a centrifugal redistribution is observed [66]. This, by countering alveolar collapse and airway closure, results in the improved gas exchange for O_2 noted with PEEP; V_D/V_T increases as high-$\dot{V}_A/\dot{Q}$ regions are produced.

MV can cause additional perturbances in the lung due to O_2 toxicity [39], interference with the ciliary activity and cellular morphology of the tracheobronchial tree [30, 50], and alterations of surface-active material [46].

Of greater clinical importance is the pulmonary barotrauma [34, 82]. Overdistension of alveolar and bronchiolar structures can lead to tissue rupture and dissection of interstitial space along bronchi and vessels, often visible on chest X-rays [5]. Subsequently, mediastinal or subcutaneous emphysema, pneumothorax, pneumoperitoneum and pneumoretroperitoneum may develop, when the leakage of gas from the lung is significant and sustained [4, 82]. This gas must be drained away if it accumulates in a sufficient volume to impair ventilation, circulation or other organ function, and when the danger of tension pneumothorax is anticipated.

Heart and circulation

Positive pressure ventilation has important effects on cardiac output and systemic blood flow (Fig. 20.4). The most important and best-known mechanisms responsible for the interference of MV with cardiocirculatory function are: (1) a decrease in venous return and cardiac filling [104]; (2) changes in RV and LV end-diastolic pressure and volumes [20, 27, 28, 74, 103, 106, 108]; (3) changes in ventricular geometry [75, 86]; (4) alterations in myocardial contractility due to reflex or humoral mechanisms [61, 93]; (5) changes in coronary artery perfusion [97]; (6) alterations in pulmonary vascular resistance [13, 15, 25, 133].

These cardiovascular side-effects can be corrected or prevented by intravascular volume expansion [104] or administration of dopamine [10, 14, 69, 89]. Their importance depends on the level of airway pressure (or intrathoracic pressure) applied, the circulating blood volume [125], the degree of pressure transmission from the alveoli to the pleural space, and the response of the myocardium and the vasomotor tone.

The distribution of the systemic blood flow to the vital organs can be altered by increasing intrathoracic pressure [93], but in man this aspect has not yet been adequately studied.

Figure 20.7 illustrates the changes in LV and RV volume and configuration in diastole and systole during IPPV and CPPV in a patient with severe ARDS. The ventricular spaces are filled with isotope-labeled red cells and the pictures are taken by gamma camera.

Central nervous system

Positive pressure ventilation can influence CNS function by the changes in pulmonary gas exchange, because $PaCO_2$, pH, and PaO_2 all have important effects on cerebral blood flow. In addition, the cerebral perfusion pressure, which is the difference between arterial and jugular venous pressure, is directly influenced by cardiac output and intrathoracic pressure. Depending on the intracranial compliance, the central venous pressure can also aggravate cerebral edema and increase intracranial pressure. All these factors, cerebral perfusion pressure, cerebral blood flow, intracranial pressure, and cerebral edema, determine the function of the nervous cell and the brain [2, 110].

These considerations and effects are of particular importance in the neurosurgical patient, after craniocerebral trauma, and in cerebral edema. In these patients close monitoring of

neurologic function, intracranial pressure, arterial and central venous pressure, and arterial blood gases is mandatory to avoid or minimize detrimental effects of MV.

Renal function

Renal function is impaired during MV when PEEP is applied [62, 85, 94]: renal perfusion, glomerular filtration, creatinine clearance, and sodium and free water clearance are all decreased. The mechanisms responsible for these changes are decreased cardiac output, decreased perfusion pressure, redistribution of intrarenal blood flow, and, increased antidiuretic hormone secretion [70, 83].

Left and right ventricular volume and function

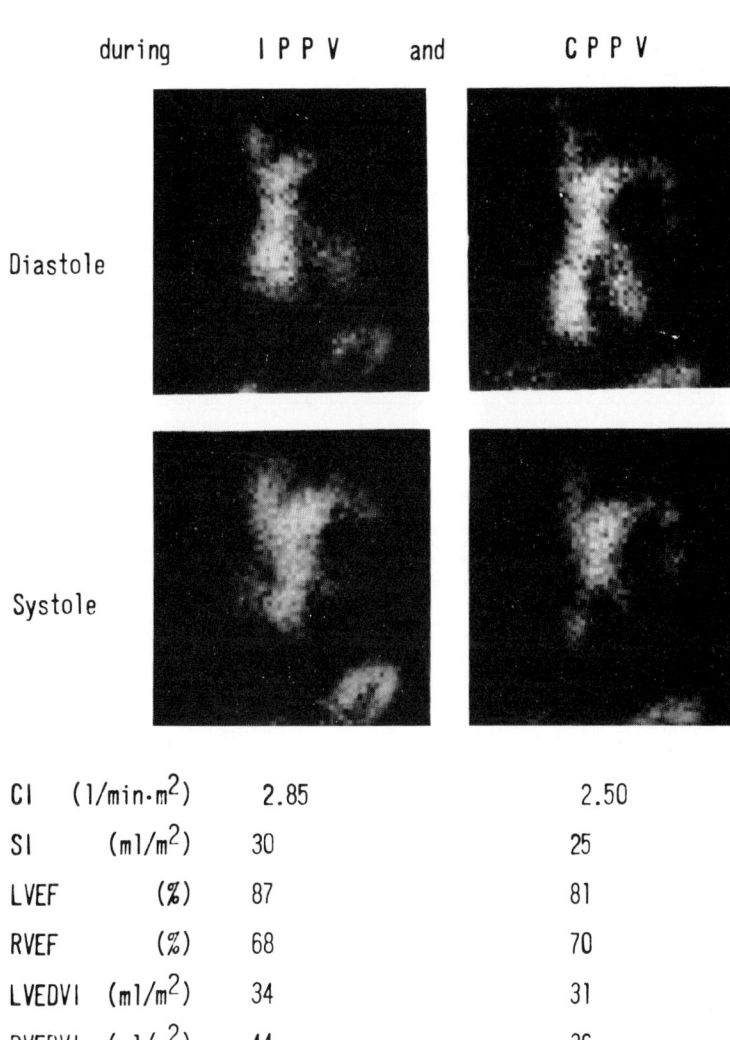

during   I P P V   and   C P P V

Diastole

Systole

Fig. 20.7. Effect of PEEP on configuration volume and ejection fraction of left and right ventricle in a patient with severe ARDS. During diastole (*upper two photographs*) PEEP is associated with a decreased LV end-diastolic volume index (*LVEDVI*) and RV end-diastolic volume index (*RVEDVI*), and a more vertical position of the heart. Cardiac index (*CI*) decreases with PEEP due to a decrease in stroke index (*SI*) whereas LV and RV ejection fractions (*LVEF* and *RVEF*) do not change significantly. These images are obtained in the 45° left anterior oblique view by gated blood pool scan utilizing red cells labelled in vivo with Tc-99 m. Courtesy of Dr. A. Righetti and Dr. C. Viquerat, Centre de Cardiologie, Genève.

		IPPV	CPPV
CI	$(1/min \cdot m^2)$	2.85	2.50
SI	(ml/m^2)	30	25
LVEF	(%)	87	81
RVEF	(%)	68	70
LVEDVI	(ml/m^2)	34	31
RVEDVI	(ml/m^2)	44	36

The consequences of the impaired renal function are mainly fluid retention and edema formation. The renal situation can be improved with intravascular volume expansion and/or administration of dopamine [10, 14, 69, 104].

Hepatic function

Clinically, hepatomegaly and jaundice are observed frequently in patients requiring prolonged ventilatory support with high intrathoracic pressures. In animals, CPPV produces a rise in pressure in the portal and hepatic veins associated with a decrease in blood flow; biliary duct pressure is also increased. The clearance of sulfobromophthalein sodium from the plasma, which is used to assess hepatocellular function, is impaired during CPPV [67, 76].

Weaning from ventilatory support

With the advent of newer techniques of ventilatory support, such as IMV and CPAP, weaning can be initiated early. Some relevant clinical and respiratory conditions must be stable and the patient's comfort has to be ensured during this phase. The respiratory criteria for the start of the weaning process are quite different from those required for extubation (Table 20.5). After short-term MV in patients presenting no serious cardiac disease, sepsis, or metabolic problems, weaning is achieved easily via IMV, CPAP, or T-piece [64]. IMV and CPAP help to improve pulmonary gas exchange and decrease the work of breathing during this period in more complex situations [6, 40, 47, 48, 100].

In the patient with cardiac failure the cardiac filling pressures must be monitored closely to avoid weaning failure and cardiac decompensation [131] due to an intolerable increase in central blood volume. Mechanical problems interfering with efficient spontaneous ventilation such as abdominal distension, incoordinate respiratory movement, pleural effusion, or pulmonary edema must be corrected as far as possible. The patients must have enough time for rest and sleep to enable them to tolerate the effort represented by spontaneous breathing in this phase. During recent years, special attention has been given to the respiratory problems caused by excessive carbohydrate intake [9, 22]. Patients treated with a large calorie intake in the form of glucose present increased rates of CO_2 production, impairing their capacity for sufficient spontaneous alveolar ventilation and delaying weaning.

Psychological factors are also important for successful weaning from ventilatory support. The patient should have no pain or dyspnea and must feel confident of close attention and

Table 20.5. Minimum criteria for initiation of weaning and for extubation

Clinical state:
  Stable cardiovascular condition
  No severe abdominal distension
  No fluid overload
  No major metabolic disturbances
  No important respiratory movement discoordination
  Adequate rest and sleeping time

	Respiratory criteria for	
	Initiation of weaning	Extubation
Vital capacity	≥ 5	≥10–15 ml/kg
Inspiratory force	≥10	≥25 cm H_2O
PEEP/CPAP required	≤15	≤ 5 cm H_2O
PaO_2 at F_1O_2 0.4	≥60	≥60 mm Hg (8kP)
pH	≥ 7.30	≥ 7.30
Respiratory frequency	<45	<35/min
Minute ventilation	<18	<10 l/min

Other important elements:
Nutrition:
  Must be adequate, but a high carbohydrate load should be avoided
Psychological factors:
  Subjective clinical state: pain, fatigue, and dyspnea must be avoided and corrected
  Continuous monitoring by nurses
  Motivation
Position, mobilization if possible
Cough, swallowing reflex in unconscious patients

help from the nursing staff; in addition, encouragement should be provided by early mobilization and frequent information on the progress of weaning.

References

1. Abramson NS, Wald KS, Grenvik A, Robinson D, Snyder JV (1980) Adverse occurrences in intensive care units. JAMA 244:1582–1584
2. Aidinis SJ, Lafferty J, Shapiro HM (1976) Intracranial responses to PEEP. Anesthesiology 45:275–286
3. Albert RK, Lakshminarayan, Kirk W, Butler J (1980) Lung inflation can cause pulmonary edema in zone I of in situ dog lungs. J Appl Physiol 49:815–819
4. Altman AR, Johnson Th (1979a) Pneumoperitoneum and pneumoretroperitoneum. Arch Surg 114:208–211
5. Altman AR, Johnson TH (1979b) Roentgenographic findings in PEEP therapy—indicators of pulmonary complications. JAMA 242:727–730
6. Annest SJ, Gottlieb M, Paloski W, Stratton H, Newell JC, Dutton R, Powers SR (1980) Detrimental effects of removing end-expiratory pressure prior to endotracheal extubation. Ann Surg 191:539–545
7. Asbaugh DG, Bigelow DB, Petty TL, Levine BE (1967) Acute respiratory distress in adults. Lancet II:1319–1322
8. Asbaugh DG, Petty TL, Bigelow DB, Harris TM, Waddell WR (1969) Continuous positive-pressure breathing (CPPB) in adult respiratory distress syndrome. J Thorac Cardiovasc Surg 57:31–41
9. Askanazi J, Nordenstrom J, Rosenbaum SH, Elwyn DH, Hyman AI, Carpentier YA, Kinney JM (1981) Nutrition for the patient with respiratory failure: glucose vs. fat. Anesthesiology 54:373–377
10. Augustin HJ, Bischoff K, Engels T (1979) Der Einfluss von Dopamin auf die Nierenfunktion während kontinuierlicher Überdruckbeatmung (PEEP). Anaesthesist 28:159–162
11. Baum M, Benzer H, Geyer A, Haider W, Mutz N (1980) Forcierte Diffusionsventilation (FDV). Anaesthesist 29:586–591
12. Baum M, Benzer H, Mutz N, Pauser G, Tonczar L (1980) Inversed ratio ventilation (IRV). Anaesthesist 29:592–596
13. Benumof JL (1979) Anesthesia and pulmonary circulation. Ann Refresher Course Lecture. Ann Meet Am Soc Anesth 227:1–14
14. Benzer H, Haider W, Kundi M, Laczkovics A, Todt W (1977) Die Kombination von kontinuierlicher Überdruckbeatmung (PEEP) und Dopamin beim postkardiochirurgischen Patienten. Herz 2:465–472
15. Berryhill RE, Benumof JL, Rauscher LA (1978) Pulmonary vascular pressure reading at the end of exhalation. Anesthesiology 49:365–368
16. Binder AS, Kageler W, Perel A, Flick MR, Staub NC (1980) Effect of platelet depletion on lung vascular permeability after microemboli in sheep. J Appl Physiol 48:414–420
17. Bland RD, Kim MH, Light MS, Woodson JL (1977) High-frequency mechanical ventilation of low-birth-weight infants with respiratory failure from hyaline membrane disease: 92% survival. Pediatr Res 11:531
18. Bø G, Hauge A, Nicolaysen G (1977) Alveolar pressure and lung volume as determinants of net transvascular fluid filtration. J Appl Physiol 42:476–482
19. Brigham KL, Bowers RE, McKeen CR (1981) Methylprednisolon prevention of increased lung vascular permeability following endotoxemia in sheep. J Clin Invest 67:1103–1110
20. Brown DR, Bazaral MG, Nath PH, Delaney DJ (1981) Canine left ventricular volume response to mechanical ventilation with PEEP. Anesthesiology 54:409–412
21. Buda AJ, Pinsky MR, Ingels NB, Daughters GT, Stinson EB, Alderman EL (1979) Effect of intrathoracic pressure on left ventricular performance. N Engl J Med 301:453–459
22. Burke JF, Wolfe RR, Mullany CJ, Mathews DE, Bier DM (1979) Glucose requirements following burn injury. Ann Surg 190:274–285
23. Butler WJ, Bohn DJ, Bryan AC, Froese AB (1980) Ventilation by high-frequency oscillation in humans. Anesth Analg (Cleve) 59:577–584
24. Caldini P, Leith JD, Brennan MJ (1975) Effect of continuous positive-pressure ventilation (CPPV) on edema formation in dog lung. J Appl Physiol 39:672–679
25. Canada ED, Benumof JL (1980) Correlates of pulmonary vascular resistance. Anesthesiology 53:S383
26. Carlon GC, Ray C, Klain M, McCormack PM (1980) High-frequency positive-pressure ventilation in management of a patient with bronchopleural fistula. Anesthesiology 52:160–162
27. Cassidy SS, Robertson CH, Pierce AK, Johnson RL (1978) Cardiovascular effects of positive end-expiratory pressure in dogs. J Appl Physiol 44:743–750
28. Cassidy SS, Eschenbacher WL, Robertson CH, Nixon JV, Blomqvist G, Johnson RL (1979) Cardiovascular effects of positive-pressure ventilation in normal subjects. J Appl Physiol 47:453–461
29. Cavanilles JM, Garrigosa F, Prieto C, Oncins JR (1979) A selective ventilation distribution circuit (S.V.D.C.). Intens Care Med 5:95–98
30. Chalon CP, Ramanathan J, Turndorf H (1980) Tracheobronchial cytologic changes during prolonged cannulation. Anesth Analg (Cleve) 59:759–763
31. Chapin JC, Downs JB, Douglas ME, Murphy EJ, Ruiz BC (1979) Lung expansion, airway pressure transmission and positive end-expiratory pressure. Arch Surg 114:1193–1197
32. Connors AF, Hammon WE, Martin RJ, Rogers RM (1980) Chest physical therapy: The immediate effect on oxygenation in acutely ill patients. Chest 78:559–564
33. Cournand A, Motley HL, Werko L, Richards DW (1948) Physiological studies of the effects of intermittent positive pressure breathing on cardiac output in man. Am J Physiol 152:162–174
34. Cullen DJ, Caldera DL (1979) The incidence of ventilator-induced pulmonary barotrauma in critically ill patients. Anesthesiology 50:185–190
35. Danek SJ, Lynch JP, Weg JG, Dantzker DR (1980) The dependence of oxygen uptake on oxygen delivery in the adult respiratory distress syndrome. Am Rev Respir Dis 122:387–395
36. Dantzker DR, Lynch JP, Weg JG (1980) Depression of cardiac output is a mechanism of shunt reduction in the therapy of acute respiratory failure. Chest 77:636–642
37. Demedts M, Clément J, Stanescu DC, Van de Woestijne KP (1975) Inflection point on transpulmonary pressure-volume curves and closing volume. J Appl Physiol 38:228–235
38. Demling RH, Duy N, Manohar M, Proctor R (1980) Comparison between lung fluid filtration rate and measured Starling forces after hemorrhagic and

endotoxic shock. J Trauma 2:856–860

39. Deneke SM, Fanburg BL (1980) Normobaric oxygen toxicity of the lung. N Engl J Med 303:76–86

40. Downs JB, Klein EF, Desautels D, Modell JH, Kirby RR (1973) Intermittent mandatory ventilation: A new approach to weaning patients from mechanical ventilators. Chest 64:331–335

41. Downs JB, Douglas ME (1980) Assessment of cardiac filling pressure during continuous positive-pressure ventilation. Crit Care Med 8:285–290

42. Edmonds HL, Spohr RW, Finnegan RF, Webb GE, Gott JP, Van Arsdall LR, Flint LM (1981) Indomethacin pretreatment in continuous positive-pressure ventilation. Crit Care Med 9:524–529

43. Egan EA, McIntyre B (1979) Lung inflation, alveolar epithelial albumin permeability, and alveolar flooding. Physiologist 22:33–37

44. Falke KJ (1980) Do changes in lung compliance allow the determination of "optimal PEEP"? Anaesthesist 29:165–168

45. Falke KJ, Pontoppidan H, Kumar A, Leith DE, Geffin B, Laver MB (1972) Ventilation with end-expiratory pressure in acute lung disease. J Clin Invest 51:2315–2323

46. Faridy EE (1976) Effect of ventilation on movement of surfactant in airways. Respir Physiol 27:323–334

47. Feely TW, Hedley-Whyte J (1975) Weaning from controlled ventilation and supplemental oxygen. N Engl J Med 292:903–906

48. Feely TW, Saumarez R, Klick JM, McNabb TG, Skillman JJ (1975) Positive end-expiratory pressure in weaning patients from controlled ventilation: A prospective randomised trial. Lancet II:725–729

49. Fewell JE, Abendschein DR, Carlson CJ, Murray JF, Rapaport E (1980) Continuous positive-pressure ventilation decreases right and left ventricular end-diastolic volumes in the dog. Circ Res 46:125–132

50. Forbes AR, Gamsu G (1979) Lung mucociliary clearance after anesthesia with spontaneous and controlled ventilation. Am Rev Respir Dis 120:857–862

51. Fredberg JJ (1980) Augmented diffusion in the airways can support pulmonary gas exchange. J Appl Physiol 49:232–238

52. Fuleihan SF, Wilson R, Pontoppidan H (1976) Effect of mechanical ventilation with end-inspiratory pause on blood gas exchange. Anesth Analg (Cleve) 55:122–127

53. Gattinoni L, Pesenti A, Rossi GP, Vesconi S et al. (1980) Treatment of acute respiratory failure with low-frequency positive-pressure ventilation and extracorporeal removal of CO_2. Lancet II:292–299

54. Gee MH, Williams DO (1979) Effect of lung inflation on perivascular cuff fluid volume in isolated dog lung lobes. Microvasc Res 17:192–201

55. Gherini S, Peters RM, Virgilio RW (1979) Mechanical work on the lungs and work of breathing with positive end-expiratory pressure and continuous positive airway pressure. Chest 76:251–256

56. Goldberg HS (1980) Pulmonary interstitial compliance and microvascular filtration coefficient. Am J Physiol 239:H189–H198

57. Gorin AB, Stewart PA (1979) Differential permeability of endothelial and epithelial barriers to albumin flux. J Appl Physiol 47:1315–1324

58. Greenbaum DM (1979) Positive end-expiratory pressure, constant positive airway pressure, and cardiac performance. Chest 76:248–249

59. Greenbaum DM, Millen JE, Eross B, Snyder JV, Grenvik A, Safar P (1976) Continuous positive airway pressure without tracheal intubation in spontaneously breathing patients. Chest 69:615–619

60. Gregory GA, Kitterman JA, Phibbs RH, Tooley WH, Hamilton WK (1971) Treatment of the idiopathic respiratory-distress syndrome with continuous positive airway pressure. N Engl J Med 284:1333–1340

61. Grindlinger GA, Manny J, Justice R, Dunham B, Shepro D, Hechtman HB (1979) Presence of negative inotropic agents in canine plasma during positive end-expiratory pressure. Circ Res 45:460–467

62. Hall SV, Johnson EE, Hedley-Whyte J (1974) Renal hemodynamics and function with continuous positive-pressure ventilation in dogs. Anesthesiology 44:452–461

63. Harf A, Lemaire F, Régnier B (1979) Physiologie de la ventilation artificielle. Revue du Praticien XXIX:3885–3898

64. Hastings PR, Bushnell LS, Skillman JJ, Weintraub RM, Hedley-Whyte J (1980) Cardiorespiratory dynamics during weaning with IMV versus spontaneous ventilation in good-risk cardiac-surgery patients. Anesthesiology 53:429–431

65. Hedenstierna G, White FC, Mazzone R, Wagner PD (1979) Redistribution of pulmonary blood flow in the dog with PEEP ventilation. J Appl Physiol 46:278–287

66. Hedenstierna G, White FC, Wagner PD (1979) Spatial distribution of pulmonary blood flow in the dog with PEEP ventilation. J Appl Physiol 47:938–946

67. Hedley-Whyte J, Burgess GE, Feely TW, Miller MG (1976) Applied physiology of respiratory care. Little, Brown, Boston

68. Heenan TJ, Downs JB, Douglas ME et al (1980) Intermittent mandatory ventilation: Is synchronization important? Chest 77:598–602

69. Hemmer M, Suter PM (1979) Treatment of cardiac and renal effects of PEEP with dopamine in patients with acute respiratory failure. Anesthesiology 50:399–403

70. Hemmer M, Viquerat CE, Suter PM, Vallotton MB (1980) Urinary antidiuretic hormone excretion during mechanical ventilation and weaning in man. Anesthesiology 52:395–400

71. Hopewell PC (1979) Failure of positive end-expiratory pressure to decrease lung water content in alloxan-induced pulmonary edema. Am Rev Respir Dis 120:813–819

72. Ilabaca PA, Ochsner JL, Mills NL (1980) Positive end-expiratory pressure in the management of the patient with a postoperative bleeding heart. Ann Thorac Surg 30:281–284

73. Ingram RH, O'Cain CF, Fridy WW (1974) Simultaneous quasi-static lung pressure-volume curves and "closing volume" measurements. J Appl Physiol 36:135–141

74. Janicki JS. Weber KT (1980) The pericardium and ventricular interaction, distensibility and function. Am J Physiol 238:H494–H503

75. Jardin F, Farcot JC, Boisante L, Curien N, Margairaz A, Bourdarias JP (1981) Influence of positive end-expiratory pressure on left ventricular performance. N Engl J Med 304:387–392

76. Johnson EE, Hedley-Whyte J, Hall SV (1977) End-expiratory pressure ventilation and sulfobromophthalein sodium excretion in dogs. J Appl Physiol 43:714–720

77. King EG, Jones RI, Patakas DA (1973) Evaluation of positive end-expiratory pressure therapy in the adult respiratory distress syndrome. Canad Anaesth Soc J 20:546–558

78. Kirby RR, Downs JB, Civetta JM, Modell JH, Dannemiller FJ, Klein EF, Hodges M (1975) High level positive end-expiratory pressure (PEEP) in acute respiratory insufficiency. Chest 67:156–163

79. Kirby RR (1980) High-frequency positive-pressure ventilation (HFPPV). Anesthesiology 52:109–110

80. Klain M, Smith RB (1977) High frequency percutaneous transtracheal jet ventilation. Crit Care Med 5:280–287

81. Kumar A, Falke KJ, Geffin B, Aldredge CF, Laver MB, Lowenstein E, Pontoppidan H (1970) Continuous positive-pressure ventilation in acute respiratory failure. Effects on hemodynamic and lung function. N Engl J Med 283:1430–1436

82. Kumar A, Pontoppidan H, Falke KJ, Wilson RS, Laver MB (1973) Pulmonary barotrauma during mechanical ventilation. Crit Care Med 1:181–186

83. Kumar A, Pontoppidan H, Baratz RA, Laver MB (1974) Inappropriate response to increased plasma ADH during mechanical ventilation in acute respiratory failure. Anesthesiology 40:215–221

84. Labrousse J, Tenaillon A, Longchal J, Chastre J, Lissac J (1979) Pression positive expiratoire optimale au cours de la ventilation artificielle. Nouv Presse Med 8:759–763

85. Laver MB (1979) Dr Starling and the "ventilator" kidney. Anesthesiology 50:383–386

86. Laver MB, Strauss HW, Pohost GM (1979) Right and left ventricular geometry: Adjustments during acute respiratory failure. Crit Care Med 7:509–519

87. Laver MB, Morgan J, Bendixen HH, Radford EP (1964) Lung volume, compliance, and arterial oxygen tensions during controlled ventilation. J Appl Physiol 19:725–733

88. Lemaire F, Simonneau A, Risara D, Tesseire B, Atlan G, Rapin M (1979) Static pulmonary pressure-volume curve, positive end-expiratory pressure ventilation and gas exchange in acute respiratory failure. Am Rev Respir Dis 119:328

89. Lemaire F, Régnier B, Simoneau G, Harf A (1980) Positive end-expiratory pressure (PEEP) ventilation suppresses the increase of shunting caused by dopamine infusion. Anesthesiology 52:376–377

90. Luce JM, Pierson DJ, Hudson LD (1981) Intermittent mandatory ventilation. Chest 79:678–685

91. Lutch JS, Murray JF (1972) Continuous positive-pressure ventilation: Effects on systemic oxygen transport and tissue oxygenation. Ann Intern Med 76:193–202

92. Malik AB, Van der Zee H, Neumann PH, Gertzberg NB (1980) Effects of pulmonary edema on regional pulmonary perfusion in the intact dog lung. J Appl Physiol 49:834–840

93. Manny J, Justice R, Hechtman HB (1979) Abnormalities in organ blood flow and its distribution during positive end-expiratory pressure. Surgery 85:425–432

94. Marquez JM, Douglas ME, Downs JB, Wu WH, Mantini EL, Kuck EJ, Calderwood HW (1979) Renal function and cardiovascular responses during positive airway pressure. Anesthesiology 50:393–398

95. Naver L, Walter S, Glöwinski J (1980) Pulmonary fat embolism treated by intermittent continuous positive airway given by face mask. Br Med J 280:1413–1414

96. Parker JC, Guyton AC, Taylor AE (1978) Pulmonary interstitial and capillary pressures estimated from intra-alveolar fluid pressures. J Appl Physiol 44:267–276

97. Pepine CJ (1977) Coronary circulatory effects of increased intrathoracic pressure in intact dogs. Chest 72:72–78

98. Perschau RA, Pepine CJ, Nichols WW, Downs JB (1979) Instantaneous blood flow responses to positive end-expiratory pressure with spontaneous ventilation.

Circulation 59:1312–1318

99. Pontoppidan H, Geffin B, Lowenstein E (1972) Acute respiratory failure in the adult. N Engl J Med 287:690–698, 743–752, 799–806

100. Pontoppidan H, Wilson RS, Rie MA, Schneider RC (1977) Respiratory intensive care. Anesthesiology 47:96–116

101. Powers SR, Dutton RE (1975) Correlation of positive end-expiratory pressure with cardiovascular performance. Crit Care Med 3:64–68

102. Powner DJ, Eros B, Genvik A (1977) Differential lung ventilation with PEEP in the treatment of unilateral pneumonia. Crit Care Med 5:170

103. Prewitt RM, Wood LDH (1979) Effect of positive end-expiratory pressure on ventricular function in dogs. Am J Physiol 5:H534–H544

104. Qvist J, Pontoppidan H, Wilson RS, Lowenstein E, Laver MB (1975) Hemodynamic response to mechanical ventilation with PEEP: The effect of hypervolemia. Anesthesiology 42:45–55

105. Remolina C, Khan AU, Santiago TV, Edelman NH (1981) Positional hypoxemia in unilateral lung disease. N Engl J Med 304:523–525

106. Robotham JL, Lixfeld W, Holland L, MacGregor D, Bromberger-Barnea B, Permutt S, Rabson JL (1980) The effects of positive end-expiratory pressure on right and left ventricular performance. Am Rev Respir Dis 121:677–683

107. Rossing TH, Slutsky AS, Lehr JL, Drinker PA, Kamm R, Drazen JM (1981) Tidal volume and frequency dependence of carbon dioxide elimination by high-frequency ventilation. N Engl J Med 305:1375–1979

108. Scharf SM, Brown R, Saunders N, Green LH, Ingram RH (1979) Changes in canine left ventricular size and configuration with positive end-expiratory pressure. Circ Res 44:672–678

109. Schmidt GB, O'Neill WW, Kotb K, Hwang KK, Bennett EJ, Bombeck CT (1976) Continuous positive airway pressure in the prophylaxis of the adult respiratory distress syndrome. Surg Gynecol Obstet 143:613–618

110. Shapiro HM, Marshall LF (1978) Intracranial pressure responses to PEEP in head-injured patients. J Trauma 18:254–256

111. Simonneau G, Lemaire F, Harf A, Safran D, Georges C, Rieuf P, Teisseire B, Rapin M (1979) Insuffisance respiratoire aiguë de l'adulte : comparaison des effets hémodynamiques et respiratoires de la pression expiratoire positive en ventilation spontanée et en ventilation artificielle. Nouv Presse Med 8:113–115

112. Sjöstrand UH (1977) Experimental and clinical evaluation of high-frequency positive-pressure ventilation. Acta Anaesthesiol Scand [Suppl] 64:1–178

113. Sjöstrand UH, Eriksson IA (1980) High rates and low volumes in mechanical ventilation—not just a matter of ventilatory frequency. Anesth Analg (Cleve) 59:567–576

114. Slutsky AS, Drazen JM, Ingram RH Jr et al. (1980) Effective pulmonary ventilation with small-volume oscillations at high frequency. Science 209:609–611

115. Staub NC (1978) Pulmonary edema due to increased microvascular permeability to fluid and proteins. Circ Res 43:143–151

116. Staub NC (1980) The pathogenesis of pulmonary edema. Prog Cardiovasc Dis 23:53–80

117. Staub NC, Ohkuda K (1978) PGE_1 reverses increased lung microvascular permeability during air emboli. Microvasc Res 15:271–272

118. Staub NC, Nagano H, Pearce ML (1967) Pulmonary edema in dogs, especially the sequence of fluid accumulation in the lungs. J Appl Physiol 22:227–240

119. Stone DR, Downs JB (1980) Collateral ventilation and PEEP in normal and edematous lungs of dogs. Anesthesiology 53:S186

120. Suter PM (1980) "Optimal" regulation of mechanical ventilation. Anaesthesist 29:163–164

121. Suter PM, Fairley HB, Schlobohm RM (1975) Shunt, lung volume and perfusion during short periods of ventilation with oxygen. Anesthesiology 43:617–627

122. Suter PM, Fairley HB, Isenberg MD (1975) Optimum end-expiratory airway pressure in patients with acute pulmonary failure. N Engl J Med 292:284–289

123. Suter PM, Brigljevic M, Hemmer M, Gemperle M (1977) Effects de la pause en fin d'inspiration sur l'échange gazeux et l'hémodynamique chez des patients en ventilation mécanique. Can Anaesth Soc J 24:550–558

124. Suter PM, Fairley HB, Isenberg MD (1978) Effect of tidal volume and positive end-expiratory pressure on compliance during mechanical ventilation. Chest 73:158–162

125. Sykes MK, Adams AP, Finlay WEI, McCormick PW, Economides A (1970) The effects of variations in end-expiratory inflation pressure on cardiorespiratory function in normo-, hypo- and hypervolaemic dogs. Br J Anaesth 42:669–677

126. Terry PB, Traystman RJ, Newball HH, Batra G, Menkes HA (1978) Collateral ventilation in man. N Engl J Med 298:10–15

127. Trichet B, Falke K, Togut A, Laver MB (1975) The effect of pre-existing pulmonary vascular disease on the response to mechanical ventilation with PEEP following open-heart surgery. Anesthesiology 42:56–67

128. Venus B, Jacobs HK, Lim L (1979) Treatment of the adult respiratory distress syndrome with continuous positive airway pressure. Chest 76:257–261

129. Venus B, Pratap KS, Op'Tholt T (1980) Treatment of unilateral pulmonary insufficiency by selective administration of continuous positive airway pressure through a double-lumen tube. Anesthesiology 53:74–77

130. Webb HH, Tierney DF (1974) Experimental pulmonary edema due to intermittent positive pressure ventilation with high inflation pressures. Protection by positive end-expiratory pressures. Am Rev Resp Dis 110:556–565

131. Wolff G, Grädel E (1975) Hemodynamic performance and weaning from mechanical ventilation following open-heart surgery. Intensive Care Med 1:99–104

132. Woolverton WC, Brigham KL, Staub NC (1978) Effect of positive pressure breathing on lung lymph flow and water content in sheep. Circ Res 42:550–557

133. Zapol WM, Snider MT (1977) Pulmonary hypertension in severe acute respiratory failure. N Engl J Med 296:476–487

134. Zapol WM, Snider MT et al. (1979) Extracorporeal membrane oxygenation in severe acute respiratory failure. JAMA 242:2193–2196

Chapter 21

Equipment for Respiratory Therapy

J. Labrousse, A. Tenaillon, and J. Chastre

In cases of severely ill patients, it was often said that 'their lives are hanging on a thread'. This expression, however, is no longer meaningful in a modern ICU, in view of the multitude of devices currently available to treat such cases. Equipment for ICUs has become increasingly complex and costly. Yet the quality of the unit depends largely on a wise selection of such equipment.

Oxygen therapy

The equipment necessary to ensure proper O_2 therapy consists of a source of O_2 and devices for its administration [8, 23, 47, 49].

Source of oxygen

High-pressure O_2 is available either in cylinders of various sizes, which are necessary when patients are moved, or from wall pipelines in ICUs. For clinical use, the O_2 must be reduced to atmospheric pressure by a regulator, and to measure the quantity delivered to the patient a flowmeter is used, which is usually incorporated in the regulator. To obtain precise control of the quantity supplied several flowmeters should be available, covering various ranges of gas flow such as 0–1.5 litres/min, 0–5 litres/min, 0–15 litres/min, and 0–50 litres/min.

When an air–O_2 mixture with a precise O_2 concentration is desired compressed air and appropriate manometers are necessary, and the required mixture can then be obtained by simply combining the two gas sources or by using a gas-mixing and -metering unit.

Administration

Basically, there are two different means of administration: one uses relatively simple devices of variable performance in which the inspired O_2 concentration (FiO_2) cannot be controlled, while the other employs more complex items which provide known accurate concentrations of O_2.

Variable performance devices

These supply to the patient a fixed O_2 flow per minute, irrespective of the volume of air with which the O_2 will be mixed. This volume varies from patient to patient, and in each patient with variations in inspiration; therefore under these circumstances, blood gas measurements have to be interpreted with some caution.

Nasal catheters. These provide the easiest method of administration, through a simple plastic catheter with a foam tip and numerous perforations. Correct positioning is most important: to limit O_2 loss the tip should be just visible beneath the soft palate. Oxygen flow rates vary between 0.5 and 15 litres/min and the O_2 must be humidified. The method has the advantage of providing continuous O_2 therapy without disturbing the patient's sleep or feeding. A few complications may arise but these are practically always due to faulty positioning of the catheter. Oxygen may be swallowed, leading to abdominal distension, ulceration of the nasal mucosa with nasal haemorrhage may occur, and erosion of the pharyngeal mucosa can lead to subcutaneous emphysema.

Simple masks. Currently manufactured masks are plastic, lightweight and disposable. Held in place by a simple rubber band, they cause practically no compression on the edge of the mask. The O_2 flow enters through the middle part and the exhaled gases escape through lateral perforations. The FiO_2 is known to vary from 35% to 55%, with O_2 flows of between 6 and 10 litres/min.

They have the disadvantage of interfering with feeding and cause excessive condensation of water. Moreover, like all masks, they may facilitate bronchial aspiration if vomiting occurs, particularly in unconscious patients, in whom they should not be used. The increase in dead space and some degree of rebreathing are not really of practical significance.

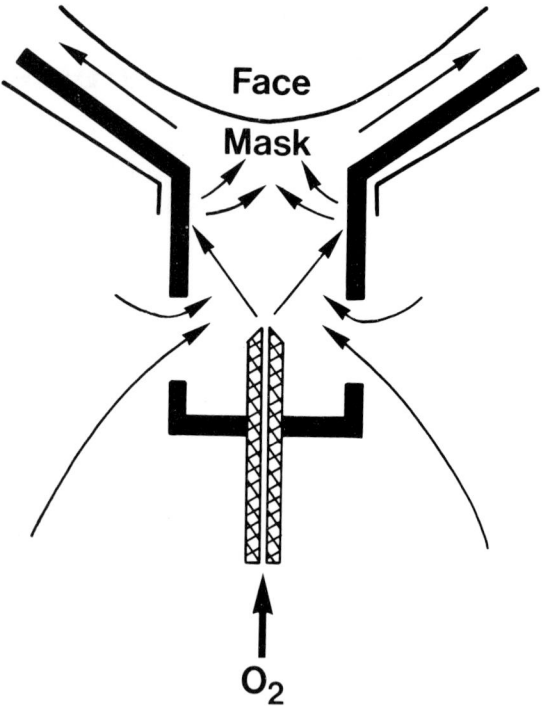

Fig. 21.1. A Venturi system.

Fixed performance devices

With these, a gas mixture with a preset FiO_2 is administered directly to the patient.

Venturi masks. The principle of Venturi masks is based on the use of a high air flow with O_2 enrichment (HAFOE). The non-airtight mask includes a Venturi system (Fig. 21.1) through which a jet of O_2 entrains a constant ratio of air to produce a fixed concentration mixture: for example, an O_2 flow of 2 litres/min entrains 50 litres of air, giving an O_2 concentration of 25% in the inhaled mixture. In the first masks designed by Campbell, the FiO_2 could be set at 24% and 35% [12], but there are now many models available, most of which are disposable, providing O_2 concentrations of 24%, 28%, 35%, 40%, 50% and 60%.

Airtight O_2 masks. These consist of three elements, an airtight, transparent plastic mask with a fixation device, a valve system which prevents mixing of inhaled and exhaled gases, and a source of O_2 including an air–O_2 mixer and a reservoir bag. These masks have the advantage of allowing a gaseous mixture of pure O_2 to be given in very small quantities, but have the same disadvantages as other masks

and are also poorly tolerated when used for long periods. Moreover, pressure from their edges is necessary to ensure an airtight seal, and this may cause skin necrosis.

Facial tents. These consist of a transparent plastic bag into which a high gas flow with a preset FiO_2 enters through one or two openings in the upper part. The gas flow ensures a constant FiO_2 and rebreathing is avoided by drainage of the exhaled gases through the lower, unsealed part of the tent. Facial tents are usually well tolerated; their main disadvantage is that they require large quantities of commercial gas mixture.

Other methods. Only two need be mentioned:

1) The O_2 tent, which has the same disadvantages as the facial tent and is now practically never used in adults.

2) *Hyperbaric O_2 in pressure tanks or chambers,* which is now no longer indicated in intensive care except for severe cases of carbon monoxide poisoning, suplhaemoglobinaemia, and methaemoglobinaemia.

Establishing and maintaining a clear airway

Airway obstruction may arise at different levels. In the upper airways [62] it may be due to tongue-swallowing, spasm of the glottis, and laryngeal oedema, whilst in the lower airways it is the result of diffuse bronchial obstruction such as might follow inhalation of food.

Establishing a clear airway will therefore require different techniques according to the level of obstruction.

Upper airways

Oropharyngeal tubes

These are rigid tubes curved according to the concave shape of the palate and long enough to lift the base of the tongue away from the posterior pharyngeal wall. When they are in place, pharyngeal secretions can be aspirated through the tube. They are used in unconscious patients to avoid tongue-swallowing and to keep the mouth open. Their theoretical advantages are somewhat outweighed by the risk of vomiting.

Nasopharyngeal tubes

These are indicated for similar reasons to those for oropharyngeal tubes, but they are inserted nasally and are often better tolerated. When a patient's mouth cannot be opened, as in tetanus, they are the only tubes that can be used.

Suction catheters

Aspiration catheters are currently manufactured in siliconized plastic, and are disposable. Depending on the manufacturer, they have a single terminal perforation and one or more lateral perforations, which help to avoid damage to the mucosa during suction. They must be long enough for oral, nasopharyngeal, and tracheal aspiration.

Lower airways

Rigid and fiberoptic bronchoscopy

In respiratory intensive care, it is usually considered to be more rational to use a rigid rather than a fiberoptic bronchoscope for removal of foreign bodies and retained bronchial secretions [4, 55, 61]. A rigid bronchoscope is more difficult to manage, however, and most physicians now prefer a fiberoptic instrument. This can be used not only for relieving obstruction but also for bronchial lavage, bronchial biopsy, and taking samples for bacteriological study. Because it is relatively small it can be inserted through a tracheal prosthesis without interrupting MV.

Endotracheal and tracheostomy tubes

Endotracheal tubes for use in adults always have an inflatable cuff to guarantee an airtight seal around the airways. They were initially made of rubber and were reusable after sterilization, but rubber tubes are poorly tolerated and repeated sterilization makes them even more irritant. They have now been replaced by disposable plastic tubes with better long-term tolerance; the tubes for nasal intubation are more flexible than the oral tubes. The most recent improvements in design and manufacture concern the cuffs [16, 21, 50]. To ensure an airtight seal of the airways, the earlier cuffs exerted a high pressure on the tracheal wall, often up to 80–150 mmHg (10–20 kPa), much greater therefore than within the tracheal mucosal vessels, which is approximately 32 mmHg (4.2 kPa). Consequently, there was a risk of ischaemia and necrosis of the mucosa and sometimes the tracheal wall. This problem has now been partially solved by the introduction of so-called 'low pressure cuffs'; to merit this description, the cuffs must be large and cylindrical and manufactured from very flexible material (Fig. 21.2). With this design their compliance is high and the pressure they exert on the tracheal wall is relatively small, averaging about

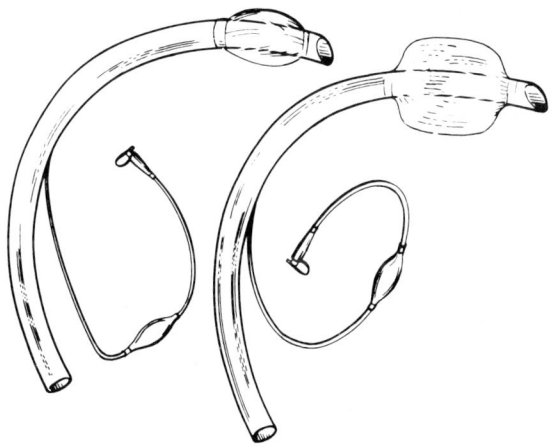

Fig. 21.2. Endotracheal tubes with inflated cuffs: *left*, conventional cuff; *right*, low-pressure cuff.

20 mmHg (2.7 kPa). Nevertheless, excessive in-flation must still be avoided and should be con-trolled with a manometer. Unfortunately, these tubes are somewhat more difficult to insert be-cause of their flexibility and the increased size of the cuff; they are also more easily expelled be-cause the greater compliance of the cuff makes it easier and more likely to slip between the vocal cords [60].

Similar design changes have occurred with tracheostomy tubes and these now incorporate 'low-pressure' cuffs. Cuff-less tracheostomy tubes are available for use during weaning from MV and for the relief of glottis obstruction.

Humidification of the airways

Alveolar air is normally 100% saturated in water vapour, the inspired air being both warmed and humidified in the nasopharynx. When the up-per airways are bypassed, artificial humidifica-tion of the inspired gases with sterile, distilled water is necessary and numerous types of humidifiers and nebulizers are available, some of which can also be used for aerosol therapy [23, 31, 35, 41, 69].

Humidifiers

Humidifiers supply water in a particulate state and are of two types:

1) Passover humidifiers, in which the air simply passes over water, and which are not very efficient
2) Bubble diffusion humidifiers, in which the air actually passes through the liquid and which are therefore much more efficient (Fig. 21.3).

The amount of water contained in a gas de-pends on its temperature. For instance, full saturation of a dry gas at 20°C requires 17 mg of water, whereas at 37°C 44 mg is needed. This is the reason why, when unheated humidifiers are used, there is a decrease in the water vapour saturation when the gas warms in the airways, and such humidifiers cannot provide more than 50%–60% relative humidity. It is therefore al-ways preferable to use heated humidifiers, bear-ing in mind that the inspired gas temperature should never exceed 41°C [69].

The 'artificial nose' is the original type of humidifier. Designed by Toremalm [71], it is fundamentally a heat exchanger, recovering

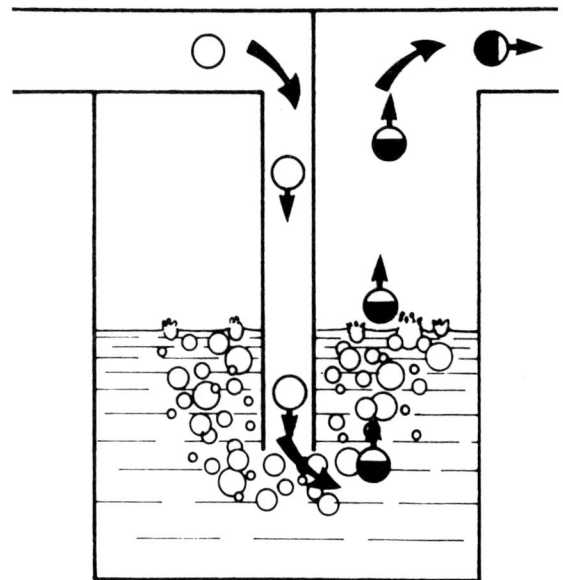

Fig. 21.3. Bubble-diffusion humidifier.

heat and humidity from the expired air and restoring them to the inspired air; the expired water condenses on an aluminium spiral (Fig. 21.4). Lightweight, disposable models are now available.

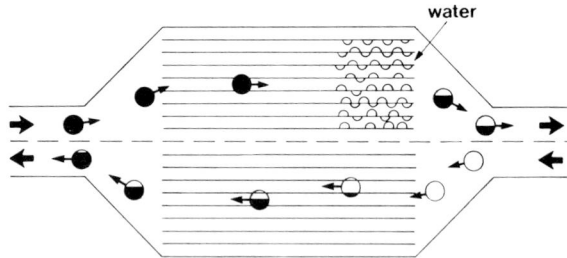

Fig. 21.4. Principle of the 'artificial nose' of Toremalm.

Nebulizers

Nebulizers deliver water in the form of droplets that together form a mist. It is important that the droplet sizes vary, and if they are to pen-etrate right into the bronchioles they must be between 0.5 and 1 μm in diameter.

1) *Nebulization by gas jet* is the simplest method. A jet of compressed gas is released through a calibrated orifice above a capillary tube that is filled by the Bernoulli effect, the orifice acts as a Venturi, and contact of the liq-uid with the gas jet disperses the liquid as a suspension of fine droplets (Fig. 21.5). Some nebulizers incorporate a heating system which makes them even more efficient.

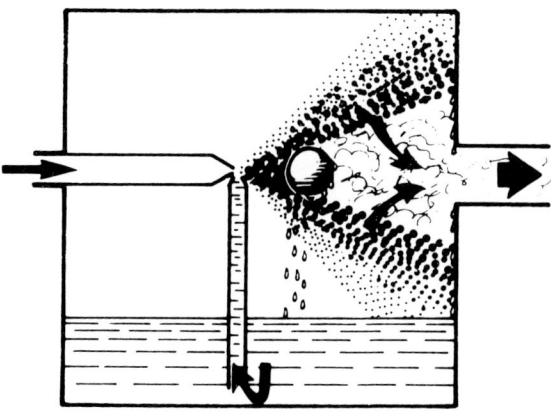

Fig. 21.5. Principle of jet nebulization.

2) *Ultrasonic nebulizers* agitate the water by means of an ultrasonic generator; the vibrations at the liquid–gas interface fragment the liquid into sufficiently fine droplets that then remain in suspension. Though very efficient, ultrasonic nebulizers are nevertheless expensive.

All types of nebulizers can be used for the administration of drugs and other therapeutic agents in the form of aerosols.

Overheating will cause burns of the respiratory tract, and highly efficient nebulizers can result in overhydration [41]. Furthermore, despite the use of sterile water, humidifiers and nebulizers remain a significant reservoir and source of pathogenic organisms, and have been responsible for isolated or even epidemics of pulmonary infection [34, 56]; regular sterilization and bacteriological control is essential.

For patients who are breathing spontaneously a constant mist should be maintained in front of the endotracheal or tracheostomy tube. With artificial ventilation humidification is easier,

since ventilators are usually equipped with an efficient humidifying device. Water levels must be checked frequently, since hot, dry gases are harmful. On the other hand, if humidification is too efficient, the ventilator tubing may become flooded and water traps should therefore also be checked regularly and the tubing emptied of water as necessary. This applies to all mechanical means of respiratory support incorporating endotracheal ventilation or any form of external body respirator.

Artificial ventilation (AV)

Mechanical ventilators

All models function by insufflating a gas mixture into the airways to replace or supplement inspiration, expiration is usually passive and, although there are many different designs, they all require a control system to release pressurized gas, an inspiratory circuit, an expiratory circuit, and a separation system to prevent the inspired and expired gases from mixing (Fig. 21.6).

Classification

Manual ventilators. These are the simplest form, where the control system is the physician himself whose hands activate a reservoir bag. The inspiratory circuit is simply a tube connected to the airways via a two-way valve, the expiratory part of which represents the expiratory circuit. Several models exist, differing in their valves or in the characteristics of the reservoir bag, which is either a concertina or a self-inflating balloon.

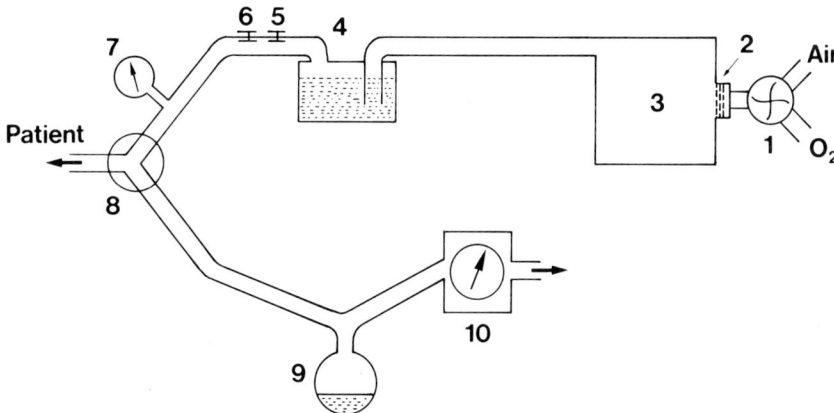

Fig. 21.6. Components of a ventilator: 1, FiO$_2$ mixer; 2, bacterial filter; 3, gas generator; 4, humidifier; 5 safety blow-off valve; 6, air-inlet valve; 7, manometer; 8, circuit separator; 9, water trap; 10, spirometer.

Although simple in appearance and principle, these devices enable a trained physician to perform practically every pattern of AV that the various manufacturers have attempted to simulate.

Automatic ventilators. In automatic devices [23, 38, 53], the *inspiratory circuit* delivers the gas mixture to the patient's airways. The flow and composition of this mixture must be set precisely with the aid of an air and O_2 flowmeter; this method does not indicate FiO_2 directly and it is therefore preferable to have an air–O_2 mixer with an automatic FiO_2 selector; some ventilators include an oximeter with an alarm. The gases must be sterile, which means that a bacterial filter should always be used for fresh air and is also recommended for industrial gases. The mixture must then be heated and humidified before delivery to the patient.

The pressure at which the gases are introduced into the airways must be controlled and a manometer should be positioned close to the airways. This usually has a needle indicator, but on some models a digital display unit indicates inspiratory, expiratory, and peak airway pressure. To avoid an excessive increase of pressure, the inspiratory circuit must be fitted with a preset blow-off valve. An air-inlet valve should also be included in case there is a marked increase in the patient's ventilatory requirements or a generator failure.

The *expiratory circuit* removes the expired gases. The expired volume is the only true reflection of the patient's actual ventilation, and it should be measured mechanically (winged spirometers, etc.) or electronically (pneumotachograph, etc.). If required, 'expired minute volume' alarms can be adapted into the circuit.

Expired gases are usually saturated with water vapour which condenses in the tubing, and some form of water trap is required in the descending portion of the tubing.

The *circuit separator* prevents mixing of the inspired and expired gases by pneumatic, electric, or electronically controlled valves of varying sophistication.

The *gas generator* is the part of the ventilator that delivers the gas mixture and determines the force of its delivery. It is powered either electrically or pneumatically (compressed gas), and in many models the source of energy is used to empty a reservoir bag (balloon, concertina) containing the gases. Electric devices accomplish this by the movement of a piston (Engström 150), a turbine (Spiromat 662), or a pump (Dieffel 70); pneumatic devices use a weight (Manley MN2, Logic 03 and 05, Ohio

CCV), a pneumatic jack (RPR), or a spring system('Servo' Ventilator 900). There are also some pneumatic devices that do not have a reservoir bag, which are traditionally known as flow generators; these function on the basis of an injector, the time this remains open determining the volume injected (Bird, Bennett, Logic, Airox-R).

The *control system* regulates the gas generator and circuit separator and effects the changeover (cycling) from expiration to inspiration. The timing of the cycling is determined by volume, pressure, flow, or time, and ventilators are commonly classified according to this mechanism.

Volume-cycled ventilator (RPR, M250). In this type the control system is based on the volume of the reservoir bag. Once a preset volume has been attained in the bag it is driven out until the entire volume has been delivered. The rate therefore depends on the magnitude of the driving pressure and the patient's airway resistance. If the ventilator is not set correctly or resistance to flow is high, the frequency diminishes and ventilation may even stop.

Pressure-cycled ventilators (Bird, Bennett, PRI and PR2, Airox VP 2000). Here the controlling parameter is the pressure in the inspiratory circuit: insufflation stops once this reaches a preset level. Tidal volume and frequency are therefore a direct function of the preset pressure level and patient's airway resistance. The main disadvantage of this type of ventilator is the inability to deliver a constant ventilation if resistance to inflation increases either from changes in the patient's condition or obstruction somewhere in the inspiratory circuit or ET tube. The cycling pressure is attained more rapidly and inspiratory time is reduced and frequency increases. By contrast, if there is a leak in the circuit a longer time will be required to reach the cycling pressure and, if the leak is large, the ventilator will slow or even stop.

Flow-cycled ventilators. In this type flow into the patient's circuit regulates the change-over and the generator is, in effect, a low-pressure flow generator. When the driving pressure reaches the insufflation pressure, the flow becomes zero and, at this point, the control system switches to expiration (Bennett, PR1 and PR2).

Time-cycled ventilators. Here, an electromechanical or logic clock regulates the change-over:

Electromechanical clocks are based on an electric engine which opens the injector mechanically or according to an electromechanical programme (Bary, SF4, SF4T, AD1); in older devices the motor variator performed this function (Engström 150, RET 104);

Logic clocks are either pneumatic with fluidic logic components (Airox-R, Logic) or electronic, with transistors (MMS 107, Bourns paediatric, Servo ventilator 900).

Mixed-cycled ventilators. The traditional classification of ventilators described above has the advantage of simplicity and also highlights the dominant function of the ventilator. Some ventilators may be classified differently, however, depending on their mode of use; for instance, the Barnet Mark III ventilator can be cycled on volume, time, or pressure, the Bourns Bear 1 on volume or time, and the Servo ventilator 900 on frequency or pressure, whilst the Bennett PR1 and PR2 ventilators are flow-cycled, but include a timing system that provides a preset frequency function.

It should be noted that almost all time-cycled ventilators can deliver the selected volume or flow of gas and they are therefore the best type of machine for use in difficult cases.

Modes of ventilation

The optimal pattern of ventilation varies from patient to patient, largely depending on the nature of the pulmonary pathology. Ventilators have therefore been designed to incorporate a range of functions and it is important to have thorough knowledge of these before making a purchase. The different use can be illustrated by considering controlled and assisted ventilation.

Controlled ventilation. Controlled ventilation completely takes over the patient's ventilation and must therefore provide a sufficient minute ventilation; this depends solely on the frequency of the ventilator and the delivered tidal volume. Time-cycled ventilators are ideally suited to this purpose; they have a wide range of frequencies (10–60/min) and in adults are usually used in the range of 14–24/min. In fact, they really only cycle on frequency and the delivery of a preset volume (generally 6–15 ml/kg) depends on their power. Usually inflation pressures vary from 10 to 35 mmHg (1.3 to 4.6 kPa), but ventilators should be available for special cases in which pressures up to 80 mmHg (10.6 kPa) may be needed.

The inspired O_2 concentration must be adjustable from 21% to 100%, and exactly monitored since high concentrations are potentially toxic.

With control of frequency, tidal volume, and inflation pressure it is possible to adequately ventilate a large number of patients; experience and better understanding of the pathophysiology of respiratory failure have shown the limits of the method, however. An unchanging ventilatory pattern may be deleterious [59] and increases in intrathoracic pressure may have unwanted haemodynamic effects, whereas in the treatment of severe hypoxaemia the method may well be inadequate.

In an attempt to overcome these problems, the ventilators have been equipped with new controls, all of which can improve ventilation. But it should be noted that in these circumstances any improvement in ventilation is often accomplished at the expense of a fall in cardiac output.

Inflation curve kinetics. With different ventilators, or sometimes with the same apparatus,

different inspiratory pressure waveforms [3, 7] can be obtained which are basically of four kinds: sine flow, squared flow, decelerated flow, and accelerated flow (Fig. 21.7). The most frequently used is the accelerated flow form, but at present there are no special criteria for choosing any one particular waveform. The only established fact is that for a given tidal volume

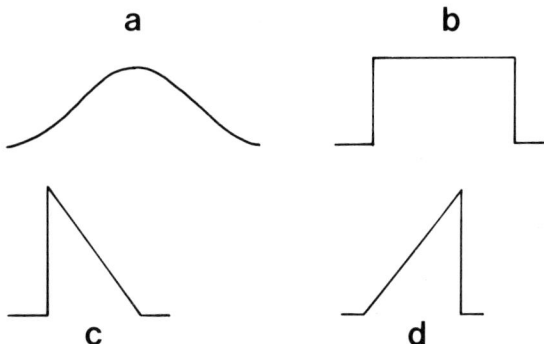

Fig. 21.7. Insufflation flow curves: a, sine flow; b, squared flow; c, decelerated flow; d accelerated flow.

the inflation pressure is lower with squared or decelerated waveforms than with the other two.

Scandinavian authors have emphasized the importance of a period of zero flow at the end of inspiration (plateau) (36), this improves the intrapulmonary distribution of gases, particularly in the case of unequally distributed respiratory pathology. The preferential distribution of gas flow to the 'healthy' areas, which offer less resistance to gas flow is avoided. Whilst supported by some workers this concept still remains controversial [29]. If required the plateau can either be then preset (Engström) or adjustable (SF4, SF4T, Servo ventilator 900, Bennet MA 1 and MA 2 , Bourns Bear 1, UV 1 Dräger . . .). A static phase at the end of inflation also provides a convenient point for the evaluation of quasi-static compliance.

Inspiration:expiration (I:E) ratio. In some ventilators, the I:E ratio is fixed, usually at approximately 1:2, which is considered to be ideal and comparable to the value in spontaneous ventilation. In others, it is adjustable to varying degrees. A reduction in the time of the inspiratory phase is designed to lessen the haemodynamic repercussions, for whilst the peak inspiratory pressure increases the mean airway pressure actually falls, so explaining the beneficial haemodynamic effect. Despite this fact, this type of control is rarely used because it has an adverse effect on ventilation [48].

An increase in the I:E ratio might theoretically improve gas exchange and reduce the peak inspiratory pressure [27]; in practice, however, a maximum I:E ratio of 50% has never been efficient with regard to ventilation and the decrease in inspiratory peak pressure only concerns its dynamic aspect (patients with high bronchial resistance), whereas its static aspect does not change for equal volumes, and depends solely on static compliance of the thorax–lung system. In addition, prolonging the inspiratory time generally increases the mean intrathoracic pressure and therefore the haemodynamic repercussions of AV. It has recently been shown, and confirmed by our experience, however, that the use of very high I:E ratios (80%), formerly considered to be dangerous, definitely improves PaO_2 in cases of severe hypoxaemia, without compromising patient ventilation [46]. These results are due to the persistance of a positive intrathoracic pressure for up to 80% of the respiratory cycle, and the technique is therefore similar to AV with PEEP.

Positive expiratory pressure. In numerous cases of acute respiratory failure, particularly in the ARDS, the dominant element is a decrease in pulmonary volume at end-expiration, probably due to oedema and/or micro-atelectasis. A simple way of increasing this volume is to maintain a positive pressure in the airways during expiration [1, 25, 68]. This can be done by two methods; either by introducing resistance to gas flow (expiration retard cap) or by blocking expiration when airway pressure falls below a predetermined level: PEEP.

By limiting expiratory flow, the expiration retard method maintains a positive pressure in the airways, which progressively decreases according to the drop in intrapulmonary volume (Fig. 21.8). Depending on frequency, a zero pressure (low frequency) or a positive residual pressure (high frequency) can be obtained at end-expiration. End-expiration pressure does not therefore reflect mean airway pressure during expiration, the level of which is actually very imprecise and often high. Moreover, this method is dangerous, since blocking expiration exposes the pulmonary alveoli to considerable excess pressure during coughing.

PEEP can be obtained by blocking expiration at a determined level in two ways: the simpler consists in passing the expired gases into the lower part of a column of water, the level of which determines the residual pressure. However, turbulence caused by gas flow sometimes makes it difficult to set precisely, and the water level has to be frequently adjusted. The safest procedure, included in all modern ventilators, uses spring (optional) or pneumatic valves (incorporated in the apparatus) which can be precisely and stably set. With these methods, airway pressure drops rapidly at the beginning of expiration and then stabilizes at the preset level, thus inducing a stable residual pressure plateau. Moreover, in the case of accidentally excessive pressure gases can be quickly evacuated. Recent studies have shown that high-level PEEP is useful in certain cases [40, 45]. But depending on the ventilator, maximal PEEP varies from 5 to 15 mmHg (0.7 to 2 kPa), only exceptionally reaching 20 mmHg (2.7 kPa).

Negative expiratory pressure. Inducing a negative

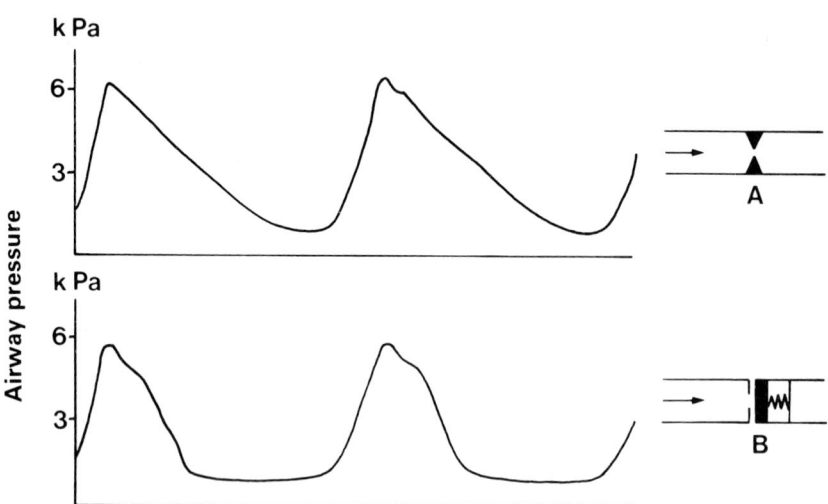

Fig. 21.8. Positive end-expiratory pressure by expiration retard cap (A) and by preset valve (B).

expiratory pressure was one of the first methods used to reduce the haemodynamic repercussions of AV [51]. The increase in intrathoracic pressure induced by AV has been known to decrease cardiac output [17]. To reduce this effect, it was suggested that airway pressure be reduced during expiration by creating active exhalation. This can be accomplished by either a pneumatic (Venturi) or a mechanical system. However, the cardiovascular benefits are doubtful [2] (except perhaps in cases of cerebral oedema) and the respiratory changes induced by this method have led to its abandonment; the fall in the airway pressure during expiration intensifies the spontaneous tendency of alveoli and bronchioles to collapse (54) and the resulting increase in closing volume may alter gas exchange.

Periodic hyperventilation: sighing. During spontaneous breathing at rest, gas distribution is inconsistent. Sighing is a means of compensating for this and is in fact a form of periodic hyperventilation. In AV the use of constant tidal volumes especially when close to physiologic values, has been held responsible for causing micro-atelectasis [59] and it has been shown that periodic increase of the intrathoracic volume decreases the risk [6, 52]. It is for this reason that an artificial sigh mechanism has been integrated into a number of ventilators; intrathoracic volume is increased periodically, either by increasing the tidal volume or by applying a positive expiratory pressure. Clinically, this method is used for the ventilation of healthy lungs during anaesthesia and in patients in coma, etc., but in the presence of lung pathology high tidal volumes and/or PEEP are usually used and these limit the usefulness of intermittent sighs.

Assisted ventilation. This term 'assisted ventilation' implies all types of AV that require some form of patient participation. Long considered to be a rehabilitation and/or weaning technique, assisted ventilation can now be used for the treatment of severe hypoxaemia.

Triggering makes ventilator frequency depend on the patient's inspiration as a stimulus, the patient thereby becoming the control system. The principle of the trigger is manometric: a constant tidal volume is delivered when the patient produces a fall in the inspiratory pressure below a preset level which can be adjusted appropriate to the clinical situation. The quality of a trigger depends on its sensitivity and response time. For a given pressure, the sensitivity is related to the compliance and volume in the inspiratory circuit: the lower the compliance

and the higher the volume, the greater is the required inspiratory effort [24]. The response time depends on the nature of the ventilator's valves and, whilst it is satisfactory with pneumatic or electronic systems, it is slow in mechanical systems where there is the risk of it becoming out of phase.

Theoretically, the advantage of triggering is to assure a more physiologic form of ventilation by reducing inspiratory pressures and avoiding any opposition between patient and ventilator. In addition, the adjustments of inspiratory effort that are possible could prepare the patient for weaning. In practice, however, it is limited by its very principle. If the patient's ventilatory frequency is too low it is dangerous, necessitating an automatic replacement system, particularly in the case of apnoea, when the ventilatory frequency is too high; it can lead to inefficient ventilation with pressure-cycled ventilators or hyperventilation with volume-cycled machines. Moreover, the technique can exhaust the patient and, in our experience, it is not very helpful in the treatment of severe hypoxaemia, but is useful in respiratory rehabilitation.

Intermittent mandatory ventilation. The principle of intermittent mandatory ventilation (IMV) is simple: it completes spontaneous patient ventilation by periodically imposing a preset ventilator-delivered tidal volume (Fig. 21.9). It should be noted that this method, which is currently being increasingly used in intensive care, has already been widely employed in the operating room by anaesthetists who periodically assisted a patient's spontaneous ventilation by manual inflation. The technique was first used in children, but is now frequently used in adults, often in association with PEEP [18, 19, 40]. The necessary circuit can easily be fitted into any ventilator by incorporating an annex circuit into the inspiratory circuit, separated from it by a valve. When the ventilator is in the expiratory phase, the patient can inhale a gas mixture through the annexed circuit, but when the ventilator inflates the connecting valve is closed and the imposed respiratory cycle can be carried out. With such a system, however, the patient's ventilation and the 'mandatory' ventilation are not synchronized, and many ventilators are now equipped with IMV systems that are synchronized by a trigger with the patient's breathing (SIMV). In the Servo ventilator 900, the Bourns Bear 1, the UV 1 Dräger, M 251, and the Bennet MA 2, the FiO_2 and ventilator alarms can also be preset, but the quality of such a system varies from one apparatus to the other, depending on the trigger

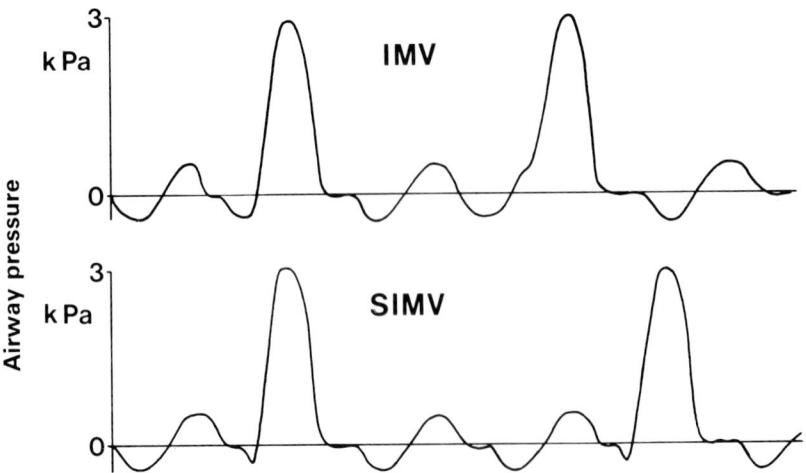

Fig. 21.9. IMV: mechanical inflation is time-cycled and starts whatever the phase of patient breathing. SIMV: mechanical inflation starts only at the beginning of spontaneous inspiration.

quality and also on the gas flow that is available during spontaneous inspiration.

The main purpose of IMV is to reduce the deleterious effects of AV. This is accomplished by reducing the number of AV cycles, which results in an overall decrease in intrathoracic pressure and thereby diminishes the haemodynamic disturbance. Thus, in severe hypoxaemia, the use of IMV and PEEP has, for the first time, improved respiratory conditions without any major cardiovascular side-effects [40]. The mandatory cycle frequency must be adjusted to maintain the $PaCO_2$ near to normal values, and can be progressively decreased during weaning when eventually only very low frequencies will be needed. The maintenance of some degree of spontaneous breathing lessens the patient's psychological dependence on the ventilator, assures some function of his ventilatory mechanisms, and therefore eventually facilitates weaning.

Mandatory minute volume. Derived from IMV, this method is an even better approach to subjecting the ventilator to patient needs. Instead of cycling on frequency, the complementary ventilation provided by the apparatus is based on mandatory minute volume (MMV). The necessary minute volume is adjusted and the patient breathes spontaneously; the ventilator acting only when this minute volume falls below the preset value. Thus, depending on his capabilities, the patient can transfer from spontaneous breathing to complete AV without the physician intervening. This method has only recently been described [37] but has already been incorporated into some ventilators (Engström Erica).

Continuous positive airway pressure. Although this type of ventilation (CPAP) does not fit into the category of AV because the patient is breathing spontaneously, it should be mentioned here for two reasons: it is often associated with new assisted ventilation techniques and is now incorporated in many ventilators, and may therefore be taken into consideration for therapy. The technique consists of providing a positive airway pressure throughout the respiratory cycle when the patient is breathing spontaneously [15, 32, 33]. It is carried out through an airtight mask or tracheal prosthesis.

A CPAP circuit is easy to fit (Fig. 21.10): it consists of an air-oxygen mixer, a high-capacitance reservoir bag, an humidifier, a T piece dividing the inspiratory and expiratory circuits and connecting to the patient, and a PEEP valve. It is also advisable to incorporate a manometer near the T piece to monitor airway pressure. This very simple circuit was not originally equipped with any form of alarm system, but manufacturers have now introduced CPAP circuits with alarms and at a relatively low cost compared to other alarm-equipped ventilators. The quality of a CPAP device depends on the gas flow and bag compliance; a good system should give only slight variations of pressure from inspiration to expiration to limit respiratory muscle work. The advantage of the method over AV with PEEP is a smaller haemodynamic disturbance for a given intrathoracic volume [63]. These effects can be further diminished by progressively decreasing the positive pressure during inspiration (decrease in flow and/or bag compliance). At the limit of this, expiratory positive airway pressure (EPAP) occurs, where

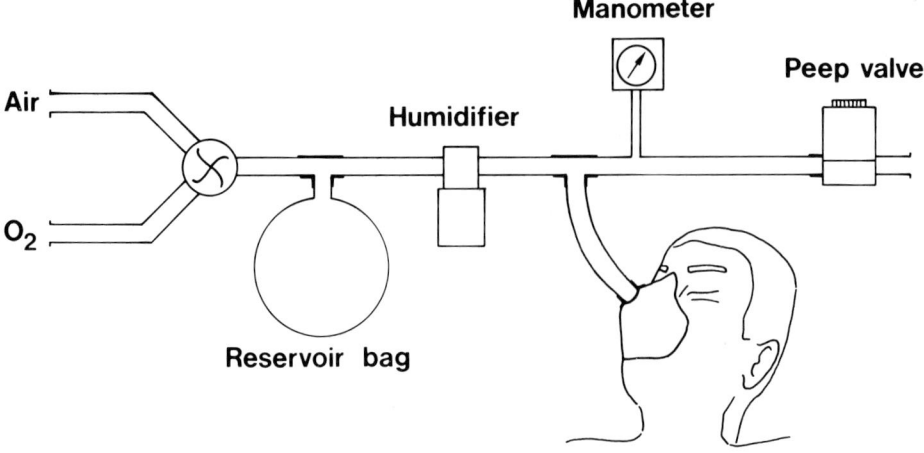

Fig. 21.10. Continuous positive airway pressure system.

only expiration is in positive pressure (Fig. 21.11). With the latter method, however, the haemodynamic advantages are counterbalanced by a considerable increase in respiratory muscle work [67].

Special forms of ventilation

The recent use of jet and high-frequency positive pressure ventilation has led to the construction of very special ventilators.

Jet ventilation. Although this method [39, 42, 58] is based on the same principle as the others, namely insufflation of a gas mixture into the airways, it differs significantly in two ways. There is no expiratory circuit and the injection of the gases is highly pressurized. The respirator basically consists of a source of highly

pressurized gas (4 bars; 400 kPa) and a manual trigger to divide up the gas flow. The inspiratory circuit is merely a small-calibre probe (generally 3.5 mm in diameter for adults) directly inserted into the airways; expiration occurs naturally. High-pressure, high-flow gas insufflation (60–100 litres/min) creates a Venturi effect, providing an air–O_2 mixture and patient ventilation: 6–20 insufflations of 2–3 s duration are generally delivered per minute. This type of AV is used mainly during laryngeal or bronchial endoscopy and pharyngolaryngeal interventions, usually in curarized patients with healthy lungs.

High-frequency positive pressure ventilation. Following experimentation aimed at reducing the haemodynamic repercussions of AV, certain teams have started to use HFPPV [9, 64, 65] in man. This method consists of injecting low tidal

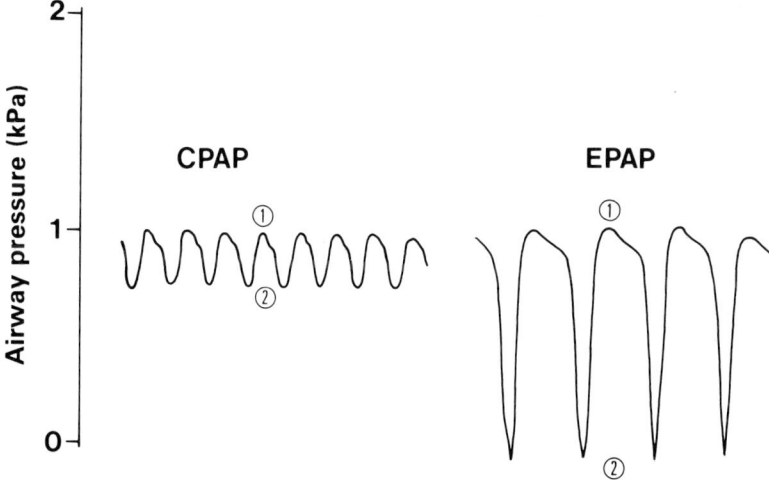

Fig. 21.11. Airway pressure curves during CPAP and EPAP: during CPAP the difference between expiratory (1) and inspiratory (2) pressure is slight; during EPAP the difference is greater, making breathing work harder.

volumes at high frequencies of between 60 and 100/min. It requires a maximal reduction of the dead space in the patient–machine system, with the probe inserted either near the carina or through the usual endotracheal prosthesis, and a ventilator with a small compressible volume and low internal compliance. There are currently only a few prototype ventilators that function satisfactorily in such conditions. These have been designed to function not only under HFPPV, but also according to the various traditional types of AV. Their characteristics, small compressible volume and low internal compliances, allow the delivery of a constant tidal volume whatever the airway resistance, which is not possible in other respirators.

The advantage of HFPPV is the reduction of intrathoracic pressure that it produces. It is particularly useful in cases of bronchopleural fistula. Nonetheless, it is still not clear how gas exchange occurs in the alveoli, especially when very high frequencies are used.

Tank and cuirass ventilators

These ventilate patients by creating a physiological pattern of breathing [53, 69]. Expansion of the chest during inspiration is obtained by providing a negative pressure around the chest, and expiration is either passive or active, if a positive perithoracic pressure is applied.

Tank ventilators

These are made up of two elements: an airtight box for the patient, and an engine powering a device that controls the cycle change-over. The I:E ratio is generally preset at approximately I:2, but the perithoracic pressure, as well as the frequency, can be adjusted. They are, however, very cumbersome and make patient care and monitoring difficult.

Cuirass ventilators

These consist essentially of a sealed cavity fitted over the thorax and abdomen, they also generate a negative pressure and are easier to manage than tank ventilators, but they are less powerful, and for identical pressure variations, their performance is approximately one third that of a tank ventilator. They were originally used only in adults, mainly for transporting patients and weaning them from tank ventilators. After being used almost solely for the

treatment of respiratory paralysis without any disorder of swallowing, their application has been extended by certain authors to the treatment of the respiratory distress syndrome, particularly in children. In these cases maintaining a constant perithoracic negative pressure is equivalent to a PEEP in endotracheal AV [13, 44, 66].

Monitoring

Taking over a patient's ventilation by an artificial mechanism, whether or not complete, requires strict monitoring [14, 22, 57, 70, 72]. To make this task easier for hospital staff, manufacturers now equip their ventilators with monitoring and alarm systems, which are becoming increasingly sophisticated due to the application of electronics and/or data processing.

Alarms

A ventilator must have at least three basic alarms indicating: (1) that the ventilator is not functioning (sector alarm); (2) that the patient is not being ventilated according to the desired norms (flow or volume alarm); and (3) that the intrathoracic pressure is incorrect (pressure alarm).

Some ventilators have a more extensive alarm system that monitors FiO_2, frequency, I:E ratio, triggering, PEEP, etc. With electronic alarms efficient correcting mechanisms are possible, including opening of the safety blow-off valve and stopping of insufflation in the case of excessive pressure (Servo ventilator 900); volume compensation in the case of leakage (Bourns); and maintenance of a PEEP level even with leakage (Bourns).

Further monitoring

In addition to the basic controls which determine their function, some ventilators possess controls for monitoring other functions. These devices may be connected to the ventilator or incorporated in it and are particularly useful for IMV, MMV, or CPAP because they indicate: patient and ventilator frequency; patient and ventilator ventilation; insufflation pressure curve; expired gas composition; quasi-static compliance; and airway resistance.

Use of increasingly sophisticated controls in the future will make it possible to completely monitor AV ranging from simple recording on a central station to computerized monitoring for processing long-term information and providing details of trends.

Care of the ventilators

It is essential to discuss problems of equipment management since they are aspects that have to be taken into consideration when choosing a ventilator.

Maintenance

To provide for continuous use of a ventilator, an adequate stock of spare parts such as disposable tubes, water traps, circuit separators, humidifiers, flexible cannula extensions, and reservoir bags should be available. This is all the more necessary when absence of the equipment during autoclave or ethylene oxide sterilization may be relatively long. An ICU should also have qualified personnel who are capable of repairing 'simple' breakdowns and who can check the reliability of the different ventilation parameters and monitors. This will require the provision of equipment for evaluating the ventilator-delivered flow, volume, and pressure.

Disinfection

In spite of the care taken by manufacturers to avoid infection by the use of sterile gases, bacterial filters, and the complete separation of inspiratory and expiratory circuits, it is essential to sterilize all ventilators after use.

A disinfection room should be set aside for the complete sterilization of ventilators with formaldehyde. A portable unit for sterilization of the internal circuits with vaporized formaldehyde (secondarily neutralized by ammonia), and an autoclave or ethylene oxide sterilization plant for the removable parts and the internal circuits should also be available.

Extracorporeal membrane oxygenation (ECMO)

In contrast to the other methods, ECMO is the only technique that can provide homeostasis in patients in acute respiratory failure without using the lungs. The principle is simple, venous blood being oxygenated by an extracorporeal circuit.

Oxygenator

As in the lungs, gas is exchanged through a membrane that separates the blood film and the gas phase [10, 20, 30, 73].

Membranes and gas phase

Two types of membrane are in use:

1) *Continuous silicone membranes*, which have an excellent permeability coefficient (very thin membranes) and are selective for CO_2, thereby limiting the risk of hypocapnia. Their main inconvenience is their great fragility.
2) *Microporous membranes* which, because they are thicker, are more resistant. They have a good permeability coefficient, but are not selective and may induce hypocapnia. Moreover, they must be used with limited pressure in the gas phase as well as in the blood phase, to avoid bubble contamination or ultrafiltration.

Blood film

The blood film [28] must be as thin as possible, since the thickness of the liquid column is an obstacle to gas exchange, particularly plasma for O_2. However, due to pressure demands, the small size of the blood channels induces a laminar flow which perturbs oxygenation. Several procedures can be used to avoid this problem: creation of obstacles in the blood compartment [10], use of helicoidal capillary tubes, changes in pressure during gas [43] or blood phase [5], etc. Whatever method is chosen, it is essential that blood flow be consistent in the oxygenator's canals to avoid the occurrence of disorders resembling an abnormal ventilation:perfusion ratio in the lungs.

Extracorporeal circuit

An extracorporeal circuit is made up of several components. *Bypass cannulae* are inserted into the patient's vessels and are connected to the oxygenator by a *tubing system*. To avoid problems of blood clotting the cannulae and tubing are generally made of silicone. *Pumps* circulate the blood in the extra-corporeal circuit and in the patient. In long-term use non-occlusive pumps seem to cause the least damage to the red blood cells [11]. A *heating system* compensates for heat loss while the blood is in the extracorporeal circuit. The circulation is kept constant by a *control system*; this is achieved either by flow control, which requires a reservoir and which increases the circuit volume, or by pressure control, which reduces the circuit capacity and eliminates any risk of the bypass cannulae collapsing.

The efficiency of such a method depends not only on the characteristics of the membrane and blood phase, but also on the exchange surface. A modular system is generally used when large surfaces are necessary and the distribution of blood flow be consistent in the various modules.

Three main techniques of bypass have been used. They differ in their haemodynamic effects and on PaO_2 in different parts of the body.

In *venovenous bypass*, blood is bypassed from the inferior vena cava and reinjected into the superior vena cava (Fig. 21.12). Extracorporeal venous output must not exceed 50% of the cardiac output. This limitation can be avoided by inserting the drainage cannula in the right atrium and the return cannula in the right ventricle. Extracorporeal flow can thus be increased up to 80% of cardiac output. Reinjection of oxygenated blood into the right-hand cavities provides the body with physiologically distributed cardiac output and maintains pulsatile flow. But the high pressure and flow in the pulmonary artery may perpetuate pulmonary oedema and RV failure [26].

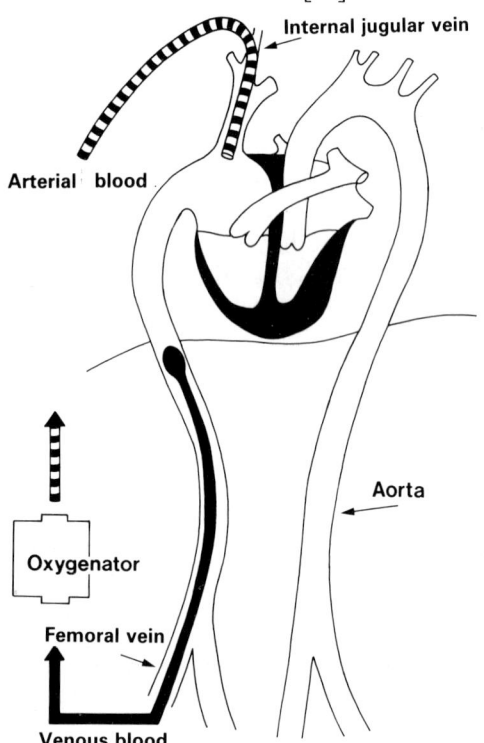

Fig. 21.12. Veno-venous bypass.

Veno-arterial bypass consists in removing the blood from the right atrium and reinjecting it into one or both femoral arteries, the axillary artery or the arch of the aorta (Fig. 21.13). It can

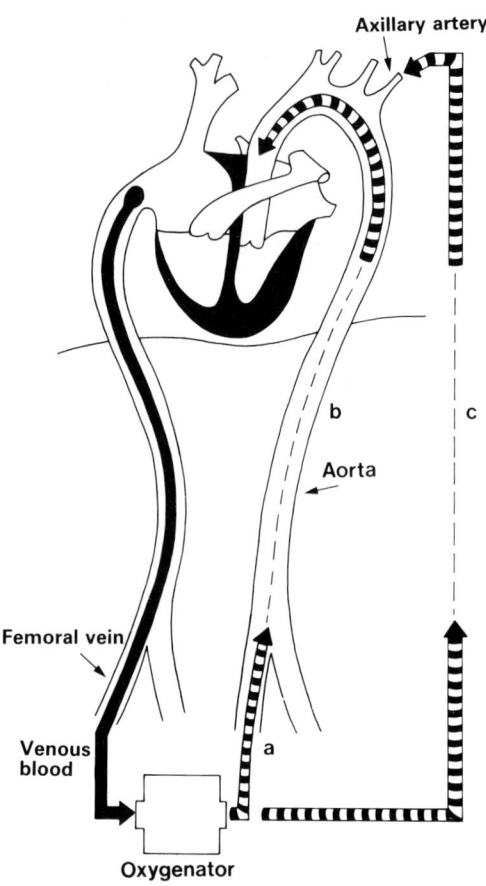

Fig. 21.13. Veno-arterial bypass.

provide a high enough extracorporeal output to permit total bypass. The reduction in pulmonary blood flow will limit pulmonary oedema but may predispose to the development of pulmonary artery thrombosis or other ischaemic lesions. In addition, the distribution of oxygenated blood depends on the site of reinjection and on the quantity of pulmonary flow that remains. To obtain adequate oxygenation of the entire body with this technique an extracorporeal output greater than 60% of cardiac output is essential, regardless of the site of reinjection.

In combined venovenous and veno-arterial bypass, blood is drained from the inferior vena cava: part of it is then reinjected into the femoral artery, and part into the right ventricle (Fig. 21.14). This technique has the combined advantages of the previous two methods and less disadvantages. Its drawback is the need for multiple vascular approaches.

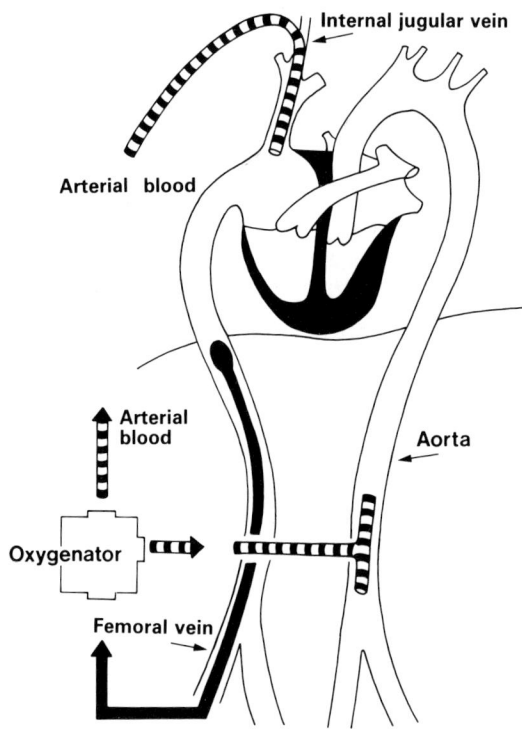

Fig. 21.14. Mixed veno-venous and veno-arterial bypass.

The applications of ECMO are limited by the complexity of the method, which requires numerous skilled personnel, the risk of infection (numerous vascular approaches), and haematological problems (cellular alterations and consumption coagulopathy). It is also worth noting that AV must be carried out simultaneously.

It is difficult, at least as far as heavy equipment is concerned, to define a standard for an ICU having to treat acute respiratory failure. Such a standard depends on various factors, including the size of the unit and its staff, its financial resources, the kind of patients treated and whether clinical research is being carried out.

Artificial ventilators are the basic apparatus for intensive respiratory care, and it seems preferable to have machines of the same brand to avoid manipulation mistakes by personnel. Certain patients sometimes require very complex AV, demanding ventilators that are capable of carrying out all the previously described modes of ventilation. These are, of course, the

most costly. For many patients whose lungs are generally healthy, however, AV can be provided by practically any ventilator. It therefore appears illogical, at least financially, for a unit treating both types of patient, to be equipped with only very sophisticated ventilators. The proportion of 'heavy' and 'low-range' ventilators thus depends on patient distribution in each unit. Whatever type of ventilator is used it must be fitted with a reliable alarm system. 'Emergency' respirators are necessary, particularly for patient transportation.

Finally, patients in intensive care often need to undergo complex diagnostic procedures, and since they are very difficult to move, the unit, or somewhere nearby, should be equipped with certain items of respiratory function equipment for; blood gas analysis, pulmonary volumes, respiratory mechanics, isotopic studies (ventilation and perfusion scintiscan with evaluation of regional $\dot{V}A/\dot{Q}$) and x-ray examinations (image intensifier, pulmonary angiography).

References

1. Ashbaugh DG, Bigelow DB, Petty TL, Levine BE (1967) Acute respiratory distress in adults. Lancet II:319–323
2. Auchincloss JH Jr, Gilbert R (1967) An evaluation of the negative phase of a volume-limited ventilator. Am Rev Respir Dis 95:66–72
3. Baker AB, Balington PCB, Collis JE, Cowie RW (1977) Effects of varying inspiratory flow waveform and time in intermittent positive pressure ventilation. Br J Anaesth 49:1207–1237
4. Barrett CR Jr (1978) Flexible fiberoptic bronchoscopy in the critically ill patient. Methodology and indications. Chest 73:746–749
5. Bellhouse BJ, Bellhouse FH, Curl CM, MacMillan TI, Gunning AJ, Spratt EH, MacMurray SB, Nelems JM (1973) A high efficiency membrane oxygenator and pulsatile pumping system and its application to animal trials. Trans Am Soc Artif Intern Organs 19:72–79
6. Bendixen HH, Hedley-White J, Chir B, Laver MB (1963) Impaired oxygenation in surgical patients during general anesthesia with controlled ventilation. N Engl J Med 269:991–996
7. Bergman NA (1969) Effect of varying respiratory waveforms on distribution of inspired gas during artificial ventilation. Am Rev Respir Dis 100:518–525
8. Bethune DW, Collis JM (1967) An evaluation of oxygen therapy equipment: experimental study of various devices on the human subject. Thorax 22:221–225
9. Borg U, Lyttkens L, Nilsson LG, Sjöstrand U (1977) Physiologic evaluation of the HFPPV pneumatic valve principle and PEEP. Acta Anaesthesiologica Scandinavica [Suppl] 64:37–53
10. Bramson ML, Osborn JJ, Main FB (1965) A new disposable membrane oxygenator with integral heat exchange. J Thorac Cardiovasc Surg 50:391–400
11. Butruille Y, Chevallet J, Granger A, Lissot J, Sausse A

(1976) Rhone–Poulenc oxygenator and associated pumping system In: Zapol WM, Quist J (eds) Artificial lungs and acute respiratory failure. Theory and practice. Hemisphere, Washington, pp 223–233

12. Campbell EJM (1960) A method of controlled oxygen administration which reduces the risk of carbon-dioxide retention. Lancet II:12–14

13. Chernick V (1970) Hyaline-membrane disease; therapy with constant lung-distending pressure. N Engl J Med 289:302–304

14. Chopin C, Chambrin MC, Robin H, Boulenguez C, Duguesne B, Vallet D, Durocher A, Gosselin B, Wattel F (1977) Determination sous ventilation assistée de la ductance globale du CO_2 et de ses composantes partielles. Problèmes techniques et intérêt pratique en réanimation respiratoire. Ann Anesthesiol Fr 18:593–602

15. Civetta JM, Brons R, Gabel JC (1972) A simple and effective method of employing spontaneous positive pressure ventilation. J Thorac Cardiovasc Surg 63:312–317

16. Cooper JD, Grillo HC (1969) Experimental production and prevention of injury due to cuffed tracheal tubes. Surg Gynecol Obstet 129:1235–1241

17. Cournand A, Motley HL, Werko L, Richards DW Jr (1948) Physiological studies on the effects of intermittent positive pressure breathing on cardiac output in man. Am J Physiol 152:162–174

18. Desautels DA, Bartlett JL (1974) Methods of administering intermittent mandatory ventilation (IMV). Respiratory Care 19:187–191

19. Downs JB, Perkins HM, Modell JH (1974) Intermittent mandatory ventilation. Arch Surg 109:519–523

20. Drinker PA (1972) Progress in membrane oxygenator design. Anesthesiology 37:242–260

21. Dunn CR, Dunn DL, Moser KM (1974) Determinants of tracheal injury by cuffed tracheostomy tubes. Chest 65:128–135

22. Duvivier C, Peslin R, Polu JM, Fringant JC (1978) Caractéristiques et performances d'un système de surveillance de la ventilation et des échanges gazeux en réanimation. Bull Eur Physiopathol Respir 14:335–346

23. Egan DF (1977) Fundamentals of respiratory therapy, 3rd edn. Mosby, Saint-Louis, p 551

24. Epstein RA (1971) The sensitivities and response times of ventilatory assistors. Anesthesiology 34:321–326

25. Falke KJ, Pontoppidan H, Kumar A, Leith DE, Geffin B, Laver MB (1972) Ventilation with end-expiratory pressure in acute lung disease. J Clin Invest 51:2315–2323

26. Fallat RJ, Hill JD, Lamy M, Ratliff J, Dietrich HP (1976) Clinical hemodynamic and gas exchange by three extracorporeal membrane oxygenation canulation methodes. In: Zapol WM, Quist J (eds) Artificial lungs and acute respiratory failure. Theory and practice. Hemisphere, Washington, pp 297–317

27. Finlay WE, Wightman HE, Adams AP, Sykes MK (1970) The effects of variations in inspiratory expiratory ratio on cardiorespiratory function during controlled ventilation in normo- hypo- and hypervolaemic dogs. Br J Anaesth 42:935–940

28. Galletti PM (1971) Blood interfacial phenomena: An overview. Fed Proc 30:1491–1493

29. Gibert C, Marsac J, Tremolieres F, Pocidalo JJ (1974) Modalités particulières de la ventilation artificielle; Bases de leur utilisation au cours des hypoxémies réfractaires. In: L'Année en réanimation médicale. Flammarion Médecine-Sciences, Paris, pp 149–175

30. Gille JP, Bagniewski A (1976) Ten years of use of extracorporeal membrane oxygenation (ECMO) in treatment of acute respiratory insufficiency. Trans Am Soc Artif Intern Organs 22:102–108

31. Graff TD, Benson DW (1969) Systemic and pulmonary changes with inhaled humid atmospheres: clinical applications, Anesthesiology 30:199–207

32. Greenbaum DM, Millen JE, Eross B, Snyder JV, Grenvik A, Safar P (1976) Continuous positive airway pressure without tracheal intubation in spontaneously breathing patients. Chest 69:615–620

33. Gregory GA, Edmunds LH, Kitterman JA, Phibb RH, Tooley WH (1975) Continuous positive airway pressure and pulmonary and circulatory function after cardiac surgery in infants less than three months of age. Anesthesiology 43:426–431

34. Grieble HG, Colton FR, Bird TJ, Toigo A, Griffith LG (1970) Fine-particle humidifiers: Source of Pseudomonas aeruginosa infections in a respiratory disease unit. N Engl J Med 282:531–535

35. Hayes B, Robinson JS (1970) Assessment of methods of humidification of inspired gas. Brit J Anaesth 42:94–104

36. Herzog P, Norlander OP (1968) Distribution of alveolar volumes with different types of positive pressure gas-flow patterns. Opuscula Médica 13:3–18

37. Hewlett AM, Platt AS, Terry VG (1977) Mandatory minute volume. A new concept in weaning from mechanical ventilation. Anaesthesia 32:163–169

38. Ivanoff S, Cazalaa JB, Weber B, et al. (1977) Respirateurs, caractères et fonctions. Agressologie 18:1–373

39. Jardine AD, Harrison MJ, Healy TEJ (1975) Automatic flow interruption bronchoscope: a laboratory study. Br J Anaesth 47:385–389

40. Kirby RR, Downs JB, Civetta JM, Modell JH, Dannemiller FJ, Klein EF, Hodges M (1975) High level positive end expiratory pressure (PEEP) in acute respiratory insufficiency. Chest 67:156–163

41. Klein EF Jr, Shah DA, Shah NJ, Modell JH, Desautel D (1973) Performance Characteristics of conventional and prototype humidifiers and nebulizers. Chest 64:690–696

42. Klein JP, Sauvage JP, Desmonts JM (1976) Intérêt de la jet-ventilation au cours des endoscopies oto-rhinolaryngologiques pratiquées sous anesthésie générale. Ann Anesthesiol 27:889–893

43. Kolobow T, Bowman RL (1963) Construction and evaluation of an alveolar membrane artificial heart-lung. Trans Am Soc Artif Intern Organs 9:238–242

44. Krumpe EP, Zidulka A, Urbanetti J, Anthonisen NR (1977) Comparison of the effects of continuous negative external chest pressure and positive end-expiratory pressure on cardiac index in dogs. Am Rev Respir Dis 115:39–45

45. Labrousse J, Tenaillon A, Longchal J, Chastre J, Lissac J (1979) Pression positive expiratoire optimale au cours de la ventilation artificielle. Application au traitement du syndrome de détresse respiratoire de l'adulte. Nouv Presse Med 8:759–763

46. Lachmann B, Haendly B, Schulz H, Jonson B (1980) Improved arterial oxygenation, CO_2 elimination, compliance and decreased barotrauma following changes of volume-generated PEEP ventilation with inspiratory/expiratory (I/E) ratio of 1:2 to pressure-generated ventilation with I/E ratio of 4:1 in patients with severe adult respiratory distress syndrome (ARDS). (abstract) Intensive Care Med 6:64 (abstr)

47. Leigh JM (1973) Variation in performance of oxygen therapy devices. Ann R Coll Surg Engl 52:3–22

48. Lindhal S (1979) Influence of end inspiratory pause on pulmonary ventilation, gas distribution and lung perfusion during artificial ventilation. Crit Care Med 7:540–546

49. Lissac J, Labrousse J, Tenaillon A, Bousser JP (1977) Aspects techniques de la réanimation respiratoire. Bailliere, Paris, p 125

50. Mackenzie CF, Klose S, Browne DRG (1976) A study of inflatable cuffs on endotracheal tubes. Pressures exerted on the trachea. Br J Anaesth 48:105–109

51. Maloney JV Jr, Handford SW (1954) Circulatory response to intermittent positive and alternating positive negative pressure respirators. J Appl Physiol 6:453–459

52. Mead J, Collier C (1959) Relationship of volume history of lungs to respiratory mechanics in anesthetized dogs. J Appl Physiol 14:669–678

53. Mushin WW, Rendell-Baker L, Thompson PW, Mapleson WW (1980) Automatic ventilation of the lungs, 3rd edn. Blackwell Scientific, Oxford London Edinburgh Melbourne, p 887

54. Nunn JF (1977) Applied respiratory physiology, 2nd edn. Butterworths, London Boston, p 524

55. Pereira W, Kovnat DM, Snider GL (1978) A prospective cooperative study of complications following flexible fiberoptic bronchoscopy. Chest 73:813–816

56. Pierce AK, Sanford JP (1973) Bacterial contamination of aerosols. Arch Intern Med 131:156–159

57. Pocidalo JJ, Tremolieres F (1979) Surveillance et optimisation de la ventilation artificielle mécanique: moyens actuels et perspectives. Bull Eur Physiopathol Respir 15:565–574

58. Poling HE, Wolfson B, Siker ES (1975) A technique of ventilation during laryngoscopy and bronchoscopy. Br J Anaesth 47:382–384

59. Pontoppidan H, Hedley-White J, Bendixen HH, Laver MB, Radford EP Jr (1965) Ventilation and oxygen requirements during prolonged artificial ventilation in patients with respiratory failure. N Engl J Med 273:401–409

60. Rippoll I, Lindholm CE, Carroll R, Grenvik A (1978) Spontaneous dislocation of endotracheal tubes. Anesthesiology 49:50–52

61. Sackner MA (1975) Bronchofiberscopy. Am Rev Respir Dis 111:62–88

62. Safar P (1965) Respiratory therapy. Davis, Philadelphia, p 419

63. Simonneau G, Lemaire F, Harf A, Safran D, Georges C, Rieuf P, Teisseire B, Rapin M (1979) Insuffisance respiratoire aiguë de l'adulte: comparaison des effects hemodynamiques at respiratories de la pression expiratoire positive en ventilation spontanée et en ventilation artificielle. Nouv Presse Med 8:113–115

64. Sjöstrand U (1977a) Review of the physiological rationale for and development of high-frequency positive-pressure ventilation—HFPPV. Acta Anaesthesiologica Scandinavica [Suppl] 64:7–27

65. Sjöstrand U (1977b) Pneumatic systems facilitating treatment of respiratory insufficiency with alternative use of IPPV/PEEP, HFPPV/PEEP, CPPB or CPAP Acta Anaesthesiologica Scandinavica [Suppl] 64:123–147

66. Stern L, Ramos AD, Outerbridge EW, Beaudry PH (1970) Negative pressure artificial respiration: use in treatment of respiratory failure of the newborn. Can Med Assoc J 102:595–601

67. Sturgeon CL, Douglas ME, Downs JB, Dannemiller FJ (1977) PEEP and CPAP cardiopulmonary effects during spontaneous ventilation. Anesth Analg 56:633–642

68. Suter PM, Fairley HB, Isemberg MD (1975) Optimum end-expiratory airway pressure in patients with acute pulmonary failure. N Engl J Med 292:284–289

69. Sykes MK, McNicol MW, Campbell EJM (1976) Respiratory failure, 2nd edn. Blackwell Scientific, Oxford London Edinburgh Melbourne, p 461

70. Tenaillon A, Longchal J, Labrousse J, Lissac J (1979) Surveillance des malades en ventilation artificielle. Rev Prat (Paris) 29:3973–3985

71. Toremalm NG (1960) A heat and moisture exchanger for post-tracheotomy care. Acta Otolaryngol (Stockh) 52:461–472

72. Wilson RS (1976) Monitoring the lung: mechanics and volume. Anesthesiology 45:135–145

73. Zapol WM, Snider MT, Schneider RC (1977) Extracorporeal membrane oxygenation for acute respiratory failure. Anesthesiology 46:272–285

Chapter 22

Respiratory Physiotherapy

Susan Lewis

The use of breathing and physical exercises in the treatment of lung disorders was first described following war wounds to the pleura, lungs and diaphragm by Cortlandt MacMahon in 1915 [14].

Modern intensive respiratory care dates from the 1952 epidemic of poliomyelitis [22, 26]; the prime role of the physiotherapist was to ensure that the patient's airways were kept clear of secretions. Today the specialized ICU physiotherapist has a more varied and challenging role; although the management of respiratory disease remains the most common problem, other conditions have also to be treated.

General management

The critically ill patient may be comatose, metabolically deranged, or hypercatabolic and therefore susceptible to pressure sores, wound breakdown, infections, and contractures from oedema or muscle spasm.

The ICU physiotherapist should be adept at both general and specific treatments, including giving ice, ultraviolet irradiation, and massage to treat pressure sores, infected wounds, oedema, and muscle spasm.

In the ICU good team-work is essential, with the nursing, medical and physiotherapy staff working in close liaison. Physiotherapy treatments are timed to be given before the patient's feeds and to coincide with their 2-hourly turns. A well organized ICU fully integrates all its staff and the nurses are instructed in and should be familiar with physiotherapy treatments [30].

Active or passive movements

These are required twice daily for all patients and can be given by the nursing or physiotherapy staff. They are essential to prevent:

1) Contractures or deformities, e.g., dropped feet: moulded splints can be made to maintain a joint in position but these must be removed twice daily so that the joint can be exercised and to prevent pressure sores developing. Blocks or sandbags can maintain a foot in dorsiflexion but should not be used if there is existing or potential extensor spasticity;
2) Venous stasis and thrombosis;
3) Muscle wasting;
4) Loss of remembrance of patterns of movement.

Some movements should be modified, e.g., following intra-aortic balloon counterpulsation. Care must be taken when the patient is turned to avoid possible kinking of the femoral line. Trunk and hip flexion should not exceed 30° [37].

Respiratory management

Different methods of treatment can be considered for use in ventilated patients (either during ventilation (IPPV) or during the 'weaning' process) or in non-ventilated, spontaneously breathing patients (either intubated with an endotracheal or tracheostomy tube or not intubated). The two essential purposes of respiratory treatment are to increase alveolar ventilation and to aid expectoration of pulmonary secretions.

Techniques used mainly to increase alveolar ventilation

Sighing for ventilated patients

This technique is advocated in some ICUs to increase tidal volume and to prevent the development of patchy consolidation.

Normally we yawn, sigh or stretch to increase our tidal volume every 10 min. Alveolar collapse may begin within 1 h of shallow monotonous tidal ventilation [35].

Sophisticated ventilators (e.g., Servo 900 or Bennett MA-1) are intended to mimic normal respiratory physiology by delivering twice the pre-set tidal volume for 3 in every 100 ventilated breaths. Patients on ventilators without a sigh mechanism (e.g., Brompton Manley), require sighing for five breaths every hour. During the day the patients generally receive 2-hourly physiotherapy.

Manual hyperinflation—bag squeezing

Bag squeezing allows hyperinflation of the lungs, usually in conjunction with chest manipulations, postural drainage, and suction (Fig. 22.1). This differs from the hand ventilation used for patients during a cardiac arrest or transfer between units, and from the sighing technique.

Uses. The aim of this technique is to keep small airways open, thus preventing sputum retention, patchy pulmonary consolidation, and lung or lobar collapse.

Unless contra-indicated or technically impossible (as with silver tracheostomy tubes) bag squeezing is performed 2-hourly in all long-term ventilated patients and some intubated and tracheostomized patients who are breathing spontaneously. It is often performed in conjunction with postural drainage, although some positions e.g., sitting erect, may be unsuitable because of the patient's condition (e.g., circulatory embarrassment).

Methods. The choice of method will depend on the equipment that is available and the patient's diagnosis [6] (Fig. 22.2).

When the *Waters' cannister* is selected, a 2-litre black rubber reservoir bag and a metal cannister are connected via a catheter mount to the intubated patient. Oxygen tubing is attached to a flowmeter set at 15 litres O_2/min. The cannister contains soda lime which absorbs the patient's expired CO_2. An adjustable one-way valve allows the operator to adapt to changing lung compliance and can enable the performance of an artificial cough. This non-rebreathing valve is designed so that spontaneous inhalation will be through the bag and not through the exhalation port. The main disadvantages are the cannister's unwieldiness, the possible inhalation of alkaline dust (hopefully prevented by wiping all the connectors before use), and the need for compressed gas at source.

The Ambu-bag is widely used for resuscitation, as it has the advantage of being filled with air or O_2 and is not so clumsy as a cannister. The

Technique

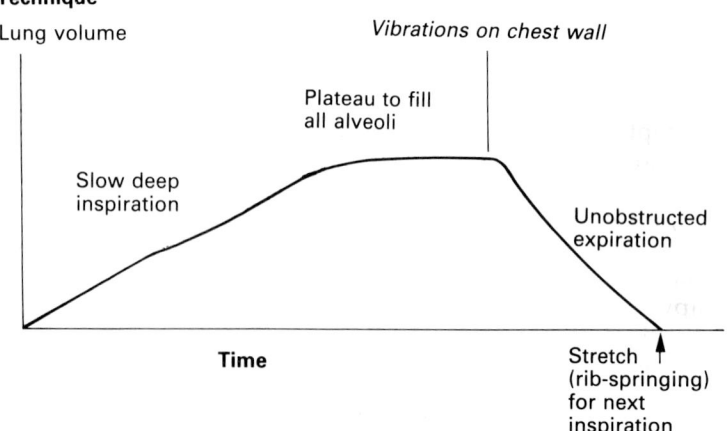

Fig. 22.1. Manual hyperinflation with chest manipulations.

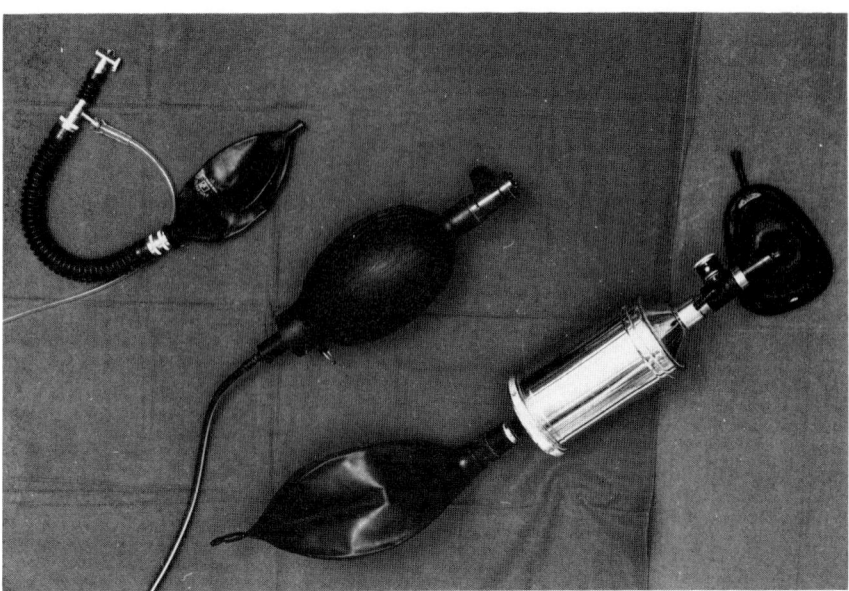

Fig. 22.2. Bag squeezing equipment (front to back): Waters' cannister; Ambu-bag; Paediatric bag.

fast recoil of the bag does not, however, realistically mimic the elastic recoil of the lungs.

With the *manual rebreathing bag* CO_2 will be rebreathed unless a high minute volume and fast flow rate are used, since the bag is incorporated in the expiratory limb of the ventilator circuit. With the ventilator on manual control, the pressure applied to the bag and therefore the lungs is shown on the ventilator dial, which is helpful in teaching. For patients who have been hyperventilated, this method is useful to raise their PCO_2 to normal levels prior to weaning.

Boyle's anaesthetic circuit is similar to the Waters' cannister and the Ambu-bag, but nitrous oxide and O_2 can be used to fill the rebreathing bag for patients in severe pain or when sedation is contra-indicated.

Contra-indication. Bag-squeezing might cause a tension pneumothorax with mediastinal shift; however, a ventilated patient with a previous pneumothorax will have a chest drain in situ, and providing this is not clamped bag-squeezing can be done if essential.

Complications. Care must be taken when bag-squeezing an emphysematous patient as bullae can easily rupture leading to a pneumothorax and surgical emphysema. The danger of causing a pneumothorax when bag-squeezing a patient with multiple fractured ribs is very great, so a chest drain is usually inserted. When this technique is used in frail, emaciated osteoporotic patients there is a risk of fracturing ribs and puncturing the lungs.

To prevent pneumothoraces in infants, an open-ended 0.5- or 0.75-litre bag is used so the inflation pressure can be constantly adjusted by the operator.

Following subclavian vein catheterization the physiotherapist must check the chest x-ray for a pneumothorax and verify that the root of the pleura has not been nicked by the central venous pressure line.

Hypoxia and hypotension may occur in conjunction with this technique. A slightly positive end-expiratory pressure can be maintained in the bag and theoretically bag-squeezing could decrease venous return and cardiac output and thus lower blood pressure. For patients in circulatory failure this could be critical and great caution must be exercised. Despite the haemodynamic disadvantages some patients require, and are very dependent on, high levels of PEEP, e.g. $+ 10$ cmH$_2$O, to maintain an adequate arterial PO_2; removal of the PEEP to allow for bag-squeezing may cause them to become hypoxic.

Bronchospasm may be caused by this treatment, and if it is severe, bag-squeezing should be stopped. To prevent bronchospasm, salbutamol can be nebulized in the ventilator circuit, via the Bird micronebulizer, prior to the physiotherapy treatment.

Bronchopulmonary fistula may occur when a patient is treated following a pneumonectomy or recent lung resection. This can be avoided by not allowing the inflation pressure to exceed the ventilating pressure.

Following bag-squeezing the patient may be tired and will have altered blood gases, so extubation and blood gas analysis should preferably be deferred for 30 min after the end of the treatment.

Intermittent positive pressure breathing (IPPB)

IPPB provides a versatile method of treating ventilated or non-ventilated, intubated or spontaneously breathing patients. The pressure-cycled ventilators most commonly used are the Bird Mark 7 or 8 or the Bennett PR2 or PV3P (Fig. 22.3). All are pressure-cycled from the inspiratory to the expiratory phase. When the machines are used for IPPB the patient initiates inspiration. A mask, mouthpiece, or catheter-mount can connect the patient to the machine; a mask is often disliked by conscious patients and has the disadvantage of depositing the nebulization on the face and in the upper respiratory tract only. Breathing head assembly sets are autoclaved or sterilized between treatments.

Mechanism of the Bird Mark 7 respirator. The patient's inspiratory effort overcomes the attraction of a magnet and metal disc. The lower the number on the inspiratory sensitivity control, the greater the distance between the magnet and the disc, and therefore the less effort is required to trigger inspiration. Inspiration continues until a pre-set pressure is reached and the attraction of another magnet and disc in the pressure chamber is overcome, thus allowing passive expiration. The rate of rise of pressure build-up in the lungs depends on the inspiratory flow rate. The lower the flow rate number, the longer and slower the build-up to reach the pre-set pressure, and vice versa. The Bird Mark 8 has the addition of a negative expiratory control.

Mechanism of the Bennett PR2 respirator. The Bennett respirator has a unique flow-sensitive valve which consists of a rotating drum supported by jewelled bearings. When the patient initiates inspiration (with a minimum 0.5 cmH$_2$O subatmospheric pressure) a pressure differential is created across the flow-sensitive valve. The drum window thus rotates open allowing gas to pass into the patient's lungs until a pre-set pressure is reached. The valve closes when the inspiratory flow is reduced to 1 litre/min, allowing passive expiration.

Uses of IPPB

Assisted ventilation: A weaning programme may consist of 10 min IPPB, 10 min spontaneous respirations, and 40 mm IPPV, the latter gradually decreasing. When self-triggering the patient feels more independent, and following prolonged IPPV with reassurance from the staff, self-confidence will return. The strength of the respiratory muscles will improve while the patient is being weaned from IPPV. During weaning, a Wright's respirometer can be left in

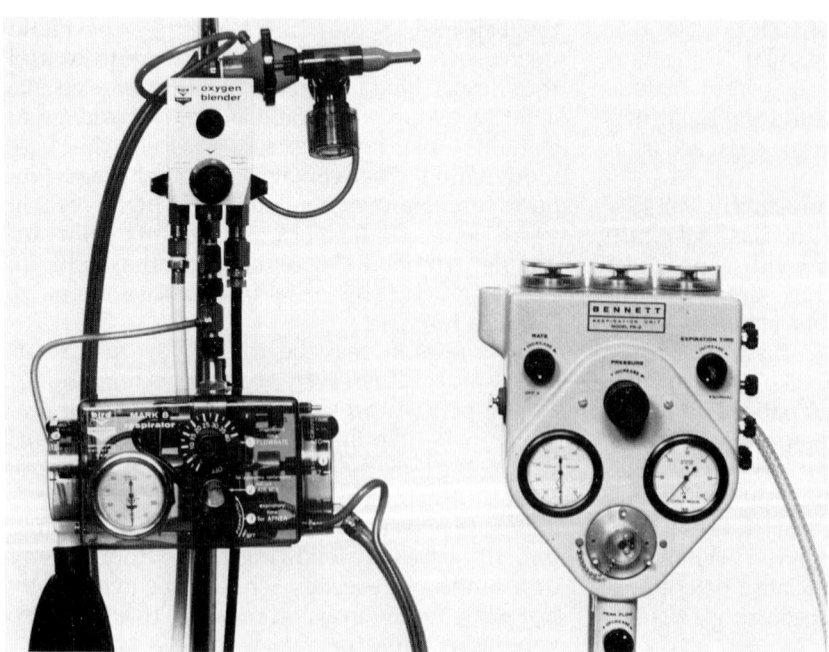

Fig. 22.3. IPPB *right*: the Bennett PR–2 respirator; *left*: the Bird mark 8 respirator, showing the breathing head assembly.

the expiratory port to measure tidal and minute volumes. Intermittent mandatory ventilation (IMV) has superseded IPPB for assisted ventilation in some centres.

To re-educate paralysed respiratory muscles, e.g., in quadraplegics; quadraplegics can be made to cough artificially during IPPB by increasing the inspiratory pressure to simulate a deep inspiration prior to the expulsive cough, aided by a stretch to the diaphragm. In patients with neuromuscular disease, e.g., muscular dystrophy, myasthenia gravis, and Guillain–Barré syndrome, IPPB can be used prophylactically to prevent patchy atelectasis. In myasthenia gravis, Bendixen [11] recommended hourly patient-triggered ventilation or bag-squeezing with a mask. If the patients are receiving anticholinesterase drugs, the vital capacity and muscle power are maximal 30 min after the drug administration, so this is the optimum time for treatment to be given.

IPPB, like IPPV, can be used prophylactically to increase tidal volume and alveolar ventilation, to assist in the removal of secretions, and to decrease the tired patient's respiratory effort and O_2 consumption.

For sputum retention or lobar collapse, IPPB is given in conjunction with postural drainage, chest manipulations, coughing or suction.

IPPB can be used *in imminent respiratory failure*, particularly at night, when patients hypoventilate and retain CO_2.

In extreme fatigue, e.g., acute severe asthma, especially in combination with retention of secretions and bronchospasm, relaxation of accessory muscles is encouraged by IPPB, and intubation and ventilation may be avoided.

Inhalation can also be achieved with this technique. When normal saline is to be inhaled, the nebulizers are never run by anhydrous gas. Normal saline is preferred to water as it is isotonic with plasma. Bronchodilators can be administered by IPPB or via a nebulizer not under pressure. If bronchospasm is present 0.5–2 ml 0.55% w/v in 10 ml strength salbutamol solution (5 mg/ml) is diluted in saline and used to fill the Bird micronebulizer to 3–5 ml or the Bennett nebulizer (using a correspondingly higher dose) to 30 ml. Antimicrobial therapy has also been attempted by inhalation: both antifungal agents and antibiotics have been given by this method, but its efficiency remains to be proven.

IPPB can be driven by Entonox for an *analgesic* effect [7].

In *LV failure* IPPB can be used to impede the formation of pulmonary oedema as a last resort prior to ventilation. This is achieved by using a retard cap to exert a constant positive airways pressure (CPAP) and reduce alveolar collapse.

Contra-indications. As for bag-squeezing, if a patient with a *pneumothorax* is given IPPB a fatal tension pneumothorax could ensue. If a chest drain is in situ and the patient has an air-leak no advantage is achieved with IPPB. Following *pneumonectomy* or *recent lung resection* with an air-leak IPPB is contra-indicated unless as a last resort prior to IPPV. This treatment should be avoided in *active pulmonary tuberculosis*, to prevent spread, and also in cases of *massive haemoptysis* and of *bronchial tumour in the proximal airways*.

In some situations IPPB should be used only with caution. In the presence of emphysema there is a danger of rupturing bullae and causing a pneumothorax, and following subclavian vein catheterization the chest x-ray must be checked to exclude a pneumothorax. Cystic fibrosis patients are very prone to pneumothoraces, and it has also been demonstrated that prolonged use of the equipment can cause an increase in residual volume [51].

Children under 5 years old are often frightened and unable to use IPPB correctly, so one should only persevere if absolutely essential, e.g., in postoperative lung collapse to prevent re-intubation.

For patients dependent upon hypoxic drive, IPPB should be run off air with added O_2 or incorporating a blender since the variable O_2 concentration (between 40% and 70%) may cause problems. However, with very strict supervision the majority of patients with COAD but without dangerous hypercapnea can tolerate high levels of O_2, and their PO_2 returns to the previous levels 5 min after treatment [45].

Some patients can become addicted to IPPB, and the number of treatments should be reduced as their condition improves.

Incentive spirometry

An incentive spirometer (IS) (e.g., Marion Laboratories Spirocare) is a controversial adjunct to physiotherapy. The patient breathes in and when his maximal inspiration equals the pre-set inspiratory value a goal is scored. The goal is advanced on a scale from 250 to 5000 cm^3. as the patient improves (Fig. 22.4)

An IS is excellent when patients are not under close supervision e.g., at night, and is also a good incentive for poorly motivated patients, especially postoperatively, to regain their

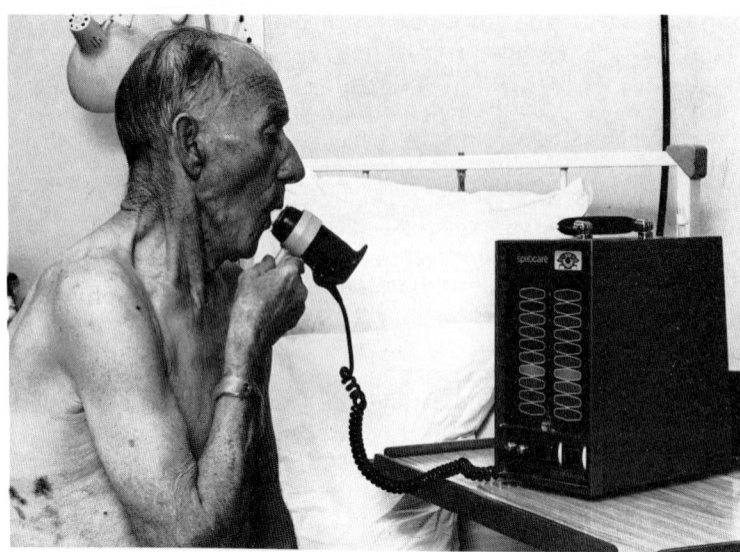

Fig. 22.4. Patient post-thoracotomy with the incentive spirometer.

pre-operative lung function [33]. The patient is instructed to achieve ten goals per hour, as once inflated alveoli remain patent for at least an hour. Some authorities [4] prefer IPPB under specialist supervision, whilst Bartlett and McConnell found higher inflation pressures with IS than IPPB [5, 38].

IS is extensively available in the United States and Canada, where the responsibility of the physiotherapist is greatly reduced. Patients receive instructions on the use of IS from the respiratory technicians who are responsible for the setting up of respiratory equipment, including ventilators. They perform all the respiratory function tests and, if necessary, administer treatment with the Bird respirator (which is now less widely used in the United States and Canada, as incorrect over-use possibly causes lung damage).

Localized breathing exercises

In conscious and non-ambulant patients there is poor ventilation to the lower lateral costal and posterior basal segments of the lungs, and therefore particular attention and encouragement are needed to prevent these areas from collapsing. Patients respond to proprioceptive impulses from the operator's hands and it appears that alveolar ventilation improves.

The patients are taught to 'hold' at maximal inspiration to allow time for all alveoli to fill. The diaphragm is the major respiratory muscle, and diaphagmatic breathing exercises are taught to all conscious patients. In sitting the abdominal viscera descends and the abdominal muscles relax. Inspiration combines flattening of the domes of the diaphragm and anterior movements of the abdominal wall. Expiration is by passive recoil. Patients are encouraged to relax their shoulders and to minimize the use of accessory muscles of respiration, thus allowing more effective ventilation for a given O_2 consumption [19, 21, 23, 34]. In unconscious patients some authorities recommended deeper inspiration by stimulating the abdominal muscles by proprioception [18].

Techniques used to aid expectoration

Normally 100 ml of fluid is produced daily by the respiratory tract. Its purpose is to assist in the elimination of infected particles by the mucociliary transport mechanism [8]. Normal clearance of bronchial secretion is achieved primarily by the action of the mucociliary escalator [46], with coughing acting as a reserve mechanism [25]. In this way bronchial toilet extends down to the 16th airway generation but the cough is ineffective beyond the 6th generation [36]. The efficacy of the cough mechanism depends largely on the peak expiratory air flow velocity generated by the patient. The patient is required to take a deep inspiration, build up a high alveolar pressure against a closed glottis, then contract the abdominal muscles and diaphragm to expel any debris. Any impairment of the mucociliary transport mechanism or ineffective coughing will lead to inadequate expectoration and sputum retention. Coughing is impaired by

1) Severe reduction in vital capacity, e.g. in marked kyphoscoliosis;
2) Laryngeal weakness or incompetence which gives rise to an ineffective hoarse bovine cough, e.g., after prolonged intubation;
3) CNS depression of the cough reflex, due to drugs or metabolic disturbances for example;
4) Pain and fear of pain, as illustrated by the frequent suppressed dry hacking expulsive efforts in pleurisy;
5) Immobility or debilitated state of a patient;
6) The presence of thick tenacious secretions and increased sputum viscosity due to dehydration, respiratory tract infection, or inadequate humidification, especially of the endotracheal or tracheostomy tubes;
7) Unstable rib cage or sternum.

Mucociliary clearance is impaired by

1) Cigarette smoking;
2) Hypothermia ($< 35°C$);
3) Hyperthemia ($> 41°C$).

Examination of the sputum often gives an indication of the diagnosis before bacteriological confirmation, e.g., bright yellow sputum usually indicates *Klebsiella*, musty green sputum often indicates *Pseudomonas*, and rusty sputum is expectorated in pneumococcal pneumonia.

Rehydration

To reduce the viscosity of the secretions the patient must be optimally hydrated.

Humidification

Alveolar air is 100% saturated with water vapour at body temperature. The amount of H_2O vapour depends on atmospheric temperature; thus to deliver absolute humidity to the patient the H_2O in the humidifier must be heated. Humidification of inspired gases prevents drying of bronchial secretions by mucosal dehydration and allows correct functioning of cilia.

A humidifier can be used in all intubated patients as a substitute nose and after any recent tracheostomi. This equipment is also useful for patients with chronic respiratory disease where ciliary action is impaired, often by smoking. Mouth breathers, debilitated patients, dehydrated or pyrexial patients can also derive benefit from humidification. It is useful postoperatively for sputum retention, as the mucosa is irritated by anhydrous anaesthetic gases. Its application is also beneficial in infants and children with tenacious secretions, in any patient receiving O_2 therapy, and in burned patients with respiratory problems, especially children with laryngeal oedema [9, 29, 54].

Humidifiers are of various types. Heat and moisture exchangers were first described by Toremalm [48]; in these where expired H_2O vapour condensed, originally on aluminium foil, and 80% of it was inspired during the next breath. Garthurs, Portex, Norbel and Thackery exchangers are now used, in which H_2O vapour condenses on metal, corrugated paper, or foam, but these involve the disadvantages of easy crusting.

In ultrasonic appliances the droplet size is controlled by a crystal, 5 μm being the best size for lung penetration [46]. Intermittent ultrasonic therapy can be used for patients with thick secretions. There is a danger of fluid overloading the patient. The water reservoir must be lower than the patient's airway to prevent aspiration.

In the hot water bath gases bubble through water heated to 65°C so it is bacteriostatic (e.g., Bennett's cascade). Bubblers, e.g., the Puritan–Bennett all-purpose nebulizer, are also used, although the heating rods are sometimes inefficient.

The Medic-Aid Solo-sphere, working on the Babington principle, which together with a baffle produces an aerosol with a particle size of 4 μm, will deliver a nearly constant 45 mg H_2O per litre of gas over a flow range of 4–60 litres/min at 100% relative humidity when measured at body temperature [48] (Fig. 22.5).

Inhalations of mucolytic agents

Tincture of benzoine or pine oil and menthol inhalations encourage deep breathing and aid expectoration of tenacious secretions, especially postoperatively. They must be carefully monitored to prevent accidental scalds. To prevent burns and to give continuous O_2 therapy, which is preferable to intermittent treatment, O_2 and inhalation can be combined by using a disposable Inspiron humidifier, tubing, and mask (Fig. 22.6).

Bronchodilators

Bronchodilators may be given to the patient in

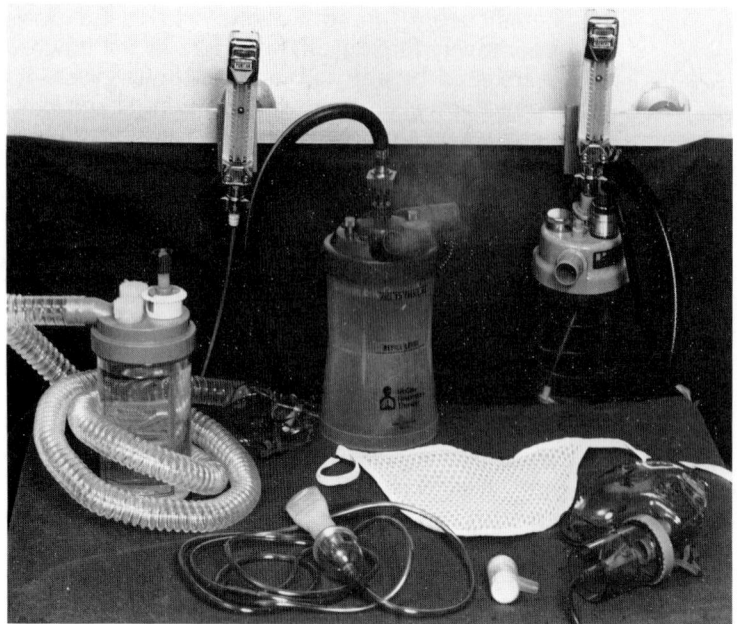

Fig. 22.5. *Left* to *right* (back row): Inspiron, Solo-sphere Puritan-Bennett; (front row): Acorn, Thackery bib, Portex, and Hudson humidifiers and nebulizers.

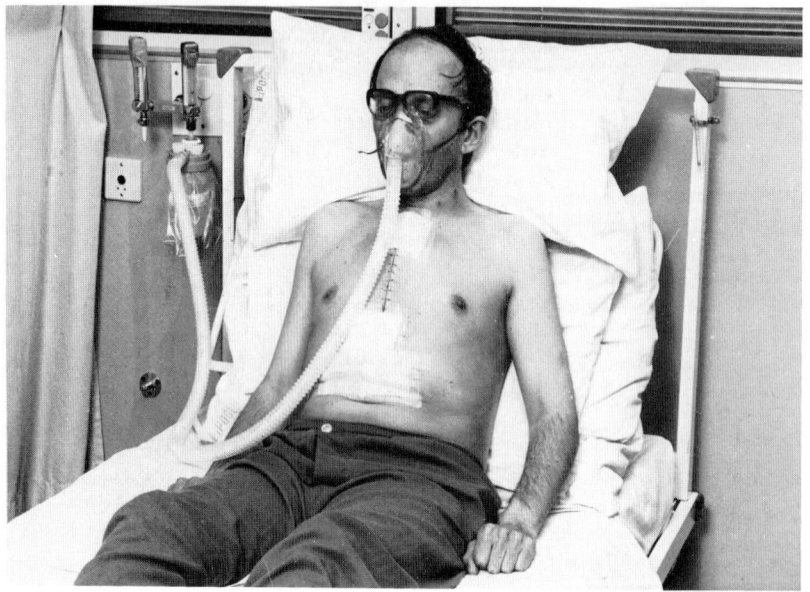

Fig. 22.6. Tinc Benz inhalation with a disposable Inspiron humidifier.

several forms, e.g., IV administration, tablets, suppositories, or as an inhalation.

Inhalation therapy delivers the drug directly to the site of action and there is increasing evidence that this is the method of choice, as a greater bronchodilator response is achieved with fewer unwanted side effects [52]. Inhalation therapy may take several forms:

1) The *aerosol* is the simplest and cheapest method of inhalation, but requires a good technique in use of the 'puffer' by the patient and so is more suitable for out-patients. Some puffers are available with a front platform 'spacer' to allow the drug to be inhaled over a number of breaths, which may be useful if the patient has no co-ordinated breathing pattern.

2) *Powdered inhalation* is available in some forms, and administered with a Rotohaler.

3) *Nebulization* Bronchodilator solution may be nebulized with a driving gas derived from an O_2 supply and flow meter, from an air compressor, or in conjunction with IBBP. If the patient is ventilated, it is possible to incorporate a nebulizer into the inspiratory circuit of the ventilator tubing to deliver a nebulized form of bronchodilation, as in the Bird micronebulizer.

Studies undertaken over recent years have shown that nebulized bronchodilators delivered in conjunction with IPPB have no particular advantage or enhanced effect over those administered by spontaneous breathing [12]. If there are no indications for the use of IPPB other than to deliver a bronchodilator, it seems an unnecessary adjunct to bronchodilator inhalation therapy [49]. It has been reported in studies of patients receiving bronchodilators with and without IPPB that those given IPPB showed an increase in tachycardia [28] and less peripheral penetration and deposition of aerosol particles than those receiving their inhalation through quiet spontaneous mouth breathing [10]. Routes of oral administration can include masks or mouthpieces, which give a more direct delivery of the bronchodilator.

Nebulizers working on Bernoulli's principle are used for the inhalation not only of bronchodilators but also of antibiotics, mucolytic agents, antifungal agents, or saline.

Analgesic gas and support

Entonox is commonly used as an analgesic gas as it relieves pain and does not cause depression of the cardiac and respiratory centres. The cylinder contains 50% O_2 and 50% nitrous oxide (N_2O). The patient inspires the gas mixture through a tightly sealed face-mask via a demand valve so the deeper the breath, the more pain relief is achieved (Fig. 22.7).

Postoperatively pulmonary complications occur in 30%–40% of patients following upper abdominal surgery, and Entonox has decreased

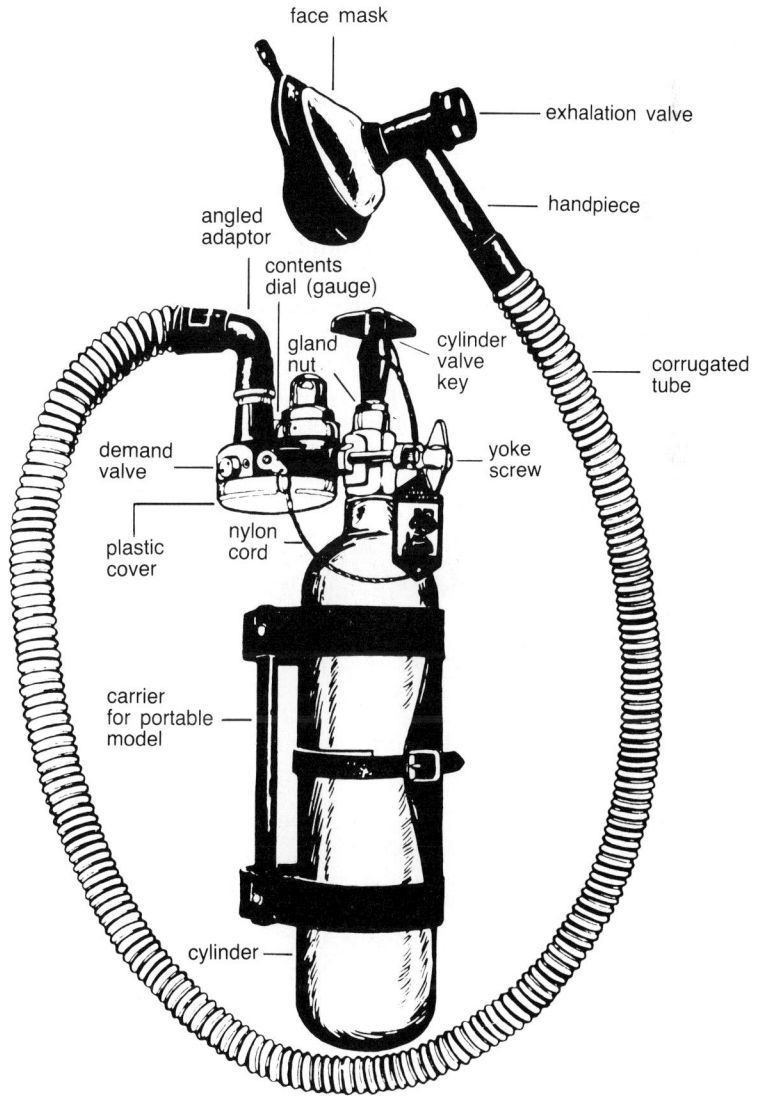

Fig. 22.7. Entonox cylinder and head-set.

hypoxaemia and pain in these cases [1, 2, 15, 16, 27]. An increased tidal volume can be achieved with analgesia and patients can co-operate to clear secretions from their chests [7]. Seal [17] recommends Entonox for mild chest injuries, continuous extradural marcain 0.5% for multiple rib fractures and IPPV for flail chests and stabilizing the chest wall, thus relieving pain.

Following surgery good incisional support is essential, e.g., cough lock for median sternotomy, and knee flexion and manual pressure for abdominal incisions (Fig. 22.8).

Postural drainage

This is the use of gravity to assist drainage of secretions into the main bronchi and trachea from where they can be expectorated or aspirated by suction. In suitable patients it is an effective method of re-expanding pulmonary segments, and preventing sputum retention, infection, and lung collapse.

The positions for postural drainage vary according to the anatomy of the bronchopulmonary tree; for a collapsed left lower lobe, for example, the patient is comfortably positioned lying on the right side and the bed is tilted 18 in [44]. The positions may be modified, e.g., following lung resection.

It is hoped that when secretions are cleared more alveoli open up and the action of surfactant is potentiated. The surface tension of surfactant lining the alveoli changes with alveolar size, thus increasing the compliance of the lung, decreasing the work-load, and promoting stability of the alveoli [20].

Contra-indications. Postural drainage is contra-indicated in cases of orthopnoea, e.g. in patients with chronic obstructive respiratory disease or cardiac failure; and where there is severe hypertension. Caution should be exercised when considering its use in neurosurgical patients; it should never be instituted following cerebro-vascular surgery, and if there is an external cerebro-spinal fluid shunt, it should be used with care and only if the drainage bottle is lowered with the head. It should never be used in a non-intubated patient without a gag reflex.

It is also contra-indicated following oesophageal surgery, where the cardiac sphincter may be incompetent. If a naso-gastric tube is in situ and the gastric contents are removed, then postural drainage under strict supervision may be possible.

Advanced pregnancy or a large hiatus hernia drainage may lead to reflux of gastric contents. During the 'running in' cycle of peritoneal dialysis, if the patient is not ventilated, excursions of the diaphragm are curtailed and the patient may become too short of breath. Following cardiac or some vascular surgery, e.g. carotid endarterectomy, postural drainage is not used routinely unless medically requested.

It should not be used in patients with severe neck or facial oedema, e.g. in cases of burns or severe surgical emphysema, nor where there are recent head injuries.

Chest manipulations

The most widely used methods of effectively clearing the lungs of secretions are the chest

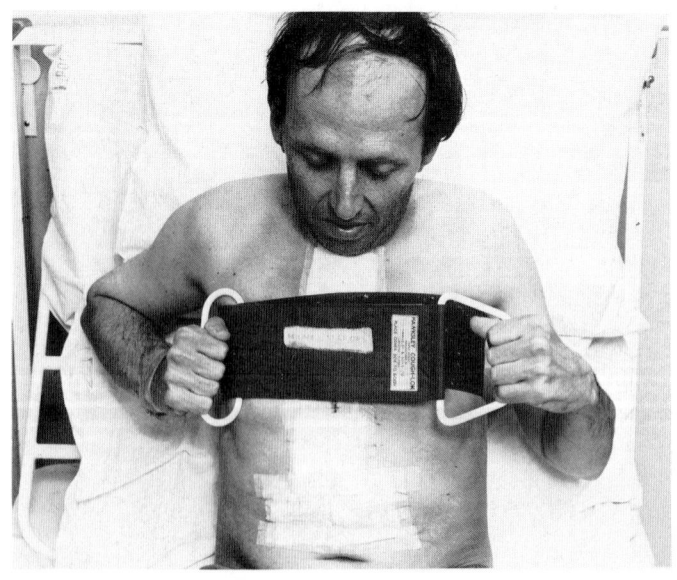

Fig. 22.8. Patient using a cough-lock following a fourth median sternotomy.

manipulations: rib-springing; vibrations or shakings; and clapping or percussion.

Rib-springing is a stretch, ideally on a mobile chest wall, at the beginning of inspiration. It was one of Lassen's original precepts and he proved that local compression of consolidated lung caused retained secretions to be squeezed along the bronchus as toothpaste is squeezed from a tube [26].

Vibrations are performed by the physiotherapist's hands throughout expiration and vary from fine to coarse shakings; they can be performed on a more rigid chest wall.

Chest percussion, or clappings, are independent of the respiratory cycle and help to loosen secretions; they are performed rhythmically with cupped hands (Fig. 22.9).

Chest manipulations are performed on all ICU patients, often in conjunction with postural drainage, bag-squeezing, and IPPB. The value of chest physiotherapy combined with postural drainage in clearing bronchial secretions was shown by Cochrane et al. [13], who proved that sputum has a detrimental effect on pulmonary function and physiotherapy can decrease airways obstruction. This was demonstrated by measuring the improved specific airways conductance in patients with copious sputum, e.g. over 30 ml per day. During the acute phase of pneumonia chest manipulations may be of no value [13].

Contra-indications. Chest manipulations should not be performed in patients with cardiovascular instability, fractured osteoporotic ribs or rib metastases. They are contra-indicated in acute asthma with severe bronchospasm, although sometimes there is an improvement with rhythmical gentle clappings. In cases of tetanus, percussion can increase unwanted spasm, and therefore the patient must be fully sedated prior to treatment. With empyema and lung abscess, percussion increases the spread of infection if no drain is in situ, and where there is acute pulmonary embolism in anti-coagulated patients, percussion leads to bruising.

If there is severe chest pain, e.g. pleurisy, a mechanical vibrator may be used in preference to the operator's hands. A foam-padded vibrator or electric tooth brush may also be used on infants or neonates. In burned patients with chest wall skin grafts a sterile foam rubber pad is used over the chest wall if vibrations are essential and respirations are not inhibited by pain [29].

Complication. Arterial gas tensions in some patients deteriorate with treatment, e.g. following mitral valve replacement, a fall in cardiac output and mixed venous oxygen tension may occur during percussion treatment [53]. The treatment must therefore be adapted to the patient's condition.

Forced expiration technique

In spontaneously breathing patients the efficiency of postural drainage is improved by using a forced expiratory technique (FET) [3]. FET or huffing from mid to low lung volumes

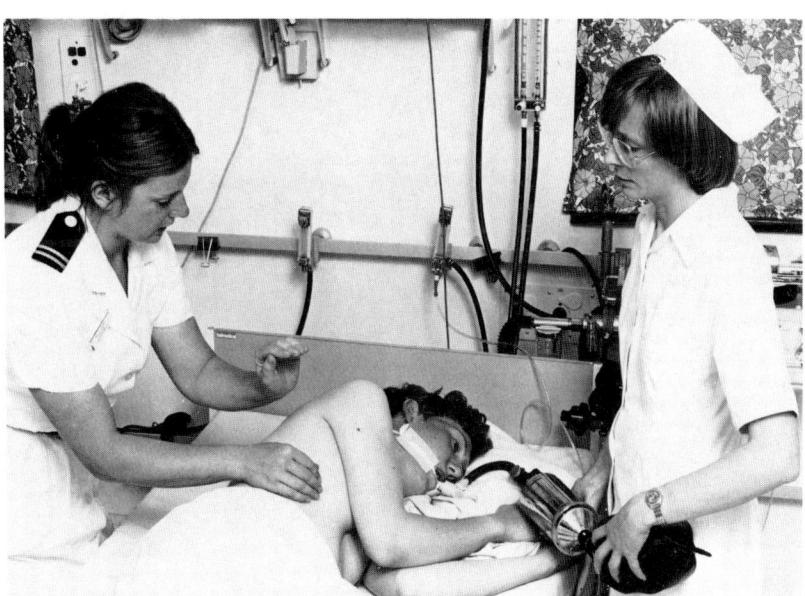

Fig. 22.9. Chest percussion to patient's right lung combined with bag squeezing via the Waters' cannister.

allows more mobilization of peripheral secretions, and should be followed by diaphragmatic breathing to prevent the occurrence of bronchospasm [40].

Suction

Any patient who is unable to expectorate pulmonary secretions efficiently requires suction. Suction should never be regarded as a last resort only for unconscious patients, and all medical personnel should be proficient in the technique. *Intubated patients.* With the suction equipment turned off a sterile catheter is introduced down the endotracheal tube or tracheostomy during inspiration (Fig. 22.10). The catheter size is critical and must not be greater than half the internal diameter of the endotracheal or tracheostomy tube to prevent the patient becoming hypoxic. For tenacious secretions or to obtain a trapped sputum specimen up to 5 ml isotonic saline or a weak solution of sodium bicarbonate may be instilled down the endotracheal or tracheostomy tubes. In infants the amount used must be added to the fluid balance chart.

Non-intubated patients. Lubricating gel is required to prevent trauma for nasal or oral routes. With one-eyed catheters on expiration a suction-release technique is preferred without rotation, to prevent tracheal invagination. During suction a cough should be achieved. Treatment should not be prolonged, otherwise the patient may become hypoxic. Combining suction with chest compression and other techniques the treatment continues until the chest is clear [24, 41, 42, 47].

During extubation. Breathing exercises and suction are essential prior to routine extubation. Following suction via the endotracheal tube as described above, the oro-pharynx must be cleared of secretions. The securing tapes of the endotracheal tube are cut and a sterile suction catheter is introduced down the endotracheal tube. Whilst the endotracheal tube is being withdrawn suction continues, aiming to keep the catheter half an inch below the tip of the endotracheal tube to remove any further secretions. The patient must then be encouraged to breathe deeply and cough frequently to prevent secretions collecting, necessitating re-intubation.

Atropine is occasionally used to reduce excessive secretions and decrease the amount of suction, required e.g. in myasthenia gravis with excessive salivation.

Contra-indications. Nasal suction should not be used in non-intubated patients following frontal head injuries if there is a cerebrospinal fluid leak; in cases of brain abscess; following nasal operations; or where there is severe epistaxis.

Complications. Hypoxia can occur in patients on high levels of PEEP to maintain a PO_2 of 60 mmHg (8.0 kPa), e.g. in shock lung syndrome. Following high cervical cord lesions prolonged suction with hypoxia may lead to bradycardia

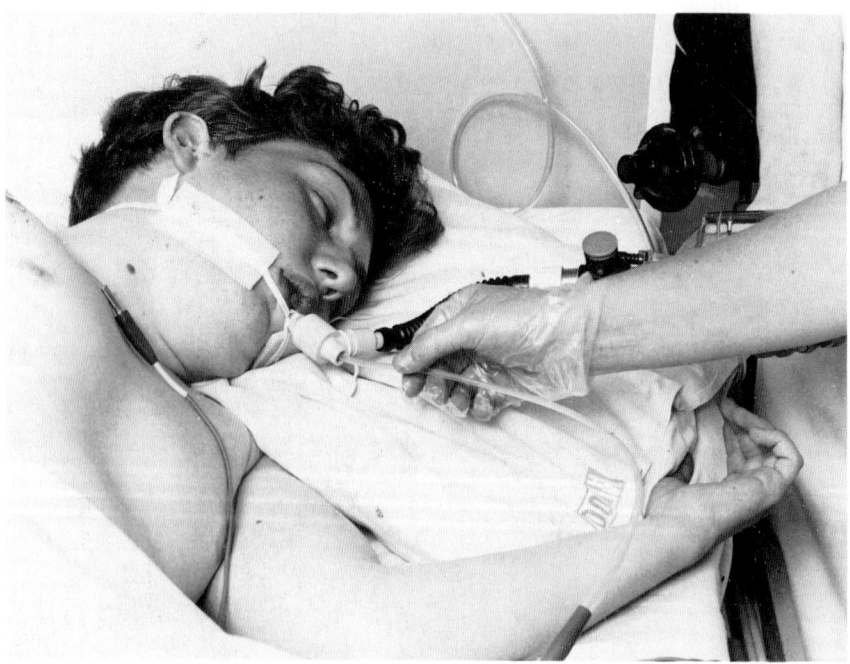

Fig. 22.10. Suction for the intubated patient.

and cardiac arrest. To prevent rebound hypoxaemia in spontaneously breathing non-intubated patients, O_2 therapy must be continued during suction. If the PO_2 is critical a cutaneous oxygen electrode can monitor constantly the PO_2 level.

It is essential to prevent trauma in patients with a bleeding diathesis.

Emphasis must be placed on sterility in immunosuppressed patients and in those with inhalation burns [54] to avoid infection.

Accurate technique is essential following oesophageal and pulmonary surgery.

There are a number of catheters available, some people still preferring red rubber sterilizable or Cudé-tip catheters for pneumonectomy patients or children. Some catheters, e.g. the Sherwood Argyle Hovercraft with multiple side holes, are less traumatic to the mucous membranes.

Although the ICU physiotherapist is responsible mainly for the respiratory care of the critically ill patient, the chest cannot be taken in isolation. The mental attitude of the patient may partly dictate the speed of recovery so all members of the team must communicate with one another and with the patient. Explanation of all physical actions and constant reassurance must be given to the patient even when treating a brain-damaged individual. Patients can become aware of their environment and orientated to time by the use of radios, clocks and dim lights at night. Visitors are encouraged and in certain cases, especially with young patients remain during treatments and can play an active role particularly by supporting and encouraging their relatives. Even ventilated patients can be mobilized to sitting in an arm-chair and therefore feel more independent (Fig. 22.11).

References

1. Alexander JI, Spence AA (1973) Apparent improvement in postoperative lung volume by using the Entonox apparatus. Br J Anaesth 45:90
2. Alexander JI, Parikh RK, Spence AA (1973) Postoperative analgesic and lung function: A comparison of narcotic analgesic regimes. Br J Anaesth 45:90
3. Barrell SE, Abbas HM (1978) Monitoring during physiotherapy after open heart surgery. Physiotherapy 64/9:272
4. Bartlett RH (1971) Post traumatic pulmonary insufficiency. In: Cooper P Nyphus L (eds) Surgery annual. Appleton-Century Crofts, New York, chap 1
5. Bartlett RH, Brennan ML, Gazzaniga AB, et al (1973) Studies on the pathogenesis and prevention of postoperative pulmonary complications. Surg Gynecol Obstet 137:925
6. Bartlett RH, Krop RH, Hanson EL, et al (1970) The physiology of yawning and the application to postoperative care. Surg Forum 21:222–275
7. Bendixen HH (1961) Myasthenia gravis: Case report and discussion. Anesth Analg (Cleve) 40:701–706
8. Bethune D (1975) Neurophysiological facilitation of respiration in the unconscious adult patient. Can Physiotherapy J 27:5
9. Brown J (1977) Respiratory complications in burned patients. Physiotherapy 63:151

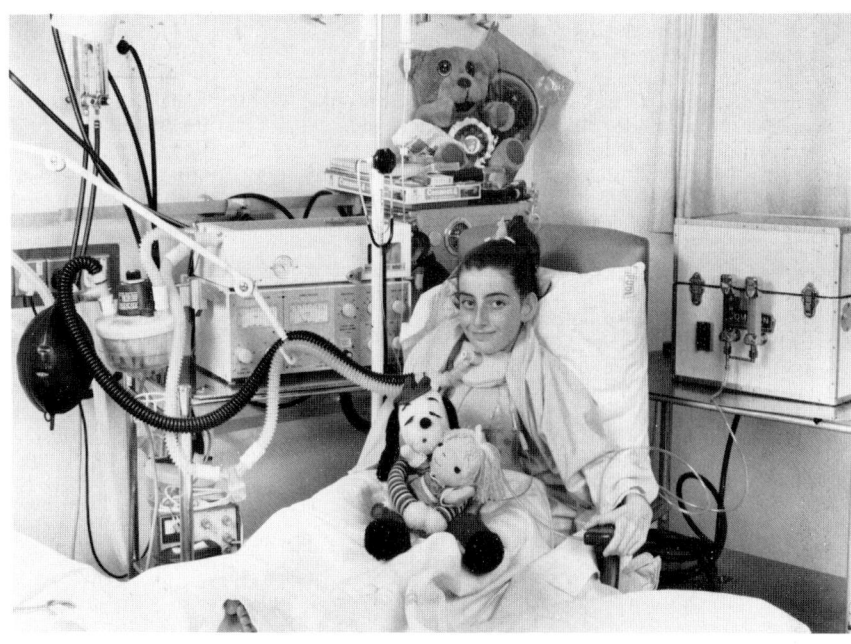

Fig. 22.11. Frances happy to be in a chair.

10. Campbell I et al (1978) Intermittent positive pressure breathing. Br Med J i:1186

11. Clement AJ, Hubsch SK (1968) Chest physiotherapy by bag-squeezing method. Physiotherapy 54:355–359

12. Cochrane GM (1979) Bronchodilators. Practitioner 223:489

13. Cochrane GM, Webber BA, Clarke SW (1977) Effects of sputum on pulmonary function. Br Med J ii:1181–1183

14. Cortlandt MacMahon (1915) Breathing and physical exercises for use in cases of wounds in the pltura, lungs and diaphragm. Lancet II:769

15. Dalrymple DG, Parbrook GD (1976) Personality assessment and postoperative analgesia. Br J Anaesth 48:593

16. Dolovich MB, Killian D, Wolff R, et al (1977) Pulmonary aerosol deposition in chronic bronchitis: IPPB versus quiet breathing. Am Rev Respir Dis 115:397

17. Egbert LD, Bendixen HH (1964) Effects of morphine on breathing pattern: A possible factor in atelectasis. JAMA 188:485–488

18. Fry D, Hyatt R (1960) Pulmonary mechanics. Am J Med 29:672

19. Gaskell D (1975) Chronic bronchitis, emphysema and asthma. In: Cash J (ed) Chest, heart and vascular disorders for physiotherapists. Faber & Faber, London, p 155

20. Gaskell DV, Webber BA (1980) The Brompton Hospital guide to chest physiotherapy, 4th edition. Blackwell, London

21. Hawkins J (1968) Movement of the diaphragm postoperatively. Lancet II:85

22. Ibsen B (1954) The anaesthetist's viewpoint on treatment of respiratory complications in poliomyelitis during the epidemic in Copenhagen 1952. Proc Soc Lond [Biol] 47:72–74

23. Innocenti D (1966) Breathing exercises in treatment emphysema. Physiotherapy 52:437

24. Keown KK (1960) A method of removing tracheobronchial secretions by the production of effective coughing. Anesth Analg (Cleve) 39:570–571

25. Kilburn KH, Durham NC (1967) Cilia and mucus transport as determinants of the responses of lung to air pollutants. Arch Environ Health 14:77

26. Lassens HCA (1953) 1952 Poliomyelitis epidemic in Copenhagen with special reference to acute respiratory insufficiency. Lancet I:37–41

27. Latimer RG, Dickman M, Clinton Day W, et al (1971) Ventilatory patterns and pulmonary complications after upper abdominal surgery determined by pre-operative and post operative computerized spirometry and blood gas analysis. Am J Surg 122:622–632

28. Lawford Jones BJM, Milledge VS, et al (1978) Comparison of intravenous and nebulised salbutamol in initial treatment of severe asthma. Br Med J

29. Leith DE (1968) Cough. Phys Ther 48:439

30. Lewis SJ (1978), Physiotherapy in the intensive care unit. In: Tinker J (ed) Intensive care. (A Nursing Times publication) MacMillan, London

31. Link W, Spaeth E, Wahle W, Penny W, Glover J (1976) The influence of suction catheter tip design on tracheobronchial trauma and fluid aspiration efficiency. Anesth Analg (Cleve) 55:290–297

32. Lloyd E, Macrae WR (1971) Respiratory tract damage in burns. Br Anaesth 43:365–378

33. Matthews LR, Doershvk C, Wise M, et al (1964) A

therapeutic regimen for patients with cystic fibrosis. J Pediatr 65:558

34. McConnel DH, Maloney JV, Buckberg GD (1974) Postoperative intermittent positive pressure breathing treatments. J Thorac Cardiovasc Surg 68:994

35. Mendelson CL (1946) Aspiration of stomach contents into lungs during obstetric anaesthesia. Am J Obstet Gynecol 52:191

36. Newhouse M, Bienstock J, Sanchis J (1976) Lung defense mechanisms. N Engl J Med 295:990–997

37. O'Rourke MF, Shepherd KM (1973) Protection of the aortic arch during intra-aortic balloon pumping. J Thorac Cardiovasc Surg 65:543

38. Pfeninger J, Roth F (1977) Intermittent positive pressure breathing (IPPB) versus incentive spirometer (IS) therapy in the post-operative period. Intensive Care Med 3:279–281

39. Plum F, Dunning MF (1956) Techniques for minimizing trauma to the tracheobronchial tree after tracheostomy. N Engl J Med 254:193–200

40. Pryor JA Webber BA, Hodson ME, Batten JC (1979) An evaluation of the forced expiration technique as an adjunct to postural drainage in treatment of cystic fibrosis. Br Med J ii:417–418

41. Rosen MT, Hullard EK (1960) The use of suction in clinical medicine. Br J Anaesth 32:486

42. Rosen MT, Hullard EK (1963) Further considerations on tracheal suction catheters. Br J Anaesth 35:125

43. Sacker M, Landa J, Greeneltch N, Robinson M (1973) Pathogenesis and prevention of tracheobronchial damage with suction procedures. Chest 64:284–290

44. Seal P (1974) Analgesia in the treatment of chest injuries. Physiotherapy 60:134

45. Starke ID, Webber BA, Branthwaite MA (1979) IPPB and hypercapnea in respiratory failure: The effect of different concentrations of inspired oxygen on blood gas tensions. Anaesthesia 34:283–287

46. Sykes MK, McNichol MW, Cambell EJM (1970) Respiratory failure. Blackwell Scientific, Oxford Edinburgh

47. Thompson BJ (1973) The physiotherapy role in rehabilitation of the asthmatic. NZ J Physiotherapy 4/4:11

48. Toremalm NG (1960) A heat and moisture exchanger for post-tracheotomy care. Acta Otolaryngol (Stockh) 52:461–472

49. Webber BA, Shenfields, Paterson JW (1974) A comparison of three different techniques for giving nebulised albuterol to asthmatic patients. Am Rev Respir Dis 109:293

50. West JB (1979) Physiological advantages of surfactant. Respiratory physiology, the essentials, 2nd edn. Blackwell, Oxford, pp 94–96

51. Wiggs S (1978) IPPB with bronchodilators and Entonox. Physiotherapy 64:43–44

52. Wijdan Al-Diaidy, Skeates SK, Hill DW, Tinker J (1977) The use of transcutaneous oxygen electrodes in intensive therapy. Intensive Care Med 3:35–39

53. William GB, Graham MD, Deborah A, Bradley BS (1978) The efficacy of chest physiotherapy and intermittent positive pressure breathing in the resolution of pneumonia. N Engl J Med 299:624

54. Wootton R, Hodgson E (1977) Physiotherapy treatment of burns with inhalation involvement. Physiotherapy 63:153

Chapter 23

Respiratory Pharmacology

François Lhoste and Peter J. Barnes

The treatment of lung conditions in the critically ill patient is mainly concerned with the urgent supply of O_2 to peripheral tissues and the removal of CO_2. This therapeutic aim can be achieved either by such physical methods as increase in the inspired O_2 concentration (FiO_2), CPAP, mechanical ventilation (MV), PEEP and their various combinations or by pharmacological methods.

During the past few years physical methods have tended to overshadow the use of drugs, because of the easy and rapid corrections of disordered physiology they permit in the most severe respiratory cases, in particular those unaffected by drugs. However, problems associated with methods of MV [15], the risk of infection with intubation and tracheostomy [8], and the subsequent difficulties of weaning [4] have resulted in a fresh interest in the use of drugs. Moreover, advances in pulmonary pathophysiology and the development of clinical investigations in the ICU have allowed better understanding of the limitations of mechanical respiratory assistance and the realization of some of its shortcomings [38]. The decrease in the blood and O_2 supply to peripheral tissues induced by the most aggressive mechanical methods (e.g., PEEP ventilation), which reduce the cardiac output, was an important stimulus to new interest in the pharmacological treatment of cardiorespiratory failure.

The purpose of this chapter is to examine the various drug approaches to the treatment of respiratory conditions in the intensive care setting.

The prime function of the lung is to exchange gas between the external environment and the blood; this exchange involves alveolar ventilation, pulmonary capillary blood flow, and their close relationship. In the normal subject, almost the entire cardiac output passes through the lungs and therefore makes close contact with the alveoli. At rest, the alveolar ventilation and the pulmonary capillary blood flow are very similar (4.5 litres/min and 5 litres/min, respectively), giving an overall ventilation:perfusion ratio $\dot{V}/\dot{Q}$ of 0.9. This overall ratio is an abstract concept, however, insofar as some alveoli will be well ventilated and poorly perfused (physiological dead space) whereas some will be well perfused and poorly ventilated (physiological shunt). The $\dot{V}/\dot{Q}$ may be greatly altered in respiratory disease, sometimes unexpectedly, because of the extreme patchiness of the pulmonary lesions and the physiological compensatory mechanisms which affect both alveoli and pulmonary capillaries.

An uneven distribution of $\dot{V}/\dot{Q}$ within the lungs nearly always results in hypoxaemia. In intensive care medicine, one of the most convenient ways of measuring the deterioration of $\dot{V}/\dot{Q}$ due to the hypoventilation of persistently perfused areas at the bedside is to measure intrapulmonary shunting (Qs/Qt) [33]. This measures the amount of blood passing through the lungs but may underestimate the extent of the non-ventilated pulmonary parenchyma, as a number of vessels have high critical closure pressures [5]. The control of both the alveolar ventilation and the pulmonary capillary flow is necessary to achieve a normal O_2 supply to the tissues.

Alveolar hypoventilation

Hypercapnia [PaCO$_2$ > 45 mmHg (6kPa)] implies inefficient ventilation, which may be due to disorders at many sites: brain, spinal cord, neuromuscular junction, respiratory muscles, thoracic cage or lungs. Alveolar hypoventilation, therefore, has many causes but these may be classified into four main groups: (1) Defects in central regulation (such as sedative overdose or Pickwickian syndrome); (2) neuromuscular deficiency (such as poliomyelitis or myaesthenia gravis); (3) disorders of the ventilatory pump [such as chronic obstructive airways disease (COAD)]; and (4) abnormalities in ventilation perfusion relationships (such as emphysema and asthma). Often several mechanisms may operate in a disease process such as chronic airways obstruction.

Treatment of alveolar hypoventilation depends on the underlying cause, and the use of pharmacological respiratory stimulants (analeptics) may not be indicated in all situations. The use of such drugs may be limited by impairment of thoracopulmonary mechanisms, as some patients with alveolar hypoventilation are already fully stimulated centrally (i.e., they already have a high drive to respiration) and further central stimulation may be deleterious by increasing O$_2$ demand.

Control of ventilation

Alveolar hypoventilation is treated primarily by MV, and pharmacological methods are less important except where mechanical methods may be deleterious, such as in terminal emphysema. Non-specific stimulants such as amphetamines, ephedrine, and theophylline act on respiratory centres but also have a generalized CNS-stimulant action which limits their clinical use. More specific respiratory stimulants were introduced, such as nikethamide, pentylenetetrazol, and bemegride, but doses capable of stimulating ventilation were very close to those causing convulsions. Furthermore, CNS stimulation resulted in increased muscular activity and so increased O$_2$ demand, and these drugs have now been largely abandoned.

Recently, with the introduction of newer, safer analeptic drugs, their role has been re-evaluated. Analeptics may be indicated in impaired ventilation secondary to sedative overdose, in cases of idiopathic respiratory depression (Pickwickian syndrome), in post-anaesthetic respiratory depression, and in acute exacerbations of COAD with hypercapnia—particularly if these are precipitated by sedatives. By the judicious use of analeptics it may be possible to avoid the use of MV.

Analeptics

Doxapram. This pyrrolidinone derivative was the first relatively selective analeptic with an acceptable margin of safety between doses causing stimulation of respiratory centres and doses causing convulsions. At low doses (0.5 mg/kg IV) doxapram appears to stimulate carotid chemoreceptors, but at higher doses stimulation of the medullary respiratory centre occurs. The onset of action is within 10 min and lasts only a few minutes with single IV injections, so it is necessary to give the drug by continuous infusion. The increase in ventilation is dependent on dose and increases linearly over the range 0.3–3.0 mg.kg^{-1}.min^{-1}, resulting in an increase in tidal volume but little increase in respiratory rate [56].

Side-effects are uncommon, but following doses of over 2 mg. kg^{-1}. min^{-1} nausea, sweating, anxiety, and hallucinations may occur. At higher doses there is an increase in systemic and pulmonary artery pressures, and rare cases of hepatic failure and gastro-intestinal (GI) haemorrhage have been reported [25]. As doxapram is metabolized by the liver, care should be taken in patients with impaired hepatic function.

Almitrine. A new analeptic, almitrine is a piperazine derivative which appears to selectively stimulate chemoreceptors in the carotid body and so cause increased ventilation. There does not appear to be any central action at the doses used and its effect is completely abolished by denervation of the carotid bodies in animals [32]. Almitrine increases ventilation by increasing tidal volume in both normals [19] and chronic bronchitics with hypercapnia [21]. When given IV the effect on ventilation may persist for several hours after discontinuation of the infusion.

When almitrine is given IV in a dose of 0.25–0.5 mg/kg over 30 min there are no significant side-effects, but at higher doses sweating and nausea have been reported. No significant elevation of PAP has been reported during infusions [54], and as the preparation is devoid of central action there is no problem of increased activation leading to increased O$_2$ consumption.

There is some evidence that almitrine may increase P$_a$O$_2$ even in patients with hypoxic respiratory failure without evidence of hypercapnia: this effect does not involve an increase in ventilation but may be due to an improvement in ventilation-perfusion matching by stimulation of receptors in the pulmonary vasculature [62].

Almitrine may prove to be a major advance in the ICU, where it may be given by infusion. An oral preparation is available for more long-term use.

Progesterone. The hyperventilation produced by progesterone has been known for many years. Medroxyprogesterone appears to stimulate ventilation by increasing the sensitivity of the respiratory centre to CO_2 in some unknown way [40]. It has no role in the acute management of hypoventilation, and the results in COPD, altitude hypoventilation, and Pickwickian syndrome are questionable.

Acetazolamide. This is a carbonic anhydrase inhibitor which induces a metabolic acidosis and thereby stimulates ventilation, but it has not proved useful in practice. There is certainly no place for it in the acute situation, and the metabolic imbalance it produces may be detrimental in respiratory acidosis [43].

Airway calibre

Much of respiratory pharmacology is concerned with increasing airway calibre. Airways obstruction may be caused by bronchial smooth muscle contraction, by swelling of bronchial epithelium, or by bronchial secretions. Bronchodilator drugs achieve their main effect by relaxing bronchial smooth muscle either directly or by inhibiting the release of bronchoconstrictor mediators from mast cells in the lung, and to a lesser extent by reducing mucosal edema and bronchial secretions.

Autonomic nervous system

Airway smooth muscle has a rich parasympathetic innervation from the vagus. Stimulation of the vagus or administration of cholinergic agonists such as acetylcholine, methacoline, or carbachol result in bronchoconstriction. Conversely, antagonists such as atropine cause bronchodilatation both in normal subjects and in patients with airways obstruction [14].

By contrast, there is no convincing evidence for direct sympathetic innervation of the airways and sympathetic nerves to the lungs are distributed mainly to blood vessels, although there is some evidence that sympathetic fibres may synapse in cholinergic ganglia and modulate parasympathetic activity [52]. However, beta-adrenergic antagonists such as propranolol, when given to patients with airways obstruction, cause increased bronchial obstruction, indicating that the airways are under a certain amount of tonic adrenergic stimulation [42]. There is good evidence for numerous beta receptors in bronchial smooth muscle, which presumably respond to circulating adrenaline and noradrenaline and to the adrenergic agonists used in therapy to produce bronchodilatation. Based on the relative potencies of agonist and antagonist drugs, beta receptors can be subdivided into beta 1 and beta 2 receptors. Bronchial smooth muscle contains predominantly beta 2 receptors [30], and it has been possible to develop agonists which are relatively beta 2-selective to minimize the cardiac stimulation resulting from beta 1 activation. Beta receptors have been alternatively classified into $beta_T$ receptors responding to the neurotransmitter noradrenaline and $beta_H$ receptors, which respond to the circulating hormone adrenaline. In the airways $beta_H$ receptors (equivalent to beta 2 receptors) predominate [1]. Alpha receptors, which mediate bronchoconstriction, have been demonstrated in the airways of patients with obstructive airways disease but not in normal human airways [28]. Alpha receptor-mediated release of mediators from pulmonary mast cells has also been demonstrated. Alpha antagonists such as phentolamine and thymoxamine have been shown to have a weak bronchodilating effect in asthmatics [47], although this could be explained by other actions of these drugs such as antihistamine effects or baroreflex stimulation of the sympathetic nervous system.

Cyclic nucleotides

Recently the measurement of cyclic nucleotides has advanced our understanding of bronchodilator mechanisms. Cyclic nucleotides are thought to be the final intracellular messengers for the control of smooth muscle tone and of the release of mediators from pulmonary mast cells. Cyclic 3′5′-adenosine monophosphate (cAMP) is formed from ATP by the enzyme adenylate cyclase, which is present in the cell membrane. Increased intracellular levels of cAMP activate protein kinases, which have the effect of reducing active myosin coupling by a mechanism involving calcium in bronchial smooth muscle cells, so producing bronchodilatation [55], and by binding calcium in mast cells, so reducing the release of bronchoconstrictor mediators such as histamine and the slow-reacting substance of anaphylaxis (SRS-A) [46]. Beta 2 adrenoceptors are closely linked to adenylate cyclase in the cell membrane and stimulation activates the enzyme, thereby producing bronchodilatation. Prostaglandins E_2 and I_2 (prostacyclin) are also known to activate adenylate cyclase directly (and are therefore bronchodilators), whereas prostaglandin $F_{2\alpha}$ inhibits the enzyme and is a bronchoconstrictor [22].

Guanyl cyclase similarly catalyses the formation of cyclic 3'5'-guanyl monophosphate (cGMP) within the cell; this has opposite effects to cAMP and produces bronchial smooth muscle contraction and increased release of mediators from mast cells. Cholinergic stimulation increases intracellular cGMP levels leading to bronchoconstriction. It is probably the balance between intracellular cAMP and cGMP levels that is important in controlling bronchial tone and mediator release, although cGMP may play a less important role as it can produce bronchodilatation in some situations.

Both cyclic nucleotides are broken down in the cell by phosphodiesterases. These enzymes are inhibited by theophyllines, which therefore cause an increase in both cAMP and cGMP levels, although the net effect is bronchodilatation. Recently the importance of the cAMP/cGMP system has been questioned as bronchodilators may directly affect calcium fluxes across smooth muscle membranes [55] (Fig. 23.1).

Bronchodilator drugs

Beta adrenergic agonists. These drugs produce bronchodilatation by stimulating beta 2 receptors in bronchial smooth muscle to produce relaxation and by inhibiting the release of mediators from pulmonary mast cells.

Adrenaline was used for many years as a bronchodilator, and it stimulates both alpha and beta receptors. The alpha-agonist action achieved by increasing systolic blood pressure may make arrhythmias more likely to occur. Theoretically, alpha receptor-mediated vasoconstriction of pulmonary arterioles should have the effect of reducing bronchial wall edema, which may contribute to airway narrowing in exacerbations of obstructive airways disease. However, there is experimental evidence that when given systemically alpha receptors on the

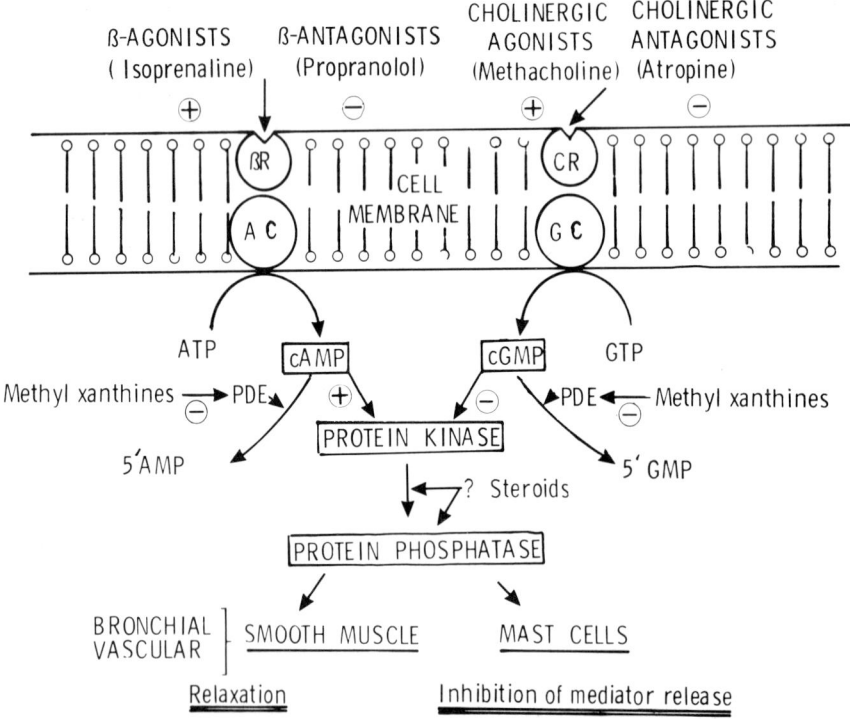

Fig. 23.1. Cyclic nucleotides in bronchial smooth muscle and pulmonary mast cells. BR, beta receptor; CR, muscarinic cholinergic receptor, AC, adenylate cyclase; GC, guanidyl cyclase; ATP, adenosine triphosphate; cAMP, cyclic 3'5' adenosine monophosphate; GTP, guanidine triphosphate; cGMP, 3'5' guanidine monophosphate; PDE, phosphodiesterase.

venous side of the pulmonary circulation are stimulated to a greater extent, causing an increase in capillary pressure and consequent worsening of bronchial edema [20]. The routine use of adrenaline in severe exacerbation should therefore be questioned as the alpha-agonist action is likely to be harmful.

Isoprenaline has no alpha-agonist activity and is a potent beta agonist producing bronchodilatation. However, it increases heart rate by stimulating cardiac beta 1 receptors. Its length of action is short as a result of breakdown by catechol O-methyl transferase (COMT). It has now been largely abandoned as it was implicated in the increase in asthma deaths in the UK in the 1960s [59] and has been succeeded by beta 2-selective agonists such as salbutamol, terbutaline, fenoterol, and rimiterol, which do not stimulate cardiac beta 1 receptors at doses that achieve significant bronchodilatation. There is little to choose between them; rimiterol is metabolized in a similar way to isoprenaline and is short-acting but salbutamol, terbutaline, and fenoterol are resistant to the action of COMT and therefore have a longer duration of action.

In the ICU these beta 2-selective agonists may be given either IV or by IPPV. There is some evidence that the IV route may be preferable in severe asthma attacks; if IPPV is used airway secretions and bronchospasm may prevent adequate distribution in the airways [66]. When they are given IV a constant infusion is preferable to a bolus injection, as less cardiac stimulation occurs. There may be an increase in heart rate as some stimulation of cardiac beta 1 receptors is likely to occur, although the tachycardia may be reflex stimulation resulting from a beta 2 vasodilator effect. There is no convincing evidence of tolerance to beta agonists in patients with airways obstruction [31].

Bronchodilators should increase alveolar ventilation and thereby increase arterial O_2 tension. However, PaO_2 has been found to fall with beta agonists as they cause increased pulmonary blood flow by vasodilatation and an increase in cardiac output [48]. If the increase in blood flow is distributed to areas of the lung which are poorly ventilated (physiological shunt), as in airways obstruction, this may cause a fall in PaO_2. This is most likely to occur if the PaO_2 is less than 60 mmHg (8 kPa), when $\dot{V}/\dot{Q}$ is likely to be most markedly disturbed: the PaO_2 should be carefully monitored in such patients during bronchodilator therapy and the inspired O_2 concentration increased if necessary. As a result of bronchodilator therapy in asthmatics the over-distended alveoli decrease in size, so relieving the mechanical compression of pulmonary vessels, which has the effect of increasing total blood flow in alveoli that are still poorly ventilated, thereby exacerbating the ventilation/perfusion mismatch [11, 45]. This provides a possible explanation for the often profound decrease in PO_2 when patients are weaned from ventilation by PEEP.

Apart from tachycardia other side-effects of beta 2 agonists may occur with IV use, such as a coarse tremor due to stimulation of beta 2 receptors in skeletal muscle. Several metabolic effects have been reported after IV beta 2 agonists, including insulin release, glycogenolysis, and lipolysis [61]. Significant falls in serum potassium may occur so it is important to monitor plasma potassium carefully in intensive care patients treated with IV beta agonists as the hypokalaemia may predispose to cardiac arrhythmias [2]. Bronchial selectivity is increased and side-effects reduced when beta agonists are given by inhalation, and for prolonged administration this is the preferred route.

Theophylline. Theophylline is a methylxanthine closely related to caffeine and is a bronchodilator. It inhibits phosphodiesterase (PDE) and therefore increases intracellular cAMP, although there is some doubt as to whether this is the mechanism of bronchodilatation since more potent inhibitors of PDE have been synthesized which have no bronchodilator effect [51]. It is possible that the theophyllines have some direct effect on calcium flux or interact with adenosine receptors on cell membranes. Theophylline itself is unsuitable for use because of low solubility, but when combined with ethylene diamine (aminophylline) it is suitable for IV use. There is a linear relationship between plasma theophylline concentration and bronchodilator effect from 5 mg/litre up to 20 mg/litre [44]. Above 15 mg/litre side-effects, including nausea, vomiting, and anxiety, may occur. Above 20 mg/litre sinus tachycardia and cardiac dysrhythmias are common and at higher levels, convulsions. Theophylline is extensively metabolized in the liver and the metabolites are excreted by the kidney. There are large interindividual differences in plasma half-life [44]. Reduced clearance occurs with age, and in congestive cardiac failure, hepatic cirrhosis, pneumonia, COAD, and hypoxaemia [49]. For this reason and because the therapeutic and toxic ranges are close it is important to measure plasma levels during prolonged IV treatment. It is safest to aim for a blood level of about

10 mg/litre which is achieved by a loading dose of 5.6 mg/kg and a maintenance infusion rate of 0.5 mg.kg^{-1}.h^{-1}. Intravenous aminophylline may have a place in the treatment of acute asthmatic attacks but the loading dose should be given slowly (over 15 min) as peak plasma concentrations may lead to cardiac arrhythmias and sudden death [7].

It is difficult to compare the effectiveness of theophylline with beta agonists, since both are usually given in an acute attack. With an adequate dosage of theophylline it is possible to achieve the same degree of bronchodilatation. As both theophylline and beta agonists increase cAMP by different proposed mechanisms it has been suggested that synergy between the two drugs may occur, but there is no good evidence for this in practice [9].

Anticholinergic drugs. Such drugs as atropine antagonize the action of acetylcholine released from vagal nerve endings at bronchial smooth muscle cells and mast cells. These drugs appear to be less effective clinically than beta agonists in asthma, but may be equally or even more active in chronic bronchitis [14]. Parenteral atropine at doses which produce bronchodilatation has unacceptable side-effects, such as reduced secretions, urinary retention, and tachycardia. The onset of bronchodilatation is slow; the peak effect may not be seen for an hour, which is a disadvantage in the acute situation.

Quaternary ammonium derivatives of atropine, atropine methyl nitrate, and ipratropium bromide do not cross the blood–brain barrier and so are devoid of central side-effects such as delirium and hallucinations, which may occur with high doses of atropine. They are not well absorbed when given PO but are effective when administered by inhalation, which increases their bronchial selectivity. In practice anticholinergic drugs are of little value in acute management of airways obstruction.

Steroids. Corticosteroids have no significant effect on the airways of normal subjects, yet they are very effective in asthma. Single dose studies in stable asthmatics produced a peak effect 5 h after IV hydrocortisone and 8 h after IV prednisolone [16], although the maximum benefit in patients may take several days to develop [13].

The dose is difficult to determine as the response is delayed and variable. Hydrocortisone 3 mg/kg every 6 h is usually adequate, and higher doses seem to produce no greater benefit as they are more likely to produce side-effects such as hypokalaemia [13]. In the ICU, hydrocortisone IV is probably preferable to methyl prednisolone, as it is more rapidly effective. Steroids are only useful in *reversible* airways obstruction, and their inappropriate use in the ICU is hazardous in view of the increased incidence of infection and metabolic disturbance.

The mode of action of steroids in relieving airways obstruction is still unclear. There is good evidence that steroids may reduce inflammatory mucosal swelling and bronchial wall edema [3], and some evidence that steroids may potentiate the effects of beta agonists in isolated bronchial muscle, and possibly in patients who have become unresponsive to isoprenaline. They may increase the intracellular production of protein kinases by increasing nuclear RNA production (explaining the delayed action), which would amplify the effects of cAMP within the cell.

Alpha blockers. Alpha antagonists such as phentolamine and phenoxybenzamine have been shown to have a weak inhibitory effect on histamine- and exercise-induced bronchospasm in asthmatics, although these actions could be explained by their antihistamine effects and by a reflex sympathetic stimulation from baroreceptors stimulated by the fall in blood pressure. These drugs have no role in the management of patients with airways obstruction, particularly as their hypotensive action is likely to be deleterious.

Anti-allergic drugs. Cromoglycate, as well as ketotifen, which may act by inhibiting the release of mediators from mast cells, have no role in the management of an acute asthmatic attack.

Antihistamines. At doses necessary to cause bronchodilatation the side-effects, such as drowsiness, are unacceptable when antihistamines are given parenterally, although there is some evidence that bronchial selectivity can be increased by inhalation. As antihistamines antagonize the effects of only one mediator released from mast cells, they are unlikely to be as effective as beta agonists since there is no antagonism of mediators such as SRS-A, which may be more important in prolonged and severe asthmatic attacks.

Bronchial secretions

Mucus. Mucus is produced by the submucosal glands and by the goblet cells of the airways. Submucosal glands are innervated by both the sympathetic and the parasympathetic nervous systems, and stimulation of both causes increased secretion of mucus and may also change its composition [17]. Atropine reduces but does not inhibit the secretory activity of submucous glands in normal subjects, but in patients with chronic bronchitis who have glandular hypertrophy there is no effect on either the volume or viscosity of sputum [37]. Beta agonists increase sputum production but this effect does not seem to be clinically important.

Several mucolytic drugs have been described which reduce sputum viscosity in vitro. Various cysteine analogues have been developed which reduce cross-linking disulphide bridges of polymeric mucus glycoproteins so that less viscous thiomonomers result, which leads to an impressive decrease in sputum viscosity in vitro. However, acetylcysteine given by aerosol and bromhexine given PO have no significant effect in patients and there are no good clinical indications for the use of these drugs [37].

Mucociliary clearance. Bronchial mucus acts as a protective barrier by trapping inhaled particles and bacteria, which are then transported by the mucociliary system to the larynx and swallowed. Clearance therefore depends on the integrity and activity of the cilia as well as on the volume and viscosity of the sputum. It has been possible to study mucus clearance in normal man by the inhalation of radiolabelled microspheres, but interpretation is difficult in the presence of airways obstruction because of the more central deposition of the particles. Beta 2 agonists, methyl xanthines, and cholinergic drugs increase mucociliary transport in normal subjects and in patients with airways obstruction [26], although the significance of this is uncertain clinically. Anticholinergic drugs slow mucociliary transport, which is a potential disadvantage in patients with airways obstruction. Mucolytic drugs such as bromhexine or mistab-

ron do not appear to increase mucociliary clearance significantly [63].

Pulmonary blood flow

Regional pulmonary blood flow (PBF) depends on three factors: vascular tone, overall pulmonary arterial blood flow (cardiac output), and left atrial pressure.

Pulmonary vascular tone

Pulmonary vessels contain smooth muscle fibres, the contractile elements of which are activated by ionized calcium [10]. Many substances and drugs are able to stimulate or inhibit the excitation–contraction coupling (Table 23.1). Hypoxia is by far the most important factor clinically in pulmonary vasoconstriction [64]. Hypoxaemia induces pulmonary hypertension due to the vasoconstriction of the pulmonary resistance vessels by a direct effect on plasma membrane permeability to calcium. A greater amount of cellular calcium has been measured in the pulmonary vascular smooth muscle of animals rendered chronically hypoxaemic [10], and this hypoxic pulmonary vasoconstriction can be inhibited by calcium antagonists in isolated lungs [41]. These results have recently been confirmed in man [57]. The local hypoxia due to regional hypoventilation causes pulmonary vessels supplying that region to constrict [24]. This reduces local perfusion to the hypoxic alveoli, thus decreasing the local shunt, and redirects the pulmonary arterial

Table 23.1. Effect of various pharmacological agents on cyclic nucleotides, bronchial smooth muscle, mast cell mediator release, bronchial mucus and mucociliary clearance, and pulmonary vessels

Agent	Effect on cyclic nucleotides	Bronchial smooth muscle	Mediator release	Mucus and mucociliary clearance	Pulmonary vessels
α Agonist (e.g., methoxamine)	? ↓ cAMP	Constrict(±)	Increase(±)	Decrease	Constrict
α and β Agonist (e.g., adrenaline)	↑ cAMP	Relax	Decrease	Decrease	Constrict
β Agonist (e.g., isoprenaline)	↑ cAMP	Relax	Decrease	Increase	Dilate
β_2 Agonist (e.g., salbutamol)	↑ cAMP	Relax	Decrease	Increase	Dilate
α Antagonist (e.g., phentolamine)	? ↑ cAMP	Relax (±)	Decrease(±)	Increase(±)	Dilate
β Antagonist (e.g., propranolol)	↓ cAMP	Constrict	Increase	Decrease(±)	No effect
Cholinergic antagonist (e.g., atropine)	↓ cAMP	Dilate	Decrease	Decrease	Dilate
Methylxanthine (e.g., aminophylline)	↑ cAMP	Relax	Decrease	Increase	Dilate
Corticosteroids	No change	Relax	No effect	Decrease	?

blood flow to better ventilated areas. The redistribution of the blood flow due to hypoxaemic vasoconstriction is therefore beneficial to the overall PaO_2. Should this vasoconstriction be overcome either by a vasodilator drug or by increased pulmonary blood flow due to a cardiotonic drug or fluid overloading, then shunting recurs or may even increase.

Overall pulmonary arterial blood flow

The overall arterial blood flow in the lungs is essentially equal to the cardiac output. The PAP depends directly on both the PVR and the cardiac output (Qc) (PAP = Qc × PVR). The cardiac output is therefore a critical factor in determining the distribution of PBF and thus of intrapulmonary shunting. Drugs which increase PBF and PAP may therefore overcome hypoxic vasoconstriction, as discussed above. This hypothesis has been confirmed in animals [39] and in man in various conditions [34, 35]. The increased intrapulmonary shunting produced by adrenergic agonists is explained at least in part by positive inotropic effects resulting in increased PBF.

Left atrial pressure

An increase in left atrial pressure is always deleterious in the presence of hypoxaemia. Even in the absence of cardiac failure, raised left atrial pressure leading to increased pulmonary capillary pressure (Pcp) will increase lung water, resulting in edema. According to Starling's law, cardiogenic alveolar edema occurs when Pcp exceeds the COP. However, in non-cardiogenic pulmonary edema where vascular endothelium may be damaged by different agents (bacteria, viruses, endotoxin, drugs, fat embolism, noxious gas inhalation, gastric juice aspiration, etc.), the increase in Pcp has a more deleterious effect on the pulmonary $\dot{Q}s/\dot{Q}t$ shunt [60].

Drugs affecting PBF

Many drugs can affect PBF. However, the response is non-specific because of the simultaneous action on cardiac contractility and on both arterial and venous peripheral vessels. In the same way it is difficult to predict, in patients with severe pulmonary conditions, the effect of these drugs on the pulmonary shunt ($\dot{Q}s/\dot{Q}t$) because of the concomitant action on both bronchial and pulmonary vessel smooth muscle fibres.

Catecholamines

The existence of alpha and beta adrenoceptors in pulmonary vessels has been well documented, and there is a marked numerical preponderance of alpha receptors [5]. Alpha stimulation results in vasoconstriction and beta stimulation in vasodilatation. A sympathomimetic drug that stimulates both alpha and beta receptors, such as adrenaline or dopamine, produces a significant increase in the pulmonary pressure owing to the stimulation of both alpha pulmonary arterial adrenoceptors and beta cardiac inotropic adrenoceptors. In experimental animals the pulmonary shunting is dependent, for the same cardiac output level, on the specific pulmonary microcirculatory effects of catecholamines.

The more alpha and beta receptors are stimulated simultaneously, the more uneven the distribution of perfusion and the greater the pulmonary shunting (Table 23.2). The shunt becomes progressively larger with isoprenaline, adrenaline, and noradrenaline [6]. In patients with ARDS similar results have been found on comparison of the effects of catecholamines [34]. $\dot{Q}s/\dot{Q}t$ was linearly correlated with PBF and inversely correlated with PVR. These two factors are crucial for pulmonary capillary recruitment. The shunt was correlated with PAP only when PVR was low, that is, when PAP and PBF varied concomitantly. $\dot{Q}s/\dot{Q}t$ was correlated with Pcp only when it varied in the same way as PBF. Conversely, phenylephrine, a pure alpha-

Table 23.2 Vascular pulmonary effects of catecholamines

Drug	Receptors[a]	CI (PBF)	PAP	PVR	Pcp	$\dot{Q}S/\dot{Q}T$
Dopamine	α, β, δ	+	+	−	+	+++
Isoprenaline	β	+	NS	−	−	++
Dobutamine	β	+	NS	NS	−	++
Phenylephrine	α	−	+	+	++	−

[a] α, alpha receptor; β, beta receptor; δ, dopaminergic receptor.

adrenergic agent which increases Pcp and decreases Qc and therefore PBF, decreased $\dot{Q}s/\dot{Q}t$, suggesting a greater effect of Qc than of Pcp on vascular recruitment.

Vasodilator drugs

All the drugs which relax smooth vascular muscle may affect the intrapulmonary distribution of PBF, especially in the case of pulmonary lesions. This is because vasodilators decrease pulmonary hypoxaemic vasoconstriction in areas with poorly ventilated alveoli.

Theophyllines. Theophyllines can produce a paradoxical worsening of PaO2 soon after their use in asthmatic subjects because of ventilation/perfusion mismatch [50]. After infusion of aminophylline, only a small reduction in perfusion to hypoxic areas of lung has been observed concomitantly with a fall in PaO2 [20]. For this reason it has been suggested that FiO2 should be increased in severe non-ventilated asthmatics.

Nitrates. Nitrates and nitroglycerine (TNG) are potent vasodilators acting on capacitance vessels and pulmonary vessels. Therefore, TNG may aggravate pre-existing intrapulmonary shunting and hypoxaemia. This fact is of particular importance in patients with chronic obstructive pulmonary disease, in whom the PaO2 is already low [29].

Sodium nitroprusside. Sodium nitroprusside is a potent vasodilator mainly used in congestive heart failure and in surgically controlled hypotension. This drug, like other vasodilators, may decrease PAP and PVR, and therefore decrease PaO2 by the worsening of $\dot{V}/\dot{Q}$ [65].

Drugs such as catecholamines and vasodilators, which alter the pulmonary circulation, usually worsen the PaO2 when used in severe respiratory failure. If they are required to treat concomitant cardiac failure, additional treatment to counteract the deleterious effect on the pulmonary shunting may be necessary. In this instance a combination of ventilation with PEEP or CPAP and inotropic drugs is indicated.

The impaired O_2 supply to the tissues due to pulmonary diseases is very often life-threatening in acutely ill patients, and therefore requires urgent and logical treatment. As both ventilation and blood flow are involved in the maintenance of a normal PaO2 and O_2 supply to the tissues, respiratory pharmacology involves both the lungs and the cardiovascular system.

Because of the effects of the ventilation/perfusion mismatch, any drug-induced change in either ventilation or perfusion may modify PaO_2. Therefore, the effect of a given drug cannot be safely anticipated; in differing situations, bronchodilatation, pulmonary vasodilation, or increase in cardiac output may be deleterious [65], or beneficial [12, 53].

In critically ill patients, the pulmonary conditions are very unstable. They are often exacerbated by multiple organ failure, such as renal insufficiency or cardiac failure. MV improves the alveolar ventilation but may sometimes decrease the cardiac output to a dangerous level [23]. This in turn may require support with drugs which, in the absence of mechanical alveolar inflation, might be deleterious [36]. Moreover, frequent changes in the drug regimen for control of the illness or alteration in the MV regimen may lead to serious changes in ventilation/perfusion mismatch. Weaning procedures, in the light of these changes, may be particularly dangerous if not carefully monitored [4].

Respiratory therapeutics therefore requires frequent assessment of both ventilation and perfusion. As both factors may change independently, it is difficult to lay down rigid therapeutic guidelines. Drugs have to be selected in the light of an individual patient's condition. Moreover, the drug metabolism and kinetics can be profoundly altered by the disease itself, leading to either toxic or ineffective blood levels [58]. Both effects and levels of drugs must therefore be carefully monitored.

Further investigations are necessary for a more complete understanding of the pathophysiology of respiratory failure and for the search for more selective drugs.

References

1. Ariens EJ, Simonis AM. (1976) Receptors and receptor mechanisms. In: Saxena PR, Forsyth RP (eds) Beta-adrenoceptor blocking agents. North-Holland, Amsterdam, pp 1–27
2. Barend N, Marlin GE (1978) Characterisation of beta-adrenoceptor subtype mediating the metabolic actions of salbutamol. Br J Clin Pharmacol 5:207–211
3. Baxter JD, Forsham PH (1972) Tissue effects of glucocorticoids. Am J Med 53:573–589
4. Beach T, Millen E, Grenvik A (1973) Hemodynamic response to discontinuance of mechanical ventilation. Crit Care Med 1:85–90
5. Bergofsky EH (1974) Mechanisms underlying vasomotor regulation of regional pulmonary blood flow in normal and disease states. Am J Med 57:378–394

6. Berk JL, Hagen JF, Tong RK, Levy ML, Martin PJ (1977) The role of adrenergic stimulation in the pathogenesis of pulmonary insufficiency. Surgery 82:366–372

7. Camatata SJ, Weil MH, Honashiro PK, Shubin H (1971) Cardiac arrest in the critically ill. I. A study of predisposing causes in 132 patients. Circulation 44:688–695

8. Cameron JL, Reynolds J, Zuidema GD (1973) Aspiration in patients with tracheostomies. Surg Gynecol Obstet 136:68–70

9. Campbell IA, Middleton WG, Mettardy GJR, Shotter MV, McKenzie R, Kay AB (1977) Interaction between isoprenaline and aminophylline in asthma. Thorax 32:424–428

10. Casteels R, Raeymaekers L, Goffin J (1973) A study of factors affecting the cellular calcium content of smooth muscle cells. Arch Int Pharmacodyn Ther, 201:191–192

11. Chick TW, Nicholson DP, Johnson RL, Jr (1973) Effects of isoproterenol on distribution of ventilation and perfusion in asthma. Am Rev Respir Dis 107:869–873

12. Colley PS, Cheney FW, Hlastala MJ (1979) Ventilation-perfusion and gas exchange effects of sodium nitroprusside in dogs with normal and edematous lungs. Anesthesiology 50:489–495

13. Collins JV, Harris PWR, Clark TJH, Townsend J (1970) Intravenous corticosteroids in treatment of acute bronchial asthma. Lancet II:1047–1049

14. Crompton GK (1968) A comparison of responses to bronchodilator drugs in chronic bronchitis and chronic asthma. Thorax 23:46–55

15. Cullen DJ, Caldera DL (1979) The incidence of ventilator-induced pulmonary barotrauma in critically ill patients. Anesthesiology 50:185–190

16. Ellul-Micallef R, Fenech FF (1975) Intravenous prednisolone in chronic bronchial asthma. Thorax 30:312–315

17. Gallagher JF, Kent PW, Passatore M, Phipps RJ, Richardson PS (1975) The composition of tracheal mucus and the nervous control of its secretion in the cat. Proc R Soc Lond [Biol] 192:49–76

18. Gilbert RP, Hinshaw LB, Kuida H, Visscher MB (1958) Effects of histamine, 5-hydroxytryptamine and epinephrine on pulmonary haemodynamics with particular reference to arterial and venous segment resistances. Am J Physiol 194:165–170

19. Guillerm R, Radziszewski E (1974) Effets ventilatoires chez l'homme sain d'un nouvel analeptique respiratoire le S2620. Bull Eur Physiopathol Respir 10:775–791

20. Hales CA, Kazemi H (1974) Hypoxic vascular response of the lung. Effect of aminophylline and epinephrine. Am Rev Respir Dis 110:126–132

21. Haunbart B, Peslin R, Bohodana AB, Jansen da Silva JM, Pino J (1979) Response ventilatoire isocapnique a l'almitrine dans l'hypercapnie chronique. Bull Eur Physiopathol Respir 15:195–205

22. Hedqvist P, Mathe AA (1977) Lung function and the role of prostaglandins. In: Lichtenstein LM, Austen KF (eds) Asthma, physiology, immunopharmacology and treatment. Academic Press, New York, pp 77–91

23. Hemmer M, Suter PM (1979) Treatment of cardiac and neural effects of PEEP with dopamine in patients with acute respiratory failure. Anesthesiology 50:399–403

24. Hughes JMB, Grant MJB, Jones HA, Davies EE (1974) Relationship between blood flow and alveolar gas tensions and aerosols. Scand J Respir Dis [Suppl] 85:17–19

25. Hunt CE, Inwood RJ, Shannon DC (1979) Respiratory and non-respiratory effects of doxapram in congenital central hypoventilation syndrome. Am Rev Respir Dis 119:263–269

26. Iravani J, Melville GN (1974) Mucociliary function of the respiratory tract as influenced by drugs. Respiration 31:350–357

27. Kaliner M, Orange RP, Austen KF (1972) Immunological release of histamine and slow reacting substance of anaphylaxis from human lung IV. Enhancement of cholinergic and alpha adrenergic stimulation. J Exp Med 126:556–567

28. Kneussl MP, Richardson JB (1978) Alpha-adrenergic receptors in human and canine tracheal and bronchial smooth muscle. J Appl Physiol 45:307–311

29. Kochukoshy KN, Chick TW, Jenne JW (1975) The effect of nitroglycerin in gas exchange on chronic obstructive pulmonary disease. Am Rev Respir Dis 111:177–183

30. Lands AM, Arnold A, McAuliff JP, Luduena FP, Brown TG (1967) Differentiation of receptor systems activated by sympathetic amines. Nature 214:597–598

31. Larsson S, Svedmyr N, Thiringer G (1977) Lack of bronchial beta adrenoceptor resistance in asthmatics during long-term treatment with terbutaline. J Allergy Clin Immunol 59:93–100

32. Laubie M, Diot F (1972) Etude pharmacologique de l'action stimulante respiratoire du S2620. Rôle des chémorécepteurs carotidiens et aortiques. J Pharm Belg 3:363–374

33. Lemaire F, Harf A, Harari A, Teisseire B, Regnier B, Atlan G, Rapin M (1975) La mesure du shunt intra pulmonaire en réanimation. Bull Eur Physiopathol Respir 11:659–681

34. Lemaire F, Gastinne H, Regnier B, Teisseire B, Rapin M (1978a) Perfusion changes modify intra-pulmonary shunting ($\dot{Q}s/\dot{Q}t$) in patients with adult respiratory distress syndrome. Am Rev Respir Dis 117:144

35. Lemaire F, Jardin F, Regnier B, Loisance D, Goudot B, Lange F, Eveleigh MC, Teisseire B, Laurent D, Rapin M (1978b) Pulmonary gas exchange during venoarterial bypass with a membrane lung for acute respiratory failure. J Thorac Cardiovasc Surg 75:839–846

36. Lemaire F, Regnier B, Harf A, Simoneau G (1979) Positive end expiratory pressure (PEEP) ventilation suppresses the increase of shunting due to dopamine infusion. Anesthesiology 52:376–377

37. Lopez-Vidriero MT, Costello J, Clark TJH, Das I, Veal EE, Reid L (1975) Effect of atropine on sputum production. Thorax 30:543–547

38. Lutch JS, Murray JF (1972) Continuous positive-pressure ventilation: Effects on systemic oxygen transport and tissue oxygenation. Ann Intern Med 76:193–202

39. Lynch JP, Mhyre JG, Dantzher DR (1979) Influence of cardiac output on intrapulmonary shunt. J Appl Physiol Res Environ Physiol 42:315–321

40. Lyons HA, Huang CT (1968) Therapeutic use of progesterone in alveolar hyperventilation associated with obesity. Am J Med 44:881–888

41. McMurtry IF, Davidson AB, Reeves JT, Grover RF (1976) Inhibition of hypoxic pulmonary vasoconstriction by calcium antagonists in isolated rat lungs. Circ Res 38:99–104

42. McNeill RS, Ingram CG (1966) The effect of propranolol on ventilatory function. Am J Cardiol 18:473–475

43. McNicol MW, Pride NB (1961) Dichlorphenamide in chronic respiratory failure. Lancet I:906–908

44. Mitenko PA, Ogilvie RI (1957) Rational intravenous doses of theophylline compounds. Br Med J ii:67–69

45. Nicholson DP, Johnson RL (1973) Effect of isoproterenol on distribution of ventilation and perfusion in asthma. Am Rev Respir Dis 103:869–873

46. Orange RP, Kaliner MA, Laraia PJ, Austen KF (1971) Immunological release of histamine and slow reacting substance of anaphylaxis from human lung. II Influence of cellular levels of cyclic AMP. Fed Proc 30:1725–1729

47. Patel KR (1976) Alpha adrenoceptor blocking drugs in asthma Br J Clin Pharmacol 2:539–540

48. Paterson JW, Shenfield GM (1974) Bronchodilators. Thorac Tuberc Assoc Rev 4:25–40
49. Powell JR, Vozek S, Hopewell P, Costello J, Scheiner LB, Riegelman S (1978) Theophylline disposition in acutely ill hospitalised patients. Am Rev Respir Dis 118:229–238
50. Rees HA, Borthwick RD, Millar JS, Donald KW (1967) Aminophylline in bronchial asthma. Lancet II:1167–1169
51. Richards AJ, Walker SR, Paterson JW, Case DE (1971) A new antiasthmatic drug (ICI 58, 301): Blood levels and spirometry. Br J Dis Chest 65:247–252
52. Richardson JB (1979) Nerve supply to the lungs. Am Rev Respir Dis 119:785–801
53. Rubin LJ, Peter RH (1980) Oral hydralazine therapy for primary pulmonary hypertension. N Engl J Med 302:69–73
54. Schrijen F, Romero Colomer P (1978) Effets hemodynamiques d'un stimulant ventilatoire (almitrine) chez des pulmonaires chroniques. Bull Eur Physiopath Respir 14:775–784
55. Schultz G (1977) Possible inter-relations between calcium and cyclic nucleotides in smooth muscle. In: Lichtenstein LM, Austen KF (eds) Asthma, physiology, immunopharmacology and treatment. Academic Press, New York, pp 77–91
56. Scott RM, Whitwam JG, Chakrabarti MK (1977) Evidence of a role for the peripheral chemoreceptors in the ventilatory response to doxapram in man. Br J Anaesth 49:227–231
57. Simonneau G, Escourrou P, Cerrina J, Raffestin B, Lockart A, Duroux P (1980) Inhibition of pulmonary hypoxic vasoconstriction by a calcium antagonist (Nifedipine). Eur J Clin Invest, Salzburg (Abstract no 204)
58. Souich P du, McLean AJ, Lalka D, Erill S, Gibaldi M (1978) Pulmonary disease and drug kinetics. Clin Pharmacokinet 3:257–266
59. Speizer FE, Doll R, Heaf P, Strang LB (1968) Investigation into the use of drugs preceding death from asthma. Br Med J ix:339–343
60. Staub NC (1978) Pulmonary oedema: Physiological approaches to management. Chest 74:559–565
61. Taylor MW, Gaddie J, Murchison E, Palmer KNV (1976) Metabolic effects of oral salbutamol. Br Med J ix:22–22
62. Tenaillon A, Labrousse J, Longchal J, Bahloul F, Lissac J (1980) Effects of almitrine on PaO$_2$ in chronic obstructive pulmonary disease with constant ventilation. (Abstract) Intensive Care Med 6:64
63. Thompson ML, Pavia D, McNicol MW (1973) A preliminary study of the effect of guaiphenesin on mucociliary clearance from the human lung. Thorax 28:742–747
64. Von Euler US, Liljestrand G (1946) Observations on the pulmonary arterial blood pressure in the cat. Acta Physiol Scand 12:301–320
65. Wildsmith JAW, Drummond GB, MacRae WR (1975) Blood-gas changes during induced hypotension with sodium nitroprusside. Br J Anaesth 47:1205–1211
66. Williams S, Seaton A (1977) Intravenous or inhaled salbutamol in severe acute asthma? Thorax 32:555–558

General References

Analeptics
Wong SC, Ward JW (1977) Analeptics. Pharmacol Ther 3:123–165
Bronchodilators
Paterson JW, Woolcock AJ, Shenfield GM (1979) Bronchodilator drugs. Am Rev Respir Dis 120:1149–1188
Tattersfield AE (1979) Airway pharmacology. Br J Anaesth 51:681–691
Bronchial mucus and mucociliary clearance
Clamp JR (ed) (1978) Mucus. Br Med Bull 34:1–97
Wanner A (1977) Clinical aspects of mucociliary transport. Am Rev Respir Dis 116:73–125
Ventilation perfusion ratio
Hughes JMB (1975) Lung gas tensions and active regulation of ventilation/perfusion ratios in health and disease. Br J Dis Chest 69:153–170
Pharmacology of the pulmonary circulation
Harris P, Heath D (1977) Pharmacology of the pulmonary circulation: Its form and function in health and disease, 2nd edn. Churchill Livingstone, London
Respiratory intensive care
Pontoppidan H, Wilson RS, Rie MA, Schneider RC (1977) Respiratory intensive care. Anesthesiology 47:96–116

Section D
Renal, Electrolyte, and Metabolic Disorders

Chapter 24

Acute Renal Failure

A. Kanfer, O. Kourilsky, J. D. Sraer, and G. Richet

There are many forms of acute renal failure (ARF), each with its own particularities but the common denominator is acute uraemia.

Acute uraemia is accompanied by certain disturbances of blood chemistry, some of which are life-threatening. The danger of these disturbances may be averted by appropriate therapeutic measures, the most important of which is dialysis. The onset of acute uraemia is frequently masked by the symptoms of the underlying condition, medical, obstetric, traumatic, or surgical, and the renal failure remains symptomless until the visceral consequences of the metabolic disorders suddenly become manifest.

Acute renal failure may occur in many diseases and syndromes; schematically there are four types:

1) *Functional or prerenal ARF*: the healthy kidney is subjected to conditions which prevent normal renal function; once these are corrected, return to normal function is, if not immediate, rapid.

2) ARF resulting from *acute tubular necrosis (ATN)* complicates acute states, generally associated with shock; it is organic, for it persists after renal haemodynamics have returned to normal, but it is spontaneously and totally reversible. It is the commonest form of ARF and has a uniform renal symptomatology. It was first described in the 1940s, and led to the invention of the artificial kidney, the starting point of modern clinical nephrology. Yet doubt still remains about the exact significance of the tubular lesions and the mechanisms involved in the onset and persistence of ARF; it is, therefore, still not possible to prevent its occurrence.

3) Organic ARF resulting from *lesions in the arteries, intra- or extrarenal, in the glomeruli or in the interstitium*: these forms of ARF may regress, but may also lead to chronic renal failure. Progression to chronic renal failure may sometimes be prevented by appropriate treatment, for often the lesions only become irreversible later in the course of the illness. Thus, much depends on early identification of the anatomical lesions, their mechanism, and their cause. It is a highly complex situation, particularly as the same aetiology may produce different forms of ARF. Septicaemia, for example, may lead to ATN from shock, to glomerular ischaemia or necrosis from angiitis, to glomerulonephritis with complement and sometimes immunoglobulin deposits, or even to pyelonephritis; each form requires its own particular treatment. Experience at Hôpital Tenon illustrates this point: 54 patients with an acute infection and ARF had a renal biopsy. The diversity of the lesions is clearly shown in (Table 24.1), and their lack of uniformity is also shown by biopsy findings in different circumstances, for example in cases of ARF with haemolytic anaemia at the end of pregnancy or post partum (Table 24.2), and in cases of ARF due to nephrotoxic drugs (Table 24.3).

4) Postrenal ARF resulting from *obstruction of the urinary tract or of the intrarenal ducts, with or without accompanying infection*.

Table 24.1. Renal biopsy findings in 54 patients with an acute infection and acute anuric uraemia (Hôpital Tenon, 1966–1979)

Acute tubular necrosis: 23
  (Septicaemia, 18; Pulmonary infection, 5)

	Extracapillary glomerulonephritis	5
	Membranoproliferative glomerulonephritis	3
Glomerular nephropathy: 17	Endocapillary glomerulonephritis	3
	Focal and segmental glomerulonephritis	3
	Miscellaneous glomerular lesions	3

  (Septicaemia, 9; Pulmonary infection, 5; Naso-pharyngeal infection, 3)

	with polymorphonuclear cells	7
Acute interstitial nephritis: 11	with round cells	3
	with tuberculous granulomata	1

  (Septicaemia, 8 – 5 of which had a urinary infection; Pulmonary infection, 2; Tuberculosis, 1)

Cortical necrosis: 2
  (Septicaemia, 1; Pulmonary infection, 1)

Myelomatous tubular nephropathy: 1
  (Pulmonary infection)

Table 24.2. Acute renal failure (ARF) with haemolytic anaemia at the end of pregnancy or post-partum. Renal biopsy findings in six patients

	Age	Time of onset of ARF	Obstetric history	Renal histology	Outcome
1	24	32nd week	Pre-eclampsia, caesarian section	Acute tubular necrosis	Recovery
2	21	32nd week	Pre-eclampsia, abruptio placentae	Acute tubular necrosis	Recovery
3	27	34th week	Abruptio placentae	Acute tubular necrosis	Recovery
4	23	22nd week	Pre-eclampsia	Thrombotic microangiopathy[a]	Permanent anuria, transplantation
5	23	12th week post-partum	Normal	Thrombotic microangiopathy[a]	Death
6	26	2nd week post-partum	Dystocia, caesarian section	Thrombotic microangiopathy[a]	Recovery

[a]Lesions corresponding to haemolytic and uraemic syndrome (see p. 446).

Table 24.3. Renal biopsy findings in 14 cases of acute renal failure following administration of nephrotoxic drugs

Acute tubular necrosis	9
Acute interstitial nephritis	5

The aim of treatment of ARF is twofold: the treatment of the acute uraemia, which is imperative for survival, and the treatment of the underlying cause and/or mechanism producing the renal lesions. When spontaneous healing is unlikely, the latter treatment is particularly important, if it is at all possible.

Treatment of acute uraemia

Signs common to all forms of ARF, irrespective of its aetiology, are (1) a sudden, steep fall in GFR, with no reduction, and sometimes an increase, in kidney size, as shown by tomography or echotomography; (2) oliguria, 20% of cases have a normal or increased urinary output; (3) a metabolic syndrome with nitrogen retention, hyperkalaemia, and metabolic acidosis; (4) possible salt and water overload; and (5) a variety of nonspecific clinical signs: normochromic normocytic anaemia, anorexia, nausea, vomiting, and neuropsychological disturbances to which the accumulation of drugs and their metabolites may contribute.

Aim of treatment

The aim of treatment is the prevention of life-threatening metabolic disturbances, namely an increase in the plasma concentrations of the nitrogenous waste products, creatinine and urea, the latter giving its name to the syndrome. Their levels should not be allowed to exceed 700 μmol/litre and 30 mmol/litre, respectively. Although these nitrogen-containing substances are not themselves very toxic, high concentrations are a warning of impending hyperkalaemia and metabolic acidosis.

Hyperkalaemia is dangerous; levels of above 6–6.5 mmol/litre are toxic to the myocardium. The rate of rise is greater when protein catabolism is intense. In the case of rhabdomyolysis, crush injuries, and muscle destruction, the danger is even greater because of the early onset of marked hypocalcaemia and acidosis, both of which aggravate the effects of hyperkalaemia on the myocardium [77, 162].

Metabolic acidosis, even after several days of anuria, is not usually very marked. Blood bicarbonate levels are in the range of 18–20 mmol/litre and pH remains between 7.32 and 7.36, because of a compensatory lowering of PCO_2. Should this compensatory mechanism become in any way impaired, however, the pH can fall in a matter of minutes to 7.20–7.10 or even less, with the danger of sudden death. This danger is increased by the inevitable hyperkalaemia resulting from immediate, acidosis-induced, transport of potassium out of the cells. The production of endogenous acids, and thus the rapidity of onset of acidosis, depends on the degree of protein catabolism and muscle involvement. Hypochloraemia and a variable increase of the unmeasured anions are customary.

Salt and water overload may present a major risk. Sodium overload is the consequence of excessive intake, as it is entirely of exogenous origin. The use of mannitol may involve the same danger, because its diffusion space is extracellular and physiologically similar to that of sodium. Overhydration may result from incorrect or inappropriate fluid treatment. To the exogenous water intake must be added endogenous water derived from cellular breakdown and the oxidation of lipids, carbohydrates, and proteins. Nowadays, this water is progressively eliminated by dialysis but prior to this it accumulated and was then eliminated during the diuretic phase, when weight loss approaching 10%–20% of the normal body weight occurred. A pure water overload has little or no haemody-namic effect but when associated with sodium (or mannitol) overload it involves a risk of hypertension and pulmonary oedema. This danger depends on several factors, principally the existence of a third fluid compartment and its mobilization, the nature of the renal involvement, the state of the cardiovascular system and, therefore, the age of the patient. Measurement of central venous and pulmonary artery pressure, and if necessary of cardiac output, enables haemodynamic risks to be evaluated and provides a guide to management.

Conservative treatment

This method is not only of historical interest, but is also of great value in preventing or delaying the onset of life-threatening complications and, when these exist, in gaining the time necessary for setting up dialysis.

Control of fluid and electrolyte intake

Theoretically, patients with ARF should receive 300–500 ml water/24 h (to compensate for imperceptible extrarenal loss), no sodium or potassium, and a minimum intake of 1500 kcal, as carbohydrates and fats, to reduce protein catabolism. These amounts have to be increased if there is any diuresis or unusual extrarenal loss.

Control of metabolic disorders before dialysis

Dangerous hyperkalaemia (>7.5 mmol/litre). The emergency treatment for this consists of (1) *calcium gluconate* (10%), 20–60 ml IV (hypercalcaemia antagonizes the effect of potassium on the heart); (2) *hypertonic glucose* (30%): a rapid infusion (in about 1 h) of 500 ml containing 30–50 units of soluble insulin (this induces intracellular penetration of potassium); (3) *Sodium bicarbonate* (isotonic 1.4%, or better still the molar, hypertonic, 8.4% solution): an intravenous infusion of 40–100 ml in 10–30 min diminishes the metabolic acidosis and increases potassium transport into the cells. The molar solution offers the advantage of reducing the infused volume and consequently the ever present risk of pulmonary oedema. (4) *Isoprenaline* infusion if there is complete atrioventricular block due to hyperkalaemia.

All these measures are usually combined as necessary, and they will lower the blood potassium level by 0.5–1 mmol/litre and improve cardiac contractility and conduction, gaining the 30–60 min necessary for setting up dialysis.

Extreme metabolic acidosis. Plasma bicarbonate ≤ 8 mmol/litre with pH ≤ 7.10 necessitates molar bicarbonate solution IV, as described above. In the case of insufficient respiratory compensation, assisted ventilation should be started and blood pH can thus be increased within minutes, which may be life-saving.

Salt and water overload. This is treated according to whether the renal failure is oliguric or not. Intravenous frusemide is indicated in recent nonoliguric ARF, after obstruction of the urinary tract has been excluded. The effectiveness of this treatment is demonstrated by a sudden increase in diuresis. In oliguric ARF, frusemide is often without effect and dialysis and ultrafiltration are then the only means of removing the salt and water overload.

Severe and malignant hypertension. This condition accompanies some forms of acute uraemia and must be treated immediately (hydralazine, 10 mg IM; sodium nitroprusside infusion IV; or IV bolus injection of diazoxide 100–300 mg). The choice of antihypertensive drug depends on the clinical context and especially on the cardiac status. These drugs, however, usually have no effect if there is salt and water retention, and treatment of the latter restores their efficacy. For this, the necessary weight loss may be in the order of several kilograms [48, 105, 147, 183].

Dialysis

Dialysis averts the dangers of the metabolic disorders associated with uraemia. It should be performed as an emergency procedure when plasma levels show a dangerous trend: creatinine ≥700 μmoles, urea ≥30 mmoles, potassium ≥5.5 mmoles, HCO_3 ≤20 mmoles, and when there is overhydration. These disorders occur 3–6 days after the onset of renal failure when protein catabolism is not dramatically increased, in 24–48 h when protein catabolism is intense, and in minutes in the presence of a mixed acidosis with hyperkalaemia and inadequate respiratory compensatory mechanisms. The department receiving such patients should have dialysis facilities permanently available, and personnel experienced in both peritoneal dialysis (PD) and haemodialysis (HD). A vascular shunt should be inserted for eventual HD, and, if this is contra-indicated it should be possible to start PD within 30 min.

Peritoneal

Peritoneal dialysis takes 30 min to set up, including the time for the preparatory creation of ascites that is necessary to avoid the risk of perforation. In a few hours, the potentially lethal metabolic abnormalities will have been corrected. This procedure entails a not insignificant risk of peritonitis, but this nearly always responds to medical treatment. PD is generally avoided immediately after abdominal surgery, and because it impedes diaphragmatic movement, it should not be used in the presence of respiratory distress unless assisted ventilation is available.

Haemodialysis

Haemodialysis requires 1–2 h preparation. This delay depends on the time spent creating vascu-

Table 24.4. Choice of method of dialysis

Haemodialysis
   Indications: Most effective method
               Hypercatabolism makes it mandatory
   Contra-indications: Cardiovascular collapse
                     Cerebrovascular accident
   Cautious use in: Advanced age
              Heart failure

Peritoneal dialysis
   Indications: Difficult vascular access
              The contra-indications of haemodialysis
              Some cases of acute pancreatitis
   Contra-indications: Abdominal distention (obstruction, etc.)
                   Peritonitis and/or progressive intra-abdominal disease (except in special circumstances, when the catheter is placed during surgery)
   Use with caution in: Diabetes mellitus (danger of hyperglycaemia)
                Previous abdominal surgery

Fluid restriction, if not associated with administration of sodium salts, will correct the hyponatraemia but deplete the extracellular volume. The primary renal H_2O retention may be due to drugs which stimulate the secretion of antidiuretic hormone or its effect on the kidney, e.g., diuretics, the chemotherapeutic agents vincristine and cyclophosphamide, the oral antidiabetic agent chlorpropamide, or the antiepileptic agent carbamazepine. When none of these causes is present, the 'inappropriate ADH syndrome' may reveal a bronchogenic carcinoma, particularly oat cell carcinoma. It has also been reported in a great variety of diseases including malignant tumours of different organs, lymphoma, chest infections, and CNS disorders. A similar syndrome may be seen in hypothyroid patients. This type of disorder is not always easy to differentiate from the dilutional hyponatraemia sometimes observed in acutely or chronically ill patients where total body sodium is normal or increased and where both sodium and H_2O excretion equilibrate with intake while serum sodium concentration remains around 130 mmol/litre. This situation, sometimes termed 'essential hyponatraemia' [16], does not require administration of sodium and, after correction of hyponatraemia by fluid restriction, the patient may complain of thirst and feel less comfortable than if the hyponatraemia is left uncorrected.

Management. Symptomatic treatment of the fluid and electrolyte disorder will always be coupled with treatment of its cause.

For *cellular overhydration with increased extracellular volume.* Severe restriction of sodium and fluid intake remains the basis of treatment. When a rapid effect is desired or in cases of refractory oedema, loop diuretics, such as ethacrynic acid or particularly frusemide, can be used, but large doses may be required. Aldactone may be used alone or in association with a loop diuretic in case of potassium depletion and signs of hyperaldosteronism. In the absence of cardiac failure, diuresis may sometimes be induced by plasma expansion with sodium-free solutes, particularly albumin or, less commonly, hypertonic mannitol. Administration of demethylchlortetracycline has been proposed to treat ascites due to cirrhosis, where it may induce both sodium and H_2O diuresis. But serum creatinine rises during treatment, and as it is not clear whether this is due to hypovolaemia or to a nephrotoxic effect of the drug, it should be used with caution. In patients with severe renal failure, dialysis will be used to deplete the patient. Dialysis, and preferably haemofiltration, have been used to deplete patients with refractory cardiac failure.

In *cellular overhydration with decreased extracellular volume* extracellular volume expansion is the primary objective. Administration of a hypertonic salt solution will attain this objective and attract fluid from the intracellular space. It can be administered as a direct IV injection of a 20% saline solution to treat a patient with convulsions. It is usually given as a continuous infusion of a 1.2%–1.4% saline solution by a central venous catheter. If hyponatraemia is corrected before the salt and H_2O deficit, volume expansion is continued with 0.9% saline or with a 5% glucose solution containing 6–8g NaCl/litre until the deficit is corrected within 24–48 h. Care should be given to avoid too rapid or excessive solute administration, which can provoke circulatory overload and pulmonary oedema, particularly in elderly patients or those with cardiac disease. Hypokalaemia is likely to develop during volume restoration requiring administration of potassium salts.

In the *inappropriate ADH syndrome* severe restriction of fluid intake with normal salt intake are often sufficient to correct the hyponatraemia. In cases where hyponatraemia is held responsible for CNS disorders, initial administration of hypertonic saline may be necessary. Simultaneous administration of a small dose of frusemide can prevent a sudden extracellular overload. When the cause of the syndrome persists, particularly in patients with malignant disease, fluid restriction may be insufficient or felt by the patient to be too constraining. Drugs having an effect antagonistic to that of antidiuretic hormone can then be proposed [25]. Demethylchlortetracycline in doses of 600–1200 mg/day decreases urine osmolality and increases water clearance within 48 h after initiation of treatment. Lithium carbonate has a similar effect but its use is limited by the CNS, GI, and myocardial disorders which it may induce. In hypothyroid patients, natraemia does not increase notably with fluid restriction but hyponatraemia is rapidly corrected by the administration of thyroid hormone.

Hypokalaemia and hyperkalaemia

Variations in plasma potassium levels can constitute a life-threatening situation requiring rapid institution of appropriate therapy.

Although the metabolic situation may be complex, the pathological significance of hypo- or hyperkalaemia can be inferred from the patient's case history, clinical status, level of plasma potassium, blood acid–base status, ECG, and renal function.

Errors in the determination of plasma potassium levels can be misleading. Falsely elevated levels may be due to muscle contraction while blood is being drawn, thrombocythaemia, diffusion out of the red blood cells (kalaemia should be measured in plasma, not serum), and particularly haemolysis. Rarely, falsely low levels may be due to dilution in vitro (when blood is drawn into a tube containing a large volume of anticoagulant) or in vivo (when blood is drawn from a vein above an infusion).

Hypokalaemia

Although hypokalaemia can be defined as a plasma potassium level below 3.3 mmol/litre, clinical symptoms usually become apparent only in patients with a plasma potassium of 3 mmol/litre or less. The chances of its being symptomatic increase with the degree of hypokalaemia, of potassium depletion when present, and the rate at which the plasma potassium level decreases. Major alterations in plasma potassium level can be found in patients with little or no symptoms when due to very progressive variations. Immediate institution of therapy is nevertheless imperative for even moderate hypokalaemia can cause dysrhythmias in cardiac patients, particularly those treated with cardiac glycosides or those with concomitant hypocalcaemia.

Potassium depletion is often, although not constantly, associated with hypokalaemia. It is defined as a loss of body potassium in excess of that corresponding to lean body mass. It should be suspected whenever the clinical situation indicates a negative potassium balance due to gastro-intestinal or urinary losses (or both). Urinary potassium excretion may help in determining whether they are of renal (>25 mmol/24 h) or of extrarenal (<10 mmol/24 h) origin. The degree of potassium depletion, and hence the amount of potassium to be administered, can be only grossly evaluated from the degree of hypokalaemia.

Clinical manifestations. Modifications of cardiac conduction are the most frequent and severe manifestations of hypokalaemia. Supraventricular tachycardia, ventricular extrasystoles 'torsade de pointe' [4] (a form of ventricular tachycardia sometimes termed 'wave bursts'), when caused by hypokalaemia, will be corrected by administration of potassium salts alone. Other ECG modifications may be clinically asymptomatic: as the degree of hypokalaemia increases, the T wave becomes broad, the ST segment is depressed, a large U wave appears and the T wave becomes flat.

Other clinical symptoms become apparent only in cases of severe hypokalaemia, usually associated with potassium depletion: increased arterial pulsatility, decreased diastolic arterial pressure (sometimes associated with a diastolic murmur which disappears during potassium repletion), orthostatic hypotension, constipation, abdominal distention, ileus and muscle paralysis.

Metabolic disturbances induced by hypokalaemia. Hypokalaemia induces metabolic alkalosis, particularly when associated with potassium and sodium depletion. It is due to a complex disturbance of renal hydrogen ion excretion. Exceptionally, hypokalaemia is found associated with metabolic acidosis due to concomitant retention of hydrogen ion and/or to loss of buffer base (as in cases of ureterosigmoidostomy malfunction). Hypokalaemia is then a sign of potassium depletion more severe than would be suspected on the degree of hypokalaemia for, during acidosis, potassium tends to move from the intracellular to the extracellular space.

Hyponatraemia during potassium depletion has been attributed both to abnormal H_2O retention by the kidney and to entry of sodium into cells [23]. Total body sodium is nevertheless increased by concomitant renal retention of sodium. Unrestricted sodium intake during potassium repletion can lead to accumulation of peripheral oedema, as sodium is transferred from the cells to the extracellular space.

Severe potassium depletion has been associated with cellular damage in the myocardium, skeletal muscles and in the renal tubules [23]. Interstitial nephritis and renal failure sometimes observed in patients with long-term potassium depletion, particularly after purgative abuse, has been attributed to potassium depletion alone; however, other pathogenic factors may be responsible, particularly urinary tract infection due to an increased susceptibility to infection [23]. Acute potassium depletion and hypokalaemia have been implicated in the pathogenesis of rhabdomyolysis induced by violent exercise [32].

Aetiology (see Table 25.2). Gastro-intestinal losses are among the most frequent cause of hypo-

Table 25.2. Causes of hypokalaemia

I. Potassium depletion
  A. Due to GI losses
    1. Vomiting
    2. Fistulas
    3. Chronic diarrhoea (malabsorption, villous papillomas, purgative abuse, cholera, Zollinger–Ellison syndrome, ulcerative colitis)
  B. Due to renal losses
    1. Diabetic ketosis
    2. Hypermineralocorticism
       Primary hyperaldosteronism
       Increased desoxycorticosterone secretion (congenital deficit in adrenal II, hydroxylase and 17-hydroxylase)
       Increased secretion of 18-hydroxycorticosterone
       Liddle's syndrome (increased tubular response to aldosterone and decreased aldosterone secretion)
    3. Secondary hyperaldosteronism
       Due to increased renin secretion
       Severe hypertension (renal artery stenosis, malignant hypertension)
       Without hypertension (Bartter's syndrome)
    4. Cushing's syndrome
    5. Drug administration
       Chronic steriod administration
       Diuretic therapy
       Treatment with large doses of certain beta-lactamines (penicillin G, carbenicillin, cefalotin)
       Excessive administration of exchange resin (in patients with renal failure)
       Chronic intake of glycyrrhizine
    6. Ureterosigmoidostomy malfunction
    7. Renal tubular acidosis
    8. Magnesium depletion
    9. Hyperlysozymaemia and hyperlysozymuria
II. Transfer of potassium from extracellular to intracellular fluid
  A. Due to an elevation of blood pH
  B. During an increase in glycogen stores
  C. In near-drowning victims (?) [5]
  D. In patients with familial periodic paralysis

---

kalaemia and potassium depletion encountered in intensive care patients. Metabolic disturbances observed in these patients are often complex, resulting from concomitant disorders in H_2O, sodium, and acid–base balance. Thus loss of gastric fluid due to pyloric stenosis will cause dehydration, sodium depletion, metabolic alkalosis, and decreased glomerular filtration. Though the quantities of potassium lost in the gastric fluid may be relatively small, potassium depletion may be severe due to urinary potassium losses induced by metabolic alkalosis and hyperaldosteronism. Major hypokalaemia in an apparently healthy woman is suggestive of long-term abuse of laxatives or of diuretics taken because she feels constipated or overweight. Urinary potassium output is low in the first case and high in the second.

During diabetic ketosis, major potassium depletion will result from urinary losses due to osmotic diuresis and hyperaldosteronism. Despite severe potassium depletion, kalaemia may be normal or elevated as a consequence of resistance to intracellular penetration of potassium ions due to the lack of insulin and to metabolic acidosis.

Hypermineralocorticism or glycyrrhizine intoxication may be suspected in a patient with hypokalaemia, metabolic alkalosis, persistent urinary potassium output, and moderately alkaline urine. The levels of plasma aldosterone and renin activity will then help distinguish between cases of primary hyperaldosteronism (elevated aldosterone, no renin activity), secondary hyperaldosteronism (elevated aldosterone and renin activity), and glycyrrhizine intoxication (low aldosterone and renin activity).

Hypokalaemia is only one of the complications of Cushing's syndrome or of long-term steroid administration.

During treatment of hypertension by thiazides or loop diuretics, serum potassium levels may decrease slightly to levels no lower than 3.5 mmol/litre, usually without potassium depletion. In most other circumstances, diuretic therapy may induce hypokalaemia due to a negative potassium balance and is often associated with metabolic alkalosis.

Hypokalaemia due to excessive urinary loss of potassium is sometimes observed in patients receiving large doses of beta-lactamines, particularly carbenicillin; when these are administered to patients with endocarditis or any form of heart disease, kalaemia should be closely monitored.

In patients with a ureterosigmoidostomy, urinary retention in the colon may cause diarrhoea and increased urea breakdown to ammonium chloride by the bacterial flora of the colon. Dehydration and loss of potassium and bicarbonate in the watery stools and reabsorption of ammonium chloride from the gut cause an increase in blood urea, metabolic acidosis and hypokalaemia with severe potassium depletion.

Increased urinary excretion in patients with proximal or distal tubular acidosis can cause potassium depletion and hypokalaemia along with acidosis.

In patients with chronic diarrhoea, malnutrition, or cirrhosis, it has recently been demonstrated that magnesium depletion with hypomagnesaemia may contribute to urinary losses of potassium and hypokalaemia.

During the course of acute monoblastic or myelomonocytic leukaemia, hyperlyzozymaemia and hyperlysozymuria can enhance renal potassium excretion and cause hypokalaemia.

Transitory hypokalaemia due to intracellular penetration of potassium may occur during acute elevations of blood pH, particularly when due to hypocapnia, or in patients treated by infusions of dextrose or dextrose and insulin without potassium salts. Concomitant potassium depletion can only be ruled out when serum potassium returns to normal levels after correction of the initiating factor.

In victims of near-drowning in soft H_2O, severe hypokalaemia causing life-threatening arrhythmia may be found, sometimes associated with metabolic acidosis. Its mechanism remains obscure but it seems, at least in part, related to hypothermia. It warrants caution in the use of diuretics or alkalinizing agents before correction of hypokalaemia [6].

Periodic attacks of intense weakness or frank paralysis of limb and trunk muscles occurring during sleep, on awakening, or after a meal, sometimes preceded by profuse diaphoresis, suggests the diagnosis of familial periodic paralysis. Hypokalaemia is transitory and is found only during the attack. Although the initiating factor remains unknown, hypokalaemia results from acute-onset intracellular penetration of potassium.

Management. Arrhythmia associated with hypokalaemia usually requires the IV administration of potassium salts. Potassium chloride is most commonly used. Citrate, propionate or lactate salts of potassium may be preferred when acidosis renders alkalinization necessary.

But rapid IV administration of potassium salts should be monitored by continuous ECG monitoring and frequent determinations of plasma potassium levels. When hypokalaemia co-exists with metabolic acidosis, potassium salts should be administered before, or at least simultaneously with, alkaline salts.

Correction of potassium depletion should be obtained progressively over a number of days. Although it has been claimed that a decrease of 1 mmol/litre in serum potassium correlates with a loss of 500 mmol body potassium, it cannot be relied upon for calculation of the amount of potassium to be administered.

In cases of mild hypokalaemia (plasma potassium between 2.5 and 3.5 mmol/litre) with no major cardiac complications, hypokalaemia can be corrected by a potassium-rich diet and oral supplementation of potassium. Potassium chloride should not be used in the form of concentrated tablets because of the possible caustic effects on the GI mucosa. The alkaline salts of potassium should not be used when metabolic alkalosis is present.

A large intake of carbohydrate, particularly when given with insulin, will slacken the rate of correction of hypokalaemia.

Associated pathogenic factors should also be attended to: correction of metabolic alkalosis and hypovolemia, discontinuation of incriminated drugs (when possible), compensation of GI losses, drainage by rectal catheterization in patients with ureterosigmoidostomy malfunction.

Hyperkalaemia

Hyperkalaemia is defined as a plasma potassium level above 5.3 mmol/litre. 9 mmol/litre is considered the upper limit compatible with life. Although levels of 7 mmol/litre or more may be observed in patients with few or no clinical symptoms, lower levels may be highly symptomatic, inducing cardiac arrhythmias and, possibly, the patient's death.

Hyperkalaemia is never coincident with any significant increase in total body potassium. Hyperkalaemia can be found in patients with depleted potassium stores when acidosis is present.

Clinical manifestations. Major myocardial conduction disturbances should be feared in patients with hyperkalaemia. The ECG shows modification of the T wave which becomes elevated, narrow, pointed and symmetrical initially in the precordial leads, but rapidly also in the other leads. These changes are constantly observed when plasma potassium levels rise above 6 mmol/litre. As potassium levels continue to rise, the P wave flattens out and may even disappear. The PR interval may increase and a Luciani–Wenckebach rhythm appear. Plasma potassium levels above 7.5 mmol/litre will induce intraventricular conduction disturbances; a uniformly enlarged QRS complex is strongly, suggestive of hyperkalaemia. An aspect of ventricular tachycardia or of ventricular flutter may ensue, preceding ventricular fibrillation. Cardiac arrest can occur suddenly. Although ECG changes are not well correlated with potassium levels, a level above 6 mmol/litre without ECG changes is suggestive of a technical error in measurement and should be checked.

Peripheral neuromuscular disturbances occur after the myocardial effects and are thus more rarely observed. These include tingling of the extremities, the tongue, the lips, and around the mouth, decreased sense of vibration and position, exceptionally generalized areflexic motor paralysis, with normal or increased response to percussion of muscles. Paralysis usually starts in the lower limbs and may affect the cranial nerves.

Laboratory findings. Biological disorders observed in patients with hyperkalaemia are associated with, rather than due to, hyperkalaemia, although recent studies have shown that renal hydrogen ion output is decreased during hyperkalaemia, due to decreased ammoniogenesis [23]. Metabolic acidosis, often associated with hyperkalaemia, tends to increase the level of plasma potassium due to the shift of potassium from the cells to extracellular fluid, but hyperkalaemia may be less frequent during acidosis due to organic acids [1a, 7].

Aetiology (see Table 25.3). Whatever the cause of hyperkalaemia, dietary potassium intake or administration of potassium salts will further increase the level of plasma potassium and may cause death.

As the kidneys normally control potassium excretion, a decrease in renal function decreases the patient's capacity to excrete a potassium load. Metabolic acidosis, usually present in renal failure, further raises the level of plasma potassium. Until recently, hyperkalaemia was the major cause of death in patients with acute or advanced chronic renal failure. Severe, life-

Table 25.3. Aetiology and prevention of hyperkalaemia

Mechanism	Clinical circumstances	Prevention and treatment
I. Decreased renal capacity for excreting potassium	Oliguric acute renal failure. Advanced chronic renal failure	Reduce dietary potassium. Do not administer potassium salts except to compensate for losses Treat metabolic acidosis
	Decreased mineralocorticoid secretion: Acute adrenocortical insufficiency Hyporeninemic hypoaldosteronism Congenital adrenal hyperplasia	Institute appropriate hormonal therapy
	Pseudohypoaldosteronism [24a]	Diuretics
	Administration of potassium-sparing diuretics	Monitor serum potassium levels
	Diabetes	Treat by adequate insulin administration
II. Release of intracellular potassium	Acidosis (metabolic or respiratory). Cellular destruction	Monitor acid–base balance and apply appropriate therapy
	Rhabdomyolysis (traumatic or non-traumatic)	Administer adequate hydration to maintain urinary output and renal function
	Acute haemolysis Initiation of chemotherapy in patients with lymphoma or leukaemia	
	Rapid transfusion of long-stored bank blood	If rapid and/or massive tranfusion is required, use recently drawn blood. Alkalinization of patient may help
	Administration of succinylcholine	Avoid succinylcholine in patients with renal failure
	Cardiac glycoside intoxication Adynamia episodica herediteria	Avoid strenuous exercise

threatening hyperkalaemia should now no longer be seen when patients are correctly managed.

Mild hyperkalaemia is frequent in patients with untreated Addison's disease and in the exceptional cases of congenital deficiency in 21-hydroxylase observed in infants. But during acute adrenal insufficiency, hyperkalaemia may become severe and is usually contemporary with extracellular dehydration and hyponatraemia. Hyperkalaemia can occur in patients receiving potassium-sparing diuretics, particularly when renal function is even mildly reduced.

During diabetic ketosis, hyperkalaemia due to metabolic acidosis and insulin deficiency is often present initially, despite potassium depletion. But in patients with severe diabetes, it may occur in the absence of ketosis. This has recently been shown to be due to hypoaldosteronism with hyporeninaemia in patients with renal failure due to diabetic nephropathy [23].

Cellular breakdown from whatever cause can liberate large quantities of potassium that are likely to induce severe hyperkalaemia when associated with metabolic acidosis and renal failure, as in patients with the crush syndrome and in cases of septic abortion with intravascular haemolysis. Both situations require emergency treatment. The risk is less in non-traumatic rhabdomyolysis, during mild haemolysis, or during the initial phase of chemotherapy in patients with leukaemia or lymphoma when renal function is normal.

Plasma potassium increases with time in bank blood, due to red cell leakage, and can reach levels of 15 mmol/litre after 2 weeks of storage; hence the danger of hyperkalaemia in patients receiving rapid and/or massive transfusions, particularly if renal function is altered.

Renal failure is a contra-indication for the use of succinylcholine as a curarizing agent because it induces a leakage of potassium from muscle cells.

In patients who have accidentally or voluntarily ingested a toxic dose of cardiac glycosides, kalaemia may be initially high due to inhibition of entry of potassium into cells. Acute hyperkalaemia due to a sudden outpouring of potassium from cells is held responsible for the attacks of paralysis observed, often consequent to muscular exercise, in patients with adynamia episodica hereditaria. During attacks, potassium and acid–base balance remain normal and there is no sign of cellular destruction. Between attacks, the patient is both clinically and metabolically normal.

Management. Severe hyperkalaemia rarely occurs if patients are correctly managed, i.e., if potassium intake is restricted in patients with severely reduced renal function and a rising plasma potassium. In such patients, plasma potassium should be closely monitored.

Severe hyperkalaemia requires urgent treatment. Infusion of a hypertonic glucose solution containing 1 u insulin/10 g glucose will acutely decrease plasma potassium levels by enhancing the intracellular transfer of potassium. The concomitant administration of an ion-exchange resin removes potassium from the body, thus preventing a rebound from occurring when the infusion is discontinued. Each gram of the resin, administered by mouth or rectally, will exchange one millimole of potassium against one millimole of sodium (or calcium, according to the resin used). Infusion of sodium bicarbonate should be preferred in patients with metabolic acidosis. But both methods induce extracellular volume expansion, which can be dangerous in patients with severe renal failure. Emergency dialysis may then be required.

Patients with mild hyperkalaemia can usually be managed by restriction of potassium intake and restoration of renal function by appropriate treatment. In patients with severe chronic renal failure, administration of an ion-exchange resin will help maintain near normal plasma potassium levels.

Hypocalcaemia and hypercalcaemia

Biological disturbances induced by variations in plasma calcium levels result from modifications of its ionized fraction. But the measurement of ionized calcium has not yet become a common laboratory procedure, thus preventing a precise estimation of its variations. Valid therapeutic conclusions can nevertheless be drawn from comparison between measured plasma calcium values and theoretical values calculated according to plasma protein levels [22]:

Ca (mmol/1) = 0.139 protein (mg%) + 1.5.

Normal values for total plasma calcium, when measured by atomic absorption spectrophotometry, range between 2.4 ± 0.1 mmol/litre (96 ± 4 mg/litre). When measured by titration, they range between 2.5 ± 0.15 mmol/litre (100 ± 6 mg/litre).

Hypocalcaemia

Clinical manifestations. A decrease in the plasma level of ionized calcium may induce clinical symptoms of increased neuromuscular excitability. In its full-blown form it will induce tetany. It is more often expressed as tetanic equivalents such as paraesthesias, numbness, muscle cramps, dysphagia, cardiac irregularities, etc. Electromyographic changes, when suggestive of tetany, can be a useful diagnostic aid in these minor forms. Shortening of the ST segment in the ECG can be observed in cases where the calcium level is below 2.1 mmol.

Clinical symptoms appear more readily when plasma ionized calcium is acutely decreased [9]. But they may also be due to hypomagnesaemia, which should be checked for in the normocalcaemic patient.

Chronic hypocalcaemia due to hypoparathyroidism may be suspected when hypocalcaemia is accompanied by dermatological symptoms (dry skin, disappearance of axillary and pubic hair, brittle nails, etc.), cataract with superficial calcifications, intracranial calcifications, etc.

Aetiology [9]. In the acutely ill patient, of the type treated in ICUs, hypocalcaemia is often due to hypoproteinaemia secondary to dilution, decreased albumin production, and/or increased albumin catabolism and loss. But in these and in other patients in whom hypoproteinaemia can be ruled out as the sole cause of hypocalcaemia, the decrease in free calcium can have any of a variety of aetiologies (see Table 25.4), the most commonly observed probably being renal failure, acute pancreatitis, and rhabdomyolysis. Diagnosis is usually oriented by the patient's case history and by clinical findings. In patients with severe renal failure, moderate hypocalcaemia (between 1.75 and 2.25 mmol/litre) is due to decreased absorption of calcium, hyperphosphataemia and phosphate retention, and to resistance of bone to parathyroid hormone [30]. In patients with abdominal pain, hypocalcaemia can support a diagnosis of acute pancreatitis. Initially attributed to intra-abdominal saponification, the mechanism of hypocalcaemia in acute pancreatitis is probably complex, involving calcitonin, glucagon and parathyroid hormone responses, and perhaps still other factors [24].

In a patient with signs of rhabdomyolysis, hypocalcaemia has been attributed to precipitation of calcium salts in soft tissues.

For patients receiving large amounts of bank blood, it has long been advised that calcium salts be administered to prevent hypocalcaemia and reduction in plasma ionized calcium, which can occur with the infusion of citrate used as anticoagulant. Recent experimental and clinical studies have shown that citrate administration is well tolerated except in cases of massive transfusion and that administration of calcium, usually in the form of calcium chloride, will often induce hypercalcaemia. The tendency among anaesthesiologists has thus been to refrain from administering calcium salts to adults except in cases of rapid, massive transfusion.

Management. Hypocalcaemia related to hypoproteinaemia alone requires no treatment. Hypocalcaemia due to a decrease in free calcium can be corrected by administration of calcium salts. Administration of calcium salts IV is required only when hypocalcaemia is symptomatic or when calcium cannot be administered PO. It can be given in the form of a 10% solution of the alkaline salt calcium gluconate (0.23 mmol/ml) or of the acid salt calcium chloride (0.45 mmol/ml). Calcium chloride should be given IV with care, to avoid tissue necrosis due to spilling in the subcutaneous tissues. If not

Table 25.4. Causes of hypocalcaemia

I. Decreased protein-bound calcium
   1. Nephrotic syndrome
   2. Hepatic cirrhosis
   3. Malnutrition
   4. Acute illness

II. Decreased free calcium
   1. Parathyroid hormone disorders
      Hypoparathyroidism
      Following parathyroidectomy
      Infarction of parathyroid adenoma
      Metastases to parathyroid glands
      Due to parathyroid dysfunction
      Pseudohypoparathyroidism due to parathyroid hormone insensitivity
   2. Vitamin D deficiency
      Dietary deficency
      Malabsorption due to small-bowel disease or to neomycin administration
   3. .Hyperphosphataemia
      Acute or chronic renal failure
      Phosphate infusions
   4. Miscellaneous
      Neoplastic disorders
      Increased skeletal activity due to osteoblastic metastases
      Calcitonin-secreting tumours
      Acute pancreatitis
      Magnesium deficiency
      Renal tubular acidosis
      Adrenal corticosteroid excess
      Treatment by glucagon, mithramycin, EDTA infusions
      Citrate intoxication (massive blood transfusions)
   5. Neonatal tetany

diluted for IV infusion, the injection should be given slowly. The total dose to be administered varies widely and depends on the clinical and biological response. In less urgent cases, hypocalcaemia can be corrected by calcium salts given PO or by a diet rich in dairy products. In patients receiving cardiac glycosides, calcium salts should be administered prudently.

Associated metabolic disorders such as hypomagnesaemia, hyperkalaemia, and alkalosis should also be corrected. In cases of vitamin D deficiency, vitamin D_3 can be administered. In patients with hepatic or renal failure, vitamin D should be given in the form of $25-(OH)\ D_3$.

Hypercalcaemia

Clinical manifestations. The degree of hypercalcaemia does not correlate with clinical manifestations, and high levels of serum calcium may be asymptomatic. When present, clinical symptoms are non-specific. Anorexia and fatiguability are frequently observed. Polyuria due to impaired renal concentrating ability induces polydipsia and is more suggestive of hypercalcaemia. In the more severe cases, other symptoms may be present: nausea, vomiting, constipation, lethargy, confusion, or even coma. Certain symptoms may be predominant during a hypercalcaemic crisis, so that the clinical setting is that of an abdominal emergency, an acute psychiatric disorder, or acute renal failure. Early alteration of myocardial function is apparent on the ECG, shortening of the QT segment being present in even mild elevations of serum calcium. But cardiovascular disturbances are not apparent unless associated hypokalaemia or cardiac glycoside administration add to the risk of cardiac arrhythmia and perhaps even cardiac arrest.

In long-standing hypercalcaemia, as may be seen in primary hyperparathyroidism, precipitation of calcium salts may provoke the formation of renal stones, nephrocalcinosis, or calcium precipitation in the cornea and conjunctiva. Precipitation in other soft tissues realising so-called metastatic calcifications may rarely be observed in cases of milk alkali syndrome or vitamin D intoxication, when elevated levels of serum phosphorus and alkalosis increase the risk of precipitation.

Metabolic disturbances. Automation of calcium measurements has increased the number of cases where hypercalcaemia is discovered fortuitously in asymptomatic or paucisymptomatic patients. But hypercalcaemia can only be asserted when plasma calcium levels are high or, when only mildly elevated, after correction for plasma protein levels.

Low serum phosphorus levels can have a variety of aetiologies but, associated with elevated urinary calcium and phosphorus excretion, a lowered serum phosphorus in the presence of hypercalcaemia strongly suggests hyperparathyroidism.

Some degree of renal failure can be secondary to dehydration in patients with acute hypercalcaemia, or occur as a complication of nephrocalcinosis and lithiasis in patients with chronic hypercalcaemia.

Metabolic alkalosis can occur as a complication of increased renal hydrogen ion excretion, due to the effect of hypercalcaemia on tubular hydrogen ion exchange [23]. But the opposite effect of parathyroid hormone probably explains the absence of alkalosis or even the metabolic acidosis of patients with primary hyperparathyroidism [23]. Relative hyperchloraemia thus becomes an indication of primary hyperparathyroidism. Hypokalaemia will decrease cardiac tolerance to hypercalcaemia and should be corrected.

Aetiology. Although hypercalcaemia is observed in a great variety of pathologic circumstances (see Table 25.5), those which lead a patient to require intensive care are usually those in which calcium levels are high and acutely elevated. The most frequently encountered are thus cases of adenocarcinoma (particularly breast and prostate) with bone metastases and of multiple myeloma. If the original disease is unknown these diagnoses should be checked out first. Primary hyperparathyroidism can sometimes lead to acute and even symptomatic elevations of plasma calcium, and should be suspected when the other obvious causes are absent. Although rarely the cause of major rises in plasma calcium, sarcoidosis should be sought when the preceding aetiologies have been ruled out. Prolonged immobilization usually causes hypercalciuria, but exceptionally leads to hypercalcaemia, and should be held responsible only after all other causes have been looked for.

Management of the acute hypercalcaemic emergency. The acute hypercalcaemic emergency or the patient whose rising level of plasma calcium puts him in danger of entering such a state is best managed in an ICU, where correction of dehydration and electrolyte disturbances can be associated with the measures aimed at lowering plasma calcium levels. To this effect, various therapeutic methods have been recommended

Table 25.5. Causes of hypercalcaemia

I. Hyperparathyroidism
  1. Primary hyperparathyroidism due to parathyroid:
    Adenoma: Sporadic
                Familial (associated with a pituitary or pancreatic tumour, a medullary cancer of the thyroid gland or a
                phaeochromocytoma)
    Hyperplasia (familial)
    Cancer
  2. Secondary hyperparathyroidism
    In patients with renal failure, hypercalcaemia appearing during the recovery phase of acute renal failure or after
    renal transplantation

II . Neoplastic hypercalcaemia
  1. Bone metastases of malignant tumours
  2. Secretion by tumours of an osteolytic
    substance (a peptide similar to PTH, prostaglandins, a steroid similar to vitamin D, an osteoclast-activating factor)
  3. Multiple myeloma
  4. Lymphoma or leukaemia

III. Action of vitamin D on bone
  1. Vitamin D intoxication
  2. Sarcoidosis
  3. Tuberculosis
  4. Berylliosis

IV. Immobilization

V. Miscellaneous
  1. Milk alkali syndrome
  2. Administration of calcium salts
  3. Administration of thiazides or lithium salts
  4. Hormonal disturbance other than hyperparathyroidism: hyper- or hypothyroidism, adrenal insufficiency
  5. Familial hypocalciuric hypercalcaemia [14]
  6. Excessive administration of vitamin A

VI. Causes found in children
  1. Maternal hypoparathyroidism
  2. Subcutaneous fat necrosis
  3. Familial parathyroid hyperplasia
  4. Idiopathic hypercalcaemia

(see Table 25.6). The choice of treatment must be adapted to suit the patient's disease and condition. If the cause of hypercalcaemia is unknown, adequate diagnostic investigations should be rapidly pursued, for aetiologic treatment should be instituted early whenever possible. This is particularly true in cases of parathyroid adenoma, where surgery is required.

Hypophosphataemia and hyperphosphataemia

Hyperphosphataemia has long been known to be a complication of various diseases, particularly of renal failure. Routine measurement of serum phosphate has revealed that hypophosphataemia is also frequent, particularly in patients being treated in ICUs [31]. In a hospital population, 2%–3% are estimated to have a de-

crease in serum phosphate at some time during the course of their stay.

Hypophosphataemia

Hypophosphataemia may or may not correlate with phosphate depletion. The distinction between the two conditions can only be inferred from experimental data extrapolated to the clinical case at hand.

Pathogenic mechanisms and aetiology. Administration of glucose will lower serum phosphate [11]. Large glucose intakes such as are now being given to patients as part of IV hyperalimentation appear to cause a redistribution of body phosphate, with a shift of phosphorus from the extracellular to the intracellular space. This pathogenic mechanism is suggested by the observation that large glucose infusions increase uptake of radioactive phosphate by the skeletal muscles and that hypophosphataemia is not induced in patients with major muscle

Table 25.6 Methods of lowering elevated levels of plasma calcium[a]

Drug	Mode of action	Mode of administration	Indications and effect	Contra-indications
Inorganic phosphate	Diminished bone resorption. Increased bone formation	IV: 1 litre solution containing 19 mmol KH_2 PO_4 and 81 mmol Na_2HPO_4 (= 100 mmol P, 162 mmol Na, 19 mmol K) infused over 6–8 h. PO: 1–3 g phosphorus/24 h	Mild hypercalcaemia or hypercalcaemia subsequent to lowering of plasma calcium by other means. During IV infusion, monitor blood pressure, urinary output, ECG, calcium levels. Progressive decrease of calcaemia	Severe hypercalcaemia (can induce precipitation of calcium phosphate in soft tissues, hypotension, pulmonary oedema, acute renal failure)
High doses of frusemide	Increased urinary output of calcium by inhibition of proximal tubular reabsorption	IV: 100 mg/hour or every 2 h. Compensation of the large volume of urine (10–15 litres/24 h) by an equal amount of IV fluid containing Na and K in the same concentration as that found in urine. Monitor patient's weight and plasma electrolytes. Duration: 1 to 3 days	Severe hypercalcaemia. Rapid decrease in plasma calcium levels	Renal failure
Mithramycin	Decreased bone resorption by inhibition of the differentiation of osteocytes into osteoclasts	IV: 25–50 µg/kg as a single injection or infused over a period of hours. Can be repeated 48 h later	Severe hypercalcaemia. Progressive decrease in plasma calcium levels over 36–48 h	Thrombocytopenia or hepatic disease (risk of bone marrow, hepatic and renal toxicity at close to therapeutic doses
Indomethacin, aspirin	Decreased bone resorption by inhibition of prostaglandin synthetase, and hence of the effects of prostaglandins on differentiation of osteocytes into osteoclasts	PO Indomethacin: 75–200 mg/24 h. Aspirin: 2–5 g/24 h. When effective, plasma calcium levels decrease over 2–3 days	Mild hypercalcaemia due to solid tumours	
Calcitonin	Decreased bone resorption and increased bone formation due to transformation of osteoclasts to osteoblasts	IV: 4 IU every 6–12 h. When effective, plasma calcium levels decrease rapidly but the effect may be transitory	Mild hypercalcaemia due to non-malignant disease	
Hydrocortisone	Decreased intestinal absorption of calcium. Effect on bone calcium metabolism?	PO: 100–200 mg/24 h. When effective, plasma calcium levels decrease over a period of days	Hypercalcaemia of sarcoidosis and vitamin D intoxication. Mild hypercalcaemia due to malignant disease	

[a]In cases of severe renal failure (serum creatinine >70 mmol/litre), peritoneal dialysis or haemodialysis must be used in patients with high levels of plasma calcium [2].

atrophy. Hypophosphataemia may follow the infusion of even moderate amounts of glucose, around 200 g/day, particularly in alcoholics with previous phosphate depletion, but also in normal subjects; in the latter it is less severe and of shorter duration. Intravenous glucose infusions, particularly in patients treated by IV hyperalimentation, are probably the most common cause of severe hypophosphataemia in severely ill patients. The decrease in serum phosphate is induced within 24–48 h after the starting of an infusion and persists until discontinuation or until it is corrected by administration of phosphate. The degree of hypophosphataemia depends on the amount of calories being given, particularly in the form of glucose [28]. Urinary phosphate decreases to very low levels due to increased tubular phosphate reabsorption.

Increased cellular uptake of phosphorus is held responsible for hypophosphataemia induced by respiratory alkalosis due to hyperventilation of any cause. Increased bone deposition of phosphate in patients with condensing bone metastases could also induce hypophosphataemia.

Phosphate depletion is rarely due to decreased dietary intake of phosphorus but may be observed in severely malnourished patients or in alcoholics. Gastro-intestinal losses can cause a negative phosphorus balance in patients with malabsorption or in patients absorbing antacids containing no phosphates over long periods of time. Urinary losses of phosphate may produce a large negative balance in patients with glycosuria, particularly during diabetic ketosis. Alcohol intake, and magnesium or potassium depletion increase urinary phosphate excretion, and all contribute to the phosphate depletion in alcoholic patients. Certain forms of congenital or acquired renal tubular dysfunction increase urinary phosphate excretion. Hypophosphataemia and increased renal phosphate excretion are, of course, among the biological signs of primary hyperparathyroidism.

Other factors may contribute to the induction of hypophosphataemia, such as liberation of catecholamines (the effect is prevented by giving a beta blocker) or circulating endogenous or exogenous insulin. A number of factors probably contribute to the genesis of the hypophosphataemia found in two-thirds of patients suffering from gram-negative septicaemic shock.

Clinical manifestations. As in other electrolyte disorders, there is no correlation between the degree of hypophosphataemia and clinical symptoms, but symptoms have been reported mainly in patients with serum phosphate levels below 0.4 mmol/litre. Furthermore, symptoms are not specific. They can be attributed to hypophosphataemia if the following conditions are combined: severe and persistent hypophosphataemia; absence of other electrolyte disturbances likely to account for the symptoms, such as potassium or magnesium depletion; and regression of the symptoms after phosphate administration. Asthenia, irritability, anxiety, and mental confusion may be the only expression of the metabolic encephalopathy. Exceptionally, if left untreated, they may precede the onset of convulsions, status epilepticus, coma, or even death. Paraesthesias and muscular fatigue can occur as the precursor of a diffuse, sensory and motor form of peripheral neurophathy. Again, if left untreated, this condition has been held responsible for acute respiratory failure (ARF). Some cases of non-traumatic rhabdomyolysis in alcoholic patients have been attributed to hypophosphataemia. Haemodynamic measurements in patients with hypophosphataemia have shown decreased myocardial contractility restored by administration of phosphate, suggesting hypophosphataemia might be a pathogenic factor of circulatory failure particularly in septic shock.

Laboratory findings. Hypophosphataemia has primarily been accused of modifying blood cell metabolism. Red blood cell metabolism is altered by the decrease in 2–3 diphosphoglyceraldehyde, which correlates with serum phosphate levels and by the decrease in erythrocyte ATP. The former increases the affinity of haemoglobin for O_2, thus potentially decreasing O_2 delivery to the tissues. The latter increases the rigidity of the red cell membrane and increases red cell destruction. Haemolytic anaemia has thus been reported when serum phosphate falls below 0.45 mmol/litre. The decrease in intracellular ATP has also been shown to decrease the chemotactic and phagocytic properties of leucocytes for serum phosphate levels below 0.35 mmol/litre. Thrombocytopenia and a bleeding tendency has been observed when ATP levels fall below 50%.

Management. Administration of phosphate is required primarily in patients receiving parenteral nutrition. Amounts of 15–25 mmol phosphate/1000 calories are considered adequate. Some solutes used for parenteral nutrition (lipid emulsions and amino acid solutions) contain phosphate in various amounts, which must be taken into account to calculate intake.

Administration of phosphate should be considered in patients with a significantly reduced serum phosphate concentration and with normal or reduced calcium levels (when serum calcium is elevated, there is a risk of precipitation of calcium phosphate in soft tissues). It has recently been recommended in patients with diabetic ketosis once the initially elevated level of serum phosphate starts to fall but it should proceed with caution to avoid inducing hypocalcemia and hypomagnesaemia [33].

Correction of hypophosphataemia requires the oral or intravenous administration of phosphate in amounts which can be determined by following the course of the serum phosphate. Caution is warranted, particularly in patients with decreased renal function in whom the serum level may rise rapidly with, even moderate, intake. Rapid correction of severe hypophosphataemia may induce a decrease in serum calcium requiring administration of calcium salts. Frequent monitoring of serum phosphate levels is desirable in severely ill patients, in ICUs.

Hyperphosphataemia

A rise in serum phosphate concentration will only be revealed by laboratory measurement, for it causes no manifest clinical symptoms.
Aetiology. Hyperphosphataemia can nevertheless be suspected in patients with renal failure in whom it starts to rise when the glomerular filtration rate falls below 20–40 ml/min and it may then attain levels above 4 mmol/litre. Hypercatabolic states, major cell destruction (during traumatic or non-traumatic rhabdomyolysis, chemotherapy of acute lymphoblastic leukemia or of large lymphomatous masses), or tissue ischemia will liberate large quantities of phosphate [19]. Serum phosphate levels rise, particularly if urinary excretion is reduced by decreased renal function. In other circumstances a rise in serum phosphate concentration is a sign of diagnostic value, as in acromegaly, hypoparathyroidism and vitamin D intoxication.
Management. In acute situations, treatment of hyperphosphataemia will be derived indirectly from maintaining or restoring the patient's circulatory status and fluid, electrolyte, and acid–base balance, thus contributing to the restoration of renal function and increasing urinary excretion of phosphate.

In patients with chronic renal failure, the rise in serum phosphate tends to decrease the plasma calcium concentration, thus constituting the primary factor of secondary hyperparathyroidism. Every effort should thus be made in such cases to maintain serum phosphate levels as low as possible (below 2.8 mmol/litre). Dietary reduction in phosphate is not always compatible with sufficient protein intake. But ingestion of phosphate chelators will help reduce the phosphate load. In patients with acute oliguric or terminal chronic renal failure dialysis will help to maintain serum phosphate levels below 2.8 mmol/litre.

Hypomagnesaemia and hypermagnesaemia

Until recently, disorders of magnesium metabolism have most often gone undetected. Their significance may appear greater in years to come, with more frequent measurements of magnesium in biological fluids and greater awareness of their clinical consequences. Magnesium and calcium metabolisms being intimately linked, it is no surprise to find that the clinical symptoms and causes of disorders of magnesium metabolism are similar to those seen in disorders of calcium metabolism.

Normal plasma magnesium concentration measured by atomic absorption photometry is 0.85 ± 0.07 mmol/litre, 0.2–0.3 mmol of which is bound to plasma protein. Of free magnesium, 80%–90% is in the ionized form. The red blood cell concentration is 0.26 ± 0.3 mmol/litre, lower than that found in other cells. The significance of variations in red blood cell magnesium values remains debated.

Hypomagnesaemia

Hypomagnesaemia is probably a frequent disorder in a variety of clinical settings. A plasma magnesium below 0.7 mmol/litre may be of clinical consequence. Magnesium depletion is probable when hypomagnesaemia is associated with a daily urinary excretion of less than 1 mmol/24 h. Magnesium depletion is often associated with other biological disorders, such as hypocalcaemia, hypophosphataemia, and hypokalaemia.
Clinical manifestations. Tetany or its equivalents are indistinguishable from these symptoms as they are seen in hypocalcaemia. Neurological symptoms may appear during severe hypo-

magnesaemia and are similar to those seen in delirium tremens. The ECG shows a lowering of the ST segment and an inverted T wave. Arrhythmias may be caused by severe magnesium depletion [23].

A hypocalcaemic state may remain uncorrected by calcium salts in the case of concomitant hypomagnesaemia. Serum calcium levels rise only after administration of magnesium.

Aetiology [15]. Prolonged parenteral feeding devoid of magnesium can cause hypomagnesaemia.

Intestinal malabsorption due to intestinal disease or to cirrhosis, or prolonged gastrointestinal losses, may cause magnesium depletion. Oral calcium supplementation competes with magnesium absorption.

A number of disease states decrease renal tubular reabsorption of magnesium causing urinary losses, eventually contributing to magnesium depletion: chronic alcoholism, renal tubular acidosis, hypercalcaemia, diabetes, hyperaldosteronism, hyperthyroidism. Use of diuretics and excessive gentamicin administration also enhance urinary excretion.

Treatment. Hypomagnesaemia during exclusive parenteral feeding can be prevented by administering approximately 10 mmol/24 h in the form of magnesium sulphate (the 15% solution contains 0.61 mmol/ml of magnesium) or magnesium chloride (the 10% solution contains 0.49 mmol magnesium/ml).

In patients with serum levels below 0.7 mmol/litre, oral magnesium supplementation, with 5–10 mmol/24 h, is usually sufficient. In case of intestinal malabsorption or in acutely symptomatic patients, parenteral administration is necessary.

In patients with renal failure, monitoring of serum magnesium levels is necessary and magnesium administration should proceed with caution.

Hypermagnesaemia

Clinical manifestations. With a rise in plasma magnesium values between 2.5 and 12.5 mmol/litre the following signs may be observed, in order of gravity: ECG modifications (increased PR interval, enlargement of the QRS complex, increased amplitude of the T wave), decreased or absent tendon reflexes, paralysis of respiratory muscles, drowsiness, coma, cardiac arrest.

Aetiology. Hypermagnesaemia is common but usually remains below 2.5 mmol/litre in patients with renal failure [15]. A mild elevation

may also be seen in patients with adrenal insufficiency or myxoedema.

Parenteral administration of magnesium salts for the treatment of toxaemia raises plasma magnesium to levels which should not exceed 3.5 mmol/litre. Fetal hypermagnesaemia may follow excessive treatment [23].

Oral administration of magnesium salts as antacids or as laxatives will raise plasma magnesium levels in patients with renal failure [15].

Treatment. Caution in the use of antacids containing magnesium in patients with renal failure is warranted. In the treatment of toxaemia, a decrease in tendon reflexes is a sign that plasma magnesium levels have reached 5 mmol/litre and that treatment should be discontinued. In most other cases, hypermagnesaemia remains asymptomatic and requires no specific treatment.

Metabolic disorders of acid–base balance

Normal acid–base equilibrium is determined by maintenance of normal $paCO_2$ values through adaptation of respiration to CO_2 production and by maintenance of whole-body buffer stores through regulation of bicarbonate reabsorption and generation in the kidney. Metabolic acidosis and alkalosis result from situations in which the renal response is inadequate to the maintenance of normal balance. Disorders of metabolic origin induce a respiratory response tending to counterbalance the original disorder. Conversely, respiratory acidosis and alkalosis induce a compensatory renal response.

Despite its apparent simplicity, the maintenance of normal acid–base balance is the result of complex mechanisms with many determinants. In pathologic conditions, a number of these determinants are often simultaneously disturbed, enhancing or compensating the original disorder.

Measurement and interpretation of the acid–base status

The acid–base status of a patient is assessed according to the values of the three variables of the Henderson–Hasselbach equation: pH, pCO_2, and bicarbonate. The three variables may be measured or two of the variables measured and the third calculated.

A number of nomograms have been proposed, either to facilitate calculation of the third variable or to take into account modifications in the buffering capacity of the body, particularly the level of haemoglobin. The nomogram proposed by Siggaard-Andersen in 1960 [29] and based on the interpolation method of Astrup, was an attempt to differentiate between the metabolic and respiratory components of the variations in acid–base balance. The concept was ultimately challenged by a number of authors, because pH values determined in vitro could not be extrapolated to in vivo values. Most authors have now adhered to the 'physiologic' approach of Schwartz and Relman [26], for whom assessment of acid–base balance is best made on clinical grounds, and on the measurement of pH, PCO_2, and plasma bicarbonate. This indeed 'allows rational evaluation of even the most complicated acid-base disorder'.

For a correct determination of acid–base status of a patient and analysis of both metabolic and respiratory determinants of the disorder, measurement should be made of the acid–base variables and of PO_2 in arterial blood drawn into a heparinized syringe immediately before. In patients with a major variation in temperature, either above or below normal, PCO_2 should be corrected for temperature. For more routine evaluation of acid–base status, acid–base values can be measured in venous blood drawn without stasis or with a minimum of stasis.

Expression of results

Following the institution of Système International (SI) units, PCO_2 should no longer be expressed in millimetres of mercury but in Pascals, and plasma bicarbonate in mmol/litre rather than in mEq/litre. For clarity and on theoretical grounds, it has been suggested that pH should be replaced as an expression of hydrogen ion status by H^+ activity in nanomoles per litre [8].

Deviations from normal values in a given patient have traditionally been expressed according to the patient's recent case history, the primary disturbance of acid–base balance being attributed to dysfunction of one of the two organ control systems, the kidney or the lung, the other tending to modify its function to keep blood H^+ concentration within normal limits. The terminology used to describe the acid–base disturbance reflects these concepts, e.g., 'metabolic acidosis with compensatory re-spiratory alkalosis' or 'metabolic alkalosis with compensatory respiratory acidosis'. The terms 'acidosis' and 'alkalosis' are used even though pH values remain within normal limits. In 1964, it was recommended by the New York Academy of Science [18], at a meeting on acid–base balance, that the terminology for acid–base disturbances remain purely descriptive. Depression or elevation of values should be termed respectively 'acidaemia' and 'alkalaemia' for pH, 'hypobasaemia' and 'hyperbasaemia' for bicarbonate, 'hypocapnia' and 'hypercapnia' for PCO_2. The disturbance is then only interpreted in the light of the patient's recent case history and clinical symptoms. This new terminology has not been adopted in the recent medical literature.

Metabolic acidosis

Metabolic acidosis is characterized by reduced whole-body buffer base, with or without increased hydrogen ion activity in the extracellular space (acidaemia), due to accumulation of acids other than carbonic acid ('non-volatile' acids) or to loss of buffer base.

Causes and mechanisms

Metabolic acidosis should be suspected in a patient presenting with one of the pathologic conditions listed in Table 25.7 along with the pathogenetic mechanism of the acidosis. In clinical practice the most frequent causes are intestinal losses, renal failure, keto-acidosis, and lactic acidosis, and they should be checked for before all others. Calculation of the anion gap may then be helpful in orienting diagnosis in the more difficult cases.

The anion gap

The anion gap [20] can be calculated as the difference between measured serum cations and anions: $(Na^+ + K^+) - (Cl^- + HCO_3^-)$. Its normal value lies between 17 and 19 mmol/litre. Since total serum cations must be equal to total serum anions, changes in the anion gap must result from a change in both unmeasured cations and unmeasured anions (unless there is a laboratory error in measurement of serum Na^+, K^+, Cl^- or HCO_3^-). Modification of the anion gap due to a change in unmeasured cations Ca^{2+} and Mg^{2+} is rarely observed clinically, as their concentrations are low in relation to that of

Table 25.7. Metabolic acidosis

General mechanism	Specific mechanism	Pathological conditions
I. Acidosis with a decrease in buffer base		
A. Gain of acid	Increased production and/or decreased elimination of endogenous noncarbonic acid	
	Ketonic acidosis (incomplete oxidation of fat)[a]	Insulin deficiency, fasting or starvation, ethanol intoxication, ketotic hypoglycaemia with hypoalaninaemia
	Lactic acidosis (incomplete oxidation of carbohydrate)[a]	Tissue hypoxia in shock or severe hypoxaemia, phenformin therapy, diabetes mellitus, cirrhosis, pancreatitis, ethanol ingestion, leukaemia, type I glycogen storage disease, fructose-1, 6-diphosphatase deficiency
	Exogenous acid[b]	NH_4Cl, arginine Cl, lysine Cl
	Incompletely identified organic acids[a]	Salicylate, methanol, ethylene glycol, paraldehyde intoxication; propionyl CoA carboxylase deficiency, methylmalonic aciduria
	Inappropriately reduced amount of bicarbonate delivered to the extracellular fluid by the kidneys[b]	Renal failure, renal tubular acidosis
B. Loss of bicarbonate	By the gastro-intestinal tract[b]	Diarrhoea, external fistulas (pancreatic, biliary, intestinal) ureterosigmoidostomy, ingestion of calcium chloride, magnesium sulphate, or cholestyramine administration
II. Acidosis without a decrease in buffer base ('dilutional acidosis')	Dilutional reduction of the concentration of bicarbonate in extracellular fluid[b]	Rapid expansion of extracellular fluid by administration of bicarbonate-free isotonic or hypertonic fluid (especially in oliguric or salt-retaining states, when renal acidification is impaired, and in infants)

[a] The anion gap is always increased in these patients often reaching high values ≥ 30 mmol/litre.
[b] The anion gap remains normal in these conditions except in severe renal failure where it rises to values usually < 30 mmol/litre. Interstitial nephritis (particularly pyelonephritis) may induce severe hypobasaemia with a normal anion gap.

sodium, and large variations in their concentration are incompatible with life. On the other hand, the unmeasured anions protein, phosphate, sulphate, and organic acids may increase in patients with metabolic acidosis.

An increase in the anion gap will be observed each time endogenous or exogenous acids pour into the circulation in a situation where the kidneys are unable to excrete all the corresponding anions (Table 25.8). The anion gap increases in patients with metabolic acidosis when capacity of the kidney to excrete both the H^+ and the corresponding anion is similarly limited; e.g. acidemia due to lactic acidosis, keto-acidosis, or phosphate and sulphate retention in patients with renal failure. The degree to which the anion gap is increased is of clinical significance. A large increase to values of 30 or 40 mmol/litre is observed in patients with acidosis due to accumulation of organic acids. In other cases, the increase is usually in the order of 10 mmol/litre or less. The anion gap may remain within normal values in patients with interstitial nephritis, particularly pyelonephritis, and in patients with renal tubular acidosis. Indeed, the capacity of the kidney to excrete even a normal acid load is reduced, causing acidosis, while it maintains its capacity to excrete the corresponding anions. In other situations, such as intestinal losses of bicarbonate, acidosis is due to loss of buffer base and not to accumulation of acid. In this case also, the anion gap remains normal. Thus, in a patient with acidosis the value of the anion gap may be an asset in the evaluation of the mechanism of the acid–base disorder (Tables 25.7 and 25.8).

Table 25.8. Increased anion gap due to increased unmeasured anion

Organic anions: lactate, ketone acids
Inorganic anions: phosphate, sulfate
Exogenous anions: salicylate, formate, nitrate, penicillin, carbenicillin, etc.
Incompletely identified anions accumulating in paraldehyde, ethylene glycol, methanol and salicylate poisoning, uraemia, hyperosmolar hyperglycaemic non-ketotic coma

Consequences of metabolic acidosis

The decrease in blood pH creates clinical and biological disturbances which are observed in patients with severe acidosis.

Clinical manifestations. A decrease in blood pH will cause generalized cellular dysfunction and is often accompanied by metabolic and circulatory disturbances which contribute to clinical symptoms.

Hyperventilation can result from an acid blood pH alone. It will then take on the aspect of Kussmaul breathing characterized by a large increase in depth and frequency of respirations with equalization of inspiratory and expiratory times, as observed in diabetic ketosis. But hypoxia and shock may be contributory factors in many circumstances. The physiological mechanism for the ventilatory response in metabolic acidosis has not been completely explained. The resultant hypocapnia is a vital device for preventing or reducing the fall in blood pH, but its efficiency decreases with increasing metabolic acidosis.

Stupor progressing to coma has been attributed to lowering of the spinal fluid pH, but this mechanism has been questioned, at least in patients with diabetic ketosis [5]. Other factors, such as hyperosmolality or high concentrations of ketones in the spinal fluid, may also have a role in the induction of cerebral dysfunction. On the other hand, the administration of bicarbonate in such patients has been accused of increasing the neurological disturbance by lowering the spinal fluid pH due to an increased local PCO_2 [5].

Lowered blood pH has also been implicated in circulatory failure; however, shock is more often the cause than the consequence of acidosis, and it is unlikely that acidosis is itself a cause of shock until blood pH reaches very low values, when cardiac arrhythmia causes circulatory collapse.

Laboratory findings. Hyperkalaemia due to the shift of potassium from the cells to extracellular fluid is the best-known of the biological effects of metabolic acidosis. It is of grave consequence in patients with acute renal failure, particularly when there is potassium influx into the circulation resulting from cell destruction or increased protein catabolism. In these circumstances the rapid rise in serum potassium levels may induce cardiac arrhythmias, cardiac arrest, and death, even with a moderate rise in kalaemia.

The haemoglobin dissociation curve is displaced toward the right with consequent increase in the quantity of O_2 available to the tissues.

The ionized fraction of plasma calcium is increased by the decrease in blood pH. This may afford some protection against hypocalcaemia due to decreased absorption of calcium from the gut such as is seen in various forms of malabsorption or to decreased absorption and increased fixation to tissue, as in renal failure. A rapid correction of acidosis in these circumstances may induce tetany.

The normal kidney reacts to metabolic acidosis with increased acid secretion and tubular reabsorption of sodium and calcium. But this response decreases quantitatively with decreasing renal function.

Finally, a decrease in blood pH will, at least theoretically, interfere with the bioavailability of drugs. In the past, it has been said to induce a resistance to certain drugs, such as insulin in keto-acidosis or catecholamines in shock. But other pathogenic factors may be operative in such circumstances, and full correction of metabolic acidosis by alkalinization is not warranted in these patients.

Management

Principles of therapy. Replacement of buffer base is required whenever blood pH is below normal or when plasma bicarbonate is significantly lowered even though blood pH is maintained within the normal range by a decrease in PCO_2. Early and full alkalinization should be instituted when acidosis is progressing rapidly, as it does in lactic acidosis. Administration of potassium may have to be started early in patients with potassium depletion coincident with metabolic acidosis, as in diabetic keto-acidosis. Although various alkaline salts (lactate, acetate, gluconate, etc.) have been used, the anion will be converted to equal amounts of bicarbonate in the body. Neither does the organic buffer THAM (tris-[hydroxymethyl]aminomethane) offer any advantage over bicarbonate. Sodium bicarbonate is administered IV as an isotonic (166 mmol/litre) or as a hypertonic (at various concentrations up to 1000 mmol/litre) solution. A hypertonic solution is used in patients with hyponatraemia and when H_2O intake has to be restricted. In less acute situations, sodium bicarbonate can be given by mouth as a 60–80 mmol/litre solution. Various formulas have been recommended to calculate the amount of bicarbonate to be given to correct the hypobasaemia ranging from 20%–60% of body weight multiplied by the variation of plasma bicarbonate desired. We have found the following formula to be effective when bicarbonate is administered rapidly.

Quantity of bicarbonate = plasma
bicarbonate ×
0.4 body wt.

But, in acute situations, it is best to calculate bicarbonate as the difference between 20 mmol/litre and the observed level of plasma bicarbonate. If endogenous acid production is continuing at an accelerated rate, the expected level of plasma bicarbonate may not be attained or sustained for a significant period of time. Inversely, metabolic alkalosis may result after cessation of production and metabolization of endogenous acids. Therapy should thus be guided by close monitoring of the patient's acid-base status.

Haemodialysis or peritoneal dialysis is advisable as a means of restoring buffer stores in anuric patients with a circulatory overload. But lactate or acetate should be replaced by bicarbonate in the exchange fluid in patients with lactic acidosis or liver failure. Dialysis may also be used to remove a drug responsible for the acidosis (such as phenformin).

Examples of patient management. The patient with diabetic keto-acidosis requires moderate initial alkalinization only in cases of severe acidosis. After early initiation of insulin administration associated with fluid and electrolyte replacement the production of keto-acids decreases and metabolism of circulating keto-acids proceeds, thus restoring buffer base. With restitution of renal function the excess acid is excreted, with further restoration of buffer base.

In cases of lactic acidosis, the increased production and decreased metabolism of lactic acid may lead to overwhelming acidosis [21]. Bicarbonate should be infused rapidly but the quantities necessary may lead to circulatory overload requiring dialysis. In cases of shock the production of acid ceases and metabolism of acid proceeds, with the correction of circulatory failure. But shock is often unresponsive to treatment in such patients. Peritoneal dialysis with fluid containing bicarbonate should then be attempted.

In anuric patients with severe acidosis, alkalinization will alleviate the disorder until dialysis is performed, but in patients with circulatory overload emergency dialysis should be started.

In patients with advanced chronic renal failure a daily intake of bicarbonate is sometimes required to maintain plasma bicarbonate levels between 20 and 25 mmol/litre. The same is true for patients with tubular acidosis.

Acidosis due to intestinal losses is best treated by replacement of losses by fluids containing electrolytes and 40 mmol sodium bicarbonate/litre PO or IV.

In a patient with ureterosigmoidostomy, potassium depletion is often coincident with acidosis. Correction of acidosis can lead to severe hypokalaemia and death. Both bicarbonate and potassium should be administered simultaneously and the effects closely monitored on the ECG and by repeated serum measurements. Treatment should include adequate fluid and electrolyte administration and rectal catheterization to prevent stagnation of urine in the rectum.

Metabolic alkalosis

Metabolic alkalosis is characterized by an increase in whole-body buffer base, with or without decreased hydrogen ion activity (alkalaemia) in the extracellular space, due to retention of bicarbonate or loss of acid from the body.

Generation, maintenance and clinical conditions

The generation of metabolic alkalosis results from an increased bicarbonate load due to infusion of alkaline salts, increased renal bicarbonate reabsorption, or loss of gastric juice [1]. These mechanisms and the corresponding clinical settings are depicted in Table 25.9. The normal kidney has a great capacity to excrete a bicarbonate load and for a state of metabolic alkalosis to be maintained renal function must be organically or functionally altered. Renal failure due to a diminished nephron mass limits the capacity of the kidney to excrete both acid and bicarbonate, but, even with a normal nephron mass, various pathological conditions enhance renal bicarbonate reabsorption and generation despite an increase in plasma bicarbonate to above normal values, thus maintaining a state of metabolic alkalosis (Table 25.10).

Therapeutic management is based on the correction of these factors. Among these, potassium deficiency stands out as a frequent cause of metabolic alkalosis.

Contraction alkalosis, although usually classified among the mechanisms of metabolic alkalosis, does not conform to the definition given above. Indeed, whole-body buffer base remains normal despite the rise in the level of plasma bicarbonate due to a decrease in extracellular volume.

Table 25.9. Metabolic alkalosis

Generation	Clinical conditions
I. Loss of acid	
Loss of gastric fluid	Vomiting or aspiration of acid gastric fluid
Loss of acid into cells and increased urinary excretion of acid	Potassium deficiency with excessive mineralocorticoid activity
Loss of acid into stool	Congenital chloride-losing diarrhoea
II. Gain of bicarbonate	
Oral or parenteral loads of bicarbonate or alkalinizing salts	Excessive bicarbonate administration, milk alkali syndrome
	Excessive administration of lactate or acetate
	Massive blood transfusions (citrate)
Conversion of accumulated metabolic acids to bicarbonate	Hypercalcaemia (?)
Increased reabsorption of bicarbonate	Post-ventilation period in a patient with chronic hypercapnia
Undue retention of bicarbonate	
III. Contraction alkalosis	

Table 25.10. Maintenance of metabolic alkalosis

I. Increased proximal bicarbonate reabsorption
  A. Increased hydrogen ion secretion
    Hypercapnia
    Potassium deficiency
    Phosphate excess (?)
  B. Diminished bicarbonate back-leak
    Reduced effective arterial blood volume
    Hypoparathyroidism with reduced AMP (?)
II. Increased distal bicarbonate reabsorption
  A. Persistent mineralocorticoid excess
  B. Potassium deficiency
  C. Hypercalcaemia
III. Diminished nephron mass

Adapted from Seldin [27].

Consequences of metabolic alkalosis

Clinical manifestations. A variety of clinical symptoms have been attributed to the elevation of blood pH. But many of these symptoms can, in fact, be due to the consequent hypokalaemia which may attain very low levels in cases of concomitant potassium depletion. They include muscle weakness, or paralysis, ileus, abdominal distension, and cardiac arrhythmias.

Tetanic manifestations and convulsions are rarely observed, in contrast to the situation in respiratory alkalosis. This may be due to the protection afforded by the hypokalaemia and the normal or elevated PCO_2 which usually accompany metabolic alkalosis.

Laboratory findings. Hypochloraemia is a natural consequence of hyperbasaemia due, in particular, to chloride loss proportional to the gain in bicarbonate, as in loss of gastric juice, or dilu-

tion of chloride, as in excessive administration of sodium bicarbonate.

Moderate hypokalaemia due to an intracellular shift of potassium usually accompanies metabolic alkalosis. But serum potassium will be further decreased by potassium depletion, whether cause or consequence of metabolic alkalosis. A high urinary excretion of potassium is an indiication that the primary disorder is a state of renal potassium losing.

Hypercapnia often accompanies metabolic alkalosis. It does not usually exceed 50 mmHg, except in patients with pulmonary insufficiency [27]. Arterial PO_2 decreases in proportion to the increase in PCO_2 independently of pulmonary malfunction.

The haemoglobin dissociation curve is displaced toward the left, thus decreasing the capacity to deliver O_2 to the tissues. The ionized fraction of serum calcium decreases and may induce tetany or even convulsions.

The bioavailability of certain drugs may be modified by the increase in blood pH alone, but also by the above concomitant disturbances.

Principles of therapy

Treatment is based on correction of the underlying pathophysiological mechanism. In the case of volume contraction, extracellular volume should be restored. Potassium salts should be administered over several days to correct any deficit. In cases of primary hyperaldosteronism, spironolactone will help to correct the potassium depletion. When drug administration, such as that of ACTH or diuretics, is held responsible it must be discontinued whenever possible.

Carbonic anhydrase inhibition with acetazolamide can be useful in post-ventilation metabolic alkalosis.

Parenteral administration of acid in the form of an arginine hydrochloride hydrochloric acid or ammonium chloride solution is rarely required. It may nevertheless be necessary in a patient with continuing loss of acid gastric juice as in pyloric obstruction. Major alkalosis should be corrected before anaesthesia.

Haemodialysis will correct alkalosis along with the other metabolic disorders in patients with severe renal failure.

References

1. Arruda JAL, Kurtzman NA (1977) Metabolic acidosis and alkalosis. Clin Nephrol 7:201–215
1a. Adrogue HJ, Madais NE (1981) Changes in plasma potassium during acute acid–base disturbances. Am J Med 71:456–467
2. Cardella CJ (1979) Role of dialysis in the treatment of severe hypercalcemia: Report of two cases successfully treated with hemodialysis and review of the literature. Clin Nephrol 12:285–290
3. Chonko A, Bay WH, Stein JH, Ferris TF (1977) The role of renin and aldosterone in the salt retention of edema. Am J Med 63:881–889
4. Dessertene F, Gourgon R, Coumel P, Fabiato A (1971) Tachycardie ventriculaire et torsades de pointe. Ann Cardiol Angeiol (Paris) 20:234–251
5. Editorial (1971) Ketones and coma. N Engl J Med 284:328–329
6. Fourrier F, Chopin C, Durocher A, Wattel F (1980) Hypokaliémie au cours des noyades en eau douce. Nouv Presse Med 9:714
7. Fulop M (1979) Serum potassium in lactic acidosis and ketoacidosis. N Engl J Med 300:1087–1089
8. Howorth PJN (1974) RIpH revisited. Lancet I:253–254
9. Juan D (1979) Hypocalcemia. Differential diagnosis and mechanisms. Arch Intern Med 139:1166–1171
10. Katz MA (1973) Hyperglycemia – induced hyponatremia. Calculation of expected serum sodium depression. N Engl J Med 289:843–844
11. Knochel JP (1977) The pathophysiology and clinical characteristics of severe hypophosphatemia. Arch Intern Med 137:203–220
12. Kokko JP (1977) The role of the renal concentrating mechanisms in the regulation of serum sodium concentration. Am J Med 62:165–169
13. Loeb JN (1974) The hyperosmolar state. N Engl J Med 290:1184–1187
14. Marx SJ, Stock JL, Attie MF, Downs RW, Gardner DG, Brown EM, Spiegel AM, Doppman JL, Brennan MF (1980) Familial hypocalciuric hypercalcemia: Recognition among patients referred after unsuccessful parathyroid exploration. Ann Intern Med 92:351–356
15. Massry SG, Seelig MS (1977) Hypomagnesemia and hypermagnesemia. Clin Nephrol 7:147–153
16. Maxwell MH, Kleeman CR (eds) (1980) Clinical disorders of fluid and electrolyte metabolism, 3rd edn. McGraw-Hill, New York
17. Mudge GH (1975) Diuretics and other agents employed in the mobilization of edema fluid. In: Goodman LS, Gilman A (eds) The pharmacological basis of therapeutics, 5th ed. Macmillan, New York, London, pp 817–847
18. Nahas G (ed) (1966) Current concepts of acid–base measurements. Ann NY Acad Sci 133: Art 1 pp 1–274
19. O'Connor LR, Klein KL, Bethune JE (1977) Hyperphosphatemia in lactic acidosis. N Engl J Med 297:707–709
20. Oh MS, Carroll HJ (1977) Current concepts. The anion gap. N Engl J Med 297:814–817
21. Park R, Arieff AI (1980) Lactic acidosis. In: Advances in internal medicine, vol 25. Year Book Medical Publishers, Chicago, pp 33–68
22. Peters JP, Van Slyke DD (1931) Quantitative clinical chemistry. Baillière, Tindall and Cox, London, Vol I p 811
23. Richet G, Ardaillou R, Amiel C, Paillard M, Kanfer A (1979) Equilibre hydro-électrolytique normal et pathologique, 4th edn. Baillière, Paris
24. Robertson GM, Moore EW, Switz DM, Sizemore GW, Estep HL (1976) Inadequate parathyroid response in acute pancreatitis. N Engl J Med 294:512–516
24a. Schambelan M, Sebastian A, Rector FCJ (1981) Mineralocorticoid resistant renal hyperkalemia without salt wasting (type II pseudo-hypoaldosteronism): role of increased chloride reabsorption. Kidney Int 19:716–727
25. Schrier RW (1978) New treatments for hyponatremia. N Engl J Med 289:214–215
26. Schwartz WB, Relman AJ (1963) A critique of the parameters used in the evaluation of acid base disorders. N Engl J Med 268:1382–1388
27. Seldin DW (1976) Metabolic alkalosis. In: Brenner BM, Rector FC (eds) The kidney. Saunders, Philadelphia, London, pp 661–702
28. Sheldon GF, Grzyb S (1975) Phosphate depletion and repletion. Relation to parenteral nutrition and oxygen transport. Ann Surg 182:683–689
29. Sigaard–Andersen O (1960) A new acid–base nomogram. Scand J Clin Lab Invest 12:177–186
30. Singer FR, Bethune JE, Massry SG (1977) Hypercalcemia and hypocalcemia. Clin Nephrol 7:154–162
31. Swaminathan R, Bradley P, Morgan DB (1979) Hypophosphatemia in surgical patients. Surg Gynecol Obstet 148:448–454
32. Vertel RM, Knochel JP (1967) Acute renal failure due to heat injury. Am J Med 43:435–451
33. Winter RJ, Harris CJ, Phillips LS, Green OC (1979) Diabetic ketoacidosis. Induction of hypocalcemia and hypomagnesemia by phosphate therapy. Am J Med 67:897–900

Chapter 26

Nutritional Failure

Harry M. Shizgal

The nutritional state is one of the major determinants of the ultimate course of a critically ill patient, especially for the patient subjected to a prolonged catabolic stress. Generally, the critically ill patient is unable to maintain an adequate oral intake of nutrients, and must rely on endogenous fuels. The body stores of carbohydrate, in the form of muscle and hepatic glycogen, are minimal. In the reference 70-kg man, there are 150 and 75 g glycogen in skeletal muscle and liver, respectively [3]. These glycogen stores are depleted within the first 24–48 h of starvation. Subsequently, the body relies on triglycerides from adipose tissue and amino acids from body protein. One of the primary functions of adipose tissue is to provide a source of endogenous calories when the supply of exogenous nutrients is inadequate. However, a labile pool of body protein is unavailable. All the proteins that are broken down during periods of starvation serve either a structural or functional role. The skeletal muscles are the major source of this protein, although the viscera are also involved in this process. This catabolism of body protein is responsible for many of the functional abnormalities associated with injury and starvation.

Normal body composition

Body weight, or total body mass, encompasses two major components; body fat (BF) and lean body mass (LBM). The LBM is equivalent to the fat-free mass and consists of the extracellular mass (ECM) and the body cell mass (BCM). As a result it is anatomically and metabolically heterogenous (Fig. 26.1). Moore et al. [18] defined the body cell mass "as that component of body composition containing the oxygen-exchanging, potassium-rich, glucose-oxidizing, work-performing tissue". It is therefore the metabolically active energy-exchanging mass of the body, and as such can serve as a reference for the metabolic activity of the body as measured by O_2 consumption, CO_2 production, caloric requirement, and work performance. The BCM is the sum of all the cellular elements of the body. It includes the cells of both smooth and skeletal muscle, the viscera, the nerve tissue, and the cellular components of those tissues with a sparse cellular population (cartilage, tendon, and adipose tissue). Skeletal muscle represents approximately 60% of the BCM, while the viscera account for 20%–30%. Red cells, and the cellular mass of adipose and connective tissue and the skeleton comprise the remainder.

The ECM is the component of the fat-free mass that surrounds the cellular mass. It is not

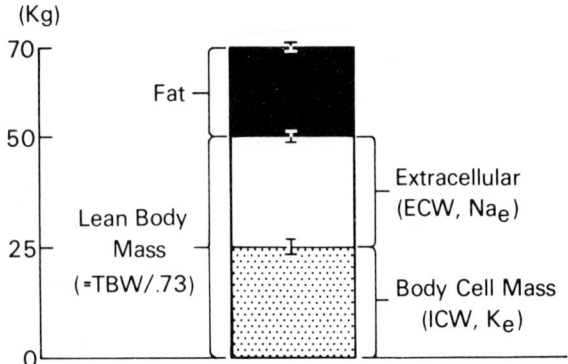

Fig. 26.1. The mean body composition of 25 normal volunteers. Total body mass in kilograms is the sum of BF and the LBM. The LBM is in turn the sum of the ECM and the BMC.

metabolically active, does not consume O_2, and does not perform work. Rather, it is largely concerned with transport and support. The fluid component of the ECM consists of plasma, interstitial, and transcellular water. Transcellular water is extracellular water that is secreted into a well-defined space such as the lumen of the gastro-intestinal tract (GI) and the cerebral, spinal, and joint spaces. The solid component of the ECM includes collagen, tendon, fascia, and the skeleton.

A variety of techniques have been employed to quantatively assess body composition. The earliest measurement involved underwater weighing to determine LBM [1]. Biologically the BCM is a more important body-compositional parameter than the LBM. As a result, the majority of the current body composition measurements involve the measurement of total body potassium to estimate the size of the cellular mass. This is because 98% of total body potassium is within the cellular compartment and the intracellular potassium concentration varies within a narrow range. Total body potassium is therefore linearly related to the size of the BCM. Total body potassium can be determined by measuring the total body content of potassium-40 by means of a whole-body counter [4]. Potassium-40, a radioactive isotope of potassium, accounts for 0.012% of all naturally occurring potassium. However, the total-body counter is an expensive installation, and its calibration remains a difficult problem.

The BCM can also be determined by measuring total-body nitrogen by means of neutron-activation analysis. This involves irradiating the subject with neutrons from either a cyclotron or a plutonium source [14, 29]. The bombarding neutrons momentarily render the nitrogen

atoms radioactive, and they decay with the emission of a gamma ray of a specific energy. Total-body nitrogen is determined by counting these gamma rays with a whole-body counter. Calibration of the counter to take account of the geometry of the subject remains a difficult problem. Moore et al. [18] employed multiple-isotope dilution to measure body composition. Potassium-42 was used to measure total exchangeable potassium (K_e), which is equivalent to total body potassium. Potassium-42 is a relatively unstable radioisotope of potassium, and decays rapidly with a half-life of 12.5 h. To overcome the difficulties associated with whole-body counting, and with the use of the rapidly decaying radioactive isotopes of potassium, a technique for the indirect measurement of potassium was developed [26].

In our laboratory, body composition is measured by multiple-isotope dilution [27], which involves the simultaneous IV injection of 10 μCi iodine-125-labelled human serum albumin (RISA), 50 μCi chromium-51-tagged autologous red cells, 8 μCi sodium-22, and 500 μCi tritiated water. Venous blood samples are obtained at 10-min intervals between 60 and 110 min and at 4 and 24 h. To correct for isotope loss during the 24-h equilibration period, all the body fluids excreted and drained during this period, are collected and counted. The red cell mass (RBC) is determined from the mean chromium-51 whole blood concentration between 60 and 110 min. The plasma (PV) and extracellular water (ECW) volumes are determined by plotting the logarithm of the plasma concentration of RISA and sodium-22, respectively, against time for the period between 60 and 110 min. Time is plotted as the independent variable. To obtain the respective volumes, the resultant straight line obtained by least-squares fitting is reverse-extrapolated to the time of isotope injection. The plasma sodium-22 specific activity at 24 h is used to obtain total exchangeable sodium (Na_e). Total body water (TBW) is determined from the plasma tritium concentration at 24 h. Appropriate corrections are made for the Donnan equilibrium and plasma water concentration. Total exchangeable potassium is determined from

$$K_e = TBW \times R - Na_e,$$

where R is the ratio of the sodium plus potassium content of whole blood divided by the water content. The validity of this measurement of K_e has been established in both man and experimental animals [26]. Additional parameters of body composition are obtained as follows:

$$BV = RBC + PV$$
$$ICW = TBW - ECW$$
$$LBM = TBW/0.73$$
$$BF = \text{Body weight} - LBM$$
$$BCM = 0.00833\ K_e$$
$$ECM = LBM - BCM$$

where BV = blood volume, ICW = intracellular water volume.

The body composition of 25 normal volunteers (15 males and 10 females) is listed in Table 26.1. Their mean body weight was 70.4 kg, of which 20.1 kg was BF. Mean BCM was 24.6 kg, with an ECM of similar size. To correct for body size, the various components of body composition are expressed as a function of TBW, which is a better measure of body size than body weight as it is linearly related to the LBM. Thus, K_e/TBW and ICW/TBW are both measures of the BCM normalized for body size, while Na_e/TBW and ECW/TBW are similarly related to the ECM. Body composition, expressed as a function of TBW, permits the comparison of individuals and groups of individuals of different body size.

Starvation and injury

During periods of either partial or total starvation, endogenous fuels are utilized to meet the daily energy requirements. Since the available glycogen stores are meagre and depleted within the initial 24 h of total starvation, the starving individual must rely on body protein and lipid [19]. During the first few days of total starvation, the normal unstressed 70-kg man breaks down approximately 75 g protein, primarily from skeletal muscle, and 160 g adipose tissue, which provides 1800 calories [3]. The amino acids released as a result of the breakdown of body protein are converted to glucose, which is required by those tissues (principally the CNS) which rely on glucose as their primary fuel. This gluconeogenesis from body protein results in a daily negative nitrogen balance of 12 g (Fig. 26.2). The normal unstressed individual adapts to starvation with an increased reliance on lipids as the major endogenous fuel, and thus gluconeogenesis from protein is decreased. As a result, the daily urinary nitrogen loss decreases from 12 g, early in starvation, to 5 g by the 4th week of starvation. This nitrogen loss represents a significant loss of BCM (Fig. 26.3). In the first few days of total starvation, the BCM decreases by 300 g/day but this loss is reduced to 125 g/day by the 4th week. The total loss of BCM during this 4-week period of total starvation (Fig. 26.4) is 5.7 kg, which in the reference 70-kg man represents 38% of his skeletal muscle mass or 23% of the BCM. It has been estimated that a loss of 50%–60% of BCM is incompatible with survival.

The traumatized patient, in contrast to the unstressed starved individual, is unable to increase his reliance on endogenous lipids, and subsequently decrease the rate of gluconeogenesis from protein. In addition, trauma causes an increase in both the resting metabolic rate and urinary nitrogen. The magnitude of this metabolic response is directly proportional to the severity of trauma. Kinney [17] has described an increase in the resting metabolic expenditure of 10% following uncomplicated elective operations, 10%–25% with multiple fractures, 20%–50% with major sepsis, (e.g., peritonitis), and 50%–125% with a major thermal burn. There is a similar increase in the

Table 26.1. Normal body composition

	Mean ± SEM	95% confidence limits Lower	Upper
Body weight (kg)	70.4 ± 2.5	45.6	95.2
Body fat (kg)	20.1 ± 1.4	6.4	33.7
Lean body mass (kg)	50.4 ± 1.9	31.8	69.0
Body cell mass (kg)	24.6 ± 1.1	14.0	35.2
Extracellular mass (kg)	25.8 ± 0.9	16.9	34.6
K_e/TBW (mmol/litre)	80.0 ± 1.0	69.9	90.1
ICW/TBW (%)	57.5 ± 1.1	47.0	67.9
Na_e/TBW (mmol/litre)	77.5 ± 0.9	68.3	86.6
ECW/TBW (%)	42.5 ± 1.1	32.1	53.0
Na_e/K_e	0.98 ± 0.4	0.75	1.22
PV/TBW (%)	7.4 ± 0.2	5.4	9.4
RBC/TBW (%)	5.0 ± 0.1	3.9	6.0
BV/TBW (%)	12.4 ± 0.2	10.4	14.4

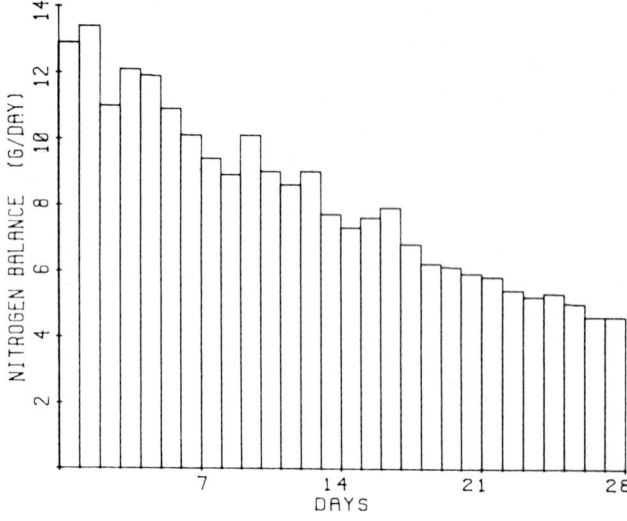

Fig. 26.2. The daily urinary nitrogen loss in a
normal unstressed 70-kg man subjected to total
starvation. Data adapted from Owen OE, Felig P,
Morgan AP, Wahren J, Cahill GF: Liver and kidney
metabolism during prolonged starvation. J Clin
Invest. 48:574–583, 1969.

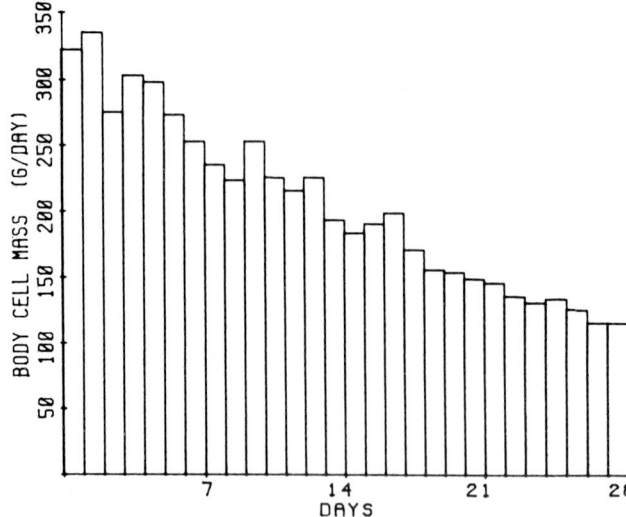

Fig. 26.3. The daily loss of BCM with total
starvation in the 70-kg man, obtained by
multiplying urinary nitrogen data (plotted in
Fig. 26.2) by 25.

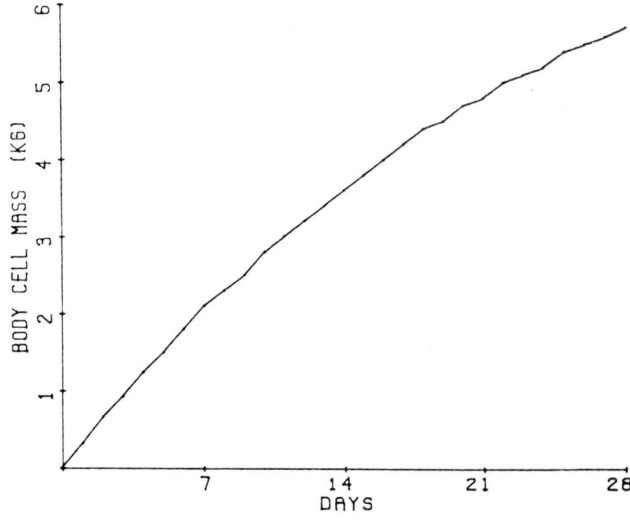

Fig. 26.4. The cumulative loss of BCM with total
uncomplicated starvation. Adapted from the data
plotted in Fig. 26.2.

daily nitrogen loss, which ranges from 10 to 15 g/day, following an uncomplicated operation of moderate severity. When injury is complicated · with sepsis, the daily nitrogen loss increases to 15–25 g/day. With severe injury and sepsis (thermal burns), it may rise to 35 g/day. These large nitrogen losses represent an extensive erosion of the BCM. Cumulative BCM losses, with various rates of nitrogen loss, are depicted in Fig. 26.5. A nitrogen loss of 10 g/day for 1 month results in a 7-kg loss of BCM, which is equivalent to 47% of the skeletal muscle mass or 28% of the BCM. A negative nitrogen balance of 30 g/day for 1 week results

in a 5.3-kg loss of BCM. At this rate, by $2\frac{1}{2}$ weeks, over 50% of the BCM is lost. Thus starvation and injury, especially when complicated with sepsis, results in a rapid erosion of the cellular mass.

The effect of moderate injury and starvation was demonstrated by body composition measurements performed before and after an elective operation of moderate severity in 19 normally nourished patients [24]. The majority of patients underwent either a gastrectomy or a colon resection. Body composition was determined pre-operatively and on the 5th post-operative day (Table 26.2). Their body

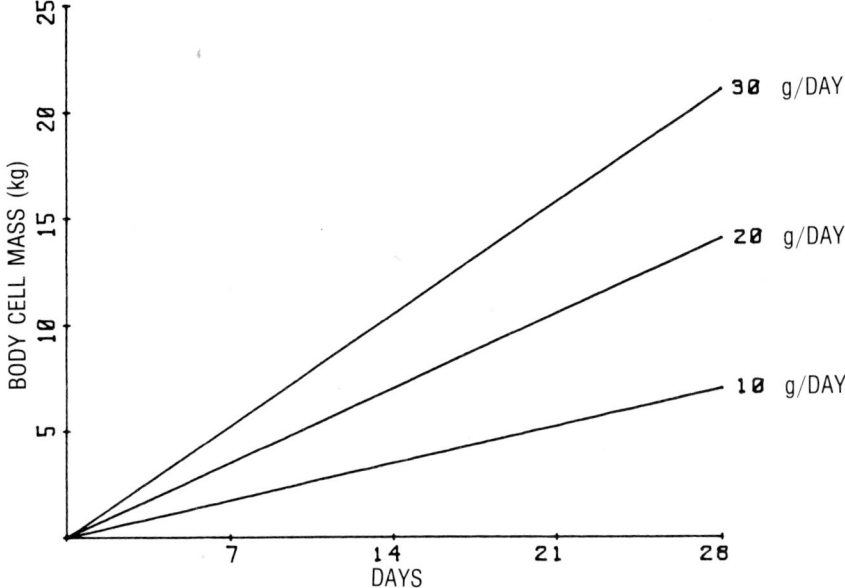

Fig. 26.5. The cumulative loss of BCM in the starved and stressed individual with nitrogen losses of 10, 20, and 30 g/day. In the reference 70-kg man the BCM is 25 kg, of which the skeletal muscle is 15 kg.

Table 26.2. Body composition following operation of moderate severity

	No.	Normal	Pre-op.	5th postop. day	Difference (kg)	(%)
Body weight (kg)	19	70.4 ± 2.5	66.2 ± 1.9	63.5 ± 1.8[a]	−2.6 ± 0.6	−3.9
Body fat (kg)	19	20.2 ± 1.4	18.2 ± 1.6	16.4 ± 1.5[a]	−1.8 ± 0.9	−9.9
Lean body mass (kg)	19	50.3 ± 1.9	48.0 ± 1.8	47.2 ± 1.6	−0.8 ± 0.6	−1.7
Extracellular mass (kg)	19	25.8 ± 0.9	24.9 ± 0.9	27.3 ± 0.9	2.4 ± 0.5	9.6
Body cell mass (kg)	19	24.7 ± 1.1	23.1 ± 1.5	19.9 ± 1.4[a]	−3.2 ± 0.6	−13.9
K_e/TBW (mmol/litre)	19	80.0 ± 1.0	78.2 ± 2.8	68.3 ± 3.1[a]		
ICW/TBW (mmol/litre)	10	57.5 ± 1.1	55.7 ± 1.9	53.5 ± 1.6		
Na_e/TBW (mmol/litre)	19	77.4 ± 0.9	77.3 ± 2.1	82.5 ± 2.2[a]		
ECW/TBW (mmol/litre)	10	42.5 ± 1.1	44.3 ± 1.9	46.5 ± 1.6		
Na_e/K_e	19	0.98 ± .02	1.04 ± .08	1.29 ± .11[a]		
PV/TBW (%)	10	7.4 ± 0.2	8.0 ± 0.6	8.1 ± 0.5		
RBC/TBW (%)	10	5.0 ± 0.1	4.4 ± 0.2	4.4 ± 0.5		
BV/TBW (%)	10	12.4 ± 0.2	12.3 ± 0.5	12.7 ± 0.7		

[a]Significantly ($P < 0.05$) different from preoperative mean by paired Student's t-test.

composition prior to surgery was normal. By the 5th postoperative day these patients had lost 1.8 ± 0.9 kg BF and 3.2 ± 0.6 kg from their BCM, which is 13.9% of their pre-operative BCM. The resected specimen accounted for a portion of this loss of cellular mass. The decrease in the BCM was accompanied by a concomitant expansion of the ECM by 2.4 ± 0.5 kg. As a result, the 3.9% (2.6 ± 0.6 kg) loss of body weight was not a good reflection of the 13.9% decrease in the cellular mass. These postoperative changes in body composition are consistent with the development of mild malnutrition.

Similar measurements were performed in 75 clinically diagnosed malnourished patients [24]. The majority had developed postoperative complications, and all had been referred for a course of total parenteral nutrition (TPN). Their body composition was characterized by a contracted BCM (Fig. 26.6). The K_e/TBW and ICW/TBW,

which are both measures of the BCM corrected for body size, were significantly different from normal (Table 26.3). This loss of cellular mass was accompanied by an expansion of the ECM (Fig. 26.6). Thus, Na_e/TBW and ECW/TBW were both significantly elevated above normal (Table 26.3).

The Na_e/K_e ratio was also significantly elevated in both postoperative (Table 26.2) and malnourished patients (Table 26.3). This ratio, a measure of the ECM expressed as a function of the BCM, is a sensitive index of the nutritional state. In normally nourished subjects the BCM and ECM are approximately equal in size and therefore the Na_e/K_e ratio approximates unity (Table 26.1). With malnutrition, this ratio increases because of the reciprocal changes in the BCM and ECM. In 25 normally nourished volunteers, the upper 95% confidence limit was 1.22. We have therefore used a $Na_e/K_e > 1.22$ to

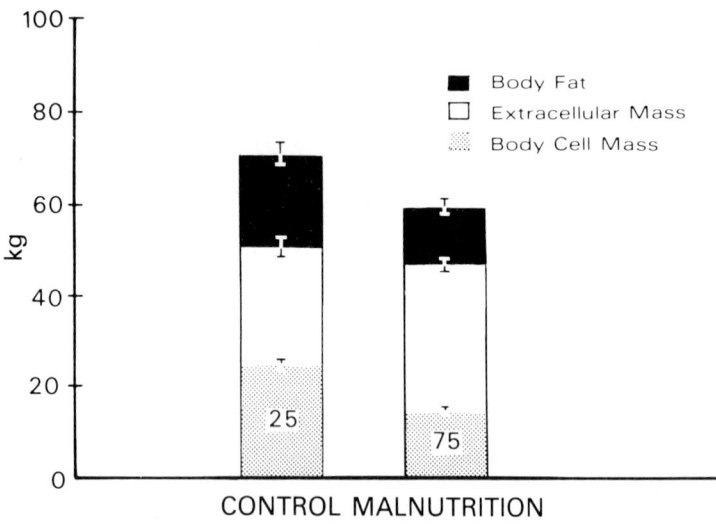

Fig. 26.6. The body composition of 25 normally nourished volunteers and 75 clinically malnourished patients. The means ($\pm$SEM) for BF, ECM, and BCM were plotted.

Table 26.3. Body composition in severe malnutrition

	Normal volunteers	Malnourished patients	Difference kg	%	$P<$
Number	25	75			
Body weight (kg)	70.4 ± 2.5	58.9 ± 1.8	-11.5	-16	0.001
Body fat (kg)	20.2 ± 1.4	12.7 ± 1.2	-7.5	-37	0.01
Lean body mass (kg)	50.3 ± 1.9	46.5 ± 1.3	-3.8	-8	NS
Extracellular mass (kg)	25.8 ± 0.9	31.9 ± 0.9	6.1	24	0.001
Body cell mass (kg)	24.7 ± 1.1	14.7 ± 0.6	-10.0	-40	0.001
K_e/TBW (mmol/litre)	80.0 ± 1.0	51.8 ± 1.2			0.001
ICW/TBW (%)	57.5 ± 1.1	49.1 ± 0.9			0.001
Na_e/TBW (mmol/litre)	77.4 ± 0.9	94.7 ± 0.9			0.001
ECW/TBW (%)	42.5 ± 1.1	50.9 ± 0.9			0.001
Na_e/K_e	0.98 ± 0.02	1.95 ± 0.08			0.001
PV/TBW (%)	7.4 ± 0.2	8.4 ± 0.2			0.01
RBC/TBW (%)	5.0 ± 0.1	3.8 ± 0.1			0.001
BV/TBW (%)	12.4 ± 0.2	12.3 ± 0.3			NS

define malnutrition. The validity of this definition of malnutrition has been confirmed by body composition measurements performed during the past several years in over 1700 patients [10].

The importance of nutritional support

The importance of nutritional support in general, and parenteral nutrition in particular, has been recognized for many years. The increased complication rate in surgical patients with protein-calorie malnutrition has been a common clinical observation. Studley [28] was one of the first to document this when, in 1936, he correlated weight loss with morbidity and mortality in a group of patients undergoing surgery for peptic ulcer disease. A mortality rate of 33% was observed in patients with malnutrition, as defined by a 20% loss of body weight. The majority of fatalities were secondary to infection. In the remaining patients, the mortality rate was 3.5%. Rhoads and Alexander [21] similarly reported an increased incidence of infection in surgical patients suffering from malnutrition. In this study, the serum albumin concentration was used to evaluate the nutritional state.

Elman was the first to emphasize the importance of parenteral nutrition. In a paper published in 1939, he emphasized that "intravenous alimentation becomes important whenever the nutritional needs of the body cannot be met by oral feeding; it becomes essential when death threatens because of nutritional deficiencies which can be remedied in no other way" [7]. Although amino acids had previously been administered IV in the experimental animal, this was the first time that amino acids were successfully infused in humans. The amino acids were obtained by the acid hydrolysis of casein, to which tryptophan and cystine were added. The importance of administering the amino acids with a caloric source was recognized by Elman. He reported that "dextrose was always added, not only because of its caloric value, but also because there is considerable evidence that the utilization of amino acids is enhanced by the presence of carbohydrate."

Despite the widespread availability of a variety of solutions of hydrolysed proteins for IV administration, TPN was not accepted as a practical method of nutritional support, primarily because its efficacy had not been demonstrated. Prior to 1967, it was generally accepted that lasting anabolism and a gain of cellular mass was not possible with parenteral nutrition alone. In 1967, at the annual meeting of the American College of Surgeons, Dudrick et al. reported normal growth and development in a group of beagle puppies who received all their nutrition by the parenteral route [5]. Since then a large number of reports have appeared in the literature testifying to the clinical benefits of TPN. The effect of TPN on the mortality associated with enteric–cutaneous fistulas is an excellent example of the importance of nutritional support. Prior to the advent of TPN, the mortality of patients with this complication was 20%–54% [6, 22]. A significant reduction in the mortality rate occurred when these patients were treated with long-term TPN [23]. This was nicely demonstrated by a retrospective review in our institution of 91 cases of small-bowel fistula [15]. Sixty-six patients were treated prior to the introduction of TPN (Table 26.4).

Table 26.4. Small-bowel fistulas

	No nutrition	Parenteral nutrition
Non-surgical closure	16	14
Surgical closure	21	9
Recurrence following surgical closure	5	
Deaths	22	2
	66	25

Twenty-two patients died (mortality rate of 33%). Non-operative closure of the fistula occurred in 18 (27%), while in 21 (32%) surgical closure was successful. In 5 (8%) a fistula recurred following an attempt at surgical closure. TPN was administered as part of the clinical treatment in 25 of the 91 patients. The fistula closed without surgery in 14 (56%) and a surgical procedure was required in 9 (36%). There were only two deaths, giving a mortality rate of 8%. Thus, the addition of nutritional support to the treatment of patients with enteric cutaneous fistulas resulted in a significant decrease in mortality. The provision of calories and amino acids prevented the patients from dying because of starvation during the period of time required for the fistula to close. Nutritional support of the critically ill patient prevents malnutrition and improves the individual's ability to repair injured tissues successfully and effectively to counteract such stressful insults as shock and sepsis.

Nutritional assessment

Nutritional support in the critically ill patient may be associated with serious, and occasionally life-threatening, complications. This is true of both enteral and parenteral nutrition. It is therefore important to identify those patients who require nutritional support.

For many years, a variety of anthropometric and biochemical measurements have been performed in epidemiological surveys to assess a population's nutritional status. These techniques have recently been applied to assess the nutritional status of the hospitalized patient. Serum albumin is commonly used to assess the nutritional state, as it is usually decreased in the presence of protein-calorie malnutrition. The excretion rate of creatinine, a breakdown product of muscle, is related to the size of the muscle mass. The 24-h excretion rate of creatinine, expressed as a function of body height, has therefore been used to measure the size of the BCM. Similarly, the weight: height ratio and the mid-arm muscle area are a measure of the BCM. An estimate of BF can be obtained by measuring the triceps skin fold.

To evaluate the reliability of the nutritional assessment obtained with these measurements, we determined the serum albumin, serum protein, mid-arm area, triceps skin fold, creatinine/height, hand strength, and weight/height in 216 hospitalized patients [9]. Body composition measurements were simultaneously performed at 2-week intervals. The population consisted of both normal and malnourished patients and morbidly obese individuals who underwent weight reduction surgery. The majority of malnourished patients received TPN.

A statistically significant correlation ($P <$ 0.001) existed between the serum albumin concentration and the K_e/TBW, a measure of the BCM corrected for body size (Fig. 26.7). However, the correlation coefficient was only 0.67 and the 95% confidence limits about the regression were wide. With a normal K_e/TBW of 80.0 mmol/litre (Table 26.1), a serum albumin concentration of 3.8 g/100 ml is obtained from the regression with 95% confidence limits of 2.6 and 5.0 g/100 ml. In our laboratory the normal range for the serum albumin concentration, as determined by electrophoresis, is 3.5–5 g/100 ml. Based on these criteria, our sample population included a number of normally nourished individuals with a subnormal serum albumin (Fig. 26.7). There were also malnourished individuals with a normal serum albumin.

Similar results were obtained with the other parameters examined. The data are summarized in Tables 26.5, where the anthropometric and biochemical parameters are tabulated in descending order of their correlation coefficients. Although all the correlation coefficients were statistically significant ($P < 0.05$), the correla-

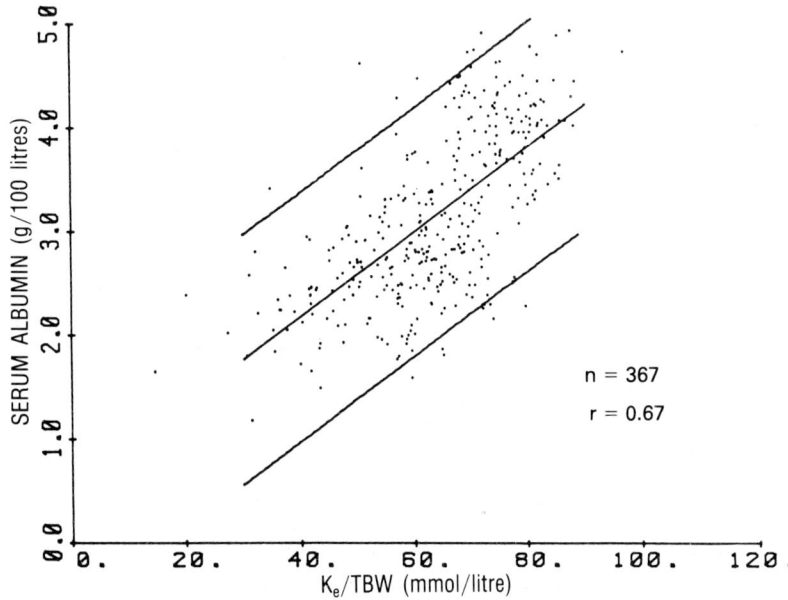

n = 367

r = 0.67

Fig. 26.7. The serum albumin concentration was correlated with the BCM, as measured by the K_e, divided by TBW to correct for body size. The resulting regressions in 367 studies were statistically significant ($P < 0.001$), with a correlation coefficient of 0.67.

tions were poor. In all instances, the 95% confidence limits were wide. In Table 26.5 the 95% confidence limits are tabulated with the mean of each dependent parameter, which represents the mid-point of each regression. The best correlation ($r = 0.82$) was obtained with the weight: height ratio, and the worst ($r = 0.37$) with creatinine:height.

Data obtained by repeating the measurements in 179 patients permitted an assessment of the ability of the anthropometric and biochemical measurements to detect changes in body composition. Sixty-nine patients were initially malnourished and experienced an improvement in their nutritional status, as indicated by an improvement in body composition (Table 26.6). Since not all the anthropometric and biochemical parameters were measured in each patient, the mean initial and final Na_e/K_e ratios were tabulated with the appropriate component of body composition. In 69 patients there was a significant increase in the BCM accompanied by a significant decrease in the mean Na_e/K_e ratio. This is indicative of an improvement in the nutritional state. In spite of this, there were insignificant changes in weight, mid-arm area, creatinine:height ratio, and hand strength. The serum albumin and total protein

concentration increased by 10%, with a corresponding 19% increase in K_e/TBW ratio. Neither the triceps skin fold nor total BF changed. Similar data were obtained in 25 normally nourished individuals who became malnourished (Table 26.7) and in 42 malnourished patients whose nutritional state deteriorated (Table 26.8).

Nutritional assessment, with the anthropometric and biochemical parameters described, is simple, inexpensive, and reproducible; provides quantitative data; and does not require specialized equipment or specially trained personnel. The presence of a statistically significant correlation between each of the parameters evaluated and the nutritional state indicates that they are accurate measures of the mean nutritional state of a population. They are therefore useful in epidemiological surveys. They are of little value in assessing an individual's nutritional state, however, because they lack sufficient sensitivity and specificity. This was demonstrated by the wide confidence limits and the failure to detect significant changes in the nutritional state.

Similar results were obtained when the nutritional state was evaluated by means of skin testing [11]. A relationship between immune

Table 26.5. Nutritional assessment

Parameter (dependent)	Body composition parameter (independent)	n	r	Mean	95% confidence limits
Weight/height (kg/m)	K_e	331	0.82	48.9	25.3 to 72.5
Tricep skin fold (mm)	Body fat	358	0.79	17.2	3.7 to 30.7
Mid-arm area (dm²)	K_e	358	0.68	0.54	0.10 to 0.98
Albumin (mg/100 ml)	K_e/TBW	367	0.67	3.2	2.0 to 4.4
Total protein (mg/100 ml)	K_e/TBW	367	0.62	6.6	5.0 to 8.2
Hand strength (kp/cm²)	K_e/TBW	86	0.45	0.41	0.03 to 0.79
Creatinine/height (mg/m)	K_e/TBW	331	0.37	7.1	−6.3 to 20.5

Table 26.6. Nutritional assessment in the malnourished patient whose nutritional state improves

Parameter	n	Initial	Final	Body composition Parameter	Initial	Final	Initial Na_e/K_e	Final Na_e/K_e
Albumin (mg/100 ml)	77	2.68 ± 0.07	3.0 ± 0.07[a]	K_e/TBW	54.3 ± 1.2	64.8 ± 1.2[a]	1.87 ± 0.09	1.39 ± 0.05[a]
Total protein (mg/100 ml)	77	6.07 ± 0.12	6.73 ± 0.10[a]	K_e/TBW	54.3 ± 1.2	64.8 ± 1.2[a]	1.87 ± 0.09	1.39 ± 0.05[a]
Weight (kg)	77	64.9 ± 2.8	66.2 ± 2.7	K_e	1764 ± 68	2159 ± 90[a]	1.87 ± 0.09	1.39 ± 0.05[a]
Mid-arm area (dm²)	68	0.44 ± 0.03	0.48 ± 0.04	K_e	1775 ± 71	2185 ± 97[a]	1.79 ± 0.07	1.36 ± 0.04[a]
Tricep skin fold (mm)	68	14.2 ± 1.07	13.2 ± 0.8	Body fat	21.9 ± 1.9	22.1 ± 1.9	1.79 ± 0.07	1.36 ± 0.04[a]
Creatinine/height (mg/m)	61	5.77 ± 0.83	5.79 ± 0.88	K_e/TBW	55.7 ± 1.3	67.3 ± 1.3[a]	1.80 ± 0.10	1.30 ± 0.05[a]
Hand strength (kp/cm²)	26	0.41 ± 0.05	0.43 ± 0.03	K_e/TBW	52.5 ± 1.9	62.0 ± 1.6[a]	1.93 ± 0.18	1.42 ± 0.07[a]

[a] Significantly ($P < 0.05$) different from initial measurement according to paired Student's t-test.

Table 26.7. Nutritional assessment in the normally nourished who develop malnutrition

Parameter	n	Initial	Final	Body composition Parameter	Initial	Final	Initial Na_e/K_e	Final Na_e/K_e
Albumin (mg%)	21	3.47 ± 0.16	3.04 ± 0.15[a]	K_e/TBW	74.5 ± 1.1	61.4 ± 1.6[a]	1.06 ± 0.03	1.51 ± 0.07[a]
Total protein (mg/100 ml)	21	7.06 ± 0.19	6.62 ± 0.25	K_e/TBW	74.5 ± 1.1	61.4 ± 1.6[a]	1.06 ± 0.03	1.51 ± 0.07[a]
Weight (kg)	21	85.2 ± 8.7	83.1 ± 6.7	K_e	2755 ± 213	2197 ± 151[a]	1.06 ± 0.03	1.51 ± 0.07[a]
Mid-arm area (dm²)	19	0.61 ± 0.11	0.62 ± 0.06	K_e	2950 ± 237	2321 ± 186[a]	1.05 ± 0.04	1.63 ± 0.10[a]
Tricep skin fold (mm)	19	22.7 ± 2.9	20.2 ± 2.0	Body fat	42.3 ± 6.6	40.3 ± 4.5	1.05 ± 0.04	1.63 ± 0.10[a]
Creatinine/height (mg/m)	15	8.03 ± 0.85	8.26 ± 1.18	K_e/TBW	74.9 ± 1.8	61.8 ± 1.2[a]	1.04 ± 0.04	1.48 ± 0.05[a]

[a]Significantly ($P < 0.05$) different from initial measurement according to paired Student's t-test.

Table 26.8. Nutritional assessment in the malnourished whose nutritional state deteriorates

Parameter	n	Initial	Final	Body composition Parameter	Initial	Final	Initial Na_e/K_e	Final Na_e/K_e
Albumin (mg/100 ml)	40	2.82 ± 0.08	2.62 ± 0.09[a]	K_e/TBW	60.2 ± 1.1	52.6 ± 1.6[a]	1.56 ± 0.05	2.00 ± 0.09[a]
Total protein (mg/100 ml)	40	6.50 ± 0.15	6.16 ± 0.15[a]	K_e/TBW	60.2 ± 1.1	52.6 ± 1.6[a]	1.56 ± 0.05	2.00 ± 0.09[a]
Weight (kg)	40	68.1 ± 3.9	68.6 ± 3.4	K_e	2074 ± 109	1856 ± 95[a]	1.56 ± 0.05	2.00 ± 0.09[a]
Mid-arm area (dm²)	38	0.45 ± 0.03	0.51 ± 0.06	K_e	2069 ± 98	1814 ± 85[a]	1.60 ± 0.05	2.02 ± 0.08[a]
Tricep skin fold (mm)	38	13.3 ± 1.6	12.7 ± 1.5	Body fat	27.7 ± 3.2	21.2 ± 2.8	1.60 ± 0.05	2.02 ± 0.08[a]
Creatinine/height (mg/m)	32	6.12 ± 1.9	6.16 ± 1.5	K_e/TBW	59.6 ± 1.2	53.4 ± 1.7[a]	1.57 ± 0.06	1.92 ± 0.10[a]
Hand strength (kp/cm²)	8	0.26 ± 0.08	0.34 ± 0.12	K_e/TBW	55.8 ± 3.4	48.1 ± 3.3[a]	1.77 ± 0.15	2.17 ± 0.19[a]

[a]Significantly ($P > 0.05$) different from initial measurement according to paired Student's t-test.

competence and the nutritional state was demonstrated in 257 hospitalized patients (459 studies) receiving TPN. These patients represent a population with a high incidence of malnutrition, in whom it is possible to measure protein and caloric intake accurately. Immune competence was assessed by skin testing with five recall antigens: purified protein derivative of tuberculosis (PPD), mumps, candidin, trichophytin, and streptokinase streptodornase. The patients were classified as normal, relatively anergic, or anergic if they reacted to at least two, one, or none of the recall antigens, respectively. Body composition measurements and skin testing were performed at the beginning and at 2-week intervals during TPN.

A relationship between the nutritional state and the response to skin testing was demonstrated (Table 26.9). A deterioration of immune competence, as indicated by the development of relative anergy or anergy, was associated with a loss of BCM, expansion of the ECM, and increase in the Na_e/K_e ratio. These changes in body composition are characteristic of malnutrition. The differences in body composition between the reactive and anergic patients were

statistically significant, although in each group there were wide 95% confidence limits about the means (Figs. 26.8 and 26.9). To demonstrate the overlap between the normally reactive and anergic patients, each group was subdivided into normally nourished and malnourished patients on the basis of the Na_e/K_e ratio (Fig. 26.10). Ninety-three (43%) of the 216 normally reactive patients were malnourished. The mean K_e/TBW of these patients was 59.7 ± 0.7 mmol/litre, which is significantly ($P < 0.001$) different from normal. Thirty-five (21.3%) of the 129 anergic patients had a normal body composition.

The reliability of skin testing to evaluate the nutritional state is similar to the reliability of the anthropometric and biochemical parameters. A statistically significant relationship exists between the response to skin testing with recall antigens and the nutritional state [11]. However, because of the large variance associated with this response it is of little value for evaluation of an individual's nutritional state. Skin testing can be reliably employed in epidemiological surveys to determine a population's nutritional state.

Table 26.9. The response to skin testing and the nutritional state

	Normal volunteers	Reactive	Relative anergy	Anergy
Number	25	216	79	164
Body weight (kg)	70.4 ± 2.5	61.9 ± 1.0	57.5 ± 1.7^a	59.0 ± 1.2^a
Body fat (kg)	20.2 ± 1.4	15.9 ± 0.7	12.8 ± 1.1^a	$12.3 \pm 0.8^{a,b}$
Lean body mass (kg)	50.3 ± 1.9	46.0 ± 0.7	45.0 ± 1.2	46.6 ± 0.8
Body cell mass (kg)	24.7 ± 1.1	19.7 ± 0.4^a	$17.5 \pm 0.6^{a,b}$	$16.6 \pm 0.4^{a,b}$
Extracellular mass (kg)	25.6 ± 0.9	26.3 ± 0.4	27.5 ± 0.8	$30.1 \pm 0.7^{a,b}$
K_e/TBW (mmol/litre)	80.0 ± 1.0	70.0 ± 0.8^a	$63.7 \pm 1.3^{a,b}$	$58.7 \pm 1.1^{a,b}$
Na_e/TBW (mmol/litre)	77.5 ± 0.9	82.5 ± 0.7	$88.3 \pm 1.4^{a,b}$	$92.6 \pm 1.1^{a,b}$
Na_e/K_e	0.98 ± 0.02	1.23 ± 0.02	$1.47 \pm 0.06^{a,b}$	$1.76 \pm 0.07^{a,b}$

[a]Significantly ($P < 0.05$) different from normal volunteers according to an analysis of variance and Scheffe's test.
[b]Significantly ($P < 0.05$) different from reactive patients according to an analysis of variance and Scheffe's test.

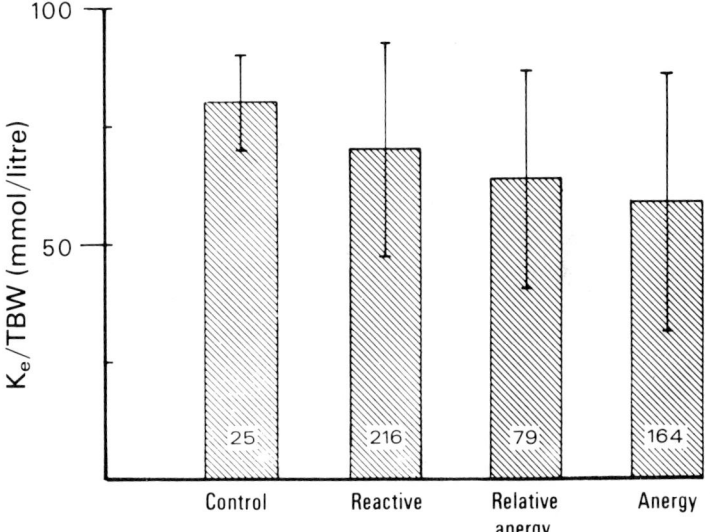

Fig. 26.8. The mean and the 95% confidence limits about the mean (*bars*) for K_e/TBW, a measure of the BCM normalized for body size. Ninety-five percent of the individual data points lie between the two confidence limits. As a result there is considerable overlap of individual data points among the three groups of patients.

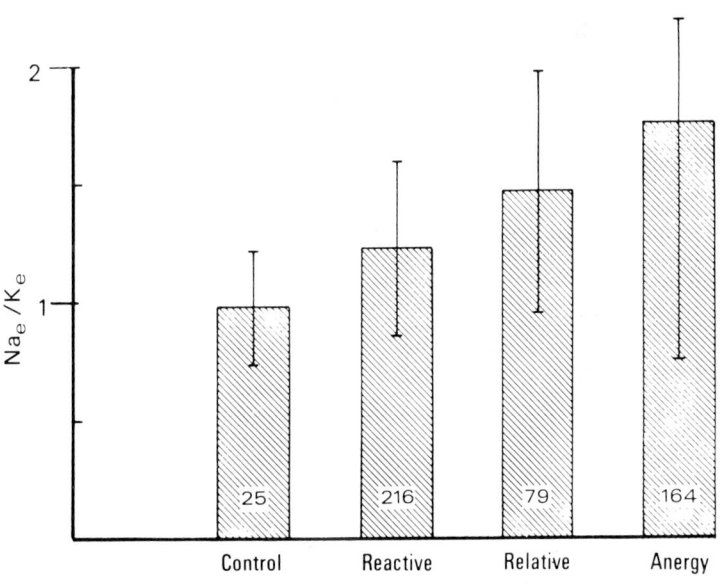

Fig. 26.9. The mean and 95% confidence limits about the mean (*bars*) for Na_e/K_e.

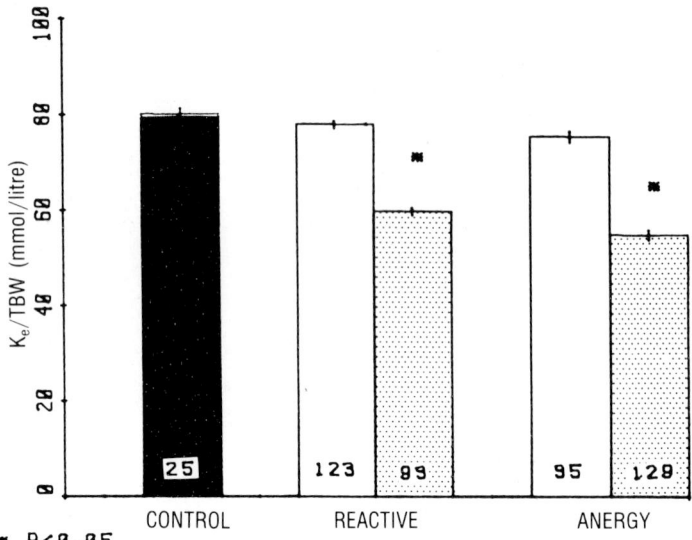

Fig. 26.10. The mean ± SEM for K_e/TBW, a measure of the BCM corrected for body size in normal volunteers and in the reactive and anergic patients who were subdivided into normally nourished (*clear histograms*) and malnourished (*stippled histograms*) subgroups.

Body composition measurements will allow an accurate and quantitative assessment of the nutritional state and determine the efficacy of nutritional support. The measurements are complex and time-consuming, and require specialized facilities and specially trained personnel. They are therefore not suitable for the routine clinical laboratory, but are ideal for research purposes.

A good history and physical examination are often all that is required to establish the requirements for nutritional support. In the majority of patients, the requirement for nutritional support is clinically obvious with no need for specialized measurements. The nature and the duration of nutritional support can also be established clinically. The patient with an obstructing oesophageal carcinoma, a history of decreased food intake, and weight loss should be nutritionally repleted before undergoing a major surgical procedure. During this period, a course of radiotherapy might be appropriate. If possible, a feeding tube should be placed in the stomach and enteric feeding instituted. Otherwise TPN should be instituted. Nutritional repletion is indicated by weight gain, loss of oedema, increased muscle strength, increased work capacity, an improvement in appetite, and a sense of well-being. In contrast, the presence of malnutrition and the need for nutritional repletion should not delay surgical intervention to drain an abscess, relieve bowel obstruction, or drain a septic biliary tract. On the other hand, the absence of malnutrition does not contraindicate nutritional support, especially for the patient in whom it is anticipated that oral intake will be inadequate for a prolonged period of time. Thus, nutritional support is indicated for the patient with an enteric cutaneous fistula even in the absence of malnutrition. For the vast majority of patients, a complete history and physical examination will provide all the information required to arrive at the appropriate decisions regarding nutritional therapy.

Nutritional support

Once it has been established that a patient requires nutritional support, a decision must be made regarding the method of administration. Either the GI tract or the IV route may be used. Nutritional support is best achieved by having a patient eat a balanced diet. However, this requires an intact GI tract and the presence of a normal appetite. An anorexic patient is usually unable to achieve an adequate oral intake. Proper dietary preparation with respect to the composition, preparation, and taste of food will result in a substantial increase in food intake only in the individual with a normal appetite. In the absence of a normal appetite it is extremely difficult to maintain an adequate oral intake. In the comatose or anorexic patient with a normally functioning GI tract, enteric tube feeding is indicated to meet nutritional requirements. A variety of feeding tubes are currently available. A feeding tube may be placed in the stomach by the nasogastric route or by a surgically fashioned gastrostomy. Similarly, tubes may be placed in either the duodenum or jejunum.

Failure to achieve an adequate dietary intake with enteric tube feeding is generally due to the development of either gastric stasis or diarrhoea. In the anorexic patient, enteric tube feeding often fails, in spite of an intact GI tract, because of gastric stasis. This may result in aspiration, one of the most serious complications of enteric tube feeding. The presence of an endotracheal tube is no assurance against aspiration. In the supine patient gastric contents easily flow past a lax oesophagogastric sphincter and up the oesophagus, with subsequent spillage around the inflated ballon. In addition, the presence of a nasogastric tube will often render the oesophagogastric sphincter incompetent.

Diarrhoea is not an uncommon complication of enteric tube feeding. Rapid GI transit is responsible for the development of the diarrhoea associated with enteric tube feeding, and may develop because of defective small-bowel absorption or because the feeding preparation irritates the gut. Inappropriate temperatures and bacterial contamination of the solution may also produce diarrhoea. Many of the enteric preparations are hypertonic. This is especially true of the chemically defined diets, which are composed of amino acids, simple sugars, and triglycerides. The amino acids are either crystalline or are derived from the hydrolysis of intact proteins. These diets require little or no digestion and produce zero residue. At the other end of the spectrum are the tube feedings which are prepared by putting cooked food through a blender. These preparations are available commercially or can easily be prepared by the hospital's dietary department. The commercial products generally provide a more complete diet, are bacteriologically sterile, and because they are less viscous are easily administered with small tubes. They do not require refrigeration and are administered at room temperature. Material prepared in the hospital kitchen for tube feeding may develop bacterial overgrowth and should therefore be refrigerated.

To minimize the complications associated with tube feeding the following protocol is followed in our institution. A small-diameter nasogastric tube, generally a paediatric feeding tube, is placed into the stomach. If the patient is to undergo a laparotomy, a gastrostomy or jejunostomy is performed. The proper placement of the feeding tube is established radiographically. Initially quarter-strength tube feeding is administered at room temperature by means of a continuous infusion pump. The initial rate is 50–75 ml/h. Over the next few days, in the absence of diarrhoea the concentration of the solution and the perfusion rate are gradually increased until the required nutritional intake is achieved. It is important that enteric tube feeding be infused at a constant rate and not as a bolus, as this often produces diarrhoea. If either diarrhoea or gastric stasis develops the infusion rate is reduced. The presence of gastric stasis is determined by aspirating the stomach at hourly intervals. Aspiration of a large volume is indicative of gastric stasis.

We generally prefer a commercially prepared tube feed to a chemically defined diet since it tastes better, is not as hypertonic, and is more economical. In the majority of patients the digestive processes are not impaired, and regular tube feeding diet is well tolerated. Furthermore, the absorption of dipeptides is more rapid than that of simple amino acids. Chemically defined diets are used in patients with deficient digestion and/or absorption (short-bowel syndrome, pancreatic insufficiency, etc.).

Parenteral nutrition is required in patients with a non-functioning GI tract and in cases where adequate nutritional support cannot be achieved by the enteric route. In our surgical ICU enteric tube feeding is seldom successful, because of gastric stasis and/or diarrhoea, and therefore the majority of patients are receiving parenteral nutrition. Parenteral nutrition is administered with either a peripheral or a central venous catheter. The latter is required for hypertonic glucose solutions. With a peripheral venous catheter an adequate caloric intake can only be achieved with the infusion of a lipid emulsion and/or large volumes of a 10% dextrose solution. In the majority of patients in our surgical ICU a central catheter is employed for nutritional support. In these patients the peripheral veins are often thrombosed and therefore inadequate as infusion sites. In addition, our experimental data indicate that these patients respond better to TPN with hypertonic dextrose than to TPN with lipid [25]. A peripheral infusion of amino acids with either 10% dextrose or a lipid emulsion has been successfully employed to maintain the BCM of normally nourished patients, but is generally inadequate in restoring a depleted BCM in a patient with pre-existing malnutrition.

Protein and caloric requirements

Although the importance of nutritional support is well established, especially for the patient subjected to a prolonged catabolic stress (extensive body burn, multiple fractures, sepsis, etc.), the protein and caloric requirements of the critically ill patient remain controversial [8, 20]. As a result, during the past several years, we have collected data to establish the protein and caloric requirements of the hospitalized patient [25]. The studies were carried out in patients receiving TNP, as these patients have a high incidence of malnutrition and their caloric and protein intake can be accurately measured. Although these studies were carried out in patients receiving TPN, the results are probably applicable to all hospitalized patients, regardless of the route used for nutritional support.

Two hundred and four patients who required TPN were randomly allocated to receive one of the following three TPN solutions (1) 2.5% crystalline L-amino acids (Travasol, Travenol–Baxter Laboratories, Canada) with 25% dextrose; (2) 5% crystalline L-amino acids (Travasol) with 25% dextrose, or (3) a 10% lipid emulsion (Intralipid, Pharmacia, Canada), which is infused with an equal volume of a solution containing 5% amino acids (Travasol) and 25% dextrose. Since the two solutions were infused at the same rate via a Y tube, the final solution administered contained 2.5% amino acids, 12.5% dextrose, and 5% lipid. There were 102, 68, and 34 patients who received the first, second, and third solutions, respectively. The number of patients in each group was unequal because the study was performed in two stages. Initially all patients referred for TPN were randomized to receive either the first or the second solution. In the second stage of the study, patients were randomized between the first and third solutions. Each patient in the first two groups received 100 ml 10% Intralipid weekly to prevent the development of an essential fatty acid deficiency.

To quantatively assess the efficacy of TPN with each solution, body composition measurements were performed at the beginning and at 2-week intervals during the course of TPN. The rate of change in the BCM was used as a measure of the efficacy of TPN. In the normally nourished individual, the BCM will not increase regardless of the caloric and protein intake, except with a special exercise programme designed specifically to increase muscle mass.

Therefore each group was subdivided according to the presence or absence of pre-existing malnutrition at the onset of each TPN period. Malnutrition was defined by the presence of an $Na_e/K_e > 1.22$.

As expected, in the normally nourished patients the BCM did not increase with any of the three solutions (Table 26.10). Body weight increased slightly, due principally to an increase in BF. Otherwise their body composition remained unchanged with TPN. In the patients with pre-existing malnutrition, TPN with each of the three solutions produced a significant improvement in body composition (Table 26.11). Two weeks of TPN with 2.5% amino acids and 25% dextrose resulted in a mean increase in body weight of 1.1 ± 0.5 kg ($P < 0.5$), due principally to a 0.9 ± 0.3 kg ($P < 0.01$) increase in BCM. Similar changes occurred in the malnourished patients receiving a TPN solution containing 5% amino acids. Two weeks of TPN with a solution in which lipids supplied 47% of the non-protein calories also resulted in a 1.0 ± 0.4 kg ($P < 0.05$) increase in BCM. This group also experienced a significant increase in BF.

Two weeks of TPN with the three solutions resulted in a similar increase in BCM. Clearly, increasing the amino acid concentration from 2.5% to 5% and infusing 47% of the non-protein calories as lipid did not appear to affect the efficiency of TPN. The latter group, however, received 15% more calories than the other two groups. To account for the different calorie, protein, and lipid intake, a multiple linear regression analysis was performed. The daily change in the BCM ($\Delta BCM/day$) was correlated with the calories per kilogram of body weight infused of carbohydrate, lipid, and protein, and with the Na_e/K_e ratio, a measure of the nutritional state. This analysis was performed on a total of 212 TPN periods by combining the data obtained in the three groups of malnourished patients. This approach is valid, as the ratio of amino acid to non-protein calories, and the ratio of lipid to carbohydrate calories were different with the three solutions. The following statistically significant ($P < 0.01$) multiple linear regression was obtained.

$$\Delta BCM = -348.5 + 4.9 \, CHO + 3.2 \, lipid$$
$$(P < 0.005) \quad (P < 0.05)$$

$$+ 4.7 \, protein + 98.7 \, Na_e/K_e.$$
$$(NS) \qquad\qquad (P < 0.001)$$

There was considerable scatter of points about the regression, as indicated by a correlation coefficient of 0.4. The correlation coefficient was improved ($r = 0.6$, $P < 0.01$) by correlating the daily change in the BCM, expressed as grams per kilogram BCM per day, with the carbohydrate lipid and protein intake, expressed as calories per kilogram BCM:

Table 26.10. The effect of TPN on body composition in normally nourished patients

	Normal volunteers	2.5% amino acid 25% dextrose		5% amino acids 25% dextrose		2.5% amino acid 12.5% dextrose 5% lipid	
		Pre	Post	Pre	Post	Pre	Post
Weight (kg)	70.4 ± 2.5	58.7 ± 1.5	59.9 ± 1.5^a	60.5 ± 2.5	62.7 ± 2.6^a	67.3 ± 7.7	68.8 ± 7.8
Body fat (kg)	20.2 ± 1.4	13.0 ± 1.2	14.6 ± 1.1^a	16.2 ± 1.9	16.0 ± 1.8	18.1 ± 4.8	19.4 ± 7.1
Lean body mass (kg)	50.3 ± 1.9	45.7 ± 1.1	45.4 ± 1.1	44.3 ± 1.5	46.7 ± 1.7^a	49.2 ± 4.0	49.4 ± 3.5
Body cell mass (kg)	24.7 ± 1.1	21.3 ± 0.6	20.6 ± 0.7	20.8 ± 0.9	21.2 ± 1.2	21.9 ± 1.7	20.8 ± 2.8
Extracellular mass (kg)	25.6 ± 0.9	24.5 ± 0.6	24.8 ± 0.6	23.5 ± 0.7	25.5 ± 0.8^a	27.3 ± 2.3	28.6 ± 1.0
K_e/TBW (mmol/litre)	80.0 ± 1.0	76.3 ± 0.8	74.1 ± 1.3^a	76.7 ± 1.2	73.6 ± 2.0^a	73.4 ± 0.7	68.1 ± 4.5
Na_e/TBW (mmol/litre)	77.5 ± 0.9	76.6 ± 0.7	78.5 ± 1.0	74.7 ± 1.3	76.2 ± 1.7	81.4 ± 2.1	81.6 ± 3.8
Na_e/K_e	0.98 ± 0.02	1.01 ± 0.02	1.10 ± 0.04^a	0.98 ± 0.03	1.07 ± 0.05^a	1.11 ± 0.03	1.23 ± 0.1
Patients	25	50		23		5	
Studies		116		50		10	
TPN periods		64		27		5	
TPN days		15.2 ± 0.7		13.6 ± 0.3		14.4 ± 0.2	
Total calories (cal/kg/day)		49.6 ± 1.4		51.8 ± 2.4		58.0 ± 6.8	
Carbohydrate (cal/kg/day)		43.7 ± 1.2		41.1 ± 1.9		27.8 ± 3.3^c	
Lipid (cal/kg/day)		0.8 ± 0.2		1.6 ± 0.2		25.0 ± 3.1^c	
Protein (g/kg/day)		1.28 ± 0.04		2.29 ± 0.12^c		1.29 ± 0.14	

[a] Significantly ($P < 0.05$) different from mean before TPN according to a paired Student's t-test.
[b] Significantly ($P < 0.05$) different from normal volunteers according to an analysis of variance and Scheffe's test.
[c] Significantly ($P < 0.05$) different from the other two groups according to an analysis of variance and Scheffe's test.

Table 26.11. The effect of TPN on the body composition of malnourished patients

	Normal volunteers	2.5% amino acid 25% dextrose		5% amino acids 25% dextrose		2.5% amino acid 12.5% dextrose 5% lipid	
		Pre	Post	Pre	Post	Pre	Post
Weight (kg)	70.4 ± 2.5	57.5 ± 1.5	58.6 ± 1.4^a	56.9 ± 1.5	57.7 ± 1.4^a	57.4 ± 2.3	59.1 ± 2.4^a
Body fat (kg)	20.2 ± 1.4	11.9 ± 0.9	12.4 ± 0.8	13.6 ± 0.9	14.4 ± 1.0	13.6 ± 1.6	15.5 ± 1.6^a
Lean body mass (kg)	50.3 ± 1.9	45.6 ± 1.1	46.2 ± 1.0	43.3 ± 1.3	43.3 ± 1.0	43.8 ± 1.5	43.6 ± 1.5
Body cell mass (kg)	24.7 ± 1.1	15.5 ± 0.5	16.4 ± 0.4^a	14.9 ± 0.5	16.1 ± 0.5^a	14.6 ± 0.7	15.6 ± 0.8^a
Extracellular mass (kg)	25.6 ± 0.9	30.1 ± 0.8	29.9 ± 0.9	28.4 ± 0.9	27.3 ± 0.7	29.2 ± 1.1	28.0 ± 1.0
K_e/TBW (mmol/litre)	80.0 ± 1.0	56.1 ± 1.1^b	$59.2 \pm 1.3^{a,b}$	56.5 ± 1.1^b	$61.1 \pm 1.2^{a,b}$	54.7 ± 1.4^b	$58.2 \pm 1.6^{a,b}$
Na_e/TBW (mmol/litre)	77.5 ± 0.9	94.6 ± 1.0^b	$91.5 \pm 1.2^{a,b}$	92.2 ± 1.11^b	$88 \pm 1.2^{a,b}$	94.1 ± 1.3^b	91.3 ± 1.3^b
Na_e/K_e	0.98 ± 0.02	1.79 ± 0.07^b	$1.66 \pm 0.06^{a,b}$	$1/71 \pm 0.06^b$	$1.50 \pm 0.05^{a,b}$	1.85 ± 0.11^b	1.70 ± 0.11^b
Patients	25	55		50		29	
Studies		151		125		81	
TPN periods		90		72		50	
TPN days		14.9 ± 0.3^c		13.8 ± 0.2		14.0 ± 0.22	
Total calories (cal/kg/day)		49.5 ± 1.4		53.6 ± 1.6		57.1 ± 2.3^c	
Carbohydrate (cal/kg/day)		43.6 ± 1.2		41.6 ± 1.2		27.4 ± 1.1^c	
Lipid (cal/kg/day)		0.8 ± 0.1		2.5 ± 0.5^c		24.4 ± 1.2^c	
Protein (g/kg/day)		1.26 ± 0.04		2.37 ± 0.07^c		1.36 ± 0.06	

[a] Significantly ($P < 0.05$) different from mean before TPN according to a paired Student's t-test.
[b] Significantly ($P < 0.05$) different from normal volunteers according to an analysis of variance and Scheffe's test.
[c] Significantly ($P < 0.05$) different from the other two groups according to an analysis of variance and Scheffe's test.

$$\Delta BCM/day = -24.0 + 0.11\ CHO + 0.07\ Lipid$$
$$\quad\quad\quad\quad (P < 0.001)\quad (P < 0.01)$$
$$\quad\quad + 0.14\ protein + 5.4\ Na_e/K_e.$$
$$\quad\quad (NS)\quad\quad\quad\quad (P < 0.001)$$

The statistical significance of the regression coefficients also improved. Nevertheless, in the subsequent discussion we have used the equation in which the caloric intake is expressed as a function of body weight. Although it is less precise, the results obtained with it are more applicable to daily clinical practice.

The multiple linear regression indicates that the restoration of the BCM is related to the caloric intake and the degree of malnutrition, and is not affected by increasing the amino acid concentration from 2.5% to 5%. With both regression equations the regression coefficient associated with carbohydrate intake was higher than the one associated with lipid intake. This indicates that in the malnourished patient with a depleted BCM, carbohydrate calories are more efficient than lipid calories. This difference is demonstrated in Fig. 26.11, where the above regression equation is used to relate the daily change in the BCM, in kilograms per day to the non-protein calories infused. The regression involves four independent parameters and one dependent parameter, and therefore a multi-dimensional space is required to plot the curve. A two-dimensional graph can be plotted by keeping several of the independent parameters constant. In Fig. 26.11, Na_e/K_e is set at 1.50

(indicative of moderate malnutrition) and the daily amino acid infusion rate is set at 1.26 g/kg body weight, the mean amino acid infusion rate in the patients who received the 2.5% amino acid solution. As illustrated in Fig. 26.11, BCM mass was maintained with a daily infusion of 36 cal/kg body weight, when all of the non-protein calories were given as carbohydrate, and 55 cal/kg body weight with the lipid solution. When 50% of the non-protein calories were carbohydrate, an infusion of 44 cal/kg body weight was required to maintain the BCM. A daily infusion of 50 non-protein calories/kg body weight resulted in a BCM increase of 69 g/day with the carbohydrate solution, and 16 g/day when 50% of the non-protein calories were lipid. These data therefore demonstrate that in these depleted malnourished patients, carbohydrate calories were far more efficient than lipid calories. An additional important consideration is the difference in cost between a carbohydrate and a lipid calorie. In our institution a lipid calorie is 1180% more expensive than a carbohydrate calorie.

The regression data also indicated that doubling the amino acid concentration did not alter the repletion rate of a depleted BCM. This is demonstrated in Fig. 26.12, where the daily change in the BCM is plotted against the caloric intake, the daily amino acid intake being either 1.26 or 2.37 g/kg body weight. These amino acid infusion rates represent the mean amino acid intake of the malnourished patients re-

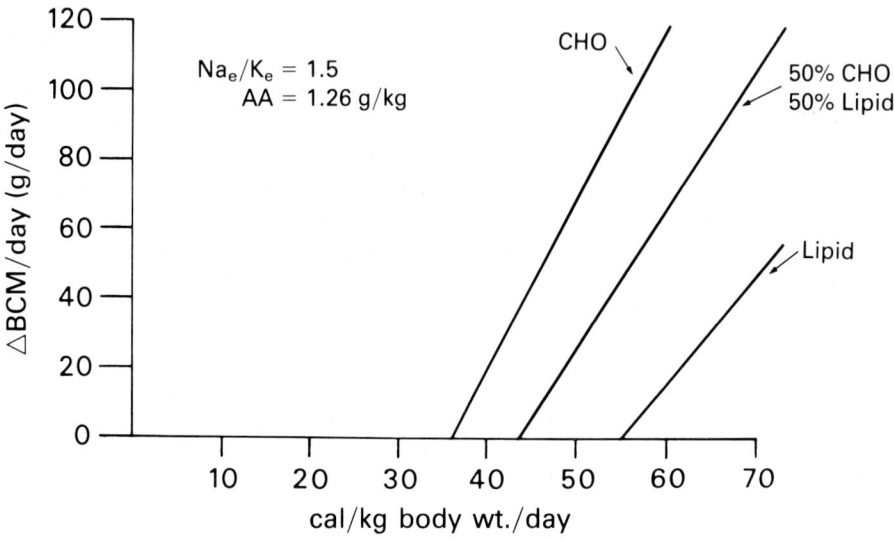

Fig. 26.11. The effect of the non-protein caloric intake on the daily change in BCM, when this intake is carbohydrate, lipid or equally divided between the two. The $Na_e:K_e$ and the amino acid intake was set at 1.5 and 1.26 g/kg/day, respectively. With carbohydrates the BCM is maintained with 36 cal/kg/day and the infusion of 50 non-protein calories kg/day the daily increase in BCM is 69 g.

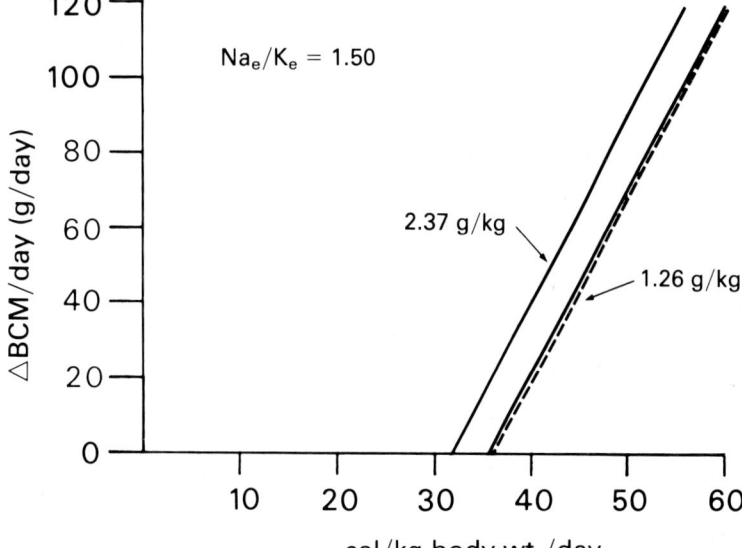

Fig. 26.12. Results of infusing solutions containing 25% dextrose with 2.5% and 5% crystalline amino acids, involving mean daily amino acid infusion rates of 1.26 and 2.37 g/kg/day. The Na_e/K_e was set at 1.5, indicative of moderate malnutrition. When the extra calories associated with the higher amino acid concentration is taken into account, the *broken line* is obtained.

ceiving the 2.5% and 5% solutions, respectively. The Na_e/K_e ratio is set at 1.50, and all the non-protein calories are carbohydrate. Increasing the amino acid concentration shifted the curve to the left and therefore, at the same caloric intake, there is a more rapid restoration of BCM. However, this apparent increased efficiency disappeared when the extra calories associated with the increased amino acid concentration were accounted for (Fig. 26.12). Wilmore, in a recent review [30], pointed out that at any level of protein intake, nitrogen balance improves as the caloric intake is increased, and with a constant caloric intake nitrogen balance improves as the protein intake is increased. However, the relationship between nitrogen balance and protein intake reaches a maximum, so that a further increase in protein intake does not result in any further improvement in nitrogen balance. In the present study the flat portion of the curve was probably achieved with the 2.5% solution. As a result, increasing the amino acid concentration above 2.5% had very little effect on the restoration rate of a depleted BCM. However, doubling the amino acid concentration in our TPN solution increased the solution cost by 84%.

The regression equation also indicated that there is a relationship between the restoration rate of a depleted BCM and the degree of malnutrition. This is illustrated in Fig. 26.13, where the daily change in the BCM is plotted against the caloric intake for increasingly more severe malnutrition, as indicated by the Na_e/K_e ratio. The three curves in Fig. 26.13 are drawn

with a daily amino acid intake of 1.26 g/kg body weight, the mean intake of the malnourished patients who received the 2.5% solution. As the severity of malnutrition increased the caloric requirements for maintenance decreased. Thus with moderate malnutrition ($Na_e/K_e = 1.5$) BCM is maintained with a caloric intake of 36 cal/kg body weight. With severe malnutrition ($Na_e/K_e = 2.5$) 16 cal/kg are sufficient for maintenance. With caloric intakes in excess of the amount required for maintenance, the restoration of the depleted BCM is more rapid in the more malnourished. Thus, with a daily infusion of 50 cal/kg body weight, the BCM increases at a rate of 69 g/day when $Na_e/K_e = 1.5$ and 168 g/day when $Na_e/K_e = 2.5$.

The restoration rate of the depleted BCM decreases continuously as the malnourished state is corrected, and becomes zero as the normally nourished state is achieved. The regression data are therefore consistent with our observation that in the normally nourished individual, TPN has no effect on the BCM. These data also emphasize the importance of a knowledge of an individual's nutritional state when analysing the results of nutritional therapy. This is true whether body composition measurements or nitrogen balance data are employed to evaluate the results of nutritional therapy. In the normally nourished, nitrogen balance will never exceed zero despite the caloric and protein intake, except with a special exercise programme designed to increase muscle mass. Thus in evaluation of the effects of nutritional support it is imperative to differentiate between the

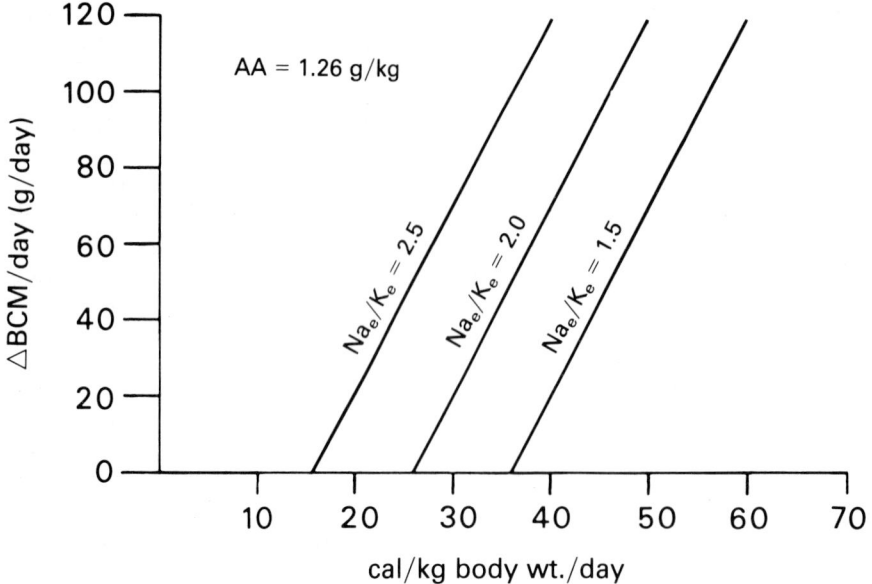

Fig. 26.13. The restoration of a depleted BCM increases as the severity of malnutrition is increased, as indicated by the higher Na_e/K_e ratio. Thus the daily infusion of 50 non-protein calories/kg gives rise to a daily BCM increase of 79 g with moderate malnutrition ($Na_e/K_e = 1.5$) and 168 g/day with severe malnutrition ($Na_e/K_e = 2.5$).

normally nourished and the malnourished individual. Otherwise the data from the normally nourished will bias the malnourished data. Lastly it is important to estimate the degree of malnutrition present, as this will affect the response to nutritional therapy.

The data described indicate that the restoration rate of a depleted BCM is related to caloric intake and the degree of malnutrition, but is not affected by increasing the amino acid intake from 1.3 to 2.4 g/kg/day. Elwyn et al. have reported a similar relationship between the restoration rate of the BCM and caloric intake [8]. In a group of BCM-depleted patients receiving TPN, they described a straight-line relationship between nitrogen balance and the daily caloric intake. Their equation had an intercept of –24.3 mg nitrogen/kg body weight and a slope of 1.4 mg nitrogen/calorie. When the mean values for the malnourished patients receiving the 2.5% solution (Table 26.11) were used, this equation predicted a mean daily positive nitrogen balance of 45 mg/kg body weight. This is equivalent to a BCM restoration rate of 64 g/day. With the same data, our regression equation predicted a restoration rate of 69 g/day. At this rate 2 weeks of TPN would therefore result in a 0.97 kg increase in the BCM, which is the actual increase measured in the malnourished patients who received the 2.5% solution for a mean of 14.7 days (Table 26.11).

Although the data described were obtained in patients receiving TPN, the conclusions are applicable to all forms of nutritional support. Thus the restoration rate of a malnourished individual is directly dependent on the caloric intake, provided the protein intake is adequate [20, 30]. There are no apparent advantages in increasing the daily protein intake to levels above 1.5–2 g/kg body weight. Carbohydrate calories are more efficient than lipid calories in restoring the malnourished individual. These data also emphasize that correction of the malnourished state is relatively slow compared with the rate at which it develops. The normally nourished individual, during the first few days of starvation, breaks down more than 300 g BCM/day. A much more rapid breakdown occurs with trauma, especially when it is complicated by sepsis. However, the BCM is only restored at a rate of 50–100 g/day in spite of large caloric intakes.

Protein sparing

In the previous section, the importance of an adequate carbohydrate intake was emphasized. This is because, in the malnourished patient, the repletion rate of a depleted BCM is related to the caloric intake, especially carbohydrate calories. However, this is not the case for the nutritional support is maintenance of the BCM. Numerous studies exist in the recent literature, which indicate that this can be achieved with an adequate intake of amino acids regardless of caloric intake [2, 12–14, 16]. To assess the protein-sparing effect of amino acid-containing solutions, a study was performed in 38 patients undergoing elective surgery of moderate severity [27]. The majority of patients underwent either gastrectomy or colon resection. All were deemed to be nutritionally normal on the basis of a clinical examination. They were randomly divided into two groups. The first group received all postoperative fluids IV as a 5% glucose solution. In the second group the postoperative fluids were administered IV as 5% casein hydrolysate (Amigen, Travenol–Baxter Laboratories, Canada). In all patients sodium chloride was added to the IV fluids as required to maintain electrolyte balance.

To assess the protein-sparing effects of the administered amino acids, body composition studies were performed before surgery and on the fifth postoperative day. The results obtained are shown in Table 26.12. By the fifth postoperative day body weight had decreased significantly ($P < 0.05$) in both groups. In patients receiving glucose, the postoperative body weight loss of 2.6 ± 0.6 kg resulted from a 0.8 ± 0.6 kg loss of LBM and a 1.8 ± 0.9 kg loss of BF. In contrast, the 2.0 ± 0.5 kg weight loss in the patients receiving IV amino acids was due entirely to a loss in BF. Their BCM did not change and the Na_e/K_e ratio remained normal following operation. The patients receiving the glucose-containing solutions experienced a significant ($P < 0.001$) loss of BCM from 23.1 ± 1.5 to 19.9 ± 1.4 kg. This 3.2 ± 0.6 kg loss includes the cellular mass of the resected specimen. The postoperative loss of BCM was accompanied by an expansion of the ECM and an elevation of

the Na_e/K_e ratio to 1.29 ± 0.11. These body composition changes are indicative of mild malnutrition. Thus the IV infusion of amino acids at a daily rate of 1.8 ± 0.2 g/kg body weight effectively prevented the malnutrition which developed in the control patients.

Blackburn and co-workers [2] were the first to report that significant protein sparing could be achieved postoperatively with the infusion of solutions containing amino acids. They originally attributed this effect to the avoidance of glucose-containing solutions. In the absence of an adequate caloric intake, the average postoperative patient must rely on endogenous fuels to meet daily energy requirements. They postulated that the infusion of glucose increased the plasma insulin concentration, which in turn inhibited the mobilization of lipid to meet this caloric deficit. This resulted in gluconeogenesis from body protein. In support of this hypothesis they reported an inverse correlation between nitrogen sparing and both the plasma glucose and insulin concentrations. A positive correlation was also present between nitrogen sparing and the plasma concentrations of both free fatty acids and ketone bodies. They therefore recommended the infusion of amino acid and the avoidance of solutions containing glucose to achieve protein sparing postoperatively. Subsequent studies have demonstrated that the protein-sparing effects of amino acid solutions are a function of the amino acids themselves and are not affected by the additional infusion of either lipids or glucose [13, 14]. Protein sparing is therefore related to the infusion of the appropriate amino acids, and not to the avoidance of glucose.

Our data and the data published in several recent reports clearly demonstrate that IV amino acids will effectively spare protein [12–14, 16]. These studies were, however, carried out

Table 26.12. Postoperative protein sparing

	Glucose		Amino acids	
	Pre-op.	Postop.	Pre-op.	Postop.
Body weight (kg)	66.2 ± 1.9	63.5 ± 1.8^a	68.1 ± 3.9	66.2 ± 3.7^a
Body fat (kg)	18.2 ± 1.6	16.4 ± 1.5^a	20.0 ± 2.1	15.9 ± 2.4^a
Lean body mass (kg)	48.0 ± 1.8	47.2 ± 1.6	48.2 ± 2.5	50.3 ± 2.4^a
Body cell mass (kg)	23.1 ± 1.5	19.9 ± 1.4^a	22.9 ± 1.5	23.8 ± 1.3
Extracellular mass (kg)	24.9 ± 0.9	27.3 ± 0.9^a	25.3 ± 1.1	26.5 ± 1.3
K_e/TBW (mmol/litre)	78.2 ± 2.8	68.3 ± 3.1^a	76.9 ± 1.4	77.8 ± 1.4
Na_e/TBW (mmol/litre)	77.3 ± 2.1	82.5 ± 2.2^a	78.6 ± 1.5	76.8 ± 1.6
Na_e/K_e	1.04 ± 0.08	1.29 ± 0.11^a	1.03 ± 0.03	1.00 ± 0.03

[a] Significantly different ($P < 0.05$) from the pre-operative mean according to a paired Student's t-test.

in normally nourished individuals who experienced trauma of moderate severity. The majority of these patients had undergone elective surgery. The results of these studies cannot therefore be extrapolated to the malnourished, the severely traumatized, or patients subjected to a prolonged catabolic stress. Further studies are required to evaluate the role of protein sparing with IV amino acids in these patients.

Our present practice is to administer amino acids IV to those patients who require nutritional support but who are not as yet candidates for TPN. This would include the severely malnourished patient who has just undergone corrective surgery and is expected to resume a normal oral intake in a few days. Because of pre-existing malnutrition and therefore a decreased reserve this individual cannot tolerate an additional loss of nutritional reserve, especially if a postoperative complication develops and the resumption of oral intake is further delayed. Protein sparing with IV amino acids is similarly indicated for the extensively traumatized patient in whom there is uncertainty regarding the return of normal GI function. In such a patient amino acids are administered until oral intake is resumed or until it is obvious that dietary intake will be unduly delayed. When it becomes obvious that there is a prolonged delay in the resumption of GI function, TPN is started. Generally therefore, protein sparing with IV amino acids is used when the indications for TPN do not exist but it is anticipated that TPN might be required. To achieve protein sparing amino acids are administered at a rate of 1.5–2.0 g/kg body weight with a solution containing 5% amino acids with 5% dextrose.

References

1. Behnke AR, Guttentag OE, Brodsky C (1959) Quantification of body weight and configuration from anthropometric measurements. Hum Biol 31:213–234
2. Blackburn GL, Flatt JP, Clowes GHA Jr, et al (1973) Protein sparing therapy during periods of starvation with sepsis or trauma. Ann Surg 177:588–594
3. Cahill GF Jr (1970) Starvation in man. N Eng J Med 282:668–675
4. Cohn SH, Dombrowski CS (1970) Absolute measurement of whole body potassium by gamma ray spectrometry. J Nucl Med 11:239–246
5. Dudrick SJ, Wilmore DW, Vars HM (1967) Long-term parenteral nutrition with growth in puppies and positive nitrogen balance in patients. Surg Forum 18:356–357
6. Edmunds LD Jr, Williams EM, Welch CE (1960) External fistula arising from the gastrointestinal tract. Ann Surg 152:445–473
7. Elman R, Weiner DO (1939) Intravenous alimentation with special reference to protein (amino acid) metabolism. JAMA 112:796–802
8. Elwyn DH, Gump FE, Munro HM, et al (1979) Changes in nitrogen balance of depleted patients with increasing infusions of glucose. J Clin Nutr 32:1597–1611
9. Forse RA, Shizgal HM (1980a) The assessment of malnutrition. Surgery 88:17–24
10. Forse RA, Shizgal HM (1980b) The Na_e/K_e ratio: A predictor of malnutrition. Surg Forum 31:89–92
11. Forse RA, Christou N, Meakins JL, MacLean LD, Shizgal HM (1981). Reliability of skin testing as a measure of the nutritional state. Arch Surg 116:1284–1288
12. Freeman JB, Stegink LD, Wittine MF, et al (1977) The current status of protein sparing. Surg Gynecol Obstet 144:843–849
13. Greenberg GR, Marliss EB, Anderson GH, et al (1976) Protein sparing therapy in postoperative patients. N Engl J Med 294:1141–1416
14. Harvey TC, Dykes PW, Chan MS, et al (1973) Measurement of whole-body nitrogen by neutron activation analysis. Lancet II:395–398
15. Himal HS, Allard JR, Nadeau JE, Freeman JB, MacLean LD (1974) The importance of adequate nutrition in closure of small intestinal fistulas. Br J Surg 61:724–726
16. Hoover HC Jr, Grant JP, Gorschboth C, et al (1975) Nitrogen-sparing intravenous fluids in postoperative patients. N Engl J Med 293:172–175
17. Kinney JM (1975) Energy requirements of the surgical patient. In: Manual of surgical nutrition. Committee on pre and postoperative care, American College of Surgeons Saunders, Philadelphia, pp 223–235
18. Moore FD, Olesen KH, McMurray JD, Parker HV, Ball MR, Boyden CM (1963) The body cell mass and its supporting environment. Saunders, Philadelphia.
19. Owen OE, Felig P, Morgan AP, Wahren J, Cahill GF (1969) Liver and kidney metabolism during prolonged starvation. J Clin Invest 48:574–583
20. Peters CP, Fischer JE (1980) Studies in calorie to nitrogen ratio for total parenteral nutrition. Surg Gynecol Obstet 151:1–8
21. Rhoads JE, Alexander CE (1955) Nutritional problems of surgical patients. Ann NY Acad Sci 63:268–275
22. Roback SA, Nicoloff DM (1972) High output enterocutaneous fistula of the small bowel. Am J Surg 123:317–322
23. Sheldon EF, Gardiner BM, Way LW, Dunphy JE (1971) Management of gastrointestinal fistulas. Surg Gynecol Obstet 133:385–389
24. Shizgal HM (1981) The effect of malnutrition on body composition. Surg Gynecol Obstet 152:22–26
25. Shizgal HM, Forse RA (1980) Protein and calorie requirements with total parenteral nutrition. Ann Surg 192:562–569
26. Shizgal HM, Spanier AH, Humes J, et al (1977) Indirect measurement of total exchangeable potassium. Am J Physiol 233:F253–F259
27. Shizgal HM, Milne CA, Spanier AH (1979) The effect of nitrogen-sparing intravenously administered fluids on postoperative body composition. Surgery 85:496–503
28. Studley HC (1936) Percent weight loss: A basic indicator of surgical risk. JAMA 106:458–460
29. Vartsky D, Ellis KG, Cohn SH (1979) In vivo measurement of body nitrogen by analysis of prompt gammas from neutron capture. J Nucl Med 20:1158–1165
30. Wilmore DW (1977) Energy requirements for maximum nitrogen retention. In: Green HL, Holliday MA, Munro HM (eds) Clinical nutrition update: Amino acids. American Medical Association, Chicago, pp 47–56

Chapter 27

Acute Liver Failure and Encephalopathy

J. De Groote

Acute liver failure is a much dreaded complication of liver diseases. It has always attracted the attention of physicians as an extreme example of the possible morbid influence of an organ on the brain. The interpretation, however, has changed over the centuries according to fluctuating medical concepts and the real significance of this brain–liver relationship has still not been elucidated.

Definition

Liver failure may be defined as a syndrome of all the symptoms which may arise because the liver fails to carry out its normal metabolic function. The most impressive and also the most dangerous features occur in the brain, which loses control over its own metabolism. A complex set of neuropsychiatric disturbances are observed, often designated hepatic encephalopathy.

This encephalopathy may arise in either 'acute' or 'chronic' liver failure, and although the mode of origin is quite different the clinical syndromes may be very similar. The acute encephalopathy is a consequence of the disturbances caused by acute failure of a previously normal liver. The chronic form is due to the inflow of 'toxic' substances in the peripheral blood through a collateral circulation, either extra- or intrahepatic, and also through the failing cirrhotic liver. It is almost impossible to separate those two forms of failure completely when discussing the metabolic events which may play a role in their pathogenesis.

Aetiology

Any lesion which produces necrosis of more than 60% of the functional liver tissue may cause acute failure; Caroli et al. [13] have shown this by morphometric studies in liver puncture biopsies. It is generally accepted that the classic hepatitis viruses can cause extensive liver necrosis and failure. They are not cytotoxic in themselves, but are eliminated, together with an hepatocyte, by an immunological mechanism, probably of the delayed type and this reaction is thought to be excessive in about 1% of patients with acute encephalopathy. A similar sequence of events may also induce coma in drug hepatitis of the indirect type, and this has been described for several drugs, including halothane, iproniazid, metahexamide, phenelzine, and hycanthone.

Direct damage is produced by a direct interference with the cellular metabolism, e.g., an overdose of acetaminophen produces an oxidized metabolite which binds glutathione and hence damages the cell. Phosphorus poisoning has always been a well-known cause of 'yellow liver atrophy'; other causes are amanita phalloides, various rat poisons, halogenated and nitrated hydrocarbons, and overdosage with IV tetracycline.

Anoxia of the hepatocyte as occurs in the Budd–Chiari syndrome, in shock, and after ligation of the portal vein and/or the hepatic artery during surgery is another cause of liver cell necrosis and experimental coma may be produced this way in animals. It is also possible experimentally to produce extensive necrosis and coma by the administration of toxic substances such as the glucosamines [26]. Recently endotoxinaemia has been proposed as a possible factor in the production of fulminant hepatic failure and it has been shown in animals that at least part of the liver necrosis in galactosamine hepatitis is due to the simultaneous action of endotoxin. Indeed Liehr et al. [52] produced fulminant necrosis in the rat liver by adding endotoxin to a low dose of galactosamine which alone only gave rise to membrane lesions. A similar mechanism involving endotoxinaemia and activated complement system may be proposed for human liver cell death complicating acute liver disease; in acute Reye's syndrome the blood levels of endotoxin correlate strongly with the EEG changes [25].

In man alcoholic hepatitis with, or even without, cirrhosis is an important cause of liver atrophy. This state is often considered to be intermediate between the acute and the chronic form of liver failure, especially when cirrhotic transformation is already present.

Pathogenesis of hepatic encephalopathy

The actual causes of the symptoms and signs of acute liver failure are still poorly understood. Many theories have been proposed, none of which completely explains all the facts. It is very likely, however, that because the situation is multi-factorial no single mechanism will fully explain all the findings and it will always be necessary to investigate the various factors involved in causing the symptoms and those that cause the death of the patient, many of which are interrelated.

One effect of acute liver damage is the release into the circulation of the liver's disintegration products, which may be toxic. In addition, the existing homeostasis may be altered by failure either of synthesis or of detoxification of various substances.

Current ideas concerning the pathogenesis of liver failure fall into three main groups.

Synthesis deficiency

The liver synthesizes a number of complex molecules that are used elsewhere in the body, in particular in the brain. Some of them are well known, such as the sterol skeleton, while others are unknown and there is only circumstantial evidence of their existence but it has been shown that brain slices can only use glucose in the presence of liver extracts [37] and, that the liver has to be included in an artificial brain perfusion system to promote the uptake of glucose [40]. Uridine and cytidine both facilitate this uptake, but parenteral infusion of these substances has not altered the course of acute hepatic failure [70].

Intoxication

Earlier experiments showed that autolysing liver cells produced toxic effects and were also capable of increasing the blood ammonia level [76, 44, 62, 80]. In fact, the most familiar of all the theories relates to this increased ammonia level. In 1896 Nencki and Zaleski [59] showed an increase of blood ammonia in animals with Eck fistulas and some years earlier the Pavlow school had demonstrated a relationship between meat feeding and coma in animals with porta caval shunts. Bessman [6] in 1955 proposed a new concept of cerebral energy deficiency based on interference by ammonia in the Krebs cycle. It was already known from the work of Krebs and his school in 1935 [45] that ammonia could be metabolized not only in the urea cycle but also via the glutamate pathway, which is active in the brain; this shunting of alpha-ketoglutarate in hyperammonaemia decreased the efficiency of the citric acid cycle in producing ATP.

There are arguments in favour of the theory of ammonia toxicity and indeed all the symptoms of hepatic coma may be produced by its administration as protein ammoniogenic amino acids, or ammonia-loaded resins. Its blood level correlates fairly well with the clinical condition: however, there is no definite proof of its direct toxicity or its mode of action. Nevertheless, most of the measures aimed at reducing the blood ammonia level do appear to have some beneficial effect on the clinical symptoms, particularly in chronic encephalopathy; the benefit is not so great in the acute state. But the action of these ammonia-lowering agents, such as neomycin or lactulose is also not clear either, and Conn [21] describes the search for the modus operandi of lactulose. Furthermore, several authors have shown that the alpha-ketoglutarate used in the metabolism of ammonia did not come from the Krebs cycle but was newly formed [23]. A vast amount has been written about O_2 consumption and ATP levels in the brain, and although there are some contradictory results most observers agree that such disturbances are probably the consequence and not the cause of the symptoms.

Other toxic substances that have been incriminated are alpha-ketoglutaramate and intermediate chain fatty acids, which when injected into experimental animals may produce liver failure-like symptoms, but the concentrations used are much higher than those found in human patients. However, it has been demonstrated that several of these agents are synergistic, so that a small increase in the concentration of each may precipitate symptoms [86].

False neurotransmitters

To transmit a message from one neurone to another, a synaptic process transferring a chemical neurotransmitter is initiated by the impulse in the presynaptic axon. Fisher and Baldessarini [34] proposed the hypothesis that neurotransmitter disturbances might explain many features of the acute liver failure syndrome. Many substances may have a central neurotransmitter function: e.g., acetylcholine, dopamine, serotonin, noradrenaline, various amino acids, and histamine; and any substance with a phenolic ring and a beta-hydroxyl group on the side chain, such as octopamine, may act as a transmitter [4]. These substances, however, are much less active than the true transmitter and are therefore designated false neurotransmitters, but they may accumulate under certain pathological conditions and profoundly disturb synaptic transmission in the brain, producing signs of coma [20].

Such a basis for the pathogenesis of hepatic coma has been suggested and indeed during acute and chronic liver failure many nitrogenous compounds, such as amines and amino acids, do accumulate and reach peripheral tissues through the liver. The normal relationship of amino acids is altered, the molar ratio of branched chain amino acids to tyrosine and phenylalanine decreases from the normal of 3–4 to approximately 1 or less; but the overall pattern in fulminant hepatic failure differs from that in the chronic form in that the branched-chain amino acids are normal or only slightly depressed while the ratio remains low because of an increase in tyrosine and phenylalanine. Tyramine, which is a precursor of dopamine and octopamine, also accumulates in the blood [65], and these false neurotransmitters, especially octopamine, are elevated not only in the brain but also in urine, blood, and muscle. This may be the result of an interference of tyramine with the metabolism of dopamine and a good correlation of octopamine levels with the depth of the hepatic failure syndrome has been found [58]. However, direct infusion of octopamine to high concentration into the lateral ventricle of the rat brain did not produce coma, even though the level of active neurotransmitters fell to about 10% [29]. Tryptophan, a precursor of serotonin, and 5-hydroxyindolacetic acid, a metabolite of it, also accumulate in liver failure, but in psychiatric patients tryptophan ingestion caused drowsiness only when levels 10 times greater than those observed in acute hepatic encephalopathy are used [67]. Livingstone et al. [53] described changes in the blood–brain barrier that permitted a relatively free passage of aromatic amino acids, and in fulminant hepatic failure their concentration in the brain approximated to that in the plasma. Chase et al. observed similar features in some of their cases, but not in others who were seemingly identical otherwise [18].

All these conflicting reports almost certainly indicate a multifactorial aetiology of the disease and more recently the beneficial effects of haemoperfusion with large-pore acrylonitrile membranes have focused attention on dialysable toxic substances. Earlier experience had shown that classic dialysis through small-pore membranes did not significantly alter the course of acute hepatic failure from which it was concluded that either the toxic substance(s) had a larger molecular weight or they were bound to some larger molecule, presumably albumin. With the advent of acrylonitrile membranes, substances with molecular weights up to about 5000 daltons could be dialysed and according to the school of Opolon a much higher proportion (up to 50%) of patients regained consciousness; however, the final mortality of around 25% remained unchanged [27].

The impossibility of altering the mortality inevitably invites speculation about irreversible liver cell necrosis and perhaps irreversible cerebral oedema due to damage to the blood–brain barrier. The factor(s) determining liver regeneration are not well understood. There is certainly a stimulus for regrowth from glucagon and insulin in the portal blood [33]. The amount of viable liver that remains may itself have an effect on regeneration; surgical excision of more than 65% of the liver does not produce more regeneration than a smaller excision and cross circulation has shown that the factor(s) responsible may be blood-borne, but they have not yet been identified.

Cerebral oedema is very frequent; in about 50% of patients it is the direct cause of death in fulminant hepatic failure [39, 61, 83]. It may occur even in those with a good degree of regeneration of the liver at the time of death. This phenomenon has been shown in many experimental situations, e.g., after hepatectomy [70] and intracranial pressure was studied by Hanid et al. [42] in an experimental model of serial hepatic infarctions in the pig. They observed a rise in intracranial pressure from 12.81 ($\pm$ SE 2.52) to 51.6 ($\pm$ 11.86) mmHg after 16 h and just prior to death. The administration of methylprednisolone during surgery prevented this rise, but had no effect when given 4 h later.

In acute liver failure, during the Reye syndrome, cerebral oedema is also a preterminal event [32]. Here it is probably due to a mitochondrial disturbance similar to that seen in the liver and muscle [64].

Signs and symptoms, function tests

The most prominent symptom of fulminant hepatic failure is impaired consciousness: hepatic coma or encephalopathy. This state is a gradation from a state of disturbed consciousness, labelled precoma or impending coma through to profound coma (Table 27.1). Hepatic encephalopathy is graded as precoma, which includes the early stages (grades 1 and 2), and true coma (grade 3). These signs of acute liver failure are not pathognomonic, however, and can all occur in other forms of metabolic encephalopathy.

The initial changes of hepatic coma are very

Table 27.1. Gradation of hepatic encephalopathy

Clinical stage	Flapping tremor	EEG
Precoma		
Grade 1: Prodromes Slowing mentation	Slight	I
Grade 2: Impending coma Drowsiness, confusion	Marked	II–III
Coma		
Grade 3: Unconsciousness	Absent	III–IV
a) Peripheral reflexes normal		
b) Peripheral reflexes abnormal		
c) Vital reflexes disturbed		
d) Decerebration		IVb to flat

subtle usually present as personality changes, with slight slowing of mentation, some euphoria or depression, and lack of attention to personal detail. As the disease develops other symptoms, such as inappropriate behaviour, mental confusion, intense euphoria or depression, and drowsiness may become prominent. At this stage the patient begins to sleep most of the time, although he is still rousable . He answers questions, but his speech becomes slow and slurred. He also writes much more slowly with an unsteady hand, and makes many mistakes. He has disturbed spatial perception and cannot copy a shape such as a square or a star; a trail test becomes more and more difficult. The repetition of these simple tests are clinically useful in following the patient's progress. During the development of the encephalopathy a flapping tremor appears which was very well described by Adams and Foley in 1949 [2]. The other motor disturbances include both pyramidal and extrapyramidal components with a rigid facies, muscle rigidity, and dysarthria [88].

Grade 3 coma may at first seem like normal sleep; the reflexes at this stage are still normal but may disappear later, and the Babinski sign may be elicited. Deeper coma is characterized first by loss of tone and later by signs of decerebration and disturbances of the vital reflexes such as the respiratory, vasomotor, and thermoregulatory reflexes.

One sign that is almost pathognomonic is hepatic foetor, a sweetish unpleasant smell due to exhalation of mercaptans [14]. In acute failure these substances escape through the liver and in chronic failure they bypass the organ through the collateral circulation. The sign therefore has a different significance in acute and in chronic encephalopathy. In the acute situation it signifies a profound metabolic disturbance and may herald other symptoms. In the chronic cirrhotic state it bears witness to an active collateral circulation, and so also indicates the potential for a chronic encephalopathy.

Biochemistry

The classic liver function tests are of prime importance in the diagnosis of liver disease, although not of the encephalopathy. There are, however, some changes that must be looked for (decrease in transaminases and total cholesterol in combination with a rise in serum bilirubin), for together they usually indicate a lack of viable tissue. A marked fall in blood coagulation also has an unfavourable prognosis (PTT <10%). This is mainly due to failure of synthesis, but utilization may also be accelerated by intravascular consumption.

On occasion, it is possible for a patient to lapse into coma and wake again without much variation in the results of the classic liver function tests; disturbances in water and electrolyte balance or other changes in extrahepatic metabolic changes may be responsible.

Retention of fluid in the abdomen as ascites and in the periphery as oedema may account for a fall in urine output and dehydration may lead to a fall in central venous pressure. The urine is usually normal except for the presence of bilirubin and its breakdown products, but frequently there is significant sodium retention and loss of potassium. This can lead to hypernatraemia and hypokalaemia. These features must be taken into account during IV therapy.

For many decades a more specific test for liver coma has been sought; in 1896 Nenchi, Pavlow, and Zaleski [59] demonstrated an increase in the arterial blood ammonia level during the neurological disturbances that developed after meat was fed to the dogs with an Eck fistula: the so-called meat intoxication (Fleischstückenvergiftung). Until now the blood ammonia has been the most reliable witness of impending coma. As already described, many authors believe that a rise in its level is at least one of the causes of coma, but many examples have shown that it is by no means the only factor, and the diagnosis of liver coma should not be discarded if it is normal. On the other hand, if it rises after bleeding it is almost diagnostic of liver disease. Some other substances may also play a role in the pathogenesis as well as in the diagnosis. An amino acid imbalance has been described with an increase in aromatic amino acids and a decrease of the branched-chain ones. Blood levels of fatty acids, pyruvic acid, and alpha-ketoglutaric acid are also elevated. All these features are roughly and statistically correlated with the degree of coma, but are much less helpful in the individual patient.

The EEG is a good indicator of the cerebral disturbances in hepatic failure but it is neither pathognomonic nor diagnostic, because the same patterns may be observed in any type of metabolic coma. Foley and co-workers [36] were the first to describe the relationship between the EEG and the fulminant hepatic failure, and Parsons-Smith et al. [63] established a practical gradation of the abnormalities. In general, the waves are initially slow and increase in voltage; later a spike and slow wave pattern appears and the voltage may again decrease at this time.

The combination of abnormal liver function tests, the clinical signs, including hepatic foetor and the EEG abnormalities, are practically diagnostic of liver coma.

Pathology

The histological changes in the liver of patients with acute failure correspond to those classically described in severe acute hepatitis. The changes are caused by tissue damage, inflammatory infiltration, and tissue reaction. Lucké and Mallory [54] wrote a good description in 1946, and Desmet et al. [28] a more recent one in 1972. The tissue alterations revealed by optical microscopy are due to liver cell necrosis causing pleomorphism and collapse of cells, and also to cholestasis. The necrosis in the severe form is always of the lobular-to-interlobular confluent type and may even encompass several lobuli, leading to massive panlobular necrosis. The remaining parenchyma is then reduced to a peripheral rim of varying width around the portal field. The most extensive necrosis is observed in the rapidly progressive cases, who die within a few days. A pleomorphic appearance of the remaining cells is a frequent finding. This feature consists of anisocytosis, anisokaryosis, liver cell plate disarray, hydropic swelling, and irregular cytoplasmic aspects. Cholestasis is practically always present. It is seen as fine and coarse bilirubin granules in the cell, and as extracellular bilirubin thrombi. In severe cases these thrombi may be found in the larger portal bile ducts. Bile retention in so-called bile lakes are also observed in severe liver necrosis, and are certainly not pathognomonic of extrahepatic obstruction.

The reticulin framework is emptied by the loss of hepatocytes, and this web-like structure may either slowly collapse with septa formation or be filled with regenerating liver cells. The development of cirrhosis in surviving patients is a rare but possible occurrence.

The inflammatory infiltration, mainly lymphocytic, is most conspicuous in the portal areas but small groups of cells are also observed in the parenchyma, especially in the necrotic zones. Some granulocytes are also present especially in connection with bile duct proliferation. Macrophages appear in the areas of necrosis and are considered to phagocytose the remaining cellular debris. Their number roughly parallels the extent of the damage. A variable degree of bile duct proliferation is always noted; the cells of these ducts may show signs of degeneration such as vacuolization and necrosis. Their extension is somehow correlated to the extent of the cholestasis and they may expand beyond the limits of the portal tract and be continuous with peripheral cell plates.

Features of regeneration are very variable and not easy to differentiate from changes due to the disease. They are, however, the keystone to the survival of the patients and are therefore more pronounced in biopsies from patients who survive. Parenchymal regeneration is characterized by the appearance of mitotic figures, multinucleated cells, two-cell-thick plates and acinar arrangements. Some of these regenerating cells may have a pseudomalignant aspect caused by nuclear hyperchromasia, budding and large nucleoli. In many cases the regeneration proceeds in a rather orderly fashion, according to the pre-existing architecture. Nodular regeneration with disturbance of the normal cellular relationship does not occur in the acute failure so often as in the so-called subacute atrophy with multilobular necrosis of the more chronic type [3].

At autopsy the liver is usually reduced in volume although there is wide variation from 400 g to 1800 g. This scatter is not correlated with other features since oedema and necrosis with loss of parenchyma may have opposing influences. The surface is rather smooth or finely wrinkled, but never nodular. The colour is variable, mostly a mottled greyish red, certainly not yellow as the old term 'yellow atrophy' might suggest. It often has a soft consistency and the cut surface is not characteristic. The landmarks may be indistinct, reminiscent of a congested spleen, or the pattern may have more nutmeg-like features that represent the macroscopic aspect of the extensive necrosis.

Treatment and prognosis

The treatment of acute hepatic failure is still an important challenge to clinical medicine. A patient with a seemingly rather benign disease may suddenly become drowsy and lapse into coma within a few hours. Although the patient may appear to have a good potential for recuperation and survival, the prognosis of hepatic failure is nevertheless gloomy. There are several conflicting studies of the mortality of acute hepatic failure, discrepancies probably arising because the series are not homogeneous, some of them containing cases of both acute and chronic hepatic failure and others being collections of published data which do not correspond to an overall random selection. Benhamou et al. [5] reviewed this question and found a survival rate of 91.7% in 24 patients published as single cases, which fell to 36.8% when a small series containing 277 patients was summated. These authors themselves obtained a survival rate of 16.7% in 60 patients. The mortality rate also seems to vary according to the period of publication and to the country of origin. For instance, Ufer et al. [80] in Germany recorded 88%; Reynolds [69] in California, 60%; and Benhamou et al. [5] in France, 85%.

The depth of coma must also be taken into account: 66% survival is expected when only grade 2 coma is reached, and the prognosis in young patients is better than in the more elderly, where the mortality can approach 100%. If a precipitant can be identified, such as the administration of sedatives, tranquillizers, or diuretics, the prognosis is usually better. Survival depends on the amount of liver necrosis and the capacity of the liver to regenerate: according to Caroli et al. [13] a loss of liver cells more than 60% of the total is never compatible with survival.

No single feature allows a reliable prediction: survival after the most extreme signs, such as decerebrate and decorticate states, has been reported [22]. We have tried to correlate a number of features on a scale of 1 to 4 for the depth of coma, EEG grade, blood ammonia concentration, transaminase level, and PTT. The worst score is 20, the best 5. Only one patient with a score of 11 died but three patients with scores of 15 survived [28]. It is therefore still very difficult, if not impossible, to predict the outcome for a single patient. Ware et al. [84a] examined the prognostic significance of the presence of bridging necrosis in liver necrosis and of other serological markers in a prospective double blind randomized trial. They were not able to identify any feature with prognostic significance.

Many forms of treatment have been used, which indicates that no one form of treatment can be considered as especially suitable for this disease. Intensive therapy should be instituted as soon as the first signs of impending coma are diagnosed. The patient with suspected hepatitis should be considered infectious and all the usual measures should be applied to prevent the spread of the disease. Special care is needed when dealing with blood, excreta, and suction fluids. There is no need for extreme apprehension when treating these comatose patients, however, because the severity of the disease is not due to the virulence of the infective agent but to the inadequate immunological response of the host. The patient should be monitored very carefully; a catheter is placed in a central vein or in the right atrium for feeding, blood sampling, and manometry. A nasogastric tube is also passed to aspirate the gastric contents and avoid the occurrence of vomiting. Alkalis may be given through this tube. Oxygen therapy may be needed to correct hypoxia, and MV for severe respiratory failure; this is an ominous sign in very deep coma and recovery from this stage is rare. Water and electrolyte balance has to be monitored with great care; hypo- and hypernatraemia are not infrequent. Hypertonic sodium should never be used. Potassium replacement is often needed, for hypokalaemia due to reduced intake, glucose feeding, and urinary loss is common. In some patients oedema and ascites formation may cause a rapid shift of fluid out of the circulation with a resulting decrease in blood pressure and urinary output. An increased circulation of vasoactive compounds may aggravate these phenomena and may lead to collapse with shock and development of the hepatorenal syndrome. Large amounts of fluid may need to be given IV to correct this situation and it seems to be more important to restore blood volume and urinary output than to avoid ascites and peripheral oedema. A good review of the treatment of acute liver failure in ICUs is given by

Ward et al. [82], but some special forms of therapy merit further discussion.

Correction of biochemical abnormalities

With different concepts of hepatic encephalopathy, many attempts have been made to correct biochemical alterations presumed to play a role in the pathogenesis of both the acute and the chronic forms. The best results, however, have been obtained in the chronic form. Several such methods are based on the ammonia theory: bowel cleansing, neomycin (4 g/daily, lactulose (30–120 ml syrup 50% daily or by enema).They all have beneficial effects in the chronic, but not in the acute condition. Other methods developed on the neurotransmitter theory have been used; infusions containing high concentrations of branched-chain amino acids and low concentrations of aromatic amino acids have been used, and especially in chronic encephalopathy a beneficial effect has been observed [75]. The application of this therapy in acute failure has yet to be subjected to a properly controlled study and it must still be considered secondary to the use of a more potent hepatic supporting or detoxifying device [35]. The effect of L-dopa on chronic encephalopathy does not seem to be corroborated in controlled studies [55, 56], and this therapy is not effective in acute failure. Bromocriptine, a specific dopamine receptor agonist, has also been used in encephalopathy, but results in the chronic state are again rather conflicting [57, 81].

Substitution therapy for clotting factors is very short-lived and should rarely be recommended. In some cases the infusion of platelet-rich plasma may be beneficial. The administration of H_2 blockers to reduce gastro-intestinal (GI) bleeding needs further testing in acute failure.

Exchange blood transfusion

This was advocated by Trey and co-workers [79] in 1966. In a small uncontrolled series they obtained good results, but few workers could confirm them. Controlled studies of exchange blood transfusion have not yielded superior results: Lewis et al. [51] observed a survival of 21% in 21 treated patients. This is exactly the same figure as the recovery rate computed by the hepatic failure surveillance study. Some authors have tried to replace the whole amount of blood from the body [48, 78], but the survival rate achieved with this more complicated procedure was no better than that yielded by conventional supportive therapy [24]. It is, however, undoubtedly true that some patients may wake during the exchange transfusion and lapse again into coma after it has finished. The strain on the quantity and quality of blood is enormous and because of the relative ease of performance plasmapheresis has been proposed as a substitute. Results with this procedure, however, are also not of any real value.

Cross circulation with human donor or excised liver

Cross circulation could offer a reasonable alternative for the failing liver. It is rather unethical to use healthy donors for this therapy, as the danger of infection is unreasonably high and no real cure or prevention exists. Summers et al. [77] used patients in irreversible coma for this purpose, with seemingly good results. Of the small series published about 80% survived, but this does not seem to be different from the survival in summated small series [5]. It is extremely difficult to find a suitable donor when hepatic failure occurs, and similar difficulties will arise when cross circulation with animals such as baboons or goats are tried on a more than experimental scale [68]. Research was therefore directed at the use of extracorporeal liver perfusion, for which many difficulties had to be overcome. Several kinds of livers have been used, including human cadaver [43] and pig [1, 85]. Although successful results have been published several drawbacks, especially the development of a severe bleeding tendency with thrombocytopenia, were reported.

Corticosteroids

As soon as corticosteroids became available their use in acute liver disease and in liver failure was considered. Indeed, one could assume that their anti-inflammatory effect might limit the amount of hepatocyte necrosis irrespective of its cause. The first attempts were published by Ducci and Katz [30] and seemed favourable. However, further studies did not confirm this early hope and increasing the dose did not produce better results. Administration before the onset of coma had no effect in preventing its development [8, 5]. Recently some controlled studies were carried out, which showed that the mortality was higher with corticosteroids than without: 9 of 48 survived with and 17 of 48 without corticosteroids [66, 68]. It is therefore unlikely that corticosteroids will be beneficial in these cases; on the contrary, their use may precipitate dangerous complications.

Haemodialysis

As it is supposed that toxic substances are circulating in acute hepatic failure, haemodialysis was used when the technique became available. At that time, as now, it was not known precisely what substances were responsible for the cerebral damage. Their passage through the membranes is purely hypothetical and it is also possible that they may be bound to protein and therefore not dialysable. If the substance is of medium or higher molecular weight it will not pass through small-pore membranes and this method, however sound it may look, is greatly hampered by our ignorance of the 'toxic' substances. The first results obtained by Kiley et al. [47] and by Nienhuis et al. [60] in chronic and acute coma were rather promising (as many first attempts!), however.

Further series collated by Benhamou et al. [5] showed recovery of 7 patients in 16 treated (43.7%), as against 36.6% in patients receiving conventional intensive care. The whole question of dialysis was taken up again by Denis et al. [27], who started to use Rhône-Poulenc (RP) polycrylonitrile (AN 69 HD) membrane with a high permeability up to molecular weights of 5 000–10 000 daltons. The rejection coefficient for albumin with a molecular weight of 65 000 is above 99% [72]. Opolon's group treated 41 patients with fulminant hepatic failure and liver coma with 180 haemodialysis periods. All cases except one were probably due to viral hepatitis. In 17 patients (43.6%) a total recovery of consciousness was observed, in 7 (17.9%) a partial recovery; of all the patients only 9 recovered completely (22.2%). The survival rate obtained by Williams' group [73, 74] is somewhat different: only one of 21 [4.8%] died after recovering consciousness. The overall survival rate was 30.8%. However, their series consisted of 29 cases of paracetamol poisoning with a survival of 44.6% and 31 with presumed viral hepatitis with a survival of 25.8%. This last figure is quite similar to all other results of different forms of treatment, except that a higher number regained consciousness. This feature may indicate lack of liver regeneration and lack of control of secondary events such as cerebral oedema.

Sorbents

Sorbents are extremely useful for separation of different molecules and are applied for purification of fluids, especially in industry. This principle was also introduced into medicine and used for the treatment of acute hepatic failure [16]. Here again the application of the method is hampered by our lack of knowledge about the substances to be removed. Therefore a broad spectrum of activity has to be looked for, which of course neglects specificity. Most often activated charcoal, initially uncoated, has been used. This material rapidly absorbs many substances, including proteins and platelets, so producing thrombocytopenia. Severe hypotension was also noted, possibly due to the release of vaso-active substances. The charcoals have now been coated with several products, e.g., acrylic hydrogel, but this reduces the rate of absorption. The first results were promising with a survival of 38% in the first 37 patients, but of the last 32 only three survived. The best survival rates were noted in the patients suffering from Paracetamol overdosage [38]. According to Chang [17], the use of albumin-cellulose nitrate-coated charcoal could improve the biocompatibility of the material. They claim a survival rate of 44% without major complications. The results of Bismuth et al. [7] are less convincing, but they were obtained mostly in drug toxification. Experimental work in rats and dogs showed prolonged survival time [19, 45].

Other exchange systems, such as the amberlite resin, have been developed and used in acute liver failure. They do not seem to give better results than charcoal. Many other systems tested, such as artificial cells [16, 17], immobilized NAD [12], adsorbed enzymes [9, 10], are still in the purely experimental phase.

Further improvement must be awaited from extended knowledge of the multifactorial intoxication. Nevertheless, even if a perfect liver substitute could be developed, the survival of the patient would still depend on the regeneration of the liver, which we also cannot control. Prevention of liver cell death will always be the best measure. The generalized use of vaccination against classic hepatitis viruses may already prevent many cases of infectious hepatitis and dramatically decrease the number of patients with acute hepatic encephalopathy. The clinician urgently needs a better understanding of fulminant necrosis of liver cells, the toxic products causing encephalopathy, and the factors governing liver regeneration. These are the keystones to the search for a more efficient therapy.

References

1. Abouna GM, Fisher LM, Still WJ, Hume DM (1972) Acute hepatic coma successfully treated by extracorporeal baboon liver. Br Med J i:23–25
2. Adams RD, Foley JM (1949) The neurological changes in the more common types of severe liver disease. Trans Am Neurol Assoc 74:217–219
3. Baggenstoss AH, Soloway RD, Summerskill WHJ, Elveback LR, Schoenfield LS (1972) Chronic active liver disease. The range of histologic lesions, their response to treatment and evolution. Hum Pathol 3:183–198
4. Baldessarini RJ, Vogt M (1971) The uptake and subcellular distribution of aromatic amines in the brain of the rat. J Neurochem 18:2519–2533
5. Benhamou JP, Rueff B, Sicot C (1972) Severe hepatic failure. In: Orlandi F, Jezequel AM, (eds) Liver and drugs. Academic Press, London, New York , p 213–228
6. Bessman SP, Bessman AN (1955) The cerebral and peripheral uptake of ammonia in liver disease with an hypothesis for the mechanism of hepatic coma. J Clin Invest 34:622–628
7. Bismuth C, Wattel F, Gosselin R, Lambert H, Genestal M, Galliot M (1979) L'hémoperfusion sur charbon activé enrobé. Expérience des centres antipoisons francais: 60 intoxications. Nouv Presse Med 8:1235–1238
8. Blum AL, Stutz R, Haemmerli UP, Schmid P, Grady GF (1969) A fortuitously controlled study of steroid therapy in acute viral hepatitis. Am J Med 47:82–92
9. Brunner G (1974) Microsomal enzymes bound to artificial carriers. In: Williams R, Murray-Lyon IM, (eds) Artificial liver support. Pitman, London, p 153–157
10. Brunner G (1978) Approaches to an artificial liver. Acta Hepatogastroenterol (Stuttg) 25:77–86
11. Cachin M, Pergola F, Guyet-Rousset P, Gavelle M (1963) Corticothérapie au cours de l'hépatite virale. Bull Soc Med Hop 114:719–731
12. Campbell J, Chang TMS (1969) The recycling of NAD+ (free and immobilized) within semi-permeable aqueous microcapsules containing a multi-enzyme system. Biochem Biophys Res Commun 69:562–569
13. Caroli J, Opolon P, Scotto J, Hadchouel P, Thomas M, Lageron A (1971) Elements du pronostic au cours des comas par atrophie hépatique aiguë. Presse Med 79:463–466
14. Challenger F, Walshe JM (1955) Foetor hepaticus. Lancet II:1239–1241
15. Chang TMS (1972a) Artificial cells. Thomas Springfield
16. Chang TMS (1972) Hemoperfusion over microencapsulated charcoal adsorbent in a patient with hepatic coma. Lancet II:1371–1372
17. Chang TMS (1975) Experience with the treatment of acute liver failure patients by haemoperfusion over biocompatible microencapsulated (coated) charcoal. In: Williams R, Murray-Lyon IM (eds) Artificial liver support. Pitman, London
18. Chase RA, Davies M, Trewby PN, Silk DB, Williams R (1978) Plasma amino acid profiles in patients with fulminant hepatic failure treated with polyacrylonitile membrane. Gastroenterology 75:1033–1040
19. Chirito E, Reiter B, Lister C, Chang TM (1977) Artificial liver: The effect of ACAC microencapsulated charcoal

haemoperfusion on fulminant hepatic failure. Artif Organs 1:76–83

20. Cohen RA, Kopin IJ, Creveling CR, Musacchio JM, Fisher JE, Crout JR, Gill JR (1966) False neurochemical transmitters. Ann Intern Med 65:347–362

21. Conn HO (1978) Lactulose: A drug in search of a modus operandi. Gastroenterology 74:624–626

22. Conomy JP, Swash MS (1968) Reversible decerebrate and decorticate postures in hepatic coma. N Engl J Med 278:876–879

23. Cooper AJL, McDonald JM, Gelbard AS, Gledhill RF, Duffy TE (1979) The metabolic fate of N-labeled ammonia in rat brain. J Biol Chem 254:4982–4992

24. Cooper GN, Karlson KE, Clowes GH, Martin H, Randall HT (1977) Total blood washout and exchange. A valuable tool in acute hepatic coma and Reye's syndrome. Am J Surg 133:522–530

25. Cooperstock MS, Tucher RP, Baublis JV (1975) Possible pathogenetic role of endotoxin in Reye's syndrome. Lancet I:1272–1274

26. Decker K, Keppler D (1972) Galactosamine induced liver injury. In: Popper H, Schaffner F (eds) Progress in liver disease. Grune & Stratton, New York, pp 183–199

27. Denis J, Opolon P, Nusinovici V, Granger A, Darwin F (1978) Treatment of encephalopathy during fulminant hepatic failure by haemodialysis with high permeability membrane. Gut 19:787–793

28. Desmet VJ, De Groote J, Van Damme B (1972) Acute hepatocellular failure. A study of 17 patients treated with exchange transfusion. Hum Pathol 3:167–182

29. Doizaki WM, Zieve L (1979) In: Popper H, Schaffner F (eds) Lethal doses of methionine, phénylalanine and tryptophan do not cause coma before death in normal rats. Grune and Stratton, New York, San Francisco, London

30. Ducci H, Katz R (1952) Cortisone ACTH and antibiotics in fulminant hepatitis. Gastroenterol 21:357–374

31. EASL study (1978) cited in Berk PD, Popper H (eds) Fulminant hepatic failure. Am J Gastroenterol 69:349–400

32. Evans H, Bourgeois CH, Comer DS, Keschamras N (1970) Brain lesions in the Reye's syndrome. Arch Pathol 99:543–546

33. Farivar M, Wands JR, Isselbacher KJ, Bucher NNL (1976) Effect of insulin and glucagon on fulminant murine hepatitis. N Engl J Med 296:1517–1519

34. Fisher JE, Baldessarini RJ (1971) False neurotransmitters and hepatic failure. Lancet II:75–79

35. Fisher JE, Freund JE, Rosen H, Yoshimura N, Bradford R, Sofio C (1978) Effect of F 080 in clinical hepatic encephalopathy: Result of phase I study. Gastroenterology 75:963

36. Foley JM, Watson CW, Adams RD (1950) Significance of electroencephalographic changes in hepatic coma. Trans Am Neurol Assoc 75:161–165

37. Gallagher CH, Judah JD, Rees KR (1956) Enzyme changes during liver autolysis. J Pathol Bacteriol 72:247–256

38. Gazzard BG, Weston MJ, Murray-Lyon IM, Flax H, Record CO, Portmann B, Langley PG, Dunlop EH, Mellin PJ, Ward MB, Williams R (1974) Charcoal haemoperfusion in the treatment of fulminant hepatic failure. Lancet I:1301–1307

39. Gazzard BG, Portmann B, Murray-Lyon IM, Williams R (1975) Cause of death in fulminant hepatic failure and relationship to quantitative histological assessment of parenchymal damage. Q J Med 44:615–626

40. Geiger A, Magnes J, Tailor AM, Veralli M (1954) Effect of blood constituents on uptake of glucose and metabolic rate of the brain in perfusion experiments. Am J Physiol 177:138–149

41. Gregory PB, Knauer CM, Kempson RL, Miller R (1976) Steroid therapy in severe viral hepatitis: A double-blind randomized trial of methyl-prednisolone versus placebo. N Engl J Med 294:681–687

42. Hanid MA, Mackenzie RL, Jenner RE, Chase RA, Mellon PJ, Trewby PN, Janota I, Davis M, Silk DBA, Williams R (1979) Intracranial pressure in pigs with surgically induced acute liver failure. Gastroenterology 76:123–131

43. Hardison WG, Norman JC (1967) Ex vivo pig liver perfusion for acute hepatic failure: Bile salt composition of pig bile during perfusion. Medicine 46:97–102

44. Heyd CC (1943) The concept of liver deaths. JAMA 121:736–737

45. Horak J, Horky J, Rabl M (1980) Haemoperfusion through activated charcoal in dogs with fulminant hepatic failure. Digestion 20:22–30

46. Hoyumpa AM, Desmond PV, Avant GR, Roberts RK, Schenker S (1979) Hepatic encephalopathy (clinical conference). Gastroenterology 76:184–195

47. Kiley JE, Pender JC, Welch HF, Welch CS (1958) Ammonia intoxication treated by hemodialysis. N Engl J Med 259:1156–1161

48. Klebanoff G, Hollander D, Cosimi AB, Stanford W, Kemmerer WT (1972) Asanguinous hypothermic total body perfusion (TBW) in the treatment of stage IV hepatic coma. J Surg Res 12:1–7

49. Krebs HA (1935) Metabolism of amino acids IV. The synthesis of glutamine from glutamic acid and ammonia and the enzymatic hydrolysis of glutamine in animal tissues. Biochem J 29:1951–1969

50. Lawrence W, Schwartz AE, Randell HT (1958) Alterations in blood ammonia in dogs following total hepatectomy and abdominal evisceration. Surg Gynerol Obstet 107:69–73

51. Lewis JD, Hussey CV, Varma RR, Darin JC (1977) Exchange transfusion in hepatic coma. Factors affecting results with long-term follow-up data. Am J Surg 129:125–129

52. Liehr H, Grun M, Seelig HP, Seelig R, Rasenack U (1978) Synergistic action of hepatocyte membrane defect and activated complement system in liver cell death. Acta Hepatogastroenterol (Stuttg) 25:105–110

53. Livingstone AS, Potvin M, Goresky CA, Finlayson MH, Hinchey EJ (1977) Changes in the blood brain barrier in hepatic coma after hepatectomy in the rat. Gastroenterology 73:697–704

54. Lucke B, Mallory T (1946) The fulminant form of epidemic hepatitis. Am J Path 22:867–945

55. Lunzer M, James IM, Weinman J, Sherlock S (1974) Treatment of chronic encephalopathy with levodopa. Gut 15:555–561

56. Michel H, Cauvet G, Granier PM, Bali JP, Andre R, Cuilleret G (1977) Treatment of cirrhotic hepatic encephalopathy by L-dopa. A double blind study of 58 patients. Digestion 15:232–233

57. Morgan MY, Jakobovits AW, James IM, Sherlock S (1980) Succesfull use of bromocriptine in the treatment of chronic encephalopathy. Gastroenterology, 78:663–670

58. Muto Y (1966) Clinical study on the relationship of short-chain fatty acids and hepatic encephalopathy. Nippon Shokakibyo Gakkai Zasshi 63:19–32

59. Nencki M, Pawlow JP, Zaleski J (1896) Ueber den Ammoniakgehalt des Blutes und der Organe und Harnstoffbildung bei der Säugetiere. Arch Exp Pathol Pharmacol 37:26–51

60. Nienhuis LI, Mulmed EI, Kelley JW (1963) Hepatic coma: Treatment emphasizing merit of peritoneal dialy-

sis. Am J Surg 106:980–985
61. Nusinovici V, Crubille C, Opolon P, Touboul JP, Darnis F, Caroli J (1977) Hépatites fulminantes avec coma. Revue de 137 cas. Complications. Gastroenterol Clin Biol 1:861–873
62. Dettel H (1948) Folgen der Leberinsuffiziens. Schweiz Med Wochenschr 78:833–834
63. Parsons-Smith BG, Summerskill WHJ, Dawson AM, Sherlock S (1957) The electroencephalograph in liver disease. Lancet I:867–871
64. Partin JC, Schubert WK, Partin JS (1971) Mitochondrial ultrastructure in Reye's syndrome. N Engl J Med 285:1339–1343
65. Rabinowitz JL, Staeffen J, Blanquet P, Vincent JD, Terme R, Series C, Myerson RM (1978) Sources of serum [14C]-octonoate in cirrhosis of the liver and hepatic encephalopathy. J Lab Clin Med 31:223–227
66. Rakela J, Acute Hepatic Failure Study Group (1979) A double blind, randomized trial of hydrocortisone in acute hepatic failure. Gastroenterology 76 abstr 1297
67. Record CO, Buxton B, Chase RA, Curzon IM, Murray-Lyon IM, Williams R (1976) Plasma and brain amino acids in fulminant hepatic failure and their relationship to hepatic encephalopathy. Eur J Clin Invest 6:387–394
68. Redeker AG, Schweitzer H, Yamahiro HS (1976) Randomization of corticosteroid therapy in fulminant hepatitis. N Engl J Med 294:728–729
69. Reynolds TB, Redeker AG, Davis P (1958) A controlled study of the effects of l-arginine on hepatic encephalopathy. Am. J Med 25:359–367
70. Rueff B, Benhamou JP (1973) Acute hepatic necrosis and fulminant hepatic failure. Gut 14:805–815
71. Saunders SJ, Terblanche J, Bosman SCW, Harrison GG, Wales R, Hickman R, Biebuyck J, Dent D, Pearce S, Barnard CM (1968) Acute hepatic coma treated by cross-circulation with a baboon and by repeated exchange transfusions. Lancet I:584–588
72. Sausse A, Granger A, Man NK, Funck-Brentano JL (1974) Un nouveau rein artificiel: Nouvel appareil associant une membrane a haute perméabilité et un bain de dialyse en circuit fermé. Nouv Presse Med 3:957–958
73. Silk DBA, Williams R (1978) Experiences in the treatment of fulminant hepatic failure by conservative therapy, charcoal haemoperfusion and polyacrylonitrile haemodialysis. Int J Artif Organs 1:29–33
74. Silk DBA, Hanid MA, Trewby PN, Avies M, Chase RA, Langley PG, Mellon PJ, Wheeler PG, Williams R (1977) Treatment of fulminant hepatic failure by polyacrylonitrile membrane haemodialysis. Lancet II:1–3
75. Smith AR, Rossi-Fanelli F, Ziparo V, James HJ, Perelle BA, Fisher JE (1978) Alterations in plasma and CSF amino acids, amines and metabolites in hepatic coma. Ann Surg 187:343–350
76. Stadie WC, Van Slyke DD (1920) The effect of acute liver atrophy on metabolism and composition of the liver. Arch Intern Med 25:693–696
77. Summers RW, Curtis SJ, Hartford CE (1970) Acute hepatic coma treated by cross circulation with irreversibly comatose donor. JAMA 214:2297–2301
78. Tobias HW, Isom W (1973) Total body perfusion in the treatment of hepatic coma secondary to fulminant hepatitis. Gastroenterology 64:157 (abstract)
79. Trey C, Burns DG, Saunders SJ (1966) Treatment of hepatic coma by exchange blood transfusion. N Engl J Med 274:473–381
80. Ufer C, Dolle W, Martini GA (1966) Ueberlebungsdauer und Prognose bei Kranken mit Leberkoma. Internist 7:43–47
81. Uribe M, Farca A, Marquez MA, Garcia-Ramos G, Guevara L, with Briones A, Gil S (1979) Treatment of chronic portal systemic encephalopathy with promocriptine: A double blind controlled study. Gastroenterology 76: 1347–1351
82. Ward ME, Trewly PN, Williams R, Strumin L (1977) Acute liver failure. Experience in a special unit. Anaesthesia 32:228–231
83. Ware AJ, D'Agostino AN, Combes B (1971) Cerebral oedema: A major complication of massive hepatic necrosis. Gastroenterology 61:877–884
84. Ware AJ, Jones RE, Shorey JW, Combes B (1974) A controlled trial of steroid therapy in massive hepatic necrosis. Am J Gastroenterol 12:130–133
84a. Ware AJ, Cuthbert JA, Shorey J, Gurian LE, Eigenbrodt EH, Combes B (1981) A prospective trial of steroid therapy in severe viral hepatitis. The prognostic significance of bridging necrosis. Gastroenterology 80: 219–224
85. Watts J, McK, Douglas MC, Dudley HAF, Gurr FW, Owen JA (1967) The use of pig liver extra-corporeal circulation in hepatic coma Br J Med ii:341–345
86. Zieve FJ, Zieve L, Doizaki WM, Gilsdorf RB (1974a) Synergism between ammonia and fatty acids in the production of coma: Implications for hepatic coma. J Pharmarol Exp Ther 191:10–16
87. Zieve L, Doizaki WM, Zieve FJ (1974b) Synergism between mercaptans and ammonia or fatty acids in the production of coma: A possible role for mercaptans in the pathogenesis of hepatic coma. J Lab Clin Med 83:16–28
88. Zillig G (1974) Neurologische und psychische Störungen bei Leber-Erkrankungen. Nervenarzt 18:297–313

Chapter 28

Acute Pancreatitis

Stephen N. Joffe and Leslie Donaldson

The incidence of acute pancreatitis varies between 50 and 100 cases per million population per annum, and in the west of Scotland it has a similar incidence to that of perforated peptic ulcer. Histological evidence of acute pancreatitis is present in 0.6% of unselected autopsy studies.

Postoperative pancreatitis, following abdominal surgery, occurs in 1%–6% of cases. Delay and difficulty in establishing the diagnosis leads to a higher mortality than primary pancreatitis. In a post-mortem study of patients dying from acute pancreatitis, 14% had postoperative pancreatitis [44]. This chapter considers various aspects of acute pancreatitis, including aetiology, pathogenesis, methods of diagnosis, current treatment, and management of the complications.

Aetiology

The aetiology of acute pancreatitis is not well understood, although there are a number of associated factors. Table 28.1 lists the available data recorded in several recent studies. Acute pancreatitis is associated with gallstones in 42% of cases and with alcohol in 34%; it is idiopathic in 17%, and a miscellaneous group accounts for 7%. These last two groups include postoperative pancreatitis, viral infections, pancreatitis associated with lipid abnormalities, drugs, hyperparathyroidism, and trauma. The variation in incidence of gallstones- and alcohol-related pancreatitis probably relates to the study of different patient populations.

Gallstone pancreatitis (42%)

In patients with gallstone pancreatitis, choledocholithiasis is present in only 20% of cases, 2% being ampullary, while 72% have stones in the gallbladder. Gallstones were recovered from a 10-day collection of faeces in 88% of patients with acute pancreatitis, as against only 11% without pancreatitis [1]. This may mean that the pancreatic duct becomes obstructed with gallstone fragments during their passage down the common bile duct. Biliary 'mud' is frequently the cause of recurrent attacks of acute pancreatitis in females with apparently normal biliary radiology [43].

Table 28.1. Review of aetiological factors, diagnosis, and complications in 1837 patients

Author	No. of cases	Country	Aetiological factors				Diagnostic amylase	Antibiotics	Mortality	Complications			Type of Study[d]
			Gall-stones	Alcohol	Idiopathic	Post-operative				Acute renal failure	Pseudo-cyst %	Abscess %	
Storcke et al. 1976	116	Sweden	43	25	18	14	N/A	N/A	Post-mortem study				Retr.
Imrie and Whyte 1975	78	UK	51	26	13	5	4 × normal	No	11.5%	6%	5%	4%	Pro.
Jacobs et al. 1977	519	USA	46	31	35 (Incl. mort. 17%)				12.9%	4.4%	2%	3%	Retr.
MRC trial 1977	257	UK	55	9	32	Exc.[c]	6 × normal	No	11%	3%	6%	4%	Pro.
Imrie et al. 1978	161	UK	52	31	13	N/A	4 × normal	No	8.7%	N/A	N/A	N/A	Pro.
Durr et al. 1978	56	Germany	34	51	9	5	2 × normal	As necessary	13%	N/A	N/A	N/A	Pro.
Ranson and Spencer 1978	450	USA	16	70	9		>200 Somogyi units	Routine	7%				Pro.
Feller et al. 1974	200	Canada	5%–6% N/A		N/A	N/A	>600 Somogyi units	Routine	6%	N/A		8.5%	

[a]UK, United Kingdom; USA, United States of America.
[b]N/A, not available.
[c]Exc., excluded.
[d]Retr., retrospective; Pro., prospective.

Alcoholic pancreatitis (34%)

The mechanism of alcohol-induced acute pancreatitis is not clearly established. It develops after 8–10 years of excessive alcohol ingestion in susceptible individuals. Overt pancreatitis occurs in 10% of alcoholic patients and endoscopic retrograde pancreatography frequently demonstrates ductal changes in these patients. At post mortem pancreatic damage is found in 17%–45% of alcoholic patients. In the majority of patients who develop acute pancreatitis with continued alcohol ingestion the condition progresses to chronic pancreatitis. Either may occur in a relapsing or recurrent form.

Idiopathic pancreatitis (17%) and miscellaneous causes (7%)

The number of patients with idiopathic pancreatitis depends on the extent to which the rarer causes have been investigated following the exclusion of alcohol and gallstones. Acute pancreatitis is found in 7% of patients with primary hyperparathyroidism, but in 30% of such patients during hypercalcaemic crisis. In 2% of patients it is attributed to a viral infection such as mumps or Coxsackie B. Hyperlipidaemia has been implicated in 1% of cases, but it is unclear whether it is a primary cause or a secondary effect. Atherosclerosis and pancreatic ischaemia probably account for a small number of cases [47]. Many drugs have been reported to produce pancreatitis. These include steroids, oestrogens, and diuretics, but it is frequently unclear whether it was the underlying disease being treated or the actual drugs that induced the pancreatitis. The incidence of pancreatitis following endoscopic retrograde cholangio-pancreatogram (ERCP) examination is between 1% and 7%, and an important but rare cause of acute pancreatitis is pancreatic carcinoma (2%).

Pathogenesis

Autodigestion is the basic pathological process, and it occurs as a result of premature activation of proteolytic enzymes, including trypsinogen, which are normally synthesized in the pancreas. Precisely how this occurs is not known, although many theories have been postulated. Activated trypsinogen (trypsin) produces a vasculitis and activates the precursors of elastase, phospholipase, lysolecithin, and kallikrein, which further damage the gland, causing a vicious circle.

Bile reflux into the pancreatic duct is associated with activation of these enzymes. The intrapancreatic ductal pressure is normally in excess of the common bile duct pressure, but it is not uncommon to see contrast material rapidly refluxing into the pancreatic duct in patients undergoing operative cholangiography, particularly if they have had an antecedent pancreatitis.

Hypoxia of the gland as a result of either local ischaemia or systemic hypoxia can precipitate acute pancreatitis [16]. In patients with ruptured abdominal aortic aneurysms the incidence of pancreatitis is closely related to the incidence of acute tubular necrosis [47]. Recent studies indicate a marked local ischaemia and reduced percentage cardiac output and O_2 consumption in experimental pancreatitis in the dog [11, 14]. Excessive stimulation of the gland by food, alcohol, or pancreatic secretagogues may be additional factors.

Symptoms and signs

Sudden and constant upper abdominal pain occurs in 90% of patients, with radiation through to the back in more than half. The pain is of variable intensity and frequently is relieved by sitting up or leaning forward. Many patients have anorexia, nausea, and vomiting, but occasional patients may have no abdominal pain. These patients frequently present in coma or shock and have a high mortality [39]. On examination tachypnoea, tachycardia, and hypotension are found, which are of adverse prognostic importance, although some patients present with transient hypertension. In 50% of patients there are abdominal guarding and reduced bowel sounds, but there is a striking discrepancy between the severity of the pain and the lack of abdominal signs.

One-third of patients have a facial flush and only rarely (1%) is there loin staining (Cullen's sign) or umbilical staining (Grey-Turner's sign). Both are associated with increased mortality and they reflect severe retroperitoneal haemorrhage. Since there are no specific signs or symptoms, diagnosis depends on laboratory investigations.

Diagnostic aids

Serum amylase

The most frequently performed laboratory investigation to confirm the diagnosis of pancreatitis is determination of the serum amylase level. There is a difference of opinion as to the degree of elevation and specificity of the hyperamylasaemia. A serum amylase level in excess of 200 Somogyi units [36], twice [19], four times [25] or six times [32] the value for the upper limit of normal, have all been mentioned as diagnostic of acute pancreatitis (Table 28.1). This makes comparisons between studies difficult. Some accept a lower serum amylase in conjunction with a 'typical' clinical presentation and course or an elevated urinary amylase.

Serum amylase is elevated in many non-pancreatic conditions. These include renal insufficiency, diabetic keto-acidosis, pneumonia, mumps, prostatic disease, perforated peptic ulcer, ectopic pregnancy, dissecting abdominal aneurysm, mesenteric infarction, peritonitis and appendicitis [41]. Fortunately, an elevated serum amylase level correlates with acute pancreatitis in about 75% of patients, but the degree of hyperamylasaemia is not related to the severity of the disease. Hyperamylasaemia of non-pancreatic origin rarely exceeds five times the upper limit of normal.

Macro-amylasaemia is due to binding between amylase and a globulin complex and is present in 1% of the normal population and does not indicate pancreatitis. The serum amylase is raised but the urinary amylase clearance and amylase: creatinine clearance ratio (ACCR) are normal. Elevated serum triglycerides can artificially depress the serum amylase level, and following serum dilution the measured amylase can increase by over 350% [10].

Amylase: creatinine clearance ratio

The ACCR is derived from the ratio of

$$\frac{\text{urine amylase}}{\text{serum amylase}} \times \frac{\text{serum creatinine}}{\text{urine creatinine}} \times 100.$$

This ratio uses both the serum and urine amylase level and is independent of the timed urine collection required with either the 4^{-h} or the 24^{-h} urinary amylase clearance measurements. Urine is voided and a simultaneous blood sample collected. The ACCR is calculated from the amylase and creatinine measurements and the normal range is between 2% and 3.1% [30, 34, 46]. An ACCR of greater than 5%–5.5% is diagnostic of acute pancreatitis [34, 46]. The ACCR may be normal during the acute phase of pancreatitis, but it may also identify cases presenting more than 36 h after the onset of pancreatitis when the serum amylase level has returned towards normal [34]. Urinary amylase activity varies considerably with the technique used to measure it, and the commonly used Phadebas kit yields higher urinary amylase levels than the sacchrogenic method [9]. In addition, the urinary creatinine value alters with time and therefore all urine samples must be freshly tested.

Amylase isoenzymes

The ideal method of diagnosing hyperamylasaemia due to pancreatic disease would be identification of the pancreatic component of the amylase isoenzymes. At present there is no satisfactory technique for the identification of these amylase isoenzymes. An alternative method is to identify the pancreatic component of the serum amylase level by a thermolability technique in which the amylase activity is measured in the serum before and after heating to 65°C. Heat destroys the salivary and pancreatic amylase components, and normal serum amylase activity is less than 50% thermolabile. In acute pancreatitis the amylase thermolability increases to more than 80% and remains elevated with the development of pancreatic pseudocysts [12, 13].

Other tests

Serum lipase closely parallels the rise of serum amylase but is no more specific. Methaemalbuminaemia was previously thought to be diagnostic of haemorrhagic pancreatitis but is also found in GI haemorrhage, tubal pregnancy, and soft tissue trauma. Deoxyribonuclease is elevated in acute pancreatitis but there is insufficient evidence indicating specificity for pancreatic necrosis.

Investigations

Straight abdominal x-ray

This is abnormal in one third of patients, showing either a sentinel or duodenal loop containing a fluid level or a distended transverse colon with no gas in the descending colon. Occasionally pancreatic calcification or gallstones may be seen, but none of these is diagnostic.

Computed axial tomography and ultrasound

These techniques make it possible to identify an oedematous mass in the head of the pancreas during the acute phase and can assist in the early detection of pancreatic pseudocysts and gallstones. Their value is being assessed.

Differential diagnosis

Acute pancreatitis can be a difficult diagnostic problem since there are no specific signs, clinical symptoms, or investigations which are pathognomonic for this disease. Within the first 2–3 h the clinical features suggest acute cholecystitis or acute peptic ulceration, at 6–8 h the presentation is that of a perforated viscus, and by 2–3 days the features may mimic an intestinal obstruction.

One must consider the diagnosis of acute pancreatitis in all patients who present with sudden shock which is not associated with abdominal pain. It must also be considered in patients who have persistent abdominal pain, ileus, fever, or shock after abdominal surgery. In postoperative pancreatitis the serum amylase

level rarely reaches the diagnostic level for primary acute pancreatitis.

Mortality

The mortality from acute pancreatitis varies from 6% to 13% (Table 28.1). This alters considerably if patients are divided into groups according to the severity of the disease. In mild pancreatitis the mortality is less than 1% [25, 36], while it increases to 23% or 28% in severe pancreatitis [25, 36].

An attempt must be made as early as possible to identify those patients with severe acute pancreatitis. These are the only patients who really require specific and urgent treatment in an attempt to reduce the mortality and morbidity. The prognostic factors which categorize the severity of the pancreatitis include the age of the patient and various routine biochemical and haematological tests given in Table 28.2 [25, 36].

While these criteria identify the patients with severe pancreatitis and indicate possible mortality, none of them directly measures the extent of pancreatic damage. Instead they reflect the systemic response of the body to the pancreatitis. More recently McMahon and Pickford [31] have found no correlation between various biochemical values and the severity of pancreatitis. They considered that an SGOT > 60 IU/litre, in the absence of a history of

Table 28.2. Prognostic factors in acute pancreatitis on admission or within 48 h[a]

Factors	Ranson and Spencer 1978	Imrie et al. 1978
Age	>55 years	>55 years
White cell count	>16 000/mm^3	>15 000/mm^3
LDH	>350 IU/litre	>600 IU/litre
SGOT	>250 units/100 ml	>100 units/litre
Plasma glucose in absence of diabetes	>200 mg/100 ml	>10 mmol/litre
Blood urea	>5 mg/100 ml	>16 mmol/litre and not responding to IV fluids
Serum calcium	<8 mg/100 ml	<2.0 mmol/litre
Arterial pO$_2$	<60 mmHg (8 kPa)	<60 mmHg (8 kPa)
Albumin	—	<32 g/litre
Estimated fluid sequestration	>6000 ml	—
Haematocrit	During the initial 48 hours, haematocrit fell by >10 percentage points	—

[a]Patients in whom less than three of the factors listed were present were considered to have mild pancreatitis, while the condition was judged to be severe when more than three of these factors were present. The mortality rose exponentially with the number of factors, to almost 100% when seven or eight were present.

excessive alcohol consumption, was indicative of gallstones.

Principles of management

The management of acute pancreatitis has two components. The first is general supportive treatment and the second consists in specific measures to prevent the complications of pancreatitis and to reduce pancreatic inflammation.

Naso-gastric intubation

Naso-gastric intubation has long been advocated in the treatment of patients with acute pancreatitis, without objective evidence of its efficacy. Its objective is to reduce gastric and duodenal distension, minimize vomiting, and decrease pancreatic exocrine stimulation.

Intravenous fluid replacement

The cornerstone of medical therapy of acute pancreatitis is adequate IV fluid replacement [3]. This is to replace the fluid sequestrated into the peritoneal cavity, retroperitoneal space, liver, and pleural cavities and to maintain renal function. IV fluids in the form of normal saline and 5% dextrose are given in a sufficient volume to maintain a urine output in excess of 30 ml/h. An indwelling urinary catheter ensures accurate measurement of hourly urine volumes. A central venous pressure catheter is obligatory in patients with severe pancreatitis, and the central venous pressure should be kept between 8 and 10 cm H_2O. In the first 48 h the patient may require large quantities of colloid, up to 6 or even 8 litres, since 30%–40% of the effective circulating plasma volume may be lost. Thereafter the patient develops a diuretic phase and care must be taken that he is not overloaded with fluid. The loss of albumin partly explains the hypocalcaemia seen in patients with severe pancreatitis. Although the serum calcium level falls, the serum ionized calcium usually remains normal [2].

Analgesics

The pain in pancreatitis can be very severe and most patients require large doses of analgesics. These may be given either IM or by IV infusion. The analgesic of choice is pethidine, since unlike the opiates it does not produce spasm of the ampulla. Some authors advocate the use of epidural anaesthesia in the treatment of pancreatitis, but we have no experience of this technique.

Inhibition of pancreatic exocrine secretion

Many authors emphasize the necessity of suppressing pancreatic exocrine secretion. A wide variety of drugs have been advocated, which include antacids, anticholinergic drugs, tranquillizers (to inhibit the cephalic phase of pancreatic secretion), glucagon, calcitonin, cimetidine, vasopressin, and diamox. However, none of these drugs has been proved to be of definite value in controlled clinical studies [18]. Indeed, there is no objective evidence that the pancreatic exocrine gland is active and secreting in acute pancreatitis. Enteral and parenteral feeding have also been advocated.

However, prevention of the renal and respiratory failure is the most important feature in the treatment of acute pancreatitis.

Treatment of respiratory failure

One-third of patients with acute pancreatitis have an abnormal chest x-ray on admission. The abnormalities include left pleural effusion, pulmonary oedema, and atelectasis [27, 28]. Serial estimations of arterial blood gases taken in acute pancreatitis reveal that almost 80% of patients have a PaO_2 below 70 mmHg (9.3 kPa) and 45% have severe arterial hypoxia, with a PaO_2 below 60 mmHg (8 kPa) [27]. Clinically these patients do not appear to be in respiratory failure. Supplementary humidified O_2 therapy is recommended for all patients over the age of 60 years and for younger patients who have a PaO_2 of less than 70 mmHg (9.3 kPa). Twice-daily measurements of arterial blood gases whilst the patients are breathing ambient air and supplementary O_2 should be continued for a minimum of 5 days so that progress and the effects of therapy can be monitored. In patients not responding to controlled O_2 therapy IPPV or PEEP may be required.

The mechanism of this ARDS is not clearly understood but is probably multifactorial. The factors involved include pleural effusion, atelectasis, retroperitoneal oedema, elevation of the diaphragm, abdominal distension with guarding, intravascular coagulation, thrombo-emboli, right-to-left shunting within the pulmonary vascular bed, reduced pulmonary surfactant, and an alteration in the oxyhaemoglobin dissociation curve to the right [18, 24, 40]. Whatever the mechanisms for this arterial hypoxia, it is associated with an increased mortality. Systemic hypoxia or hypercapnia can produce a 50% reduction in pancreatic blood flow in the normal dog, which may partially explain the detrimental effect of systemic hypoxia seen in man [6].

Treatment of renal complications

Half the patients with acute pancreatitis have proteinuria, microscopic haematuria, and pus cells in the urine, indicating a nephropathica pancreatica. Rising blood urea and serum creatinine are adverse prognostic signs. Accordingly its prevention with high volume IV fluid replacement is indicated. In patients not responding to fluid replacement and whose urine volume is less than 30 ml/h, bolus treatment with IV plasma (500 ml), mannitol (20 g) or frusemide (80 mg) is often beneficial. Established acute renal failure is treated by peritoneal dialysis, which itself may have a therapeutic role in the management of severe pancreatitis [36]. Haemodialysis is required if patients are still failing to respond. The incidence of acute renal failure secondary to acute pancreatitis is only 4%, but it is itself associated with an increased mortality. When it is combined with ARDS requiring artificial ventilation nearly all patients die.

Pancreatic encephalopathy

Psychotic disturbance in the form of disorientation, confusion, delirium, and hallucinations occurs in 12% of patients. This psychiatric disturbance may be due primarily to pancreatitis or, more probably, reflects either systemic hypoxia or delirium tremens subsequent to alcohol withdrawal. It requires no specific therapy.

Haematological abnormalities

Thrombocytopenia, hypofibrinogenaemia, and fibrinogen degradation products are found in acute pancreatitis, suggesting intravascular coagulation [33, 37]. The haematological abnormalities do not vary with the aetiology of the pancreatitis [33].

Venous thrombosis

Deep venous thrombosis is common in acute pancreatitis and may be associated with the hypercoagulability state [37]. Pulmonary micro-thrombo-embolism could account for some of the respiratory complications, and venous thrombosis is prominent in the peripancreatic tissues and splenic vein in patients dying from acute pancreatitis. In patients undergoing laparotomy and pancreatic resection for acute pancreatitis, there is a sharp demarcation between healthy and necrotic tissue [29, 35].

Specific medical treatment

Many drugs inhibit pancreatic exocrine function and have been advocated in the management of acute pancreatitis. However, as mentioned, none of these drugs is of proven value. A variety of other specific treatments have been advocated and will now be considered.

Anti-enzyme preparations

A vast and contradictory literature has built up on the usefulness of the anti-kallikrein drug aprotinin (Trasylol) since its introduction in 1950. The more recent double-blind prospective clinical studies of this drug [25, 32], in which aprotinin was given in initial doses of 500 000 KIU and then 200 000 KIU four times a day for 5 days, have failed to demonstrate any reduction in mortality compared with standard conservative treatment. It may, however, have a place in the prevention of pancreatitis if given prophylactically in patients undergoing pancreaticobiliary surgery.

Inhibitors of plasminogen activation

Epsilon aminocaproic acid (EACA) and the more potent p, aminomethyl benzoic acid (PANBA) inhibit activation of plasminogen and in high concentrations also plasmin and trypsin. Some authors noted an increased mortality in animals given EACA in treatment of their experimental pancreatitis, and in humans it is considered as ineffective as aprotinin. Accordingly their use is not currently recommended [18].

Improvement of pancreatic microcirculation

Both direct and indirect experimental and clinical studies suggest a reduction in pancreatic blood flow in acute pancreatitis [16]. In man, the clear demarcation between normal and inflamed pancreas suggests a vascular aetiology

[29, 45]. Blood flow studies in dogs have demonstrated a 72% reduction in pancreatic blood flow at 3 h, associated with a selective reduction in the percentage of the cardiac output to the gland and a fall in the pancreatic O_2 consumption. These were all in the presence of normal arterial blood gas values [11, 14].

This suggests that pancreatic injury could be minimized in acute pancreatitis if stasis and thrombosis within the pancreatic microcirculation was prevented and a satisfactory blood flow maintained. While there are no clinical data to prove the value of anti-aggregant drugs such as fibrinolysin, heparin, and dextran 40, there is animal evidence to show that all these drugs reduce the mortality in experimental pancreatitis [22, 23] and improve the pancreatic blood flow and O_2 uptake [11, 14]. Post-ganglionic sympathectomy has been shown also to maintain pancreatic blood flow and reduce mortality in experimental pancreatitis [48].

Antibiotic therapy

The routine use of prophylactic antibiotics in the treatment of acute pancreatitis has been advocated [3, 5, 20]. The antibiotics are given to prevent secondary chest infection and possibily to reduce the incidence of pancreatic abscess formation. However, prospective clinical trials in the United States, where alcohol-induced pancreatitis predominates, have shown that prophylactic antibiotics failed to reduce the mortality, sepsis rate, or incidence of pancreatic abscess formation [8, 21]. In Britain, gallstones are the most common aetiological factor, and the infection which commonly co-exists may cause a higher mortality and septic complication rate. This is not confirmed by the United Kingdom studies in which prophylactic antibiotics were not given and the mortality and complication rates were similar [25, 26, 32]. There is at present insufficient objective evidence for the use of prophylactic antibiotics in patients with acute pancreatitis.

Surgical treatment

According to Babb [4], there are four possible indications for surgery in patients with acute pancreatitis:

Diagnostic laparotomy

This is undertaken when there is uncertainty about diagnosis and there is a suspicion of a surgically correctable lesion. It is controversial whether such a laparotomy has a detrimental effect on the mortality from pancreatitis, but it seems reasonable to avoid such laparotomies whenever possible.

Biliary tract surgery

The removal of gallstones from the gallbladder and common bile duct is clearly indicated in patients who have suffered an attack of acute pancreatitis. The timing of this operation is under review. It should not be undertaken during the acute phase of the disease unless the patient develops a progressive obstructive jaundice with a deteriorating clinical situation and gallstones have been clearly demonstrated by ultrasound. Even in these cases a decompressing cholecystostomy may be the optimum procedure.

Early specific surgery

A laparotomy may be undertaken within 24 h if there is progressive clinical deterioration with signs of peritonitis. This involves the removal of necrotic tissue and slough around the pancreas and can be associated with a gastrostomy, decompression of the biliary tract, feeding jejunostomy, and insertion of drains into the lesser and greater sac. Some authors even advocate a partial or near-total pancreatectomy [29, 35]. Since the main purpose of early surgery is removal of necrotic tissue, this type of treatment is not suitable for the majority of patients presenting with oedematous pancreatitis. The main question arising at present is the identification of patients with a marked pancreatic necrosis who would benefit from such procedures. The use of prognostic factors may be beneficial in the future, but at present there is no indication for the routine use of this type of surgery in patients with severe pancreatitis, and the results of controlled trials are awaited. It must be appreciated that early surgery of this type is associated with considerable morbidity and mortality by the nature of the underlying disease process.

Surgical correction of abdominal complications

This includes treatment of pseudocysts or pancreatic abscesses, which usually are not apparent until towards the end of the second week.

Management of complications

Pancreatic pseudocyst

A pancreatic pseudocyst is a collection of fluid and debris rich in pancreatic enzymes, which is situated in the region of the pancreas. It does not have an epithelial lining and it is usually associated with disruption of the pancreatic ductal system [47]. The incidence of pseudocyst formation is about 4% and it is found particularly in patients with alcoholic pancreatitis.

The majority of patients complain of abdominal pain and weight loss. An abdominal mass is only palpable in 50% of cases. The serum amylase level is elevated in 33%–78% of patients, but often it fluctuates around the upper limit of normal and the amylase thermolability remains abnormal [13].

Diagnosis was formerly made by means of a barium meal, which reveals a deformity of the stomach or duodenum. The CAT scanner and ultrasound have assumed more importance, as they can differentiate between an inflammatory mass in the head of the pancreas, a developing pseudocyst, or a pancreatic abscess. These investigations can also quantify the size of the lesion and its anatomical location, and indicate whether it is single, lobulated, or multiple (multiple lesions occur in 20% of patients) [17]. Serial studies of the cyst by ultrasonography show its natural history, whether it is increasing or regressing in size, and its pre-operative localization.

In 70% of patients with pseudocysts, the cysts will mature and either resolve spontaneously or require surgical decompression. However, in 30% significant complications occur [42]. These take the form either of infection, which results in a pancreatic abscess, or of erosion into a blood vessel, particularly the splenic vessels, producing severe bleeding. The cyst may also rupture into the peritoneal cavity or into the lumen of the bowel. Pseudocysts which are less than 4 cm in size on ultrasonography in an asymptomatic patient should be followed with serial scans, and if they have not resolved completely by 3 months should be considered for a drainage procedure [38]. In patients with a pseudocyst that is greater than 6 cm in size or is displacing the intestinal tract or associated with a complication, surgery is required. In general terms the more mature cysts are easier to treat and are associated with reduced mortality. Pseudocysts may be drained into the nearest viscus, which is preferred, either by cysto-gastrostomy or into a defunctioned loop of jejunum. In complicated cases good results are now obtained, with a mortality of 6% and a recurrence rate of 11%.

Pancreatic abscess

Sudden deterioration, pyrexia, abdominal distension, or intestinal obstruction, especially if associated previously with a pseudocyst, indicates a pancreatic abscess. Radiological gas is occasionally seen in the retrogastric region, indicating infection in the lesser sac [4]. Treatment takes the form of an exploratory laparotomy with drainage of the infected material and insertion of multiple drains. Postoperatively the patient requires prolonged parenteral or enteral feeding and the condition is associated with an 18% mortality [7].

References

1. Acosta JL, Rossi R, Ledesma CL (1977) The usefulness of stool screening for diagnosing cholelithiasis in acute pancreatitis. A description of the technique. Dig Dissci 22:168–172
2. Allam BF, Imrie CW (1977) Serum ionized calcium in acute pancreatitis. Br J Surg 64:665–668
3. Anderson MC (1969) Review of pancreatic disease. Surgery 66:434–449
4. Babb RR (1976) The role of surgery in acute pancreatitis. Dig Dissci 21:672–676
5. Baker RJ (1972) Acute surgical diseases of the pancreas. Surg Clin North Am 52:239–255
6. Broadie TA, Devedas M, Rysavy J, Leonard AS, Delaney JP (1979) The effect of hypoxia and hypercapnia on canine pancreatic blood flow. J Surg Res 27:114–118
7. Camer SJ, Tan EGC, Warren KW, Braasch JW (1975) Pancreatic abscess. A critical analysis of 113 cases. J Surg 129:426–431
8. Cameron JL, Howes R, Zuidema GD (1975) Antibiotic therapy in acute pancreatitis. Surg Clin North Am 55:1319–1324
9. Donaldson LA, Joffe SN (1977) Amylase creatinine clearance ratio in pancreatitis. 73:1462–1463
10. Donaldson LA, McIntosh W (1977) A cause of misleading serum amylase concentrations in acute pancreatitis. Scott Med J 22:151–153
11. Donaldson LA, Schenk WG Jr (1979) Experimental acute pancreatitis. The changes in pancreatic oxygen consumption and the effect of dextran 40. Ann Surg 190:728–731
12. Donaldson LA, McIntosh WB, Brodie MJ (1977) Amylase thermolability in body fluids. Scand J Gastroenterol 12:637–639
13. Donaldson LA, Brodie MJ, McIntosh WB, Joffe SN (1978) Amylase thermolability as a screening test for pancreatic pseudocysts. Br J Surg 65:413–415
14. Donaldson LA, Williams RW, Schenk WG Jr (1978)

Experimental pancreatitis—effect of plasma and dextran on pancreatic blood flow. Surgery 84:313–321

15. Donaldson LA, Joffe SN McIntosh W (1979) Serial serum amylase levels in patients with pancreatic pseudocysts. Scott Med J 24:13–16

16. Donaldson LA, Joffe SN, Schenk WG Jr (1980) Acute pancreatitis ischaemia or hyperaemia? Medical Hypothesis 6: in press

17. Duncan JG, Imrie CW, Blumgart LH (1976) Ultrasound in the management of acute pancreatitis. Br J Radiol 49:858–862

18. Durr HK (1979) Acute pancreatitis. In: Howat and Sarles (eds) The exocrine pancreas. Saunders, London Philadelphia and Toronto, pp 352–401

19. Durr HK, Maroske D, Zelder O and Bode JCh (1978) Glucagon therapy in acute pancreatitis. Report of a double-blind trial. Gut 19:175–179

20. Feller JH, Brown RA, Toussaint GPM, Thompson AG (1974) Changing methods in the treatment of severe pancreatitis. Am J Surg 127:196–201

21. Finch WT, Sawyers JL, Schenker S (1976) A prospective study to determine the efficacy of antibiotics in acute pancreatitis. Ann Surg 183:667–671

22. Gerber PU, Meyer WH Jr, Farrell JJ (1962) Experimental pancreatitis and fibrinolysin. Am Surg 28:445–447

23. Goodhead B (1969) Acute pancreatitis and pancreatic blood flow. Surg Gynecol Obstet 129:331–340

24. Greenburg AG, Terlizzi L, Peskin GW (1977) Oxyhaemoglobin affinity in acute pancreatitis. J Surg Res 22:561–565

25. Imrie CW, Benjamin IS, Ferguson JC, McKay AJ, Mackenzie I, O'Neill, Blumgart LH (1978) A single-centre double-blind trial of Trasylol therapy in primary acute pancreatitis. Br J Surg 65:337–341

26. Imrie CW, Ferguson JC, Murphy D, Blumgart LH (1977) Arterial hypoxia in acute pancreatitis. Br J Surg 64:185–188

27. Imrie CW, Whyte AS (1975) A prospective study of acute pancreatitis. Br J Surg 62:490–494

28. Jacobs ML, Daggett WM, Civetta JM, Vasu MA, Lawson DW, Warshaw AL, Nardi GL, Bartlett MK (1977) Acute pancreatitis: Analysis of factors influencing survival. Ann Surg 185:43–51

29. Jonsell G, Boutelier P (1979) Observations during treatment of acute necrotizing pancreatitis with surgical ablation. Surg Gynecol Obstet 148:385–386

30. Marten A, Beales D, Elias E (1977) Mechanism and specificity of increased amylase/creatinine clearance ratio in pancreatitis. Gut 18:703–708

31. McMahon MJ, Pickford IR (1979) Biochemical prediction of gallstones in an attack of acute pancreatitis. Lancet II:541–543

32. MRC Multicentre Trial (1977) Death from acute pancreatitis. MRC multicentre trial of glucagon and aprotinin. Lancet II:632–637

33. Murphy D, Imrie CW, Davidson JF (1977) Haematological abnormalities in acute pancreatitis. A prospective study. Postgrad Med J 53:310–314

34. Murray WR, Mackay C (1977) The amylase/creatinine clearance ratio in acute pancreatitis. Br J Surg 64:189–191

35. Norton L, Eiseman B (1974) Near total pancreatectomy for hemorrhagic pancreatitis. Am J Surg 127:191–195

36. Ranson JHC, Lackner H, Berman IR, Schinella R (1977) The relationship of coagulation factors to clinical complications of acute pancreatitis. Surgery 81:502–511

37. Ranson JHC, Spencer FC (1978) The role of peritoneal lavage in severe acute pancreatitis. Ann Surg 187:565–573

38. Ravelo HR, Aldrete JS (1979) Analysis of forty-five patients with pseudocysts of the pancreas treated surgically. Surg Gynecol Obstet 148:735–738

39. Read G, Braganza JM, Howatt HT (1976) Pancreatitis—a retrospective study. Gut 17:945–952

40. Reinitz ER, Motoyama E, Smith GTW, Kerstein MD (1977) Pulmonary sequelae of experimental pancreatitis. J Surg Res 22:566–579

41. Salt WB, Schenker S (1976) Amylase—its clinical significance: A review of the literature. Medicine 55:269–289

42. Sankaran S, Walt AJ (1975) The natural and unnatural history of pancreatic pseudocysts. Br J Surg 62:37–44

43. Smith R, Williams R and Cotton PB (1976) Gallstone pancreatitis with normal biliary radiology. Br J Surg 63:861–863

44. Storck G, Pettersson G, Edlund Y (1976) A study of autopsies upon 116 patients with acute pancreatitis. Surg Gynecol Obstet 143:241–245

45. Thal AP, Perry JF Jr, Egner W (1957) A clinical and morphological study of forty-two cases of fatal acute pancreatitis. Surg Gynecol Obstet 105:191–202

46. Warshaw AL, Fuller AF (1975) Specificity of increased renal clearance of amylase in the diagnosis of acute pancreatitis. N Engl J Med 292:325–328

47. Warshaw AL, O'Hara PJ (1978) Susceptibility of the pancreas to ischemic injury in shock. Ann Surg 188:197–201

48. Goodhead G, Wright PW (1969) The effect of postganglionic sympathectomy on the development of haemorrhagic pancreatitis in the dog. Ann Surg 170:951–960

Chapter 29

Acute Gastro-intestinal Lesions and Acute Mesenteric Ischaemia

J. R. Le Gall and P. L. Fagniez

I. Acute Gastro-intestinal Lesions

Gastro-intestinal (GI) bleeding may be the cause of admission to an ICU or a complication occurring in a patient hospitalized for another problem. In the first group, endoscopy allows the diagnosis in 95% of cases [36]. The second group will be described here, with especial reference to acute gastroduodenal lesions and acute mesenteric ischaemia in critically ill patients.

Definition

Acute gastroduodenal lesions embrace the whole range of mucosal abnormalities, from submucosal haemorrhage and erosion to multiple ulceration. They may be found in the oesophagus, stomach, and duodenum after some form of injury to the patient [2], shock of any aetiology, intracranial disease, burns, or malignant diseases. Complication of haemorrhage or perforation may occur [6].

Eight major risks have recently been identified by Priebe [24]: major operative procedures, respiratory failure, sepsis, renal failure, peritonitis, multiple trauma, hypotension, and jaundice. Fulminant hepatic failure constitutes a ninth risk factor, for it is complicated by acute gastroduodenal lesions in almost all cases [17].

Aetiology

The extensive use of endoscopy enables sequential observations to be made of the gastric and duodenal mucosa after acute injuries:

1) Recent studies have shown that acute lesions are found in 100% of patients with *multiple organ injury or severe trauma*. Ischaemia and erosions develop in the fundus of the stomach within 6 h of injury and in more seriously ill patients spread to the whole stomach during the following 48 h [16]. In patients who are recovering healing may be completed within 2–4 days, and the reason why all such patients do not bleed is probably related to the regenerative capacity of the gastric mucosa, which renews the gastric lining every few days [16].

2) To determine the incidence of acute gastroduodenal lesions during *severe sepsis,* Le Gall et al. [13] performed prospective endoscopies in critically ill patients. In all the septic patients there were abnormalities of the mucosa, while in non-septic patients gastroscopies showed either superficial lesions or normal mucosa. Furthermore, the gastroduodenal lesions became worse as the sepsis persisted, and improved dramatically when focal infection and septicaemia were eradicated.

3) Early and serial examination of *patients with head injuries* showed acute lesions, mainly in the stomach, in 35 of 47 cases (75%) [9]. Erosive gastritis was observed in 78% of cases, oesophagitis in 12%, and duodenitis in 10%. Cushing's ulcers, which occur in association with intracranial trauma or tumours and following craniotomy, are associated with very high acid outputs and high levels of gastrin in the plasma and they are therefore probably of a different origin [28, 37].

4) After *burns,* particularly when they affect more than 30% of the body surface, multiple acute superficial erosions develop in the fundus of the stomach within the first few days. Czaja et al. [3] performed systematic endoscopies in severely burned patients and found duodenal erosions in 82% and gastric erosions in 83.3%; these progressed to ulcers in the same area some 72 h later. Such acute ulcers occurring in burned patients are often called Curling's ulcers [2].

5) *Erosive gastritis* secondary to ingestion of a variety of *drugs* and *alcohol* is seen very frequently with the greater availability of gastroscopy: Aspirin may induce gastric and duodenal ulcers, when given PO or IV [4].

Pathology

Acute ulcers or stress ulcers are round or oval ulcerations, usually less than 1 cm in width with sharply demarcated borders, without peripheral oedema; they are more than 5 mm in depth and destroy the muscularis mucosae. They may or may not be haemorrhagic; bleeding follows erosion of small vessels or large arteries such as the gastroduodenal. They are usually located in the fundus of the stomach and the first part of the duodenum.

In fact acute ulceration is only one stage in the development of acute gastroduodenal lesions, which are almost always multiple and disseminated. Direct observation of the mucosa by endoscopy has led to the description of four stages, which are in increasing order of severity: stage I, extensive erythematous purpuric macular lesions; stage II, discrete and superficial erosions; stage III, one or several gastric or duodenal ulcers without bleeding; and stage IV, one or several gastric or duodenal ulcers with bleeding [13].

Specific changes in the eroded areas include necrosis of superficial epithelium with underlying haemorrhage and infiltration with polymorphs. Tissue destruction may extend to the serosa as deep ulceration, and in submucosal vessels organized thrombus is occasionally found [29].

Pathogenesis

Three factors, usually working together, may be involved in the pathogenesis of acute gastroduodenal lesions: the presence of acid, ischaemia, and disruption of the gastric mucosal barrier [31].

Presence of acid

In 1970, serially collected gastric juice from patients in coma due to neurological damage was studied [25]. On the 1st day, acid secretion was lower than normal, but by the 6th day it had risen to a peak value similar to that observed in duodenal ulcer. In 1973, a study of acid output on the day after trauma showed a low value, which increased later, particularly when there was an intracranial lesion [15]. Czaja et al. [3] found that duodenal ulcers only developed when acid secretion exceeded 3.1 mmol/h. In all these studies severe haemorrhage occurred preferentially with high acid output.

Nevertheless, active secretion of acid on the luminal surface of the stomach is associated with an equal amount of an alkaline tide of bicarbonate on the serosal surface or in the gastric venous blood [12]; the importance of this secretion in mucosal protection against luminal acid has recently been specified. When rabbit gastric mucosa is stimulated with histamine the alkalinization of the lamina propria prevents the marked decrease in intramural pH that is provoked by the luminal acid and so prevents ulceration [11].

Ischaemia

Gastric ischaemia secondary to shock, burns or trauma precedes the formation of acute ulcers [11]. Selective infusion of a vasodilator such as isoprenaline into the arterial blood vessels of the stomach protects the mucosa against ulceration [27]. Kivilakso et al. [12] have studied the pH of the lamina propria of rabbits during haemorrhagic shock: a significant decrease in pH occurring during shock was prevented by buffering. The critical determinant of ulceration during shock could be the impaired capacity of the mucosa to remove the influx of acid rather than the tissue hypoxia [12].

Mucosal barrier

Back diffusion of acid into the gastric wall occurs normally but is restricted by the mucosal membrane. Agents such as aspirin, bile salts, and alcohol, which break this barrier, increase the back diffusion [4]. Mucosal blood flow seems to be a major factor in preserving the integrity of this barrier. An increase of back diffusion of hydrogen ions is observed after haemorrhagic shock. Ischaemia probably initiates the damage and then the back diffusion of acid perpetuates it. Impairment of the buffering capacity of the mucosa, rather than tissue anoxia, might be the main pathogenic factor that leads to ulceration during haemorrhagic shock [12]. A deficiency of mucus also seems to be a factor that predisposes to acute ulcers [30], whilst stimulation of its production increases mucosal resistance [12].

Clinical features

The studies of Kamada et al. [9] and of Pruitt et al. [25] showed that 4%–15% of critically ill patients required transfusion of over 1000 ml blood. However, since the use of nutritional therapy, either IV or by naso-gastric tube, has become more widespread, the incidence of GI bleeding seems to have been dramatically reduced [5, 14].

Czaja et al. [3] reported a higher incidence of bleeding between the 4th and the 10th days in burned patients and Priebe et al., studying 75 critically ill patients, observed that the incidence of bleeding increased with the number of risk factors, particularly when there were three or more [24].

It seems that the incidence of bleeding compared with the frequency of acute ulceration is less than 10% [2]. With systematic endoscopy in critically ill patients, Le Gall et al. found acute lesions in 75% of patients without any clinical signs of bleeding [13] and the incidence of bleeding increased with the duration of these acute lesions, i.e., the duration of the primary illness responsible for the stress lesions.

Some acute ulcers may perforate into the peritoneal cavity but no epidemiologic data have so far been published about the incidence of perforation, as against the incidence of acute ulcers.

In practice, endoscopy is the method of choice to identify the site of bleeding, although some authors consider it to be a useless exercise since there are no clear guidelines for treatment once bleeding has occurred [2]. Indeed, the finding of one or more stress ulcers may mean that a remote septic focus has to be looked for and eradicated if the bleeding is to be stopped.

As previously mentioned, the incidence of acute GI bleeding in seriously ill patients does appear to be decreasing [8, 26]. McElwee et al. [22] reported only one patient with major gastroduodenal haemorrhage in over 750 patients treated for thermal injuries since 1975. In another series, the introduction of enteral nutrition could have been a significant factor in reducing the incidence of gastroduodenal bleeding from 7.4% to 2.3% [14].

Treatment of acute gastroduodenal bleeding

Usually acute gastroduodenal lesions are symptomatic of other abnormalities, such as haemorrhagic shock, sepsis, intracranial lesions, or fulminant hepatic failure. Therefore, the treatment has to be considered in two parts: treatment of the underlying cause, which is the more important, and symptomatic treatment.

Treatment of the underlying cause

If the risk factors are not controlled symptomatic treatment is usually ineffective and in a patient who is haemorrhaging the first step is to find the cause or causes of the bleeding.

Sepsis seems to be the most frequent and important factor [16] and when symptomatic therapy with cimetidine failed to increase the pH of the gastric juice above 4, severe sepsis was found in 9 of 11 cases [19]. The occurrence of an acute ulcer in an apparently well-controlled patient with no neurological signs of illness is almost invariably associated with a septic focus [13]. Other risk factors have to be controlled as far as possible. Hastings et al. [8] indicated that patients with renal failure, jaundice, and hypotension are at greater risk of developing acute ulcers and bleeding.

Usually when the cause of the acute lesion is treated the mucosa heals rapidly and specific treatment is not necessary [35].

Symptomatic treatment

Miscellaneous methods

Bleeding may stop after sedation and adequate transfusion. Some methods, such as gastric lavage with iced saline, selective angiographic techniques with vasopressin infusion, and embolization, have not been subjected to controlled studies [2]. Electrocoagulation and laser coagulation have been used, but would be difficult to apply in diffuse gastritis [10].

Antacids

Antacids have been widely used for the treatment of stress ulcer bleeding [30]. When instilled at hourly intervals through a nasogastric tube to maintain the pH of the gastric secretions above 7.0, they stopped bleeding in 89% of patients with endoscopically proven haemorrhagic gastritis. Nevertheless, bleeding recurred if the pH fell to 5.0. Similarly, antacid treatment of seven at-risk bleeding patients in a control group was effective in all cases [30].

H_2-receptor antagonists

H_2-receptor antagonists such as cimetidine and metiamide are now increasingly used to treat acute bleeding. In 1978, 27 patients with acute bleeding in an ICU were treated with H_2-receptor antagonists and in 24, i.e., 88%, the bleeding was controlled [21]. H_2-receptor antagonists were effective in all the 23 patients

described by MacDougall et al. [17], in spite of severe liver failure in 12 of them. Metiamide was successfully used to treat 14 bleeding episodes in 11 critically ill patients with acute gastritis, but its use was unsuccessful in two patients in whom chronic ulcers were responsible for the bleeding [20].

Surgical treatment

Surgical treatment of acute ulcers is only performed when haemorrhage persists in spite of treatment of the underlying cause and antacid therapy or when the ulcer perforates.

When an acute ulcer erodes the gastroduodenal artery, healing will not occur even though the cause of the ulcer has been eradicated. In this situation, oversewing of the ulcer combined with vagotomy and pyloroplasty is usually sufficient [15]. However, the rebleeding rates for vagotomy and pyloroplasty are higher than those reported for vagotomy and gastric resection (40% versus 13%) [29].

In perforated stress ulcers the operative procedure depends upon the site of perforation and the duration of the peritonitis. Simple closure has been advocated for both duodenal and gastric perforations but it seems wiser to add some form of acid-reducing procedure [35], although proximal gastric vagotomy is time-consuming and does not seem to be beneficial [15].

Preventative treatment

Preventative treatment of acute gastroduodenal bleeding in patient at risk has been tried in numerous studies, both experimental and clinical.

Experimental studies

To study septically induced acute gastric erosions and the role of cimetidine, Belliveau et al. [1] developed a reproducible septic canine model in which four different bacteria plus canine gallbladder bile were instilled intraperitoneally. Oral cimetidine given 24 h prior to induction of the peritonitis prevented the induction of acute erosions even though blood cultures were positive.

The combination of cimetidine and carbenoxolone sodium has been used in the prevention of experimental restraint stress ulcer in rats [33]. The number of ulcers decreased substantially in the group receiving either cimetidine or carbenoxolone for at least 2 days before stress. Used in combination, these two drugs were efficient after half a day of pretreatment; antacids were as efficient as the two combined drugs. Cimetidine might act by decreasing gastric acid secretion, i.e., the aggressive factor, while carbenoxolone increases mucosal resistance, i.e., the defensive factor, by stimulating the production of gastric mucus and increasing the longevity of the gastric epithelial cells [7].

Clinical studies

Two major groups of drugs have been proposed for the prevention of stress ulcer bleeding: antacids and cimetidine-type drugs.

Cimetidine or metiamide. In 75 patients with fulminant hepatic failure, two controlled trials [18, 20] showed that antacids given every 4 h had no significant effect. The gastric pH was maintained above 5 in only 35% of cases, whereas this was easily achieved with the histamine H_2-receptor antagonists metiamide or cimetidine administered IV at a rate of 100 mg/h. Only 1 patient of 36 receiving these drugs bled, compared with 13 (54%) of the 24 controls. In the antacid-treated group 3 of the 13 patients bled, as against 6 of the 12 controls.

But cimetidine is not always so effective [19]. In 11 of 34 at-risk patients in whom the intention was to keep the gastric pH level above 4, cimetidine failed. Of these 11 patients, 9 had positive blood cultures or clinical infection. Martin et al. concluded that it is possible to identify a high-risk group of patients who may not respond to cimetidine treatment.

Antacids. Hastings et al. [8] studied 100 critically ill patients at risk in a controlled, randomized trial. The first group of 51 patients received antacid prophylaxis. Titration, checked hourly, kept the pH of gastric fluid above 3.5. In the first group 2 patients bled, as against 12 in the second group ($P < 0.005$). The antacid used was either aluminium hydroxide or Mylanta II[1], which contains magnesium. The intragastric instillation of antacid had to be made every hour, except if the pH of the gastric content was 3.5 or greater. Minor complications were observed in 29% of the patients receiving antacids: diarrhoea, gross regurgitation, and elevated serum magnesium levels were noted. Importantly, in the non-antacid group, the incidence of severe bleeding on mortality was no higher than in the antacid group, and if antacids are to be effective they are extremely time-consuming for the nurses, requiring virtually a nurse-to-patient ratio of 1:1.

[1]Stuart Pharmaceuticals, Division of ICI United States Inc., Wilmington, DE 19897.

As cimetidine is easier to administer than antacids, the same group performed a randomized trial of antacid versus cimetidine in 75 critically ill patients [24]. The first group received 300 mg cimetidine IV every 6 h, and the second received 30 ml antacid intragastrically every hour. Gastric pH was titrated above 3.6. Bleeding occurred in 7 of 38 cimetidine-treated patients but in none of 37 antacid-treated patients ($P < 0.01$). They concluded that cimetidine does not protect seriously ill patients from bleeding and that antacid is better for this purpose.

Two important questions have therefore to be posed:

Why were the antacids inefficient in the study in patients with hepatic failure? [20] Probably this was because they were only given every 4 h; this dosage schedule is unlikely to produce continuous protection of mucosa.

Why were H_2-receptor antagonists less effective than antacids in preventing gastric bleeding in critically ill patients?

If acid plays an essential role in the formation of stress ulcer, recent investigations have shown that the secretory state of the mucosa appears to play an important part in the protection of the mucosa [12]. A non-secreting mucosa, such as one inhibited by burinamide, an H_2-receptor antagonist, is more sensitive to the deleterious effects of intraluminal acid. Actively secreting gastric mucosa produces bicarbonate, which protects against ulceration [11].

Cimetidine may be ineffective in preventing acute ulcers in man because it impairs the secretory state of the mucosa, decreases the intracellular buffering capacity, and inadequately reduces the intraluminal acidity.

The numerous clinical studies that have been carried out on the prevention of stress ulcer do leave some questions unanswered. Not all the studies have used gastroscopy, so they cannot reveal whether the treatment prevented stress ulceration or only the resulting bleeding. Solem et al. [32] indicated that a prophylactic antacid regimen does not prevent mucosal injury but does prevent bleeding. McElwee et al. [22] studied the effectiveness of cimetidine versus antacids in burned patients by systematic gastroscopy and showed that in both groups the frequency and distribution of minor gastric abnormalities remained high (78%), and was similar to that reported for patients not receiving any form of prophylaxis. Preventative measures seemed to reduce the severity of the disease rather than eradicate it. In all these studies bleeding was detected by the guaiac test on three consecutive samples of naso-gastric aspirate. No mention was made of transfusions, and overall the patients who did not receive antacids or cimetidine did not fare any worse than those who did; the death rate was identical in both groups.

In burn centres or in neurosurgical units the effect of alkali-therapy could have been brought out much more dramatically. Menguy [23] concluded recently in an editorial in the *New England Journal of Medicine*: "the neutralization of the milieu bathing the gastric mucosa ... should be a part of the treatment of patients with any acute illness and three or more risk factors associated with stress ulcers."

References

1. Belliveau P, Vas S, Himal HS (1978) Septic induced acute gastric erosion. The role of cimetidine. J Surg Resp 24:264–271
2. Croker JR (1979) Acute gastro intestinal bleeding in the critically ill patient. Intensive Care Med 5:1–4
3. Czaja AJ, McAlhany JC Pruitt BA (1974) Acute gastroduodenal disease after thermal injury and endoscopic evaluation of incidence and natural history. N Engl J Med 291:245–253
4. Davenport HW (1964) Gastric mucosal injury by fatty and acetylsalicylic acids. Gastroenterology 46:245–253
5. Deysine M, Katzka D (1977) Prevention of experimental gastric stress bleeding by intravenous hyperalimentation. Intensive Care Med 3:156
6. Fogelman MJ, Gravey JM (1966) Acute gastroduodenal ulceration incident to surgery and disease. Am J Surg 112:651
7. Glass GBJ (1976) Mucus and gastric injury. In: Belk IT (ed) North American Symposium on carbenoxolone. Excerpta Medica, Princeton, pp 32–47
8. Hasting PR, Skillman JJ, Bushnell LS, Silen W (1978) Antacid titration in the prevention of acute gastrointestinal bleeding. A controlled, randomized trial in 100 critically ill patients. N Engl J Med 298:1041–1045
9. Kamada T, Fusamoto H, Kawano S, Noguchi M, Hiramatsu K, Masuzawa H, Sato N (1977) Acute gastroduodenal lesions in head injury. Am J Gastroent 68:249–253
10. Kiefharer P, Nath H, Monitz K (1977) Endoscopic controle of massive gastro-intestinal hemorrhage by irradiation with a high-power neodynium yag laser. Prog Surg 15:140–144
11. Kivilaakso E, Fromm D, Silen W (1978a) Relationship between ulceration and intramural pH of gastric mucosa during hemorrhagic shock. Surgery 84:70–78
12. Kivilaakso E, Fromm D, Silen W (1978b) Effect of the acid secretory state on intramural pH of rabbit gastric mucosa. Gastroenterology 75:641–648
13. Le Gall JR, Mignon FC, Rapin M, Redjemi M, Harari A, Bader JP, Soussy CJ (1976). Acute gastroduodenal lesions related to severe sepsis. Surg Gynecol Obstet 142:377–380
14. Levy E, Malafosse M, Huguet C, Liégeois A, Loygue J (1977) Prophylaxie des hémorragies gastroduodenales graves post-operatoires par la réanimation entérale continue hypernutritionnelle précoce. Intensive Care Med 3:155
15. Lewis FA (1973) Gastroduodenal ulceration and haemorrhage of neurogenic origin Br J Surg 69:279
16. Lucas CE, Sugawa C, Riddle J, Rector F, Rosenberg B, Walt AJ (1971) Natural history and surgical dilemma of "stress" gastric bleeding. Arch Surg 102:266–273
17. MacDougall BRD, Bailey RJ, Williams R (1977a) H₂ receptor antagonists and antacids in the prevention of acute gastro-intestinal hemorrhage in fulminant hepatic failure. Two controlled trials. Lancet I:617–619
18. MacDougall BRD, Bailey RJ, Williams R (1977b) Histamine H₂ receptor antagonists in the prophylaxis and control of acute gastro-intestinal hemorrhage in liver disease. Cimetidine. Excerpta Medica, pp 329–336
19. Martin LF, Staloch DK, Simonowitz DA, Patchen Dellinger E, Max MH (1979) Failure of cimetidine prophylaxis in the critically ill. Arch Surg 114:492–496
20. McDonald AS, Steele BJ, Bottomley MG (1976) Treatment of stress-induced upper gastro-intestinal hemorrhage with metiamide. Lancet I:68–70
21. McDonald AS, Pyne DA, Freeman A (1978). Upper gastro-intestinal bleeding in the intensive care unit. Can J Surg 21:81–85
22. McElwee HP, Stirineck KR and Levin BA (1979) Cimetidine affords protection equal to antacid in prevention of stress ulceration following thermal injury. Surgery 86:620–626
23. Menguy R (1980) The prophylaxis of stress ulceration. N Engl J Med 302:461–462
24. Priebe HJ, Skillman JJ, Bishnell LS, Long PC, Silen W (1980) Antacid versus cimetidine in preventing acute gastro intestinal bleeding. A randomized trial in 75 critically ill patients. N Engl J Med 302:426–430
25. Pruitt BA, Foley ED, Moncried JQ (1970) Cushing's ulcer: a physiopatho logical study of 323 cases. Ann Surg 172:523–530
26. Richardson JD, Avst JB (1977) Gastric devascularization: a useful lavage procedure of massive hemorrhagic gastritis. Ann Surg 185:649–655
27. Ritchie WP Jr, Shearburn LW (1977) Influence of isoproterenol and cholestyramine on acute gastric mucosal ulcerogenesis. Gastroenterology 73:62–65
28. Skillman JJ, Silen W (1970) Acute grastroduodenal "stress" ulcerations barrier disruption of varied pathogenesis? Gastroenterology 59:478–482
29. Silen W, Skillmann JJ (1979) Stress ulcers in gastrointestinal surgery. Year Book Medical Publishers Chicago, pp 949–952
30. Simonian SJ, Curtis LE (1976) Treatment of hemorrhagic gastritis by antacid. Ann Surg 184:429–432
31. Smith P, O'Brien P, Fromm D, Silen W (1977) Secretary state of gastric mucosa and resistance to injury by exogenous acid. Am J Surg 138:81–85
32. Solem LD, Strate RG, Fisher RP (1979) Antacid therapy and nutritional supplementation in the prevention of Curling's ulcer. Surg Gynecol Obstet 148:367–370
33. Strauss RJ, Stein TA, Mandell C, Wise L (1978a) Cimetidine, carbenoxolone sodium and antacids for the prevention of experimental stress ulcers. Arch Surg 113:858–862
34. Strauss JR, Stein TA, Wise L (1978b) Prevention of stress ulcerations using H₂ receptor antagonists. Am J Surg 135:120–125
35. Stremple JR, Mori H, Lev R, Glass GBJ (1973) The stress ulcer syndrome. Curr Probl Surg (April):36–42
36. Vilar HV, Fenker RH, Watson LC, Thompson JC (1977) Emergency diagnosis of upper gastro-intestinal bleeding by endoscopy. Ann Surg 185:367–374
37. Watts CL, Clark K (1969) Gastric acidity in the comatose patients. J Neurosurg 30:107–110

II. Acute Mesenteric Ischaemia

Acute mesenteric ischaemia occurs much more often than is suspected in such patients. The symptoms are ill defined and uncommon; the clinician very often does not think of the diagnosis and the prognosis can be improved only by an aggressive therapeutic approach.

Ischaemia and necrosis of the intestine are due either to obstruction of mesenteric vessels by emboli or atherosclerotic disease, or to intensive vasoconstriction. The latter is described as 'non-occlusive mesenteric infarction' or 'low-flow-state infarction'. Regardless of the mechanism of infarction it seems likely that earlier diagnosis and treatment would offer the best means of improving the dismal prognosis of this condition.

Pathophysiology

Whatever the cause of the ischaemia, the end-result is the same, namely haemorrhagic necrosis [17]. Marston [14] found histological evidence of changes in mucosal cells after occlusion of the superior mesenteric artery (SMA) in dogs. Brown et al. [7], using the electron microscope, found some changes within 10 min and extensive changes within 30 min.

Haemorrhagic necrosis comprises extensive submucosal oedema, some interstitial oedema and haemorrhage, and little inflammatory infiltration except in the colon [8]. The mucosal cells lose their ability to produce mucus and become permeable to bacteria and other toxic substances [6].

The extensive submucosal haemorrhage has a thumb-print appearance in barium studies, whereas mucosal destruction is seen as superficial ulceration [4]. When the muscular layer is involved, an initial hyperperistaltism is followed by marked distension with disordered mobility [4].

Guidelines are available to predict the degree of ischaemic damage on the basis of the duration or the cause of the ischaemia. A normal patient with occlusion of the SMA tolerated 4 h of complete gut ischaemia with no subsequent need for bowel resection [26], and in patients, undergoing embolectomy within 30 h of the embolization it should be possible to avoid bowel resection [26].

Aetiology

Non-occlusive mesenteric infarction

This represents the course of more than one half of the cases of acute mesenteric ischaemia [11] and both general and local factors are implicated in its aetiology.

General factors

A *decrease in cardiac output* for any reason is the major cause. Digitalis toxicity has been implicated as a causative factor, the splanchnic arterioles being major sites of constriction by cardiac glycosides [21].

Either *hypovolaemic or septic shock* may be associated with non-occlusive bowel infarction, but this is uncommon since the human bowel is not a primary or common focus of shock injury. Diuretic agents may be an inciting factor, when a massive extracellular volume deficit is induced [22], a packed cell volume above 48% may have represented dehydration that led to increased blood viscosity and consequent reduction in intestinal perfusion.

Local factors

Atherosclerotic narrowing of the mesenteric vessels is frequent in elderly patients and often facilitates the decrease of blood flow to the intestine.

The role of *bacteria* in intestinal ischaemic injuries has been mentioned with special reference to the colon. They may add another vascular factor through the release of vaso-active substances.

Distension proximal to *obstructive lesions of the colon* may impair microvascular flow and lead to non-occlusive infarction.

Both oral contraceptives [13] and enteric-coated potassium chloride tablets may be associated with intestinal lesions of indistinct pathophysiology [10].

Arterial emboli

Arterial emboli in the SMA usually arise from a cardiac mural thrombus secondary to myocardial infarction or from an atrial thrombus associated with rheumatic mitral valve disease. This last situation accounted for 14% of patients reported by Aakus and Ottinger [1, 16]. Unusual emboli arising from bronchogenic carcinoma, left atrial myxoma, proximal aortic wall, and aortic valvular prostheses have been reported.

Atherosclerotic obstructions of the SMA

All the acute SMA thromboses occur against the background of atherosclerosis of the aorta and mesenteric arteries. Angiography reveals evidence of severe aortic atherosclerosis, occlusion of the SMA at its origin, and slight but inadequate development of collateral flow. Many patients with complete occlusion of the gut vessels are asymptomatic, however, and others only become symptomatic when two of the three arteries are diseased.

Acute venous occlusion

In most series this occurs in less than 10% of the cases [16]. The causes include polycythaemia, carcinoma, portal hypertension, sepsis, tumour compression, and the use of oral contraceptives. In one study, those women taking oral contraceptives who suffered from small-bowel ischaemia and infarction were usually of blood group A and cigarette smokers [10]. Many of them presented with a history of symptoms over 2 weeks or more, and at operation some of the cases appeared to be reversible. Selective SMA angiography showed spasm of the major SMA branches with prolongation of the arterial phase, failure of the fine arterial branches to empty, and opacification of the thickened wall with extravasation of dye into the lumen.

Distribution

Lesions are encountered in both the small and the large bowel, but the ileum is the site most frequently and severely involved. Short or long segments and single or multiple lesions may be seen.

Two patterns of distribution are more frequent than any others. When the major trunk of the SMA is narrowed, infarction affects the supplied segment of the intestine and lies between the proximal jejunum irrigated from the coeliac axis through the artery of Riolan and the terminal ileum supplied by a marginal artery from the inferior mesenteric artery. The second pattern is that seen in patients with ischaemic colitis where the lesions tend to be localized to the splenic flexure and proximal descending colon.

In non-occlusive infarction there is a tendency for the involvement to be superficial, with only the mucosa undergoing infarction, but full-thickness infarction is by no means uncommon.

Clinical presentation

Acute mesenteric ischaemia can be suspected on the basis of the history and physical examination.

Pain is present in 75%–98% of cases. Periumbilical or colicky at its onset, the pain rapidly becomes severe, diffuse, and continuous. According to Williams [26], one of the characteristics is the lack of significant abdominal abnormalities even when the pain is unbearable; the possibility of infarction may be eliminated in patients without pain [15]. With perforation, the usual clinical signs of a perforated viscus are found and early bacterial invasion from the left side of the colon may suggest localized peritonitis without actual perforation.

Severe abdominal distension occurs after a few hours, and a fever develops. Diarrhoea and bloody stools are frequent [3]. If a pre-operative abdominal paracentesis is performed bloody fluid is usually obtained [15]. Adynamic dilatation follows full-thickness infarction, the abdomen becoming quiet and non-tender. Perforation alters the clinical course later by provoking diffuse peritonitis or localized abscesses.

The systemic effects of bowel infarction are hypotension and metabolic acidosis, due to massive loss of blood, plasma, and intracellular fluid into the infarcted tissue and intestinal lumen [9, 12]. Bacterial invasion or release of vaso-active substances may play a role and patients suffering from underlying cardiac disease usually do not readily tolerate such cardiovascular and metabolic disturbances.

Careful examination of the case history can reveal symptoms of chronic ischaemia resulting from SMA obstruction existing before the acute infarction, such as postprandial pain and weight loss. Diarrhoea and an accentuated gastrocolic reflex may be features in narrowing of the inferior mesenteric artery.

The laboratory finding are: high haematocrit due to dehydration, ischaemia, and sepsis. Blood urea and the serum amylase are occasionally elevated and proteinuria and haematuria have been noted. Elevations of serum oxaloacetic transaminase, glutamic pyruvic transaminase, lactic dehydrogenase and creatine phosphokinase are usual.

Radiological examination is of limited value [24] if only the plain abdominal films are used. Specific findings, such as intramural gas and gas in the portal system, are rare and later features. The non-specific signs can include a gas-less abdomen and diffuse small-bowel distension with fluid levels.

Barium studies may demonstrate submucosal haemorrhage, seen as indentations of thumb-print type, superficial ulceration; distension and motor abnormalities may also be seen. The major value of thumb-printing has been in establishing the diagnosis of ischaemic colitis, but it can be seen in other segments of the bowel and in other syndromes [15].

Diagnosis

Mesenteric angiography is essential to define the specific causes of gut ischaemia. It can be carried out even in very sick patients with a minimum of delay or danger [1, 5, 16]. Despite the risk of producing changes in SMA flow, cardiac output, and diastolic blood pressure, the specific information obtained by far outweighs the potential disadvantages [18]. The first study should be a flush aortogram with the patient in a lateral position, so that the proximal part of the coeliac axis can be visualized together with the SMA and the inferior mesenteric artery. This aortogram is followed by selective angiography to demonstrate the exact position of any arterial blockage, occlusion, or spasm and to show the extent of any collateral circulation or evidence of venous occlusion [18]. Nevertheless, when there is no occlusion of the visceral arteries and the clinical picture is consistent with intestinal ischaemia, it is assumed that non-occlusive mesenteric ischaemia is present.

In SMA embolism the embolus is located in the middle colic artery in 55% of cases, but can occlude the SMA (18%), the right colic artery (16%), or the ileocolic artery (7%). The arteriogram shows the occlusion and lack of any collateral flow [19].

Arteriographic findings in acute venous occlusion are seen on selective SMA arteriography as spasm of the major SMA branches with prolongation of the arterial phase, failure of the fine arterial branches to empty, and failure of the portal system to opacify.

In non-occlusive mesenteric ischaemia, arteriography documents the lack of obvious organic occlusive lesions of the major arteries or veins. Poor filling of the distal mesenteric arteries and evidence of mucosal damage suggests a decreased splanchnic flow. Occasionally slight narrowing of the SMA or occlusion of the inferior mesenteric artery is found in association with the spasm, but the latter is clearly the dominant lesion.

Treatment

Effective therapy demands that the specific cause of the gut ischaemia be defined. Some form of immediate corrective vascular procedure is mandatory in dealing with an SMA embolus; resection is urgently required for venous occlusion, while early operation is contra-indicated in non-occlusive cases.

In *SMA emboli* embolectomy should be performed where possible, without resection. A second look should then be undertaken 6–8 h later [26]. This permits appreciation of the patency of the vascular repair and the need if any, for removal of a non-viable bowel. The results are encouraging, since survival after 5 days of occlusion has been reported [18].

The proper treatment of *atherosclerotic obstruction* is immediate surgical relief of the obstruction by means of bypass via a venous or prosthetic graft, with a second look a few hours later [18]. Mortality is clearly high, over 60%, because the patients usually have diffuse atherosclerosis.

The treatment of *acute venous occlusion* is prompt surgical resection of all the involved gut together with its mesentery. The involved segment can be delineated during operation because the mesentery is oedematous and its veins extrude clot when opened. Prognosis is better than with other causes, the mortality being about 20%.

Non-occlusive mesenteric ischaemia differs from ischaemia secondary to major vessel occlusion in that emergency surgery is not warranted [25]. There is no vascular occlusion to be corrected and anaesthesia may worsen gut perfusion. Non-operative measures are aimed at reversing the underlying cause, at correcting the systemic and metabolic effects of infarction, and at relieving the vasospasm. Correction of hypovolaemia and acidosis is carefully monitored and large volumes of fluid should be infused whenever possible; antibiotics active against Gram-negative and anaerobic organisms, such as gentamicin, should be given together with metronidazole and penicillin for the relief of spasm, for which purpose local measures seem to be the most effective.

Angiographic examination must include multiple injections of contrast material. An initial flush aortogram detects aneurysms, dissection, emboli, and other occlusions and evaluates the collateral circulation. Selective angiography then detects emboli, thrombosis, or mesenteric vasoconstriction in the SMA or its branches.

If an embolus or mesenteric vasoconstriction is found, Boley et al. [4] recommend the injection of a single bolus of a vasodilator (papaverine) through the SMA catheter, followed by a repeat angiogram to provide better visualization of the peripheral circulation and to show the effect of the papaverine infusion. Papaverine (60 mg) used as the bolus may be substituted by tolazoline (25 mg), which has a more rapid effect. Tolazoline is not recommended for infusion, however, because it is less effective and not as safe as papaverine, which is infused through the SMA catheter at a rate of 30–60 mg/h with a constant infusion pump; some workers prefer to infuse glucagon into the SMA for periods of 12–24 h [23].

Recent experimental studies by Adar and Salzman [2] have tested the hypothesis that angiotensin might be responsible for a selective decrease of blood flow in the SMA during dehydration or cardiac tamponade, because such an effect is mimicked by angiotensin II. Also, saralazin, an inhibitor of angiotensin II, and SQ 208, an agent which prevents conversion of angiotensin I to angiotensin II, both improve the changes in SMA flow and resistance produced by dehydration. Perhaps in the future intra-arterial infusions of papaverine will be unnecessary if inhibition of angiotensin II can be accomplished by the IV route.

A preliminary period of non-operative treatment must achieve maximal reversal of the vasospasm to enable the true extent of intestinal involvement to be ascertained by gross observation at the time of the subsequent operation. A second-look operation must be avoided in these critically ill patients, and intra-arterial papaverine should be continued from the time of the initial operation for up to 24–48 h after.

Prognosis

The survival rate reported up to 1973 was about 20%–30% [16, 26]. Using an aggressive approach, with earlier and more liberal use of angiography and intra-arterial infusion of papaverine for the relief of vasoconstriction in both occlusive and non-occlusive acute mesenteric ischaemia, Boley et al. [4] reported a survival rate of 54%. In 85% of the surviving patients a normally functioning GI tract was obtained and in 17 of the 19 survivors no bowel excision or only limited excision of less than 3 ft. of small intestine was performed.

References

1. Aakus T, Braband G (1967) Angiographie in acute superior mesenteric arterial insufficiency. Acta Radiol [Diagn] Stockh 6:1–12
2. Adar R, Franklin A, Spark RF, Rosoff CB, Salzman EW (1976) Effect of dehydration and cardiac tamponade on superior mesenteric artery flow: Role of vaso-active substances. Surgery 79:534–548
3. Aldrete JS, Han SY, Laws HL, Kirklin JW (1977) Intestinal infarction complicating low cardiac output states. Surg Gynecol Obstet 144:371–375
4. Boley SJ, Schwartz S, Lash J (1963) Reversible vascular occlusion of the colon. Surg Gynecol Obstet 116:53–60
5. Boley SJ, Sprayregan S, Siegelman S, Veith FJ (1977) Initial results from an aggressive roentgenological and surgical approach to acute mesenteric ischemia. Surgery 82:848–855
6. Bounous G, Sutherland NG, Mc Ardle AH (1969) The prophylactic use of an elemental diet in experimental haemorrhagic shock and intestinal ischemia. Ann Surg 166:312–343
7. Brown RA, Chiv C, Scott HJ (1970) Ultrastructural changes in the canine mucosal cell after mesenteric arterial occlusion. Arch Surg 101:290–297
8. Dawson MA, Schaeffer JW (1971) The clinical cause of reversible ischemic colitis. Gastroenterology 60:577:580
9. Ende N (1958) Infarction of the bowel in cardiac failure. N Engl J Med 258:879
10. Hoyle M, Kennedy A, Prior AL, Thomax GE (1977) Small bowel ischemia and infarction in young women taking oral contraceptive and progestational agent. Br J Surg 64:533–537
11. Jackson BB (1963) Occlusion of the superior mesenteric artery. Monograph in American lectures in surgery. Thomas, Springfield, pp 1–141
12. Kangwalklai K, Saadat S, Bella E, Enquist IF (1973) Space studies during occlusion of the superior mesenteric artery. Surg Gynecol Obstet 137:263–266
13. Lescher TJ, Bombeck T (1977) Mesenteric vascular occlusion associated with oral contraceptive use. Arch Surg 112:1231–1232
14. Marston A (1964) Patterns of intestinal ischemia. Ann R Coll Surg Engl 35:150–181
15. Ottinger LW (1974) Non-occlusive mesenteric infarction. Surg Clin North Am 54:689–698

16. Ottinger LW, Austen WG (1967) A study of 136 patients with mesenteric infarction. Surg Gynecol Obstet 124:251–261
17. Pierce GE, Brockenbrough EC (1970) The spectrum of mesenteric infarction. Am J Surg 119:233–239
18. Recek C, Kren V, Fixa B, et al (1968) Selective mestericography as a guide to diagnosis and treatment of acute superior mesenteric artery occlusion. J Cardiovasc Surg (Torino) 9:184–189
19. Reiner L, Jimenez FA, Rodrigues FL (1963) Atherosclerosis in the mesenteric circulation: Observations and correlations with aortic and coronary atherosclerosis. Am Heart J 66:200–209
20. Rob C (1966) Surgical diseases of the coeliac and mesenteric arteries. Arch Surg 93:21–32
21. Shanbour LL, Jacobson ED (1972) Digitalis and mesenteric circulation. Dig Dis Sci 17:826–827
22. Sharefkin JB, Silen W (1974) Diuretic agents: Inciting factor in non occlusive mesenteric infarction. JAMA 229:1451–1453
23. Silen W (1979). Nonocclusive intestinal infarction. Gastrointestinal surgery. Year Book Medical Publishers, Chicago, pp 587–592
24. Thomchik FS, Wittenberg J, Ottinger LW (1970) The roentgenographic spectrum of bowel infarction. Radiology 96:249–260
25. Viken JK (1973) Recovery from acute intestinal ischemia without bowel resection. JAMA 226:776–777
26. Williams LF (1971) Vascular insufficiency of the intestines. Gasteoenterology 61:757–777

Haematological Disorders

Chapter 30

Disorders of Haemostasis

Samuel J. Machin

Physiology of haemostasis

The process of haemostasis involves protecting blood flow through a virtually closed circuit of blood vessels at various pressures and re-establishing vascular patency if any segments become occluded. Haemostatic reactions can be classified into several overlapping and sequential events: localized vasoconstriction at the site of injury, platelet adhesion to exposed sub-endothelial basement membrane and collagen fibres, formation of a platelet aggregate or plug, activation of the coagulation cascade leading to formation of fibrin which reinforces the platelet plug, and finally activation of the fibrinolytic system which digests the haemostatic plug and allows growth of new vascular endothelial cells to complete the repair process [56]. Also a complex system of physiological inhibitors and feed-back control mechanisms exists to control and limit any excessive or inappropriate activation of the haemostatic system [4].

Following injury vasoconstriction is transient, lasting less than 1 min, and seems to have little influence on the rate of bleeding. The lumen is not even reduced below two-thirds of its original diameter. The mechanism of vasoconstriction is unclear but is probably related to neurogenic contraction of the vessel wall and the release of

various humoral substances, such as serotonin and thromboxane A_2, from activated platelets.

The various blood components are not activated to any significant extent by the healthy vascular endothelial surface. After injury platelets adhere to the damaged subendothelial structures which are exposed. Platelet adhesion is also influenced by the von Willebrand factor, a high-molecular-weight plasma protein component of the factor VIII molecule, and circulating red blood cells. The precise manner in which the von Willebrand factor influences adhesion is unknown, but patients with von Willebrand's disease who are deficient in this factor have defective platelet adhesion [8] and prolonged bleeding times [45]. Also the physiological role of intracellular von Willebrand's factor in vascular endothelial cells [35], megakaryocytes and platelets [7] has not yet been determined. Injured red cells locally release adenosine-5-diphospate (ADP), which could activate platelets and induce adhesion [10]. With increasing red cell counts and whole blood viscosity more platelets are forced against the vessel wall surface, thus promoting their adhesion. This contributes significantly to the increased thrombotic tendency observed in polycythaemia rubra vera [11].

After adhesion to subendothelial structures, platelets lose their discoid shape and form lengthy pseudopods which spread out over the damaged vessel surface. There seem to be specific platelet membrane receptors for the physiological inducers of aggregation, such as ADP, thrombin, and collagen. These induce a contractile process by releasing calcium ions from storage sites, which leads to activation of platelet actomyosin and thrombasthenin. Changes in platelet membrane shape and configuration now occur so the membrane develops coagulation-promoting properties [54].

The contacting platelets then align together into, at first, a rather loose and reversible aggregate and later into a larger irreversible plug.

Increased levels of cytoplasmic calcium ions activate phospholipase A_2, which liberates fatty acids, most importantly arachidonic acid, from platelet membrane-bound phospholipids. Arachidonic acid is transformed by cyclooxygenase into endoperoxides and thence into thromboxane A_2. Thromboxane A_2 released locally is a most potent stimulator of platelet aggregation and vasoconstriction. The platelet-dense and α-granules then secrete their contents locally by exocytosis. These include ADP, which acts as a chemical messenger to promote growth of the aggregate, serotonin, a local vasoconstrictor, a mitogenic factor [51], which stimulates proliferation of smooth muscle in the vessel wall and various lysosomal enzymes. Two other release proteins, β-thromboglobulin, of unknown biological activity, and platelet factor 4, can now be measured by sensitive radioimmunoassays [40, 44], and they may allow assessment of any excessive platelet aggregation and release which is occurring in vivo.

The coagulation mechanism, which consists of a multicomponent enzyme system of pro-enzymes, co-factors and inhibitors, is activated by contact with the negatively charged damaged endothelial surface (the intrinsic pathway) and local release of tissue thromboplastin (the extrinsic pathway). This leads to the formation of fibrin, which consolidates the platelet plug. The coagulation reaction is shown schematically in Fig. 30.1. The complex interaction of factor XII and high-molecular-weight kininogen, which are adsorbed onto the negatively charged endothelial surface, and the binding of prekallikrein and factor XI to high molecular-weight kininogen leads to the activation of factor XI [62]. Then follows a series of conversions of inert precursors into active serine proteases, leading to fibrin formation. Diffusion of tissue juices into the circulation will activate the extrinsic pathway by converting factor VII into factor VIIa, which subsequently activates factor X.

Two main clotting reactions are accelerated by phospholipid micelles on the platelet surface; firstly the interaction of activated factor IXa with factor VIII to activate factor X, and secondly that of activated factor Xa with factor V to form thrombin from prothrombin. Factors VIII and V are not serine proteases but play a role in orienting clotting factors on the platelet surface so as to accelerate proteolysis of factor X and prothrombin, respectively. Platelets may also actually trigger coagulation by directly activating factor XI and factor X.

The digestion of fibrin depends on activation of the fibrinolytic enzyme system [23] and subsequently the defect in the vessel wall is repaired by regrowth of healthy endothelial cells. Plasminogen circulates as an inactive pro-enzyme and is converted by various different activators to the active serine protease, plasmin. The fibrinolytic pathway is shown schematically in Fig. 30.2. Several different pathways of plasminogen activation exist.

Vascular activator, which is released by vascular endothelial cells into the bloodstream, is the main physiological activator, and higher levels are released by various stimuli such as venous occlusion, vaso-active agents, exercise, and hyperpyrexia. Tissue activator, particularly rich in the uterus and prostate, is not normally released into the bloodstream but becomes available locally after extensive trauma and extravascular fibrin deposition. The renal parenchymal cells synthesize and release a urinary activator, urokinase, which is excreted continously in the urine and is probably important in maintaining patency of the urinary tract. Other activating systems include a factor XII-mediated pathway which follows activation of the intrinsic coagulation system and is interrelated with co-activation of kallikrein–kinin and complement systems [58].

Physiological levels of plasma activators are rapidly inactivated by anti-activators and are also degraded in the liver. Only at the site of thrombus formation is plasminogen converted to plasmin in appreciable amounts. Any plasmin that is released into the general circulation is rapidly inactivated by complex formation with antiplasmins [19]. Plasmin hydrolyzes fibrin into soluble split products and brings about gradual thrombus dissolution.

To prevent uncontrolled activity in blood of the large number of interrelated reactions leading to fibrin formation a powerful natural system of coagulation inhibitors exists. Anti-thrombin III is the major inhibitor of thrombin but also inhibits activated factor IXa, Xa, XIa,

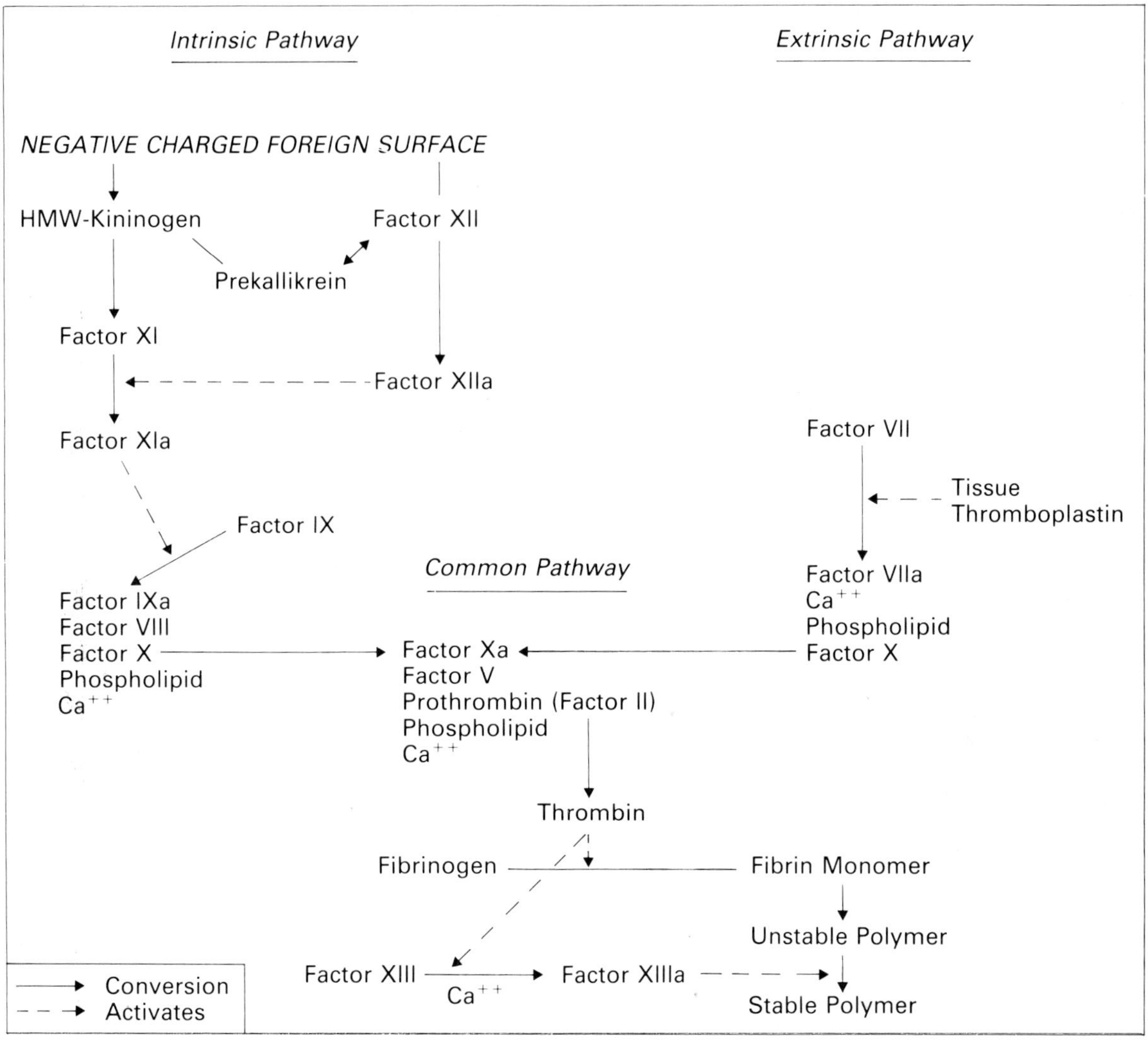

Intrinsic Pathway   Extrinsic Pathway

NEGATIVE CHARGED FOREIGN SURFACE

HMW-Kininogen   Factor XII

          Prekallikrein

Factor XI

       ← – – – – – – – Factor XIIa

Factor XIa

                                                      Factor VII
          Factor IX
                          Common Pathway   ← – – Tissue
                                                            Thromboplastin

Factor IXa   Factor VIIa
Factor VIII   Ca^{++}
Factor X ──────────→ Factor Xa ←────────── Phospholipid
Phospholipid   Factor V   Factor X
Ca^{++} Prothrombin (Factor II)
                       Phospholipid
                       Ca^{++}

                       Thrombin

          Fibrinogen ────────┐────────── Fibrin Monomer

                                         Unstable Polymer

┌─────────────────┐   Factor XIII ──────→ Factor XIIIa – – – →
│ ──→ Conversion │   Ca^{++} Stable Polymer
│ – –→ Activates   │
└─────────────────┘

Fig. 30.1. Blood coagulation process.

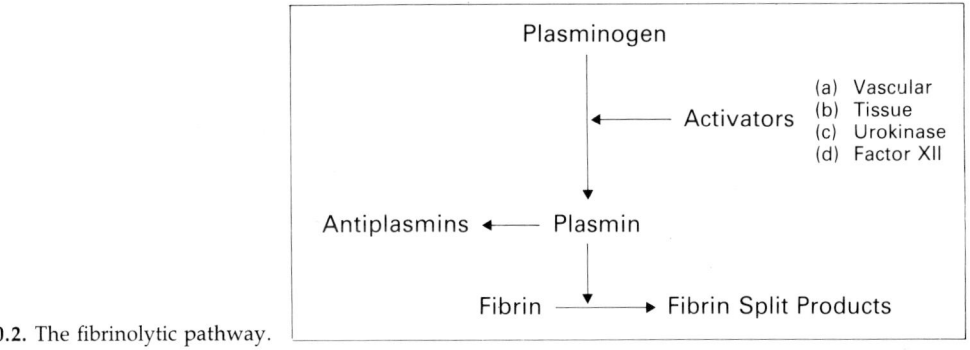

                       Plasminogen

                                                    (a) Vascular
                          ←────────── Activators   (b) Tissue
                                                    (c) Urokinase
                                                    (d) Factor XII

       Antiplasmins ←──── Plasmin

                       Fibrin ────→ Fibrin Split Products

Fig. 30.2. The fibrinolytic pathway.

kallikrein, and plasmin [55]. Heparin binds to antithrombin III and alters its molecular configuration so that inhibition of thrombin and factor Xa in particular are markedly accelerated [50]. The other main plasma thrombin inhibitors are α_2-macroglobulin and α_2-antitrypsin. As

well as these inhibitory agents it seems likely that both coagulation pathways can control their own activity to some extent by a series of feedback mechanisms.

The healthy endothelial cells of the vessel wall are able to synthesize from arachidonic acid and release into the circulation prostacyclin, a potent vasodilator and the most potent natural inhibitor of platelet aggregation yet described [65]. Prostacyclin, which is also produced in the lungs, binds to specific platelet membrane receptors and activates membrane-bound adenylate cyclase, which produces increased levels of cAMP. This inhibits platelet aggregation, the release reaction, and thromboxane A_2 synthesis. Thus the vessel wall controls excessive platelet activation by prostacyclin production and can activate the fibrinolytic system locally by release of plasminogen activator from endothelial cells if excess fibrin is deposited. These two control mechanisms emphasize the important complex interactions between the blood and vessel wall which help to maintain vascular integrity and patency [63].

Clinical and laboratory approach to haemostatic disorders

The haemostatic process is carefully balanced so that haemorrhage is promptly arrested and inappropriate thrombosis does not occur. The causes of haemostatic failure are numerous and it is useful to have a standardized approach to the clinical and laboratory diagnosis of any bleeding tendency.

The initial problem is to determine whether bleeding is due to a local factor, such as a peptic ulcer, or to an underlying haemostatic abnormality. Often a mild abnormality only becomes apparent after trauma or a local precipitating lesion. Any bleeding disorder may be inherited or acquired. This may result from one of the following mechanisms, as shown in Table 30.1.

Table 30.1. Pathogenesis of haemostatic failure

1 Thrombocytopenia
2 Functional platelet abnormality
3 Blood vessel defect
4 Coagulation factor(s) defect
5 Excess fibrinolysis
6 Combined defect

A careful clinical history and physical examination should be undertaken, and special care must be taken in patients with multisystem disease to recognize any bleeding tendency. In particular, continual oozing from venepuncture

and drip sites, extensive petechiae and purpura at pressure areas, and steady blood loss from drainage tubes are often signs of impending haemostatic failure. Often the cause of the bleeding will then be strongly suspected but laboratory tests are always required to make a precise diagnosis and to define the severity of any abnormality.

Initially a series of simple screening tests which are easy to perform and give reliable results should be undertaken. A suggested screening procedure is given in Table 30.2.

Table 30.2. Screening tests for a bleeding tendency

For Platelet Disorders
1 Bleeding time
2 Platelet count
3 Fresh blood film inspection

For Vascular Disorders
1 Bleeding time
2 Torniquet test (Hess)

For Coagulation Disorders
1 Prothrombin time
2 Kaolin partial thromboplastin time
3 Thrombin time
4 Fibronogen assay

The normal range for each test performed in the particular laboratory involved should be known before any results can be interpreted. If the screening tests suggest an abnormality, further specialized investigations, such as coagulant and immunological factor assays or platelet aggregation studies should be carried out to define precisely the defect and its severity. The technical details of these tests are described in detail elsewhere [2, 22].

Most patients with an inherited disorder present in childhood, often with a family history of a bleeding tendency and excessive bleeding in response to minor operations, dental extractions, or trauma. However, mild defects may sometimes not present until adult life, often as a result of major trauma or operative procedure. If an inherited disorder is suspected no effort should be spared to investigate other family members who might also be affected.

A simple screening programme which is likely to detect an on-going thrombotic process or individuals who are at greater risk of developing thrombosis in the near future, the so-called prothrombotic state, is more difficult to define. The thrombotic factors to be considered include the vessel wall endothelium, blood flow, platelets, red cells, white cells, and the coagulation and fibrinolytic systems.

Platelet disorders

Excessive bleeding due to a deficiency in the circulating platelet mass or abnormal platelet function can usually be controlled by prolonged local pressure. Generally platelet bleeding starts immediately after the initiating event, but once controlled it does not recur. In comparison, bleeding primarily due to coagulation factor deficiency is not controlled by prolonged pressure but continues with a slow but steady loss of unclottable blood and large friable non-functioning fibrin clots. This type of bleeding classically occurs up to several hours after the initial trauma and if untreated will, in severe cases, continue unabated for prolonged periods. Surgical bleeding, in the presence of a normal haemostatic system, is usually more dramatic, with a much faster initial rate of blood loss, and is never generalized.

The peripheral platelet count and the bleeding time are the first-line basic laboratory tests of platelet involvement in the haemostatic process. If the results of these two tests are within normal limits it is almost certain that a platelet defect is not responsible for excessive clinical bleeding. The normal range for the peripheral platelet count in children and adults is $150-400 \times 10^9$/litre. The standard laboratory procedure for counting platelets is by phase-contrast microscopy after suitable dilution of anticoagulated whole blood [12]. The accuracy of this procedure is probably only about $\pm 15\%$, however, and all abnormal results should be verified by careful inspection of a freshly stained peripheral blood film. In recent years several automated machines have improved the accuracy of platelet counting to some extent, but they occasionally produce wildly abnormal results (usually counting low values as normal or high) which may be very misleading clinically. For example, machines which count platelets following the lysis of red cells in whole blood count intracellular red cell inclusions of the same size range as platelets, such as Howell–Jolly bodies and malaria parasites. Also paraproteinaemias and collagen disorders may sometimes cause a falsely high count.

Although a platelet count of 150×10^9/litre is the lower limit of the normal range, spontaneous bleeding due to thrombocytopenia alone is unlikely to occur until the count is below 50×10^9/litre and usually does not occur until it has fallen below 20×10^9/litre. However, in the presence of a localized or generalized infection, serious platelet bleeding can occur when the count is at a higher level. Spontaneous platelet bleeding usually starts initially from the mucous membranes, especially the mouth and gums, often being exacerbated by poor oral hygiene, or as skin purpura around areas of local pressure such as tight socks around the ankles or under the application site of a sphygmomanometer cuff.

There are several methods for performing a bleeding time test (Ivy, Duke, and template methods), all of which rely on the time taken for a standard skin incision of small subcutaneous vessels to stop bleeding. The normal range for the particular test performed by each laboratory should be clearly stated along with the result. A prolonged bleeding time occurs when the platelet count falls below approximately 100×10^9/litre or, if found in the presence of a normal or raised platelet count, is suggestive of a platelet function defect.

Thrombocytopenia may occur as a result of diminished bone marrow production, excessive peripheral utilization or destruction, or excessive peripheral pooling in an enlarged spleen. A bone marrow aspirate and trephine section will provide an assessment of megakaryocyte number and their form. Decreased platelet production due to a reduction in the megakaryocyte mass is a feature of aplastic anaemia and malignant infiltration of the marrow by leukaemia or secondary carcinoma. In severe megaloblastic anaemia impaired megakaryocyte production and release of platelets rather than a reduction in megakaryocyte number is responsible for diminished marrow platelet production. Increased peripheral utilization or destruction is associated with increased marrow megakaryocyte production of platelets.

Excess utilization occurs in on-going disseminated intravascular coagulation (DIC) when continuing thrombus formation with platelet involvement causes thrombocytopenia due to the marrow being unable to compensate fully for the high platelet turnover.

Thrombotic thrombocytopenic purpura and the haemolytic uraemic syndrome, which are probably different spectra of the same pathological process, present with widespread intravascular hyaline thrombi consisting mainly of platelets and fibrin, thrombocytopenia, and a microangiopathic haemolytic anaemia. Thrombocytopenia is caused by continuing platelet activation and utilization, and a deficiency of prostacyclin seems responsible. Plasma transfusions or intensive plasma exchange often halt the excessive platelet activation by supplying a missing or deficient plasma factor that is essential for prostacyclin release from the vessel wall or are effective by removing a toxic factor or inhibitor to the vessel wall [15].

Increased peripheral destruction is caused by immune mechanisms. The platelet membrane is coated by IgG auto-antibodies and premature platelet destruction occurs by phagocytosis in macrophages mainly in the spleen and liver. It is now possible to detect these antibodies directly on the platelet surface membrane or free in the plasma [27, 66]. Plasma levels of antibodies are an unreliable indicator of clinical severity and disease progression. However, levels bound to the platelet surface have been found to be more helpful. In vivo platelet lifespan measurements with the patient's own platelets labelled with Cr^{15} or indium^{111} oxide will show reduced survival curves. Normal platelet lifespan is approximately 10 days in the peripheral circulation but in severe immune thrombocytopenia it may be reduced to only a few hours. Three main forms of immune platelet destruction are recognised clinically. Acute thrombocytopenia occurs in children and is usually self-limiting. It often follows a few days after an acute viral or bacterial infection, and platelets are probably destroyed due to interaction with antigen–antibody complexes related to the infective agent. Chronic immune thrombocytopenia is often primary and idiopathic. However, the idiopathic variety is a diagnosis of exclusion from associated diseases such as systemic lupus erythematosus and chronic lymphatic leukaemia, which may also develop platelet auto-antibodies that react with some, as yet undetermined, basic part of the platelet membrane. The third type is drug-induced thrombocytopenia, where the drug or one of its metabolites combines with a plasma protein to form an antigen. The antibody to this antigen forms an immune complex which is adsorbed secondarily onto the platelet surface, leading to premature platelet destruction. As soon as an offending drug is withdrawn the platelet survival and count recover gradually over the next 10 days.

The normal-sized adult spleen, weighing 150–200 g, pools about 30% of the total peripheral platelet mass, which exchanges freely with the platelets in the circulation. When a spleen becomes pathologically enlarged the percentage of pooled platelets increases considerably and, especially if the bone marrow reserve capacity to increase platelet production is impaired, severe thrombopenia will result.

A platelet function disorder should be suspected in patients with abnormal skin or mucous membrane bleeding in whom the bleeding time is prolonged despite a normal platelet count. These disorders may be primary, due to platelet dysfunction, or secondary to a recognised clinical condition. Platelets adhere to different surfaces, aggregate, secrete locally their granular contents and later play a role in clot retraction. Isolated and combined defects of an inherited or acquired nature have been described for each of these physiological functions [31].

Platelets adhere to collagen or non-collagenous subendothelial surfaces. For adhesion to collagen a co-factor is not required. Patients with Erlers–Danlas syndrome, who have an inherited abnormal collagen structure, have a bleeding tendency due to the inability of their normal platelets to adhere to their own defective collagen [36]. Adhesion to non-collagen structures depends on an interaction between platelets and the divalent cations, fibrinogen, and von Willebrand's factor. Binding of von Willebrand factor to a platelet membrane receptor seems necessary for normal adhesion. Defective adhesion will occur in patients with absent or abnormal fibrinogen, von Willebrand's disease, and a platelet membrane defect. There is a group of giant platelet syndromes which have a reduced sialic acid and glycoprotein I membrane content, large circulating platelets and a variable degree of thrombocytopenia. These syndromes, commonly known as the Bernard–Soulier syndrome, have abnormal adhesion due to absence of the platelet membrane receptor to the von Willebrand factor. In the laboratory these disorders can be recognized by defective platelet adhesion to a standardized glass bead column or an everted damaged rabbit aorta in a perfusion chamber. Ristocetin-induced aggregation depends on the interaction between ristocetin, von Willebrand factor, and the platelet membrane receptor. Defective ristocetin aggregation occurs in patients with Bernard–Soulier syndrome and approximately 80% of cases of von Willebrand's disease cases.

After adhesion has occurred in vivo, collagen, thrombin and ADP bind to specific receptors on the platelet membrane and activate an enzyme system which releases free arachidonic acid from membrane-bound phospholipids. Arachidonic acid in turn is converted into unstable endoperoxides by cyclo-oxygenase, which are precursors of thromboxane A_2 and other prostaglandins. The endoperoxides initiate the release reaction of the α and dense granules and thromboxane A_2 is the most potent inducer of further platelet aggregation. These reactions are shown schematically in Fig. 30.3. Probably two other aggregating mechanisms which are independent of arachidonic acid metabolism exist. These are activated by collagen and high-dose thrombin and seem dependent on the availability of free intracellular calcium ions and the recently described PAF (platelet-activating factor) [25].

Thrombasthenia (Glanzmann's disease) is an inherited deficiency of glycoproteins II and II in the platelet membrane which results in absent aggregation to ADP and collagen, although adhesion and ristocetin-induced aggregation are normal. Presumably ADP and collagen membrane receptors are missing as a result of the membrane abnormality.

Inherited deficiency of cyclo-oxygenase or thromboxane synthetase enzymes occur very rarely [24] but acquired cyclo-oxygenase deficiency is the most commonly occurring acquired platelet defect. Aspirin (acetylsalicylic acid) irreversibly inhibits cyclo-oxygenase by acetylation of the enzyme [52]. As circulating platelets are unable to synthesize new proteins, the defect produced by a single dose of aspirin lasts for the remainder of the platelet's lifespan. Thus in clinical practice, after only 300 mg aspirin a platelet function defect and an increased bleeding tendency lasts for between 4–7 days until the bone marrow megakaryocytes have released sufficient unaffected platelets into the circulation. Many drugs, particularly indomethacin and other nonsteroidal anti-inflammatory agents, inhibit cyclo-oxygenase activity, but they inactivate the enzyme in a reversible manner so that the increased bleed-ing tendency only lasts for 12–24 h after drug ingestion. Aggregation defects can be assessed by the response of platelet-rich plasma to various aggregation inducers in an aggregometer. The pattern of platelet aggregation can be followed by the change in light transmission detected by a photoelectric cell as aggregation occurs [9].

There are two groups of inherited release defects, known collectively as storage pool disease. One is associated with absent dense granules and their ADP content and the other has a failure of the dense granules' release mechanism despite normal numbers of granules.

Bleeding in certain frequently occurring clinical conditions may be associated with platelet function abnormalities. In uraemia, disturbances in adhesion and aggregation are often found [29]. This disorder is probably multifactorial. Certain dialysable substances may coat the platelet surface and inhibit function. Recently evidence of increased amounts of a plasma factor which stimulates prostacyclin release from the vessel wall has been reported [49]. Prostacyclin inhibits aggregation by binding to a specific membrane receptor, which raises intracellular cAMP levels. Raised cAMP levels inhibit thromboxane A_2 synthesis.

The abormalities in myeloproliferative disorders are quite heterogeneous [68]. Various intrinsic defects, including enzyme abnormalities, may occur due to abnormal platelet production from the malignant megakarycoyte clone. Polycythaemia, due to a raised red cell mass, or thrombocytosis may paradoxically present simultaneously with thrombosis and bleeding.

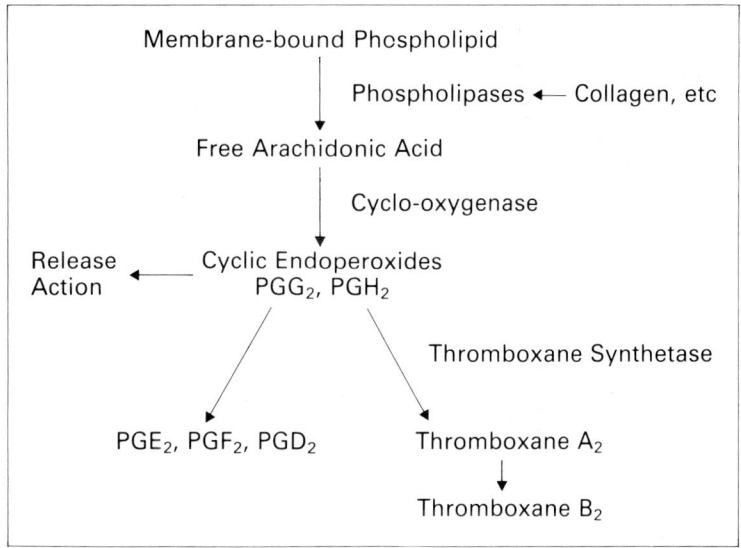

Fig. 30.3. Platelet arachidonic acid metabolism.

Increased blood viscosity causes sluggish blood flow and a thrombotic tendency; while membrane defects may result from partially activated platelets or excessive buffeting in the circulation and result in a haemorrhagic tendency. The polycythaemia associated with congenital heart disease, especially when the haematocrit exceeds 0.60, may be associated with thrombocytopenia and a membrane defect. Together they present a considerable haemostatic risk, especially if cardiac bypass surgery is contemplated.

Coating of the platelet surface with gamma globulin in patients with hypergammaglobulinaemia interferes with platelet adhesion and aggregation. This occurs in Waldenstrom's macroglobulinaemia, multiple myeloma and system lupus erythematosus. Impaired platelet function has also been reported in scurvy, pernicious anaemia, liver disease, and valvular heart disease and in patients receiving infusions of low-molecular-weight dextrans and hydroxyethyl starch.

Thrombocytosis becomes clinically important at platelet counts above 800×10^9/litre. With increasing counts above this, the risk of widespread thrombosis, particularly arterial lesions, increases considerably. Thrombocytosis may be primary, due to a haematological malignancy involving the marrow megakaryocytes, or secondary to certain reactive processes. Secondary causes include the acute phase reaction after major trauma or operative procedures, myocardial infarction, collagen disorders, lymphomatous diseases and splenectomy. It is important to reduce any raised counts as quickly as possible by treating the primary condition. Until the disease is controlled platelet removal on a cell separator, reduction of marrow production with busulphan, and inhibition of platelet function with aspirin will reduce the thrombotic risk.

Platelet transfusions, preferably as platelet concentrates rather than as fresh blood, are the cornerstone for the emergency treatment of uncontrollable platelet bleeding. To control bleeding it is usually satisfactory to raise the platelet count above 50×10^9/litre. However, several problems associated with the use of platelet infusions should be remembered. Platelet concentrates only contain viable functioning platelets for 48–72 h after collection. There is still controversy as to the best way to store platelets before infusion, and in Britain this varies at different transfusion centres. Platelets stored at 4°C [57] function immediately after infusion but have only a short-lived effect

for about 24 h, whereas if stored at 22°C [64] it is several hours after infusion before they all function satisfactorily but they retain useful activity for up to 72 h. Obviously, 4°C storage is better for therapy of acutely bleeding episodes and 22°C storage better for prophylactic support of non-bleeding thrombopenic patients. Continued prophylactic support of chronic thrombopenic patients (i.e., aplastic anaemia, pancytopenia during remission induction for acute leukaemia) will eventually lead to the formation of platelet allo-antibodies and non-effectiveness of random platelet infusions. These patients then require platelet support from HLA and platelet-specific antigen compatible donors (usually a sibling). In patients with inherited platelet membrane defects it is essential to limit platelet transfusions to serious bleeding episodes only or to major operations. They are very prone to form antibodies against the part of the membrane they are deficient in, and once this occurs effective platelet transfusions become impossible. Patients with an auto-immune thrombopenia are generally unresponsive to platelet infusions. In life-threatening situations, however, they may be helpful in conjunction with immunosuppressive therapy, plasma exchange, and splenectomy. Fever, infection, and hypersplenism will all increase platelet transfusion requirements to achieve satisfactory haemostasis.

Steroid therapy is helpful in immune conditions as it reduces the rate of destruction of antibody-coated platelets by the reticuloendothelial system. However, in some non-immune conditions steroids may also lessen clinical bleeding without raising the platelet count, possibly by improving vascular integrity.

Coagulation defects

Results of the three basic laboratory screening tests for the coagulation system usually suggest the nature of any deficiency. The significance of each test is shown in Table 30.3. The partial thromboplastin time is more sensitive to factor XII, XI, IX, and VIII abnormalities than the later factors of the common pathway and, like the prothrombin time, is especially insensitive to fibrinogen (factor I) deficiency. If a prolonged partial thromboplastin time is found by repeating the test with a 50:50 mixture of patient plasma and normal plasma it can be shown whether the abnormality is caused by factor deficiency or

Table 30.3. Sensitivity of coagulation screening tests to factor deficiency

Test	Detect abnormalities
Prothrombin time	VII, X, V, II, I
Partial thromboplastin time	XII, XI, IX, VIII, X, V, II, I
Thrombin time	I, raised FDPs, circulating heparin

Table 30.4. Relationship of factor VIII coagulant level to bleeding tendency in classic haemophilia

Plasma factor VIII (% of normal)	Bleeding tendency
>50	None. Normal range
25–50	Only after major trauma or surgery. Otherwise asymptomatic
5–25	After minor surgery and dental extractions
1–5	Severe after minor injury. Occasional spontaneous haemarthroses
0	Severe and frequent spontaneous bleeding and after trivial injury

an inhibitor, usually IgG in nature, which is inactivating one of the coagulation proteins. A factor deficiency will be significantly corrected by the normal plasma, whereas if an inhibitor is present very little correction of the prolonged time will occur. The nature and degree of any suggested deficiency should be ascertained by specific assays of the biological activity of the factors involved.

Coagulant factor defects can be produced in several ways. There may be reduced or absent synthesis of the coagulation protein, or a qualitatively abnormal molecule may be produced which is deficient in the biological, active part of the molecule only. Defects can also arise from excess peripheral utilization or loss, and inactivation can occur by way of circulating antibodies or inhibitors. All the coagulation factors apart from factor VIII are synthesized in the liver. The factor VIII antigen is synthesized in endothelial cells and acquires coagulant activity in the circulation, probably by forming a complex with a small-molecular-weight substance.

Congenital coagulation disorders

Deficiency of every coagulation factor has been described, but all are rare disorders except haemophilia, Christmas disease (haemophilia B), and von Willebrand's disease [5, 13]. Haemophilia and Christmas disease are transmitted as sex-linked recessive traits and von Willebrand's disease usually as an autosomal dominant trait; all the others are believed to be autosomal recessive.

Classic haemophilia results from the synthesis of an abnormal molecule which has deficient or absent biological activity but raised levels of immunological reactive material and normal platelet function [6]. Clinical severity correlates very well with the degree of deficiency of biological coagulant activity. The relationship of factor VIII activity to bleeding tendency is shown in Table 30.4. Therapy consists of replacing factor VIII material so as to allow normal haemostasis and healing to occur after trauma or to cover any operative or dental

procedures which are to be undertaken. Severe haemophiliacs who experience frequent spontaneous and often crippling bleeding episodes may now benefit from regular prophylactic replacement therapy. As factor VIII has a half-life in vivo of only 10–14 h, twice-daily infusions are needed to provide adequate treatment. Cryoprecipitate prepared from fresh blood and lyophilized concentrates from newer fractionation procedures are now available for replacement therapy. The concentrates have several advantages which include greater purity, known content of factor VIII activity in a small volume, and ease of administration which makes self-administered and home therapy possible. For effective haemostasis a level of 15%–20% is required but a level of 50%–60% must be maintained after major trauma and surgery. Severe haemophiliacs who have had repeated exposure to blood products are at a great risk of developing viral hepatitis, chronic liver disease, and allo-antibodies to red cell, platelet, HLA and serum protein antigens [38, 42]. Approximately 5%–10% will develop factor VIII inhibitors and become resistant to therapy with cryoprecipitate and lyophilized concentrates. Bleeding episodes in these patients may become very difficult to manage and therapy with steroids, immunosuppressive agents, intensive plasma exchange, bovine or porcine factor VIII preparations, or very high doses of human factor VIII concentrate may be required [47].

The clinical problems associated with Christmas disease (factor IX deficiency) and the relationship of bleeding tendency to the degree of factor deficiency are similar to classic haemophilia. However, factor IX has a half-life in the circulation of approximately 24 h and factor IX replacement therapy is readily available with fresh-frozen plasma and factor IX concentrates.

Von Willebrand's disease is characterized by a

prolonged bleeding time, reduced platelet adhesion and a reduction in factor VIII coagulant and immunological antigen activity [43]. Classic von Willebrand's have a parallel reduction in all three plasma VIII activities, but recently several variants have been described which may have normal antigen content but altered electrophoretic activity and abnormal platelet adhesion. Some of these patients have a reduced carbohydrate content of the factor VIII molecule, which prevents normal platelet adhesion and ristocetin aggregation. Rarely acquired forms of von Willebrand's disease may develop in patients with auto-immune disorders [33]. They can form antibody that precipitates part of the factor VIII molecule or blocks the expression of normal platelet adhesion. These patients usually have a lymphomatous process or a collagen disorder. Cryoprecipitate is more effective in treating bleeding episodes than factor VIII concentrates and, unlike patients with classic haemophilia, the effective half-life of infused factor VIII is approximately 24 h.

All the other deficiencies should be easily identified by the screening tests, and therapy depends on maintaining a factor level necessary for haemostasis and wound healing. Fresh-frozen plasma is a readily available source of replacement therapy and the frequency of infusions depends on the half-life of the particular factor in the circulation. Only factor XIII deficiency will not be detected by the basic screening procedures and this usually presents as renewed bleeding 2–3 days after the initial clot has formed. Factor XIII deficiency is diagnosed by abnormal solubility of a fibrin clot in $5\,M$ urea.

Vitamin K deficiency

Vitamin K, a fat-soluble vitamin, is required by the liver for synthesis of factors II (prothrombin), VII, IX, and X. The natural K vitamins are synthesized by intestinal bacteria and are present in green plants. As they are fat-soluble they require bile for absorption and are not stored in the body to any extent.

Vitamin K acts at a post-ribosomal site and causes the carboxylation of glutamyl residues at the amino end of the molecule [14]. This enables the factors to bind to a phospholipid surface in the presence of calcium ions and activate the next part of the coagulation cascade. In vitamin K deficiency the liver synthesizes an abnormal protein which is unable to bind to phospholipid surfaces despite having the same immunological and amino acid composition as the normal protein. These immunologically detectable proteins are known as PIVKAs—protein induced by vitamin K absence or antagonism—and may themselves even inhibit coagulation [32].

However, in liver disease when the synthesis of all proteins is diminished, PIVKAs are not produced. When vitamin K becomes deficient the activity of the dependent factors decreases according to their circulating half-life (factor VII 2–4 h, factor IX 25 h, factor X 40 h, and factor II 60 h).

In haemorrhagic disease of the newborn, functional immaturity of the liver and reduced stores of vitamin K, because the infant's gut is sterile and maternal milk contains virtually no vitamin K, leads to a mild decrease of the vitamin K-dependent factors for the first 3–5 days of life. A small dose of up to 1 mg vitamin K_1 at birth will prevent any bleeding tendency, but larger amounts may cause a haemolytic anaemia due to glycolytic enzyme deficiencies, especially in the premature infant.

Vitamin K malabsorption will occur in obstructive jaundice due to the absence of bile. Various malabsorption syndromes such as sprue, prolonged diarrhoea, cystic fibrosis, and medication with large doses of mineral oil may also result in vitamin K deficiency. Intestinal sterilization will decrease the bacterial production of vitamin K. This is seen in patients receiving antibiotics to sterilize the colon prior to gastrointestinal surgery or during long-term parenteral feeding in combination with gut-sterilizing antibiotics. Especially if the patient has previously had a poor diet, severe vitamin K deficiency may develop. In these circumstances the deficiency can be easily corrected by 10 mg vitamin K_1 IV at weekly intervals.

Oral anticoagulants of the coumarin and inandione derivatives probably inhibit the action of vitamin K in the carboxylation of glutamyl residues of factors II, VII, IX, and X at a post-ribosomal site [59]. Many patients receiving long-term oral anticoagulants are taking various other drugs, some of which may potentiate or antagonize oral anticoagulants [67]. This may cause fluctuating control and serious bleeding may occur spontaneously if the prothrombin time becomes grossly prolonged. An IV dose of vitamin K_1 takes 6 h before any synthesis of biologically active factors occurs. So to control acute bleeding immediately, an infusion of fresh-frozen plasma or prothrombin complex concentrate is required.

Occasionally, psychiatrically disturbed patients may be encountered who are secretly taking oral anticoagulants themselves. They usually have a previous history of thrombosis and are often associated with one of the para-medical professions. Despite an unexplained prolonged prothrombin time and fluctuating bleeding problems, they deny vigorously taking any drugs and go to great lengths to conceal and ingest their supply of tablets. If necessary, to prove drug ingestion the drug concentration in the blood may be measured [30].

Liver disease

Bleeding is a frequent complication of liver disease. As the circulating survival times of the clotting factors are much shorter than those of the other plasma proteins synthesized by the liver, laboratory clotting tests and specific factor assays give a most reliable index of the current state of liver cell synthesis. The vitamin K-dependent factors decrease first, and with more severe liver disease factor V activity falls. As factor V is not vitamin K-dependent, depression of factor V indicates liver synthetic failure rather than malabsorption of vitamin K. With more severe disease fibrinogen levels decrease and, in some cases, an abnormal fibrinogen molecule with defective fibrin polymerization is synthe-sized. It has been shown that in acute liver failure factor VII coagulant levels are an accurate prognostic indicator. In a small series patients whose level fell below 8% all died, whilst those with activity exceeding 8% survived.

The liver also degrades activated clotting fac-tors and the fibrinolytic enzymes. The failure to degrade activated clotting factors in liver dis-ease may trigger off disseminated intravascular coagulation (DIC). Impaired breakdown of the fibrinolytic enzymes may result in abnormally excessive fibrinolysis. Surprisingly, factor VIII levels are often raised in liver failure due to the fact that it is synthesized mainly outside the liver and impaired clearance of activated factor VIII molecules by damaged liver cells may occur.

Thrombocytopenia commonly occurs due to hypersplenism secondary to cirrhosis and portal hypertension. Excessive alcohol intake may depress platelet production and occasionally functional platelet abnormalities have been reported.

Major bleeding complications are usually due to gastro-intestinal haemorrhages related to portal hypertension. The management of any underlying coagulation defect involving the temporary correction of any abnormality may improve the chances of recovery of liver cell function. Infusions of fresh-frozen plasma and

platelet concentrates will control haemorrhage due primarily to coagulation disorders for a short time. The use of prothrombin complexes instead of fresh-frozen plasma has been associ-ated with thrombo-embolic complications due to the presence of activated coagulation factors and should not routinely be used [37]. How-ever, the Oxford product appears much safer and no adverse thrombotic effects have been reported.

Disseminated intravascular coagulation

Episodes of DIC result from intravascular activation of the coagulation system, with resultant widespread deposition of altered fibri-nogen and platelets mainly in the microcircula-tion. In the majority of patients the process of diffuse DIC produces no clinical symptoms but evidence of excess consumption of coagulation factors and platelets can be demonstrated by laboratory tests. However, in some patients the epidose is severe enough to give rise to a generalized haemorrhagic state and/or end-organ failure following blockade of the micro-vasculature by thrombus formation. The organ most liable to ischaemic damage is the kidney, but the brain, heart, and adrenals can also sustain severe ischaemic changes. Underlying triggering mechanisms are numerous but DIC may be initiated in three basic ways [17]:

1) Stimulation of the coagulation process by release of tissue factors into the blood-stream. This occurs, for example, follow-ing surgical trauma, during an acute intravascular haemolytic episode, or dur-ing dissemination of malignant tissue.
2) Induction of platelet aggregation, which occurs in septicaemia, viraemia, and im-mune complex diseases and also by thrombin, which forms whenever the coagulation process is activated.
3) Severe endothelial injury of the vessel wall, which occurs in patients with exten-sive burns, widespread vasculitis, infec-tions, prolonged hypotension, acidosis, and hypoxia and activates both intrinsic and extrinsic coagulation pathways.

It is likely that more than 60% of clinical cases of DIC have a strong association with septicaemic infections, Gram-negative bacteria being the most frequent micro-organism; but other agents including viruses, fungi, tubercle bacilli, and Rickettsia have also been clearly responsible. Partial blockage by fibrin of the microcircula-tion, particularly in the kidney, may cause damage to red cells as they pass through the obstructed vessels. Strands of fibrin act rather like a fine-mesh sieve and passing red cells are traumatized, leading to distorted microcytic red cells and an intravascular haemolytic process which has been called micro-angiopathic haemolytic anaemia.

In the acute state of DIC it is essential to demonstrate the abnormal laboratory parameters accurately and quickly. Ideally the screening tests should be available 30 min after the laboratory receives the sample. To demonstrate depletion or consumption of clotting factors and platelets and the degree of the process a thrombin time, prothrombin time, fibrinogen assay, platelet count and haemoglobin estimation will give all the necessary information. The abnormalities are reflected by a prolonged thrombin time, hypofibrinogenaemia and thrombocytopenia. On these values therapy can be initiated and the progress of the consumptive coagulopathy monitored by frequent repeat estimations of these simple screening tests. Although patients will also often have a decreased level of prothrombin, factor V, and factor VIII, specific coagulation factor assays, apart from a fibrinogen level, are of limited value in acute DIC [26]. A fibrinogen level below 1.0 g/litre and a platelet count below 100×10^9/litre are regarded as almost diagnostic. Following activation of the coagulation system and intravascular thrombosis, there is usually a localized secondary increase in fibrinolytic activity, leading to the formation of plasmin which degrades fibrin and fibrinogen progressively. Secondary fibrinolysis causes increased levels of circulating fibrin complexes and fibrin split products. A serum fibrinogen/fibrin degradation product (FDP) assay, which the provision of commercial kits has made readily available as a rapid screening technique, is usually raised above 100 μg/ml in acute DIC. However, some patients with severe DIC have no elevation of FDPs, due to inhibition of their fibrinolytic response, and they usually have a poor outcome due to irreversible organ failure. The thrombin time is prolonged by a deficiency of clottable fibrinogen, elevated serum FDPs which act as anticoagulants, or the presence of circulating heparin. This acts as a practical guide to the bleeding significance of raised FDPs and a low fibrinogen level. A prolonged thrombin time more than double the control time is usually indicative of impending overt clinical bleeding.

The management of acute DIC is extremely controversial and several widely different approaches are currently advocated. The first essential, if at all possible, is to eliminate the precipitating factors. In particular, all antibiotics must be given IV and shock should be vigorously treated to avoid excess vascular stasis. If the bleeding diathesis is severe enough to warrant replacement therapy platelet concentrates, fresh-frozen plasma and cryoprecipitate (which also contains fibrinogen) should be given. Volume expanders, such as dextrans, should not be used as they may exacerbate bleeding but human plasma protein fractions which contain 5% albumin can be safely given. The various factor IX concentrates and fibrinogen preparations should also not be used because of potential thrombogenicity. Excessive fibrinogen and platelet therapy may lead to their rapid consumption and further exacerbate microvasculature thrombosis. Frequent repetition of the basic laboratory screening tests should be undertaken and the response of the thrombin time, fibrinogen assay, and serum FDP level used to determine when future replacement therapy is required. The use of heparin in DIC remains particularly controversial and there are many reports of benefit and marked deterioration in the literature. As a general guideline I only advocate its use after a satisfactory trial of replacement therapy has failed to alleviate clinically severe bleeding and/or thrombosis. I begin with a low-dose continuous IV infusion of 500 u/h, increasing the dose hourly by 500 u if no improvement of the clinical condition or serial laboratory results ensues.

Associated low levels of antithrombin III occur in acute DIC, which will make heparin therapy relatively ineffective. Infusions of antithrombin III or complexed antithrombin III–heparin may well be the therapy for severe DIC in the future.

Problems associated with blood transfusion

When the patient's blood volume is replaced by the administration of large quantities of stored bank blood in a short period of time, haemorrhagic manifestations may well follow [20].

Bank blood that has been stored for more than 24 h contains no functioning platelets, concentrations of factors V and VIII of approximately 10%, and of factor XI of about 20%. If a transfusion equal to the blood volume of the patient is given, a significant dilutional thrombocytopenia and clotting-factor deficiency develop. These must be corrected by an infusion of platelet concentrates and fresh-frozen plasma or clotting concentrates. Bank blood may precipitate DIC due to a combination of partial activation of clotting factors during storage and breakdown of platelets, leucocytes, and red cells releasing thromboplastic substances into the blood. There is also evidence that platelet function may be impaired in patients receiving massive transfusions [39].

Occasionally severe post-transfusion thrombocytopenia develops about 1 week after a transfusion [18]. This is a self-limiting process due to the formation of platelet antibodies against infused platelet antigens with secondary destruction of the patient's own platelets as a result of attachment to the antigen–antibody complexes.

The use of dextrans or hydroxyethyl starch as volume expanders after severe blood loss are associated with haemostatic disorders. Haemodilution is common to all colloidal plasma expanders, but even small doses of low-molecular-weight dextrans inhibit platelet function with a maximum effect about 4 h after infusion. Higher doses precipitate factor VIII and give an acquired von Willebrand's type of syndrome [48] and also inhibits the fibrinolytic system so fibrinolysis is retarded [16]. If higher molecular-weight dextrans are used coagulation factors are also affected resulting in prolonged coagulation times. However, the various gelatin solutions do not interfere with any aspect of coagulation even when very high clinical doses are used [34].

Inhibitors of coagulation

The physiological inhibitors of coagulation, in particular antithrombin III, play an important role in controlling a balance in haemostasis. Several various techniques are available to study the concentrations of inhibitors and the clinical importance of decreased levels of antithrombin III has recently been recognized [46]. Reduced levels of antithrombin III below 80% have been reported in liver disease, DIC, nephrotic syndrome, during the postoperative period, and in a small percentage of women taking oral contraceptives containing oestrogens. Values below 80% signify a hypercoagulable state and a considerable risk of developing a thrombo-embolic episode. Several families with a congenital deficiency of antithrombin III with levels of 40–60% have been reported [28]. The clinical features are multiple episodes of venous thrombosis and embolism. If a patient's antithrombin III level is decreased before heparin therapy, this may lead to a further fall and may even exacerbate a thrombotic tendency. It is hoped that in the near future antithrombin III concentrates will be readily available for infusion to patients with deficient levels and on-going thrombosis.

In a number of clinical conditions acquired circulating inhibitors or anticoagulants may inhibit specific coagulation factors, most frequently factor VIII, and cause a bleeding tendency. This occurs in 5%–10% of patients with classic haemophilia but very rarely in the other inherited deficiencies. Circulating anticoagulants may occur in systemic lupus erythematosus, rheumatoid disease, multiple myeloma, pregnancy, and old age. Bleeding is rarely troublesome and therapy of the underlying disease usually corrects any bleeding problems.

Vascular disorders

A diagnosis of a vascular defect is usually suspected when bleeding is confined to the skin and mucous membranes and the standard laboratory screening tests show no abnormality. The tourniquet (Hess) test is usually positive and occasionally the bleeding time may be prolonged. Bleeding is usually minor with an easy bruising tendency and spontaneous bleeding from small vessels, and is commonly seen in clinical practice. The underlying defect is in the vessels themselves, which may be structurally weak or suffer damage due to inflammatory or immune processes, or in the supporting connective tissue.

Hereditary haemorrhagic telangiectasia is transmitted as an autosomal dominant trait and is clearly an inherited vascular abnormality. These patients have multiple telangiectasis, which are abnormal dilatations of capillaries and arterioles, usually found on the skin and mucous membranes around the nose and mouth. The lesions blanch on pressure and become more numerous with advancing age, and they bleed easily because of vascular wall thinness and contract poorly, so that bleeding tends to be prolonged. Treatment consists of local pressure but if bleeding becomes persistent oestrogens or cautery may control bleeding from the nasal mucosa. Chronic mucosal blood loss will precipitate chronic iron deficiency and persistent gastro-intestinal lesions may be very difficult to control.

Vascular endothelium damage can be associated with infections, drug reactions, and the Henoch–Schönlein syndrome, which is a hypersensitivity reaction involving inflammatory changes in the capillaries and small arterioles [21]. Paraproteinaemias can cause vascular purpura by directly injuring endothelial cells as well as causing platelet and coagulation factor disorders. In contrast, purpura and bruising in patients with Cushing's syndrome, excess cortiocosteroid therapy, senile purpura, and vitamin C deficiency are due to loss of perivascular supporting tissue. Vitamin C is necessary for normal collagen formation and a deficiency state may develop in severe starvation or in babies who have been breast-fed for prolonged periods without vitamin supplements. High levels of steroids cause loss of subcutaneous tissue so that small vessels are very friable, especially to mild trauma of a shearing nature. In senile purpura atrophy of collagen fibres, mainly on the extensor surfaces of the hands and arms, causes thin, inelastic skin and the skin vessels also tear and bleed easily with slight shearing strains.

Simple easy bruising is a very common but benign disorder, usually seen in women who are otherwise healthy. They develop small, painful, circumscribed bruises on the legs and trunk probably due to increased vessel fragility. It is an important condition only because of its frequency and cosmetic effects and other more serious disorders can be excluded by a normal coagulation screen.

Excessive pathological fibrinolysis

In certain conditions inappropriately large quantities of plasminogen activator are occasionally released into the circulation and may induce a bleeding tendency. This initially presents as progressive bleeding at sites of trauma, postoperative wound areas and venepunctures and, if severe and uncontrolled, generalized haemostatic failure may develop. Excess activator converts plasminogen to plasmin, which digests clotting factors before it can be inactivated by antiplasmins. For example, as a result of extensive tissue trauma following burns, postoperatively (especially after prostatic operations), or in patients with disseminated neoplasms, large amounts of tissue activator may

be released. Plasminogen activators are inactivated by the liver but in chronic liver disease impaired inactivation may also produce excessive bleeding. Thrombolytic therapy with streptokinase or urokinase infusions for acute thrombotic lesions may cause bleeding in up to 25% of patients, usually at sites of skin incisions and venepunctures, and severe bleeding occasionally necessitates cessation of treatment. Both agents act by generating plasmin from plasminogen [3]. Excess fibrinolysis is recognized by a prolonged thrombin time, due to decreased fibrinogen levels and raised FDPs. The euglobin clot lysis time, which is a measure of fibrinolytic potential of a patient's plasma to lyse a clot, is shortened considerably below the normal range.

Local release of excess activator may occur in the renal and urogenital tracts and be responsible for chronic blood loss. Primary menorrhagia in particular may be precipitated in this way. Antifibrinolytic agents, such as epsilon aminocaproic acid (EACA) and tranexamic acid, are inhibitors of plasminogen activation. They have proved effective in controlling clinical bleeding due to excessive fibrinolysis, especially in patients who have undergone prostatic surgery or have urinary tract bleeding or primary menorrhagia.

Antithrombotic therapy

Thrombosis occurs when there is a breakdown in the protective mechanisms of the haemostatic process leading to an intravascular deposit of fibrin and the blood cellular elements. Arterial thrombi in high flow systems are mainly composed of platelet aggregates and fibrin strands, whereas venous thrombi in low flow systems are a mixture of red cells, fibrin, and platelets and are commonly found in valve cusps or venous sinuses in the deep leg veins. The basis of prevention and therapy of thrombosis depends considerably on the use of anticoagulants which inhibit fibrin formation, drugs which inhibit platelet function and agents with fibrinolytic activity to digest formed fibrin.

Heparin

Heparin is a negatively charged sulphated mucopolysaccharide with a molecular weight of between 6000 and 30 000. It is undoubtedly an effective drug for prophylaxis and therapy of venous thrombo-embolism [61].

For prophylaxis an injection of 5000 u SC every 8–12 h has been shown to be effective [1] and laboratory monitoring is not required. Whether combining the heparin injections with 0.5 mg dihydroergatamine or the use of synthetic heparin analogues which have a more specific anti-Xa effect will reduce the incidence of thrombosis even further in high-risk groups (i.e., elective hip replacement operations) has yet to be proved by clinical trials.

For therapy of a thrombotic episode 40, 000–60,000 u every 24 h by continuous IV infusion for 6 days, followed by oral anticoagulation, seems the treatment of choice. However, even in patients with a normal haemostatic mechanism the incidence of haemorrhage is 10% [53]. To avoid high plasma levels of heparin some form of laboratory monitoring is required to maintain levels between 0.2 and 0.6 u/ml. The simplest method is to keep the thrombin time between two and four times the control value.

Oral anticoagulants

The vitamin K antagonists are not effective antithrombotic agents until at least 48 h after therapy has started. Their effect is delayed until all the circulating clotting factors (II, VII, IX, and X) have been cleared and this is dependent on prothrombin, which has the longest circulating half-life. If a large loading dose is given the patient runs a considerable risk of haemorrhage due to acute deficiency of factor VII, which has the shortest half-life of only 2–4 h.

In view of this, anticoagulation should be started cautiously and controlled by prothrombin time estimations aiming to maintain a therapeutic range between two and four times the control value. Numerous factors, including drugs, diet, and malignant disease may frequently interfere with anticoagulant control, and regular monitoring of the prothrombin time is essential to prevent over or underdosage.

Thrombolytic therapy

Certain patients who are acutely ill and have developed severe peripheral venous thrombosis, major pulmonary embolus or obstructive arterial disease and are unfit for surgery may be suitable for thrombolytic therapy in addition to standard anticoagulation [41]. Both streptokinase and urokinase accelerate lysis but in so doing produce a generalized lytic state with its risk of bleeding. The shortened euglobin clot lysis time reflects fibrinolytic activity and the decrease in plasma fibrinogen levels and the appearance of FDPs represent plasmin action. The optimal duration of therapy is probably 72 h, and once a lytic state exists the dosage should be kept constant unless serious bleeding occurs. Administration of fresh-frozen plasma and fibrinolytic inhibitors will restore normal haemostasis.

Antiplatelet drugs

Platelet hyperactivity contributes significantly to the pathogenesis of several disease states, including valvular heart disease, coronary artery disease, atherosclerosis, the closure of arteriovenous shunts, and recurrent venous thrombo-embolism. Laboratory evidence of hyperfunction is suggested by shortened platelet survival, thrombocytosis, spontaneous platelet aggregation, increased plasma levels of β-thromboglobulin and platelet factor 4, and circulating platelet aggregates.

The combination of aspirin, a cyclo-oxygenase inhibitor, and dipyridamole, a phosphodiesterase inhibitor which raises platelet cAMP levels, has been shown to have an antithrombotic effect. There is considerable controversy about the correct aspirin dosage but a small amount (approximately 300 mg twice a week) seems the most effective. A higher dosage regimen will also block vessel wall cyclo-oxygenase and reduce prostacyclin release, and thus possibly enhance any thrombotic tendency.

Sulphinpyrazone has been shown to reduce closure of arteriovenous shunts and the frequency of sudden death after acute myocardial infarction. Its mode of action has not been determined. Recently infusions of prostacyclin have been shown to effect a symptomatic improvement of severe obstructive peripheral arterial lesions [60], but its exact therapeutic role remains to be determined.

References

1. An International Multicentre Trial (1975) Prevention of fatal post-operative pulmonary embolism by low doses of heparin. Lancet II:45–51
2. Austen DEG, Rhymes IL(1975) A laboratory manual of blood coagulation, 1st edn. Blackwell, Oxford
3. Bell WR, Meek AG (1979) Guidelines for the use of thrombolytic agents. N Engl J Med 301:1266–1270

4. Bennett B (1977) Coagulation pathways: Interrelationship and control mechanisms. Semin Haematol 14:301–318

5. Biggs R (1978) The treatment of haemophilia A and B and von Willebrand's disease, 1st edn. Blackwell, Oxford

6. Bloom AL (1977) Physiology of factor VIII. In: Recent advances in blood coagulation, vol 2. Churchill Livingstone, Edinburgh, pp 141–181

7. Bloom AL, Giddings JC, Wilks CJ (1973) Factor VIII on the vascular intima: Possible importance in haemostasis and thrombosis. Nature 241:217–219

8. Borchgrevink CF (1960) A method for measuring platelet adhesiveness in vitro. Acta Med Scand 168:157–164

9. Born GVR (1962) Aggregation of blood platelets by adenosine diphosphate and its reversal. Nature 194:927–929

10. Born GV, Bergquist D, Arfors KE (1976) Evidence for inhibition of platelet activation in blood by a drug effect on erythrocytes. Nature 259:233–235

11. Boughton BJ, Corbett WEN, Ginsburg AD (1977) Myeloproliferative disorders: A paradox of in vivo and in vitro platelet function. J Clin Pathol 30:228–234

12. Brecher G, Cronkite EP (1950) Morphology and enumeration of human blood platelets. J Appl Physiol 3:365–377

13. Brinkhaus KM, Hemker HC (1975) The handbook of haemophilia, 1st edn. Excerpta Medica, Amsterdam

14. Brozovic M (1976) Oral anticoagulants, vitamin K and prothrombin complex factors. Br J Haematol 32:9–12

15. Byrnes JJ, Liam ECY (1979) Recent advances in thrombotic thrombocytopenic purpura. Semin Thromb Hemostas 5:199–212

16. Carlin G, Saldeen T (1978) Influence of dextran 70 on the action of the primary fibrinolysis inhibitor. Thromb Res 12:681–686

17. Cash JD (1977) Disseminated intravascular coagulation. In: Recent advances in blood coagulation, vol 2. Churchill Livingstone, Edinburgh, pp 293–312

18. Cimo PL, Aster RH (1972) Post transfusion purpura. Successful treatment by exchange transfusion. N Engl J Med 287:290–294

19. Collen D, Wiman B (1978) The fast acting plasmin inhibitor in human plasma: (Editorial review) Blood 51:563–569

20. Collins JA (1976) Massive transfusion. Clin Haematol 5:201–227

21. Crean JJ, Grumpel JM, Peachey RDG (1970) Schönlein–Henoch purpura in the adult. Q J Med 39:461–484

22. Dacie JV, Lewis SM (1977) Practical haemotology, 5th edn. Churchill, London

23. Davidson JF (1977) Recent advances in fibrinolysis. In: Recent advances in blood coagulation, vol 2. Churchill Livingstone, Edinburgh, pp 9–122

24. Dechavanne M, Lagarde M, Byron PA (1976) Thrombocytopathie avec déficit en cyclooxygenase. Nouv Rev Fr Hematol 16:421–426

25. Demopoulos CA, Pinckard RN, Hanahan DJ (1979) Platelet-activating factor. J Biol Chem 254:9355–9358

26. Deykin D (1970) The clinical challenge of disseminated intravascular coagulation. N Engl J Med 283:636–641

27. Dixon R, Rosse W, Elbert L (1975) Quantitative determination of antibody in idiopathic thrombocytopenic purpura. N Engl J Med 292:230–237

28. Egeberg O (1965) Inherited antithrombin deficiency causing thrombophilia. Thromb Haemost 13:516–530

29. Evans EP, Branch RA, Bloom AL (1972) A clinical and experimental study of platelet function in chronic renal failure. J Clin Pathol 25:745–753

30. Gover PA, Ingram GIC, Cork MS, Holland L, Hopkins RP, Callaghan P, Barkhan P, Shearer MJ (1976) Bleeding from self administration of phenindione: A detailed case study. Br J Haematol 33:551–564

31. Hardisty RM (1977) Disorders of platelet function. Br Med Bull 33:207–212

32. Hemker HC, Veltkamp JJ, Loeliger EA (1968) Kinetic aspects of the interaction of blood clotting enzymes. Thromb Haemost 19:346–363

33. Ingram GIC, Kingston PJ, Leslie J, Bowie EJW (1971) Four cases of acquired von Willebrand's syndrome. Br J Haematol 21:189–200

34. International Forum (1979) To which extent is the clinical use of dextran, gelatin and hydroxyethyl starch influenced by the incidence and severity of anaphylactoid reactions? Vox Sang 36:39

35. Joffe EA, Hayer LW, Nachman RH (1974) Synthesis of von Willebrand factor by cultured human endothelial cells. Proc Natl Acad Sci USA 71:1906–1910

36. Karaca M, Cronberg L, Nilsson IM (1972) Abnormal platelet-collagen reaction in Ehlers-Danlos syndrome. Scand J Haematol 9:465–471

37. Kasper CK (1973) Postoperative thromboses in haemophilia. N Engl J Med 289:160–161

38. Levine PM, McVerry BA, Attock B (1977) Health of the intensively treated hemophiliac, with special reference to abnormal liver chemistries and splenomegaly. Blood 50:1–9

39. Lim RC, Olcott C, Robinson AJ, Blaisdell FW (1973) Platelet response and coagulation changes following massive blood replacement. J Trauma 13:577–582

40. Ludlam CA, Moore S, Bolton AE, Pepper DS, Cash JD (1975) The release of a human specific protein measured by a radio immunoassay. Thromb Res 6:543–548

41. Marder V (1979) The use of thrombolytic agents: Choice of patient, drug administration, laboratory monitoring. Ann Intern Med 90:802–808

42. McVerry BA, Machin SJ (1979) Incidence of alloimmunization and allergic reactions to cryoprecipitate in haemophilia. Vox Sang 36:77–80

43. Meyer D (1977) von Willebrand's disease. In: Recent advances in blood coagulation, vol 2. Churchill Livingstone, Edinburgh, pp 183–218

44. Moore S, Pepper DS, Cash JD (1975) Platelet antiheparin activity. Biochim Biophys Acta 379:370–384

45. Nilsson IM, Blombäck M, von Francken I (1957) On an inherited autosomal hemorrhagic diathesis with antihemophilic globulin deficiency and prolonged bleeding time. Acta Med Scand 159:35–42

46. Odegård OR, Abildgaard U (1978) Antithrombin III: Critical review of assay methods: Significances in health and disease. Haemostasis 7:127

47. Penner JA, Kelly PE (1975) Management of patients with factor VIII or IX inhibitors. Semin Thromb Hemostas 1:386–399

48. Raasch RH (1979) Effect of dextran 70 on factor VIII activity. Am J Hosp Pharm 36:89–97

49. Remuzzi G, Livio M, Cavenaghi AE, Marchesi D, Mecca G, Donati MB, de Gaetano G (1978) Unbalanced prostaglandin synthesis and plasma factors in uraemic bleeding. Thromb Res 13:531–541

50. Rosenberg RD (1978) Heparin, antithrombin and abnormal clotting. Annu Rev Med 29:367–378

51. Ross R, Glomset JA, Kariya B, Harker LA (1974) A platelet dependent serum factor that stimulates the proliferation of arterial smooth muscle cells in vitro. Proc Natl Acad Sci USA 71:1207–1210

52. Roth GJ, Majerus PW (1975) The mechanism of the effect of aspirin on human platelets. J Clin Invest 56:624–632

53. Salzmann EW, Deykin D, Shapiro RM, Rosenberg RD (1975) Management of heparin therapy—controlled

prospective trial. N Engl J Med 292:1046–1051

54. Schick PK, Kurica KB, Chacko GK (1976) Location of phosphatidylethanolamine and phosphatidylserine in the human platelet plasma membrane. J Clin Invest 57:1221–1226

55. Seegers WH (1978) Antithrombin III: Theory and clinical implications. Am J Clin Pathol 69:299–359

56. Sixma JJ, Wester J (1977) The haemostatis plug. Semin Haematol 14:265–299

57. Slichter SJ, Harker LA (1976) Preparation and storage of platelet concentrates. Br J Haematol 34:403–412

58. Stormorken H (1977) Activation and interaction of some defence systems. In: Recent advances in blood coagulation, vol 2. Churchill Livingstone, Edinburgh, pp 35–58

59. Suttie JW (1977) Oral anticoagulant therapy: The biosynthetic basis. Semin Haematol 14:365–374

60. Szezeklik A, Skowinski S, Gluszko P, Nizankowski R, Szezeklik J, Gryglewski RJ (1979) Successful therapy of advanced arteriosclerosis obliterans with prostacyclin. Lancet I:1111–1114

61. Thomas DP (1978) Heparin in the prophylaxis and treatment of venous thromboembolism. Semin Haematol 15:1–17

62. Thompson RE, Mandle RT, Kaplan AP (1977) Association of factor XI and high molecular weight kininogen in human plasma. J Clin Invest 60:1376–1380

63. Thorgeirsson G, Robertson AL (1978) The vascular endothelium—pathobiologic significance. Am J Pathol 93:803–848

64. Valeri CR (1976) Circulation and haemostatic effectiveness of platelets stored at 4°C or 22°C. Transfusion 15:195–202

65. Vane JR, Bergström S (1979) Prostacyclin, 1st edn. Raven Press, New York, p 12

66. Von dem Born AEK, Verheught FWA, Oosterhof F, von Riesz E, Brutel de la Riviere A, Engelfreit CP (1978) A simple immunofluorescent test for the detection of platelet antibodies. Br J Haemat 39:195–208

67. Von Preiss R (1979) Arzneimittelinteraktionen mit oralen Antikoagulantien. Dtsch Gesundh Wochenschr 34:673–686

68. Weinfeld A, Bronelög I, Kutti J (1975) Platelets in the myeloproliferative syndrome. Clin Haematol 4:373–392

Chapter 31

Blood and Blood Products

N. Duedari and P. Mannoni

Advances in methods of blood or plasma collection, cell separation and preservation, and new techniques for plasma or cell fractionation have made blood component therapy available in all hospitals with a transfusion service. This has emphasized the unjustified wastage of whole blood, which is in short supply, and has highlighted the preservation and quality of all blood components. There is no witchcraft in blood at all, and blood transfusion is no more and no less than substitution therapy [45].

However, replacement is used in pathological situations in which the lack of one or more blood constituents is only one of a number of features observed in the patient. With a better knowledge of the physiological role of each cellular or plasma constituent, it should now be possible to give the patient only the necessary product to prevent or treat qualitative or quantitative defects of blood function. It is now necessary to delineate the particular defects.

The methods of collection and preservation are, in some ways, different for each cell population and for plasma components [28]. To date we do not know how to preserve whole blood, that is, how to maintain the viability and function of each component at a level that is compatible with efficient post-transfusion recovery. Therefore specific techniques have been developed to preserve red cells, platelets, granulocytes, and plasma derivatives. In this respect, supportive therapy must be selective and adapted to the clinical and biological status of the patient. Moreover the therapeutic effect should be assessed according to clinical improvement, and quantified by measuring the biological post-transfusion recovery of the injected component as often as is deemed necessary.

The problems involved in massive blood transfusion are in part common with those encountered in any transfusion of blood products. Some of them are, however, more specific, and relate to the large quantities of blood infused in a short period of time; massive transfusion is defined as the infusion of 50% or more of the patient's blood volume within a period of 6 h.

Liquid preserved blood induces a 'storage lesion' and the potential toxicity or defects in preserved blood assume greater clinical significance in massive transfusion than in low volume transfusion. It is therefore necessary to appreciate defects which arise during blood preservation and their relevance to the resuscitative process. Table 31.1 summarizes the main indications for transfusion and stresses the most important parameters involved in the quality of the red blood cells. Tables 31.2–31.4 show the main characteristics of the various blood derivatives.

Table 31.1. Main purposes of blood transfusion

1. To increase oxygen transport.
    1.39 ml O_2 may be carried by 1 g hemoglobin
2. To increase tissue release of oxygen.
    Importance of 2,3 DPG red cell level, of the quality of the red cell membrane; ATP and pH relationship
3. To correct or maintain blood volume
4. To treat or prevent selective defects.
    Red cells, platelets, granulocytes, coagulation factors

Table 31.2. Blood derivatives used for O_2 transport and blood volume correction

	Main component	Contaminated by:	Volume	Maximum storage duration
Red cell concentrates (packed cells)	Red cells (hematocrit 70%–80%)	Plasma Leucocytes Platelets Preservative solution (ACD or CPD)	Total: 200–300 ml Red cells 150–220 ml	ACD–packed cells: 7 days at 4°C CPD–packed cells: 10 days at 4°C CPD–Adenine 28–35 days
Cryopreserved red cells	Red cells (hematocrit 80%)	NaCl Glycerol	170–250 ml 150–220 ml	Several years at −80°C, −150°C, or −196°C 12–48 h after thawing and washing
Poor leucocyte red cells	Red cells (hematocrit 80%)	Plasma Lymphocytes Platelets	150–200 ml	12 h after preparation at 4°C
Washed red cells	Red cells	Leucocytes (Plasma and platelets removed)	150–250 ml	12 h after preparation
FFP	Plasma	Anticoagulant Platelets	200–250 ml	6–12 months below −30°C 6–24 h after thawing
Albumin	Albumin	IgA $\alpha2$ macroglobulin Na: 500 mg/100 ml	10 ml 50 ml	Several years at 4°C

Table 31.3. Blood products used for the prevention or treatment of infection

	Main component	Contaminated by:	Volume	Optimal storage duration
Polyvalent immunoglobulins (IM and IV)	IgG	Plasma proteins	50 ml (IV) 5% 10 ml (IM) 16%	Several years at 4°C
IgGAM	IgG, IgA, IgM		10 ml (IM) 6.6%	Several years at 4°C
Specific immunoglobulins			1–10 ml	Several years at 4°C
Single donor granulocyte concentrate	Granulocytes	Platelets	300–500 ml $2\text{–}4 \times 10^{10}$ granulocytes	Up to 12 h

Storage lesions of red cell concentrates

Most whole blood or packed cells are stored at 4°C in plastic bags which contain 400–450 ml donor blood and about 60 ml acid citrate dex-trose (ACD) or citrate phosphate dextrose (CPD) solution [30]. Currently 21 days' storage is permissible, although extension of this period is under negotiation in some countries [28].

For many years whole blood has been the standard product against which other blood products are measured [26]. Red cell concen-

Table 31.4. Blood derivatives used for the correction of coagulation defects

	Main component	Contaminated by:	Volume	Optimal duration
Platelet concentrates	Platelets	Plasma Leucocytes Red cells	20–50 ml (0.7×10^{11} platelets)	2 days at $20°C \pm 2°C$
FFP	All coagulation factors	ACD CPD	200–250 ml	6–12 months at $-30°C$ 6–12 h after thawing
Cryoprecipitate	Factor VIII	Fibrinogen Factor XIII	20 ml (80–150 U)	12 months at $-80°C$
Factor VIII concentrate	Factor VIII	—	20 ml (400–1000 U)	Several years at 4°C
Factor IX concentrate (PPSB)	Factors II, VII, IX and X		10 ml, corresponding to 200 ml FFP	Several years at 4°C
Fibrinogen	Factor I	Plasma protein	100 ml (2–3 g)	Several years at 4°C

trates (packed red blood cells) are made by removing, after centrifugation, two-thirds to three-quarters of the plasma. In this way less anticoagulant, phosphate, and potassium are present for the same volume of hemoglobin. To date, packed red blood cells are widely used in many countries to restore an acute loss of blood [43, 54, 65]. This approach has led to the possibility of developing specific procedures for the preservation of red cells and for the preparation of other blood components such as platelet concentrates, fresh frozen plasma (FFP), or albumin.

Oxygen transport function (Fig. 31.1)

During liquid preservation many alterations occur within the red cell [4, 63] (Table 31.5). In 1962, it was demonstrated that the red cell hemoglobin capability to load and unload oxygen was regulated mainly by a glycolytic intermediate in the red cell: 2,3 diphosphoglycerate (2,3 DPG) [5]. Red cell 2,3 DPG has been shown to be linked to the blood oxygen transfer function according to the relation:

$$Hb\ O_2 + 2,3\ DPG \rightleftharpoons Hb - 2,3\ DPG + O_2$$

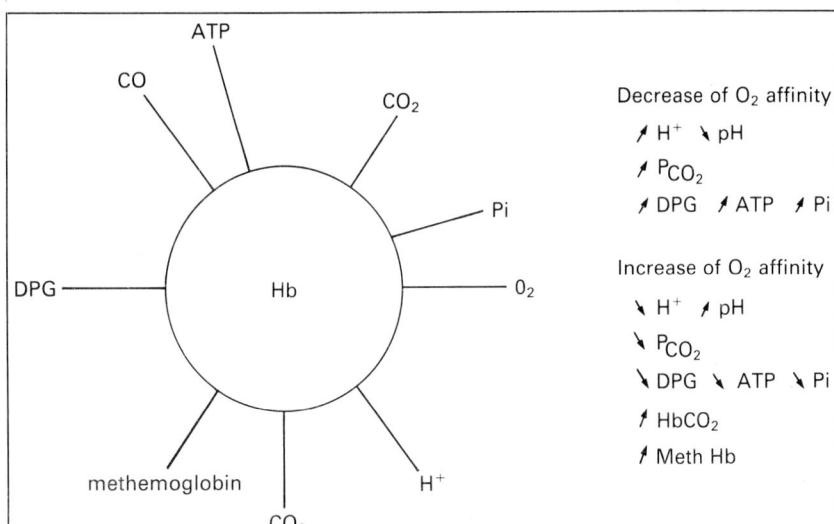

Fig. 31.1. The binding of different components to hemoglobin modifies its oxygen affinity.

Table 31.5. Changes during preservation of ACD blood at 4°C

	Days				
	0	7	14	21	28
pH	6.97	6.89	6.79	6.68	6.65
ATP level (%)	100	90	80	60	30
2,3 DPG (%)	100	40–60	10	10	0
P_{50} mmHg	26	22	17	15	15
Plasma Na (mmol/liter)	145	149	154	147	151
Red cell Na (mmol/liter)	3	7	14	18	
Plasma K (mmol/liter)	4	9	17	23	30
Red cell K (mmol/liter)	90	73	65	62	
Post-transfusion red cells (%)	100	98	85	70	65

This equilibrium depends almost exclusively on the oxygen and 2,3 DPG concentrations [25]. A fall in 2,3 DPG is accompanied by a fall in the P_{50} value of the oxyhemoglobin dissociation curve, i.e. an increased oxygen affinity [7]. Conversely, an increase in 2,3 DPG concentration involves a lower hemoglobin affinity for O_2 [8], with a shift of the dissociation curve to the right (Fig. 31.2).

2,3 DPG is produced, along with 3-phosphoglycerate, in the anaerobic Embden–Meyerhof pathway from the common substrate 1,3 diphosphoglycerate in the Rapoport–Luebering shuttle [5]; it undergoes conversion to 3 phosphoglycerate and thus acts as a bypass to

the phosphoglycerate kinase step. Hence, the two pathways compete for the common substrate producing either ATP or 2,3 DPG (Fig. 31.3).

The regulatory mechanism is complex and can occur in several ways [66]. 2,3 DPG concentration may be changed secondarily to a direct effect upon the rate of overall glycolysis [19, 48]. One of the most important parameters is pH since the glycolytic pathway is pH sensitive [49]: in acidosis the rate is decreased, and this leads to a diminished 2,3 DPG concentration. Conversely, alkalosis stimulates glycolysis and increases the 2,3 DPG concentration [6]. These

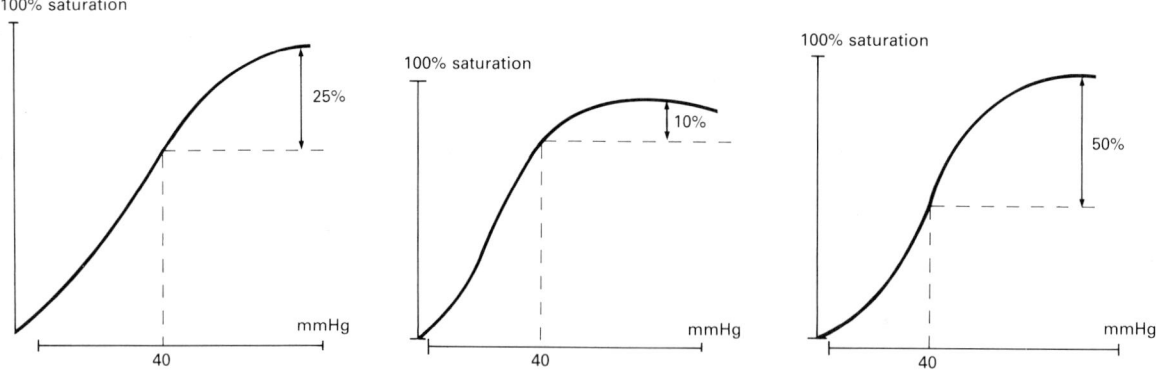

Fig. 31.2. Relation between the released oxygen and oxyhemoglobin dissociation curve (ODC) at the same pressure. **A** In ODC normal position, about 25% of the oxygen is delivered. **B** With a shift of the ODC to the left, only 10% of the oxygen is delivered. **C** When the shift of ODC is to the right, release is more effective—about 50%.

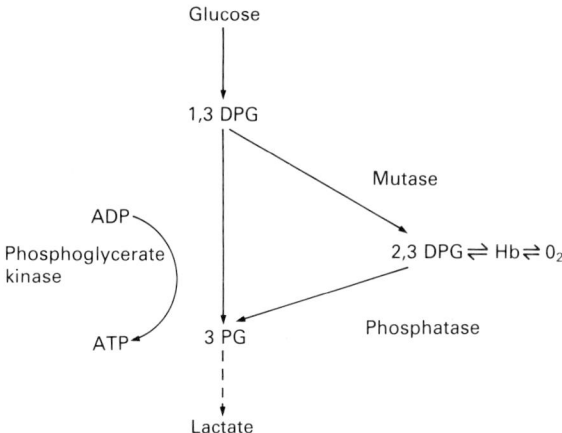

Fig. 31.3. Rapoport–Luebering shuttle.

effects of pH may be mediated by an enzyme, phosphofructokinase, which is an early step in glycolysis and is pH dependent.

Since adequate oxygen transport by blood is obviously imperative for tissue survival [12], and since the 2,3 DPG level appears essential for the delivery and the release of the red cell oxygen, the red cells used particularly ·in massive transfusion, must have a high level of 2,3 DPG [13, 53].

ATP level and survival

The post-transfusion survival of red cells is related primarily to their ATP level [45, 48]. This falls more slowly during storage than does the 2,3 DPG level. Two weeks after collection, 90% of the original ATP level is still conserved in CPD red cells. Therefore, these red cell organic phosphates, ATP and 2,3 DPG, can be conveniently used as markers to the quality of preserved red cells in terms of functional viability.

These modifications in organic phosphate levels are reversible after infusion but at least 24 h are required for the in vivo restoration of red cell oxygen transport and release function [9, 10].

In massive transfusion, the infusion of red cells with a decreased capacity to deliver oxygen places patients in jeopardy who cannot increase their blood flow and who need an immediate maximization of oxygen transport and release for tissue viability [20, 34]. The supplementation of preserved red cells with inosine, pyruvate, glucose, adenine and inorganic phosphate can help to maintain or improve both the post-transfusion survival and oxygen-transport function of the red cells during periods of storage at 4°C [1, 14, 18, 47, 51].

Other storage changes

Electrolytes. As shown in Table 31.5, in blood stored at 4°C the active transport of potassium and sodium across the red cell membrane is almost halted and intracellular and extracellular concentrations tend to come into equilibrium. With an increase of storage time lactic acid, plasma hemoglobin and inorganic phosphate also increase [4, 15, 45].

Platelets. Whole blood stored for longer than 2 days in liquid preservative should be considered to be devoid of functioning platelets. Moreover, storage of platelets at 4°C further impairs platelet function, even if a high proportion of the original number may still be present [28, 44].

Clotting factors. With the exception of the labile factors V and VIII, clotting factors deteriorate slowly during the storage of whole blood. By the end of the 21-day shelf life, factors V and VIII are low enough to have clinical significance [32, 45]. It is worth noting that some factors (IX, X, XI) may be activated spontaneously during storage of whole blood, while thromboplastins generated from platelet destruction are present in the supernatant plasma [42].

Toxic factors—the microaggregates. Platelet and white cell aggregates develop within a few hours to 1 week after storage, according to the anticoagulant solution being used. After the first week of storage in liquid preservation, the aggregates range in size from 10 to 160μm and may exceed 140 000 per cubic millimeter of blood. These microaggregates are undesirable debris thought to be capable of obstructing the pulmonary microcirculation and impairing pulmonary function [11, 17, 41, 47].

Effect on preservation of removal of supernatant plasma

If most of the supernatant plasma is removed from whole blood and the packed cells are stored, their viability is almost as well maintained as in whole stored blood (Fig. 31.4). FFP is valuable especially when kept at −30°C to −40°C and all coagulation factors are maintained at almost the 100% level; at −20°C, about half the factor VIII activity disappears in 4 months [45].

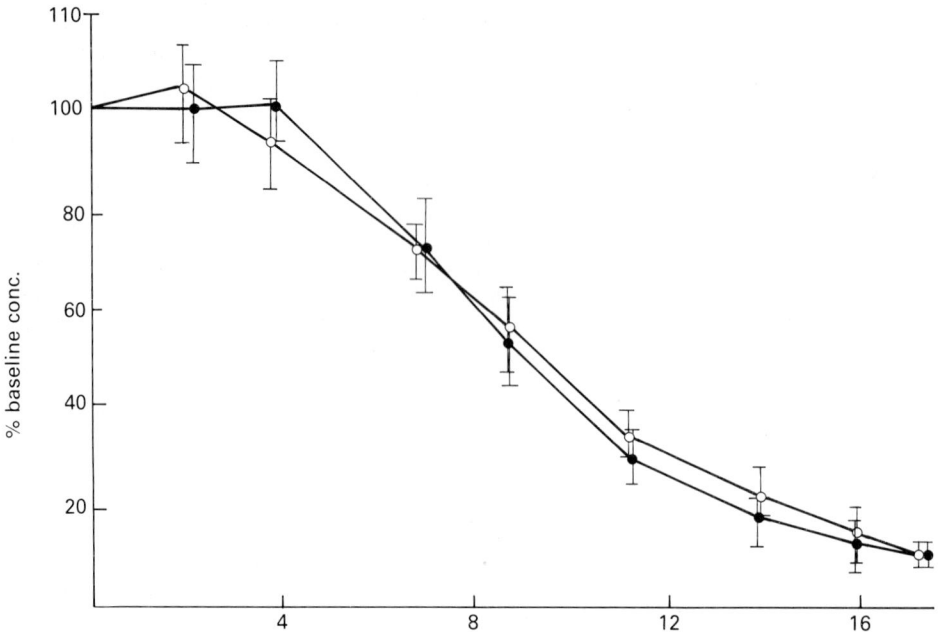

Fig. 31.4. 2,3 DPG values diminish during liquid storage in CPD preservative, equally in packed cells or whole blood. The data are expressed as a percentage of initial 2,3 DPG values. *Open circles,* whole blood values; *filled circles,* packed cell values.

Supportive therapy

Massive transfusion is defined clinically as the infusion of 50% or more of the patient's blood volume within a 6-h period. Blood which is transfused within an hour or two of taking, without having been refrigerated, is undoubtedly far better for restoring intravascular volume after acute blood loss. The definition of 'fresh blood' varies; much emotionalism and little documented benefit surround the use of fresh blood of any definition [26]. There is little, if any, quantitive scientific data to support its use when the appropriate component can be identified by proper testing and given in the required amount. Although there is no disadvantage in fresh blood itself, the need to test it before transfusion means that it must be kept for some hours before it can be safely used [27, 42]. Because blood in liquid preservation develops storage lesions, defects in preserved blood assume greater clinical significance in massive transfusions than in low-volume elective transfusions [16]. In massive transfusions there are three vital considerations: to be sure that oxygen transport and release functions are preserved in the infused cells; to restore intravascular volume and haemodynamic status; and to avoid iatrogenic complications (Table 31.6).

Table 31.6. Some uses of blood and components

Purpose	Component/process used
Maintaining tissue oxygenation	Red cells with normal or elevated 2,3 DPG level
Maintaining microcirculation	Hemodilution Red cells with normal or elevated ATP level
Maintaining efficient intravascular volume	Red cells Crystalloid solutions Colloid solutions Plasma protein fraction
Controlling hemostasis	FFP Platelet concentrates Specific treatment of DIC
Controlling acidosis and maintaining alkalosis and electrolyte balance	Electrolytic solutions Calcium?
Maintaining constant patient temperature	Blood warmers
Maintaining pulmonary circulation	Filtered blood; thawed and washed blood

Functional and viable red cells (rejuvenated cells)

The commonly used preservative, CPD, gives red cells approximately 10 days of relatively normal oxygen-carrying capacity (Fig. 31.4). Recent technical advances have made possible the routine biochemical treatment of red cells to increase 2,3 DPG and ATP levels rather than simply restoring them to normal. This biochemical modification, called rejuvenation, is usually done prior to freeze preservation [43, 61, 62].

However, freeze preservation is not absolutely necessary, although washing the biochemically modified red cells before transfusion is obligatory to remove the potentially toxic additives [55]. Preserved red cells with elevated levels of 2,3 DPG and ATP can be prepared by incubation with solutions containing pyruvate [47], inosine [1], glucose [30], phosphate, and adenine. Such biochemically modified cells have an improved ability to deliver oxygen to tissues immediately upon transfusion [59, 67]. Recent studies have demonstrated that the oxygen transport function of preserved red cells influences myocardial function in patients undergoing emergency surgery for repair of abdominal aneurysms [20, 21]. These studies indicate that myocardial performance was improved when red cells were able to release oxygen at high oxygen tension [67].

While it is generally difficult to obtain sufficient quantities of biochemically modified red cells for massive transfusion, the use of red cells with at least normal 2,3 DPG and ATP levels is obligatory.

Hemodilution

Crystalloid solutions can correct certain acid–base disorders; 5% dextrose in lactated Ringer's solution is frequently used. Colloid solutions may also be used for volume expansion, but protein solutions may actually increase interstitial dehydration by causing absorption of tissue fluid into the intravascular space. One gram of albumin will mobilize 17.2 ml of extravascular fluid; when albumin is used, crystalloids may be alternated to neutralize this 'sponge' effect [3, 35, 37, 64].

Hemodilution is now a fairly common practice in major institutions that routinely perform massive transfusion and trauma surgery. The choice of the dilution solution depends on each patient's clinical and metabolic status. Its use permits rapid adjustments of treatment on the basis of the hematocrit or other metabolic changes [39, 42, 54].

Plasma protein fraction (PPF) may be used to restore colloid osmotic pressure. There has been considerable controversy regarding the use of

this product or crystalloid solutions in recent years. Some of the current evidence suggests that, in most instances, crystalloid solution is equally effective, and it is certainly cheaper.

Hemostasis

The practice of empirically transfusing FFP and platelets at specified intervals has its advocates. The circumstances at different institutions may make this the most practical mechanism of handling massive transfusions. If this preventative infusion is set up, however, many patients will be overtransfused and supplies of certain components, e.g. platelet concentrates, may be exhausted, and be unavailable for other patients who require them [28].

The purpose of component therapy is to replace deficits selectively using the highest concentration of the missing component in the lowest volume. Different diseases and individual variations between patients require different management strategies of coagulation support. A wide range of pre-existing inherited and acquired conditions influence hemostasis and the response to trauma or surgery (Table 31.7). In addition, shock plays a most important

Table 31.7. Pre-existing diseases influencing coagulation

Inherited coagulopathies
    Hemophilia
    Von Willebrand's disease
    Christmas factor deficiency
    Congenital afibrinogenemia

Thrombocytopenia and platelet function abnormalities
    Hypersplenism
    Aplasia
    Cancer chemotherapy

Liver disease
    Cirrhosis

Iatrogenic
    Anticoagulant therapy
    Infectious diseases

role in coagulation disorders since the reduced blood flow and acidosis that accompany it appear to cause consumption of coagulation factors. The exact mechanism of this disseminated intravascular coagulation (DIC) is postulated but not proven [38, 50]. The complex nature of shock and the various complicating factors of surgery and transfusion may potentiate the consumption of procoagulants and worsen the bleeding [58].

The coagulation disorders in massive transfusion are mainly due to dilution; procoagulants in people without pre-existing coagulopathies are present in quantities far exceeding those necessary for hemostasis.

In moderate degrees of dilution, it is doubtful if the dilutional effect, by itself, will cause sufficient diminution of procoagulants to cause iatrogenic bleeding [46]. In some institutions, open heart surgery patients are transfused with previously frozen red cells suspended in saline, or with CPD liquid-preserved cells, and thus receive no, or little, procoagulants or platelets. In addition, the non-blood pump prime causes a 50% or greater dilution of plasma procoagulants even before any transfusions are administered. Clotting studies in such patients are no more abnormal than in patients receiving fresh-frozen plasma and platelets and transfusion requirements are no greater. Therefore, severe coagulation abnormalities during transfusion cannot be routinely attributed to dilution [43, 54, 59].

Marked dilution of platelets during massive transfusion has generally been accepted as a common occurrence but there are large variations in the platelet counts that are offered as the necessary minimum level to support surgical hemostasis, and some authors suggest that platelet counts in excess of 80 000/mm^3 may be necessary for hemostasis with surgically induced bleeding. Obviously, there are wide individual differences in platelet requirements, especially when DIC is present.

When platelet infusions are required, platelet concentrates, available from most blood banks, contain $6-7 \times 10^{10}$ platelets stored in 20–50 cc of plasma obtained from a single donor. Currently, platelets can be stored up to 72 h in CPD but are usually used within 24 h of collection. The proper treatment of transfusion-related thrombocytopenia is the administration of 8–10 platelet concentrates in an adult patient (an increase of 50 000 per cubic millimeter is obtained by the infusion of one platelet concentrate/7 kg body weight) [44].

The need for FFP, or cryoprecipitate, is gauged by screening tests such as the prothrombin, partial thromboplastin, and thrombin times. When needed, cryoprecipitate may be used as a source of fibrinogen [45].

Other toxic factors

Thermal load. Rapid infusion of large quantities of stored blood at 4°C frequently causes a fall in body core temperature. A fall of less than 1°C can greatly increase oxygen consumption and cardiac output by causing shivering. A further decline in temperature also impairs platelet function and may contribute to bleeding complications. Citrate metabolism also suffers in hypothermia and increases the potential for hypocalcemia during massive transfusion. Prevention of hypothermia is achieved by warming the blood before administration and several types of blood warmer are now available [24].

The effects of the potential citrate intoxication and hypocalcemia are hypotension and left ventricular impairment. In general, most normothermic adults can withstand an infusion of large quantities of stored blood without requiring supplemental calcium [36]; but if needed, supplemental ionized calcium should be administered.

Microaggregates. Recent clinical studies indicate that the problem of microaggregates is still equivocal [52]. All the commercially available microfilters have specific advantages and disadvantages. In active bleeding, it is essential that microfilters do not hamper the adequate rate of transfusion. Buffy-coat-poor red cell concentrates contain substantially fewer microaggregates than conventional stored whole blood units. The use of microfilters may be contraindicated in fresh blood transfusion because they retain viable platelets [29, 40].

Protocol for supportive therapy

Our routine protocol may be summarized as follows:

When the loss of blood is less than the total blood volume, red cells and hemodilution are used, with FFP if needed. In larger volume loss, special precautions are necessary. Functional and viable red cells are infused immediately, and hemodilution and administration of FFP are carried out. Specific hemostatic treatment is sometimes useful [28, 42, 60].

Compatibility hazards

The peril to the patient with significant hypovolemic shock is delay in instituting transfusion. Patient survival depends on the speed with which a blood bank responds to an urgent, unexpected request for blood.

Blood bank policies must establish procedures for emergency issue of blood when there is no time for compatibility testing. Under certain conditions, group-specific blood may be issued, and in other situations group O blood may be preferable. In addition, guidance should be given for the switching of blood types when massive transfusion is required. When a specimen is obtained for submission to the blood bank, patient identification procedures must be rigorous. Often, this is a time of maximal confusion, particularly if several seriously injured patients are being treated. A clerical identification error can result in one or even two hemolytic transfusion reactions. In a previous review, we found 13 out of 27 ABO-related incompatibilities were due to errors in identification of the patient [23, 56].

If the patient's clinical condition necessitates immediate transfusion, blood may be issued before completion of routine tests. Approximately 3–5 min are required to determine ABO and Rh groups. Carried to an extreme, one or two units of group O Rh (D)-negative red cells could be issued immediately and then the ABO and Rh grouping performed so that subsequent units of blood could be group specific. If a patient has received group O 'Universal donor' blood, the decision to change back to group-specific blood is based on the presence or absence of anti-A or anti-B antibodies in the recipient's circulating blood.

The type and antibody screen have been demonstrated as a safety procedure, especially when associated with cross-matching [2]. Testing should be performed even if several units of a nonspecific blood group have been issued. As seen in Table 31.8 [22], about 50% of antibodies,

Table 31.8. Circumstances of detection of anti-RH (E) and anti-Kell (K) antibody

	Anti-E	Anti-K
Screening[a]	42	50
Post-transfusion control	97	112
Discovered when post-transfusion hemolytic reaction occurs	30	32
Total	169	194

[a]Supposedly untransfused patients.

initially present, may be responsible for an acute hemolytic reaction increasing the gravity of the patient's condition.

When a bleeding patient has received a large-volume transfusion in a short period of time, the composition of his circulating blood will be altered profoundly. Thus a pretransfusion specimen is no longer representative of his circulating blood. Continued testing for compatibility after exchange of one blood volume becomes of dubious benefit to the patient. Under these conditions, confirmed ABO compatibility may be sufficient and the cross-matching procedure can be reduced to an immediate spin.

References

1. Akerblom O, de Verdier CH, Garby L, Högman C (1968) Restoration of defective oxygen transport function of stored red blood cells by addition of inosine. Scand J Clin Lab Invest 21:245–249
2. Bacher LB (1981) Type and screen, seven steps to success. American Association of Blood Banks 34th meeting. Transfusion 21:584
3. Ballinger WF, Rutherford RB, Zuidema GD (1973) The reanimation of hypovolemic shock in the management of trauma. Saunders, Philadelphia, p 70
4. Bartlett GR, Barnet HN (1960) Changes in the phosphate compounds of the human red blood cell during blood bank storage. J Clin Invest 39:56–61
5. Bellingham AJ, Grimes AJ (1973) Red cell 2,3 diphosphoglycerate (Editorial). Br J Hematol 25:555–561
6. Bellingham AJ, Detter JC, Lenfant C (1971) Regulatory mechanisms of hemoglobin oxygen affinity in acidosis and alkalosis. Clin Invest 50:700
7. Benesch R, Benesch RE (1969) Intracellular organic phosphates as regulators of oxygen release by hemoglobin. Nature (Lond) 221:618–622
8. Beutler E (1969) A "shift to the left" or a "shift to the right" in the regulation of erythropoiesis. Blood 33:396
9. Beutler E, Wood L (1969) The in vivo regeneration of red cell 2,3-diphosphoglycerate (DPG) after transfusion of stored blood. J Lab Clin Med 74:300–304
10. Beutler E, Muel A, Wood LA (1969) Depletion and regeneration of 2,3-diphosphoglyceric acid in stored red blood cells. Transfusion 9:109–114
11. Bredenberg CE (1977) Does a relationship exist between massive blood transfusions and the adult respiratory distress syndrome? If so, what are the best preventive measures? Vox Sang (Basel) 32:311
12. Broennle AM, Tung CK, Buchman B, Laver MB (1970) Oxyhemoglobin dissociation following massive transfusion in man. Fed Proc 29:473
13. Bunn HF, May FH, Kocholaty WF, et al. (1969) Hemoglobin function of stored blood. J Clin Invest 48:311–321
14. Chanutin A (1967) The effect of the addition of adenine and nucleosides at the beginning of storage on the concentrations of phosphates of human erythrocytes during storage in acid-citrate-dextrose and citrate-phosphate-dextrose. Transfusion 7:120–132
15. Chanutin A, Curnish RR (1962) Effect of organic and inorganic phosphates on the oxygen equilibrium of human erythrocytes. Arch Biochem Biophys 121:96–102
16. Collins JA (1974) Problems associated with the massive transfusions of stored blood. Surgery 75:274–295
17. Connel RS, Swank RI (1973) Pulmonary microembolism after massive transfusion. Ann Surg 177:40
18. Dawson RB Jr, Ellis TJ (1970) Hemoglobin function of blood stored at 4°C in ACD and CPD with adenine and inosine. Transfusion 10:113–120

19. Dawson RB Jr, Kocholaty WF (1971) Hemoglobin function in stored blood. VI. The effect of phosphate on erythrocyte ATP and 2,3 DPG. Am J Clin Pathol 56:656–660

20. Dennis RC, Vito L, Weisel RD, et al. (1975) Improved myocardial performance following high 2,3-diphosphoglycerate red cell transfusion. Surgery 77:741

21. Dennis RC, Hechtman HB, Berger RL, et al. (1978) Transfusion of 2,3 DPG enriched red blood cells to improve cardiac function. Ann Thorac Surg 26:17–26

22. Desaint C, Duedari N, Mannoni P (1977) Alloimmunisation post-transfusionnelle. Standardisation des techniques transfusionnelles. Symposium held at Jouy en Josas. Fenwal, Paris

23. Duedari N, Desaint C (1977) Causes et origines des accidents par incompatibilité ABO. Standardisation des techniques transfusionnelles. Symposium held at Jouy en Josas. Fenwal, Paris.

24. Dybkjaer E, Elkjaer L (1964) The use of heated blood in massive blood replacement. Acta Anaesth Scand 8:271–278

25. Finch AC, Lenfant C (1972) Oxygen transport in man. N Engl J Med 286:407–415

26. Fresh blood. A myth or a real need? (1976) International Forum (Holländer LP, ed). Vox Sang (Basel) 31:368–379

27. Gauthier-Lafaye JP, Otteni JC (1971) Complications de la transfusion massive, solutes de substitution, rééquilibration métabolique. Librairie Aruette, Paris, p. 111–134

28. Genetet B, Mannoni P (1978) La transfusion. Flammarion, Paris

29. Gervin AS, Mason KG, Wright CB (1975) The filtration limits of ultrapore filters. Surgery 77:186–193

30. Gibson JG 2nd, Rees SB, McManus TJ, et al. (1957) A citrate-phosphate-dextrose solution for the preservation of human blood. Am J Clin Pathol 28:569–578

31. Glover JL, Smith R, Yaw P, Plawecki R, Link W (1976) Intraoperative autotransfusion: an underutilized technique. Surgery 80:474

32. Hardisty RM, Ingram Gi (1965) Bleeding disorders: investigation and management. Blackwell, Oxford

33. Hemotherapy in trauma and surgery (1979) Technical workshop (Barnes A Jr, ed). American Association of Blood Banks, Washington D.C.

34. Holsinger JW, Salhany JM, Eliot RS (1973) Physiologic observations on the effect of impaired blood oxygen release on the myocardium. Adv Cardiol 9:81–97

35. Howland WS, Schweizer O (1965) Diagnosis and therapy of physiologic changes occurring during shock and massive transfusion. In Orkin LR (ed) Management of the patient in shock. Clinical Anaesthesia. Davis

36. Howland WS, Schweizer O, Boyan CP (1964) Massive blood replacement without calcium administration. Surg Gynecol Obstet 118:814–818

37. Kopriva CJ, Ratliff JL, Fletcher JR, Fortier NL, Valeri CR (1972) Biochemical and hematological changes associated with massive transfusion of ACD-stored blood in severely injured combat casualties. Ann Surg 176:585–589

38. Larrieu MJ (1969) Le syndrome de coagulation intravasculaire. Acta Inst Anesth 17:93–105

39. Litwin MB, Smith LL, Moore FD (1959) Metabolic alkalosis following massive transfusion. Surgery 45:805–813

40. Lundsgaard-Hansen P (1980) Introduction. Symposium on micro-filtration of blood and pulmonary function. Vox Sang 39:46–59

41. McNamara JJ, Burran EL, Larson E, et al. (1972) Effect of debris in stored blood on pulmonary microvasculature. Ann Thorac Surg 14:133

42. Mannoni P, Vernant JP (1972) Transfusions massives. Réanimation et médecine d'urgence. Expansion scientifique Francaise, Paris, pp 247–262

43. Mannoni P, Genetet B, Beaujean F, Fauchet R (1975) A new transfusional protocol in extracorporeal circulation. XIV Congress of International Society of Blood Transfusion. Helsinki, [Abst]

44. Mannoni P, Rodet M, Beaujean F (1976) Transfusion de plaquettes. Rev Franc Transf Immuno-Hémato 19:489

45. Mollison PL (1974) Blood transfusion in clinical medicine, 3rd ed, Blackwell, Oxford

46. Moriau M, Masure R, Hurlet A, et al. (1977) Haemostasis disorders in open heart surgery with extracorporeal circulation. Vox Sang (Basel) 32:41

47. Oksi FA, Travis SF, Miller LD, Delivoria-Papadopoulos M, Cannon E: (1971) The in vitro restoration of red cell 2,3-diphosphoglycerate levels in banked blood. Blood 37:52–58

48. Rapoport S (1969) Regulation of concentration of DPG and ATP in red blood cells. Forsvarsmedicin 5:168

49. Rorth M (1970) Dependence of oxyhemoglobin dissociation and intraerythrocytic 2,3 DPG on acid-base status of blood. I. In vitro studies on reduced and oxygenated blood. Red cell metabolism and function. In Brewer GJ (ed) Advances in Experimental Medical Biology, Vol. 6, p 57

50. Scott R, Crosby WH (1954) Changes in the coagulation mechanism following wounding and resuscitation with stored blood; a study of battle casualties in Korea. Blood 9:609–621

51. Seman ER, Chapman RG, Finch CA (1962) Adenine in red cell preservation. J Clin Invest 41:351–359

52. Solis RT, Gibbs MB (1972) Filtration of the microaggregates in stored blood. Transfusion 12:245–250

53. Spector JI, Zaroulis CG, Pivacek L, et al. (1977) Physiologic effects of normal- or low-oxygen affinity red cells in hypoxic baboons. Am J Physiol 232:H79–H84

54. Streiff F (1974) Réanimation hématologique et apport transfusionnel. Actualités transfusionnelles. Proceedings of the 9th International Congress on Blood Transfusion, 1973. Masson, Paris, p 14–47

55. Strumia MM, Strumia PV (1971) Transfusion of long stored whole blood or washed red blood cells incubated with adenine and inosine. Transfusion 11:258–265

56. Taswell HF, Sonnenberg CL (1981) Blood bank errors: classification on frequency [Abst], American Association of Blood Banks meeting, Nov. 1981. Transfusion 21:620

57. Telischi M, Patel AR, Zafar M, et al. (1977) Microaggregate counts in frozen-preserved erythrocytes: Effects of washing in three blood processors and filtration. Blood 50:743–748

58. Treat H, Aggeler PM, Robinson AJ, Blaisdelle FW (1969) Intravascular coagulation in the surgical patient. Its significance and diagnosis. Am J Surg 118:281–291

59. Valeri CR (1975) Blood components in the treatment of acute blood loss: Use of freeze-preserved red cells, platelets and plasma proteins. Anesth Analg 1:54

60. Valeri CR (1976) Blood banking and the use of frozen blood products. Chemical Rubber Co Press, Cleveland

61. Valeri CR, Zaroulis CG (1972a) Cryopreservation and red cell function. In: Progress in transfusion and transplantation (Schmit PJ, ed). American Association of Blood Banks, Washington DC, pp 343–365

62. Valeri CR, Zaroulis CG (1972b) Rejuvenation and freezing of outdated stored human red cells. N Engl J Med 287:1307–1313

63. Valtis DJ, Kennedy AC (1954) Defective gas-transport function of stored red blood cells. Lancet, i, 119–125

64. Vourch G, Radiguet De La Bastaie P, Triner L, et al. (1970) La place des solutés sodés équilibrés dans le traitement de l'hémorragie. Anesth Analg Reanim 27:737

65. Wilson RF, Mammene, Walt A (1971) Eight years of experience with massive blood transfusions. Trauma 11:275–286

66. Wranne B, Woodson RD, Detter JC (1972) Bohr effect interaction between H^+, CO_2 and 2,3-diphosphoglycerate in fresh and stored blood. J Appl Physiol 32:749

67. Zaroulis CG (1979) The importance of red cell 2,3 DPG in transfusion therapy. In: Hemotherapy. (Barnes A Jr, ed). American Association of Blood Banks, Washington DC, pp 43–55

Chapter 32

Plasma Substitutes

K. Messmer

By definition, plasma substitutes aim to replace a fluid which is colloidal in nature by virtue of its content of different species of highly specialized proteins. In plasma, albumin is present in the highest concentration and has the highest colloid osmotic power of all the plasma proteins.

Infusion solutions without colloid molecules cannot be considered as plasma replacing fluids, although they might be used for short-term volume replacement. Establishment and maintenance of normovolaemia with crystalloids exclusively, however, requires volumes 2.5–4 times the actual volume lost.

While the maintenance of a normal plasma colloid osmotic pressure (COP) is no guarantee of normovolaemia, a low COP allows significant shifts of fluid into the interstitial compartment.

To minimize the risks of fluid overload and edema, especially interstitial pulmonary edema, we strongly advocate the replacement of acute plasma losses by colloid solutions that provide a predictable and long-lasting volume expansion. In addition to the colloid, sodium and water have to be given to replace daily losses and extracellular fluid deficits.

Volume replacement with plasma substitutes is limited by the dilution it produces of the cellular and plasma components of the recipient's blood. Based on a large number of studies of pre- and intra-operative normovolaemic haemodilution it seems that most patients will safely tolerate haemoglobin levels of 8–10 g/100 ml without a reduction in O_2 delivery to the tissues if cardiac output can be increased. In the presence of coronary or myocardial disease, however, this degree of dilutional anaemia cannot be tolerated [21]. In these and many of the conditions found in critically ill patients with higher O_2 demands higher levels of haemoglobin are needed.

Physicochemical characteristics of plasma substitutes

Albumin, with a molecular weight of 69 000 daltons, is the ideal colloid osmotic molecule. Since all the molecules of an albumin solution are of identical weight the ratio between average molecular weight ($\bar{M}_w$) and average molecular number ($\bar{M}_n$) reaches unity and indicates monodispersity of the solution. Colloid molecules of weights below 50 000 daltons, which is the threshold size for the glomerular membrane, are rapidly excreted by the kidney [8].

For technical reasons artificial colloid solutions cannot be prepared in a monodispersed form; all such solutions are polydispersed and contain a mixture of different molecules whose weights are distributed in a Gaussian fashion around the arithmetic mean molecular weight ($\bar{M}_w$). To assess the intravascular persistence of artificial colloids it is therefore essential to know

Table 32.1. Artificial colloids for plasma volume substitution[a]

Colloid	Generic name	Colloid content	$\bar{M}_w$	$\bar{M}_w : \bar{M}_n$	Intervascular persistence (h)	Remarks
Dextran (Dx)	Dx 60[b]	6 g%	60 000	2.0	6	Antithrombotic effect
	Dx 70	6 g%	70 000	1.85	6	Antithrombotic effect
	Dx 40	10 g%	40 000	1.4	2–3	Antithrombotic effect
Starch (HES)	HES 450/0.7	6 g%	450 000	6.3	6	∅
	HES 200/0.5	10 g%	200 000	—	2–3	∅
	HES 40/0.5	6 g%	40 000	2.0	2–3	∅
Gelatin	Urea-linked gel	3.5 g%	35 000	2.3	2–3	Diuretic effect
	Modified fluid gelatin (MFG)	4 g%	35 000	2.2	2–3	
	Oxypolygelatin	5.5 g%	30 000	1.5	2–3	Diuretic effect

[a]According to data from literature and manufacturers.
[b]Dx 60: $\bar{M}_w$ 60 000, available in Germany and Austria; properties nearly identical to those of Dx 70.

the molecular weight of the majority of the molecules as well as the distribution of their molecular weights. The degree of polydispersity is given by the ratio of $\bar{M}_w$ to $\bar{M}_n$ (Table 32.1). This term enables predictions to be made for any colloid solution concerning its volume expansion effects and intravascular persistence.

The water-retaining capacity, or colloid osmotic power, of colloid solutions depends upon the $\bar{M}_w \bar{M}_n$ ratio and the colloid content of the solution. For human albumin it amounts to 17 ml/g. Solutions with a higher tonicity than plasma (hyperoncotic colloid solutions) attract water from the interstitial space, and infusion of these solutions results in an expansion of the plasma volume at the expense of the interstitial fluid volume. This might be desirable if edema is present, but should be avoided in dehydrated patients.

The physicochemical properties (average molecular weight, average molecular number and colloid content of the solution) of colloids determine how effective they are in restoring deficits in the plasma volume. Predictions based upon these characteristics have been verified in numerous experimental and clinical studies [8, 10, 19].

Natural colloids

Of the various natural colloids prepared from human plasma or placenta, the 4% pasteurized protein solution (PPS, PPL, Plasmanate) and 5% human serum albumin (HSA) are highly suitable for plasma volume replacement. With normal capillary permeability both solutions will yield a volume effect roughly equal to the volume infused.

Human plasma protein solutions

For volume replacement, only pasteurized plasma protein solutions which are free from the risk of transmitting hepatitis, especially hepatitis NonA/NonB, should be used. If both plasma substitution and replacement of plasma clotting factors are needed then fresh frozen plasma (FFP) is the solution of choice, and the risk of hepatitis transmission is accepted.

Human albumin solutions

In contrast to the plasma protein preparations, HSA solutions contain practically no proteins other than the albumin. They are available as both isotonic (5%) and hypertonic (20% and 25%) solutions.

Because of their excellent volume effect, HSA solutions are used in some centres for intra- and postoperative volume replacement. However, all natural plasma protein solutions are in short supply and extremely expensive, and neither plasma protein solution nor HSA should be routinely used for volume replacement. Both should be reserved for those patients with a combination of hypovolaemia and significant hypoproteinaemia (plasma protein content <5 g/100 ml). Intra-operative blood loss should never be replaced with protein solutions before the surgical bleeding has been controlled. The body's pool of exchangeable albumin amounts to 3.5–4.5 g/kg body wt, with about 40% in the intravascular and 60% in the extravascular space. This provides for an influx of albumin from the extravascular space in the case of volume and protein losses. Therefore, volume replacement does not necessarily require plasma proteins to maintain colloid COP, but can be adequately performed with artificial colloids.

Whilst hypo-albuminaemia (albumin < 3.5 g/ 100 ml) is a clear indication for albumin substitution, the use of albumin as a primary resuscitation fluid is a matter of heated debate. Several groups have attempted to establish whether or not the acute respiratory distress syndrome (ARDS) can be prevented by the early infusion of HSA. In injured patients without hypoproteinaemia HSA was no better than other colloids or crystalloids [30, 31, 33].

Risks of natural colloid solutions

Protein and albumin solutions, even when treated by pasteurization, β-propiolactone or ultraviolet radiation to destroy the hepatitis viruses, are still not free from risks. For all the different preparations adverse reactions have been reported. Anaphylactoid reactions of varying degrees of severity do occur, and although they are rare they might be fatal. The overall incidence of severe reactions with hypotension or cardiac arrest is < 0.1% [27, 29]. Genetic polymorphism of the albumin molecule, the formation of noxious albumin aggregates, and the use of stabilizers have all been identified as causes of albumin incompatibility [27, 29].

The reactions to plasma proteins can occur during the first infusion or after multiple infusions. The symptoms range from mild skin reactions to fatal hypotension or cardiac arrest. Recently, Wells and King [35] have demonstrated that reactions to FFP, whole blood, or human immunoglobulins can be due to immunodeficiencies (high titres of anti-IgA antibodies in the recipient). Severe hypotension following infusion of plasma protein solution might originate from the activation of Hageman factor fragments, triggering production of bradykinin in the recipient [2, 7, 20]. It should be stressed that the hypotension that is caused by Hageman factor fragments and activation of the kininogen–kinin system calls for rapid volume expansion but the additional infusion of plasma protein solution might worsen the situation [6]. Since preventive means are not available it is strongly suggested that only plasma protein solutions which have been screened for the absence of Hageman factor fragments or kinins are used.

Artificial colloids

Table 32.1 shows the relevant data on the solutions most frequently used in clinical practice. The number of types varies considerably in different countries. Differences exist in terms of the source and manufacturer of the colloid, the $\bar{M}_w \bar{M}_n$ ratio, the colloid content, and the concentrations of non-colloidal solutes. The following discussion is therefore restricted to representative colloid solutions based on dextran, gelatin, or hydroxyethyl starch. (For further details the reader is referred to the monographs of Gruber [8] and Lutz [19].)

An analysis of the literature reveals substantial differences in the advantages and disadvantages of various artificial colloids. Many of the controversies are caused by failure to define the precise physicochemical characteristics of the colloid in question, which are undoubtedly the most important criteria on which comparisons of the efficiency: risk ratio will be based. It should be stressed that the artificial colloids have definite advantages over the plasma protein solutions: they are effective in restoring plasma volume, the solutions are stable and readily available, and they are relatively very cheap. For these reasons they should be used for volume replacement in patients without significant hypoproteinaemia.

Dextrans

Dextrans are high-molecular-weight polysaccharides consisting of glucose molecules mainly connected by 1.6 glucosidic linkages. The clinically used dextrans are obtained by hydrolytic fractionation. Dextran 70 (Macrodex) and dextran 40 (Rheomacrodex) are the most important and most frequently used preparations. The 6% solution of dextran 70 exerts a colloid osmotic effect expressed as a water-retaining capacity per gram of the non-diffusing polymer in vivo of 20–25, which is higher than that of albumin or plasma proteins; therefore it seems to be particularly suitable for plasma replacement and maintenance of the intravascular volume over a relatively long period of time [8, 10, 19].

Dextran 40, with an average molecular weight of 40 000, is available as a 10% solution which, compared with plasma, is strongly hyperoncotic. Hence the initial volume effect of dextran 40 is about twice the volume infused. However, because of a lower $\bar{M}_w$, it is more rapidly excreted and 3–4 h after infusion the gain of intravascular volume is only equal to the volume infused. The initial volume expansion is due to transcapillary shift of fluid from the interstitial compartment. Therefore as a general rule saline and dextran 40 solution should be given in identical volumes to avoid dehydration. The colloid–osmotic power pulls interstitial fluid into the intravascular space, preferentially at the venous end of the microcirculation. Microcirculatory flow is therefore rapidly restored as a result of the additional haemodilution that takes place in the postcapillary venules which, in terms of red cell aggregation and stasis, are the most vulnerable parts of the microcirculation. This local dilutional effect depends upon the colloid–osmotic pressure gradient across the capillary membrane and is thus not specific for dextran 40.

While volume replacement is the main indication for using dextran 70, dextran 40 is preferred in situations of disturbed microcirculatory flow, such as prolonged shock and hyperviscosity syndromes [10].

The dextrans are completely excreted or metabolized after a short period of storage in the cells of the reticuloendothelial system. Both have antithrombotic properties due to a decrease of platelet adhesiveness, depression of factor VIII activity, increased susceptibility of thrombi to fibrinolysis, and finally to improved blood flow [1, 9]. These are different from their influence on the clotting mechanism, and changes in blood coagulation are only seen when a dose of 1.5 g/kg body wt per day is exceeded. Both dextran preparations have been used to good effect for the prophylaxis of postoperative deep vein thrombosis and pulmonary embolism [9, 11]. Finally, dextrans involve a risk of anaphylactoid reactions.

Gelatin

Gelatin was the first artificial colloid to be used clinically for plasma replacement and now three preparations, differing in the source of the raw material, the method of production, and the physicochemical properties of the gelatin, are commercially available (Table 32.1).

The key difference from dextran 70 and high-molecular-weight hydroxyethyl starch is the lower average molecular weight, which enables the molecules to pass readily across the glomerular membrane. Therefore the intravascular persistence of gelatin solutions is less marked than that of identical volumes of dextran 70 or HES. Nevertheless, normovolaemia can be achieved if, initially, higher amounts of gelatin

are infused; to maintain normovolaemia infusions are needed more frequently. Apart from the dilutional fall in red cell mass, there is no limit to the quantity of gelatin solution that can be given [18]. There is no specific effect of gelatins on the blood clotting mechanism, nor do they have any antithrombotic properties [18].

Hydroxyethyl starch

Hydroxyethyl starch (HES) is manufactured from amylopectin and consists of hydroxyethylated glucose molecules linked by α 1.4 bindings. At present three preparations are commercially available.

High-molecular-weight hydroxyethyl starch (HES 450/0.7)

The average molecular weight of this 6% solution is 450 000 in vitro; the degree of substitution is 0.7, which means that seven of ten glucose molecules are substituted by hydroxyethyl groups. Depending upon the degree of hydroxyethylation, the initially very large molecules are rather rapidly degraded in vivo, by serum α-amylase, to molecules with weights of around 70 000. Consequently the intravascular volume effect is comparable to that of dextran 70. An expansion of the plasma volume in excess of the infused volume has been reported, but was not observed in our own experiments [14, 22]. Jesch et al. [14] were the first to report an increase in serum α-amylase concentration following starch infusion. This effect has apparently no pathogenic importance, but has to be remembered in order to avoid a false diagnosis of pancreatitis. The elimination of HES 450/0.7 follows a different pattern from that of dextran 70/60 [4]. It is stored in the reticuloendothelial cells of the liver for a rather prolonged time [22], and in an attempt to overcome this problem starch preparations with lower $\bar{M}_w$ and faster elimination patterns are currently under examination [22, 32]. Apart from a dilutional effect, HES 450/0.7 does not influence the clotting system and antithrombotic properties have never been demonstrated.

Medium-molecular-weight hydroxyethyl starch (HES 200/0.5)

Only recently a new preparation of HES with a $\bar{M}_w$ of 200 000 and a degree of hydroxyethylation of 0.5 (HES 200/0.5) has been introduced.

With 10 g HES/100 ml this solution is hyper-oncotic, and yields an expansion of the circulating volume comparable to that of the 10% dextran 40 solution [12]. Few clinical studies are available as yet, and the potential advantages of this solution cannot be judged.

Low-molecular-weight hydroxyethyl starch (HES 40/0.5)

HES 40/0.5 provides a volume effect comparable to that of gelatin preparations. The claim for an intravascular persistence identical with that of dextran 70 was not corroborated by studies of isovolaemic haemodilution [22]. During isovolaemic haemodilution with gelatin solution, however, the COP was maintained in the normal range but fell significantly with progressive haemodilution by HES 40/0.5. Therefore, because the COP is decreased, this starch preparation does not meet the requirements of a colloidal plasma substitute. As with other HES preparations, serum α-amylase in the plasma increases in response to infusions of HES 40/0.5; this phenomenon is due to the formation of an HES-amylase complex (macro-amylase) [15].

Adverse effects of colloidal plasma substitutes

Adverse effects may be encountered after infusion of any of the colloids mentioned, and these are itemized below.

1) *Fluid overload* can be prevented by estimating the volume loss and by adjusting the infusion volume and speed to the actual cardiopulmonary situation while the patient is closely monitored.

2) *Dilution of plasma clotting factors* may affect haemostasis (Chap. 30). Dextran, when infused in doses >1.5 g/kg body wt per day can cause clinically significant disturbance of haemostasis but oozing after the recommended dose probably indicates improved capillary flow rather than a disturbance of haemostasis.

3) *Disturbances of renal function* have been reported after infusion of dextran 40 in patients with incipient or established renal failure or severe dehydration. It should be possible to avoid these by observing the contra-indications for hyperoncotic colloid solutions and by giving additional crystalloid solutions where necessary.

4) None of the colloids, including human serum albumin and plasma proteins, is free from the risk of *anaphylactoid reactions*. The majority of these are mild and affect mainly the skin (flushing erythema, etc.); severe reactions with fatal outcome following irreversible hypotension or cardiac arrest have been reported, however. Even though the general incidence of these reactions is low by comparison with the adverse reactions of whole blood or other drugs, the possibility of a fatal outcome calls for special awareness and early diagnosis of this imminent risk.

The reported incidence of anaphylactoid reactions due to colloids varies considerably in the literature. This can be explained on the basis of conceptual differences: retrospective studies in general give lower figures and the highest incidences have been found in prospective, randomized trials [5, 13, 27].

a) The incidence of *dextran-induced anaphylactoid reactions* (DIAR) ranges from 0.07% to 1.1% [11, 28]. Cardiac arrest was observed with a higher frequency than with plasma protein, starch, or gelatin. In recent years it has been shown that dextran-reactive antibodies (DRA) arising in response to immunization with bacterial polysaccharides that cross react with dextran are widely distributed in the normal human population with titres ranging from 0 to 2048 as determined by passive haemagglutination. On the basis of the immunologic findings DIARs can be classified as antibody-dependent and -independent types. DIARs of grades III–IV (life threatening hypotension, cardiac and/or respiratory arrest) have been found to be mediated by dextran-reactive antibodies of the IgG class. A very close correlation between the IgG titres of dextran-reactive antibodies and the severity of the DIAR was apparent [25]. Upon infusion of dextran solutions the dextran-reactive antibodies combine with the dextran molecules to form noxious immune complexes which activate the complement system and trigger the release of vaso-active mediators which finally cause the clinical symptoms. By the pre-injection of a high dose of monovalent hapten-dextran, which blocks the binding sites of the circulating antibodies, the formation of noxious immune complexes can be prevented, and as a consequence the clinical manifestations of dextran incompatibility fail to appear [23, 25].

The concept of hapten inhibition of DIAR was recently introduced into clinical medicine, and led to a highly significant reduction in the overall incidence of anaphylactoid and anaphylactic reactions to dextran. Life-threatening reactions can be prevented in the large majority of patients at risk if 20 ml hapten–dextran is injected IV prior to the infusion of dextran 40 or 70 [16, 23, 24, 26].

b) The incidence of *anaphylactoid reactions to gelatin* clearly depends upon the type of the gelatin preparation. The figures vary from 0.05% to about 10% [18, 28]. Life-threatening and fatal reactions have also been reported. Histamine release has been identified as the cause of most of the anaphylactoid reactions to gelatin [17, 34]. Consequently, blocking of histamine receptors (H_1 and H_2) by antagonists has been applied as a prophylactic measure and current clinical studies do indeed reveal a prophylactic effect for the infusion of urea cross-linked gelatin [17, 34]. Whether prevention of anaphylactoid reactions to other gelatin preparations can be obtained by the same principle has not yet been demonstrated.

c) *HES preparations* are used less often than preparations of dextran and gelatin. Therefore reports on side-effects are limited in number. The studies available do indicate, however, that anaphylactoid reactions to HES occur with an incidence of about 0.1% [29]. Life-threatening reactions also occur, but they seem less frequent than with dextran [3]. The mechanism of the reactions to HES is unknown and prophylactic measures are therefore not available.

The clinician has to accept the occurrence of these untoward anaphylactoid reactions when using colloid solutions. Their incidence is low, however, and they should not be regarded as a contra-indication for the use of any of the colloids. Anticipation and rapid diagnosis are of paramount importance to enable resuscitation.

References

1. Åberg M, Hedner U, Bergentz SE (1978) Effect of dextran on factor VIII (antihemophilic factor). Ann Surg 189:243–247
2. Alving BM, Hojima J, Pisano JJ, Mason BL, Buckingham RE, Mozen MM, Finlayson JS (1978) Hypotension associated with prekallikrein activator (Hageman Factor Fragments) in plasma protein fraction. N Engl J Med 299:66–70
3. Beez M, Dietl H (1979) Retrospektive Betrachtungen der Häufigkeit anaphylaktoider Reaktionen nach Plasmasteril^R und Longasteril^R. Infusionstherapie 6:23–26
4. Boon JC, Jesch F, Ring J, Messmer K (1976) Intravascular persistence of hydroxyethyl starch in man. Eur Surg Res 8:497–503
5. Collins JA, Larcan A, Litwin MS, Lutz H, Ring J, Thorén L, Tschirren B (1979) To which extent is the clinical use of dextran, gelatin and hydroxyethyl starch influenced by the incidence and severity of anaphylactoid reactions? (International Forum). Vox Sang 36:39
6. Colman RW (1978) Paradoxical hypotension after volume expansion with plasma protein fractions. N Engl J Med 299:97–98
7. Combridge DS, Wesley ED (1979) Plasma protein fraction: the disappearance of kinin from the solution on storage. Transfusion 19:599–600
8. Gruber UF (1969) Blood replacement. Springer, Berlin Heidelberg New York
9. Gruber UF (1975) Dextran and the prevention of postoperative thromboembolic complications. Surg Clin North Am 55:679–696
10. Gruber UF, Sturm V, Messmer K (1976) Fluid replacement in shock. In: Ledingham I McA (ed) Shock, clinical and experimental aspects. Excerpta Medica/American Elsevier, Amsterdam, p 231–256
11. Gruber UF, Saldeen T, Brokop T, Eklöf B, Erikson J, Goldie I, Gran L, Hohl M, Jonsson T, Kristersson S, Ljungström KG, Lund T, Maartman Moe H, Svensjö E, Thomson D, Torhorst I, Trippestad A, Ulstein M (1980) Comparison of the incidence of fatal pulmonary embolism with dextran 70 and low dose heparin prophylaxis. An international multicenter trial. Br Med J 280:69–72
12. Harke H, Pieper C, Meredig I, Rahman S, Rüssler P (1980) Rheological and clotting investigations after the infusion of HES 200/0.5 and dextran 40. Anaesthesist 29:71–77
13. Isbister JP, Fisher M McD (1980) Adverse effects of plasma volume expanders. Anaesth Intensive Care 8:145–151
14. Jesch F, Kloevekorn WP, Sunder-Plassmann L, Seifert J, Messmer K (1975) Hydroxyläthylstärke als Plasmaersatzmittel. Untersuchungen mit isovolämischer Hämodilution. Anaesthesist 24:202–209
15. Köhler H, Kirch W, Weihrauch TR, Prellwitz W, Horstmann HJ (1977) Macroamylasemia after treatment with hydroxylethyl starch. Eur J Clin Invest 7:205–211
16. Laubenthal H, Peter K, Hedin H, Richter W, Messmer K (1980) Specific hapten inhibition for prevention of dextran-induced anaphylactoid reactions. Clinical results. Europ Surg Res 12 [Suppl 1]:68–69
17. Lorenz W, Doenicke A, Dittmann I, Hug P, Schwarz B (1977) Anaphylactoid reactions following administration of plasma substitutes in man. Prevention of side-effects of Haemaccel by premedication with H_1- and H_2-receptor antagonists. Anaesthesist 26:644–648
18. Lundsgaard-Hansen P, Tschirren B (1978) Modified fluid gelatin as a plasma substitute. Prog Clin Biol Res 19:227–257
19. Lutz H (1980) Plasmaersatzmittel, 3rd edn. Thieme, Stuttgart New York
20. McMillin RD, Hood TR, Griffen WO (1978) Systemic anaphylaxis secondary to the use of 5 percent plasma protein fractions. Am J Surg 135:706–707
21. Messmer K (1975) Hemodilution. Surg Clin North Am 55:659–678
22. Messmer K, Jesch F (1978) Volumenersatz und Hämodilution durch Hydroxyäthylstärke. Infusionstherapie 5:169–173
23. Messmer K, Ljungström KG, Gruber UF, Richter W, Hedin H (1980a) Prevention of dextran-induced anaphylactoid reactions by hapten inhibition. Lancet I:975
24. Messmer K, Seemann C, Hedin H, Richter W, Peter K (1980b) Anaphylaktoide Reaktionen nach Dextran: II) Tierexperimentelle und klinische Ergebnisse der Prophylaxe durch Hapten-Hemmung. Allergologie 3:59–66
25. Richter W, Hedin H, Ring J, Kraft D, Messmer K (1980a) Anaphylaktoide Reaktionen nach Dextran: I) Immunologische Grundlagen und klinische Befunde. Allergologie 3:51–58

26. Richter W, Hedin H, Messmer K (1980b) Ist die Hap-
    tenhemmung bei der Infusion von Dextranlösungen
    wirksam? Anaesthesist 29:444–445
27. Ring J (1978) Anaphylactoid reactions. Springer, Berlin
    Heidelberg New York (Anesthesiology and intensive
    care medicine, vol 111)
28. Ring J, Messmer K (1977) Incidence and severity of
    anaphylactoid reactions to colloid volume substitutes.
    Lancet I:466–469
29. Ring J, Richter W (1980) Wirkungsmechanismus un-
    erwünschter Reaktionen nach Hydroyäthylstärke (HÄS)
    und Humanalbumin. Allergologie 3:79–86
30. Shires GT, Bergentz SE, Gruber UF, Baxter Ch, Moss GS
    (1980) Colloids or not for resuscitation? In: Allgöwer M,
    Harder F (eds) State of the art of surgery 1979/80.
    Springer, Berlin Heidelberg New York, p 84–85

31. Shoemaker WC, Hauser CJ (1979) Critique of crystalloid
    versus colloid therapy in shock and shock lung. Crit
    Care Med 7:117–124
32. Thompson WL, Bloxham DD, Rudnick MS (1977) New
    short-persistence hydroxyethyl starch (HES-S). Inten-
    sive Care Med 3:206
33. Virgilio RW, Rice CL, Smith DE, James DR, Zarins CK,
    Hobelman CF, Peters RM (1979) Crystalloid versus
    colloid resuscitation: Is one better? A randomized clini-
    cal study. Surgery 85:129–139
34. Watkins J, Milford Ward A (1978) Adverse response to
    intravenous drugs. Academic Press, London/Grune &
    Strutton, New York
35. Wells JV, King MA (1980) Adverse reactions to human
    plasma proteins. Anaesth Intensive Care 8:139–144

Section F

Endocrine Disorders

Chapter 33

Diabetic Coma

T. D. R. Hockaday

Any article on this starts best with prevention, by early diagnosis of the newly evolving disease, by wise management of the inevitable fluctuations of glucose control in the diagnosed patient, or by such early admission to hospital that a short spell of IV fluid and 2 or 3 days' adjustment of insulin dosage are all that is necessary: all in contrast to the complicated and demanding medical, nursing, and laboratory care required by the seriously ill 'hyperglycaemic', whether or not they are neurologically 'comatose'. Any such severely ill patient represents a failure of community health care, either of education or of practice, at all stages from a diabetic's relative or landlady through health visitors, district nurses, general practice receptionists, and family doctors to the hospital doctors.

This account first describes an orthodox approach to hyperglycaemic emergencies, in the conventional order of pathogenesis, precipitating causes, diagnosis, prognosis, treatment and complicating factors. In a shorter, second section, certain controversial issues are discussed less dogmatically, for we probably do not yet know the best approach, for instance, to the osmolality of the infused fluid, or whether IV phosphate is of help. Finally there is a didactic action list.

Hyperglycaemic emergencies

Classification

A diabetic patient may be in coma because of a metabolic disturbance related to his diabetes, or from any of the processes that may equally affect non-diabetics, e.g., subarachnoid haemorrhage. The relevant metabolic disturbances are:

(1) *Keto-acidotic hyperglycaemic* coma: this is the classic diabetic coma, though happily few patients are now admitted completely unconscious. A quantitative definition demands that the sum of the blood concentrations of 3-hydroxybutyrate and aceto-acetate exceed 3 mM [12], or alternatively 5 mM [2], in addition to the clinical criterion of a patient ill enough to require emergency treatment with IV fluids and insulin. Keto-acidosis may occur with remarkably little hyperglycaemia, as reported from Scotland, possibly particularly in association with high ethanol intake, but more likely because of wise self-treatment by trained diabetics with insulin, perforce unaccompanied by necessary IV fluids.

(2) *Hyperglycaemic non-ketotic coma*, with or without hypernatraemia. The original phrase

'hyperosmotic non-ketotic' diabetic coma is unfortunate, despite the cheerful abbreviation HONK, because nearly all hyperglycaemic emergency patients are hyperosmolar, whether or not ketotic, because of high glucose concentrations and usually an elevated blood urea. The distinguishing features are really (a) the degree of ketosis and the accompanying acidosis, and (b) whether there is hypernatraemia from a disproportionate loss of water compared with sodium; typically, plasma sodium is low on admission, due to at least partial osmotic compensation for the hyperglycaemia. When plasma sodium is normal or high, it therefore implies disproportionate loss of water compared with sodium, at least from the extracellular fluid (ECF). An arbitrary numerical estimate of this can be obtained from the formula (observed plasma sodium) − (expected plasma sodium), as calculated with an arbitrary assumption of normal plasma sodium concentration as 140 mM by

$$\text{Observed } [Na] - \left[140 - \frac{(\text{mM Glucose} - 5)}{2} \right].$$

Though often around 5, this factor may be as high as 40. It is simpler, and almost as useful, to consider the plasma sodium alone, to be surprised if it is over 135 mM, to be perturbed if above 145, to consider altered management from 150, and to worry about the prognosis if it is above 155 mM.

Hyperosmolality may be reckoned to be substantially present above 330 mosmol/litre, but it is not uncommon for it to exceed 360. Although no single factor closely predicts the depth of the cerebral lesion, this does so better than any other easily measured (or 'calculated') factor [7], and perhaps almost as well as the technically elaborate, purely research measurement of reduced uptake of O_2 by the brain [15].

(3) *Other metabolic factors* that can complicate the picture:

a) *Lactic acidosis* can occur in non-diabetics or normoglycaemic diabetics, and it always denotes a failure of the hepatic uptake and metabolism of lactate to glucose, to triglyceride, and to CO_2. An entirely healthy liver can cope with any possible increase in peripheral formation of lactate, but often hepatic failure is accompanied by some increase in peripheral production. The commonest precipitant of acute lactic acidosis is a sudden failure of proper arterial supply to the liver, particularly if some other hyperlactacidaemic agent is present, such as ethanol or phenformin (a hypoglycaemic biguanide). Phenformin used to make diabetics particularly prone to lactic acidosis, due to its inhibition of hepatic gluconeogenesis, but happily it is little prescribed in Europe now, and was never licensed in the United States of America. Lactic acidosis is reckoned to be present if blood lactate exceeds 5 or 7 mM, and the metabolic causes are separated from the hypoxic by reversal of the latter on improvement of the O_2 supply.

b) *Uraemia* may result from diabetic nephropathy, but equally from any other cause of renal failure in a diabetic. As usual, one cannot really be numerically 'hard and fast', but the dehydration and impaired circulation of uncontrolled diabetes rarely lift the blood urea above 25 mM if renal function was previously normal. Uraemia will be associated in varying degrees with acidosis, hyperphosphataemia and hyperkalaemia.

c) *Toxification, e.g., by ethanol or salicylates* can be confusing; salicylates stimulate ventilation, while ethanol may mask the smell of ketones on the breath, and delayed hypoglycaemia is one of its diverse metabolic effects.

Pathogenesis

Although every patient in acute hyperglycaemic illness has a shortage of effective insulin action, other factors may be important in determining the severity of the illness. A previously undiagnosed patient may give a history of severe thirst and polyuria for several weeks, while known diabetics may be reasonably fit with blood glucose values as high as 35 mM. It probably requires a mathematical analysis akin to 'catastrophe theory' to pinpoint factors whose sudden change precipitates the critical illness. They probably include (1) cumulative loss of water and salts from osmotic diuresis and 'neutralization' of urinary 'ketones' with their comparatively low pK of 5.5 for 3-hydroxybutyrate; this will affect both intra- and extra-cellular spaces, and we have very little knowledge of how potassium deficiency, for instance, affects intermediary metabolism within a cell; (2) changes from the increasing mobilization of intracellular proteins for hepatic gluconeogenesis, especially as body fat decreases; and (3) increasing stimulation (?how) of secretion of the many catabolic hormones including catecholamines, cortisol, growth hormone, prolactin, and glucagon, all with hyperglycaemic and lipolytic actions.

Our ignorance is reflected in the precipitation of keto-acidosis by strenuous exercise. This has a beneficial, hypoglycaemic effect in healthier diabetics, but on the margin of ketosis it may initiate severe trouble, either by overtaxing an already compromised circulation or by substrate consumption, and so cause an increase in lipolysis and consequent ketonaemia, with further acidaemia and loss of cations in the urine.

The essential features of insulin lack are removal of the usual inhibitory influences on adipose tissue lipolysis and hepatic gluconeogenesis, with an accompanying failure of protein anabolism, and so mobilization of peripheral protein as a fuel for that gluconeogenesis. Insulin lack may well increase hepatic ketogenesis and reduce peripheral utilization of 'ketone bodies', but the essential cause of the ketosis is the unbridled lipolysis and consequent high plasma free fatty acid concentration.

High concentrations of the 'catabolic' hormones are present in keto-acidosis, and they oppose insulin, the only unequivocally anabolic hormone. Probably it is not an increase in any single hormone that is essential for ketoacidosis, though doubtless there are others whose role is still to be defined, e.g., dopamine, with its action in increasing insulin resistance. Their quantitative importance will remain uncertain until the extent of their increase in non-hyperglycaemic illnesses, e.g., fever, shock, is compared with that seen in keto-acidosis.

On presentation, plasma 'free' insulin concentrations in keto-acidosis vary from very low to values found in normals at a normal glucose concentration. Very probably these latter patients have some increase in the resistance to insulin's action; but however fever or extreme acidosis act to produce this, a major cause of such resistance is a relative failure of glucose and insulin (and perhaps O_2) to reach the relevant cells, because the average distance between a cell and the nearest patent capillary has increased so much (and an inverse-square law is involved in nutrient supply by diffusion through the ECF). Although there have been conflicting reports, a careful study in Barcelona, in which C-peptide concentrations were used to assess insulin secretion, showed patients with non-ketotic hyperglycaemic coma to have higher C-peptide concentrations than those with keto-acidosis. This highly useful measurement avoids the previous criticism of measurement of immuno-reactive insulin with antibodies which cross react with pro-insulin, which may well be secreted in some of these patients, as whatever residual beta-cell

activity remains will be working to maximum capacity.

Other attempts to describe critical differences between ketotic and non-ketotic diabetic coma have failed on analysis of many metabolites and hormones, but the increasing liability to non-ketotic coma in the elderly makes one suspect that older patients are more likely to need urgent treatment for dehydration before they have reached ketosis. The ability of their kidneys to concentrate the urine may well be impaired, and some may lack the ability to obtain as much fluid as they wish when they feel thirsty, while others may not be so sensitive to the development of thirst in face of hyperosmolality. Undoubtedly, the fluid drunk to quench the increasing thirst of developing diabetes may influence things, and either high-sucrose fluids such as many lemonades or a high osmolar solution such as milk may influence the outcome. It is also possible (though there is no evidence of this) that the sympathetic division of the autonomic nervous system is less active in the elderly, making lipolysis less rapid.

The exact role of the high circulating concentrations of the catabolic hormones is uncertain, but these will affect cell metabolism to exacerbate the metabolic disturbances of diabetes, as well as having their own effect on the circulation.

Presenting features and precipitating causes

All patients in hyperglycaemic coma or precoma have been unwell for many hours (if not days) and are markedly dehydrated, to an extent readily appreciable from decreased skin turgor, and quite beyond the dryness of the tongue that can easily develop from mouth breathing, as in pneumonia. Ketotic patients have two further features: the typical odour of ketosis on their breath, and the marked overbreathing or air hunger, because of their acidosis. The sweet, sickly smell of ketosis ('rotten apples') is detected by different people to very different degrees, and perhaps a fifth of modern medical students are unable to detect it at all, while the range of sensitivity is wide among the remainder. Hence, it is important during training to learn how easily one can appreciate this odour. Happily, though, such hyposmia can be easily remedied by bedside tests. If urine is available (which it often is not in the comatose and dehydrated patient), it can be tested for ketone bodies by Ketostix or Acetest. But, more usefully, a semi-quantitative impression of the ketone-body concentration can be obtained by testing plasma with Ketostix [1]. In this case 5 ml heparinized blood is centrifuged and a Ketostix dipped into the supernatant plasma. A reading of 1+ corresponds to approximately 1 mM aceto-acetate. The usefulness of this is limited by its lack of reaction with 3-hydroxy-butyrate. In health the concentrations of these two ketone bodies may well be equal, but 3-hydroxybutyrate becomes predominant in ketosis, and the iller (with impaired circulation) the patient is, the higher its ratio to aceto-acetate is likely to be. Exceptionally, it will be as much as 20 or even 30, and so a 1+ Ketostix reading could be obtained with a ketone body concentration as high as 21 mM or, worse, a negative result might be obtained when there are as many as 10 mM ketone bodies present. The method is sensitive to acetone, but at a much lower level than for aceto-acetate, and this further complicates its precise quantitative interpretation.

If the Ketostix test is negative and air hunger is nonetheless present, the possibilities are (1) acidosis from uraemia, when the patient may be known already to have advanced nephropathy; (2) lactic acidosis, in which case it may be necessary to perform an emergency blood lactate analysis, which is perfectly possible within 1 h; or (3) an overstimulated respiratory centre, e.g. due to salicylate toxification or damage to the fourth ventricle (or related nervous pathways), as in subarachnoid haemorrhage or meningitis. This will produce an alkalaemia of respiratory origin, and so determination of the arterial pH will readily separate it from the acidaemia of the metabolic disturbances.

None of these three cardinal features of dehydration, ketosis, and overbreathing is present in hypoglycaemic coma, in which, in addition the history may be as short as 30 min (assuming, of course, that there is a history from a bystander).

Keto-acidotic patients often have a history of 1 or 2 days of vomiting (or nausea, and certainly anorexia), sometimes accompanied by diarrhoea. They will have the usual history (particularly when previously undiagnosed) of thirst, polyuria, and weight loss. Occasionally, and more often in younger than in older patients, there will be abdominal pain, usually diffuse but sometimes with a particular focus, as in the right iliac fossa or right hypochondrium. While

tenderness on examination usually accompanies this abdominal pain, there may be guarding or even rigidity, as well as absent or grossly diminished bowel sounds, so that occasionally young patients are operated on as abdominal emergencies when they have diabetic coma. Detection of glycosuria or hyperglycaemia, or of keto-acidosis, should prevent this error.

However, infection is a great precipitant of keto-acidosis, and it is always possible that a known diabetic will be precipitated into diabetic coma by abdominal sepsis. Although it is always a worrying situation, in practice the management is clear, namely, treatment of the diabetic keto-acidosis, since operation before this has at least partially resolved is unduly dangerous. Treatment of the keto-acidosis includes fluid replacement, gastric aspiration, and antibiotics against infection, so is not misdirected should appendicitis, etc., be present (even if it is not ideal). If the abdominal signs are entirely due to keto-acidosis, they will improve within 4–6 h, and so continued observation will vindicate a conservative approach.

As stated, infection is an important precipitant of keto-acidosis, and the patient should be carefully examined for signs of it, to exclude a collection of pus deep to an apparently small foot ulcer, an ischiorectal or perinephric abcess, or an early pneumonia. Several features make infection more difficult to detect than usual. First, presumably because of the severe dehydration, the usual physical signs may be masked. Thus, bronchial breathing and bronchophony may not be found as usual over the consolidated lung. Again, a polymorphonuclear leucocytosis as high as 30 000 per mm^3 with 95% polymorphs may result from the 'stress' (presumably high plasma cortisol) of ketosis alone while, even when there is a well-established pyogenic infection body temperature may be normal or even low for as long as 4–8 h after the start of treatment. When the history points to a purely metabolic development of the emergency illness, and there is no indication on examination or from fever, there is no likely benefit from prescribing antibiotics, but it is a good rule always to consider them and to have a fairly low threshold for their use (but only after specimens have been drawn for blood culture).

Sterile inflammation as from a cardiac infarct can also precipitate hyperglycaemic emergencies, and it must be remembered that cardiac infarction in diabetics is pain-free perhaps three or four times more often than in non-diabetics.

In diabetics already under treatment with

insulin, a mistaken reduction in its dose is an important precipitant of coma. The commonest error is to stop or greatly reduce insulin administration because of a vomiting illness which prevents intake of food. The patient's argument has two errors, namely the assumption that insulin is needed only to metabolize ingested food, and the disregard of the diabetogenic influence of infection. The proper preventative measure is to persist with as substantial a calorie intake as possible, if necessary in the form of sugared drinks, and to change from long-acting to frequent SC injections of short-acting insulin, varying the dose according to the results of home glucose tests. However, this is of course a time when the patient is least able to do such tests, and so it is crucial that a relative or friend should help or, if no-one is available, that help is sought from the medical services. Occasionally, an undue reduction in insulin dosage is deliberate, usually in the same way that non-lethal doses of sedatives or narcotics are taken by 'pseudocides', though occasionally the intent will be more serious.

Diagnosis

This is based on the presenting features just described and re-emphasized in Table 33.1. As dehydration is the only reliable physical sign of non-ketotic hyperglycaemic coma, any patient (and particularly an elderly patient) who is confused or stuporose must have a bedside blood glucose determination, e.g., with Dextrostix or Boehringer 20/800 Glycemie Stix, unless there is some other well-established

cause of their trouble. Even then a laboratory glucose determination can be useful (urine can equally well be tested, providing it is available and providing the cardiac output is not so low that the normal resorptive capacity of the renal tubules for glucose is extracting all the filtered load from a very small glomerular filtration rate despite hyperglycaemia. Thus, with gross cardiac upset such as results from a ruptured interventricular septum, one may have sugar-free urine and a blood glucose of 30 mM).

The cardinal features of dehydration, ketosis, and overbreathing are the basis of recognition of the more classic keto-acidotic coma. The trickiest differential is probably that from 'piqure' diabetes, as described by Claude Bernard as a consequence of severe irritation of the medulla oblongata which, presumably through massive discharge of the sympathetic division of the autonomic nervous system, produces a short-lived but severe hyperglycaemia (easily up to 30 mM), together with hyperventilation from excessive action of the respiratory centre (giving a respiratory alkalosis as described above). There is also often a mild ketosis from lack of food intake, perhaps exacerbated by vomiting and dehydration. The hyperglycaemia will resolve spontaneously within 8–24 h and, if the start of the fall coincides with an injection of insulin, severe hypoglycaemia may easily occur. It is tempting, too, to repeat the insulin injection, as the first will not have produced the lightening of consciousness usual in a successfully treated keto-acidotic. Neck rigidity is highly likely to be present with the central nervous system lesion, but it does occur (at least to the extent of 'meningism') in perhaps 5% of confused but not unconscious diabetics. These are generally restless and the meningism is part

Table 33.1. Differential diagnosis

	Dehydration	Hyper-ventilation	Ketosis	Plasma Sodium	pH
Keto-acidotic	+++	+++	+++	↓	↓
Non-ketotic, usual	+++	−	−	↓	N
Non-ketotic, hypernatraemic	+++	−	−	↑	N
Medulla oblongata irritation	+	+++	+	N	↑
Uraemia	+	+++	−	N	↓
Lactic acidosis	+	+++	+	N	↓
Hypoglycaemia	−	−	−	N	N

N, normal

of an overall resistance to examination as well as their general high muscle tone. It may be necessary (though one never does this readily) to give a small IV injection of diazepam, perhaps with 2 mg in the syringe, but given so slowly that there is a chance for a smaller amount to render the patient sleepy and relaxed, albeit for just a few moments, but long enough to check that the neck rigidity then resolves. Occasionally keto-acidotic patients are so restless that a longer-acting agent such as IM paraldehyde may be necessary.

Uraemia or lactic acidosis also causes hyperventilation, as mentioned, as does salicylate overdosage, but the latter will not be accompanied by hyperglycaemia unless the patient is a diabetic, and ketosis should not be present.

Hypoglycaemia should give no difficulty, providing one remembers that such patients lack all three cardinal features of the keto-acidotic, and of course it is now readily recognized by the bedside solid-state tests for blood glucose.

Prognosis

This depends upon the age and selection of the patients considered. The most useful study is still that of Zieve and Hill [23, 24], even though it was reported in the 1950s; enough antibiotics were available then for their findings to be highly relevant still.

As can be seen from Table 33.2 (from their study), when individual factors are considered the most important is age, followed by the precipitating or associated illness. The most significant biochemical measurement is the blood urea, ahead of blood glucose or the degree of acidosis, and this almost certainly reflects the overriding importance of the maintenance of an adequate circulation, something we shall emphasize strongly in discussing treatment. When the interaction between indi-

vidual factors is considered, age disappears and the associated illness becomes dominant, followed by the depth and duration of coma. This is because older patients are more likely to have more severe associated illnesses, as well as longer and deeper comas. Again, the leading biochemical feature is the blood urea, with blood pressure also registering, and the (very unimportant) association by which a lower rather than a higher blood glucose is a disadvantage (once all the interactions are allowed for) may again reflect the importance of an adequate circulation. Thus, if the circulation is inadequate, or the patient is generally very ill in other ways, the liver is not fit enough to carry out the excessive gluconeogenesis that is the driving force behind the hyperglycaemia.

Such considerations underlie the mortality of 5%–10% found for hyperglycaemic ketotic coma in hospitals admitting the general medical emergencies from an area, while the prognosis for non-ketotic coma is even worse, presumably because of its predominance among the elderly and the high probability that it will be associated with severe generalized illness. In an absolute sense, though, it is not only the elderly who die in the United Kingdom. The multicentre study organized by the British Diabetic Association and collated by Tunbridge [21] concluded that some 75 patients under 50 years of age die from hyperglycaemic coma annually. Very roughly, a third of these deaths may be ascribed to shortcomings in the patient, a third to problems in the health services outside hospitals, and a third to problems of management following admission to hospital. In any series of coma cases the ratio of known to newly diagnosed diabetics is informative, as it tells something of the relative efficiency of education of the diabetics attending general practitioner or hospital clinics as against education of the laity at large, together with the efficiency of primary health care.

Wherever particular attention is paid to patients with diabetic coma, the results are likely

Table 33.2. Prognosis of keto-acidosis, as relative risk of factors taken separately and allowing for their interactions

Separate		With interactions allowed for	
Age	31	Associated condition	139
Lower blood pressure	28	Degree of unconsciousness	68
Associated condition	24	Depth of coma	10
Blood urea	23	Blood urea	10
Degree of unconsciousness	18	Lower blood pressure	3
Depth of coma	17	Lower blood glucose	1

to improve, though naturally this has never been shown in a controlled way; but many special studies, even in those including general emergencies, show mortality rates nearer to 5% than to 8% or 10%. Some very estimable studies have been reported, namely those by Harwood [10] and by Malins and colleagues [6]. These were both compiled in the early 1950s. The American series combined the advanced understanding of IV fluid treatment gained in World War II with higher doses of insulin than had been usual in the 1930s, and the good results achieved were ascribed (perhaps incorrectly) to this latter factor, without enough credit given to the improved fluid and salt infusion. At any rate, that study was very influential in instituting an era of treatment of keto-acidosis by large doses of insulin.

More recent trends towards lower insulin dosage have not been proven to give better results, and the improvement seen during the 1960s in some reports is more probably due to better understanding of the need for adequate potassium replacement and to background improvement in general medical care (such as introduction of further antibiotics). However, it has been well established by several studies that the prognosis is not adversely affected by the lower doses of insulin.

Pathophysiology

To summarize this briefly, it is dominated by: (1) Disinhibition through inadequate insulin action of hepatic gluconeogenesis and adipose tissue lipolysis. The high levels of plasma free fatty acids fuel excessive ketone body production in the liver, and lack of insulin also reduces their effective utilization in the periphery. Providing the circulation remains adequate, peripheral glucose utilization is not much less than usual (because the hyperglycaemia compensates for the reduced action of insulin in the insulin-sensitive tissues); and (2) loss of water and sodium and potassium from the body, with average deficits of 5 litres water and 300–500 mM of both sodium and potassium. The deficit of these is likely to be greater in ketotic than in non-ketotic patients. The loss of water and sodium reduces the circulating blood volume, and so there is likely to be an increased distance from any given cell to the nearest patent capillary. The difficulty of proper O_2 supply to cells may be increased through re-

duced liability of oxyhaemoglobin to dissociation in the periphery, should a left shift of the dissociation curve of oxyhaemoglobin from the reduced erythrocyte concentration of 2, 3-diphosphoglycerate override any right shift from acidosis. However, some histotoxic factor may prevent the usual uptake of O_2 in both the arm and the brain [15, 19].

Another important consideration is the behaviour of central nervous system tissue in face of plasma hyperosmolality, when this is due to a natural substance, such as urea or glucose. Changes occur within the neurones that increase the intracellular osmolality, as by generation of 'idiopathic osmoles' (as shown in animals by Arieff [4]). The persistence of these despite improvement of the composition of the plasma as treatment proceeds may predispose to cerebral oedema.

Hyperglycaemic states are sometimes associated with an increased liability to aggregation of the formed elements of the blood, whether as thrombus or clot, or occasionally a widely disseminated intravascular coagulation [20, 22].

Treatment

The aim of treatment is to restore the metabolism of the body to normal. This involves more than addition of the missing substances (e.g., insulin, sodium, water, potassium) as though the body were one large black box. Above all, it means restoring an adequate circulation, so that necessary substances are transported near enough to deficient cells to be of use, and so that all the struggling organs are linked together. The second principle is that during correction one may see exposed compensatory mechanisms previously set in chain by the initial deviations from normal, and finally acting to derange the 'milieu intérieur'. This no doubt is why we are still uncertain of the optimal rate of correction of many of the abnormalities.

Water and sodium

As stated, there is likely to be a deficiency of 5–7 litres water in an adult, and around 500 mM sodium. Although the plasma sodium concentration is usually reduced, there is typically a greater shortage of water than of sodium compared with the consequences of a loss of normal saline from the body; in other words, the apparently correct replacement fluid is nearly always a more hypotonic solution than IV physiological saline (0.9% sodium chloride solution, 154 mM sodium).

Such a solution will expand the circulating volume and the ECF faster than would hypotonic saline, and water will enter cells more slowly than from a weaker solution. The dehydration and desalination are severe and require prompt correction. Physiological saline 500 ml should be given IV in the first 15 min and the next litre should be infused over the following hour. Thereafter, a customary rate of fluid infusion would be 1 litre/2 h, to a total of some 5 litres. Occasionally, and perhaps particularly in the elderly, such an infusion rate is excessive for the cardiac function, as shown by a rise in the jugular venous pressure or developing pulmonary oedema. Careful watch should be kept for these as an indication to slow the infusion, and if there is any doubt a central venous cannula should be inserted to measure the pressure continuously. Some advocate this routinely, but I am against it, as it is rarely necessary and provides another risk of introducing infection into devitalized tissues. If such a catheter is inserted, it should be removed as soon as the need for it has passed, with improvement in the patient's circulation, the metabolism of cardiac cells, and the rate of fluid infusion. In the occasional patients who develop 'disseminated intravascular coagulation' (DIC, see below), coarse crepitations occur at the lung bases about 4–8 h after the start of insulin therapy, with a simultaneous drop in oxygenation of the blood passing through the lungs. This should not be mistaken for pulmonary oedema, and certainly the DIC crepitations are nearly always much coarser. If artificial ventilation is given for the hypoxia, the lung compliance is found to be high.

Half-normal physiological saline is recommended only when there is relative or absolute hypernatraemia. In any case, it should not be started until enough normal saline has been given at least substantially to repair the circulation (e.g., after 3 litres). Then, if the entry plasma sodium was above 145 mM, or the 1-h value above 150 mM, I recommend use of 'half-normal' saline for the next 2 litres fluid, and indeed as long as the concentration remains above 150, until solutions containing glucose are introduced.

Glucose IV (as in 4% glucose in N/5 saline) should be commenced when the blood glucose has dropped below 15 mM, and some adjustment in the rate of insulin administration will then be necessary.

The essential first aim of the IV saline is to restore the circulation, for only thereafter will intracellular dehydration be repaired. One is looking, therefore, for slowing of the sinus tachycardia and increase in pulse pressure and mean blood pressure, with increased warmth of the hands and a smaller difference between the temperature of either the periphery of the limbs or the nose and the core (which itself, of course, may be low on entry to hospital). If the circulation does not seem adequate after 1 h 30 min of normal saline (or if it has not at least improved substantially), agents that expand the plasma volume should be considered. Thus, we recommend sending blood for grouping initially, for then at this later stage one can request that two units of blood are cross-matched, though initially using dextran to expand the circulation. If there is any possibility of abnormal coagulation, blood should be sent to assess this before dextran is started, as it upsets several of the assays involved.

Insulin

Flux of glucose into cells occurs readily at the high extracellular concentrations present, providing the necessary relatively small amounts of insulin are present, and the main objects of insulin treatment are (1) to inhibit hepatic gluconeogenesis, so that the glucose concentration can drop through peripheral utilization of glucose by the body cells, and (2) to inhibit adipose tissue lipolysis, so that there is no longer so large a flux of free fatty acids from the periphery to the liver, where they are converted into aceto-acetate and 3-hydroxybutyrate. Again, the main fall in ketone body concentration will then come from peripheral utilization, and the essential aim is to prevent their further formation.

Plasma concentrations around 60–80 mU insulin/litre are more than adequate to ensure these aims (which would probably be achieved at concentrations around 20 mU/litre providing the circulation were good). Such concentrations are readily achieved by frequent or even continuous administration of relatively small amounts of insulin, most directly by an IV injection of a loading dose of 5 IU insulin, followed by continuous IV infusion of 6 U/h [17]. If there are any difficulties in doing this efficiently, it may be more suitable to provide insulin by hourly IM injections. Such injections must indeed be IM rather than SC, for absorption from the subcutaneous site will be slow, particularly early on when the circulation is poor. We recommend initial injection of 20 IU of insulin, and then 5 IU hourly thereafter [3]. Such hourly IM injections can be changed either to IV administration or to SC injections (once adequate rehydration has occurred).

There are many other ways of giving insulin adequately, and many patients have recovered, for example, with intermittent (even hourly) boluses of IV insulin. However, this is an inefficient mode of insulin administration, in that much of the insulin present at the initial very high plasma concentrations will be broken down without adding anything to its action. With such a regimen there must inevitably be a highly erratic tissue insulin concentration, which may or may not perturb metabolism. The only identified metabolic differences [3] between the present, relatively small amounts of insulin administered and the old classic high-dose regimens are (1) the plasma potassium fell to a lower level with the high doses (for a given rate of IV potassium administration), involving a greater risk of dangerous cardiac arrhythmia, and (2) blood lactate rose further on the high-dose regimen, on average by 1.5 rather than 0.5 mM, though the effect was never nearly enough to precipitate lactic acidosis. (Nonetheless it did increase a strong organic anion at a time of marked acidosis, when all treatment is directed at reducing the acidosis.)

The rate of fall of glucose and of ketone bodies is the same with both high- and low-dose insulin regimens, as one is watching the rate of peripheral utilization of these compounds once their central formation has been abolished. Indeed, the main advantage of these newer insulin regimens is the accompanying loss of anxiety as to just how much insulin should be given in successive doses. Equally, there is no point in straining to find the lowest dose of insulin that will be just adequate (or, much more worryingly, just inadequate) to deal with the metabolic defect. Hence, it is best not to drop below the concentrations mentioned, though smaller amounts are certainly adequate to deal with milder cases of diabetic keto-acidosis.

It is essential to know that enough insulin is being given, and this is best checked by measurement of the blood glucose 1 h after the start of insulin. Indeed, the fall in the first hour gives a surprisingly good prediction of the rate of fall of glucose during the next 3–5 h, though one would certainly check it chemically 5 h after the start of insulin and, if there is any doubt about the patient's progress, it should be checked 3 h after insulin is started. It is unusual for these amounts of insulin not to be associated

with a rate of fall of the blood glucose of at least 3 mM/h, but occasionally there seems to be 'resistance' to insulin's hypoglycaemic effect. This is most likely either when there is still an inadequate circulation or when there is some complicating factor, such as a pyogenic infection, pregnancy, or chronic administration of a glucocorticoid. Thus, double the amounts of insulin mentioned above were needed by a pregnant patient with systemic infection from active pyelonephritis, and by a chronic rheumatoid arthritic being treated with glucocorticoids who also had a bacterial infection.

Potassium

Surprisingly, the timing and amount of potassium replacement remain contentious, even though the greater attention given to this is one of the more important developments in treatment of keto-acidosis during the last 20 years. However, although the reasons for early and adequate potassium infusion were argued at the turn of the decade [11], a recent review [18] still states: "I prefer to delay the start of (potassium) treatment until the (serum) level has fallen to about 4.5 mM or less." Patients presenting with diabetic keto-acidosis have a gross total body deficit of potassium (around 500 mM), and a major action of insulin is to increase tissue potassium uptake. Once insulin treatment has been started, therefore, it is safe to give potassium, providing that both the potassium and the insulin will reach their target tissues. The only contra-indication to early potassium supplementation is, therefore, so grossly inadequate a circulation that potassium added to the small circulating blood volume does not reach near enough to cells for its uptake to be increased effectively by the equally limited circulating insulin. It is also perhaps only in patients with such inadequate circulation that there is a real risk of acute renal tubular necrosis, which with its 10 days or so of anuria (or gross oliguria) made potassium administration unduly hazardous until the development of peritoneal or haemodialysis.

Even though a quarter of the patients admitted with diabetic keto-acidosis have a plasma potassium above the normal range, we recommend that infusion of plasma potassium should be started once a rapidly running saline infusion and insulin treatment are under way; in other words, within a few minutes of IV insulin and about 10 min after IM insulin, excluding only those with marked failure of the peripheral circulation. Blood will have been sent for plasma potassium assay before insulin was given, and only 1 g potassium chloride (13 mmol potassium) is given in the first hour, after which the initial potassium concentration should be available. At this stage, another plasma potassium should be sent, for, as with insulin, the change during the first hour is very instructive as to future developments, and the dose of potassium can be altered accordingly. If plasma potassium is between 3 and 4 mM, the rate of IV infusion can be increased to 26 mM/h, while if it is below 3.0 at least 39 mM/h should be given.

Under the influence of resalination and insulin, plasma potassium may fall fast, perhaps particularly from high values. Thus, it may drop from 6.4 mM to 5.2 mM in the first hour, even if 13 mmol potassium is given during that time.

This approach supersedes attempts to decide when to start potassium infusion according to whether or not urine flow has commenced, or whether the blood glucose has fallen sufficiently. There also seems no need to withhold potassium until the plasma level has dropped below 4.5 mM. Certainly one cause of death in patients otherwise faring well has been cardiac arrhythmia from a low plasma potassium some 4–6 h after the start of insulin treatment, particularly if bicarbonate was liberally infused, just as hyperkalaemia may precipitate a cardiac catastrophe before treatment starts.

A low plasma potassium concentration on entry is more likely in newly diagnosed diabetics (when kaliuresis will usually have been longer lasting than in patients already treated with insulin), and particularly if they have been treated with a thiazide or similar diuretic. The tendency of these agents to cause potassium loss in the urine is magnified by the preceding osmotic diuresis from heavy glycosuria. Such patients may well require 400–600 mmol potassium in the first 12 h of treatment.

Plasma potassium should be measured 1 and 5 h after the start of treatment as well as initially, and if there is any doubt about the progress of potassium replacement, it should also be measured 3 h after treatment started. Another guide to potassium status comes from the ECG, with particular reference to the T waves, for if these are flattening or becoming inverted a low plasma potassium is a possible explanation, while large peaked T waves should limit IV potassium. However, T wave changes can also be influenced by acidosis, so they are not an unambiguous guide to the potassium levels.

Oral potassium should be started as soon as fluids are taken orally, initially as a constituent of the fluids, whether these be meat soups, fruit juice, or even milk, and later as definite supplements, but only when solid food is being taken. Potassium is usually given IV as the chloride, but may also be administered as a hydrogen phosphate salt.

Observations during treatment with the old, high-dose insulin regimens (T. D. R. Hockaday and K. G. M. M. Alberti, 1973, unpublished work) showed that the drop in plasma potassium correlated inversely with the amount of potassium infused over the first 5 h, and from this relationship one could estimate that if no potassium at all had been given, plasma potassium would fall by an average of 2.0 mM in this time, while if the aim was to prevent any change in the entry level, on average 110 mM potassium was needed in that time.

Observations over the first 12–24 h also showed how great the loss of potassium could be in urine, despite a deficit of total body potassium, no doubt because of the impaired renal funtion in this acute metabolic upset. As might be expected, the patients with lower entry plasma potassium concentrations lost relatively the least potassium in the urine and conserved the most added potassium.

There is a smaller drop in plasma potassium concentration with the newer, low-dose insulin regimens. In practice, this is reckoned one of their advantages, but one could argue theoretically that the faster intracellular potassium is replaced, the better.

Bicarbonate

This is also a contentious facet of treatment. The advantage of giving bicarbonate is to speed the reversal of metabolic acidosis, which may well be so severe as to impair tissue function and to distress a conscious patient via severe overventilation. However, there are disadvantages, namely, first a risk of precipitating hypokalaemia with possible consequent cardiac arrhythmia, and second the possibility of causing a leftward shift in the dissociation curve of oxyhaemoglobin, so that O_2 is less readily supplied to the peripheral tissues. This is because, perhaps surprisingly, the dissociation curve is approximately normal on admission in most patients, despite the marked acidosis which, by the Bohr shift, would be expected to move the curve to the right. However, that shift is approximately balanced by a decrease in red cell 2, 3-diphosphoglycerate [8]. If the metabolic acidosis is too rapidly corrected, the curve will shift to the left, as the 2, 3-diphosphoglycerate defect is not corrected until 24–72 h after treatment starts. Third, it is easy with bicarbonate to end with a metabolic alkalosis and, though this is rarely severe enough to be any threat to health, it shows how easy it is to give excess bicarbonate.

The main process correcting the acidosis is the oxidation of the ketone bodies in the periphery coincident with inhibition of their further formation in the liver, once insulin has checked excessive lipolysis. As their blood concentration falls, so the acidosis will disappear, even if bicarbonate has not been given. Interestingly, the drop in concentration of organic acids is faster than the spontaneous rise in bicarbonate concentration of the plasma, and usually a mild hyperchloraemic acidosis occurs for a short while during replacement therapy. This harmless tendency will intensify as more sodium chloride is used as the replacement fluid rather than sodium bicarbonate.

Bicarbonate should not be given so long as the peripheral circulation is grossly deficient, for it will almost certainly reduce O_2 delivery to the periphery. However, once some saline has been given, if arterial pH is below 7.1, it is probably wise to reduce the acidosis, with 100 mmol bicarbonate over 20 min if pH is below 7.0, and 50 mmol in that time if it is between 7.1 and 7.0. Such bicarbonate should be accompanied by an extra 13 mM potassium chloride/100 mmol bicarbonate. Once it has been given, it is necessary to wait another 60–90 min before further measurement of arterial pH to decide by the same criteria whether a second dose of bicarbonate is needed.

General care

As well as general nursing care of the comatose patient, e.g., a mostly semi-prone position, with chest massage and regular turning, one of the most important requirements in patients comatose enough to have lost their cough reflex is early aspiration of the stomach. This is done with a thin (Ryle's) nasogastric tube and is particularly important because these patients are liable to gastric dilatation and stasis, so that, should they vomit, a large quantity of acid gastric juice may be aspirated into the lungs, with a consequent chemical pneumonitis (Mendelsohn's syndrome). It is easy to neglect this move until too late, with all the rush to establish IV infusion, take ECG recordings, and obtain blood for analysis.

Relatively early urethral catheterization is recommended by some, but I believe this outmoded advice. The successful resolution of hyperglycaemia is much better followed by blood than urine analysis; IV potassium therapy no longer awaits demonstrations of substantial urine production; and the rare development of anuria (or severe oliguria) from 'lower nephron nephrosis' is no longer the major disaster it was before the modern ways of handling acute renal failure were developed. The risk of unduly zealous catheterization is introduction of bacteria along with trauma to devitalized tissues, and so infection takes root in a way that would not occur if the same organisms had been implanted on healthy tissue. Once established, urinary tract infection may remain a recurrent problem, and it is regrettable if this stems from unduly hasty and unnecessary intervention. It is not surprising if only a small amount of urine forms in a grossly dehydrated and initially hypotensive patient, even with the osmotic diuresis of hyperglycaemia, and there seems no cause for anxiety if urine has not been passed for at least 8–10 h after IV fluid was started. Earlier catheterization is, of course, indicated if a taut and distended bladder makes the patient restless.

An ECG should be done within the first hour, and either the patient should be left on a cardiac monitor or the recording should be repeated after 3 h of treatment, to help monitor ionic changes, particularly of potassium.

Routine observations of a comatose patient, such as level of consciousness, state of the pupils, pulse and respiration rate, and blood pressure, are all of vital concern. It cannot be emphasized too much that the object of treatment is to improve these and that, while biochemical measurements give a most useful guide to what the clinical state is likely to be in the near future, this is less important than what the clinical state actually is, should this be deteriorating.

About a fifth of the patients have an arterial O_2 tension of 60 mmHg (8 kPa) or less on admission [2], and they are relatively less cyanosed than would be expected if there is a left shift in the O_2 dissociation curve. Such patients should be supported with an O_2 mask (either 28% or 100%, though the latter should never be used for too long a period continuously.) Oxygen should be started as soon as arterial blood has been obtained for gas analysis, but stopped if the O_2 tension is found to be adequate. If it is low, the O_2 should be continued either until the patient's conscious state has clearly improved, or until repeat arterial testing 1–2 h later (necessary to check the progress of the acidosis) indicates improvement in the level.

Antibiotics

There is no likely benefit in giving these in the absence of bacterial infection, but it may be difficult to detect such infection. Hence, it is very reasonable to have a low threshold for suspecting infection, but this is unlikely to be important, for instance, in a newly diagnosed diabetic with a history of increasing thirst, polyuria, and weight loss over several weeks. As mentioned previously, a careful search should be made for pyogenic infection, and in any case urine should be centrifuged and examined for cells and organisms as soon as it is available. If a staphylococcal infection is suspected, a combination of flucloxicillin and fucidic acid may be recommended, but otherwise a mixture of flucloxicillin and ampicillin, or alternatively one of the cephalosporins may be used. If a severe gram-negative septicaemia is suspected, treatment will be by gentamicin and metronidazole together with cloxacillin.

Controversial topics

Anticoagulants

At post-mortem examination, many hyperglycaemic patients are found to have scattered small ante-mortem thromboses, particularly in small vessels of the intestine but often also intracranially. How often these vascular blockages are important is highly debatable. Occasionally, they dominate the clinical picture, as in DIC, but most workers feel this is a very rare complication. Usually they are both relatively small in amount compared to the total circulation and also pre-agonal in timing. Apart from this, there remains the tragic occurrence in a minority of surviving patients of major vascular occlusions occurring under cover of keto-acidosis, as with the sudden development of hemiplegia or a mesenteric thrombosis. Such major occlusions are commoner in the elderly, and so loom particularly large in the prognosis of the non-ketotic patients.

All this had led to recommendation of routine anticoagulation, whether by heparin or inhibition of prothrombin synthesis. A study by Gale and Tattersall in Nottingham of diabetic deaths among patients over 60 showed only some 20%–25% to have vascular occlusion as a major contributant to the fatal outcome. That leaves one asking whether routine anticoagulation for all is worthwhile for the sake of this substantial minority, and also what would be its risks for the remainder. Most physicians straddle the fence by prescribing anticoagulants for the patients reckoned at greatest risk, namely those with a past history of venous thrombosis or obvious factors predisposing to it, such as marked varicose veins. Again, the markedly obese and particularly those in the deepest coma (and so likely to lie still longest) are often treated with anticoagulants, while any history or current evidence of bleeding is a marked contra-indication.

Disseminated intravascular coagulation should only be diagnosed from accepted haematological evidence of (1) decreased platelet count, (2) decreased prothrombin concentration with increased cephalin–cholesterol time, and (3) decreased fibrinogen with increased fibrin degradation products. There may be evidence of spontaneous bleeding or just of multiple vascular blocks. Such coagulation can occur in the pulmonary vessels and may be indicated by coarse basal crepitations with scattered opaque areas on the chest x-ray. These do not show the distribution of pulmonary oedema from high left atrial pressure, nor is there other evidence of this, such as Kerley's B lines or diversion of blood flow to the upper lung. If DIC is present, particularly with bleeding, heparin should be given and its effect followed haematologically.

Osmolality of IV fluid

In severely ill patients, there is a risk of cerebral oedema [15, 22]. It is not known whether this is due primarily to poor supply or utilization of O_2 for either cytotoxic or ischaemic reasons, or whether it relates more to the relative osmolalities of the intra- and extracellular fluids (there almost certainly is a cerebral ECF). We have already argued that physiologically normal (isotonic) saline is preferable to weaker solutions, and more boldly Irsigler [13] has argued that sometimes a hyperosmolar solution should be infused; he described recovery of some notably ill patients so treated. This approach is based on observations in young children with non-diabetic hypernatraemia (from vomiting and diarrhoea) in whom unduly rapid correction of the hyperosmolality can cause cerebral oedema. One generalization is that, if the osmolar gap between cerebrospinal fluid and serum exceeds 7 osmol/kg water, clinical trouble may develop [14].

There seems much logic in Irsigler's argument, though to carry through his ideas in routine practice would mean complicating management by recurrent lumbar puncture. Again, it is uncertain how often use of these concentrated fluids would yield a real advantage, though it is a commonplace that many conscious patients in pre-coma become less alert a few hours after the start of treatment, though this may be merely a result of fatigue. This is a problem perhaps best worked out by experiment on animals, and certainly it has been previously shown [9] that, if hypotonic solutions are infused IV the CSF pressure may rise noticeably in dogs with experimental ketoacidosis [5]. All this questions the rationale for using half-normal physiological saline if plasma sodium is above 150 mM. It is possible that the traditionally poor results in non-ketotic coma patients are partly dependent upon use of such dilute fluids, and it is probably important to withhold them, however high the plasma sodium, until the circulation has recovered largely towards normal and gross dehydration has disappeared.

Intravenous phosphate

The plasma concentration of inorganic phosphate is notably low in patients with ketoacidosis, and it is uncertain whether its IV infusion would speed recovery. Too much inorganic phosphate will cause a drop in plasma calcium, so care must be taken in its administration. However, it can be readily given as potassium phosphate. Although this has been shown to speed recovery of the low erythrocyte 2, 3-diphosphoglycerate concentration, randomized studies of phosphate infusion have failed to demonstrate clinical benefit or indeed even speedier recovery of the O_2 tension in the blood at which haemoglobin is 50% oxygenated [16]. Hence, the general opinion is against the further complication of phosphate infusion.

Speed of recovery

The optimal rate of recovery of the various blood factors we measure as a guide to the progress of coma patients is unknown. While the rate of administration of insulin would have to be reduced substantially to retard the rate of fall of blood glucose, the plasma potassium concentration appears more susceptible to alteration around the dose levels of insulin now used. To answer the question theoretically, we need to know the dose–response curve for insulin for each separate function in each of the many organs involved. The practical answer should come with adequate non-invasive methods of assessing organ function.

Action list

1. Clinical diagnosis. Bedside blood glucose and plasma ketones. Send blood for glucose, urea, sodium, potassium assay and haematological report + blood culture + blood group
2. 'Normal' saline IV (500 ml in 15 min, then 1 litre in 1 h, then 1 litre every 2 h)
3. Insulin, either IV (5 IU stat and 6 IV/h) or IM (20 IU stat and 5 IV/h)
4. Narrow (e.g., Ryle's) nasogastric stomach tube to aspirate stomach (if cough reflex lost)
5. ECG. Establish basic observations, e.g., pulse
6. Add potassium to IV line (13 mmol [1 g Pot. Chloride] in first hour)
7. Arterial blood for pH and pO_2 assay. Consider need for O_2 and/or IV bicarbonate treatment (with latter, wait for at least 1 litre saline to have been given, then give 50 mM over 20–30 min if pH < 7.1, and 100 mM if pH < 7.0, giving an extra 13 mM potassium/100 mM bicarbonate)
8. Consider antibiotic treatment
9. Obtain initial biochemical results. Decide on rate of further potassium. Consider need for plasma or blood transfusion. Send blood for further glucose, sodium, and potassium assay (1 h after start of insulin)
10. From results (9) check adequate glucose fall and adjust insulin dose if necessary. Reconsider rate of IV potassium
11. If entry and 1 h plasma sodium values too high (e.g., 1 h sodium above 150 mM), consider use of half-normal physiological saline after 3 litres normal saline has been given
12. Consider anticoagulants
13. Watch for need for IV glucose, when oral fluids can be started, and when hourly IM insulin can cease

References

1. Alberti KGMM, Hockaday TDR (1972) Rapid blood ketone body estimation in the diagnosis of diabetic ketoacidosis. Br Med J II:565–568
2. Alberti KGMM, Hockaday TDR (1977) Diabetic coma: reappraisal after five years. Clin Endocrinol Metab 6:421–455
3. Alberti KGMM, Hockaday TDR, Turner RC (1973) Small doses of intramuscular insulin in the treatment of diabetic coma. Lancet II:515–522
4. Arieff AI, Kleeman CR (1973) Studies on mechanisms of cerebral oedema in diabetic comas. Effects of hyperglycaemia and rapid lowering of plasma glucose in normal rabbits. J Clin Invest 52:571–583
5. Clements RS Jr, Prockop LD, Wiregrad AI (1971) Increased cerebro-spinal fluid pressure during treatment of diabetic ketosis. Lancet II:671–675
6. Fitzgerald MG, O'Sullivan DJ, Malins JM (1961) Fatal diabetes ketosis. Br Med J I:247–250

7. Fulop M, Tannenbaum H, Dreyer N (1973) Ketotic hyperosmolar coma. Lancet II:635–639

8. Guest GM, Rapoport S (1939) Role of acid-soluble phosphorus compounds in red blood cells. Am J Dis Child 58:1072–1089

9. Habel AH, Simpson H (1976) Osmolar relation between cerebro-spinal fluid and serum in hyperosmolar hypernatraemic dehydration. Arch Dis Child 51:660–666

10. Harwood R (1951) Diabetic acidosis, results of treatment in 67 consecutive cases. N Engl J Med 245:1–9

11. Hockaday TDR (1971)) Diabetic comas. Postgrad Med J 47: [Suppl] 376–381

12. Hockaday TDR, Alberti KGMM (1972a) Diabetic coma. Br J Hosp Med 7:183–192

13. Hockaday TDR, Alberti KGMM (1972b) Diabetic coma. Clin Endocrinol Metab 1:751–788

14. Irsigler K, Kaspar L, Bruneder H, Lageder H (1977) Kein freies Wasser bei der Therapie des 'Coma diabeticum hyperosmolare'. Therapiekontrolle durch Vergleich von Serum und Liquor. Dtsch Med Wochenschr 102:1655–1661

15. Kety SS, Polis BD, Nadler CS, Schmidt CF (1948) The blood flow and oxygen consumption of the human brain in diabetic acidosis and coma. J Clin Invest 27:500–510

16. Kitabchi AE, Fisher JN (1981) Insulin therapy of diabetic keto-acidosis: physiologic versus pharmacologic doses of insulin and their routes of administration. In: Brownlee M (ed) Diabetes mellitus, vol. 5. Wiley, Chichester, pp 99–149

17. Page MM, Alberti KGMM, Greenwood R, Gumaa KA, Hockaday TDR, Lowy C, Nabarro JDN, Pyke DA, Sonkson PH, Watkins PJ, West TET (1974) Treatment of diabetic coma with continuous low dose infusion of insulin. Bri Med J II:687–690

18. Pyke DA (1980) Diabetic ketoacidosis. J R Soc Med 73:131–134

19. Schecter AE, Wiesel BH, Cohn C (1941) Peripheral circulatory failure in diabetic acidosis and its relation to treatment. Am J Med Sci 202:364–378

20. Timperley WR, Preston FE, Ward JD (1974) Cerebral intravascular coagulation in diabetic ketoacidosis. Lancet I:952–956

21. Tunbridge M (1981) Factors contributing to deaths of diabetics under fifty years of age. Lancet II:569–572

22. Young E, Bradley RF (1967) Cerebral oedema with irreversible coma in severe diabetic ketoacidosis. N Engl J Med 276:665–669

23. Zieve L, Hill E (1953a) Descriptive characteristics of patients with moderate or severe diabetic acidosis: relation to recovery or death. Arch Intern Med 92:51–62

24. Zieve L, Hill E (1953b) Prognosis in moderate or severe diabetic acidosis. Arch Intern Med 92:63–74

Chapter 34

Endocrine Emergencies

Peter Daggett

Acute disturbances involving hormonal mechanisms are uncommon, but when they do occur rapid diagnosis and treatment are essential. They produce typical clinical syndromes when they present de novo, but in patients who are already unwell because of another condition their features may be masked. Investigations are therefore important in establishing a diagnosis and can be divided into two groups. First those which can be carried out rapidly and at any time, so that a clinical impression can be supported in the emergency situation and second those more sophisticated studies which may take many days to perform and which are used to confirm the diagnosis, so that long-term management can be planned. This chapter will concentrate on clinical features and practical management of endocrine emergencies, with a brief discussion of relevant investigations.

Thyroid

Thyroid crisis (thyroid storm)

These terms are used to describe a condition in which there is an exaggeration of the usual features of hyperthyroidism, accompanied by some manifestations not found in the uncomplicated disease. It may be the presenting form of the disorder or arise in patients already known to be hyperthyroid, but it does not occur when adequate treatment is being given. There is nearly always a complicating illness which precipitates the crisis, and on the basis of the mechanism involved, 'surgical' and 'medical' crises have been differentiated [45]. Surgical crisis is said to result from manipulation of the thyroid gland leading to release of hormones into the bloodstream, but as the condition can follow procedures not involving the thyroid, it is more likely that it is anaesthesia rather than surgery which is responsible. Medical crisis may be precipitated by any major stress, including injuries, childbirth, diabetic keto-acidosis, myocardial infarction, and severe infections. In practice the division between surgical and medical crisis is unhelpful, as the pathogenesis of the two is probably similar and the clinical features and treatment certainly are! It is worth noting that the administration of a therapeutic dose of radioactive iodine to an untreated thyrotoxic patient can lead to a crisis, probably by producing irradiation thyroiditis [13]. Iodine in contrast media can have a similar effect [6]. The clinical picture is variable, but pyrexia is always present and may be extreme. A goitre is the rule and since thyroid crisis is virtually confined to cases of Graves' disease: it is smooth and accompanied by a bruit or thrill. In young patients neuropsychiatric features are prominent, with severe tremor, anxiety, and confusion. This state may mimic mania, and if not treated leads to stupor and convulsions, followed by death from exhaustion. In all patients there is tachycardia, but in older age groups cardiovascular manifestations may dominate the clinical picture. These include the development of atrial fibrillation or other rhythm disturbances and cardiac failure, which is refractory to treatment and may be fatal. Abdominal symptoms may occur at any age and epigastric pain with vomiting can develop early in the course of the illness [52]. Later there may be severe diarrhoea and liver dysfunction, sufficient to cause jaundice.

Apathetic thyroid crisis

This uncommon form is very difficult to diagnose unless the patient is already known to be hyperthyroid. The subjects are elderly and have few features of thyroid overactivity, apart from evidence of substantial weight loss and tachycardia. There is seldom a large goitre, and instead of the usual restless energy these patients are lethargic. The temperature, however, is raised, but even this sign is less marked than in a typical crisis. It may be that the victims of this form have passed through an active stage un-noticed and have reached this state from exhaustion. This view is supported by their tendency to die suddenly and unexpectedly.

The physiological mechanism leading to thyroid crisis is obscure. In many cases the levels of thyroid hormones recorded are little different from those in uncomplicated hyperthyroidism [9]. This may mean that a lesser proportion than usual of thyroxine (T_4) and tri-iodothyronine (T_3) are bound to plasma proteins, or alternatively, that tissue sensitivity to the effects of thyroid hormones has become increased. At present there is insufficient information to be certain which mechanism is operating and very little about the factors which bring about any changes between the normal and crisis states. The measurement of the serum concentrations of thyroid hormones is not useful in distinguishing severe hyperthyroidism from thyroid crisis, but is helpful in confirming the diagnosis of thyroid overactivity in patients presenting de novo in crisis. There is no current method for making these measurements which is sufficiently rapid to be useful in initial management. Treatment must therefore be started on clinical grounds, but 20 ml blood should first be taken into plain glass tubes, so that analysis can be made later.

Treatment

This aims to prevent further thyroid hormone synthesis, to block release from the gland of stored hormone, and to antagonize the effects of hormones already circulating. A recent additional approach has been to remove circulating hormones by several methods, which have included dialysis [38], plasmapheresis [39], and resin haemoperfusion [12]. These techniques have not been widely used, however, and are not recommended. Prevention of synthesis of new hormones can be achieved by interfering with thyroidal iodide trapping or with the formation of iodotyrosines. The first of these could be achieved with potassium perchlorate, but it is more effective to interfere with the formation of iodotyrosines, for which purpose propylthiouracil is the most rapidly acting drug [1]. Inhibition of the release of stored hormones can be produced by some monovalent ions. Lithium has been suggested for this purpose [49], but in the acute situation the well-tried action of inorganic iodine is best. The iodide ion stops the hydrolysis of the thyroglobulin storage complex and brings about a rapid fall in the circulating level of thyroid hormones. The effect is only temporary, however, and starts to wear off after about 14 days (some would say less). The peripheral actions of circulating thyroid hormones can be antagonized by drugs which act on adrenergic receptors, although there is no convincing evidence of sympathetic overactivity in hyperthyroidism. Propranolol is the best tried of the beta adrenergic antagonists, but despite some reports [37] is not effective in the prevention or treatment of thyroid crisis on its own [26]. Chlorpomazine has alpha adrenergic antagonist properties [32] but its chief use in patients with a thyroid crisis is as a sedative and to lower temperature [84].

Synopsis of treatment

1) Propylthiouracil PO: 150 mg every 6 h.
2) Either saturated potassium iodide solution PO: 10 drops every 8 h in milk; or potassium iodide IV: 200 mg diluted to 500 ml in 0.9% saline, infused over 2 h, twice daily.
3) Propranolol: either PO, 40 mg every 8 h; or by slow IV injection, 1 mg as required.
4) Chlorpromazine by IM injection: 25–50 mg every 4–8 h.
5) Tepid sponging, treatment of heart failure and general supportive measures, depending on the patient's condition.

The IV route for drugs should only be used if the patient is unable to assimilate medicines by mouth.

Myxoedema coma

This, the most profound stage of hypothyroidism, arises when a severely myxoedematous person encounters a stress that requires additional energy which cannot be provided at the low metabolic rate. Precipitating factors include major injury, an abdominal catastrophe, myocardial infarction, cerebrovascular accident and infections, particularly urinary. Myxoedema coma occurs only in patients who are completely untreated, as even a small amount of thyroid hormone replacement is sufficient to raise the metabolic rate enough to prevent its development. It is seen mainly in the elderly and is rare in patients aged less than 60 years old. The reason for its predilection for older age groups is uncertain, but may be merely a reflection of the solitary life led by many old people, which results in a failure to recognize the hypothyroidism in its earlier stages. In addition, the presentation may be atypical in the very old [44]. Not all patients with this condition are comatose, but the conscious level is, by definition, depressed to some degree. The clinical features include the typical myxoedematous facial appearance and sallow complexion, bradycardia, and tendon reflexes which may be so slowed as to appear absent. The last is due in part to hypothyroid myopathy [2] and in part to hypothermia. Peripheral oedema is found and there may be effusions into any of the serosal body cavities. Pericardial effusion in particular is common, resulting in enlargement of the cardiac silhouette on a chest X-ray and, possibly, in signs of tamponade [78]. Many patients hypoventilate, leading to CO_2 retention and respiratory acidosis [11]. The typical picture is completed by hypothermia in the majority of cases, although this is not invariable [61]. If treatment is not started, progressive carbon dioxide narcosis, hypotension and hypothermia cause further lowering of the conscious level and death within a few hours [88]. In rare cases ileus [86] or convulsions [87] may occur.

Measurement of the serum level of thyroxine (T_4) and tri-iodothyronine (T_3) cannot usually be made sufficiently rapidly to be helpful in the acute situation, and is in any case a poor guide on its own. This is because low levels of thyroid hormones are commonly found in sick old people, even if their thyroid gland has previously been normal. To confirm a diagnosis of myxoedema coma, in due course the serum level of the thyroid-stimulating hormone (TSH) must be measured. This will be high in patients with primary hypothyroidism, but normal or low in all other situations. These specific estimations can be carried out on the serum from 10–20 ml blood, which should be collected before therapy is started. In addition to the hormonal abnormality there are frequently associated biochemical features. Arterial blood gas analysis shows acidosis, due to a combination of a raised CO_2 content [11] and a lowered bicarbonate, the latter being due to accumulation of lactic acid. Hyponatraemia is usual [29] and may be severe; it results from enhanced activity of the anti-diuretic hormone (ADH) [76]. Finally hypoglycaemia should be sought, as when present, the outlook is specially poor [61]. Abnormalities of serum enzymes may be shown, but these can be due to the hypothyroidism itself [20] and are not useful for diagnostic purposes.

Treatment

Replacement of thyroid hormones is, paradoxically, the least important aspect in the treatment of this dangerous state. Precipitating factors should be looked for and treated. Infection should be suspected if no cause can be found and consideration given to the use of broad-spectrum antibiotics, after collection of sputum, urine, and blood for bacteriological examination. The patient should be nursed in a unit where careful attention can be given to the cardiac rhythm during rewarming, for which purpose a 'space blanket' is best. Fluids should be infused under the control of measurements of the central venous pressure (CVP) using 0.9% saline supplemented if necessary, with 1.8% saline if the plasma sodium level is below 120 mmol/litre. The strong saline should be administered in quantities of 500 ml over 4 h, but the CVP should not be allowed to exceed +8 cmH₂O. The aim is to raise the plasma sodium level to 125 mmol/litre and it must be stressed that large volumes of 1.8% saline are *not* needed. Hypoglycaemia is treated in the usual way with a bolus of 50% dextrose solution, but a watch must be kept because hypoglycaemia may recur after the initial treatment. Corticosteroids should be given for two reasons. First, the adrenal cortex shares in the general hypo-metabolism and may not be able to respond to stress. Second, exceptionally, there may be associated auto-immune primary hypo-adrenalism, or the thyroid disorder may be secondary to hypopituitarism. Hydrocortisone is used in a dose of 100 mg 6-hourly, given IV. Several regimens for specific thyroid hormone replacement have been described. Thyroxine has been used in small, large, and 'total replacement' doses [42], but has two disadvantages. First, it is a pro-hormone, which must be converted in the body into the active hormone T_3. Second, it has a half-life in the circulation of about 7 days in normal subjects, but this is prolonged in hypothyroidism and if there is excessive acceleration of metabolism there may be long-lasting cardiovascular difficulties. The transition from T_4 to T_3 cannot be made efficiently in critically ill patients, and it is therefore logical to use T_3 itself in the treatment of myxoedema coma. If possible it should be given by mouth or nasogastric tube, because parenteral solutions must be prepared specially and are potentially hazardous; it can if necessary be given IV. Large doses of thyroid hormones are not required and are dangerous; they should not be used. The dose of T_3 is built up very slowly and a change made to T_4 when the patient is better [33]. (T_3 has a half-life in the circulation of less than 2 days; 20 μg T_3 is equivalent to 100 μg T_4.)

Synopsis of treatment

1) Re-warm with a space blanket. Monitor ECG.
2) Use CVP to restore fluid balance. Infuse 1.8% saline if plasma sodium is below 120 mmol/litre; give 500 ml in 4 h, then check whether sodium is above 125 mmol/litre. Repeat if necessary. Give 50-ml bolus of 50% dextrose if plasma glucose is low. Observe closely and repeat if necessary.
3) Hydrocortisone 100 mg 6-hourly IV as a bolus.
4) Broad-spectrum antibiotics, after collection of relevant samples.
5) Artificial ventilation if $PaCO_2$ exceeds 60 mm or rises progressively under observation.
6) Oral/nasogastric T_3, 5 μg daily. Increase by 5 μg daily every 5th day and change to T_4 1 week after reaching a daily dose of 20 μg.

Thyroid eye disease

This term is preferred to describe the condition which is also known as infiltrative ophthalmopathy, exophthalmic ophthalmoplegia and endocrine exophthalmos. Although there may be eye signs in hyperthyroidism from any cause, severe thyroid eye disease occurs only in Graves' disease, in which condition it may be associated with pretibial myxoedema and, rarely, with acropachy of the fingers. Thyroid eye disease is believed to be caused by stimulation of retro-orbital tissues by a circulating immunoglobulin, leading to hypertrophy, infiltration by lymphocytes, and oedema [15]. In its severe form thyroid eye disease causes proptosis, conjunctival oedema (chemosis), and interference with external ocular muscles. Vision may be threatened by corneal exposure leading to ulceration, or by damage to the optic nerve leading to a fall in acuity. There is often gross swelling of the conjunctiva at this stage, complicated by prolapse between the retracted lids and infection. Inability to close the lids adequately over the cornea, or reduction in visual acuity should be regarded as emergencies which must be treated at once.

Corneal exposure can be treated in the first instance by the regular instillation of lubricant drops. Reduction in visual acuity is a much more sinister development and blindness may follow quite quickly if action is delayed.

Treatment

The aim is to reduce rapidly the bulk of the retro-orbital tissues. External irradiation of the orbits [19] may be effective, but this treatment cannot always be given at once. Large doses of steroids combined with diuretics are as effective, and in sufficient quantities, make emergency surgical decompression unnecessary in almost all cases (P. MacFaul, 1979, personal communication). Three approaches for the latter procedure have been used; from above, through the anterior cranial fossa; from the side, through the lateral orbital wall; and from below, through the maxillary antrum. The last of these has been the most widely employed, but may result in infection or imbalance of the extraocular muscles. Recently, attempts to remove the stimulating immunoglobulin have met with some success, especially if combined with immunosuppressive therapy [16].

Synopsis of treatment

1) Nurse the patient in a sitting position.
2) Prevent exposure keratitis with instillations of 1% hypromellose eye drops, every 1–2 h. Consider lateral tarsorraphy.
3) Frusemide PO 80 mg daily, with a potassium supplement.
4) Dexamethasone PO 20 mg daily. Reduce after 2 days to 16 mg daily, and then by 4 mg per day every 3 days if the situation is improving. Reduction from 4 mg daily should be over a period of 3–6 months.

5) Assess visual acuity at least once every day. Consider orbital decompression if it falls during the above regimen.

N.B. This condition must be managed jointly by ophthalmologist and physician.

Acute swelling of the thyroid gland

This may be due to an acute inflammatory process or to haemorrhage into an abnormal area of the gland. It is not usually sufficient to cause immediate danger, but respiratory difficulty may arise if the thyroid is very large or in the retrosternal position.

Acute inflammation

This may be subdivided into suppurative, subacute non-suppurative, and irradiation-induced. Suppurative thyroiditis may complicate any septicaemic illness, but is rare. *Staphylococcus aureus* is most commonly involved, other well-described causes being streptococci and *Salmonella typhi* [8]. Severe pain characterizes this condition, usually with tenderness localized to part of the gland only. It differs from the subacute disease in that it is often possible to image the gland with radionuclides, the scan showing an area of poor uptake. Antibiotic treatment is usually curative [36]. Subacute thyroiditis is not uncommon but is seldom dramatic. The name 'De Quervain's disease' is usually applied, but some prefer to use a term based upon the typical histological finding of giant cells [82]. The cause is presumed to be viral, mumps virus being implicated most often [28]. The gland is swollen and uniformly tender, and the pain is referred to the throat or angles of the jaw. Systemic upset of varying degree is the rule. Investigations show a raised ESR, and with the evolution of the disease a rising titre of antibodies against a virus may be shown. The specific feature is attributable to inflammatory damage to the gland, resulting in the release of stored hormone, despite an inability to take up new iodine. Thus, the circulating levels of T_4 and T_3 are raised (perhaps accompanied by clinical evidence of hyperthyroidism), but the uptake of radioactive iodine by the gland is low or absent. Aspirin is the best analgesic for the sore throat, given in conventional doses and combined with gargles and bed rest. In severe cases prednisone should be given by mouth in a dose of 10 mg every 6 h, followed by a reduction in dosage over a period of a month. The disease runs a self-limiting course, although

relapses may occur. Long-term thyroid dysfunction is unusual [81]. Irradiation-induced thyroiditis occurs in patients given a therapeutic dose of radioactive iodine, but only in about 20% of cases is it sufficient to cause tenderness or swelling. It is only dangerous when there is a retrosternal thyroid, in which case even minor swelling can lead to tracheal compression.

Haemorrhage

This may occur into a solitary cyst or part of a nodular goitre. It causes acute, painful, but self-limiting enlargement of part of the gland. It is usually without significance, but must be distinguished from acute inflammation. Ultrasound scanning is the best method of making the distinction.

Retrosternal thyroid

It is very rare for the thyroid to be wholly and truly intrathoracic, and the term 'retrosternal goitre' usually implies downward enlargement of a normally sited gland. If further enlargement occurs, the tissues within the rigid thoracic inlet become compressed, leading to several clinical features. There may be dyspnoea with stridor, dysphagia, and venous obstruction, but it is the tracheal compression which is life-threatening. The problem can arise spontaneously, but may be precipitated by treatment of associated hyperthyroidism. Radioactive iodine is the most dangerous in this respect because of resultant thyroiditis, but any action which causes the serum TSH level to rise can cause enlargement of the gland. The diagnosis of retrosternal goitre is made easily on plain X-rays and radionuclide scans of the upper mediastinum. The treatment is surgical, electively if there is no compression, but as an emergency if there is respiratory embarassment. In the latter situation, the patient must be nursed in the sitting position while awaiting surgery, and dexamethasone 5 mg IV may be given to reduce swelling.

Adrenal

Addisonian crisis

This is the end-result of bilateral destruction of the adrenal cortices and its clinical features follow from deficiency of both glucocorticoids and mineralocorticoids [40]. Like many other endocrine emergencies it is usually precipitated by some complicating factor, which may be infection, trauma, or a surgical procedure. It is in addition likely to develop following salt loss caused by excessive sweating, which may occur during unaccustomed exposure to a warm climate [50].

Glucocorticoid deficiency results in weakness and malaise, abdominal discomfort, a tendency to infection, and fasting hypoglycaemia. It also allows the unrestrained secretion of ACTH by the pituitary gland, leading to pigmentation of the skin. This is seen best over the knuckles and in the palmar creases, inside the mouth next to the teeth, and in recent scars, but occasionally this important sign is absent [31]. The immediate threat to life results from deficiency of mineralocorticoids, which allows excessive amounts of sodium and water to be lost in the urine. It is shown by dehydration, evidence of weight loss, and hypotension with tachycardia. This combination of symptoms and signs demands urgent treatment, but some investigations can be arranged during preparation of an IV infusion. Hyponatraemia and hyperkalaemia are usually present, with elevation of the blood urea concentration due to dehydration. Hypoglycaemia is common and there may be hypercalcaemia [21]. The diagnosis is confirmed by the finding of a low plasma cortisol associated with a high ACTH level, but the results of these investigations will only be available at a much later time. Before commencing treatment, 30 ml heparinized blood should be obtained and centrifuged at once: 5 ml plasma should be stored for the measurement of cortisol and the remainder of the sample frozen at once, pending analysis for the labile hormone ACTH. An alternative diagnostic approach based on a modified adrenal stimulation test has been described by Mattingly et al. [55], but is more complex than the protocol suggested here.

Treatment

Correction of the salt and water deficiency is life-saving, and for this purpose 0.9% saline is used. Glucocorticoid replacement is best given as hydrocortisone (preferably the hemisuccinate), but prednisolone (NOT prednisone) can be used. If adequate saline is given, specific mineralocorticoid replacement is not needed, but some authorities recommend the use of aldosterone IM. The older mineralocorticoid deoxycorticosterone acetate (DOCA) is no longer used. Incidental precipitating illnesses should

be treated at the same time (see section: 'Myxoedema coma').

Synopsis of treatment

1) Give 0.9% saline, 1 litre in 30 min then 1 litre in 1 h followed by 1 litre in 3 h.
2) Give hydrocortisone hemisuccinate, 100 mg IV every 4 h. After 24 hours, change if possible to oral hydrocortisone, 20 mg every 8 h. If the patient cannot take drugs orally, the IV dose should be reduced to 50 mg every 4 h.
3) Give aldosterone, 0.5 mg IM, as a single dose.
4) Treat the precipitating cause. Consider broad spectrum antibotics.

Iatrogenic steroid deficiency

Corticosteroids are widely used in all branches of medicine and the syndrome which results from their sudden withdrawal is, therefore, relatively common. Their glucocorticoid effect, exerted through the hypothalamus, causes inhibition of ACTH release from the pituitary gland and this brings about dormancy of the cortisol-secreting tissues of the adrenal cortex. If this situation continues for long enough atrophy of these tissues occurs, but aldosterone, which is independent of ACTH, is unaffected. The syndrome of iatrogenic steroid deficiency is thus a consequence of glucocorticoid deficiency alone. It usually arises within 24 h of stopping or reducing steroid therapy, but will also follow failure to increase steroid dosage at times of unusual stress. General malaise and anorexia are followed by abdominal discomfort and symptoms of postural hypotension. These features are often accompanied by a low pyrexia, the cause of which is unknown. If ignored, the picture starts to resemble that in Addisonian crisis, but dehydration is less prominent and pigmentation is of course absent. The treatment of this condition involves infusion of 0.9% saline and administration of hydrocortisone in the same way as for Addisonian crisis. It should however be preventable by education of patients and care when reducing steroid dosage.

Suppression of the hypothalamo-pituitary-adrenal (HPA) axis is unlikely to occur in less than 2 weeks, no matter how large a dose of glucocorticoid is used. After this time suppression is increasingly likely and after a long period (variously estimated as between 2 and 10 years) there will be adrenal atrophy so severe as to be irreversible. Accordingly, the longer the duration of steroid therapy the more gradual should be the reduction in dose. If treatment has been given for more than 8 years it is unlikely that adrenal cortical recovery will ever occur, even if injections of exogenous ACTH are given. It is recommended that in this circumstance a small dose of glucocorticoid should be continued indefinitely.

Glucocorticoids—some relevant facts

1) The combined daily production of cortisol from both adrenal cortices under unstressed conditions is 12–30 mg. The daily requirement of an adult after a bilateral adrenalectomy is 20–30 mg hydrocortisone PO.
2) Equivalent glucocorticoid effects of some common steroids are as follows:

Hydrocortisone	1.0
Cortisone acetate	0.8
Prednisone	5.0
Prednisolone	6.0
Dexamethasone	20–30

   (There is individual variation.)
3) Cortisone must be converted in the body to hydrocortisone, and prednisone to prednisolone before they are active. These conversions may not be possible in severely ill patients.

Waterhouse–Friedrichsen syndrome

This syndrome is usually regarded as a complication of meningococcal septicaemia [53], but a similar condition can arise in other forms of overwhelming infection, notably pneumococcal. The cardinal pathological feature is haemorrhagic infarction of the adrenal glands, starting in the medulla but bursting out to destroy the cortex [68]. This 'adrenal apoplexy' is not, however, the only life-threatening aspect of the disorder. The illness starts abruptly with rigors and severe headache, but the temperature need not be raised and may even be low. An extensive purpuric rash soon appears on the limbs and on the trunk, but the purpuric areas often coalesce. The patient sinks rapidly into a shock-like state with tachypnoea, but consciousness is preserved until late in the course of the disease. There may be evidence of meningitis or encephalitis, but this is not necessary to make the diagnosis. Death follows within a few hours, from cardiovascular collapse or abnormal bleeding, the latter being due to disseminated intravascular coagulation (DIC) [27]. Biochemical investigations are unhelpful in diagnosis, but

may show the electrolyte disturbances of hypoadrenalism (see section: 'Addisonian crisis') and evidence of renal impairment. Haematological studies are essential, however, to detect DIC at a stage when it can be treated and to show the leucopenia which is the rule in this condition. Blood cultures must be taken and unless there is evidence of abnormal bleeding, a lumbar puncture may be performed.

Treatment

As soon as blood cultures have been obtained, treatment with penicillin in high dosage must begin. If the patient is allergic to penicillin, chloramphenicol should be used, and in either case it is generally advised that a sulphonamide be given as well. Fluid balance should be restored with 0.9% saline, CVP being monitored constantly if possible. Hydrocortisone is given as for cases of Addison's disease, although the evidence for steroid deficiency in this condition is poor. Treatment is given for DIC in the usual way (Chap. 30).

Synopsis of treatment

1) Benzylpenicillin, 2 mega-units IV every 2 h.
2) Sulphadiazine, 1.5 g IV every 4 h.
3) Hydrocortisone, 100 mg IV every 4 h.
4) 0.9% saline according to measurements of CVP.
5) Treat associated DIC.
6) Sulphonamide prophylaxis PO for attendants.

Acute hypercortisolism

This condition may arise in severe and long-standing Cushing's syndrome due to adrenal or hypothalamo-pituitary disease and in the syndrome of ectopic production of ACTH. In the latter case, the source is most often oat cell bronchial carcinoma and the patient may already be very unwell on account of this. The clinical problems which result from very high circulating levels of cortisol are related to the duration of the syndrome. When it has been present for many months there will be features of Cushing's syndrome, the most serious of which are muscle wasting and osteoporosis. When the condition is of recent onset, as will be the case in the ectopic ACTH syndrome, only the biochemical features will be found. The principal metabolic effects of severe hypercortisolism are the induction of glucose intolerance and of hypokalaemia, the latter dominating the clinical picture. It causes profound muscular weakness and cardiac arrhythmias [63] and may interfere with the ability of the kidney to concentrate the urine. The plasma cortisol level may be as high as 2000 nmol/litre, but the ACTH level will depend upon the aetiology of the syndrome. If there is an adrenal tumour the level will be low, if there is a hypothalamo-pituitary lesion it may be normal or slightly raised, but if there is ectopic production values in excess of 200 ng/ml may occur [67].

Treatment

Any surgical intervention in patients with un-treated severe hyper-cortisolism is likely to be fatal and treatment must be medical in the first instance. Urgent correction of the hypokalaemia is required, but this can sometimes be achieved with oral medication. If cardiac arrhythmias are troublesome, however, potassium can, with caution be given IV. The cause of the metabolic abnormality should then be dealt with, by re-ducing cortisol synthesis. The best means of achieving this is to interfere with 11-beta-hydroxylase activity in the adrenal cortex, with oral metyrapone [46]. This manoeuvre lowers the plasma cortisol concentration acutely and can precipitate collapse unless replacement ster-oids are given at the same time.

Synopsis of treatment

1) Potassium supplement, either PO as Sando K, four tablets 6-hourly or IV under ECG control: 80–100 mmol potassium should be added to 1 litre 5% dextrose and infused by burette over 12 h.
2) Metyrapone (Metopirone), 500 mg every 6 h PO, increasing to 750 mg or 100 mg every 6 h if the response is inadequate.
3) Hydrocortisone, 20 mg every 6 h PO. This may be given at the same time as the mety-rapone to prevent a hypo-adrenal collapse.

Steroid psychosis

This is a consequence of glucocorticoid excess and can take several forms. It may develop in patients with Cushing's syndrome or compli-cate exogenous steroid medication [77]. In the former case depression is prominent and may persist for long after the underlying disease has been successfully treated. By contrast the thera-

peutic use of steroids is more likely to produce euphoria than depression, and the syndrome resolves quickly when treatment is withdrawn. It is interesting that some steroids are more prone to cause psychiatric problems than others, dexamethasone being particularly likely to produce difficulties. The effect of exogenous steroids is generally dose-related, but some pa-tients are especially sensitive; it is not possible to identify these cases beforehand. Pre-existing psychiatric illness does not necessarily get worse and is not a contra-indication for steroid treatment. The psychiatric syndrome associated with steroids may include hypomania, a toxic confusional state and a schizophrenia-like ill-ness. Treatment of steroid psychosis should depend upon the dominant feature, but in all cases the most important step is to reduce the circulating concentration of glucocorticoid. In the case of exogenous steroid medication, the dose should be reduced or a change made to a different drug. In the case of Cushing's syn-drome, treatment with metyrapone may be con-sidered (see section: 'Acute hypercortisolism').

Phaeochromocytoma

This tumour, which may occur at any point along the sympathetic chain, can cause attacks of life-threatening hypertension or cardiac arrhythmias, due to release of adrenaline and noradrenaline. These crises are the only emergencies related to catecholamines, there being no syndrome of adrenal medullary insuf-ficiency. Of all phaeochromocytomas, 90% are within the adrenal glands, the next commonest site being the organ of Zuckerkandl (situated at the fusion of the two sympathetic chains, over the front of the sacrum), but they may occa-sionally occur in the thorax or elsewhere in the abdomen and pelvis, including the bladder wall. In about 10% of cases there may be a tumour in more than one site and in 10% of all cases, the phaeochromocytoma behaves as a malignant neoplasm.

The synthesis of catecholamines from tyro-sine involves a series of enzymatic steps, the last of which leads to adrenaline and is brought about by the enzyme phosphoethanolamine-N-methyl-transferase (PNMT), which requires a high concentration of steroids to function. A suitable environment is only provided within the medulla [43], so that adrenaline production elsewhere is minimal. When a phaeochromocy-toma arises outside the adrenal it secretes only noradrenaline. If it develops within the adrenal, either noradrenaline or adrenaline may be produced, but the latter usually predominates.

Noradrenaline has agonist actions which are principally alpha-adrenergic, and when this hormone predominates hypertension without tachycardia is the rule. Adrenaline on the other hand has beta-adrenergic properties in addition, and when this predominates there is tachycardia with the hypertension. In the latter case, rather than elevation of the blood pressure, there may be postural hypotension consequent upon peripheral vasodilatation. Other symptoms commonly found in patients with a phaeochromocytoma are pulsating headache, peripheral paraesthesiae, pallor during attacks, feelings of impending doom, and constipation. Diarrhoea may occur if the tumour is one which makes the neurotransmitter vaso-active intestinal peptide (VIP) in addition to catecholamines. The hypertension and tachycardia are paroxysmal, but a background of moderately elevated blood pressure is quite common. There are no specific signs in this condition, but there may be stigmata of neurofibromatosis (café-au-lait spots and cutaneous nodules), a disorder which is sometimes complicated by a phaeochromocytoma.

The best means of confirming the diagnosis is to show that the plasma level of one or both catecholamines is elevated [7]. This investigation requires 20 ml heparinized blood, and the plasma must be separated and frozen as quickly as possible. Results of this, or the more widely used measurement of urinary excretion of vanilmandelic acid (VMA) cannot usually be obtained rapidly. It is possible, however, to perform a screening test on the urine, which will be positive if large amounts of catecholamines are present [30].

A number of techniques have been applied to the localization of phaeochromocytoma [25]. They include intravenous pyelography (IVP), arteriography, computerized axial tomography (CAT or EMI scan), ultrasonography, and multiple venous sampling [60], but full discussion is outside the scope of this chapter. After localization the tumour should be removed if possible.

Treatment

The medical management of these patients is directed towards reducing or eliminating hypertensive and arrhythmic episodes. It *must* be commenced well in advance of any surgical procedure or invasive investigation, preparation for 3 weeks being desirable. This is to allow the cardiovascular system to equilibrate after alpha- and beta-adrenergic blockade. Treatment must be started with an alpha-adrenergic antagonist first to prevent a hypertensive crisis, which can be precipitated by beta-adrenergic antagonists alone [66]. Phentolamine is a short-acting alpha-adrenergic antagonist which can be given IV in an emergency and which is so effective that it has been used in a therapeutic test for phaeochromocytoma. Phenoxybenzamine has a half-life in the circulation of 6–8 h and is generally given PO in the preparation for surgery. Propranolol is the most effective beta-adrenergic antagonist in this condition and is generally given PO, although it can be given IV if necessary (see section: 'Thyroid crisis'). Prolonged treatment with these drugs allows the contracted plasma volume to expand, thereby preventing the hypotensive collapse which can occur immediately after removal of the phaeochromocytoma [70]. A number of drugs are available to control the blood pressure during hypertensive crises which occur despite this preparation. Sodium nitroprusside (Chap. 15) by infusion is probably the best [14], and may be given safely to patients prepared with alpha- and beta-adrenergic antagonists. This type of treatment requires close monitoring, which includes continuous measurement of the intra-arterial blood pressure and central venous pressure.

Synopsis of treatment

A) Emergency management when first diagnosed

1) Phentolamine, 5–10 mg IV. This will lower blood pressure rapidly but its effect will last only for 10–30 min.
2) Propranolol, 1 mg IV. This can be used for severe tachyarrhythmia.

B) Preparation for surgery
Alpha-adrenergic antagonists *must* be given before beta antagonists. This regimen should be started at least 3 weeks before planned surgery and at least 1 week before planned contrast radiology (except for IVP. For this investigation, it is sufficient to have phentolamine on hand).
1) Phenoxybenzamine, 10 mg every 8 h PO.
2) Propranolol, 20–40 mg every 6 h PO.

C) Management of crises occurring despite 'adequate' preparation
During surgery and contrast radiology, continuous measurement of intra-arterial blood pressure is mandatory.

1) Give sodium nitroprusside in carefully controlled infusion of 0.01% solution. This agent may cause precipitous fall in blood pressure, but its effect ceases almost at once when the infusion is stopped.
2) Propranolol, 1 mg IV for dangerous tachycardia.

Pituitary

Hypopituitary crisis

A state of crisis progressing to coma may occur when patients who are hypopituitary are subjected to unusual stress (see section: 'Myxoedema coma'). It may in addition develop acutely, following pituitary apoplexy (see below). The syndrome combines features of deficiency of thyroid hormones and of glucocorticoids, due respectively to impaired production of TSH and of ACTH. There is also evidence of hypogonadism secondary to absence of gonadotrophins, but mineralocorticoid production, which is independent of ACTH, is normal.

The immediate threat to life is caused by glucocorticoid deficiency, manifested by anorexia, vomiting, hypotension, and fever. The patient usually appears well nourished, but the skin is soft and there is little body hair. Thyroid hormone deficiency is shown by inappropriate bradycardia and slow relaxation of the tendon jerks, but other feures of hypothyroidism are minimal or absent. In patients who are known to have a disease of the pituitary gland the diagnosis can be made easily. In cases presenting de novo, however, it may be very difficult to identify the condition on clinical grounds, but a clue may be provided by investigations. Hypoglycaemia is common and may be the principal cause of unconsciousness [57]. Hyponatraemia is the rule and may be severe [17]; it is believed to be dilutional in nature. In contrast to Addisonian crisis the plasma potassium concentration is not raised, because aldosterone production is normal. The diagnosis of hypopituitarism can be confirmed subsequently by measurement of the plasma concentrations of pituitary trophic hormones and of the appropriate target organ hormones; both would be expected to be low in this condition. Before starting treatment, 20 ml blood should be collected into heparinized tubes and 20 ml into plain tubes, for the measurement of thyroxine, TSH, cortisol and ACTH (see section: 'Addisonian crisis').

Treatment

This must be started at once, glucocorticoid replacement being the most urgent need. This must be given before thyroid hormones, to prevent a worsening of the situation, which could follow acceleration of the metabolic rate [18]. Fluid replacement is required by IV infusion in most cases, for which purpose 0.9% saline is usually appropriate. In the presence of severe hyponatraemia (a plasma level below 115 mmol/litre), however, stronger saline may be needed. In some patients glucocorticoid replacement unmasks diabetes insipidus, which should be treated in the usual way. As in other endocrine emergencies a precipitating cause must be sought and treated.

Synopsis of treatment

1) Hydrocortisone, 100 mg every 6 h IV. Change to oral route, 20 mg every 8 h when the patient is improved. Mineralocorticoids are *not* needed.
2) Restore fluid balance with 0.9% saline infusion under CVP control. Glucose is often needed in addition, provided by dissolving 100 ml. 50% dextrose solution in each litre of saline.
3) Give tri-iodothyronine by mouth or nasogastric tube, 10 μg daily. Increase to 10 μg every 12 h after 1 week. Glucocorticoids *must* be given before thyroid hormones.

Pituitary apoplexy

This term is used to describe acute haemorrhagic infarction of a pituitary tumour [85] and is distinct from post-partum necrosis [74]. It may be the presenting feature of a pituitary tumour or occur in a patient already known to have an adenoma. This may be secreting growth hormone [10], prolactin, or ACTH, but in some cases the tumour is apparently functionless. Sudden expansion of the gland distorts the meninges, giving rise to headache which may mimic subarachnoid haemorrhage. Acute chiasmatic compression can cause blindness [69] and damage to oculomotor nerves frequently results in eye movement disorders. The diagnosis is supported by finding an abnormal sella turcica on skull x-ray and blood staining or xanthochromia of the CSF.

Hypopituitary crisis may complicate this condition and treatment with glucocorticoids should be started as soon as the diagnosis is made (see section: 'Hypopituitary crisis'). Neurosurgical decompression of the sella turcica is required if the vision is compromised.

Acute enlargement of a prolactinoma in pregnancy

The prolactin-secreting pituitary tumour (prolactinoma) causes infertility, but conception can be induced by treatment with dopamine agonists or by surgery, resulting in a lowering of the circulating prolactin concentration [5]. Pregnancy causes enlargement of prolactin-secreting adenomas, as a consequence of the high oestrogen levels. This can give rise to chiasmatic compression during the pregnancy [48], which if left untreated may lead to blindness. If a visual field defect is found as a result of the regular monitoring of a pregnant patient who has been treated for a prolactinoma, three courses of action are possible. First, the tumour can be removed at a formal decompressive operation. Second, the tumour can be shrunk with interstitial irradiation from a rod of yttrium[90] introduced by the trans-sphenoidal route. Third, an attempt can be made to reduce the bulk of the tumour with oral bromocriptine. There is good evidence that this drug not only lowers the plasma concentration of prolactin, but that it also inhibits the growth of the tumour and even makes it smaller [79]. There is no evidence that bromocriptine is teratogenic and it has been recommended that it should be reintroduced, if a visual field defect occurs during pregnancy [83]. If the visual field defect gets worse or other signs of tumour enlargement occur during bromocriptine treatment, consideration should be given to decompression.

Synopsis of treatment

1) Start bromocriptine in a dose of 2.5 mg PO daily, taken after supper. Increase dose by 2.5-mg increments every 3 days, until a daily dose of 15 mg is reached.
2) Monitor visual fields twice weekly and measure plasma prolactin concentration once weekly. If either index deteriorates, particularly the former, consider transfrontal or trans-sphenoidal decompression.

N.B. All patients who have conceived after treatment of any kind for a prolactinoma should have visual fields plotted and plasma prolactin measured monthly. They must report any headache or visual disturbance at once.

Acute diabetes insipidus

Of the many causes of diabetes insipidus, only head injury and neurosurgery are likely to cause the acute onset of the condition. In these situations a check should be made routinely for polyuria, so that the diagnosis can usually be made with ease at an early stage. Dehydration may develop rapidly in patients who are unconscious or who have associated damage to thirst mechanisms, but treatment should be deferred until the diagnosis has been confirmed biochemically. This is particularly important when the cause of the syndrome is unclear, because injudicious use of anti-diuretic agents can result in water intoxication. Before commencing treatment, the following steps should be taken:

1) Exclude or correct associated hyperglycaemia.
2) Measure the osmolality of plasma and a urine sample obtained simultaneously. In diabetes insipidus, the plasma osmolality is usually above 310 mosmol/kg and may exceed 350 mosmol/kg. The urinary osmolality is usually below 200 mosmol/kg and may be less than 100 mosmol/kg.

Formal tests for diabetes insipidus may be carried out at a later date if necessary [23].

Treatment

Once diagnosis, based upon the clinical setting, large urine volumes, and inappropriate osmolalities, has been made, specific treatment should be started. The older preparations have been superseded by a synthetic analogue of the antidiuretic hormone, desamino-D-8-arginine vasopressin (DDAVP or desmopressin). This substance can be given by nasal instillation, SC, or IM [24]. When the urine flow has been slowed down, an infusion of 5% dextrose should be adjusted so that the plasma osmolality is maintained within the normal range. Failure to modify the rate of infusion can result in water intoxication, particularly if 5% dextrose is used in place of saline. If serial measurements of osmolality cannot be made, the plasma sodium concentration is a useful guide to therapy.

Synopsis of treatment

1) Do not treat until the diagnosis is established.
2) Give DDAVP, 1 μg IM. The effect of this lasts for 8–24 h. In some patients doses of 2 or 4 μg are needed to control the polyuria.

3) Rehydrate with 5% dextrose, adjusting the rate of infusion to keep pace with the urine flow and maintain plasma osmolality in the range 270–300 mosmol/kg *or* plasma sodium concentration in the range 135–145 mosmol/kg.

Minerals

Severe hypercalcaemia

Hypercalcaemia is a common finding on biochemical screening, but in the early stages is associated only with mild and non-specific symptoms. Severe hypercalcaemia on the other hand is rare, but usually declares itself on account of its associated clinical features [62]. Symptoms become increasingly likely at plasma calcium concentrations above 3 mmol/litre (12 mg/dl) and almost invariable above 4 mmol/litre (16 mg/dl). Hypercalcaemia causes changes in the kidney at first bringing about tubular damage and polyuria, but progressing to impairment of overall function and frank renal failure [4]. There is in addition the risk of ureteric obstruction due to calculus formation when the abnormality is long-standing.

The principal symptom, then, is polyuria with thirst [51], but other prominent complaints are lethargy, general malaise, abdominal discomfort, and constipation. Occasionally there is deafness, conjunctivitis (due to calcium deposition in the cornea), and profound weakness due to a neuromyopathy. Physical signs of hypercalcaemia per se are few, but include band keratopathy, hypotonia of the muscles, and loss of tendon reflexes. There may of course be evidence of the underlying disease process in addition to these specific features. Cardiac dysfunction is not apparent clinically, but shortening of the $Q-T_c$ interval on the ECG is common [71]. Although there are many conditions which may be associated with hypercalcaemia, only three are likely to cause the severe form. These are carcinoma, especially of the breast and bronchus, myelomatosis, and primary hyperparathyroidism. The following investigations are required to clarify the diagnosis and guide treatment:

1) Measurement of the plasma concentration of phosphate and alkaline phosphatase. In primary hyperparathyroidism phosphate is low and phosphatase moderately elevated; in carcinoma phosphate is normal and phosphatase markedly elevated; in myelomatosis phosphate is normal and phosphatase usually normal. These rules are a guide and do not apply if there is renal impairment.
2) Marrow examination. As a means of diagnosing myelomatosis this is the most likely test to give a rapid result, but serum and urine must of course be screened for abnormal proteins.
3) Radiographic skeletal survey. This may show bony abnormalities in any of the three conditions, each with specific features. In an emergency, however, views of the skull and hands are the most likely to yield diagnostic information. A chest X-ray may show a primary carcinoma and should always be included.
4) Assessment of renal function. The blood urea concentration may be used as a guide in the acute situation, but the creatinine clearance is more reliable.

Treatment

Urgent treatment is required for plasma calcium levels in excess of 3.5 mmol/litre (14 mg/dl) because of the risk of rapidly progressing renal damage. A diuresis must be established with the aim of achieving a urine output of at least 3 litres daily. This single step will confer substantial protection on the kidneys while other therapeutic action is taken. Large doses of systemic steroids will lower the calcium concentration over the course of 1–3 days but will not be effective in primary hyperparathyroidism. In this case urgent exploration of the neck may be required [73], with the aim of removing an adenoma but if one cannot be found, subtotal parathyroidectomy may be performed. A further useful manoeuvre in severe hypercalcaemia is to give phosphate. Intravenous phosphate [54] may cause metastatic calcification and is not recommended. The principal side-effect of oral phosphate is diarrhoea [80], but this is not usually serious. Several other forms of treatment have been described, but are seldom needed. They include the use of the hormone calcitonin in high doses [3] and the cytotoxic agent mithramycin [75], the latter being particularly effective in cases due to carcinoma. When all else fails, dialysis has been advocated.

Synopsis of treatment

1) Establish a urine output of 3–4 litres daily by giving an infusion of 0.9% saline and IV

frusemide. A potassium supplement may be needed.

2) Hydrocortisone, 200 mg every 4 h IV. When the patient is improved change to oral prednisone 15 mg every 6 h. Add cimetidine if there is indigestion or a history of peptic ulcer.
3) Phosphate as oral Phosphate Sandoz, two tablets dissolved in water every 6 h.
4) In refractory cases:
   a) Exploration of the neck if primary hyperparathyroidism is suspected;
   b) Mithramycin if there is evidence of carcinoma.

Acute hypocalcaemia

The clinical features of hypocalcaemia are caused by a reduction in the plasma concentration of ionized calcium. This may result from alkalosis, both metabolic and respiratory. The former may complicate prolonged vomiting or be associated with hypokalaemia, while the latter, which is commoner, is caused by hyperventilation. It is assumed that alkalosis will be considered and corrected before taking further action. The alternative cause of a reduction in the ionized calcium concentration is a low total calcium level. When the latter falls the percentage of calcium bound to plasma proteins also falls, so that the ionized calcium concentration remains almost normal until the hypocalcaemia is very severe. In practice, clinical features of hypocalcaemia are not usually found with a total calcium concentration exceeding 2 mmol/litre (8 mg/dl) and are uncommon until the level is below 1.5 mmol/litre (6 mg/dl). Hypocalcaemia of this severity is most often caused by deficiency of parathyroid hormone (PTH), but it may occur in acute pancreatitis [56] and after surgery for thyrotoxicosis, even if the parathyroid glands are unharmed [72]. The commonest cause of hypoparathyroidism is the deliberate or accidental removal of the parathyroid glands. Their anatomy and number are so variable that the inadvertent removal of all functioning parathyroid tissue is not uncommon. Idiopathic hypoparathyroidism is rare [65], although it may be commoner than once thought in the elderly [34]. Deficiency of ionized calcium enhances neuromuscular excitability. This is shown by the painful muscular spasms which may occur in the hands and feet (tetany) and the twitch of the mouth which can be produced by tapping the facial nerve within the parotid gland (Chvostek's sign). In severe cases there may be a grand mal convulsion. Personality disturbances may be found, verging on psychosis. This is most likely when the condition has been long-standing and in this case, there may be cataract, papilloedema and intracranial calcification in addition. Other features are rare, but there may be prolongation of the Q–T_c interval on the ECG. The diagnosis is confirmed by measurement of the plasma calcium level.

Treatment

After exclusion of alkalosis calcium ions should be given. The least irritant preparation is calcium gluconate, but calcium chloride is effective and widely used. The dose may need to be repeated several times during the day but if the condition persists, additional measures are needed. Calcium replacement can be continued orally and a vitamin D preparation should be added. Dihydrotachysterol in a dose of 1 mg daily may be employed, but 1-alpha-hydroxycholecalciferol is more reliable [64]. The natural hormone 1:25-dihydroxycholecalciferol may prove to be better still.

Synopsis of treatment

1) Consider and correct alkalosis.
2) Calcium gluconate, 10 ml 10% or 20% solution, given IV over 5–10 min. Repeat in 15 min if there is no response. In refractory cases, re-check plasma calcium concentration and arterial pH and measure the plasma magnesium concentration. For persistent true hypocalcaemia, infuse calcium as gluconate, 20 ml 10% solution in 1 litre 0.9% saline in 4 h.
3) Change to oral calcium after 24 h, two tablets of Calcium Sandoz every 6 h.
4) 1-alpha-Hydroxycholecalciferol, 1 μg PO. Start after 24 h if tetany continues on the above regimen.

N.B. Calcium and vitamin D therapy must be monitored by frequent estimations of the plasma calcium concentration. Measurement of ionized calcium is not needed for clinical purposes.

Magnesium problems

Disorders of magnesium metabolism have only recently been recognized. This ion has physiological properties which in some contexts resemble those of calcium and in others, those of potassium. The total body magnesium content of a 70-kg man is about 200 mmol, over 50% of which is in the skeleton. The plasma magnesium level is a poor indicator of total body reserves and is maintained within a narrow range of 1.4–1.8 mmol/litre.

Hypomagnesaemia

Abnormally low plasma concentrations of magnesium may occur in chronic states of diarrhoea, alcoholism, thiazide diuretic usage [58] and after the therapeutic irrigation of certain body cavities [47]. In addition, hypomagnesaemia often co-exists with hypocalcaemia from any cause, in which case it predisposes to tetany [22]. Pure magnesium deficiency is more likely to cause other neurological features, including grand mal convulsions, nystagmus and bulbar symptoms [35]. In addition, there may be cardiac arrhythmias [59].

Treatment

Oral administration of magnesium ions is not possible, because of their purgative action. Parenteral therapy must therefore be given if there is evidence of hypomagnesaemia. All magnesium salts irritate the tissues, the chloride being the best for clinical use. An infusion should be given of 20 mmol Mg^{2+} in 1 litre 0.9% saline over 2–4 h.

Hypermagnesaemia

This is virtually confined to patients with severe renal impairment. It results in lethargy, ataxia and eventually, cardiac arrest in diastole [41]. The clinical features are so vague that it is very difficult to make the diagnosis without first measuring the plasma magnesium concentration.

Treatment

The most effective treatment is haemodialysis, peritoneal dialysis being the second choice. There is at present no other useful therapeutic step.

References

1. Abuid J, Larsen PR (1974) Tri-iodothyronine and thyroxine in hyperthyroidism. Comparison of the acute changes during therapy with anti-thyroid agents. J Clin Invest 54:201
2. Astrom KE, Kugelberg E, Muller R (1961) Hypothyroid myopathy. Arch Neurol 5:472–482
3. Behn AR, West TET (1977) Emergency treatment with calcitonin of hypercalcaemia associated with multiple myeloma. Br Med J i:755
4. Benabe JE, Martinez-Maldenado M (1978) Hypercalcaemic nephropathy. Arch Intern Med 138:777–779
5. Bergh T, Nillius SJ, Wide L (1978) Clinical course and outcome of pregnancies in amenorrhoeic women with hyperprolactinaemia and pituitary tumours. Br Med J i:875
6. Blum M, Kranjaz T, Park CM (1976) Thyroid storm after cardiac angiography with iodinated contrast medium in a patient with a previously autonomous nodule of the thyroid. JAMA 235:2324–2325
7. Bravo EL, Tarazi RC, Gifford RW, Stewart BH (1979) Circulating and urinary cathecholamines in phaeochromocytoma New Engl J Med 301:682
8. Brenizer AG (1951) Suppurative strumitis caused by Salmonella Typhosa: Ann Surg 133:247
9. Brooks MH, Waldstein SS, Bronsky D (1975) Serum tri-iodothyronine in thyroid storm: J Clin Endocrinol Metab 40:339–441
10. Brooks MR, Baylis PH, Heath DA (1977) Diabetes insipidus and panhypopituitarism after pituitary infarction in acromegaly. Br Med J ii:369
11. Buchanan KD, McKiddie M, Reid M (1967) Respiratory acidosis in hypothermic myxoedema coma. Postgrad Med J 43:114
12. Burmann KD, Yeager HC, Earle JM (1975) Resin haemoperfusion, a potential new treatment for thyroid storm. Proceedings of the Seventh International Thyroid Conference, Boston, p 54
13. Cruetzig H, Kallfelz I, Haindl J (1976) Thyroid storm and iodine 131 treatment. Lancet 2:145
14. Daggett PR, Verner I, Carruthers M (1978) Intraoperative management of phaeochromocytoma with sodium nitroprosside. Br Med J 2:311
15. Dandona P, EL Kabir (1970) The effect of the injection of exophthalmic sera on the Harderian gland of the guinea pig. Clin Sci Mol Med 38:2p
16. Dandona P, Marshall NJ, Bidey SP, Nathan A, Havard CWH (1979) Successful treatment of exophthalmos and pre-tibial myxoedema with plasmapheresis. Br Med J i:374–376
17. Davis BB, Bloom ME (1969) Hyponatraemia in pituitary insufficiency. Metabolism 18:821
18. de Groot CJ, Stanbury JB (1975) The thyroid and its diseases. Wiley, London, p 456
19. Donaldson SS, Bagshaw MS (1972) Supervoltage orbital radiotherapy for Grave's ophthalmopathy. 48th Meeting of the Americal Thyroid Association 1972, p 55
20. Doran GR, Wilkinson JH (1975) The origin of the elevated activities of creatine kinase and other enzymes in the sera of patients with myxoedema. Clin Chim Acta 62:203–211
21. Downie WW, Gunn A, Paterson CR (1977) Hypercalcaemic crisis as a presentation of Addison's disease. Br Med J 1:145–146
22. Durlach J (1977) Magnesium in normocalcaemic tetany. Neurology (NY) 27:1181
23. Edwards CRW (1975) Diabetes insipidus In: Lant AF (ed) Proceedings of the Eleventh Symposium on Advanced Medicine. Pitman Medical, London, pp 276–288
24. Edwards CRW, Kitau MJ, Chard T, Besser GM (1973) Vasopressin analogue DDAVP in diabetes insipidus. Br Med J 3:375
25. Engelman K (1977) Phaeochromocytoma. Saunders, Philadelphia, pp 769–797 (Clinics in Endocrinology and metabolism, vol 6/3, pp 769–799)

26. Eriksson M (1977) Propranolol does not prevent thyroid storm. N Eng J Med 296:263–264

27. Evans RW, Glick B, Kimball F, Loebl M (1969) Fatal intravascular consumption coagulopathy in meningococcal sepsis. Am J Med 46:910

28. Eyland E, Sheba C (1957) Mumps virus and subacute thyroiditis evidence of a causal association. Lancet 1:1062

29. Forrester CF (1963) Coma in myxoedema. Arch Intern Med 111:734

30. Gitlow D, Bretani L, Ralzan A, Gribetz D, Dziedic S (1970) Diagnosis by qualitative and quantitative determination metabolites in urine. Cancer 25:1377

31. Goodwin TJ (1973) Addison's disease without pigmentation. Postgrad Med J 49:305–308

32. Gordon M (1967) Psychopharmacological agents, vol 2. Academic Press, New York

33. Graham JJ, Harding PE (1977) A case of myxoedema coma successfully treated by low dose oral tri-iodothyronine. Aust NZ J Med 7:163–168

34. Graham K, Williams BO, Rowe MJ (1979) Idiopathic hypoparathyroidism: A cause of fits in the elderly. Br Med J i:1460

35. Hamed IA., Lindeman RD (1978) Dysphagia and vertical nystagmus in magnesium deficiency. Ann Intern Med 89:222–223

36. Hazard JB (1955) Thyroiditis: A review. Am J Clin Pathol 25:289

37. Hellman R, Kelly RL, Mason WD (1977) Propranolol for thyroid storm. N Eng J Med 279:671–672

38. Hermann J, Kruskemper HL, Grosser KD (1971) Peritonealdialyse in der behandlung der thyrotoxischen crise. Dtsch Med Woschenschr 96:742

39. Hermann J, Hilger P, Kruskemper HL (1973) Plasmpheresis in the treatment of thyrotoxic crisis. Acta Endocrinol [Suppl] (Copenh) 173:22

40. Himathongkam T, Newmark SR, Greenfield M, Dluhy RG (1974) Acute adrenal insufficiency. JAMA 230:1317–1318

41. Hollinrake K, Thomas PK, Willis MR (1970) Observations on the plasma magnesium levels in patients with uraemic neuropathy under treatment with periodic haemodialysis. Neurology (NY) 20:939

42. Holvey DN, Goodner CJ, Nicoloff JT, Dawbrig JT (1964) Treatment of myxoedema coma with intravenous thyroxine. Arch Intern Med 113:89

43. Hung W, Migeon CJ (1968) Hypoglycaemia in a two-year-old boy with ACTH deficiency (Probably isolated) and adrenal medullary unresponsiveness. J Clin Endocrinol Metab 28:146

44. Impallomeni MG (1977) Unusual presentation of myxoedema coma in the elderly. Age Ageing 6:71–77

45. Ingbar W (1978) Thyroid storm or crisis. In: Werner SC, Ingbar SH (eds) The thyroid. Harper & Row, London, p 800

46. Jeffcoate WJ, Rees LH, Tomlin S (1977) Metyrapone in long-term management of Cushing's syndrome. Br Med J ii:215–217

47. Jenny DB, Goris GB, Urwiller RD, Brian R (1978) Hypermagnesaemia following irrigation of the renal pelvis. Cause of respiratory depression. JAMA 240:1378–1379

48. Lamberts SWJ, Seldenrath HJ, KWA HG, Birkenhager JC (1977) Transient bitemporal hemianopia during pregnancy after treatment of galactorrhoea amenorrhoea syndrome with bromocriptine. J Clin Endocrinol Metab 44:180

49. Lazarus JH, Addison GM, Richards RA, Owen (1974) Treatment of thyrotoxicosis with lithium carbonate Lancet II:1160

50. Liddle GW (1974) The Adrenals. In: Williams RH (ed) Textbook of endocrinology. Saunders, London, pp 233–322

51. Lins LE (1978) Reversible renal failure caused by hypercalcaemia. A retrospective study. Acta Med Scand 203:309–314

52. Mackin JF, Canary JJ, Pittman CS (1974) Thyroid Storm and its management. N Engl J Med 29:1396–1398

53. Martland HS (1944) Fulminating meningococcal infection with bilateral adrenal haemorrhage (the Waterhouse-Friedrichsen syndrome). Arch Pathol 37:147

54. Massry SG, Muellere E, Silverman AG, Kleeman CR (1968) Inorganic phosphate treatment of hypercalcaemia. Arch Intern Med 121:307

55. Mattingly D, Sheridan P (1978) Simultaneous diagnosis and treatment of acute adrenal insufficiency. Lancet I:432–433

56. McMahon MJ, Woodhead JS, Hayward RD (1978) The nature of hypocalcaemia in acute pancreatitis. Br J Surg 65:216–218

57. Merimee TJ, Felig P (1971) Glucose and lipid homeostasis in the absence of human growth hormone. J Clin Invest 50:574

58. Moore MJ (1978) Thiazide-induced hypomagnesaemia. JAMA 240:1241

59. Moore MJ, Flink EB (1978) Magnesium deficiency as a cause of serious arrhythmias. Arch Intern Med 138:825–826

60. Moss S, Greenbaum R, Sever PS (1978) Pre-operative localization of a phaeochromocytoma using plasma noradrenaline concentrations in multiple site samples. Proc R Soc Med 73:139

61. Nickerson JF, Hill SR, McNeil J, Barker S (1960) Fatal myxoedema, with and without coma. Ann Intern Med 53:475

62. O'Doriso TM (1978) Hypercalcaemic crisis. Heart Lung 7:425–434

63. O'Riordan JLH, Blanshard GP, Moxham A, Nabarro JDN (1966) Corticotrophin-secreting carcinomas. Q J Med 35:137

64. Parsons V (1977) The use of 1 alpha hydroxyvitamin D in the management of patients undergoing parathyroidectomy. Clin Endocrinol (Oxf) [suppl] 7:223s–224s

65. Philipson B, Angelin B, Christenson T, Einarsson K, Leijd B (1978) Hypocalcaemia with zonular cataract due to idiopathic hypoparathyroidism, with a note on the incidence of severe hypocalcaemia in health screening. Acta Med Scand 203:223–226

66. Pritchard BNC, Ross EJ (1966) Use of propranolol in conjunction with alpha blocking drugs in phaeochromocytoma. Am J Cardiol 18:394

67. Rees LH, Ratcliffe JG (1974) Ectopic hormone production by non-endocrine turmours. Clin Endocrinol (Oxf) 3:263–299

68. Robbins SL (1967) Textbook of pathology. Saunders, London, p 1233

69. Robinson JL (1972) Sudden blindness in pituitary tumours. J Neurosurg 36:83

70. Ross EJ, Pritchard BNC, Kaufman L, Robertson AIG, Harries BJ (1967) Pre-operative and operative management of patients with phaeochromocytoma. Br Med J i:191

71. Rumancik WM, Denlinger JK, Nahrwad ML, Falk RB (1978) The QT interval and serum ionized calcium: JAMA 240:366–368

72. Schaefer SD, Fee WE (1978) Thyroid Surgery: Surgical and metabolic causes of hypocalcaemia. Acta otolaryngol (Stockh) 104:263–266

73. Schweitzer VG, Thompson NW, Herness JK, Nishiyama RH (1978) Management of severe hypercalcaemia

caused by primary hyperparathyroidism. Arch Surg 112:1233–1234

74. Sheehan HL, Standfield JP (1961) The pathogenesis of post-partum necrosis of the anterior lobe of the pituitary gland. Acta Endocrinol (Copenh) 37:479

75. Singer FR, Neer RM, Murray TM (1970) Mithramycin treatment of intractable hypercalcaemia due to parathyroid carcinoma. N Engl J Med 283:634–636

76. Skowsky WR, Kikuchita (1978) The role of vasopressin in the impaired water extretion of myxoedema. Am J Med 64:613–621

77. Smith CK, Barish J (1972) Psychiatric disturbance in endocrinologic disease. Psychosom Med 34:69–86

78. Smolar EN, Rubin JE, Avramides A (1976) Cardiac tamponade in primary myxoedema and review of the literature. Am J Med Sci 272:345–352

79. Sobrinho LG, Nunes MCP, Santos MA, Mauricio JC (1978) Radiological evidence for regression of prolactinoma after treatment with bromocriptine. Lancet 2:257

80. Thalassinos N, Joplin GF (1968) Phosphate treatment of hypercalcaemia due to carcinoma. Br Med J iv:14

81. Volpe R (1978) Subacute (non-suppurative) thyroiditis. In: Werner SC, Ingbar SH (eds) The thyroid. Harper & Row, London

82. Volpe R, Johnston MW (1957) Subacute thyroiditis: A disease commonly mistaken for pharyngitis Can Med Assoc J 77:297

83. Wass JAH, Thorner MO, Charlesworth M, Moult PJA, Dacie JE, Jones AE, Besser GM (1979) Reduction of pituitary tumour size in patients with prolactinomas and acromegaly treated with bromocriptine with and without radiotherapy. Lancet II:66

84. Webster RA (1965) Effects of mephenesin and chlorpromazine on motor nerve discharges in the rabbit. Br J Clin Pharmacol 25:566

85. Weisberg LA (1977) Pituitary apoplexy: Association of degenerative change in pituitary adenoma with radiotherapy and detection by CT scanning. Am J Med 63:109

86. Wells I, Smith B, Hinton M (1977) Acute ileus in myxoedema. Br Med J 1:211–212

87. Woods KL, Holmes GK (1977) Myxoedema coma presenting in status epilepticus. Postgrad Med J 53:46–48

88. Zwillich CW, Ierson DJ, Hofeldt FD (1975) Ventilatory control in myxoedema and hypothyroidism. N Engl J Med 292:662–665

Section G

Trauma

Chapter 35

Multiple Injuries

Harry M. Delany and Arnold W. Berlin

Definition of multiple injury

Allgower, in a report on infection and trauma, defines 'polytrauma' as injury to any body cavity (head, thorax, or abdomen) together with one or more major fractures of long bone and pelvis or vertebrae [1]. Allgower states that extensive soft tissue damage may be substituted as equivalent to a major fracture. This definition is restrictive and excludes serious injury to two body cavities without fractures or extensive soft tissue injury. Multiple system injury of any type should be considered multiple trauma. The most appropriate definition of multiple trauma is the presence of injury to more than one body area or system. The currently popular indices of injury severity do not define multiple trauma but do provide a formula to relate the magnitude of injury to the prognosis of the patient. As an example, severity of injury measured by the injury severity score (ISS) is a function of the square of the three most seriously involved body areas categorized according to the extent of injury to an individual area (AIS) [10].

The presence of CNS trauma and other system injury is associated with a high mortality and morbidity. The mortality rate for chest and abdomen or pelvic injuries is 36%. For CNS and chest injuries it is 50%, and for CNS and abdomen or pelvic injury it is 55% [2]. The contribution of craniocerebral trauma to the overall mortality for a series of injuries in San Francisco was reported by Baker et al. [8] (Fig. 35.1 and Tables 35.1 and 35.2). Over 50% of the patients died of primary brain injury. The other major cause of death was blood loss due to major cardiac, vascular, or liver injury. Multiple injury is characteristic of the injuries sustained by victims of military conflict. Heaton states that for 3154 patients in World War II the injury-to-patient ratio was 1.55 [30]. Feltis stated that in Vietnam the ratio was 1.67 injuries per patient [26]. The experience with multiple injuries at the North Central Bronx Hospital in New York City for the period between March 1978 and March 1980 on a general surgical ward is typical for an urban American hospital. There were 504 patients admitted with the primary diagnosis of trauma. One hundred and ten patients, or

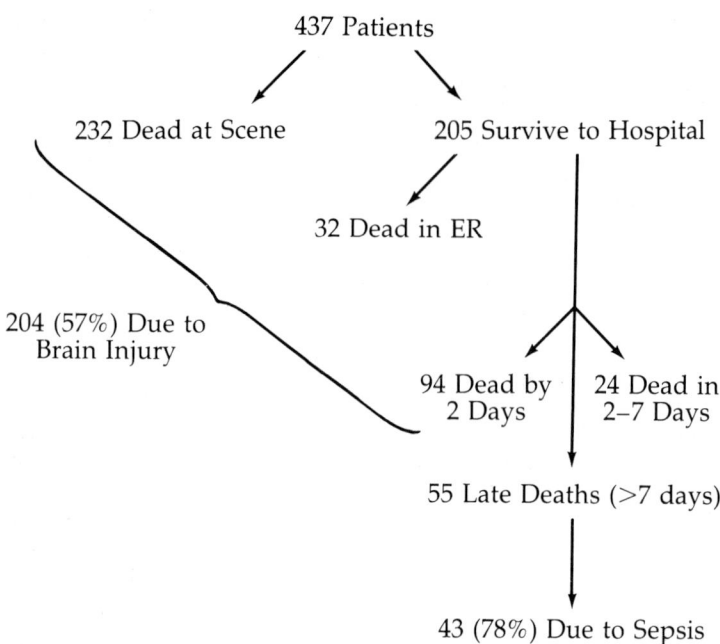

Fig. 35.1. Outcome and duration of survival in 437 patients who died from trauma in San Francisco in 1977. ER, emergency room. From Baker et al. [8].

Table 35.1. Mechanisms of injury in 437 patients dying of trauma in San Fransisco in 1977

Mechanism	Patients No.	Percentage
Gunshot wound	140	23.0
Fall or jump	122	27.9
Motor vehicle accident	52	11.9
Stab wound	35	8.0
Assault	33	7.7
Burn	29	6.6
Pedestrian struck by motor vehicle	26	5.9
	437	100

Data from Baker et al. [8].

Table 35.2. Causes of death in 437 patients dying of trauma in San Fransisco in 1977

Cause	Patients No.	Percentage
Brain injury	219	50.1
Heart or aortic injury	76	17.4
Hemorrhage	51	11.7
Sepsis	43	9.8
Lung injury	24	5.5
Burn	15	3.4
Liver injury	9	2.1
	437	100

Data from Baker et al. [8].

21.8%, suffered multiple injuries defined as multiple system, region, or organ injuries. There were 42 deaths in the 504 patients overall and 20 deaths (47%) occurred in patients with multiple trauma. Eighteen deaths were in patients with gunshot wounds, and 16 patients suffered blunt injuries. Eight deaths were recorded in patients with stab wounds.

A review of both military and civilian trauma experience reveals a number of similarities. The rapid transport of the injury victim has influenced the correlation between the condition of patients at the time of arrival at a trauma treatment center and prognosis. The resuscitation of the trauma patient is often rapid and successful in a modern setting. Yet the initially stable patient may expire at some later time from several complications of serious multiple injury. Trauma to several organs and systems has secondary effects compounding the problems produced by the specific injuries. Pulmonary insufficiency, fat embolism, negative nitrogen balance, vulnerability to sepsis, and multiple organ failure are such late effects. It is of great interest that the civilian and military trauma experience has resulted in a high mortality in the severely injured patient shortly after arrival at the treatment facility. Fifty-six percent of deaths occurred in the first 24 h after arrival, with a 33% mortality in the operating room in Vietnam [26]. A similar rising death rate during the early interval of resuscitation has been described in civilian trauma. In Baker's review of deaths from trauma in San Francisco, 53% of the patients were dead at the scene of the injury before transport could be accomplished, 7.5% of patients died in the emergency room, and 39.5% died in the hospital [8]. McNamara and Stremple reviewed the causes of death following combat injury in an evacuation hospital in Vietnam and found death was caused by hemorrhage, pulmonary insufficiency, and sepsis [45]. Forty-seven percent of patients in their series died shortly after admission. In a further review, this group appeared to be so severely injured that survival seemed remote. Pulmonary insufficiency was the cause of death in the majority of patients thought to be potentially salvageable. It is clear from this study that rapid and adequate volume resuscitation is quite important in the resuscitation of the military casualty; however, there is a potentially definable group that will go on to expire despite all available standard efforts.

With continuing improvements in the transport of civilian patients as in the combat situation, no doubt we will progressively narrow the time interval between injury and resuscitation. Only limited progress can be made in getting the victim to the hospital or trauma center, and a better definition will be obtained either by scoring indices or other measures to specify the patient who is beyond resuscitation. Baker states that only 1.3% of patients with an ISS greater than 60 lived longer than 1 week, while 6.2% of 289 patients with scores of 30–60 lived more than 1 week [8]. To achieve progress in reducing the mortality and morbidity for civilian trauma will require better treatment at the accident site, education of paramedics and physicians in advanced trauma life support, accident prevention, better automobile design for safety, enforcement of speed limits, and gun control.

Multiple system and multiple organ injury

The mortality and morbidity for multiple injury is much greater than for single organ trauma except for the involvment of critical organs, the heart, the great vessels, or the CNS. Exsanguination from the aorta, vena cava, or major blood vessels or destruction of the brain or high spinal cord can produce almost immediate demise of the injured patient. Injury to multiple organs in a given system without injury to other systems or body areas has not always been considered to be multiple trauma, but certainly should be included in this category. Most studies in multiple injury have focused on civilian blunt injury vehicular trauma, with less attention to assault-related injuries. However, the importance of injuries unique to the 'urban' environment has been described in a number of studies [23]. Several reports link specific individual organ injuries with association of other abdominal organ trauma. Multiple viscera involvement with blunt abdominal trauma was described by Kleinart et al. in 1961 [38]. They stated that the mortality rate with one organ involved was 8% with two organs, 38% and with three or more organs, 70%. With abdominal penetrating injuries a similar pattern of escalating mortality rate has been reported by Wilson et al. [71]. Feltis reviewed a surgical experience in a combat zone and found that patients with three organs injured suffered a 24.4% mortality, while patients with four or more organs injured suffered an 81.8% mortality [26]. Intraabdominal organ injury and associated extraabdominal organ injury can occur in a very significant percentage of cases. In a report by Steele and Lim on splenic injury, 116 of 183 patients (63%) with blunt injury involving the spleen had 291 associated injuries [66]. There were 67 intraabdominal associated injuries and 224 extraabdominal associated injuries. In their description of 58 patients with penetrating injuries involving the spleen, 41 of the patients had 118 associated injuries. In a large review of liver trauma by Defore et al., the correlation between the number of associated injuries and mortality was described [22]. Of the 1590 patients, 596 had isolated hepatic injuries. This represents approximately one-third of the series. The mortality for this group of patients was 4.4%. For patients with liver injury and three associated injuries, the mortality was 25.4%, and for patients with five or more injuries the mortality was 72.9%. In a report on blunt injuries to the small intestine by Cerise et al., 20 patients were described [18]. There were 11 associated abdominal organ injuries and 14 extraabdominal associated injuries. Colon injuries occur with a significant mortality and morbidity. The report from the Charity Hospital between 1972 and 1974 established the significant increase in this type of injury and the increasing incidence of associated injuries with trauma to the colon. The relatively high incidence of associated injuries with pancreatic trauma was described by White and Benfield [70]. There were associated injuries in 49 of the 63 patients reported with pancreatic trauma between 1965 and 1971 by their group. Of the six patients that died in their series, all were multiple trauma victims.

Clinical assessment and injury severity indices

The categorization of the severity of disease of acutely ill patients at the time of arrival in an emergency room for initial assessment by ambulance personnel, has currently focused on trauma. A number of injury severity indices have been described and correlated with mortality and biochemical variables (Table 35.3).

Table 35.3. Trauma-related scoring systems

Trauma index (IT)
Modified trauma index
Abbreviated injury scale (AIS)
Comprehensive injury scale
Injury severity score (ISS)
Therapeutic intervention scoring system
Cumulative illness rating score
Anatomic index

Although most of the available indices are imprecise and depend to a large extent on subjective assessment, the refinement of this form of categorization provides emergency services personnel and trauma medical trainees with an appreciation of the significance of one form of system injury and its relationship to another and the additive effect of multiple system trauma. The general principle that head and neck, abdomen, and chest are highly vulnerable regions for serious life-threatening injury and that cardiovascular instability or multiplicity of injury with major open fractures further increase the severity of the injury is incorporated into most trauma assessment scoring systems [14].

A sequence of proper clinical evaluation for purposes of defining treatment priorities is valuable in the education of trauma care personnel. However, some of the structured evaluation systems reach a level of considerable complexity and therefore will only have value for retrospective evaluation, comparative data studies, and clinical research. In an emergency with an acutely injured patient, time is not available for detailed injury categorization. The categorization for hospitalization at an appropriately staffed hospital is one use for simple trauma indices that may justify the time taken to make relatively simple determinations. As the regionalization of trauma services become more widespread, decisions for transport must be based on the patient's immediate condition. An example of a simplified system is the field categorization of trauma patients developed by the American college of Surgeon's Committee on Trauma [2]. Lindsay's trauma index and Ogawa's modification of the trauma index are other relatively easy systems for prehospital categorization [42, 50] (Table 35.4).

The relative value of the various currently described indices is reviewed by Cayton [17]. The trauma index gives numerical scores to region, type of injury, cardiovascular status, respiratory status and consciousness. Thus, the body area involved, the etiology of the trauma, and the condition of the patient measured by clinical evaluation and assessment of mental status are all integrated in the derived numerical score [36]. Unfortunately, the system is only numerical in the region-type injury and blood pressure values. Evaluation of the respiratory status and level of consciousness is not quantitated. The abbreviated injury scale is a numerical score for individual injuries [21]. When the AIS is used the injury is categorized by body area including head or neck, face, chest, abdominal or pelvic contents, extremities or pelvic girdle and general severity (1, minor; 2, moder-

Table 35.4. Modified trauma index for prehospital categorization of trauma patients

	Score 1	3	5	6
Region	Extremities	Back	Chest	Head and neck, abdomen
Type of injury	Laceration	Contusion	Stab wound	Blunt missile
Cardiovascular status	External hemorrhage	BP 60–100 P 100–140	BP < 60 P > 140	Absent pulses P < 55
Respiratory status	Chest pain	Dyspnea	Cyanosis	Apnea
Level of consciousness	Drowsy	Stupor	Semi-coma	Deep coma

Data from Ogawa and Sugimoto [50].

ate; 3, severe, not life-threatening; 4, severe, life-threatening, survival probable; 5, critical, survival uncertain). The comprehensive injury scale includes the category for threat to life, permanent impairment and treatment. The ISS is derived from the abbreviated injury score and can be determined by using the sum of the squares of the highest AIS values in each of the three most severely injured parts of the body [10]. The range of scores is 0–75. The therapeutic intervention scoring system and the cumulative illness rating scale are comprehensive illness scales that are not primarily indices of trauma [17].

The reliability of several of the injury score

systems has been confirmed in clinical study. The AIS and the ISS correlate with mortality (Figs. 35.2 and Fig. 35.3; Table 35.5) [9, 10]. The ISS has been confirmed as reliable in relationship to a number of other clinical criteria. In terms of the time period between injury and mortality, patients with ISS below 50 had the best potential for survival. Most of the patients that died in this group were alive 1 h after injury. Baker, in 1976, reported confirmation of the value of the ISS in comparing the data from 1033 hospital in-patients treated in the Birmingham Accident Hospital and 2128 highway injuries at eight Baltimore hospitals [9]. A correlation of the ISS with disability and mortality

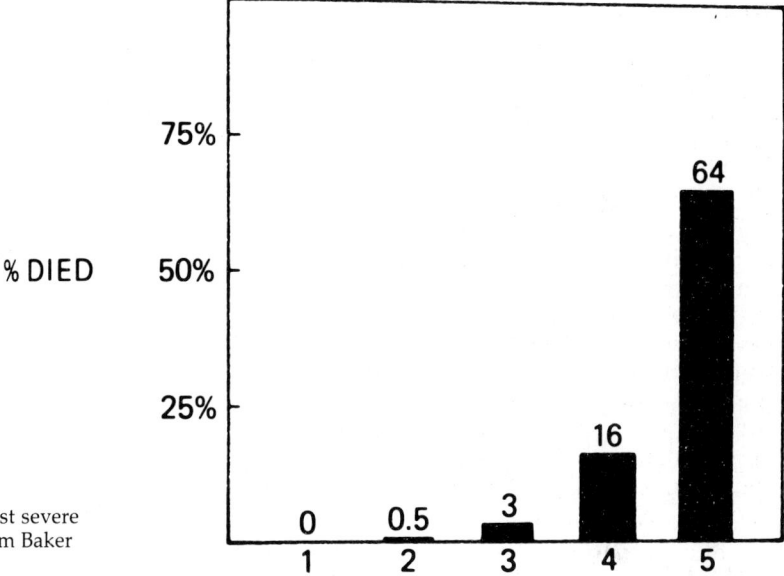

Fig. 35.2. Mortality by AIS grade of most severe injury included in the calculations. From Baker et al. [10].

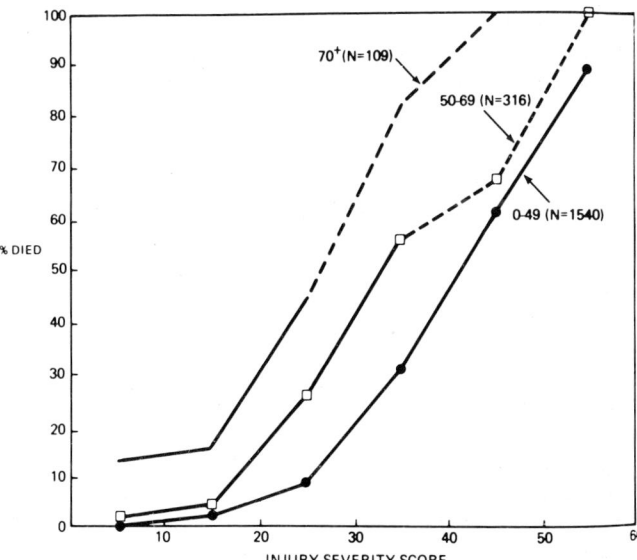

Fig. 35.3. Mortality by ISS for three age groups. Patients who were dead on arrival are excluded from calculations. *Dotted lines* connect points based upon fewer than ten persons. From Baker et al. [10].

Table 35.5. Outcome of multiple trauma by AIS grade of most severe injury in 2128 patients

AIS grade of most severe injury	Dead on arrival	Died later[a]	Admitted Survived	Unknown	Total No.	Percentage
1	0	0	80	1	81	4
2	0	2	437	1	440	20
3	6	23	997	20	1046	49
4	13	30	229	3	275	13
5	93	80	97	3	273	13
Unknown	1	0	12	0	13	1
Total no.	113	135	1852	28	2128	
Total %	5	6	88	1	100	100

Data from Baker et al. [10].
[a]Includes 34 patients who were alive on arrival but died before admissions procedures were completed.

was demonstrated. Oppenheim studied the ISS in relationship to initial blood metabolite concentrations in subsequent biochemical changes in 33 injured patients [51]. The study was designed to determine whether biochemical variables have a direct and predictable relationship to injury severity. At 4 h post injury, severity related directly to blood lactate, pyruvate, and alanine. In 19 patients, daily nitrogen, histidine and 3, methylhistidine excretion was measured for 7 days. Only total urinary nitrogen was clearly related to injury. A recent report by Champion introduced the anatomic index (AI) [19]. Despite the good correlation of the ISS with several injury parameters, the categorization of patients according to the ISS system depends on subjective determination of the injury severity. Champion substitutes the probability of mortality for individual injuries for the use of the abbreviated injury score. He further utilizes the ICDA or international classification of disease-adapted code as part of the system. In his report the ISS is compared to the AI for accuracy, and the AI predicts more death than the ISS. The AI overpredicts mortality rate, while the ISS underpredicts mortality rate (Table 35.6). The most valid suggested advantage of the AI is that it utilizes the classification system that is familiar to most hospital and medical records personnel and is easily adapted to computer use. Although injury severity scores and classification systems have not been used in most hospitals, the current study of these systems will ultimately effect area-wide, nation-wide, and eventually international correlation of data on injury. As subjective interpretation is replaced by accurate description and numerical classification, trauma care resources will be more appropriately distributed.

Systemic effects of multiple trauma

The sequence of hemodynamic and metabolic changes that occur following multiple trauma and the resuscitation of the multiple trauma patient are complex. These phenomena precipitate a score of secondary and tertiary reactions that contribute to the ultimate outcome for the patient. Despite the use of appropriate immediate measures for trauma patient resuscitation and initially good immediate response, some patients die after days or weeks of heroic critical care efforts. The appearance of sepsis, pulmonary insufficiency, multiple system organ failure, and stress bleeding are common terminal complications in the course of the multiple trauma victim.

Several subtle effects of massive trauma include changes in coagulation parameters, impaired host defense by a depressed reticuloendothilial system function, immunologic deficiency, hypoxemia with elevated free fatty acid levels in the blood, and impaired hepatic function reflected as hyperbilirubinemia in patients with hypotension [39, 49, 58, 60]. Sepsis is a frequent complication for the multiple injury patient who fails to respond to therapeutic measures late in the course of management. Despite the availability of potent and highly specific antibiotic preparations, the demise of the injury patient often relates to systemic infection. Fry et al. recently reported a study of 553 surgical patients at risk of multiple organ failure following major surgery [27]. Three hundred seventy-eight patients had emergency surgery for traumatic injuries, and 175 patients had emergency procedures for reasons other than

Table 35.6. Index performance in all patients in a large sample and in critically injured patients

| | All patients | | | | | |
| | ISS[a] | | | AI[b] | | |
	Predicted/ lived	Predicted/ died	Totals	Predicted/ lived	Predicted/ died	Totals
Lived	1086	4[c]	1090	1070	20[d]	1090
Died	45[e]	19	64	29[f]	35	64
Totals	1131	23	1154	1099	55	1154
	Critically injured patients					
	ISS[g]			AI[h]		
	Predicted/ lived	Predicted/ died	Totals	Predicted/ lived	Predicted/ died	Totals
Lived	84	3[j]	87	77	10[k]	87
Died	19[l]	18	37	11[m]	26	37
Totals	103	21	124	88	36	124

Data from Champion et al. [19].
[a]ISS total misclassification rate in all patients $= (4 + 49)/1154 = 4.7\%$.
[b]AI total misclassification rate in all patients $= (20 = 29)/1154 = 4.2\%$.
[c]False-positive rate $4/1090 = 0.37\%$.
[d]False-positive rate $20/1090 = 1.83\%$.
[e]False-negative rate $45/64 = 70.3\%$.
[f]False-negative rate $29/64 = 45.3\%$.
[g]ISS total misclassification rate in critically injured patients $= (3 + 19)/124 = 17.7\%$.
[h]AI total misclassification rate in critically injured patients $= (10 + 11)/124 = 10.97\%$.
[j]False-positive rate $3/87 = 3.4\%$.
[k]False-positive rate $10/87 = 11.5\%$.
[l]False-negative rate $19/37 = 51.4\%$.
[m]False-negative rate $11/37 = 29.7\%$.

trauma. The criterion for defining system organ failure was hypoxia requiring respiratory assisted ventilation for at least 5 days post operation or until death from pulmonary failure, and that for renal failure, serum creatinine levels of greater than 2 mg/dl. In patients with pre-existing renal disease, renal failure was defined as doubling of the admission creatinine. Hepatic failure was defined as a serum bilirubin level greater than 2 mg/dl with elevation of the SGOT and LDH to twice the normal values. Stress bleeding was considered the requirement for two units of blood replacement therapy within 24-h period from upper GI bleeding secondary to stress ulceration. In the analysis of the results of Fry's study, it was noted that for organ failure involving single organ systems, renal failure carried the highest mortality (72%) and liver failure carried the lowest (53%). The evaluation of multiple system organ failure (MSOF) revealed a progression of mortality with the number of organs involved from 30% for a single organ to a uniformly fatal outcome if there was four-organ failure (Tables 35.7 and

35.8). The major contribution of sepsis to the development of MSOF is demonstrated in the fact that all patients with failure of three or more organs had sepsis. Fifty-five patients died post-operatively and infection was the cause of death in 32. The etiology of infection in Fry's series was principally pulmonary or abdominal.

The importance of the vulnerability of the multiple injury patient to bacterial invasion and sepsis relates to several effects of massive trauma. The catabolic effects of hypermetabo-

Table 35.7. Incidence and mortality of postoperative organ failure by organ system in 553 patients[a]

System	No. of patients	No. dead	Mortality (%)
Lung	42	28	67
Liver	47	25	53
Kidney	39	28	72
Stress bleeding	17	10	59

Data from Fry et al. [27].
[a]Patients who underwent emergency operations

Table 35.8. Incidence and mortality of multiple organ failure in 553 patients[a]

Organ failures	No. of patients	No. dead	Mortality (%)
1	46	14	30
2	20	12	60
3	13	11	85
4	5	5	100
Multiple[b]	38	28	74

Data from Fry et al. (27).
[a]Patients who underwent emergency operations.
[b]Two or more organ failures.

lism and immune deficiency may both contribute to the development of systemic infection [40]. Reticuloendothelial system function deficiency demonstrated in the trauma patient is not clear in its influence of resistance to bacterial invasion. It seems reasonable to suppose that the effect of high blood levels of microaggregates and dysfunction in reticuloendothelial clearance capacity would reduce host defense. Effeney studied 48 patients with multisystem injury or nonseptic surgical illness [24]. In this study he relates intravascular coagulation to post injury sepsis (Tables 35.9 and 35.10). Massive transfusion is a factor in the introduction of platelet clumps, dead cells, and other particulate matter to the fibrin and platelet microemboli released by the syndrome of disseminated intravascular coagulation. Apparently some disseminated intravascular coagulation is common,

Table 35.9. Relationship of intravascular coagulation and post injury sepsis in 48 patients with multisystem injury or nonseptic surgical illness

Degree of coagulation	No. of patients	No. of infections	Survivors without infection
Severe	21	15 (71%)	1 (5%)
Moderate	16	10 (63%)	6 (27%)
Minimal	11	1 (9%)	10 (91%)

From Effeney et al. [24].

with extensive soft tissue injury and release of large amounts of thromboplastin. The supporting evidence for the theory that sepsis results from tissue injury and subsequent impairment of host defense includes evidence that blood opsonic protein (alpha 2 globulin) shows a rapid drop following injury [57]. Lymphocyte functions are inhibited by fibrin degradation products. The consumption of complement associated with intravascular coagulation impairs immune response. Leukocyte function has been demonstrated to be reduced in trauma victims, most of the substantial data recorded in burn patients [7]. It has further been suggested that blockade of accessory cells can affect the bacterial T cell interaction and modify immune activation.

Despite continuing and expanding confusion in the study of pulmonary failure in trauma and stress, the concepts of sepsis and infused debris in the etiology of respiratory insufficiency are still well established. Polk has suggested that the two concepts may be related in that a more active neutrophil population is aggregated in the pulmonary capillary bed and the resulting decrease in the circulating population of the neutrophils may affect resistance to infection [54].

Many studies have demonstrated an accelerated catabolism associated with multiple trauma, a systemic effect that is well known [47]. In addition to the catabolism associated with the initial stress of trauma, the multiple secondary problems of infection, fever, and the demands of wound healing, compound the negative nitrogen balance of multiple injury. The need for nutritional support in the form of early enteral and parenteral administration of protein and sufficient calories as carbohydrates and fats has gained increased attention as being fundamental to the support of the multiple trauma patient. The rapid development of protein calorie malnutrition as a result of profound negative balance will affect the patient response to infection, wound healing and respiratory function. Although the routine surgical patient will rarely require extraordinary nutritional sup-

Table 35.10. Location of infection versus intravascular coagulation (IVC) in 48 patients with multisystem injury or nonseptic surgical illness

Degree of IVC	Pneumonia	Septicemia	Peritonitis	Abscess	Urinary tract	Total
Severe ($n = 15$)	14	5	6	5	3	33
Moderate ($n = 10$)	9	4	0	0	0	13
Minimal ($n = 1$)	1	0	0	0	0	1

From Effeney et al. [24].

port, the massively injured patient needs such support. Trauma to the abdomen, thorax, and extremities usually affects a patient's ability to ingest an adequate diet. Aside from the mechanical interference with alimentation caused by GI injuries, the pain of major chest and extremity trauma and the effects on mood and appetite of analgesics will further prevent adequate enteral nutritional support. The aggressive use of nasogastric, jejunal, peripheral, or central-line IV techniques for feeding should be considered.

Early clinical considerations in multiple trauma patient management

In the initial management of the injured patient, many critical decisions must be made quickly, based only on clinical impression or incomplete laboratory data. Often aggressive therapeutic maneuvers must be instituted parallel with or before diagnostic procedures. Injured patients should be divided into three groups based on clinical status at arrival in an emergency medical service facility, as recommended by Steichen et al. [67]. The first group contains the 'lifeless' patients, so named because they do not have detectable vital signs and do not show signs of life. The next group are patients who arrive with systemic hypotension or shock. The third category is the group of patients who have suffered severe injury but do not have hypotension or other clinical signs of severe hypovolemia.

Therapeutic maneuvers must be instituted immediately for the lifeless patient. Treatment should be initiated purely on the basis of history and physical examination. The patient presenting in shock also needs immediate resuscitation. However, the tempo is less urgent and diagnostic maneuvers can often be conducted concurrently. The approach to the patient presenting in shock should be aggressive in determining the source of blood or fluid loss or circulatory compromise and in treatment of the condition. A patient suffering severe injury but not in shock and without signs of other circulatory or respiratory compromise presents a problem in diagnosis. In this situation the surgeon must anticipate the development of abrupt changes in the patient's clinical status.

A list of priorities for treatment must be established and routinely followed for the man-

agement of the injured patient and the sequence should begin with the most life-threatening and proceed to the progressively least serious (Table 35.11). The preparation and training of

Table 35.11. Priorities in management of multiple trauma

Impairment of airway or breathing
  Injuries of head and neck
    Facial fractures
    Tracheal injuries
    Intracranial injuries
    Injuries to cervical spine
  Injuries of the chest
    Simple pneumothorax
    Hemothorax
    Tension pneumothorax
    Sucking wounds
    Flail chest
Hypotension
  Hemorrhagic
    External bleeding
    Intrathoracic
    Intraperitoneal
    Retroperitoneal
    Fractures
  'Mediastinal'
    Tension pneumothorax
    Pericardial tamponade
  Other
    'Irreversible'
    Myocardial infarction
Neurosurgical trauma
  Brain
  Cord
Injuries producing peritonitis:
Ruptured intra- or retroperitoneal viscus
Burns
Lower GU tract (urethra, bladder)
Peripheral vascular
Musculoskeletal
Cold exposure

personnel for surgical and medical emergency services should include emphasis on a consistent routine in the approach to the problem of multiple severe injury. It has been recommended by Hopkins that formal algorithms may be helpful [33] (Fig. 35.4). The injuries of highest priority cause major compromise of the respiratory and circulatory status of the patient. The next injury group involves trauma that may threaten the life of the patient in the period following hospitalization but will not require immediate aggressive therapeutic effort. This latter group is typified by injuries to the CNS or injuries producing peritonitis or burns. Injuries of the lowest priority involve threat to the integrity of function of a portion of the body not essential to the survival of the patient, e.g., peripheral vascular or musculoskeletal injuries.

Throughout the initial resuscitation of any

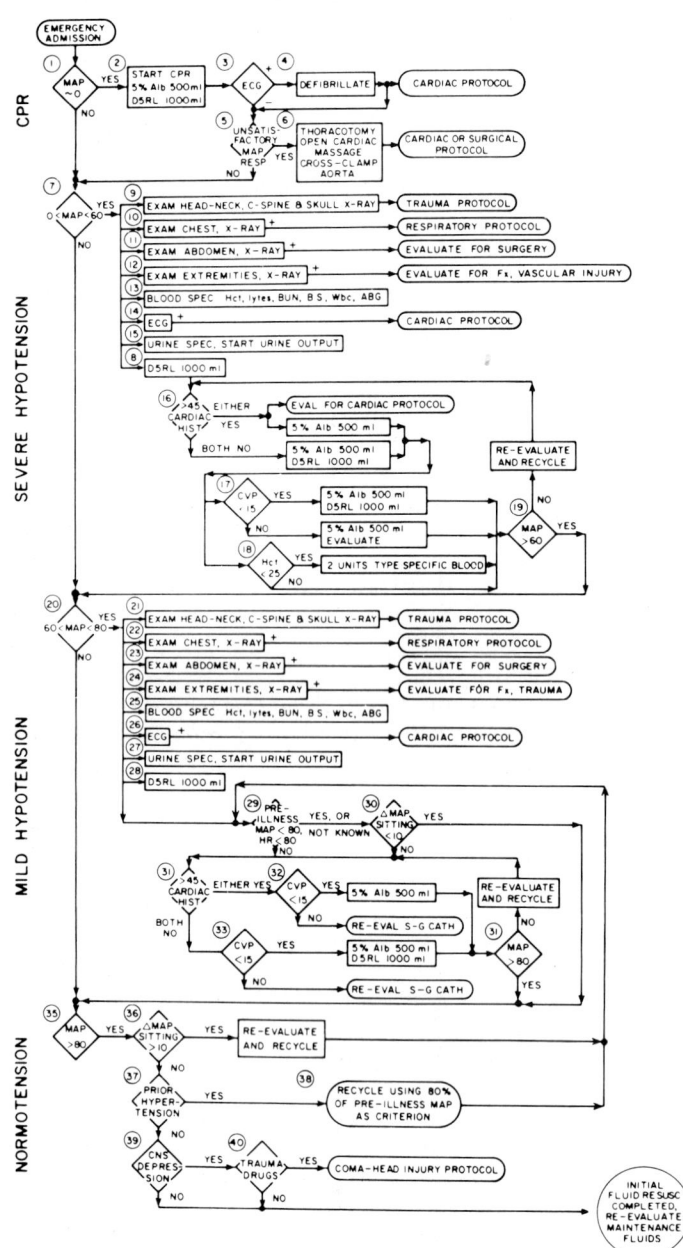

Fig. 35.4. Diagrammatic representation of an algorithm showing each step in a resuscitation procedure. *CPR*, cardiopulmonary resuscitation; *MAP*, mean arterial pressure; *Alb*, albumin; *D5RL*, 5% dextrose in lactated Ringer's solution; *Fx*, fractures; *lytes*, serum electrolytes; *B.S.*, blood glucose; *ABG*, arterial blood gas; *HR*, heart rate; *S-G Cath*, Swan-Ganz catheterization; *CVP*, central venous pressure. From Hopkins et al. [33].

trauma patient, injury to the cervical spine must be suspected [20]. When such a suspicion exists, lateral cervical spine films should be taken at the earliest possible opportunity. Until that time the patient must be managed as if an injury to the cervical spine is present, avoiding flexion and hyperextension of the neck. In many major hospitals members of both the emergency room staff and surgical staff are available to assist in the resuscitation of the trauma victim. When adequate staff is available several problems can be managed concurrently [73].

The senior, most experienced member of the team should assume responsibility for directing the resuscitation. It is important for this person to maintain a continued awareness of the progress of the resuscitation effort. They must be attentive to details, including a check that the blood bank and the radiology department are notified of the emergency, and should be aware of the rate and type of IV fluids administered. It is the senior surgeon's responsibility to decide when the patient is transfused, when the patient should be intubated, whether a chest tube should be inserted, whether the patient should have a paracentesis, and most of all, whether the patient should go to the operating room and when.

Specific priorities in management of the multiply injured

Airway and ventilation

Injuries that impair breathing have the highest and most urgent priority. The primary therapeutic effort should be directed at insuring a secure, patent airway and achieving adequate ventilation. Recognition of ventilatory insufficiency is of prime importance and involves both physical examination and laboratory studies. Patients who demonstrate restlessness, tachypnea, agitation, or cyanosis must be considered for immediate ventilatory support. Arterial blood gases should be obtained, but it is sometimes necessary to initiate therapy on the basis of the clinical impression alone.

The simplest technique for airway management is often the best. If possible, an oropharyngeal or nasopharyngeal airway combined with Ambu bag ventilation should be employed first. Intubation hastily performed by inexperienced personnel may produce trauma to the larynx. When the attempt at intubation is unsuccessful or prolonged it may delay the effective ventilation of patients who are already hypoxic. A mask should be utilized until the patient is well ventilated and then alternative techniques used under controlled circumstances [4]. These techniques include endotracheal intubation by the oral or nasal routes, and emergency cricothyroidotomy or tracheostomy.

The injuries that most often interfere with respiratory function are trauma to the head, neck and chest: these are divided into those that physically block the airway and those that interfere with the mechanical process of ventilation. The airway may be occluded by a foreign body or secretion and can sometimes be cleared manually or with suction. Active bleeding into or from the oropharanx may justify the prompt use of an endotracheal tube. However, if secretions or bleeding obscure proper visualization of the larynx, some form of emergency laryngotracheal access should be obtained either by formal tracheostomy or cricothyroidotomy, as recently suggested by Boyd [13]. Facial bone fractures may also cause airway obstruction. A bilateral mandibular ramus fracture may cause occlusion of the airway by posterior displacement of the tongue. In this situation simple traction on the jaw and/or tongue in the forward direction will open the airway. An airway splint or mouthpiece should then be inserted.

Neck injuries which have produced displacement and compression of the airway secondary to bleeding or with penetrating injury directly violating the trachea may compromise ventilation. An expanding mass in the neck should be managed by prompt endotracheal intubation, if possible. Emergency tracheostomy in the presence of massive hemorrhage into the substance of the neck may be very difficult. Respiratory obstruction associated with crepitus in the neck suggests injury to the trachea or larynx and may be more safely managed by neck exploration and emergency tracheostomy. In some injuries involving the larynx and trachea it may be impossible to pass an endotracheal tube beyond the injury and attempting to do so will produce further damage.

A second category of injuries that impair respiratory function interfere with the mechanics of ventilation; examples are flail chest, simple pneumothorax, sucking thoracic wounds, and tension pneumothorax. According to Symbas, a flail chest is defined as multiple fractures of three or more adjacent ribs or one fracture with costochondral separation or with a fracture of the sternum [68]. A segment of unstable chest wall is created that moves paradoxically during respiration. Paradoxical motion and concurrent shifts of the mediastinum decrease tidal volume.

The size of the injured flail chest wall segment will determine whether the patient's condition is stable without treatment or whether there is hypoventilation and respiratory insufficiency. The current management of this problem is sequential repeated evaluation of the patient's respiratory status. If clinical evidence of respiratory distress exists or blood gas determinations demonstrate hypoventilation, endotracheal intubation with positive pressure breathing is indicated. If the flail chest does not lead to respiratory compromise, then the complications of the use of mechanical ventilation (MV) may be avoided [61].

A sucking wound results from an opening in the chest wall. The lung collapses due to the atmospheric pressure in the pleural space and the opening, if large enough, competes with the trachea for ventilatory exchange. In addition, if the wound behaves like a flap valve, allowing air to enter the pleural space during inspiration but preventing it from escaping during expiration, a tension pneumothorax develops. For a sucking chest wound the proper treatment consists in the application of an occlusive vaseline dressing to the wound and drainage of the pleural space with a thoracostomy tube.

High transection of the spinal cord is an injury which will impair the mechanics of ventilation causing paralysis of intercostal muscles and the diaphragm. In this situation adequate ventilation must be assured by mask or endotracheal intubation.

Shock

Hypotension must be managed quickly and aggressively. Diagnostic maneuvers are begun as soon as feasible, but the resuscitation effort must be initiated on the basis of the available clinical and laboratory data.

The majority of hypotensive multiple injury patients are hypovolemic from blood loss. However, hypotension may be the result of other factors. The most common form of non-hypovolemic hypotension is 'pump' failure, as in tension pneumothorax, pericardial tamponade, or myocardial infarction. The occurrence of myocardial infarction in a patient driving a car may cause an accident and severe injury. In hypovolemic patients, coronary hypoperfusion can cause myocardial infarction, and an initial period of hemorrhage and hypovolemia becomes complicated by cardiogenic shock. Similarly, any patient subjected to prolonged hypotension may prove refractory to resuscitation. This form of hypotension has been termed intractable or irreversible shock and may be due to continued hypoperfusion with accumulation of toxic products and failure of energy metabolism at the cellular level [56].

Assessment of the patient with multiple injuries

Physical examination

A very rapid initial examination of the trauma patient must be performed. While the vital signs are being determined, the airway is secured and ventilatory support begun if needed. The patient should then be inspected for gross signs of severe injury, such as sucking wounds of the chest or massive external hemorrhage. Findings suggesting internal injury should be noted, such as penetrating wounds, external contusions, abrasions, or hematomas. For appropriate examination, the patient must be completely undressed and thoroughly inspected. The head

should be examined for swelling or lacerations. If abnormalities are present they should be probed with the gloved hand feeling for skull fractures. The pharynx is inspected for injury or obstruction and the tympanic membranes viewed for signs of hemotympanum. The neck should be inspected for penetrating injury, swelling, or distention of the neck veins. The neck should also be palpated for subcutaneous crepitus or spinal tenderness, and the trachea palpated for shift from the midline position. The chest is examined for contusions, areas of paradoxical motion, tenderness or subcutaneous crepitus. Physical examination of the abdomen in the multiply injured patient may be unreliable. Serious retroperitoneal or intraperitoneal pathology may not produce dramatic findings on physical examination. For example, the presence of intraperitoneal blood is quite variable in its manifestations, ranging from severe peritoneal irritation to absence of significant findings [20, 73]. In addition, CNS injury to either brain or spinal cord may blunt the clinical response to peritoneal reaction. For this reason, more objective techniques for assessing the abdomen have been developed [16, 69].

There are several important special considerations in the physical examination. The diaphragm rises to the nipple line and penetrating wounds at or below this level may involve subdiaphragmatic structures. The status of bowel sounds should be assessed. Loss of bowel sounds may be an important indication of intraabdominal injury [62]. Kehr's sign is pain at the tip of the shoulder from diaphragmatic irritation and can be elicited by palpation deep in the left upper quadrant [43]. In blunt injury of the perineum in the male, injury to the urethra may occur. The classic triad suggesting urethral trauma is blood at the urethral meatus, 'floating' prostate detected on rectal examination, and inability to void spontaneously. The presence of blood on rectal examination suggests a colorectal injury. Of course, the bladder should be catheterized as both a diagnostic and therapeutic procedure, and the urine checked for blood. If urethral injury is suspected, a urethrogram should be performed by a catheter placed at the meatus before forceful insertion of a Foley catheter to avoid tearing the injured urethra [54].

Thoracostomy and paracentesis

Invasive techniques aid in identifying the source of major hemorrhage from the chest and abdomen. The presence of decreased breath sounds associated with hypotension or respiratory distress should be treated with prompt insertion of a thoracostomy needle or tube. Penetrating wounds in the region of the heart or mediastinum accompanied by shock or hypotension unresponsive to fluid resuscitation is an indication for emergency thoracotomy. A pericardiocentesis may be indicated in diagnosis and treatment of pericardial tamponade. In this situation, pericardial drainage may be performed as a temporary measure prior to thoracotomy [15]. If life-threatening chest injury is suspected therapeutic efforts should be accomplished promptly and without waiting for a preliminary chest x-ray.

Abdominal paracentesis with lavage has been proven to be over 95% accurate in the diagnosis of intraabdominal bleeding [69]. A catheter with multiple openings is inserted through the infraumbilical midline and any intraperitoneal fluid withdrawn. A peritoneal dialysis-type catheter or modification is used and may be inserted percutaneously or via a minilap [41]. A return of gross blood is considered positive. If blood is not returned, 1 litre normal saline for adults or 15 ml per kg body weight for children is infused into the peritoneal cavity then siphoned by gravity. Although interpretations may vary, a red cell count of 50 000–100 000 cells cm^3 is considered positive for a significant abdominal injury [25, 34]. A WBC count in the lavage fluid of >500 ml or elevation of the peritoneal fluid amylase are also considered positive findings [25]. Abdominal x-rays should be performed before paracentesis and lavage to avoid incorrect interpretation of pneumoperitoneum.

At the Albert Einstein College of Medicine we favor the liberal use of paracentesis and lavage as a diagnostic technique in the multiply injured, for the following reasons: (1) Physical examination can be inaccurate in evaluating the abdomen in the multiply injured, especially in the patient with neurological injury: (2) the test can be performed quickly and safely, with a low morbidity [25]; and (3) the results are accurate and reliable for identifying blood in the peritoneal cavity. Several large studies have shown a total false-positive and -negative rate of less than 4% [25, 69].

x-Ray examination

The presence of fracture of the first rib is of special significance. This structure is well protected and strong force is required to cause a fracture [37]. A patient with a fracture of the first rib is at high risk for associated injuries of the mediastinum and great vessels. Inspection of the lung fields may reveal pneumo- or hemothorax as well as parenchymal pathology. Interstitial infiltrates that are present on admission usually represent pulmonary contusion. Careful attention should be given to the x-ray appearance of the mediastinal structures. An enlarged heart shadow may represent a pericardial effusion or tamponade. A widened superior mediastinum is a most important finding, and may be due to a hematoma arising from rupture of the aorta or other mediastinal vascular structure. Additional findings that should suggest a traumatic aortic aneurysm are obliteration of the aortic nob, depression of the left main stem bronchus, and displacement of a nasogastric tube to the right and posteriorly [72]. Deceleration aortic injury usually occurs at the aortic isthmus, the relatively fixed point just distal to the take-off to the left subclavian artery. The tear may be of the intima, intima and media, or the entire wall. Of patients with this injury, 80%–90% die at the scene of accident [37]. Surviving patients have a mediastinal hematoma contained by adventitia or pleura. Suspicion of aortic injury must be high, because over 90% of the hematomas will rupture within minutes to hours following admission. Aortography must be performed promptly if the patient's condition can be stabilized for the procedure.

x-Ray pictures of the abdomen may show enlargement of the hepatic or splenic shadows suggesting a hematoma. Extraluminal peritoneal air indicates laceration or perforation of a viscus. Air bubbles in the supracolic compartment of the abdomen may be caused by rupture of the retroperitoneal duodenum. The radiologic appearance of the vertebral column should be inspected for fractures, especially if the patient has sustained a fall. An x-ray of the pelvis should be taken in patients who have sustained blunt injury. Fractures of the pelvic bones, especially of the posterior arch, are associated with significant bleeding and retroperitoneal hematomas [52].

x-Ray pictures of the skull may document fractures although neurosurgical intervention is currently dictated by CT scanning or cerebral angiography. For genitourinary (GU) tract injury, a 'one-shot IVP' may be obtained [19]. This one-shot study may yield valuable information, such as the location and the function of the patient's kidneys or injury to a portion of the GU tract.

ECG

Myocardial contusion has been recognized as an important entity in the multiply injured patient [59]. It occurs in between 15% and 75% of cases of blunt injury to the sternum and chest wall. A 12-lead ECG should be performed to look for myocardial injury. The only evidence of myocardial contusion may be the presence of an arrhythmia. Sinus tachycardia and atrial arrhythmia are most common in this situation. Other ECG findings range from nonspecific ST and T-wave changes to frank injury current.

The outlined scheme for diagnosis for the multiple injury patient can be clinically applied in a very short time. The more stable the clinical condition of the patient, the more diagnostic effort can be applied, and the more accurate the diagnosis. Nonetheless, it is important to emphasize that the institution of treatment of the hypotensive patient with multiple injuries assumes priority over diagnostic studies.

Treatment of the patient with multiple injuries

Basic cardiopulmonary resuscitation

Standard techniques for cardiopulmonary resuscitation should be applied in the presence of cardiac arrest [4]. For trauma patients the resuscitation technique may require modification because with hypovolemia and cardiac arrest, cardiac function may be more effectively assisted by open-chest cardiac massage than by a closed-chest technique.

Intravenous access

The multiply injured patient must have several large-bore intravenous catheters inserted as soon as possible. Large-bore catheters inserted into a peripheral vein are satisfactory for infusion but these veins may be collapsed or inaccessible in the patient in shock. One can also utilize the central veins, cannulated via either supra, infraclavicular or femoral routes.

Fluid resuscitation

Rapid and adequate circulatory volume expansion is the most important principle of resuscitation in the management of patients suffering hypovolemic hypotension. A blood volume loss of >25% will produce a BP of 70–90 and a pulse rate of 110–130. A volume loss of 50% will produce a BP of 0–50 or 'no BP' [46]. Therefore, a 70-kg adult male presenting with a BP of 50 mmHg may be assumed to have lost as much as 2500 cm^3 blood. An IV infusion should be started and continued rapidly until there is evidence of a response measured by improved vital signs. Red cells must be replaced as soon as possible. The predominant use of blood is in the form of component therapy. Therefore, red cells are transfused initially, with clotting factors given separately as needed. In the lifeless patient it may be justified to start type O-negative blood as soon as possible; otherwise type-specific red cells are used. There is controversy as to the other types of fluid to be given prior to the blood and as added volume to the blood transfusion. The use of serum protein-containing solution is favoured by some [64, 65]. It is felt that colloids provide higher serum oncotic pressure and do not rapidly extravasate from the vascular system. Therefore, in theory, the patient's volume will be restored more efficiently and for a longer period of time. In addition, it is argued that maintaining fluid in the vascular compartment will prevent the development of posttraumatic adult respiratory distress syndrome. Advocates of the use of so-called crystalloid or balanced salt solutions, such as Ringer's lactate, maintain that although more fluid is required, crystalloids are satisfactory for volume replacement and do not predispose to development of adult respiratory distress syndrome [44]. Studies of the problem have failed to demonstrate a difference in pulmonary parameters, light or electron microscopy of lung substance, or measurements of lung water in animals resuscitated with shed blood and either crystalloid or colloid solutions [32, 48]. Shires has shown an advantage in favor of balanced salt solution over colloids in resuscitating dogs subject to hemorrhagic shock [63]. The explanation is that when an organism is subjected to hemorrhagic shock the interstitial space becomes depleted of sodium and water, and interstitial fluid is lost into the vascular space in an attempt to re-establish volume. However, sodium and water from the interstitium have also been shown to enter the cells during hemorrhagic shock. The end-effect is a severely shrunken interstitial fluid compartment depleted of salt and water. Resuscitation with a balanced salt solution has been shown to replete this important compartment.

Crystalloid is inexpensive. It is an effective volume expander and has the advantage of restoring the interstitial space, and it does not predispose to an increase in lung water. Our preference is for the use of balanced salt solutions in combination with packed red cells in the resuscitation of hemorrhagic shock.

Medication

Sodium bicarbonate

Metabolic acidosis is a common complication of severe trauma. It is generally a lactic acidosis resulting from tissue underperfusion. Acidosis is of some benefit to the hypotensive trauma patient, in that metabolic acidosis shifts the oxyhemoglobin dissociation curve to the right, increasing oxygen release in the underperfused tissue. When the serum pH is greater than 7.25, buffer does not have to be given. Below this level sodium bicarbonate should be administered. If a patient suffers cardiac pulmonary arrest, 1 mmol sodium bicarbonate/kg is given initially, and repeated every 10 min until cardiac function returns [4].

Diuretics

Oliguria in the trauma patient is invariably the result of renal hypoperfusion secondary to hypovolemia. The proper therapy to increase urine output is to restore circulating blood volume. Mannitol is a drug that both increases glomerular filtration rate and expands blood volume, and can be considered for use in this situation. Potent loop diuretics, such as frusemide or ethacrynic acid, should not be used. Their effect would be further dehydration of the already volume-depleted patient. If urine output does not improve after adequate restoration of circulating blood volume, acute tubular necrosis (ATN) may have developed. A diagnosis of ATN is established if the urine is iso-osmotic with plasma, has high urine sodium concentration, and has red cells and tubular casts. In early ATN, diuretics do not reverse the syndrome but may convert low- to high-output renal failure [12]. Since the management of high-output failure is easier, a dose of frusemide may be indicated in suspected early ATN, but 'beating' the kidneys with massive doses of diuretics to reverse or prevent ATN is not warranted.

Vasopressors

Vasopressors such as noradrenaline, which increase vascular tone via sympathetic alpha vasoconstriction, are absolutely contraindicated in a patient with hypovolemic hypotension. A patient of this type is already physiologically vasoconstricted and further pharmacologic vasoconstriction combined with the volume-contracted state magnify the effects of ischemia on the brain, heart, kidney, and viscera. On the other hand, some patients initially in hypovolemic shock may progress to 'irreversible' shock or may suffer a myocardial infarction [55]. A complicating component of shock in this situation can be pump failure, in which case the use of cardiotonic drugs would be indicated. It is imperative to be aware of the volume and cardiac status of the patient, and 'blind' use of vasoconstrictor drugs without this information is improper.

Specific management problems

External blood loss

Massive external bleeding is invariably well controlled by direct manual pressure. The use of a constricting tourniquet on an extremity is contraindicated. A tourniquet may be ineffective in controlling arterial bleeding and will compress veins, producing increased venous hemorrhage. On occasion, pressure must be maintained in a bleeding wound while the patient is taken to the operating room.

Abdomen

If peritonitis or intraabdominal blood loss is present then exploratory laparotomy is indicated. An exception to this rule may be blood loss associated with a pelvic fracture. Although grossly positive peritoneal lavage in this situation is treated by laparotomy, a microscopically positive tap may not indicate intraperitoneal bleeding. In this instance clinical judgment must be exercised when deciding upon laparotomy [35]. Any patient who has sustained abdominal trauma with rapid blood loss and unstable vital signs despite rapid transfusion should be taken directly to the operating room. Laparotomy should not be performed in the emergency department unless that area is equipped as a formal operating room.

Retroperitoneum and kidney

Most patients with trauma to the kidney can be managed nonoperatively. A patient suspected of having an injury to the kidneys should have an IVP. A renal vascular injury should be suspected if there is nonvisualization of either kidney on IVP. Angiography should be performed, and the results will indicate whether the injury can be corrected surgically. Late filling or frank extravasation of contrast material in a stable patient can be managed expectantly.

Pelvis

Fracture of the pelvis is frequently associated with multiple injuries and is often accompanied by massive retroperitoneal bleeding [52]. Several new techniques for management of bleeding from pelvic fracture are available. Initially, external compression and tamponade can be attempted by the application of the MAST or military anti-shock trousers [11]. If pelvic bleeding continues, angiography should be performed and endovascular occlusion of the bleeding vessels used. Embolization can be performed with Gelfoam or autogenous clots via the angiography catheter [6]. If nonoperative techniques for controlling bleeding are unsuccessful and transfusion requirement exceeds 8 to 10 units, surgical exploration of the pelvic retroperitoneum is indicated. Direct surgical control of the bleeding vessels is often very difficult. Although of questionable value, in this situation hypogastric artery ligation or even packing of the pelvis may be performed [53]. Earlier exploration may be indicated with complete sacroiliac joint disruption associated with massive bleeding. This injury may suggest a tear of the iliac vein [29].

Chest

The prompt recognition and treatment of injuries is crucial to the survival of the injured patient. An x-ray examination of the chest is necessary in all severely injured patients. If there are decreased breath sounds, hypotension, or respiratory distress, or if a chest x-ray picture demonstrates a pneumo-, hydro-, or hydropneumothorax, a needle is immediately placed into the thorax and followed by insertion of an intercostal catheter.

Simple pneumothorax results from air in the pleural space causing collapse of the lung. The air may be introduced from the outside or escape from a hole in the lung or airway. There is a loss of function in the collapsed lung but no disturbance of cardiovascular physiology. Most simple pneumothoraces are well tolerated.

A tension pneumothorax causes collapse of the ipsilateral lung and pushes the mediastinum to the opposite side. There is compression of the contralateral lung and distortion of the great vessels with impaired venous return to the heart. There is decreased cardiac filling, elevated CVP, respiratory distress and hypotension. This sequence is easily reversed by insertion of a needle to vent the tension, converting a tension to a simple pneumothorax. The placement of an intercostal catheter is sufficient treatment for simple pneumothorax and the majority of hemothoraces.

Bleeding from the chest most often comes from low-pressure pulmonary circulation, and re-expansion of the lung is all that is required to tamponade the bleeding. While the lung is 'down' bleeding may continue into the chest until the lung is re-expanded. The initial insertion of the chest tube may result in return of large volumes of blood. With the tube in place, a chest x-ray should be taken to determine whether there has been complete evacuation of the hemothorax and expansion of the lung. From this time on, the rate of blood loss through the catheter should be carefully recorded. Thoracotomy is recommended when blood loss through the chest tube exceeds 300–500 cm^3/h for 2–3 h or is greater than 200 cm^3/h for 5 h [37]. Bleeding of this severity is usually from a systemic artery, such as an intercostal or internal mammary artery. Bleeding from these vessels is under systemic pressure and not controlled by expansion of the lung. A thoracotomy is also indicated if a clotted hemothorax occurs or an increasing hemothorax is shown on subsequent chest x-ray pictures. The occurrence of massive initial chest tube drainage (greater than 2 liters) may be an indication for immediate thoracotomy if the patient does not rapidly respond to initial volume replacement [37]. An immediate emergency room thoracotomy should be considered on the lifeless patient with a penetrating thoracic wound when suspicion of a cardiac or major vessel injury is high. Salvage of such lifeless patients is reported [5].

Mediastinum

Mediastinal injury may produce hypotension in two ways. Injury of the heart or great vessels may produce massive and sudden blood loss or pericardial tamponade. The latter occurs when a small wound in the pericardium does not allow the escape of blood from the pericardial sac. Bleeding results in the rapid increase in pressure in the nondistensible pericardium, with obstruction of venous return to the heart and subsequent impaired filling of the cardiac chambers, decrease in cardiac output, and hypotension. Pericardial tamponade must be suspected in chest wounds when hypotension is associated with an elevation in the central venous pressure. Although pericardiocentesis may be helpful in diagnosis and even act as a temporizing maneuver, the definitive treatment of pericardial tamponade is immediate thoracotomy, release of the tamponade, and control of hemorrhage [15]. Although rare, injury to the esophagus should be suspected if there is radiologic evidence of pneumomediastinum. The diagnosis of esophageal injury can be confirmed by water-soluble contrast esophagram. Esophageal perforation requires early drainage of the area and direct suture repair of the injury.

References

1. Allgower M Durig M, Wolff G (1980) Infection and trauma. Surg Clin North Am 60:133–144
2. American College of Surgeon's Committee on trauma. (1980) Field categorization of trauma patients and hospital trauma index. Bull ACS 65 2:28–33
3. American College of Surgeon's Committee on Trauma (1980) Instructor's Manual: Advanced trauma life support course. ACS, New York
4. American Heart Association (1975) Advanced cardiac support instructor's manual. AMA, Dallas
5. Asfaw I, Arbolo A (1977) Penetrating wounds of the pericardium and heart. Surg Clin North Am 57:37–49
6. Athanasoulis CA (1980) Therapeutic applications of angiography. N Engl J Med 302:1121
7. Baker CC, Miller CL, Trunkey DD (1979) Predicting fatal sepsis in burn patients. J Trauma 19:641–648
8. Baker CC, Oppenheimer L, Stephens B, Lewis FR, Trunkey DD (1980) Epidemiology of trauma deaths. Am J Surg 140:144–150
9. Baker SP, O'Neil B (1976) The injury severity score: An update. J Trauma 16:882–885
10. Baker SP, O'Neill B, Haddon W Jr, Long WB (1974) The injury severity score: A method for describing patients with multiple injuries and evaluating emergency care. J Trauma 14:187–196
11. Batalden DJ, Wickstrom PH Ruiz E, Gustilo R (1974) Value of the G-Suit in patients with severe pelvic fracture. Arch Surg 109:326–328
12. Beck CH (1980) Acute renal failure: Prevention and amelioration. Delivered at 8th Annual Intensive Care Symposium. University of Miami
13. Boyd AD, Romita M, Colon A, Fink S, Spencer F (1979) A clinical evaluation of cricothyroidotomy. Surg Gynecol Obstet 149:305–308
14. Boyd DR, Lowe RJ, Baker RJ, Nyhus LM (1973) Trauma registry. New computer method for multifactorial evaluation of a major health problem JAMA 223:422–428
15. Breaux EP, Dupont JB Jr, Albert HM, Bryant LR, Schecter FG (1979) Cardiac tamponade following penetrating mediastinal injuries: Improved survival with early peri-

cardiocentesis. J Trauma 19:461–466
16. Carnevale N, Baron N, Delany HM (1977) Peritoneoscopy as an aid in the diagnosis of abdominal trauma: A preliminary report. J Trauma 17:634–641
17. Cayten CG, Evans W (1979) Severity indices and their complications for emergency medical services research and evaluation. J Trauma 19:98–102
18. Cerise EJ, Scully JH (1970) Blunt trauma to the small intestine. J Trauma 10:46–50
19. Champion HR, Sacco WJ, Lepper RL, Atzinger EM, Copes WS, Prall RH (1980) An anatomic index of injury severity. J Trauma 20:197–202
20. Cloward RB (1980) Acute cervical spine injuries. CIBA Symposium 32:1
21. Committee on medical aspects of automotive safety (1972) Rating the severity of tissue damage II: The abbreviated scale. JAMA 220:717–720
22. DeFore WW, Mattox KL, Jordon GL Jr, Beall AC (1976) Management of 1,590 consecutive cases of liver trauma. Arch Surg 111:493–497
23. Delany HM (1974) Physical injury and urban trauma: An overview. J Nat Med Assoc 66:12–15
24. Effeney DJ, Blaisdell WM, McIntyre KE, Graziano CJ (1978) The relationship between sepsis and disseminated intravascular coagulation. J Trauma 18:689–695
25. Engrav LH, Benjamin CI, Strate RG, Perry JF Jr (1975) Diagnostic Peritoneal Lavage in blunt abdominal trauma. J Trauma 15:854
26. Feltis JM (1970) Surgical experience in a combat zone. Am J Surg 119:275
27. Fry DE, Pearlstein J, Fulton RL, Polk HC (1980) Multiple system organ failure: The role of uncontrolled infection. Arch Surg 115:139–140
28. Griswold RA, Collier HS (1961) Collective review: Blunt abdominal trauma. Surg Gynecol Obstet 112:309–329
29. Hawkins L, Pomerantz M, Eisman P (1970) Laparotomy at the time of pelvic fracture. J Trauma 10:619–623
30. Heaton LD (1966) Military surgical practices of the United States army in Vietnam. Current Prob Surg Year Book Publishers
31. Heideman M, Kaijser B, Gelin LE (1978) Complement activation and hematologic, hemodynamic and respiratory reactions early after soft tissue injury. J Trauma 18:696–700
32. Holcroft JW, Trunkey J (1975) Extravascular lung water following shock in the baboon. Ann Surg 180:408–417
33. Hopkins J, Shoemaker W, Greenfield S, Chang, McAuliff T, Sproot R (1980) Treatment of surgical patients with and without an algorithm. Arch Surg 115:745–750
34. Hornyake SW, Shaftan GW (1979) Value of 'inconclusive lavage' in abdominal trauma. J Trauma 19:329–333
35. Hubbard SG, Bivins B, Sachatello CR, Griffin WO (1979) Diagnostic errors with peritoneal lavage in patients with pelvic fractions. Arch Surg 114:844–849
36. Kirkpatrick JR, Youmans RL (1971) Trauma index: An aid in the evaluation of injured victims. J Trauma 2:711–714
37. Kirsh MM, Sloan H (1977) Blunt chest trauma: General principles of management, 1st edn. Little Brown
38. Kleinert AE, Romero J (1961) Blunt abdominal trauma. Review of cases admitted to a General Hospital over a 10 year period. J Trauma 1:226–247
39. Lahivi B, VuWallack R (1977) The early diagnosis and treatment of fat embolism syndrome: A preliminary report. J Trauma 17:956–959
40. Law DK, Dudrick SJ, Ahdow NL (1974) The effects of protein calorie malnutrition on immune competence of the surgical patient. Surg Gynecol Obstet 139:257–266
41. Lazarus H, Nelson JA (1979) Technique for peritoneal

lavage without risk or complications. Surg Gynecol Obstet 149:889–892

42. Lindsey D (1980) Teaching the initial management of major multiple system trauma. J Trauma 20:160–162

43. Lowenfels AB (1966) Kehr's Sign. A neglected aid in ruptures of the spleen. N Engl J Med 274:1019

44. Lucas C, Ledgewood A, Higgins D, Weaver D (1980) Impaired pulmonary function after albumin resuscitation from shock. J Trauma 20:446–451

45. McNamara JJ, Stremple JF (1972) Causes of death following combat injury in an evacuation Hospital in Vietnam. J Trauma 12:1010–1012

46. Moore FD (1966) Metabolic care of the surgical patient. Saunders, London, p 195

47. Moore FD (1980) Energy and the maintenance of the body cell mass. J Parenteral and Enteral Nutrition 4:228–260

48. Moss G (1972) An argument in favor of electrolyte solution for early resuscitation. Surg Clin North Am 52:3–16

49. Nixon JR, Brock-Utne JG (1978) Free fatty acid and arterial oxygen changes following major injury: A correlation between hypoxemia and increased free acid levels. J Trauma 18:23–26

50. Ogawa M, Sugimoto T (1974) Rating severity of the injured by ambulance attendants. J Trauma 14:934–937

51. Oppenheim WL, Williamson DH, Smith R (1980) Early biochemical changes and severity of injury in man. J Trauma 20:135–140

52. Pacey J, Forward W, Preto AJ (1971) Peritoneal tap and lavage in patients with blunt abdominal trauma. Their contribution to surgical decisions. Can Med Assoc J 105:365

53. Patterson FP, Morton KS (1973) The cause of death in fractures of the pelvis with a note on treatment by ligation of the hypogastric (internal iliac) artery. J Trauma 13:849–856

54. Polk HC (1980) Further clarification of the pathogenesis of pulmonary failure in human. Surg Gynecol Obstet 150:727

55. Pontes JE (1977) Urologic injuries. Surg Clin North Am 57:77–95

56. Rodman GH (1980) Irreversible shock: Fact or fancy?

Delivered at the 8th Annual Intensive Care Symposium, University of Miami.

57. Saba TM (1979) Reversing multiple organ failure. J Trauma 19:993–886

58. Sarfeh JI, Balint JA (1978) The clinical significance of hyperbilirubinemia following trauma. J Trauma 18:58–62

59. Saunders CR, Doty DB (1977) Myocardial contusion. Surg Gynecol Obstet 144:595–607

60. Scovill WA, Saba TM, Kaplan JE et al (1976) Deficits in reticuloendothelial humoral control mechanisms in patients after trauma. J Trauma 16:898

61. Shackford S, Zarins C, Rice CL, Virigilio RW (1976) The management of flail chest: A comparison of ventilatory and nonventilatory treatment. Am J Surg 132:759–762

62. Shaftan GW (1960) Indications for operation in abdominal trauma. Am J Surg 99:657–664

63. Shires GT, Canizaro PC (1973) Fluid resuscitation in the severely injured. Surg Clin North Am 53:1342–1358

64. Shoemaker WC (1977) Choice of replacement fluids in shock. Hospital Physician 13:27–37

65. Skillman JJ, Restall S, Salzman E (1975) Randomized trial of albumin vs electrolyte solutions during abdominal aortic operations. Surgery 78(3):291–303

66. Steele M, Lim RC (1975) Advances in management of splenic injuries. Am J Surg 130:159–169

67. Steichen FM (1972) The emergency management of the severely injured. J Trauma 12:786–790

68. Symbas PN (1969) The chest wall and thoracic duct. In: Martin JD Jr (ed) Trauma to the chest and abdomen. Thomas, Springfield, Ill., p 159

69. Thal E, Shires GT (1973) Peritoneal lavage in blunt abdominal trauma. Am J Surg 125:64–69

70. White PH, Benfield JR (1972) Amylase in the management of pancreatic trauma. Arch Surg 105:158–163

71. Wilson H, Sherman R (1961) Civilian penetrating wounds of the abdomen. Factors in mortality and differences from military wounds in 494 cases. Ann Surg 153:639

72. Wiot JF (1975) The radiologic manifestations of blunt chest trauma. JAMA 231:500–503

73. Wright L Delany HM (1976) Calls & Carts speed trauma treatment. The Surgical Team 5–6, pp 44–46

Chapter 36

Head Injuries

David J. Price

General information

In the last decade our understanding of pathophysiological changes following head injury has increased considerably, but application of this knowledge still remains confined to relatively few centres in the world. As there is no known treatment to promote recovery from damage already sustained at or immediately after injury our principle efforts should be directed to the prevention of secondary damage.

Unfortunately, many patients with severe head injuries die or become disabled entirely as a result of late treatment of complications. Early detection and correction of these secondary events demands a high level of intensive management, which is often only available within a hospital's ICU.

Incidence

When considering the overall strategy, it is important to realize that only one in every 130 patients seen by a doctor after head injury will require intensive care. In England and Wales, 9 people per 100,000 population die in a year as a direct result of severe head injury, 4 of these before reaching hospital [73]. Fifteen patients

per 100,000 population a year probably require some degree of head injury intensive care.

In many countries, the incidence of severe trauma [110] could be 2 or even 3 times higher. Man, in creating the motor vehicle, has released a new form of violence on himself. Fortunately, with improvements in road and car design, implementation of speed limits, penalties against those who drink and drive, and the use of seat belts and crash helmets, the incidence of fatal head injuries in road accidents has been slowly and steadily falling since 1967 [40, 62]. Despite this encouraging evidence of some reduction in unnecessary carnage on the roads, intensive care specialists throughout the world are faced with the challenge of attempting to achieve further reductions of both mortality and morbidity in this significant group of patients, who have an average age of less than 30.

Economy

The cost of head injury intensive care should never be underestimated, as it entails a drain on hospital resources and personnel. Very few units treat more than 100 head-injured patients in a year and in a general ICU this number might account for up to 25% of patient days. It is essential to attempt to select those patients who are most likely to benefit, and the admission policy must be based on the aim of preventing secondary brain damage from occurring during recovery from the initial impact injury. This involves the detection and treatment of cerebral shift, hypoxaemia, and ischaemia.

Neuropathologists have emphasized the strong evidence that this secondary brain damage contributes significantly to mortality, and presumably morbidity. These facts alone justify efforts to reduce the number of deaths in patients admitted to hospital.

Components of intensive care

The three essential components of intensive care for victims of severe injury to the head are neuromonitoring, provision of assisted ventilation, and the control of intracranial hypertension. The first is mandatory; the others are not entirely without risk and therefore should be applied only when specifically indicated.

Pathophysiology

Craniospinal buffering capacity

Within the fixed-volume adult cranium there are four components. These are the brain substance, interstitial fluid, intravascular blood and cerebrospinal fluid. Any change in the volume of one of the components needs to be offset by a reciprocal change in another to keep the total volume of the contents constant and therefore the intracranial pressure (ICP) stable. In fact, the spinal CSF compartment behaves as a compensatory reservoir-like buffering mechanism and allows drainage of CSF from the cranium to prevent pressure rises. In the almost fixed volume of the spinal axis, such displacement is only made possible by transfer of an equal volume of blood from the large spinal epidural plexuses. Figure 36.1 is a simplified diagram of the components of the cranial and spinal compartments.

An understanding of the effects of available buffering capacity is best gained by examining the pressure-volume relationship. If saline is injected into an intracranial balloon and ICP measured after each increment in volume, a curve (Fig. 36.2) is produced. Initially, the increments have little influence on the pressure, but as the buffering capacity is gradually used up, the change in pressure response increases steeply. The shape of the curve is determined

by the combined influence of visco-elastic properties of the brain parenchyma and the CSF bulk flow dynamics.

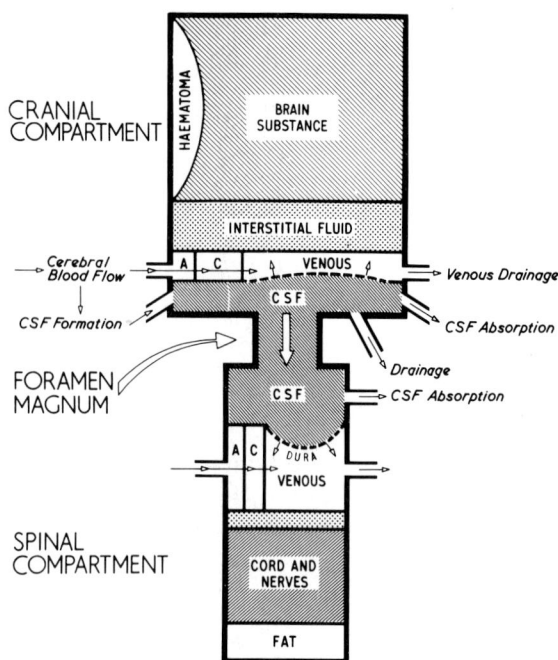

Fig. 36.1. A diagrammatic representation of the cranial and spinal compartments with expulsion of CSF through the foramen magnum and displacement of blood from extradural venous plexuses. This pressure-buffering mechanism provides protection of the brain substance during expansion of a haematoma, but when it is exhausted, the ICP rises steeply.

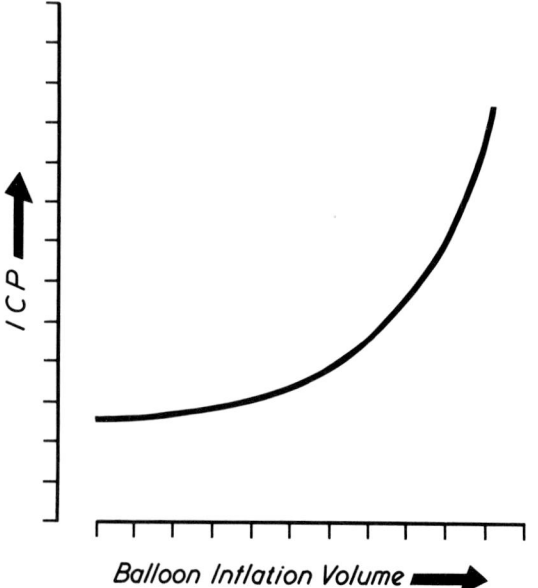

Fig. 36.2. A graph of the ICP of an animal on inflation of an extradural balloon. As the buffering capacity is exhausted the rate of rise in pressure increases alarmingly.

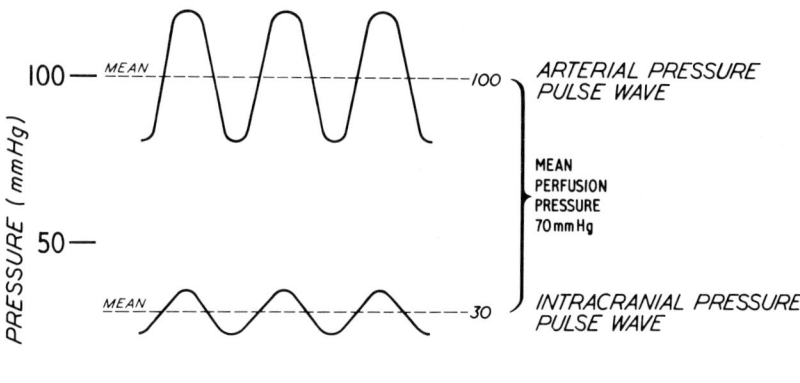

Fig. 36.3. The mean perfusion pressure is the difference between arterial pressure and ICP.

The aim of ICP monitoring is to provide the earliest warning of any inadequacy of this buffering capacity. Whilst it is gradually used up, there is a sequence of four events, the last of which, although tolerated for short periods by a normal brain, has a devastating effect on a brain that is already partly damaged. These events are as follows:-

1) A 'silent' decrease in the total buffering space available.
2) Decreasing compliance recognized by a rise in the ICP pulse wave amplitude.
3) An increase in mean ICP.
4) A reduction in cerebral perfusion.

Treatment should prevent the fourth event from occurring by therapy of the first three [79].

Cerebral perfusion pressure

The intimate relationship between ICP and cerebral blood flow hinges on the fact that intracranial venous pressure has to increase simultaneously with a rise in intracranial pressure to prevent venous collapse. This difference in pressures is usually only 3 or 4 mmHg (0.4 or 0.5 kPa). As the ICP is more easily measured than the venous pressure, it is usual in clinical practice to approximate the perfusion pressure as mean arterial pressure minus mean ICP (Fig. 36.3). This overall index of cerebral perfusion presumes the absence of both tissue pressure differences within the brain substance and arterial pressure gradients along the intracranial arterial tree. This presumption does not usually apply in the first few days after severe injury.

Intracranial hypertension

Definition

In most reports mean ICP levels of 15 or 20 mmHg (2 or 2.7 kPa) have been taken as thresholds for definition of intracranial hypertension [45, 61]. Miller et al. [69] chose 10 mmHg (1.3 kPa), defending this on the grounds that pressures of less than 10 mmHg (1.3 kPa) can be unequivocally accepted as normal. They also showed that when they analysed the outcome of 98 patients who, on admission, were unable to obey simple commands and had no intracranial haematoma, there was a surprisingly significant difference in the outcome between those patients with pressures on admission of less than 11 mmHg (1.5 kPa) and those with pressures between 11 and 20 mmHg (1.5 and 2.7 kPa) on admission (Fig. 36.4).

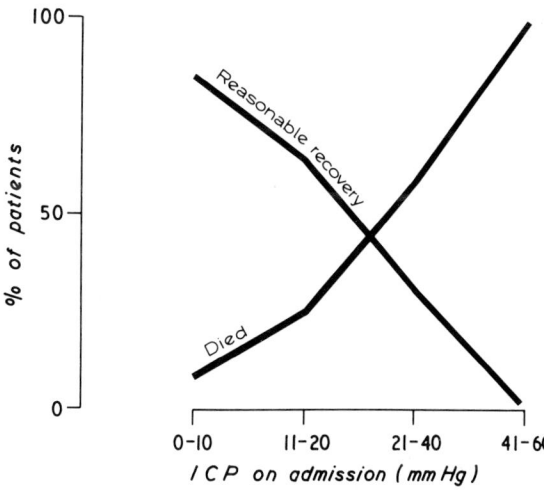

Fig. 36.4. The correlation between ICP on admission of a group of 98 severely head-injured patients and outcome.

Incidence

Clinical measurements of ICP in head injuries
have mostly been made in a heterogeneous
group of patients over varying duration and
often starting several hours or even days
after injury. The true incidence can therefore
only be determined in a population of clearly
defined severity and monitored on arrival at the
Emergency Department.

In a series of 158 such patients first seen in
coma (with no eye opening, no verbal response,
and no obedience to commands) 62% had a
persistent elevation of mean ICP above
20 mmHg (2.7 kPa) [71]. Those patients with
entirely normal computer tomography (CT)
scans, however, had only a 2% risk of developing elevated pressure in the first 24 h but this
rose to 8% within the first 3 days and 17%
within 5 days [51]. In a British series of 151
patients who died following head injury, 125
(83%) had autopsy evidence of uncontrolled
ICP as shown by secondary haemorrhage or infarction of the brain stem [4].

ICP gradients

In the normal brain, pressure is equally distributed throughout the cranial cavity and any
apparent gradients are only related to gravity
[109]. In a recently traumatized brain, very high
gradients develop around intracerebral haemorrhages of any size, beneath surface haematomas
and within areas of abnormally low density
seen on the CT scan. If interstitial fluid measurements are made within such areas [72], the
gradients are seen to develop rapidly, and then
as the plasticity of the brain allows further shifts
over a period of hours they dissipate, resulting
in an overall rise in pressure as measured by a
surface sensor. Figure 36.5 is a diagrammatic
representation of an area of contusion, causing
serious reductions in perfusion pressure in and
immediately adjacent to it.

The aim of treatment in the patients without
surgically removable haematoma is to reduce
this pressure, as measured at the brain surface,
to less than 20 mmHg (2.7 kPa) to provide a
more rapid alternative gradient dissipation
mechanism to that of further hazardous shift of
brain substance. At the same time, perfusion in
the surrounding areas of brain is restored more
rapidly.

Impact injury

When the head is subjected to an impact injury,

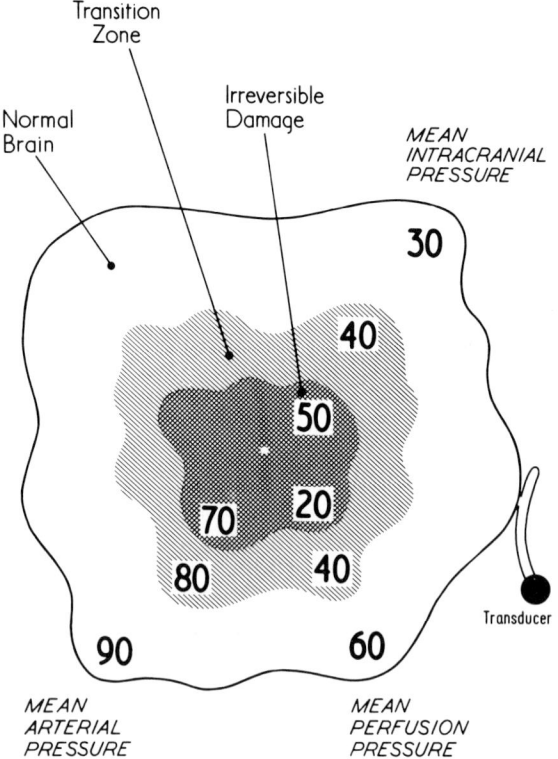

Fig. 36.5. A highly simplified diagram showing arterial,
intracranial and perfusion pressure gradients in and around
a small area of haemorrhagic cerebral contusion. A subdural
transducer measuring a pressure of 30 mmHg implies an
adequate perfusion pressure of 60 mmHg, but in the transition zone of potentially recoverable brain tissue it is dangerously low at 40 mmHg, and can only be increased
by artificially reducing the pressure as measured in the
subdural space.

the dissipation of kinetic energy may be confined almost entirely to the bone to cause a
fracture or it may be transmitted to the brain to
disrupt neurones or intracranial vessels. As
high kinetic energy injuries are associated with
an increased incidence of primary brain damage and a greater risk of developing secondary
complications, it is essential to ascertain the
circumstances of the accident to help anticipate
these problems.

Complications

There are no known methods of repairing brain
already damaged from primary impact injury,
and all management is therefore directed to the
early detection and treatment of secondary complications.

Cerebral vasodilatation

An increase in cerebral blood flow can raise the

ICP dramatically to above 40 mmHg (5.3 kPa) within seconds [53]. This is caused by a transient imbalance between the flow of blood into and out of the cranial cavity, resulting in a sudden increase in cerebral blood volume (CBV). The reason why this occurs in some severely injured patients and not in others is unknown, but it is more common in children [14].

Grubb et al. [35] confirm that in Rhesus monkeys with intact autoregulation, the CBV responds inversely to changes in cerebral perfusion pressure. With increasing ICP following head injury, the fall in perfusion pressure produces an increase in CBV which further exacerbates the intracranial hypertension. In the traumatized human brain, there are zones of hypovolaemia and hypervolaemia associated with areas of ischaemia and intracerebral haemorrhage [55]. It is when hypervolaemia predominates that it generates a high ICP.

There is no evidence to suggest that this vicious circle is initiated by a hypertensive episode as the cerebrovasculature's ability to maintain a steady blood flow during fluctuations in blood pressure (autoregulation) is preserved at this early stage. It is more likely to be due to localised ischaemia causing vasodilatation (Fig. 36.6).

Cerebral oedema

There is some evidence [91] to suggest that significant extravasation of fluid does occur during the development of focal ischaemia. This process is entirely different from conventional cerebral oedema formation due to permeability changes in the vessel walls. Post-traumatic oedema results from transient transmural pressure increases between the mean capillary hydrostatic pressure and the surrounding mean interstitial pressure. Shulman [100] suggested a simple equation derived from the Starling filtration–absorption hypothesis:

FLUID MOVEMENT = k(CAPILLARY
BLOOD
PRESSURE
− INTERSTITIAL
PRESSURE − 25).

If fluid movement proves positive, extravasation occurs and if negative, absorption. Within minutes of injury, reactive vasodilatation at the sites of contusion occur, raising the capillary hydrostatic pressure and producing extravasation of fluid. It has been shown in animal experiments [11] that mannitol, if given within minutes of injury, can prevent this process, but this is clinically impractical. A few minutes later, the interstitial pressure rises and equilibrium is established with cessation of fluid movement. These zones are often visible on a CT scan as low-density areas. Nakatani et al. [72] have confirmed that gradients between interstitial pressures within these zones and surrounding areas resolve gradually over the course of days as the oedema propagates from the contusions in repeated waves of fluid through the brain to produce more generalized intracranial hypertension.

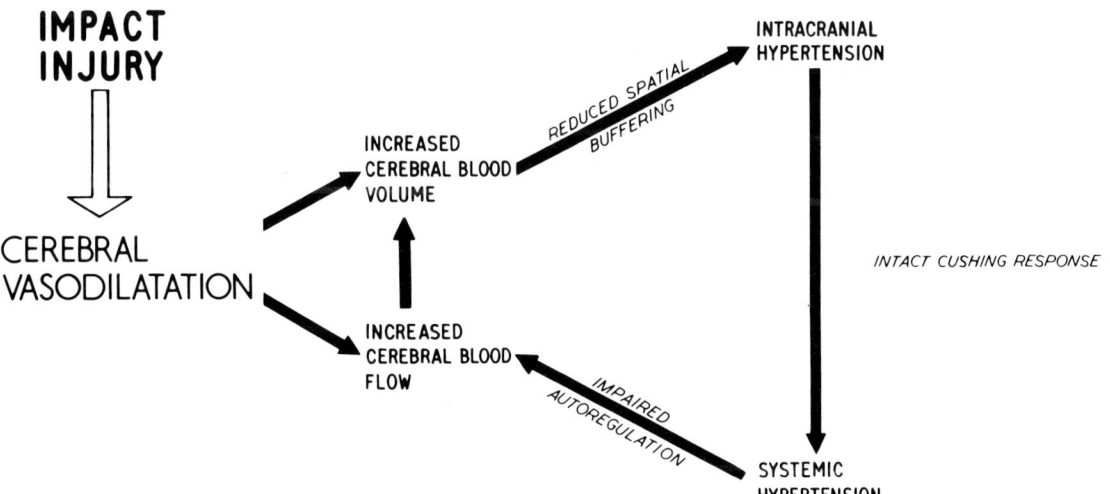

Fig. 36.6. Volume, flow, and pressure responses to cerebral vasodilation. Autoregulation usually becomes impaired at a later stage.

Ischaemic brain damage

Graham et al. [34] reported the incidence of secondary diffuse or focal ischaemic damage in patients dying as a result of non-missile injuries. In a full neuropathological study of 151 brains, well-established ischaemic damage was assessed as severe in 25% and moderately severe in 34%. As 40% of the series had experienced a lucid interval, it seemed unlikely that cytological changes had occurred at impact. Statistically significant correlations were found between ischaemic brain damage and an episode of either hypoxia or raised ICP. From the nature of the brain damage, they concluded that this secondary event was more commonly due to focal or diffuse areas of high interstitial pressure reducing the cerebral perfusion pressure. They emphasized that under such conditions variations in systemic arterial pressure may be very crucial and arterial hypotension was seen to be a frequent contributing factor, as shown by the high incidence of lesions in the artery boundary zones [3]. In a selected group of fatally head-injured patients, a correlation was seen between the presence of vasospasm seen at angiography and ipsilateral ischaemic brain damage [63]. This spasm is presumably a response to ischaemia creating a vicious circle reducing the intra-arterial pressure and jeopardising perfusion to create more ischaemia (Fig. 36.7).

When a middle cerebral artery was occluded permanently in an awake primate, the minimum local flow threshold for irreversible damage was reported to be 17–18 ml/100 g/min [48]. In a comprehensive study of comatosed head injured patients, Overgaard et al. [74] demonstrated a similar critical 20 ml/100 g/min threshold of regional CBF for survival of cortical function, with potential recovery of responsive communication interaction with the environment. They attributed the ischaemia in the fronto-parietal 'watershed' areas to uncontrolled elevations of ICP.

Brain shifts

Lateral distortion

Lateral distortion is produced by a unilateral supratentorial mass lesion shifting intact brain across the midline. The four most common causes of such mass effect following trauma are extradural haematoma, subdural haematoma, expanding haemorrhages in areas of contusion, and unilateral brain swelling. Shifts in excess of 10 mm cause neuronal stretching, but unlike the sudden stretching caused at impact injury, changes over a period of hours are fortunately rather less likely to cause irreversible damage.

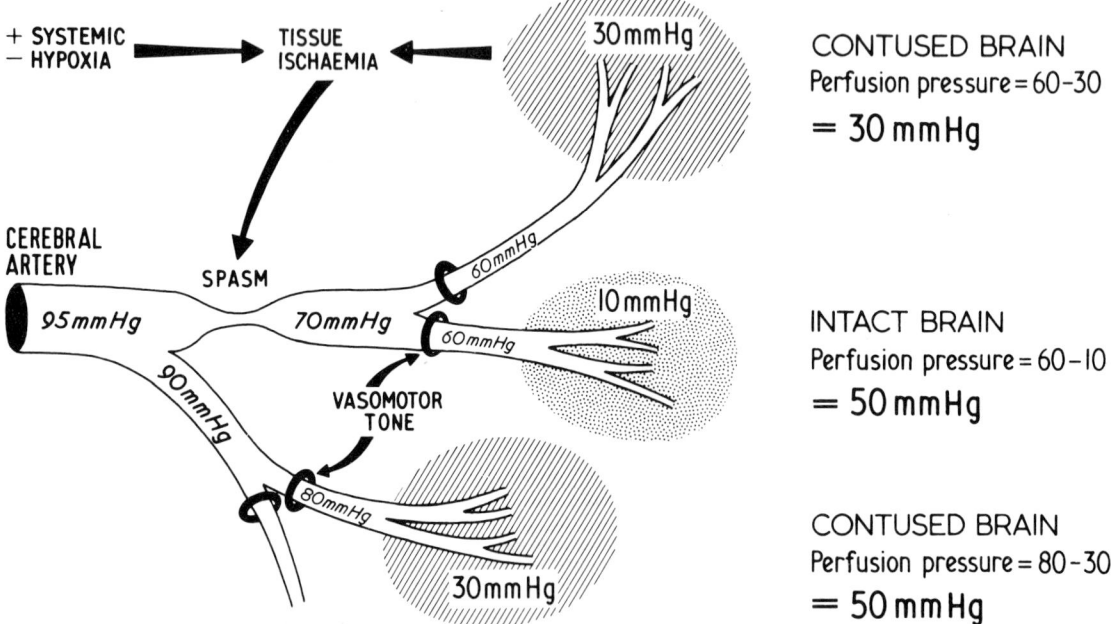

Fig. 36.7. Intravascular and interstitial pressure in contused brain with or without arterial spasm. This example shows spasm causing the focal perfusion pressure to fall from 50 mmHg to 30 mmHg.

During the accumulation of a mass lesion, the adjacent brain tissue is often subjected to very high tissue pressure with focal reduction in perfusion pressure and blood flow. If surgery is delayed, shifting of brain substance away from the lesion is nature's only available alternative mechanism for dissipation of the pressure gradients (Fig. 36.8). The falx cerebri is a relatively

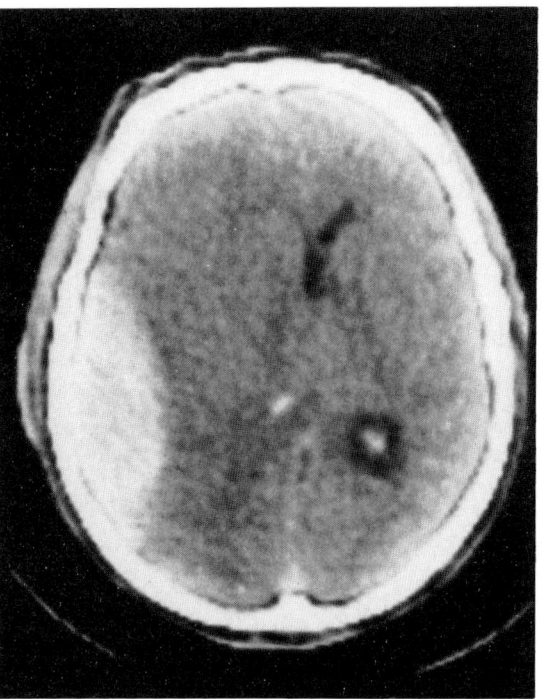

Fig. 36.9. A CT scan of a patient with a left parietal extradural haematoma causing midline shift and ventricular distortion.

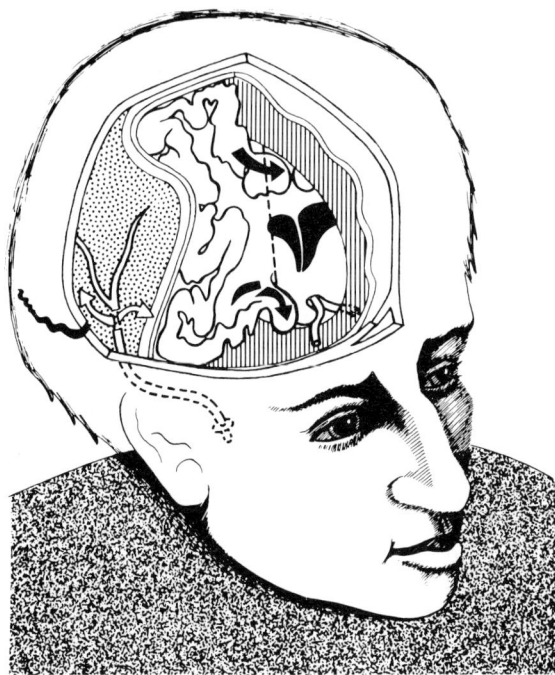

Fig. 36.8. An extradural haematoma causing compression of the underlying brain; brain substance has shifted laterally beneath the falx and downwards through the tentorial hiatus, compressing the third nerve. The ipsilateral ventricle is compressed and the contralateral ventricle dilated.

fixed structure and acts as a barrier allowing tissue to herniate beneath it and generate a local band of high tissue pressure and permanent damage to the corpus callosum. On the CT scan, the ventricle on the side of the compressing lesion is usually smaller than normal and the contralateral ventricle is dilated (Fig. 36.9).

Transstentorial shift

Experimental work in monkeys has shown that when a small temporal extradural balloon is continuously expanded, pressure gradients across the tentorium develop [24]. When the supratentorial ICP rises above 40 mmHg (5.3 kPa) the pressure at the tentorium itself becomes so high that perfusion of the brain

stem is impaired, and if this impaction through the tentorial hiatus is not immediately corrected infarction is inevitable. These experiments have shown that transtentorial impaction, as measured by the tentorial pressure transducers, begins to develop before the pressure gradient, suggesting that the obstruction of CSF flow to the arachnoid space on the surface of the brain stem causes the gradient.

As the IIIrd cranial nerves traverse the arachnoid space at the hiatus, clinical evidence of compression is easily recognized by the dilatation and reduced responsiveness to light of one or both pupils.

Figure 36.10 gives an outline of the pathological implications of head injury with or without concurrent impairment of pulmonary function. Points at which therapeutic intervention may be required are indicated.

Monitoring

For any traumatized patient the principle organ of damage should attract the highest monitoring attention. In an ICU receiving direct head injury admissions, 48% of these have other major systemic injuries also requiring early recogni-

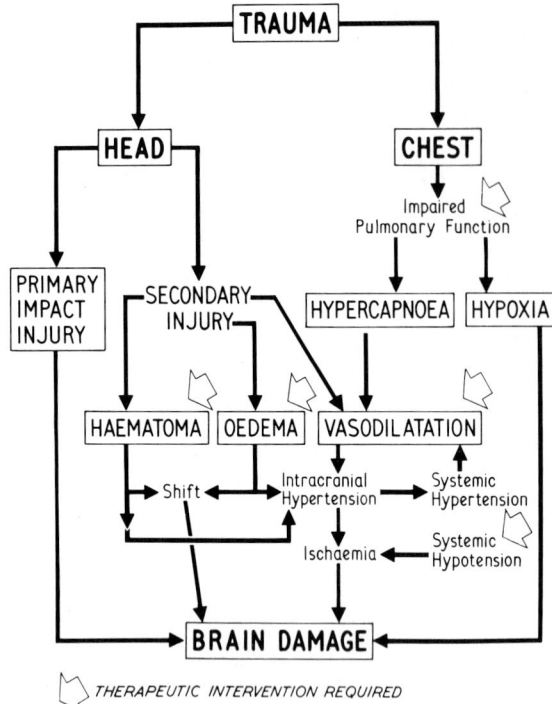

Fig. 36.10. Severe trauma often involves both head and chest. This diagram shows the closely associated pathophysiological consequences.

tion and treatment [71]. It is reasonable to suggest that a significant proportion of the nurses' monitoring duties should be concerned with the frequent assessment of brain function. Unfortunately, very few ICUs achieve a realistic balance, whether measured in terms of nursing effort, number of parameters, or total number of discrete points within each parameter or even of designated surface area on the chart. The number of discrete points for each parameter in a typical general ICU chart is given in Table 36.1.

Although neurological monitoring is essential for the evaluation of treatment and the measurement of progress, its main function is the preservation of life by providing an early warning of potentially treatable complications. The most common secondary event is the development of an intracranial haematoma and a typical sequence during haematoma expansion is listed in Table 36.2.

Haematoma risk

It has always been generally believed that once clinical deterioration is occurring, delay in evacuation of the blood clot reduces the changes of recovery substantially. The management of patients with head injuries aims to prevent

Table 36.1. Number of discrete points for each parameter in a typical intensive care chart used for head injury management

Physiological monitoring	
Pulse	70
Systolic blood pressure	40
Diastolic blood pressure	26
Respiratory rate	20
Respiratory type	4
Temperature	50
	210

Neurological monitoring	
Level of consciousness	5
Hemiparesis	3
Pupil reaction	3
Pupil size	5
Intracranial pressure	50
	66

Table 36.2. A common sequence of events during the expansion of an extracerebral haematoma

	CT scan	Ultrasound shift	Clinical observation
1. Ventricular asymmetry	*		
2. Midline shift	*	*	
3. High-density surface lesion	*	*	
4. Deteriorating level of consciousness	*	*	*
5. Unilateral pupillary dilatation	*	*	*
6. Unilateral pupillary fixation	*	*	*
7. Bilateral pupillary fixation	*	*	*
8. Respiratory depression	*	*	*

* detectable.

secondary brain damage and it is therefore paradoxical to wait for it to develop before instituting treatment.

In a review of 116 patients who were known to have talked before dying after head injury and were transferred to a neurosurgical unit

[94], 50 died as a direct result of delays in evacuation of haematoma. This single avoidable factor proved to be more common than all the other factors combined, and in a quarter of these cases the delay occurred within the neurosurgical ward. Sometimes there was a delay because the patient's coma was attributed to alcohol excess or to a cerebrovascular accident [27]. More often than this there was a failure to recognize the deterioration from its onset or to appreciate its rate when it had already occurred. Of 168 patients admitted to primary care hospitals and subsequently dying, delayed haematoma evacuation accounted for unnecessary deaths in 55 [38].

The early recognition of patients at risk has become an essential component of management. The need for prompt evacuation was emphasized by Mendelow et al. [66] and Fig. 36.11 shows the delay in time from the first recorded observation of deteriorating consciousness to evacuation of the haematoma correlated with the outcome. A similar conclusion is reached by Seelig et al. [98], who discovered a mortality resulting from acute subdural haematomas to be 3 times higher if evacuation is delayed beyond 4 h.

Level of consciousness

A structured method of measuring level of consciousness with the prime purpose of early detection of deterioration must have all the following characteristics:

1) An optimum balance between sensitivity and complexity
2) Minimal inter-observer error
3) 'At-a-glance' detection of trend
4) Precision of terminology to enable nurses to use it after minimal training

When a scale for detection of deterioration in level of consciousness is considered, its effectiveness in this respect must be quantified.

Cranswick et al. [20] compared the effectiveness of eight scales used in a series of 60 patients with deteriorating consciousness level. Figure 36.12 shows their results, with the rather disturbing conclusion that cruder scaling systems give a dangerously false sense of security as even a 4- or 5-point fall in a 0–50 scale may be completely missed and not detected until even further deterioration has occurred. The well-structured 12-point Glasgow Coma Scale [105] with its three-component sub-scores, failed to detect the initial deterioration in almost 60% of patients. Scales with more than 30 points miss initial deterioration in less than 10% of patients and the sensitivity advantages beyond a 40-point scale are minimal.

A compromise between complexity and sensitivity has to be reached, and a 34-point scale measuring seven aspects of consciousness has been designed for use in emergency departments, ICUs, and neurosurgical and general wards [82] (Fig. 36.13). In hospitals without a resident neurosurgeon, it is unwise to expose patients at significant risk of developing a com-

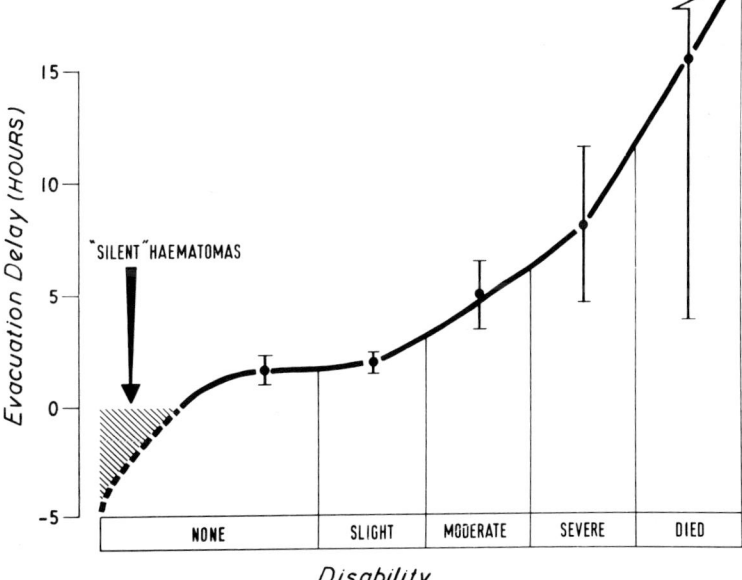

Fig. 36.11. A series of 83 patients with extradural haematoma was allocated into five outcome groups. The mean time lapse from clinical deterioration to evacuation was calculated for each group and is shown on this graph. With the advent of CT scanning and ultrasound, a proportion of patients may have diagnosis and treatment of 'silent' haematomas before the onset of clinical deterioration.

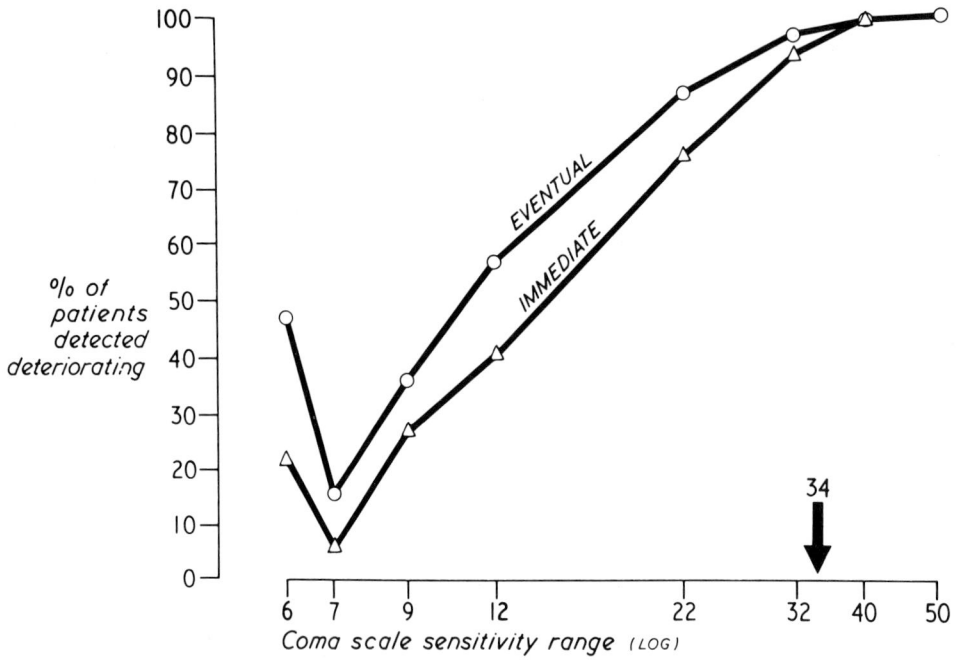

Fig. 36.12. Graphs taken from coma scale data relating to 100 patients who deteriorated by 4 or 5 points on a 0–50 scale. Each fall was replotted onto a selection of scales with ranges of between 6 and 40 points. The percentage of patients detected to be deteriorating by each of the scales rises steeply with increasing range, but beyond an optimum of 34 points there is minimal advantage in terms of sensitivity.

plication to unnecessary delays by using in-adequate methods of monitoring consciousness level.

Computerized ultrasound

When CT scanners became widely available, it was presumed that they would simplify haema-toma detection before clinical deterioration. Pa-tients at risk require serial scans every few hours, and for those receiving treatment in an ICU for head and other injuries, this is imprac-tical. Ultrasound scanning with small comput-erized equipment for the measuring of midline shift is easy for radiographers or nursing staff (Fig. 36.14). Unlike the CT scanner its useful-ness is not invalidated by restless patients, and it can be very easily repeated. When this in-formation is considered together with clinical data, an accurate risk level can be obtained [96]. If the risk is increasing and time allows, a CT scan can then be used to find the exact site prior to surgical evacuation. These clinical data in-clude a careful measurement of level of con-sciousness, hemiparesis, and pupil reaction and the presence or absence of a fracture.

A patient admitted to an ICU with multiple injuries, but who has recovered consciousness, has a 0.3% risk of developing an intracranial haematoma if he has no skull fracture, but the risk rises to 6.9% with a fracture [46]. A similar patient with a fracture, but no ultrasound mid-line shift has a 1% risk but with a 4-mm midline shift, this rises to 85% [96]. With increasing reliance on computerized ultrasound measure-ments of midline shift, a higher proportion of patients have evacuation of their extradural haematomas before the onset of deterioration of consciousness. A recent series indicated that 42% had surgery before any deterioration [97].

Pupil size and reaction

The pupil size is best measured in millimetres with a transparent rule, and a bright torch should always be used to test the response of the pupils to light both directly and consensu-ally. Changes in pupil size and reaction to light usually signify a late stage in a deteriorating patient, and remedial action should have pre-vented this from ever occurring. In common with most other brain stem function tests, pupil signs depend on the combined integrity of the afferent and efferent components of the reflex arc in addition to the nuclei and interconnecting neurones within the brain stem itself. Destruc-tion of the optic nerve can be detected by testing consensual pupil reaction. If a pupil fails to react

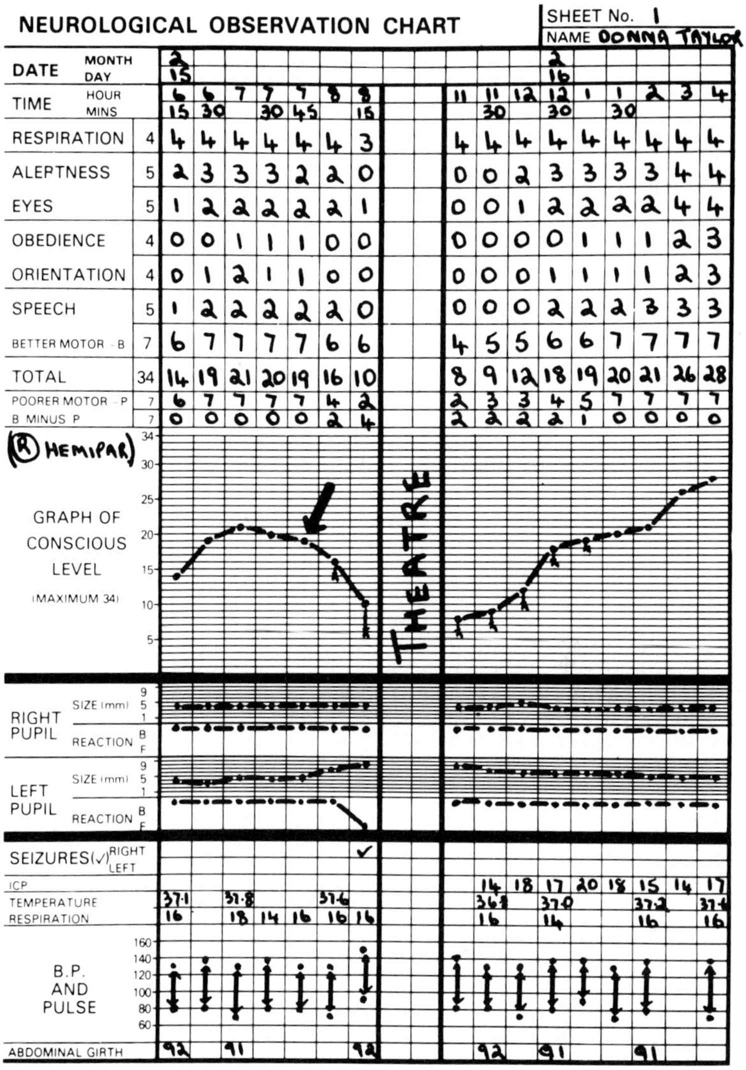

NEUROLOGICAL OBSERVATION CHART

SHEET No. 1
NAME DONNA TAYLOR

Fig. 36.13. An example of a structured neurological chart showing changes in level of consciousness and in pupils before and after evacuation of a left temporal extradural heamatoma. The high sensitivity of the coma scale alerts the nurse to small changes indicating the need for more frequent observations and repeat investigations at the time marked by the *arrow*.

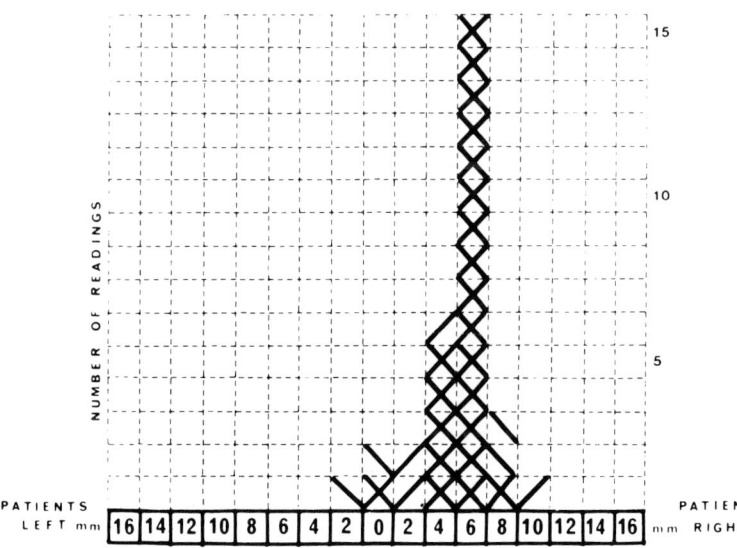

MIDLINER

Fig. 36.14. The results of a series of ultrasound measurements of midline shift taken from a restless patient over a 5-min period and presented as a histogram. This shows a median of 6 mm of shift from left to right, which proved at operation to be due to a rapidly expanding extradural haematoma.

to light either directly or consensually, it could be due either to impact injury to the 3rd cranial nerve or to stretching or compression of that nerve by herniation of the temporal lobe uncus through the tentorial hiatus as a result of increasing intracranial compression (Fig. 36.8). Pupil signs remain one of the most useful brain stem function tests, as they are both easy to repeat and unaffected by relaxants and non-narcotic sedatives.

Other brain stem tests

All other brain stem tests, including the oculocephalic or oculovestibular reflexes, are useful predictive indicators but they have no practical monitoring use.

Hemiparesis

Motor response is an important component of most coma scales and if the score for motor response on the weaker side is compared with that on the stronger side, the difference gives an indication of the degree of paresis.

ICP monitoring

Methods

Over the years an aura of mystique has developed around the technique of ICP monitoring, and yet this physiological signal is no different from any other. An external transducer connected by hydraulic transmission to a device inserted through a burr hole into the ventricle or subdural space is the traditional method [79].

Transducers for screw insertion into the burr hole are available commercially and prove reliable, but the saline-filled urethral catheter for insertion into the subdural space remains the simplest to implant and remove (Fig. 36.15).

Indications

Both the risk of developing a haematoma and intracranial hypertension of other causes are enhanced by the severity of coma. The deeper the coma, the higher the incidence of both complications. It is for this reason that a summated Glasgow coma score of less than 8 is often considered an indication for ICP monitoring. The four main indications are therefore:

1) Necessity for ventilation (Table 36.3)

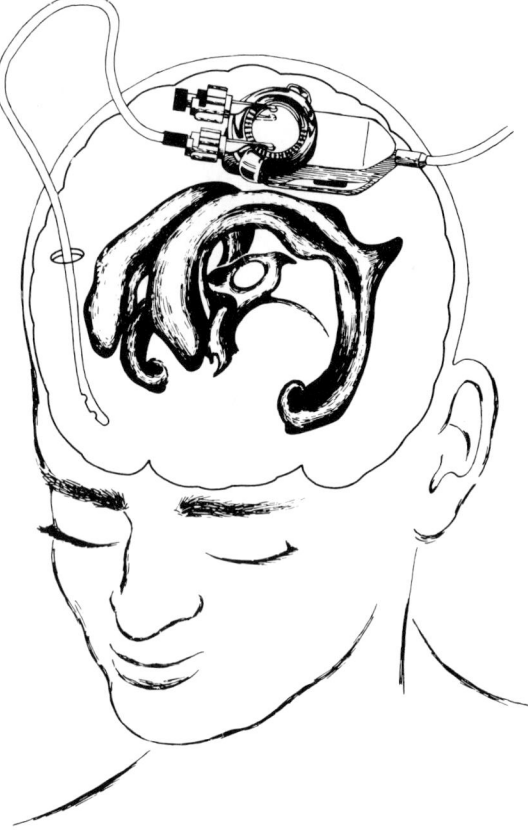

Fig. 36.15. A conventional transducer with disposable plastic dome and hydraulic catheter link for subdural pressure measurements.

2) Glasgow coma score less than 8

3) After decompressive surgery

4) Presence of a small intracerebral haematoma on a CT scan.

Table 36.3. Indications for controlled ventilation

1. Mean ICP higher than 15 mmHg (2 kPa)
2. PO_2 with oxygen mask less than 75 mmHg (10 kPa)
3. PCO_2 greater than 45 mmHg (6 kPa)
4. PCO_2 less than 26 mmHg (3.5 kPa)
5. Severe chest or facial injuries
6. Repeated seizures
7. Coma causing inadequate protection of the airway with intubation only tolerated with muscle relaxation and sedation

EEG monitoring

Continuous monitoring of the EEG by simple low-cost filtered amplifiers provides some additional warning of ischaemia due to either inadequate perfusion or hypoxia [90, 103]. It is no alternative to blood gas or ICP monitoring, as a reduction in level of signal occurs only when insult on cellular metabolism has already occurred. For patients with status epilepticus supported by elective ventilation it becomes indispensable, as there is no other way of monitoring the effectiveness of anticonvulsant treatment to ascertain the optimum required dosage [75, 80]. Its other practical use is to record the time of onset of electrical silence in those patients who die. This aids appropriate timing of the essential tests of cerebral death, which are primarily clinical [43, 83].

Associated pulmonary insufficiency

The cerebro-pulmonary relationship

This two-way interactive relationship between brain and lungs has been well recognised in head injured patients for many years. William Buchan [15] noted that the co-existence of head injury and lung 'inflammation' usually resulted in a fatal outcome. At the end of the last century [54] it was observed that death after head injury was due to respiratory arrest rather than cardiac failure, and it was suggested that if respiration could be supported, survival might be possible.

To provide supportive therapy for one organ while ignoring the needs of the other is potentially dangerous and it is for this reason that severe head injuries are best managed jointly between neurosurgical and anaesthetic staff in an ICU.

Incidence of hypoxaemia

The incidence of severe hypoxaemia in comatose head-injured patients reflects the quality of the airway control at the accident site, in the ambulance, and in the receiving room. If hypoxaemia is arbitrarily defined as any period of time during which a PO_2 of less than 60 mmHg (8 kPa) is recorded, an incidence of 37% was found in a series of 225 comatose head-injured patients on admission to ICU [71]. It is so common in the comatose patients that it should be presumed until proven otherwise. Similar findings in other countries emphasize the need for routine blood gas analysis at admission [49].

In 1977, an analysis of 116 patients who died despite the fact that at one time after injury they had been sufficiently conscious to talk was published [94]. In this retrospective study of the records, airway obstruction was found to have made a certain contribution to death in eight patients, and uncontrolled epilepsy with presumed hypoxia in a further seven.

Causes of associated pulmonary insufficiency

1) Central respiratory depression
2) Inadequate airway protection
3) Aspiration of gastric contents
4) Neurogenic shunting
5) Pulmonary oedema
6) Pulmonary infection
7) Fat embolism syndrome
8) Trauma

Neurogenic pulmonary insufficiency

Neurogenic pulmonary insufficiency is well recognized but difficult to explain, quantify, and treat. It may be produced by perfusion of poor or non-ventilated alveoli or by the opening of normal anatomical arteriovenous anastomoses or simply by redistribution of flow through preferential channels [65]. Transient respiratory arrest within the first few seconds of head injury impact may have caused diffuse micro-atelectasis producing inadequate ventilation in some areas. Some of the mixed venous blood passes through the lung without oxygenation to mix in the left heart with normally oxygenated blood and cause arterial hypoxaemia. This venous admixture is equivalent to a right-to-left shunt and therefore, despite inhalation of high concentrations of oxygen, the arterial oxygen tension is not affected. Other areas of lung hyperventilate to compensate, allowing excretion of CO_2 to preserve normocapnea. Chest x-ray changes lag 12–14 h behind arterial gas alterations, making this a poor initial diagnostic tool [49].

Treatment. Intubation and ventilation with a large tidal volume should reverse an atelectatic state by re-expansion of the alveoli, but in practice this is only partly efficient, and if the shunt exceeds 15% in patients over the age of 50 a fatal outcome is said to be virtually inevitable [26]. Although animal studies have suggested that methyl prednisolone might be effective in this condition [112], studies of the effect of bolus doses of this steroid on patients with major trauma showed a rise rather than a fall in shunting, and there was an overall fall in arterial oxygenation [60].

Pulmonary oedema

Overwhelming pulmonary oedema with classic pink frothy foam emerging from the endotracheal tube is fortunately not commonly seen in an ICU. In a series of 86 severe head injuries requiring elective ventilation, however, it was observed in 7 [26]. Approximately 20% of patients dying of massive head injury in the absence of resuscitative measures show acute pulmonary oedema at autopsy [1]. Experimental work [23] re-affirmed Cushing's law [21] that systemic diastolic blood pressure will usually rise to a level greater than that of ICP. When the ICP was artificially elevated, a rise in pulmonary venous pressure followed the expected rise in systemic blood pressure, and this was in turn followed by a rise in pulmonary arterial pressure (PAP). If the pulmonary venous pressure rise was dramatic and became greater than that in the pulmonary artery for some seconds, the pulmonary capillary pressure rose so high that it exceeded the oncotic pressure of the plasma and massive pulmonary oedema was inevitable. If, in addition to the high ICP, the head injury is severe enough, and particularly if the hypothalamus is involved, it has been postulated that a sudden centrally mediated surge of sympathetic outflow produces an intense generalized but transient vasoconstriction [108]. This causes a sudden shift of blood from the high-resistance systemic circulation to the low-resistance pulmonary system. This flow then opens up arteriovenous anastomoses, aggravating hypoxaemia by causing a shunt; this in turn reduces cardiac contractility and output and further increases the pulmonary venous congestion, exacerbating pulmonary oedema [12].

In ten patients with pulmonary oedema [22] there had been a preceding sudden rise in ICP, and it was emphasized that the only hope of relief depended upon an immediate drastic reduction in this pressure. Other measures, such as positive pressure respiration, are only palliative and temporary.

Pulmonary infection

It is naive to suggest that antibiotics prevent ventilated patients from developing pulmonary infection. It could be claimed that those at the highest risk would include patients with chest injuries, with suspected aspiration of gastric contents and with atalectasis, and that these conditions might merit antibiotics. Pus cells are found in the secretions from almost all patients after 24 h of ventilation, but even the isolation of pathogens with pus from the trachea and bronchi does not indicate true pulmonary parenchymal infection. The treatment of bacteriology reports rather than patients can lead to a gross misuse of these drugs, with serious consequences. It has been shown [76] that prophylactic antibiotics in comatose patients increases their chances of developing pneumonia by some three times. In a neurosurgical unit where a severe outbreak of *Klebsiella* pulmonary infection caused unnecessary deaths, the only effective treatment was to completely abandon the use of all antibiotics in all patients, including those producing copious purulent sputum [88]. This drastic measure eradicated the *Klebsiella* and also dramatically reduced the overall incidence of pulmonary infections caused by other pathogens.

Influence of hypoxia

Although the normal brain may withstand moderate degrees of hypoxia for long periods with no lasting effects, severely traumatized brain with focal areas of ischaemia are intolerant of even transient falls in PO_2. Histological evidence of ischaemic brain damage, often with a known preceding period of hypoxia, was found in 138 of 151 brains [34]. In a small matched series of patients who had survived after recovering from coma lasting at least a week [87], those who had suffered hypoxia were less than 30% as likely to return to their normal work as those with no recorded hypoxia. An unmatched series of 150 patients transferred to a British neurosurgical unit in coma was reported. Of those seen to be cyanosed on arrival, only 17% eventually made a good recovery compared to 34% in those not cyanosed [30]. Additional systemic hypotension further influenced the morbidity and indeed, in this small group, no patients made a good recovery. In a similar series from the United States, 225 patients with severe head injury were treated with more enthusiastic intensive care. Of their hypoxic group, 44% made a good recovery compared with 65% in those with a PO_2 in excess of 60 mmHg (8 kPa) [71]. Other workers confirmed the close correlation between persisting hypoxia and outcome [26, 70].

Intracranial hypertension

The ability to measure the ICP accurately has in the past been heralded as a fascinating opportunity to follow intracranial events continuously after head injury. Such retrospective analysis of the physiological signal is meaningless, however, unless the prime indication for such measurement is anticipation and prevention of dangerous rises in pressure. This is particularly important during the first few days following injury, before the pressure gradients within the brain substance have dissipated. Of 158 patients admitted to an ICU in coma, 62% had an ICP above 20 mmHg (2.7 kPa) [71]. Such a level of risk in this group of patients makes ICP monitoring mandatory. The highest incidence of raised ICP was 70% in those after evacuation of haematoma as compared with 29% in those without a haematoma.

Clinical significance

Cause of death

It is easy to assume that increased ICP must eventually harm the brain and that it must therefore be beneficial to reduce it. By this logic, treating the pressure becomes an end in itself. If a large volume of already injured brain is the source of the hypertension, then raised ICP is merely an epiphenomenon and reducing the pressure will procure no benefit. Neuropathologists provide autopsy evidence [2], however, that in a high proportion of patients, the raised pressure is the cause of significant secondary damage and they imply that treatment would have been beneficial. In a series of 160 patients with severe brain trauma 48 died, and nearly half of these had severe intracranial hypertension that was considered in retrospect to be the ultimate cause of death [69]. A later report from the same centre indicates a mortality of 18% in patients found with an ICP consistently less than 20 mmHg (2.7 kPa) compared with 26% in those with pressure rising above this level but reducible with treatment. In the smaller group of patients with irreducible intracranial hypertension, the mortality was 92% [71].

As an indication of a developing haematoma

In the absence of CSF leakage, an ICP of less than 10 mmHg (1.3 kPa) virtually excludes the possibility of a haematoma.

As an indication for surgical evacuation of an intracranial haematoma

It is now over two centuries since Percival Pott [78] first pointed out that intracranial haematomas can be present in the absence of clinical deterioration.

In a group of 36 patients with ICPs above 30 mmHg (4 kPa) on admission, 27 had mass lesions requiring surgery [69]. A rising pressure therefore provides a moderately useful warning of a developing haematoma but is not an adequate alternative to serial ultrasound or CT examinations. Experience in the last decade with the CT scanner has shown that intradural haematomas are much more common than we have realized [92, 102] and their presence does not necessarily indicate immediate evacuation. Galbraith et al. [28] suggested that intradural haematomas should be removed early in those patients with pressures rising above 20 mmHg (2.7 kPa), and this information proved a better predictive indicant of imminent deterioration even than the measure of midline shift.

Artificial increase of the intracranial buffering capacity

ICP would remain within its normal range if the buffering capacity were adequate. Principles for controlling it depend on the ability to increase the compensatory capacity artificially, either by improving the natural mechanism or by introducing new ones. The ability to transfer venous blood out of the cranium is enhanced by artificially lowering total blood volume with diuretic agents. The volume of interstitial fluids is reduced by mannitol [68] and the cerebral blood flow can be decreased either directly by hypocapnoea or indirectly by lowering the demand for blood flow with barbiturates or Althesin. Such a fall in flow results in a reduction in the size of the intracranial vascular compartment.

Steroids

Steroids are highly effective in reducing the cerebral oedema due to disturbances of capillary permeability in the tissues surrounding brain tumours and abscesses. As the mechanism for production of oedema in head injuries is not related to pathological changes within the capillary walls, it is not surprising that steroids even in high doses influence neither the ICP nor the eventual outcome [17, 32, 36, 77].

Unlike mannitol, they have no effect on the volume of normal interstitial fluid within the brain, the absorption of propagated post-traumatic oedema, or the intracranial blood volume.

Mannitol and frusemide

A 20% solution of mannitol is the most widely used agent. Its three-fold action accounts for its effectiveness in the majority of head-injured patients. It directly reduces the normal interstitial fluid volume, it accelerates the absorption of oedema fluid during its propagation from contused areas by creating an osmolar gradient and it very effectively reduces blood viscosity. The viscosity changes are due to the combined influence of increased red cell deformability and reductions in haematocrit, red cell blood volume and aggregation [16]. They allow a freer passage of red cells through the microcirculation and enhance tissue perfusion. This may account for the rise in cerebral blood flow [44]. A rigid maintenance of fluid balance is essential, and maximal effect can be expected within 40 min of a bolus infusion [24]. Such an infusion of a hyperosmolar solution should not be administered too rapidly as a sudden movement of free water from the cells causes active vasodilatation resulting in reduced perfusion pressure due to the transient hypotension [18, 47]. If more than 1 litre a day is required, serum osmolality should be measured and not allowed to rise above 310 mosmol. After 48 h of treatment, hypokalaemia and hyponatraemia may develop and require correction. Frusemide is both a diuretic and an inhibitor of CSF production [91]. Its effect on electrolyte balance and osmolality has been reported to be less than of mannitol in the short term [19].

Dosage. The conventional dosage of a single bolus ranges between 1 and 2 g/kg body weight [37]. This is a useful guide for the first dose, but calculation of the optimum timing and volume of subsequent infusions is more difficult. The dosage depends on the fall of pressure required, the preceding trend, the effectiveness of the last dose, an estimate of the residual circulating mannitol and even the current position on the pressure–volume curve. Adherence to such criteria is too demanding for the staff of a busy ICU. Unless computerized closed-loop techniques are used [86, 89] (Fig. 36.16) it is necessary to have recourse to the only practical alternative of inspired guesswork. If its effectiveness falls, it is necessary to improve its activity by administering frusemide (Lasix) at a

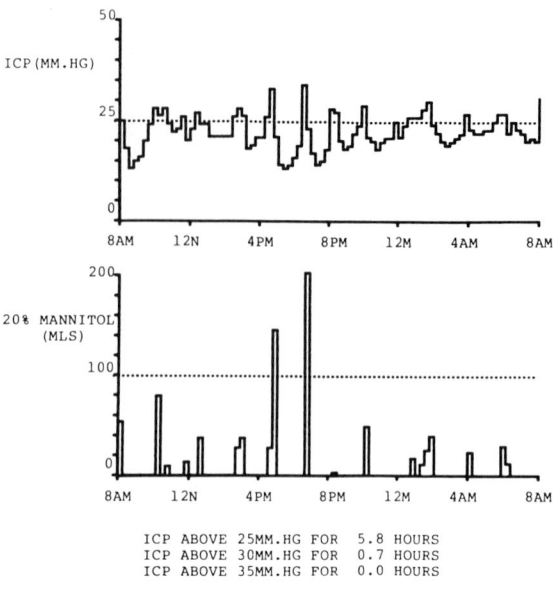

Fig. 36.16. A computer record of mean ICP and mannitol infused. The closed-loop system was programmed to instigate treatment at 25 mmHg, which was considered an acceptable threshold some 5 days after injury.

dose of 0.7 mg/kg [85]. If there is then no response and a haematoma has been excluded, a hyperaemic state should be immediately presumed and treated with a cerebral blood flow supressant.

Cerebral blood flow suppressants

Both alphaxalone-alphadalone (Althesin) and barbiturates produce a decrease in ICP by inhibiting cerebral metabolism and its demand for cerebral flood flow [50]. The fall in flow to uninjured areas of the brain then reduces the intracranial blood volume to provide more buffering space and hopefully improves perfusion through damaged tissue. For those patients with post-traumatic hyperaemia these drugs provide the only hope of control. In high doses, both drugs share the problem of causing systemic arterial hypotension by peripheral vasodilatation. This effect has to be combatted with plasma infusions or vasoconstrictor agents. Failure to prevent the mean arterial pressure from falling below 90 mmHg (12 kPa) precipitates further reductions of perfusion pressure in contused areas. This treatment demands continuous arterial and central venous pressure surveillance and some workers even advise cardiac monitoring with Swan–Ganz catheters [67]. There is no substantive evidence that either drug, even in EEG suppressing doses, affords the human protection from ischaemia following head injury, and any suggestion that there are advantages other than for reduction of ICP are purely speculative.

Pentobarbitone. Barbiturate therapy in a comatose patient is no minor undertaking. It should only be applied within the confines of an experienced, well-supervised and well-instrumented ICU. Until its precise indications and efficacy have been well defined, this treatment should only be used when simpler methods based on osmotic agents and ventilation have been meticulously employed and proved ineffective [67].

Marshall et al. [64] suggested 100-mg dose increments over a period of 20 min to a total of 3–5 mg/kg followed by 1–2 mg/kg supplement every 1 or 2 h to maintain an ICP below 15 mmHg (2 kPa), a mean blood pressure in excess of 70 mmHg (9.3 kPa), a body temperature around 34°C, and a serum barbiturate level between 2.5 and 4 mg/dl. Most patients require 30–60 mg/kg per day. Unfortunately, blood levels give little indication of brain tissue concentration, and it is advisable to use EEG monitoring to show burst suppression or loss of electrical activity [67].

Althesin. In recent years, barbiturates have been less favoured as clearance from fatty tissues is slow, causing difficulties with maintenance dosage and delays in diagnosing brain death in those who prove to be resistant to all therapy. Althesin, with its shorter half-life, appears to be a safer and easier agent to use. This drug may be given by 2–4 ml bolus injections, which usually produces a fall in ICP within 10 min [111] or continuously at an initial rate of 10 ml/h, increasing to a maximum of 35 ml/h in adults until control is achieved.

CSF drainage

If pressure rises above 40 mmHg (5.3 kPa) it can be seen from the pressure–volume curve (Fig. 36.2) that a significant fall in pressure will result from the removal of a relatively small volume of CSF from the ventricle. Unfortunately, head-injured patients usually have smaller ventricles than normal, as fluid has already been displaced from them as part of the buffering mechanism. The introduction of a ventricular catheter by anterior approach into a slit-like frontal horn is therefore often difficult but a lateral approach to the broader 'target' of the trigone rarely fails. Only a small volume can be aspirated and minimal negative pressure should be used to avoid choroid plexus obstruction.

Surgical decompression

Three methods of surgical decompression are used singly or in combination to achieve a fall in intracranial hypertension and correction of brain shift. (1) Haematomas usually require urgent evacuation. (2) External decompression by removal of a large bone flap provides a small increase in buffering space. (3) Less eloquent areas of contused brain may be excised to provide more space, and hopefully to remove a source of oedema propagation. Britt and Hamilton [10] indicated that for patients with acute subdural haematomas, both mortality and morbidity were reduced if they were treated with large external decompressions in addition to haematoma evacuation.

Controlled ventilation

The powerful mechanisms that regulate the transport of metabolites to and from the brain cells have been well recognized for many years. They provide a reciprocal interaction between respiration, cerebral blood flow and ICP.

Changes in cerebral blood flow

Ischaemic brain produces hydrogen ion release in the form of lactic acidosis and causes local hypercarbia which leads to arterial vasodilatation of those reactive undamaged vessels supplying normal brain [52] (Fig. 36.17). This 'steal phenomenon' [104] diverts blood away from the damaged areas, increasing the intravascular volume by enhancing blood flow through the normal brain, producing hypervolaemic zones around contusions which in turn transmits a higher interstitial pressure to the damaged areas and exacerbates the ischaemia. This hydrogen ion release reaches the ventricular CSF and induces hyperventilation to correct the local hypercarbia and normalize brain tissue pH [59]. As CO_2 is the most rapidly diffusing component of the CSF buffering system its washout is the most effective means of achieving this. Unfortunately, as the clearance of excess lactic acid from the pH is slow, this chemical transmitter feedback compensatory system causes unnecessary prolongation of hyperventilation. If the PCO_2 is then allowed to fall below the normal range, the reversed steal phenomenon causes even further problems. The arteries supplying undamaged brain constrict in response to the hypocapnoea, and blood flow is diverted through the non-reactive and paralysed vessels supplying the damaged areas. This torrential flow is catastrophic, as it gives rise to sudden expansion of injured areas often with haemorrhage and further ischaemia causing distortive damage to the previously normal surrounding brain (Fig. 36.17).

The aim of controlled ventilation is to steer a careful course between hypercapnoea and hypocapnoea, and the maintenance of PCO_2 between 26 and 30 mmHg (3.5 and 4.0 kPa) has been accepted by most workers as a reasonable compromise. The majority of researchers have shown in both experimental and clinical studies that it results in an overall lowering of mean ICP [92, 95] for a limited period.

Indications for IPPV

Ventilation should not be used indiscriminately as a form of treatment unless specifically indicated [6]. Table 36.3 gives an example of a list of indications. Figure 36.18 shows the place of ventilation as a component of management for some head-injured patients.

Medication

An appropriate regimen of muscle relaxants with sedation and, if necessary, analgesia is best selected according to personal preferences.

Frequent chest physiotherapy, tracheal toilet and, if necessary, bronchoscopic lavage and PEEP [25, 99] may all help to maintain an

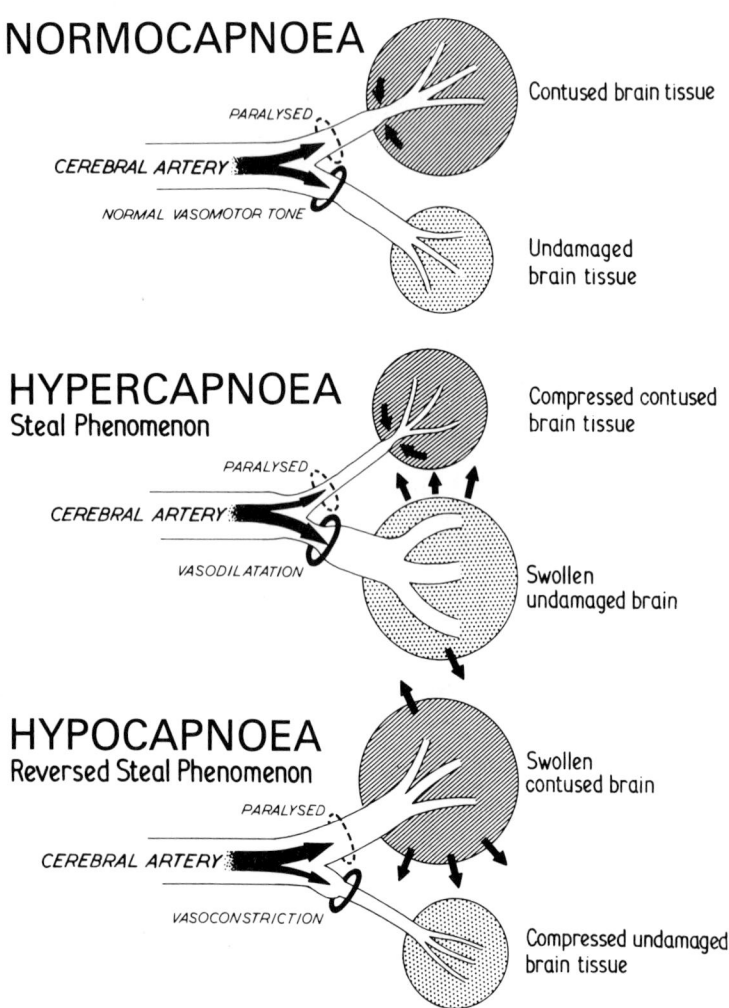

Fig. 36.17. Changes in distribution of blood flow to contused and undamaged brain in response to variations in PCO_2.

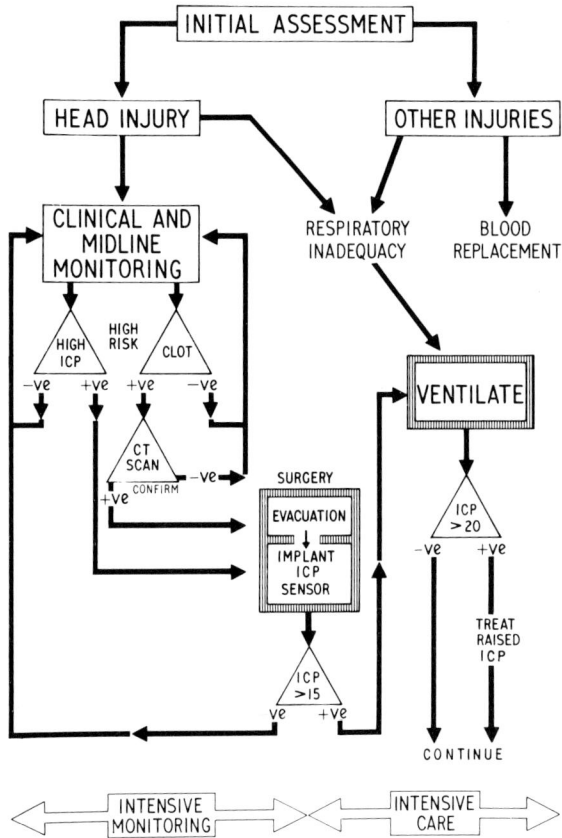

Fig. 36.18. An overall plan for intensive monitoring and treatment, emphasizing the importance of repeated assessment of risk factors and outlining the indications for ICP monitoring throughout ventilation therapy.

adequate PO$_2$. If they cause any more than a transient rise in ICP, 'premedication' with an ICP-controlling agent or CSF drainage is indicated.

Prediction

An increasing interest in the prediction of outcome from severe head injury has developed over recent years. The potential advantages are threefold—economy, keeping relatives well informed, and evaluation of new treatment regimens.

Economy

The cost of intensive care in terms of drainage of a hospital's financial and staffing resources should never be underestimated [101]. When resources are limited, therefore, it might be thought reasonable to suggest that those patients with the least chances of good recovery should have their initial active treatment withdrawn. This requires a management decision within an hour or two of injury. When faced with an individual patient, anything less than 100% certainty of death or persisting severe disablement is ethically difficult to accept in most countries, as there is then always that lingering doubt of a chance of reasonable recovery.

Several workers have attempted to define a group of patients with an inevitable chance of dying or making a very poor recovery [39, 84]. As might be expected, they have failed to achieve any useful certainty levels within the critical first 6 h except in those patients who had already developed early unequivocal evidence of brain stem death. It should be emphasized that patients admitted in deep coma with bilateral unreacting pupils may survive with no residual disability [13, 84], and patients admitted with severe continuous extensor posturing may recover sufficiently well to resume normal activities [9]. Either a misplaced pessimistic approach or simply an indecisive policy in initial management so often results in unnecessary mortality and morbidity. Prediction requires a substantial data base collected over several years and the potential influence of any recent advance in therapy has to be excluded. Even if complete (100%) certainty becomes feasible shortly after injury it is unlikely that the necessary rejection of the possibility that new methods of treatment might influence outcome will be accepted by the medical profession.

Informing relatives

Presuming that attempts to predict eventual outcome should not influence our initial management, such attempts may help relatives to understand the severity of the injury. In practice, however, they will naturally have even more difficulties than we do in translating the percentages appertaining to a group of patients into the future prospects of one individual. Fortunately, over the first few days after injury, both the proportion of patients on whom prediction can be made and the level of certainty steadily increase [41, 84].

Evaluation of new treatment

It has been suggested [39] that the results of new treatment in relatively small numbers of patients can be conveniently evaluated by comparing each outcome with that predicted for individuals with more conventional treatment. The statistical principles are valid provided that the population of both the old data base and that of the new series have distinct clearly defined and controlled treatment regimes. As yet, no data base includes all the necessary factors that influence outcome and there have been no attempts to standardize and control the quality of treatment regimens. When such a data base eventually becomes available it may well prove to be a convenient tool for evaluation of new methods of management.

Is intensive care of head injuries worthwhile?

The reduction of mortality by intensive care is not enough if patients are merely kept alive with severe disabilities or in a persisting vegetative state. There is in fact very little evidence to support the belief that there has been an overall decrease in mortality throught the world in the last 50 years. Only in the 1970s were any serious attempts made to correlate outcome with initial neurological status and management regimen [57]. Langfitt has also pointed out the pitfalls in interpreting outcome and the dangers of attributing success to a particular therapeutic approach without careful matching of the two populations [58].

The introduction of the Glasgow Coma Scale in 1974 [105] proved an important step forward. Although the scale is too insensitive for the hour-to-hour detection of early deterioration of head-injured patients, it is now an internationally accepted standard for comparative studies. It is tempting to simplify the scale by adding up the three component scores but they are non-parametric and this therefore introduces inaccurate presumptions [106].

Evaluating the effectiveness of intensive care

Several recent studies have attempted to evaluate the effectiveness of individual components of intensive care. The outcome of patients with or without hypoxia [87], with or without steroids [17, 32, 36, 77] with or without ventilation [33], and with or without aggressive ICP control [7, 8, 13, 31, 64, 71, 93] have been published. All

the workers cited selected only a few of the clinical factors influencing outcome in their comparisons, failing to compare 'like with like.' Their conclusions were therefore relatively meaningless, although most were fully aware of the very serious limitations implicit in studies of this nature. As the outcome in the more severely injured patients is poorer it could be expected that those who received more intensive treatment would also be those who are more likely to fail to recover.

In an attempt to overcome this dilemma, Jennett together with colleagues from three countries standardized a method of assessing their patients with particular reference to the severity of injury [42, 107]. The considerable effort required to evaluate a series of over 1000 patients also unfortunately failed to yield any valid conclusion, as some of the crucial indicators of severity influencing outcome were excluded from the analysis [56]. The treatment regimens were reviewed retrospectively without predefinition. There was inevitable therapeutic assortment with no attempt to compare the influence of one clearly defined therapeutic 'package' with that of another.

Table 36.4 shows the more powerful factors influencing outcome. Some of these could not be included in Jennett's study as the subgroups would be too small and no attempts at matching were made. One of these relevant factors is the time after injury that selection for inclusion into the study is made [5]. In a series of 462 patients recorded as in coma with fixed dilated pupils within minutes of injury, immediate admission of all these patients would have resulted in a mortality rate of 95%. If however, admission to

Table 36.4. Major factors influencing outcome following severe head injury: A minimum inclusion requirement for comparative studies.

Pre-accident
 1. Age
 2. Possible influence of drugs

Impact
 3. Initial depth of coma, including motor activity
 4. Initial pupil signs
 5. Initial eye movements
 6. Other injuries
 7. Time from injury to inclusion into comparative study
 8. Extent of contusions seen on CT scan

Secondary events
 9. Severity and period of hypoxia
10. Severity and period of systemic hypotension
11. Severity and period of intracranial hypertension
12. Type of haematoma
13. Size and expansion rate of haematoma
14. Delay in evacuation of haematoma

---

a specialist centre had been delayed for 24 h, the selection by death would have apparently improved the mortality by reducing it to 65% [81]. If this single factor alone is ignored, a statistical analysis merely shows that patients treated very early have a higher mortality than those who have survived a delay in treatment, as the more severely injured of that group have already been excluded by their death. It was therefore not surprising to find in Jennett's work that patients selected for inclusion in the study late and given less intensive care had an apparently lower mortality than those who were included early and treated aggressively [42].

A study accurately comparing two groups of head-injured patients differing only in treatment regimes would be a mammoth task. In the light of the more recent neuropathological evidence [2, 34, 63] it would now be unethical to mount a controlled trial to compare outcome in patients with and without effective treatment for cerebral ischaemia, hypoxia or brain shift.

References

1. Abrams JS, Deane RS, Davis JH (1976) Pulmonary function in patients with multiple trauma and associated severe head injury. J Trauma 16:543–549
2. Adams JH, Graham DI (1976) The relationship between ventricular fluid pressure and the neuropathology of raised intracranial pressure. Neuropathol Appl Neurobiol 2:323–332
3. Adams JH, Brierley JB, Connor RCR, Treip CS (1966) The effects of systemic hypotension upon the human brain—clinical and neuropathological observations in 11 cases. Brain 89:235–268
4. Adams JH, Graham DI, Scott G, Parker LS, Doyle D (1980) Brain damage in fatal non-missile head injury. J Clin Pathol 33:1132–1145
5. Becker DP, Miller JD (1978) Neurosurgical forum on head injury management. J Neurosurg 48:492–493
6. Becker DP, Vries JK, Young HF, Ward JD (1975) Controlled cerebral perfusion pressure and ventilation in human mechanical brain injury: Prevention of progressive brain swelling. In: Lundberg N, Ponten U, Brock M (eds) Intracranial pressure vol II. Springer, Berlin Heidelberg New York, pp 480–484
7. Becker DP, Miller JD, Ward JD, Greenberg RP, Young HF, Sakalas R (1977) The outcome from severe head injury with early diagnosis and intensive management. J Neurosurg 47:491–502
8. Bowers SA, Marshall LF (1980) Outcome in 200 consecutive cases of severe head injury treated in San Diego County: a prospective analysis. Neurosurgery 6:237–242
9. Bricolo A, Turazzi S, Alexandre A, Rizzuto N (1977) Decerebrate rigidity in acute head injury. J Neurosurg 47:680–698
10. Britt RH, Hamilton RD (1978) Large decompressive craniotomy in the treatment of acute subdural haematoma. Neurosurgery 2:195–200
11. Brown FD, Johns L, Jafar JF, Crockard HA, Mullan S (1979) Detailed monitoring of the effects of mannitol following experimental head injury. J Neurosurg 50:423–432
12. Brown RS, Shoemaker WC (1973) Sequential hemodynamic changes in patients with head injury: evidence for an early hemodynamic defect. Ann Surg 177:187–192
13. Bruce DA, Schut L, Bruno LA, Woods JH, Sutton LN (1978) Outcome following severe head injuries in children. J Neurosurg 48:679–688
14. Bruce DA, Alavi A, Bilaniuk L, Dolinskas C, Obrist W, Uzzell B (1981) Diffuse cerebral swelling following head injuries in children: the syndrome of "malignant brain oedema." J Neurosurg 54:170–178
15. Buchan W (1828) Domestic medicine. Williams, Exeter, p 256
16. Burke AM, Quest DO, Chien S, Cerri C (1981) The effects of mannitol on blood viscosity. J Neurosurg 55:550–553
17. Cooper PR, Moody S, Kemp Clark W, et al. (1979) Dexamethasone and severe head injury. J Neurosurg 51:307–316
18. Cote CJ, Greenhow DE, Marshall BE (1979) The hypotensive response to rapid intravenous administration of the hypertonic solutions in man and in the rabbit. Anesthesiology 50:30–35
19. Cottrell JE, Robustelli A, Post K, Turndorf H (1977) Furosemide- and mannitol-induced changes in intracranial pressure and serum osmolality and electrolytes. Anesthesiology 47:28–30
20. Cranswick T, Smith BJ, Coulter LJ, Cowell MM (1979) Recherche d'une échelle de coma de sensibilité optimale. Le Journal de l'Infirmière de Neurochirurgie 23:16–20
21. Cushing H (1901) Concerning a definite regulatory mechanism of the vasomotor centre which controls blood pressure during cerebral compression. Bull Johns Hopkins Hosp 12:290–292
22. Ducker TB (1968) Increased intracranial pressure and pulmonary edema. 1. Clinical study of 11 patients. J Neurosurg 29:112–117
23. Ducker TB, Simmons RL (1968) Increased intracranial pressure and pulmonary edema. 2. The hemodynamic response of dogs and monkeys to increased intracranial pressure. J Neurosurg 29:118–122
24. Ferrer E, Vila F, Isamat F (1980) Mannitol response and histogram analysis in raised ICP. In: Schulman K, Marmarou A, Miller JD, Becker DP, Hochwald GM, Brock M (eds) Intracranial pressure, vol iv. Springer, Berlin Heidelberg New York, pp 647–649
25. Frost EAM (1977) Effects of positive end-expiratory pressure on intracranial pressure and compliance in brain-injured patients. J Neurosurg 47:195–200
26. Frost EAM, Arancibia CU, Shulman K (1979) Pulmonary shunt as a prognostic indicator in head injury. J Neurosurg 50:768–772
27. Galbraith S (1976) Misdiagnosis and delayed diagnosis in traumatic intracranial haematoma. Br Med J i:1438–1439
28. Galbraith S, Teasdale G (1981) Predicting the need for operation in the patient with an occult traumatic intracranial haematoma. J Neurosurg 55:75–81
29. Gennarelli TA, Czernicki Z, Segawa H, et al. (1980) ICP in experimental head injury. In: Shulman K, Marmarou A, Miller JD, Becker DP, Hochwald GM, Brock M (eds) Intracranial pressure, vol iv. Springer, Berlin Heidelberg New York, pp 28–32

30. Gentleman D, Jennett B (1981) Hazards of inter-hospital transfers of comatose head-injured patients. Lancet II:853–855

31. Gobiet W (1977) Advances in management of severe head injuries in childhood. Acta Neurochir (Wien) 39:201–210

32. Gobiet W, Bock WJ, Liesegang J, Grote W (1976) Treatment of acute cerebral edema with high dose of dexamethasone. In: Becks JWF, Bosch DA, Brock M (eds) Intracranial pressure, vol III, Springer, Berlin Heidelberg New York, pp 231–235

33. Gordon E (1979) Nonoperative treatment of acute head injuries: The Karolinska experience. Int Anesthesiol Clin 17:181–199

34. Graham DI, Adams JH, Doyle D (1978) Ischaemic brain damage in fatal nonmissile head injuries. J Neurol Sci 39:213–234

35. Grubb RL, Raichle ME, Phelps ME, Ratcheson RA (1975) Effects of increased intracranial pressure on cerebral blood volume, blood flow and oxygen utilization in monkeys. J Neurosurg 43:385–398

36. Gudeman SK, Miller JD, Becker DP (1979) Failure of high-dose steroid therapy to influence intracranial pressure in patients with severe head injury. J Neurosurg 51:301–306

37. James HE (1980) Methodology for the control of intracranial pressure with hypertonic mannitol. In: Shulman K, Marmarou A, Miller JD, Becker DP, Hochwald GM, Brock M (eds) Intracranial pressure, vol IV. Springer, Berlin Heidelberg New York, pp 653–655

38. Jeffreys RV, Jones JJ (1981) Avoidable factors contributing to the death of head injury patients in general hospitals in Mersey Region. Lancet II:459–461

39. Jennett B (1979) Severe head injury: Prediction of outcome as a basis of management decisions. Int Anesthesiol Clin 17:133–152

40. Jennett B, MacMillan R (1981) Epidemiology of head injury. Br Med J 282:101–104

41. Jennett B, Teasdale G, Minderhoud J, Heiden J, Kurze T (1979) Prognosis in series of patients with severe head injury. Neurosurgery 4:283–289

42. Jennett B, Teasdale G, Fry J, Braakman R, Minderhoud J, Kurze T (1980) Treatment for severe head injury. J Neurol Neurosurg Psychiatry 43:289–295

43. Jennett B, Gleave J, Wilson P (1981) Brain death in three neurosurgical units Br Med J 282:533–539

44. Johnston IH, Harper AM (1973) The effect of mannitol on cerebral blood flow. An experimental study. J Neurosurg 38:461–471

45. Johnston ILH, Jennett B (1973) The place of continuous intracranial pressure monitoring in neurosurgical practice. Acta Neurochir (Wien) 29:53–63

46. Jones JJ, Jeffreys RV (1981) Relative risk of alternative admission policies for patients with head injuries. Lancet II:850–853

47. Jones RM, Nahrwold ML, de Rosayro AM, Hill AB (1981) Cardiovascular responses and changes in plasma cation levels associated with infusion of hyperosmolar urea solutions. Anesth Analg 60:641–645

48. Jones TH, Morawetz RB, Crowell RM, et al. (1981) Thresholds of focal cerebral ischaemia in awake monkeys. J Neurosurg 54:773–782

49. Katsurado K, Yamada R, Sugimoto T (1973) Respiration insufficiency in patients with severe head injury. Surgery 73:191–199

50. Keaney NP, McDowall DG, Pickerodt VWA, et al. (1978) Time course of the cerebral circulatory response to metabolic depression. Am J Physiol 234(1):74–79

51. Kishore PRS, Lipper MH, Becker DP, Domingues Da Silva AA, Narayan Raj K (1981) Significance of CT in head injury: Correlation with intracranial pressure. Am J Radiol 137:829–833

52. Klatzo I (1967) Neuropathological aspects of brain oedema. J Neuropathol Exp Neurol 26:1–14

53. Kobrine AL, Timmins E, Rajjoub RK, Rizzoli HV, Davis DO (1977) Demonstration of massive traumatic brain swelling within 20 minutes after injury. J Neurosurg 46:256–258

54. Kramer SP, Horsley V (1897) The effects produced on the circulation and respiration by gun-shot injuries of the cerebral hemispheres. Philos Trans R Soc Lond [Biol] 188:223–256

55. Kuhl DE, Alavi A, Hoffman EJ, et al. (1980) Local cerebral blood volume in head-injured patients. J Neurosurg 52:309-320

56. Lancet (1980) Managing severe head injury—doing more and faring worse? Lancet I:1229

57. Langfitt TW (1978a) Measuring the outcome from head injuries. J Neurosurg 48:673–678

58. Langfitt TW (1978b) Outcome index for head injured patients. J Neurosurg 49:777–778

59. Leusen IR (1954) Chemosensitivity of the respiratory centre. Influences of changes in the H^+ and total buffer concentrations in the cerebral ventricles on respiration. Am J Physiol 176:45–51

60. Lozman J, Dutton RE, English M (1975) Cardiopulmonary adjustments following a single high dosage administration of methylprednisolone in traumatised man. Ann Surg 181:317–324

61. Lundberg N, Troupp H, Lorin H (1965) Continuous recording of the ventricular fluid pressure in patients with severe acute traumatic brain injury. A preliminary report. J Neurosurg 22:581–590

62. McDermott F (1978) Control of road trauma epidemic in Australia. Ann R Coll Surg Engl 60:437–450

63. Macpherson P, Graham DI (1978) Correlation between angiographic findings and the ischaemia of head injury. J Neurol Neurosurg Psychiatry 41:122–127

64. Marshall LF, Smith RW, Shapiro HM (1979) The outcome with aggressive treatment in severe head injuries. II. Acute and chronic barbiturate administration in the management of head injury. J Neurosurg 50:26–30

65. Maxwell JA, Goodwin JW (1973) Neurogenic pulmonary shunting. J Trauma 13:368–373

66. Mendelow AD, Karmi MZ, Paul KS, Fuller GA, Gillingham FJ (1979) Extradural haematoma: effect of delayed treatment. Br Med J i:1240–1242

67. Miller JD (1979a) Barbiturates and raised intracranial pressure. Ann Neurol 6:189–193

68. Miller JD (1979b) The management of cerebral oedema. Br J Hosp Med 21:152–164

69. Miller JD, Becker DP, Ward JD, Sullivan HG, Adams WE, Rosner MJ (1977) Significance of intracranial hypertension in severe head injury. J Neurosurg 47:503–516

70. Miller JD, Sweet RC, Narayan R, Becker DP (1978) Early insults to the injured brain. JAMA 240:439–442

71. Miller JD, Butterworth JF, Gudeman SK et al. (1981) Further experience in the management of severe head injury. J. Neurosurg. 54:289–299

72. Nakatani S, Koshino K, Mogami H, Sawada Y, Sugimoto T (1980) Brain interstitial fluid pressure measurement in head injury patients. In: Shulman K, Marmarou A, Miller JD, Becker DP, Hochwald GM, Brock M (eds) Intracranial pressure, vol IV. Springer, Berlin Heidelberg New York, pp 39–44

73. Office of Population Censuses and Surveys (1976) Mortality statistics: Review of the Registrar-General on deaths in England and Wales. HMSO, London

74. Overgaard J, Mosdal C, Tweed WA (1981) Cerebral circulation after head injury. Part 3: Does reduced regional cerebral blood flow determine recovery of brain function after blunt head injury? J Neurosurg 55:63–74

75. Partinen M, Kovanen J, Nilsson E (1981) Status epilepticus treated by barbiturate anaesthesia with continuous monitoring of cerebral function. Br Med J 282:520–521

76. Petersdorf RG, Curtin JA, Hoeprich PD, Peeler RN, Bennett IL (1957) A study of antibiotic prophylaxis in unconscious patients. N Engl J Med 257:1001–1009

77. Pitt LH, Kaktis JV (1980) Effect of megadose steroids on ICP in traumatic coma In: Shulman K, Marmarou A, Miller JD, Becker DP, Hochwald GM, Brock M (eds) Intracranial pressure, vol IV Springer, Berlin Heidelberg New York, pp 638–640

78. Pott P (1768) Observations on the nature and consequences of those injuries to which the head is liable from external violence. London, p 106

79. Price DJ (1980a) Intracranial pressure monitoring. British Journal of Clinical Equipment 5:92–98

80. Price DJ (1980b) The efficiency of sodium valproate as the only anticonvulsant administered to neurosurgical patients. In: Parsonage MJ, Caldwell ADS (eds) The place of sodium valproate in the treatment of epilepsy. Academic Press, London Toronto Sydney, pp 23–34

81. Price DJ (1981) Difficulties in evaluating the effectiveness of intensive care in head injury management. Crit Care Med 9:151

82. Price DJ (to be published) A practical coma scale for monitoring head injuries. In: Wilson DH, Marsden AK (eds), Progressive care of the acutely ill and injured, John Wiley & Sons, Chichester

83. Price DJ (to be published) The confirmation of death. In: Farman JV (ed) Anaesthesia for transplant surgery. Exerpta Medica, Amsterdam

84. Price DJ, Knill-Jones R (1979) The prediction of outcome of patients admitted following head injury in coma with bilateral fixed pupils. Acta Neurochir [Suppl] (Wien) 28:179–182

85. Price DJ, Mason J (1981) An attempt to rationalise the medical management of intracranial hypertension. Br J Anaesth 53:310

86. Price DJ, Mason J (to be published) Automated prophylaxis of postoperative and posttraumatic intracranial hypertension. In: Brock M (ed) Modern neurosurgery, vol. I. Springer, Berlin Heidelberg New York

87. Price DJ, Murray A (1972) The influence of hypoxia and hypotension on recovery from head injury. Injury 3:218–224

88. Price DJ, Sleigh JD (1970) Control of infecton due to *Klebsiella aerogenes* in a neurosurgical unit by withdrawal of all antibiotics. Lancet II:1213–1215

89. Price DJ, Dugdale RE, Mason J (1980) The control of ICP using three asynchronous closed loops. In: Shulman K, Marmarou A, Miller JD, Becker DP, Hochwald GM, Brock M (eds) Intracranial pressure, vol IV. Springer, Berlin Heidelberg New York, pp 395–399

90. Prior PF (1979) Monitoring cerebral function. Elsevier, Amsterdam

91. Reulen HJ, Graham R, Spatz M, Klatzo I (1977) Role of pressure gradients and bulk flow in dynamics of vasogenic brain oedema. J Neurosurg 46:24–35

92. Roberton FC, Kishore PRS, Miller JD, Lipper MH, Becker DP (1979) The value of serial computerized tomography in the management of severe head injury. Surg Neurol 12:161–167

93. Rockoff MA, Marshall LF, Shapiro HM (1979) High-dose barbiturate therapy in humans: A clinical review of 60 patients. Ann Neurol 6:194–199

94. Rose J, Valtonen S, Jennett B (1977) Avoidable factors contributing to death after head injury. Br Med J ii:615–618

95. Rossanda M, Collice M, Porta M, Boselli L (1975) Intracranial hypertension in head injury. Clinical significance and relation to respiration. In: Lundberg N, Ponten U, Brock M (eds) Intracranial pressure, vol II. Springer, Berlin Heidelberg New York, pp 475–479

96. Salem F, Price DJ (to be published) Monitoring of head injured patients In Brock M (ed.) Modern neurosurgery I, Springer-Verlag, Berlin, Heidelberg, New York

97. Salem F, Price DJ (to be published) Single indicants for prediction of the risk of head injured patients developing an intracranial haematoma. J Neurosurg

98. Seelig JM, Becker DP, Miller JD, Greenberg RP, Ward JD, Choi SC (1981) Traumatic acute subdural hematoma. N Engl J Med. 304:1511–1518

99. Shapiro HM, Marshall LF (1978) Intracranial pressure responses to PEEP in head-injured patients. J Trauma 18:254–256

100. Shulman K (1965) Small artery and vein pressures in the subarachnoid space of the dog. J Surg Res 5:56–61

101. Skillman JJ (1974) Ethical dilemmas in the care of the critically ill. Lancet II:634–637

102. Snoek J, Jennett B, Adams JH, Graham DI, Doyle D (1979) Computerised tomography after recent severe head injury in patients with acute intracranial haematoma. J Neurol Neurosurg Psychol 42:215–225

103. Stidham GL, Nugent SK, Rogers M (1980) Monitoring cerebral electrical function in the ICU. Crit Care Med 8:519–523

104. Symon L (1968) Experimental evidence of intracerebral steal following CO_2 inhalation. Scand J Clin Lab Invest 22:46–51

105. Teasdale G, Jennett B (1974) Assessment of coma and impaired consciousness: A practical scale. Lancet II:81–84

106. Teasdale G, Murray G, Parker L, Jennett B (1979a) Adding up the Glasgow Coma Score. Acta Neurochir. [Suppl.] (Wien) 28:13–16

107. Teasdale G, Parker L, Murray G, Jennett B (1979b) On comparing series of head injured patients. Acta Neurochir [Suppl] (Wien) 28:205–208

108. Theodore J, Robin ED (1975) Pathogenesis of neurogenic pulmonary oedema. Lancet II:749–751

109. Troupp H, McDowall DG (1976) Patient management: Summary. In: Beks JWF, Bosch DA, Brock M (eds) Intracranial pressure, vol III. Springer, Berlin Heidelberg New York, pp 279–280

110. United Nations Organization (1975) Demographic year book 1973. UNO, Geneva

111. Versari P, Vecchi G, Arosio M, Collice M, Rosanda M (1980) Effect of Althesin on intracranial hypertension in patients with severe head injury. In: Shulman K, Marmarou A, Miller JD, Becker DP, Hochwald GM, Brock M (eds) Intracranial pressure, vol IV. Springer, Berlin Heidelberg New York, pp 610–612

112. Wilson JW (1972) Treatment or prevention of pulmonary cellular damage with pharmacological doses of corticosteroid. Surg Gynecol Obstet 134:675–681

Chapter 37

Acute Cervical Spinal Cord Injuries

Maurice S. Albin and Maciej F. Babinski

Because of the significant mortality, CNS effects, and often overwhelming physiological responses from other organ systems, this report will deal with some of the critical care management problems associated with acute cervical cord trauma (ACCT).

Epidemiological data from many countries [27, 64, 80] appear to indicate that the etiological factors [19, 50, 53, 87] causing spinal cord injury (SCI) are (in order of increasing to decreasing incidence) vehicular accidents, falls (job- and not-job-related), and sports activities. Within the latter group, diving injuries [86] appear to predominate. It appears that there is a much higher incidence of SCI in the male; that the majority of patients range between 15 and 35 years of age; that younger and middle-aged persons are targeted with occupational injuries; that there is a considerable increase in falls at home as age increases; and within this group of older patients (>50 years) suffering SCI from falls, there appeared to be a high percentage of cervical SCI without bony injury. Identification of incidence rates of SCI had been difficult to resolve because of a nonexistent or nonfunctional reporting system [2, 22, 29, 43, 45, 55, 62, 65, 71, 74, 99, 107]. During the past two decades the 'tip' as well as a portion of the 'base' of the iceberg appears to be coming into view with incidence rates ranging from 12.4 to 53.4 per million population [11, 23] being reported from different countries and localities. Because of the great advances made in the care and rehabilita-

tion of the patient with SCI, longevity times for the paraplegic and quadriplegic have increased tremendously. The increasing worldwide incidence of SCI resulting from vehicular accidents (e.g., the leading cause of death in Venezuela during 1979), combined with better medical care and longer survival, carries with it the implication that this type of holocaust will inevitably cast a severe strain on the medical economy of the more affluent nations, let alone those countries with scarcer resources. First-year hospital cost factors of those with ACCT range from 35 000 to 50 000 dollars [102], and it is estimated that medical costs during the lifetime of a paraplegic in the United States probably will average about one half-million dollars [27, 64, 80]. The solution to the familial, personal, and socioeconomic tragedy that characterizes the patient with SCI probably lies in the preventive aspects of the problem—better informed and safety-educated individuals; better designed vehicles with more energy-absorbing passive and active restraining systems; augumented industrial safety measures and above all, legal and social deterrents to the combination of alcohol and vehicular usage. From the treatment aspect we must think in terms of a logical flow pattern encompassing initial identification of the individual with ACCT, retrieval and transportation to a designated SCI treatment center; initial evaluation and diagnosis at this hospital center and triage to the special ICU or to the operating theater.

Physiopathology and therapy in SCI

The past decade has changed much of our thinking related to acute SCI. We formerly thought of acute spinal trauma as irreversible and hopeless, and concentrated our efforts on improving the functional ability of the patient with this type of lesion by bettering the rehabilitation process. Albin et al. [5–10] and White et al. [104–106] gave impetus to our new understanding of the physiopathology of SCI by reviving and modifying the impact injury animal model first developed by Allen [16] and studied by Freeman and Wright [42] in 1953. Albin's and White's groups indicated that the acute cord lesion has progressively developed time-dependent characteristics involving primarily the gray matter vascularity; that up to a point in time (4.0 h) it was possible to arrest this destructive process by localized spinal cord hypothermia; and that it was possible to use somatosensory cortically evoked responses (SER) [47] to test the completeness of the lesion. These findings have been verified in elegant histological studies [17, 32–35, 46, 100, 101]. Changes in O_2 tensions have also been indicated [37, 60], and in addition the sensitivity of the SER as a diagnostic and prognostic tool has been shown [36, 81, 85]. Lewin et al. [67] and Eidelberg et al. [38] implicated changes in Na^+ and K^+ in the injured spinal cord secondary to tissue edema and necrosis, while Kakari et al. [60] thought the release of lysosomal enzymes was important in the development of the lesion. An important development in our understanding of this pathological process involving SCI was made by Osterholm and Matthews [76–78], who described an increase in norepinephrine in the gray matter of the contused spinal cord and noted that blocking norepinephrine synthesis by alpha-methyltyrosine could prevent lesion expansion. Although this finding was not corroborated by other investigators [25, 26, 30, 73], they can be credited with opening the area of SCI to neurochemical evaluation.

In terms of the dynamics of experimental impact injury, the trauma can bring with it mechanical destruction of neuronal elements and/or hemorrhage, a decreased vascular perfusion, and lowering tissue PO_2, edema, and necrosis. The criticality of the time dependence has been recently shown by Albin et al. [12]. Inhibition of axoplasmic transport (with tritiated leucine) can be seen 2 h after injury, with a marked block occurring 4 h after trauma and complete inhibition at 6 h.

Therapeutic modalities evaluated in the experimental animal have involved localized selective hypothermia as described by Albin et al. [5, 6–8, 10], White et al. [104], Ducker and Hamit [37], Kelly et al. [60], Hansebout et al. [52], and Kucher and Hansebout [66]. Tator and Deecke [94] did not find spinal cord hypothermia effective against balloon compression injury and thought that normothermic perfusion was helpful. On the other hand, Thienprasit et al. [96] found localized cord cooling useful against balloon compression injury, while Albin and White [4] found normothermic perfusion valueless against the impact injury preparation. The hyperosmotic agents have been used without indication that they are effective. Ducker and Hamit [37] and Black and Markowitz [21] noted the efficacy of the glucocorticoids in experimentally injured animals. Osterholm and Mathews [79] reasoned that steroids depress post-injury catecholamine metabolism and accumulation when they found steroids effective against experimental impact injury, but the steroidal norepinephrine depression was less striking than that observed with localized hypothermia of the spinal cord. Hyperosmotic agents have been shown by Joyner and Freeman (urea) [58] and by Richardson and Nakamura (mannitol) [83] in experimental animals to have a beneficial effect. Hyperbaric oxygenation (three atmospheres) has also been used by Hartzog et al. [54] on baboons with impact injury and resulted in improvement compared with controls. Other experimental therapies reported have been the use of vasopressors to maintain adequate perfusion; epsilon-aminocaproic acid by Naftchi et al. [73] for cell membrane stabilization and the use of dimethyl sulfoxide by de la Torre et al. [31].

The application of therapies mentioned above is difficult to evaluate in the human unless a standardized, randomized study with rigid selection criteria is effected. The primary difficulty involves getting the patient as rapidly as possible to a hospital center equipped to initiate therapy. Although dexamethasone and other glucocorticoids have been used clinically over the years for SCIs, no substantial data have emerged to indicate their benefit. Similarly, the use of hyperosmotic agents in trauma have not established their efficacy. Clinically, spinal cord cooling has been used with inconsistent results in humans [1, 24, 63, 70, 100]. Our own experience has been hampered by difficulties in delivering and evaluating the patient to begin cooling within the 4-h time frame. We have also found that our original estimation of the caloric gradient required to reduce the intrinsic spinal cord temperature to 10°C or below was not large enough. Dr. Robert J. White and I thought that by increasing the flow rate of the inflow perfusate to 1300 ml/min (entering at 3°C), it would be possible to reach 10°C rapidly. In the first case of human cooling reported by us, it was not found possible to go below 17°C in the cervical area with flows of 600 ml/min. In the clinical trials reported in the literature, criteria for patient selection, perfusion flows, and temperature and duration of cooling have varied from one report to another. At the University of Pittsburgh, we noted in one patient that cord temperature at the C_6–C_7 vertebral level could not be lowered below 17°C with a perfusion flow of 1300 ml/min. This signifies that adequate cord temperature reduction (to 10°C) has not been obtained and maintained in the clinical cases of SCI where selective hypothermia has been used. Using an in vitro heat sink simulating the mass and caloric output of three segments of the cervical cord, we found that a flow of at least 2000 ml/min was needed to reach 10°C when the perfusate entered between 3° and 5°C. Because of both the experimental and clinical data, it is felt that a standardized, randomized cooperative clinical study of localized cooling should be initiated to evaluate spinal cord injury therapy. Selection criteria should ensure that only those patients with a complete lesion (as indicated by neurological evaluation and abolition of somatosensory evoked responses) and patients where cooling can be initiated within 4 h after injury are included. Incomplete lesions should be excluded as well as those with a pulped or lacerated spinal cord.

That spinal cord cooling might be effective with the above-mentioned criteria can be noted in a 16-year-old female with a cord injury complete at the T_{12}–T_{11} vertebral level who had a posterior laminectomy and institution of localized hypothermia within 3 h after injury. The perfusate entered at 3°C at a flow rate of 2000 ml/min and was carried out for 3.0 h [3]. Good function returned within 3.0 days and the patient was back to preinjury neurological levels by the end of the 1st week after cooling, being able to ambulate well again.

Initial response, retrieval systems, and clinical overview

We have noted the need for transporting the patient with SCI as rapidly as possible to a specialized unit because of the important time factor [2, 15, 40, 57, 95]. That rapid evacuation can be efficacious in limiting the progression of neurological damage is demonstrated by the experience of Gregg and Wilmot [49] in Eire, where a special 'flying squad' of a physician and nurse are helicoptered to the scene of the accident, the patient retrieved by helicopter on a specially designed stretcher, and transported with the team to the National Rehabilitation Centre in Dublin [48]. The high percentage of incomplete cervical cord lesions indicates the effectiveness of this approach. Coordination of ground air ambulance service is best exemplified by the Swiss Air Rescue Unit, where all spinal cord injury cases are transported to a spinal cord center, the average time elapsed being 50 min instead of 4 h with a conventional ambulance system [51]. It is obvious that rapid safe transportation to a unit specialized in care of the patient with SCI is one of the keys to successful therapy. Protocols should be developed on a geographical basis to standardize evacuation and delivery of the patient to a specialized center. Similarly, standards for SCI centers should be delineated and coordinated with air and highway transportation.

Whether the patient with a SCI is first seen by a flying squad or a paramedically staffed ambulance unit, the patient should be immobilized on a spine board with the head and neck placed in a neutral position. All comatose patients and/or patients with multiple trauma should be treated as if a cord injury has occurred. Ventilatory evaluation must be made and assistance given where needed. The primary early cause of death among cervical cord victims is usually respiratory failure. Training of emergency medical technicians in ventilatory management of these types of patients and recognition of neurological symptoms is critical. Adequate equipment, including spine boards, collars, ventilating bags and masks, IV solutions, and volume expanders should be considered part of normal operations. A centralized communications system with operational control handled by an emergency medical service assistance group allows for optimal triage and the opportunity to interpose specialist consultation when needed. If we are to have any hope of preventing the incomplete cervical cord lesion from becoming complete, let alone of salvaging the patient with multiple trauma, including head and cord injury, then we must move into these modern systems of integrated communication and command [95]. The parochialism involved in mandating that local ambulance services transport patients to the nearest hospital (even though it has minimal facilities to take care of these acute problems) must give way to extrication and transportation to the unit with optimal facilities for acute care, in this case, the SCI center [23].

The essential purpose of the first response is to extricate, identify, and move the patient with a cord lesion to the appropriate medical institution and maximally support the cardiovascular and pulmonary system without exacerbating existing neurological damage. Attempts at reduction should not be made at the scene of the accident (or anywhere) without adequate diagnostic studies.

A flow pattern with documentation of movement and frequent neurological checks should be carried out since the patient may be taken to many different service areas of the hospital—emergency room, radiology, patient unit, or operating theater. Unfortunately, few hospitals have adopted the regular practice of moving the patient from the ambulance to a special frame (Stryker or modification).

As mentioned earlier, respiratory complications are not uncommon in cervical and high thoracic cord injuries, especially when complicated with associated injuries [88, 97]. Cervical cord lesions may develop an ascending level because of increasing spinal cord edema which can compromise ventilation considerably. The patient with acute traumatic tetraplegia demands instant and close ventilatory monitoring and care. With a complete lesion, there will be total intercostal paralysis; with lesion at or below the level of the 6th cervical segment, the diaphragmatic innervation is intact. If the level is at the 5th cervical segment, there is a partial diaphragmatic innervation and with a level at or above the 4th cervical segment, the diaphragm is deprived of its major segmental nerve supply and function is grossly impaired. In these cases ventilatory assistance is mandatory and the rapid, careful placement of an endotracheal tube may be life-saving. The combination of a high cervical injury with inadequate ventilation can lead to a decreased vital capacity, retention of secretions, increased PCO_2, decreased PO_2, increased dead space, anoxia, vasoconstriction, respiratory failure, and pulmonary edema—a leading cause of death in acute traumatic tetraplegia. The availability of the fiberoptic bronchoscope has facilitated many aspects of pulmonary care in these patients as well as making the placement of the endotracheal tube both easier and safer.

Associated injuries are very common in pa-

tients with spinal cord trauma, the incidence ranging from 25% to 65%. In general, head injuries are the most common severe associated injury with a cervical cord injury; and then comes chest injury with a serious injury to the thoracic spine. No part of the body is immune when trauma has occurred, and two or more associated injuries are not uncommon. A thorough neurological examination, with attention to ventilatory problems, evaluation of 'silent areas' such as the chest, head, and abdomen; the use of x-rays of chest, skull, abdomen, and long bones; placement of nasogastric and urinary catheters will all be helpful in delineating this possibility, providing one always starts off with a high index of suspicion.

Cardiovascular responses may be triggered when sudden, traumatic complete cord transections initiate a state of 'spinal shock' with the cord ceasing to function below the level of the lesion. Compromises of the sympathetic outflow from the T_1 to the L_2 segments can significantly affect the blood pressure. Transections above T_1 can cause a blood pressure fall to 40 mmHg. The other symptoms of this type of autonomic blockade are bradycardia, hypothermia, and psychic disturbances. Moving and tilting the patient precipitously in this condition could be hazardous because the compensatory mechanism for postural changes is lost. The combination of spinal shock and hemorrhage from other associated injuries can indeed be dangerous. Transfusions should be given judiciously and fluids should be titrated with a CVP or Swan–Ganz line. Urinary output and fluid intake must be quantitated continuously, and since the patient in spinal shock becomes poikilothermic, external heat should be regulated to ensure normothermia.

Diagnosis [40, 95]

Neurological evaluation

This is of fundamental importance, and input into the initial neurological evaluation should be documented by the time and description of injury and repeated examinations as the patient with a SCI progresses from initial contact in the emergency department to definitive treatment. The neurological examination should be complete, including grading of motor function, sensory loss, reflexes, cranial nerves, fundi, pupillary changes, and extraocular movements.

Radiological studies

These should encompass an initial lateral cervical spine, including C_7 and T_1, with special views taken if needed. Early gas myelography has been used to delineate compromising bone fragments and intraspinal disks impinging on the cord. Tomograms and the recent employment of computerized axial tomography (CAT) have helped to delineate the lesioned cord.

Somatosensory evoked response (SER)

This is a noninvasive diagnostic tool [36, 81] that has become an important diagnostic method which may also have prognostic value [85]. The technique involves stimulation of a peripheral afferent nerve and use of a scalp electrode to record from the underlying contralateral somatosensory cortex. A signal averager analyzes these evoked responses. In general, in patients with complete motor and sensory loss below the spinal cord lesion SER is absent. On the other hand, the presence or return of the SER may be an indication for hopeful prognosis and may even precede clinical improvement.

Critical care components of ACCT

Cardiopulmonary problems

Pulmonary dysfunction with acute respiratory failure is frequently seen in patients with ACCT and figures prominently as a major cause of mortality [88, 89, 97]. This may be due to intercostal paralysis and the inability of the diaphragm to compensate for lack of rib cage expansion [20]. Other important factors concern themselves with the inability of the quadriplegic to remove bronchial secretions because of the low expiratory reserve volumes with reduced maximal expiratory pressures; a change in chest cage movement with the maximal motion occurring in the upper part of the chest, little movement in the upper part of chest, little movement in the lower portion, and sucking in of the lower ribs when maximum breaths are taken; an increase in the work of breathing has been found in quadriplegics because of the decreased compliance necessitating augmented ventilation and increased expenditure of energy [28, 41, 44, 79, 90]. The critical mechanism concerning ventilatory failure appears to be alveolar hypoventilation [20], which is due to the high extrapulmonary resistances to breathing necessitating an inordinate increase in work. When the diaphragm becomes the sole muscle of ventilation the resistances also occur because of the incorporated movements of the abdominal viscera.

Pulmonary evaluation

This must be a continuous ongoing procedure in the patient with ACCT, since an unstable spine with improperly handled patient movement and a small cephalad increase in spinal cord edema may be enough to change a patient's position from low to high quadriplegia, with potential severe ventilatory dysfunction. Thus, the total baseline evaluation including the neurological, cardiovascular, and pulmonary systems, should be done as completely and as rapidly as possible after the patient's entering the basic triage unit (emergency room or specialized care unit). This of course becomes even more difficult in the comatose patient or one with associated injuries. Nevertheless, the ventilatory rate, tidal volume, pattern of ventilation, and chest auscultation should be carried out immediately, with appropriate radiological procedures as needed and arterial blood gas tests to assess gas exchange and metabolic responses.

It has been noted that changes in lung volumes [28] and pulmonary function occur in the quadriplegic, with reductions in vital capacity, total lung capacity, expiratory reserve volume, and an increased residual volume. Flow-volume loop studies [41] have shown that the forced vital capacity in the quadriplegic is considerably reduced in the sitting position, being much lower than in the supine or Trendelenburg position. Pulmonary volumes should be obtained as soon as clinically feasible and serve as a guide to the patient's ventilatory status [94].

Cardiovascular responses

The patient with ACCT will manifest some degree of spinal shock characterized by bradycardia, arterial hypotension, and increased venous capacitance [72]. For the most part, this is due to the transection interrupting the control of the sympathetic outflow and responses. Because of the transection and lack of sympathetic control, the patient also becomes poikilothermic. Since most patients with ACCT have some manifestation of spinal shock, we often assume that the immediate result of transection is the development of bradycardia, hypotension, and changes in venous capacitance. A large body of experimental evidence has been developed during the past two decades to indicate that the immediate response to acute cervical cord transection is a transitory marked arterial hypertension, and bradycardia with brady-arrhythmias lasting 10–30 min [8, 39, 61, 84]. Recent experimental work has shown that a significant transitory rise in intracranial pressure (ICP) with an increase in brain water and extra-vascular lung water (EVLW) also accompanies early ACCT. Paradoxically, although the arterial hypertension can be blocked by phentolamine, an alpha blocker, the rise in ICP and EVLW is not totally attenuated. This may be a significant finding, since pulmonary edema has been reported associated with ACCT [13, 15].

These abnormal cardiopulmonary responses render these patients extraordinarily sensitive to volume loading, drugs, anesthetics [98], and the stresses of emergency management and surgery. Under these conditions, information concerning the cardiovascular status can be obtained by means of adequate monitoring techniques. This includes the ECG and indwelling catheter for arterial blood pressure; a catheter in the right atrium or superior vena cava for measuring CVPs. Unfortunately, the CVP may not be an adequate guide for determining the need for volume replacement, since we do not have an indication of the dynamics of the left side of the heart and normal CVPs have been noted in face of a failing left heart. Fortunately, the development of the Swan–Ganz catheter [93] allows us to look at right atrial (RA), pulmonary artery (PA), and pulmonary capillary wedge pressure (PCWP) and to assess cardiac output (CO) by means of the thermodilution technique. This flow-directed balloon-tipped catheter is relatively easy to insert, provides critical management information in these patients, and has become almost routine in our unit. Physiological profiles relating to systemic vascular resistance, stroke volumes, work of the heart, intrapulmonary shunting, cardiac indices, etc. can easily be obtained with this system. A knowledge of the PCWP, colloid oncotic pressure (COP) and osmolarity allows one to evaluate some of the factors in the development of pulmonary edema and provide a baseline for therapeutic management.

Other monitoring would include temperature, electrolytes, chemistries for renal function, and either continuous or discontinuous bladder catheterization for urine volumes and analysis.

The combination of acute head injury and ACCT might also necessitate the use of ICP monitoring if intracranial hypertension is suspected. This may indeed become important in view of the finding [13, 14] relating to the initial rise in ICP following experimental ACCT since it has also been shown that acute rises in ICP may trigger pulmonary edema of centrogenic origin [68, 72, 82].

General management concepts

Basic treatment philosophy must be oriented to move the patient with ACCT as rapidly and directly as possible to the definitive treatment area (preferably a SCI center) to 'interrupt auto-destructive pathophysiologic processes to prevent post-traumatic ischemia and infarction of the spinal cord' [95].

A specialized unit or center is important because of the need to concentrate and commit the critical technical and human resources at such a strategic place. At such a unit, the neuroradiological facilities would include equipment for myelography, tomography and a CAT scanner. The last has become an important diagnostic tool for looking at the spinal cord in depth and enabling disc protusions to be recognized. Similarly, somatosensory evoked potentials have been shown to have both diagnostic and prognostic value in SCI. This is especially true in the unconscious or uncooperative patient.

Spinal immobilization has become the sine qua non of management for the unstable spine. Immobilization can be accomplished early in evacuation by means of a spine board or tongs applied by the medical team. In the hospital unit, halo traction devices have become extremely popular and replaced skull traction with tongs in many institutions. Spinal immobilization can also be accomplished by operative fusion anteriorly or posteriorly, with and without the use of devices (like the Harrington rod) for external fixation [40, 95].

Anesthesia

Because airway management is critical in the patient with cervical cord injury (actual or suspected), an overall 'philosophy' should be developed. This includes supplying all areas where emergency intubation is to be accomplished with essential equipment, including endotracheal tubes, conventional laryngoscope blades, apparatus for ventilation [18, 92] and the fiberoptic bronchoscope. We regard the last two items as important aids to solving a problem which has often been considered insuperable.

Patients with suspected or real cervical cord injury should have the head and cervical spine immobilized and in some adequate type of traction. In general, this means that the normal extension–flexion maneuvers involved in intubation will not be possible. It is our practice to intubate these patients while awake after adequate sedation with fentanyl–droperidol or fentanyl–diazepam. It is equally important to inform the patient what is to be done and the reasons for these maneuvers. Because of the problem of spinal shock, we believe that adequate monitoring is mandatory in operative procedures and in the ICU management of these cases. This includes direct measurement of arterial blood pressure (radial artery catheter); monitoring of central venous pressure, pulmonary arterial and wedge pressure; ECG; minute volume, tidal volume, airway pressure and urinary output; use of a nerve stimulator to estimate the condition of the neuromuscular junction; facilities for rapid determination of blood gases, hematocrit, and serum and/or urine osmolalities and electrolytes; and temperature. The existence of any physiological conduction along spinal cord pathways can be monitored during surgical procedures on cord and spine by stimulation-recording computerized averaging (somatosensory cortically evoked responses).

In general, our anesthetic technique utilizes diazepam–fentanyl–thioamylal induction, intubation under pancuronium, and maintenance with narcotic–N_2O–pancuronium. As mentioned previously, a large proportion of these cases are intubated awake under sedation with maintenance as noted above. Fluid and blood replacements are monitored and limited because loss of sympathetic tone easily allows fluid overload and pulmonary edema. Frequent arterial blood gas sampling can give an evaluation of the adequacy of tissue perfusion, and hence the rush to bring the patient's blood pressure to normotensive levels by the infusion of large volumes of colloids, crystalloids, and blood should be avoided. We intubate these patients with soft plastic tubes having prestretched cuffs, using a pressure-limiting balloon for cuff regulation. Because of the well-known hazard involving excessive potassium release from denervated muscle after succinylcholine administration (even in fresh SCIs), we choose to use a nondepolarizing agent for muscle relaxation [91]. Suctioning the patient with ACCT can become a problem because of the

cardiovascular responses involved due to spinal shock. Severe bradycardia and cardiac arrest have been reported during tracheal suction exacerbated by hypoxia. In these patients good preoxygenation is important, and if this does not prevent the bradycardia the use of IV atropine is indicated [69, 103].

References

1. Acosta-Rua G (1970) Treatment of traumatic paraplegic patients by localized cooling of the spinal cord. J Iowa Med Soc 60:326
2. Albin MS (1978) Resuscitation of the spinal cord. Crit Care Med 6:270
3. Albin MS, Bunegin L (1978) Flow rates and cord temperatures during selective spinal cord hypothermia. Fed Proc 37:109–601
4. Albin MS, White RJ, (1973) Evaluation of normothermic spinal cord perfusion after impact injury. Proceedings of the Society for Neurosciences's Third Annual Meeting, November 1973
5. Albin MS, White RJ, Donald DE, et al (1961) Hypothermia of the spinal cord by perfusion cooling of the subarachnoid space. Surg Forum 12:188
6. Albin MS, White RJ, Locke GE, et al (1966) Spinal cord hypothermia by localized perfusion cooling. Nature 210:1059
7. Albin MS, White RJ, Locke GE, et al (1967) Localized spinal cord hypothermia: Anesthetic effects and application to traumatic injury. Anesth Analg (Cleve) 46:8
8. Albin MS, White RJ, Taslitz N (1967) Initial cardiovascular responses following cervical cord transection. Anat Rec 157:347
9. Albin MS, White RJ, Acosta-Rua G, et al (1968) Study of functional recovery produced by delayed localized cooling after spinal cord injury in primates. J Neurosurg 29:113
10. Albin MS, White RJ, Yashon D, et al (1969) Effects of localized cooling in spinal cord trauma. J Trauma 9:1000
11. Albin MS, Aronica MJ, Black WA Jr, et al (1978) Report, Spinal Cord Injury Task Force, Health Advisory Council, Department of Health, Commonwealth of Pennsylvania. Pennsylvania Medicine 81:29
12. Albin MS, Helsel P, Bunegin L, et al (1978) Axoplasmic transport patterns after experimental spinal cord crush injury. Anat Rec 190:603
13. Albin MS, Bunegin L, Helsel P, Babinski M, Marlin AE (1979) Intracranial pressure and cardiovascular responses to experimental cord transection. Crit Care Med 7:127
14. Albin MS, Bunegin L, Wolf S, Babinski M, Ison R (1980a) Phentolamine does not attenuate the intracranial pressure (ICP) rise after experimental spinal cord transection. Proc FASEB 39(3):9–959
15. Albin MS, Hung TK, Babinski M (1980b) Spinal Cord Injury — Epidemiology, emergency care and acte care: Advances in physiopathology and treatment. Curr Probl Surg 17:190
16. Allen AR (1911) Surgery of experimental lesion of spinal cord equivalent to crush injury of fracture dislocation of spinal column. A preliminary report. JAMA 57:878

17. Assenmacher DR, Ducker TB (1971) Experimental traumatic paraplegia: The vascular and pathologic changes seen in reversible and irreversible spinal cord lesions. J Bone Joint Surg [Am] 53:671

18. Babinski M, Smith RB, Klain M (1980) High-frequency jet ventilation for laryngoscopy. Anesthesiology 52:178

19. Bedbrook GM (1979) Spinal injuries with tetraplegia and paraplegia. J Bone Joint Surg [Br] 61:267

20. Bergofsky EH (1964) Mechanism for respiratory insufficiency after cervical cord injury. Ann Intern Med 61:435

21. Black P, Markowitz RS (1971) Experimental spinal cord injury in monkeys: Comparison of steroids and hypothermia. Surg Forum 22:409

22. Bosch A, Stauffer ES, Nickel VL (1971) Incomplete traumatic quadriplegia, a ten year review. JAMA 216:473

23. Botterell EH, Joosse AT, Kraus AS, et al (1975) A model for the future care of acute spinal cord. Ann R Coll Phys Surg Can 8:193–218

24. Bricolo A, Dalle-Oro G, DaPian R, et al (1976) Local cooling in spinal cord injury. Surg Neurol 6:101

25. Bunegin L, Albin MS, Jannetta PJ (1976) Catecholamine responses to experimental spinal cord impact injury. II. Fate of intravenous 3H-NE. Exp Neurol 53:281

26. Bunegin L, Albin MS, Jannetta PJ (1976) Catecholamine responses to experimental spinal cord impact injury. I. Intrinsic spinal cord synthesis rates. Exp Neurol 53:274

27. Carter RE (1977) Etiology of traumatic spinal cord injury: Statistics of more than 1100 cases. Tex Med 73:61

28. Carter RE (1979) Medical management of pulmonary complications of spinal cord injury. Adv Neurol 22:261

29. Cheshire DJE (1968) The complete and centralized treatment of paraplegia. Paraplegia 6:59

30. De la Torre JC, Johnson CM, Harris LH, et al (1974) Monoamine changes in experimental head and spinal cord tissue: Failure to confirm previous observations. Surg Neurol 2:5

31. De la Torre JC, Johnson CM, Goode DJ, et al (1975) Pharmacologic treatment and evaluation of permanent experimental spinal cord trauma. Neurology 25:508

32. Dohrmann GJ, Wagner FC, Bucy PC (1971) The microvasculature in transitory traumatic paraplegia. An electron mircoscopic study in the monkey. J Neurosurg 35:263

33. Dohrmann GJ, Wagner FC, Bucy PC (1972) Transitory traumatic paraplegia: Electron microscopy of the early alterations in myelinated nerve fibers. J Neurosurg 36:407

34. Dohrmann GJ, Wick KM, Bucy PC (1972) Blood flow patterns in the intrinsic vessels of the spinal cord following contusion. An experimental study. Trans Am Neurol Assoc 97:189

35. Dohrmann GJ, Wick KM, Bucy PC (1973) Spinal cord blood flow patterns in experimental traumatic paraplegia. J Neurosurg 38:42

36. Donaghy RMP, Numoto M (1969) Prognostic significance of sensory evoked potential in spinal cord injury. Proceedings of the Spinal Cord Injuries Conference 17:251

37. Ducker TB, Hamit HF (1969) Experimental treatments of acute spinal cord injury. J Neurosurg 30:693

38. Eidelberg E, Sullivan S, Brigham A (1975) Immediate consequences of spinal cord injury: Possible role of potassium in axonal conduction block. Surg Neurol 3:317

39. Eidelberg EE (1973) Cardiovascular response to experimental spinal cord compression. J Neurosurg 38:326

40. Fever H (1976) Management of acute spine and spinal cord injuries. Old and new concepts. Arch Surg 111:638

41. Forner JV, Lombart RL, Valdizan-Valledor MC (1975) The flow volume loop in tetraplegics. Paraplegia 15:245

42. Freeman LW, Wright TW (1953) Experimental observations of concussion and contusion of the spinal cord. Ann Surg 137:433

43. Frey CF, Huelke DF, Gikas PW (1969) Resuscitation and survival in motor vehicle accidents. Trauma 9:292

44. Frost ER (1979) The physiopathology of respiration in neurosurgical patients. J Neurosurg 50:699

45. Gehrig R, Michaelis LS (1968) Statistics of acute paraplegia and tetraplegia on a national scale. Paraplegia 6:93

46. Goodkin R, Campbell JB (1969) Sequential pathologic changes in spinal cord injury, a preliminary report. Surg Forum 20:430

47. Gossman M, White RJ, Taslitz N, et al (1968) Electrophysiological responses immediately after experimental injury to the spinal cord. Anat Rec 160:473

48. Gregg TM (1967) Organization of a spinal injury unit within a rehabilitation centre. Paraplegia 5:163

49. Gregg TM, Wilmot CB (1964) The flying squad and the paraplegic unit (preliminary report). Paraplegia 2:15

50. Griffiths ER (1980) Spinal injuries from swimming and diving treated in the Spinal Department of Royal Perth Rehabilitation Hospital: 1956–1978. Paraplegia 18:109

51. Hachen GJ (1974) Emergency transportation in the event of acute spinal cord lesion. Paraplegia 12:33

52. Hansebout RR, Kuchner EF, Romero-Sierra C (1975) Effects of local hypothermia and of steroids upon recovery from experimental spinal cord compression injury. Surg Neurol 4:531

53. Hardy AG (1977) Cervical cord injury without bony injury. Paraplegia 14:296

54. Hartzog JT, Fisher RG, Snow C (1969) Spinal cord trauma: Effect of hyperbaric oxygen therapy. Proceedings of the Spinal Cord Injury Conferences 17:70–71

55. Heil HL (1971) Spinal cord injuries. J Neurosurg 35:251

56. Holmstrom F, Babinski MF (1980) Spirometry in acute spinal cord injury. Crit Care Med 4:253

57. Hung TK, Albin MS, Brown TD, et al (1975) Biomechanical responses to open experimental spinal cord injury. Surg Neurol 4:271

58. Joyner J, Freeman LW (1963) Urea and spinal cord trauma. Neurology 13:69

59. Kakari S, Diaz A, DeCrescito V, et al (1974) On the role of lysosomes in the pathogenesis of traumatic paraplegia. Presented at the Fifth Annual Meeting of the American Society for Neurochemistry, New Orleans, March 1974

60. Kelly DL Jr, Lassiter RL, Calogero JA, et al (1970) Effects of local hypothermia and tissue oxygen studies in experimental paraplegia. J Neurosurg 33:554

61. Kerr FWL (1964) Blood pressure responses in acute compression of the spinal cord. J Neurosurg 21:485

62. Key AG, Retief PSM (1970) Spinal cord injuries: An analysis of 300 new lesions. Paraplegia 7:243

63. Koons DD, Gildenberg PL, Dohn DF, et al (1972) Local hypothermia in the treatment of spinal cord injuries: Report of seven cases. Cleve Clin Q 39:109

64. Kraus JF (1978) Epidemiologic features of head and spinal cord injury. Adv Neurol 19:261

65. Kraus JF, Franti CE, Riggins RS, et al (1975) Incidence of traumatic spinal cord lesions. J Chronic Dis 28:471

66. Kuchner EF, Hansebout RR (1976) Combined steroid and hypothermia treatment of experimental spinal cord injury. Surg Neurol 6:371

67. Lewin MG, Hansebout RB, Pappius HM (1974) Chemical characteristics of traumatic spinal cord edema in

cats. J Neurosurg 40:65

68. Malik AB (1977) Pulmonary vascular response to increase in intracranial pressure: Role of sympathetic mechanisms. J Appl Physiol 42:335

69. Mathias CJ (1976) Bradycardia and cardiac arrest during tracheal suction-mechanisms in tetraplegia patients. Eur J Intensive Care Med 2:147

70. Meachem W, McPherson W (1973) Local hypothermia in the treatment of acute injuries of the spinal cord. South Med J 66:95

71. Meinecke FW (1968) Frequency and distribution of associated injuries in traumatic paraplegia and tetraplegia. Paraplegia 5:196

72. Meyer GA, Berman IR, Doty DB, et al (1971) Hemodynamic responses to acute quadriplegia with or without chest trauma. J Neurosurg 34:168

73. Naftchi NE, Demeny M, Decrescito V, et al (1974) Biogenic amine concentrations in traumatized spinal cords of cats: effects of drug therapy. J Neurosurg 40:52

74. Nyquist RH (1965) Mortality in spinal cord injuries. Follow-up report. Californian Medicine 103:417

75. Ohry A, Molho M, Rozin R (1975) Alterations of pulmonary function in spinal cord injured patients. Paraplegia 13:101

76. Osterholm JL, Mathews GJ (1971) Treatment of severe spinal cord injuries by biochemical norepinephrine manipulation. Surg Forum 22:415

77. Osterholm JL, Mathews GJ (1972) Altered norepinephrine metabolism following experimental spinal cord injury. P 1. Relationship to hemorrhagic necrosis and post-wounding neurological deficits. J Neurosurg 36:386

78. Osterholm JL, Mathews GJ (1972) Altered norepinephrine metabolism following experimental spinal cord injury. 2. Protection against traumatic spinal cord hemorrhagic necrosis by norepinephrine synthesis blockade with alpha methyl tyrosine. J Neurosurg 36:395

79. Osterholm JL, Mathews GJ (1972) Effect of hypothermia and steroids upon spinal NE metabolism. Presented at the 40th Annual Meeting of the American Association of Neurological Surgeons, Boston, April, 1972

80. Peerless SJ, Schweigel JF (1974) The medical and economic fate of twenty-nine industrial spinal cord-injured patients. Paraplegia 12:145

81. Perot PL (1973) The clinical use of somatosensory evoked potentials in spinal cord injury. Clin Neurosurg 20:367

82. Poe RH, Reisman JL, Rodenhouse TG (1978) Pulmonary edema in cervical spinal cord injury. J Trauma 18:71

83. Richardson HD, Nakamura S (1971) An electron microscopic study of spinal cord edema and the effects of treatment with steroids, mannitol and hypothermia. Thirty-ninth Annual Meeting of the American Association of Neurological Surgery, Houston, April 1971

84. Rowe SE, Perot PL (1979) Pressor response resulting from experimental contusion injury to the spinal cord. J Neurosurg 50:58

85. Rowed DW, McLean JAG, Tator CH (1978) Somatosensory evoked potentials in acute spinal cord injury: Prognostic value. Surg Neurol 9:203

86. Scher AT (1978) The high rugby tackle—an avoidable cause of cervical spinal injury? S Afr MEd J 53:1015

87. Shrosbree RD (1979) Spinal cord injuries as a result of motorcycle accidents. Paraplegia 16:102

88. Silver JR (1963) The oxygen cost of breathing in tetraplegic patients. Paraplegia 1:204

89. Silver JR, Gibbon NOK (1968) Prognosis in tetraplegia. Br Med J iv:79

90. Silver JR, Maulton A (1969) The physiological and pathological sequelae of paralysis of the intercostal and abdominal muscles in tetraplegic patients. Paraplegia 7:131

91. Smith RB, Grenvik A (1970) Cardiac arrest following succinylcholine in patients with central nervous system injuries. Anesthesiology 33:558

92. Smith RB, Klain M, Babinski M (1980) Limits of high-frequency percutaneous transtracheal jet ventilation using a fluidic logic controlled ventilator. Can Anaesth Soc J 27:351

93. Swan HJC, Ganz W, Forrester J, Marcus H, et al (1970) Catheterization of the heart in man with use of a flow-directed balloon-tipped catheter. N Engl J Med 283:447

94. Tator CH, Deecke L (1973) Value of normothermic perfusion, hypothermic perfusion, and durotomy in the treatment of experimental acute spinal cord trauma. Neurosurgery 39:52

95. Tator CH, Rowed DW (1979) Current concepts in the immediate management of acute spinal cord injuries. Can Med Assoc J 121:1453

96. Thienprasit P, Bantli H, Bloedel JR, et al (1975) Effect of delayed local cooling on experimental spinal cord injury. J Neurosurg 42:150

97. Tribe CR (1963) Causes of death in the early and late stages of paraplegia. Paraplegia 1:19

98. Troll GF, Dohrmann GJ (1975) Anaesthesia of the spinal cord-injured patient: Cardiovascular problems and their management. Paraplegia 13:162

99. U.S. Department of Health Education and Welfare, Public Health Service (1973) Impairments due to injury in the United States, 1971. National Center for Health Statistics, Washington (Vital and health statistics series 10, no 87)

100. Wagner FC Jr, Taslitz N, White RJ, et al (1969) Vascular phenomena in the normal and traumatized spinal cord. Anat Rec 163:281

101. Wagner FC Jr, Dohrmann GJ, Bucy PC (1971) Histopathology of transitory traumatic paraplegia in the monkey. J Neurosurg 35:272

102. Webb SB Jr, Berzins E, Wengardner TS, Lorenzi ME (1978) First-year hospitalization costs for the spinal cord patient. Paraplegia 15:311

103. Welply NC, Mathias CJ, Frankel HC (1975) Circulatory reflexes in tetraplegics during artificial ventilation and general anaesthesia. Paraplegia 13:172

104. White RJ, Albin MS (1970) Spine and spinal cord injury. In: Gurdijian ES, Lange WA, Patrick LM, Thomas LM (eds) Impact injury and crash protection. Thomas, Springfield, pp 63–85

105. White RJ, Albin MS, Harris LS, et al (1969) Spinal cord injury: sequential morphology and hypothermic stabilization. Surg Forum 20:432

106. White RJ, Yashon D, Albin MS, et al (1972) The acute management of cervical cord trauma with quadriplegia. Presented at the 40th Annual Meeting of the American Association of Neurological Surgeons, Boston, April 1972

107. Wilcox NF, Stauffer ES, Nickel VL (1970) A statistical analysis of 423 consecutive patients admitted to the Spinal Cord Injury Center, Rancho Los Amigos Hospital, 1 January, 1964–31 December, 1967. Paraplegia 8:27

Chapter 38

Care of Burns

Richard D. Goodenough and John F. Burke

In the United States alone, there are 2 million significant burn injuries each year. Of these persons, 6%–7% are hospitalized, 70 000 require intensive care, and 12 000 die [31, 52]. It has been estimated that 80% of these injuries could have been prevented [52].

Thermal burns may be the result of hot liquids (scalds), flame, and contact with hot objects. Electrical, chemical, and ionizing radiation are special types of burn injuries. These injuries occur in varying depths and are classified as partial- or full-thickness cutaneous injuries. There may also be significant injury to the deeper tissues.

A severe burn is an acute injury with a protracted, debilitating course [18, 61]. While the care of this acute injury has been much improved, progress aimed at minimizing the persistence and significance of the burn insult has been much slower. There is little theoretical disagreement that thermally killed skin should be treated as are other surgical wounds [19, 44]; that is, clean wounds may be promptly excised and autografted. As the size of the burn injury increases, different strategies become necessary to implement this goal. However, current systems of burn care have been developed, to the extent that all patients may be treated by these methods. This chapter attempts to define a unified method of burn care that begins at the time of hospitalization and proceeds through the critical period of the illness.

Initial assessment and therapy of the thermally injured patient

Initial assessment

The initial assessment of the burned patient requires the careful and thoughtful attention of a knowledgeable physician. The majority of such patients are first seen with thermal trauma alone, although multiply injured patients are not rare. Presentation at the most expedient medical facility is the norm, so that the responsibility for initial care and triage is incumbent upon that facility [69].

Initial therapy and physical examination are undertaken immediately. Adequate venous access is attained while the need for immediate pulmonary or cardiovascular resuscitative efforts is evaluated. Often, a prudently placed central venous catheter will be helpful in the future management of the patient. This central venous line may also be converted to a flow-directed right heart catheter by means of the Seldinger technique.

Respiratory and/or cardiac arrest are treated as in other critical care situations with tracheal intubation, closed-chest massage, administration of cardiotonic agents, mechanical ventilation (MV), and ventricular defibrillation as necessary. The multiply injured patient may require cervical spine stabilization, control of bleeding, and expert thoracoabdominal, neurological, and orthopedic evaluation and care. Errors of omission can certainly be made when one focuses only on the thermal aspects of trauma. For this reason, ongoing evaluation is important after the patient is initially stabilized and leaves the emergency suite.

The assessment of pulmonary status also includes the possibility of impending airway obstruction due to thermal and chemical injury. While it is uncommon for thermal damage to occur in the lower airways, expectorated soot, nasopharyngeal or laryngeal erythema, stridor, singed nasal vibrissae, and a history of being confined with steam or the products of combustion (smoke), all connote the serious possibility of respiratory injury [6]. Arterial blood gases [38] and carboxyhemoglobin levels are frequently obtained with the initial hematologic and chemistry profiles. Carboxyhemoglobin levels below 15% suggest low-grade poisoning, and are probably unimportant [91]. Chest and any other x-ray examinations indicated and urinalysis upon indwelling urinary catheterization are performed. Other laboratory examinations are individualized to the patient's needs. It should be noted that normal blood gases and chest x-rays do not clear the patient of pulmonary injury. If suspicion of a developing injury exists, then these tests, and physical examinations, should be serially performed.

The pertinent medical history is obtained. This includes the specific details of the trauma as well as baseline pulmonary, cardiac, renal, metabolic, and other disease states. Allergies and current medications are also noted. Thorough physical examination is then completed. The patient's weight and height are recorded. The burn size is then measured and recorded as accurately as possible. This measurement of burn size will include attention to depth, location, and special anatomic considerations. These considerations include facial and perineal burns or patterns of burn suggestive of child abuse. Charts and tables are readily available for burn size calculations [52] (Table 38.1).

There are special considerations in chemical and electrical injuries. The chemical agent, its concentration, and previous efforts at first aid are of note. Concomitant thermal injury is also noted. White phosphorus requires special underwater handling to prevent oxidation, but is usually seen only in wartime. In the case of all other chemical burns, especially those to the

Table 38.1. Estimation of percentage body surface burned

Area	Body percentage by age (years)					Burn distribution		% Total
						% second degree	% third degree	
	0–1	1–4	5–9	10–15	Adult			
Head	19	17	13	10	7			
Neck	12	2	2	2	2			
Ant. trunk	13	13	13	13	13			
Post. trunk	13	13	13	13	13			
R. buttock	$2\frac{1}{2}$	$2\frac{1}{2}$	$2\frac{1}{2}$	$2\frac{1}{2}$	$2\frac{1}{2}$			
L. buttock	$2\frac{1}{2}$	$2\frac{1}{2}$	$2\frac{1}{2}$	$2\frac{1}{2}$	$2\frac{1}{2}$			
Genitalia	1	1	1	1	1			
R. upper arm	4	4	4	4	4			
L. upper arm	4	4	4	4	4			
R. lower arm	3	3	3	3	3			
L. lower arm	3	3	3	3	3			
R. hand	$2\frac{1}{2}$	$2\frac{1}{2}$	$2\frac{1}{2}$	$2\frac{1}{2}$	$2\frac{1}{2}$			
L. hand	$2\frac{1}{2}$	$2\frac{1}{2}$	$2\frac{1}{2}$	$2\frac{1}{2}$	$2\frac{1}{2}$			
R. thigh	$5\frac{1}{2}$	$6\frac{1}{2}$	$8\frac{1}{2}$	$8\frac{1}{2}$	$9\frac{1}{2}$			
L. thigh	$5\frac{1}{2}$	$6\frac{1}{2}$	$8\frac{1}{2}$	$8\frac{1}{2}$	$9\frac{1}{2}$			
R. leg	5	5	$5\frac{1}{2}$	6	7			
L. leg	5	5	$5\frac{1}{2}$	6	7			
R. foot	$3\frac{1}{2}$	$3\frac{1}{2}$	$3\frac{1}{2}$	$3\frac{1}{2}$	$3\frac{1}{2}$			
L. foot	$3\frac{1}{2}$	$3\frac{1}{2}$	$3\frac{1}{2}$	$3\frac{1}{2}$	$3\frac{1}{2}$			
Total								

Adapted from Lund CC, Browder NC (1944) *Surg Gynecol Obstet* 79:352–358, by permission of *Surgery, Gynecology and Obstetrics*.

eyes, copious, long-term irrigation of the affected part with water is the rule of common sense.

Electrical burns and electrocutions are frought with complications such as vascular injury leading to thrombosis or hemorrhage, neurologic deficit, cardiac arrest, and muscular damage with its attendant myoglobinuria and compartmental syndromes.

Cold water soaks may be used on small, partial-thickness injuries for means of pain control [6]. Care should be taken to prevent hypothermia, however, Morphine may be administered to the conscious patient if there are no obvious contraindications. Small amounts of morphine IV are appropriate.

In burns effecting greater than 15%–20% of body surface area (BSA), nasogastric suction should be instituted at this point. Paralytic ileus frequently accompanies thermal trauma, so that gastric decompression becomes important in the prevention of aspiration. As will be discussed later, enteral nutritional therapy should only be provided through soft, small-bore tubes. The possibility of tracheoesophageal fistula must also be considered when concomitant tracheal intubation is present.

The burn wound should be cleansed and debrided. Sterile precautions are applied. Topical therapy should then begin and the wound should be covered with a sterile dressing. Tetanus prophylaxis is given, depending on the patient's immunization status. It may be necessary to administer both active and passive prophylactic measures [82].

Approximate criteria for the transfer of a burn patient to a burn center exist. Burns involving greater than 20% of the BSA or 10% full-thickness BSA should be transferred to a facility with burn specialists [6, 69]. Similarly, patients at the extremes of age or those with severe pulmonary and electrical injuries are best attended by personnel with a significant amount of experience in this type of care.

Fluid therapy

Fluid resuscitation is the cornerstone of therapy in acutely burned patients. It is the condition necessary for life-saving in all major burns [15, 75, 88]. The two indispensable components of fluid resuscitation are sodium and water [88], although there is much current discussion involving electrolyte concentration and the inclusion of other constituents, e.g., colloid. The ultimate goal of fluid therapy is the maintenance of vital functions without the accrual of long-term deleterious effects [18, 76].

A widely used fluid replacement formula is the revised Parkland formula and is reasonable for resuscitation of small to moderate thermal burns in low risk patients. In its present state, it recommends the fluid needs for the first 24 h after the burn [6]. In adults, 2 ml lactated Ringer's solution/kg body weight per 1% of body surface burn is given. In children, 3 ml/kg per 1% burn is given. One half of the calculated amount is given in the first 8 h, and the remainder is given over the next 16 h. A urine output of 30–50 ml/h in adults, or 1 ml/kg/h in patients weighing less than 30 kg is the most frequently followed parameter of successful replacement [6, 18]. Although this regimen is satisfactory for the treatment of small thermal burns, no empirical formula can accurately estimate fluid needs in large burns [75]. Supplementary fluid may be necessary. In addition to resuscitation of extensive injury, resuscitation of injury in the elderly or very young requires special attention to the loss of plasma proteins. It is well to maintain an albumin concentration of greater than 3 g/100 ml throughout this period of fluid shift. To maintain the plasma oncotic pressure close to the normal range, it is often best to intervene with colloid support early in the first 24 h after the burn injury. Colloid, in our view, is best given as fresh-frozen plasma.

Cardiac output is depressed in large burns [75]. There has been considerable interest in the identification of a myocardial depressant factor (MDF) [10] although the data on MDF thus far are inconclusive [75]. This low-flow state parallels a decrease in intravascular volume, which has been attributed to the extravasation of plasma at sites of thermal injury. The measurement of cardiac output and intravascular volume will therefore be important in many burn patients. Also, pulmonary wedge pressure is more reliable than central venous pressure as an indicator of intravascular volume [2]. These considerations make the Swan–Ganz catheter a very useful tool in the care of the seriously burned patient.

The loss of capillary integrity is probably reversed 24 h after the burn [75], and there is considerable discussion at present on the systemic effects of vasoactive substances [31]. The prostaglandins and kinins may generalize this leaky capillary syndrome, and thereby prevent colloid from remaining, preferentially, intravascular. This has been the general argument against using any type of colloid in the immediate postburn period.

There is, however, a difference in cardiac output and pulmonary vascular resistance, when colloid is used in the immediate postburn period [7, 18, 75]. Also, echocardiography has shown a more rapid return in left ventricular (LV) end-diastolic filling with colloid administration [75, 76]. The lack of consensus in immediate colloid therapy is attested by the global differences in therapy. Initial resuscitation includes dextran in Germany and Denmark, albumin in Sweden, and hypertonic saline in the Netherlands [7]. Similarly, there has been some interest in hypertonic resuscitation in the United States, based on theoretical concerns [43]. The data necessary to compare isotonic and hypertonic therapies, however, seem equivocal thus far [75, 88].

Currently, we use fluid resuscitation in adults with greater than 15% BSA burn and children with greater than 10% BSA burn. Therapy is begun immediately upon hospital admission. The fluid initially employed in small and moderate-sized burns is lactated Ringer's solution. It is continued for the first 24 h. However, colloid is frequently added in the first 24 h if the patient's circulatory response is inadequate or urinary output is unsatisfactory. Colloid therapy is therefore begun as a function of the patient's response to resuscitation. Infants, the aged, and patients with large burns will require colloid sooner [18]. The fluid status of these patients therefore needs to be closely followed. Daily measurements of fluid and electrolyte balance should include serum electrolytes, serum osmolality, serum proteins and body weights [75]. Therapy is individualized to each patient, by means of the integration of physical measurements, laboratory values, and clinical acumen.

Inhalation injuries

The respiratory injuries of burn patients are a heterogenous group of pulmonary complications. These may be divided into (1) asphyxia, (2) pharyngeal-glottic and upper airway injuries (i.e., problems of upper airway obstruction), and (3) respiratory bronchiol-alveolar injury (i.e., gas exchange problems).

Asphyxia

There are 3000–4000 deaths from carbon monoxide (CO) poisoning in the United States each year [40]. The majority of these die at the scene of the accident. Death occurs from a combination of decreased available hemoglobin (due to

carboxyhemoglobin generation) and decreased P_{O_2}. The target organs are the brain and myocardium. These victims, therefore, present with myocardial ischemia and neurologic depression [31]. Pharyngeal and tracheobronchial injury may or may not co-exist. Treatment consists of oxygenation and ventilation as necessary.

With the increasing use of polymers containing nitrogen comes the probability of increasing exposure to cyanide in fires. Cyanide is normally metabolized to thiocyanate, which contributes to tissue ischemia. It should be noted that chronic cyanide exposure is also present in cigarette smokers. Therefore, the awareness of a patient's smoking history and the presence of burning plastics should alert the physician to the possibility of cyanide toxicity [91].

Glottic and airways injuries

Upper airway injuries may be a combination of thermal and chemical damage. They may present early as airway obstruction and/or later as tracheobronchial infection (1–2 weeks). With the exception of superheated steam, few gases possess sufficient heat capacity to carry thermal damage below the trachea [63]. The difficulty in caring for patients with airway injury is a result of the variable presentation and insidious onset of symptoms. Injury may occur in as many as one-third of burn patients [65, 66].

Upper airway injuries are best diagnosed by clinical suspicion and bronchoscopy. As previously noted, facial flame burns and the history of smoke exposure in an enclosed space suggest that damage may have occurred. The production of sooty sputum and the development of stridor herald the possibility of airway obstruction and denote significant airway insult. The diagnosis becomes evident via indirect laryngoscopy or fiberoptic bronchoscopy [66]. Chest x-ray and arterial blood gases may initially be normal. The knowledge of developing upper airway edema may allow early therapy with humidified air, but nasotracheal intubation is often required until the edema subsides [66]. Tracheostomy should be avoided in almost all cases because of the high incidence of pulmonary aspiration infection from the tracheostomy, which is accompanied by high mortality [37].

Respiratory bronchiol-alveolar injury

Respiratory bronchiol-alveolar injuries are usually chemical in nature and are often delayed hours to days in presentation. The products of combustion inhaled may include such irritants as hydrochloric acid, sulfuric acid, phosgene, various aldehydes, and acrolein [31]. The time interval between exposure and symptoms may be protracted. Here again, early diagnosis would be helpful in managing these patients. The recent use of [133]xenon lung scanning [67], ventilation/perfusion lung scans, and pulmonary function tests seem promising in this regard [1, 71]. The sequelae of pulmonary chemical injuries are the adult respiratory distress syndrome (ARDS), pulmonary infection, and pulmonary fibrosis [11].

The treatment of acute pulmonary injuries and their respiratory complications is entirely symptomatic. Because little is known about the mechanisms of injury or repair, therapy necessarily becomes supportive. There is consensus of opinion against the continuous use of corticosteroids in the early postburn period (i.e., 3 days or longer [74]). Therefore, while experimental evidence supports the use of steroids immediately after aspiration injury, evidence is lacking for clinical effectiveness in inhalation burn injury. We routinely give a single bolus of steroids immediately upon admission when a respiratory injury is suspected, if the patient is seen within the first 4 h of injury. The consensus against preventive (prophylactic) antibiotics is less developed [74]. Bacteriologic surveillance should be employed, along with maximal pulmonary physiotherapy [31, 66, 69, 74]. However, MV is frequently required in the treatment of respiratory bronchial-alveolar inhalation injury. Finally, it should be noted that the combination of respiratory injury and cutaneous burn has a much higher risk of mortality than either alone [11].

Escharotomy and fasciotomy

Impairment of distal circulation may result from circumferential burn injuries. With the development of firm, noncompliant eschar and the resultant underlying edema, a syndrome of vascular compromise may occur. In addition, the depth of the burn may extend into an anatomic compartment, and the resultant edema may produce a true compartment syndrome.

Escharotomy is the axial incision of this nonyielding eschar. It is indicated when severe vascular compromise is present. The signs of cyanosis, impaired capillary bed refilling, and developing distal neurologic deficit are, unfortunately, inconsistently present [75]. While

their presence is suggestive of compromise, these signs should be verified by means of the ultrasonic flow probe (Doppler instrument). If distal pulses are documented, then elevation of the involved extremity and 'expectant' therapy[1] are indicated [75, 80].

When objective vascular compromise occurs with either eschar or compartment syndromes, formal escharotomy and, if necessary, fasciotomy should be performed. Also, stiff eschar of the thorax may compromise ventilatory mechanics and should be incised when functionally present [80]. Escharotomy requires no anesthesia, is carried out on the ward, and should extend the length of the eschar. Extension of the incision across the joints is necessary when the overlying skin is involved. Adequate incision is evidenced by the separation of the overlying eschar and appearance of subcutaneous tissue [75]. Adequacy of incision is ultimately judged by the return of blood flow. Escharotomy of the hands and fasciotomy, when necessary, should be performed only by experienced surgeons [69].

Primary excision and wound closure

It has long been appreciated that the likelihood of infection in damaged skin increases, with increasing time since injury [19, 28, 44]. Bacterial colonization and invasive infection may be retarded by the appropriate use of topical agents, though they do not correct the defect in host defense, sterilize the wound, or eliminate the probability of infection [44, 64]. The ideal method of treating a burn injury is removal of the devitalized tissue and replacement with viable skin [21, 24, 26].

While there is consensus [44] on the validity of this theoretical approach there is limited compliance [33, 78]. Recently, evidence to support the practice of early excision and prompt wound closure in all patients with deep dermal and full-thickness burns has become more compelling. While large, controlled series comparing early excisional therapy with more traditional care have not been performed, a large

---

[1] 'Delaying,' and harmless treatment administered to minimize symptoms while awaiting the emergence of a more characteristic picture of the disease process or its resolution — 'wait and see.'

childrens' series and the ongoing care of a large adult burn population lead us to believe that early excision and closure of burns is the routine treatment mode of choice [21, 24, 26].

Excision

'Primary' excision of deep dermal and full-thickness burn wounds implies that excision is the cornerstone of the therapeutic scheme. Excision may be performed in two ways, depending upon the depth of injury [55]. When the burn depth extends into the subcutaneous fat and covers a large area, fascial excision becomes appropriate [50]. This may be carried out with a scalpel, electrocautery or a laser instrument [9, 24, 55]. The advantage of the coagulating instruments is that they minimize blood loss at the expense of a small amount of tissue injury. In skilled hands this leads to adequate hemostasis, the prerequisite of graft adherence [24]. When the injury is subfascial, adequate fasciotomy and debridement of muscle and fascia must be performed to eliminate devitalized tissue, prevent compartment syndrome, and insure graft take [75].

For injury levels that are not uniform in depth, sequential (tangential) eschar excision is undertaken [24]. A guided free-hand knife removes successive layers of approximately 6/1000ths of an inch. This approach is repeated until punctate capillary bleeding is present in all areas of the wound. This denotes viable tissue that will accept graft and allows a sculptured wound excision, depending on local depths of injury [42, 51]. Again, hemostasis is of paramount importance and is attained through the judicious use of electrocautery, pressure, and topical thrombin. Brisk bleeding may occur, so that each small area should be excised and controlled individually, before being left for the next [24].

It should be noted that wound excision could theoretically be replaced by eschar debridement if the appropriate debriding agent existed [49]. The ideal agent would be a painless enzyme that would hydrolyze eschar down to a clean, graftable surface. At present, several agents are being investigated, although none has yet received significant clinical trial.

Wound closure

The wound must be immediately closed if overall clinical success is to be achieved. In larger burns, this requires adequate planning of the source of graft. In recent history, the choices of closure material have become autograft, allograft (homograft), and artificial materials [103]. Ultimately, the wound must be closed with autograft material. However, this is not immediately possible in deep burns involving over 35%–45% of BSA, depending on the distribution of remaining donor sites [24]. Therefore, the successful treatment of the massively burned patient by prompt excision and immediate closure, is only possible through the temporary use of allograft and artificial skin.

We have divided the size of burn injury into three categories, based on the methods needed for closure [21, 26] (Table 38.2): (1) Full- and deep partial-thickness burns involving less than 35% of BSA are closed entirely with autograft. When the burn BSA approaches 35%, the use of special donor sites, such as the scalp and soles of the feet, becomes necessary; (2) Burns of 35%–70% of BSA are too large to be immediately closed by the available donor tissue, and are closed with autograft supplemented with allograft; (3) Massive burns, in which the deep component of burn covers more than 70% of BSA, require autograft plus the temporary transplantation of allograft or artificial skin.

Table 38.2. Scheme for burn excision and wound closure based on burn size

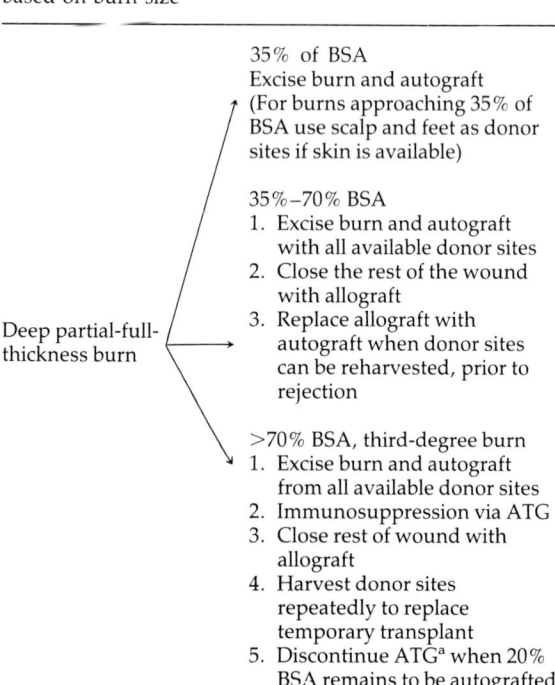

Deep partial-full-thickness burn

35% of BSA
Excise burn and autograft
(For burns approaching 35% of BSA use scalp and feet as donor sites if skin is available)

35%–70% BSA
1. Excise burn and autograft with all available donor sites
2. Close the rest of the wound with allograft
3. Replace allograft with autograft when donor sites can be reharvested, prior to rejection

>70% BSA, third-degree burn
1. Excise burn and autograft from all available donor sites
2. Immunosuppression via ATG
3. Close rest of wound with allograft
4. Harvest donor sites repeatedly to replace temporary transplant
5. Discontinue ATG[a] when 20% BSA remains to be autografted

[a]Antithymocyte globulin.

Immunosuppression allows this temporary transplantation by prolonging allograft survival to the time required for repeated harvesting of limited donor sites. In this way, the entire wound is autografted [22, 23].

Choosing from these methods as a function of the size of injury, the first autograft and excision is performed as soon as the patient has achieved cardiovascular stabilization [24]. This may be achieved within hours of the injury, although the first operation is frequently performed during the second to fourth postburn days for logistic reasons. In this early period, the patient's overall physiology is nearest to normal. The presence of pulmonary or other trauma is only a relative contraindication to operation and must be judged in each case. The extent of each excision is limited to about 20% of BSA plus the harvesting of 15% of BSA donor sites. This harvest provides enough meshed autograft to close the excised area immediately [21, 24]. Excision is repeated at 1- to 3-day intervals until all of the deep dermal or full-thickness injury is removed.

We initiate wound closure in all burn patients by using the available autograft first. In the 35%–70% group, the rest of the wound is closed with allograft. Cadaver or live donor allografts allow ingrowth of budding capillaries, but are immunologically rejected from about 2 weeks after the graft. The allograft is removed and replaced with autograft harvested from regenerated donor sites at about 14 days. Adequate regeneration of donor sites routinely occurs prior to complete rejection of autograft [21, 26]. Therefore, through the use of autograft, allograft, and skin meshing, early excision of over twice the area of the available donor site is routinely successful [23, 24].

In massive burns, immunosuppression allows the use of allograft for extended periods of time [22, 24, 30, 48, 93]. With the patient in a bacteriologically controlled environment [25], antithymocyte globulin is given just prior to the first procedure, when the excised area will be closed with allograft. The initial dose is 10 mg/kg body wt. T cell suppression is titrated by T cell rosette methods [102] to 10% of the presuppression T cell level. Daily IV maintenance doses are given in conjunction with the antihistamine diphenhydramine (2 mg/kg) and with methylprednisolone (0.5 mg/kg) to avoid any febrile response. Immunosuppression allows early excision of the whole of a massive burn injury with immediate auto- and allografting. Immunotherapy is continued until the available donor sites have been harvested sufficient times to replace all but 20% transplanted allograft [22, 23].

In the treatment of massive burns, the areas first grafted should be those with the most promise of success. The anterior trunk, flanks, and back are closed before the extremities [24]. Judicious use of skeletal traction is frequently necessary after grafting of an appendage. Joint function must always be of concern.

Design and development of an artificial skin has been attempted by many workers over the last several years [103, 104]. Currently, a promising laminate of nonimmunoreactive collagen–glycosaminoglycan (GAG) complex and semipermeable silastic rubber sheet has been tested in clinical trials. Collagen–GAG performs as a biodegradable template for the formation of new dermal tissue [103, 104]. This may help to minimize wound contracture and eventual scar formation, as well as the need for immunosuppression in massive injury. We have had preliminary success with the use of this artificial skin and will continue its evaluation in patients with greater than 70% of BSA full-thickness and 80% of BSA total burn.

The adjuncts that allow the above therapy are hypotensive anesthesia [24], the bacterially controlled nursing unit (BCNU) [25], topical 0.5% $AgNO_3$ [64], intensive nutritional care [59], and excellent anesthesia, nursing, and technical staffs. In addition, blood and skin banking are necessary to hold and process tissue [14]. Antibiotic use is limited to anti-β streptococcal therapy (penicillin G in moderate dose) for the 3 days after admission, perioperative (preventive) use [15–17], and the treatment of specific sepsis [24].

In summary, a therapeutic system of burn care has been developed that allows primary excision and immediate wound closure of all deep dermal and full-thickness burns. Burn patients are placed in one of three categories as a function of the technical methods needed to close their wounds. Small burns are excised in toto and immediately grafted. Larger burns are closed with the available autograft and supplemented with temporary allograft closure until the donor sites regenerate. Massive burns require the temporary transplantation of allograft and immunosuppression or artificial skin. Through the use of these modalities, a burn care system can be fashioned for each patient. In this way, the principles of devitalized tissue removal and clean wound closure are followed to improve survival and shorten illness in burned patients.

Metabolic changes and nutritional requirements

Seriously burned patients exhibit two striking phases in their response to injury. Sir David Cuthbertson aptly labelled these ebb and flow [35]. The initial cardiovascular changes, known as 'burn shock,' are present at the time of medical presentation. These changes represent the ebb phase. Provided that fluid resuscitation is adequate, this phase will end by 24–48 h after the burn injury. The flow phase will then ensue as a chronic hypermetabolic response to thermal injury and will only be completed with closure and healing of the burn wound [26].

Ebb phase

During the ebb phase, the classic changes of burn shock encompass major decrements in cardiac index, loss of capillary integrity in the area of the burn (and possibly in the lungs) [57] and the consequent loss of intravascular volume [75]. Hypometabolism, as judged by O_2 consumption, is the rule [98]. Major losses in the red cell mass may also occur due to direct thermal injury to red cells. Plasma proteins are significantly lost in concert with plasma oncotic pressure. A redistribution of the available blood flow is mediated by the sympathetic nervous system to the vital organs [12, 75, 81, 98]. Despite a lack of consensus, the myocardium is probably depressed [98].

In addition, the ebb phase presents major hormonal and substrate changes. Catecholamines, corticosteriods, glucagon, antidiuretic hormone and aldosterone are all increased [68, 98]. The insulin level falls as does its peripheral effectiveness; the 'insulin resistance' of trauma and sepsis [92]. Hyperglycemia, lipolysis and lactate release all reflect the effects of shock at the tissue level [98].

Flow phase

As the cardiovasculature is stabilized and the tissue metabolic deficits repleted, the patient enters the flow phase with a 'resurgence of vitality' [35]. This is an extended period evidenced by increased O_2 consumption, substrate demand, cardiac output, hyperthermia, and eventual healing of the wound [98]. Malnutrition and sepsis become the two major obstacles to successful passage of this stage.

Overall metabolic requirements

Although a hypermetabolic response in burn patients is the rule, metabolic rates greater than 100% above normal basal rates in severely burned patients are unusual (G. T. Royle et al., 1981, unpublished work). The exact reasons for this hypermetabolic response are unclear at present. We know that higher ambient temperature and combined adrenergic blockade will lower the metabolic rate towards normal [13, 95]. We also know that there are faster rates of protein synthesis and breakdown in this state [45], and so suspect that large amounts of energy are used and heat produced in the formation of the peptide bond in protein synthesis. Futile cycling of substrates has also been implicated (e.g., glucose → glucose-6-phospate → glucose) with net energy usage but no change in glucose [97, 98, 100]. It is less clear whether decreasing evaporative water loss will lower the metabolic rate [84, 105]. It is also unclear whether this hypermetabolic response is adaptive or deleterious. In this light, it should be noted that serious burn sepsis tends to depress the metabolic rate [94, 95].

Fluid, blood product, and pharmacologic support of the ebb crisis have previously been discussed. Ebb phase therapy is directed toward cardiovascular homeostasis, not nutritional support. However, the nutritional support of severely burned patients during the hypermetabolic flow phase is of interest. This interest lies in several factors. Firstly, rapid weight loss is common in this hypermetabolic setting unless nutrients are adequately supplied [29, 62]. The traditional nitrogen balance techniques are still the best available as a yardstick of success [46, 54]. A 20% weight loss is thought to define increased mortality rates in surgical patients, and 40% is thought to be uniformly lethal [58, 59]. Impaired wound repair and immunocompromise occur with protein calorie malnutrition [59]. The exact defects in the immune system seem myriad, although impaired neutrophil function, decreased opsonization and hypogammaglobulinemia have been identified as key defects [3, 72]. The state of nutrition has a major effect on these host-resistance factors [3, 72].

The goals of nutritional therapy should then be to supply the body with adequate amounts of substrate in the forms most appropriate for energy production and biologic synthesis [59, 87]. However, energy expenditure is variable in patients with the same burn size as measured by consumption [53; G. T. Royle,

1981, unpublished work]. In our experience, the hypermetabolism of large burns increases energy use to 50% above basal in adults treated in an uncontrolled thermal environment and to 30% above basal in children treated in an environment controlled for heat and humidity [25]. As noted above, this increase rarely exceeds 100% over the basal. The difference between adult and child may in part be due to the differences in the ambient temperature of their care setting (G. T. Royle, 1981, unpublished work).

Caloric requirements

The calculation of energy requirements can be based upon several recommendations. While there is no consensus at present for the seriously burned patient, we use the Harris–Benedict equation [4, 39, 53, 86] based on the 50th percentile of ideal body weight to calculate the daily basal energy expenditure (Table 38.3). The patient is then supplied with twice this calculated caloric amount [59]. This will supply the active and hypermetabolic daily requirements of a seriously ill, bedridden burn patient.

There are many questions about substrate usage in burned patients. Glucose oxidation to CO_2 is increased from normal levels to 40%–50% of the substrate oxidized following serious burn injury in patients who are supported with moderate amounts of glucose [27]. It has been shown that glucose oxidation can be increased via progressively larger glucose infusions of up to 5 mg/kg/min. This will maximize the CO_2 produced directly from glucose to about 50% of CO_2 produced [27]. Glucose infusions above this point do not increase glucose oxidation [98–100]. Fatty hepatocellular changes, large insulin requirements [101] and increased CO_2 production due to lipogenesis from glucose [27] may also be noted. Therefore, exogenously supplied glucose is successfully used for energy production up to 5 mg/kg/min in acutely ill burn patients [27].

Plasma free fatty acids (FFA) are elevated in trauma and are assumed to be a major energy source, although this is not yet proven [59, 98]. However, carbohydrate, below 5 mg/kg/min, appears to be a necessary caloric source to achieve nitrogen sparing [59, 98]. Exogenous glucose delivery above 5 mg/kg/min spares no additional nitrogen, and produces the problems of increased CO_2 production and fatty liver, as already noted. The additional required calories not supplied by 5 mg/kg/min of glucose should be provided as exogenous fat.

Table 38.3. Determination of daily caloric need in severely burned patients

Flow sheet

1. Measure patient height
2. Obtain 50th percentile ideal body weight for height from ideal body weight table[a]
3. Calculate basal metabolic rate (BMR) from the ideal weight[b]

   BMR = 66.47 + 13.75 (wt) + 5.0(ht) − 6.76(A) for males

   BMR = 55.10 + 9.56   (wt) + 1.85(ht) − 4.68(A)   for females

   where,

   wt = 50th percentile ideal body weight in kilograms

   ht = height in centimeters

   A = age in years
4. Caloric need = Calculated BMR × 2

[a]Documenta Geigy (1970) Scientific Tables, 7th edn. Ciba-Geigy, Basle, p 712.
[b]Adapted from reference [40].

Substantial protein intake is necessary to provide adequate nutritional support in the burned patient, although the exact level has not yet been determined adequately [59]. We do know, however, that there are large increases of nitrogenous loss in wound fluid and urine after burn injury [46]. While a net loss of muscular protein occurs, its magnitude and determinants are complex [8, 59, 68, 98]. Increased rates of protein synthesis and breakdown have been measured in children and adults [45]. These patients can be maintained in positive nitrogen balance with the administration of 2.5 g protein/kg body wt/day, provided that the caloric intake is adequate [45]. We, therefore, have accepted 2.5 g/kg/day as a first approximation of protein need for all burn patients. patients.

Vitamins and trace elements

Nutritional considerations must also include vitamins and trace minerals. Vitamin C is known to play a role in collagen synthesis and wound healing, and may undergo increased losses in severe thermal stress [59]. The exact requirements, however, are unknown. Vitamin A, which may protect against stress ulceration [83], vitamins E and K, folate, pyridoxine, biotin, thiamin, and B_{12} all need to be provided. Zinc has also been proposed to be important in wound healing [59].

Table 38.4. Micronutrients supplied with total parenteral nutrition

Vitamins	
B complex (Berocca C)	1 ml daily
C	550 mg daily
Folic acid	0.5 mg/litre
Multivitamins (B group, A, D, E) MVI	3.5 ml weekly
C (additional)	800 mg weekly
Electrolytes	
Potassium	12 mmol/liter
Sodium	21 mmol/liter
Magnesium	8 mmol/liter
Calcium	4.5 mmol/liter
Phosphorous	13.4 mmol/liter
Chloride	16 mmol/liter
Trace elements	
Zinc	1.0 mg/liter
Copper	0.5 mg/liter
Manganese	0.2 mg/liter
Chromium	0.005 mg/liter
Iodide	0.028 mg/liter

Enteral diets, with the exception of the elemental regimens, probably contain adequate vitamins and trace minerals. These are frequently supplemented with an oral multivitamin preparation plus extra vitamin C on a daily basis in burn patients [59]. Parenterally fed patients require much stricter attention to replacement of minerals and vitamins [5, 70]. Zinc, magnesium, selenium, chromium, and copper deficiencies may occur in burn patients receiving total parenteral nutrition (TPN) for long periods, and must be provided [59]. Our standard TPN solution includes the vitamins and minerals listed in Table 38.4. Iron, vitamin B_{12}, and vitamin K are provided PO or IM, beginning after 10 days of TPN. It should be understood that these amounts are estimates to initiate therapy and should be modified in accord with frequent blood chemistry results and future research in this area.

Delivery

The modes of nutritional delivery are via the oral route, tube feeding, peripheral IV alimentation, and central TPN. The method chosen should make it possible to deliver the calculated nutritional requirements at the least risk and discomfort to the patient [34, 59]. Burned patients who require nutritional therapy other than regular diet are those with greater than 20% burn; preburn malnutrition due to disease, alcoholism, drug abuse, or morbid obesity; other major injuries; systemic complications of burning; and those whose weight loss is greater than 10% of preburn weight [87].

The oral route of delivery should be the first choice. This may be supplemented by tube-feeding a meal replacement formula or blenderized, home-made diet through a soft, small-diameter tube. We have had much success with the use of a powdered egg, Polycose, and vegetable oil formula madeup in the dietetics department. Intragastric tube positioning is usually adequate. The complications of tube feeding are pulmonary aspiration, hyperosmolar GI symptoms, hyperglycemia, fluid excess, and electrolytic imbalance [59]. Unfortunately, postburn ileus due to recent anesthesia, sepsis, or associated injury may exclude or severely limit use of the enteral route. TPN is then necessary, with its attendant risks. With TPN, the risk of the induction of sepsis is greater than normal due to the burn wound, necessitating frequent site changes and immediate removal when sepsis supervenes [26]. The technical and metabolic complications of TPN are well known.

In summary, our current practice is to institute nutritional support immediately after cardiovascular stabilization is achieved. Nutritional therapy is used for the burn patients indicated above. The basal energy requirements are calculated using the Harris–Benedict equation based on the 50th percentile of the patient's ideal body weight. The resultant figure is then doubled, providing the 24-h calorie requirement for an acutely ill, supine patient. Protein is delivered at about 2.5 g/kg/day and carbohydrate at 4–5 mg/kg/min. At least 10% of the calories should be in the form of essential fatty acids (EFA) to prevent EFA deficiency. The remaining calories are supplied as fat. Trace minerals and vitamins are supplied. It should be realized that these are guidelines and are individualized to the patient's needs as appropriate.

Bacteriology and infection control

Seventy-five percent of burn mortality in hospitalized patients is at least partially attributable to bacterial infections [72]. While tremendous strides have been taken in fluid resuscitation and cardiovascular support, the remainder of burn therapy has not yet advanced to uniform treatment or success in major burn injury [72]. Nonetheless, noteworthy changes in the bacteriologic picture have occurred.

The principle burn wound pathogens have changed from the Gram-positive cocci to *Pseudomonas aeruginosa*, the Gram-negative rods, and fungi [72]. By the 1940s the incidence of β-hemolytic streptococcus infection had dropped from 40% to 2% in burn patients [41]. This may have been attributable to the application of penicillin cream [41]. Many physicians now give prophylactic oral penicillin for 3–5 days after admission to prevent erysipelas [60].

The burn wound becomes colonized in the first few days [64]. This occurs both via auto- and cross-contamination [25]. Auto-contamination is commonly due to the Gram-negative rods of the GI tract. A burn wound infection becomes a systemic illness when this colonization escapes the control of the host defenses. Escape may occur at any time after colonization takes place. As in other surgical procedures, however, burn wound manipulation may be the antecedent factor [60]. For this reason, perioperative preventive (prophylactic) antibiotics are usually given in the excision of contaminated burn wounds [26, 60]. These are given in such a way that tissue antibiotic levels are adequate at the time of excision and are discontinued when the patient's physiology returns to baseline [15–17], usually in less than 24 h.

Full therapeutic courses of antibiotics are given for proven burn wound infections or other culture proven infections [60]. There is, however, no full agreement on when to employ parenteral antibiotics in the therapy of burn wound infection [72]. The commonly used parameters are: the positive blood culture, the positive burn wound biopsy, and clinical evidence of systemic infection or deterioration. The shortcomings of these diagnostic modalities are well known [90]. Bacteremia and fungicemia may occur despite negative blood cultures [77]. By the same token, there is no end-point as to when a biopsy is positive. Quantitative, full-thickness, biopsy cultures which grow greater than 10^5 organisms per gram of tissue, and have histologic sections which reveal large numbers of eschar-related or invasive organisms, should be considered positive [77].

Topical antimicrobial therapy

The advent of topical antimicrobial therapy as presently practiced, occurred in the 1960s. It has been shown to improve survival in patients with burns less than 60% of BSA [79]. Topical agents may act by preventing colonization, delaying colonization, and minimizing the bacterial density as colonization occurs [60]. The three agents presently in frequent use are silver nitrate, silver sulfadiazine, and mafenide acetate. There is at present no consensus on which is the most effective of these three [72]. Each agent has its own untoward effects and should be considered prior to implementation. In addition, there is some consideration of the efficacy of mafenide in the treatment of established burn infections because of its superior tissue penetration [60].

Our current system of care utilizes 0.5% $AgNO_3$ as topical agent. It has a wide antibacterial spectrum [64] and allows for expeditious excision of the wound. The major systemic effect of $AgNO_3$ is electrolyte leaching from the burn surface [73]. Sodium replacement is often necessary. Adequate sodium repletion is present when urinary sodium levels are above 40 mmol/liter [20].

Our system of infection control also includes the BCNU [25]. This is a series of strict isolation units for individual patients, with transparent walls, filtered air, laminar flow and temperature/humidity control. This method results in markedly lowered rates of patient cross-contamination [25].

Much current research centers on depressed host defense via immunologic changes. Studies have shown that several areas of immunocompetence are impaired. These include the complement system, opsonization, and phagocytosis by macrophages and neutrophils [3]. The causative mechanisms of impaired immune function may be nutritionally or traumatically induced, although this is, at present, conjecture. Tests of immunocompetence have had some success predicting fatal sepsis [10]. Current research also includes the development of polyvalent pseudomonal vaccines and non-specific immunopotentiators [3, 56].

In summary, the infectious complications of burn injury have changed as therapeutic methods have arisen. The current mainstays of therapy include specifically indicated systemic antibiotics, topical antimicrobials, and mechanical isolation techniques. Immunologic intervention and appraisal will become important as our knowledge of these modalities increases.

Complications

As we have just discussed, the most frequent complications facing the burned patient are bacterial in origin. At least three-quarters of burn deaths include an infectious component. Of these, frank septicemia and bronchopneumonia contribute to mortality most often, with roughly equal incidence [90]. Acute pyelonephritis occurs less commonly, followed by the rare presentation of meningitis, enterocolitis, and gas gangrene [90].

Burn sepsis

Burn wound sepsis may be due to any of the previously discussed pathogens and is the main source of septicemia. But, pneumonia, urinary tract infection, and venous catheter infections are also frequently found as sources of sepsis and septic complications [90]. Their identification results from continuing clinical suspicion and thorough surveillance methods.

Treatment of the septic wound requires the physician's careful judgment. Systemic antibiotics, defined by culture data, become necessary when septicemia supervenes [82]. These should be continued until the full course required to eradicate the pathogen has been administered. It may also be necessary to use multiple antibiotics when a major septic catastrophe occurs. The mechanical measures of wound care also take on increased importance. Subeschar abscesses should be unroofed and drained adequately. Extensive wound manipulation may result in exacerbated sepsis due to increased bacteremia, but frequent changes of biological dressings and removal of obviously necrotic eschar are beneficial [82]. With these specific points in mind, care of the septic burn patient should follow the same tenets as the care of other septic patients.

Pulmonary

Bacterial bronchopneumonia, most commonly due to the same organism as has colonized the burn wound, occurs frequently, and usually accompanies inhalation injury. As already mentioned, long-term prophylactic corticosteroids are detrimental, and preventive antibiotics probably ineffective, after inhalation injury [65, 66, 74]. Daily sputum cultures are appropriate in the susceptible patient and will dictate the choice of antibiotic if pneumonia occurs [66]. Attention to pulmonary therapy and toilet is also indicated.

Pulmonary embolism has been noted in the burn setting, although the incidence is probably low [69, 90]. It seems to be more likely in older patients. The embolic pathogenesis is the same

as in the other patients, although thermal injury may acutely cause showers of microthrombi to the lungs and other organs [90]. There is no consensus on the need to prophylactically anticoagulate the asymptomatic burn patient [69].

Pulmonary edema may occur with parenchymal inhalation injury or fluid overload [66, 69, 90]. Close attention is given to arterial PO_2, respiratory mechanics, and the administered fluid load. Intubation, positive end-expiratory pressure (PEEP), and pharmacologic intervention may become necessary. When pulmonary edema occurs immediately after the burn, extensive parenchymal damage is present and portends a guarded prognosis [66].

Atelectatic changes, aspiration pneumonitis, and respiratory embarrassment due to thoracic eschar may also occur. Atelectasis and aspiration are prevented and treated as in other hospitalized patients. The possibility of thoracic escharotomy must be entertained in patients so injured [80].

Renal

Acute renal failure is not an uncommon complication of thermal injury [82, 89, 90]. It may be secondary to hypoperfusion and hypoxia during the ebb state of trauma and may be exacerbated by precipitation of free hemoglobin from RBC attrition or myoglobin in crush or electrical injuries. Alkalization of the urine is therefore appropriate in these settings. These insults may also be superimposed on preexisting renal compromise. Oliguric or nonoliguric acute tubular necrosis can be the end-result, with the attendant clinical problems of acute renal failure.

As mentioned, acute pyelonephritis may be an infectious complication. Renal abscess may occur secondary to bacteremic seeding. It should also be kept in mind that the aminoglycosides possess nephrotoxicity, and therefore may add a renal insult when employed.

Cardiovascular

Congestive heart failure occurs either in the acute phase of burn injury or during the mobilization of edema [75, 82, 90]. Patients with underlying cardiac atherosclerosis may also be prone to infarction. Endocarditis may be a complication of burn sepsis and should be kept in mind as a less frequent cause of the signs of infection. The use of digitalis and antiarrhythmics may become necessary in specific situations.

Gastrointestinal

Curling first noted the association between bleeding duodenal ulcers and burn injury in 1842 [32]. The incidence of diagnosed gastric or duodenal ulceration in burn patients was about 10% in 1970 [31]. Subsequent prospective studies with upper endoscopy showed that three-quarters of severely burned patients develop identifiable mucosal erosions by 72 h after the burn [36]. One half of these became frank ulcerations. Ulcer-related complications, however, have markedly decreased in the last 5 years, probably due to the advent of continuous tube feeding [69] and exact control of gastric acidity via antacid therapy.

The pathophysiology of the initial mucosal injury appears to be related to mucosal hypoxia leading to susceptibility to normal concentrations of gastric acid [47]. This hypoxia may be due to submucosal arteriovenous shunting immediately after injury [47]. Knowledge of the frequency of occurrence of these lesions would prescribe the use of antacids and/or cimetidine unless tube feedings maintain a neutral gastric pH [31, 52, 69].

The other notable GI complication is impaired motility. Acute gastric dilatation and intestinal paralytic ileus are frequently seen [90]. These are probably the result of frequent anesthesia, sepsis, and fluid overload [90]. Ileus frequently limits the success of oral alimentation.

Neurologic

Burn encephalopathy includes a wide range of cerebral compromise syndromes. Necropsy at the end-stage of this encephalopathic picture reveals cerebral edema and uncal or cerebellar herniation [90]. Fortunately, this end of the neurologic spectrum is seldom seen.

Etiologic possibilities for burn encephalopathy include water intoxication, acute hypertension, drug narcosis, septicemia, hyperpyrexia, and dehydration [90]. Expert neurological evaluation and care should be obtained when the origin of encephalopathy is unclear.

References

1. Agee RN, Long JM, Hunt JL, Petroff PA, Lull RJ, Mason AD, Pruitt BA (1976) Use of ^{133}Xenon in early diagnosis of inhalation injury. J Trauma 16:218–224
2. Aikawa N, Martyn JAJ, Burke JF (1978) Pulmonary artery catheterization and thermal dilution cardiac output determination in the management of critically burned patients. Am J Surg 135:811–817
3. Alexander JW (1979) Immunological responses in the burned patient. J. Trauma 19:887–889
4. Altman PL, Dittmer DS (1968) Metabolism. Federation of American Societies for Experimental Biology Bethesda, p 344
5. AMA Department of Foods and Nutrition (1979) Guidelines for essential trace element preparations for parenteral use. JAMA 241:2051–2054
6. American College of Surgeons, Committee on Trauma (1979) Assessment and initial care of burn patients. ACS, Chicago
7. Arturson G (1979) Types of resuscitation therapy. J Trauma 19:873
8. Aulick HL, Wilmore DW (1979) Increased peripheral amino acid release following burn injury. Surgery 85:560–565
9. Auth DC (1979) Techniques for burn wound debridement. J Trauma 19:926
10. Baker CC, Miller CL, Trunkey DD (1979) Predicting fatal sepsis in burn patients. J Trauma 19:641–648
11. Bartlett RH (1979) Types of respiratory injury. J Trauma 19:918–919
12. Baxter CR (1974) Fluid volume and electrolyte changes of the early postburn period. Clin Plast Surg 1:693–709
13. Birke G, Carlson LA, von Euler US, Liljedahl SO, Plantin LO (1972) Studies on burns. XII. Acta Clin Scand 138:321–333
14. Bondoc CC, Burke JF (1971) Clinical experience with viable frozen human skin and a frozen skin bank. Ann Surg 174:371–382
15. Burke JF (1961) The effective period of preventive antibiotic action in experimental incisions and thermal lesions. Surgery 50:161–168
16. Burke JF (1973) Preventive antibiotic management in surgery. Annu Rev Med 24:289–294
17. Burke JF (1975) Preventive antibiotics in surgery. Postgrad Med 58:65–68
18. Burke JF (1979a) Fluid therapy to reduce morbidity. J Trauma 19:865–866
19. Burke JF (1979b) The benefits of prompt excision. J Trauma 19:924
20. Burke JF, Bondoc CC, Morris PJ (1968) Metabolic effects of topical silver nitrate therapy in burns covering more than fifteen percent of the body surface. Ann NY Acad Sci 150:674–681
21. Burke JF, Bondoc CC, Quinby WC (1974a) Primary burn excision and immediate grafting: A method shortening illness. J Trauma 14:389–395
22. Burke JF, May JW, Albright N, Quinby WC, Russell PS (1974b) Temporary skin transplantation and immunosuppression for extensive burns. N Engl J med 290:269–271
23. Burke JF, Quinby WC, Bondoc CC, Cosimi AB, Russell PS, Szyfelbein SK (1975) Immunosuppression and temporary skin transplantation in the treatment of massive third degree burns. Ann Surg 182:183–197
24. Burke JF, Quinby WC, Bondoc CC (1976) Primary excision and prompt grafting as routine therapy for the treatment of thermal burns in children. Surg Clin North Am 56:477–494
25. Burke JF, Quinby WC, Bondoc CC, Sheehy EM, Moreno HC (1977) The contribution of a bacterially isolated environment to the prevention of infection in seriously burned patients. Ann Surg 186:377–387
26. Burke JF, Quinby WC, Bondoc CC (1978) Early excision and prompt wound closure supplemented with immuno-suppression. Surg Clin North Am 58:1141–1150
27. Burke JF, Wolfe RR, Mullany CJ, Mathews DE, Bier

DM (1979) Glucose requirements following burn injury. Ann Surg 190:274–285

28. Cope O, Langohr JL, Moore FD, Webster RC (1947) Expeditious care of full thickness burn wounds by surgical excision and grafting. Ann Surg 125:1–22

29. Cope O, Nardi GL, Quijano M, Rovit RL, Stanbury JB, Wight A (1953) Metabolic rate and thyroid function following acute thermal trauma in man. Ann Surg 137:165–174

30. Cosimi AB, Burke JF, Russell PS (1978) Transplantation of skin. Surg Clin North Am 58:435–451

31. Cuono CB (1980) Early management of severe thermal injury. Surg Clin North Am 60:1021–1033

32. Curling TB (1842) On acute ulceration of the duodenum in cases of burn. Medico–Chirurgical Transactions (London) 25:260–281

33. Curreri PW (1979) Hard questions on excision J Trauma 19:931–933

34. Curreri PW, Luterman A (1978) Nutritional support of the burned patient. Surg Clin North Am 58:1151–1156

35. Cuthbertson DP (1932) Observations on the disturbance of metabolism produced by injury to the limbs. Q J Med 1:233–246

36. Czaja AJ, McAlhany JC, Pruitt BA (1974) Acute gastroduodenal disease after thermal injury: an endoscopic evaluation of incidence and natural history. N Engl J Med 291:925–929

37. Eckhauser FE, Billote J, Burke JF, Quinby WC (1974) Tracheostomy complicating massive burn injury. A plea for conservatism. Am J Surg 127:418–423

38. Greenburg AG, Frank H, Peskin GW (1976) The left-shifted oxyhemoglobin curve in the burn patient. J Trauma 16:573–578

39. Harris JA, Benedict FG (1919) A biometric study of basal metabolism in man. Carnegie Institution, Washington (Publication no. 279)

40. Horovitz JH (1979) Abnormalities caused by smoke inhalation. J Trauma 19:915–916

41. Jackson DM (1979) Burns: McIndoe's contribution and subsequent advances. Ann R Coll Surg Engl 61:335–340

42. Janzekovic Z (1970) A new concept in the early excision and immediate grafting of burns. J Trauma 10:1103–1108

43. Jelenko C (1979) Fluid therapy and the HALFD method. J Trauma 19:866–867

44. Jurkiewicz MJ (1979) Consensus summary on excisional therapy. J Trauma 19:933–934

45. Kien CL, Young VR, Rohrbaugh DK, Burke JF (1978) Increased rates of whole body protein synthesis and breakdown in children recovering from burns. Ann Surg 187:383–391

46. Kinney JM (1979) Protein metabolism in burned patients. J Trauma 19:900–901

47. Kitajima M, Allsop JR, Trelstad RL, Burke JF (1978) The experimental studies on stress ulcer of the stomach following thermal injury with special reference to H+ back diffusion and microcirculation. Gastroenterol Jpn 13:175–183

48. Koumans RKJ, Burke JF (1969) Skin allografts and immunosuppression in the treatment of massive thermal injury. Surgery 66:89–96

49. Levenson S (1979) Debriding agents. J Trauma 19:928–930

50. Levine BA, Sirinek KR, Pruitt BA (1978) Wound excision to fascia in burn patients. Arch Surg 113:403–407

51. Levine BA, Sirinek KR, Peterson HD, Pruitt BA (1979) Efficacy of tangential excision and immediate autografting of deep second-degree burns of the hand. J Trauma 19:670–673

52. Lloyd JR (1977) Thermal trauma: therapeutic achievements and investigative horizons. Surg Clin North Am 57:121–128

53. Long CL (1979) Energy expenditure of major burns. J. Trauma 19:904–906

54. Long CL, Schaffel N, Geiger JW, Schiller WR, Blakemore WS (1979) Metabolic response to injury and illness: estimation of energy and protein needs from indirect calorimetry and nitrogen balance. Journal of Parenteral Nutrition 3:452–456

55. MacMillan B (1979) Determining the depth of injury. J Trauma 19:927

56. Markley K (1979) Burned patients and immunoregulation. J Trauma 19:891–892

57. Martyn JAJ, Burke JF (1979) Is there a selective increase in pulmonary capillary permeability following cutaneous burns? Chest 76:374–375

58. Mason AD (1979) Weight loss in burned patients. J Trauma 19:903–904

59. Molnar, JA, Wolfe RR, Burke JF (1981) Metabolism and nutritional therapy in thermal injury. In: Schneider HA, Anderson CE, Coursin DB (eds): Nutritional support in medical practice, 2nd edn. Harper & Row, Hagerstown

60. Monafo WM (1979) An overview of infection control. J Trauma 19:879–880

61. Montgomery BJ (1979) Consensus for treatment of the "sickness patients you'll ever see". JAMA 241:345–346

62. Moore FD (1970) The body weight burn budget: basic fluid therapy for the early burn. Surg Clin North Am 50:1249–1265

63. Moritz AR, Henriques FC, McLean R (1945) The effects of inhaled heat on the air passages and lungs: an experimental investigation. Am J Pathol 21:311–321

64. Moyer CA, Brentano L, Gravens DL, Margraf HW, Monafo WW (1965) Treatment of large human burns with 0.5% silver nitrate solution. Arch Surg 90:812–867

65. Moylan JA (1979) Diagnostic techniques and steroids. J Trauma 19:917

66. Moylan JA, Chan CK (1978) Inhalation injury-an increasing problem. Ann Surg 188:34–37

67. Moylan JA, Wilmore DW, Mouton DE, Pruitt BA (1972) Early diagnosis of inhalation injury using ^{133}Xenon lung scan. Ann Surg 176:477–484

68. Munro HN (1979) Hormones and the metabolic response to injury. N Engl J Med 300:41–42

69. Munster AM (1980) The early management of the thermal burns. Surg 87:29–40

70. Nicholalds GE, Meng HC, Caldwell MD (1977) Vitamin requirements in patients receiving total parenteral nutrition. Arch Surg 112:1061–1064

71. Petroff PA, Hander EW, Clayton WH, Pruitt BA (1976) Pulmonary function studies after smoke inhalation. Am J Surg 132:346–351

72. Polk HC (1979) Consensus summary on infection. J Trauma 19:894–896

73. Polk HC, Tessler RH (1968) Sodium transit across burn wounds treated with silver nitrate solution(0.5%). Ann NY Acad Sci 150:682–685

74. Powers SR (1979) Consensus summary on smoke inhalation. J Trauma 19:921–922

75. Pruitt BA (1978) Advances in fluid therapy and the early care of the burned patient. World J Surg 2:139–150

76. Pruitt BA (1979) The effectiveness of fluid resuscitation. J. Trauma 19:868–870

77. Pruitt BA, Foley FD (1973) The use of biopsies in burn patient care. Surgery 73:887–897

78. Pruitt BA, McManus WF (1980) Surgical management of burns. Contemporary Surgery 16:11–16

79. Pruitt BA, Moylan JA (1972) Current management of thermal burns, In: Hardy JD, (ed): Advances in surgery, vol 6. Yearbook Medical Publishers, Chicago

80. Pruitt, BA, Dowling JA, Moncrief JA (1968) Escharotomy in early burn care. Arch Surg 96:502–507

81. Pruitt BA, Mason AD, Moncrief JA (1971) Hemodynamic changes in the early postburn patient: the influence of fluid administration and of a vasodilator (Hydralazine).

82. Quinby WC, Burke JF (1979) Treatment of burns. In: Cave EF, Burke JF, Boyd RJ (eds) Trauma management. Yearbook Medical Publishers, Chicago pp 1137–1162

83. Rai K, Courtemanche AD (1975) Vitamin A assay in burned patients. J Trauma 15:419–424

84. Roe CF, Kinney JM, Blair C (1964) Water and heat exchange in third-degree burns. Surgery 56:212–220

86. Sargent DW (1961) An evaluation for basal metabolic data for children and youth in the United States. US Department of Agriculture, Washington (Home economics research report no. 14)

87. Schumer W (1979) Consensus summary on metabolism. J Trauma 19:910–911

88. Schwartz SI (1979) Consensus summary on fluid resuscitation. J Trauma 19:876–877

89. Sevitt S (1965) Renal function after burning. J. Clin Pathol 18:572–578

90. Sevitt S (1979) A review of the complications of burns, their origin and importance for illness and death. J Trauma 19:358–369

91. Symington IS, Anderson RA, Oliver JS, Thomson I, Harland WA, Kerr JW (1978) Cyanide exposure in fires. Lancet II:91–92

92. Thomas R, Aikawa N, Burke JF (1979) Insulin resistance in peripheral tissues after a burn injury. Surgery 86:742–747

93. Whelchel JD, Cosimi AB, Burke JF, Bondoc CC, Morrell RM, Wortis HH, Russell PS (1975) Treatment of extensively burned children with skin allografts and antithymocyte globulin. Transplant Proc 7:765–769

94. Wilmore DW (1974) Nutrition and metabolism following thermal injury. Clin Plast Surg 1:603–619

95. Wilmore DW, Long JM, Mason AD, Skreen RW, Pruitt BA (1974) Catecholamines: mediator of the hypermetabolic response to thermal injury. Ann Surg 180:653–669

96. Wilmore DW, Orcutt TW, Mason AD, Pruitt BA (1975) Alterations in hypothalamic function following thermal injury. J Trauma 15:697–703

97. Wolfe RR (1979) Burn injury and increased glucose production. J Trauma 19:898–899

98. Wolfe RR (1981) Acute versus chronic response to burn injury. Circ Shock 8:105–115

99. Wolfe RR, Burke JF (1978) Effect of glucose infusion on glucose and lactate metabolism in normal and burned guinea pigs. J Trauma 18:800–805

100. Wolfe RR, Durkot MJ, Allsop JR, Burke JF (1979) Glucose metabolism in severely burned patients. Metabolism 28:1031–1039

101. Wolfe RR, O'Donnell TF, Stone MD, Richmond DA, Burke JF (1980) Investigation of factors determining the optimal glucose infusion rate in TPN. Metabolism 29:892–900

102. Wortis HH, Cooper AG, Brown MD (1973) Inhibition of human lymphocyte rosetting by anti-T sera. Nature 243:109–110

103. Yannas IV, Burke JF (1980) Design of artificial skin. I. Basic design principles. J Biomed Mater Res 14:65–81

104. Yannas IV, Burke JF, Gordon PL, Huang C, Rubenstein, RH (1980) Design of skin II. Control of chemical composition. J Biomed Mater Res 14:107–132

105. Zawacki BE, Spitzer KW, Mason AD, Johns LA (1970) Does increased evaporative water loss cause hypermetabolism in burned patients? Ann Surg 171:236–240

Chapter 39

Electrical Injury

Charles E. Hartford

Electricity causes a unique multifaceted and fascinating but at times devastating injury, which can result in instant death. Otherwise, even with massive tissue destruction, there is an excellent chance of surviving an electrical accident. Survival from high-voltage injury is characterized by a high incidence of permanent disabling sequelae.

Brief historical perspective

Although man has been exposed to death and injury from lightning during his entire existence, the first known electrical shock from a man-made source occurred in 1749, when the current from an inadvertently discharged Leyden jar traversed the bodies of two Dutch physicists [54]. Direct current was the earliest (1849) form of commercial electricity. However, in 1881, Westinghouse, using the alternating current induction motor invented by Tesla and the transformer invented by Stanley, developed an alternating current power transmission system which could be used commercially to deliver inexpensive electrical power [11]. The first recorded accidental electrocution occurred in Lyons, France, in 1879, when a carpenter was killed by the current from a 250-V alternating current dynamo [51]. Deaths from electricity followed in Scotland in 1880 and in Buffalo, New York, USA, in 1881 [11]. In 1890, the State of New York first used electricity to impose the death penalty [51]. Ventricular fibrillation from electricity was described in 1899 [79].

Incidence, cause, and death rate

During the 20th century in Western industrialized nations, the development and wide use of relatively cheap hydroelectric power has been associated with a rapid increase in both fatal and nonfatal electrical accidents. In the United States there were 670 electrical deaths in 1914, 989 in 1960, over 1000 in 1965 and now approximately 1500 each year [65]. During 1977, 2400 patients with electrical shock were treated in emergency departments of United States hospitals. Approximately 3%–6% of patients admitted to burn care facilities have sustained electrical injury. Skoog [85] noted that in Sweden during the first half of the 20th century the incidence of electrical accidents paralleled the rise in production of electrical power. However, in the early 1950s, because of the implementation of stringent regulations governing electrical installations and the development of safer electrical appliances, there has been a substantial reduction in the incidence of injury in spite of a continued rise in the production of electrical energy.

Most electrical accidents are preventable. Men at work are at great risk of high-voltage (arbitrarily greater than 1000 V) accidents [42]. Frequent causes of injury include installation of antennas, repair of commercial electrical equipment and high-voltage lines, and operation of machinery that comes in contact with high-voltage wires. Inadvertent contact with downed commercial lines, attempts to rescue victims of accidental electrocution, climbing of electrical poles or towers by young athletically gifted males, and young adults at play or mischief in electrical train yards are common causes of high-voltage accidents not related to work [16]. The peak incidence of high-voltage electrical injury is late in the second and in the third decades of life. In the home, young children are at risk not only of dying but of sustaining a nasty burn of the lip and mouth from sucking or chewing on a defective electrical cord or on the female end of an energized plug; there is enough electrolyte in the saliva to complete the electrical circuit. Adults of either gender are at risk of dying of ventricular fibrillation from 60-cycle house current [37], even with no external wound. Operating an electrical appliance while taking a bath is a frequently cited cause. Domestic electricity is the source of two-thirds of the fatal electrical accidents in Great Britain [59] and one-fourth of those in the United States. Each year in the United States lightning causes 150–300 deaths [22].

Even patients are not exempt from the dangers of electricity. There is a growing body of publications [8, 9, 14, 90] about the hazards of improperly grounded or used and defective electrical equipment, including that used for electrocautery, monitoring, and even diathermy, which can cause either ventricular fibrillation or burns. There is no absolutely safe level of current [93].

Pathogenesis

When a part or all of the body is interposed between two conductors of different potentials, an electrical circuit is completed, allowing current to flow through the tissues.

$$\text{Ohm's law, I (amperes)} = \frac{\text{V (Volts)}}{\text{R (ohms)}},$$

applies. The current (amperage) to which the tissues are exposed is directly proportional to the voltage delivered and inversely proportional to the resistance (ohmage) of the tissues. Since the amount of current required for physiologic effect is proportional to the frequency of alternating current and since impedance (resistance) of tissues varies widely, it is useful to measure physiological changes relative to current flow. In response to increasing levels of current flow, sensation is produced, then contraction of muscle, fibrillation, defibrillation, and finally tissue injury from heat [81].

Although a variety of conditions affect perception of current, such as the kind of electrode used, wave form of the current, the hertz (H_z) value, and the part of the body on which the current is applied, a current level of approximately 1 mA can be detected by humans [25]. While the first perception of direct current is warmth, that of alternating current is tingling. With increasing levels of current the sensation is increasingly more noxious.

Alternating current causes tetanic contraction of muscles, which may be so severe as to freeze the victim to the current source, prolonging exposure. This is a factor that makes alternating current more dangerous than direct current. A human male can be trapped with a hand-to-hand 60-cycle current of 16–20 mA [25, 27]. This is referred to as the 'let-go' current. It is lower for women. The let-go current increases as the frequency increases. Prolonged transthoracic exposure to tetanic levels of current may cause asphyxiation by holding the muscles of respiration in the contracted state [53]. The respiratory muscles may be slow to recover and consequently prolonged artificial ventilation is often needed following electrical shock, even when circulatory function was not compromised or has been restored.

Ventricular fibrillation is thought to be responsible for most deaths from electricity. There is an extensive list of publications about fibrillation [26, 37, 38, 55, 56, 79]. Fibrillation of cardiac muscle is most frequently caused by 60-Hz low-voltage house current with the heart being exposed to approximately 300 mA [37]. Among dogs, a current of 7.5 A or above never caused ventricular fibrillation [55]. Alternating current of 10 A or more 'defibrillates' the heart [55]. 'Defibrillation' current actually produces contraction of the myocardium. The contraction is sustained until current flow ceases; then the heart muscle relaxes, after which the muscle often resumes rhythmic contraction. Direct current is used to defibrillate hearts in clinical situations.

Currents above myocardial fibrillation levels cause contraction of the myocardium. These levels of currents also produce burn injury, often of catastrophic extent [7, 16, 30, 42, 85]. The typical injury is a contact conductive injury with deep necrosis involving underlying muscle and often bone (Figs. 39.1, 39.2, 39.4, 39.9, and 39.12). The injury is caused by heat. For practical purposes, living tissues obey Joule's law [43]: $J = I^2 RT$, where heating (J) is proportional to the power dissipated multiplied by the time duration; I is the current that passes through the tissues in amperes; R is the resistance of the tissues in ohms, and T is the duration of contact in seconds.

Resistance of tissues changes as currents flow through [45]. As electrical current is applied to skin, an electrical insulator of variable but relatively high impedance (the calloused palm may have a resistance of 1 000 000 Ω, normal skin 5000 Ω, and moistened skin as little as 1000 Ω [77]), there is a slow rise in amperage, representing a progressive decrease in skin resistance (Fig. 39.3) [45]. If the current is discontinued the skin recovers its resistance. If the application of

current is continued, however, there is a rapid rise in amperage coinciding with complete breakdown of skin resistance (Fig. 39.3) [45]. This signals unimpeded flow of current through

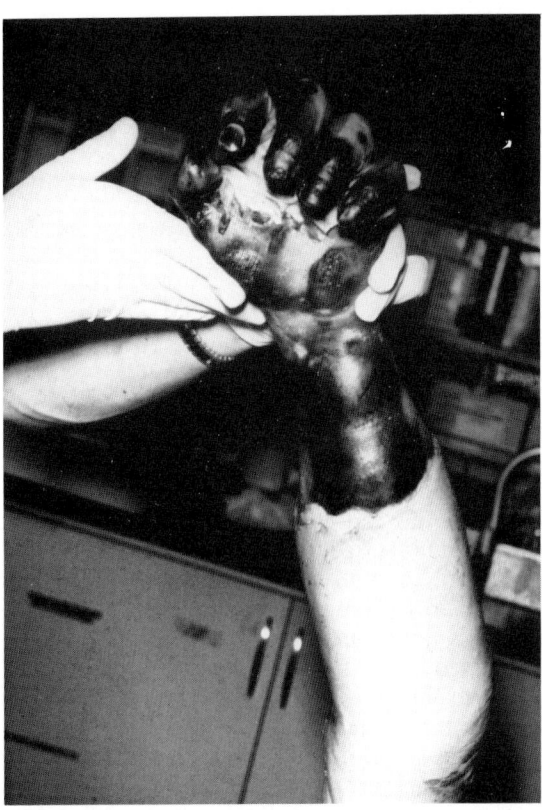

Fig. 39.2. High-voltage electrical contact wound 1 week after injury. Extensive abscess was found within muscle compartment of forearm. Amputation through arm was required.

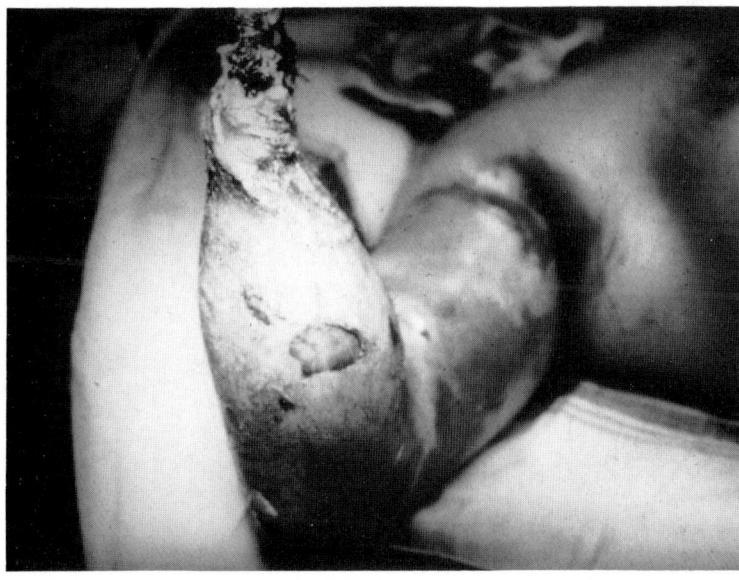

Fig. 39.1. Entry wound from high-voltage electrical contact involving bone and resulting in immediate autoamputation at wrist. Muscle necrosis in both forearm and arm necessitated surgical amputation through shoulder.

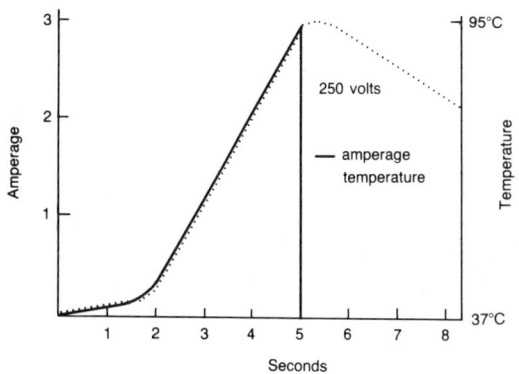

Fig. 39.3. Relationship of amperage, temperature, and time. See text. From Hunt et al. [45].

the internal tissues of the body. Although isolated tissues have different levels of impedance, the internal milieu of the body acts as a single uniform resistance. Living tissues act as a volume conductor and the current moves as a wave through gel [94]. The amperage continues to rise rapidly until the current arcs, resulting in an instantaneous and precipitous fall in the amperage to zero (Fig. 39.3) [45]. Once the current arcs there is cessation of current flow through the tissues and no additional heat is generated [45]. There is an inverse relationship between the voltage and the time necessary for the current to arc.

The tissue temperature attained before the current arcs is critical in determining the extent of injury. The rise in tissue temperature parallels the slow and then rapid rise in amperage, peaks as arcing occurs, and then slowly dissi-

pates (Fig. 39.3) by conduction, convection, and radiation [45]. Tissue temperatures in excess of 60°C are associated with muscle damage [81]. The severity of tissue damage decreases as the distance from the contact site increases. As the voltage increases the chance of and extent of tissue damage increases. While exposure to household currents of 440 V and below, usually 110 V, are capable of producing tissue necrosis (Fig. 39.8), it is seldom as massive as that seen with exposure to commercial currents, which are usually greater than 1000 V. Factors that increase current density, e.g., good electrode contact, which delays arcing, and small diameter of the portion of the body in contact with electrode, increase the extent of tissue damage [81].

In most electrical accidents, the initial point of contact is an extremity. As current flows from an extremity into the torso there is a huge increase in cross-sectional area, resulting in dissipation of current. Therefore, it is unusual to have enough current flow through the internal tissues of the torso to produce sufficient heat to cause heat necrosis of internal organs. However, a viscus may be damaged if it is adjacent to a contact point and enough heat has been produced to extend to the organ.

Current flows through the body to a grounding contact point where the current exits causing, depending largely on local conditions, a variety of wounds (Figs. 39.4–39.6).

When the current arcs, temperatures up to 4000°C are produced [81]. This heat causes cutaneous flash burns or ignites the clothing, exposing the victim to flame burns.

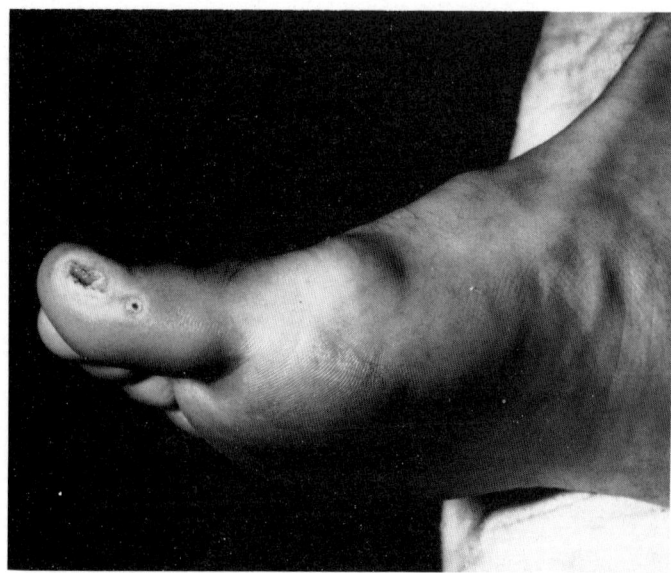

Fig. 39.4. Wound of electrical exit; a current mark.

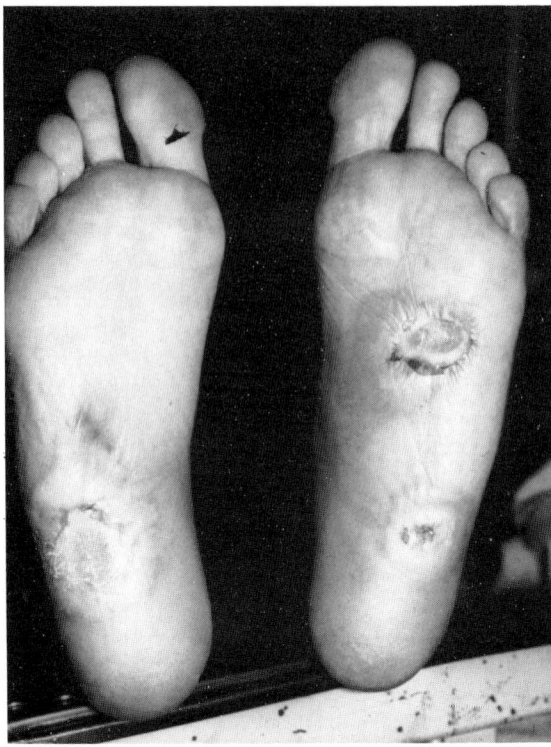

Fig. 39.5. Wounds of high-voltage electrical exit. No deep necrosis to skin.

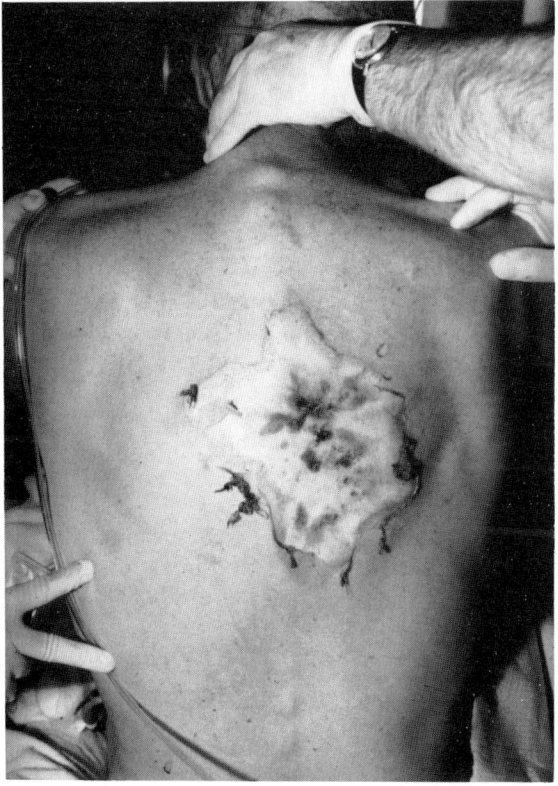

Fig. 39.6. Wound of high-voltage electrical exit. No underlying muscle necrosis.

Initial treatment

Those who witness accidental electrocution must exercise great caution so they do not sustain injury as well. Unless an insulated prod, such as a wooden pole, can be used to dislodge the victim, the rescue effort must be delayed until the current can be interrupted.

If circulatory or ventilatory insufficiency or both exist, cardiopulmonary resuscitation must be instituted immediately. If there is circulatory failure of cardiac origin, one must determine whether the cause is from ventricular fibrillation or cardiac asystole and treat the patient accordingly. At times, because of the residual effect of electricity on the muscles of respiration, ventilatory support will need to be continued for a time beyond the restoration of circulation [53]. These efforts are important, because once the patient reaches a hospital the mortality rate is low even in the presence of massive tissue injury. Most reported mortality rates are below 10%, and some are around 5% [42, 47]. In most instances, by the time the patient is admitted to a hospital the respiratory and cardiac problems have been resolved.

Wounds need no first aid other than to extinguish and remove any source of heat.

It was Artz [6] who publicized the finding that the response to high-voltage electrical injury resembled crush injury more than the response to an ordinary burn and that formulae used to estimate the volumes of fluid required to prevent burn shock were *not* applicable to this group of patients. There is no effective means by which the amount of fluid sequestered into or in response to necrotic or injured muscle can be estimated. At times, with massive injury, the fluid shift is immediate and prodigious. The net result of this shift of fluid is oligemia.

With death of muscle, myoglobin enters the circulation [10]. Although free hemoglobin from destruction of red blood cells also occurs with electrical injury, the amount is quite low relative to that of myoglobin. Whereas haemoglobin is bound to available circulating haptoglobin and cleared slowly from the plasma, myoglobin is excreted rapidly. Urine the color of port wine or reddish black indicates the presence of urinary hemochromogens. Blondheim et al. [12] have described a simple test for myohemoglobinuria. The concentration of myoglobin in the urine may be as high as 6 g/100 ml. Baxter [10] reported that in his experience, if myoglobinuria was present for more than 6 h, the patient required a high amputation of one or more extremities or a resection of a large mass of muscle, or both.

These pigments, together with oligemia and the accompanying metabolic acidosis, present a set of circumstances in which the incidence of acute renal failure is high, a clinical fact reported by many workers [18, 30, 42, 72, 78]. Nonetheless, if timely and appropriate therapy is given to replenish sequestered fluid, the incidence of acute renal insufficiency should be low [10].

Intravenous fluid therapy with an isotonic balanced salt solution is to be instituted as soon as possible. The initial rate of infusion should be rapid enough to relieve the systemic manifestations of shock and to establish urine flow. In the presence of pigmenturia, the rate of infusion is to be maintained at a sufficiently fast rate to insure flow of urine in excess of 100 ml/h until the pigment is cleared. Urine should be examined microscopically to make sure the abnormal color is not from red blood cells in the urine. In the absence of pigmenturia or after the pigment has been cleared, urine output in the range of 30–50 ml/h for adults is certainly acceptable.

With myoglobinemia there is a high incidence of severe metabolic acidosis [10]. It is essential that this be corrected and that the pH of arterial blood be maintained above 7.35. Hemochromagens produce an alkaline urine and therefore urine pH cannot be used to monitor therapy. Baxter [10] reported the need to administer as much as 200–400 mmol sodium bicarbonate per hour during the first several hours after injury, to attain and maintain an acceptable arterial blood pH. It may be advantageous to add the sodium bicarbonate to the balanced salt solution.

In this clinical setting it has been suggested that mannitol [10], given either as an intermittent bolus or as a constant infusion, and other diuretics may be helpful in reducing the chance of acute renal failure. It has also been suggested that if pigmenturia is unusually massive or prolonged (2–3 days) it may be helpful to resect large portions of necrotic tissue to reduce the myoglobin load on the kidney [6]. Although I have not found any of these techniques necessary, they might be considered in unusual clinical circumstances.

If acute renal failure does supervene, this fact needs to be recognized as promptly as possible and measures taken to prevent circulatory overload. As soon as convenient, hemodialysis should be done and the patient immediately taken to the operating room for the removal of all necrotic tissue [42]. Resolution of the renal failure can be expected if infection can be prevented.

Wounds caused by electricity and their management

There are a variety of wounds which result from exposure to electricity. By careful inspection, one can, with reasonable certainty, ascertain whether the patient sustained a high- or low-voltage accident, the sites of electrical entrance and exit and whether or not the patient sustained an arc flash burn or flame burn from arc ignition of clothing.

Low-voltage contact wounds

Wounds produced by low-voltage household current are usually small and involve the hand; many do not require surgical treatment. Most of these wounds can be allowed to slough and heal spontaneously. Occasionally debridement or excision and a skin graft or local flap will be needed. This kind of wound confirms exposure to electricity.

The wound that results from a child sucking or chewing on an energized electrical cord may vary from a small nondeforming injury of the vermillion portion of the lip (Fig. 39.7) to a mutilating wound [69, 71] involving the commissure, a large portion of one or both lips, orbicularis oris muscle, the buccal sulcus, tongue, alveolar ridge, and teeth. If the wound is deep enough to involve the labial artery, hemorrhage from it is almost inevitable. This may be a reason to admit the child to the hospital.

There are three treatment options. The first is to allow the wound to heal by second intention and reconstruct the residuum after the tissues become supple [52, 57]. While this has been the method most frequently employed, it may now be the least desirable for all but minimal injury which does not involve the commissure. Severe untreated perioral electrical burns allowed to heal spontaneously lead to unsightly microstomia, dental deviation and drooling due to obliteration of the buccal sulcus. A second approach, early repair, is exemplified by the recommendation of Ortiz-Monasterio [69]. For those with injury of more than one-third of either lip, involving the commissure or deep wounds involving muscle, he advocates exci-

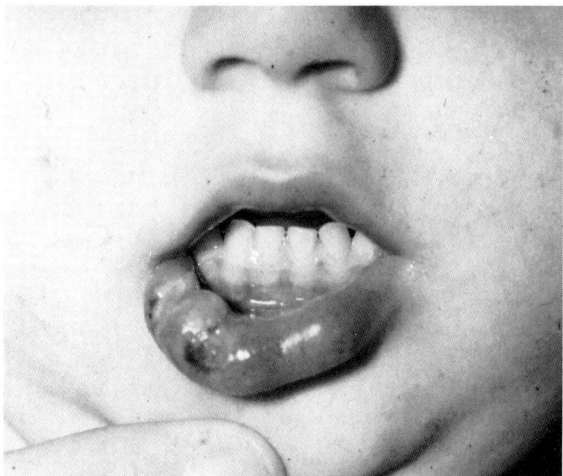

Fig. 39.7. Limited low-voltage contact wound of lip from sucking on the female plug of an energized electrical extension cord.

sion of necrotic tissue and repair with a forked-tongue flap 2 weeks after injury. He contends that one cannot accurately determine the extent of necrosis until that time has passed. Other local flaps and plastic procedures may be just as applicable or preferred [34, 48]. Thompson et al. [89] contend that there is no difference in end-result between those repaired by early and late methods. The most recent innovation, which shows considerable promise, involves the use of a fabricated orthodontic retainer with acrylic posts smoothed and contoured to fit the commissure and positioned to prevent contraction of the mouth as the tissues heal by second intention [58, 80]. The retainer is inserted after the slough has been removed and is worn continuously until the scar tissue has matured, usually 6–8 months. Results have been encouraging and when the device has been worn properly for a sufficient duration there has not been any need for late reconstructive procedures. Many more cases are needed before the efficacy of this technique can be definitively assessed.

High-voltage contact wounds of electrical entry and exit

These wounds have unmistakable characteristics (Figs. 39.1, 39.2, 39.4–39.6, 39.8, 39.9, and 39.12). At the site of electrical entry, most often on an extremity, the wound is usually leathery, charred, dry, depressed, insensitive and extensive. The necrosis typically involves muscle contiguous with the surface wound and may extend into bone. It is not unusual to have muscle necrosis and injury extend far beyond

the edge of the contact wound and lie under unburned skin. If there is swelling beyond the contact wound, the muscle has usually been injured. When joints, e.g., fingers, wrists,

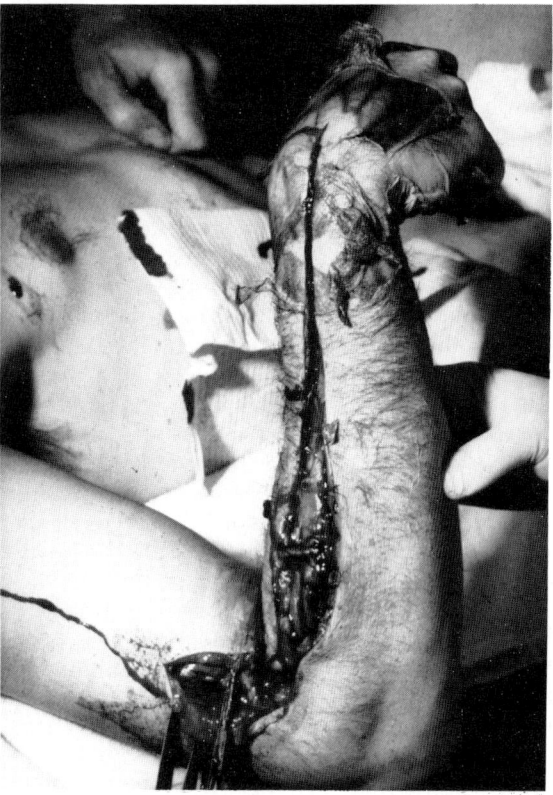

Fig. 39.8. High-voltage electrical wound. Elbow, wrist, and hand held immobile in flexion, indicating necrosis of muscles that activate these joints.

Incision for fasciotomy produced no bleeding in the skin and subcutaneous tissue of the forearm and exposed necrotic muscle. In the arm bleeding was produced in the subcutaneous tissue, but underlying muscles were necrotic. Amputation through the shoulder was eventually done.

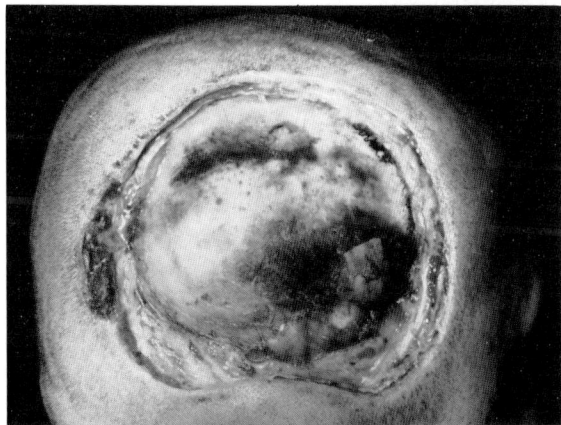

Fig. 39.9. High-voltage contact wound of head with necrotic scalp and periosteum removed, uncovering nonviable calvarium.

elbows, etc., are held immobile in flexion, it can be assumed that the flexor muscles which activate those joints have been coagulated while in the contracted position (Fig. 39.8). Flexion is produced because of the tetanic stimulation of alternating current and flexors are stronger than extensors. The muscle cells are then destroyed by heat and relaxation of the muscle fibers cannot occur.

All who have cared for patients with high-voltage injury have found necrotic muscle adjacent to bone with overlying viable muscle. Necrosis occurs at this site because the high impedance of bone causes increased production of heat in the immediate periosseous tissues [75]. Nonetheless, the periosseous necrotic tissue is always contiguous with the contact wound of the surface.

In high-voltage electrical accidents it is not unusual to have a contact wound of the scalp. This wound may initially be overlooked on a cursory examination. Furthermore, the wound may extend to involve one or both tables of the calvarium (Figs. 39.9 and 39.10). In the usual instance, only the outer table is necrotic because, it is believed, the vascular diplöe is responsible for dissipating the electrical current, the heat, or both [85]. When both tables are destroyed, necrosis of underlying brain may occur as well [65].

The hand is a frequent initial contact point. With alternating current, when the palm touches the energy source the wrist is flexed violently, resulting in wounds of both the palm and the volar aspect of the forearm just proximal to the wrist [85] (Fig. 39.12). It is not unusual to have a limited wound of the palmar aspect of the hand with destruction of the volar compartment of the forearm. The dorsal compartment may or may not be spared.

There may be additional wounds of the antecubital fossa and axilla, sites of decreased impedance from moisture. Although these wounds may look innocent, there may be underlying muscle necrosis.

After the current has traversed the body it accumulates in the subcutaneous tissue at one or several grounding or exit sites, often in the feet. The current bursts through causing several kinds of wounds. The first, a small, dry, full thickness wound known as a 'current mark' (Fig. 39.4). These wounds usually need no operative treatment. The necrotic tissue sloughs spontaneously and the wound heals by second intention. There are larger wounds of electrical exit which are depressed, well demarcated, yellow or white, leathery, and insensitive

(Figs. 39.5 and 39.6). While muscle necrosis may underlie these exit wounds, the extent and incidence are much less than at the wounds of electrical entrance.

Burns

Electricity can produce additional wounds of the skin by two mechanisms, both by heat. First, as the current arcs, temperatures up to 4000°C are generated which may cause flash burns [81]. Second, the arcing current may ignite the clothing, exposing the victim to flame burns, which at times are extensive.

Management of large wounds of electrical contact

As soon as IV fluid therapy is initiated and the patient thoroughly examined, all areas of electrical entrance and exit which are leathery are incised to determine the depth of injury [42] (Fig. 39.8). We also incise areas of deep burn caused by flame. In the presence of either muscle injury or an elevation of the tissue pressure to 40 mmHg or above, the incision is extended to open and decompress the entire fascial compartment. Before one decides not to decompress a swollen limb injured by electricity, the tissue pressure should be measured. While there are a number of ways to do this, the technique described by Whitesides et al. [96], is simple, direct, and reliable, and it can be performed with equipment readily available in any hospital. The escharotomy–fasciotomy should prevent extension of the injury caused by Volkmann's ischemia.

If there is no injury to muscle, the wound is managed as any thermal burn. Excisional treatment, as advocated by some workers, may still be indicated. If dead muscle is found, plans are made for further exploration of the wound and debridement with the patient anesthetized [28, 42, 49, 64, 95]. Timing of this procedure is controversial. There are those who advocate long delay [26, 57, 61, 68], and some workers even advocate allowing spontaneous sloughing of necrotic tissues. The point at issue is the difficulty of determining the demarcation between viable and nonviable tissues when these injuries are debrided early [44, 76]. On the other hand, in the presence of necrotic muscle the patient is at great risk for clostridial and bacterial infection [6, 10, 30, 73] (Fig. 39.2). Nothing is gained by delaying removal of irreparably damaged muscle. Delay invites additional tissue loss from invasive infection as well as the systemic sequelae of sepsis. In addition, the catastrophic complication of hemorrhage from rupture of a large artery is prevented by removal of the necrotic portion of the vessel [42].

In the usual instance, operative treatment is delayed until fluid resuscitation is completed. If the injury is of limited extent, i.e., involves only one extremity, the excision may be further delayed to the end of the first week to allow complete spontaneous demarcation. Should several large areas and/or multiple extremities be involved, however, the author prefers to begin surgical treatment after 36–48 h.

The operation is begun with the excision of all skin with full-thickness injury and underlying subcutaneous tissue to fascia. The author prefers to leave areas of skin with partial-thickness burns, even when they may eventually provide the skin covering of flaps. Then each fascial compartment is systematically explored. As dead muscle is found, it is excised until bleeding contractile muscle is encountered. If there is any question about the viability of a piece of tissue, it is not removed.

All who have attempted early excision of muscle injured by high-voltage electricity have had the frustrating experience of leaving muscle which was thought to be viable but on reinspection several days later finding it to be obviously necrotic. In the original cutting of this tissue, blood vessels bleed, but bleeding from the muscle itself was not as brisk as one would have hoped. To add to the confusion, the muscle may have contracted somewhat when stimulated. This muscle then died. This has led to the concept of progressive muscle necrosis or progressive vascular thrombosis. It is the author's contention that during the original accident these cells were either irrevocably damaged or injured to such an extent that subsequent conditions were unsatisfactory to permit ultimate survival of these cells.

Several techniques have been employed to try to identify precisely the extent of the soft tissue that is either dead or irrevocably injured. Detection of arterial blood flow either by physical examination or by the Doppler ultrasound technique does not guarantee viability of surrounding tissues, because in this clinical setting large blood vessels may be open and temporarily transmit blood through necrotic tissue even when the wall of the blood vessel is also necrotic [21].

Arteriograms may be helpful in assessing the presence and extent of injury [46]. Findings include complete occlusion, partial occlusion, narrowing, irregularity, and beading of the arteries and a decrease in visualization of nutrient muscle branches. Occasionally however, a normal arteriogram in the presence of muscle necrosis limits the usefulness of this procedure.

In electrical injury, muscle blood flow studies based on the Xenon-133 washout technique have shown precise correlation between muscle blood flow of less than $1.00 \text{ cm}^3/\text{min}$ per 100 g tissue and histopathologic confirmation of muscle necrosis [21]. But the need for sequential studies and studies at multiple sites limits the usefulness of this technique.

Quimby and co-workers [76] advocate the use of frozen-section microscopy to aid in determining whether the appropriate level of resection has been reached. While this technique shows promise, it requires a pathologist with experience; for instance, the presence of cross striations in skeletal muscle is an unreliable mark of viability.

Technetium-99m stannous pyrophosphate scintigraphy has been used to detect and localize both large and focal areas of skeletal muscle necrosis following high-voltage electrical injury [44]. Muscle damage is identified by an increased cellular uptake of the radionucleotide, indicating perfused but injured muscle that is not yet necrotic. The authors emphasize that tissue should not be removed unless it is obviously nonviable. It is probable that the most appropriate use of this technique among patients with electrical injury will be to detect undebrided necrotic tissue in the presence of clinical sepsis of unknown focus.

Even with the use of one or more of these techniques, the surgeon still has to make a decision based on experience as to which tissue is nonviable before it is removed. Furthermore, if a piece of tissue is not viable, that fact will become obvious with time.

Necrotic muscle often extends beyond the level of excised skin and subcutaneous tissue. In these instances, incisions need to be made to expose deep tissues adequately. These incisions should not be made indiscriminately, but with eventual closure of the wound in mind.

During debridement, nerves that are structurally intact should not be removed. To preserve their integrity, they should be covered with viable soft tissues. Arteries must also be covered in this manner. If this is not done, necrosis of the vessel will occur and the artery will eventually rupture. Large arteries which require ligation should be ligated in a viable segment with nonabsorbable suture. A section of the artery just distal to the point of ligation should be submitted for pathological examination to determine its state of viability.

Amputation is resorted to only after it has been found that the necrosis of soft tissue is circumferential and of such extent that viable soft tissues, including flaps, are not available to cover vital structures. Amputation stumps should initially be left open, and closed subsequently only when one confirms that there is no remaining necrotic tissue.

It is the author's opinion that the duration of each procedure should be limited to no more than 2 or 2.5 h. If there is extensive necrosis it is safer to do a series of operations, anesthetizing the patient every 2–3 days until all necrotic tissue is removed, rather than to do it all in one procedure.

Uninflated tourniquets should be placed on the proximal part of all injured extremities. If massive bleeding should occur, it can easily be stopped by inflating the tourniquet until the bleeding can be controlled with adequate exposure in the operating room.

Management of nonviable calvarium

The first step is to remove all necrotic soft tissue. There are two ways of dealing with the nonviable bone.

The first involves the removal of all nonviable bone either by excision or by spontaneous sequestration aided by drilling multiple holes into the bone and piecemeal removal over several months (Fig. 39.10) [30, 36, 60, 85]. Since in many instances only the outer table is nonviable, the vascular diploë soon forms excellent quality granulation tissue. At this point the wound can be closed by one of several techniques [15, 35, 60]. Although applying a split-thickness skin graft is the simplest method, the resulting defect is unsightly and nonhair bearing (Fig. 39.11). A variety of local, distant, or even free flaps may be used. When the bony defect extends to dura, a flap of some kind is required before a bone graft or synthetic bony substitute, e.g., acrylic, is used to restore the hard protective covering of the brain. Caffee [19] repaired a bony defect by placing split bony ribs under omentum vascularized by microvascular techniques and covered with a split-thickness skin graft.

The second method utilizes a flap moved to cover the nonviable bone immediately after all necrotic soft tissue has been removed [97]. The dead bone is gradually replaced by viable bone from the periphery by creeping substitution. The author has successfully employed this technique. A bone scan should be obtained to prove a perfusion defect in the skull. To insure success, it is absolutely essential that *all* injured and necrotic soft tissue be removed, that the nonviable bone be covered in its entirety, and that the wound be closed completely. In the author's case, a bone scan done 6 months later showed a substantial decrease in the volume of nonperfused bone.

Management of electrical wounds of the hand

Since a large majority of patients have deep wounds of the hand, a comment about management of wounds at this site is in order.

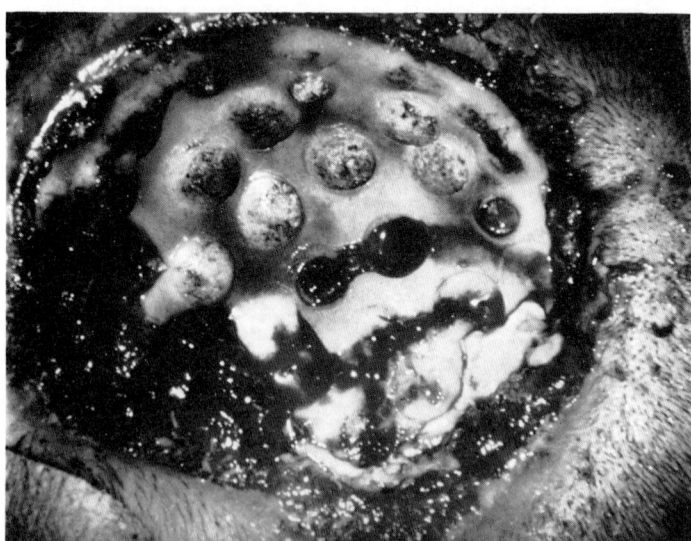

Fig. 39.10. Same wound as in Fig. 38.9, depicting holes drilled through nonviable outer table of calvarium into diploë to aid in sequestration of necrotic bone.

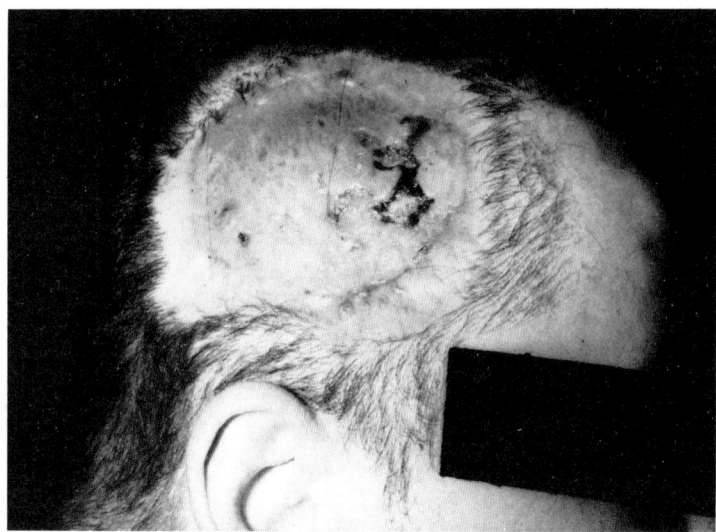

Fig. 39.11. Same wound as in Figs. 38.9 and 38.10, showing viable skin graft on inner table of calvarium. The unsatisfactory cosmetic result is obvious.

Most workers agree that wounds of 1 cm or less in area are best treated by allowing the necrotic tissue to slough and the wound to heal by second intention [18]. While a number of authors have advocated allowing large deep wounds of the hand to demarcate and slough spontaneously [24, 57, 61, 62, 68], this approach may be complicated by invasive infection and is conducive to excessive cicatrization and stiffness and contractures of joints, all detrimental to restoration of optimal hand function [70]. On the other side, the advocates of early excision maintain that, with experience, particularly by the end of 1 week, the nonviable tissue can be identified and should be excised [28, 49, 64, 70]. Some even use a tourniquet [70]. After the debridement is completed, several days should elapse before the surgeon commits the wound to closure by delayed primary closure, skin graft, or flap. By this approach and with a good quality of occupational therapy, optimal early restoration of hand function can be attained.

In instances in which there is limited destruction of the hand with extensive destruction of the volar compartment of the forearm but sparing of the dorsum, amputation should not be done early (Fig. 39.12). After careful and complete excision of all necrotic tissue, if the blood supply of the hand is lost it may be restored

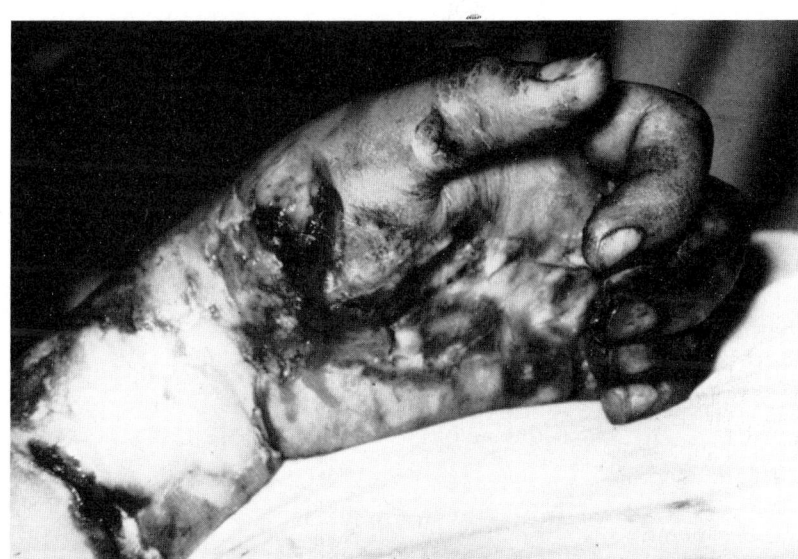

Fig. 39.12. High-voltage electrical contact wound of hand, with arc to volar aspect of wrist. Limited destruction of hand with extensive destruction of volar compartment of forearm; dorsal compartment spared.

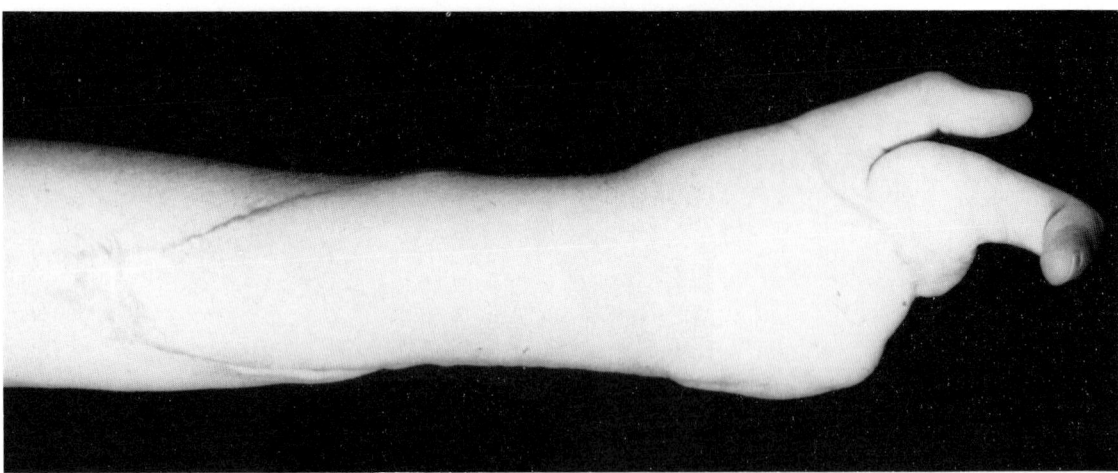

Fig. 39.13. Same patient as in Fig. 38.12. After excision of all necrotic tissue, a flap was used to provide full thickness of skin coverage. Subsequently, reinnervation by nerve graft and transfer of tendons restored hand to limited but useful function.

with an autogenous vein graft. This repair can be protected either with a flap or by burying the forearm into the abdominal wall. Reinnervation of the hand and tendon transfers are done later to restore the hand to limited but useful function (Fig. 39.13).

Infectious complications

Since patients with wounds caused by electricity are prone to develop tetanus, they should receive appropriate prophylaxis against this disease.

In the presence of necrotic muscle there is a substantial risk of clostridial myositis [6, 10, 30, 73]. For this reason, it has been recommended that patients receive systemic penicillin until all dead muscle has been removed [1]. It has also been suggested that mafenide be the topical antibacterial agent of choice, because it has specific activity against clostridium species and it penetrates eschar in an effective concentration [66]. While these adjuncts may be used, the key to prevention of clostridial myositis is the timely removal of necrotic muscle.

As long as necrotic tissue remains, the possibility of local and systemic sepsis from a variety of gram-negative bacteria and *Staphylococcus aureus* exists. The key to successful prevention and treatment of infection is removal of necrotic tissue. Systemic antibiotics are used as adjuncts in the treatment of infection and not as definitive therapy. Only when all the necrotic tissue has been removed will the patient become afebrile and be relieved of other manifestations of sepsis.

Visceral injuries and their treatment

Injury to bone

There are several causes of bony injury from electrical accidents [10, 13, 17, 30]. First, the accident may initiate a fall which results in one or more fractures. Second, the violent tetanic contraction of muscles stimulated by alternating current may cause avulsion fractures or dislocations. The shoulder joint is apparently the most frequent site of the latter complication [13, 17]. Victims of electrical accidents must be carefully examined for these injuries and appropriate roentgenographic studies obtained.

At times, sufficient heat is produced in the contact wound of entry to cause heat necrosis of bone (Figs. 39.1 and 39.9). The bones of the hand and skull are the most frequent sites.

While the necrotic bone may sequester, small rounded densities in bone, resembling 'pearls' or 'wax drippings', have been described and are believed to be a residual of heat injury to bone [13]. Acro-osteolysis, periosteal reaction, osteochondritis, joint change and, among children, impairment of bone growth following damage to epiphyses have all been reported as sequelae of electrical injury [13].

Injury to the heart

The relationship of electrical current to ventricular fibrillation and cardiac asystole, their importance in determining outcome, and the principles of treatment of these conditions have been described earlier in this chapter.

Many patients who reach the hospital after an electrical accident have a wide variety of ECG abnormalities and arrhythmias [87]. The most frequent ECG change is a nonspecific change in the ST–T wave segment and the most frequent troublesome arrhythmias are among the atrial fibrillation-flutter group [10, 30, 42]. Arrhythmias are to be treated as any arrhythmia would be, regardless of cause. Following an electrical accident, cardiac activity should be monitored until 48 h after the ECG has reverted to normal. The overwhelming majority of patients have no permanent cardiac sequelae.

It is believed that electricity can cause a myocardial infarct. If this does occur, it probably does not result from the direct effect of the electrical current, but rather is a complication of hypoxia or poor myocardial perfusion following respiratory arrest, ventricular fibrillation, or cardiac asystole.

Injury to other viscera

Because of the large cross-sectional area of the torso compared with an extremity, as electrical current passes from the latter to the former the substantial decrease in current density virtually eliminates the possibility of generating enough heat to cause necrosis of viscera [75]. If necrosis of one of these organs does occur, the organ is contiguous with a deep contact wound. Bronchopleural [42], urinary bladder [20] and bowel fistulae [4, 84] have been reported.

Full-thickness injury of the abdominal parities must be approached aggressively to prevent evisceration. The necrotic tissue must be completely removed and the integrity of the abdominal cavity restored. A synthetic mesh, such as marlex, may be required.

Focal coagulation necrosis of the liver [67], pancreatitis [40, 67], necrosis of the gallbladder [86, 88], and gallstones [10] have been reported following electrical injury. While these changes do not result from heat, and are probably related to the passage of electrical current, the exact causal mechanism is not known.

Neurological injury

A striking feature of electrical injury is the pot pourri of neurological manifestations that may occur [83]. These may be temporary or permanent, immediate or delayed, effects of heat or of electrical current, affect the peripheral or central nervous systems, and involve the motor, sensory, or autonomic nervous system or any combination of these. Virtually any neurological sequelae can occur. Therefore, it is imperative that a careful neurological examination be accurately recorded as soon as practical after injury and that neurological follow-up be done conscientiously. In general, the neurological effects are maximal at the time of injury and recovery is complete. But recovery may arrest at any point and latent neurological effects, while rare, nevertheless do occur.

Central nervous system

In general, as the voltage increases so do the neurological sequelae. Nonetheless, cardiac and respiratory arrest and the direct effects of trauma, such as a fall, initiated by the electrical accident may cause CNS injury.

Among those exposed to high-voltage electricity, the incidence of unconsciousness is quite high [42, 83]. The duration of unconsciousness varies, but in most instances lasts for only several minutes, at times for several hours, and rarely for a day or more. The patient may then emerge through a period of manic hyperkinetic behavior and even have convulsions, then go on to complete and permanent neurological recovery [23]. Often the patient complains of a headache, which is usually transient, and amnesia for the accident, which may be permanent. Unconsciousness of delayed onset does occur and is probably caused by cerebral edema [83].

If the patient is not rendered unconscious he or she may experience a loud bang and temporary tinnitus, deafness, disorders of vision including hallucinatory flashes, aphasia, agonizing pain, paralysis, and apraxia [23, 33, 83]. In spite of frequent contact wounds of the head, even with necrosis of calvarium heat destruction of the brain is unusual, but it does occur [65] and may occasionally be the seat of an abscess.

While complete recovery is the rule, after restoration of consciousness a great variety of neurological manifestations may be encountered and recovery may be incomplete. The residua vary, may be patchy in their distribution, and may include deficits in the motor, sensory, or autonomic nervous systems and may affect any level [83].

Delay in onset of neurological sequelae, while unusual, is well documented [3, 33, 83]. In the author's personal series of 59 cases of high-voltage accidents there was not a single case. Caution about making the diagnosis of a latent neurological dysfunction must be expressed because a deficit may go undetected until ambulation is attempted [87].

A wide range of residual neurological manifestations has been described, including: generalized or focal spasticity, hemiplegia or hemiparesis, aphasia, striatal syndromes, brain stem syndromes, seizure disorders, cerebellar dysfunction, Parkinsonism, choreoathetosis, disorders of cranial nerve function, disorders of autonomic nervous system function, amnesia, vestibular disorders, psychoneuroses or psychoses, impotence, partial or complete transection of the spinal cord at any level, spinal atrophic palsies, hematomyelia, spastic paraplegia or quadriplegia, and amyotrophic lateral sclerosis–like syndromes [10, 23, 83].

The mechanisms by which these lesions occur are not precisely known, but probably do not involve the production of heat. Morphological changes in the brain and spinal cord do occur and while a variety of changes have been reported, focal petechial hemorrhages and other vascular and perivascular changes, thrombi, chromatolysis of neurons, and demyelination are the most common [23]. Also, the mechanism by which latent neurological manifestations are initiated is unknown.

Peripheral nerves

In most instances, destruction of peripheral nerves is by heat [91]. The ulnar and median nerves are the most frequently involved because of their proximity to wounds of electrical contact. Any peripheral nerve or plexus may be involved, however.

Ugland [92] studied the function of peripheral nerves traversed by electricity but not damaged by heat, and concluded that while there is loss of function it is transient, and complete recovery can be expected. Nonetheless, peripheral neuropathy progressing for several years after injury may occur [91]. The cause is thought to be perineural scarring or neural ischemia, or both. Sequential arteriograms showing progressive neural arterial lesions tend to substantiate this concept [74].

Eye

Although the injurious effect of electricity may occur in any portion of the eye [82], the classic and most frequent effect is the development of a cataract [32]. The earliest recorded cataract resulting from electricity was in 1722, and occurred in a patient exposed to lightning [63]. Cataracts resulting from man-made electricity have been reported since 1905 [29].

Alternating current, direct current, and lightning produce indistinguishable cataracts [39]. The exact cause of these cataracts is not known, but is probably related to a change in permeability of the capsule of the lens [63]. As a result of his experimental work, Long [63] reported that electricity had to pass through the eye, and the application of electricity that caused the typical cataract was not associated with any significant increase in intraocular temperature near the lens. Furthermore, cataracts produced by heat are morphologically different from those caused by electricity [63].

Cataracts have been reported with a variable incidence. DiVincenti, et al. [26] reported one case in a review of 65 patients, whereas Baxter [10] found 12 among 45 patients injured by over 5000 V.

The overwhelming majority of cataracts follow high-voltage alternating current accidents with a contact wound of the head, especially if it is close to the eye. But they have been reported after a 200-Volt shock [2] and with the current entering the body as far away from the eye as an extremity [39]. The changes in the lens usually occur earliest, and are more severe in the eye closer to the wound of the head. A cataract may occur unilaterally. Most cataracts are discovered after the patient complains of a decrease in vision. While some have been discovered within 1 month after injury, the peak incidence is at 2-6 months; but they have been found as late as 19 months after injury. Long [63], in examining several patients shortly after injury, found classic changes in the lens before visual acuity decreased. Although the cataract may be completely formed in several weeks, progression may occur as long as 3 years after the accident [63]. In rare instances the opacities of the lens disappear [63].

The morphological changes, generally worse when the voltage is greater, usually occur in the anterior capsule and subcapsular region and consist of multiple vacuoles of variable size and punctate, irregular linear or scale-like grayish opacities [63]. Posteriorly located opacities occur but the nucleus is usually clear.

Additional ocular manifestations of electrical injury include unilateral or bilateral optic neuritis with optic atrophy, central scotoma, ring scotoma, field constriction, color vision loss, visual disturbances without observable changes in the fundus, photophobia, blepharospasm, unilateral or bilateral complete blindness, nystagmus, decreased fusion as a result of injuries to optical parts of the CNS [63], night blindness [39], choroiditis, cyclitis, dislocation of the lens [2], thermal, ultraviolet and infrared damage from electrical arcs [63], and complete destruction of the eye from a contact injury.

In patients who are hospitalized because of an electrical injury, examination should include a slit-lamp examination by a competent opthalmologist as soon as the patient's condition permits, and certainly before discharge. Subsequently, this examination should be repeated if there is a complaint of decrease in visual acuity. Medicolegally, one should not exclude the possibility of occurrence of a cataract for 2 years, or the stability of the cataract until 3 years after the injury.

Permanent residual deficits of function

Among individuals who survive low-voltage accidents the incidence of residual permanent effects is low, and these effects are most often related to small residual scars. An exception to this is electrical injury of the mouth among children.

The situation is much different for individuals who have sustained high-voltage injury. The high incidence of residual deficits remains the most depressing facet of treatment of this group of patients. Virtually all patients injured by high voltage are young productive men. In the author's personal series of 56 patients injured by high-voltage electricity, one-half were left with one or more significant deficits. This is not a unique experience [10, 30, 42, 87]. These deficits include: one or more amputations of major extent (defined as an amputation beyond the long, ring, and/or little finger or any or all toes; about one-third of the patients are so afflicted); loss of a large amount of soft tissue, resulting in a significant deficit of function, e.g., removal of the volar compartment of a forearm; neurological deficits; cataracts; and loss of a vital organ, e.g., an eye.

Lightning injury

Considering the frequency of electrical storms, the incidence of injury and death from light-

ning [5] is quite low; 150–300 deaths in the United States each year.

Static electricity is produced in clouds by the collision of particles of ice carried upward and downward by drafts. This results in a large negative charge at the bottom of the cloud, which then discharges as a bolt of lightning to the positively charged earth. Estimates of the amperage generated range betwen 12 000 and 2 000 000.

When the victim is struck by lightning, a wound of entrance and exit may be produced and the violent contraction of skeletal muscles may cause the victim to be thrown several feet. The burns of the skin often have a spidery, aborescent pattern with redness and blistering, as though the skin were splashed with boiling water. There may be acute and residual neurological, vascular, and cardiac sequelae.

Hanson and McIlwraith [41] emphasize that apnea, absence of cardiac activity, and fixed and dilated pupils immediately after lightning injury should not be used as indicators of death, and these individuals should be appropriately resuscitated.

It is also well recognized that following lightning injury, limbs that are mottled, paralyzed, pulseless, and cold may later show signs of adequate perfusion after fluid resuscitation has re-established blood flow in the limb. Therefore, it should be emphasized that in this clinical setting, fasciotomy should be delayed.

Beyond these aspects of care, treatment consists of general supportive measures including fluid resuscitation, tetanus prophylaxis, antibiotics for the specific indication of infection, nutritional support, and topical antibacterial therapy. If there is muscle necrosis, it should probably be excised as soon as the patient's general condition permits.

References

1. Aaron H (ed) (1976) The choice of antimicrobial drugs. Med Lett Drugs Ther 18:9–16
2. Adams AL, Klein M (1945) Electrical cataract. Notes on a case and review of literature. Br J Ophthalmol 29:169–174
3. Alexander L (1938) Electrical injury to the central nervous system. Med Clin North Am 22 [Suppl 3]:663–688
4. Almgard LE, Libjedahl SO, Nylen B (1965) Electric burns of the abdomen. Acta Chir Scand 130:550–559
5. Apfelberg DB, Masters FW, Robinson DW (1974) Pathophysiology and treatment of lightning injuries. J Trauma 14:453–460

6. Artz CP (1967) Electrical injury simulates crush injury. Surg Gynecol Obstet 125:1316–1317
7. Artz CP (1979) Electrical injury. In: Artz CP, Moncrief JA, Pruitt BA Jr (eds) Burns: A team approach. Saunders, Philadelphia, pp 354–362
8. Atkin DH, Orkin (1973) Electrocution in the operating room. Anesthesiology 38:181–183
9. Battig CB (1968) Electrosurgical burn injury and their prevention. JAMA 204:1025–1209
10. Baxter CR (1970) Present concepts in the management of major electrical injury. Surg Clin North Am 50:1401–1418
11. Bernstein T (1975) Theories of the causes of death from electricity in the late nineteenth century. Med Instrum 9:267–273
12. Blondheim SH, Margoliash E, Shafrir E (1958) A simple test for myoglobinuria. JAMA 167:453–454
13. Brinn LB, Moseley JE (1966) Bone changes following electrical injury. Semin Roentgenol 97:682–686
14. Brown BH, Johnson SG, Betts RP, Henry L (1977) Burns threshold to radio frequency leakage currents from surgical diathermy equipment. Biomedical Engineering 1:277–281
15. Brown JB, Fryer MP (1957) Reconstruction of electrical injuries, including cranial losses with preliminary report of cathode ray burns. Ann Surg 146:342–356
16. Burke JF, Quinby WC Jr, Bondoc C, McLaughlin E, Trelstad RL (1977) Patterns of high tension electrical injury in children and adolescents and their management. Am J Surg 133:492–497
17. Burrows HJ (1936) Three cases of fractures resulting from electric shock. Br J Surg 24:159–165
18. Butler ED, Gant TD (1977) Electrical injuries, with special reference to the upper extremities. A review of 182 cases. Am J Surg 134:95–101
19. Caffee HH (1980) Scalp and skull reconstruction after electrical burn. J Trauma 20:87–89
20. Chari PS, Bapna BC, Balakrishnan C (1978) Electrical burn causing a urinary bladder fistula. Case report. Plast Reconstr Surg 61:446–448
21. Clayton JM, Hayes AC, Hammel J, Boyd WC, Hartford CE, Barnes RW (1977) Xenon-133 determination of muscle blood flow in electrical injury. J Trauma 17:293–298
22. Coleman TH (1969) Deaths from lightning. Penn Med 72/3:56–58
23. Critchley M (1934) Neurological effects of lightning and of electricity Lancet I:68–72
24. Dale RH (1954) Electrical accidents: A discussion with illustrated cases. Br J Plast Surg 7:44–66
25. Dalziel CF (1954) The threshold of perception currents. Transactions of the American Institute of Electrical Engineering 73:625–630
26. Dalziel CF, Lee WR (1968) Re-evaluation of lethal electric currents. IEEE Transactions on Industry and its General Applications 4:467–476
27. Dalziel CF, Ogden E, Abbot CE (1943) Effect of frequency of let-go currents. Transactions of the American Institute of Electrical Engineering 62:745–750
28. Davies MR (1959) Burns caused by electricity: A review of seventy cases. Br J Plast Surg 11:288–300
29. Desbrieres, Bargy M (1905) Un cas de cataracte due à une discharge electrique industrielle. Ann Ocul 133:118
30. DiVincenti FC, Moncrief JA, Pruitt BA Jr (1969) Electrical injuries; A review of 65 cases. J Trauma 9:497–507
31. Dosseter JB, Drummond JA, Allen AC, Celis TT, Baxter HA (1967) Prolonged oliguric renal failure after electric burns. Plast Reconstr Surg 40:67–71
32. Duke-Elder S (1954) Textbook of ophthalmology. Mosby, St Louis, p 6423

33. Farrell DF, Starr A (1968) Delayed neurological sequelae of electrical injuries. Neurology 18:601–606
34. Fleury AF (1959) Electric burns of the lips: A modified plan of treatment. Am Surg 25:328–331
35. Gardner WG (1948) Electrical burn of the brain. J Neurosurg 5:90–94
36. Gatewood JW, McCarthy NH (1957) The treatment of electrical burns of the skull. Am J Surg 93:525–532
37. Geddes LA, Baker LE (1968) Principles of applied biomedical instrumentation. John Wiley & Sons, New York
38. Geddes LA, Baker LE (1971) Response to passage of electric current through the body. Med Instrum 5:13–18
39. Geeraets WJ, Nooney TW Jr (1973) Retinal injury due to electric current. A clinical study. Ann Ophthalmol 5:265–268
40. Glazer AM (1945) Pancreatic necrosis in electric shock. Arch Pathol Lab Med 39:9–10
41. Hanson GC, McIlwraith GR (1973) Lightning injury: Two case histories and a review of management. Br Med J iv:271–274
42. Hartford CE, Ziffren SE (1971) Electrical injury. J Trauma 11:331–336
43. Hemingway A, Stenstrom WK (1932) Physical characteristics of high frequency current. JAMA 98:1446–1455
44. Hunt JL, McManus WF, Haney WP, Pruitt BA Jr (1974) Vascular lesions in acute electrical injuries. J Trauma 14:461–473
45. Hunt JL, Mason AD, Masterson TS, Pruitt BA Jr (1976) The pathophysiology of acute electric injuries. J Trauma 16:335–340
46. Hunt J, Lewis S, Parkey R, Baxter C (1979) The use of technetium-99m stannous pyrophosphate scintigraphy to identify muscle damage in acute electric burns. J Trauma 19:409–413
47. Hunt JL, Sato RM, Baxter CR (1980) Acute electric burns: Current diagnostic and therapeutic approaches to management. Arch Surg 115:434–438
48. Hyslop VB (1957) Treatment of electric burns of the lip. Plast Reconstr Surg 20:315–317
49. Hyslop VB, Miller EW (1955) The treatment of electric burns. J Int Coll Surg 23:481–486
50. Jackson FE, Martin R, Davis R (1965) Delayed quadriplegia following electrical burn. Milit Med 130:601–605
51. Jex-Blake AJ (1913) The Goulstonian lectures on death by electric currents and lightning. Br Med J i:425–430; 492–498; 548–552; 601–603
52. Kazanjian VH, Roopenian A (1954) The treatment of lip deformities resulting from electric burns. Am J Surg 88:884–890
53. Keesey JC, Letcher FS (1970) Human thresholds of electric shock at power transmission frequences. Arch Environ Health 21:547–552
54. Kouwenhoven WB (1949) Effects of electricity on the human body. Electrical Engineering 68:199–203
55. Kouwenhoven WB (1964) The effects of electricity on the human body. Bull Johns Hopkins Hosp 115:425–446
56. Kouwenhoven WB, Hooker DR, Langworthy OR (1932) The current flowing through the heart under conditions of electric shock. Am J Physiol 100:344–350
57. Kragh LV, Erich JB (1961) Treatment of severe electric injuries. Am J Surg 101:419–427
58. Larson TH (1977) Splinting oral electrical burns in children: Report of two cases. J Dent Child 44:382–384
59. Lee WR (1961) A clinical study of electrical accidents. Br J Ind Med 18:260–269
60. Lewis D (1918) Electric burns causing necrosis of skull. Ann Surg 67:149–151
61. Lewis GK (1950) Burns from electricity. Ann Surg 131:80–91

62. Lewis GK (1958) Electrical burns of the upper extremities. J Bone Joint Surg [Am] 40:27–40
63. Long JC (1963) A clinical and experimental study of electric cataract. Am J Ophthalmol 56:108–133
64. McLaughlin CW Jr, Coe JD (1954) Management of electric burns. Arch Surg 68:531–537
65. Mills W Jr, Switzer WE, Moncrief JA (1966) Electrical injuries. JAMA 195:852–854
66. Moncrief JA, Lindberg RB, Switzer WE, Pruitt BA Jr (1966) The use of a topical sulfonamide in the control of burn wound sepsis. J Trauma 6:407–419
67. Newsome TW, Curreri PW, Eurenius K (1972) Visceral injuries, an unusual complication of an electrical burn. Arch Surg 105:494–497
68. Nunn L (1957) Severe electrical burns. Northwest Med 56:691–694
69. Ortiz-Monasterio F, Factor R (1980) Early definitive treatment of electric burns of the mouth. Plast Reconstr Surg 65:169–176
70. Peterson RA (1966) Electrical burns of the hand: Treatment by early excision. J Bone Joint Surg [Am] 48:407–424
71. Pitts W, Pickrell K, Messengill R (1969) Electrical burns of lips and mouth in infants and children. Plast Reconstr Surg 44:471–479
72. Platts MM, Rozner L (1966) Survival after high tension electrical burns complicated by acute tubular necrosis. Br Med J i:781–782
73. Poate WJ, Macafee AL (1962) Gas Gangrene following electrical burns: A report of two cases. Br J Plast Surg 15:17–19
74. Poten B, Erickson U, Johansson S, et al (1970) New Observations on tissue changes along the pathway of current in an electrical injury. Scand J Plast Reconstr Surg 4:75–82
75. Pruitt BA Jr (1979) The burn patient: I. Initial care. Curr Probl Surg 16:1–55
76. Quinby WC, Burke JF, Trelstod RL, Caulfield J (1978) The use of microscopy as a guide to primary excision of high-tension electrical burns. J Trauma 18:423–431
77. Pearl FL (1933) Electric shock: Presentation of case and review of literature. Arch Surg 27:227–249
78. Rouse RG, Dimick AR (1978) The treatment of electrical injury compared to burn injury: A review of pathophysiology and comparison of patient management protocols. J Trauma 18:43–47
79. Prevost JL, Battelli F (1899) Death by electric currents (alternating current). C R Acad Sci [D] (Paris) 128:668–670
80. Ryan JE (1979) Prosthetic treatment for electrical burns to the oral cavity. J Prosthet Dent 42:434–436
81. Sances A Jr, Larson SJ, Myklebust J, Cusick JF (1979) Electrical injuries. Surg Gynecol Obstet 149:97–108
82. Sautter AC (1911) Electric injuries of the eye. Ophthalmol Rec 20:238
83. Silversides J (1964) The neurological sequelae of electrical injury. J Can Med Assoc 91:195–204
84. Shinha JK, Roy SK (1976) Perforation of the caecum caused by electric burn. Br J Plast Surg 29:179–181
85. Skoog T (1970) Electrical injuries. J Trauma 10:816–830
86. Smith J, Rank BK (1946) Case of severe electric burns with unusual sequence of complications. Br J Surg 33:365–368
87. Solem L, Fischer RP, Strate RG (1977) The natural history of electrical injury. J Trauma 17:487–492
88. Taylor PH, Pugsley LO, Vogel EH (1962) The intriguing electrical burn. J Trauma 2:309–326
89. Thompson HG, Jukes AW, Farmer AW (1965) Electric burns to the mouth in children. Plast Reconstr Surg 35:466–477
90. Tomlin PJ, Newell JA (1975) Unusual diathermy hazard. (Letter) Br Med J i:681
91. Ugland OM (1966) Electric injuries to peripheral nerves in animals: A preliminary report. Acta Chir Scand 131:432–437
92. Ugland OM (1967) Electrical burns: A clinical and experimental study with special reference to peripheral nerve injury. Scand J Plast Reconstr Surg [Suppl] 2:1–74
93. Watson AB, Wright JS, Loughman J (1973) Electrical thresholds for ventricular fibrillation in man. Med J Aust 1:1179–1182
94. Weeks AW, Alexander L (1939) The distribution of electrical current in the animal body: An experimental investigation of 60-cycle alternating current. J Indust Hyg 21:517–525
95. Wells DB (1929) The treatment of electric burns by immediate resection and skin graft. Ann Surg 90:1069–1078
96. Whitesides TE Jr, Haney TC, Harada H, Holmes HE, Morimoto K (1975) A simple method for tissue pressure determination. Arch Surg 110:1311–1313
97. Worthen EF (1971) Regeneration of the skull following a deep electrical burn. Plast Reconstr Surg 48:1–4

Chapter 40

Drowning and Near-Drowning

Barbara B. Tabeling and Jerome H. Modell

Worldwide, 140 000 [30] persons drown each year. Since victims of near-drowning are not reported routinely, their numbers are unknown; but it is estimated there are approximately eight near-drowned victims for each fatality [56].

Nearly half of those who drown are less than 20 years of age [34], the highest incidence being in the second decade of life [49]. In most studies, over 75% of the victims are male, [28, 43, 46] and 35% are accomplished swimmers [34].

Since most persons who drown or nearly drown are young, healthy individuals who have the capacity for a long and productive life, it is imperative that effective therapy begins promptly after the accident.

Definitions

Webster's dictionary defines the word 'drown' as 'to suffocate by submersion, especially in water' [61]. Not all persons who drown aspirate water. Approximately 10% die from asphyxia secondary to laryngospasm or breath-holding [9]. For those who do aspirate, the type and the quantity of fluid will vary and will influence the character of the lesion. Fresh water, seawater, or brackish water may all have a variety of contaminants that can play a role in the course of the disease.

'Near-drowned' is a term applied to those who survive submersion, at least temporarily [34]. 'Near-drowned without aspiration' describes patients who experience asphyxia secondary to breath-holding or to laryngospasm without aspiration of fluid. In one study, approximately 12% of the patients fell into this category [43]. 'Near-drowned with aspiration' describes those persons who survive, at least temporarily, after aspirating some of the fluid in which they were submerged.

'Delayed death subsequent to near-drowning' describes patients who survive the initial resuscitation but die later during therapy. These patients usually succumb to unrecognized pulmonary insufficiency, to secondary bacterial infection of the lung, or to CNS damage from hypoxia or from increased intracranial pressure (ICP).

Of recent concern has been the effect of water temperature on survival [5, 6, 16]. Several reports of complete recovery after prolonged submersion in very cold water emphasize the necessity of initiating resuscitation after such an incident and of continuing resuscitation until there is in-hospital documentation that the victim is not salvageable. The longest reported submersion with successful recovery was 40 min in icy water [58]. A 'diving reflex' is thought to occur when the face is submerged in cold water (less than 20°C) [22, 26]. This neurogenic reflex produces bradycardia and vasoconstriction which effectively shunt blood to the heart and brain, thus prolonging the duration of submersion possible without irreversible damage to the CNS. In addition, hypothermia may occur, which would reduce O_2 consumption and would protect against hypoxic injury to the brain.

Many experiments have been performed to delineate the pathophysiology of drowning and near-drowning. These studies have provided many guidelines for therapy. It must be remembered, though, that each case is different and therapy ultimately must be individualized.

Physiologic changes

Respiration and acid-base

The most consistent injury in the near-drowned victim is pulmonary insufficiency and related blood gas and acid–base changes. In 1931, Cot demonstrated that 10% of drowned victims died without evidence of fluid aspiration [9]. More recently, Modell et al. reported that 12% of near-drowned victims they treated did not aspirate [43]. Experimental work with dogs to simulate the effects of laryngospasm without aspiration, i.e., tracheal obstruction, has demonstrated the pHa decreased by approximately 0.05 u/min and $PaCO_2$ increased approximately 6 mmHg (0.8 kPa)/min; however, PaO_2 fell rapidly from an average control value of 92 mmHg (12.3 kPa) before tracheal obstruction to 40 mmHg (5.3 kPa) after 1 min of obstruction, to 10 mmHg (1.3 kPa) after 3 min, and to 4 mmHg (0.5 kPa) after 5 min. After 5 min of tracheal obstruction, 80% of these animals were successfully resuscitated by a brief period of intermittent positive pressure ventilation (IPPV) [41].

Persons who hyperventilate before swimming to increase their time under water enter the water hypocarbic. Since hypoxia is a minor respiratory stimulant in healthy individuals, they can consciously override this impulse to breathe. As the degree of hypoxia progresses, they lose consciousness before the CO_2 threshold for breathing has been reached. Then, respiration and aspiration occur.

If adequate ventilation and circulation are reestablished before cerebral damage occurs, near-drowned victims who do not aspirate may require no further therapy. This is in marked contrast to the patient who aspirates significant quantities of water and in whom profound, persistent hypoxemia requires aggressive and prolonged therapy. Hypercarbia and a combined respiratory and metabolic acidosis frequently accompany the hypoxemia [37]. Reestablishment of spontaneous ventilation or institution of mechanical ventilation (MV) rapidly reverses the respiratory component of the acidosis, but metabolic acidosis may persist secondary to hypoxemia, cardiovascular depression or both. The metabolic acidosis frequently requires sodium bicarbonate (IV) for correction.

The severity of acidemia and hypoxemia found on initial analysis of arterial blood does not reliably predict the patient's ultimate outcome, as patients treated with severe hypoxemia and acidosis have lived and patients with near-normal pHa and PaO_2 when admitted to the hospital have died [14, 28, 43, 46].

The mechanism of hypoxemia after aspiration of fresh water is different from that after aspiration of seawater. After freshwater aspiration, the fluid is absorbed rapidly into the circulation and transient hypervolemia occurs [36]. However, the surface tension properties of pulmonary surfactant extracted from the lungs are altered such that the minimal surface tension reached at maximal compression of the surfactant film is higher than normal [20]. This results in unstable alveoli producing areas of low but finite ventilation-to-perfusion ratios as well as areas of atelectasis [40]. After seawater aspiration, the primary pathology is fluid-filled but perfused alveoli producing a large intrapulmonary shunt [38, 40]. Since seawater is hypertonic, fluid is drawn into the alveoli from the vascular space. When dogs aspirate 22 ml seawater/kg body wt, an average of 33 ml/kg can be drained from their lungs by gravity after 5 min, whereas virtually none can be recovered after aspiration of an equal quantity of fresh water [42]. After seawater aspiration, a reduction in the amount of surfactant has been demonstrated, although what remains has normal compression characteristics [20]. Both types of aspirate reduce pulmonary compliance [25] and cause pulmonary edema.

At autopsy, the lungs of rats which aspirated small quantities of fresh water showed no changes on light microscopy. When similar volumes of seawater were aspirated, lung weight increased and intra-alveolar hemorrhages occurred [24]. When large quantities of fresh water were aspirated, electron microscopy revealed widening of the alveolar septa, collapse of the capillaries, decrease in the number of red blood cells, enlargement of the endothelial and septal cell nuclei, swelling of the mitochondria, and obliteration of the cell outlines. With similar volumes of aspirated seawater, these changes were less pronounced, and the septal and endothelial nuclei were small and dark. In addition, structural integrity was preserved [51]. Thus, the variable pathological response of humans after drowning may relate to the volume and the toxicity of the fluid aspirated. Frequently, hyperexpansion of the lungs, with areas resembling acute emphysema, is seen in both humans and animals soon after drowning [18, 31]. This is thought to represent rupture of alveoli secondary to a wide fluctuation in airway pressure generated by violent ventilatory efforts against a closed glottis or obstruction from a column of water during submersion.

At autopsy, the lungs of patients who die after surviving for 12–72 h frequently show evidence of bronchopneumonia, multiple abscesses, mechanical injury, and deposition of hyaline material in the alveoli [18]. Fuller reported that 70% of drowned humans show evidence of having aspirated particulate matter such as vomitus, mud, sand, and algae [17, 18]. Butt et al. could not demonstrate any consistent permanent abnormality in the results of pulmonary function tests or in the arterial oxygenation of patients recovered from near-drowning [3].

Studies of dogs that aspirated 22 ml seawater or fresh water/kg body wt have demonstrated the efficacy of positive end-expiratory pressure (PEEP) to reduce intrapulmonary shunt and to improve arterial oxygenation. After seawater aspiration, intrapulmonary shunt and PaO_2 consistently improved with either spontaneous ventilation with continuous positive airway pressure (CPAP) or MV with PEEP [42]. After freshwater aspiration, the response of some dogs to spontaneous ventilation with CPAP was a marked reduction in intrapulmonary shunt and an improvement in arterial oxygenation, while other animals improved little unless they were also mechanically ventilated [2]. This may have been due to the surfactant changes that occur after freshwater aspiration, resulting in the need for MV to inflate collapsed alveoli before PEEP or CPAP could maintain alveolar inflation in some animals. Since pulmonary surfactant has normal compression characteristics after seawater aspiration, spontaneous ventilation with PEEP or CPAP could be expected to maintain alveolar inflation and to restore more normal ventilation-to-perfusion ratios without the addition of MV. Observations during the treatment of humans who have aspirated fresh water or seawater are consistent with these animal studies [42, 43].

Cardiac output, measured after dogs aspirated fresh water, decreased significantly when ventilation was controlled mechanically, and decreased further when 15 cmH_2O PEEP was applied. Animals that breathed spontaneously did not have a significant reduction in cardiac output until 15 cmH_2O CPAP was applied, and the decrease was not as severe as when controlled MV (CMV) and PEEP were applied [2]. Recent studies of near-drowned dogs treated with CMV and PEEP in our laboratory have shown that, when cardiac output is supported by supplemental fluid administration, intrapulmonary shunt remains low while cardiac output increases and, thus, O_2 delivery is improved.

Cardiovascular system

Studies of dogs totally submerged in fresh water suggest that death should occur secondary to ventricular fibrillation [59, 60]. However, this is rarely reported in humans [43], probably because humans rarely aspirate enough water to cause the degree of hyponatremia thought necessary to produce ventricular fibrillation.

The cardiovascular changes that occur subsequent to near-drowning in either seawater or fresh water primarily result from arterial hypoxemia and acidosis. While variations in electrolytes or blood volume could contribute, less than 15% of drowning victims aspirate enough water to cause significant changes in these parameters [35].

Bradycardia, frequently seen both in near-drowned humans and in experimental animals [36, 38] may occur secondary to a reflex, such as the diving reflex [22], or may occur on the basis of hypoxemia. Often, intense vasoconstriction is also present, due to hypoxemia, catecholamine release, hypothermia, the diving reflex, or a combination of these factors. Because of this, it may be difficult to determine at the scene of the accident whether spontaneous cardiac activity is present or whether asystole has occurred.

In dogs, cardiac output falls immediately after freshwater aspiration in association with bradycardia, hypotension, and increased systemic vascular resistance [2]. In survivors, these parameters return toward normal over the ensuing 30 min. Cardiac output may then fall in response to MV, PEEP, or CPAP during the course of therapy [2]. This is probably on the basis of an absolute or a relative reduction in the effective circulating blood volume due to redistribution of fluids and losses of fluid secondary to pulmonary edema. In such cases, cardiac output can be restored to normal by increasing the intravascular volume with supplemental fluids.

A number of ECG changes can occur secondary to drowning and near-drowning; these include bradycardia, tachycardia, loss of P waves, ST elevation, changes in T wave amplitude, increased PR interval, AV dissociation, widening of the QRS complex, premature ventricular contractions, ventricular tachycardia, ventricular fibrillation, and asystole [36–38, 59]. Correction of hypoxemia, acidosis, hypothermia, and hypovolemia should result in return of the ECG toward normal.

Arterial blood pressure has been reported as normal, increased, or decreased after near-drowning [37, 38, 52, 59] and may vary with the time elapsed since the episode. Central venous pressure (CVP) rises briefly after aspiration of small amounts of fresh water or seawater, then rapidly returns to normal [36, 38]. After aspiration of larger volumes of fresh water, an elevated CVP may persist, but it ultimately will return to normal or will even fall below normal [37]. After large amounts of seawater are aspirated, CVP increases transiently and then rapidly decreases secondary to decreased circulating blood volume [37, 38]. After freshwater aspiration, pulmonary artery pressure and pulmonary artery occlusion pressure are elevated transiently. Systemic vascular resistance and pulmonary vascular resistance both increase after freshwater aspiration and remain elevated after other parameters have returned to normal [2]. Repletion of circulating blood volume by fluid administration returns resistances to normal (personal observation).

Electrolytes and blood volume

Early studies of animals drowned by total immersion suggested that significant electrolyte and blood volume changes occurred. Swann et al. found that, when dogs drowned in fresh water, there was a marked increase in blood volume in association with a severe reduction in the concentration of serum sodium and chloride. After seawater drowning, dogs showed a reduction in blood volume associated with an elevation in serum sodium and chloride concentrations [59, 60]. It was recommended that these findings be applied to the management of near-drowned patients, although marked changes in electrolyte concentrations generally were not seen clinically [17, 33]. Subsequently, it was found at autopsy that serum electrolyte concentrations were either normal or only mildly deranged in 85% of drowned humans which suggests that they had aspirated 22 ml water or less per kilogram of body weight [35].

Studies with this quantity of fluid aspirated by dogs revealed that, after freshwater aspiration, serum electrolyte concentrations reflected the volume of fluid aspirated at three minutes, but that these values returned to normal within 10–60 min of aspiration without therapy. Furthermore, ventricular fibrillation occurred commonly after the aspiration of 44 ml or more of fresh water/kg, but did not occur after the aspiration of 22 ml/kg or less. Serum potassium concentration increased in animals aspirating 22 ml fresh water/kg or more, but usually returned to normal within 10 min. Blood volume increased in proportion to the amount of water aspirated, with maximal changes occurring 3 min after aspiration [36].

After seawater aspiration, serum sodium and chloride concentrations in dogs were maximally elevated after 3 min. While these values returned toward normal during the ensuing hour, they were still mildly elevated after that. Blood volume decreased within 5 min of aspiration [38]. Since these studies, further reports on large numbers of near-drowned victims have confirmed the paucity of severe abnormalities in serum electrolytes at the time of admission to the hospital [14, 36, 38].

Hematology

Hemoglobin and hematocrit concentrations usually are normal after humans near-drown [14, 39, 43]. Similar findings have been demonstrated in dogs after aspiration of either fresh water or seawater except when very large volumes are aspirated [36–38]. Gross hemolysis is evident after animals aspirate large quantities of freshwater, but not seawater [37]. Humans who near-drown in fresh water usually have plasma hemoglobin levels that are normal or slightly elevated. Levels as high as 500 mg/100 ml have been reported, but these patients did not suffer renal damage secondary to elevated plasma hemoglobin [17, 39].

There are few large series in man or animals regarding white blood cell count after near-drowning. Available case reports [17, 19, 21, 32, 52] indicate that the white blood cell count is frequently elevated. In one reported case, neutrophil function studies were found to be normal [19]. Similarly, there are few reports of platelet counts or of clotting function after near-drowning. A single case of disseminated intravascular coagulation in a patient who had profound hypoxemia, acidosis and hemolysis resulting from near-drowning has been reported [10]. While masses of agglutinated platelets have been found at autopsy in larger blood vessels, particularly in the lung [18], definitive studies are necessary before conclusions can be drawn.

Renal function

Significant renal dysfunction secondary to near-drowning is seldom reported [23, 29]. In the largest series in which some type of renal abnormality was noted, Fuller found that 12 of 50 near-drowned humans had transient albuminuria, cylinduria or both, thought to be secondary to renal hypoxia. One patient also had an elevated blood urea nitrogen which returned to normal in a few days. At autopsy, another victim was found to have acute tubular necrosis, but this was believed to be secondary to prolonged hypotension rather than to hemolysis [18]. Fuller also reported two cases with hemoglobinemia and hemoglobinuria, one after seawater and the other after freshwater near-drowning. Neither was associated with renal dysfunction [18]. Modell et al. reported a patient with a hemoglobinemia of 500 mg/100 ml without evidence of renal dysfunction [39]. Several cases of hemoglobinuria without renal damage also have been reported [27, 45, 50]. Significant renal dysfunction seems unlikely if oxygenation, acid–base balance, and intravascular volume are maintained.

Central nervous system

Since the advent of sophisticated pulmonary and cardiovascular monitoring and therapy, survival after the pulmonary injury of near-drowning has improved [8, 17, 43, 44]. Recent attention has focused on the significant morbidity and mortality associated with the CNS damage resulting from near-drowning. Peterson gave a very pessimistic outlook, as 21% of the children he reported suffered brain damage [48]. All evidence suggests that the etiology of such brain damage is either cerebral hypoxia or increased ICP secondary to anoxic injury and cerebral edema [17, 18, 30].

A number of studies have attempted to correlate death or serious neurological sequelae with information that can be obtained in the emergency department, including initial arterial pH, initial arterial O_2 tension, initial temperature recorded, initial EEG, initial electrolyte concentrations, age, duration of submersion, history of the promptness and duration of resuscitative measures, level of consciousness on admission, and need for MV [8, 14, 28, 43, 44, 46, 48]. Many of these factors correlate poorly with ultimate outcome. Low arterial pH and documentation of CPR in the emergency department seemed to correlate with outcome, but neither was absolute [28, 44]. When one large series was divided into adults and children [44] it appeared that age may be a significant factor in patients who survived with brain damage. This may be because the heart of a child is more amenable to resuscitation than an adult's after prolonged hypoxia, whereas the brain is not.

Recently, two authors each reported a large retrospective series of patients in such a manner as to compare the two more adequately [8, 44]. In these studies, level of consciousness on admission to the emergency department was correlated with outcome. Of 121 patients reported by Modell et al. [44], all the 61 who were alert when admitted recovered with no neurological sequelae, even though many had suffered respiratory and cardiac arrest. Patients with blunted consciousness (described as lethargic, semicomatose, combative, or confused) either survived with no sequelae (90%) or died secondary to pulmonary insufficiency (10%). Of the 29 patients who were comatose when admitted, 55% recovered with no neurological dysfunction, 10% had brain damage, and 34% died. Overall, 87% survived with apparently normal brain function, 2% survived with brain damage, and 11% died. When children were analyzed separately, those who were awake when admitted survived with normal function. When the level of consciousness was blunted, one patient died but all others survived to function normally. Of the comatose children, 44% survived with normal function, 17% survived with brain damage, and 39% died. In this study, no specific protocol for brain resuscitation was carried out, although many of the comatose patients were hyperventilated and received steroids as treatment for brain edema.

Conn's study of 96 children produced similar results [8]. Fifty-three percent were awake and 6% had blunted levels of consciousness on admission; all survived with normal brain function. Thirty-nine patients (41%) were comatose; and of these, 17 survived with normal function, 9 survived with brain damage, and 13 died. Overall, 77% of the 96 patients survived with normal function, 9% survived with brain damage, and 13.5% died.

Conn further designated the comatose patients as decorticate, decerebrate, or flaccid. Sixty-six percent of decorticate and 56% of decerebrate patients survived with normal function, whereas only 14% of the flaccid patients survived normally. Eighteen of Conn's comatose patients received aggressive brain resuscitation consisting in hyperventilation, dehydration, active cooling, muscle paralysis, steroid and barbiturate therapy, and ICP monitoring [7, 8]; whereas six additional patients received some, but not all, of these measures. Ten of the 18 patients treated with all the measures, who were decorticate or decerebrate on admission, survived with normal function, and one survived with brain damage. Of the seven flaccid patients treated with the complete regimen, one survived with normal function and six died. Five of the patients treated with some, but not all, of the measures were decorticate or decerebrate on admission. Three survived normally, one died and one was brain damaged. The one flaccid patient so treated lived but was brain-damaged. While this study suggests that aggressive brain resuscitation may enhance normal survival, in a joint editorial Conn and Modell recommend a large prospective study to confirm this [5a].

Pearn [47] reported that 70 of 75 patients who were apneic or unconscious when retrieved from the water survived with normal brain function; the remaining five died in spite of intensive therapy. At this time, these reports should be taken optimistically and a guess as to ultimate outcome should not be a factor in determining whether to initiate or to discontinue resuscitation. In fact, as the basic cardiopulmonary resuscitation technique becomes more widespread among the lay public and emergency transport systems become more sophisticated, there may be a further reduction in the number of near-drowned persons who die or who have serious cerebral damage.

Treatment

At the scene of the accident

Since all evidence points to hypoxia as the major cause of morbidity and mortality from near-drowning and drowning, first aid for the victim should be aimed at restoring adequate O_2 delivery as rapidly as possible after the accident. The victim must be removed from the water quickly; if this is not feasible, ventilation of apneic victims should begin in the water if possible. Some apneic patients may still have an effective cardiac output, and early ventilation will help restore myocardial and cerebral oxygenation. In the absence of sophisticated equipment, mouth-to-mouth and mouth-to-nose ventilation are the most effective modes of emergency ventilation available [55].

Time should not be wasted in attempting to drain water from the lungs [53]. Studies have demonstrated that, after 3 min, no water can be drained from the lungs of animals that aspirated fresh water [40]; similar results are reported in humans [53]. While fluid can be drained from the lungs of animals when they have aspirated large volumes of seawater [42], observations in humans suggest that few aspirate such volumes [35]. Besides delaying cardiopulmonary resuscitation, attempting to drain the lungs or the stomach may result in regurgitation and aspiration of stomach contents.

Once effective ventilation has begun, the patient must be evaluated for evidence of spontaneous cardiac activity. While some cardiac output may be present without a palpable pulse, if a pulse is not palpable the rescuer must assume that the heart has stopped. Closed-chest massage must begin at once. The rescuer must continue basic cardiopulmonary resuscitation until spontaneous ventilation and circulation are restored or until he can be relieved or is no longer able to continue [1].

If a patient near-drowns without aspiration, the prognosis with treatment is excellent. These patients usually respond promptly to cardiopulmonary resuscitation and may not require further therapy. If cerebral hypoxia is prolonged, however, an altered sensorium may be present. If aspiration has occurred, the pulmonary insult may be quite severe. Hypoxemia may be profound even after restoration of spontaneous breathing and circulation [39, 43]. The patient's appearance can be misleading and may not accurately indicate the degree of hypoxemia. Since there is no certain way of determining at the scene of the accident whether aspiration has occurred or hypoxemia is present, all victims should be taken to a hospital for further evaluation.

Since hypoxemia and acidosis cause the most significant pathology after near-drowning, maneuvers to correct these abnormalities must be prompt. Supplemental O_2, in the highest concentration possible, should be given when first available, whether at the scene, in transit to the emergency department, or in the hospital itself. If the patient is awake and breathing spontaneously, O_2 may be given by face mask. For patients who remain apneic or asystolic, MV with a high concentration of O_2 should replace mouth-to-mouth breathing. These patients, as well as those who are breathing spontaneously but are unconscious, are at risk of aspirating gastric contents and, thus, their airways require special attention. If a patent airway is not maintained, artificial ventilation may overdistend the stomach, which frequently is already distended by water swallowed during the accident [18, 31]. This may lead to pulmonary aspiration of gastric fluid or restriction of ventilation.

Endotracheal intubation is required for arrested and comatose patients for airway protection and for MV. As advanced cardiac life-support training becomes more common among emergency medical technicians, this intervention may be performed at the scene of the accident or during emergency transport. If endotracheal intubation is not feasible, an esophageal obturator airway may be used.

Similarly, other advanced resuscitative maneuvers should be performed as soon as facilities and trained personnel are available. These include the placement of a large-bore IV catheter for fluid and drug therapy and the application of an ECG to determine whether treatment is needed for arrhythmia. If the rescue vehicle has trained personnel and if consultation by radio with a physician is possible, drug therapy (e.g., sodium bicarbonate) may be advised.

While it has been demonstrated that PEEP improves ventilation-to-perfusion ratios and decreases intrapulmonary shunting in both experimental animals and near-drowned humans [2, 42, 43, 54], this therapeutic modality is usually not available outside the hospital.

At the hospital

Supplemental O_2 should be continued until measurement of oxygen tension in arterial blood demonstrates that O_2 is no longer needed. In addition, arterial blood should be analyzed for CO_2 tension and pH. Since the results of these tests will guide further therapy, they should take priority over other laboratory tests. The level of consciousness should be ascertained and, if necessary, the airway should be protected. If other measures, such as placement of an IV catheter, have not already been performed, they should now be implemented.

Intrapulmonary shunting after near-drowning is quite variable, but can exceed 70% of the cardiac output of both man and experimental animals [2]. Use of PEEP and CPAP can reduce intrapulmonary shunting under such conditions [2, 42, 54]. The amount of PEEP or CPAP necessary to provide the least intrapul-

monary shunt and the optimal O_2 tension and cardiovascular function must be individualized for each patient. The optimal level is that which produces the lowest intrapulmonary shunt without adversely affecting cardiac output [12, 13]. If needed to improve arterial oxygenation and shunting in a patient who is alert and not hypercarbic, up to 12 mmHg (1.6 kPa) CPAP can be delivered through a tight-fitting face mask. For the patient who is comatose, who is not capable of maintaining normocarbia, or who requires higher levels of CPAP, an endotracheal tube should be used. Mechanical ventilation can then be added as needed. Intermittent mandatory ventilation (IMV) can be adjusted to maintain minute ventilation while allowing the patient to continue breathing spontaneously. If necessary, CMV can be instituted.

After dogs aspirate fresh water, MV and PEEP have been demonstrated to lower intrapulmonary shunt more consistently than spontaneous ventilation with CPAP [2]. Although it has not been proved in a controlled situation, adding a few breaths per minute to a given level of CPAP may improve ventilation-to-perfusion ratios. Thus, if the desired effect is not achieved with spontaneous breathing and CPAP, adding mechanical breaths may be advantageous.

There often is concern that increasing PEEP may cause a significant reduction in cardiac output, especially if MV is combined with PEEP. However, this reduction usually is due to hypovolemia. If intravascular volume is adequately maintained, cardiac output can be maintained. In fact, as PEEP increases and oxygenation improves, cardiac output may actually increase [12].

Pulmonary edema frequently occurs with both freshwater and seawater aspiration, and is best treated by titrating CPAP or PEEP to the optimal level. Once achieved, this level should not be lowered rapidly or terminated abruptly, since pulmonary edema can recur within seconds. Suctioning of the pulmonary edema fluid is inappropriate and dangerous to the patient, because recurrent pulmonary edema, hypoxemia, and atelectasis will result. When the patient is being treated with high levels of PEEP or CPAP, suctioning should only be performed when necessary to remove mucus plugs.

Bronchospasm may occur after near drowning. When mild, this may be treated with an aerosol of a bronchodilating agent. More severe cases may require an IV infusion of aminophylline.

Initially, correction of metabolic acidosis with

sodium bicarbonate may be necessary, as approximately 70% of patients have a significant metabolic acidosis on admission [43]. As oxygenation improves and cardiovascular stability is achieved, it is usually unnecessary to continue administration of bicarbonate.

Some patients may incur other trauma besides near-drowning. This is particularly true after a diving accident, since a cervical spine fracture with quadriplegia may result. When the history of the accident is unknown, special attention must be given to the possibility of other life-threatening injuries. Appropriate physical examination, roentgenograms, and laboratory tests are indicated.

Once the patient is stabilized, complete blood cell count, serum electrolyte concentrations, and urinalysis are essential laboratory tests. While these tests are usually normal, they may reveal other pathology and will help to determine appropriate intravenous fluid therapy. A complete ECG should be obtained. While it should never be relied upon solely for evaluating pulmonary insufficiency, a chest roentgenogram often helps in evaluating the patient's progress. Severe hypoxemia may be present even when the chest roentgenogram appears normal [43]. More frequently, the chest roentgenogram reveals pulmonary edema, atelectasis, or infiltrates secondary to aspiration [17, 18, 43].

Further monitoring and therapy

All near-drowned patients should be monitored in the hospital. The patient who is asymptomatic and who has normal arterial blood gases on admission may be ready for discharge after 12–24 h. If so, a follow-up visit several days later should be arranged. Patients who exhibit only mild hypoxemia requiring low concentrations of supplemental O_2 may require brief hospitalization; however, they should be monitored closely in case the hypoxemia increases.

Patients with significant hypoxemia or with an abnormal level of consciousness require admission to an intensive care unit and frequent measurements of vital signs (blood pressure, pulse rate, respiratory rate, and temperature). In addition, ECG monitoring and careful recording of fluid intake and output are necessary. An arterial catheter can be used for accurate blood pressure recording and for blood sampling to facilitate measurement of pHa, PaO_2, and $PaCO_2$. A central venous catheter may be helpful, but it only allows measurement of pressures proximal to the right atrium. When high levels of PEEP or CPAP are necessary or when cardiovascular function is unstable, a pulmonary artery catheter is very useful for measuring cardiac output and pulmonary artery occlusion pressure. The latter reflects left heart filling pressure, and the catheter permits sampling of mixed venous blood for determination of intrapulmonary shunt. While there is some risk and expense involved with such a catheter, the benefits of knowing accurately the effects of CPAP and PEEP, volume status, and cardiac function may in fact reduce morbidity and shorten hospitalization.

Ventilatory support should be directed toward providing an acceptable PaO_2 and intrapulmonary shunt with the lowest amount of supplemental O_2. In addition to the risk of O_2 toxicity with high inspired O_2 concentrations, absorption atelectasis may convert an area with low ventilation-to-perfusion ratios into one of absolute shunt [11].

There is controversy in the literature regarding pharmacologic doses of corticosteroids and prophylactic antibiotics for near-drowned victims. One of the authors (JHM) recommended these drugs on an empirical basis in 1968 [39]. After reviewing the cases of 121 near-drowned victims treated by him and his associates, however, he has withdrawn this recommendation [44]. In animal studies, pharmacologic doses of corticosteroids did not improve oxygenation or survival after freshwater aspiration [4]. Furthermore, Wynne et al. [62] have shown that corticosteroids may interfere with pulmonary healing after aspiration of foodstuff. Secondary pulmonary infection is a frequent complication in the near-drowned victim with prolonged hospitalization. Because pneumonia caused by organisms resistant to prophylactic antibiotics occurs in some patients, such prophylaxis is no longer recommended. Instead, gram stains and cultures of the sputum should be checked carefully. When the patient develops evidence of pulmonary infection, such as fever, leukocytosis, and infiltrates revealed by chest roentgenograms, then appropriate antibiotic therapy should be instituted, based on sputum culture and sensitivity testing. Infection frequently manifests on the second or third day in hospital, a time when pulmonary edema is resolving. Then, vigorous pulmonary toilet in addition to antibiotic therapy is appropriate.

When these principles are applied, normal survival should result in more than 90% of the patients who either are alert or have a blunted level of consciousness when admitted [8, 44]. The prognosis for comatose patients is not so clear-cut. Specific measures for brain resuscitation must be considered, although a prospective study of near-drowned victims is necessary to evaluate such measures. Elevated ICP secondary to brain edema may respond favorably to moderate hyperventilation [$PaCO_2$ approximately 30 mmHg (4 kPa)], this effect being secondary to reduced cerebral blood flow [57]. Pharmacologic doses of corticosteroids have been advocated to treat cerebral edema [15]. These measures are generally accepted by most physicians who treat comatose patients. Barbiturate therapy, hyperoxia, hypothermia, and dehydration have also been suggested for cerebral resuscitation [8]. Hypothermia and barbiturate therapy are thought to reduce cerebral metabolism. Hyperoxia is thought to improve O_2 diffusion into the brain, although this has never been soundly proved. In determining whether any of these techniques should be used, one must weigh the potential risks against the anticipated advantages for each patient. Even those who advocate such therapy agree that these measures should be reserved for comatose patients and are unnecessary and may only complicate therapy for those who are alert or who have blunted sensorium on admission [5a, 8, 44].

In summary, prompt resuscitation and therapy aimed at alleviating hypoxemia are crucial for near-drowned persons. The pathophysiology is related to the type and the volume of fluid aspirated. The most frequent significant injury is to the lung, although hypoxemia and acidosis secondary to this may result in damage to other organs. Each victim must be thoroughly evaluated in the emergency department and closely observed during the ensuing hours. Further therapy, as outlined, depends on the severity of the lesion. Patients who are alert or who have a blunted level of consciousness have an excellent prognosis when therapy is directed toward the pulmonary lesion, cardiovascular stability, and the maintenance of intravascular volume. Comatose patients may require special measures to recover brain function, but the benefit from them has not as yet been fully evaluated prospectively.

References

1. American Heart Association (1974) Standards for cardiopulmonary resuscitation (CPR) and Emergency Cardiac Care (ECC). JAMA 227:833–868
2. Bergquist RE, Vogelhut MM, Modell JH, Sloan SJ, Ruiz BC (1980) Comparison of ventilatory patterns in the treatment of freshwater near-drowning in dogs. Anesthesiology 52:142–148
3. Butt MP, Jalowayski A, Modell JH, Giammona ST (1970) Pulmonary function after resuscitation from near-drowning. Anesthesiology 32:275–277
4. Calderwood HW, Modell JH, Ruiz BC (1975) The ineffectiveness of steroid therapy for treatment of freshwater near-drowning. Anesthesiology 43:642–650
5. Conn AW (1979) Near-drowning and hypothermia (editorial). Can Med Assoc J 120:397–400
5a. Conn AW, Modell JH (1980) Current neurological considerations in near-drowning. (Editorial) Can Anaesth Soc J 27:197–198
6. Conn AW, Edmonds JF, Barker GA (1978) Near-drowning in cold fresh water: Current treatment regimen. Can Anaesth Soc J 25:259–265
7. Conn AW, Edmonds JF, Barker GA (1979) Cerebral resuscitation in near-drowning. (Symposium on the Chest) Pediatr Clin North Am 26:691–701
8. Conn AW, Montes JE, Barker GA, Edmonds JF (1980) Cerebral salvage in near-drowning following neurological classification by triage. Can Anaesth Soc J 27:201–210
9. Cot C (1931) Les Asphyxies Accidentelles (submersion, electrocution, intoxication, oxycarbonique) Etude clinique, therapeutique, et preventive. Editions medicales N Maloine, Paris
10. Culpepper RM (1975) Bleeding diathesis in freshwater drowning. Ann Intern Med 83:675
11. Douglas ME, Downs JB, Dannemiller FJ, Hodges MR, Munson ES (1976) Change in pulmonary venous admixture with varying inspired oxygen. Anesth Analg (Cleve) 55:688–695
12. Downs JB, Modell JH (1977) Patterns of respiratory support aimed at pathophysiologic conditions. ASA Refresher Courses in Anesthesiology 5:71–85
13. Downs JB, Klein EF Jr, Modell JH (1973) The effect of incremental PEEP on PaO_2 in patients with respiratory failure. Anesth Analg (Cleve) 52:210–215
14. Fandel I, Bancalari E (1976) Near-drowning in children: Clinical aspects. Pediatrics 58:573–579
15. Fishman RA (1975) Brain edema. N Engl J Med 293:706–711
16. Fleetham JA, Munt PW (1978) Near-drowning in Canadian waters. Can Med Assoc J 68:914–917
17. Fuller RH (1963a) The clinical pathology of human near-drowning. Proc R Soc Med 56:33–38
18. Fuller RH (1963b) The 1962 Wellcome prize essay. Drowning and the postimmersion syndrome. A clinicopathologic study. Milit Med 128:22–36
19. Gauto A, Majeski JA, Alexander JW (1979) Drowning and near-drowning: Current concepts and neutrophil function studies. South Med J 72:690–692
20. Giammona ST, Modell JH (1967) Drowning by total immersion. Effects on pulmonary surfactant of distilled water, isotonic saline, and sea water. Am J Dis Child 114:612–616
21. Gilfoil MP, Carvajal HF (1977) Near-drowning in children. Tex Med 73:39–44
22. Gooden BA (1972) Drowning and the diving reflex in man. Med J Aust 2:583–587
23. Grausz H, Amend WJC Jr, Early LE (1971) Acute renal failure complicating submersion in seawater. JAMA 217:207–209
24. Halmagyi DFJ (1961) Lung changes and incidence of respiratory arrest in rats after aspiration of sea and fresh water. J Appl Physiol 16:41–44
25. Halmagyi DFJ, Colebatch HJH (1961) The drowned lung. A physiological approach to its mechanism and management. Aust NZ J Med 10:68–77
26. Hunt PK (1974) Effect and treatment of the diving reflex. Can Med Assoc J 111:1330–1331

27. King RB, Webster IW (1964) A case of recovery from drowning and prolonged anoxia. Med J Aust 1:919–920

28. Kruus S, Bergstrom L, Suutarinen T, Hyvonen R (1979) The prognosis of near-drowned children. Acta Paediatr Scand 68:315–322

29. Kvittingen TD, Naess A (1963) Recovery from drowning in fresh water. Br Med J 5341:1315–1317

30. Miles S (1968) Drowning. Br Med J iii:597–600

31. Miloslavich EL (1934) Pathological anatomy of death by drowning. Am J Clin Pathol 4:42–49

32. Modell JH (1963) Resuscitation after aspiration of chlorinated freshwater. JAMA 185:651–655

33. Modell JH (1966) Serum electrolyte changes during drowning and near drowning. Bulletin of Pathology (Dec.):304, 311

34. Modell JH (1971) Pathophysiology and Treatment of Drowning and Near-Drowning. Thomas, Springfield, pp 4, 8–9

35. Modell JH, Davis JH (1969) Electrolyte changes in human drowning victims. Anesthesiology 30:414–420

36. Modell JH, Moya F (1966) Effects of volume of aspirated fluid during chlorinated fresh water drowning. Anesthesiology 27:662–672

37. Modell JH, Gaub M, Moya F, Vestal B, Swarz H (1966) Physiologic effects of near drowning with chlorinated fresh water, distilled water and isotonic saline. Anesthesiology 27:33–41

38. Modell JH, Moya F, Newby EJ, Ruiz BC, Showers AV (1967) The effects of fluid volume in seawater drowning. Ann Intern Med 67:68–80

39. Modell JH, Davis JH, Giammona ST, Moya F, Mann JB (1968a) Blood gas and electrolyte changes in human near-drowning victims. JAMA 203:337–343

40. Modell JH, Moya F, Williams HD, Weibley TC (1968b) Changes in blood gases and A-aDO$_2$ during near-drowning. Anesthesiology 29:456–465

41. Modell JH, Kuck EJ, Ruiz BC, Heimlich H (1972) Effect of intravenous vs. aspirated distilled water on serum electrolytes and blood gas tensions. J Appl Physiol 32:579–584

42. Modell JH, Calderwood HW, Ruiz BC, Downs JB, Chapman R (1974) Effects of ventilatory patterns on arterial oxygenation after near–drowning in sea water. Anesthesiology 40:376–384

43. Modell JH, Graves SA, Ketover A (1976) Clinical course of 91 consecutive near-drowning victims. Chest 70:231–238

44. Modell JH, Graves SA, Kuck EJ (1980) Near-drowning: Correlation of level of consciousness and survival. Can Anaesth Soc J 27:211–215

45. Munroe WD (1964) Hemoglobinuria from near-drowning. J Pediatr 64:57–62

46. Orlowski JP (1979) Prognostic factors in pediatric cases of drowning and near-drowning. JACEP 8:176–179

47. Pearn JH, Bart RD Jr, Yamaoka R (1979) Neurologic sequelae after childhood near-drowning: A total population study from Hawaii. Pediatrics 64:187–191

48. Peterson B (1977) Morbidity of childhood near-drowning. Pediatrics 59:364–370

49. Press E, Walker J, Crawford I (1968) An interstate drowning study. Am J Public Health 58:2275–2289

50. Rath CE (1953) Drowning hemoglobinuria. Blood 8:1099–1104

51. Reidbord HE, Spitz WU (1966) Ultrastructural alterations in rat lungs. Changes after intratracheal perfusion with freshwater and seawater. Arch Pathol 81:103–111

52. Rivers JF, Orr G, Lee HA (1970) Drowning. Its clinical sequelae and management. Br Med J ii:157–161

53. Ruben A, Ruben H (1962) Artificial respiration. Flow of water from the lung and the stomach. Lancet I:780–781

54. Ruiz BC, Calderwood HW, Modell JH, Brogdon JE (1973) Effect of ventilatory patterns on arterial oxygenation after near-drowning with fresh water: A comparative study in dogs. Anesth Analg (Cleve) 52:570–576

55. Safar P, Escarraga LA, Elam JO (1958) A comparison of the mouth-to-mouth and mouth-to-airway methods of artificial respiration with the chest-pressure arm-lift methods. N Engl J Med 258:671–677

56. Schuman SH, Rowe JR, Glazer HM, Redding JS (1976) The iceberg phenomenon of near drowning. Crit Care Med 4:127–128

57. Severinghaus JW, Lassen N (1967) Step hypocapnea to separate arterial from tissue PCO$_2$ in the regulation of cerebral blood flow. Circ Res 20:272–278

58. Siebke H, Breivek H, Rod T, Lind B (1975) Survival after 40 minutes' submersion without cerebral sequelae. Lancet 1:1275–1277

59. Swann HG, Brucer M (1949) The cardiorespiratory and biochemical events during rapid anoxic death. VI. Freshwater and sea water drowning. Tex Rep Biol Med 7:604–618

60. Swann HG, Brucer M, Moore C, Vezien BL (1947) Freshwater and sea water drowning: A study of the terminal cardiac and biochemical events. Tex Rep Biol Med 5:423–437

61. Webster's New Collegiate Dictionary (1979). Merriam, Springfield, p 347

62. Wynne JW, Reynolds JC, Hood CI, Auerbach D, Ondrasick J (1979) Steroid therapy for pneumonitis induced in rabbits by aspiration of foodstuff. Anesthesiology 51:11–19

Chapter 41

Snakebites

J. A. M. White

Venomous snakes are found throughout the world, but the many fatal cases of snakebite recorded annually are caused by a few highly dangerous species. In Southern and Central Africa there are about 150 species of snakes but only about 10% secrete a potentially lethal venom [2].

Identification

Precise identification of the snake after an attack is possible in about 40% of urban and 20% of rural series [5]. Fortunately it is only important following suspected bites by dangerous species, because specific therapy with a potential morbidity may be indicated. Identification of reptile species by members of the public is notoriously inaccurate and may be difficult in hospital even

with the aid of pictorial charts, because the head of the snake is frequently damaged or missing (Table 41.1).

Three groups of indigenous snakes are responsible for nearly all fatal cases in the subcontinent (Table 41.2) [4]. The relative importance of each group differs in urban and rural practice over the large land area. Even if the snake cannot be identified, rational immediate care can be given provided a careful history is taken and a full clinical examination is carried out with a limited number of special investigations. The time of the attack and the circumstances under which the injury was sustained have an important bearing on initial care.

The *time lapsed* between injury and arrival at hospital has a considerable influence on the clinical picture, prognosis, and management. With the exception of the rare attacks by the gaboon adder (*Bitis gabonica*) and the black

Table 41.1. Groups of snakes responsible for 251 cases of snakebite seen in the University of Natal, Addington Hospital, 1973–1979

Group		% Total
Small adders	164	65.4
Non-venomous snakes	40	16.0
Large adders	18	7.1
Elapid snakes	16	6.3
Venomous colubrid snakes	13	5.2
	251	100.0

Table 41.2. Groups of snakes responsible for 1067 cases of fatal snakebite seen at the University of Natal, 1957–1963

	% Mortality
Black mambas	100
All elapid snakes	25
Puff adders	5.2
All adders	2.0
All venomous snakes	2.4

From Visser and Champan [4].

Table 41.3. Recognition of snake groups by clinical sequelae of bite

	Non-venomous snakes	Small adders	Large adders snakes	Venomous colubrid	Cobra	Mamba
Ragged wound	++	0	0	0	0	0
Fang marks	0	+	++	++	+	+
Rapid local reaction	0	++	+++	0	0	0
Spreading local bruising	0	+	+++	0	0	0
CNS signs	0	0	+	0	±	++
Peripheral nerve paresis	0	0	0	0	++	+++
Cardiac lesions	0	0	0	0	±	++
Peripheral circulatory failure	0	0	++	0	±	++
Delayed bleeding tendency	0	0	0	+++	0	0

mamba (*Dendroaspis polylepis*), it takes some time for the full clinical picture caused by venom injection to develop. Observation in hospital is advised after all bites by potentially venomous snakes, because first aid measures may modify or aggravate the effects of venom injection and abortive attacks by dangerous species may modify the clinical picture.

Fang marks may be difficult to recognize because they are obscured by local swelling or may be atypical, e.g., mere scratches. Fang marks are not irrefutable proof that venom has actually been injected. The whole clinical picture must be taken into account in making a diagnosis and planning management. If there are no significant symptoms or signs other than fang marks on arrival in hospital it is usually wise to observe the patient very carefully and avoid therapeutic measures carrying a significant morbidity, e.g., use of specific anti-venoms.

Prognosis

Few species of Southern African snakes secrete a potentially lethal venom, and even fewer are naturally aggressive reptiles. Small children are most exposed to these species, and injury by dangerous species is commoner in rural than urban areas. Lack of education and access to well-equipped hospitals contribute to higher rural death rates, but inappropriate general and local treatment methods contribute to morbidity and mortality rates. There are other important factors governing prognosis.

Species responsible for attack

Although there is a risk of secondary infection and tetanus after all snakebites, the major risk to patients bitten by non-venomous species of snakes is inappropriate local and general therapy, e.g., use of tourniquets and anti-venoms.

Venom composition is significantly different in closely related species belonging to the same group of venomous snakes, e.g., ringhals (*Haemachatus haemachatus*) and cobras. Following an attack by black or green mambas (*Dendroaspis angusticeps*) there are significant differences in the clinical picture and prognosis. These are probably related to known differences in the chemical composition of the two indigenous mamba species. Similar differences exist in the venom composition of the numerous indigenous adders and three local venomous colubrid snakes.

Venom dose injected

The general and local effects of injected venom tend to be more severe in small children because the dose–mass ratio is high (Table 41.3). Many factors influence the dose of venom actually delivered through a fang mark (Table 41.4).

Site of injury

Eye injuries caused by spitting elapid snakes are not associated with systemic venom absorption.

Centrally situated bites are more dangerous because local treatment is more difficult to apply in immediate care and venom absorption is

Table 41.4. Factors causing variation in venom effects caused by groups of venomous snakes

Avoiding action	Fang penetration
Protective clothing	Capacity of sacs
Dose–mass ratio	Species differences
Immediate care	

more rapid. Direct IV venom injection is often rapidly fatal. Venom is absorbed more rapidly after subfascial injection into muscle than from fatty tissue.

Distal bites are fortunately much more common than proximal limb injuries. The numerous adder species do not rear to strike as elapid snakes do (Table 41.1).

First aid measures

Spread of venoms has been studied by isotope labelling. Absorption through the lymphatic and venous systems is rapid and is increased by using the limb. Adder venoms contain hyaluronidase, and spread rapidly by permeation. These studies suggest that local measures, such as sucking on the fang marks, incision of the bite, and locally applied chemical antidotes, are likely to be quite ineffective and may cause needless morbidity [5]. Tourniquets prevent the spread of cytotoxic adder venom at the expense of maintaining a high local concentration and may further impair tissue viability.

Antivenoms should only be used strictly according to the instruction pamphlet issued with each package by the manufacturer. These preparations require careful storage and are inactivated by consistent exposure to high environmental temperatures.

Susceptibility of the victim

In most regions of Africa, 80% of those bitten are children. A high dose–mass ratio of venom may lead to death before medical aid is available. Although mortality rates have fallen dramatically in the last decade (Table 41.2), inadequate or incorrect care of the adder and elapid bites immediately after injury is still responsible for deaths that might otherwise be avoided.

Reactions to the equine protein of antivenoms are usually mild, but serious anaphylactic reactions are seen and are more likely to occur in patients previously treated with equine sera or suffering from allergic disorders.

Non-venomous snakes

In hospital practice in a large urban area over a 7-year period (Table 41.1), bites by non-venomous snakes have made up 16% of our

cases. As the population density rises the numbers of highly venomous snakes declines, but the numerous non-venomous snakes and small adders survive in urban areas. These two groups of snakes were responsible for 81.4% of the attacks in our series.

Diagnosis

No attempt was made at accurate identification of the many species of non-venomous snakes that inflict a relatively minor injury. Among the non-venomous species identified were grass snakes and the large mole snake (*Pseudaspis cana*), because these snakes bear superficial resemblance to local dangerous species.

This group of snakes *do not have fangs*. Their numerous small teeth may be embedded in the small ragged wound and may be recognized under magnification in a good light. There is minimal reaction around the wound and the general reaction is caused by fear and anxiety because of the similarity between some of these snakes and dangerous species.

Treatment

Wounds should be carefully cleansed under local anaesthesia and foreign matter removed. Recent wounds may be sutured under antibiotic cover and tetanus prophylaxis given. Reassurance of frequently hysterical victims may be supplemented by administration of a tranquilliser.

Viperidae

During the period 1973–1979 adder bites made up 72.5% of our series derived largely from a densely populated urban area. Bites by small adders made up 65.4% of our patients. In the rural areas puff adder bites are more common, but made up only 7.1% of our cases. No bites by the indigenous Berg adder (*Bitis atropos*) were seen. The dangerous saw-scaled viper (*Echis carinatus*) is not indigenous to Southern or Central Africa.

Positive identification of the adder responsible for the attack is more frequent in urban practice. The two large indigenous adders are easily recognized by the lay public. Over 80% of our cases of injury by small adders were caused by common night adders (*Causus rhombeatus*) or burrowing adders (*Actractaspis bibronii*).

Adder venoms of indigenous species differ significantly from those of Indian and Northern African species. These venoms are cytotoxins and there are important differences in the effects produced by the venoms of small and large adders in this region.

Small adders

Common night adders are not strictly nocturnal snakes. Bites are found mainly on the feet or ankles of those who do not wear shoes or the hands of snake collectors. Burrowing adders live in burrows, holes, pipes and conduits. Bites are usually seen on the hands of children and workmen. The snake gives no warning hiss before striking, often with a sideways raking action, to give a single fang mark or scratch. Other species of adders occur throughout the subcontinent but many have vestigial fangs and venom sacs.

The effects of these venoms are highly variable, and fortunately none should be fatal with appropriate care. Their venoms are cytotoxins that evoke a brisk and painful inflammatory reaction around the fang marks. These are tiny and the paired puncture wounds are set close together (less than 1.5 cm apart). The swelling spreads proximally and distally and is maximal in 48 h. In patients who have not been treated by tourniquets tissue necrosis is rare, but is occasionally seen after burrowing adder bites. Local subcutaneous bleeding is minimal but more extensive in burrowing adder bites. Systemic disturbance is minimal. Neurological signs and disturbance of the coagulation mechanism do not occur.

Berg adders are common in our mountains but bites are rare. The local reaction is more severe and may be followed by a transient ophthalmoplegia (paralysis of ocular movement, strabismus, and pupillary changes) with nausea, vomiting, and loss of taste and smell. These effects may persist for some weeks but paralysis of respiratory muscles does not occur. Saw-scaled vipers cause a serious consumption coagulopathy for which treatment with a specific antivenom is required.

Diagnosis

It is not difficult to make the diagnosis from the history and local signs. Precise identification is not essential because specific therapy is not required. Serological tests have not been performed for precise identification.

Treatment

Local. Management should be entirely conservative, because none of these snakes inflicts a lethal injury and serious injury can be caused by ill-advised interference. Incision, tourniquet application, topical applications, and local antivenom injection should NOT be employed. The affected area should be elevated and kept at rest. A firm supporting bandage should be applied to control troublesome lymphoedema.
General. Simple analgesics and antihistamines may be given but there is no indication for steroid therapy. The patient should be covered by antibiotic therapy and given tetanus prophylaxis. Antivenom therapy should NOT be used. The venoms of these snakes are no longer used by the South African Institute for Medical Research (S.A.I.M.R.) in the preparation of their *polyvalent antivenom.*

Large adders

Gaboon adders are indigenous to the forest areas of the region and are bred in captivity for the export market. These large and colourful adders may bite their handlers, inflicting a very grave and formerly fatal injury. Puff adders are more common in rural areas and inflict grave injuries on children. Both species have large and erectile front fangs that are widely separated in the diamond-shaped heads and connected to large venom sacs. These species do not rear to strike. Fang marks are almost invariably at or below ankle level (Table 41.2). The clinical picture produced by injection of their venoms is very different from that caused by small adders (Tables 41.3 and 41.4).

The venoms of these large adders are potent cytotoxins and may be deeply injected into the tissues through the long fangs. They spread by permeation in the tissues and are rapidly absorbed through the lymphatic and venous systems. Puff adder venom (Table 41.5) contains proteases (causing endothelial disruption, cell lysis, capillary disruption, and dissolution of blood clots), phosphatidases (causing haemolysis), and hyaluronidase (causing rapidly swelling oedema). Subfascial injection causes

Table 41.5. Effects of large adder venom

Cytotoxic effect
Absorption from tissues
Blood volume deficit
Organ damage

tense oedema of muscle compartments and this may extend into the large fascial spaces of the abdominal and chest cavities. Although serious central effects (loss of consciousness, respiratory and circulatory depression with sudden death) may follow injection of gaboon adder venom or direct IV injection of either venom, the serious effects of bites by these large adders may be closely correlated with the dose–mass ratio (Table 41.4), the extent of the local lesion, and secondary effects produced by incorrect immediate care.

The release of chemical fractions (histamine, kinins, and prostaglandins) from the extensively damaged tissues may cause secondary changes in the endothelium of the capillaries of vital organs, e.g., brain, heart, lungs, and kidneys. The lesions are similar to those found following serious closed injuries of large muscle masses. Loss of plasma and whole blood into the tissues is maximal in the first 24 h but continues for 48–72 h. A considerable blood volume deficit may ensue and cause poor perfusion of vital organs, endothelial damage by chemical fractions incompletely cleared from the pulmonary circulation, and secondary organ failure.

Skin necrosis is usually limited and superficial but may be very extensive in neglected, infected, and incorrectly treated patients, e.g., patients treated by prolonged tourniquet application, injection locally of contaminated antivenom, and wide fasciotomy. Regional adenitis is common, but transient in most cases.

Thrombosis of deep calf veins may be shown on phlebography and may be associated with persisting brawny oedema, but embolism is very rare. Occlusion of major vessels is rare and is usually a complication of prolonged tourniquet application.

Diagnosis

Local signs considered together with the history normally permit a firm diagnosis to be made. These snakes are easily identified and the local reaction to venom injection follows rapidly. Fang marks are deep and widely spaced but a side-strike may produce only a deep scratch mark. These snakes do not rear, and usually strike at the ankle or foot. The extent of limb oedema, blistering, erythema, and subcutaneous haemorrhage (Table 41.3) is considerable, and within a few hours the whole limb may be involved with later extension to the trunk.

General signs of massive venom injection may include rapid loss of consciousness and respiratory and cardiac depression, but this is exceptional and is seen mainly after the rare gaboon adder bites. An insidious general deterioration is much more common, and is accompanied by signs of increasing peripheral circulatory failure and deteriorating cerebral, pulmonary, and renal function. Secondary thrombocytopenia follows increased platelet consumption but a generalized bleeding tendency is very rare in attacks by indigenous vipers, in contrast to the picture following venom injection by saw-scaled vipers and Malayan species. Renal failure is a grave indication of organ damage and carries a serious prognosis. Secondary infection of damaged tissues causes rapid general deterioration.

Treatment

The conservative regimen of local and general care advocated for bites by the small adders is adopted.

Tourniquet application during immediate care may accentuate damage to muscles, vessels, and nerves, and possibly contribute to the development of renal tubular necrosis. Tourniquets must be released, but every effort should be made to maintain a high renal tubular flow. Careful assessment of the vascular and neural damage is required. Decompression of the calf compartments by linear incision or fibulectomy is not routinely employed in major injuries by these snakes because the general effects of possible secondary infection may be very serious.

Skin necrosis may eventually require limited excision and skin grafting but its eventual extent is usually more limited than originally estimated.

Polyvalent antivenom (S.A.I.M.R.) is used with suitable precautions against serum reactions in the immediate care of bites by our two indigenous adders. Following the routine administration of 100–200 mg hydrocortisone hemisuccinate, 20–40 ml (adults) or 2–3 mg/kg (children) is given slowly IV after dilution in 200 ml 5% dextrose. In the experience of those who have treated these patients immediately after a bite, adequate antivenom therapy modifies the general and local effects of venom injection. However, there is usually a long delay before these patients are seen in hospital, and under these circumstances the lesion is already well established. Antivenom therapy is then much less effective and is no longer used as part of the treatment protocol.

Intravenous fluid therapy is used to restore the circulating blood volume and urine output as rapidly as possible and to maintain tissue perfusion throughout the phase of fluid extravasation into the tissues. The need is greatest in the first 24-h period but must be continued for 72 h or more. Fluid therapy should be similar to that employed in extensive closed injuries of the limbs and shoulder and pelvic girdles. Respiratory, renal, and cardiac function should be closely monitored and anaemia corrected with red cell concentrates.

Drug therapy should be similar to that employed in small adder bites. Late administration of steroids in pharmacological dosage does not influence the course of the injury.

Elapidae

Ringhals, many cobra species, and two types of mambas are found in Southern Africa. In the last decade the number of attacks has declined and these injuries formed only 6.3% of our current series.

Although the above snakes belong to the same group, there are considerable differences in the chemical structure of their venoms and subsequent clinical signs from those produced by the venoms of Indian cobras. There is wide species variation in the effect of venom injection on humans and small experimental animals. The presence of chemical fractions in indigenous elapid venoms cannot be accurately correlated with the lesions found in patients. Ringhals injuries are the least serious and mambas inflict the most serious injury. All venoms of dangerous indigenous elapid snakes are used in the preparation of modern S.A.I.M.R. polyvalent antivenom.

Elapid venoms contain phosphatidases, but haemolysis and spontaneous bleeding are not features of bites by indigenous species. Cardiotoxins directly depress the vasomotor centre, decrease peripheral arterial tone, interfere with neural conduction in the myocardium and depress myocardial activity to cause profound circulatory failure not attributable to hypoxia caused by respiratory failure. Neurotoxins of indigenous venoms affect the central and peripheral nervous systems.

Alpha-bugaratoxins [1] are small-molecular-weight proteins (Table 41.6) that can bind tem-

Table 41.6. Important toxins in elapid venoms

| Phosphatidase |
| Cardiotoxins |
| Neurotoxins |

porarily to the membrane of acetylcholine (AC) receptor plates in striated muscle. Subsequent failure of neural transmission is a transient curare-like non-depolarizing neuromuscular blockade that responds for short periods to anticholinesterase drugs. Cobra venom labelled with iodine-131 is used to identify end-plates in experimental myasthenia gravis [3] and has been shown not to produce any permanent effect on these structures. After administration of elapid venoms the severity, duration, and extent of the muscular paralysis is highly variable. Peripheral nerve paresis is uncommon after ringhals bites, and venom injection affects mainly the CNS to cause non-specific symptoms and signs of a transient nature. Following cobra bites the dominant lesion is a muscular paralysis. Effects on the CNS, heart, and circulation may be minimal but death may follow from respiratory paralysis. In victims of mamba attacks, the onset of paralysis is more rapid (15–30 min) and the duration is more prolonged. In patients treated after cobra and green mamba bites by assisted ventilation without administration of antivenom, spontaneous recovery of paralysed muscle occurs in 12–72 h. The eye muscles (pupillary changes, ptosis, and strabismus), muscles of facial expression, and pharyngeal musculature tend to be affected selectively in the first instance with subsequent involvement of the muscles of respiration to cause interference with the cough reflex, aspiration, and death from hypoxia. Peripheral muscles are affected but the diaphragm is more resistant. Difficulty with swallowing saliva, aspiration, and progressive hypoventilation progress more slowly after cobra than mamba bites. The paralysis may pursue a fluctuating course with dangerous relapse after apparent initial improvement.

Anticholinesterase drugs potentiate the effect of AC release at nerve endings, and prostigmine (2 mg) will retard the progress of paresis. Its muscarine-like effects may be blocked with atropine (0.6 mg). The effect of these drugs is transient and repeated administration may accentuate the blockade. Prostigmine is a water-soluble drug, does not penetrate the CNS, and cannot affect the effect of elapid venoms on the CNS.

Diagnosis

Elapid species are frequently accurately identified by the victim because the appearance of these snakes is characteristic. Only experts can differentiate the many cobra species and green mambas may be mistaken for boomslangs. The clinical picture varies with the mode of attack, elapid species responsible, dose–mass ratio and the efficiency of immediate care (Table 41.7).

Eye injuries. Ringhals and certain cobras can spit venom onto the face and eyes accurately from a distance of many feet. In this region chemical conjunctivitis is the commonest injury inflicted by ringhals. *Naja mossambica (M'fezi)* is a cobra that can spit venom into the eye without rearing because it has a characteristically shaped venom aperture on its front fangs. Systemic effects of venom absorption do not occur after eye injuries and antivenom therapy is not indicated. Swelling persists for many days after these extremely painful injuries, but permanent damage does not occur after appropriate therapy.

Elapid bites. Elapid snakes have small fangs fixed in the front of the upper jaw of the relatively small head. The fang marks are therefore small and set close together. In contrast to the local injury caused by the small adders, there is little or no reaction to the bite and little pain but local paraesthesia may follow. A strike is not synonymous with a bite, because the small fangs may fail to penetrate the clothing or protective footwear. Bites may be found on any part of the body, because these are mostly long and slender snakes that rear to strike.

General effects. Venom absorption after labelling with isotopes is as effectively retarded by limb immobilization and firm compression bandaging (55 mmHg pressure) as by the dangerous expedient of tourniquet application [3]. Absorption of venom through the superficial veins and lymphatics is rapid, but deep subfascial injection, as in bites by large adders, does not occur. Elapid fangs are short and have a subterminal aperture.

Table 41.7. Effects of elapid venoms[a]

Conjunctivities
Minimal local lesions
'Myasthenia'
Central CNS lesions
Circulatory changes

[a]There is marked species variation in the effects of these venoms.

Dose–mass ratios are variable, and are highest in black mamba bites because these snakes have proportionately the largest venom sacs. The wide variation in the severity of the general effects of elapid bites may be partly dose-related.

Prodromal effects (headache, nausea, vomiting, malaise, and vertigo) may follow within minutes of venom injection and may be the only general effects of ringhals bites. The relatively mild effects of ringhals venom on the CNS contrasts with the severe effect of black mamba venom on the brain, circulatory system, and peripheral nerves. Following injection of cobra venom, the onset of the general effects may be delayed and further retarded by antivenom injection during immediate care with its dominant effect on the peripheral nerves.

Progressive muscular weakness presents with a clinical picture of 'myasthenic crisis', but the ocular, facial, and 'bulbar' features are dominant. In attacks by cobras CNS excitation, depression of consciousness, and cardiac depression may be completely absent.

Central nervous lesions are prominent and early in attacks by black mambas, with fits, hallucinations, severe headache, and loss of consciousness followed by spreading paralysis. The venom acts centrally on the vasomotor centre and directly on the heart to impair the circulation. Black mamba venom causes a more severe, widespread, and prolonged effect on the patient than green mamba venom or those of the many cobra species, and may have to be countered by specific therapy for up to 7 days in survivors of the initial effects.

Haematological changes are not seen after bites by indigenous elapid species.

Immediate transfer to a major hospital under skilled supervision, with facilities in transit for pharyngeal suction, maintenance of airway patency, and ventilatory assistance is recommended after all elapid bites. Relapse after initial improvement is common and skilled management may be required for long periods. The great fall in the mortality rate of elapid injuries (Table 41.2) is largely attributable to the greater availability of critical care facilities.

Treatment

Local. Tourniquets should never be used in the treatment of any form of snakebite, because they are a potent cause of serious morbidity in the hands of the untrained. It is fortunate that their application by the lay public is usually ineffective. The safer method of immobilization with limb compression is preferred in immediate care of recent elapid bites.

Cleanse the wound by washing away surface venom and taking care to avoid contamination of the eyes. Local anaesthetic agents should be instilled into the swollen conjunctival sacs after injuries caused by spitting snakes. The eyes should be irrigated with sterile water, saline, or dilute antivenom (1:10), but there is no clear advantage in using antivenom. This should be followed by application of an ophthalmic antibiotic ointment to the eyelids under a sterile ophthalmic dressing. A sterile dressing is applied to bites on the limbs after cleansing with appropriate precautions against tetanus and other forms of secondary infection.

General. It is rare for a doctor to see victims of elapid bites soon after an injury. Before instituting antivenom therapy it is essential to be sure from the history and local and general examination that the bite has in fact been inflicted by an elapid snake and that the general signs of venom injection, albeit in the prodromal stages, are present.

Antivenom administration is an integral part of the immediate therapy of elapid bites and should be carried out strictly in accordance with the recommendations of the manufacturer.

Polyvalent antivenom (S.A.I.M.R.) is a high-titre preparation of equine immunoglobulins produced by repeated injection of increasing doses of the venoms of two indigenous large adders, ringhals, common indigenous cobras, and two mamba species into horses. Minor reactions to the foreign protein of the antivenom are not uncommon, but serious reactions are rare. Appropriate drugs to counter anaphylactic reactions should always be available before even the first test dose (0.1 ml 1:10 dilution) is given. Hydrocortisone hemisuccinate (100–200 mg) is given routinely before antivenom administration. Administration IV (40–80 ml) of a dilute solution of the antivenom in 5% dextrose by slow infusion is preferred, but the total dose given to victims of black mamba may exceed 200 ml over 7 days. It is unwise to use antivenom therapy in attacks in which there is no general evidence of venom injection, and great care must be exercised in patients with a history of allergic disorders or previous exposure to equine sera.

Meticulous monitoring of these patients is mandatory, because the course of the neurological lesions and the circulatory changes is unpredictable. Relapse after initial response to therapy is not uncommon.

Ventilatory assistance with maintenance of a secure airway and adequate oxygenation is the cornerstone of modern care of injuries by elapid snakes with respiratory signs. In institutions with the appropriate facilities for long-term assisted ventilation and monitoring, respiratory support has been used without antivenom therapy in treating bites by cobras and green mambas complicated by respiratory paralysis. In these injuries the CNS and circulation are minimally affected in well-oxygenated patients and spontaneous recovery of muscle power may be expected in 12–72 h. This form of care is not advised after black mamba bites.

Circulatory support with deep sedation and ventilatory assistance may be required for many days after black mamba bites. In the previous decade (Table 41.2) these injuries were uniformly fatal, but recovery under expert care may be expected in those who survive to reach a major critical care unit.

Colubridae

Among the many indigenous colubrid snakes, boomslangs (*Dispholidus typus*) and vine or bird snakes (*Thelotornis capensis*) of the sub-family *Boiginae* are highly venomous. Natal black snakes (*Macrelaps microlepidus*) are mildly venomous. These snakes are shy and non-aggressive; they rarely bite unless handled.

Boomslangs ('tree snakes') are highly venomous and have fixed fangs in the rear of the upper jaw below the eye level. Their colour is highly variable and their green form resembles that of a green mamba. On being threatened they may inflate the head and neck to resemble a cobra with its hood. Vine snakes secrete a similar venom but are less dangerous, and the local black snake causes only a mild haemorrhagic injury.

Boomslang venom is an extremely potent haemotoxin (Table 41.8), and sudden death has followed direct IV injection. The fang marks are usually found on the hands and are deep paired

Table 41.8. General effects of venomous colubrid snakes (boomslangs)

Delayed consumption coagulopathy
Depletion of factors X, V, and VIII
Secondary thrombocytopenia
Spontaneous bleeding

puncture wounds, but scratch marks may follow a tangential blow. The venom is a digestive enzyme (modified saliva) and is injected deeply into the tissues in determined bites. These snakes have a tendency to 'hang on' and may have to be plucked off the victim. During venom injection a 'chewing action' may be associated with laceration around the fang marks. There is little or no reaction around the local injury. After a variable latent period of several hours, during which there may be vague and non-specific prodromal symptoms, spontaneous bleeding from the eyes or gums or into the gastro-intestinal and urinary tracts reveals the presence of a generalized bleeding disorder. If immediate treatment is not instituted widespread haemorrhage occurs, with bleeding into the subcutaneous tissues, fascial planes, body cavities, and muscle masses. The venom is a potent activator of the coagulation mechanism with the formation of microthrombi throughout the capillary bed and a consumption coagulopathy. Activation of factor X with thrombocytopenia, low levels of factors V and VIII, increased fibrinolysis, and fibrinogen depletion are found in coagulation studies.

Diagnosis

The history is usually clear, but patients may present with or without an established bleeding disorder. During the latent period of several hours, there is little or no general disturbance or bleeding from the fang marks. Boomslang antivenom is extremely difficult to prepare, because these snakes cannot be 'milked' of their venom. The antivenom must be specifically ordered from the South African Institute of Medical Research. It is a highly allergenic preparation and should only be used for boomslang bites in which there has been proven venom injection.

Laboratory tests performed during the latent period in patients affected by venom injection will be abnormal. There is prolongation of the clotting time, levels of fibrin-degradation products are elevated, and the blood may be nearly incoagulable before the onset of frank bleeding. The mere presence of boomslang fang marks does not mean that the snake has actually injected a significant dose of venom.

Widespread spontaneous bleeding confirms the diagnosis, because no other indigenous snake except the vine snake causes a general bleeding tendency. Saw-scaled viper venom (*Echis carinatus*) causes a similar bleeding tendency, but these snakes are found only in North and West Africa. The effects of vine snake venom are similar but less severe. Laboratory tests are used to monitor antivenom and blood component therapy.

Treatment

Transfer to a major hospital under skilled supervision is advised, because control of the bleeding disorder requires access to a coagulation laboratory, use of a potentially dangerous specific antivenom, and access to blood components. Polyvalent antivenom is ineffective and must not be given. During immediate care the specific antivenom should not be given without good evidence of venom injection and after full precautions have been taken against serious reactions. Serious problems have been seen in patients to whom the specific antivenom has been given without precautions for tentative bites and scratch marks without proof that venom has actually entered the circulation. No antivenom has been prepared against vine snake venom.

Blood component therapy is essential in boomslang and vine snake bites. Standard transfusion of whole blood or packed cells is ineffective. Depletion of the stable and labile coagulation factors should be corrected by infusion of fresh freeze-dried plasma in preference to the fresh-frozen variant. Platelet transfusion may be indicated in patients with severe thrombocytopenia, and low-titre heparin therapy may be used to potentiate the action of antithrombins. Restoration of the red cell mass should be carried out with freshly drawn blood, and suitable precautions taken against circulatory overload.

Specific antivenom therapy is not available for injuries caused by vine and black snakes. Prior to infusion of a loading dose of 10–20 ml antivenom diluted in 200 ml 5% dextrose, 200 mg hydrocortisone hemisuccinate should be given and drugs must be available to counter anaphylactic reactions. Further antivenom therapy may be required over 5–6 days to control the bleeding tendency during blood component therapy, as indicated by repeated coagulation studies.

References

1. Havard CWH (1977) Use of cobra venom in experimental myasthenia gravis. Br Med J i:1008

2. Reitz CJ (1979) Poisonous South African snakes. Department of Health, Pretoria, p 53
3. Sutherland W (1979) Absorption of elapid venom. Lancet I:1078
4. Visser J Chapman DS (1978) Snakes and snakebite. Purnell, London, p 12
5. White JAM Goodwin NM (1979) Resuscitation manual. Natal Blood Transfusion Service, Pinetown, Natal, section 15

Section H

Neurological Disorders

Chapter 42

Coma

Marialuisa Bozza-Marrubini

Definitions

Coma, the 'deep sleep' of ancient Greeks, is currently defined in neurology as 'unarousable unresponsiveness' [120]. Other definitions are all centered on the abolition of consciousness and on defects in the arousal mechanisms (Table 42.1). In the care of critically ill patients the term 'coma' is commonly used in the broader sense of a disturbance in consciousness, with all its physiopathological consequences. "Impaired or decreased consciousness reflects severe brain dysfunction, and coma means *brain failure* [our italics], just as uremia means renal failure" [120].

Coma defined as brain failure is a concept that is most appropriately used in the identification of cerebral pathological conditions requiring resuscitation and intensive care. "Brain failure . . . [is] an uncompensated cerebral disturbance of self-regulating mechanisms which leads to loss of body homeostasis" [79]. The concept implies that the brain is the central regulatory system of all vital functions; that such a system may also fail in cases with disturbances in consciousness that are not coma in a neurological sense.

Brain failure is both the starting point and the final link of a vicious circle in which impairment of consciousness for whatever reason—trauma, disease, or poison—leads to failure of

Table 42.1. Definitions of coma

1. The absence of any psychologically understandable response to external stimulus or inner need (Medical Research Council Brain Injuries Committee 1941; Rowbotham [133])
2. A state of prolonged unconsciousness from which it is difficult or impossible to rouse a person due to disease, injury, poison, etc. (The American College Dictionary. Random House, New York, 1952)
3. Coma is a complete loss of consciousness from which one cannot be aroused by various stimuli (Encyclopaedia Britannica, 1959)
4. A distinguishing characteristic of coma . . . is that external stimulation fails to produce arousal (Fazekas and Alman [52])
5. Coma designates states in which psychological and motor responses to stimulation are either completely lost (deep coma) or reduced to only rudimentary reflex responses (moderately deep coma) (Plum and Posner [120])
6. A state of complete loss of consciousness from which a patient cannot be aroused even by powerful stimulation (Dorland's Illustrated Medical Dictionary 25th edn. Saunders, Philadelphia London, 1974)
7. Sleeplike, unarousable unresponsiveness, without evidence of psychological awareness of self or environment (Bates et al. [5])
8. Typical features of coma are the abolition both of consciousness and of behavioural arousal (Masson and Henin [98])
9. A state of complete loss of consciousness from which the patient cannot be aroused by ordinary stimuli . . . a state of complete unresponsiveness to the environment (De Jong [46])

the vital functions, and this in turn may aggravate brain failure or even be the direct cause of brain damage.

The basic treatment of coma is designed to prevent or break this vicious circle; this outlook represents a challenge for the theory and practice of intensive care. Doctors treating patients in coma must have a wide knowledge of the physiology and pathology of the nervous system; they are called upon to solve difficult problems in diagnosis, evaluation of severity, and prediction of the outcome; therapy involves both the correction of the cause of coma and the support of vital functions; in many instances the latter is the only treatment possible.

Physiopathology

"Full conscious behaviour depends on the physiological interaction between arousal systems located in a normal brain stem and the extensive neuronal population of the intact cerebral hemispheres" [119]. Functional or anatomical disruption of this physiological interaction leads to changes in the conscious state ranging from minimal reduction of the contents of consciousness to deep coma. According to Plum and Posner [120], therefore, the pathological processes that impair consciousness are:

Conditions that lead to extensive cortical lesions or to diffuse neuronal or synaptic depression of the cerebral hemispheres;

Conditions that depress or destroy the ascending reticular activating system of the diencephalon, the midbrain, and the upper part of the pons.

A wide spectrum of specific causes may lead to coma or progressing defects of consciousness. The most common diagnoses in patients admitted to an ICU in coma are head injury, brain tumour, stroke, subarachnoid haemorrhage, and some of the secondary metabolic encephalopathies [120], i.e., meningitis and encephalitis, exogenous poisoning, metabolic, and hypoxic/ischaemic encephalopathy. All the factors leading to coma impair neural activity in the crucial areas of the brain through one or more of the following pathological mechanisms:

1) Changes in the turnover and balance of central chemical neurotransmitters;
2) Changes in neuronal metabolic activity due to: exogenous and endogenous toxins; O_2 lack; cerebral blood flow changes uncoupling perfusion from tissue metabolic demands; lack of substrate; abnormalities of ionic, osmolar and acid–base environment of the CNS; primary cell membrane damage with cytotoxic oedema (free-radical reactions, toxins);
3) Destruction of neurones and axons by mechanical forces, by viral and bacterial invasion or by mechanisms listed under 2).

A major common pathway of the different mechanisms underlying coma is the interference with the O_2 supply to the nervous tissue.

Neuronal hypoxia may be caused not only by any type of general or focal hypoxia or ischaemia, but also by perfusion defects and non-homogeneities resulting from intracranial hypertension, brain oedema, no-reflow *after* temporary ischaemia, loss of autoregulation and CO_2 reactivity. Hypoxia leads, in sequence, to a shift to anaerobic glycolysis, a block in energy-producing processes, a block in biosynthetic and osmotic cellular work, and tissue acidosis and hyperosmolarity.

These events provoke most of the mechanisms listed above, neurotransmitter changes, perfusion defects, oedema and neuronal death, representing steps of progressive and eventually irreversible damage.

Clinical examination

The clinical examination of a comatose patient must include:

1) Assessment of the functional conditions of the respiratory and circulatory systems with correction *as first priority* of any deficit menacing brain oxygenation and perfusion. In coma the dangerous lower limits of hypoxia and hypotension may be very near normal readings;
2) A general physical examination, complemented by specific laboratory data, to reveal any relevant extracranial pathology;
3) A neurological examination to identify the cause of coma (not treated here) and to obtain basic information on the patient's initial condition so that changes with time or in response to therapy can be judged.

Step 3 can be accomplished correctly only if the confusing effects on neural activity caused by changes in the vital functions are eliminated (see step 1); the possible effects of alcohol [120, 134] taken before the onset of coma or of drugs given in the early stages of treatment are duly taken into account; and other non-responsive states than coma, such as psychogenic unresponsiveness or a locked-in syndrome, are ruled out.

The neurological examination of a patient in coma is much simpler than the full neurological examination, because the patient's co-operation is absent or reduced to a few rudimentary motor responses. Indeed, in comatose states very few relevant data are available. The majority are based on the patient's responses to three sets of stimuli, i.e., acoustic/verbal, pain, and the specific stimuli required to elicit the ocular and pupillary reflexes.

Table 42.2 presents a neurological profile, partly derived from recent work [5, 153], and consisting of five categories of observations. For each category the observations and responses are graded approximately from best to worst.

Table 42.2. Neurological examination of comatose patients

Spontaneous motor activity	
Normal	Seeking and changing comfortable positions and sleep postures
	Eye opening, blinking and orientating gaze
Absent	(Test for motor responses)
Pathological	Tremors, myoclonus
	Choreo-athetosis
	Focal convulsions
	Generalized convulsions
	Status epilepticus
	Extensor spasms, opisthotonus
Responses	
Verbal	Orientated speech
	Confused conversation
	Inappropriate speech
	Incomprehensible sounds
	No speech
Motor	Obeying commands
	Localizing pain
	Withdrawing from pain
	Abnormal flexion
	Abnormal extension
	None
Reflexes	
Pupillary to light (photomotor reflex)	Present
	Sluggish or doubtful
to pain (ciliospinal reflex)	Absent
Vestibulo-ocular (cold caloric test)	Normal (rapid nystagmus toward non-irrigated ear)
	Tonic conjugate (toward irrigated ear)
	Dysconjugate or minimal
	None

Some relate to the conscious state and are needed to mark the end-point between consciousness and coma both in an initially worsening patient and during recovery. The terms used to describe the motor responses have been carefully tested and selected among synonyms as having unequivocal meanings for a wide range of observers [153, 155].

Although the clinical and prognostic significance of the observations and responses differs according to the cause of coma, the neurological profile in Table 42.2 is valid in any type of coma and can be used as a basis for any type of classification.

Classification

A classification system is required for coma

1) To assess initial severity and compare it with subsequent progress and outcome
2) To evaluate the response to treatment and to guide further treatments
3) To compare different treatments and to compare results from different centres
4) To select features that may be of prognostic significance.

The coma classifications proposed in the last 20 years can be schematically divided into two groups: coma scales and scoring systems, each reflecting a basic difference in the approach to the problem. The coma scales are based on synthesis, since the neurological symptoms, which are assumed to be related, are combined into abstract wholes, the coma levels. The scoring systems, on the contrary, are analytic; the symptoms are all assumed to be independent and are accordingly considered and scored separately [20a].

Coma scales

Coma, together with minor impairment of consciousness, is classified in different 'levels', 'degrees', 'stages', or 'grades'; each level is characterized by a fixed constellation of more or less clearly defined neurological signs to form a scale, with steps indicating progressive brain dysfunction. In some instances [4, 27] the scale follows anatomical–clinical correlations, usually derived from the rostral–caudal deterioration syndrome described by Plum and Posner [120]. Some examples of the coma scales proposed are schematically presented in Table 42.3, to dem-

Table 42.3. Coma scales

Clinical signs	Rowbotham [133]	Reed et al. [126]	Mollaret and Goulon [105]	Bozza–Marrubini [18]	Matthew and Lawson [99]	Subczynsky [152]	Bricolo et al. [27]	Barge et al. [4]	Cooper et al. [44] (Grady modification)	Obrist [112]
Year	1949	1952	1959	1961	1967	1975	1975	1978	1979	1979
Awake	Mild or moderate confusion	0	Coma vigile [coma vigil]	1		10	Hemispheric syndrome	Corticosubcortical syndrome	0–1	1
Arousable by voice; answering questions					I	9–6			2	2
Obeying orders	Severe confusion			2		8–7				
Responses to painful stimulation:	Semi-coma		Coma typique [typical coma state]	3	II	5	Diencephalic syndrome (pupillary reflex +; cold caloric test (c.c.t.), conjugate deviation)		3	3
Localizing (purposeful)					III					
Withdrawal (semi-purposeful)		1				4		Diencephalic syndrome (pupillary and ocular reflexes ++)		
Abnormal flexion (decorticate rigidity, non-purposeful)				4		3	Uncal syndrome (anisocoria; c.c.t., dysconjugate deviation)		4 (Corneal and ocular reflexes – –)	4
Abnormal extension (decerebrate rigidity)		2	Coma carus [deep coma]	5 Pupillary reflex + / 6 Pupillary reflex –		2	Mesencephalo-pontine syndrome (pupillary reflex sluggish or absent; c.c.t., dysconjugate deviation)	Diencephalo-mesencephalic syndrome (pupillary and ocular reflexes ++) Mesencephalic syndrome (pupillary and ocular reflexes –)		
No response	Coma Deep tendon reflex and corneal reflex + or –	3 Reflexes –	Coma dépassé [brain death]	7 Both pupils fixed	IV		Bulbar syndrome (pupillary and ocular reflexes –)	Bulbar (reflexes –)	5 (Reflexes –)	
Severe insufficiency of vital functions and of autonomic responses		4				1	Coma dépassé (pupillary and ocular reflexes –)			

reflexes: present + absent –

onstrate that despite the ample differences in the number of levels or degrees, some end-points between successive levels are remarkably similar.

Table 42.3 shows also that some scales are too simple overlooking important differences either at the deeper or at the lighter levels of coma; while others are too detailed and complicated, with frequent overlapping of relevant clinical signs between two or more levels. In the Bozza-Marrubini scale [18, 19] (Fig. 42.1) progressive impairments of consciousness are classified in seven levels. True coma is represented from level three onwards; the difference between one level and the next is marked by the presence or absence of an objective neurological symptom. The steps indicating each level are: *speech* in answer to verbal stimuli (level 1); ability to *obey simple orders* (level 2); *response to pain*: *localization* (level 3); *flexion without localization* (level 4); *bilateral extension*, with ocular and pupillary reflexes still *present* at least on one side (level 5); abnormal extension or flexion and *bilateral abolition of ocular and pupillary reflexes* (level 6); and *no response*, with ocular and pupillary areflexia, apnoea, circulatory collapse, poikilothermia and polyuria (level 7, coma dépassé).

Coma scales have a number of limitations. Each scale is specific for a given type of coma. In addition, the continuum of responsiveness, ranging from full consciousness to deep coma, is split into and reduced to a static pigeon-hole system, and focal signs and other localising differences are not taken into account. Scoring systems (Table 42.4) have been devised to overcome these drawbacks.

Scoring systems

Each category of neurological signs considered relevant is explored independently; the type of response is evaluated following a hierarchy of progressive functional impairments and is accordingly graded by a numerical score.

Jouvet was the first to devise a coma classification based on a scoring system [75, 76], four categories of responses being explored: perceptivity (P), aspecific reactivity (R) to a verbal stimulus, motor reactivity (D), and autonomic responses (V) to pain. The result is a variable ranging between P1, R1, D1, V1 (indicating full consciousness) and P5, R3, D4, V2 (corresponding to global unresponsiveness).

A similar approach has been adopted by Overgaard et al. [115], by Goulon [60], in the code system by Ommaya and Sadowsky [113],

and in the Munich Coma Scale [30]. These systems differ mainly in the number of functions explored, the most extensive and accurate being Goulon's classification, while in the Munich Coma Scale the main concern is with using measurable stimuli.

The most widely accepted classification currently available is the Glasgow Coma Scale [153], which, like the Munich one, is in fact a scoring system, despite its name. Three different aspects of behavioural response are examined: eye opening, best motor response, and verbal response. Each response is given a number (high for normal and low for impaired response) so that (see Table 42.4) if the figures given for a patient are added up, numbers ranging between 3 and 15 express the patient's responsiveness. The scores obtained for each behavioural response can also be recorded on a time graph, together with other variables, such as pupillary size and reactivity, ocular reflexes, differences between left and right, intracranial pressure (ICP), and vital signs (see for instance charts devised by Marsh et al. [93] and by Marshall [94]).

This aspect of the Glasgow system is particularly valuable. A coma scale can provide only single 'snapshots' of the patient's status but, since coma is not a static but a dynamic condition, the information thus obtained is insufficient and fragmentary. With the Glasgow Coma Scale a most successful attempt has been made to obtain a dynamic record of the comatose patient's condition, i.e., to transform the snapshot into a film. A similar approach was used in Bouzarth's 'neurosurgical watch sheet' [17].

The Glasgow Coma Scale was originally developed mainly for the study of brain injuries; Bates et al. [5] have extended its use to non-traumatic coma by increasing the number of functions explored from three to eleven.

Outcome scales

As well as the coma scale, the Glasgow workers developed a practical scale for the assessment of outcome after severe brain damage [71, 72]. The five exclusive outcome categories of the scale are:

1) *Death*, with an indication of the need to subcategorize deaths occurring after patients have regained consciousness;
2) *Persistent vegetative state*, to describe patients who remain unresponsive and speechless for weeks or months until death;

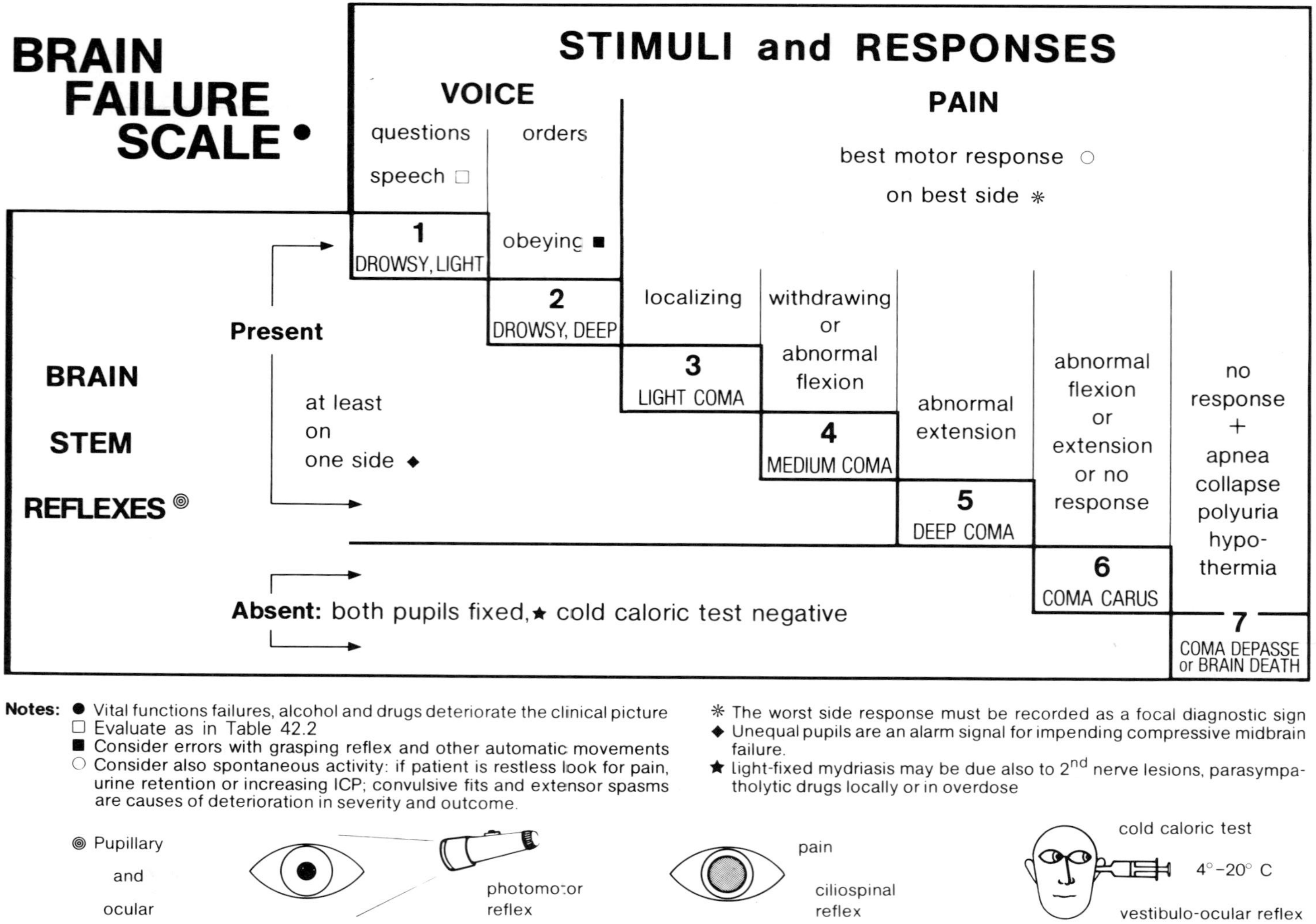

BRAIN FAILURE SCALE ●

STIMULI and RESPONSES

VOICE

questions □ speech
orders
best motor response ○
on best side ✳

PAIN

Present

1 DROWSY, LIGHT

obeying ■

2 DROWSY, DEEP

localizing

3 LIGHT COMA

withdrawing
or
abnormal
flexion

4 MEDIUM COMA

abnormal
extension

5 DEEP COMA

abnormal
flexion
or
extension
or no
response

6 COMA CARUS

no
response
+
apnea
collapse
polyuria
hypo-
thermia

7 COMA DEPASSE
or BRAIN DEATH

BRAIN STEM REFLEXES ◎

Present at least on one side ◆

Absent: both pupils fixed, ★ cold caloric test negative

both pupils fixed, ★ cold caloric test negative

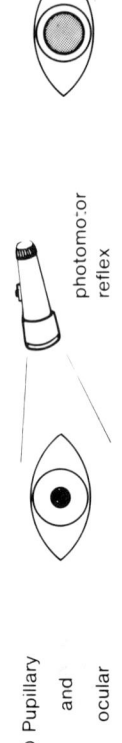

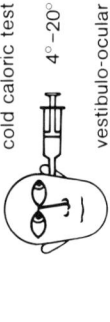

pupillary
and
ocular

photomo-or
reflex

pain
ciliospinal
reflex

cold caloric test
4°–20° C

vestibulo-ocular reflex

Notes:
● Vital functions failures, alcohol and drugs deteriorate the clinical picture
□ Evaluate as in Table 42.2
■ Consider errors with grasping reflex and other automatic movements
○ Consider also spontaneous activity: if patient is restless look for pain, urine retention or increasing ICP: convulsive fits and extensor spasms are causes of deterioration in severity and outcome.

✳ The worst side response must be recorded as a focal diagnostic sign
◆ Unequal pupils are an alarm signal for impending compressive midbrain failure.
★ Light-fixed mydriasis may be due also to 2nd nerve lesions, parasympatholytic drugs locally or in overdose

◎ Pupillary and ocular

Fig. 42.1. Bozza-Marrubini brain failure scale.

Table 42.4. Scoring systems

Jouvet (1961, 1969)		Overgaard et al. (1973)	
Function explored	Score	Function explored	Score
	1 2 3 4 5	*Consciousness levels* (C):	
Perceptivité [perceptivity] (P):		Awake	C I
Ordre écrit [written instruction]	+ − − − −	Somnolent	C II
Orientation [orientation]	+ + − − −	Semi-coma or sopor	C III
Ordre verbal [spoken instruction]	+ + + − −	Coma	C IV
Clignement à la menace [eyelid flicker on threat]	+ + + + −		
Réactivité non spécifique [non-specific reactivity] (R):		*Motor pattern* (M):	
Orientation [orientation]	+ + −	Normal coordination	M 1
Éveil [arousal]	+ − −	Typical decerebrate rigidity	M 2
		Atypical decerebrate rigidity	M 3
Réactivité motrice à la douleur [motor response to pain] (D):		Hypotonia	M 4
Mimique [signs]	+ − − −		
Eveil [arousal]	+ + − −	*Pupillary reflexes* (OD):	
Retrait [withdrawal]	+ + + −		Present +
			Absent −
Réactivité végétative [vegetative reactivity] (V):			
Respiration [breathing]	+ −		
Vasomotricité [vasomotor tone]	+ −		
Rithme cardiaque [cardiac rhythm]	+ −		
Pupilles [pupillary response]	+ −		

Score range (from full consciousness [x]	x	P1	R1	D1	V1	x	C I	M1	OD+
to deep coma [xx])	xx	P5	R3	D4	V2	xx	C IV	M4	OD−

Table 42.4. Scoring systems (continued)

Glasgow Coma Scale (Teasdale and Jennett 1974) Function explored	Score	Munich Coma Scale (Brinkmann, et al. 1976) Function explored	Score	Goulon et al. (1977) Function explored	Score
Eyes		*Susceptibility to stimulation*		*Reaction to nociceptive stimuli*	
Open:				I Adaptive reaction	1
Spontaneously	4	No response to any stimulus	0	II Inappropriate reaction	2
On spoken command	3	Response to:		III No reaction; spontaneous	
On pain	2	Electrical stimulus (E)		respiration preserved	4
No response	1	electric shocks, 1–10 mA,		*EEG reactivity*	
Best motor response		600–1200 V, 5 s	1	I To sound	1
To spoken command: obeys	6	Tactile stimulus (T)		II Only to pinching	4
To painful stimulus:		nylon hair, diameter		III Non-reactive	4
Localizes pain	5	0.05 mm 30 s	2	*Mydriasis* and absence of	
Flexion withdrawal	4	Acoustic stimulus (A)		spontaneous reflex eye	
Flexion, abnormal	3	siren g d B, 300–1000 Hz,		movements	
(decorticate rigidity)		20 s, 30 cm from ear	3	No	0
Extension	2	Optical stimulus (O)		Yes	2
(decerebrate rigidity)		flashlight 6000 Lux,		*Decerebration signs*	
No response	1	10 flashes in 1 s,		No	0
Best verbal response		10 cm from eyes	4	Yes	2
Oriented and converses	5	*Reactivity* (to the above stimuli)		*Autonomic signs*	
Disoriented and converses	4	No reaction	0	No	0
Inappropriate words	3	Motor	1	Yes	2
Incomprehensible sounds	2	Signs	2	*Convulsions*	
No response	1	Orientation	3	No	0
		Communication	4	Yes	1

Score range	x 15		x 4–4		x 2
	xx 3		xx 0–0		xx 15

3) *Severe disability*, to describe patients who are dependent for daily support by reason of mental and/or physical disability (conscious but disabled); the patients who have recovered to the point where they can maintain self-care within their room or home should also be included in this group;

4) *Moderate disability*; this term is used to indicate patients who, even though suffering from varying degrees of speech, memory, intellectual, psychological, or motor deficits, are independent even outside their room or home insofar as daily life is concerned, i.e., disabled but independent;

5) *Good recovery*; patients recovering to this point resume a normal life within the family and their social group, even if they suffer from minor neurological or psychological deficits. Working activity is not considered an exclusive and reliable index of this type of recover, since return to work may be grossly influenced both in a positive and in a negative sense by local socio-economical circumstances.

The definition of the outcome categories also presupposes a definition of the time interval after which it can reasonably be assumed that no further change in the patient's conditions will occur. Bond [16] and Jennett et al. [74] demonstrated that after brain injury most of the recovery occurs in the first 6 months; this limit is shorter, 1 month, for non-traumatic coma [5].

Results

The improved general understanding arising from the increased use of uniform methods and of a common language in reports about coma has already led to some valuable results.

In the last 5 years many papers have been published, (a) presenting statistically significant data on mortality and outcome rates, (b) identifying reliable prognostic indices, and (c) comparing treatments in reports of correctly controlled clinical trials.

Provided the cases were described by clear and unequivocal criteria, the specific type of coma classification adopted was relatively unimportant. The use of the Glasgow Coma and Outcome Scales led to observations from different centres and from different countries being pooled to form fairly homogeneous patient populations [5, 74, 154]. But remarkably similar death and other outcome rates, and significant consistencies in severity and negative prognosis factors, were found even in series of patients classified by widely differing systems, such as the Glasgow and the Overgaard scoring systems and the Bozza-Marrubini and the Bricolo coma scales [6].

In contrast, Frowein [56] analyzing a number of reports on brain injuries in which no homogeneous criteria were used to define the patient population, found an 'extraordinary discrepancy' in the mortality rates.

Selection of coma scales and scoring systems

Experience gained in recent years suggests that coma scales and scoring systems must be used in different circumstances and for different purposes. Being synthetic, coma scales are most suitable for classification of cases into various levels of initial severity, especially when this classification is required to analyse statistical correlations with outcome scales.

For this purpose they cannot be replaced by the Glasgow scoring system; indeed, in comparison with coma scales the information given by the total score of the Glasgow coma scale is of limited value, since widely different clinical pictures can give the same final score [20a].

Scoring systems are especially valuable for recognizing the relative value of individual signs and of their combinations in predicting outcome; being numerical they are the ideal basis for sophisticated computer data processing. It has already been stated that scoring systems are at present the best method available for monitoring and recording the clinical course of all types of coma. They are also the only possible system for the classification of toxic coma. In toxic coma, constellations of unique clinical features do exist, but their main significance is diagnostic, i.e., they are typical for a specific poison. Evaluation of severity, of the clinical course, and of the result of treatments can be obtained only by scoring all the relevant clinical signs separately by using a suitable variant of the scoring systems described.

Prognosis

In recent years, the thrust of clinical research has been increasingly directed towards statistical evaluation of outcome rates and their earliest possible prediction. The psychological and socio-economical causes of this trend have been repeatedly pointed out [40, 80b].

Many experts believe that the expensive and

necessarily limited resources of ICUs and of rehabilitation services should not be deployed for prolonged treatment of patients who remain permanently unconscious until they eventually die. Withdrawal of artificial life-support systems in such 'hopeless' cases is a major ethical and medical problem [60]. Although the discussion of this issue lies outside the scope of this chapter, it must nonetheless be pointed out that the first and most important step in determination of prognosis at present seems to be the earliest possible identification of patients in whom the outlook is hopeless, however well they are cared for.

Severity factors and negative prognostic indices

No single neurological sign has an absolute value in prognosis.

Ocular reflexes

The most powerful predictive index is the oculovestibular reflex; its absence is associated with a very high rate of unfavourable outcomes (death, persistent vegetative state, or severe disability) in all the types of coma considered [5, 28, 70, 73, 74, 86, 87, 121]. This test is more reliable than the oculocephalic test since the caloric response may be preserved when the oculocephalic reflexes are lost [31]. According to Poulsen and Zilstorff [123], in brain injuries a definite relationship can be found between progressive impairment of this reflex response and the type of outcome. These workers also point out that in the first 20–24 h of coma the oculovestibular reflex pattern shows a high variability, stabilizing only 1–3 days after injury; a single caloric test is then of reliable prognostic value.

The length of the reflex response suppression is certainly a very important factor, but this point has been neglected by most workers; only Plum and Caronna [121] and Bates et al. [5] state that in non-traumatic coma persistent abolition of the oculovestibular response *for 24 h to 3 days* implies a grave prognosis (death or persistent vegetative state in 97%–100% of such cases).

Pupillary reflexes

Pupillary reflexes have practically the same value as the caloric test; for the correct evaluation of the prognostic significance of their suppression the time factor is of paramount importance; according to Bozza-Marrubini [19] the prolonged bilateral abolition of the light reflex (provided hypoxia and shock with adrenergic hyperactivity have been corrected and autonomic effects of drugs or lesions of the 2nd and 3rd cranial nerves have been excluded) is a certain sign of irreversible coma.

The period of observation required to reach a completely reliable prognosis is limited to a few hours following postanoxic encephalopathy or stroke, and may be as long as 7–10 days for brain injuries. Bates et al. [5] and Price and Knill-Jones [124] specify a 3-day interval, after which persisting absence of the photomotor reflex leaves no hope of good recovery or only moderate disability. The statistical evaluation made in 1000 cases of brain injuries by the Glasgow team [70] and a long-term study by Levin et al. [86] seem to suggest a higher prognostic value of the ocular reflexes than the pupillary light reflex. Unfortunately, these workers also failed to take account of the time factor in reflex response impairment.

Extensor spasms and rigidity

So-called decerebration—the presence of spontaneous or provoked bilateral extensor spasm and/or rigidity of limbs and trunk—has been associated in the past with virtual certainty of a fatal outcome in any type of coma.

Recent reports demonstrate that at least one in four patients with brain injuries presenting this sign may survive, and at least one in ten may even regain consciousness with minimal or no permanent disability, provided pupillary and/or ocular reflexes are retained. The outlook is much better in young people (under 20), and especially in children [6, 28, 74, 87, 115, 132, 159].

In other types of coma, e.g., postanoxic encephalopathy or stroke, this may be a much more negative sign; in all cases, however, its negative prognostic significance increases with time, patients with brain injuries and extensor responses lasting more than 2 weeks seldom surviving without severe disabilities. In non-traumatic coma Bates et al. [5] found that of patients with extensor posturing 24 h after the onset of coma fewer than 8% achieved moderate disability or good recovery. This sign, however, can no longer be considered by itself a sure index of irreversible brain stem damage [28]; as a prognostic sign, it is of lesser importance than ocular and pupillary reflexes.

Other motor responses

Of the other abnormal motor responses, abnormal flexion has a limited predictive value, while the absence of any response is followed by death or persistent vegetative state in over 90% of cases.

Age

Age by itself has no absolute predictive value [121]; mortality due to the primary cerebral lesion seems to be independent of age [34]; but extracerebral complications of coma and their related mortality increase progressively with age.

Duration of coma

The length of coma is a critical factor in non-traumatic coma: Bates et al. [5] state that most of their 310 patients were either awake or dead within a week. In postanoxic encephalopathy a 3-day coma is the maximum compatible with chances of recovery without severe disability. Patients who are awake or at least have localizing motor responses to pain within 1 h after resuscitation from cardiac arrest have a 100% probability of full neuropsychical recovery [162]. The chances of good recovery steadily fall with increasing duration of coma, being less than 10% for patients remaining in coma more than 6 and less than 24 h, and becoming practically zero for postanoxic–ischaemic comas lasting over 24–48 h [5, 7, 147, 156].

Early treatment of patients resuscitated after cardiac arrest with high doses of barbiturates [22, 107] hampers the evaluation of this factor, even if continuous EEG or CFM recording makes it possible to monitor the drug effects.

The length of post-traumatic coma is also linked with the chances of recovery but on a much longer time-scale; therefore, this time factor is of very limited value for early prediction of outcome in brain injuries.

Combined factors

The possibility of early and correct prediction is greatly increased if the most significant factors are considered together.

Many reports point to a combination of abnormal motor posturing, impaired or absent ocular reflexes, and bilateral absence of the pupillary light responses as having a strongly adverse significance. Yet, both Becker et al. [6]

and Bruce et al. [31] state that 15%–45% of patients with this adverse combination of signs may still make a good recovery or be only moderately disabled. This statement may be misleading: a higher proportion of positive results has been observed in children, in whom, as already stated by Carlsson et al. [34] and by Bruce et al. [31], cerebrovascular changes and brain swelling with little or no parenchymal damage may give clinical signs so severe as to suggest brain stem damage or diffuse brain injury. The lower mortality and better outcome in children in relation to the clinical signs could thus be merely apparent. In adults the reported favourable outcomes [6, 23] have occurred as a rule in patients with transient vascular changes or with mass lesions promptly operated upon. Indeed, in the same report by Becker et al. [6], of ten patients with this adverse combination of signs and *without mass lesion*, eight died and two survived either severely disabled or in a persistent vegetative state.

Time course of adverse signs

It must be emphasized again that the prognostic significance of adverse signs and of their combinations can be fully appreciated only if their time course is duly taken into account. For instance, in patients with mass lesions leading to severe neurological signs, immediate operation is the rule and this, besides radically changing the intracranial condition, may lead to prompt regression of the worst signs.

Obviously, the same prognostic value cannot be attributed to a combination of signs lasting a short time and regressing after correction of their cause and to the same signs persisting a long time and unresponsive to any treatment.

Effectiveness and accuracy of outcome predictions

The existence of combinations of signs having strong prognostic significance may explain why predictions based on the use of coma scales may have about the same *effectiveness* (defined by Jennett [70] as the proportion of patients for whom outcome can be confidently predicted) as those obtained by computer processing of data given by scoring systems. Indeed, by use of the Glasgow scoring system coupled with Bayesian probability statistics [74] in a series of 600 cases it was possible to distinguish between a poor outcome (dead or vegetative) and a more favourable one (severely disabled or better) in

60% of patients 2–3 days after the onset of traumatic coma and in 68% 4–7 days after the onset of coma; over 90% of these predictions were correct and most of the errors were optimistic [70].

Using the Bozza-Marrubini coma scale and observing the coma levels during the first 3 days after a brain injury, Levati [85] and Bozza-Marrubini et al. [20a] were able to distinguish the same two outcomes in 71% and in 100% of two different groups of 100 consecutive cases. In both studies 90% of the predictions were correct at 6 months. No pessimistic errors were made. Some optimistic errors were due to patients who succumbed to extracranial complications after having recovered consciousness. Obrist et al. [112] found that with 36 cases with head injuries the Glasgow Scoring System and a simple four-step coma scale were equally effective in predicting outcome.

Additional data assisting prognosis

The above data show that an early and correct prediction of outcome, if based on clinical signs only, is possible in a high proportion of individual cases but *not in all*. To increase the effectiveness and the accuracy of prediction it therefore seems necessary to complete the information given by the clinical signs with prognostically significant additional data.

Some changes in physiological variables recorded during coma due to brain injury have been shown to be correlated with poor outcomes: arterial hypertension [115] or hypotension [132], spontaneous hyperventilation and hyperthermia [159], low arterial PO_2 persisting despite respirator treatment [128, 132].

Intracranial pressure monitoring

Intracranial pressure (ICP) monitoring may be a guide to therapy in brain injuries, but there is no general agreement about its prognostic value: a high ICP has been considered a poor prognostic sign by Vapalahti and Troupp [161] and by Langfitt [81], especially when combined with signs of midbrain dysfunction [43], but the reverse (normal ICP = good prognosis) is not true and the researchers mentioned are agreed that the level of ICP has no constant relation with a specific outcome.

Recently Pitts et al. [118], however, have found a good correlation between ICP and outcome in their series of severe brain injuries.

According to Fleisher et al. [55] a positive response to specific antihypertensive treatments does not change the bad prognostic significance of an initially high ICP, while Rockoff et al. [127] and Bruce et al. [32] believe that a good outcome can be expected when a stable reduction of ICP is obtained.

Cerebral blood flow

Cerebral blood flow, although positively correlated with the level of consciousness, seems to have little value in predicting outcome in brain injuries owing to wide variations in initial measures [112].

Although Langfitt [81] suggested the inclusion of a set of criteria given by CT scan among data to be recorded for the comparison of brain injuries, to date the prognostic value of such criteria has not been studied in any type of coma, with the single exception of acute CO poisoning. Sawada et al. [137] have shown that in patients poisoned by CO, detection by CT scan of bilateral areas of low density in the globus pallidus is an early and reliable index of poor outcome.

Electroencephalograph

The EEG, a 'final common denominator' of cerebral perfusion and oxygenation, continuously reflects changes in cortical function and should therefore be the most comprehensive and reliable index of cerebral state in unconscious patients [37, 126]. Its value in prognosis has been the subject of much debate, however.

Visual rating scales of single EEG recordings repeated during the first 12 h of coma were found to be a good index of the chances of survival or death both in adults and in children resuscitated after cardiac arrest, with an accuracy in the order of 80% [116].

The application of discriminant function techniques to a system of EEG assessment and coding by a high number of variables increased the accuracy of prediction in the same type of patients to a confidence level better than 99.8% [13, 125]. A similar method enabled Thomassen et al. [157] to estimate with a fair degree of accuracy the length of survival of patients in coma after cardiac arrest. In other types of structural brain damage single and short-term EEG recordings seem of little value.

Besides high-voltage delta activity, the most frequent pattern recorded during coma, a whole series of other abnormal wave forms can be observed, including a rhythmic activity of low amplitude within the alpha range ('alpha coma'), which can be distinguished from the pattern obtained in normal waking subjects only by the absence of response to any stimulus [53, 88, 140]. Attempts to classify these polymorphous patterns failed to give reliable prognostic criteria, so that many clinicians were led to believe that EEG studies had no place in the assessment of comatose states. Polygraphic studies [8, 9, 25, 26, 36] however, yielded evidence that *continuous* EEG recording could provide much information of relevant prognostic value. In particular, the maintenance or early return of typical sleep patterns could be correlated with a favourable prognosis and quick recovery, while 'biphasic' or 'monophasic' activity unidentifiable with sleep implied severe cerebral damage. The EEG pattern was especially valuable in evaluating the chances of recovery of patients with clinical signs of midbrain dysfunction (mesencephalic syndrome, [3, 4, 27]), a condition generally considered of very uncertain prognosis.

These studies, however, did not lead to the routine use of EEG monitoring in ICUs until recent technical developments enabled the clinician to overcome the well-known drawbacks and difficulties of conventional EEG recording and interpretation.

The cerebral function monitor (CFM) has been gradually introduced into clinical practice since 1971: it is a small portable apparatus with only two recording electrodes, which gives a filtered and compressed single-channel trace at 6–30 cm/h, and is therefore suitable for recordings lasting hours, days, and even longer.

Clean records indicating voltage and variability of cerebral electrical activity can be obtained in the electrically hostile environment of the ICU without interfering with the usual nursing and therapeutic procedures or with other types of monitoring. Artefacts are either automatically excluded or indicated on a separate trace. The interpretation of the records is simple to learn, even for doctors who are not EEG experts.

Prior [125, 125a] described typical features of CFM tracings in comatose patients (Fig. 42.2). The analysis of five key features of the tracing (steady, rising, falling, fluctuating, and reactive to stimuli) enable the clinician to add to any type of coma scale or scoring system information of high discriminatory power for diagnosis and early prediction of outcome in comatose patients.

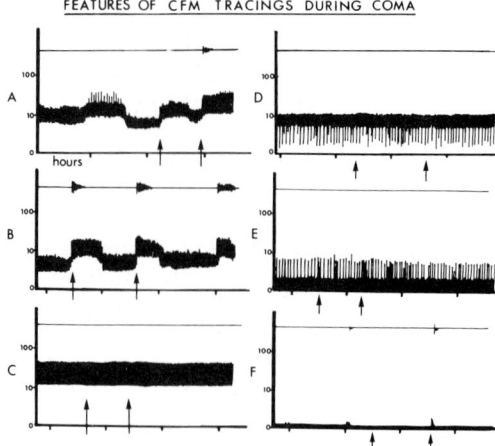

FEATURES OF CFM TRACINGS DURING COMA

Fig. 42.2. Diagrammatic representation of typical features of CFM tracings in comatose patients. *Arrows* indicate stimuli. A Smoothly fluctuating tracing with features resembling sleep changes and cerebral and scalp muscle responses to a stimulus; B Abrupt alterations in level, both stimulus-induced and spontaneous, with associated scalp muscle response; C Monotonous trace without response to stimuli; D Saw-tooth trace resembling a comb with the teeth pointing downwards zero; E Lower level saw-tooth trace with the lower level (minimum voltages present) at zero and resembling a comb with the teeth pointing upwards; F Sustained zero level tracing. Tracings of type A suggest a good outcome; B suggests brain stem dysfunction; C–F, all tracings with no fluctuation or any response to stimuli, are bad prognostic signs, except in drug-induced coma or profound hypothermia.

(Reproduced by kind permission of the Author and Editor from: P.F. Prior: Monitoring cerebral function. Elsevier/North Holland Biomedical Press, Amsterdam, 1979, p. 198.)

Personal experience [106] (Fig. 42.3) and further work in progress in the same hospital fully confirm Prior's assumptions for both traumatic and non-traumatic coma. In toxic coma awakening can be predicted long before the clinical signs show any favourable change; the same applies to coma due to brain injury (see Fig. 7.15 in Prior's book [125a]) and to postanoxic encephalopathy.

Other electrophysiological monitoring techniques, such as the Fast Fourier Transform of the EEG assembled into a compressed spectral array or the study of the brain stem evoked responses [29, 151], are still at a research and development stage. The use of these expensive, often computer-based and highly sophisticated monitoring systems is still confined to selected research centres. Their inclusion in the routine bedside assessment of coma therefore seems remote at present.

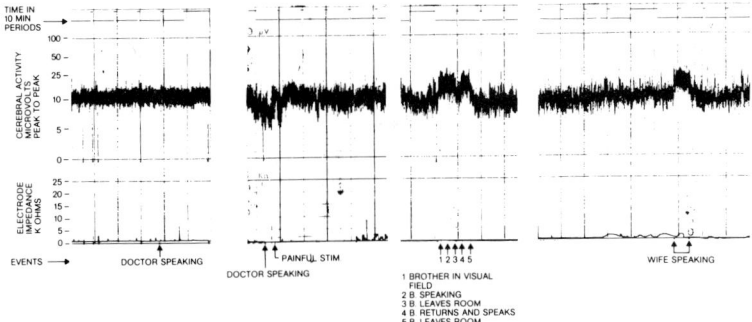

Fig. 42.3. Cerebral function monitor tracing in a 48-year-old man with a typical locked-in syndrome due to basilar artery thrombosis. While the neurological picture at first sight closely mimicked a deep unresponsive coma, the CFM trace showed reactivity to psychologically significant auditory and visual stimuli. Further neurophysiological studies demonstrated that the patient was conscious; during the course of his illness he also gained the ability to communicate with an eyelid code system.

Therapy

General and universally accepted principles

The general principles of treatment of coma are outlined in Table 42.5. These lines are followed in most centres with only minor differences on a few points, such as the use of prolonged nasotracheal intubation versus early tracheostomy.

The basic philosophy of intensive care is the correction and maintenance of body homeostasis. This principle means that correct intensive care for coma patients also implies the causal therapy of some secondary metabolic encephalopathies, as hypoglycaemic, hyper- or hypo-osmolar coma, keto-acidotic coma, hypercapnic coma and the like.

Points debated

In the last 20 years a number of therapeutic procedures have been proposed as adjuncts to the general supportive care of coma (Table 42.6). Most of them are based on recent knowledge of brain biochemistry and circulation in the different pathological conditions underlying coma. And for most of them there is

Table 42.5. General principles of management in comatose patients

1. Prevent respiratory obstruction and pulmonary complications by:
   Positioning of patient and chest physiotherapy
   Artificial airways
   Efficient and sterile humidification of inhaled gases
   Frequent oropharyngeal and tracheobronchial toilet
   Controlled ventilation or CPAP
   Point debated: prolonged nasotracheal intubation versus early tracheostomy

2. Monitor and maintain 'optimal' blood gas levels by O_2 therapy and/or artificial ventilation
   Points debated: Definition of 'optimal' blood gas levels in brain failure and indications of hyperoxia and hypocapnia;
           Management of spontaneous hyperventilation (see Table 43.6 and discussion in text)

3. Monitor and maintain MAP within optimal range for brain perfusion by:
   Blood volume expansion with appropriate fluids
   Dopamine infusion to correct non-hypovolemic hypotension
   Clonidine 150–300 µg to correct hypertensive crises

4. Monitor and maintain normal body temperature by:
   Antipyretics (acetylsalicilic acid, aminophenazone 10–20 mg/kg
   Vasodilating drugs (chlorpromazine 0.2–0.5 mg/kg: beware of hypotension/tachycardia)
   Surface cooling (for discussion of artificial hypothermia see text)

5. Monitor and maintain water–electrolyte balance and caloric protein intake according to intensive care standards
   Haemodilution may improve brain microcirculation
   A moderately negative water balance may contribute to reduction of ICP

6. Sedate:
   Restlessness with benzodiazepines (first exclude/treat rising ICP, urine retention, pain, respiratory insufficiency)
   Convulsive fits with barbiturates   } in resistant cases also
   Extensor spasms with benzodiazepines } give muscle-blocking drugs
   Maladaptation to respirator with diazepam, meperidine, phentanyl, barbiturates, curarization

Table 42.6. Therapeutic procedures aiming at correction of specific cerebral pathologic mechanisms

1. Neurotransmitter changes
   Physostigmine in central anticholinergic syndrome
   Diazepam, barbiturates in central cathecholamine excess[a]
   L-Dopa in prolonged coma with decreased dopamine turnover[a]

2. Neuronal metabolic changes
   'Awakening' drugs[a]
   Hypocapnia (PaCO$_2$ 25–35 mmHg, 3,3–4,7 kPa) for tissue acidosis[a]
   Hyperoxia (PaO$_2$ 200–400 mmHg, 26, 7–53, 3 kPa) for reduced O$_2$ availability (oedema)[a]
   Glucose for lack of substrate
   Corticoids, barbiturates for free radical membrane damage[a]
   Hypocapnia, barbiturates for capillary flow inhomogeneity[a]

3. Increased ICP and brain oedema
   Exclude surgically treatable mass lesions VFP monitoring essential
   Corticoids in standard or mega-doses[a]
   Osmotic dehydration with 20% mannitol (or 10% glycerol) 1–10 ml/kg (serum osmolality not >330 mosmol/litre)
   Diuretics (frusemide 0.5–1.5 mg/kg, max. 10 mg/kg per 24 h)
   Ventricular CSF drainage
   Hypocapnia (PaCO$_2$ not < 20 mmHg, 2, 7 kPa)[a]
   Barbiturates, alphaxolone–alphadolone (monitor EEG and plasma levels)[a]

4. Toxic neuronal or synaptic load
   Specific therapy (e.g. naloxone in opiate poisoning; neomicine to reduce hyperammoniaemia)
   Special depuration procedures: forced diuresis, peritoneal/haemodialysis, haemoperfusion (e.g., in barbiturate coma)

[a]Points debated: for discussion and drug doses see text

as yet no definite proof of their actual value in modifying the pathological process, the clinical course of coma, and its final outcome. As stated by Langfitt [82], published data suggest that the decrease in mortality from head injury in the last 50 years has been no more than 10%–15%, and this decrease may simply be due to the improvements in early and intensive care, including laboratory and instrumental diagnosis, monitoring, nursing and medical care in spe cially organized and equipped units. Similar considerations apply to any other type of coma. The special therapeutic approaches proposed differ from basic intensive care in being more or less 'aggressive' instead of simply supportive; many of them, in fact, imply a more or less substantial increase in risk and in the cost of an already highly sophisticated and complex treatment. Their value and indications must, therefore, be carefully evaluated. The most important recent contributions in this respect are summarized in Table 42.6 and some of them are discussed below.

'Awakening' drugs

The use of CNS stimulants and analeptics has long been obsolete, even in cases of poisoning by barbiturates and other CNS depressants.

No sound statistical evidence has been put forward to date for the claimed favourable effects in comatose states of other 'metabolic activating' drugs such as centrophenoxine (mec-

lofenoxate) or cytidine disphosphocholine [35, 50, 91]. In a single controlled clinical trial [19] centrophenoxine has been shown to have no useful activity. On the other hand, when coma is due to alteration in the turnover of brain neurotransmitters, specific pharmacological therapy has been demonstrated to be feasible and effective.

Physostigmine, an anticholinesterase crossing the blood–brain barrier, can reverse the neurological syndrome (coma, hallucinations and pathological motor activity) that results from an overdose of atropine or other belladonna drugs, phenothiazines, tricyclic antidepressants, and antihistamines [20] in a matter of minutes. The clinical results of treatment with the dopamine precursor L-dopa in prolonged coma and in the apallic syndrome have, however, been disappointing [2, 122].

Corticosteroids

Dexamethasone is currently used in almost all the coma states that are due to structural brain damage. The prevention or reduction of brain oedema is assumed to be the beneficial effect of corticosteroids.

Corticosteroid treatment of perifocal oedema associated with primary and metastatic tumours and with abscesses has proved so effective that, since its introduction, emergency surgery for sudden neurological deterioration and coma is seldom required. On the other hand, although corticosteroids are nearly always used in human brain injuries, stroke, and postanoxic and other secondary metabolic encephalopathies, no report has yet demonstrated that this treatment significantly improves the clinical course and the outcome in these conditions [141]. Demopoulos et al. [47] have given a theoretical explanation for this different activity.

Recent carefully controlled studies [44, 61, 117] have demonstrated that neither standard (0.4 mg/kg in first 24 h; 0.2 mg/kg/24 h for 6 days) nor mega-doses (2.5 mg/kg in first 24 h; 1.5 mg/kg/24 h for 6 days) of dexamethasone have an appreciably favourable influence on high ICP or on the clinical course and outcome of brain-injured patients.

Reviewing critically previous literature, Cooper et al. [44] also showed that the positive results claimed by other researchers, e.g., Gobiet et al. [57] and Faupel et al. [51] could not be maintained when careful statistical analysis was applied to the reported data. Similarly, both experimental and clinical studies failed to demonstrate that corticosteroids could alter the course of experimental ischaemic, cytotoxic or vasogenic brain oedema or that they could improve the clinical course of experimental ischaemic cerebral injury or of human ischaemic infarction [1, 65, 68]. The possible beneficial effects of mega-doses of corticosteroids in stroke has not yet been investigated.

An increased incidence of extracerebral complications (gastro-intestinal lesions, exacerbation of diabetes, infections) linked with the use of corticosteroids has been suspected, but not definitely demonstrated with either brain injuries or stroke [1, 44]. A recent necroscopy study on patients who died from cerebrovascular disease demonstrated a significantly higher incidence of gastro-intestinal lesions when corticosteroids had been used [114].

No definite data are available on the effectiveness of steroid treatment in metabolic coma and in encephalitis; some benefit may be obtained in Herpes simplex encephalitis [24].

Mechanical ventilation and hyperventilation

The use of mechanical artificial ventilation in comatose states at the earliest sign of pulmonary dysfunction, whether neurogenic or due to chest trauma, atelectasis, or infection, is now a generally accepted principle. This procedure can reduce mortality from early and delayed pulmonary complications, once the most frequent cause of extracerebral deaths in comatose states [92].

Brain injuries. Artificial *hyperventilation* with moderate hypocapnia [$PaCO_2$ 20–30 mmHg (2.7–4 kPa)] and high O_2 tension [PaO_2 above 120 mmHg (16 kPa)] was advocated by Rossanda [129, 130] and by Gordon [58, 59] as a therapeutic procedure that could directly improve the intracerebral status by increasing the O_2 supply to the nervous tissue, correct cerebral microcirculatory maldistribution and nervous tissue acidosis, and reduce ICP. Spontaneous hyperventilation, a phenomenon frequently observed in the course of coma, apparently does not achieve these effects, and it very soon leads to exhaustion in severely ill patients.

Both the authors quoted maintain that in their experience hypocapnia with hyperoxia, prolonged until patients begin to recover consciousness, reduces mortality, especially from brain injury, without increasing the proportion of patients who remain in a persistent vegetative state or become severely disabled. The evidence so far produced is either indirect and based on CSF biochemical studies and regional cerebral blood flow measurements, or based on retrospective comparisons with untreated cases [58, 59, 130–132]. Jennett [70] compared a number of published case studies on brain injuries which were remarkably similar as regards the features in the patient population that are known to have an influence on outcome, and found that the death rates were all nearly equal, with slight fluctuations ranging from 48% to 52%, despite the differences in management, including artificial hyperventilation. However, Becker [6], comparing the same series with his own clinical experience in 148 cases, all of whom were treated with artificial hyperventilation, found that the mortality rate (32%) and the favourable outcome rate (57%) of his group were significantly better than those of the other series reported.

Work in progress in Milan [128] has given results consistent with Becker's data and with the previous observations by Rossanda and Gordon, showing that the use of hyperventilation is followed by a steady decline in mortality in brain injuries and in other coma cases.

Many other clinicians believe that in brain injuries, 'optimal' levels of PaO_2 and $PaCO_2$ should be obtained and maintained by artificial ventilation whenever necessary [66, 94]; hyperventilation is considered a valuable means of controlling ICP by Shapiro [141], by Becker et al. [6], by Marsh et al. [93], by Bruce et al. [31], and by many others.

In line with previous studies [83], Cold et al. [41, 42] have shown that the non-homogeneous regional blood flows due to loss of autoregulation and CO_2 reactivity in the acute phase of brain injury could be corrected by hypocapnia; they were not able to determine, however, whether adaptation of CSF pH values made it possible to maintain this effect until the vascular response to CO_2 returned to normal.

Stroke. Early experimental studies [150] demonstrated that hyperventilation could protect the brain from focal ischaemia and suggested that this procedure could be used in man for improving the clinical course and outcome of stroke due to cerebral infarction. Subsequent experiments [103] and carefully controlled clinical trials [38] failed to substantiate this assumption and indicated also that, at least in elderly patients with cerebrovascular disease, prolonged artificial ventilation could have some adverse effects, the most prominent of which was a significantly increased rate of pulmonary complications.

Metabolic and postanoxic encephalopathies. Since intracranial hypertension is frequent in some metabolic encephalopathies, e.g., Reye's syndrome, moderate hyperventilation might be beneficial in these cases, especially when associated with barbiturates, a treatment that already requires per se some type of ventilation support.

It may be worthwhile mentioning that in experiments on the treatment of postanoxic encephalopathy, prolonged immobilization and artificial ventilation in animals was nearly as effective as high-dose barbiturate treatment in reducing neurological damage [15].

In conclusion, controlled hyperventilation is not thought to be detrimental, and may be beneficial in most coma cases, especially when intracranial hypertension and regional vascular changes are prominent features of the underlying pathology. The main exception is coma due to cerebrovascular disease: results are disappointing in these patients and adverse effects of prolonged artificial ventilation make its use inadvisable.

A matter in debate is how long controlled hyperventilation should be maintained. Indeed, early adaptation of cerebral acid–base balance and circulation occurs when hypocapnia is maintained [38, 39, 138, 139]. Therefore the metabolic and vascular effects of hypocapnia may be effaced within a few days. After prolonged hyperventilation weaning from the respirator should be very gradual to avoid rebound phenomena [66].

Hypothermia

The cerebral metabolic rate reduction obtained by moderate and deep hypothermia has been used for many years in cardiovascular and in neurological surgery.

The therapeutic use of hypothermia in comatose states has been proposed in the past on the basis of experimental data recorded in focal brain ischaemia [80a]. Good clinical results have also been claimed with the use of artificial hibernation [104]. Subsequent experimental and clinical research, however, have failed to confirm the earlier assumptions, and at present there is no proof that the possible beneficial effects of hypothermia may outlast the period of reduced body temperature [103, 145].

On the other hand, induction and maintenance of hypothermia require heavy medication and close control of the physiological parameters of the patient. During the rewarming phase acid–base shifts and changes in cerebral metabolism and blood flow may cause detrimental effects [151].

The therapeutic role of cooling patients in coma seems at present to be confined to the control of hyperthermia [66], while the risks and technical difficulties of controlled hypothermia far outweigh its possible benefits. Shapiro [141, 143], however, believes that this technique alone or in combination with barbiturates, with additive effects both on cerebral metabolism and on ICP [62, 63, 80, 102], may still be considered for selected uses.

Barbiturates

Until recently barbiturates were used in coma mainly for the treatment of status epilepticus and of similar convulsive conditions. Shapiro et al. [142] introduced their use in neuroanaesthesia in 1973 for the rapid intra-operative reduction of ICP. Since then barbiturates have been proposed as a therapeutic agent for a number of different neuropathological conditions, such as the secondary encephalopathies, stroke, and brain injuries. The rationale for their use in each of these conditions has been the subject of much research and speculation [146].

Experimental data. Barbiturates reduce the O_2 consumption of the brain in proportion to the depression of functional activity without altering the neuronal energy charge potential [144]. When functional activity is abolished the metabolic rate is reduced to about 50% and no further decrease can be obtained even if the doses administered are increased to two or more times the dose that gives the maximal functional depression [101, 111]. Barbiturates constrict cerebral vessels and reduce cerebral blood flow and ICP [95]. The effect is similar to that given by hypocapnia. Like hypocapnia they tend to correct non-homogeneity of regional blood flow modified by injury or by previous regional or general hypoxia–ischaemia [12, 21, 77, 145].

Barbiturates stabilize cellular membranes and may act as free radical scavengers [48, 49, 54, 160] and inhibitors of fatty acid peroxidation [90]; they accelerate the fall of brain free fatty acids increased after ischaemia and can quench excessive neurotransmitter turnover in cathecolaminergic neurones such as occurs in hypoxia or hypercapnia or after brain injury [10, 11, 33, 45, 67, 78, 80a, 108, 110]. Hakim and Moss [64] and Kofke et al. [77] showed also that barbiturates enhance glucose utilization for reactions essential for cellular viability in preference to energy-producing processes.

A number of experiments have shown that both pentobarbitone and thiopentone, administered in doses from 3 to 120 mg/kg either before or shortly after the occlusion of a major cerebral artery, significantly reduced the size of the cerebral infarct in many animal species (see tables in Hoff [65]), and attenuated ischaemic brain oedema [84].

The choice of a correct experimental model of global cerebral ischaemia–anoxia is very important [69] when therapy of post-circulatory-arrest encephalopathy has to be evaluated, especially because post-insult supportive care of the animals may have a relevant influence on morbidity and final outcome.

Using a carefully controlled monkey model [109] the Pittsburgh group demonstrated that barbiturates, administered in high doses (90–120 mg/kg) shortly after global and prolonged (16 min) arrest of the brain blood circulation, significantly reduced the degree of neuronal damage and especially of the functional deficits [14, 136].

These results have not been confirmed in dogs by Snyder et al. [148, 149]; differences in species sensitivity to the cardiovascular effects of high doses of barbiturates and differences in supportive care may account for the therapeutic failures observed.

Clinical results. Human experience with the use of barbiturates both in stroke and in post-circulatory-arrest encephalopathy is limited: several unexpected good recoveries have been reported [22, 65, 107], but the results of a planned controlled clinical trial [135] have not yet been published.

It seems, however, to have been proved that barbiturate treatment with doses as high as 30 mg/kg and more can be tolerated by patients in coma even shortly after resuscitation from cardiac arrest; artificial ventilation is always necessary and vasopressors may be required to counteract the depressive effects of the higher doses in the more susceptible patients [22].

Like hypocapnia, barbiturates seem to be mostly advisable in the types of coma in which high ICP, regional non-homogeneity of flow, or neuronal hyperactivity is a known or assumed feature of the underlying pathology, e.g., in brain injuries with intracranial hypertension and/or signs of brain stem involvement, acute post-hypoxic–ischaemic encephalopathy, and Reye's syndrome.

Prolonged therapy (3–5 days) with moderate doses of phenobarbitone, pentobarbitone or thiopentone seems in general preferable to treatment with a single high-dose bolus. The doses advised range from 3 to 10 mg/kg as an initial bolus, followed by 0.5–3 mg/kg/h to maintain plasma levels between 2.5 and 7 mg/100 ml [32, 127]. According to McGraw and Howard [100] pentobarbitone has a longer-lasting action on ICP than thiopentone; thiopentone has a negligible effect if used in a continuous drip infusion; it should be used in bolus injections only for the control of peak increases in ICP.

ICP monitoring and EEG or CFM continuous recording are the best guides to dosage; depression of the brain electrical activity to a trace with burst suppression is advised; the end-points for barbiturate administration are an ICP below 20 mmHg and a flat EEG [32].

Using this method in severe brain injuries and in children with Reye's syndrome, Bruce et al. [32] and the San Diego group [96, 97, 127] have obtained good control of ICP when other methods (hyperventilation, mannitol, and hypothermia) had failed, with a high proportion of good recoveries and a reduction in mortality. Only temporary effects were obtained in severe focal cerebral ischaemia and in post-anoxic encephalopathy.

References

1. Anderson DC, Cranford RE (1979) Corticosteroids in ischaemic stroke. Stroke 10:68–71

2. Bareggi SR, Porta M, Selenati A, Assael BM, Calderini G, Collice M, Rossanda M, Morselli PL (1975) Homovanillic acid and 5-hydroxyindole-acetic acid in the CSF of patients after a severe head injury. Eur Neurol 13:528–544

3. Barge M, Ohanessian J, Baum L, Benabid AL, Chirossel JP (1977) Valeur diagnostique et prognostique des réflexes du tronc cérébral dans les comas post-traumatiques graves. Neurochirurgie 23:227–238

4. Barge M, Ohanessian J, Garrel S, Benabid AL, Chirossel JP (1978) Le stade mésodiencéphalique des traumatismes craniens graves. Neurochirurgie 24:33–36

5. Bates D, Caronna TJ, Cartlidge NEF, Knill-Jones MB, Levy DE, Shaw MB, Plum F (1977) A prospective study of non-traumatic coma: methods and results in 310 patients. Ann Neurol 2:211–220

6. Becker DP, Miller JD, Ward JD, Greenberg RP, Young HF, Sakalas R (1977) The outcome of severe brain injury. J Neurosurg 47:491–502

7. Bell JA, Hodgson JHF (1974) Coma after cardiac arrest. Brain 97:361–372

8. Bergamasco B, Bergamini L, Doriguzzi T, Fabiani D (1968a) EEG sleep patterns as a prognostic criterion in post-traumatic coma. Electroencephalogr Clin Neurophysiol 24:374–377

9. Bergamasco B, Bergamini L, Doriguzzi T (1968) Clinical value of the sleep electroencephalographic patterns in post-traumatic coma. Acta Neurol Scand 44:495–511 (1968b)

10. Berntman L, Dahlgren N, Siesjö BK (1979a) Cerebral blood flow and oxygen consumption in the rat brain during extreme hypercarbia. Anesthesiology 50:299–305

11. Berntman L, Carlsson C, Siesjö BK (1979b) Cerebral oxygen consumption and blood flow in hypoxia: Influence of sympathoadrenal activation. Stroke 10:20–25

12. Bidabe-Renou AM, Constant P, Caille JM, Vernet J (1978) Vasoréactivité des infarctus cérébraux aux barbituriques et autres anesthésiques intraveineux. Ann Anesthesiol Fr 19:821–826

13. Binnie CD, Prior PF, Lloyd DSL, Scott DF, Margerison JH (1970) Electroencephalographic prediction of fatal anoxic brain damage after resuscitation from cardiac arrest. Br Med J iv:265–268

14. Bleyaert AL, Nemoto EM, Safar P, Stezoski SW, Mickell JJ, Moossy J, Rao GR (1978a) Tiopental amelioration of brain damage after global ischaemia in monkeys. Anesthesiology 49:390–398

15. Bleyaert AL, Safar P, Stezoski SW, Nemoto EM, Moossy J (1978b) Amelioration of postischaemic brain damage in the monkey by immobilization and controlled ventilation. Crit Care Med 6:112–113

16. Bond MR (1975) Assessment of the psychosocial outcome after severe head injury. In: Outcome of severe CNS damage. Ciba Foundation Symp 34, Elsevier Excerpta Medica, Amsterdam, pp 141–155

17. Bouzarth WF (1968) Neurosurgical watch sheet for craniocerebral trauma. J Trauma 8:29–31

18. Bozza-Marrubini M (1961) Rianimazione. I. Alterazioni del sensorio. In: Bozza-Marrubini M, Rossanda M, et al (eds) Anestesia e rianimazione nella chirurgia e nella traumatologia del sistema nervoso centrale. Minerva Anestesiol 27:365–430.

19. Bozza-Marrubini M (1964) Resuscitation treatment of the different degrees of unconsciousness. Acta Neurochir (Wien) 12:352–365

20. Bozza-Marrubini M, Boselli L, Ghezzi R, Iato E, Selenati A (1979) Physostigmine salicilate as an antidote in poisoning by drugs with central anticholinergic activity. Experience in 52 cases. In: Okonek S, Fülgraff G, Frey R (eds) Humantoxicologie. Fischer, Stuttgart New York, p 85–94

20a. Bozza-Marrubini M, Ghezzi R, Iato E, Scaiola A, Selenati A, Toso A (1981) Methodology of coma classification. Crit Care Med 9:151

21. Branston NM, Hope DT, Symon L (1979) Barbiturates in focal ischemia of primate cortex: Effects on blood flow distribution, evoked potential and extracellular potassium. Stroke 10:647–53

22. Breivik H, Safar P, Sands P, Fabritius R, Lind B, Lust P, Mullie A, Orr M, Renck H, Snyder JV (1978) Clinical feasibility trials of barbiturate therapy after cardiac arrest. Crit Care Med 6:228–44

23. Brendler SJ, Selverstone B (1970) Recovery from decerebration. Brain 93:381–392

24. Brennan RW (1978) Resuscitation from metabolic coma and encephalitis. Crit Care Med 6:277–283

25. Bricola A, Turella G (1973) Electroencephalographic patterns of acute traumatic coma: diagnostic and prognostic value. J Neurol Sci 17:278–285

26. Bricolo A, Gentilomo A, Rosadini G, Rossi GF (1968) Long-lasting post-traumatic unconsciousness. A study based on nocturnal EEG and polygraphic recording. Acta Neurol Scand 44:512–532

27. Bricolo A, Battistini N, Bergamini L, Columella F, Loeb C, Mingrino S, Rossi GF, Terzian H (1975) A proposal for the clinical classification of acute coma due to organic cerebral lesions. J Neurosurg Sci 19:113–119

28. Bricolo A, Turazzi S, Alexandre A, Rizzuto N (1977) Decerebrate rigidity in acute head injury. J Neurosurg 47:680–98

29. Bricolo A, Turazzi S, Faccioli F, Odorizzi F, Sciaretta G, Erculian P (1978) Clinical application of compressed spectral array in long-term EEG monitoring of comatose patients. Electroencephalogr Clin Neurophysiol 45:211

30. Brinkmann R, Von Cramon D, Schulz H (1976) The Munich Coma Scale (MCS). J Neurol Neurosurg Psychiatry 39:788–793

31. Bruce DA, Gennarelli TA, Langfitt TW (1978) Resuscitation from coma due to brain injury. Crit Care Med 6:254–269

32. Bruce DA, Raphaely RA, Swedlow D, Schut L (1980) The effectiveness of iatrogenic barbiturate coma in controlling increased ICP in 61 children. In: Shulman K, Marmarou A, Miller JD, et al (eds) Intracranial Pressure, vol iv. Springer, Berlin Heidelberg New York, pp 630–632

33. Calderini C, Carlsson A, Nordström CH (1978) Influence of transient ischemia on monoamine metabolism in the rat brain during nitrous oxide and phenobarbitone anaesthesia. Brain Res 157:303–310

34. Carlsson CA, Von Essen C, Lofgren J (1968) Factors affecting the clinical course of patients with severe head injuries. 1. Influence of biological factors. 2. Significance of posttraumatic coma. J Neurosurg 29:242–251

35. Castellano F, Perna E, Liguori R, Petrone G (1973) Contributo al trattamento del coma cerebrale traumatico con la citidin-difosfocolina (CDP-colina). Rass Internaz Clin Terap 53:63–88

36. Chatrian GE, White LE, Daly D (1963) Electroencephalographic patterns resembling those of sleep in certain comatose states after injuries of the head. EEG Clin Neurophysiol 15:272–280

37. Chiappa KH, Burke SR, Young RT (1979) Results of electroencephalographic monitoring during 367 carotid endarterectomies. Use of a dedicated minicomputer. Stroke 10:381–388

38. Christensen MS (1976) Prolonged artificial hyperventilation in cerebral apoplexy. Acta Anaesthesiol Scand [Suppl] 62:1–24

39. Christensen MS, Boderson P, Oleson J (1973) Cerebral apoplexy (stroke) treated with or without prolonged artificial hyperventilation: 2 CSF acid base balance and intracranial pressure. Stroke 4:620–31

40. Ciba Foundation (1975) Outcome of severe damage to the central nervous system. Elsevier Excerpta Medica, North Holland (Symposium no. 34)

41. Cold GE, Jensen FT, Malmros R (1977a) The cerebrovascular CO_2 reactivity during the acute phase of brain injury. Acta Anaesthesiol Scand 21:222–31

42. Cold GE, Jensen FT, Malmros R (1977b) The effects of $PaCO_2$ reduction on regional cerebral blood flow in the acute phase of brain injury. Acta Anaesthesiol Scand 21:359–67

43. Collice M, Versari P, Vecchi G, Scornajenghi A, D'Angelo V (1980) Role of ICP monitoring in patients suffering from severe brain injuries. In: Shulman K, Marmarou A, Miller JD (eds) Intracranial pressure, vol IV. Springer, Berlin Heidelberg New York, pp 17–19

44. Cooper PR, Moody S, Clark K, Kirkpatrick J, Maravilla K, Gould AL, Drane W (1979) Dexamethasone and severe head injury. A prospective double-blind study. J Neurosurg 51:307–316

45. Corrodi H, Fuxe K, Lidbrink P, Olsson L (1971) Minor tranquilizers, stress and central catecholamine neurons. Brain Res 29:1–16

46. De Jong R (1979) The neurologic examination, 4th edn. Harper & Row, Hagerston

47. Demopoulos HB, Milvy P, Kakari S, Ransohoff J (1972) Molecular aspects of membrane structures in cerebral edema. In: Reulen HJ, Schürmann K (eds) Steroids and brain edema. Springer, Berlin Heidelberg New York, p 29:39

48. Demopoulos HB, Flamm ES, Seligman ML, Power R, Pietronigro D, Ransohoff J (1977a) Molecular pathology of lipids in CNS membranes. In: Jöbsis FF (ed) Oxygen and physiological function. Professional Information Library, Dallas Texas, pp 491–508

49. Demopoulos HB, Flamm ES, Seligman ML, Jørgensen E, Ransohoff J (1977b) Antioxidant effects of barbiturates in model membranes undergoing free radical damage. Acta Neurol Scand 56 [Suppl] 64:152–153

50. Espagno J, Trémoulet M, Gigaud M, Espagno CH (1979) Etude de l'action de la CDP-choline dans les troubles de la vigilance post-traumatique. La Vie Médicale 3:195–196

51. Faupel G, Reulen HJ, Muller D (1977) Double-blind study on the effects of dexamethasone on severe closed head injury. In: Pappius H, Reulen H (eds) Second International Workshop on cerebral edema, Montreal, 1976. Springer, Berlin

52. Fazekas JF, Alman RW (1962) Coma. Biochemistry, physiology and therapeutic principles. Thomas, Springfield, p 3

53. Fischgold H, Mathis P (1959) Obnubilations, comas et stupeurs. Masson, Paris

54. Flamm ES, Demopoulos HB, Seligman ML, Ransohoff J (1977) Possible molecular mechanisms of barbiturate-mediated protection in regional cerebral ischemia. Acta Neurol Scand 56 [Suppl 64]: 150–151

55. Fleischer AS, Payne NS, Tindall GT (1976) Continuous monitoring of intracranial pressure in severe closed head injury without mass lesions. Surg Neurol 6:31–4

56. Frowein RA (1976) Classification of coma. Acta Neurochir (Wien) 34:5–10

57. Gobiet W, Bock WJ, Liesegang J, Grote W (1976) Treatment of acute cerebral edema with high dose dexamethasone. In: Beks JWF, Bosch DA, Brock M (eds) Intracranial pressure, vol III. Springer, Berlin Heidelberg New York, pp 231–235

58. Gordon E (1971a) Controlled respiration in the management of patients with traumatic brain injuries. Acta Anaesthesiol Scand 15:193–208

59. Gordon E (1971b) The acid-base balance and oxygen tension of the cerebrospinal fluid, and their implications for the treatment of patients with brain lesions. Acta Anaesthesiol Scand [Suppl] 34:1–36

60. Goulon M, Gajdos P, Margent P, Raphael JC, Barois A, Combes A, Grosbuis S, Levy-Alcover M, Gastinne H (1977) Neurological problems in intensive care. In: Neurology. Proc 11th World Congress of Neurology, Amsterdam, 1977. Excerpta Medica, Amsterdam Oxford, pp 283–298 (International Congress series no. 434)

61. Gudeman SK, Miller JD, Becker DP (1979) Failure of high-dose steroid therapy to influence intracranial pressure in patients with severe head injury. J Neurosurg 51:301–306

62. Hägerdal M, Welsh FA, Keykhah MM, Perez E, Harp JR (1978) Protective effects of combinations of hypothermia and barbiturates in cerebral hypoxia in the rat. Anesthesiology 49:165–169

63. Hägerdal M, Keykhah M, Perez E, Harp JR (1979) Additive affects of hypothermia and phenobarbital upon cerebral oxygen consumption in the rat. Acta Anaesthesiol Scand 23:89–92

64. Hakim AM, Moss G (1976) Cerebral effects of barbiturate-shift from energy to synthesis metabolism for cellular viability. Surg Forum 27:497–499

65. Hoff JT (1978) Resuscitation in focal brain ischemia. Crit Care Med 6:245–253

66. Horton JM (1976) The anaesthetist's contribution to the care of head injuries. Br J Anaesth 48:767–771

67. Huger F, Patrick G (1979) Effect of concussive head injury on central catecholamine levels and synthesis rates in rat brain regions. J Neurochem 33:89–95

68. Ito U, Ohno K, Suganuma Y, Suzuki K, Inaba Y (1980) Effect of steroid in ischemic brain edema. Analysis of cytotoxic and vasogenic edema occurring during ischemia and after restoration of blood flow. Stroke 11:166–172

69. Jackson DL, Dole WP (1979) Total cerebral ischemia: A new model system for the study of post cardiac arrest brain damage. Stroke 10:38–42

70. Jennett B (1979) Severe head injury: Prediction of outcome as a basis for management decisions. In: Trubuhovic RV (ed) Management of acute intracranial disasters. Little Brown, Boston, p 133–152

71. Jennett B, Bond M (1975) Assessment of outcome after severe brain damage. A practical scale. Lancet I:480–484

72. Jennett B, Plum F (1972) The persistent vegetative state after brain damage: A syndrome in search of a name. Lancet I:734–737

73. Jennett B, Teasdale G (1977) Aspects of coma after severe head injury. Lancet I:878–81

74. Jennett B, Teasdale G, Braakman R, Minderhoud J, Knill-Jones R (1976) Predicting outcome in individual patients after severe head injury. Lancet I:1031–4

75. Jouvet M (1961) Essai de classification des troubles chroniques de la conscience post-traumatiques. In: Wertheimer P, Descotes J (eds) Traumatologie cranienne. Masson, Paris, p 75–83

76. Jouvet M (1969) Coma and other disorders of consciousness In: Vinken PJ, Bruyn GW (eds) Handbook of clinical neurology, vol 3. North Holland, Amsterdam, pp 62–79

77. Kofke WA, Nemoto EM, Hossmann KA, Taylor F, Kessler PD, Stezoski SW (1979) Brain blood flow and metabolism after global ischemia and post-insult thiopental therapy in monkeys. Stroke 10:554–60

78. Korf J, Aghajanian GK, Roth RH (1973) Increased turnover of norepinephrine in the rat cerebral cortex during stress. Role of the locus coeruleus. Neuropharmacology 12:933–8

79. Kugelmass IN (1962) Foreword. In: Fazekas JF, Alman RW (eds) Coma, biochemistry physiology and therapeutic principles. Thomas, Springfield, p VI

80. Lafferty JJ, Keykhah MM, Shapiro HM, Van Horn K, Behaz MG (1978) Cerebral hypometabolism obtained with deep pentobarbital anesthesia and hypothermia (30° C). Anesthesiology 49:159–164

80a. Lancet (1963) Coma with injury to chest. (Editorial) Lancet I:1151

80b. Lancet (1973) Predicting outcome after severe brain damage. (Editorial) Lancet I:523–524

81. Langfitt TW (1976) The incidence and importance of intracranial hypertension in head injured patients. In: Beks JWF, Bosch DA, Brock M (eds) Intracranial pressure, vol III. Springer, Berlin, pp 67–72

82. Langfitt TW (1978) Measuring the outcome from head injuries. J Neurosurg 48:673–8

83. Lassen NA, Palvalgyi R (1968) Cerebral steal during hypercapnia and the inverse reaction during hypocapnia observed by the 133 xenon technique in man. Scand J Clin Lab Invest [Suppl] 102:XIII D

84. Lawner P, Laurent J, Simeone F, Fink E, Rubin E (1979) Attenuation of ischemic brain edema by pentobarbital after carotid ligation in the gerbil. Stroke 10:644–47

85. Levati A (1977) Possibilità di prognosi precoce nel traumatizzato cranioencefalico. Importanza del livello di coma e dell'età. Thesis, University of Milan

86. Levin HS, Grossmann RG, Rose JE, Teasdale G (1979) Long-term neuropsychological outcome of closed head injury. J Neurosurg 50:412

87. Levy D, Bates D, Caronna J, Cartlidge N, Knill-Jones R, Shaw D, Plum F (1978) Recovery from nontraumatic coma. Ann Neurol 4:169–170

88. Loeb C, Rosadini G, Poggio GF (1959) Electroencephalograms during coma. Neurology 9:610–9

89. MacIver IN, Frew IJC, Matheson JG (1958) The role of respiratory insufficiency in the mortality of severe brain injuries. Lancet I:390–3

90. Majewska MD, Stroznajder J, Lazarewicz J (1978) Effect of ischemic anoxia and barbiturate anesthesia on free radical oxidation of mitochondrial phospholipids. Brain Res 158:423–34

91. Mannelli A, Silvestri A, Conti-Bizzarro C, Bonagura A (1973) Trattamento di alcuni casi di coma di origine traumatica con la CDP colina. Incontri Anest Rianim e Scienze affini 8:209–232

92. Marrubini G (1966) Anatomia patologica nel traumatizzato cranio-encefalico, In: Panel sulla rianimazione in neurologia e neurochirurgia. Minerva Anestesiol 32:449–477

93. Marsh ML, Marshall LF, Shapiro HM (1977) Neurosurgical intensive care. Anesthesiology 47:149–163

94. Marshall M (1979) Neuro-anaesthesia. Edward Arnold, p 35

95. Marshall LF, Shapiro HM (1977) Barbiturate control of intracranial hypertension in head injury and other conditions: Iatrogenic coma. Acta Neurol Scand [Suppl] 56/64:156–7

96. Marshall LF, Shapiro HM (1980) Barbiturates for intracranial hypertension: A ten year perspective. In: Shulman K, Marmarou A, Miller JD et al. (eds) Intracranial Pressure, vol IV. Springer, Berlin Heidelberg New York, pp 627–629

97. Marshall LF, Shapiro HM, Rauscher A, Kaufman NM (1978) Pentobarbital therapy for intracranial hypertension in metabolic coma. Reye's syndrome. Crit Care Med 6:1–5

98. Masson M, Henin D (1979) Les comas. Encycl Méd Chir, Paris. Neurologie 17023 A–1012

99. Matthew H, Lawson AAH (1975) Treatment of common acute poisonings. Churchill Livingstone, Edinburgh London New York, pp 18–19

100. McGraw CP, Howard G (1980) Effects of barbiturates on intracranial pressure and the amount of mannitol required to control the intracranial pressure. In: Shulman K, Marmarou A, Miller JD, et al (eds) Intracranial pressure, vol IV. Springer, Berlin Heidelberg New York, pp 633–635

101. Michenfelder JD (1974) The interdependency of cerebral functional and metabolic effects following massive doses of thiopental in the dog. Anesthesiology 41:231–6

102. Michenfelder JD (1978) Hypothermia plus barbiturates. Apples plus oranges? Anesthesiology 49:157–158

103. Michenfelder JD, Milde JH (1977) Failure of prolonged hypocapnia, hypothermia, or hypertension to favorably alter acute stroke in primates. Stroke 8:87–91

104. Michon P, Larcan A (1961) Agression et réanimation en médecine interne. Masson, Paris, 397

105. Mollaret P, Goulon M (1959) Le coma dépassé. Rev Neurol (Paris) 101:3

106. Mombelli F, Sargenti L, Levati A, Livini M, Stern M, Bozza-Marrubini M, Iato E (1979) Il CFM (Cerebral Function Monitor) un nuovo strumento per la valutazione dell'attività funzionale cerebrale in anestesia e rianimazione. Anestesia e Rianimazione 20:241–60

107. Mullie' A, Lust P, Penninckx J, Vanhove L, Miranda R, Hainaux M, Spincemaille J (1978) Utilization clinique du thiopental dans l'encephalopathie postischemique. Rapport preliminaire. Ann Anesthesiol Fr 19:833–41

108. Nemoto EM (1978) Pathogenesis of cerebral ischemia-anoxia. Crit Care Med 6:203–214

109. Nemoto EM, Bleyaert AL, Stezoski SW, Moossy J, Gutti RR, Safar P (1977) Global brain ischemia: A reproducible monkey model. Stroke 8:558–564

110. Nemoto EM, Shiu GK, Gilbertson JR, Alexander H (1980) Brain free fatty acids after transient global brain ischemia with postinsult thiopental therapy. In: Shulman K, Marmarou A, Miller JD (eds) Intracranial Pressure vol IV. Springer, Berlin Heidelberg New York, p 307–311

111. Nilsson L, Siesjö BK (1975) The effect of phenobarbitone anaesthesia on blood flow and oxygen consumption in the rat brain. Acta Anaesthesiol Scand [Suppl] 57:18–24

112. Obrist WD, Gennarelli TA, Segawa H, Dolinskas CA, Langfitt TW (1979) Relation of cerebral blood flow to neurological status and outcome in head injured patients. J Neurosurg 51:292–300

113. Ommaya AK, Sadowsky D (1966) A system of coding medical data for punched-card machine retrieval. J Trauma 6:605–617

114. Ottonello GA, Primavera A (1979) Gastrointestinal complication of high-dose corticosteroid therapy in acute cerebrovascular patients. Stroke 10:208–10

115. Overgaard J, Christensen S, Hvid-Hansen O, Haase J, Land A, Hein O, Pedersen KK, Tweed WA (1973) Prognosis after head injury based on early clinical examination. Lancet II:631–635

116. Pampiglione G, Harden A (1968) Resuscitation after cardiocirculatory arrest. Prognostic evaluation of early electroencephalographic findings. Lancet I:1261–1267

117. Pitts LH, Kaktis JV (1980) Effect of megadose steroids on ICP in traumatic coma. In: Shulman K, Marmarou A, Miller JD, et al (eds) Intracranial pressure vol IV. Springer, Berlin Heidelberg New York, pp. 638–642

118. Pitts LH, Kaktis JV, Juster R, Heilbron D (1980) ICP and outcome in patients with severe brain injury. In: Shulman K, Marmarou A, Miller JF, et al. (eds) Intracranial pressure vol IV. Springer Verlag, Berlin Heidelberg New York, p 5–9

119. Plum F (1972) Organic disturbances of consciousness In: Critchley M, O'Leary J, Jennett BW (eds) Scientific foundations of neurology. Heinemann Med Books, London, p 193–201

120. Plum F, Posner JB (1966) The diagnosis of stupor and coma. Blackwell Scientific Publications, Oxford

121. Plum F, Caronna JJ (1975) Can one predict outcome of medical coma? In: Outcome of severe damage to the central nervous sytem. Elsevier/Excerpta Medica, North Holland, 121–136 (Ciba Foundation Symposium no. 34)

122. Porta M, Bareggi SR, Selenati A, Assael BM, Beduschi A, Morselli PL (1973) Acid monoamines metabolites in ventricular and lumbar cerebrospinal fluids of patients in post-traumatic coma. J Neurosurg Sci 17:230–237

123. Poulsen J, Zilstorff K (1972) Prognostic value of the caloric-vestibular test in the unconscious patient with cranial trauma. Acta Neurol Scand 48:282–292

124. Price DJ, Knill Jones R (1977) Prognosis of severe head injury in 150 patients with coma and bilateral fixed pupils. Intensive Care Med 3:167

125. Prior PF (1973) The EEG in acute cerebral anoxia. Excerpta Medica, Amsterdam

125a. Prior PF (1979) Monitoring cerebral function. North Holland, Elsevier

126. Reed CE, Driggs MF, Foote CC (1952) Acute barbiturate intoxication: A study of 300 cases based on a physiologic system of classification of the severity of the intoxication. Ann Intern Med 37:290–303

127. Rockoff MA, Marshall LF, Shapiro HM (1979) High-dose barbiturate therapy in humans: A clinical review of 60 patients. Ann Neurol 6:194–199

128. Rossanda M (to be published) Basi fisiopatologiche e problemi clinici della rianimazione in neurochirurgia. In: Damia G et al (eds) Trattato enciclopedico italiano di anestesia, rianimazione, terapia intensiva, tossicologia d'urgenza e terapia del dolore. Piccin, Padova

129. Rossanda M (1968) Prolonged hyperventilation in treatment of unconscious patients with brain injury. Scand J Clin Lab Invest [Suppl] 102:XIII E

130. Rossanda M, Di Giugno G, Corona S, Bettinazzi N, Mangione G (1966) Oxygen supply to the brain and respirator treatment in severe comatose states. Acta Anaesthesiol Scand 3 [Suppl XXIII]:766–74

131. Rossanda M, Boselli L, Castelli A, Corona C, Erminio F, Nardini M, Porta M, Villa C (1972) Effects of changes in PaCO$_2$ on rCBF, cerebral oxygenation and EEG in severe brain injuries. Eur Neurol 8:169–173

132. Rossanda M, Selenati A, Villa C, Beduschi A (1973) Role of automatic ventilation in treatment of severe head injuries. J Neurosurg Sci 17:265–70

133. Rowbotham GF (1949) Acute injuries of the head. Livingstone, Edinburgh, pp 123–125

134. Rutherford WH (1977) Diagnosis of alcohol ingestion in mild head injuries. Lancet I:1021–1023

135. Safar P, Nemoto E (1978) Brain resuscitation. Acta Anaesthesiol Scand [Suppl] 70:60–74

136. Safar P, Bleyaert A, Nemoto EM, Moossy J, Snyder JV (1978) Resuscitation after global brain ischemia anoxia. Crit Care Med 6:215–227

137. Sawada Y, Takahashi M, Ohashi N, Fusamoto H, Maemura K, Kobayashi H, Yoshioka T, Sugimoto T (1980) Computerised tomography as an indication of long-term outcome after acute carbon monoxide poisoning. Lancet I:783–784

138. Severinghaus JW (1965) Role of cerebrospinal fluid pH in normalization of cerebral blood flow in chronic hypocapnia. Acta Neurol Scand [Suppl] 14:116–120

139. Severinghaus JW, Lassen N (1967) Step hypocapnia to separate arterial from tissue PCO$_2$ in the regulation of cerebral blood flow. Circ Res 20:272–78

140. Sganzerla EP, Bordone G (1979) Attività EEG alfa-simile nel coma dopo arresto cardiocircolatorio. Anestesia e Rianimazione 20:267–275

141. Shapiro HM (1975) Intracranial hypertension. Therapeutic and anesthetic considerations. Anesthesiology 43:445–71

142. Shapiro HM, Galindo A, Wyte SR, Harris AB (1973) Rapid intraoperative reduction of intracranial pressure with thiopentone. Br J Anesth 45:1057–1062

143. Shapiro HM, Wyte SR, Loeser J (1974) Barbiturate augmented hypothermia for reduction of persistent intracranial hypertension. J Neurosurg 40:90–100

144. Siesjö BK (1978) Brain metabolism and anaesthesia. Acta Anaesthesiol Scand [Suppl] 70:56–59

145. Simeone FA, Frazer G, Lawner P (1979) Ischemic brain edema: Comparative effects of barbiturates and hypothermia. Stroke 10:8–12

146. Smith AL (1977) Barbiturate protection in cerebral hypoxia. Anesthesiology 47:285–293

147. Snyder BD, Ramirez-Lassepas M, Lippert DM (1977) Neurologic states and prognosis after cardiopulmonary arrest: 1. A retrospective study. Neurology 27:807–811

148. Snyder BD, Ramirez-Lassepas M, Sukum AI (1978) Failure of pentothal to protect from anoxic cerebral injury. Stroke 9:99

149. Snyder BD, Ramirez-Lassepas M, Sukum P, Fryd D, Sung JH (1979) Failure of thiopental to modify global anoxic injury. Stroke 10:135–141

150. Soloway M, Nadel W, Albin MS, White RJ (1968) The effect of hyperventilation on subsequent cerebral infarction. Anesthesiology 29:975

151. Steen PA, Soule EH, Michenfelder JD (1979) Detrimental effect of prolonged hypothermia in cats and monkeys with and without regional cerebral ischemia. Stroke 10:522–529

152. Subczynski J (1975) State of consciousness scoring system. J Neurosurg 43:251

153. Teasdale G, Jennett B (1974) Assessment of coma and impaired consciousness. A practical scale. Lancet II:81–84

154. Teasdale G, Jennett B (1976) Assessment and prognosis of coma after head injury. Acta Neurochir (Wien) 34:45–55

155. Teasdale G, Knill-Jones R, Van Der Sande J (1978) Observer variability in assessing impaired consciousness and coma. J Neurol Neurosurg Psychiatry 41:603

156. Thierry AM, Javoy F, Glowinsky J, Kety SS (1968) Effects of stress on the metabolism of norepinephrine, dopamine and serotonin in the central nervous system of the rat. I Modifications of norepinephrine turnover. J Pharmacol Exp Ther 163:163–171

157. Thomassen A, Sørensen K, Wernberg M (1978) The prognostic value of EEG in coma survivors after cardiac arrest. Acta Anaesthesiol Scand 22:483–490

158. Thomassen A, Wernberg M (1979) Prevalence and prognostic significance of coma after cardiac arrest outside intensive care and coronary units. Acta Anaesthesiol Scand 23:143–148

159. Toole JF, Barnes RW (1979) Neurological monitoring

techniques. Stroke 10:467–470

160. Trop D (1978) Effets métaboliques des barbituriques sur le cerveau anoxique: le piégeage des radicaux libres. Ann Anesthesiol Fr 19:815–820

161. Vapalahti M, Troupp H (1971) Prognosis for patients with severe brain injuries. Br Med J iii:404–407

162. Willoughby JO, Leach BG (1974) Relation of neurological findings after cardiac arrest to outcome. Br Med J iii:437–439

Chapter 43

Cerebral Oedema

C. Thurel, J. L. Ragguenea, A. A. Habib,
and A. Levante

An early definition of brain oedema, given in 1874 by Bucknill and Tucke [3], was: "... a state in which the tissue of the organ is permeated by water or serosity". The primary characteristic of cerebral oedema is therefore the abnormal extravascular accumulation of fluid in the brain, in either the intracellular or the extracellular compartment. Accompanying the increase in brain tissue water is an increase in tissue bulk. Although oedema produces increases in tissue bulk, it must not be confused with other processes which alter bulk and which may coexist, such as vascular congestion, increased cerebral blood flow and hydrocephalus.

Cerebral oedema complicates many neurological conditions, such as head injuries, neoplasms, and infections, and its recognition and treatment are of great practical importance, particularly in those conditions (abscesses, malignant tumours) which can provoke its widespread formation. In such circumstances the volume occupied by the accumulated water may be many times that of the mass itself, and the intracranial pressure (ICP) may rise to dangerous levels. Neurosurgeons often refer to cerebral oedema as swelling, because oedema only becomes of neurosurgical concern if it is associated with an increase in volume.

Pathogenesis

It is now generally accepted that there are two basically different forms of cerebral oedema, cytotoxic and vasogenic [13]. These two types may occur as distinct entities, they may coexist, or one may lead to the other [12, 13].

Cytotoxic oedema

In this type the crucial pathogenic event is related to disturbances of cellular metabolism and ionic transport. The initial event is the loss of ions, mainly potassium, from the cells, and a gain by them of sodium and chloride ions from the extracellular space (ECS). Water uptake by the cells is osmotically coupled to these ionic shifts and causes swelling of the cells, shrinking of the ECS, and an increase in tissue fluid osmolality. This form of cerebral oedema is generalized, and anatomically the main characteristic is the integrity of both the basement membranes and the capillary endothelial cells. Water passes from the circulation into the tissues under the influence of osmotic gradients. It may be caused by organic tin compounds or hexachlorophene poisoning, or water intoxication.

Vasogenic oedema

Formation

In vasogenic oedema [22, 24, 25, 28] the main event is some degree of vascular damage; the causative factors affect cerebrovascular permeability and so disturb the blood–brain barrier (BBB).

A host of factors affect cerebrovascular permeability and regardless of the nature of the insult (trauma, tumours, etc.), the BBB is temporarily 'broken', and fluid proteins and electrolytes extravasate through the damaged vessels. Biochemical studies have shown that the oedema fluid is an exudate of plasma, with a lower protein content than plasma but equal sodium and chloride content. The site and method of leakage of the oedema fluid has been extensively studied in a cold injury model and the results can be summarized as follows:

a) The extravasation of fluid with a composition similar to that of plasma is restricted to the area of cortical injury.
b) Vessels outside this area, but within the territory of the oedema, do not show an increase in permeability.
c) The driving force for the extravasation of fluid seems to be the capillary transmural pressure gradient, i.e., the difference between the intravascular and interstitial fluid pressure (IFP).
d) The speed and extent of spread of the fluid is influenced by haemodynamic factors. Both factors can be diminished by reducing the systemic blood pressure. Conversely, an acute increase in arterial pressure produces a dramatic increase of oedema formation.
e) The duration of the vascular injury and the extent of the breakdown of the BBB play a major role in determining the magnitude of the fluid leak.

Spread

Seepage of fluid first occurs focally in the area of the lesion, and when it gains access to the ECS it then spreads throughout this, particularly in the white matter. It then crosses the brain and reaches the ventricular surface on about the third day. From then on, great lakes of oedema fluid accumulate beneath the ependyma, suggesting that the resolution of vasogenic oedema might occur through discharge into the ventricular CSF and, in fact, it is very likely that the CSF fluid does represent an important pathway for its elimination from the brain.

Electron microscopic and physiological studies with extracellular tracer substances have shown that in vasogenic oedema the ECS is significantly enlarged and provides the pathway for the movement of oedema fluid. The two possible mechanisms of spread are diffusion and bulk flow, processes that are markedly different:

a) Bulk flow (also known as convective or volume flow) is the type of fluid movement produced by either hydrostatic or osmotic pressure gradients acting singly or together.
b) Diffusion is the random movement or mixing of a solute within a system. Nett movement is the result of solute concentration gradients that exist between various regions of the system.

The cold-induced model of vasogenic oedema indicates that bulk flow rather than diffusion is the main mechanism of spread of oedema through the white matter.

This conclusion is based upon the following observations: (1) Substances of diverse molecular weights, ranging from sucrose to large protein molecules, spread from the site of injury at the same speed, suggesting bulk movement. (2) The distances actually travelled by various substances were greater than those theoretically possible by diffusion. (3) Measurements of interstitial fluid pressure (IFP) at various distances from the lesion showed the presence of increased IFP in the area of the lesion and a decreasing pressure along the oedema pathway towards the normal tissue. (4) The increase in local IFP (resulting from the extravasation of oedema fluid) and the development of pressure gradients through the tissue is the result of two opposing forces: the hydrostatic pressure of the circulation and the resistance to this offered by the small extracellular channels and intermingled structure of the brain parenchyma. (5) As a result of the increase in IFP the ECS enlarges. At first a relatively large increase in IFP is required to cause the ECS to dilate. This initial steep increase may be considered as a 'safety factor' which protects the brain tissue against oedema in minor injuries of the BBB. However, once the IFP increases above the 'structural force' of tissue resistance, the volume increase per change in pressure (compliance) occurs, slowly at first and then very rapidly. (6) The spread of oedema can be significantly reduced by using hexachlorophene to induce intracellular brain oedema before the cold lesion; this reduces the size of the ECS and increases the resistance to flow of the oedema fluid. (7) White matter is normally nourished patient, in whom the aim of affected to a greater extent than grey matter, presumably because of structural differences. (8) Developing oedema spreads from the lesion through the white matter and towards the ventricle, as has been confirmed by CT scan.

Resolution

One of the major mechanisms for resolution of vasogenic oedema is the movement of extracellular fluid into the CSF across the ventricular ependyma. Clearance of fluid into the CSF 'sink' is related to the pressure gradient between the IFP in the oedematous tissue and CSF pressure. Thus, changes in ventricular fluid pressure directly affect the amount and rate of this clearance. This explains the therapeutic effects of such drugs as acetozolamide and frusemide, which lower intraventricular pressure by reducing the rate of CSF production.

Finally, both pressure gradients and bulk flow play a major role in the dynamics of formation, and of resolution, of brain oedema.

Oedema associated with ischaemia

In some cases, the distinction between vasogenic and cytotoxic oedema is not simple, and in any study of the pathogenesis of cerebral oedema the most difficult form to characterize is the oedema that is associated with ischaemia [7, 10, 27]. Ischaemic brain oedema is predominantly of the cytotoxic type, starting with an intracellular accumulation of water. This abnormal water uptake causes swelling of the affected parenchyma cells and intensifies the ischaemia.

The first phase develops before there is any change in the BBB and is probably related to disturbance of the sodium-potassium ionic pump; accumulation of lactic and monoamino acids as a result of altered brain metabolism; and changes in brain osmolality.

In the second phase, protein leaks through the BBB and a vasogenic component is introduced. In addition to the increased permeability of the BBB, increased vesicular transport (pinocytosis) that is seen in the post ischaemic period may also play a major role in the progression of this type of oedema.

Clinical aspects

It is not possible to distinguish the clinical effects of cerebral oedema [19, 27] from those conventionally associated with a raised ICP or with disturbances and shifts of the brain substance.

Its presentation is quite variable, and so long as the compensatory capacity is not exhausted there may be no symptoms. This is particularly true in patients with benign intracranial hypertension (pseudo-tumour cerebri) which is related to generalized cerebral oedema. This condition occurs most frequently in young adult females with obesity or following withdrawal of steroid therapy and in association with hypervitaminosis A. In young children it is often associated with middle ear disease and sinus thrombosis. In some cases, ICP of over 1000 mmH$_2$O has been measured without any evidence of neurological dysfunction.

Monitoring techniques

The detection of intracranial events that threaten cerebral homeostasis remains a difficult problem because of the complex functional and structural arrangement of the central nervous system (CNS). Important aspects of neurological and neurosurgical monitoring are a combination of appropriately timed CT scans and, in some cases, continuous ICP recording.

Computerized axial tomography

The CT scan has opened a new era in the study of cerebral oedema in man, since it is the first non-invasive method which can directly diagnose 'cerebral oedema', define its extent, assess the efficiency of treatment and finally visualize the dynamic process of its formation and resolution (Fig. 43.1) [5, 14, 21].

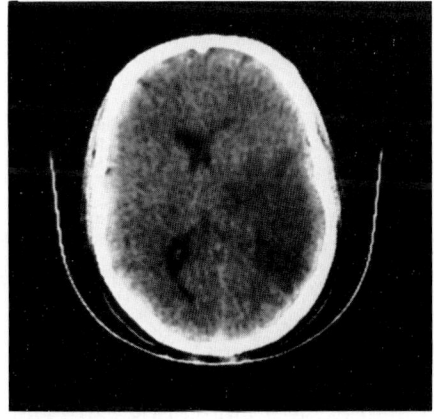

Fig. 43.1. Peritumoral brain oedema.

Direct visualization of cerebral oedema is possible, because the differential absorption of x-rays in soft tissues can be distinguished with high resolution. Cerebral oedema appears in the CT scan as an area of low density (radiolucency) because of an increase in the water content of the tissue. The density of oedematous tissue is variable, however, and this may be a reflection of the differing protein contents of the oedema fluid.

In most cases, areas of diminished density occurring around tumours, haemorrhages, or abscesses can be confidently interpreted as oedema, but in the presence of cerebral infarction it is difficult to distinguish oedema from the infarcted tissue. Care must also be exercised in interpreting the density values on a plain scan. A region may have a low average density due to loss of tissue or changes in composition, rather than to an increase in fluid content. Only when the clinical situation and the scan picture are well defined is it safe to interpret a low-density area as oedematous.

A CT scan does not provide direct information of ICP or blood flow dynamics, at least as far as morphological or compartmental changes are taken into consideration. The consequences of an increase in tissue mass too often lead to a plausible but unproven conclusion of increased ICP but in this respect three important points have been well demonstrated by simultaneous measurement of ICP and CT scanning: (1) Narrow or even closed ventricles can be observed in patients with a normal ICP. In other words, there is no reliable relationship between the morphological picture and the level of the ICP. (2) ICP may be normal despite a grossly abnormal CT scan, including significant midline shift and widely dilated ventricles. (3) No patients with a normal CT scan have had increased ICP.

Intracranial pressure monitoring

Though the CT scan can provide rapid and accurate information about cerebral oedema, it is no use for the study of its main consequence and major risk, namely the rise in ICP [11, 16]. Recent advances in monitoring have considerably improved the ability to detect and to record increases in ICP. Such measurements also facilitate calculation of the overall cerebral perfusion pressure (arterial pressure–ICP) and may be a forewarning of the likelihood of impending cerebral ischaemia.

In critically ill patients, particularly those with severe head injuries, ICP monitoring can be of great value. In such cases measurement of the ventricular fluid pressure (VFP) for periods that might range from 48 h to 10 days is of practical use, and in spite of the risk of infection, a ventricular catheter seems to be the method of choice because it provides a route for the drainage of CSF. In patients in whom there is an acute rise in pressure, the combination of immediate diagnosis (by continuous monitoring of ICP) and immediate treatment (by controlled drainage of CSF) may be life-saving. In addition, in cases with protracted intracranial hypertension due to cerebral oedema, the continuous drainage of CSF for a period of days results in a lowering of intraventricular pressure, which can directly affect the amount and rate of clearance of cerebral oedema into the CSF sink.

Finally, any patient who develops an increase in ICP that cannot be immediately explained by changes in blood gases or other easily remediable causes merits prompt re-investigation by CT scan or arteriography. Direct measurements of total and regional cerebral blood flow (CBF) complement these monitoring methods, but their cost and complexity limit their application to a few centres.

Treatment

The goals of all forms of treatment of intracranial hypertension are to secure the supply of O_2 and glucose to the entire brain and to relieve the brain tissue of any mechanical stress.

All patients with severe brain damage, in particular those in coma, are threatened by a number of extracranial disturbances which may influence the intracranial dynamics and jeopardize the O_2 supply to the brain tissue. The most important of these are airway obstruction, respiratory failure, hypotension, hypovolaemia, and anaemia. So before any attempt is made to elucidate the often complicated pattern of cause and effect in the pathogenesis of increased ICP, the primary consideration is to ensure that the substrates essential for continued cerebral metabolism are available. To this end, the airway must be clear; the arterial PO_2 should be maintained within normal limits; and the mean arterial pressure should be kept well above 60 mmHg, since this is the lower limit for autoregulation in normal patients.

The next stage in management of the patient in whom an increased ICP is suspected is to determine whether or not the pressure really is increased, and if so, its cause and to what extent the increase is responsible for any deterioration in the patient's condition.

Finally, if it is decided to try to reduce the ICP resulting from cerebral oedema, then the basis of all methods is to increase the space available for functioning brain, either by increasing the effective volume of the cranial cavity (mechanical decompression) or by reducing the volume of one (or more) of its constituents.

Cerebral decompression

Surgical decompression of the brain by large bilateral craniotomies was performed by Cushing in an attempt to relieve pressure on the vital centres. Nowadays, this procedure is seldom, if ever, carried out for that purpose. Nevertheless, particularly in severe head injuries, the presence of a significant shift of the midline structure (>5 mm) may necessitate surgical intervention. The operation is directed at the evacuation of blood clots and necrotic tissue, but on completion of the procedure, in the presence of severe brain swelling, some surgeons prefer to leave the dura open, not to replace the bone flap, and, in some cases, even to resect one frontal lobe or the anterior 5 cm of either temporal lobe.

Cerebral decompression may also be necessary or useful, as a temporary measure, after the technically difficult removal of a benign tumour (meningioma), when a period of brain swelling (or oedema) may be expected. Since the advent of hypertonic solutions, massive craniotomies are now rarely done and one can probably say that patients who are unresponsive to medical therapy have probably reached the neurological point of no return.

What is more, although craniotomy has successfully reduced ICP in most injured patients, it must be appreciated that the driving force for the formation of oedema fluid is the difference between intravascular and interstitial pressure. Decompression of the brain by bone removal probably results in a reduction of IFP, and therefore enhances the formation of oedema.

Steroid therapy

During the last decade, corticosteroids have been used extensively for the treatment of cerebral oedema, although their value has been the subject of much debate. Currently, however, there is a widespread conviction that steroids are the most effective drugs for this condition [2, 6, 8, 15, 18, 23].

During the last few years, dexamethasone, a semi-synthetic steroid, has become the most commonly used steroid in neurosurgical practice and numerous studies have demonstrated that it significantly reduces the quantity of vasogenic oedema and reduces a high ICP. In addition to the various other glucocorticoids, aldosterone has also been shown to reduce cerebral oedema [26].

The mode of action of steroids in this context is not universally agreed and in fact their beneficial effects may stem from several different mechanisms.

1) One factor is *reduction of the increased capillary permeability.* Steroids appear to correct a functional derangement, perhaps by stabilizing cell membranes and influencing local enzymes, with resultant decrease in transcellular water and electrolyte shifts. In this respect, direct effects upon the transport of sodium, potassium, and fluid across cell membranes, and a stabilizing effect upon lysosomal activity appear to be of great importance.

2) They may *improve neuronal function* by improving CBF and by restoring autoregulation in the oedematous tissue, both of which result in a decrease in transcapillary leakage.

3) They have been reported to *reduce the rate of CSF production.*

Whatever the mode of action, the influence of steroids is variable and the response differs considerably in various cerebral diseases.

Oedema associated with cerebral tumours

The response to steroid therapy in patients with cerebral metastases and gliobastomas is often dramatic [2, 8]. In astrocytomas and other more slowly growing tumours such as meningiomas, the results are less spectacular. Continuous monitoring of ICP in patients with supratentorial tumours has demonstrated that dexamethasone significantly lowers the level of ICP, decreases the amount and duration of A waves, and markedly reduces fluctuations in ICP. This last effect (barostabilization) reduces variation of cerebral perfusion pressure (CPP) and leads to a more uniform blood supply, with a possible improvement in cerebral metabolism and clinical symptoms. In patients with tumours in the posterior fossa, blockage of the CSF pathways is the main cause of intracranial hypertension (obstructive hydrocephalus). A decrease in CSF production achieved with dexamethasone should effectively improve the intracranial buffering capacity. Finally, there is evidence that some tumours undergo a reduction of their size for reasons other than reduction in oedema content.

The dose commonly used for treating peritumour cerebral oedema is 12 mg initially and then 4 mg 6-hourly, but this should be increased in patients with severe oedema. The duration of treatment varies from patient to patient but in all cases, particularly if the patient has been receiving long-term steroid therapy, the dosage must be reduced gradually to avoid recurrence of cerebral oedema and to allow restoration of adrenocortical function.

Oedema associated with cerebral abscesses

Death from brain abscesses is caused by a failure to control the rising ICP due to the associated cerebral oedema. Steroids are very effective in reducing this form of cerebral oedema, and when administered simultaneously with appropriate antibiotics they do not seem to depress the host's resistance to the primary infection. In some patients with acute abscess this combination therapy may even allow the postponement of surgical intervention until encapsulation of the abscess has occurred.

Oedema in severe head injury

Although experimental studies have provided evidence of a beneficial effect of steroids on cerebral oedema following brain injury, their clinical use in severe closed head injuries continues to be a debatable issue [5]. However, well-documented data have, in fact, demonstrated the existence of a dose-dependent effect of dexamethasone on ICP. The efficacy seems to depend on two main factors: (1) The earlier the administration, the better the results; (2) only very high doses are likely to reduce mortality, improve the neurological course, and affect the final outcome.

In such critically ill patients, the recommended doses at present are 100 mg IV initially, then 100 mg IM after an interval of 6 h, and then 4 mg IM every 4 h for 8–10 days. Not surprisingly with this high-dose regimen, concern has been expressed about possible side-effects.

Oedema in acute cerebral infarction

For reasons that are not yet fully understood it appears that corticosteroids may help prevent or decrease the oedema that is associated with abnormalities of the BBB to protein tracers. Such abnormalities do not appear for quite some time after the onset of acute cerebral ischaemia, and this may explain the relative ineffectiveness of corticosteroids in the treatment of ischaemic cerebral oedema.

Diuretics

The agents used for osmotherapy (mannitol, urea, etc.) are potent diuretics; but they lower ICP essentially by their osmotic effect across the BBB and not by their renal action. It has also been shown that frusemide, acetazolamide, and ethacrynic acid [20] curtail CSF production by the choroid plexus and are remarkably effective in reducing cerebral oedema.

This effect is readily understandable when we remember that these diuretics, especially acetazolamide, cause a reduction of the rate of CSF production by some 40%–70%, with a subsequent reduction of ICP. This reduction of ICP further enhances the clearance of oedema fluid at the tissue–ventricular interface. Since dexamethasone and the diuretics probably have differing modes of action, it has been suggested that their suppressive effects on cerebral oedema might be additive. This has proved to be true, at least as far as peritumour oedema is concerned, and for some authors [15] the combination of diuretics and steroids is the first major change in cerebral oedema therapy since dexamethasone was introduced for its treatment in 1959.

This new regimen for peritumour cerebral oedema has been studied in detail [18]: patients with brain tumours were treated with dexamethasone 4 × 4 mg IM for 4–6 days and frusemide 3 × 40 mg PO for 2–4 days. The results were evaluated by CT scan and by measurement of the water and electrolyte content of biopsies removed during craniotomy. Serial CT scans showed an impressive diminution of peritumour oedema, a reduction in the shift of midline structures (septum pellucidum, pineal body, third ventricle) and the re-opening of compressed ventricles. The time required for resolution of oedema varied considerably, however, and was possibly related to the nature of the tumour in individual cases.

The results may be summarized as follows: The decrease in oedema with combined therapy is more pronounced than with either steroids or diuretics alone; and this regimen has proved to be highly effective in peritumour cerebral oedema, particularly in malignant tumours; meningiomas showed little, if any, response.

This combined therapy also seems to be the treatment of choice for benign intracranial hypertension.

Finally, it should be stressed that this combined therapy represents an interesting approach to enhancing the natural resolution of oedema, but clinical data concerning the improvement of neurological function must be collected before it can be accepted as a routine regimen.

Osmotherapy

From the time of the well-known work of Weed and McKibben in 1919 [29], osmotically active agents have been used to treat cerebral oedema or, more precisely, to reduce increased ICP and brain bulk. The principle governing the use of hypertonic solutions is the creation of an intravascular osmotic gradient so that water passes from the brain tissue into the bloodstream. To be effective the agent must remain within the intravascular compartment and not pass across the BBB. The duration of its effect depends upon the rate of disappearance of the drug from the vascular compartment and the rate at which it diffuses into the brain, reducing the osmotic gradient between blood and brain. It therefore appears that in oedema associated with brain injury, the decompression effect of hypertonic infusions results from osmotic withdrawal of water from normal rather than oedematous tissue, and the beneficial effects must be attributed to a general decompression from a decrease in the bulk of normal tissue. In cases of severe head injuries when lesions or disturbances of the BBB are diffuse, osmotherapy may in fact have adverse effects. Hypertonic solutions increase blood volume and arterial pressure. In severe brain lesions autoregulation is disturbed and transmission of the rise in arterial pressure may further increase the ICP. Furthermore, when there are widespread lesions of the BBB, the hypertonic solutions pass into the oedematous tissue and reverse the osmotic gradient, leading to a rebound phenomenon. Hence osmotherapy is only useful if a rapid decompression is required in those patients who are in a critical condition as a result of a high ICP.

Of the various drugs available, mannitol (25%) is the most widely used; it is given IV in dosages ranging from 1 to 4 g/kg body weight (average 1.5 g/kg). For optimal effect rapid administration over a period of 20–30 min is necessary, and its effect begins after 10–20 min, is maximal between 1 and 2 h, and gradually declines over 6 h. Rebound phenomena occur but are minimal. Recently, the long-term, intermittent administration of mannitol (25%) in lower doses (0.3 g/kg IV every 6 h) has proved adequate in the treatment of cerebral oedema. These smaller doses prevent the development of circulatory overload and hypernatraemia from dehydration.

Glycerol is an hypertonic agent that may be given PO (0.5–0.7 g/kg every 3–4 h). It has minimal rebound phenomena, is non-toxic, and can be given repeatedly over long periods. It has been shown to be effective in the treatment of oedema following stroke, but its greatest promise lies in the treatment of benign intracranial hypertension and of those patients with inoperable tumours in whom prolonged osmotherapy is required.

Urea, because of the risks of serious rebound phenomenon, is no longer used.

Restriction of fluid intake

Drastic dehydration has been reported as a treatment for intracranial hypertension in severe head injuries [1]. The method consists in curtailing water intake for the first few days, or restricting it to 250 ml per day, a volume needed for administration of drugs. As a result of this, hyperosmolarity of the plasma develops on about the third day, together with hypernatraemia and functional renal failure. These changes were always reversible after restoration of normal water intake, but the efficiency of this regimen is questionable; a view expressed by Gordon is that 'a negative fluid balance will never diminish brain oedema, but it could endanger the circulation, including the cerebral circulation and the renal function' [9].

The current opinion on this procedure is that while fluid overload should be rigorously avoided after a severe cerebral insult, patients do require a basic water intake (1500–2000 ml for a normal adult). Fluid restriction should be used with caution if hyperosmolar agents, diuretics, or dexamethasone are being given.

Other measures

Hyperventilation

Cerebral blood flow is exquisitely sensitive to the arterial CO_2 tension ($PaCO_2$). During hyperventilation the fall in $PaCO_2$ leads to constriction of cerebral vessels, reduction of CBF, and a consequent reduction in ICP. Lowering the $PaCO_2$ by 1 mmHg (0.13 kPa) decreases ICP by

5%. The prerequisite for this effect is the presence of sufficient healthy brain to respond to the hypocapnia by means of vasoconstriction. The maintenance of $PaCO_2$ between 25 and 30 mmHg (3.3 and 4 kPa) and PaO_2 above 100 mmHg (13.3 kPa) promotes the maximal lowering of ICP. A $PaCO_2$ of less than 20 mmHg (2.7 kPa) intensifies the degree of cerebral vasoconstriction causing ischaemic oedema and a rise in ICP. In addition to this specific action, it is likely that part of the beneficial effect of controlled hyperventilation is due to an improved O_2 supply, particularly in unconscious patients, who are frequently hypoxaemic. The dangers of hypercapnia and arterial hypertension may also be avoided.

Hypothermia

In man, moderate hypothermia has had a considerable vogue as a treatment for head injuries and other lesions that might cause cerebral oedema. The rationale is based on the reduction of the brain's metabolic requirements at lower temperatures, with a resulting protective effect upon damaged but potentially recoverable cells or metabolic systems, and also on the demonstrated reduction in ICP, which is due, in part, to a reduced CBF. The clinical results have not been as striking as anticipated, however, and consequently hypothermia has been largely abandoned. Nonetheless, the need to avoid hyperpyrexia is widely recognized.

Hyperbaric oxygenation

Hyperbaric O_2 may reduce ICP by reducing cerebral volume in a manner similar to hyperventilation. However, high PO_2 values are themselves dangerous and in the absence of clear-cut benefits in cerebral oedema the high monetary costs and potential medical risks preclude its general use.

Barbiturate therapy

Barbiturates have been shown to reduce the formation of cerebral oedema following experimental cryogenic cortical lesions. The mechanisms of this action are probably complex and a number of theories explaining the protective effect of barbiturates on the brain have emerged, namely

a) Reduction of the brain's metabolic requirements
b) Reduction of ICP and consequent increased CPP

c) Reduction in the absolute level of arterial pressure and limitation of its fluctuation in response to noxious stimuli
d) Increase of cerebrovascular resistance in healthy areas of the brain and shunting of blood towards ischaemic regions that have a fixed low vascular resistance, also improving development of collateral flow
e) Protection against cerebral ischaemia (by controlling the co-enzyme and the free radical, and by retarding lipid peroxidation).

References

1. Benabid AL, Baud A, Rougement J de, Barge M, Chirossel JP (1979) Drastic dehydration as treatment of intracranial hypertension in severe head injuries. (Symposium on intracranial pressure). Neurosurgery 4/5:459
2. Brock M, Wiegand H, Zillig C, Zywietz C, Moc P, Dietz H (1976) The effect of dexamethasone on intracranial pressure in patients with supratentorial tumors. In: Pappius HM, Feindel W (eds) Dynamics of brain edema Springer, Berlin Heidelberg New York, pp 330–336
3. Bucknill JC, Tuke DH (1874) A manual of psychological medecine, 3rd edn. Churchill, London, p 587
4. Cantu RC, Amir Ahmadi H, Pricto C (1968) Evaluation of the increased risk of gastro-intestinal bleeding following intracranial surgery in patients receiving high steroid dosages in the immediate post-operative period. International Surgery Digest 50:325
5. Clasen RA, Hucmman MS, Pandolfi S, Laing I, Jacobs J (1976) Computed tomography of vasogenic edema. In: Pappius HM, Feindel W (eds) Dynamics of brain edema Spring, Berlin Heidelberg New York, pp 278–282
6. Faupel G, Reulen HJ, Muller D, Schurmann K (1976) Double blind study on the effects of steroids on severe closed head injury. In: Pappius HM, Feindel W (eds) Dynamics of brain edema. Springer, Berlin Heidelberg New York pp 337–343
7. Fujimoto T, Walker JJ, Spatz M, Klatzo I (1976) Pathophysiologic aspects of ischemic edema. In: Pappius HM, Feindel W (eds) Dynamics of brain edema. Springer, Berlin Heidelberg New York pp 171–180
8. Galilich JH, French LA (1961) Use of dexamethasone in the treatment of cerebral edema resulting from brain tumors and brain surgery. American Practitioner 12:169–176
9. Gordon E, Ponten U (1975) The non-operative treatment of severe head injuries. In: Winken PJ, Bruyn GW (eds) Handbook of clinical neurology, vol 24/II. North Holland, Amsterdam Oxford/American Elsevier, New York, pp 599–626
10. Hossmann KA (1976) Development and resolution of ischemic brain swelling. In: Pappius HM, Feindel W (eds) Dynamics of brain edema. Springer, Berlin Heidelberg New York, 218–227
11. Janny P (1950) La pression intra-crânienne chez l'homme. Thèse :Faculté de Médecine, Paris (Reprinted: Clermont reproduction, Clermont-Ferrand 1972)
12. Katzman R, Pappius HM (1973) Brain electrolytes and fluid metabolism. Williams & Wilkins, Baltimore, pp 366–408

13. Klatzo I (1967) Neuropathological aspects of brain edema. J Neuropathol Exp Neurol 24:1
14. Lanksch W, Oettinger W, Baethmann A, Kazner E (1976) CT findings in brain edema compared with direct chemical analysis of tissue samples. In: Pappius HM, Feindel W (eds) Dynamics of brain edema. Springer, Berlin Heidelberg New York
15. Long DM, Maxwell R, Choi KS (1976) A new therapy regimen for brain edema. In: Pappius HM, Feindel W (eds) Dynamics of brain edema. Springer, Berlin Heidelberg New York, pp 292–300
16. Lundberg N (1960) Continuous recording and control of ventricular fluid pressure in neurosurgical practice. Acta Psychiatr Neurol Scand 36 [Suppl 149]:1–193
17. Marsh ML, Marshall LF, Shapiro HM (1977) Neurosurgical intensive care. Anesthesiology 47:149–163
18. Meinig G, Aulich A, Wende S, Reulen HJ (1976) The effect of dexamethasone and diuretics on peritumor brain edema: Comparative study of tissue water content and CT. In: Pappius HM, Feindel W (eds) Dynamics of brain edema. Springer, Berlin Heidelberg New York, pp 301–305
19. Miller D, Adams H (1972) Physiopathology and management of intracranial pressure. Heinemann Medical, London, pp 308–324 (Scientific foundations of neurology)
20. Miyazaki Y, Suematsu K, Nakajama J (1969) Effects of ethacrynic acid on lowering of intracranial pressure. Arzneim Forsch 19:1961
21. Penn RP (1969) Cerebral edema and blood volume in man measured by CT scan. In: Pappius HM, Feindel W (eds) Dynamics of brain edema. Springer, Berlin Heidelberg, pp 288–292
22. Reulen HJ (1976) Vasogenic brain oedema. Br J Anaesth 48:741–752
23. Reulen HJ, Hadjimos A, Hase U (1973) Steroids in the treatment of brain edema. In: Schurmann K, Brock M, Reulen HJ, Voth D (eds) Advances in neurosurgery I. Springer, Berlin Heidelberg New York, p 92
24. Reulen HJ, Graham R, Spatz M, Klatzo I (1977) Role of pressure gradients and bulk flow in dynamics of vasogenic brain edema. J Neurosurg 46:24–35
25. Reulen HJ, Tsuyumu M, Tack A, Fenske AR, Prioleau GR (1978) Clearance of edema fluid into cerebrospinal fluid. A mechanism for resolution of brain edema. J Neurosurg 48:754–764
26. Schmiedek P, Oettinger W, Baethmann A, Enzenbach R, Marguth F (1974) Aldosterone. A new therapeutic principle for the treatment of cerebral oedema in man. Acta Neurochir (Vienna) 30:59–68
27. Spatz M, Fujimoto J, Go GK (1976) Transport studies in ischemic cerebral edema. In: Pappius HM, Feindel W (eds) Dynamics of brain edema. Springer, Berlin Heidelberg New York pp 181–186
28. Stern WE (1972) The cerebral edemas. Heinemann Medical, London, 289–296 (Scientific foundations of neurology)
29. Weed LH, McKibben PS (1919) Experimental alteration of brain bulk. Am J Physiol 48:531 (Reprinted 1965: J Neurosurg 22:404)

Chapter 44

Brain Resuscitation

P. Safar

Following breakthroughs in respiratory resuscitation in the 1950s and in cardiac resuscitation in the 1960s, there has been since 1970 a logical extension of cardiopulmonary resuscitation (CPR) to cardiopulmonary-cerebral resuscitation (CPCR) [62, 63]. Although the term 'brain resuscitation' was introduced in the 1970s, clinical developments in the evaluation, care and resuscitation of patients with cerebral trauma and ischemic stroke began in the 1920s. Examples of this progression are the neurosurgical ICUs of Walter Dandy and Harvey Cushing; osmotherapy for brain edema [32]; intracranial pressure (ICP) monitoring [39, 42]; therapeutic hypothermia [59, 60]; and pharmacologic hibernation [38]. Only recently, however, has the ability to prevent the sequence of brain damage by treatment initiated *after* cardiac arrest been demonstrated [9, 70].

Brain injury produced by cardiac arrest, ischemic stroke, other anoxic states, or head injury has a profoundly damaging effect on the patient, on his family, and on society. The potential socioeconomic importance of brain resuscitation combined with critical care triage (i.e., 'letting die' those with irreversible severe brain damage [25]) is illustrated by an estimated potential saving of billions of dollars spent on hospitalization, care in nursing homes, and loss in productivity.

Confusion and controversy have arisen because of incautious conclusions drawn from comparisons of experimental results of different animal models, treatment regimens, and post-insult management [26, 41, 64]. First, one must keep in mind these sometimes subtle, but nonetheless practically important differences between the kinds of injury produced in the brain by ischemia, anoxia, hypoglycemia, anemia, trauma, hemorrhage, metabolic or toxic abnormalities, inflammation, tumor or different combinations of these processes. Secondly, with ischemic insults, there are important distinctions between global ischemia (as in cardiac arrest or shock states) and the focal ischemia of transient or permanent embolic or thrombotic occlusion with infarction. Thirdly, there are important differences between reduced blood flow (as in shock) and total cessation of blood flow (as in cardiac arrest). Fourth, the most commonly overlooked distinction is that between *protection*, i.e., measures instituted before and usually continued during an insult [23, 72], and *resuscitation*, i.e., measures initiated after an insult [9, 70]. The fifth differentiation, related to the fourth, is that between the direct effect of the primary insult itself (e.g., cardiac arrest) and complex secondary changes after the start of reperfusion, which add to the initial damage but also offer an opportunity for therapeutic intervention. Sixth, to evaluate new treatments one should use clinically important variables which indicate nonviability, such as performance disability days or months post-insult; and histopathologic quantitation of cell necroses. In contrast, measurement of apnea time, pupil signs, EEG changes, CBF, brain metabolism, and brain and CSF chemical composition during or early after the insult, usually obtained in short-term experiments, although scientifically useful for the study of mechanisms, do not give conclusive answers to the question of brain viability as influenced by therapy.

Brain resuscitation measures for use after cardiac arrest are based on still incomplete knowledge of pathophysiologic mechanisms. The presently standard and other, still controversial, measures to be summarized in this chapter will remain in a state of flux for many years to come (Table 44.1). We will focus on global brain ischemia, but will also briefly mention the pathophysiology and management of other types of brain insults toward the end of the chapter. In spite of similarities in mechanisms, treatment that is effective in one of these conditions may not be effective in others [64, 66].

Pathophysiology

Sudden *complete* cessation of brain circulation results in depletion of available oxygen and in unconsciousness within about 10 s [61, 75, 76]; and in depletion of brain glucose and adenosine triphosphate within about 5 min [46, 75, 76]. Energy failure causes leaking cell membranes with predominantly intracellular edema. Vasogenic interstitial edema, common after cerebral trauma or encephalitis, is less pronounced and late after ischemic anoxia. Complete circulatory

arrest for more than about 5 min with standard post-arrest therapy has resulted, in animals and man, in neurologic deficit and scattered neuronal necroses [9, 14, 21, 22, 52, 81]. With use of some of the brain resuscitation measures to be described subsequently, the limit of 5 min is now being extended [9, 12, 70].

This author's hypothesis is supported by Negovski's 'post-resuscitation disease' [50]; Ames' 'no-reflow phenomenon' [4]; and Hossman's finding that some cerebral neurons can electrically recover even after 60 min of circulatory arrest [30]. Our hypothesis is as follows: (1) After global brain ischemia *without* reperfusion (as in experimental decapitation), homogeneously distributed neuronal changes can be detected by electron microscopy after 5–7 min of circulatory arrest; these changes become clearly irreversible only after about 60 min of circulatory arrest [21, 22]. (2) After global brain ischemia *with* reperfusion later than 5–7 min, multifocal necroses with an inhomogeneous distribution develop. Reperfusion seems to provoke secondary changes which evolve into miliary microscopic infarcts [4, 9, 14, 52]. The probable causative factors include transient vasoparalysis, accompanied and followed by multifocal hypoperfusion from blood cell sludging, tissue edema, and vasospasm; hypermetabolism (perhaps related to catecholamine release); tissue acidosis, release of free chemical radicals which tend to damage membranes; and varying degrees of intra- and extracellular edema [35, 53] — all of which lead via multiple positive feedback loops to multifocal neuronal death [51, 64]. These secondary changes can be intensified by failure of function in noncerebral organ systems, some of which may be treated separately with survival benefit to the brain [9,

Table 44.1. Summary of present knowledge of measure for brain resuscitation after various insults

Treatment	Acute ICP rise Animal	Man	Cardiac arrest Animal	Man	Brain infarct Animal	Man	Trauma, edema Animal	Man	Toxic, metabolic, inflammatory Animal	Man
Moderate hypertension	?	?	(+)	?	(+)	(+)	—	—	?	?
Severe hypertension	—	—	—	—	—	—	—	—	—	—
Hemodilution (IV)	?	?	(+)	?	+	(+)	(+)	?	?	?
Heparinization	?	?	(+)	?	—	—	—	—	?	?
Thiopentone—high dose	+	+	(+)	?	+	?	+	(+)	?	(+)
Thiopentone—conventional dose	+	+	0	?	+	?	(+)	(+)	?	(+)
Immobilization, contr. vent.	+	+	(+)	?	(+)	?	(+)	(+)	?	(+)
Osmotherapy	+	+	?	?	(+)	?	(+)	(+)	?	(+)
Hypothermia	+	+	(+)	?	+	?	+	(+)	?	(+)

Adapted from Safar [25a, 66, 68].
?, not known; 0, no effect shown; —, may increase brain damage; (+), may reduce brain damage; +, reduces brain damage.

12, 70]. There is no clinical method available at this time to quantitate the permanent loss of neurons.

On the basis of the identified changes mentioned above, potentials for saving injured or threatened neurons after ischemic–anoxic insults lie in combating cerebral edema and acidosis, accumulation of free chemical radicals, accumulation of brain amines, and multifocal hypoperfusion with hypermetabolism.

Although sudden complete ischemia seems to lead immediately to a shift of fluid from the extracellular into the intracellular compartment of the brain, it may not cause a rise in ICP unless the insult is very prolonged and severe, and a critical mass of brain tissue becomes edematous. Cerebral edema decreases intracranial compliance (the added CSF volume tolerated without sustained rise in ICP) before it gives a sustained increase in ICP, as CSF must first be displaced before ICP rises. A noninvasive method for recognizing cerebral edema before it raises ICP is needed. CT scanning looks promising.

Following reperfusion after various periods of circulatory arrest, total CBF is increased for 15–30 min [80], due to acidosis-induced vasoparalysis. Many microscopic brain areas, however, do not seem to reperfuse [4]. Thereafter, total CBF declines to and remains significantly below prearrest levels for reasons not fully understood, but in part because of tissue edema and vasospasm [51, 80].

In circulatory shock, i.e., *incomplete* temporary global brain ischemia, CBF autoregulation usually maintains CBF and consciousness as MAP decreases to about 50 mmHg. Below this level, delirium or coma may ensure. With MAP below about 30 mmHg and CBF below about 20% of normal, the pupils may dilate and the viability of neurons becomes doubtful. In circulatory shock states, CNS depression does not correlate well with reduction in blood volume or cardiac output; it correlates well, however, with reduction in cerebral perfusion pressure (CPP), i.e., ICP minus MAP (mean arterial pressure). Reduction in O_2 transport may become critical even when hypotension is only moderate, when hypoxemia is present as well. Brain damage secondary to hypoxemia or trauma can make prolonged hypovolemic shock irreversible; and maintaining cerebral perfusion can increase survival from shock [37]. The brain in shock has not yet been studied adequately.

A trickle of CBF can result in worse neuronal damage than complete ischemia, presumably due to a greater accumulation of acids in the presence of glucose transport [75]. Low perfusion (but more than a trickle of blood flow) e.g., 10%–20% of normal CBF, as presumably produced by standard closed-chest CPR, while incapable of restoring consciousness, seems to be able to sustain neuronal viability at least for a short time [85]. However, during CPR one cannot rely on it [8]. Open-chest direct cardiac massage seems to produce blood flows above this critical level [2, 3, 8, 18]. Reliable measurements of CBF, cerebral metabolic rate, and neuronal viability during CPR have not yet been recorded.

The normal brain tolerates hypoxemia better than ischemia. When arterial PO_2 is reduced to 30 mmHg (4 kPa) or less during normal perfusion pressure, cerebral lactic acidosis develops; cellular death does not occur unless hypoxemia is more severe or associated with severe hypotension. Hypoxemia is common in comatose patients, due to aspiration, shock lung, or neurogenic pulmonary edema. The latter condition is poorly understood, but presumably follows a massive sympathetic discharge that overloads the pulmonary vascular bed; this can be triggered by intracranial hypertension, cerebral hypoxia, or hypothalamic lesions [88].

The pathophysiology of cerebral trauma with space-occupying lesions, contusions, and petechial hemorrhages [15, 49, 58], of ischemic stroke with its central necrotic focus and surrounding 'trouble zone' [28], and that of encephalitis [44, 48] are beyond the scope of this chapter.

Standard measures for brain-oriented life-support

Early after an acute cerebral insult, in the comatose patient, extracranial complications (hypoxemia, hypercarbia, hypotension, severe hypertension, hyperthermia, uremia, sepsis) can worsen the neurologic deficit [11, 12, 22b, c]. Optimizing these extracranial variables to benefit the brain can ameliorate the deficit [10, 22b, c]. Thus, several accepted measures have evolved from experimental evidence or clinical experience which, when used immediately after restoration of spontaneous circulation following cardiac arrest (or after re-oxygenation following head injury) might salvage neurons [25a]. These measures should be initiated immediately after the insult and be sustained throughout the period of unresponsiveness, i.e., for at least 2–7 days (Table 44.2) [22b, c, 62, 63, 68].

Table 44.2. Standard measures of brain-oriented life-support. Guidelines for management of coma following global ischemia–anoxia [67, 68]

Rule out mass lesion (clinical findings, angiography, CAT scan)
1. Control mean arterial pressure (MAP)
   (a) Brief mild hypertension (MAP 110–130 mmHg) for 15 min immediately after restoration of the circulation (optional)
   (b) *Maintain normotension* or slight hypertension throughout coma (MAP 90–110 mmHg) (after trauma MAP 60–90 mmHg)
2. Immobilization: controlled ventilation: some degree of neuromuscular blockade
3. IV anesthesia for deafferentation or prevention/control of seizures e.g., thiopentone or pentobarbitone 2–5 mg/kg + 1–2 mg/kg every 1–2 h, max. 30 mg/kg (blood level 2–4 mg/dl); or diphenylhydantion 7 mg/kg IV.
4. Blood gases and acid–base status
   Arterial PCO_2 25–35 mmHg (3.3–4.7 kPa) maintained by controlled ventilation if necessary
   Arterial pH 7.3–7.6
   Arterial PO_2 over 100 mmHg (13.3 kPa)
5. Steroids (optional)
   Methylprednisolone 5 mg/kg followed by 1 mg/kg every 6 h; or dexamethasone
   1 mg/kg followed by 0.2 mg/kg every 6 h
   Short-term for 2–5 days
6. Blood variables
   Hematocrit 30%–40%; electrolytes normal
   Plasma colloid osmotic pressure over 15 mmHg (albumin over 3 g/100 ml)
   Serum osmolality 280–330 mosmol/liter
   Glucose 100–300 mg/100 ml
7. Fluids: alimentation
   No dextrose in water
   Use dextrose 5%–10% in 0.25%–0.5% NaCl IV
   30–50 ml/kg/24 h (100 ml/kg per 24 h in infants) + potassium
8. Maintain normothermia or mild hypothermia
   (Short-term hypothermia optional; long-term hypothermia not recommended)
9. Monitor ICP (only if a safe technique is established)—optional after CPR, but recommended after head injury
10. Control increases in ICP to <15 mmHg by:
    Further hyperventilation [$PaCO_2$ 20 mmHg (2.7 kPa)]
    CSF drainage (if ICP catheter)
    Mannitol 0.5g/kg; plus 0.3 g/kg per hour short-term
    Diuretic (e.g., frusemide)
    Thiopentone or pentobarbitone 2–5 mg/kg IV, repeat as needed (See 3)
    Hypothermia, 30°–32°C, short-term (relaxant, anesthesia, vasodilation)
11. Evaluate insult, coma, outcome [33, 67, 68, 87]

Respiratory care can greatly influence intracranial dynamics. For example, coughing and straining must be avoided, as they can cause a dangerous rise in intracranial blood volume and ICP and thereby worsen brain edema. Personnel must be skilled in rapid tracheal intubation, particularly in restless, comatose patients at risk from aspiration.

Control of *posture* is important. In accident victims, the head must be manipulated with caution to avoid aggravating any cervical spinal cord injury. Anteflexion and lateral rotation must be absolutely avoided. Flexion or torsion of the neck should be avoided, also because it may compress the neck veins. The head-down position should be avoided, because it increases arterial, venous, and intracranial pressures. The supine position is preferred to the sitting position, as the latter may produce postural hypotension and cerebral hypoperfusion.

Arterial blood pressure (Table 44.2) should be controlled to avoid both hypotension [4, 12, 30], as defined in terms of the individual patient, and severe hypertension [11]. After cardiac arrest, normotension, i.e., MAP of about 100 mmHg, or mild sustained hypertension may be beneficial. After head trauma, when there is a breakdown of the blood-brain barrier, normotension or mild hypotension is preferable. Possibly a brief period of moderate hypertension not exceeding MAP of 150 mmHg may be beneficial immediately after spontaneous circulation is restored after cardiac arrest. This brief hypertensive bout often occurs inadvertently, secondary to the adrenaline used during CPR. It may help restart microcirculatory blood flow in the presence of sludging. On the other hand, severe hypertension increases cerebral blood volume and ICP, can cause cerebral edema and hemorrhage, and can result in an augmented post-ischemic neurologic deficit [11].

Neuromuscular blockade achieved with a curare-like agent such as pancuronium allows prolonged immobilization, which facilitates control of arterial pressure and blood gases, and thereby may ameliorate brain damage [10, 22c].

If the neuromuscular block is partial, rather than complete, one can recognize recovery of consciousness and lateralizing neurologic signs, so as not to miss a mass lesion, such as an epidural or subdural hematoma, which calls for emergency craniotomy.

Treatment or prevention of seizures and also of noxious afferent stimuli, restlessness and straining, may all require a CNS depressant. Thiopentone or pentobarbitone in conventional anesthetic doses, which do not depress the cardiovascular system, would be one choice. Other choices include diphenylhydantoin (Dilantin, phenytoin [1, 17]) and diazepam. Other IV anesthetics that are known to decrease cerebral activity and metabolism and ICP may be used empirically, but, only barbiturates have so far been studied for their ability to ameliorate brain damage in reproducible animal models, and none have been studied in controlled clinical trials. Whether deafferentation by analgesia alone, such as is obtained with nitrous oxide [16], can help to reduce brain damage after ischemic insults has not yet been examined. Other volatile anesthetics, which vasodilate, are not recommended.

Prompt control of seizures is essential to prevent injurious hypermetabolism [31a, 75]. A muscle relaxant can be used first to facilitate ventilation and oxygenation (which may be discontinued intermittently to permit periodic neurologic assessment); and subsequently, EEG seizures must also be blocked pharmacologically with one of the drugs mentioned above (barbiturate, phenytoin, diazepam).

Tracheal intubation and mechanically controlled ventilation should be used to maintain arterial PCO_2 at 25–35 mmHg (3.3–4.7 kPa) arterial PO_2 over 100 mmHg (13.3 kPa), and arterial pH between 7.3 and 7.6 Moderate controlled hyperventilation throughout coma might decrease ICP, counteract cerebral acidosis, and improve intracerebral blood flow distribution through the 'reverse steal effect' of donating CBF to troubled areas by constricting reactive vascular beds. Prolonged controlled hyperventilation seems to increase survival rates in patients following head injury, but does not unequivocally decrease neurologic damage [24].

The use of *corticosteroids* following acute cerebral insults with coma is controversial [65]. Studies of steroids in animal models or uncontrolled clinical situations have given inconclusive results. Potentially beneficial effects of corticosteroids have been identified at the cellular level: activation of the sodium–potassium pump, stabilization of lysosomal membranes, prevention of the release of lytic enzymes, and stabilizing mitochondria and capillary walls [54, 56, 57]. There are no reports showing that steroid therapy can augment cerebral edema or cause irreversible brain damage. The only complications feared with steroid medication, namely stress ulceration, uncontrollable infection, and decreased wound healing, have not been proven to result directly from short-term steroid medication. Beneficial effects of corticosteroids are best documented for brain tumor, less well documented for inflammation, and least for ischemic stroke and trauma. Their effects after cardiac arrest have not yet been studied under controlled conditions. If steroids are used after acute brain insults, they are only adjunctive as one part of a combination of brain resuscitation measures.

Hematologic variables must be controlled (Table 44.2). Maintenance of an optimal hematocrit, electrolytes, osmolality, oncotic pressure, and glucose values must be assured. For maintenance hydration dextrose in water should be avoided, as it can worsen cerebral edema. A continuous infusion of dextrose 5%–10% in 0.25%–0.5% sodium chloride is preferred. Intravenous or intragastric alimentation should start soon after arrest if the patient remains comatose.

Normothermia should be maintained unless hypothermia is chosen as a therapeutic method. Hyperthermia increases cerebral metabolism and edema, intensifies signs of brain injury, and seems to add permanent neurologic damage at core temperatures over about 41 °C, and it must therefore be avoided and rapidly corrected if it occurs.

A rise in ICP cannot be recognized reliably by clinical means and has to be measured directly. Lumbar CSF pressure may not reflect ICP and lumbar puncture can be extremely hazardous in the presence of an increased ICP. The hollow skull screw [89] is favored in cases of medical coma and the ventricular catheter [42] in cases of head trauma. ICP monitoring is more often indicated in coma following head injury or encephalitis than after cardiac arrest.

Even serious increases in ICP may escape clinical detection. High ICP pressure waves can occur suddenly and unexpectedly, probably due to transient increases in intracranial blood volume. Prolonged or sustained increases in ICP in patients with altered consciousness should be avoided, since they can add to the ischemia by decreasing CPP. In the presence of acute intracranial pathology, a rapid sustained rise in ICP can lead to venous congestion, cerebral edema, brain displacement, brain herniation, and brain death. With the exception of such severe events, moderate transient increases in ICP in patients with head injury could not be correlated with outcome [49]. After moderate global ischemic–anoxic insults (cardiac arrest), however, cerebral edema is rarely severe enough to increase ICP. If there is initial neurologic improvement followed by secondary deterioration (usually on the second day post-arrest), however, ICP may rise and should be monitored and controlled, where facilities for safe, atraumatic, aseptic ICP monitoring are established.

ICP monitoring and control have become increasingly common for the management of intracranial emergencies. Monitored increases in ICP are used to titrate measures for its reduction (Table 44.2) such as further hyperventilation, ventricular CSF drainage, use of osmotic or loop diuretics, anesthesia (e.g., barbiturate), corticosteroids, or hypothermia.

While short-term (12–72 h) low-dose osmotherapy with mannitol or glycerol continues to be used, intracranial hypertension is increasingly controlled with anesthetic doses of IV thiopentone or pentobarbitone, particularly when the need for treatment extends beyond 24 h. When large doses of osmotic agents are used for controlling ICP, rebound edema may be a major complication and this limits their usefulness [32, 39] and anesthetic doses of barbiturate (2–5 mg/kg prn) usually suffice for ICP reduction [15, 44, 58, 73].

Although the ICP-reducing measures listed in Table 44.2 were developed from experience with patients after brain surgery or head injury, they are also appropriate for some patients with encephalitis, cardiac arrest, or stroke. ICP monitoring also assists in the detection of circumstances that may inadvertently increase ICP (e.g., tracheal suction, change of body position). Needless to say, suspected mass lesions, such as hemorrhage or tumor, must be investigated promptly by angiography or CAT scanning. These tests are usually not needed in cases of cardiac arrest clearly of noncerebral origin.

One must recognize and reverse a rise of ICP before the diencephalic changes lead to compression and displacement of the midbrain as evidenced by hyperventilation, fixed dilated pupils, and disappearing ciliospinal, oculovestibular, and oculocephalic reflexes. Decorticate rigidity may progress to decerebrate rigidity. Finally, tentorial herniation due to supratentorial ICP rise and axial displacement, either symmetrically or unilaterally, can rapidly lead to medullary herniation, with hypoventilation, tachycardia, progressive arterial hypotension, dilated fixed pupils, and apnea.

Specific (controversial) measures for brain resuscitation

The reader is encouraged to be critical when evaluating the literature on this subject. For a treatment to be of *proven* value after cardiac arrest, in a controlled animal model of global brain ischemia or cardiac arrest, there must be a statistically significant reduction in the functional neurologic deficit and the extent of histopathologic necrosis, after a period of post-ischemic life-support and control of extracranial organ function long enough to give the lesions chance to mature, i.e., at least 4–7 days [68]. Short-term observations and animal models without post-insult life-support only give suggestive evidence. At present the controversial therapies include hypothermia, attempts to promote reperfusion, and the use of anesthetics such as barbiturates, in large doses.

Therapeutic *hypothermia* after ischemic brain injury reduces the rate of brain metabolism, the magnitude of cerebral edema, and the size of experimental infarcts [59, 60]. The effect of hypothermia after global brain ischemia remains to be examined, however, and it has not gained wide acceptance because of the difficult management problems it entails, especially if prolonged beyond 24 h. It is also associated with a variety of undesirable side-effects, such as cardiac arrhythmias, increased blood viscosity with reduced tissue blood flow [45, 84], increased susceptibility to infection, and stress ulceration. The protective effect of hypothermia is unquestioned [74], while its resuscitative effect needs to be restudied.

In patients with a healthy cardiovascular system (e.g., children after drowning) moderate short-term hypothermia is justified, involving reduction of body temperature to 30–32°C for not more than 6–12 h post-insult [59, 74, 84].

To *promote reperfusion* [70, 71] a combination of measures such as sustaining a moderate degree of hypertension with vasopressors and moderate normovolemic hemodilution with plasma substitutes [34] may benefit cerebral recovery [70]. Severe hypertension in the post-ischemic stage is deleterious, however [11], and currently, the value of heparinization is uncertain [71, 86].

Barbiturates had not been studied for their brain resuscitation potential after complete global brain ischemia until the work of Bleyaert and associates in 1975–1978 in Pittsburgh [9]. These studies, in monkeys, were based on a model of global brain ischemia with a high-pressure neck tourniquet combined with induced hypotension plus long-term post-ischemic intensive care. The studies were inspired by the promising results of Yatsu [91] with methohexitone in experimental global anoxia, and of Smith and Hoff [28, 29, 78] with thiopentone after experimental focal ischemia. Amelioration of focal ischemia was later confirmed by Levy [40], Michenfelder [47], and others. In experimental animals with middle cerebral artery occlusion the pre- and post-insult use of large or anesthetic doses of thiopentone or pentobarbitone can reduce the size of the infarct [28, 29, 47, 78]. Also, thiopentone has been shown to reduce ICP in neurosurgical patients [73].

In Bleyaert's experiments [9] an IV loading dose of thiopentone (90 mg/kg) given between 5 and 65 min after the start of reperfusion (the dose which Smith had found to be effective in focal ischemia [78]) decreased the scores for neurologic deficit at 7 days post-ischemia, from control values of 50% (vegetative state) to 0% (no brain damage) in five Rhesus monkeys [9]. Less impressive, but still significant, was the reduction in neurologic deficit when thiopentone was given 15 min after the ischemic insult (5 monkeys). No significant reduction was seen when the delay was 30 or 60 min. The delayed administration of a larger dose was partially effective (5 monkeys) [9], although the histopathologic scores and neurologic deficit scores were significantly lower with early barbiturate loading. These studies [9] were recently repeated [22b, c], since the original animal series were small, the control studies were not concurrent with the barbiturate studies, and several experiments were excluded, because the large dose of thiopentone caused cardiac arrest in the post-ischaemic animals; blood levels rose as high as 20 mg/dl. Monkeys without brain ischemia tolerated these large loading doses much better, however, and only developed a mild transient hypotension without any of the lethal tachyarrhythmias seen after brain ischemia [22a]. Non-cardiotoxic doses of thiopentone given slowly, to produce blood levels of only 2–4 mg/dl, [22a], as well as the previously used thiopentone loading protocol [9], (which

gave near 0% neurologic deficit in 10/27 Rhesus monkeys), did not ameliorate brain damage in pigtail monkeys [22 b].

Barbiturates are known to reduce cerebral metabolic rate [90] and edema formation [77] and to suppress seizure activity, implying a protective influence on survival. There is also evidence to suggest that barbiturates exert a beneficial effect through a blockade of noxious stimuli by anesthesia [75] and prolonged immobilization [10]. There are other possible mechanisms of barbiturate action that have not yet been fully documented, such as scavenging free chemical radicals evolved during ischemia [19]; altering metabolic pathways [27]; and suppressing catecholamine-induced hypermetabolism [36, 51].

Thiopentone loading (as tolerated up to 30 mg/kg) given within 10–50 min of restoring the circulation after cardiac arrest, is now under controlled clinical study [19a, 66]. Clinical feasibility trials showed promising results, but also demonstrated the risk of thiopentone loading rearresting the heart [13]. It should be remembered that the circulatory depressant effects of large doses of thiopentone or pentobarbitone are considerable [20, 43, 55] and the risk: benefit ratio of this treatment has not yet been determined. The optimal dosage, blood levels, and timing of barbiturate administration are still not known. When large doses were used for 1–2 days, pulmonary complications and intractable bradycardia were noted.

Negative results with barbiturates [22b, 31, 79, 83] include failures to show a neuron-saving effect. This may be due to species difference [9, 22b] or differences in post-ischemic life support [79, 83]. There has been no report so far that barbiturates worsen cerebral outcome. Michenfelder postulates that barbiturates reduce ischemic brain damage only by depression of cellular activity and metabolic rate [46, 82, 83], which would make this treatment effective only against incomplete focal ischemia and not against the complete ischemia following cardiac arrest, when there is no metabolism. In a mouse model of alveolar anoxia, he showed that an anesthetically inactive isomer of a barbiturate failed to prolong breathing time [82]. This model, however, is not a measure of post-ischemic changes in terms of viability of neurons. Michenfelder's hypothesis can nonetheless explain a beneficial action of barbiturates when given after complete global brain ischemia, because the treatment is given to ameliorate the secondary changes following ischemia and not to treat the initial insult.

(These secondary changes are multifocal areas of incomplete ischemia.)

Barbiturates do not benefit the brain primarily by reducing ICP: in Bleyaert's experiments ICP was not increased [9]; in Reye's syndrome ICP controlled by barbiturates [44] gave better outcome than osmotherapy and hypothermia [48]; and increases in ICP do not necessarily correlate with a bad outcome following head injury [49].

Meanwhile, *conventional* anesthetic doses of thiopentone or pentobarbitone (2–5 mg/kg IV followed by 1–2 mg/kg every 1–2 h to a maximum of 30 mg/kg), which do not depress the circulation and which require only small amounts of vasopressors and plasma volume expansion, may be clinically indicated—to sedate, suppress seizures, facilitate controlled ventilation, reduce brain stress, and normalize a monitored rise of ICP [66]. But even this less controversial treatment should only be used by clinicians skilled in the administration of anesthetics, and only for those patients who are comatose following global or focal ischemic–anoxic insults [68].

Barbiturate anesthesia for protection against anticipated brain ischemia during neurosurgical and cardiothoracic surgical procedures also seems to be justified [13]. A combination of moderate hypothermia and conventional doses of barbiturates should be considered. We do *not*, however, at this time recommend the use of large loading doses of barbiturates outside controlled clinical studies. After head injury or encephalitis, administration of prophylactic barbiturates without ICP monitoring is controversial. In shock states with coma, cardiovascular stabilization has priority, since barbiturates may precipitate cardiac arrest in association with hypovolemia.

Since barbiturates suppress neurologic function and the usual clinical signs are removed, careful diagnostic evaluation is necessary. Physicians and the public should be made aware of the fact that benefit can be expected from barbiturate therapy only if it is started soon after the insult.

Other measures, including the use of CNS depressants, should be examined. For 'putting the injured brain to rest' after cardiac arrest or trauma, diphenylhydantoin or etomidate, both of which depress arterial pressure less markedly than barbiturates, deserve study in controlled animal models. Other measures that past studies and clinical impression suggest might be beneficial and which deserve investigation include hemodilution combined with moderate hypertension, osmotherapy, normalization of CSF pH, free radical scavengers which do not depress MAP or the CNS, calcium blockers, vasodilators, hypertonic glucose, high-energy phosphates, and many anesthetic drugs [1, 17, 38, 62, 64]. Volatile anesthetics such as halothane, however, which reduce metabolism but increase CBF, intracranial blood volume, and ICP, do not seem to be beneficial [78].

In the future, treatment for ischemic brain insults will probably not consist of one agent (e.g. barbiturate), but rather will include some CMR depressant as part of a combined pharmacologic and physiologic scheme of therapy.

Miscellaneous insults

In acute focal ischemia (stroke) the patient usually remains conscious with a focal neurologic deficit. Only massive infarcts are likely to produce edema leading to an increase in ICP, coma, and brain death. The collateral circulation influences the size of the infarct by maintaining viable neurons in the tissue which surrounds the eventually necrotic center [28]. Blood pressure should be maintained at normotensive or mildly hypertensive levels. There is suggestive evidence that moderate hemodilution, hyperventilation, and steroid therapy applied within minutes of the onset of paralysis or aphasia may reduce the damage. There is experimental evidence that barbiturates, even in conventional doses [47, 78], as well as hypothermia [59] decrease the infarct size. The value of heparinization has not been documented.

In *head injury* [15, 39, 58], the blood–brain barrier is damaged, which results in vasogenic interstitial edema and multifocal hemorrhages, particularly in contused areas of the brain. Therefore, blood pressure should be kept normal or slightly below normal. After a space-occupying lesion requiring surgical intervention has been ruled out, anesthetic doses of barbiturate have been used extensively for ICP reduction, prevention of convulsions and post-insult protection against ischemia and edema [15, 58]. Prophylactic barbiturate loading in coma, after head injury, however, should await controlled clinical documentation [25a, 49].

In encephalitis and a variety of encephalopathies [63], lack of animal models and the difficulty in performing controlled clinical trials (because of the small number, variety, and severity of cases), has forced clinicians to try therapies that have been found to be effective in brain ischemia and trauma.

Cessation of resuscitation

Brain death, when suspected, should be certified, and this should be followed by withdrawal of all life-support [7, 25]. Criteria for determining brain death should follow international guidelines and practices [25a].

Persistent vegetative state (apallic syndrome, social death) with an active EEG and some intact reflexes, must be clearly distinguished from brain death. The decision to discontinue extraordinary means of life-support in this condition is a medical one. It should be made by an experienced physician, usually the patient's primary physician, in consultation with relevant specialists, and should consider the patient's previously expressed wishes, the family's attitude, and the quality of life to be expected at best. One must not ask relatives to make the decision.

While the criteria for brain death certification are objective and reliable, proof with 100% reliability in a given patient that the vegetative state is irreversible is usually not possible with presently available methods. Thus, the hopelessness of the situation must often be determined on the basis of published predictive criteria, clinical experience, and judgment. Research into reliable predictive criteria in the early stages after CPR should be given high priority.

While brain death certification calls for withdrawal of *all* life-support measures, 'letting die' calls for discontinuation of only extraordinary measures [25]. These may be defined differently in different communities, but in most industrialized countries extraordinary measures include mechanical ventilation, arrhythmia control, and all types of life-supporting drugs and do not include IV fluids, alimentation, and airway control; available resources are finite everywhere.

Evaluation of results

To assess the value of different forms of treatment after acute brain insults one should attempt to assess: (1) the severity of the insult; (2) prognostic criteria such as the state of consciousness and cranial nerve reflexes soon after the insult; and (3) the ultimate outcome, in terms of the patient's performance capability.

The severity and duration of the *insult* influence the outcome, particularly in ischemic–anoxic brain injury. Additional factors are the adequacy of resuscitation, the underlying disease, and secondary complications. The severity of traumatic brain insult is in itself almost impossible to quantitate. However, the severity of a global ischaemic–anoxic insult, like cardiac arrest, can be estimated retrospectively on the spot by interviewing bystanders, relatives, and ambulance and other health care personnel. We recommend estimating 'arrest time' and 'hypoxia time' (Table 44.3), i.e., duration of severe hypotension, hypoxemia or anemia; hypoxia time includes CPR time [13, 19a, 68].

The depth of *coma*, at least so long as the patient is in the ICU after a cerebral insult, can easily be monitored by using the Glasgow Coma Scoring System [87]. It was designed for cases of

Table 44.3. Estimation of global ischemic–anoxic insult (Pittsburgh Cardiac Arrest form) [67, 68]

(1) *Hypoxia time prior to arrest*
    Time of severe hypotension, severe hypoxemia, or severe anemia   . . . . min

(2) *Arrest time*
    Time without spontaneous or artificial pulse in large arteries. Must *not* include CPR time   . . . . min

(3) *CPR time*
    Equals time of CPR-ABC, performed during absence of spontaneous pulse   . . . . min

(4) *Hypoxia time after arrest*
    Time of severe hypotension, hypoxemia or anemia following restoration of spontaneous circulation   . . . . min

(5) *Total insult time*
    Sum of [1], [2], [3] and [4]:   . . . . min

Repeated arrests and repeated restoration of spontaneous circulation within one resuscitation effort should be stated as the sum of all times without circulation (total arrest time) and all times of hypotension, hypoxemia and anemia (one total hypoxia time), the latter irrespective of whether it occurred before, during or after the first arrest or subsequent repeat arrest.

head injury, to quantitate the depth of CNS depression with a simple 15-point scale (coma with brain death = 3 points; patient conscious and neurologically normal = 15 points). A Pittsburg modification for all types of coma, which employs a 35-point scale (coma with brain death = 7 points; patient conscious and neurologically normal = 35 points), is under investigation at present [68].

In assessment of the depth of coma, rapid recovery of eye and upper airway reflexes should be considered good prognostic signs. Poor (but not hopeless) prognostic signs, on the other hand, include progressive deterioration of reflexes after initial partial recovery; absence of the oculocephalic or oculovestibular reflexes at 6–12 h post-arrest; and continuing unconsciousness and nonreactivity of the pupils [5]. Pupil size, eye and lid movements, and time to return of spontaneous breathing are less reliable indicators.

The *outcome* after emergency resuscitation, in terms of quality of life, expressed as what the patient is likely to be able to do (performance capability) should be evaluated. The Glasgow outcome categories 1 (best) through 5 (worst) [5, 33] provide a simple mechanism for delineating patients' performance capabilities after head injury. The Pittsburgh group modified the Glasgow system for use after *all* types of cerebral insults, by separating cerebral from overall performance categories (CPC, OPC) (Table 44.4) [67, 68]. Briefly, a cerebral performance category (CPC) or overall performance category (OPC) 1

means a normal status without disability; 2 means slight disability, but conscious; 3 means severe disability and conscious; 4 means coma or vegetative state without brain death; and 5 means brain death. For example, a conscious, mentally active, bedridden, post-CPR patient with severe heart disease would have a CPC of 1 and an OPC of 3. Differences in CPC and OPC are for categories 1, 2, and 3, while categories 4 and 5 are determined by the cerebral status only.

These categories should be assessed upon discharge from the ICU, and periodically thereafter up to 1 year. Particular interest in the evaluation of cerebral resuscitation measures is due to the best cerebral performance category which the patient achieves post-resuscitation.

Preservation of brain function should be the central concern in the management of patients during and after emergency resuscitation efforts, as the status of the brain will determine the quality of life subsequent to recovery. Brain damage after ischemic–anoxic insults such as cardiac arrest and resuscitation is partly the result of the initial insult and partly the result of post-resuscitative changes, which are treatable. Physicians must keep informed about current developments in brain resuscitation.

Brain death and the presence of a persistent vegetative state must be determined meticulously to allow 'safe' and ethical withdrawal of extraordinary support measures from the patient. In making these determinations,

Table 44.4. Cerebral and overall performance categories (Glasgow–Pittsburgh 1978 [33, 67, 68])

(A) *CEREBRAL PERFORMANCE CATEGORIES*
Evaluate only cerebral performance capabilities. Estimate *potential* performance if non-cerebral organ systems were (are) normal.
   CPC 1. Good cerebral performance: Conscious, alert, able to work, might have mild neurologic or psychologic deficit.
   CPC 2. Moderate cerebral disability: Conscious, sufficient cerebral function for independent activities of daily life. Able to work in sheltered environment.
   CPC 3. Severe cerebral disability: Conscious, dependent on others for daily support because of impaired brain function. Ranges from ambulatory state to severe dementia or paralysis.
   CPC 4. Coma or vegetative state: Any degree of coma without the presence of all brain death criteria. Unawareness, even if appears awake (vegetative state) without interaction with environment; may have spontaneous eye opening and sleep awake cycles. Cerebral unresponsiveness.
   CPC 5. Brain death: Apnea, areflexia, EEG silence [25].
      CPA A. Under the effect of anesthetic (CNS depressant or relaxant).
(B) *OVERALL PERFORMANCE CATEGORIES*
Reflects cerebral *plus* non-cerebral status.
Evaluate *actual* overall performance.
   OPC 1. Good overall performance: Healthy, alert, capable of normal life, CPC 1.
   OPC 2. Moderate overall disability: Conscious, CPC 2, or moderate disability from non-cerebral systems dysfunction alone, or both. Performs independent activities of daily life, but is disabled for competitive work.
   CPC 3. Severe overall disability: Conscious. OPC 3, or severe disability from non-cerebral organ systems dysfunction alone, or both. Dependent on others for daily support.
   OPC 4. Coma or vegetative state: Same as CPC 4.
   OPC 5. Brain death: Same as CPC 5.

---

premature action must be avoided. The current expansion of cardiopulmonary resuscitation for 'hearts too good to die' [6] to cardiopulmonary–cerebral resuscitation for 'brains too good to die' [62, 63, 68] can make resuscitation a positive force in human evolution. To accomplish this, critical care physicians should participate widely in epidemiologic evaluation research of resuscitation results in general and brain resuscitation trials in particular [19a, 25a, 67, 69].

References

1. Aldrete JA, Romo-Salas F, Jankovsky L, Franatovic Y (1979) Effect of pre-treatment with thiopental and phenytoin on postischemic brain damage in rabbits. Crit Care Med 7:466–470
2. Alifimoff JK, Safar P, Bircher N, Stezoski W, Barbati R (1980a) Cardiac resuscitability after closed-chest, MAST-augmented and open-chest cardio-pulmonary resuscitation (CPR). Anesthesiology 53:S151
3. Alifimoff JK, Safar P, Bircher N, Stezoski W, Barbati R (1980b) Cerebral recovery after prolonged closed-chest, MAST-augmented and open-chest cardiopulmonary resuscitation (CPR) Anesthesiology 53:S147
4. Ames A, Wright RL, Kowada M, Thurston JM, Magno G (1968) Cerebral ischemia. II. The no-reflow phenomenon. Am J Pathol 52:437–465
5. Bates D, Caronna TJ, Cartlidge NEF, Knill-Jones RP, Levy DE, Shaw DD, Plum F (1977) A prospective study of non-traumatic coma: Methods and results in 310 patients. Ann Neurol 2:211–220
6. Beck CF, Leighninger DS (1960) Death after a clean bill of health. JAMA 1974:133–135
7. Beecher H (1968) A definition of irreversible coma. JAMA 205:337–390 (Report of the Harvard Medical School Ad Hoc Committee to Examine the Definition of Brain Death)
8. Bircher N, Safar P (1981) Comparison of standard and "new" closed-chest CPR and open-chest CPR in dogs. Crit Care Med 9:384–385
9. Bleyaert AL, Nemoto EM, Safar P, Stezoski SW, Mickell JJ, Moossy J, Rao GR (1978) Thiopental amelioration of brain damage after global ischemia in monkeys. Anesthesiology 49:390
10. Bleyaert AL, Safar P, Stezoski SW, Nemoto EM, Moossy J (1978) Amelioration of post-ischemic brain damage in the monkey by immobilization and controlled ventilation. Crit Care Med 6:112
11. Bleyaert AL, Sands PA, Safar P, Nemoto EM, Stezoski SW, Moossy J, Rao GR (1980a) Augmentation of postischemic brain damage by severe intermittent hypertension. Crit Care Med 8:41–47
12. Bleyaert AL, Safar P, Nemoto E, Moossy J, Sassano J (1980b) Effect of post-circulatory-arrest life-support on neurological recovery in monkeys. Crit Care Med 8:153–156
13. Breivik H, Safar P, Sands P, Fabritius R, Lind B, Lust P, Mullie A, Orr M, Renck H, Snyder J (1978) Clinical feasibility trials of barbiturate therapy after cardiac arrest. Crit Care Med 6:228–244
14. Brierley JB, Meldrum BS, Brown AW (1973) The threshold and neuropathology of cerebral anoxic-ischemic cell change. Arch Neurol 29:367–374
15. Bruce DA, Gennarelli TA, Langfitt TW (1978) Resuscitation from coma due to head injury. Crit Care Med 6:254–269
16. Carlsson C, Hagerdal M, Kaasik AE, Siesjo BK (1977) A catecholamine-mediated increase in cerebral oxygen uptake during immobilization stress in rats. Brain Res 119:223–231
17. Cullen JP, Aldrete JA, Jankovsky L, Romo-Salas F (1979) Protective action of phenytoin in cerebral ischemia. Anesth Analg (Cleve) 58:165–169
18. Del Guercio LRM, Feins NR, Cohn JD, Coomaraswamy RP, Wollman SB, State D (1964) Comparison of blood flow during external and internal cardiac massage in man. Circulation 30:63
19. Demopoulos HB, Flamm ES, Seligman ML, Jorgensen E, Ransohoff J (1977) Antioxidant effects of barbiturates in model membranes undergoing free radical damage. Acta Neurol Scand 56 [Suppl 64]:152–153
19a. Detre K, Abramson N, Safar P et al. (1981) Collaborative randomized clinical study of cardiopulmonary-cerebral resuscitation. Crit Care Med 9:395–396
20. Etsten B, Li TH (1955) Hemodynamic changes during thiopental anesthesia in humans. J Clin Invest 34:500–509
21. Garcia JH, Kalimo H, Kamijyo Y, Tanaka J, Trump BF (1977a) Cellular events during partial cerebral ischemia. I. Electron microscopy of feline cerebral cortex after middle-cerebral artery occlusion. Virchows Arch [Cell Pathol] 25:191–206
22. Garcia JH, Kalimo H, Kamijyo Y, Tanaka J, Trump BF (1977b) Cellular events during partial cerebral ischemia. II. The ultrastructure of "brain death." Virchows Arch [Cell Pathol] 25:207–220
22a. Gisvold SE, Safar P, Alexander H, Thompson M (1981) Cardiovascular tolerance of thiopental anesthesia for brain resuscitation in monkeys. J Cerebral Blood Flow Metab 1 [Suppl 1]:S264–S265
22b. Gisvold SE, Safar P, Hendrickx HHL, Alexander H (1981) Thiopental treatment after global brain ischemia in monkeys. Anesthesiology 56:A97
22c. Gisvold SE, Safar P, Alexander H, Bleyaert A, Stezoski SW, Bron K (1981) Controlled ventilation after global brain ischemia in monkeys. Anesthesiology 56:A99
23. Goldstein A, Wells BA, Keats AS (1966) Increased tolerance to cerebral anoxia by pentobarbital. Arch Int Pharmacodyn Ther 161:138–143
24. Gordon E (1971) Controlled respiration in the management of patients with traumatic brain injuries. Acta Anaesthesiol Scand 15:193–208
25. Grenvik A, Powner DJ, Snyder JV, Jastremski MS, Babcock RA, Loughhead MG (1978) Cessation of therapy in terminal illness and brain death. Crit Care Med 6:284–291
25a. Grenvik A, Safar P (eds) (1981) Brain failure and resuscitation. Churchill Livingstone, New York
26. Gurvitch AM (1974) Determination of the depth and reversibility of post-anoxic coma in animals. Resuscitation 3:1
27. Hakim AM, Moss G (1976) Cerebral effects of barbiturate. Shift from energy to synthesis metabolism for cellular viability. Surg Forum 27:497–499
28. Hoff JT (1978) Resuscitation in focal brain ischemia. Crit Care Med 6:245–253
29. Hoff JT, Smith AL, Hankinson HL, Nielsen SL (1975) Barbiturate protection from cerebral infarction in primates. Stroke 6:28–33
30. Hossmann KA, Kleihues P (1973) Reversibility of ischemic brain damage. Arch Neurol 29:37–384

31. Hossman KA, Takagi S, Sakaki S (1977) Barbiturate loading following prolonged ischemia of the cat brain. Acta Neurol Scand 56 [Suppl 64]:376–377

31a. Ingvar M, Siesjö B (1981) Cell damage in sustained seizures: rule of local cerebral blood flow and local metabolic rate. J Cerebral Blood Flow Metab 1 [Suppl 1]: S98–S99

32. Javid M (1958) Urea—new use of an old agent. Reduction of intracranial and intraocular pressure. Surg Clin North Am 38:907–928

33. Jennett B, Bond M (1975) Assessment of outcome after severe brain damage: A practical scale. Lancet I: 480–484

34. Jurkiewicz J (1977) The effect of haemodilution on experimental brain edema. European Journal of Intensive Care Medicine 3:167

35. Klatzo I (1967) Neuropathological aspects of brain edema. J Neuropathol Exp Neurol 26:1–14

36. Kofke WA, Nemoto EM, Stezoski SW, Kessler P, Safar P (1977) Cerebral blood flow (CBF) and metabolism (CMR) after 16 minutes of global brain ischemia (GBI) in monkeys. Fed Proc 36:588 (abstract #1669)

37. Kovach AGB, Sandor P (1976) Cerebral blood flow and brain function during hypotension and shock. Ann Rev Physiol 38:571–596

38. Laborit H, Huguenard P (1954) Practice of hibernation therapy in surgery and medicine (French), Masson, Paris

39. Langfitt TW (1973) Increased intracranial pressure. In: Youmans JR (ed) Neurologic surgery. Saunders, Philadelphia, pp 443–495

40. Levy DE, Brierley JB (1979) Delayed pentobarbital administration limits ischemic brain damage in gerbils. Ann Neurol 5:59–64

41. Lind B, Snyder J, Kampschulte S, Safar P (1975) A review of total brain ischaemia models in dogs and original experiments on clamping the aorta. Resuscitation 4:19–31

42. Lundberg N (1960) Continuous recording and control of ventricular fluid pressure in neurosurgical practice. Acta Psychiatr Neurol Scand 36 [Suppl 149]:1–193

43. Lundy JS, Adams RC (1942) Pentothal sodium intravenous anesthesia. US Army Medical Bulletin 63:90–98

44. Marshall LF, Shapiro HM, Rauscher A, Kaufman NM (1978) Pentobarbital therapy for intracranial hypertension in metabolic coma: Reye's syndrome. Crit Care Med 6:1–5

45. Michenfelder JD (1977) Failure of prolonged hypocapnia, hypothermia or hypertension to favorably alter acute stroke in primates. Stroke 8:87–91

46. Michenfelder JD, Theye RA (1970) The effects of anesthesia and hypothermia on canine cerebral ATP and lactate during anoxia produced by decapitation. Anesthesiology 33:430–439

47. Michenfelder JD, Milde JH, Sundt TM (1976) Cerebral protection by barbiturate anesthesia. Use after middle cerebral artery occlusion in Java monkeys. Arch Neurol 33:345–350

48. Mickell JJ, Cook DR, Reigel DH, Painter MJ, Safar P (1976) Intracranial pressure monitoring in Reye–Johnson syndrome. Crit Care Med 4:1–7

49. Miller JD (1979) Barbiturate and raised intracranial pressure. (Editorial) Ann Neurol 6:189–193

50. Negovskii VA (1974) Introduction: reanimatology—the science of resuscitation. In: Stephenson HE (ed) Cardiac arrest and resuscitation. Mosby, St Louis, pp 3–27

51. Nemoto EM (1978) Pathogenesis of cerebral ischemia-anoxia. Crit Care Med 6:203–214

52. Nemoto EM, Bleyaert AL, Stezoski SW, Moossy J, Rao GR, Safar P (1975) Global brain ischemia. A reproducible monkey model. Fed Proc 34:384

53. Pappius HM, Feindel W (ed) (1976) Dynamics of brain edema. Springer, New York

54. Prados M, Strowger B, Feindel W (1945) Studies on cerebral edema. II. Reaction of brain to exposure to air: Physiologic changes. Arch Neurol Psychiatr 54:290–300

55. Price H (1960) General anesthesia and circulatory homeostasis. Physiol Rev 40:187–218

56. Reulen JH (1972) Steroids in brain edema. Springer, New York

57. Rovit RL, Hagan R (1968) Steroids and cerebral edema: The effects of gluco-corticoids on abnormal capillary permeability following cerebral injury in cats. J Neuropathol Exp Neurol 27:277–299

58. Rockoff MA, Marshall LF, Shapiro HM (1979) High-dose barbiturate therapy in humans: A clinical review of 60 patients. Ann Neurol 6:194–199

59. Rosomoff HL (1957) Hypothermia and cerebral vascular lesions. II. Experimental middle cerebral artery interruption followed by induction of hypothermia. Arch Neurol Psychiatr 78:454–464

60. Rosomoff HL, Shulman K, Raynor R, Grainger W (1960) Experimental brain injury and delayed hypothermia. Surg Gynecol Obstet 110:27–32

61. Rossen R, Cabat H, Anderson JP (1943) Acute arrest of cerebral circulation in man. Arch Neurol 50:510–528

62. Safar P (ed) (1977) Advances in cardiopulmonary resuscitation: Proceedings of the Wolf Creek conference, 1975. Springer, New York, pp 177:207

63. Safar P (1978) Brain resuscitation. Crit Care Med 6:199–291 (Symposium issue)

64. Safar P (1979a) Pathophysiology and resuscitation after global brain ischemia. Int Anesthesiol Clin 17:239–284

65. Safar P (1979b) Steroids in brain insults. (Abstract) Proceedings, I Pan-American Congress on Critical Care Medicine, Mexico City, September 23–27, 1979. Excerpta Medica, Amsterdam 499:78

66. Safar P (1980a) Amelioration of postischemic brain damage with barbiturates. Current concepts of cerebrovascular disease. Stroke 15:565–568

67. Safar P (1981b) Cardiopulmonary cerebral resuscitation. A manual for physicians and paramedical instructors. Laerdal, Stavanger (for World Federation of Societies of Anaesthesiologists). Saunders, Philadelphia

68. Safar P (1981c) Resuscitation after brain ischemia. In: Grenvik A, Safar P (eds) Brain failure and resuscitation. Churchill Livingstone, New York, pp 155–184

69. Safar P, Grenvik A (1977) Organization and physician education in critical care medicine. Anesthesiology 47:82–95

70. Safar P, Stezoski W, Nemoto EM (1976) Amelioration of brain damage after 12 minutes cardiac arrest in dogs. Arch Neurol 33:91–95

71. Safar P, Bleyaert A, Nemoto E, Stezoski W (1980) Treatment of hypoperfusion after global brain ischemia in dogs and monkeys. Hypertension, hemodilution, heparinization. Circ Shock 7:200–201 (Abstract 35)

72. Seeley SF, Essex HE, Mann FC (1936) Comparative studies on traumatic shock produced experimentally under ether and under sodium amytal anesthesia. Ann Surg 105:332–338

73. Shapiro HM, Galindo A, Wyte SR, Harris AB (1973) Rapid intra-operative reduction of intracranial pressure with thiopentone. Br J Anaesth 45:1057–1062

74. Siebke H, Rod T, Breivik H, Lind B (1975) Survival after 40 minutes submersion without cerebral sequelae. Lancet I:1275–1277

75. Siesjo BK (1978) Brain energy metabolism. Wiley, New York

76. Siesjo BK, Carlsson C, Hagerdal M, Nordstrom CH (1976) Brain metabolism in the critically ill. Crit Care Med 4:283–294

77. Smith AL, Marque JJ (1976) Anesthetics and cerebral edema. Anesthesiology 45:64–72

78. Smith AL, Hoff JT, Nielsen SL, Larson CP (1974) Barbiturate protection in acute focal cerebral ischemia. Stroke 5:1–7

79. Snyder BD, Ramirez-Lessepas M, Sukhum P, Fryd D, Sung JH (1979) Failure of thiopental to moderate global anoxic injury. Stroke 10:135–141

80. Snyder JV, Nemoto EM, Carroll RG, Safar P (1975) Global ischemia in dogs: Intracranial pressure, brain blood flow and metabolism. Stroke 6:21–27

81. Steegmann AT (1968) Neuropathology of cardiac arrest. In: Mickler J (ed) Pathology of the nervous system. McGraw-Hill, Newark, pp 1005–1029

82. Steen PA, Michenfelder JD (1978) Cerebral protection with barbiturates: Relation to anesthetic effect. Stroke 9:140–142

83. Steen PA, Milde JH, Michenfelder JD (1979a) No barbiturate protection in a dog model of complete cerebral ischemia. Ann Neurol 5:343–348

84. Steen PA, Soule EH, Michenfelder JD (1979b) Detrimental effect of prolonged hypothermia in rats and monkeys with and without regional cerebral ischemia. Stroke 10:522–529

85. Steen PA, Michenfelder JD, Milde JH (1979c) Incomplete versus complete cerebral ischemia: Improved outcome with a minimal blood flow. Ann Neurol 6:389–398

86. Stullken EH, Sokol MD (1976) The effects of heparin on recovery from ischemic brain injuries in cats. Anesth Analg (Cleve) 55:683–687

87. Teasdale G, Jennett B (1974) Assessment of coma and impaired consciousness. A practical scale. Lancet II:81–84

88. Theodore J, Robin ED (1975) Pathogenesis of neurogenic pulmonary edema. Lancet II:749–751

89. Vries JK, Becker DP, Young HF (1973) A subarachnoid screw for monitoring intracranial pressure. J Neurosurg 39:416–419

90. Wechsler RL, Dripps RD, Ketty SS (1953) Blood flow and oxygen consumption of the human brain during anesthesia produced by thiopental. Anesthesiology 12:308–314

91. Yatsu FM, Diamond I, Graziana C, Lindquist P (1972) Experimental brain ischemia: Protection from irreversible damage with a rapid-acting barbiturate (methohexital). Stroke 3:726–732

Chapter 45

Brain Death or Coma Dépassé

M. Goulon, P. Babinet, and N. Simon

The terms 'brain death' and 'coma dépassé' are unanimously considered to signify the patient's death.

Diagnosis of brain death must not be subject to any uncertainty, since there are only two alternatives once it has been established: discontinuation of artificial ventilation so as not to prolong a hopeless situation and transplantation of one or several organs, provided the donor has no transmissible disease and the organs are functionally normal.

The problems of brain death are now relatively straightforward; but this situation represents the results of many studies that have established the necessary criteria for its diagnosis.

Historical aspects

In 1959, at the 23rd International Neurological Meeting, P. Mollaret and M. Goulon [18] gave the first description of 23 patients with a pathological state they then called coma dépassé. They chose this term because this new, previously undescribed, state extended beyond the deepest form of coma. 'Total and definitive abolition of vegetative functions is added to the abolition of the funtions of relation.' It was a consequence of the progress made in the fields of cardiorespiratory resuscitation, because only the use of artificial ventilation made it possible to observe coma dépassé.

The controversy thus rose as to 'the ultimate frontiers of life, and further to the determination of the hour of legal death.' The frontier between life and death was assessed in new terms: no longer was the exact moment of death the instant when the heartbeat and circulation stopped, but it now extended over a more protracted period, a few hours or a few days, during which time the function of organs other than the brain—already dead—were artificially maintained, rather like a heart–lung preparation in a physiological experiment.

Since the first published study, other names have been suggested for this state: brain death, brain stem death, acute necrotic anencephaly, deanimated state, oltrecoma, and irreversible coma; of all these terms, however, the two synonymous expressions that are currently accepted are brain death and coma dépassé.

Since 1959 numerous studies have attempted to define the diagnostic elements of brain death and eliminate the states that might mimic the condition [3, 8, 11, 12, 30]. New methods have been described to add further confirmation to the diagnosis, and it has been shown that potentially reversible states due to drug overdosage and deep hypothermia must be definitively excluded before the possibility of brain death can be considered.

The implications of a diagnosis of brain death are of social rather than individual interest, since it means that organs can be used for transplantation into living recipients whose lives may depend on this. Transplantations are now regulated in France by laws and decrees. Similar regulations are in force in most other countries.

Elements of diagnosis

Brain death, i.e., the death of the brain and therefore of the person, must be diagnosed with absolute certainty.

Two conditions must be met:

1) The four fundamental signs (see below) must be present whatever the aetiology or other clinical signs;
2) These fundamental signs must persist for a time sufficient to exclude a state that might simulate brain death.

The four fundamental signs

1) Complete abolition of consciousness and of any spontaneous movement.

2) Abolition of any reactivity in the territory of the cranial nerves. No blinking on menace, no reaction to noise or to noxious stimulation (pinching or pinpricking) in the trigeminal territory; loss of the corneal reflex. Absence of ocular movements as well as oculocephalogyric and oculovestibular reflexes. The ciliospinal reflex is abolished. The pupils are bilaterally dilated or in the mid-position and have lost their response to light. Swallowing and gag reflexes are lost.

3) Abolition of spontaneous respiration. Before this is assessed the patient must be ventilated on room air. With PCO_2 of 40 mmHg (5.3 kPa), ventilation is discontinued for at least 3 min, during which time there must be no respiratory movements. Another technique consists of pure O_2 ventilation for 1 h, followed by interruption of artificial ventilation while O_2 flow is maintained; this creates a hypercapnic state without concomitant hypoxia [17], and is considered less dangerous. Absence of respiratory movements in the presence of hypercarbia is considered as the positive response.

4) Flat EEG. Performance of the EEG must be technically perfect. Each recording must last at least 10 min at normal amplitude, then at double and maximal amplitude. The recording electrodes must be set 10 cm apart with inter-

electrode resistances between 10 and 10 000 Ω. One pair of electrodes is placed on the back of the hand, 6 or 7 cm apart so as to record any electrical artefact from the patient or his surroundings that might interfere with interpretation of the EEG. A simultaneous recording of the ECG and the EEG is desirable, because of frequent interference between the two signals. In brain death the trace is linear and flat in every lead, and verbal and painful stimulations do not affect it; persistence of low-voltage activity has been described in adults [15] and children [1] with all the other signs of brain death, but the EEG activity eventually ceased. The persistence of minimal electrical activity without any clinical reactivity is possibly the ultimate manifestation of the progressive disappearance of cerebral neurones. In cases where there is any reason for doubt other investigations would be justified, however. If these investigations cannot be performed or if their results are not clear-cut, brain death cannot be diagnosed.

For us the four fundamental signs must be present before it is possible to make the diagnosis of brain death. When the fundamental clinical signs are present, however, the need for an EEG recording is now disputed. Following the Conference of the Royal Colleges and Faculties of the United Kingdom [14] it is now accepted in Britain that an EEG is not essential for the diagnosis of brain death but does have diagnostic value at an earlier stage in the care of patients with severe cerebral damage [22]. The Harvard criteria for brain death have also indicated that in those situations where EEG monitoring is not available, the absence of cerebral function can be determined by clinical assessment [2, 11, 21]. But it is our view and that of others [24] that there must be at least two flat EEG records made 6 h apart to provide graphical certainty of the diagnosis of cerebral death and so present medicolegally incontrovertible documentation.

Other related clinical signs

In almost all cases, as stated in the early papers on the subject [18], muscle tone is flaccid and the deep tendon and cutaneous reflexes are abolished, whereas idiomuscular responses can persist. Sphincter tone is absent and there is no reaction to nociceptive stimulation applied on any part of the body.

The circulation is maintained although supportive measures may be required [4]; the heart rate is generally slow, between 40 and

60 beats/min, and is not modified by eyeball compression, carotid sinus massage, or IV atropine. Haemodynamic measurements have revealed hypovolaemia, low cardiac output, and low peripheral resistance. Temperature regulation is abnormal and the body temperature progressively falls at normal room temperature, but can rapidly rise in response to warming. Diabetes insipidus may occur as a consequence of destruction of the hypothalamo-hypophyseal tract; it can be controlled with posterior pituitary extracts.

In some cases one or more tendon reflexes and uni- or bilateral extensor plantar responses may be present [7]. In others various flexion responses can be elicited and percussion of the heel or knee may provoke slow contractions and relaxation of agonist and antagonist muscles. Several authors [7, 12] noticed that painful skin stimulation, such as squeezing of a nipple or even a light touch on the skin, can cause various reflex reactions such as abdominal muscle contraction, abduction or adduction of an arm, and turning of the head towards the side of stimulation. These responses indicate the persistence or reappearance of spinal cord activity, and their extent and distribution show the levels of the cord that are involved [9]. It must, however, be stressed that the presence of these spinal 'reflexes' does not affect the diagnosis of brain death if the four fundamental signs are present.

Exclusion of drug overdosage and hypothermia

The clinical and electrical signs of brain death can be mimicked for a few hours by deep hypothermic states, either accidental or provoked, and by severe drug overdosage with CNS depressants. The prognosis is of course entirely different in these circumstances if treatment is given before respiratory or cardiac arrest occurs and causes cerebral hypoxia. In 1967, Goulon et al. reported seven cases of coma due to drug overdosage with transient loss of vegetative function [6]. They were seen in deep unresponsive coma: respiration was abolished and blood pressure could only be maintained with large measures of support. The body temperature was around 30°C and the EEG recorded periods of electrical silence of 2–25 s. All the patients recovered after several days. Some had suffered cardiac arrest, and were treated with immediate external cardiac massage. Identical cases have been reported by others [28], which emphasize the need to exclude the presence of CNS-depressant drugs in the blood or urine.

The consequences of hypothermia must also be taken into account. Weiss and Arfel [29] reported a patient who was operated on under hypothermia and who completely recovered after 1 h 45 min of electrical silence on the EEG. Nouailhat et al. [19] reported the case of a young man who fully recovered after being found apparently dead, without detectable respirations or pulse and with a body temperature below 20°C. He had been exposed to cold in a public park for over 12 h after ingesting barbiturates in a suicide attempt.

Complementary investigations

These investigations are of physiopathological rather than diagnostic interest.

For *carotid and vertebral artery angiography*, in brain death, the contrast material is arrested at the base of the skull and there is no filling of the intracerebral vessels. This circulatory deficiency is the result of severe intracranial hypertension, and is an adequate and precise means of diagnosing brain death [9]. Unlike the EEG this test gives no false-positive results in the case of reversible drug intoxication. But cerebral angiography is not always feasible and should only be performed in doubtful cases being considered for transplantation.

Isotopic cerebral angiography is very similar to the preceding investigation and the absence of a cerebral circulation is evident if the extracranial circulation is eliminated. Its limitations relate to the availability of isotopic cameras [5].

Non-invasive techniques have been suggested, namely:

Circulation time between the subclavian vein and the retina is determined by retinal fluoroscopy. A circulation time of over 30 s is said to be consistent with a diagnosis of brain death [16].

In *electroretinography* with white light, the positive b wave disappears in the event of brain death [16].

In an *echoencephalogram* the pulsated echo-wave related to the systolic pulse penetrating the brain is abolished [26].

Doppler sonography shows that the flow in the common carotid artery is inverted [31].

Other investigations proposed include:

The arteriovenous O_2 content difference between arterial and jugular venous bulb blood is diminished because there is no O_2 consumption by the brain [25].

A deep EEG via fine bipolar electrodes inserted near the thalamus gives a flat record in brain death, but the method is difficult and of little practical interest.

Enzymatic activity and lactic acid content of CSF [27] show characteristic differences in brain death.

A CT scan may show cerebral lesions and cerebral oedema but is of little value for the diagnosis of brain death [3].

Aetiology and evolution

Brain death may follow various direct brain insults, such as head injury, haemorrhage, encephalitis, etc., or may be secondary to anoxia of circulatory or respiratory origin.

The causes of cerebral death in 180 patients in an ICU in a 10-year period were [7]:

Cerebrovascular accidents	50
Bacterial or viral infection of the brain	39
Poisoning	21
Acute respiratory failure	17
Trauma	17
Cardiac arrest	14
Encephalopathies, tumours	8
Gas embolism	6
Drowning	2
Electrical injury	2
Blood transfusion accident	1
Drug addiction	1

The interval between the brain lesion and the occurrence of the fundamental signs of brain death is variable, but generally short. In a report of 33 cases it was less than 24 h in ten and more than 5 days in eleven. In nine cases, although the clinical features were present, low-voltage EEG activity was observed for several hours before the record became flat [7]. Once cerebral death is established, full supportive measures can only sustain cardiac activity for a few days at the most. In the 33 cases mentioned the heart stopped after less than 24 h in nine, and only in eight did cardiac activity persist for longer than 72 h. Times varying from 48 h to 14 days have been observed by other workers [3, 10, 13, 20].

Somatic death thus occurs relatively quickly after cerebral death, and the critical intervening state can only be maintained with the comprehensive supportive facilities of a modern ICU.

Published criteria for brain death

France

A statement on cerebral death was referred to in the official *Memorandum no. 67 of 24 April 1968*, issued by the *Ministry of Social Affairs*. It insists especially on the artificial maintenance of respiration by a mechanical ventilator and on the absence of any spontaneous or provoked EEG signs during a sufficiently long period of recording in a patient not rendered hypothermic and to whom no sedative drugs have been administered. Only the concordance of the clinical and EEG signs can establish that this state is irreversible; if one sign is missing the subject cannot be declared brain-dead. The law leaves the responsible physician free to judge in each particular case for how long the fundamental signs of brain death must be present. Obviously the observation period can be shorter in cases of brain death due to direct brain injury (trauma or massive haemorrhage) than in cases of secondary anoxia.

Brain death is pronounced after the consultation of two physicians, one of whom must be the head of a Department or Hospital Unit or his duly authorized representative, assisted if necessary by an EEG specialist. Once brain death has been recognized, cardiovascular support is withheld. In cases where the patient is to serve as an organ donor for transplantation after death has been certified, resuscitation is maintained to avoid premature interruption of blood flow to the organs concerned.

United States

The Harvard Ad Hoc Committee for the Definition of Brain Death in August 1968 recommended four criteria:

1) "Absence of receptivity and responsivity . . . Even the most intensely painful stimuli evoke no vocal or other response.

2) "No movements or breathing: Observation by physicians over a period of at least 1 h is adequate to satisfy the criteria of no spontaneous muscular movements or spontaneous respiration or response to stimuli . . . The total absence of spontaneous breathing may be established by turning off the respirator for 3 min and observing whether there is any effort on the part of the subject to breathe (this requires that CO_2 tension be normal and that the patient be breathing room air for 10 min before the test).

3) "No reflexes . . . The pupils will be fixed and dilated and will not respond to a direct source of bright light . . . Ocular movement (in response to head turning and to irrigation of ears with iced water) and blinking are absent. There is no evidence of postural activity (decerebrate or other). Swallowing, yawning, vocalizing are in abeyance . . . Corneal and pharyngeal reflexes are absent . . . As a rule the stretch or tendon reflexes cannot be elicited . . .

4) "Flat EEG. Great confirmatory value attaches to the flat or isoelectric EEG . . . There shall be no EEG response to noise or to pinching. All the above tests shall be repeated at least 24 h later with no change. The validity of such data as indications of irreversible cerebral damage depends on the exclusion of two conditions; hypothermia (temperature below 90°F, 32.2°C) and CNS depressants, such as barbiturates."

In 1977, the *North American Collaborative Study* proposed the following set of criteria [12]; it is essential that all appropriate diagnostic and therapeutic procedures have been performed. Before brain death can be diagnosed the following must be present for 30 min at least 6 h after the onset of coma and apnoea: (1) Coma with cerebral non-responsivity; (2) apnoea; (3) dilated pupils; (4) absent cephalic reflexes; (5) electrocerebral silence. Confirmation lies in the absence of cerebral blood flow.

United Kingdom

A statement on the diagnosis of brain death was issued by the Conference of the Medical Royal Colleges and their Faculties in the United Kingdom on 11 October 1976 and considered that the following conditions should all exist:

1) The patient is *deeply comatose*, and: (a) There should be no suspicion that this state is due to depressant drugs . . . This is of particular importance in patients whose primary cause of coma lies in the toxic effects of drugs followed by anoxic cerebral damage; (b) Primary hypothermia as a cause of coma should have been excluded; (c) Metabolic and endocrine disturbance that can cause or contribute to coma should have been excluded.

2) The patient is being *maintained on a ventilator* because spontaneous respiration had previously become inadequate or had ceased altogether. Relaxants (neuromuscular blocking agents) and other drugs should have been excluded as a cause of respiratory inadequacy or

failure. Immobility, unresponsiveness, and lack of spontaneous respiration may be due to the use of neuromuscular blocking drugs, and the persistence of their effects should be excluded by eliciting spinal reflexes (flexion or stretch) or by showing adequate neuromuscular conduction with a conventional nerve stimulator. Equally, persistent effects of hypnotics and narcotics should be excluded as the cause of respiratory failure.

3) There should be no doubt that the patient's condition is due to *irremediable structural brain damage*. The diagnosis of a disorder which can lead to brain death should have been fully established.

Tests to confirm brain death are necessary. All brain stem reflexes should be absent, and in particular: (a) The pupils are fixed in diameter and do not respond to sharp changes in the intensity of incident light; (b) there is no corneal reflex; (c) the vestibulo-ocular reflexes are absent. These are absent when no eye movement occurs during or after the slow injection of 20 ml ice-cold water into each external auditory meatus in turn, clear access to the tympanic membrane having been established by direct inspection. This test may be contra-indicated on one side or the other by local trauma; (d) no motor responses within the cranial nerve distribution can be elicited by adequate stimulation of any somatic area; (e) there is no gag reflex or reflex response to bronchial stimulation by a suction catheter passed down the trachea; (f) no respiratory movements occur when the patient is disconnected from the mechanical ventilator for long enough to ensure that the arterial CO_2 tension rises above the threshold for stimulating respiration.

Other considerations:

1) Repetition of testing: It is customary to repeat the tests to ensure that there has been no observer error. The interval between tests must depend on the primary condition and the clinical course of the disease. This is a matter for medical judgment, and repetition time must be related to the signs of improvement, stability, or deterioration that present themselves.

2) Integrity of spinal reflexes: It is well established that spinal cord function can persist after insults that irretrievably destroy brain stem function. Reflexes of spinal origin may persist or return after an initial absence in brain death patients.

3) Confirmatory investigations: It is now widely accepted that EEG is not necessary to

diagnose brain death. Indeed, this view was expressed from Harvard in 1969, only a year after the original Harvard criteria were published. Electroencephalography has its principal value at earlier stages in the care of patients, when the original diagnosis is in doubt. When EEG is used the strict criteria recommended by the Federation of EEG Societies must be followed. Other investigations, such as cerebral angiography or cerebral blood flow measurements, are not required for diagnosis of brain death.

Death and transplantation

The French law of 22nd December 1976 stipulates that an organ can be taken for therapeutic or scientific purposes from the body of a person who did not signify willingness for this during his or her lifetime; but in the case of a minor or a mentally deficient person the permission of the legal guardian must be obtained. The decree of 31 March 1978, however, is more restrictive and gives the relatives the right to testify that a person in a state of cerebral death was opposed to the taking of his or her organs. A memorandum on this subject on 3 April 1978 requires the next of kin to prove the will of the person concerned. The physicians who establish a record of cerebral death specify the means of diagnosis used, and the precise date and hour of their examinations. The surgeons performing the transplantation give a precise written statement of the operation and the findings related to the body and the organs. In no case may the same person certify brain death and perform the transplantation. If the dead person is liable to be submitted to a legal enquiry (crime, suicide, accidents at work, occupational disease) or is receiving a veteran's pension no transplantation should be performed.

A similar attitude has been advocated by the Committee on Moral and Ethics of the Transplantation Society of the United States (cited in [3]).

There are many restrictions to the taking of organs for transplantation, and these combined with the frequent refusal of the next of kin and the unsuitability of some organs because of age or disease of the donors mean that the number of organs available for transplantation is very low compared with the number of patients with brain death. Beecher [2] reported 9 donors out of a total of 1069 cerebral deaths, and in another study [3] only 25% of a series of brain deaths yield organs for transplantation. In 1978, of 20 adults admitted to our own ICU with brain death only 2 could be used as organ donors. The other 18 could not be used for donation, because of opposition from the family in one case and for medical and legal reasons in the other 17. In France, a total of 565 organs were taken for transplantation in 1978; most of the donors were patients who had suffered stroke or head injury after previously being in good health.

The criteria of cerebral death must be rigorously met to prevent any possibility of misdiagnosis. A time factor must be added to the clinical and paraclinical signs, during which the signs must remain unchanged. Brain death must not and cannot be confused with deep coma, where spontaneous respiration and movements persist, but there may be greater diagnostic difficulty in profound coma following drug overdose and hypothermia, and these must be excluded.

Coma dépassé was described in 1959. At that time the necessary surgical and biological knowledge had been acquired to perform transplantations of organs from voluntary living donors and of cadaver organs from patients who were brain-dead. These achievements have given rise to remarkable and well-established progress and opened new fields of medical thought, and have also intensified the responsibilities of physicians.

References

1. Ashwal S, Schneider S (1979) Failure of EEG to diagnose brain death in comatose children. Ann Neurol 6:512–517
2. Beecher HK (1969) After the definition of irreversible coma. N Engl J Med 281:1070–1071
3. Black P McL (1978) Brain death. N Engl J Med 299:338–344, 299:393–401
4. Cartier F, Chevet D, le Polles R, Launois B (1974) La fonction rénale des comas dépassés. Ann Anesthésiol Fr 15:21–25
5. Goodman JM, Heck LL (1977) Confirmation of brain death at bedside by isotope angiography. JAMA 238:966–968
6. Goulon M, Nouailhat F, Levy Alcover MA, Dordain G (1967) Comas toxiques avec sidération végétative d'évolution favorable. Rev Neurol (Paris) 116:297–317
7. Goulon M, Nouailhat F, Babinet P (1971) Le coma dépassé. Ann Med Interne (Paris) 122:479–486
8. Grenvik A, Powner DJ, Snyder JV (1978) Cessation of therapy in terminal illness and brain death. Crit Care Med 6:284–291

9. Gros C (1972) Les critères circulatoires et biologiques de la mort du cerveau. Neurochirurgie 18:9–48
10. Ibe K (1971) Clinical and pathophysiological aspects of the intravital brain death. Electroencephalogr Clin Neurophysiol 30:272–279
11. Journal of the American Medical Association (1968) A definition of irreversible coma. JAMA 205:337–340 (Report of the Ad Hoc Comittee of the Harvard Medical School to Examine the Definition of Brain Death)
12. Journal of the American Medical Association (1977) An appraisal of the criteria of cerebral death: A summary statement, a collaborative study. JAMA 237:982–986
13. Korein J, Maccario M (1971) On the diagnosis of cerebral death: A prospective study on 55 patients to define irreversible coma. Clin Electroencephalogr 2:178–199
14. Lancet (1976) Diagnosis of brain death. Lancet II:1069–1970 (Conference of Royal Colleges and Faculties of the United Kingdom)
15. Levy-Alcover MA, Babinet P (1970) Etudes des relations chronologiques entre l'installation du tableau clinique du coma dépassé et la persistance d'une minime activité EEG. Rev Neurol (Paris) 122:411–415
16. Mantz JL, Lobstein A, Jaeger A, Mack G, Tempe JD (1974) L'oeil dans le diagnostic de la mort cérébrale. Ann Anesthesiol Fr 15:95–100
17. Milhaud A, Ossart M, Gayet H, Riboulot M (1974) L'épreuve de débrancher en oxygéne. Test de mort cérébrale. Ann Anesthesiol Fr Spécial III:73–78
18. Mollaret P, Goulon M (1959) Le coma dépassé. Rev Neurol (Paris) 101:3–15
19. Nouailhat F, Gajdos Ph, Rainhorn JD (1973) Hypothermie des intoxications médicamenteuses. In: Goulon M and Rapin M (eds) Réanimation et médecine d'urgence. Expansion Scientifique, Paris, pp 25–46
20. Ouaknine G, Kosary IZ, Braham J (1973) Laboratory criteria of brain death. J Neurosurg 39:429–433
21. Powner DJ, Fromm GH (1979) The electroencephalogram in the determination of brain death. N Engl J Med 300:502
22. Scott DF, Prior PF (1979) Prediction of brain damage by electroencephalography. N Engl J Med 300:1219
23. Silverman D, Masland RL, Saunders MG, Schwab RS (1970) Irreversible coma associated with electrocerebral silence. Neurology 20:525
24. Sweet WH (1978) Brain death. N Engl J Med 299:410–412
25. Torda TA (1976) Cerebral arterio-venous oxygen difference: A bedside test for cerebral death. Anaesth Intensive Care 41:148–150
26. Uematsu S, Walker AE (1974) A method for recording the pulsation of the midline echo in clinical brain death. Johns Hopkins Med J 135:383–390
27. Voisin C, Wattel F, Scherperel P (1975) Enzymes in the cerebro-spinal fluid in diagnosis of brain death. Resuscitation 4:61–67
28. Warter G, Mantz JM, Metais P, Hamman B, Kurtz D (1963) Coma prolongé (10 jours) par intoxication massive au phénobarbital (25 g). Apnée prolongée (4 jours). Respiration artificielle. Guérison. Presse Med 71:1409–1411
29. Weiss J, Arfel G (1960) Séquences électriques de l'hypothermie profonde. Rev Neurol (Paris) 108:220–222
30. Wertheimer P, Jouvet M, Descotes J (1959) A propos du diagnostic de la mort du systéme nerveux dans les comas avec arrêt respiratoire traités par respiration artificielle. Presse Med 67:87–88
31. Yoneda S, Nishimoto A, Nukada T (1974) To and fro movement and external escape of carotid arterial blood in brain death cases: A Doppler ultrasonic study. Stroke 5:707–713

Chapter 46

Status Epilepticus

François Nouailhat, Jean-Louis Bourdain, and
Christian Brun-Buisson

Self-limiting seizures are the commonest presentation of chronic epilepsy, but persistent or repetitive fits have an ominous portent, and demand an urgent search for some underlying cerebral or systemic disorder. Whilst the term *status epilepticus* is widely used and accepted, *convulsive status* would actually be a more appropriate description for recurring motor seizures that occur in a variety of conditions, many of which are not truly epileptic.

It is widely acknowledged that persistent seizures are a frequent medical emergency in both children and adults, and that many cases require intensive care. In our experience from 1975 to 1979 [75], 119 of 2000 patients (5.95%) were admitted to an ICU because of intractable convulsions. Moreover, as the practice of intensive care grows, repetitive fits due to a multiplicity of factors are being encountered with increasing frequency in critically ill patients.

As the result of supportive management and the use of potent anticonvulsant drugs, singly or in different combinations, most fits can now be brought under control and the initial outcome of status epilepticus (SE) has dramatically improved. Enthusiasm should nevertheless be tempered, because the eventual prognosis still, of course, depends mainly on the nature of the underlying disease.

Status epilepticus and its variants

Etat de mal was the term initially introduced into the literature by Calmeil [12], after he had heard asylum patients using it among themselves to describe the condition now referred to as status epilepticus. The International League against Epilepsy has adopted Gastaut's definition [31], which encompasses every process that is characterized by seizures so prolonged or frequent as to create a fixed or persistent epileptic condition. This implies that SE is quite protean in its presentation, embracing the wide spectrum of epilepsy. Within the field of critical care, however, it may be considered under the following headings.

Generalized SE

The most typical form of SE is major or grand mal status, which shows the features of grand mal seizures, namely tonic and clonic convulsions involving the whole of the body, which persist or recur without intervening intervals of consciousness. Autonomic dysfunction may rapidly supervene and the condition then becomes life-threatening. Generalized SE can often differ from this complete presentation, however. Exhaustion or structural lesions in the CNS may partially terminate the convulsions, which may then become purely clonic, asymmetrical, or shifting in location; these features are commonly seen in critically ill patients [74]. In some cases, its only expression may be loss of consciousness with spasmodic twitching or flickering of the eyes, and it must always be remembered that cessation of seizures may in fact indicate a worsening of the patient's condition [103].

Grand mal status is quite rare in infants, and as Aicardi and Chevrie [3] have emphasized, convulsions before the age of 4 are predominantly or solely unilateral, and mainly of the clonic type (*hemiclonic status*). On the other hand, it is difficult to differentiate tonic status from the peculiar seizures of the epileptic encephalopathies of the West and Lennox–Gastaut syndromes.

Partial SE

Of its many types only the motor forms require differentiation. They present as repetitive focal twitchings occurring at various sites with varying rates of progression. Sometimes they are Jacksonian in type, with retention of consciousness and a tendency to stereotype. Kozevnikov's *epilepsia partialis continua*, is a special form characterized by unremitting myoclonic jerks confined to a discrete part of the body and occurring in the intervals between partial motor seizures.

Partial status may become generalized with loss of consciousness, and it is then indistinguishable from grand mal status. The EEG is of the utmost importance for the identification of a focal discharge.

Again in infants or children, the picture can be misleading with short-lived seizures whose presenting features are jerking of the limbs, face or eyes, staring spells, or simply changes in respiratory pattern [21].

Myoclonic status

Unremitting myoclonic twitches are seen almost exclusively in degenerative, hypoxic, toxic, and metabolic encephalopathies [14]. Myoclonic status is a rather ill-defined entity that is frequently seen in intensive care but which, on occasions, cannot be distinguished from clonic seizures, with which it may, in fact, be associated. The twitches may be generalized or localized, rhyth-

mic or disorganized, infrequent or occurring in bursts and they may arise spontaneously or be triggered by movement or various stimuli. Consciousness is variably affected, depending on the context in which the twitches develop.

Non-convulsive status

Although on the fringe of the subject, epileptic twilight states must be remembered because of the risk of their misdiagnosis. These behavioural disturbances can fluctuate from mild confusion, with stereotyped movements, to almost complete unresponsiveness [8, 27, 56]. The EEG is instrumental in making a correct diagnosis differentiating petit mal status, with diffuse spike-wave activity at three per second, from psychomotor status with discharges that are limited to the temporal lobes.

From a therapeutic point of view, we still agree with those authors who have retained the distinction between SE, as originally described, and *serial seizures*. As a continuous, convulsive, comatose state, SE demands immediate treatment, whereas serial seizures of either a generalized or a focal nature do not constitute such a grave emergency, insofar as the patient reverts to his pre-existing level of consciousness between the fits. When serial seizures become more frequent, these should of course be considered as impending SE.

Conditions and causes

Discovering the causative or precipitating factors of SE is an integral part of its management. The problem is somewhat different when it occurs in a known epileptic or arises in a patient without any previous history of epilepsy, or supervenes on an advanced disease.

Status in chronic epilepsy

The onset of status is a rather unusual event in adult epileptics. Janz [43] has recorded an incidence of 1.6% in cryptogenic epilepsy and this increased some sixfold in symptomatic epilepsy. It is, therefore, essential to search for provoking factors.

Severe stress, trauma, loss of sleep, fasting, or heavy drinking are all possibilities, but it should also be borne in mind that the patient may have failed to take prescribed drugs properly. Certain conditions such as pregnancy, hepatic failure, and renal failure and occasionally certain forms of therapy such as antibiotics, interfere with the absorption and metabolism of anti-epileptic drugs [29, 81]. On occasions high concentrations of hydantoin can cause continual seizures [48, 49]. Measurement of plasma levels of the drugs is helpful in clarifying these various situations.

Another frequent event is that of an intercurrent infection, most commonly in the respiratory tract, about which Hunter [42] advanced the hypothesis of an 'internal withdrawal'. Febrile convulsions in children are discussed below.

All these factors may act in combination, and however obvious they may appear a complete clinical and biochemical investigation is essential. If no obvious aetiological factor emerges, especially when the blood levels of the anticonvulsants are found to be adequate, all other possibilities should be thoroughly considered. Finally, the development of SE may herald a phase of rapid decline in the progression of an uncontrolled deteriorating epilepsy [78].

Status in patients with no previous history of epilepsy

In adults without any prior history SE is a very unusual presenting feature. With advancing years its occurrence increasingly (in 70%–80% of cases) signifies serious underlying disease [13, 78]. On the other hand, children often develop convulsive status as their first ictal manifestation irrespective of its cause. In a survey of 239 cases in infants and children, Aicardi and Chevrie [3] recorded status as the initial feature in 77% with idiopathic epilepsy and a similar figure for symptomatic convulsions. Fever is commonly present at the onset, and the clinical picture is rather similar to that of simple febrile convulsions except for the duration of the fits and the prognosis. In infants, however, the incidence of encephalopathic or metabolic disorders is higher. Any isolated incident of status should, therefore, give rise to a search for the cause (Table 46.1).

First it is essential to look for any clinical or radiological sign of head injury. In adults, early post-traumatic status is an ominous sign, while in children, however, it can occur after relatively minor trauma and does not necessarily indicate an intracranial lesion if consciousness returns quickly without any neurological deficit [36]. In cases of recent, severe trauma other mechanisms, such as meningitis, hypoxia, or fat embolism, should be considered. Convulsive

Table 46.1. Causes of convulsive status

Febrile convulsions in children
Cryptogenic epilepsy
Chronic encephalopathies
  Birth injury, epileptic encephalopathies
  Post-traumatic epilepsy
  Alcoholic encephalopathy
  CNS inflammatory and degenerative diseases
  Dialysis encephalopathy
Primary acute brain injuries
  Head trauma
  Space-occupying lesions
    Primary and metatastic tumours, brain abscess
  Cerebrovascular accidents
    Subarachnoid and intracerebral haemorrhage
    Arterial thrombosis, embolism, thrombophlebitis
    Hypertensive encephalopathy
  Eclampsia
  Air and fat embolism
Exogenous toxins
  Ethanol, methanol, glycols, lead poisoning, organophosphates, organochlorates, fluorides, methyl bromide etc.
  MAO inhibitors, imipramine and related compounds, amphetamine, lithium
  Xanthines, atropine, piperazine, isoniazid, bismuth salts
  Hypoglycaemic agents
  Antibiotics (penicillins, colistin, nalidixic acid)
Withdrawal syndromes
  Alcohol, drug abuse
Systemic and metabolic disorders
  Anoxia
  Sepsis, renal failure, hepatic failure
  Hypoglycaemia
  Hypocalcaemia, hypomagnesaemia
  Hypo- and hypersomolar states
  Metabolic and respiratory alkalosis
  Porphyrias
  Aminoacidopathies, pyridoxine deficiency and dependency

status may also be the first feature of late post-traumatic epilepsy due to cerebral scarring.

Space-occupying lesions are the major cause of SE in organic brain disease and must be excluded, especially when the episode is followed by post-ictal paralysis. Tumours involving the frontal lobes and those associated with marked brain swelling are more likely to trigger seizures [43, 78].

Inflammatory disease, meningitis, or encephalitis are possible causes, and must be excluded; a lumbar puncture is indicated if there is the slightest suspicion and should be performed with all the usual precautions.

In patients over 40 years of age cerebrovascular disease features is an important cause [13]. Subarachnoid haemorrhage and hypertensive encephalopathy are likely causes of fits but great caution should be exercised before implicating a stroke, even where the fits are coincidental with a neurological deficit. In such cases associated factors such as cerebral oedema or osmolar abnormalities should always be looked for [28, 74]. Nonetheless, serial seizures however sometimes denote transient ischaemic attacks due to emboli [6, 68, 83]. Air embolism may follow abortion or certain diagnostic procedures and is a possible indication for hyperbaric O_2 treatment [34, 73].

A wide range of drugs taken in overdosage can cause SE, especially antidepressant drugs. Withdrawal symptoms from alcohol or drugs may present as myoclonic or convulsive status in non-epileptics. A thorough inquiry into medication and possible exposure to toxins either at home or at work should be made, and during physical examination, needle puncture marks should be looked for. In all cases the possible toxic effects of the drugs have to be considered in relation to the state of renal and hepatic function.

The increasing variety of causes of convulsive status [13, 14, 74, 87] indicates the importance of the various metabolic and systemic disorders.

Status in systemic disorders

These give rise to any form of status but, as previously mentioned, clonic and myoclonic twitchings in varying sites are the most commonly observed while focal seizures are occasionally misleading. Among the many conditions that are likely to induce fits in critically ill patients, severe infection and renal failure, with their metabolic disturbances and drug intolerance, feature prominently.

Hypoglycaemia is a cause of seizures, especially in premature infants, but must be excluded at any age.

Electrolyte imbalance is also of major concern in paediatrics, and sodium, calcium, and magnesium levels must be carefully considered [33, 52, 93]. In infants severe diarrhoea with its associated problems of rehydration is a common cause. Likewise, in adults water intoxication can arise from inadequate sodium replacement or inappropriate secretion of ADH and is indicated by profound hyponatraemia [35, 74]. Hyperosmolar states (acute dehydration; non-ketogenic hyperglycaemia) and metabolic or respiratory alkalosis are other possibilities.

The mechanisms of seizures encountered in sepsis are not clear, but in addition to shock, renal failure, and various metabolic disorders, the possibility of subclinical meningitis should always be borne in mind. In the critically ill, hepatic and renal failure contribute to the

already complex biological changes and reinforce the potential cerebral toxicity of certain drugs, such as antibiotics or aminophylline. Patients undergoing dialysis are especially at risk because of rapid changes in osmolality and drug concentrations and also other as yet unclear factors (e.g., aluminium intoxication).

Anoxic encephalopathy is usually seen after resuscitation from cardiac arrest or acute asphyxia. It presents typically as myoclonic status affecting mainly the axial and proximal muscles. In our experience [74], it is quite rare in carbon monoxide poisoning or during acute exacerbations of chronic lung disease unless associated with electrolyte imbalance or problems of mechanical ventilation [46, 86]. Conversely, seizures are likely to occur during ischaemic anoxia in gas embolism. Convulsive syncope has to be borne in mind: serial seizures of unexplained origin demand ECG monitoring, which might reveal a paroxysmal arrhythmia. Finally, despite all available means of investigation, no cause can be found in 20%–25% of cases.

Pathophysiology

Convulsive status has long been considered to be the major cause of death in epileptics, with a mortality rate of around 50%. Nowadays death rarely results from the actual fits provided the patient is correctly managed. Severe brain damage can, however, still occur following severe or prolonged seizures.

Earlier observers have emphasized the similarity between the cerebral lesions of anoxia and epilepsy. In children dying following status, Norman [72] found anoxic ischaemic changes affecting neurones, particularly in the deeper layers of the neocortex, cornu ammonis, basal ganglia, and cerebellum. Cerebral atrophy also occurs, as demonstrated by serial radiographic studies [2]. Apart from fatalities, possible neuropsychiatric sequelae of status are a major concern in children, especially in infants under 6 months of age in whom mental and/or neurological disability has been recorded in more than 50% of cases [3, 38]. In adults, Rowan and Scott [87] have also described sequelae in 26% of cases.

The question arises as to whether the lesions are the consequence of a primary cellular metabolic disturbance or whether they are solely the result of systemic problems that accompany protracted seizures. Grand mal status obviously creates the conditions for severe hypoxia with repeated apnoeic spells, bronchial hypersecretion, inhalation of vomitus, cardiac dysrhythmias, hypotension, hyperthermia, and dehydration providing a formidable list of possibilities. Clinical and experimental data also indicate that the high O_2 requirements of neurones cannot be adequately met despite an increased blood flow [23, 60, 62]. Hypercarbia and accumulation of lactic acid from neuronal hypoxia and muscular activity promote an acute acidosis which adversely affects the brain and promotes further fits.

Under such conditions cerebral oedema is likely to develop, and Trubuhovich [93] has reviewed the causative factors, which include increased CBF and loss of circulatory autoregulation, impairment of cerebral venous drainage, neuronal hypoxia, cerebral lactic acidosis, and alterations of the blood–brain barrier [53]. Rats subjected to prolonged seizures exhibit marked swelling of astroglial processes [20]. Thus in acute prolonged seizures cerebral oedema is presumably responsible for irreversible brain damage.

Although intensive care and vigorous therapy can now reduce the mortality and morbidity directly due to the fits, the prognosis varies mainly in relation to the causes and mortality rates are still as high as 20%–40%, depending on the age and type of patients reviewed.

Management

The management of SE aims to control the seizures and support the patient's vital functions. Meanwhile, any remedial underlying disorder must be looked for, after which metabolic stabilization must be ensured at the post-ictal state. Finally, attention should be turned to long-term control.

General measures

The patient in convulsions must be protected from physical harm without excessive restraint, which might cause soft-tissue and bone injuries. He or she should be placed supine on a flat surface with the head turned to the side and all tight clothing removed from around the neck.

It is advisable to avoid any manoeuvres that act as nociceptive stimuli; in particular, introducing anything into the mouth with the mistaken intention of preventing tongue biting increases the risk of causing inhalation. In the unconscious patient a plastic incompressible airway can be firmly taped to the face to allow the careful introduction of a suction catheter. A distended bladder should be relieved by catheterization. Transfer to an ICU should be carried out as quickly as possible, all necessary precautions being taken during transfer.

Any sign of trauma (head, neck, eye globes, dislocation of shoulder, limb fractures) should be recorded.

Anticonvulsant drugs

Although there are many, no single one has proved entirely satisfactory in every case. This accounts for the numerous drug regimens and the somewhat empirical advice to use the drug with which one is most familiar. Choice is made more difficult because none of the regimens has ever been subjected to controlled clinical trials. A better understanding has however, been achieved following recent studies on the pharmacokinetics of anticonvulsants which provide the basis for more rational treatment [1, 10, 17, 21, 82, 85, 100].

The prerequisites for anticonvulsants in the treatment of SE are: (1) Rapid penetration into and steady retention within the brain tissue to ensure a prompt and prolonged effect; (2) minimal interference with consciousness so that neurological assessment can still be made; (3) minimal respiratory and haemodynamic side-effects, although the former can be managed with MV when available; (4) blood levels that are easy to measure.

The IV route is usually essential, absorption after IM administration being unreliable. The nasogastric route is too slow, and may be hampered by vomiting or paralytic ileus. The rectal route is convenient for some drugs, however, especially in children.

As a general rule, the dosages must be tailored to the age and body weight of the patients. In the presence of known or suspected renal or hepatic disease, the drugs should be administered very cautiously. Blood pressure and ECG monitoring are advisable to enable any cardiotoxic effects to be recognized.

Although clinical assessment is of paramount importance, continued EEG recording is very helpful in severe status, because electrical discharges may persist in spite of controlled motor activity. The recommended treatment schedules and dosages are summarized in Table 46.2.

Table 46.2. Recommended schedules for usual regimens

Drugs *Trademark*	Route	Dosage and rate		Precautions
		Adults	Children	
Diazepam *Valium*	IV	5–10 mg (5 mg/mn)	0.25(initial dose)–0.50 mg/kg	Slow (~2 min) separate injections, repeated as needed every 20–60 min Look out for respiratory and circulatory depression Decrease if hepatic failure occurs
	Rectal		0.5 mg/kg	
Clonazepam *Rivotril*	IV	1–2 mg (1 mg/mn)	0.25–0.50 mg	
Phenobarbitone *Luminal* *Gardenal*	IV	5 mg/kg (60 mg/mn)	5–10 mg/kg 10–20 mg/kg (infants)	Slow IV injection (~5 mn) Use only glass syringe Respiration and blood pressure control Decrease if renal failure occurs
	IM	5 mg/kg	5–10 mg/kg	
Thiopentone *Pentothal*	IV	*Initial dose* 2.5% aqueous solution: 25–100 mg (30–120 s) until convulsions cease *Maintenance* 0.2% drip Start with 1 ml/min 1–2 (up to 4) g/24 h	No available data	Mechanical respiration at hand Blood pressure control Large venous line, check site of injection for extravasation Electrically controlled rate of infusion Make sure of gastric emptying Decrease if hepatic or renal failure occurs
Amylobarbitone *Amytal* *Eunoctal*	IV	5–7 mg/kg (50 mg/min)		
Diphenylhydantoin *Dilantin*	IV	50 mg/min, up to 1 g or 18 mg/kg	100–200 mg over 5 min or 10 mg/kg	Slow injection with close blood pressure control and ECG monitoring Do not mix with other drugs Contra-indicated if heart disease and to be used with care in elderly patients
Chlormethiazole *Heminevrin*	IV	1.5% Drip, started with 50–100 drops/min, then regulated as needed for seizure control; 0.5–0.7 g/h		Look out for fluid load Monitor site of injection (phlebitis)
Sodium valproate *Depakene* *Depakine*	Rectal or gastric	200–800 mg every 6 h		Measure blood concentration (100–150 µg/ml)
Paraldehyde	Rectal		0.3–0.4 ml/kg repeated at hourly intervals × 3, then spaced	Tenfold dilution in oil Avoid plastic material

Benzodiazepines

The use of diazepam was first advocated in 1965 by Gastaut et al. [30] for the treatment of SE. Since then numerous reviews have confirmed its rapid effect in most forms of status, particularly the generalized and myoclonic types [51, 69, 80, 88]. Following IV administration the brain concentration reaches a maximum within 1 min and then falls rapidly, with a half-life of some 15 min [10, 82].

Thus its major limitation is the short-lived action, and clinical use has shown that while diazepam is usually successful in stopping seizures within a few minutes it does not provide a long-lasting anticonvulsant effect. The recurrence of seizures requires repeated boluses, and in protracted status its efficiency may progressively decrease or even disappear [74, 88].

Respiratory and circulatory depression has been reported, particularly in children, when high doses are used or when it has been given with phenobarbitone [9, 19, 37, 101]. Such side-effects are nevertheless rare, provided diazepam is injected slowly into a large vein.

The IV route is recommended in adults with a dosage schedule of 10 mg over 2 min, repeated as necessary in 20–60 min; high cumulative dosage may require ventilatory assistance. Though its relative insolubility in water theoretically precludes the dilution of diazepam, continuous IV infusion has been used (20–50 mg in 500 ml saline or glucose), provided other drugs are not given via the same line [39]. The IM route is inadvisable because of slow and unpredictable absorption. In children the parenteral form of diazepam can be administered rectally; this is well tolerated and effective, blood concentrations being achieved nearly as quickly as when the IV route is used [1, 24]; this route is very useful in paediatric practice, where venous access can be very difficult. Of the other benzodiazepines that have been used, clonazepam is the most impressive [32, 45]. However, except for a tenfold lower dosage and a rather more prolonged action, its characteristics do not actually differ from those of diazepam. It may, however, succeed in severe seizures of epileptic encephalopathies in which other anticonvulsants have failed [32].

Because of their rapid effect and potency and fair margin of safety, benzodiazepines are accepted as the first-line drugs for treatment of SE of a wide variety of causes.

Barbiturates

These are sometimes regarded as rather poor drugs for the treatment of SE, but there is no good foundation for this opinion.

Phenobarbitone. Delay in achieving therapeutic levels excludes phenobarbitone as a first-line drug for convulsive status. Indeed, adequate concentrations are not reached in the grey matter for about 30 min after an IV injection [85]. It provides anticonvulsant effects for hours after administration, however, and therefore still deserves consideration as a maintenance drug. Many paediatricians continue to favour phenobarbitone, particularly in neonates [21, 50, 52].

It can be given either IV or IM according to a general schedule of 5 mg/kg for adults, a loading dose being preferred to repeated small doses. A daily dosage of up to 1000 mg is advocated by some workers [70]. In neonates, Lockman et al. [50] found that therapeutic levels could be achieved by IV or IM administration of 16–23 mg/kg.

Depression of consciousness, respiration, and circulation appears more commonly when phenobarbitone is given shortly after a benzodiazepine [80], but in every case attention should be paid to blood pressure.

Short-acting barbiturates. Though these are usually used IV for hypnotic or anaesthetic purposes, they also have an anticonvulsive action in doses lower than those normally producing sleep. The rapid penetration of the CNS makes them quite suitable for the emergency control of seizures, but untoward respiratory and circulatory effects are a major concern.

Some authors recommend sodium amylobarbitone because of its predictable and rapid effect without depressant effects when doses of 5–7 mg/kg are injected slowly; its action lasts for at least 1 h [26, 101].

Others use sodium thiopentone, which was tried by obstetricians in 1950 for the convulsions of eclampsia [54, 61, 76]; in 1967 it was advocated by Brown and Horton [11] as the 'most effective and simplest method for controlling status epilepticus'. Despite some controversy it is now accepted by many as an alternative for the emergency control of intractable seizures [33, 44, 75, 93]. The peak brain concentration is reached within 30 s after IV injection [25], but a single dose is evanescent and the maintenance of therapeutic levels requires a continuous infusion. Seizures usually cease with an initial dose of 25–100 mg, which is definitely lower than the dose that produces apnoea. For maintenance purposes a dilute solution of thiopentone is given as a drip, the rate being adjusted according to clinical and, if possible, EEG results. A daily dosage of 1–2 g for 24–72 h usually succeeds in controlling the status without altering the pre-existing state of consciousness, but it must sometimes be increased up to 4 g/24 h, at which dose MV may be required. After the infusion is stopped the blood concentration decreases rapidly. Thus its ultrashort action allows a readily adjustable titration and this seems preferable to the cumulative doses of long-acting drugs that may increase the degree of coma.

The regimen obviously cannot be carried out in a general ward, for thiopentone has a potential for causing laryngospasm and circulatory collapse, and it also facilitates gastric regurgitation, while extravasation into the tissues may cause tissue necrosis. In our experience no major adverse effects have been observed, but this has required constant supervision and facilities must be immediately at hand to assist depressed respiration [7].

An additional advantage in using barbiturates for the treatment of severe convulsive status might be related to their protective effect against cerebral hypoxia, which is a matter of growing interest [92]. Animal work indicates the presence of an increased tolerance to focal ischaemia, severe hypotension, circulatory arrest, and asphyxia under barbiturate anaesthesia [41, 63, 64, 67, 71], and most pertinent in this connection are the preliminary clinical trials in which barbiturates have been shown to produce a reduction of ICP and cerebral oedema [57, 58, 90, 91]. The dosage required, however, remains a matter of debate and is likely to be higher than that needed for a mere anticonvulsant effect.

Diphenylhydantoin

Since the encouraging report by Murphy and Schware in 1956 [65], sodium diphenylhydantoin IV has been commonly advocated in the English literature as a basic regimen for SE in adults [93, 98, 99, 103].

It is credited with the absence of respiratory depression and with not significantly altering the level of consciousness, but all users emphasize its potential for cardiac toxicity. The risk appears to be mostly related to pre-existing heart disease [94, 104], and its use is absolutely contra-indicated in marked bradycardia, conduction disorders, and severe arteriosclerosis, which generally enforces caution with its use in the elderly. A slow rate of injection, blood pressure control, and ECG monitoring are mandatory.

It has been shown that large doses prolong the half-life of phenytoin [17] but, although IV injection can achieve therapeutic levels within a few minutes, the necessary slow rate of injection—not faster than 50 mg/min—prevents the onset of a predictable effect for 20–30 min. Instead of repeated administration, Cranford et al. [18] favour a single loading dose of 18 mg/kg, which is effective in maintaining serum levels above 10 μg/ml for 24 h. This regimen is well tolerated except for hypotension, which can always be reversed by decreasing the rate of infusion. These authors conclude, from their experience with 139 cases, that diphenylhydantoin is effective in controlling seizures

in patients who are not suffering from acute disorders of the CNS.

The drug is poorly and inadequately resorbed from an IM depot [89]. The use of phenytoin in children and even more in infants appears controversial. An IV dosage of 10 mg/kg is suggested, but without firm basis [21, 52].

Chlormethiazole

Though often omitted from general reviews, this derivative of the thiazole nucleus of thiamine, first experimented with in France [79], deserves better consideration. It was used initially as a sedative in states of alcohol withdrawal, but it also proved to be a useful adjunct to the standard treatment of refractory SE [39, 74, 75]; it is also advocated by obstetricians in pre-eclamptic toxaemia and eclampsia [22, 40].

Because of its short half-life it must be given by continuous infusion, which is run rapidly at first until convulsions stop, and then regulated as needed, usually with a mean hourly dosage of 0.5–0.7 g. No serious impairment of consciousness or depression of respiration has been encountered, but thrombophlebitis at the site of injection is frequent.

In our experience, chlormethiazole either alone or in association with other anticonvulsants often succeeds in controlling a convulsive or myoclonic status which has proved refractory to standard regimens.

Others

The marked stupefying action of IV paraldehyde together with problems in its administration (chemical reactions with plastic) and possible side-effects (sclerosis of veins, intramuscular abscess, permanent nerve injury, gastro-intestinal bleeding with gastric or rectal administration, acute pulmonary oedema) tend now to cause it not to be used, despite a potent anticonvulsant action. Sometimes, however, it still merits consideration for seizures in which alcohol is a factor [103], and it is still used by some paediatricians as an adjunctive drug [21, 52].

Chloral hydrate by the rectal or IV route (in association with sodium bromide) has depressant effects but it might still be considered for convulsions in acute porphyria, where most anti-epileptic drugs, especially the barbiturates, are contra-indicated.

Though it is only available for enteral administration, several reports have recently drawn attention to the possible use of sodium valproate for intractable convulsions [4, 5, 47, 55, 84, 95]. When it is given either via the naso-gastric route or rectally as lipid-based sup-positories, plasma levels reach the therapeutic range within hours, but with a loading dosage complete control has been obtained in cases of refractory convulsive or myoclonic status.

1-5-Hydroxytrytophan (5HTP), a precursor of serotonin, in combination with a decarboxylase inhibitor, is worth a trial in intractable post-anoxic myoclonus [96]. More recently piracetam has been successfully used in the same condi-tion [92a].

Acetazolamide has been reported to potenti-ate benzodiazepines in infants [97].

As for general anaesthesia, whenever it is considered, thiopentone is to be preferred for reasons given earlier. Lidocaine seems some-what hazardous and curarization only serves to give a false sense of accomplishment.

Supportive management

Protracted convulsions can seriously impair res-piration, circulation, and blood chemistry. It is thus of prime importance that homeostasis be promptly restored, to avoid brain damage and to reduce the side-effects from the acute administration of drugs. On occasion effective oxygenation and correction of metabolic dis-turbance have controlled seizures when drugs have hitherto failed [75, 93].

Respiratory support

Grand mal status makes it especially urgent to maintain or restore the patency of the airway and to compensate for depressed respiration. Nasotracheal intubation is the safest method; it allows clearing of the bronchi, correction of oxy-genation, and respiratory assistance with IPPV. It also prevents inhalation and enables a safe intragastric route to be established.

Circulatory support

The management of circulatory collapse de-pends chiefly on the correction of hypoxia, hypovolaemia, and electrolyte imbalance.

In special situations where hypertension is a causative factor, namely hypertensive enceph-alopathy and eclampsia, the arterial pressure should be promptly reduced by appropriate means. Chlorpromazine, hydralazine, beta-blocking agents, or diazoxide may be indicated, to be given under haemodynamic control (Chap. 14).

Thermal control

Hyperthermia is of special concern in children with febrile convulsions, but it can also result from any prolonged generalized seizure. When severe it may itself contribute to cerebral dam-age [59], and it should therefore be vigorously reduced. Fanning, tepid sponging, axillary ice-packs, and antipyretics via the nasogastric or rectal route are the usual means for achieving this.

Metabolic stabilization

A blood sample should be taken at the onset for the determination of glucose and electrolytes. Whenever hypoglycaemia is suspected, dex-trose 30%, 1–2 ml/kg, should be given im-mediately.

Acid–base disorders can be more properly appraised once ventilation is controlled and convulsions have been controlled. Actually, lac-tic acidosis clears spontaneously and premature titration with sodium bicarbonate would result in undesirable metabolic alkalosis [77]. Should acidosis persist correction is required.

Caution should be observed in replacing fluids, and a relative restriction is desirable in view of the large amount of fluid likely to be given with the IV medication. Osmolar balance should be constantly looked for.

Energy substrate is provided as glucose, and parenteral vitamin B complex is required espe-cially in alcoholics.

Prevention and treatment of cerebral oedema

Whether linked to the underlying cerebral con-dition or secondary to the prolonged convul-sions, brain swelling should be counteracted in its early stages to prevent irreversible deterio-ration [21, 93]. Possible measures include generous sedation, hypothermia, controlled hyperventilation with a negative expiratory pressure, steroids and, when the situation is very grave, osmotic agents (Chap. 43).

For severe convulsive status, we consider a high-dosage thiopentone infusion (about 4 g/24 h for adults) with controlled ventilation the best tentative regimen.

Guidelines for therapy

Because SE covers quite different entities, the treatment prescribed obviously cannot be stand-ardized but should rather conform to the degree of emergency.

A bolus dose of a benzodiazepine, however, is admittedly the preliminary measure which usually succeeds in curtailing the fits. Even if only temporary, this curtailment allows time to deal with the initial needs, i.e., inserting a well-secured venous line, taking blood samples, and intubating when necessary.

The need for glucose should then be considered and, in children in particular, the need for calcium, magnesium, or pyridoxine.

Further treatment depends on the type and frequency of seizures. Whenever a continuing cerebral insult is present and generalized seizures recur shortly after injection of benzodiazepines, one should change to other drugs.

Our choice for adults is thiopentone, because of its immediate efficiency, fair tolerance, preserved consciousness, and adjustable infusion rate, which prevents the overtreatment of patients that can occur with long-acting drugs. This regimen seems to be especially indicated in the presence of asphyxia or after cardiac arrest.

When facilities for a safe thiopentone prescription are not met, a loading dose of phenobarbitone or phenytoin must be considered. Although we have no experience of the later, its cardiac side-effects should not be underestimated.

In serial seizures and partial status where the condition is not life-threatening, large doses of IV drugs other than the benzodiazepines do not seem to be advisable, since a conscious patient is desirable for neurological evaluation; more importantly the patient should be given treatment that will prevent the seizures from becoming generalized. The oral route is often suitable; initially use of twice the calculated daily dose may hasten the attainment of a therapeutic concentration [21, 103].

The fact remains that failure to control seizures is still encountered. This may happen with patients whose epilepsy is poorly controlled in spite of heavy maintenance therapy and in whom there is a trend towards shorter half-lives and more rapid clearance of drugs; Cranford et al. [18] emphasized this for phenytoin, and we have also noticed it with thiopentone [7]. It happens more frequently in acutely ill patients whose seizures result from intermingled clinical and metabolic factors. This may be the place for chlormethiazole or sodium valproate.

Non-convulsive status usually responds to IV diazepam, which may thus be the key to diagnosis.

Finally, eclampsia is a peculiar condition in which one must avoid using anticonvulsants which have a significant action on the fetus in utero or a carry-over effect in the neonatal period, as is the case with diazepam in large doses. Chlormethiazole or thiopentone in small increments may be better choices [22, 40]. Relevant to this is experimental work indicating that fetal distress in monkeys is often ameliorated by administration of phenobarbitone to the mother before delivery by caesarean section [15].

Long-term control

One should be aware that once interrupted by pharmacological means SE is not necessarily over. This obviously depends on the cause and its possible treatment.

The last step of management is to prevent further fits by switching to the oral route of drug administration as soon as possible. In patients who are still intubated, a nasogastric tube provides the route for starting early maintenance therapy. Drugs that can rapidly achieve therapeutic levels on enteral administration, such as sodium valproate and carbamazepine, are preferable to phenytoin or phenobarbitone, which require several days. Measurements of the concentration of drug in the blood are mandatory at this stage.

A difficult problem is to decide on maintenance therapy following febrile SE in children. Because this is the most severe presentation in the spectrum of febrile convulsions, most paediatricians agree in considering it as a predictor of epilepsy which makes preventive therapy advisable [2, 66, 102].

References

1. Agurell S, Berlin A, Ferngren H, Hellström B (1975) Plasma levels of diazepam after parenteral and rectal administration in children. Epilepsia 16:277–283
2. Aicardi J, Baraton JA (1971) A pneumoencephalographic demonstration of brain atrophy following status epilepticus. Dev Med Child Neurol 13:660–667
3. Aicardi J, Chevrie JJ (1970) Convulsive status in infants and children. A study of 239 cases. Epilepsia 11:187–197
4. Barnes SE, Bland D, Cole AP (1976) The use of sodium valproate in a case of status epilepticus. Dev Med Child Neurol 18:236
5. Barois A, Babinet P (1978) La réanimation dans les affections neurologiques. In: Kleinknecht D (ed) Principes de réanimation médicale. Flammarion, Paris, pp 407–411

6. Barolin GS, Scherzer E, Schnaberth G (1971) Epileptische Manifestationen als Vorboten von Schlaganfällen: "Vaskuläre Präkursive Epilepsie". Fortschr Neurol Psychiatr 39:199–216
7. Baud JM (1980) Traitement de l'état de mal épileptique par le thiopental sodique. A propos de 31 cas. Thèse, Paris
8. Belfasky MA, Carwille S, Miller P, Waddell C, Boxley-Johnson J, Delgado-Escueta AV (1978) Prolonged epileptic twilight states: Continuous recordings with naso-pharyngeal electrodes and videotape analysis. Neurology (Minneap) 28:239–245
9. Bell DS (1969) Dangers of treatment of status epilepticus with diazepam. Br Med J i:159–161
10. Bouker HE, Celesia GG (1973) Serum concentration of diazepam in subjects with epilepsy. Arch Neurol 29:191–194
11. Brown AS, Horton JM (1967) Status epilepticus treated by intravenous infusions of thiopentone sodium. Br Med J i:27–28
12. Calmeil LF (1824) De l'épilepsie. Didot, Paris, p 13
13. Celesia GG (1976) Modern concepts of status epilepticus. JAMA 235:1571–1574
14. Celesia GG, Messert B, Murphy MJ (1972) Status epilepticus of late adult onset. Neurology (Minneap) 22:1047–1055
15. Cockburn F, Daniel SS, Dawes GS (1969) The effect of pentobarbital anesthesia on resuscitation and brain damage in fetal rhesus monkeys asphyxiated on delivery. J Pediatr 75:281–289
16. Courpotin C, Girardet JP (1976) Convulsions d'origine métabolique. Vie Médicale 57:891–896
17. Cranford RE, Leppik IE, Patrick B, Anderson CB, Kostik B (1978) Intravenous phenytoin: Clinical and pharmacokinetic aspects. Neurology (Minneap) 28:874–880
18. Cranford RE, Leppik IE, Patrick B, Anderson CB, Kostik B (1979) Intravenous phenytoin in acute treatment of status epilepticus. Neurology (Minneap) 29:1474–1479
19. Dalen JF, Evans GL, Banas JS, Brooks HL, Paraskos JA, Dexter L (1969) The hemodynamic and respiratory effects of diazepam. Anesthesiology 30:259–263
20. De Robertis E, Alberici M, Rodriguez de Lores Arnaiz G (1969) Astroglial swelling and phosphohydrolase in cerebral cortex of metrazol convulsant rats. Brain Res 12:461
21. Dodson WE, Prenski AL, De Vivo DC, Goldring S, Dodge PR (1976) Management of seizure disorders: Selected aspects. J Pediatr 89:527–540
22. Duffus GM, Tunstall ME, Mc Gillivray I (1968) Intravenous chlormethiazole in pre-eclamptic toxemia in labour. Lancet I:335–337
23. Duffy TE, Howse DC, Plum F (1975) Cerebral energy metabolism during experimental status epilepticus. J Neurochem 24:925–934
24. Dulac O, Aicardi J (1978) Interêt du diazepam rectal dans le traitement d'urgence des convulsions de l'enfant. In: Journées Parisiennes de pédiatrie, Flammarion, Paris, pp 468–471
25. Dundee JW (1956) Thiopentone and other thiobarbiturates. Livingstone, Edinburgh, pp 223–229
26. Eadi MJ (1975) The management of epilepsy. Med J Aust 2:49–51
27. Engel J, Ludwig BI, Fetell M (1978) Prolonged partial complex status epilepticus. Neurology (Minneap) 28:863–864
28. Faris AA, Poser CM (1964) Experimental production of focal neurologic deficit by systemic hyponatremia. Neurology (Minneap) 14:206–211
29. Fincham RW, Wiley DE, Schottelius DD (1976) Use of phenytoin serum levels in a case of status epilepticus. Neurology (Minneap) 26:879–881
30. Gastaut H, Naquet R, Poiré R, Tassinari LA (1965) Treatment of status epilepticus with diazepam. Epilepsia 6:167–182
31. Gastaut H, Roger J, Lob H (1967) Les états de mal épileptiques. Masson, Paris
32. Gastaut H, Catier J, Dravet C, Roger J (1969) Mise en évidence par une méthode de screening des propriétés anti-épileptiques exceptionnelles d'une benzodiazépine nouvelle. Rev Neurol (Paris) 120:402–407
33. Ginsberg PL, Fischer KC, Richey ET (1976) Status epilepticus: Clinical, electrial and therapeutic considerations in a general hospital population. Neurology (Minneap) 26:342
34. Goulon M, Rapin M, Barois A, Nouailhat F, Grosbuis S, Kernbaum S (1969) Embolies gazeuses probables au cours d'insufflation pour coelioscopie. Presse Med 77:1035–1038
35. Goulon M, Babinet P, Raphael JC (1970) Hyponatrémie et systême nerveux. In: Goulon M, Rapin M (eds) Réanimation et médecine d'urgence. Expansion Scientifique, Paris, pp 55–90
36. Grand W (1974) The significance of post-traumatic status epilepticus in children. J Neurol Neurosurg Psychiatry 37:178–180
37. Greenblatt DJ, Koch-Weser J (1973) Adverse reactions to intravenous diazepam: A report from the Boston collaboration drug surveillance program. Am J Med Sci 266:261–266
38. Harrison RM, Taylor DC (1976) Childhood seizures: A 25-year follow-up. Lancet I:948–951
39. Harvey PKP, Higenbottam TW, Loh L (1975) Chlormethiazole in treatment of status epilepticus. Br Med J ii:603–605
40. Hibbard BM, Rosen M (1977) The management of severe pre-eclampsia and eclampsia. Br J Anaesth 49:3–9
41. Hoff JT, Smith AL, Hankinson HL (1975) Barbiturate protection from cerebral infarction in primates. Stroke 6:28–33
42. Hunter RA (1959) Status epilepticus. History, incidence and problems. Epilepsia 1:162–188
43. Janz D (1961) Conditions and causes of status epilepticus. Epilepsia 2:170–177
44. Jennett WB (1977) Introduction to neurosurgery, 3rd edn. Heinemann, London, pp 268–271
45. Ketz E, Bernoulli C, Siegfried J (1973) Klinische und hirnelektrische Prüfung von Clonazepam unter besonderer Berücksichtigung des Status epilepticus. Acta Neurol Scand [Suppl] 49/53:47–53
46. Kilburn KH (1966) Shock, seizures and coma with alkalosis during mechanical ventilation. Ann Intern Med 65:977–984
47. Lance JW, Anthony M (1975) Sodium valproate in the management of intractable epilepsy: Comparison with clonazepam. Proc Aust Assoc Neurol 12:55–60
48. Lascelles PT, Kocen KS, Reynolds EH (1970) The distribution of plasma phenytoin levels in epileptic patients. J Neurol Neurosurg Psychiatry 33:501–505
49. Levy LL, Fenichel GM (1965) Diphenylhydantoin-activated seizures. Neurology (Minneap) 15:716–722
50. Lockman LA, Kriel R, Zaske D, Thompson T, Virnig L (1979) Phenobarbital dosage for control of neonatal seizures. Neurology (Minneap) 29:1445–1449
51. Lombroso CT (1966) Treatment of status epilepticus with diazepam. Neurology (Minneap) 16:629–634
52. Lombroso CT (1974) The treatment of status epilepticus. Pediatrics 53:536–540
53. Lorenzo AV, Schirahige I, Liang M, Barlow CF (1972)

Temporary alteration of cerebrovascular permeability to plasma protein during drug-induced seizures. Am J Physiol 223:268–277

54. McIntosh RR (1952) The significance of fits in eclampsia. J Obstet Gynaecol Br Cwlth 59:197–201

55. Manhire AR, Espir M (1974) Treatment of status epilepticus with sodium valproate. Br Med J iii:808

56. Markland ON, Wheeler GL, Pollack SL (1978) Complex partial status epilepticus (psychomotor status). Neurology (Minneap) 28:189–196

57. Marsh ML, Marshall LF, Shapiro HM (1977) Neurological intensive care. Anesthesiol 47:149–163

58. Marshall LF, Shapiro HM, Rausher A, Kaufman NM (1978) Pentobarbital therapy for intracranial hypertension in metabolic coma. Reye's syndrome. Crit Care Med 6:1–5

59. Meldrum BS, Brierley JB (1973) Prolonged epileptic seizures in primates. Ischemic cell change and its relation to ictal physiologic events. Arch Neurol 28:10–17

60. Meldrum BS, Vigouroux RA, Brierley JB (1973) Systemic factors and epileptic brain damage. Prolonged seizures in paralyzed artificially ventilated baboons. Arch Neurol 29:82–87

61. Menon MKK (1953) Some observations on the treatment of eclampsia with sodium thiopentone. J Obstet Gynaecol Br Cwlth 60:710–714

62. Meyer JS, Gotoh F (1965) Cerebral metabolism during epileptic seizure in man. Trans Am Neurol Assoc 90:23–29

63. Michenfelder JD, Midle J, Sundt T (1976) Cerebral protection by barbiturate anesthesia. Arch Neurol 33:345–350

64. Moseley JI, Laurent JP, Molinari GF (1975) Barbiturate attenuation of the medical course and pathologic lesions in a primate stroke model. Neurology (Minneap) 25:870–874

65. Murphy JT, Schwar RS (1956) Diphenylhydantoin sodium used parenterally in control of convulsions. JAMA 160:385–388

66. Nelson KB, Ellenberg JH (1976) Predictors of epilepsy in children who have expressed febrile convulsions. N Engl J Med 295:1029–1033

67. Nemoto EM, Frinak S, Talyor E (1979) Post-ischemic brain oxygenation with barbiturate therapy in rats. Crit Care Med 7:339–345

68. Nick J, Nicolle MH, Bakouche P, Mignot B, Reignier A (1970) L'épilepsie révélatrice de l'insuffisance circulatoire cérébrale chronique. A propos de 16 observations cliniques. Rev Neurol (Paris) 122:291–296

69. Nicol CF (1975) Status epilepticus. JAMA 234:419–420

70. Nicol CF, Tutton JC, Smith BH (1969) Parenteral diazepam in status epilepticus. Neurology (Minneap) 19:332–343

71. Nilsson L (1971) The influence of barbiturate anesthesia upon the energy state and upon acid–base parameters of the brain in arterial hypotension and asphyxia. Acta Neurol Scand 47:233–253

72. Norman RM (1964) The neuropathology of status epilepticus. Med Sci Law 4:47–51

73. Nouailhat F, Dordain G (1969) Les embolies gazeuses. In: Goulon M, Rapin M (eds) Réanimation et médecine d'urgence. Expansion Scientifique, Paris, pp 183–212

74. Nouailhat F, Levy-Alcover MA, Babinet P, Sanchez MF (1971) Les états de mal convulsifs. In: Goulon M, Rapin M (eds) Réanimation et médecine d'urgence. Expansion Scientifique, Paris, pp 257–280

75. Nouailhat F, Bourdain JL, Baud JM (1979) Anti-épileptiques et état de mal. La Revue du Praticien 29:4513–4517

76. Browne O'D (1950) The treatment of eclampsia. J Obstet Gynaecol Br Empire 57:573–582

77. Orringer CE, Eustache JC, Wunsch CD, Gardner LB (1977) Natural hystory of lactic acidosis after grand-mal seizures. A model for the study of an anion-gap acidosis not associated with hyperkaliemia. N Engl J Med 297:796–799

78. Oxbury JM, Whitty CWM (1971) Causes and consequences of status epilepticus in adults. Brain 94:733–744

79. Poire R, Royer P, Degreave M, Rustin C (1963) Traitement des états de mal épileptiques par le CTZ base (dérivé de la fraction thiazolique de la vitamine B1) Etude électro-clinique. Rev Neurol (Paris) 108:112–125

80. Prensky AL; Raff MC, Moore MJ, Schwar RS (1967) Intravenous diazepam in the treatment of prolonged seizure activity. N Engl J Med 276:779–784

81. Ramsay RE, Strauss RG, Wilder J, Willmore LJ (1978) Status epilepticus in pregnancy: Effect of phenytoin malabsorption on seizure control. Neurology (Minneapolis) 28:85–89

82. Ramsay RE, Hammond EJ, Perchalski RJ, Wilder BJ (1979) Brain uptake of phenytoin, phenobarbital and diazepam. Arch Neurol 36:535–539

83. Rohmer F, Collard M, Kurtz D, Warter JM, Coquillat G (1975) Les crises épileptiques au cours de la pathologie artérielle cérébrale Données cliniques. Rev Neurol (Paris) 131:661–669

84. Rollinson RD, Gillican BS (1979) Postanoxic action myoclonus responding to valproate. Arch Neurol 36:44–45

85. Roth LJ, Barlow CF (1961) Drugs in the brain Autoradiography and radio-assay techniques permit analysis of penetration by labeled drugs. Science 134:22–31

86. Rotheram EB, Safar P, Robin ED (1964) CNS disorder during mechanical ventilation in chronic pulmonary disease. JAMA 189:993–996

87. Rowan AS, Scott DF (1970) Major status epilepticus. A series of 42 patients. Acta Neurol Scand 46:573–584

88. Sawyer GT, Webster DD, Schult LJ (1968) Treatment of uncontrolled seizure activity with diazepam. JAMA 203:913–918

89. Serrano EE, Wilder BJ (1974) Intramuscular administration of diphenylhydantoin. Arch Neurol 31:276–278

90. Siesjo BK, Carlsson C, Haggerdal M (1976) Brain metabolism in the critically ill. Crit Car Med 4:283–294

91. Smith AL, Marque JJ (1976) Anesthetics and cerebral edema. Anesthesiology 45:64–72

92. Smith AL (1977) Barbiturate protection in cerebral hypoxia. Anesthesiology 47:285–293

92a. Terwinghe G, Daumerie J, Nicaise C, Rosillon O (1978) Effet thérapeutique du piracetam dans un cas de myoclonies d'action post-anoxique. Acta Neurol Belg 78:30–36

93. Trubuhovich RV (1979) Management of severe or intractable convulsions including eclampsia. Int Anesthesiol Clin 17:201–238

94. Unger AH, Aklaroff HK (1978) Fatalities following intravenous use of sodium diphenylhydantoin for cardiac arrhythmias. JAMA 200:335–336

95. Vajda FJE, Mihaly GW, Miles JL, Donnan GA, Bladin PF (1978) Rectal administration of sodium valproate in status epilepticus. Neurology (Minneap) 28:897–899

96. Van Woert MH, Rosenbaum D, Mowieson J, Bowers MB (1977) Long-term therapy of myoclonus and other neurologic disorders with 1-5-hydroxytryptophan and carbidopa. N Engl J Med 269:70–75

97. Vidailhet M (1974) Traitement d'urgence des convulsions du nourisson. La Revue du Praticien 26:911–924

98. Wallis W, Kutt H, Mc Dowell F (1968) Intravenous

diphenylhydantoin in treatment of acute repetitive seizures. Neurology (Minneap) 18:513–524

99. Wilder BJ, Ramsay E, Wilmore LJ (1977) Efficacy of intravenous phenytoin in the treatment of status epilepticus. Ann Neurol 1: 511–518

100. Wilensky AJ, Lowden JS (1979) Inadequate serum levels after intramuscular administration of diphenylhydantoin. Neurology (Minneap) 23:318–324

101. Wilkinson HA (1977) Treatment of status epilepticus. JAMA 237:26–27

102. Wolf SM (1979) Controversies in the treatment of febrile convulsions. Neurology (Minneap) 29:287–290

103. Wolpow ER (1978) Neurologic emergencies. In: Wilkins EW (ed) MGH Textbook of emergency medicine, Williams & Wilkins, Baltimore, pp 277–281

104. Zoneraich S, Zoneraich O, Siegel J (1976) Sudden death following intravenous diphenylhydantoin. Am Heart J 91:375–377

Chapter 47

Psychiatric Aspects of Intensive Care

Paul Bowden

All catastrophic events are associated with psychological sequelae. Those affected include persons involved in riot, parents who lose a child, the victims of violence, and those who face impending death. Just as the social world and individual life are connected, so a person's emotional and physical health are linked with his environment through the medium of psychosomatic disorders. These are a heterogeneous group of illnesses in which psychosocial events can be shown to have a direct relationship on the production of the symptoms and signs of an otherwise apparently physical disorder. Whatever the circumstances, the variety of physical and psychological responses to threats is limited and, as far as the mind is concerned, determined largely by pre-existing personality. The changes that occur in psychological functioning with alterations in the internal and external environment are exaggerated both in individuals primed with drugs and in those with metabolic changes that impair cerebral functioning.

This chapter outlines the psychological responses of the vulnerable patient to the uniquely stressful setting of the ICU. The stresses and their human responses are not particular to that environment but are encountered in many other situations. Thus, one of the correlates of stress to be found in the ICU is the fear of death, which has been described in a situation uncontaminated by other influences. The reaction shown by 64 French male criminals to the death penalty is not unlike that observed in patients in the critical care setting and the similarity illustrates the stereotyped nature of the human organism's response to stress [17]. In most of the condemned the response was of panic, which ended with a despairing struggle with the executioner; 18 remained 'calm and courageous'; 4 showed 'nervous excitement and extreme loquacity'; 12 were 'cynical and theatrical' and 5, 'indifferent' to their fate.

An important correlate of stress in the ICU is that of restricted environmental stimulation. This factor alone produces a multiplicity of responses which vary depending on personality differences and the level of arousal [51]. Thus, sensory deprivation induces disorders of perception in the form of hallucinations of sound, vision, touch, and movement. Reduced vigilance also occurs and this affects motor functioning; co-existent cognitive impairment is evinced by restricted powers of concentration, which in turn influence memory. In addition sensory deprivation causes time to be underestimated and it vastly increases susceptibility to influence from external sources.

Psychological response to stress

In vitro

Anxiety and fear

The acute reaction to stress may be predominantly a disturbance of emotion with combinations of fear, anxiety, and depression; a disturbance of consciousness; a psychomotor disturbance ranging from agitation to stupor; or a disturbance of reality in the form of psychosis.

Anxiety is a common emotion and it is not surprising that it is frequently met with in intensive care. It should be remembered that an anxiety reaction is a normal response and that its purpose is to stimulate behaviour with the intention of achieving equilibrium in the internal and external environments. In contrast, an anxiety state, or pathological (or morbid) anxiety, occurs when there is no corresponding external threat, or where the stimulus is above the optimum level that can be tolerated, or if tolerance is reduced by one or more of a wide variety of factors. Whether reaction or state, anxiety is unpleasant and is usually associated with senses of foreboding and bodily discomfort. The physiological symptoms of anxiety include weakness, dizziness, malaise, insecurity, and irritability, and, more cognitively, dread and a threat of imminent loss of control—panic. Somatic symptoms commonly occur with palpitations, dyspnoea, chest pain, paraesthesia, headache, tremor, fatigue, sweating, flushes, dry mouth, and frequency. Anxiety shows an individuality in its determinants, and a particularity of both personality traits and personally significant stresses are important in its aetiology.

Lader [38] has proposed a general model of anxiety whereby a continuous interaction of past experience and genetic endowment produce internal drives. At any time internal and external stimuli are monitored and evaluated for possible degrees of threat. If danger is perceived CNS arousal ensues which remains coordinated and integrated at all but extreme levels. The resultant affect that is experienced depends on the level of consciousness at which the threat is perceived; if it is conscious, it is experienced as fear; if it is subconscious, it is experienced as anxiety.

Fear is a response to a recognized external source of danger and the subjective experience ranges from uneasiness to intense dread. A sympatheticomimetic response occurs to prepare the subject for fight or flight.

Depression

Where there is an excessive preoccupation with traumatic experiences depressive neuroses occur, sometimes in combination with anxiety. There are also situation-specific depressive adjustment reactions, which may be brief or prolonged depending on the provoking stress. In the longer term a reactive depressive psychosis can develop which exhibits a range of affective disturbances, from minimal change to severe misery, gloom, and wretchedness. Anxiety is usually present and thinking and action are slowed. Delusional ideas and depersonalization experiences can arise from the mood disorder. Thoughts can be self-reproachful, hypochondriacal, and paranoid, the latter often taking the form of feeling shunned by others because of moral worthlessness. Sensory deceptions, particularly illusions, are not uncommon. Sleep is disturbed and there is loss of appetite. Retardation may progress to stupor.

Psychomotor disturbance and changes of consciousness

Other reactive states include excitation and confusion. In this latter condition there is clouding of consciousness with disorientation and reduced accessibility, accompanied sometimes by motor excitement and violence. Alternatively the reaction may be marked by paranoid attitudes, sometimes including delusions related to stressful situations.

Psychoses

Disturbance of affect (varieties of excitation or depression) can be associated with schizophrenia-like illnesses. Abnormal mental experiences may lead to explanatory delusions, and disturbances of perception and thinking can occur (schizo-affective psychoses).

In vivo

The above-mentioned states represent the repertoire of psychological response that is available in theory. In practice several factors prevent its manifestation in these pure forms and the observer is often faced with admixtures of one or more conditions. Furthermore, observers with different conceptual backgrounds will formulate disorders according to their bias, which may reflect any discipline in psychiatry. Other difficulties arise because of a lack of reliability and validity in psychiatric classification, so that often it is not possible to adduce the incidence of mental disorder with any accuracy, or to relate one study to another. These methodological failings are epitomized by the application of labels in the following studies: 'emotional disturbance' [46]; 'acute psychotic episodes' [55]; 'psychotic reaction' [40] and 'post-operative psychosis' [39].

A good descriptive classification of the variety of psychological reactions in critically ill patients is to be found in the report of Kiely [33]. He describes the acutely fearful patient who lies pale and nauseated, seeming limp and powerless. Tensions and anxiety are shown by tremulousness and jerky movements, increased activity and apprehensiveness. The depressed patient appears sad, his thoughts are guilty and full of self-condemnation. Sleep is disturbed and helplessness may be combined with a form of resistance called 'negativism'. A less retarded form of depression has been described [53] in a patient who was unco-operative, confused, agitated, and sometimes violent, and who appeared to be harbouring the wish to die.

Another way of looking at responses to the ICU situation is to describe patterns of behaviour which represent psychological defences to stress rather than being primarily a manifestation of illness. In this context the purpose of the defence is to protect the ego (self) from the perceived danger. Using this dynamic model Lee and Ball [41] list four responses in CCU patients. First, the obsessive compulsive defence, where the patient deals with stress by attempting to structure the situation, place it in order, systematize it, and study its conditions minutely in order to subjugate it. Here mastery of the environment is an attempt to control the source of anxiety. Second, the repressive defence, where the patient puts the problem out of his mind and looks to the staff to be firm and controlling. The third form of defence is dependent, and here the staff are made wholly responsible for the patient and his behaviour. Sometimes the dependence is severe and the patient behaves regressively by returning to some behaviour characteristic of an earlier stage of development. The fourth response is shown by the hyperintendent patient, who denies fear and hopelessness and throws himself wholeheartedly into an involvement in his own treatment.

Psychological response to impaired cerebral functioning

In vitro

The first major division of organic psychiatric illness is an organic reaction which may be either acute or chronic. Delirium is a form of organic reaction. It is not specifically associated with any one particular cause. Lishman [42] has described delirium as:

> ...a syndrome of impairment of consciousness along with intrusive abnormalities derived from the fields of perception and affect. Thus consciousness is not merely quantitatively reduced, but also qualitatively changed. Typically the patient becomes preoccupied with his own inner world, which is distorted by illusions, hallucinations and delusions, and by powerful affective changes derived therefrom or more directly from dysfunction of specific brain systems. Though conscious awareness of external events is impaired, arousal is high enabling these productive symptoms to occur, and accordingly psychomotor activity is usually increased in the form of restless and excited behaviour. Delirium commonly fluctuates in intensity and content and manifests a continuously changing clinical picture.

In that delirium is usually short lived, its features will be those of the acute organic reaction (synonyms: acute brain syndrome, acute confusional state, acute organic psychosis, acute psycho-organic syndrome). Lishman [42] has detailed the aetiology and the clinical picture. The causes include degeneration, space-occupying lesions, trauma, infection, vascular disease, epilepsy, metabolic and endocrine disturbances, hypoxia, and vitamin deficiency. There is usually an abrupt onset and whilst personality and background may affect the intensity and type of experience, the reaction is usually stereotyped. A global impairment of cognitive processes (thinking, attending, perceiving, and remembering) is associated with a reduced awareness of the environment, and drowsiness. Fluctuations and the existence of lucid intervals is an important sign, with deterioration during periods of reduced stimulation, such as at night. Muddled thinking, neglect of appearance, and amnestic periods are also characteristic.

Psychomotor behaviour is reduced and speech is usually affected, although hyperactivity and noisiness can occur. In the latter states jerky and repetitive movements are seen. Thinking becomes disorganized and there is an inability to distinguish between the internal and the external world. Subjective experiences obtrude into awareness; delusions of persecution are common. Defects in attention, comprehension, and perception lead to a disturbance of registration and defective retention impairs new learning. These memory defects lead to disorientation in time. False memories and confabulations occur. Disorders of perception lead to misinterpretations and illusions which, when combined with the memory disturbances, lead to faulty orientation in place. Hallucinations are usually visual and may be complex and colourful. Apathy is the commonest emotional state but labile and extreme emotions can be seen.

The majority of delirious states are reversible but some progress to a chronic organic brain syndrome. Impairment of memory, a change in personality, and the exaggeration of long-standing personality traits are characteristic. Inappropriate behaviour, restlessness, and withdrawal may be combined with self-neglect. Intellectual flexibility is lost with disordered thinking, and judgement may be impaired. Together with general memory impairment and emotional shallowness, explosiveness and lability of speech are seen.

In vivo

Because the effects of stress often occur in association with delirium it is important to be aware that secondary reactions may mask delirium and give the false impression of a purely psychological illness. In addition, depressive, paranoid, schizophrenic, phobic, or hysterical clinical pictures may predominate although they are purely a reaction to the underlying cognitive impairment.

In the early days of critical care it was thought that the high incidence of delirium after cardiotomy pointed to the existence of an ICU syndrome. A lucid interval was recognized between the operation and the appearance of mental disorder and this led to the belief that the environment played some part in its development. The delirium was characterized by disorders of perception in the form of illusions, followed later by hallucinations of vision and hearing. Paranoid delusions and disorientation were also thought to occur [16, 24, 37, 40]. Because delirium was manifested at a time when psychological equilibrium was largely restored it was related to the intensive care experience itself, but the observation that the physical state and the use of sedatives precluded any communication in the immediate post-operative period prompted Gilman [19] and later Tufo et

al. [54] to argue that the lucid interval was an artefact and, furthermore, that its existence could not be used to suggest an environmental aetiology for the post-operative delirium.

Cognitive impairment can be tested by asking questions regarding year, month, or asking the patient to count backwards, or to repeat series of digits in reverse order. Some patients do not show a global reduction in cerebration but only a selective loss of spatial orientation and hallucinosis. It has ben suggested that this latter form of delirium is not found in the presence of metabolic disorder but where cerebral malfunctioning is a result of loneliness, isolation, or sleep deprivation [32].

Incidence

There has been a growing awareness of the effects of stress and impaired cerebral functioning on patients receiving intensive care. This has led to changes in milieu that make the whole experience less frightening. Attention has been paid to allowing uninterrupted sleep, the provision of windows, and privacy. Monitoring equipment is made as unobtrusive as possible and vital signs are no longer communicated as auditory or visual signals that are discernible to the patient. Heller et al. [24] suggested that the steps taken to reduce stress in critical care had contributed to the reduced incidence of delirious states in the 1960s. Another change which has influenced the incidence of psychological disorder is that crude assessments have been replaced by sophisticated longitudinal studies which identify discrete disorders using more reliable standardized diagnostic criteria.

In 1955 Bliss and Rumel [7] reported a 35% incidence of psychological disorder after mitral surgery and over the next 16 years many similar studies were published. All were subject to the same methodological limitations and many subscribed to the view that cardiotomy itself represented a unique physical and psychological insult. Matarazzo et al. [46] showed a 68% incidence of psychological disorder following mitral commissurectomy and Blachy and Starr [5] found a 57% incidence of delirium after surgical procedures on the heart and great vessels. Gilman [19] and Kornfeld et al. [37] found similar incidences of delirium after open-heart surgery; 34% and 38% respectively. Weiss [55] reported a 50% incidence of psychosis after cardiotomy but in the latter part of the 1960s Lazarus and Hagens [40] and Rubinstein and Thomas [48] were reporting even lower rates, around 30%, and in 1971 Layne and Yudofsky [39] found that less than 15% of his patients exhibited signs of a post-operative psychosis. No doubt the trend towards a reduction in the incidence of severe mental disorder was in part due to an improvement in milieu but it was also related to a reduction in the mortality of patients as the most seriously ill are likely to have the greatest degree of mental disturbance. In the area of survival, matters have improved to the extent that by 1977 Tomlin [53] was able to report a mortality of only 14% in an ICU.

After surgery

In general the coronary care ward will be a less stressful environment than the ICU and, furthermore, its patients will be less subject to those disturbances of the body's internal environment that influence cerebral functioning.

Two well-designed studies suggest that delirium is the commonest post-operative psychological disturbance. Egerton and Kay [16] examined 60 survivors of an original sample of 90, the majority of whom had open heart surgery. Thirty-six percent were delirious postoperatively and a further 10% were depressed; in one individual the depression was of psychotic intensity. The delirious group were normal at follow-up 3 months later although in two of the cases the depression persisted. The second study was by Rubinstein and Thomas [48], who examined 36 cardiotomy patients postoperatively. Delirium was present at some time in 31%, depression in 5%, and one patient developed a schizophrenic reaction. In a different vein Tufo et al. [54] emphasized the neurological sequelae of open heart surgery: of the 100 cases examined nearly one-half developed focal neurological signs followed by behavioural abnormalities. At the time of discharge, 15% showed persisting signs of cerebral damage.

Coronary care and resuscitation

Hackett et al. [22] described the psychological morbidity in a consecutive series of 50 patients in a CCU: 40 were anxious, 29 depressed, and 5 delirious. The small CCU that was the background to the study of Dominian and Dobson [14] obviously provided a more agreeable environment: only 6 of 74 consecutive male patients, admitted with their first myocardial infarction, found the ward anxiety provoking.

Druss and Kornfeld [15] described the sequelae of cardiac arrest, the survivors of which are known to have a high incidence of organic brain dysfunction. A comparative group was chosen from patients with heart disease. The only difference between the group was that those who had been resuscitated subsequently experienced nightmares of violence. These dreams have been said to have a cathartic function which purges the subject of unpleasant memories [8]. All patients treated in the monitor unit showed long-standing emotional problems including insomnia, irritability, and a morbidly cautious restriction of activities far beyond that considered necessary on physical grounds [15].

In summary, transient delirium is not uncommon after cardiothoracic surgery and it is determined largely by a variety of disequilibria in physical systems. The psychological residue of resuscitation is related to the amount of organic deficit secondary to brain damage. Affective disorders are the hallmark of the CCU patient and they can produce persistent abnormalities of mind.

Risk factors

Certain characteristics, whether related to the individual (demographic or psychological), the environment, or the procedures to which the patient is subjected, will influence the development of both stress reactions and delirium. These factors are not connected with the mental abnormality in a casual manner; most are associated and interdependent.

Demographic

Blachy and Starr [5] noted that the frequency of all psychiatric symptoms tended to increase with age. This finding was confirmed by Layne and Yudofsky [39], who studied cardiotomy patients and the subjects of other major vascular surgery. The mean age of the patients who became psychotic after surgery was significantly higher than those who remained mentally stable. Both Heller et al. [24] and Morse and Litin [47] made similar observations. Three studies suggest that children are particularly resilient to psychological complications [16, 37, 40]. It has also been suggested that men are more likely to develop post-operative psychoses [39].

Psychological

Some patients admitted to an ICU will have taken an overdose of drugs or attempted to harm themselves in other ways. A proportion of these patients will have severe mental illness that will manifest itself as they regain consciousness. Alcoholics show a high incidence of accidental injury and they are particularly prone to suicide attempts, so they are likely to be over-represented in ICU populations.

An early description of the link between pre- and post-operative mental state was provided by Bliss and Rumel [7], who noted that a patient who developed schizophrenia after valvotomy was known to have been psychotic before surgery. It has been suggested by others [10] that individuals with coronary disease have abnormal personalities before they enter critical care. They have been described as exhibiting traits of passivity and suppressed hostility, with chronic restlessness and anxieties about imminent death. Indeed, a pre-existing abnormal response to stress has been linked to heart disease [31]. Those who do exhibit signs of psychiatric disturbance after surgery on the heart and great vessels have an unusually high mortality [5].

Egerton and Kay [16] showed that patients who developed delirium after open heart surgery were significantly more likely to have a family history of schizophrenia and paranoid psychosis. A careful study by Rubinstein and Thomas [48] confirmed that patients with pre-operative psychological disorder had a greater chance of developing delirium; however, these authors did not find an increased mortality in this group. Thus, there is agreement that some mental abnormalities and personality traits are associated with the development of types of physical disease, that subjects with a history of psychosis, or a propensity to psychosis (e.g. family history), are more vulnerable post-operatively, and it is possible that post-operative mental abnormality increases both morbidity and mortality from physical complications.

Whether the same is true of neurosis is more contentious. This is probably because both dissociation, which produces a separation of cognitive and emotional functioning, and the defence mechanism of denial come into effect to reduce situational anxiety. Matarazzo et al. [46] reported that those who developed psychological reactions to mitral surgery scored within the normal range on several measures of neuroticism. Weiss [55] believed that ego strength (considered to represent an individual's capacity for resourcefulness and an estimate of stability) was significantly and inversely related to the likelihood of a psychological reaction following open heart surgery. Dominian and Dobson [14] showed that there is no relationship between a patient's attitude to the unit and measures of anxiety and various personality characteristics. An explanation for these seemingly paradoxical findings was provided by Layne and Yudofsky [39] who found that on a simple anxiety rating those with the lowest scores developed post-operative psychoses more frequently, suggesting that this group relied heavily on denial. Denial is a psychological mechanism of defence by which painful experiences, impulses, or aspects of the self are not consciously acknowledged [49]. The validity of studies on neuroticism and the post-operative state will depend on the degree to which psychological assessments overcome this defence mechanism and accurately reflect the individual's response to his predicament.

Neurotic reactions have been described in almost all patients with serious heart disease [12], and it is not surprising that the atmosphere of critical care augments these anxieties. Helplessness, humiliation, and distortion of body image are hardly conducive to a sense of well-being. Dobson et al. [13] revealed something of the patients' anxieties in a study of 20 survivors of cardiac resuscitation following myocardial infarction. Although the patients were not usually informed of the arrest by the medical staff the majority had been aware of what happened and had a good understanding of the implications: most often their spouse told them. Six patients remembered the start and end of the arrest and five specifically remembered external cardiac massage. Initial anxiety was experienced by all patients and in five there were unsatisfactory adjustments with persisting physical disability and mood disorder. The spouses found it difficult to know how to treat the patients and most felt that simple explanation and discussion would have helped them in their task.

Environmental

Reduced stimulation, social isolation, and physical confinement are the characteristics of clinical sensory deprivation [27]. A similar group has been defined by Suedfeld [51] and its aetiology labelled 'iatrogenic restricted environmental stimulation'. Clinically these patients are to be found amongst the quarantined, those subject to eye surgery, those nursed in a protected environment, as well as the occupants of ICUs. Whatever the milieu, the effects are similar and subjects show reduced concentration, impaired memory, disorientation, suspiciousness, and helplessness. There is also an increased frequency of vivid and unusual dreams.

For the patient in critical care, movement is often restricted because of pain, catheters, intravenous lines, and monitoring equipment. Although the environment is dramatic there is a monotony of light and noise and these effects might be enhanced by the use of analgesics and sedatives. Sleep deprivation and interruption of what sleep there is, is associated with a dramatic reduction in rapid eye movement (REM) sleep [30]. To compound these assaults an endotracheal tube or tracheostomy might render the patient speechless.

One of the most important studies of the ICU environment was reported by Wilson [56]. This author compared 50 consecutive surgical patients treated in a unit without windows and a further 50 similar patients in a unit with windows. Over twice as many episodes of delirium were seen in the windowless unit, and the incidence was even greater in uraemic or anaemic patients. Zubek [57] has stressed that exhaustion, disorientation, confusion, and delirium abound in an atmosphere of sensory deprivation. The homologous stimulation, solitude, confinement, isolation, and invariant input predispose to illusions and hallucinations, and there is deterioration in intellectual performance with an increased susceptibility to influence and stimulus-seeking behaviour. (In this setting perceptual disorder, e.g. hallucinations, could be understood as an attempt to provide stimulae in order to maintain arousal.)

Lazarus and Hagens [40] emphasized that particular attention must be paid to prevent interruption of sleep and Kornfeld [36] stressed the necessity for the usual day-awake, night-asleep pattern. One article [8] warned that while some individuals appeared to remain calm and perceive their predicament in detail, others developed a fear of such intensity that awareness became clouded and behaviour incoherent. Hewitt [25] reported that nasopharyngeal suction was particularly unpleasant and stressful. Blacher [4] interviewed 12 apparently normal patients after cardiotomy. Eight had suffered major psychological disorder but they had managed to hide it from the medical and nursing staff because of the anxiety evoked by such symptoms in both patient and staff.

Although the witnessing of the death of a fellow patient in a CCU is associated with the physiological signs of fear and anxiety, Grace [20] has written that he has never witnessed a metastatic cardiac arrest. Jarvinen [28] suggested that certain situations are uniquely stressful; thus, a visit from relatives could produce anginal pain after myocardial infarction, and the stress evoked by ward rounds could be lethal. Jewitt et al. [29] proposed that severe pain, tissue damage, and circulatory disturbances could all result in increased sympathoadrenal activity and that the extent of this response is linked to mortality after myocardial infarction. Klein et al. [34] and Thompson and Sloman [52] both correlated the emotional changes that occur at the time of transfer to a general ward with increased urinary catecholamine excretion.

Procedural

Two uncontrolled studies suggest that patients are particularly prone to adverse psychological reaction after mitral valvotomy [7, 43]. These findings were confirmed in a controlled study [46] but the view that surgery to the mitral valve is uniquely damaging has been challenged [37]. The latter study implicated the degree of postoperative incapacity, the length of pre-surgery illness, and the severity of operative trauma with the development of delirium. It also showed that increased time on bypass and the manipulation of two valves as opposed to one increased the probability of a post-operative delirious state. A careful study by Heller et al. [24] added that the severity of the post-operative state was also important in the development of delirium. A high incidence of psychosis and other abnormal mental states has been described in patients after heart transplantation although the recipients had been screened for mental abnormalities beforehand [45]. Tomlin [53] has described how weaning from a ventilator can be particularly stressful and lead to a regressive 'terror' neurosis, hypervigilant anxiety, and depression. Withdrawal from IPPV is part of the process of critical care but other events take place that are avoidable. Abramson et al. [1] showed a significantly higher mortality in those ICU admissions subject to 'adverse occurrences' during their treatment. Failure of equipment sustaining respiration and cardiovascular function was usually due to human error rather than equipment malfunction. Other mistakes arose because of poor communication or the improper administration of medication.

Decreased cerebral blood flow has been causally associated with the development of post-operative organic and delirious states and this can occur in more than one-third of those undergoing open heart surgery [19]. Furthermore, clinical and pathological findings showed that such cerebral ischaemia was most often due to emboli. A prospective study [54] compared pre- and post-operative states on three parameters, neurological, behavioural, and psychometric. Of 100 patients subject to open heart surgery, 43% of survivors developed behavioural abnormalities preceded by focal neurological signs. Intellectual functioning was impaired in all those affected and 15% still had signs of neurological damage at the time of discharge. The presence of dehydration and hyponatremia [16], and albuminuria, alkalosis, anaemia, azotaemia, hyperchloraemia, hypokalaemia, and leucocytosis [47] also predisposes to the development of delirium.

In summary, children are apparently protected from developing mental abnormality but risk increases with age. Those who are unable to communicate are especially vulnerable. Immobility, sleep loss, and an environment that provides unchanging sensory input foster anxiety, psychosis, and delirium; while those events that do occur tend to increase stress. The length of pre-operative disability, the extent of surgery, and the post-operative condition are directly related to psychological morbidity. Persisting psychological symptoms and neurological defects are associated with the presence of post-operative brain damage and with cerebral ischaemia secondary to inadequate perfusion or embolization. Biochemical imbalance sensitizes the brain to adverse influences. The incidence of delirium and psychosis is greater in those with a history of psychosis; but no clear association has been shown to exist between pre-existing neurotic disorders and the development of abnormal mental states.

Staff

The staff involved in critical care are an elite but they have a high psychological morbidity [18] that can lead to suicide [53]. A South African study [44] showed that what is stressful to staff is socially based. Thus, in a comparison of black and white ICU nurses, it was shown that the latter found the pressure of time and coping with the relatives most stressful while in the former an incomplete understanding of machines was most anxiety provoking. (These findings were explained on the grounds that the majority of homes in Soweto, where the black nurses lived, did not have electrical appliances.)

Being a separate community, ICU personnel turn to each other for emotional support. Their apparent competence can promote antagonisms with other medical groups, and this reinforces the pressure to maintain intense peer group loyalties. The patients too are special: there is an overwhelming preponderance of first admissions, a high percentage of deaths, and few discharges home. Rewards are elusive and cures may be only partial. The strength of the nurse–patient relationship is increased by a serious illness which leads to a long stay in the unit, but which is accompanied by a greater likelihood of death. Pain and grief are common events and separation and reattachments frequent. To avoid repeated traumatic losses staff sometimes employ emotional distancing techniques so that a business-like veneer hides a defensive withdrawal from contact with both colleagues and patients. The nurse who gives immediate attention and is cheerful, kind, and tender will be disturbed by the rapid change in the population, which impedes the development of relationships and intense emotional interaction. Kornfeld [36] stressed that nursing staff may even be reluctant to call for advice or help for fear that such a request would be interpreted as evidence of inadequacy.

Baxter [3] believes that a psychiatrist can be useful in helping reduce tensions but warns that unit meetings will depend on the quality of existing staff relationships and should arise out of a desire of the staff to explore anxiety, fear, and guilt. In the apparently chauvinistic hierarchy of male doctors and female nurses it will be necessary for all staff to feel that they have a say in important decisions, for example, weaning from IPPV, and in these circumstances group meetings can be a major vehicle for reducing stress [2]. An example of the types of problem that can arise has been described by Hay and Oken [23] who noted the propensity of senior staff to displace their own guilt at not being able to save their patients onto their juniors in the form of a hypercritical and overzealous approach.

Staff must be adequately trained for positions of authority and they must know the extent of their responsibilities. From an emotional viewpoint the work is concerned with conflict. There is a conflict between the staff's role in the development of individual relationships with patients and the maintainence of an objective attitude to, for example, the patient as a potential organ donor. Again, on the one hand a nurse is expected to emanate sympathy, on the other he or she firmly guides the patient from a position of regressed dependence and total reliance, to some sort of independence. Mistakes can be life threatening and repetitive exposure to death and dying poses threats of personal failure [23]. For the patients there may be a credibility gap between the service and the people it serves [31]. It appeared from one study that the most seriously ill (i.e. those with the longest stays) and the lowest socioeconomic groups found their environment least assuring [14]. Presumably this last category had greater difficulty in comprehending their environment, and hence came their anxiety.

Ethics

For some, critical care represents the epitome of medical nemesis whereby the epidemic of modern health care has resulted in the expropriation of health for the purpose of callous medical expansionism [26]. With this view in mind Guthrie [21] saw the 'life-saving' therapy as the blood-letting, drugging, and insomnia of a terror- and torture-filled political prison, indeed, as a maximum security ward where ethical principles are challenged because previous limitations of morality are transformed. The intensivists' ability to reverse, retard, or accelerate processes of death puts them in a very powerful position [11].

Those involved in critical care become arbiters of the welfare state, selecting and rejecting individuals for the ultimate benefit, life. One question must be asked: who and in what circumstances is to decide, 'In a situation of limited resources how is care to be distributed?'. Cohen [11] argues that although the right to life cannot be over-ridden for the sake of social utility, this precisely is the decision made by intensivists. He states that since the purpose of intensive care medicine is to treat, diagnose, and maintain patients with potentially reversible life-threatening impairment of organ systems, it excludes those who are not salvageable. Furthermore, 'salvageability' will be considered in the light of the risk of permanent impairment

of organ systems; and the final decision is affected by considerations of social convenience.

Management

Relatives

All staff should be aware of their crucial role with regard to the relatives who, in their anxiety, will exploit any inconsistency in the information they have been given. An appreciation of their sense of helplessness is most important.

Patients

Procedures that involve the patient should be discussed in simple language. Staff should attempt to provide privacy without isolation so that patients do not inadvertently witness others' suffering. Monitoring equipment should not be visible or audible to the patient. Cassem and Hackett [9] recommend support through the medium of psychiatric intervention applied by a variety of techniques including medication, explanation, confrontation, and anticipation. These authors purport to show that the expected mortality of a group who received psychiatric treatment was reduced three-fold.

Klein et al. [34] have warned that the period of transfer from critical care is most important. Patients should be prepared for a sort of adolescent crisis as they emerge from a situation of dependency, handicapped sometimes by physical disability. Urgent transfer should be avoided because it represents rejection, and patients should retain some contact with staff from the ICU.

Physical treatments

Schroeder [50] reminds us that the whole effort of the intensivist must be directed to treating the admitting disease, but the success of this venture will depend on the way this task is tackled. Sometimes the prescription of psychotropic medication will be necessary but it will only be an adjunct to other psychological methods of treatment. The benzodiazepines are useful as both anxiolytics (diazepam), and hypnotics and sedatives (nitrazepam), but these preparations can cause confusion. The tricyclic antidepressants have a hypotensive effect and they have been associated with the development of cardiac arrhythmias and heart block. In consequence, they are usually contra-indicated in the treatment of depression in critical care. Blachy and Semler [6] advocate the use of electroconvulsive therapy where depression is so severe that treatment is mandatory.

The antipsychotic 'neuroleptics' are used both to quieten disturbance, whether due to physical or psychological causes, and in severe anxiety. These drugs belong to three groups: phenothiazines, such as chloromazine, pericyazine, fluphenazine; thiozanthenes (flupenthixol); and butyrophenones (haloperidol, primozide). All share common unwanted effects, but to varying degrees, and the selection of a particular drug will depend on the route of administration and the disorder requiring treatment. The neuroleptics mask depression and they can have a hypotensive effect. Hypothermia-like reactions are sometimes seen. Movement disorders in the form of dystonias or akathisias occur and they may be combined with parkinsonian-like reactions. The latter conditions usually respond to treatment with anticholinergics. Finally, withdrawal from drugs or alcohol can be facilitated by the use of chlormethiazole but there can be problems of dependency if its use is prolonged.

References

1. Abramson N, Silvasy K, Grenvik A, Robinson D, Snyder V (1980) Adverse occurrences in intensive care units. JAMA 244:1582–1584
2. Asken M (1979) Psychological stress in the ICU affects both patients and staff. Pa Med 82:40–42
3. Baxter S (1974) Psychological problems of intensive care. Br J Hosp Med ll:875–885
4. Blacher R (1972) The hidden psychosis of open heart surgery. JAMA 222:305–308
5. Blachy P, Starr A (1964) Post-cardiotomy delirium. Am J Psychiatry 121:371–375
6. Blachy P, Semler H (1967) Electroconvulsive therapy of three patients with aortic valve prosthesis. Am J Psychiatry 124:223–236
7. Bliss E, Rumel W (1955) Psychiatric complications of mitral surgery. AMA Arch Neurol Psychiatr 74:249–252
8. British Medical Journal (1967) Leading article: Life after death. Br Med J iv:693–694
9. Cassem N, Hackett T (1971) Psychiatric consultation in a coronary care unit. Ann Intern Med 75:9–14
10. Cleveland S, Johnson D (1962) Personality patterns in young males with coronary disease. Psychosom Med 24:600–610
11. Cohen C (1977) Ethical problems of intensive care. Anesthesiology 47:217–227
12. Connolly J (1974) Stress and coronary artery disease. Br J Hosp Med 11:297–302
13. Dobson M, Tattersfield A, Adler M, McNicol M (1971) Attitudes and long term adjustment of patients surviving cardiac arrest. Br Med J iii:207–212
14. Dominian J, Dobson M (1969) Study of patients' psychological attitudes to a coronary care unit. Br Med J iv:795–798
15. Druss R, Kornfeld D (1967) The survivors of cardiac arrest. JAMA 201:291–296
16. Egerton N, Kay J (1964) Psychological disturbances associated with open heart surgery. Br J Psychiatry 110:433–439
17. Ellis H (1890) The criminal, Scott, London, pp 128–129
18. Gardham J (1969) Nursing in the intensive care unit. JAMA 208:2337–2338
19. Gilman S (1965) Open heart operation. N Engl J Med 272:489–498
20. Grace W (1969) Terror in the coronary care unit. Am J Cardiol 22:746.
21. Guthrie R (1971) Maximum security ward. New York: Farrar, Straus and Girouz
22. Hackett T, Classem N, Wishnie N (1969) Detection and treatment of anxiety in the coronary care unit. Am Heart J 78:727–730
23. Hay D, Oken D (1972) Psychological stresses in intensive care unit nursing. Psychosom Med 34:109–118
24. Heller S, Frank K, Malm J, Bowman D, Harris P, Charlton M, Kornfeld D (1970) Psychiatric complications of open heart surgery. N Engl J Med 283:1015–1020
25. Hewitt P (1970) Subjective follow-up from a surgical intensive therapy ward. Br Med J iv:699–673
26. Illich I (1977) Limits to medicine. Pelican, Aylesbury, p 41
27. Jackson C (1979) Clinical sensory deprivation: a review of hospitalised eye-surgery patients. In: Zubek J (ed) Sensory deprivation: Fifteen years of research. Appleton, New York, pp 332–373
28. Jarvinen K (1955) Can ward rounds be a danger to patients with myocardial infarction? Br Med J i:318–320
29. Jewitt D, Reid D, Thomas M, Mercer C, Valori C, Shillingford J (1969) Free noradrenaline and adrenaline excretion in relation to development of cardiac arrhythmias and heart failure in patients with acute myocardial infarction. Lancet i:635–641
30. Jones J, Hoggart B, Withey J, Donaghue K, Ellis B (1979) What patients say: a study of reactions to an intensive care unit. Intensive Care Med 5:89–92
31. Journal of the American Medical Association (1971) Editorial. Intense emotions in an intensive care ward. (1971) JAMA 216:1017–1018
32. Katz N, Agle D, De Palma R (1972) Delirium in surgical patients under intensive care. Arch Surg 104:310–313
33. Kiely W (1976) Psychiatric syndromes in critically ill patients. JAMA 235:2759–2761
34. Klein R, Kliner V, Zipes D, Troyer W, Wallace A, Durham N (1968) Transfer from a coronary care unit. Arch Intern Med 122:104–108
35. Kornfeld D (1969) Psychiatric aspects of patient care in the operating suite and special areas. Anesthesiology 31:166–171
36. Kornfeld D (1969) Psychiatric view of the intensive care unit. Br Med J i:108–110
37. Kornfeld D, Zimberg S, Malm J (1965) Psychiatric complications of open heart surgery. N Engl J Med 273:287–290
38. Lader M (1975) Psycho-physiological aspects of anxiety. Medicine 2nd series, 10:429–432
39. Layne O, Yudofsky S (1971) Postoperative psychosis in cardiotomy patients. N Engl J Med 284:518–520

40. Lazarus H, Hagens J (1968) Prevention of psychosis following open heart surgery. Am J Psychiatry 124:1190–1195
41. Lee R, Ball P (1975) Some thoughts on the psychology of the coronary care unit patient. Am J Nurs 75:1498–1501
42. Lishman W (1978) Organic psychiatry. Blackwell, Oxford, pp 11–23
43. Little R, Pearson M (1954) Combined insulin coma and electro-convulsive therapy following cardiac surgery. Am J Psychiatry 110:786–787
44. Lochoff R, Cane R, Buchanan N, Cox H (1977) Nursing staff stress in an intensive care unit. S Afr Med J 52:961–963
45. Lunde D (1969) Psychiatric complications of heart transplants. Am J Psychiatry 126:369–373
46. Matarazzo R, Bristow D, Reaume R (1963) Medical factors relevant to psychological reactions in mitral valve disease. J Nerv Ment Dis 137:380–388
47. Morse R, Litin E (1969) Postoperative delirium: A study of etiologic factors. Am J Psychiatry 126:388–395
48. Rubinstein D, Thomas J (1969) Psychiatric findings in cardiotomy patients. Am J Psychiatry 126:360–369
49. Ryecroft C (1968) A critical dictionary of psychoanalysis. Nelson, London, pp 29–30
50. Schroeder H (1971) Psycho-reactive problems of intensive therapy. Anaesthesia 26:28–35
51. Suedfeld P (1980) Restricted environmental stimulation. Wiley, New York, pp 416–439
52. Thompson P, Sloman G (1971) Sudden death in hospital after discharge from coronary care unit. Br Med J iv:136–139
53. Tomlin P (1977) Psychological problems in intensive care. Br Med J ii:441–443
54. Tufo H, Ostfeld A, Shekelle R (1970) Central nervous system dysfunction following open heart surgery. JAMA 212:1333–1340
55. Weiss S (1966) Psychological adjustment following open heart surgery. J Nerv Ment Dis 143:363–368
56. Wilson L (1972) Intensive care delirium. Arch Intern Med 130:225–226
57. Zubek I (1969) Sensory deprivation. Appleton, Century, Crofts, New York, p 286

Section I

Acute Poisoning and Disturbances of Temperature Regulation

Chapter 48

The Principles of Management of Acute Poisoning

Chantal Bismuth

The management of acutely poisoned patients represents between 5% and 30% of the activity of multidisciplinary ICUs throughout the world. In recent years the incidence of accidental poisoning has increased, but the most significant rise has occurred in intentionally self-administered poisoning: a suicidal, impulsive, manipulative act undertaken to secure redress for an intolerable situation, or an increasing tendency, in young adults and teenagers to try drugs for 'kicks'.

The overall management of a poisoned patient has three stages:

(1) Obtaining, where necessary, specific information from a poisons information service; (2) assessing the patient for intensive supportive or specific therapy; and (3) securing psychiatric and/or social welfare advice.

The second of these stages will be considered in this chapter and in Chapter 49.

Accuracy of diagnosis

Clinical diagnosis [3, 4, 8]

Often the circumstantial evidence leaves little doubt that a patient has taken poison. This is particularly so in patients with self-poisoning who, before becoming drowsy or losing consciousness, intimate what they have done. It will also be evident in the determined suicide who takes elaborate precautions to avoid premature discovery but who leaves a suicide note.

It is important to remember that acute toxicity may occur by routes other than ingestion or inhalation. Some toxic substances such as weed-killers and certain insecticides may be readily absorbed through the skin or in the eye. Poisonous chemicals produced for industrial use may also be absorbed in these ways, and acute salicylate overdosage has occurred from the use of salicylic acid ointment on extensive skin lesions.

The characteristic associated clinical signs in the most common adult poisonings are summarized in Table 48.1. In many cases, however, several drugs are taken, and therefore the clinical features are not specific.

Role of the laboratory [1, 2, 11]

The only conclusive means of providing a definite diagnosis of poisoning is by laboratory analysis of specimens of blood, gastric aspirate, or urine [5, 10].

The methods of screening that are readily available are valuable in two other ways: (1) in cases where toxicity is delayed, they allow a prediction to be made. Knowledge of the initial blood level has been demonstrated to be very valuable for the prognosis of poisoning with such preparations as paraquat, or paracetamol; (2) in situations where drugs are being removed they enable the efficacy of the method to be assessed.

Table 48.1. Signs characteristically associated with the commonest forms of poisoning in adults

Clinical state (adults)	Mortality in ICUs(%)	Poison	Frequency (per 100 patients)	Associated clinical signs
Unconscious	< 1	Barbiturates	40	Skin blisters, depressed respiration, hypothermia
	<1	Methaqualone	3	Hypertonicity, extensor plantar responses, myoclonia
	<1	Carbamates	3	Circulatory failure
	0	Benzodiazepines	18	None
	1	Opiates	3	Pin point pupils, depressed respiration, puncture wounds
	1	Trichlorethylene	2	Evocative smell, hyperexcitability ECG
	1	Phenothiazines	15	Hypothermia
	0	Alcohol	5	Evocative smell, flushing, vomiting, hypothermia
	15	Carbon monoxide	5	Hypertonicity, extensor plantar responses, myolysis, pulmonary oedema
	0	Chloralose	2	Myoclonia
Encephalo-pathy	2	Tricyclic drugs	17	Anticholinergic signs, arrhythmias and conduction disturbances
	15	Organophosphates	1	As opiates, but more pronounced bradycardia, muscular fasciculation
	1	Salicylates	5	Flushing, sweating, tinnitus, deafness, hyperventilation
	17	Digitalis	3	Vomiting, sagging of the ST segment bradycardia, AV block, ventricular tachycardia
	20	Heavy metals	1	Diarrhoea, acute renal failure, encephalopathy
	0	Anticholinergic drugs	7	Dilated pupils, rashes, tachycardia, mental confusion
Conscious	15	Paracetamol	1	Delayed (24–48 h) hepatic failure
	17	Colchicine	2	Vomiting, diarrhoea, circulatory failure, marrow aplasia, later alopecia
	15	Corrosives	3	White burns of the buccal mucosa, greyish burns of the lips, fibrinoly-sis, circulatory shock
	60	Paraquat	1	Initial burns of digestive tract, acute renal failure, delayed lethal pulmonary fibrosis

Individual variations in response to drugs [7, 13]

These include differences in the intestinal absorption and activity of drug metabolites, various affinities for receptors, hepatic enzymatic induction [6], acquired tolerance, and differences in immuno-allergic reactions to drugs.

Overall, there is no doubt that the initial clinical assessment of the patient is most important. But it must be remembered that in certain cases, (e.g., paraquat paracetamol) the patient admitted in a good clinical condition may subsequently die. This prognosis can be predicted at an early stage if the dose ingested or the initial plasma level of the drug is known.

In addition, the comatose phase of poisoning has a better prognosis, statistically, than the non-comatose so long as the coma is not the result of cerebral hypoxia: mortality is less than 1% for toxifications with hypnotic drugs [15], as against 5% for non-comatose toxifications even in spite of the impressive initial clinical state of the first type of poisoning [12].

Basic principles of medical treatment

Intensive supportive therapy

Assessment of the patient

Comatose poisoning [10]. Unconsciousness is the main feature in 70% of cases of acute poisoning. Its initial assessment is of paramount importance, not only to determine the patient's presenting condition from which his progress may then be judged, but also to decide upon the treatment required. Frequent accompanying signs are depression of respiration; hypotension, which may be severe and if prolonged can lead to renal damage; and hypothermia with specific J waves in the ECG (Fig. 48.1) (C. Bismuth, 1980, unpublished work).

The adequacy of ventilation should be measured in an objective manner by means of arterial blood gases and acid–base status. It is worth remembering that in acute poisoning body metabolism is often depressed, particularly if hypothermia is present and the $PaCO_2$ is often lower than might have been expected. The presence of severe hypoxia is indicative of additional pulmonary pathology: infection, atelectasis, aspiration, or oedema (Table 48.2).

Clinical assessment of peripheral circulatory failure in acute poisoning is often difficult, since the typical features of shock may not be apparent in the presence of central nervous depression and hypothermia. Tissue perfusion is what really matters and, unless the type of toxification is known and the mechanism of hypotension readily appreciated, haemodynamic study must be undertaken. This makes it possible to assess any cardiogenic (e.g., meprobamate poisoning) or vasodilator factor (e.g., arsenic poisoning).

Hypothermia may be considered to exist if the rectal temperature falls below 36°C. Hypothermia contributes to shock, acidaemia, and hypoxia, and it is essential to monitor body temperature with a low-reading rectal thermometer.

Each patient has to be assessed by taking account of all these factors. In addition, it is necessary to consider the state of hydration and to measure the plasma urea and electrolytes, together with the acid–base status, since these may have an important bearing on treatment.

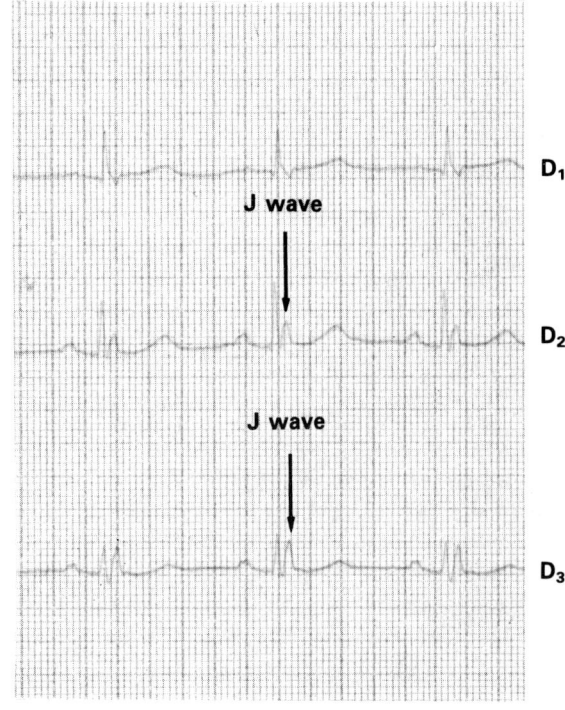

Fig. 48.1. ECG in phenobarbitone intoxication, showing J wave. Temperature 32°C.

Table 48.2. Hypoxaemia in acute poisoning

Mechanism	Aetiology
CNS depression	Barbiturates, opiates, hypnotics, organophosphate compounds
Muscular paralysis	Curares, strychnine, organophosphate compounds, convulsant drugs
Pulmonary oedema	Overload poisoning, particularly with carbamates, inhalation pneumonia NH_4Cl, opiates, SH_2, C1H, salicylates
Bronchial hypersecretion	Anti-cholinesterase agents, chloralose, prolonged coma
Atelectasis	Protracted coma
Altered affinity of haemoglobin	Carbon monoxide, methaemoglobinaemia, aniline, nitrous compounds
Pulmonary fibrosis	Inhalation pneumonia, paraquat

Non-comatose poisoning. This carries a greater risk than comatose poisoning, and many of the features have a delayed onset. The clinical evaluation must therefore be particularly careful. The most frequent organ failures are cardiac (Table 48.3), renal (Table 48.4), and hepatic (amanita phalloides, carbon tetrachloride, paracetamol, paraquat). Agranulocytosis may occur with colchicine, amidopyrine, and benzene poisoning, and also after exposure to irradiation.

The presence of a metabolic acidosis in these cases may suggest the particular poison concerned: convulsants, ethylene glycol, methanol, cyanides, isoniazid, or strong acids.

Emergency measures

Some emergency measures are the administration of antidotes, respiratory and circulatory support, and treatment of fits.

Antidotes. Few specific antidotes are available. (Table 48.5). Even when these are available they may themselves cause serious toxic effects, and so their use must be reserved for when the primary poisoning is severe. Physostigmine, for example, can cause convulsions, bronchospasm, and bradycardia. Analeptic drugs other than true pharmacological antidotes should never be given for the treatment of sedative and hypnotic drug overdosage. In most cases, therefore, treatment must be directed towards the support of vital functions.

Respiratory assistance. Endotracheal intubation is essential if there is a risk to the airways in patients in deep coma. Assisted ventilation will be necessary. Respiratory support is rarely needed for longer than 1 week unless there have been pulmonary or neurological complications.

The aim of ventilation is to maintain the PaO_2 within physiological limits.

Analeptic drugs given to stimulate the respiratory centre have made no impact on the mortality of acutely poisoned patients.

Circulatory assistance. Shock in poisoned patients should not be treated until a clear airway has been established and hypoxia corrected, since these measures alone may improve the circulation. In addition, if there has been a sustained fall in blood pressure, arterial blood pH, $PaCO_2$ and standard bicarbonate should be determined and corrected if necessary. Cardiac arrhythmias contributing to a diminished cardiac output that fails to respond to these efforts should be corrected.

Table 48.4. Acute renal failure in poisoning

Type of nephrotoxicity	Agent
Direct	Heavy metals
	Antifreeze (ethylene glycol)
	Haemolysing agents (included methaemoglobinaemia) { aniline chlorates
	Analgesics (paracetamol, Glafénine, indomethacin)
	Antibiotics (Colistine, Cephalosporin)
	Herbicides (paraquat, morfamquat)
	Solvents (carbon tetrachloride)
Indirect (hypovolaemia)	Sweating: salicylates
	Vomiting, diarrhoea: heavy metals, colchicine, mushroom poisoning
	Polyuria: diuretics
	Rhabdomyolysis: the most common cause of renal failure in comatose cases

Table 48.3 Cardiotoxic agents

Drug	Delayed toxicity	Mortality	ECG modifications
Digitalis	Several days	17%	Bradycardia, bigeminal rhythms, AV conduction disturbances, ventricular tachycardia and fibrillation
Digoxin	24 h	10%	As for digitalis
Chloroquine	2–6 h	10%	AV and IV conduction disturbances, ventricular fibrillation
Ajmaline	2–8 h	10%	AV and IV conduction disturbances, ventricular fibrillation
Tricyclic antidepressants	3 days	2%	AV and IV conduction disturbances, ventricular fibrillation, sinus tachycardia, ventricular arrhythmias
Anti-cholinergic drugs	48 h	0	Sinus tachycardia
Quinidine	3 days	1%	As for chloroquine
Meprobamate	48 h	<1%	None (inotropic effect)
Beta blockers	48 h	0%	Sinus bradycardia, AV conduction disturbances

Table 48.5. Antidotes for the treatment of acute poisoning

Poison	Specific therapy
Opium alkaloids	Naloxone (Narcan)
Paracetamol	Cysteamine, N-acetylcysteine, Acetylcysteine
	Methionine
Cyanide	Dicobalt edetate (Kelocyanor)
	Hydroxycobolamine
Organophosphorous compounds	Pralidoxime + atropine
Heavy metals	
Iron	Desferrioxamine
Arsenic } Mercury }	Dimercaprol (BAL)
Copper } Lead }	{ Penicillamine
	{ Dimercaprol (BAL)
	{ Calcium disodium edetate (EDTA)
Methanol	4-Methyl pyrazole (not yet
Ethylene glycol	commercially available)
Methaemoglobinaemia	Methylene blue
Coumarine anticoagulants	Vitamin K
Anticholinergic drugs	Physostigmine

The circulatory failure is not due to any one single mechanism: and the respective roles of hypovalaemia vasodilation or myocardial insufficiency must be ascertained.

A hypothermic patient is nearly always hypotensive, and shock with oliguria is a constant feature, with body temperatures below 32°C. Both plasma expanders (risk of pulmonary oedema) and positive inotropic drugs (risk of arrhythmias) must be withheld until the central temperature reaches 32°C. Above this temperature, (especially with carbon monoxide and alcohol) the PaO_2–PvO_2 difference sometimes increases, indicating metabolic needs in excess of the reduced cardiac output.

It is important to recognize that in toxification with hypnotics, although the circulating blood volume may be diminished, these patients are seldom dehydrated and in fact, they frequently have an excess of tissue fluid. If plasma expansion restores the circulating blood volume, therefore, it is possible that during the period of recovery, the patient may develop circulatory overload with acute pulmonary oedema. Acute poisoning, therefore, is perhaps one of the few indications for the use of vasopressors in the treatment of shock [10]. The regimen recommended by Mathew and Lawson [10] is metaraminol 5 mg by deep IM injection, which may be repeated if necessary at 20-min intervals on two occasions. Only if this is ineffective should plasma expanders be given. The central venous pressure should be monitored in every case.

If the mechanism of shock is still unclear after an accurate clinical assessment a haemodynamic study will provide a better guide to therapy. In case this is not available, adrenergic drugs, of the dopamine or dobutamine types have often proved to be efficient, for tissue perfusion as well as for their positive inotropic effect.

Convulsions. Seizures are observed in three circumstances:

1) After *poisoning with convulsant drugs* (Table 48.6). some of which have specific forms of treatment, such as glucose after insulin, calcium after EDTA, and pyridoxine for isoniazid poisoning. In the non-specific cases, the benzodiazepines, together with assisted ventilation if necessary, are usually effective.

Table 48.6. Types of poisoning associated with convulsions (according to frequency)

Tricyclic antidepressants
Chloralose
Strychnine
Isoniazid
Amphetamines
Theophylline (child)
Malignant hyperthermia
Lithium
Hypocalcaemic drugs
Hypoglycaemic drugs
Bismuth (chronic)
Arsenic (acute)
Baryum (soluble salts)
Methyl bromide
Ethylene glycol
Pentetrazol
Picrotoxin

(2) After a severe hypoxic episode, which usually indicate a poor prognosis.

(3) Convulsions may be due to physical dependence on the drug, e.g., alcohol, barbiturates, or tranquilizers. This is not uncommon, and the physician must be aware of the phenomenon for an accurate diagnosis to be possible. Treatment with benzodiazepines is usually effective, the re-introduction of the causal psychotropic drug in diminishing doses may prevent recurrence (C. Bismuth, 1980, unpublished work).

General care

Hypothermia. Significant hypothermia exists when the rectal temperature is below 35°C. Hypothermia contributes to shock, acidaemia, and hypoxia, and therefore requires careful management. Occasionally, in severe hypothermia with a rectal temperature below 30°C, the body metabolism becomes very sluggish and further heat loss will result. Severe cardiac arrhythmias appear around 26°C and ventricular fibrillation might precede death. Hypotension is constant in hypothermia and should be respected: Plasma expanders and adrenergic drugs are not indicated and are dangerous. Several methods are available for active rewarming: warm bathing at 40°C; warmed blankets; heating the air for inspiration; immersion of the forearm in water at 43°C; and peritoneal dialysis.

In no case must hot water bottles ever be prescribed. Rewarming is considered efficient and safe if the body temperature rises by 1°C every hour.

Fluid and electrolyte balance. If the patient is unconscious for longer than 12 h, IV infusion of 2 litres of 10% dextrose with 1 g Na Cl and 2 g KCl/litre is usually all that is necessary. It is always helpful to have an IV infusion set up at an early stage, in case of cardiac arrest or arrhythmias.

Nursing care. It is generally agreed that the chances of recovery from a severe overdosage depend largely on the standard of nursing care. This involves frequent turning of the patient to prevent skin pressure sores, full passive movements of all limbs, and percussion of the chest. Nursing care is particularly important when the patient is starting to show positive features of recovery. During this stage MV may be withdrawn, endotracheal tubes may be removed, and some patients may develop withdrawal convulsions or become violent and abusive. All these stages require expert nursing care and vigilance for signs of relapse.

Provided there is meticulous care of the mouth and airway, together with frequent turning and physiotherapy, routine prophylactic antibiotics to prevent respiratory infection are not required. Antibiotic therapy should be reserved for situations where there are clear clinical or radiological signs of infection.

Elimination of poisons

Prevention of absorption

From the skin

In this pattern, often of industrial, contamination (insecticides, pesticides, alcohol, cyanide, phenols, oxalic and strong acids, strong alkalis, etc.) immediate and copious irrigation of the skin is the best way to prevent further absorption. The same procedure is advised for the eyes if they have been affected by caustic substances.

From the gastro-intestinal tract

Prevention of further gastric absorption [10]. Evacuation of the stomach can be achieved by inducing vomiting or performing gastric lavage. Neither of these objectives should be attempted in poisoning with paraffin, kerosene, or corrosives. Vomiting should only be provoked if the patient is conscious and lying on his side with the head dependent; children should be placed in the 'spanking' position. Various ways of producing vomiting have been suggested, and a quite effective one still is stimulation of the patient's pharynx by introduction of a finger or spoon handle. Various drugs, including apomorphine and syrup of ipecacuanha, have been recommended, especially for children. Apomorphine may cause protracted vomiting and shock and should be avoided. Syrup of ipecacuanha is advocated in a dosage of 15 ml followed by 200 ml water and is of value, especially for children, provided its limitations are understood. There is an average delay of about 18 min in the onset of its effect, and on occasion it may produce undesirable toxic effects after absorption. Finally, although effective vomiting may be produced, it is impossible to know whether the majority of the poison has been eliminated. Therefore, if the substance ingested is particularly dangerous, gastric lavage may still be required.

Gastric aspiration and lavage is not advisable outside hospital. The dangers associated with this procedure are inadequately recognized and its limitations not fully appreciated. Vomiting and inhalation of gastric content are frequent complications in inexperienced or careless hands, and therefore it is essential that the patient be placed in the semi-prone position with the head dependent. It should only be carried out if the patient has an adequate cough reflex or is sufficiently unconscious to permit protection of the airway with a cuffed endotracheal tube. This procedure is of great value in the majority of solid poisons if ingestion has occurred within 6 h of admission. Exceptions to this include poisoning with anticholinergic drugs, where a delay of 8 h is permissible, and perhaps in the deeply unconscious and severely ill patient who is already intubated and in whom gastro-intestinal activity may be markedly slowed. Normal saline should generally be used. Exceptions to this are shown in Table 48.7 [10]; if these additives are not readily available the procedure should not be delayed and water used. If the patient has been seen very shortly after ingestion of the poisoning, activated charcoal given PO may effectively reduce the severity of poisoning. This is particularly the case with acute aspirin overdosage but also with barbiturate, glutethimide, propoxyphene, ethchlorvynol, and kerosene. It also inactivates syrup of ipecacuanha and so the two should not be given together.

Gastric aspiration and lavage are too often incorrectly performed. The position of the patient is most important. It is essential that he or she be placed in the head-down position and turned on the left side for the whole of the procedure. Although technically simple, there is always the danger of aspiration, and suction apparatus must be immediately available at all times. An adequate size of tube, passed through the mouth, must be used. This should be of a sufficient bore to make it unlikely that it will enter the patient's trachea, and to permit removal of tablet material and semi-solid food particles.

Once the tube is securely in the stomach, aspiration is performed with a Dakin's syringe. Lavage is then carried out with 300-ml portions of saline (38°C) and continued until the recovered fluid is clear. This may often require large volumes of lavage fluid. In child-ren, appropriately smaller sizes of tubes and volumes of fluid should, of course, be used.
Induced diarrhoea. The use of magnesium sulphate or hyperosmolar solutions (mannitol) to provoke diarrhoea has been shown to be less effective in removal of poisons (C. Bismuth, 1980, unpublished work).
Interruption of the enterohepatic cycle. This can be achieved with cholestyramine and has been shown to reduce paracetamol absorption and shorten the half-life of digoxin in the blood.

Hepatic elimination

Most poisons are metabolized in the liver. The microsomal enzymatic induction produced by the chronic absorption of certain drugs (phenobarbitone, hydantoines, organochlorate compounds, alcohol) increases this degradation but these effects are not indicated in acute toxicology. Nonetheless, the importance of hepatic metabolism must be noted.

The contribution of metabolism to the removal of drug can be calculated from the lowering in plasma levels of the drug and its distribution space (given in pharmacological works of reference; that for meprobamate, for example, is 75% of body weight). The amount of drug removed by diuresis/dialysis must be excluded from the calculation.

Pulmonary elimination

Volatile substances are eliminated via the lungs.

Table 48.7. Occasions when the lavage fluid should be other than warm water and the various substances which should be left in the stomach on completion of lavage[a]

Poisoning	Lavage fluid	Substances left in stomach at end of lavage
Cyanide	25% Medium thiosulphate	200 ml of freshly made mixture of two solutions: (a) 6% sodium carbonate; (b) 15.8% ferrous sulphate in 3% citric acid
Iron	2 g desferrioxamine to 1 litre of warm water	5 g desferrioxamine in 50 ml water
Glutethimide (Doriden)	Equal quantities water an castor oil.	50 ml caster oil
Opiate	Dilute potassium permanganate. One solution tablet dissolved in 3½ litres of warm water	Nil. Make sure potassium permanganate has all been removed by lavage with warm water
Bleach (containing sodium hypochlorite)	2.5% sodium thiosulphate	50 ml milk of magnesia or 100 ml 2.5% sodium thiosulphate
Oxalic acid	1% calcium gluconate	100 ml 1% calcium gluconate.
Phenol, cresol, lysol	Mixture of 2 to 1 warm water and castor oil	50 ml castor oil
Phosphorus	0.1% copper sulphate in water	50 ml 0.1% copper sulphate in water
Paraquat		500 ml suspension containing 3 g Fuller's earth and 5 g magnesium sulphate (Poison Control Centers)

From Matthews and Lawson [10].
[a]Note that further urgent treatment should not be delayed while the substances recommended are being prepared.

The most frequently encountered of these are chlorinated solvents (trichlorethylene) and alcohol. Measurement of the quantities eliminated is possible only in specialized units.

Renal elimination

Principle of the method

The quantity of a drug excreted via the kidneys increases with weak protein or lipid binding; high plasma levels; large urinary outputs (enhanced with osmotic diuresis); solubility in water; and rising urinary pH in the case of poisonings with weak acids (slow-acting barbiturates, salicylates), where the ionized form of the drug is not reabsorbed through the tubule.

Lowering the urinary pH, whilst of theoretic value in cases of poisoning with weak bases such as tricyclic antidepressants, quinine, quinidine, ajmaline, nicotine, and chloroquine (often very severe) has no practical value, since degradation of these drugs takes place essentially in the liver.

Osmotic diuresis

The greater the amount of unchanged or pharmacologically active form of the drug excreted by the kidney, the greater will be the success of this method.

Osmotic diuresis is contra-indicated when the poison in its active form is known not to be excreted by the kidney; in cardiovascular failure; when renal function is impaired; when the poison produces pulmonary oedema; and when there are no facilities for monitoring plasma electrolyte levels.

Neutral osmotic diuresis as produced by a hypertonic solution of mannitol, and dextrose 10% with addition NaCl and KCl is no longer used for most of the drugs that it was proposed for (phenothiazines, meprobamate, benzodiazepines) which are metabolized predominantly in the liver or excreted by the kidney as inactive metabolites.

Alkaline osmotic diuresis is achieved with bicarbonate, mannitol and dextrose 10%, with a KCl supplement (2 g per litre) infused IV at a rate of 6 litres per day for women and 8 litres per day for men; it is indicated in cases of poisoning with slow-acting barbiturates or salicylates.

Saline diuresis is achieved with alternate administration of mannitol in 0.9% saline and of dextrose 10% with IV KCl supplement (1 g per litre); this procedure enhances elimination in poisoning with bromide and lithium.

Exchange transfusion

This procedure can be useful in the presence of haemolysis, particularly with methaemoglobinaemia (aniline, sodium and potassium chlorates) and for extraction of poisons that involve a high mortality, when their plasma distribution is maximal (phosphorus, methanol).

Dialysis

Peritoneal

The value of this procedure in a particular case demands a knowledge of the properties of the poison in question. This is somewhat difficult to acquire, for a number of reasons. The peritoneal surface is not an inert colloid membrane, but a cellular structure possessing specialized properties of selective transudation, so that there are several characteristics of the substances that influence their passage through this membrane. These include the molecular weight, the degree of ionization, and the extent and character of protein or lipid binding. The relative pH of the blood and of the dialysate, and the concentration gradient between the two will also influence the rate at which dialysis is possible. For example, in acute phenobarbitone poisoning a blood level of 150 mg/litre (650 μmol/litre) is not uncommonly found, and there is therefore a favourable gradient, whereas the toxic level of imipramine is in the region of 1 mg/litre (3.15 μmol/litre), providing a very poor and ineffective gradient.

The dialysate may be made hypertonic to increase the recovery of water-soluble poison, or the pH, albumin or lipid content may be altered to encourage a particular poison in the blood to enter the dialysate. For example, in acute phenobarbitone poisoning, if the dialysate is made alkaline and albumin is added the recovery of active drug may be considerably increased. A further virtue of peritoneal dialysis is that acid–base and electrolyte imbalance may also be corrected by appropriate adjustments in the constitution of the dialysing fluid.

The efficacy of peritoneal dialysis is less than that of haemodialysis but it can be extended over several days, and is about the same as forced diuresis, increasing the daily extraction of drugs by a factor of 2.

Haemodialysis

As with peritoneal dialysis it is an absolute requirement for the efficacy of this treatment that the poisons and any toxic metabolites (e.g., ethylene glycol, metabolite oxalic acid; methanol, metabolite formic acid) are dialysable. The procedure is more efficient than forced diuresis and peritoneal dialysis in the great majority of cases, but lasts only 6–12 h. It must be performed in units where appropriate facilities are available which often entails significant delays before the treatment can be initiated.

Haemoperfusion

Forced diuresis, peritoneal or haemodialysis, and exchange transfusion have marked limitations. In view of this, attempts have been made in recent years to develop alternative and safer methods of increasing elimination of toxic substances from the body after absorption has occurred.

Principle [10]. The capacity of charcoal to absorb toxins and drugs such as salicylate, barbiturates and glutethimide has been recognized for many years. Yatzidis was the first to describe the use of haemoperfusion (HP) over charcoal for the treatment of patients with severe barbiturate poisoning [17]. Severe complications were encountered with this treatment, including charcoal embolization with long-term cerebral and other effects, important electrolyte disturbances, marked thrombocytopenia and leucopenia, fibrinogen loss, and pyrexial reactions. These earlier methods were not considered suitable for general clinical use and in an effort to overcome these complications anion-exchange resins were used in place of charcoal; despite the development of an uncharged resin, Amber-

lite XAD-2, however, similar complications persisted.

Attempts were made to eliminate these problems by coating the charcoal with various substances, including cellulose acetate, collodion with and without albumin, nylon, glutaraldehyde-cross-linked albumin, and various hydrogels. In recent years a successful coating has been achieved with acrylic hydrogel. This has resulted in a marked reduction in the frequency and severity of harmful side-effects from charcoal HP, with a relatively small impairment in the rate of absorption but not the absorptive capacity of the charcoal.

In vitro, HP with coated charcoal has been tested for quite a range of common drugs with good results. In vivo, however, the results are much less clear-cut.

Method. A suitable HP circuit is shown in Fig. 48.2. The charcoal columns are now available commercially in packs and ready for use as Haemocol, Absorba-gambro, Haemodetoxifier, Reby, Hemopur, etc. This column contains 150–300 g 5–10 mesh coconut shell charcoal, which is coated with an acrylic hydrogel to a thickness ranging from 25 Å to 5μm. The charcoal is housed in a double conically shaped casing of polypropylene with 600-μm meshes at each end, which is sterilized by steam autoclaving.

The circuit is set up as shown, with specially manufactured and shortened haemodialysis lines to connect the arteriovenous shunt to the HP column. A roller pump is included in the arterial line to produce an upward flow through the column of about 200 ml/min. Two litres of

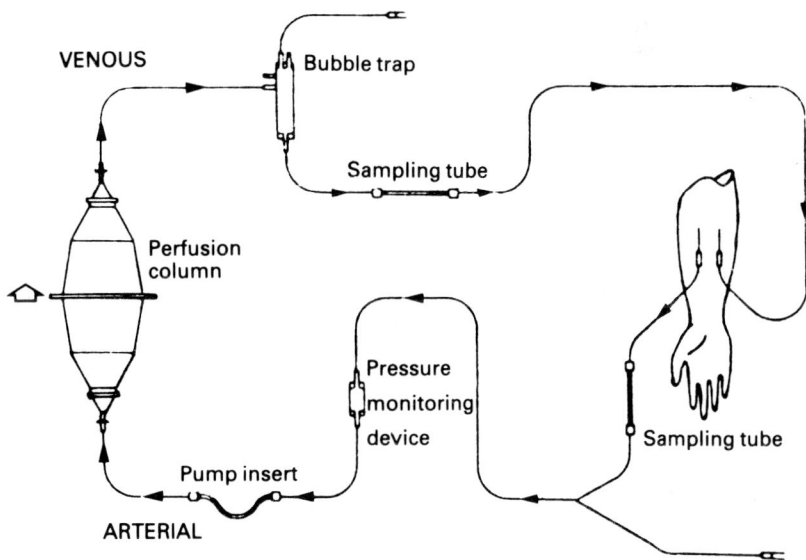

Fig. 48.2. Diagram of a haemoperfusion circuit. From Vale J, Rees AJ, Widdop B, Goulding R (1975) Br Med J i:5.

0.9% saline are run through the circuit before use, and the circuit is then left primed with saline containing heparin 1.0 unit/ml.

When HP is started, a bolus of 5000 units heparin is injected into the arterial line and heparinization is continued by administering an infusion of 0.9% saline containing 1000 units heparin per ml, at a rate to produce a plasma heparin concentration of 2.5–5.0 units per ml. A rate of infusion of one drop in 5 s is usually the maximum required, and this rate can be controlled by means of a roller pump. At the end of perfusion the blood in the circuit is returned to the patient by washing through 5.0% dextrose.

A monitor may be included in the circuit to alarm and stop the blood pump if the level in the bubble trap falls suddenly or if there is a sudden decrease of pressure in the arterial line fistula.

Results [9, 16]. There are two possible clinical situations in acute poisoning, in which HP might be valuable.

In cases of massive poisoning with sedative drugs (barbiturates, meprobamate, bromides, lithium) the mortality is nil with agressive supportive management. These drugs have a high extracellular distribution and the effectiveness of HP is therefore relatively good: between 7% and 20% of the ingested dose can be recovered. Whether these results can be judged satisfactory, life-saving, or insignificant is largely a matter of opinion.

Massive poisoning with cytoplasmic poisons (such as paraquat, amanita phalloides, acetaminophen) or cardiotropic drugs with high mortality (tricyclic compounds, anti-arrhythmic drugs) is a further indication; the use of HP in these cases is extremely attractive in view of the remarkably high clearance. Unfortunately, the extracellular distribution of these drugs is weak and the total excreted amount is low.

Finally anecdotal reports of good results of HP in the literature and the wider use of this costly method have given no critical assessment taking into account the pharmacokinetics of the drugs.

Immunotherapy

It may appear premature to describe a new method for the elimination of drugs for which there are still only strong experimental bases, and little clinical evaluation is available.

The major problem concerning the removal of drugs is to promote the movement of the intoxi-

cant from the intracellular into the extracellular space, however. Cellular accumulation explains the relative failure of dialysis. It appears, however, that this problem might be resolved by the injection of antitoxic antibodies. For example, in digitalis intoxication [14] antibodies of bovine origin are available, and in the future it may be possible to use monoclonal antibodies.

These antibodies increase the blood levels of the drugs to over ten times the initial levels, with secondary urinary elimination in 3 or 4 h. The overall effect is cellular depletion of the drug, as indicated by the quick clinical and biological recovery of patients.

References

1. Albert A (1973) Selective toxicity: The physico-chemical basis of therapy, 5th edn. Halstead, New York
2. Brown SS (1977) Clinical chemistry and chemical toxicology of metals. Elsevier, Amsterdam
3. Casarett LJ, Doull J (1975) Toxicology: The basic science of poisons. Macmillan, New York
4. Dukes MNG (1980) Meyler's side effects of drugs. Excerpta Medica, Amsterdam Oxford
5. Frejaville JP, Bismuth C, Conso F (1981) Toxicologie clinique et analytique, 2e éd. Flammarion, Paris
6. Gelehrter TD (1976) Enzyme induction. N Engl J Med 294:522–537; 589–595; 646–651
7. Gillette JR, Pang KS (1977) Theoretic aspects of pharmacokinetic drug interactions. Clin Pharmacol Ther 22:623–639
8. Goodman LS, Gilman A (1975) The pharmacological basis of therapeutics. Macmillan, New York
9. Kennedy RM, Courtney JM, Gaylor JDS, Gilchrist T (1977) Artificial organs. Macmillan, London
10. Matthew H, Lawson AAH (1979) Treatment of common acute poisonings, 4th edn Churchill Livingstone, Edinburgh
11. Mitchell FL, Young DS, Brown SS (1979) Chemical diagnosis of disease. Elsevier/North Holland, Amsterdam
12. Park J, Proudfoot AT (1977) Seven years review of coma patients admitted to the regional poisoning treatment centre, Royal Infirmary, Edinburgh. Acta Pharmacol Toxicol 41 [Suppl II]:516
13. Smith SE, Rawlins MD (1973) Variability in human drug response. Butterworths, London
14. Smith TW, Haber E, Heatman L, Bitler VP (1976) Reversal of digoxin intoxication with digoxin-specific antibodies. N Engl J Med 294:797–800
15. Vale SA (1977) The epidemiology of acute poisoning. Acta Pharmacol Toxicol 41 [Suppl II]:443–458
16. Winchester JF, Gelfand MC, Knepshield SH, Schreiner GE (1977) Dialysis and hemoperfusion of poisons and drugs—update. Trans Am Soc Artif Intern Organs 23:762–842
17. Yatzidis DA (1964) A convenient hemoperfusion microapparatus over charcoal for the treatment of endogenous and exogenous intoxications. Proc Eur Dial Transplant Assoc 1:83

Chapter 49

Management of Specific Poisonings

Chantal Bismuth

Psychotropic drugs

Barbiturates

Although they have no place in therapy except as anticonvulsants, barbiturates are still extensively prescribed and constitute the major cause of death in acute ingestant poisoning. Traditionally, the barbiturate drugs are divided into four classes and their main properties and hazards are shown in Table 49.1 [20].

Treatment. Aggressive supportive therapy is the basis of the management of acute barbiturate poisoning (see Chap. 48). Provided the regimen is applied with sufficient vigour and attention and analeptic drugs are avoided, at least 98% of patients will be treated successfully [18].

Of course the logical approach to the treatment of any poisoning is to try to remove it from the body and in recent years the use of different methods to increase the elimination of these drugs have been advocated (Table 49.2).

Assessment of the benefits of such methods entails balancing the benefits of a rapid return to normal homeostasis against complications of the treatment; for example high renal clearances of phenobarbitone obtained with lactate (1 *M* solution) and urea (5 *M* solution) diuresis were accompanied by a high mortality rate due to hyperosmolar states, and this method was therefore discontinued. In addition, slow-acting barbiturates, where a benefit can be expected from this method, must be differentiated from the other barbiturates which are degraded in the liver, where no benefit can be expected. An exception should be made for haemoperfusion (with coated charcoal or uncharged resin), which has proved to be more effective for medium- and short-acting barbiturates. Only cases of massive intoxication should be selected for the special methods of removal: it is inappropriate to introduce another possible hazard to a patient who could recover with simpler and less aggressive methods of treatment (assisted ventilation and alkaline osmotic diuresis—see Chap. 48). It is essential to bear in mind the possibility of multiple-agent poisoning; this will interfere with the barbiturate poisoning but the frequency is generally underestimated. The complications, such as respiratory or circulatory problems, must not be considered as additional indications for drastic methods of elimination, but as indications for immediate clinical surveillance.

Tranquillizers

Carbamates

Meprobamate is quickly absorbed and fairly rapidly metabolized, much more quickly than

Table 49.1. Classification of the barbiturates

	Duration of therapeutic effect	Official name	Metabolism	Intoxication	Risks	Plasma levels[a] causing deep coma when present alone
Long-acting	12–24 h 12–24 h	Barbitone Phenobarbitone	Renal excretion	Long-lasting coma	Atelectasis, respiratory depression, inhalation, hypothermia, cutaneous blisters, rhabdomyolysis	>200 (>862) Epileptic: >180 (>776) Non-epileptic: >100–120 (>431–517)
Medium-acting	8–10 h	Butobarbitone Allobarbitone Amylobarbitone	Renal excretion + hepatic degradation			>80 (>345)
Short-acting	6–8 h 4–6 h 4–6 h	Pentobarbitone Cyclobarbitone Quinalbarbitone	Hepatic degradation	Short-lasting coma	Apnoea, negative inotropic effect, vasodilatation	>25 (>108)
Anaes-thetics (ultra-short-acting)	3–4 h 1 h 1/4 h	Hexobarbitone Thiopentone Methohexitone	Hepatic degradation			?

[a]Plasma levels are given first as mg/litre, followed by μmol/litre in parentheses.

Table 49.2. Various rates of renal and other clearances in phenobarbitone poisoning

Spontaneous	1 ml/min
Saline diuresis	2.5 ml/min
Mannitol diuresis	4 ml/min
Alkaline diuresis	4 ml/min
Alkaline osmotic diuresis	6 ml/min
Peritoneal dialysis	7 ml/min
Prusemide	8 ml/min
Lactate + urea diuresis	17 ml/min
Haemodialysis	27–50 ml/min
Haemoperfusion	50–80 ml/min

either barbiturates or glutethimide. Even after a large overdosage, most of the drug will have been excreted or inactivated within 48 h.

Deep coma is to be anticipated, if the plasma level is over 100 mg/litre (458.7 μmol/litre) and levels of 200 mg/litre (917.4 μmol/litre) can cause cardiac failure. Consciousness may be retained with plasma levels of up to 120 mg/litre (550.4 μmol/litre). The plasma levels of hexapropymate are some ten times lower than plasma levels of meprobamate with equivalent clinical states.

Clinical features. The degree of coma is variable; muscle weakness and incoordination, respiratory depression, hypotension, cardiogenic shock, and hypothermia are signs of poisoning. Drug dependence may exist after prolonged treatment with meprobamate. Withdrawal features, such as convulsions, may therefore be observed.

Treatment. Intensive supportive therapy is usually all that is required. In cases with cardifferent methods of elimination. It must be remembered in this evaluation that diuresis, peritoneal dialysis, and hepatic metabolisms are effective throughout the day, whilst other [17], dopamine and dobutamine have all proved successful.

The hepatic pathway of metabolism is predominant in removal of the drug. Tables 49.3 and 49.4 show the comparative effects of the different methods of elimination. It must be remembered in this evaluation that diuresis, peritoneal dialysis, and hepatic metabolism are effective throughout the day, whilst other methods of dialysis are discontinuous.

Benzodiazepines [5, 20]

These compounds are frequently used as mild tranquillizers and night sedatives. They are also commonly prescribed with antidepressant drugs for the management of certain depressive illnesses, and so, they are often available to a group of the population who are prone to take an overdosage of drugs; not surprisingly, therefore acute overdosage is common.

Table 49.3. Some different routes of excretion in meprobamate removal following ingestion of 45 g

Meprobamate	Diuresis	Haemoperfusion	Hepatic metabolism
mg/h	177 ± 23.4	672 ± 167	482 (Plasma disappearance rate: 5.2%/h)
% of excretion/h	14	50	36
% of ingested drug/h	0.4	1.5	> 1
Removal (mg/day)	4250	3350	11560
Removal %/day[a]	22	18	60

[a]Derived value obtained by using 75% of body weight as the distribution space for the drug and by excluding the contribution of diuresis and haemoperfusion. Adapted from Maddock RK, Bloomer HA (1967) JAMA 201:999.

Table 49.4. Meprobamate intoxication (30 g): Effects of different methods of elimination

Meprobamate	Diuresis	Peritoneal dialysis	Hepatic metabolism[a]
mg/h	110	68	330
% of ingested dose/h	0.36	0.22	1.1%
Removal: mg/day	2640	1630	7920
% of ingested dose/day	8.6	5.3	26.4
Removal: %/day	21.5	13.5	65

[a]From Maddock RK, Bloomer HA (1967) Jama 201:999–1003
(meprobamate mg/litre ÷ 0.218 = μmol/litre)

Absorption of benzodiazepines from the gastrointestinal tract tends to be rather slow; several hours elapse before peak blood levels are reached after oral administration. Plasma levels then fall slowly and the excretion of the drug in the urine may continue for several days. Less than 5 per cent of the ingested dose is recovered in the urine as unaltered drug.

Clinical features. The effects are surprisingly mild and there is no authenticated report of death from these drugs. As many as 100 tablets of nitrazepam may be taken with remarkably little effect.

There is drowsiness, with possible coma in very rare instances. Dizziness, ataxia, and slurred speech may be present. Hypotension is rare and respiratory depression occurs infrequently and is not severe. Withdrawal features such as mental confusion and convulsions may be observed after prolonged treatment.

Treatment. Intensive supportive therapy is all that is required. Osmotic diuresis, peritoneal dialysis, and haemodialysis are ineffective. Charcoal HP has been reported to increase the elimination of absorbed benzodiazepines but is never indicated, as the patient is seldom more than drowsy unless other drugs have also been taken.

Antidepressant drugs

Monoamine oxidase inhibitors [10, 20]

These drugs are now infrequently used for the treatment of depressive illness and are therefore an uncommon cause of acute poisoning. Patients may present with the toxic effects of these drugs either because of acute overdosage per se, or because of interactions that may occur when the drugs are given in therapeutic dosage but in association with certain other drugs or with particular items of diet.

Cerebral excitation, which may be followed by coma and severe hyperthermia, occurs when monoamine oxidase (MAO) inhibitors are combined with morphine or other opium alkaloids, anaesthetics and antihistamines, imipramine and its congeners, antiparkinsonian drugs, and reserpine or methyldopa. The action of guanethidine may be antagonized, whilst when they are taken with other hypotensive agents, such as phenothiazines and thiazide diuretics, the hypotensive effects may be enhanced. The association of MAO inhibitors with sympathomimetic drugs such as amphetamine, ephedrine, noradrenaline, and adrenaline evokes adverse reactions including hypertensive crises.

There is also a well-recognized association of toxicity of MAO inhibitors with eating certain cheeses, especially Cheddar and Camembert; broad beans have also been implicated. This is particularly true for patients treated with tranylcypromine. The substance in the cheeses that has been implicated as the provocative factor is tyramine. Monoamine oxidase inhibitors also appear to prolong and potentiate the action of anaesthetics, opiates, barbiturates, alcohol, and insulin. These many possibilities result in severe upset to the patient and although there may not have been an actual overdosage the condition can legitimately be regarded as acute poisoning.

Monoamine oxidase inhibitors are readily absorbed from the gastro-intestinal tract and rapidly excreted as the acid metabolite, but their effects are prolonged due to irreversible inhibition of the enzyme. Enzyme function takes weeks to return to normal. Hydrazine MAO inhibitors must first undergo cleavage before the drug becomes active. Non-hydrazine MAO inhibitors can combine directly with the enzyme.

Clinical features. Drug and food interaction can cause headache; fever; hypertensive crisis with possible intracranial haemorrhage or hypotension; cerebral excitation and convulsions; loss of consciousness; and cardiac arrhythmias.

Acute overdosage of MAO inhibitors usually causes coma with hypotension due to vasodilatation. Convulsions and hyperthermia are rare, but the latter may be associated with rhabdomyolysis (C. Bismuth, 1980, unpublished work).

Treatment. The basic principles of intensive supportive therapy should be followed, but a number of important precautions must be observed:

1) Metaraminol and other sympathomimetic agents must not be given for the treatment of hypotension. Plasma expanders should be given by IV infusion.

2) Chlorpromazine is the drug of choice for cerebral excitement, but if convulsions occur diazepam should be given IM or IV.

3) Hypertensive crises should be treated by administering a short-acting hypotensive agent such as pentolinium (0.25 mg IM) or phentolamine 5 mg IV followed by phenoxybenzamine 100 mg in 200 ml 5% dextrose IV over 90 min.

4) Hyperthermia may be corrected by cooling with a damp sheet and a fan, but if severe, Dantrolene 25–400 mg/day is highly effective.

5) Forced diuresis and peritoneal dialysis are probably ineffective but haemodialysis can be considered for very severely poisoned patients.

Tricyclic compounds [9, 10, 20]

Acute poisoning with these drugs is common and the incidence is increasing. It now accounts for 9% of all deaths from toxic solids and liquids and therefore presents a major challenge. This is particularly so since no specific treatment has yet been found. Inevitably they are prescribed for patients who are most likely to indulge in self-poisoning or to attempt suicide, and the risk of overdosage is high, especially during the latent period of 14 days or so before many of the tricyclics become effective. Tricyclic compounds are prescribed frequently for the treatment of enuresis in children and many of the preparations are dispensed as pleasantly flavoured syrups which are attractive to youngsters, and as a result overdosage is common.

Tricyclic compounds are absorbed rapidly and quickly become firmly bound to proteins and enter the tissues, so that blood levels are always relatively low. Efficient detoxification occurs in the liver, and very little active drug appears in the urine. Elimination occurs rapidly and 24 h after ingestion scarcely any of the parent drug remains in the tissues. The therapeutic blood level is near 0.1 mg/litre and the toxic blood level is around 1 mg/litre (mg imipramine/litre $\div$ 0.317 = μmol/litre; μg amitriptyline/litre $\div$ 277 = μmol/litre).

Clinical features. Anticholinergic effects produced are dryness of the mouth, dilated pupils, urinary retention, absent bowel sounds, and atrial tachycardia.

Neurological effects are also seen. A state of hyper-reflexibility with an extensor plantar response progresses to tonic–clonic convulsions amounting to status epilepticus; ataxia may be pronounced in children.

Hallucinations, usually visual, are common and persist for some days after the other features have disappeared. Rapid speech is characteristic. There may be some impairment of consciousness and respiratory depression, but deep coma is rare.

Cardiac effects of tricyclic overdosage are atrioventricular block, bundle branch block, and intraventricular conduction disturbances.

These features appear 1–2 h after taking the overdose and seldom last longer than 18–24 h, but sudden deaths have been reported up to 6 days after the ingestion of the tricyclic drug and have been presumed to be due to sudden arrhythmias.

Treatment. Gastric aspiration and lavage is of value if performed within 12 h of ingestion. In the case of imipramine derivatives (but not of amitriptyline derivatives), potassium bichromate added to the gastric lavage solution turns from green to violet as long as the lavage is productive [9]. Supportive therapy is all that is necessary in the vast majority of patients. Even marked sinus tachycardia may be beneficial by virtue of its over-drive pacing effect. Forced diuresis, peritoneal dialysis, charcoal HP, haemodialysis are ineffective in view of the firm tissue binding of these drugs and the very low blood levels.

Physostigmine has been widely advocated, but it is in fact not indicated in the acute stage of the intoxication; indeed it might be dangerous, promoting epilepsy and cardiac disturbances (bradycardia and cardiac failure) [26]. Its administration can be useful when anticholinergic activity with mental confusion persists for several days after the initial cardiac risks: physostigmine or eserine 1 mg can then dramatically reverse the anticholinergic encephalopathy.

To control convulsions, diazepam (Valium) 10 mg IV is the treatment of choice. If diazepam is ineffective, sodium phenobarbitone 200 mg IM should be given. The treatment of cardiac disturbances should be prompt. Anticholinesterase agents are only effective for anticholinergic tachycardia. Hypotension with low central venous pressure is best treated with plasma expanders. Bundle-branch block might respond to molar sodium lactate infusions (400 ml with KCl added). In certain cases it is only of value if the patient has a metabolic acidosis, but in our experience it has a specific effect upon intracardiac conduction disturbances [9, 10]. Shock associated with major cardiac disturbances, might respond to inotropic drugs. Extracorporeal circulation has been proposed for desperate cases.

Lithium [20, 25, 27]

Lithium salts are now increasingly used in the treatment of manic depression, and overdosage is therefore always a potential risk.

Lithium is a monovalent cation and together with sodium and potassium, belongs to the group of alkali metals. It is readily absorbed from the gut and is not bound to plasma proteins. It passes readily from the blood into the tissues and rapidly equilibrates, but there may be considerable accumulation in liver, muscle, brain, and kidney in competition with sodium ions. The features of toxicity are particularly likely to occur in patients who are being treated with lithium and who are then given a regimen that can promote salt depletion, such as dietary salt restriction and diuretics. Also, during pregnancy the renal clearance of lithium increases markedly and plasma levels of the drug may fall, but after delivery the reverse happens rapidly and the blood levels may reach toxic values without any change in the dosage.

Therapeutic blood levels are around 1 mmol/litre, and toxic symptoms are likely to appear with levels above 2 mmol/litre.

Clinical features. Just above the therapeutic level polyuria, thirst, vomiting and diarrhoea occur and even at relatively low doses, patients can show gross agitation and violent behaviour, sometimes very marked. After large doses, coma is observed, but without respiratory depression. Hypertonia, involuntary movements, and long-lasting convulsions are rare.

Treatment. Intensive supportive therapy is necessary. Saline diuresis can be started, but in view of associated changes in sodium and potassium balance, close monitoring of plasma electrolytes is mandatory. Approximately 12% of patients taking lithium develop a syndrome reminiscent of diabetes insipidus due to failure of the kidney to respond to antidiuretic hormone. The resulting hyperosmolarity of the plasma will be worsened by an additional sodium load. In such circumstances treatment with chlorothiazide may be valuable. If hypertonicity occurs convulsions can be anticipated and diazepam should be given IM. Pentothal may be required to control established convulsions.

Peritoneal dialysis and haemodialysis are likely to be effective, but may have to be repeated as lithium is withdrawn from tissue stores, but in our experience, which is supported by laboratory data, saline diuresis is as effective as the more sophisticated methods of removal. When a state of hyperosmolality exists, however, haemodialysis is to be preferred in the more seriously ill patients.

Neuroleptic drugs

Phenothiazines [9, 20]

The most effective tranquillizers are in this group, and they tend to be the drugs most frequently prescribed for the treatment of psychoses.

The phenothiazines are well absorbed from the gastro-intestinal tract and from parenteral sites. About 70% of an administered dose is rapidly taken up by the liver and there is a very active enterohepatic circulation. The biological half-life of the phenothiazines is very long, and various metabolites, or even free drug, may be detected in the urine 6–12 months after treatment has been stopped. Approximately half the metabolites of the phenothiazines are found in the urine and the remainder in the faeces. Even in severe overdosage the blood levels of these drugs are very low and are measured in micrograms per 100 millilitres.

Clinical features. Loss of consciousness, Parkinsonism with muscle rigidity, tremor, and increased limb reflexes, dyskinesia, including torticollis, facial grimacing, abnormal eye movements, possibly with oculogyric crises, and akathisia, with marked restlessness may all occur. These extrapyramidal effects are particularly marked in young children and can last a long time.

Hypotension, may be severe and is due to a combination of myocardial depression, vasodilatation resulting from inhibition of centrally mediated pressor reflexes, and peripheral and ganglionic adrenergic blockade.

Tachycardia is usually secondary to the hypotension. Various arrhythmias may develop, which are sometimes resistant to the usual methods of treatment; cardiac arrest may occur. The common ECG changes are prolongation of the Q-T interval and blunting of the T waves. Except in the most severe overdosage, respiratory depression is uncommon. Hypothermia is usual and may be severe, but on occasions, the patient may be slightly hyperthermic with phenothiazines; in exceptional cases, 'malignant' hyperthermia may develop with rhabdomyolysis.

Treatment. Intensive supportive therapy is the basis of treatment. Methods of treatment designed to increase the removal of these drugs, such as haemodialysis, are ineffective. Dyskinesia should be treated by repeated injections of benzhexol hydrochloride or erybenzatropine. Malignant hyperthermia must be treated (Dantrolene, 25–400 mg/day).

Since phenothiazines are adrenergic blocking agents, they provide some protection against the deleterious effects of circulatory shock. In particular, in addition to having a direct diuretic action there is evidence that they prevent the fall of renal blood flow even when the systemic blood pressure is low. For these reasons strenuous efforts to elevate the blood pressure are not necessary, provided the patient has an adequate urine volume.

Attempts should be made to treat cardiac arrhythmias with the appropriate drug, and if there is accompanying severe hypotension this should be corrected, with plasma expanders, as this facilitates the correction of arrhythmias.

Butyrophenones [9]

These are practically never the sole intoxicant. Overdosage is marked by extrapyramidal syndromes, often hyperkinetic, with neuromuscular reactions: motor restlessness, dystonia, akathisia, opisthotonos, oculogyric crisis, rhythmical involuntary movements of tongue, jaw, or mouth (protrusion of the tongue, puffing of cheeks, puckering of the mouth, chewing movements, torticollis).

Such manifestations of overdosage must not be misinterpreted as hysteria. In our experience, they generally respond to repeated IM administration of ethybenzatropine. A malignant neuroleptic syndrome is possible, and responds to Dantrolene.

Non-barbiturate hypnotics

Bromides

The bromide salts are steadily losing favour in therapeutics, but their presence in sedative mixtures occasionally results in their being taken in overdosage. The fatal dose is probably only a few grams, but death very seldom occurs because the drug almost always causes vomiting.
Clinical features. Nausea and vomiting, depression of respiration, and muscular weakness and paralysis are all clinical features; impaired consciousness develops with a plasma level of above 600 mg/litre.
Treatment.
1) Gastric aspiration and lavage.
2) Intensive supportive therapy.
3) Intravenous infusion of alternating 500 ml normal saline and 1000 ml 5% dextrose at a rate of 1000 ml every 3 h until the blood bromide level is below 60 mg per 100 ml. To each 500 ml of the infusion regimen 0.5 g KCl (13 mmol/litre) should be added. Close biochemical monitoring is essential.
4) Intravenous frusemide 80 mg, repeated in 4 h. Regimens with added diuretics such as frusemide or ethacrynic acid and mannitol have been found to be successful, but biochemical control is even more important and the patients must be fully hydrated at the start of treatment.
5) In patients with cardiac or renal failure, haemodialysis is effective.

Methaqualone

This quinazolone compound has been extensively used in Europe for a number of years. It is available compounded with diphenhydramine as Mandrax; addiction and misuse are common. In France, because of these addictive effects, its prescription is now in accordance with 'Tableau B', legislation that has considerably decreased its consumption. The antihistamine component does not appear to contribute significantly to its toxicity.

Methaqualone is readily absorbed after oral administration, and the hypnotic effect is manifest within 30 min. Only 2% of unaltered drug is excreted in the urine.
Clinical features [9, 20]. Depression of consciousness may be severe, with hypertonia, increased limb reflexes, and myoclonia. Extensor plantar responses and papilloedema may be found and convulsions may occur. Dilated pupils are frequent. There is a danger of inhalation pneumonia. Severe respiratory depression is rare. Tachycardia is common, and in severe cases acute myocardial damage may result even in patients without previously known coronary vascular disease. Potentially dangerous intoxication is indicated by blood levels of methaqualone greater than 30 mg/litre in patients who do not have tolerance to the drug. The pyramidal signs described are striking and offer a useful indication of this particular type of overdosage. Such signs do occur in other poisonings as for example, by tricyclic compounds, but methaqualone intoxication should always be thought of when these features are present.
Treatment. Intensive supportive therapy has proved satisfactory [21]. Osmotic diuresis is not effective, since only 2% of the active drug is excreted in the urine. Even haemodialysis is ineffective except in severely ill patients whose methaqualone blood level is greater than 100 mg per litre. More recently charcoal HP has been reported to remove significant quantities of methaqualone.

Glutethimide [5, 20]

Glutethimide is poorly soluble in water but much more soluble in alcohol. The ingestion of alcohol together with the tablets therefore greatly facilitates absorption from the stomach. Since the preparation is also readily soluble in fat, it is rapidly stored in tissues and then only slowly released into the bloodstream. It is metabolized in the liver and a hydroxy metabolite reaches high plasma levels as glutethimide levels fall. This metabolite has been shown to be at least as toxic to mice as the parent drug, which probably explains why plasma levels of glutethimide do not correlate with the clinical course. Fluctuation of the level of consciousness so often seen in glutethimide poisoning might also be attributable to the production of a toxic metabolite.

Clinical features. The general features of overdosage are similar to those of barbiturate poisoning but certain differences require emphasis: The depth of coma may vary considerably, with periods of partial arousal. This fluctuation occurs in overdosage with several hypnotic drugs, but is most marked in glutethimide poisoning. The exact cause is uncertain but factors to be considered include the production of a toxic metabolite, the erratic absorption from the intestine as shock improves, the release from tissue stores, and the significant anticholinergic action of the drug.

Episodes of sudden apnoea may occur, which are probably due to an acute rise in ICP since papilloedema is often present at the time. The pupils tend to be dilated and unresponsive to light.

Hypotension may be severe and disproportionate to the degree of unconsciousness and myocardial damage due to a direct toxic effect of the drug may also be present. Severe and persistent metabolic acidosis may occur.

A plasma level of 30 mg/litre (4.6 μmol/litre) or more is associated with severe poisoning unless the patient is tolerant to the drug.

Treatment. Intensive supportive therapy is necessary. If gastric aspiration and lavage are undertaken the lavage fluid should consist of a mixture of equal quantities of castor oil and water shaken together; 50 ml castor oil should be left in the stomach on completion of lavage.

Sudden episodes of apnoea can be prevented (or if present, treated) by giving 500 ml 10% dextrose over the next 4 h. This should be given when there is any suspicion of raised ICP.

Although commonly advocated for the treatment of poisoning with this agent, haemodialysis is relatively ineffective even in serious overdoses, as the recovery of active drug will not exceed more than one or two tablets. There is evidence, however, that the addition of soya bean oil to the dialysis fluid will augment the amount of drug recovered, but even then the amount is probably not significant. It is important that the dialysis should be continued for at least 2 h after the patient regains consciousness, otherwise there may be a relapse into deep coma with subsequent release of drug from fat depots.

Forced diuresis and peritoneal dialysis are not effective and the place of charcoal HP is debatable in patients who do not respond adequately to intensive supportive therapy.

Cardiotropic drugs

Digitalis

Digoxin (characteristics shown in Table 49.5) represents 80% of the prescriptions for digitalis in Anglo-Saxon countries, while digitoxin (Table 49.5) represents 80% of prescriptions of digitalis in Latin countries. Therapeutic overdoses must be considered quite separately from acute poisoning, since their prognosis is nearly always benign following reduction of the dose. The problems in suicidal overdosage are quite different. For digoxin, μg drug/litre ÷ 0.781 = nmol/litre; while μg digitoxin/litre ÷ 0.765 = nmol/litre.

Prognosis. The average mortality of digitalis poisoning is about 18% following doses of above 15 mg, and reaches 95% following ingestion of quantities of over 35 mg. Mortality is 10% in patients between 20 and 25 years and 40% in those over 60 years.

The patient's cardiac state: long-standing cardiac failure, coronary disease, valvular disease, or even isolated cardiomegaly constitute high risks.

The rise in the plasma potassium level in the first 24 h for digoxin, and in the first 48 h for

Table 49.5. Metabolic differences between the two glycosides

	Digitoxin	Digoxin
Gastro-intestinal absorption	90%–100%	60%–85%
Enterohepatic cycle	+++	0
Protein binding	+++	0
Peak effect	4–12 h	1–5 h
Plasma half-life	5–7 day	36 h
Excretory pathway	Hepatic	Renal
Plasma concentration (radioimmunology)		
Therapeutic concentration (μg/litre)	15–35	1–2
Toxic concentration (μg/litre)	> 40	> 2.5
Lethal concentration (μg/litre)	> 100	> 10

digitoxin, due to inhibition of the membrane ATPase pump by digitalis is strongly correlated with the clinical course, as is shown in Table 49.6 [2]. A single ECG recording is misleading as severe deterioration in the cardiac state or rhythm may occur very suddenly.

Clinical features. Nausea and vomiting are constant features; diarrhoea also occurs, though less frequently. Drowsiness, mental confusion and even psychosis have been observed, and functional renal failure is frequent.

ECG signs merits continuous ECG monitoring: four types of abnormality are described and are often associated. Sinus bradycardia with sagging of the ST segment and T wave inversion can be considered as signs of digitalis ingestion but not of toxicity. There may be varying degrees of atrioventricular block, leading in severe cases to cardiac arrest.

Ectopic beats, particularly ventricular, are common, but atrial flutter, coupled rhythm, ventricular tachycardia, and ventricular fibrillation can occur. Features of cardiogenic shock have been observed in the absence of major arrhythmias and in subjects with a healthy myocardium; its pathogenesis is still debatable but the negative inotropic action of high doses of digitalis is probably the cause.

Treatment [9]. Intensive supportive therapy is necessary. Gastric aspiration and lavage, if indicated, should be undertaken with care as any further increase in vagal tone may predispose to cardiac arrest.

Bradycardia should be treated with atropine sulphate, 0.5 mg IV, repeated as necessary, often for as long as 4 days. Hyperkalaemia does not respond to IV glucose and insulin; IV aldosterone antagonists are probably more efficient as their intracellular potassium penetration persists even when the membrane ATPase is inhibited.

Table 49.6. Serum potassium concentration in 68 patients with acute digitoxin intoxication

Serum potassium concentration, mmol/litre	No. of patients	No. of deaths
< 5.00	41	0
5.00–5.50	10	2
5.50–7.40	7	4
> 7.40	10	10
	68	16

Personal unpublished data. (Patients who received diuretics or potassium infusions and those who had metabolic acidosis or circulatory failure were excluded from this study.)

Hypokalaemia may be present in severely poisoned patients who have previously received diuretic therapy. In such cases intracellular potassium depletion is even more pronounced. It should be treated by cautious IV infusion of 30 mmol potassium chloride in 200 ml 5% dextrose. This should be continued until either the ECG or the plasma potassium level is normal.

Demand cardiac pacing is highly desirable in the light of the possibility of atrioventricular block. Lignocaine 100 mg IV as a bolus followed by infusion of lignocaine (500 mg in 500 ml) is the most effective treatment for ventricular ectopic beats (VEBs) and ventricular tachycardia. In spite of several claims, digoxin cannot be removed via dialysis or HP: plasma concentration–time curves with and without HP are indistinguishable.

Reports concerning digitoxin removal are rare, but in our own experience, coated charcoal HP does not remove a significant amount of drug. The results of amberlite HP appear more encouraging. The administration of digoxin-specific antibodies dramatically reverses toxification with digitoxin and with digoxin [28] (Chap. 48, section: *Immunotherapy*).

Anti-arrhythmic drugs

Quinine, quinidine and chloroquine

Quinine and quinidine [9, 20] are chemically optical isomers. Quinine has been used mainly as an antimalarial; it is also a constituent of many so-called tonics and is often prescribed to prevent night cramps. It also has an ill-deserved reputation as an abortifacient and may be taken in deliberate overdosage to produce what is thought will be a really effective abortion. Quinidine, which is a potent cardiac depressant, is used in the treatment of cardiac arrhythmias. Both substances are taken occasionally in episodes of self-poisoning and may also be accidentally swallowed by children.

Chloroquine (amino-quinoleine) will be studied with these two drugs: it has as marked an antimalarial activity as quinine and anti-arrhythmic properties comparable to those of quinidine.

Clinical features. Absorption is rapid but fortunately is lessened by the almost inevitable vomiting which these drugs cause. Both drugs may cause cinchonism; 'singing' in the ears, deafness, blurred vision, headache and dizziness soon occur. Collapse with impairment of consciousness, shallow, rapid breathing, and fast pulse with low blood pressure may follow. Cardiac arrhythmias and arrest may occur. ECG changes include prolongation of the QT interval, widening of the QRS complex, and flattening of the T waves.

Blurring of vision, dilated pupils or annular scotoma, and deafness may persist for several days whilst, in rare instances, blindness may be permanent. Fundal examination may reveal marked constriction of the retinal vessels, the appearances resembling those of occlusion of the central retinal artery. Debate continues as to the mechanism of the visual loss. It is thought to be due either to a direct toxic effect on the ganglion cells of the retina or to quinine-induced vasoconstriction and consequent retinal damage. The rapid response to stellate ganglion block mentioned below strongly supports the latter view.

Acute intravascular haemolysis may occur, the first warning of which may be a reduced urine output.

Treatment. Intensive supportive therapy is needed and careful observation of the heart rate and rhythm is essential. The major cardiac hazards for chloroquine occur as early as 1 h after absorption: cardiac arrest or ventricular fibrillation have been observed during gastric lavage and this procedure should always be preceded by ECG monitoring. The acute risks do not last longer than 24 h.

If widening of the QRS complex is severe, infusion of molar sodium lactate solution (with KCl) may be effective.

If the negative inotropic action is predominant, a positive inotropic agent such as dopamine or dobutamine must be given. If ventricular fibrillation occurs external cardiac massage and electrical defibrillation are necessary. Stellate ganglion block may produce dramatic relief of the visual impairment. The degree of visual improvement is in inverse proportion to the duration of the blindness. Unfortunately this measure is not always effective but should be tried when there is severe impairment of vision.

Acute haemolysis requires treatment with hydrocortisone IV together with the treatment of any degree of associated acute renal failure. Because both quinine and quinidine are largely protein-bound, peritoneal dialysis and haemodialysis are not likely to recover a significant amount of the drugs. Quinine and its congeners are largely metabolized in the liver so that less than 5% of an administered dose appears unaltered in the urine.

Other anti-arrhythmic drugs

There are various other anti-arrhythmic drugs in use, e.g., ajmaline, aprindine, disopyramide, lignocaine, mexilitine, and phenytoin, the most dangerous of these is undoubtedly ajmaline; this powerful anti-arrhythmic drug is often prescribed to anxious subjects for the treatment of tachycardia or palpitations. Consequently it is widely available in people's homes in certain countries, and the overall mortality (misuse for children, suicide for adults) reaches some 20%. A ban on its prescription for emotional cardiac disturbances would therefore practically abolish this very high mortality.

In acute intoxication all the anti-arrhythmic drugs mentioned have the same cardiac effects, namely: sinus bradycardia, atrioventricular block, prolongation of the QT interval, widening of the QRS complex, and depression of myocardial contractility. The treatment is the same as that proposed for quinidine.

Beta-adrenergic blocking agents [9, 20]

These drugs are now commonly prescribed for a wide variety of conditions including hypertension, angina pectoris, thyrotoxicosis, cardiac arrhythmias, anxiety, and migraine. Their availability for self-poisoning is therefore very substantial and overdosage by drugs of this type is relatively common.

They reduce cardiac output by inhibiting sympathetic drive to the heart and increase airways resistance by blocking sympathetically induced bronchodilatation. Tremor is reduced by the inhibition of beta receptor activity in skeletal muscle. These drugs also vary pharmacologically insofar as some have intrinsic sympathomimetic activity in varying degrees, whereas others have a membrane-stabilizing (quinidine-like) action with or without intrinsic sympathomimetic effects.

Clinical features. The patient may complain of marked lassitude and be drowsy but any greater impairment of consciousness should suggest overdosage with an additional sedative or hypnotic. Hallucinations and nightmares are rare.

Bradycardia may be severe, with hypotension and cardiac failure; peripheral vasospasm with Raynaud's phenomenon is sometimes found.

Bronchospasm may also be severe and can occur in previously healthy patients, although it is particularly likely when the patient has had previous asthma or bronchitis. Respiratory depression may result from severe circulatory impairment or from the central effects of the drug.

Erythematous and psoriasiform rashes sometimes occur. There is in fact a wide individual variation in response to beta blockers. Some patients may show little or no ill effect after taking large doses, whereas others may be seriously ill after small doses. In spite of their many risks, mortality attributable to these drugs is practically zero even at high doses, when they are the only drug in subjects with healthy myocardium (C. Bismuth, 1980, unpublished work). This can be explained by the fact that an adrenergically blocked heart works as a denervated heart, with an automaticity that permits survival: the beta-adrenergic blockade appears as a self-limiting phenomenon and the quinidine-like action is not life-threatening.

Treatment. Intensive supportive therapy may have to be continued for several days. Gastric aspiration and lavage should be performed within 4 h of ingestion. In view of the possible severity of the cardiac and respiratory effects, continuous cardiac and ventilatory support is desirable. Ideally, all patients affected by severe overdosage should have a pacing catheter inserted. Severe bradycardia should be treated with atropine 1–2 mg IV. Transvenous electrical pacing may be of value, but it is not always effective. Isoprenaline is not efficient in the case of beta-adrenergically blocked hearts.

IV glucagon has been reported to be of value, and in severe overdosage it should be given at an early stage Glucagon is considered to activate myocardial adenylcyclase by a different mechanism from beta-adrenergic catecholamines, and its inotropic effect is not blocked by drugs such as propanolol [33]. Severe bronchospasm usually responds to salbutamol inhalation.

Analgesic agents

Salicylates [20]

Salicylate poisoning usually arises from an overdose of aspirin itself or some preparation containing it. When compound tablets containing aspirin, phenacetin, and codeine are taken in overdose, the most important toxic features are those of salicylism. The standard aspirin tablet contains 500 mg acetyl salicylic acid. Tablets specially prepared to be palatable to children contain smaller amounts, e.g., 230 mg or 100 mg, and children often take these in overdose believing them to be sweets. Methylsalicylate is very toxic when ingested since it is readily absorbed and has a high salicylate content.

Diagnosis and assessment of severity. It is a common misconception that patients suffering from acute salicylate poisoning become unconscious. In adults this is very rare. Drowsiness must be regarded as a dangerous sign. On the other hand drowsiness or even convulsive coma are more frequent in children.

Since the adult patient is likely to be conscious the diagnosis is not difficult. Patients frequently exaggerate or understate the number of tablets taken, however, and although salicylate poisoning is evident, both from the patient's history and from the somewhat characteristic clinical findings, a precise assessment of its severity may be difficult. This is because the features of salicylism and other symptoms and signs of overdosage may all be present at quite low plasma levels but on the other hand may be quite unimpressive in severe poisoning. Immediate blood analysis is therefore of great value, not only in confirming the diagnosis but also in assessing the severity of the overdosage. A plasma salicylate level of 500 mg/litre (3.125 mmol/litre) (mg salicylate/litre $\div$ 160 = mmol/litre) or more indicates moderate or severe poisoning, and intensive forced diuretic therapy must be started. If, however, the salicylate has been ingested more than 12 h previously a considerable quantity of active drug may have been taken up by the tissues and the plasma level may be misleadingly low. In these circumstances, the arterial blood pH, blood gases, and plasma potassium level are better indications of the severity of the poisoning.

Clinical features. The following clinical features of moderate to severe salicylate poisoning are usually found in an adult who has ingested 50 or more standard aspirin tablets, provided that the patient has not vomited: Mental alertness and restlessness; roaring in the ears, deafness, and blurring of vision; hyperventilation as the result of a direct stimulating effect on the respiratory centre, with both the rate and the depth of breathing increased; hyperpyrexia and profuse perspiration; epigastric pain and vomiting; dehydration; reduced urinary output, the concentrated acid urine containing albumin and, in the initial stages, large numbers of renal tubular cells.

The clinical features in children differ somewhat in that they tend to be more sensitive to the toxic effects of salicylate than adults. There is less tendency to mental stimulation and so drowsiness commonly occurs.

Laboratory findings. In all patients there is a mixed acid–base disturbance with respiratory alkalosis and metabolic acidosis. The major complications of this poisoning occur when the acidosis predominates.

In adults, respiratory alkalosis tends to persist for many hours, with a blood pH close to normal despite the increased metabolism and the presence of salicylic acid, which might be thought to predispose to acidaemia. Respiratory acidosis occurs as a terminal event.

A shift of potassium from the extracellular space occurs and there is also some increase in the renal excretion of potassium; both of these contribute to the development of hypokalaemia. The plasma salicylate level is usually 500 mg/litre (3.125 mmol/litre) or more. Hypoprothrombinaemia occurs, but is rarely sufficiently severe to require treatment. Reduction in the number and effectiveness of the platelets also occurs but seldom results in a bleeding tendency.

In children the initial respiratory alkalosis is more rapidly followed by the onset of a metabolic acidosis, which becomes the dominant acid–base abnormality. Hypokalaemia is less of a problem but hypoglycaemia may be severe.

Complications. Drowsiness and even unconsciousness may follow sustained acid–base disturbances, especially in children. Circulatory collapse is rare, although pulmonary oedema has been seen [14]. Respiratory depression is a common cause of death with plasma salicylate levels of over 1000 mg/litre (31.25 mmol/litre).

Treatment [20]. The management of salicylate poisoing is directed chiefly towards the removal of salicylate from the body. Gastric aspiration and lavage should always be performed irrespective of the time that has elapsed since ingestion.

In mild cases, where there is usually little vomiting, the patients should simply be encouraged to drink liberal quantities of alkaline solutions. In more seriously ill patients (plasma salicylate levels above 300 mg per litre in children and above 500 mg per litre in adults), positive steps must be taken to increase elimination of the salicylate. Many treatment regimens have been advocated and include water diuresis, osmotic alkaline diuresis, peritoneal dialysis, haemodialysis, charcoal HP, and exchange transfusion. Haemodialysis is the most effective method, and although peritoneal dialysis has been used as an alternative, alkaline diuresis is a simple and more effective technique. The toxicity of salicylates is due to the amount of free salicylate present and there is general agreement that the urinary excretion of the free form of the drug increases in relation to the alkalinity of the urine. Various treatment regimens are available to achieve this, but with one exception, all may provoke acute changes in acid–base and electrolyte balance and require close biochemical monitoring. The most effective method for removing salicylate is osmotic alkaline diuresis.

Hypertonic solutions and IV diuretic drugs (acetazolamide) have been added to these regimens in an effort to promote a greater flow of urine, but patients with acute salicylate overdosage may already be severely dehydrated and these preparations are not always useful.

In the potentially lethal situation where the patient has a marked metabolic acidosis, this must be corrected with IV sodium bicarbonate before the full forced diuresis regimen, since these patients are liable to acute pulmonary oedema.

If forced diuresis cannot be undertaken, peritoneal dialysis or haemodialysis will be effective. It is sometimes said that haemodialysis is mandatory if the salicylate level exceeds 1 g/litre. As speed in initiating treatment is so important, however, it is better to use osmotic alkaline diuresis in the first place whilst an artificial kidney is being prepared; if satisfactory diuresis is achieved the artificial kidney may subsequently not be required. Hypoglycaemia occurs, but is corrected in severely ill patients by using dextrose in the diuretic regimen.

In severe poisoning over-breathing and profound alkalosis may be so great that physical exhaustion is produced. In these exceptional circumstances, breathing should be maintained by assisted respiration.

Phenacetin [20]

Numerous proprietary brands of analgesic tablets are mixtures of several drugs, and most of them contain aspirin and phenacetin. Toxic effects may result from the misuse of these preparations by people treating themselves for minor ailments; self-poisoning episodes may also occur. Acute poisoning is therefore not uncommon, and although the major features of analgesic overdosage are due to the salicylate in the tablets phenacetin toxicity may be a significant factor.

Phenacetin is rapidly absorbed from the alimentary tract and passes quickly from the blood into the tissues. The liver is the main site of metabolism of the drug, and the major metabolite is paracetamol, which is excreted in the urine as the glucuronide derivative. A small amount of phenacetin is converted to para-phenecitidin, however, and this derivative is mainly responsible for the methaemoglobinaemia (rarely above 1 g/100 ml), which may be seen in phenacetin overdosage.

As there is considerable variation in response to phenacetin, and as it is a drug to which habituation builds up, assessment of the severity of poisoning is largely dependent on clinical signs. The clinical picture is similar to that which may occur with paracetamol. For the reasons given, methaemoglobinaemia may also be present. If it exceeds 1 g/100 ml its treatment is the same as for chlorate poisoning (see section: *Herbicides, sodium chlorate*).

Paracetamol [16, 20]

There is a wide individual variation in tolerance to paracetamol (acetaminophen), but in an adult serious toxicity usually results from the ingestion of more than 20 tablets each containing 500 mg paracetamol. Liquid preparations for children are also available and contain 120 mg paracetamol in 5 ml. Paracetamol is combined with other potent analgesics, including dextropropoxyphene, phenylbutazone, dihydrocodeine, and aspirin. These combinations may make acute poisoning with them difficult to assess as, quite apart from the individual toxicity of the drugs involved, there may be important changes in the absorption and metabolism of paracetamol. Dextropropoxyphene, for example, tends to slow both the absorption and metabolism of the paracetamol. The most serious complication of acute paracetamol overdosage is hepatic failure, and before effective treatment was developed, in 1973, acute liver necrosis occurred in about 20% of patients with this form of poisoning and a significant number died.

Paracetamol is rapidly absorbed from the stomach and upper intestinal tract and is then metabolized quickly in the liver to form glucuronide and sulphate conjugates. Only 4% is excreted unchanged in the urine. The rate of metabolism is remarkably constant in normal subjects, but it has been shown that in patients who develop hepatic damage, the metabolism is slow. This suggests that the liver damage occurs rapidly after ingestion and that the slow metabolism is a result rather than a cause of the liver damage. Liver biopsy reveals acute centrilobular necrosis, but in most patients regeneration occurs rapidly with no permanent sequelae. Abnormalities in liver function tests are not fully developed for 3–5 days after ingestion, but in survivors they have usually returned to normal within 1–3 weeks. The major biochemical abnormalities are a prolongation of the prothrombin time and rises in various enzyme levels. Severe hepatic failure occurs in the most seriously poisoned patients about 3–7 days after ingestion.

The liver damage has recently been shown to be due to the formation of a highly reactive intermediate alkylating metabolite, which binds to vital live cell macromolecules. The amounts of this metabolite formed with therapeutic doses or even small overdoses of paracetamol are rapidly inactivated by conjugation with hepatic glutathione. Toxic doses of paracetamol, however, cause a depletion of glutathione, and if it falls below 30% of normal, hepatic necrosis becomes likely. Administration of glutathione itself is ineffective therapeutically, but precursors such as cysteine, methionine, and cysteamine have been shown to prevent or reduce paracetamol-induced hepatic necrosis. The precise mechanism by which these substances impart this protection is not certain. Cysteamine and cysteine can restore depleted glutathione and may act either as precursors or as alternative substrates for the toxic metabolite. Cysteamine may also inhibit the microsomal oxidation of paracetamol.

Assessment of the severity of poisoning. The early clinical features are non-specific and abnormalities in liver function are delayed for several days. Plasma paracetamol levels provide a reliable means of assessment and valuable indications of prognostic significance. Plasma concentrations of less than 100 mg/litre (mg/litre ÷ 151 = mmole/litre) at 4 h after ingestion exclude the danger of liver damage, whereas if the level is above 300 mg per litre at 4 h severe liver necrosis can be anticipated. It has been shown that the plasma paracetamol half-life is the most reliable method of predicting subsequent liver damage, but as this involves measurement of serial blood samples resulting in an inevitable delay, this method is of limited practical value. A treatment reference graph has been developed which is designed to overcome these problems. This is a semilogarithmic graph relating plasma paracetamol levels to time since ingestion (Fig. 49.1) and patients with values above the 200 line have a 60% risk of developing liver damage and specific treatment with cysteine, cysteamine or

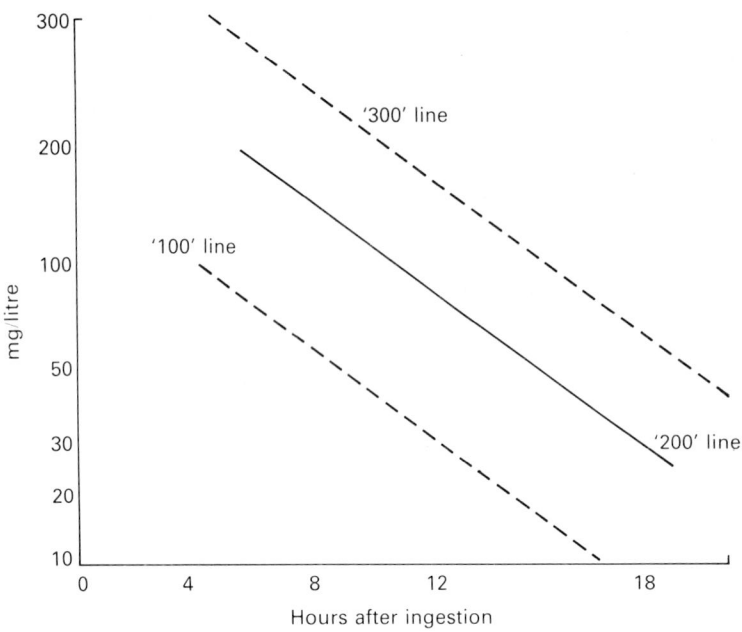

Fig. 49.1. Plasma paracetamol concentrations in relation to the time after overdosage as a guide to prognosis. Specific therapy is indicated in patients with values above the 200 line (mg/litre ÷ 151 = mmol/litre.) Prescott LF (1978) Hlth Bull 36:204.

methionine is indicated (see below). The 300 and 100 lines indicate relatively higher or lesser risks of severe complications. Tests taken less than 4 h after ingestion are unreliable because of probable further absorption.

Clinical features. Toxic effects in the first 24 h after ingestion are non-specific and include nausea, vomiting, pallor, and perspiration. There may then be a period of apparent improvement prior to the onset of the other features.

In patients with liver damage, tenderness in the right hypochondrium may develop after 36–48 h. Liver enlargement, icterus, and other evidence of impaired liver function are not uncommon. In view of the dangers of liver dysfunction this should be specifically sought and monitored by biochemical testing in all patients with plasma paracetamol levels above the 200 treatment line.

Massive overdosage may result in direct toxic damage to the myocardium together with peripheral vasodilatation and severe shock. Tubular necrosis is usual in severe forms before clinical hepatic failure.

Hyperthermia appears if the patient develops extensive skin reactions. Erythema and urticaria are quite common features, occasionally together with mucosal lesions. Hypoglycemia, tends to occur a few days after ingestion. Metabolic acidaemia may be severe. Acute heamolytic anaemia, if severe, may result in acute renal failure. Bleeding tendency due to hypoprothro-binaemia and deficiency of other clotting factors may occur.

Treatment. Various forms of therapy have been advocated for paracetamol overdosage, but most have proved ineffective in preventing the hepatic necrosis which is the most serious toxic effect. Antihistamines and corticosteroids may even increase the toxicity of paracetamol and should not be used. Osmotic diuresis, charcoal HP, and haemodialysis do produce good clearance values for paracetamol, but in practice the renal excretion of the drug and metabolites is so rapid that these methods of treatment are of very doubtful value. Ingestion of activated charcoal or cholestyramine is of doubtful value since these substances fail to delay the absorption of paracetamol significantly even when given very quickly after a small dose of the poison.

The following regimen is at present the most effective means of treatment: intensive supportive therapy is essential. When the plasma paracetamol level is above the 200 line or where the plasma half-life is longer than 4 h, specific forms of treatment are indicated, but to be effective these must be given within 10 h of ingestion. Cysteamine hydrochloride, 2.0 g IV over 10 min followed by three 400 mg doses can reduce and even prevent liver necrosis. This large dose of cysteamine may cause cutaneous vasodilatation, nausea, vomiting, and drowsiness, which can last for 48 h. In view of the dangers of paracetamol poisoning, these side-effects are considered by many to be acceptable, but because of them, alternative forms of treatment have been sought in recent years.

L-Methionine, 5.0 g in 5% dextrose IV over 10 min followed by 5.0 g in 300 ml 5% dextrose infused over 4, 8, and 8 h has also been shown to be effective. Side effects similar to those of cysteamine have been observed with methionine treatment, but they are less severe and of shorter duration.

N-Acetylcysteine has recently been shown to be more effective and less toxic than the above two treatments and is now the treatment of choice for the prevention of paracetamol hepatotoxicity [24]. An initial dose of 150 mg/kg is given IV over 15 min and is followed by an infusion of 50 mg/kg in 500 ml 5% dextrose in 4, 8, and 8 h (total 300 mg/kg in 20 h).

This drug is well tolerated and has no significant side-effects. Administration PO may achieve higher levels in the liver than those obtained after IV administration [23]. It is more easily available, but vomiting in these patients limits its use and the unpleasant odour of the drug favours digestive intolerance. The doses are identical, being repeated if vomiting occurs. The drug can also be administered by gastric tube or diluted in coca cola or fruit juice.

Infusions of sodium bicarbonate IV may be necessary to correct metabolic acidosis, and IV glucose may be required to correct hypoglycaemia. If haemolysis is severe, corticosteroids and blood transfusion may be necessary. Hypoprothrombinaemia may be corrected by vitamin K and occasionally other clotting factors may have to be given to counteract severe bleeding tendencies. In addition to the basic supportive treatment, haemodialysis may be required for acute renal failure.

Glafenine [12]

Glafenine, or glyceryl-amino-phenaquine, is used as an analgesic in many countries. A few cases of acute renal failure induced by acute haemolysis, and acute interstitial nephritis due to hypersensitivity accidents, have been reported. The most frequent accidents result from direct nephrotoxicity of the drug. Some 28 cases of oliguric renal failure, usually following the ingestion of high doses with the intention of committing suicide, have been published. The course is usually benign and recovery is easily obtained. Renal biopsy specimens showed interstitial infiltration in the patients in whom biopsies were performed. There remains some doubt about an actual nephrotoxic mechanism,

however, for in some cases the amount of glafenine absorbed hardly exceeded the usual dose. An increased number of eosinophils was also noted in a few cases. However, the administration of large amounts of glafenine (≥300 mg/kg) to rats induced proximal tubule necrosis, which was actually dose-dependent. At present, both mechanisms appear to operate in humans: a) direct renal toxicity with high doses; b) immunoallergic renal failure if occurring with therapeutic doses.

Colchicine [3, 9]

Still largely used as an analgesic in gouty arthritis, colchicine has a new therapeutic indication in familial Mediterranean fever, and this increases the store of the drug available in families.

Colchicine is rapidly absorbed after oral administration, but large amounts of the drug and its metabolites enter the intestinal tract in the bile and intestinal secretions. This fact, plus the rapid turnover of intestinal epithelium, probably explains the prominence of intestinal manifestations in colchicine poisoning. Administered IV, colchicine rapidly leaves the blood and is distributed in a space larger than that of the body water. The kidney, liver, spleen, and intestinal tract contain high concentrations of colchicine, but it is apparently absent from heart, skeletal muscle, and brain. The drug can be detected in leucocytes for at least 9 days after a single IV dose.

It is partially deacetylated in the liver, and most of the drug and its metabolites are eliminated in the faeces. In normal individuals, 10%–20% of the drug is excreted in the urine, partly unchanged. In patients with liver disease, hepatic uptake and elimination are reduced and a greater fraction of the drug is excreted in the urine.

The acute toxicity of colchicine is strictly dose-dependent and very similar to the accidents observed with vincristine or after total body irradiation. At doses under 0.5 mg/kg body weight, the symptoms are those of vomiting, diarrhoea, gastric and intestinal dilatation (sometimes necessitating surgical intervention), with water and electrolyte depletion and signs of disseminated intravascular coagulation. At doses of 0.5–0.8 mg/kg the same digestive problems occur, together with blood dyscrasias and marrow aplasia, increasing the risks of both infections and haemorrhage. This aplasia lasts for 4–6 days, and not infrequently is associated with various forms of polyneuritis and inappropriate ADH secretion. Transitory alopecia always follows marrow aplasia. With doses up to 1 mg/kg, death usually occurs from cardiogenic shock within 72 h, with dramatic signs of disseminated intravascular coagulation and pulmonary involvement.

Treatment. There is no specific treatment. Colchicine appears to be easily dialysed in vitro, but unfortunately its intravascular content is too small for dialysis to be effective. Gastric lavage is the only efficient method of removing the drug. Hypovolaemic circulatory failure and functional renal failure should be prevented by correct alkalinization and rehydration during the period of diarrhoea. Patients with marrow aplasia must be kept in a half-sterile atmosphere, with careful bacteriological surveillance. Leucocyte transfusions may be necessary in cases of uncontrolled infection, and platelet transfusions in cases of haemorrhage.

The most useful antibiotics appear to be the combination of carbenicillin (efficient even in the absence of granulocytes) and of gentamicin. For patients intoxicated with more than 1 mg/kg, heparin might be used with careful monitoring of the blood coagulation. Positive inotropic drugs such as dopamine and dobutamine appear promising (C. Bismuth, 1980, unpublished work).

Heavy metals [4]

Iron salts [20]

There are a multitude of different therapeutic preparations of iron on the market, most of which are for oral administration. Acute iron poisoning in children is therefore common and is an important cause of death in the younger age groups. All preparations of iron are dangerous but some, such as ferrous gluconate, are considered rather less toxic.

Iron preparations are readily absorbed from the gastro-intestinal tract. Dilute solutions are mildly astringent, but when the concentration is high, as in acute overdosage, such solutions have marked corrosive properties. Necrosis and perforation of the stomach and bowel may occur and subsequent stricture formation is not infrequent.

The excretion of iron is normally very limited and most of an excess is ultimately taken up as apoferritin by the reticulo-endothelial system (RES). An improvement in the management of acute iron poisoning has resulted from the introduction of desferrioxamine, a potent iron-chelating agent, which greatly restricts its absorption and enhances its excretion. The diagnosis of this poisoning may be confirmed by measuring iron levels in the plasma and gastric aspirate.

Clinical features. These are more severe in young children, but this type of poisoning is potentially dangerous in all age groups.

Stage 1. After ingestion of the overdose, symptoms may appear either very rapidly or not for several hours. The predominant initial features are those of acute gastric disturbance, with epigastric pain, nausea, and vomiting. Haematemesis is frequently evident but the vomit may be black in colour, due to the presence of iron in solution. The patient is usually pale or sometimes a curious grey colour. If gastro-intestinal haemorrhage is severe, a state of shock will develop. Respiration and pulse rate are usually rapid.

Stage 2. An interval of hours to even several days may elapse during which there are no further signs and symptoms. This may give rise to a mistaken impression that all is well, until frequent black and offensive stools are passed. Signs of acute encephalopathy may then appear, including severe headache, confusion, delirium, convulsions, and loss of consciousness. Respiration becomes deep and rapid, and circulatory collapse may occur.

Stage 3. In severe acute overdosage, death usually occurs in stage 2, but even if the patient survives this crisis recovery cannot be assured. Acute liver necrosis may develop, as evidenced by the apperence of jaundice; this sometimes progresses to hepatic coma and death. If jaundice is noted full assessment of liver function must be made. Oliguria and even anuria may develop, and these carry a poor prognosis. A level above 90 μmol/litre (mg iron/litre $\times$ 17.92 = μmol/litre) in a toddler and above 143 μmol/litre in an adult within 4 h of ingestion indicates severe poisoning.

Treatment. Treatment is a matter of urgency. When there is a reasonable suspicion that an overdose has been taken, it is better to act swiftly rather than wait for the chemical confirmation of a high plasma iron level. The basic principles of symptomatic treatment must be followed, according to intensive supportive therapy. In addition the following procedure should be undertaken: Gastric aspiration and lavage should always be performed except when the patient is severely shocked. Lavage should be carried out with appropriate volumes of a solution of desferrixoamine 2 g in 1 litre warm water. Following lavage 10 g desferrioxamine dissolved in 50 ml water should be left in the stomach. This substance is not absorbed, but will chelate any free iron in the stomach and intestine. The chelated ferrioxamine is also poorly absorbed and iron absorption is therefore effectively blocked.

Parenteral desferrioxamine (2 g in 10 ml water in an adult and 1 g in 5 ml water in a child) should be injected IM. In addition an IV drip should be set up, so that desferrioxamine may be given by continuous infusion at a rate of no more than 15 mg/kg per hour. The maximum dose by this route is 80 mg/kg per 24 h. The IM injection of 2 g desferrioxamine should be repeated at 12-h intervals, depending on an adequate urinary flow, as otherwise the chelate ferrioxamine is not excreted and may cause toxic effects in its own right. If oliguria or anuria occurs, therefore, haemodialysis or peritoneal dialysis must be started urgently.

Desferrioxamine IV has been reported to cause hypotension. This complication usually occurs if the desferrioxamine has been administered too rapidly or in too high a dose. The regimen of treatment and in particular the doses per unit body weight described here are designed to reduce these complications to a minimum.

Arsenic [9]

Acute poisoning may arise from the ingestion of arsenic in weedkillers, rodenticides, insecticides, or even medicines such as vaginal pessaries. In America arsenical pesticides cause more deaths in children than any other type of pesticide, and of the heavy metals arsenic is the second commonest cause of death. Organic arsenicals are less likely to cause poisoning than inorganic derivatives. The acute toxic dose of the trivalent inorganic salt is about 100 mg.

The chief toxic effects usually become apparent within 1 h of ingestion but may be delayed for up to 12 h.

Clinical features. The clinical signs and symptoms are constriction in the mouth and throat, severe gastro-enteritis, with copious watery stools which may contain blood, and jaundice which may appear after 2 days. Cardiovascular findings comprise tachycardia and hypotension, with a hyperkinetic circulation.

Oliguria or anuria may develop and marrow hypoplasia is not rare. Headache, irritability, muscular weakness, mental confusion, convulsions, and coma are often delayed for 3–9 days. Polyneuritis may develop as a late feature in severe cases who have survived the initial insult. Complete recovery may take longer than a year.

Treatment. It is important to confirm the clinical diagnosis by detecting arsenic in blood and urine. Intensive supportive therapy is necessary and treatment with dimercaprol should be initiated at once, without waiting for evidence of renal involvement: 4 mg/kg IM every 4 h for 48 h, followed by 3 mg/kg twice daily for 8 days constitutes the maximum recommended dosage. These injections are painful and locally irritant, and should therefore be given in different sites successively.

Correction of dehydration may require copious fluids IV together with conventional measures to correct electrolyte imbalance. Renal damage may be severe and require peritoneal or haemodialysis. The blood levels of arsenic, compared with the amount ingested, are too low for dialysis to eliminate the drug.

Mercury [20]

Acute mercury poisoning commonly results from the ingestion of mercuric chloride or mercuric cyanide, and less often of mercurous chloride (Calomel) as, even in large doses, this form of mercury is poorly absorbed. Mercuric chloride (corrosive sublimate) is used as a strong disinfectant and is highly toxic; the fatal dose can be as little as 500 mg. Acute mercury poisoning may also occur as a result of industrial accidents due to the inhalation of mercury vapour. Occasionally it may be encountered following absorption of mercury-containing ointments through the skin. Mercury in its metallic form is not toxic when taken by mouth, as it is not absorbed. The hazard from swallowing parts of a broken thermometer is that of the glass and not the mercury. Metallic mercury poisoning may arise, however, from the use of the metal as a seal in syringes for withdrawing specimens for blood gas analysis. Accidents may occur as a result of faulty technique allowing metallic mercury to enter the circulation.

In the past 20 years the use of organic mercury compounds as fungicides has resulted in mercury poisoning in whole communities as a result of people eating coated cereals. As a consequence of industrial waste containing methylmercury, being carelessly discharged into the sea, poisoning has occurred from eating contaminated fish [1].

Clinical features. The patient has a grey appearance and complains of pain in the mouth or pharynx. At the onset salivation is marked and there may be nausea, vomiting, thirst, and severe colic with bloody stools. A metallic taste with stomatitis and proctitis is an indication of the predominant elimination of mercury via the digestive tract.

Hypotension and shock are often related to initial hypovolaemia and oliguria or anuria can develop within 48 h of ingestion. Tubular necrosis is usual when the plasma level is around 1 mg/litre during the first 24 h.

If the poisoning is by inhalation, pneumonitis may result with associated tachypnoea and hypoxia. It is the main cause of death in this mode of poisoning. In addition there may be lethargy or excitement, hyperreflexia, and tremor. Muscle weakness can be severe, together with ataxia. Peripheral sensory changes may also occur, with auditory and visual disturbances; blindness may result from severe poisoning and headache, dysarthria, and mental disturbances may also occur. The chronic neurological complications, particularly after ingestion of methylmercury, may not become manifest for up to 6 weeks after ingestion. In the acute encephalopathy, high doses of mercury have usually been ingested (several grams) and plasma levels exceed several milligrams in the first 24 h.

Treatment. Intensive supportive therapy is necessary. In poisoning by ingestion gastric lavage should be done if possible, with 250 ml 5% solution of sodium formaldehyde sulphoxylate, and a further 100 ml should be left in the stomach after lavage. This substance reduces bivalent mercuric ions to the much less soluble mercurous form and so the absorption of the mercury is reduced.

Dimercaprol (BAL) should be given at once, as for arsenic poisoning, and stopped if anuria develops. Oliguria or anuria should be treated by routine medical measures initially, but if these fail peritoneal dialysis or haemodialysis may be necessary. Following inhalation, intensive respiratory care may be required. Hydrocortisone 100 mg every 6 h IV may prevent or reduce the pulmonary complications.

Prognosis. The tragic neurological symptoms which occur especially after ingestion of organic mercury compounds are often permanent, particularly in young children. If the exposure to mercury has been of short duration and the poisoning of moderate or mild degree, the chance of good recovery is high although it may take up to 2 years.

Phosphorus [9, 20]

Phosphorus may be encountered in two distinct forms, the red granular one which is not poisonous, and the highly toxic, yellow waxy, fat-soluble and water-insoluble form. Yellow phosphorus is used in fireworks and matches and in rodent and insect poisons; poisoning is usually by ingestion, but skin and lungs may be sites of absorption.

Clinical features. The main toxic effects are on the liver, leading to acute hepatic failure. Nausea, vomiting, and profuse diarrhoea are common. The liver is enlarged and tender; jaundice and acute liver failure may follow. Hypotension and shock may be features. Hypoprothrombinaemia and a marked acidosis can be found. Oliguria and anuria may follow and the urine may contain red cells.

Delirium and coma are usually terminal features.

Treatment. Gastric aspiration and lavage have to be done with 0.1% copper sulphate in water. Exchange blood transfusion should be considered in the first 8 h and intensive supportive therapy is essential. Phosphorus burns must be thoroughly washed with 1% copper sulphate solution in water. Hepatic and renal failure require supportive treatment.

Alcohols and glycols

Methanol [9, 15, 20]

Methyl alcohol (wood alcohol; methanol) can produce serious poisoning, both by inhalation and by ingestion. Most cases of methanol poisoning result from unintentional ingestion by individuals who use the substance in the course of their work, but it is also contained in certain home-made beverages and in antifreeze, paint removers, and varnish. It is much more toxic than ethyl alcohol because it is metabolized to formic acid or formaldehyde, both of which severely inhibit essential metabolic processes:

$$CH_3-OH \rightarrow H-CHO^+ (H_2O + O_2) \rightarrow$$
$$H.COOH + H_2O_2$$

The enzymatic oxidation of methanol proceeds at one-fifth the rate of the corresponding reaction with ethanol. Hence in the treatment of poisoning by methanol, the administration of a product that saturates alcohol dehydrogenase (such as ethanol or 4-methyl-pyrazole) slows the rate of accumulation of toxic products. Methylated spirit contains only 5% methanol and 95% ethanol and, contrary to common opinion, is toxic due to its ethanol content rather than methanol.

Clinical features. Since methanol is distributed in the tissues according to their water content, a high concentration is found in the vitreous body and the optic nerve, and the consequent impairment of vision is a characteristic feature of methanol poisoning. Because one of the principle metabolites is formic acid, severe metabolic acidosis occurs.

The signs and symptoms to expect are headache, nausea, and vomiting, with severe abdominal pain; blurring of vision, which may lead to blindness; dilatation of pupils and papilloedema; acidotic breathing; initial restlessness followed by loss of consciousness, varying in degree; blood levels of methanol above 1 g per litre indicate severe poisoning.

Treatment. Gastric aspiration and lavage should be performed within 4 h of ingestion of the poison. The metabolic acidosis must be treated energetically with IV infusions of sodium bicarbonate. Ethyl alcohol (50%), 1 ml/kg should be given PO at once, followed by 0.5 ml/kg every 2 h for 5 days. This treatment, which is the subject of some controversy in adults, is dangerous for children. The administration of 4-methyl-pyrazole is still experimental, although promising. If there is impaired vision and the response to these measures is unsatisfactory, haemodialysis or peritoneal dialysis is essential. Haemodialysis is the preferred method, since it will reduce the blood levels of formic acid and formaldehyde more rapidly [15]. Haemodialysis is indicated at the outset, if the blood methanol concentration exceeds 1 g per litre, if severe metabolic acidosis occurs, or if the mental, visual or funduscopic complications of methanol poisoning are present. Dialysis should be continued until the blood level falls to below 250 mg per litre. Peritoneal dialysis should be used only if haemodialysis is not readily available, as it is less effective in removing methanol. Coated charcoal does not extract alcohols.

The metabolism of methanol is slow, and there is therefore a considerable risk of recurrence of the toxic features even after a successful period of treatment. The patient should be kept under close observation for several days before recovery is considered complete.

Ethanol [9, 20]

This a frequent cause of acute poisoning. Ethyl alcohol is frequently taken with other drugs in self-poisoning, and in children cutaneous friction can lead to absorption.

The fatal dose is difficult to ascertain because of individual tolerance (the result of habituation), but the equivalent of about 600 ml pure ethyl alcohol, consumed in 1 h, may be lethal.

Ethyl alcohol is rapidly absorbed from the upper gastro-intestinal tract and is distributed in the tissues according to their water content. The main effect is that of a CNS depressant and it is always metabolized in less than 20 h, so that coma lasts less than 1 day.

Clinical features. These are varied and include inebriation; facial flushing; muscular incoordination; blurred vision, and impaired reaction time. Excitement is due to loss of inhibitions, and in severe cases impairment of consciousness precedes coma. A blood alcohol of 0.8 g/litre (g alcohol/litre ÷ 0.046 = mmol/litre) will produce recognizable features of drunkenness, while a level of 5 g per litre is dangerous to life. A high degree of tolerance may develop in people habituated to ethyl alcohol, however, and clinical assessment of this poisoning is therefore essential. In children severe hypoglycaemia and metabolic acidosis may be present.

Treatment. Gastric aspiration and lavage are important and in very severe poisoning peritoneal dialysis or haemodialysis may be necessary. Infusion of 200 g fructose (500 ml 40% solution) IV over a 30-min period is of value as it has been shown to increase the rate of fall of blood ethanol levels by about 25%. This may cause symptoms of retrosternal and epigastric discomfort and, more important, acidaemia, which should be corrected by administration of an alkali. Alcohol withdrawal will be discussed with other drug addictions.

Glycols [9]

It is not uncommon for anti-freeze containing ethylene glycol and diethylene glycol (propylene-glycol is not toxic) to be ingested by mistake (these solutions have an alcoholic taste) or in suicide attempts. Ethylene glycol has two metabolic pathways:

$$\begin{matrix} CH_2OH \\ | \\ CH_2OH \end{matrix} \rightarrow \begin{matrix} CH_2OH \\ | \\ CHO \end{matrix} \rightarrow \begin{matrix} CH_2OH \\ | \\ COOH \end{matrix} \rightarrow \begin{matrix} CHO \\ | \\ CHO \end{matrix} \rightarrow$$

$$\xrightarrow{\text{major pathway}} CO_2-H-COH-CO_2$$

$$\xrightarrow{\text{minor pathway}} \begin{matrix} CO_2H \\ | \\ CO_2H \end{matrix} \quad \text{oxalic acid}$$

The oxalic acid combined with calcium might provoke severe metabolic acidosis, renal oxalosis and sometimes cardiac and cerebral oxalosis. The half-life of ethylene glycol is around 4–5 h, but the administration of substances saturating alcohol dehydrogenase slows it. It is estimated that ethylene glycol will form 2–3 g oxalic acid and the absorption of 50 ml can be fatal, but survival has been recorded after the ingestion of 500 ml. The average mortality is about 40%. (mg Glycol/litre $\div$ 62 = mmol/litre.)

Clinical features. A metabolic acidosis in the absence of a circulatory failure or anoxia but associated with anuria and fits is very suggestive of this form of poisoning. Myocardial failure and prolonged coma are less common.

Blood levels of ethylene glycol are rarely available; crystals of oxalates might be detected in the urine in the initial stages. Oxalates can be found in blood or urine.

Treatment. Evacuation of the gastro-intestinal tract must be as complete as possible. Early and prolonged haemodialysis is essential (amberlite or charcoal HP is inefficient). The metabolic acidosis, however pronounced, is usually easily corrected with sodium bicarbonate. Survival after prolonged coma with careful control of fits is observed in ICUS with increasing frequency. Ethyl alcohol, or preferably methyl pyrazole, should be administered within the first few hours, as for methanol poisoning.

Household products

Corrosives [9]

Strong acids or alkalis are an increasing problem in acute toxicology. The initial mortality is due to shock and perforation of the bowel, with later deaths due to superimposed infection and secondary necrosis. There is now general agreement on approaches to the treatment of poisoning with corrosives. Certain measures should be undertaken within the first 10 h. The mouth and pharynx need careful examination and a rapid fiberoptic gastroscopy should be carried out. Antibiotics are given and surgical advice is obtained at an early stage. Gastric lavage, gastric intubation, and steroids should be avoided. A metabolic acidosis is common (even after absorption of alkalis), and a fibrinolytic tendency may develop. Secondary measures will depend on the results of early fibroscopy. The need for parenteral feeding will be established on considerations of the findings at gastroscopy. Surgical procedures, such as enterotomy if the lesions are localized to the upper GI tract, or limited resections, may be rapidly required. At a later date reparative surgery or resection of strictures may be necessary.

Carbon monoxide [9, 20]

The major source of carbon monoxide is town gas, but it is found in significant quantities wherever incomplete combustion occurs, particularly in the exhaust fumes from motor vehicles. It is therefore a common toxic agent and the risks of exposure are considerable. In recent years many household gas supplies have been converted from coal gas to natural gas, which is not in itself toxic except in very high concentration, when it may cause asphyxiation. Carbon monoxide poisoning may still occur, however, when inappropriate appliances are used due to the incomplete combustion of natural gas.

Carbon monoxide itself is a colourless, odourless gas with an affinity for haemoglobin that is 200 times that of O_2; as the result of the conversion of haemoglobin to carboxyhaemoglobin the O_2-carrying power of the arterial blood is diminished and hypoxia results.

There is also evidence that carbon monoxide may have a direct toxic effect on the myocardium.

Mechanisms of intoxication. Carbon monoxide poisoning generates hypoxia due to the reaction: $HbO_2 + CO_2 \rightarrow HbCO + O_2$.

Carbon monoxide (CO) combines with haemoglobin to form carboxyhaemoglobin, at the rate of 1.34 ml CO/g haemoglobin. This combination is reversible but the affinity of Hb for CO is 200 times stronger than that for O_2 and, at equilibrium, one part of CO per 1500 parts of air (800 ppm) converts 50% of Hb to HbCO. The severity of hypoxia depends on the physical activity, the need for O_2, and the Hb concentration of the patient. Generally, a concentration of 0.1% of CO in the inspired air is symptomatic as the proportion of HbCO to Hb stays lower than 10%.

Exposure to 0.5% CO for 1 h with moderate physical activity involves a carboxyhaemoglobinaemia of 20%, and the subject will complain of headaches. When it reaches 30%–50% of carboxyhaemoglobinaemia dizziness will occur. After exposure for 1 h to concentrations of 10% of CO in the inspired air the carboxyhaemoglobinaemia is 50%–80% and when death occurs, the haemoglobin conversion is always ≥66% (blood level above 8 ml/100 ml).

Laboratory investigations. CO can be detected in air by means of a Dräger apparatus or, preferably, an ONERA analyser. Colorimetric spectrography or the ONERA analyser can be used for its detection in blood. The normal blood level of CO is 0.10–0.4 ml/100 ml; this can rise to 1.5 ml/100 ml blood in acute poisoning (ml CO/100 ml ÷ 2.24 = mmol/litre).

CO is very rapidly eliminated, and if a normal blood level is measured more than 3 h after exposure this cannot be taken to indicate that CO poisoning has not occurred.

Clinical features. The cerebral effects range from dizziness and mental confusion to deep coma. Features of agitation frequently occur when cerebral oedema is present, and therefore they are often associated with papilloedema, hypertonia, intensified peripheral limb reflexes, and possibly extensor plantar responses. Hyperpyrexia may be considerable. The sequelae of the damage to the CNS can be tragic.

The incidence of myocardial damage is much more frequent than would be suspected on clinical grounds. It may result in tachycardia, various arrhythmias, hypotension, and shock. Acute myocardial infarction may develop. Myocardial ischaemia, but not necessarily actual infarction, is almost invariable in severe CO poisoning at any age.

In severe poisoning the marked degree of hypoxia initially provides a powerful stimulus to the respiratory centre, and the patient may therefore have a rapid respiratory rate. Acute congestion and oedema of the lungs may occur and failure of the respiratory centre may follow. Patients with moderate or severe CO poisoning have marked nausea and vomiting, and faecal incontinence is common.

The pink colour of the skin is due to carboxyhaemoglobin and is uncommon in clinical practice, but when present it indicates a severe degree of poisoning. Its absence by no means excludes the diagnosis. Cyanosis and skin pallor are much more frequent. Bullous eruptions may occur in CO poisoning, being localized in sites of external pressure, but the factor that predisposes to the formation of blisters is skin hypoxia. Hypoxic rhabdomyolysis is frequent with the possibility of acute renal failure.

Treatment. The patient must be removed from exposure to the poisonous atmosphere. The principles of intensive supportive therapy apply to poisoning due to CO as they do in any case of poisoning. Care of the respiratory tract is of particular importance. In patients who have ceased to breathe spontaneously, 100% O_2 should be given, together with assisted respiration. Even when the patient is breathing spontaneously, however, the respiratory centre may still be depressed by hypoxia resulting from a high carboxyhaemoglobin level. In these circumstances removal of the CO from the circulating blood is an emergency matter and the respiratory stimulant effect of the mixture of 95% O_2 and 5% CO_2 is a valuable addition to the treatment.

Hyperbaric O_2 markedly increases the elimination of CO.

Anti-rust products [9]

The toxic constituents in antirust products are fluorhydric acid and oxalic acid, both of which are powerful corrosives and chelating agents of calcium. Fluorhydric acid has a direct toxic effect on the myocardium; oxalic acid combined with calcium can produce renal oxalosis with acute renal failure.

The mortality from this form of poisoning is around 15%. Burns of the upper GI tract are assessed by rapid fiberoptic gastroscopy. Perforation of the GI tract is responsible for 50% of the deaths.

Marked hypocalcaemia may occur, together with arrhythmias and shock. Cardiac arrest is the second most frequent cause of death. Replacement of calcium must be prudent and slow; direct IV injection of a calcium salt can be dangerous; a micrometric syringe must be used and the patient carefully monitored throughout.

An intractable metabolic acidosis suggests perforation or impending shock rather than being specifically related to the toxic agents.

Industrial intoxicants

Cyanide [9, 20]

Although poisoning by hydrogen cyanide is uncommon this substance and its salts are extensively used in the chemical industry. Cyanide poisoning may arise from the inhalation of hydrocyanic acid vapour and by percutaneous absorption, as well as by ingestion. Extensive use of sodium nitroprusside presents a new medical hazard [32]. Cyanide inhibits cytochrome B, one of the enzymes necessary for O_2 transport at cellular level. It is one of the most rapidly acting poisons and death from asphyxia may occur within a few minutes, though it may be delayed for a number of hours. Ferrocyanides are not intoxicants.

Clinical features. The speed of onset of symptoms and signs obviously depends on the quantity of cyanide absorbed. The initial features following exposure to a low concentration in air or when small amounts are swallowed on a full stomach often mimic those of anxiety. This may cause considerable difficulty in diagnosis and a careful history should always be taken. Headache, dyspnea, vomiting, ataxia, and loss of consciousness occur gradually. If a large amount is absorbed the features appear very rapidly, and the patient becomes deeply unconscious. The smell of bitter almonds is not necessarily present. The skin remains pink unless breathing has ceased, even though respiration is markedly depressed. The blood pressure may be too low to be recorded. The limb reflexes are absent and the pupils are dilated. Metabolic acidosis is constant and pulmonary oedema is present in one out of five cases with coma. The patient may continue in this state for several hours, but so long as the heart sounds are audible there are good grounds for expecting recovery. Blood cyanide levels of 3 mg/litre (1000 mg $\div 26 = 38.5$ μmoles) are associated with severe toxicity. Survival has been recorded with peak levels of 5 mg/litre. Sequelae of anoxia appear to be more frequent than with other hypoxic agents.

Treatment. The purposes and effects of treatment are summarized in Table 49.7 [11].

In view of possible secondary effects it is wise to be cautious before deciding to administer antidotes for cyanide poisoning. Patients who think they may have been exposed to cyanide are almost always anxious, but in mild exposures simple reassurance with careful observation may be all that is required. In this regard it should be remembered that the body has natural detoxification mechanisms, and it has been suggested that up to 50% of absorbed cyanide is inactivated within 1 h of exposure.

If the poisoning is due to inhalation, the patient should be removed from the contaminated atmosphere and should be given artificial respiration with 100% O_2. An initial IV injection of Kelocyanor 600 mg is given over 1 min if there is no doubt of the diagnosis, as cyanide neutralizes the possible toxicity of this chelating agent. In any case, Hydroxocobalamin (4 g IV) can be administered. Its high cost and its brief duration of action restrict its use.

If poisoning is due to ingestion, in addition to the above measures gastric aspiration and lavage should be carried out and 300 ml 25% sodium thiosulphate should be left in the stomach.

The agents that induce methaemoglobin now appear obsolete as clinical experience accumulates with newer therapeutic approaches.

Carbon tetrachloride [9, 20]

Carbon tetrachloride is highly toxic to all types of cells, but especially to those of the liver and kidney. If taken with alcohol, absorption is considerably increased. It may also be absorbed by sniffing for 'kicks' or by accidental inhalation during professional use.

Clinical features. The signs and symptoms of acute toxicity are similar whether the agent has been inhaled or ingested, but in the latter case the GI upset is more marked. Sore throat, nausea, vomiting, and severe abdominal colic are common and headache, dizziness, stupor, and convulsions may occur, leading to loss of consciousness. Bradycardia with hypotension is usually present, but there is also a tendency to serious ventricular arrhythmias. Hepatic and renal disorders are frequent. After 2–3 days liver necrosis and acute tubular necrosis may appear. In very severe poisoning, however, these features may occur in the first 12 h.

Treatment. Contaminated clothing must be removed. If the poison has been ingested gastric-aspiration and lavage are necessary. Intensive supportive therapy and treatment of acute renal and hepatic failure should be given if required.

Trichloroethylene [9, 20]

This form of intoxication is frequent and follows either ingestion (self-administered for suicide attempt or professional error) or inhalation ('sniffing' or professional exposure).

Poisoning with industrial trichloroethylene is characterized by the smell of the solvent, deep and prolonged coma, persistence of trichloroacetic acid in the urine (as much as 10 days after ingestion), risk of cardiac arrhythmias (hypoxia makes these more likely), corrosive vomiting

Table 49.7. Proposed antidotes for cyanide poisoning

Agent	Mechanism	Potential toxicity	Current availability	Present indication	Estimated utility
Amyl nitrite	Forms methemoglobin (met-Hb) as step 2	Difficult to achieve antidotal levels without cardiovascular collapse	Cyanide antidote package	Obsolete	$-$ (A) $--$ (H)
Sodium nitrite	$NaNo_2 + Hb \rightleftharpoons Met\text{-}Hb$ $Met\text{-}Hb + CN \rightleftharpoons$ cyanmet-Hb	Tachycardia, vomiting, Hypotension, severe methaemoglobinaemia, hypoxia, vascular collapse	Cyanide antidote package	Obsolete	$+++$ (A) ? (H)
Sodium thiosulphate	$Na_2S_2O_3 + CN \xrightarrow{rhodanese} SCN + Na_2SO_4$	None known	Cyanide antidote package	Associated with hydroxocobalamine (Hepatrol)	$++$ (A) $+?$ (H)
Oxygen	Increased O_2 content of arterial blood may reverse CN binding with cytochromes. Potentiates activity of sodium nitrite and sodium thiosulphate.	Oxygen toxicity unlikely; when used for 48 h with $FiO_2 < 50\%$	Assisted ventilation	Life-saving procedure	$+++$ (A) $+++$ (H)
Cobalt salts including edelate	Chelates cyanide	Significant loss of Ca^{2+} Mg^{++}, plus intense purging	Edetate cobalt (Kelocyanor, France)	Efficient in certain poisoning, dangerous if no poisoning	$++$ (A) ? (H)
Hydroxocobalamin[a]	$OH\text{-}B_{12} + CN \rightleftharpoons CN\text{-}B_{12}$	None known	See nonproprietary names and trademarks listing	Efficient, atoxic, associated with thiosulphate (Hepatrol)	$+++$ (A) $++$ (H)

[a]Since the molecular weight of Hydroxocobalamin is 1346 g/mole, and one mole of cyanide is neutralized by one mole of Hydroxocobalamin, large amounts are needed for antidotal use. Thus 100 mg KCN would require approximately 1800 mg Hydroxocobalamin. (H), human studies or cases; (A), animal studies.

and diarrhoea. After poisoning with household trichloroethylene, which is rarely a pure substance, liver necrosis and in exceptional cases renal tubular necrosis have been observed in addition to the features mentioned above. Liver toxicity has been most frequently attributed to a state of enzymatic induction in affected patients, leading to the formation of a highly reactive intermediate, an alkylating metabolite that binds to vital cell molecules.

Chromatographic analysis of household solutions that are alleged to be pure trichloroethylene always reveals other carbon derivatives, such as tetrachloride or tri- and tetrachloroethane, all of which are hepatotoxic [6]. It seems therefore that hepatotoxicity cannot be definitely attributed to trichloroethylene unless the solution has been analysed.

The treatment combines assisted ventilation with non-specific anti-arrhythmic therapy.

Petroleum distillates [20]

Kerosene is irritant to the GI tract and, if absorbed, depresses the CNS. Aspiration into the lungs is a particular danger. On account of its low surface tension and high vapour pressure even a few millilitres of kerosene entering the respiratory passage will spread throughout the lungs, resulting in severe pneumonitis. Kerosene is not readily absorbed after ingestion.
Clinical features. Mild poisoning following inhalation causes symptoms resembling alcoholic inebriation. More severe poisoning produces nausea, vomiting, and diarrhoea. If inhaled or aspirated, intense pulmonary congestion and chemical pneumonitis occur. Headache, blurring of vision, vertigo, and tinnitus are rare. Restlessness, excitement, incoordination, disorientation, and delirium may deteriorate into coma and convulsions.

Respiratory failure is the most usual mode of death in the rare cases that are fatal.

Treatment. It is vital to prevent aspiration into the lungs. Therefore emesis and gastric aspiration should not be attempted. The one exception to this is when the patient is so deeply unconscious as to permit endotracheal intubation, following which gastric aspiration and lavage may be performed. Absorption of ingested kerosene can be slowed by giving 250 ml liquid paraffin PO. If there is any suspicion of chemical pneumonitis hydrocortisone 100 mg should be given IM at 6 h intervals for 48 h, together with benzylpenicillin in full dosage for 7 days. Respiratory depression may need appropriate treatment.

Pesticides

Rodenticides [9]

See Table 49.8.

Herbicides [9, 20]

Chlorates

Sodium or potassium chlorate salts are contained in many gargles and lozenges. Sodium chlorate is also used as a weed killer. The potentially fatal dose in an adult is approximately 15 g. The chief effects are irritation of the alimentary system. Severe methaemoglobinaemia may occur (up to 8 g/100 ml). Renal and circulatory damage are likely after ingestion of a large quantity.
Clinical features. Nausea, vomiting, abdominal colic, and diarrhoea occur; the corrosive effect is proven by fiberoptic gastroscopy. An initial state of confusion may be followed by coma.

Haemoglobin is present in the urine: acute tubular necrosis is frequent and is generally

Table 49.8. Rodenticides

Constituent	Clinical features	Treatment
Strychnine	Medullary irritation; convulsions. Apnoea	Assisted respiration; anti-convulsivants
Arsenic	See section: *Arsenic*	See section: *Arsenic*
Chloralose	Coma with convulsions bronchorrhoea	Assisted respiration; benzodiazepines
Coumarin derivatives	Fall in prothrombin time, haemorrhage	Vitamin K_1
Thallium	Digestive problems; Guillain–Barré-like syndrome. Alopecia	Absorption with prussian blue (250 mg/k per day). Mannitol diuresis
Barium (soluble salts)	Diarrhoea. Paralysis (reversible)	Supportive
Phosphorus	See section: *Phosphorus*	See section: *Phosphorus*
Cyanides	See section: *Cyanide*	See section: *Cyanide*

preceded by severe shock. Haematological investigation reveals evidence of methaemoglobinaemia, haemolysis, and raised serum potassium.

Treatment. Intensive supportive therapy is required. If cyanosis is severe, methylene blue 25 ml 1% solution should be given by slow IV injection and may be repeated. Haemodialysis or peritoneal dialysis is valuable in severe poisoning and hepatic and renal failure may require conventional treatment.

Exchange transfusion is required if there is profound hypoxia, severe shock and severe haemolysis.

Paraquat [9, 20]

This herbicide, chemically a dipyridilium, is highly toxic in the concentrated liquid form that is supplied to farmers. It has the unique property of being inactivated by contact with soil. The brown liquid concentrate usually contains 20% of the active substance. The granular preparation is available for domestic use and contains much weaker concentrations of paraquat. The granules are dissolved in water prior to application to the weeds.

The acute toxic effects may be divided into local and systemic features. Severe corneal and conjunctival inflammation may follow accidental splashing of paraquat concentrate in the eyes. The irritation develops gradually over several hours and is usually at a peak within 24 h. Healing may be slow, but with proper care complete recovery can be expected even in severe cases. Skin irritation and even blistering may result from contact with either the concentrated or the dilute forms of paraquat. If the skin is intact there is no significant absorption, but if the skin is broken and in contact with contaminated clothing a significant degree of absorption can occur, with subsequent systemic features. Nose bleeding and sore throats may follow inhalation of spray mist or dust containing paraquat.

Systemic clinical features usually follow ingestion of the poison. An oral dose of approximately 2–3 g paraquat is likely to be fatal if untreated. This amount is contained in 10–15 ml undiluted Gramoxone or 80–120 g of the granular preparations.

In humans, only 1%–5% of an ingested dose is absorbed from the gut.

Clinical features. A burning sensation in the mouth and abdomen is noticed at the time of ingestion and after a few hours painful ulceration of the lips and tongue appears. Marked nausea, sweating, and vomiting may occur, although even in patients who have taken a lethal dose the early signs and symptoms may be remarkably mild. Digestive burns must be assessed by early endoscopy. Tremors and convulsions may occur.

Some days after ingestion (sometimes up to a week) dyspnoea with pulmonary oedema may develop. This is due to a relentless proliferative alveolitis and bronchiolitis with resultant pulmonary fibrosis and death. This is such an important complication of paraquat poisoning that respiratory function tests should be monitored from the beginning of the poisoning. Chest x-ray examination may reveal a granular appearance in the lung fields. Other causes of pulmonary oedema should always be considered and evidence of respiratory infection sought.

Acute tubular necrosis is frequent.

If the poisoning follows the ingestion of a large amount of paraquat concentrate severe shock may develop within a few hours. This is probably due to widespread tissue damage and is resistent to treatment.

Laboratory findings. This form of poisoning is potentially very serious and vigorous treatment should be commenced immediately in all patients in whom it is suspected. It should never be delayed for laboratory confirmation.

A fast measurement of the blood level of paraquat within the first 24 h (by radioimmunology) enables a precise diagnosis (Fig. 49.2) to be made and provides a sensitive guide for evaluating new forms of therapy.

Treatment. Following exposure of the eyes (or skin), immediate and copious irrigation should be given for 10–15 min, followed by antibiotic eye drops. At a later stage, when corneal and conjunctival regrowth is complete, resolution of any granulation tissue can be attempted by instilling steroid eye drops. Toxic effects following inhalation are almost always mild, and apart from simple symptomatic treatment, removal from exposure is usually all that is required.

After absorption the stomach should be emptied as thoroughly as possible at the earliest opportunity after ingestion. As a first aid measure, therefore, vomiting should be induced, and the patient should be sent to hospital as quickly as possible. In hospital, careful gastric aspiration and lavage should be performed as soon as possible, leaving 500 ml adsorbent suspension containing 30 g Fuller's Earth and 5 g magnesium sulphate for each 100 ml water in the stomach. Bentonite (7 g) may be used in

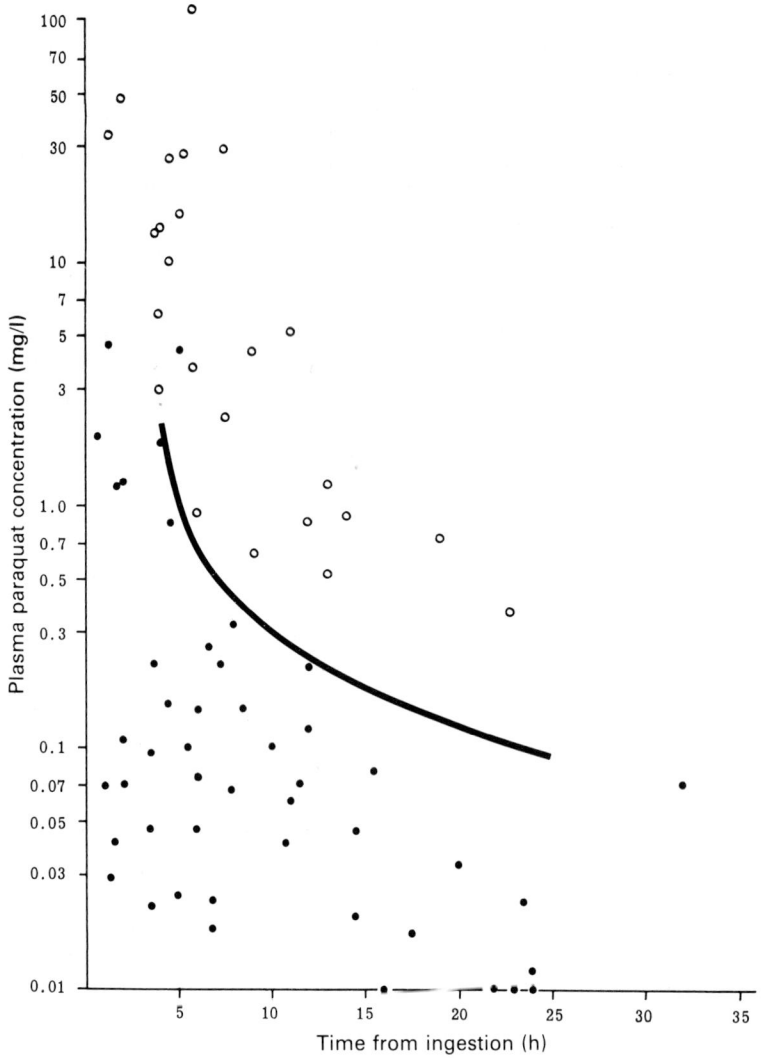

Fig. 49.2. Plasma paraquat concentrations on admission related to time from ingestion for 71 patients admitted within 35h. The *line* arbitrarily separates fatal cases (*open circles*) and survivors (*closed circles*). (1 mg = 3.9 μmol; mg/litre ÷ 0.257 = μmol/litre). Proudfoot AT et al. (1979) Lancet II:330–332.

place of Fuller's Earth, although it is less effective [31].

The purgative effects of magnesium sulphate may cause severe diarrhoea and fluid loss which may require specific treatment with fluid and electrolyte replacement. If analysis confirms paraquat poisoning the oral administration of 30% Fuller's Earth suspension 200–500 ml should be repeated at 2 h intervals for 24 h after ingestion, and then every 4 h for the second 24 h. Magnesium sulphate is given as required to ensure adequate elimination of the adsorbent form from the GI tract.

Intensive supportive therapy is necessary and immediate forced diuresis, combined with charcoal HP, should be performed in an effort to keep the blood levels of paraquat as low as possible (in an attempt to reduce or even prevent severe pulmonary damage) [31].

Haemodialysis is ineffective, which is surprising for a substance that is excreted in considerable quantities in the urine. It may be because paraquat is actively secreted by the renal tubules or because it is adsorbed by the dialysis membrane. The need for parenteral feeding is decided in accordance with the findings at gastroscopy. If respiratory difficulties arise, O_2 therapy should be avoided as far as possible, since it can make the lung damage worse. When O_2 administration is unavoidable, it has been suggested that the O_2 concentration should be reduced by adding nitrogen to achieve an O_2 tension of 52–60 mmHg (7–8 kPa). Various methods of therapy have been tried to arrest or reverse the pulmonary changes due to paraquat [7]. At the present time the most promising appears to be the administration of liposomal-super-oxide dismutase and glutathione-peroxidase, but it is still only experimental.

Insecticides

Organophosphorus compounds [9, 20]

These insecticides are highly toxic and it seems likely that the incidence of poisoning with them will increase, as organosphosphorus compounds are being used as substitutes for DDT following the ban on organo-chlorinated substances in some countries. Poisoning usually occurs from cutaneous absorption, or rarely, by ingestion or inhalation. Their toxicity is essentially due to the inhibition of cholinesterase; the consequent damage can be severe and may not be reversible unless the patient is treated within a few hours. Neurological upsets occur also due to the stimulant action of organic phosphates on sympathetic ganglia and cerebral centres [33].

Clinical features. Symptoms appear, usually, within 2 h of exposure. The diversity of clinical features can lead the physician to think of other pathological conditions, especially respiratory or alimentary disease. Delay in diagnosis can be life-threatening.

Bronchospasm and bronchorrhoea are usual, and acute pulmonary oedema is rare. Respiratory arrest is the usual cause of death. Sweating, lacrimation, headache, restlessness, ataxia, muscle weakness, fibrillary twitching, emotional lability, confusion, and convulsions are often misleading. The pupils may be constricted. Salivation is an important symptom. Nausea, vomiting, colic, and diarrhoea may occur. Retrosternal tightness, bradycardia, hypotension, peripheral circulatory failure are severe features. Blood cholinesterase will be less than 30% of normal. This is particularly the case in patients who are exposed to organophosphorus insecticides on a chronic basis. On occasion, when individuals are accidentally exposed for a short time, the cholinesterase may be mildly elevated; this is thought to be due to a compensatory protective mechanism.

Treatment. Further exposure must be prevented by wearing rubber gloves and removing contaminated clothing immediately, then washing the skin thoroughly with soap and water. Ethyl alcohol must be used for the final swabbing. Gastric aspiration and lavage should be carried out if poison has been ingested.

Intensive supportive therapy is necessary, with particular emphasis on the maintenance of respiration. Atropine sulphate 2 mg should be given IV and repeated at 5–10 min intervals until atropinization is achieved. Thereafter, it is essential to continue an effective dosage for at least 2 or 3 days. Atropine must not be given to a cyanosed patient, in case ventricular fibrillation is induced. It is not unusual for 50 mg atropine to be required in the first 24 h and as much as 1.5 g has been given to a child in the course of 1 day.

Pralidoxime is a specific reactivator of cholinesterase and should be used in addition to atropine. A dose of 30 mg/kg (i.e. above 1–2 g) IV should be injected at a rate not exceeding 500 mg per min, and repeated every 30 min if necessary. After injection of pralidoxime, the effect of atropine may become more evident and a reduction in the dosage schedule of the latter may be necessary.

Pralidoxime unfortunately does not cross the blood–brain barrier, and so cholinesterases in the brain remain inactivated for days and even weeks, psychic disturbances being exhibited by affected patients. An alternative preparation that does cross the blood–brain barrier and acts more quickly than pralidoxime with fewer side-effects is obidoxime (Toxogonin). This may also be combined with atropine with a good therapeutic response.

If sedation or control of convulsions is required short-acting barbiturates may be used, but with the greatest caution. Aminophylline, morphine, and phenothiazines are contraindicated. Plasma cholinesterase injections are only currently available in specialized centres.

Drug addiction

Alcohol, barbiturates and benzodiazepines represent by far the most frequent causes of hospitalisation for addiction, because of overdosages as well as withdrawal accidents.

Physical dependence on barbiturates and benzodiazepines is currently the most frequent cause of insomnia, mental confusion or convulsions, observed in Intensive Care Units.

Narcotics offer the same double aspect of addiction and withdrawal accidents.

Clinical features and narcotic addiction. Pin-point pupils are typical and may dilate with naloxone (0.4 mg IV). Transitory elation gives way to anxiety and restlessness. Loss of libido is frequent. Marked anorexia, constipation and severe weight loss are frequent. Icterus is often due to serum hepatitis from sharing syringes.

Abscesses, bruises, and septic thrombophlebitis at injection sites on the backs of the hands or in the cubital fossae are to be found. Septicaemia and tetanus are not rare. In overdosage, death may be due to prolonged apnoea or pulmonary oedema [8] (hypersensitivity, reaction to an additive, or similar to those observed during altitude hypoxia). Inhalation and bacterial pneumonias are rare. Naloxone electively reverses the respiratory depression but not the pulmonary oedema. In fact, during hospitalization, assisted respiration is safer.

Withdrawal effects. In the early stage, running nose and eyes, constant sneezing, gooseflesh, perspiration, vague aches and pains, and dilated pupils are among the withdrawal effects. Anxiety, restlessness, and aggression are common. The later 'cold turkey' stage is characterized by nausea, vomiting, abdominal pain, diarrhoea, limb cramps, sleeplessness, and further agitation leading to collapse.

Treatment. Naloxone and its slow-release form naltrexone are indicated, for diagnosis, therapy, and long-term aversion.

If it is considered necessary, withdrawal symptoms may be prevented with methadone 10–20 mg. The dose may be repeated in 1–2 h; this will control symptoms for 12 h. Clonidine has been recently introduced to prevent withdrawal symptoms and its effect emphasizes the importance of alpha receptors in physical dependence on opiates [29].

References

1. Amin-Zaki L, Mayeed MA, Clarkson TW, Greenwood MR (1978) Methylmercury poisoning in Iraqui children: Clinical observations over two years. Br Med J i:613–615
2. Bismuth C, Gaultier M, Conso F, Efthymiou ML (1975) Hyperkalemia in acute digitalis poisoning: Prognostic significance and therapeutic implications. Clin Toxicol 62: 153–162
3. Bismuth C, Gaultier M, Conso F (1977) L'aplasie médulaire de la colchicine à propos de 20 cas. Nouv Presse Med 6:1625–1629
4. Brown SS (1977) Clinical chemistry and chemical toxicology of metals. Elsevier/North Holland, Amsterdam
5. Chazan JA, Garella S (1971) Glutethimide intoxication. Arch Intern Med 128:215–219
6. Conso F, Efthymiou ML, Garnier R, Fournier E (1980) Intérêt de la toxicovigilance: Exemple de certains trichlorethylénes du commerce. Arch Mal Prof 41:198–200
7. Douze JMC, Van Heijst ANP (1977) Intensive oxygen therapy after paraquat intoxication, a real danger. Acta Pharmacol Toxicol 41 [Suppl II]:241–245
8. Duberstein JL, Kaufman DM (1971) A clinical study of an epidemic of heroin intoxication and heroin-induced pulmonary oedema. Am J Med 51:704–715
9. Frejaville JP, Bismuth C, Conso F (1980) Toxicologie clinique et analytique, 2e ed. Flammarion, Paris
10. Gaultier M, Conso F (1978) Toxicology of psychotropic drugs and its management. In: Clark WG, Giudice J (eds) Principles of psychopharmacology. Academic Press, New York, p 467
11. Graham DL, Haman D, Theodore J, Rabin ED (1977) Acute cyanide poisoning complicated by lactic acidosis and pulmonary oedema. Arch Intern Med 127:1051–1055
12. Hamburger J, Crosnier J, Grunfeld JP (1979) Nephrology. Wiley, New York. [Edition française: (1979) Néphrologie. Flammarion Médecine et Sciences, Paris]
13. Heber HW, Geissler R, Past D (1977) Hemoperfusion and hemodialysis in Cabromal intoxication. Acta pharmacol Toxicol 41 [Suppl II]:78–84
14. Hormaechea E, Carlson RW, Rogove H, Uphold J, Hemming RS, Weil MH (1979) Hypovolemia, pulmonary oedema and protein changes in severe salicylate poisoning. Am J Med 66: 1046–1050
15. Keyran-Karizarni H, Tannenberg AM (1974) Methanol intoxication. Arch Intern Med 134:193–196
16. Lechat P, Lagier G, Boiteau J (1978) Le paracétamol. Thérapie 33:551–585
17. Lhoste F, Lemaire F, Rapin M (1977) Treatment of hypotension in meprobamate poisoning. N Engl J Med 296:1004
18. Matthew H (1971) Acute barbiturate posioning. Excerpta Medica, Amsterdam
19. Matthew H (1974) Are there safer hypnotics than barbiturates? Lancet I:224
20. Matthew H, Lawson AAM (1979) Treatment of common acute poisonings, 4th edn. Churchill Livingstone, Edinburgh
21. Matthew H, Proudfoot AT, Brown SS, Smith ACA (1968) Mandrax poisoning: Conservative management of 116 patients. Br Med J ii:101–102
22. Okonek S, Baldamus CA, Hofmann A, Schuster CJ, Bechstein PB, Zoller B (1979) Two survivors of severe paraquat intoxication by continuous hemoperfusion. Klin Wochenschr 57:957–959
23. Peterson RG, Rumak BH (1977) Treating acute acetaminophen poisoning with acetyl cysteine. JAMA 237:2406–2407
24. Prescott LF, Parls J, Ballantyne A, Adriacussens P, Proudfoot AT (1977) Treatment of paracetamol (Acetaminophen) poisoning with N-acetylcysteine. Lancet II:432
25. Robaglia JL, Jouglard J (1976) Les effets indésirables du lithium. Masson, Paris (Coll Med Leg Toxicol Med No 93)
26. Sangster B, Landberg P (1980) The usefulness of physostigmine in clinical toxicology. Paper presented at a joint meeting of WHO, and the Association of Poison Control Centres, Copenhagen
27. Saran BM, Gaind R (1973) Lithium. Clin Toxicol 6:257–269
28. Smith TW, Haber E, Heathman L, Bitter VP (1975) Reversal of digoxin intoxication with digoxin specific antibodies. N Engl J Med 294:797–800
29. Solomon H, Snyder MD (1979) Receptors, neurotransmitters and drug responses. N Engl J Med 300: 465–472
30. Steyn DG (1977) Further developments in the treatment of poisoning with alkylphosphates (organosphosphate). Insecticides. Poisons Committee, State Department of Health, Pretoria, S Africa

31. Vale JA, Chrome P, Volans GN, Widdop B, Goulding R
    (1977) The treatment of Paraquat poisoning using oral
    sorbents and charcoal haemoperfusion. Acta pharmacol
    Toxicol 41 [Suppl II]:109–117
32. Vesey CJ, Cole PV, Simpson PJ (1976) Cyanide and
    thiocyanate concentrations following sodium nitroprus-
    side infusion in man. Br J Anaesth 48:651–660
33. Ward DE, Jones B (1976) Glucagon and beta-blocker
    toxicity. Br Med J ii:151

Chapter 50

Accidental Hypothermia

B. Regnier and A. Harari

Since the first half of the twentieth century, hypothermia has been extensively investigated. In an excellent review, Swan [87] outlined the beneficial effects of hypothermia that had already been mentioned in ancient medical texts. Our current knowledge of the subject comes from its clinical applications in cancer, psychiatry, and above all, in cardiac, vascular, and neurosurgery and transplantation.

In the future it is possible that the fascinating field of hypothermia will have other applications. Nevertheless, the problem of hibernation still poses significant problems because the tolerance of membrane phospholipids and cold-labile enzyme systems currently limit the viability of organisms in deep hypothermia even though a basic cell metabolism persists.

Accidental hypothermia is common but much of our understanding of its pathophysiology is derived from induced hypothermia. In addition to its clinical features, it is important to examine the epidemiology, the prevention, and the management; these aspects have been reviewed in the book of MacLean and Emslie-Smith [46], and in this chapter we will only consider accidental hypothermia in adults.

Aetiology

As a rule, two factors are associated in the causation of accidental hypothermia: first, exposure to the cold environment and second, disorders interfering with the thermoregulatory mechanisms. Depending upon the countries, the relative importance of these in reported cases varies with exposure predominating in the colder areas.

Exposure

Mountain casualties and cold water immersion are the commonest causes of exposure hypothermia, and in addition to other injuries and drowning, hypothermia alone is responsible for many deaths each year. Numerous reports especially from mountaineering societies and military establishments, have provided knowledge of the features, prevention, and management of this form of hypothermia [6, 36, 68].

Cold environment

In mountains, hypothermia can develop quickly and it is worth emphasizing that the frequency of exposure hypothermia is paradoxically higher in warm climates than in cold countries where awareness of the problem results in adequate prevention.

The factors that favour the onset of hypothermia include cold environment; contact with snow or wet clothes, which both increase heat loss by conduction; exercise and wind, which increase loss by convection; and poor clothing insulation, especially of the legs, which are often badly protected by non-waterproof trousers [68]. On the other hand, heat production compensates to some extent for heat loss, but the metabolic rate has to be markedly increased and this depends upon the exercise capacity of the particular individual. In addition, in cold environments, the O_2 intake has been found to be twice the level expected for a similar degree of exercise carried out in warm air [68]. It is obvious therefore that so long as heat loss exceeds heat production the body temperature will fall, and this in itself will produce abnormal behaviour with a reduction in exercise and hence reduction of heat production. Body cooling accelerates and the individual usually sits or lies down, the hypothermia continuing its relentless progression.

Immersion

The rate of heat loss in water is approximately 25 times that in air of the same temperature, and the annual incidence of immersion hypothermia is increasing. This is probably due to the use of lifejackets which prevent drowning [27]. The rate of body cooling depends on several factors: the temperature of the water, the insulation of the body, the movements of the subject, the individual body build, and the level of training (capacity to increase metabolic rate). Below a water temperature of 20°–21°C, heat loss is likely to exceed heat production; in this respect it is noteworthy that 50% of the Atlantic Ocean is below 20°C, and moreover in Britain and the north of France, mean water temperature varies between 8° and 15°C throughout the year, river temperatures commonly falling to 5°–10°C in the winter [46]. Clothing, even if not waterproofed, protects against cold immersion. For instance, an unclothed man will die after 20–30 min immersion in water at 5°C, and after 1.5–2 h at 15°C, but if conventionally clothed he will survive for 40–60 min at 5°C and 4–5 h at 15°C [36].

Subcutaneous fat is also a very good insulator, and therefore most women and fat men will cool more slowly than thin men.

Finally, cutaneous vasoconstriction is very efficient in preventing heat loss, and the skin blood flow has been shown to vary as much as 0.2–3.5 litres/min. Exercise invariably increases heat loss due to a redistribution of the warmed water layer surrounding the body and to an increase in blood flow toward the superficial tissues [27].

Nevertheless, in spite of these known facts, it is difficult to predict a tolerance time according to the temperature of the water. Thus, even in water below 10°C an obese woman, provided she keeps still, can preserve her central body temperature. By contrast, the core temperature of a thin man swimming in water at 15°C can drop to 34°C within 1 h.

Accidental causes

Many disorders may facilitate the onset of accidental hypothermia and they are summarized in Fig. 50.1 according to their mode of interference with the regulation of body temperature. The mechanisms basically include decrease in heat production, increase in heat loss, and impairment of the neural control of thermoregulation.

Neurological disorders

A wide variety of neurological lesions are involved. Coma is often associated with hypothalamic dysfunction, and may of course lead to a degree of cold exposure, resulting, for example, from lying on snow or, more commonly, the floor of a non-heated room. The commonest causes of coma associated with hypothermia include stroke, drug intoxication following either overdose or self-poisoning, and acute ethanol intoxication; barbiturate self-poisoning is frequently involved. Encephalitis, hypothalamic disease, hyperosmolarity, and ketoacidosis are less frequent. Lesions of the spinal cord result in paralysis, with loss of both shivering and control of vasomotor activity, and in some cases, perception of cold can be abolished.

Increased heat loss

Poor insulation increases heat loss and both ethanol and drug intoxication commonly produce vasodilatation. In this context, it is of practical interest to recall that alcohol should not be given to hypothermic mountaineers or immersed patients, because despite the pleasant feeling of warmth engendered, heat loss ensues and accelerates the fall in body temperature. In the elderly and malnourished loss of the subcutaneous layer of fat decreases the degree of insulation. Heat loss is also increased from extensive areas of erythrodermia.

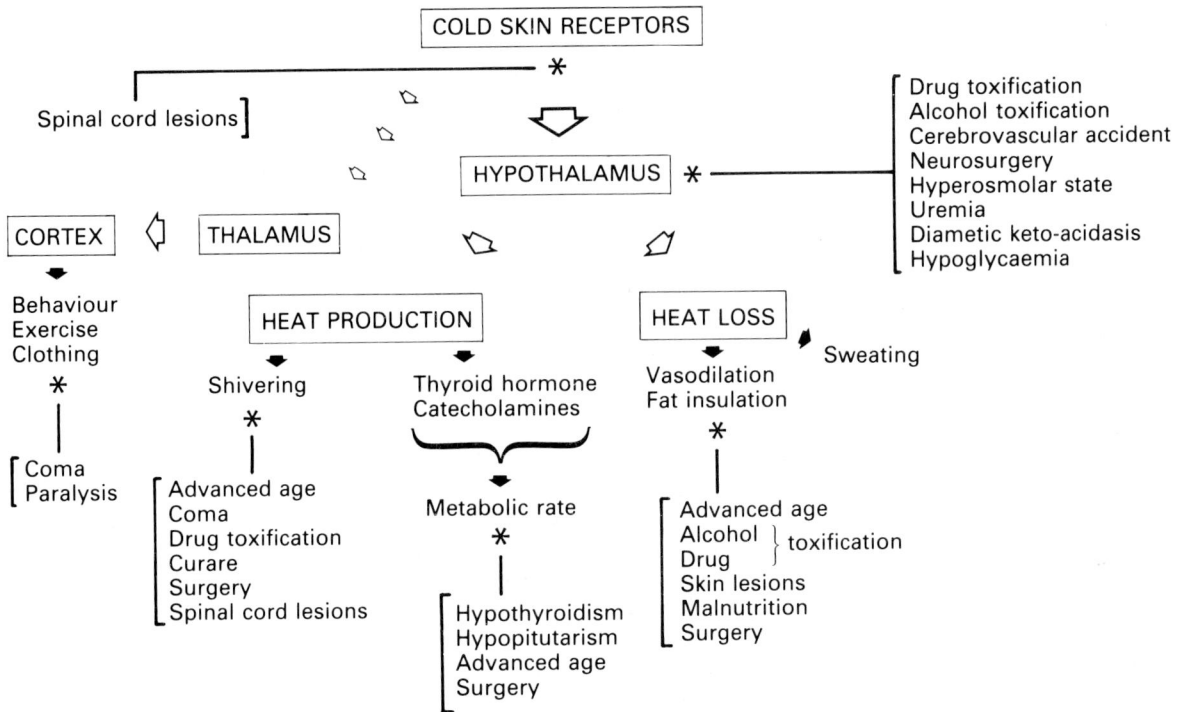

Fig. 50.1. *Disorders predisposing to accidental hypothermia.* Both the cortex (via the thalamus) and the hypothalamic centres are connected to cold skin receptors. Cold stimulation leads to increased heat production while heat loss is reduced. Heat production depends upon shivering, exercise, and metabolic rate. Heat loss is accounted for by vasodilatation and sweating.

Decreased heat production

A decrease in heat production can result from either a fall in metabolic rate, or a reduction in muscular activity. Myxoedema, hypopituitarism, and malnutrition are all associated with a decreased metabolic rate. Impairment of shivering is usual in spinal cord lesions, hypothalamic disorders, and curarized patients, and may be common in the elderly. Lack of mobility due to paralysis or other causes will interfere substantially with heat production.

Sepsis

Hypothermia may result from Gram-negative septicaemia, and if it is sustained it usually implies a grave prognosis [38].

Associated disorders

As mentioned, drug and ethanol intoxication are among the commonest causes of hypothermia, and dysfunction of the hypothalamus, vasodilatation, and coma, all combine to make the core temperature fall.

In the elderly a depressed metabolic rate, reduced fat insulation, muscular inactivity, impaired shivering, and cutaneous vasoconstriction together with inadequate social provisions all predispose to hypothermia [9, 10]. Epidemiological studies have shown that as many as 2.5%–3.6% of elderly patients admitted to hospital had body temperatures below 35°C [67].

In the operating room, many factors favour a fall in body temperature. Anaesthesia impairs hypothalamic function, inhibits shivering, and is generally associated with vasodilatation. Large quantities of cold blood or its substitutes may be infused, and wide exposure of the peritoneum, especially if washed with cold solutes, contributes to enhance the loss of heat.

Clinical features

Much of the clinical picture has been accurately reported in several publications [17, 18, 34, 41]. The clinical presentation depends upon both the depth and the duration of hypothermia, and it must be remembered that any underlying disorder will impose its own symptoms and signs.

Common clinical thermometers only measure temperatures above 34°C, and therefore when the rectal temperature is found to approach 34°C it is appropriate to use specially designed low-reading thermometers, since otherwise severe hypothermia may be missed.

From a diagnostic and prognostic point of view, hypothermia can be classified according to its degree, although the duration is also important. At temperatures above 33°C only mild manifestations are seen which do not cause any problems, since thermoregulatory mechanisms are still able to compensate. Below 29°–30°C, neurological and cardiovascular dysfunction are severe and life-threatening, and the regulatory systems becomes inactive. Temperatures between 29° and 33°C constitute an intermediate zone. Below 27°–28°C, hypothermia can mimic death and if historical information is lacking it may be impossible to distinguish hypothermic cardiac arrest from death [16]: "No-one is dead until warm and dead" [28]. MacLean considers that the only criterion for death is "the failure to revive on rewarming" [46]. Neurological manifestations become obvious at about 33°C, when dysarthria and slowness of understanding and speaking are first noted. At 30°C the patient becomes stuporous, dysarthria increases, voluntary movements become infrequent, slow, delayed, and sometimes incoordinated. Physical examination reveals hypertonicity, sluggish tendon reflexes (Fig. 50.2) and flexor plantar responses. Below 27°C, consciousness is abolished, there is no longer any voluntary movement, hypertonicity is more pronounced, tendon reflexes and plantar response disappear, pupillary light reaction is lost, and the pupils may be dilated or constricted. Nevertheless, there is no consistent relationship between body temperature and clinical findings during either cooling or rewarming. In this respect, patients as cold as 28°C have been reported with only mild neurological changes, and it is likely that both the rate of cooling and the duration of hypothermia play a role in determining the physical findings. Cardiac and circulatory activity are depressed in proportion to the fall in temperature. Initially, there is marked cutaneous vasoconstriction affecting both small arteries and veins, which accounts for the cold, purple skin prevalent on the hands and feet. The heart rate gradually falls, but as with the neurological changes it is not possible to predict heart rate from temperature. It commonly reaches 30–40 beats/min at about 28°–29°C, and 10 beats/min at 25°–26°C. At lower temperatures rates as low as 1–3 beats/min have been reported. Arterial pressure is initially normal, but below 30°C it begins to fall and the pulse weakens. Systolic and mean arterial pressure decrease more than the diastolic. At very low

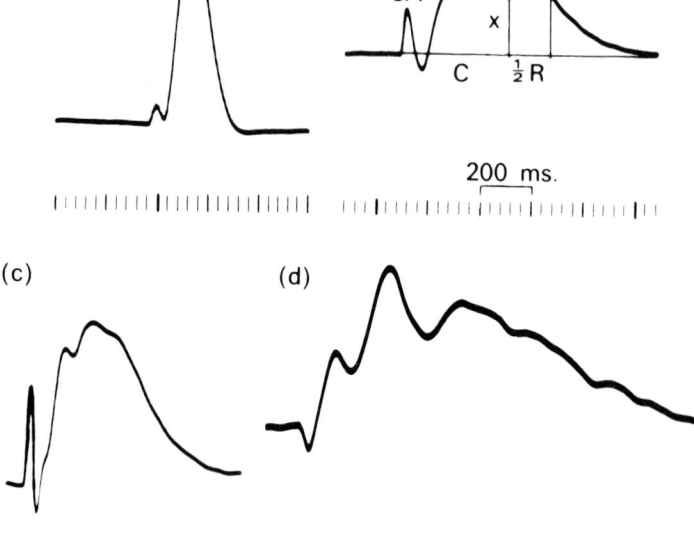

Fig. 50.2. *Achilles tendon reflex in hypothermia and myxoedema.* **a** Euthyroid, euthermic; **b** Euthyroid, hypothermic; **c** Hypothyroid, euthermic; **d** Hypothothyroid, hypothermic. *SA*, stimulus artefact; *PC*, peak contraction; *C*, contraction time; $\frac{1}{2}R$, half-relaxation time. From MacLean and Emslie-Smith [46].

temperatures (25°–28°C) the arterial pressure is no longer measurable and the pulse is impalpable. Below 33°–34°C respiration is slow and shallow, with a rate commonly ranging from 10–15 beats/min and occasionally less [17].

Pathophysiology

Sufficient knowledge is now available to enable us to understand most of the clinical findings in hypothermia, and to formulate a rational programme of treatment. Nevertheless, correct analysis must attempt to distinguish the consequences of thermoregulation from the direct effects of cold on the various systems. The initial clinical and physiological changes result from both the decreasing temperature and the thermoregulatory adjustments. Thereafter, when core temperature falls below 29°C, thermoregulation is inhibited and the changes seen reflect the direct consequences of the cold. Moreover, in much of the published experimental data it is important to separate the effects of anaesthesia from those of a falling temperature.

As a rule, all biological functions slow with cooling, and each process has a temperature coefficient which determines the degree of reduction. The Q10 is the magnitude of the decreased activity for a 10°C drop in temperature. For instance, the Q10 is 3 in metabolic and rhythmical processes and 2 in contractile processes, whereas physical processes, such as diffusion, have a Q10 of 1 [46].

Metabolic changes

The metabolic rate, expressed as the oxygen consumption ($\dot{V}O_2$), gradually decreases with core temperature. Nevertheless, Thauer showed that changes related to cooling were associated with changes induced by thermoregulation (Fig. 50.3). In unanaesthetized animals, $\dot{V}O_2$ initially increases and shivering occurs to increase heat production. But as core temperature decreases thermoregulation is inhibited, and $\dot{V}O_2$ falls markedly to values identical with the $\dot{V}O_2$ measured in anaesthetized animals [88]. These results are similar to those found in man by Rosomoff [76]. Thus $\dot{V}O_2$ is reduced by 25% at 32°C, 50% at 28°C, 75% at 20°C, and nearly 90% at 10°C (Fig. 50.3). Our own data, recorded in accidental hypothermia support the experimental findings. $\dot{V}O_2$ calculated from cardiac index

and arteriovenous O_2 difference was decreased by 25%–30% at 32°C and 42% at about 30°C [30]. Moreover, we compared these data with $\dot{V}O_2$ recorded in hypothermic myxoedema and as shown in Fig. 50.4, $\dot{V}O_2$ was more depressed in myxoedematous patients even when they were warmed.

Neurological changes

Hypothermia depresses the metabolic rate of the brain and spinal cord [49]. The utilization of glucose and the production of lactic acid are reduced. The prevention of brain hypoxia is strikingly illustrated by the case of a boy who was accidentally submerged for 40 min in a frozen river and who subsequently completely recovered [82].

It is generally recognized that hypothermic neurological changes are similar to those of general anaesthesia. The amplitude of the EEG begins to decrease between 32°C and 36°C, but the frequency is only slightly affected.

These alterations occur first in the occipital and parietal areas, and then in the frontal region. Slow delta waves of large amplitude can be seen at about 30°C, and as the temperature falls further, delta and theta waves become more frequent, with disorganization at about 20°–25°C. Paroxysmal spike activity can be seen at 20°C, but electrical activity eventually disappears at about 17°C [49, 61].

In the peripheral nervous system the conduction velocity gradually decreases. Tendon reflex responses are considerably slowed and muscular contraction and relaxation are equally prolonged. Thus direct muscle percussion elicits a very slow, palpable response. MacLean showed that both myxoedema and hypothermia prolong the contraction and the relaxation phases of the Achilles tendon reflex, but myxoedema prolongs the relaxation phase more than the contraction phase (Fig. 50.2) [46].

Respiratory changes

Changes in the mechanical properties of the lung and in the pulmonary circulation remain questionable. Lung compliance has been found to be decreased [15] or unchanged [66, 77]. Similarly, studies of dead space volume remain controversial [15, 51, 66]. Alveolocapillary transfer [31, 60] and the respiratory responses to hypoxaemia or acidosis [5], however, are generally considered to be depressed, but this is probably not of great practical significance. By

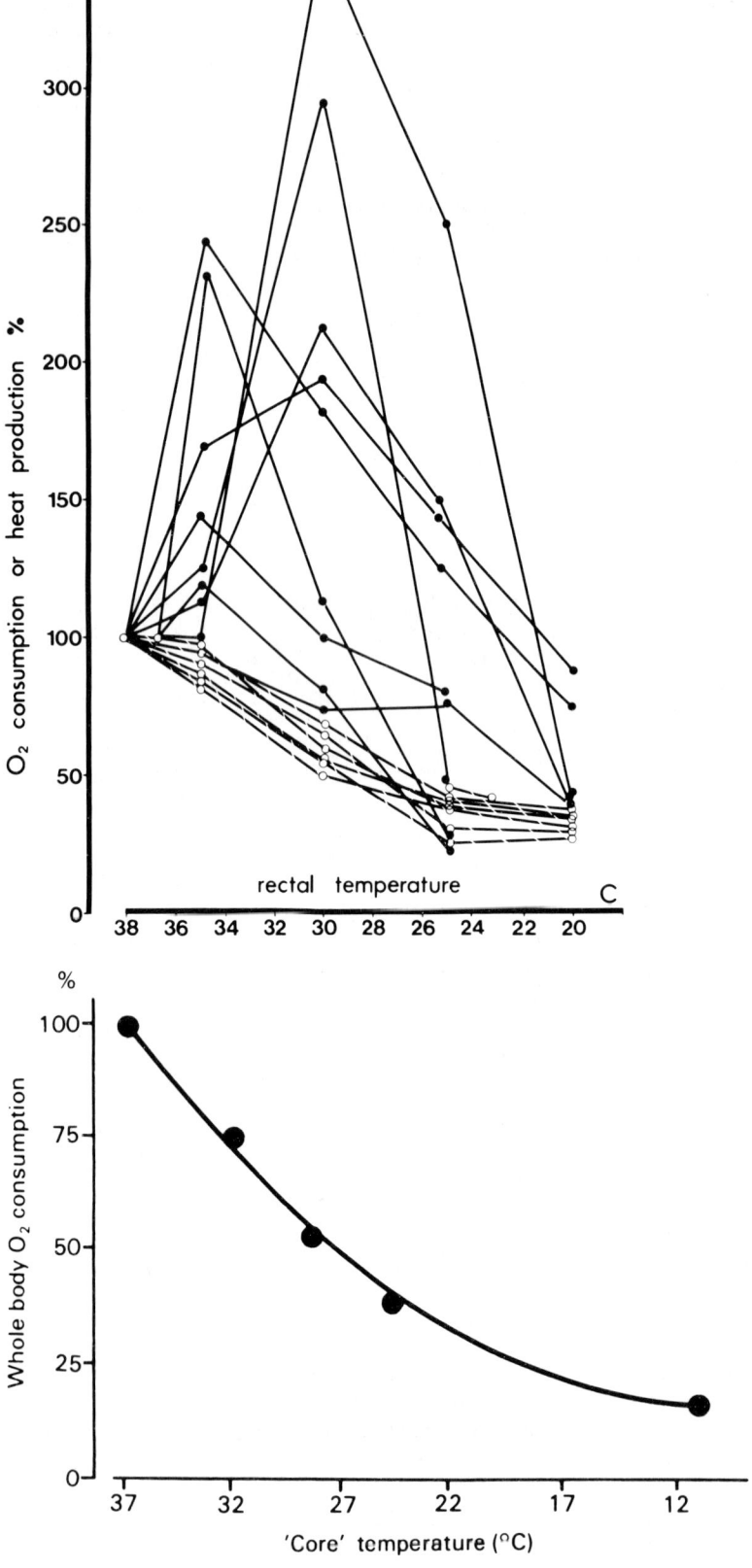

Fig. 50.3. *Metabolic rate in hypothermia.* The upper part of the figure, from Thauer [88], shows that $\dot{V}O_2$ gradually fell with body temperature in anaesthetized animals (*circles* and *dotted lines*). By contrast, in unanaesthetized animals the VO_2 increased dramatically as rectal temperature began to fall. But at 25°C, the VO_2 abruptly dropped to the same values as in anaesthetized animals at 20%C (*closed circles and solid lines*) The *lower* part of the figure, from Maclean and Emslie-Smith [46], shows the mean metabolic rate related to core temperature.

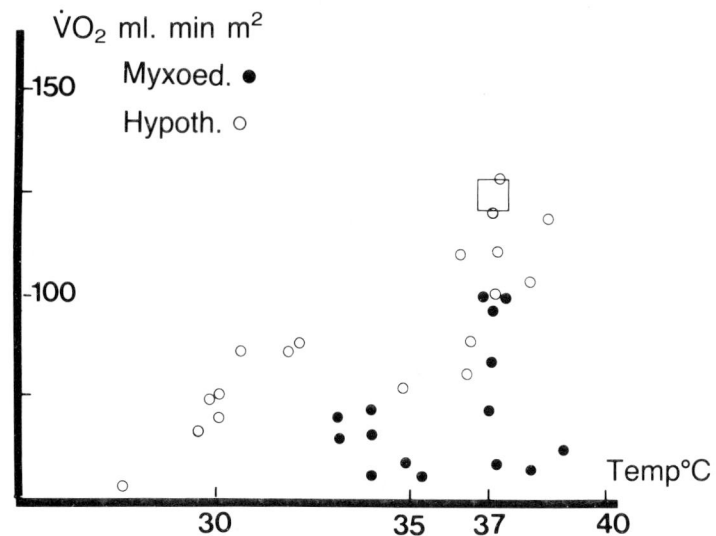

Fig. 50.4. *Oxygen consumption in hypothermia.* Patients suffering from accidental hypothermia (*open circles*) compared with patients with hypothermic myxoedema (*closed circles*). For the same core temperature the myxoedema patients showed a greater depression of metabolic rate. The *square* represents the resting normal value.

contrast, it is of interest to note the prevalence of ventilation abnormalities and of secondary bronchopulmonary infection [52, 72]. Many clinical studies have revealed such complications, usually arising during or after rewarming. Changes in arterial O_2 and CO_2 tension are still debated. Respiratory rate and tidal and minute volume are all reduced but are still adequate to meet the demands of both O_2 requirement and CO_2 elimination. The fundamental question relates to the laboratory determination of these blood gas tensions. Temperature markedly affects gas tensions in a sealed sample of blood, and the laboratory measurements are performed at electrode temperatures of 37°–38°C: Fig. 50.5 shows the magnitude of these changes. A PO_2 of 100 mmHg (13.3 kPa) and a PCO_2 of 40 mmHg (5.3 kPa) measured at 37°C become, respectively, 50 and 22.5 mmHg (6.7 and 3 kPa) at 25°C, and 126 and 47 mmHg (16.8 and 6.3 kPa) at 41°C. Conversely, if normal values of 100 and 40 mmHg (13.3 and 5.3 kPa) are required at the patient's temperature, laboratory values should be, respectively, 130 and 56 mmHg (17.3 and 7.5 kPa) for a patient at 30°C, and 155 and 71 mmHg (20.7 and 9.5 kPa) for a patient at 25°C.

If corrected to the patient's temperature, the arterial PO_2 is constantly lowered [48, 51, 58, 70] and values as low as 25–50 mmHg are common. There are several reasons for this hypoxaemia, such as decreased alveolar ventilation and an increased arteriolar–alveolar gradient related either to decreased gas transfer or to an imbal-ance of ventilation to perfusion [52]. Nevertheless, there is no evidence to suggest that such a low PaO_2 has detrimental effects. It is argued that, owing to the decreased tissue O_2 requirements, a low PaO_2 can achieve correct O_2 delivery, which is also facilitated by increased O_2 solubility. Both the inconstancy of increases in blood lactic acid [58], and normal AV O_2 differences [5, 30] are further indicators that the hypoxaemia is well tolerated and that there is no need to correct the gas tensions. Nevertheless, if indeed the hypoxaemia is tolerable it must also be emphasized that there are many factors that can abruptly disturb the delicate equilibrium. For instance, shivering (which is not always evident clinically) will suddenly and markedly increase O_2 demand. Active rewarming also results in a rapid rise in metabolic rate, greatly exceeding that at the same temperature during cooling [73]. Lastly, there is probably a wide variation in the demands of the various tissues which makes a low PO_2 more or less well tolerated, it is therefore important to ensure a high PaO_2 when rewarming is started.

There is a wide scattering of reported arterial PCO_2 values in hypothermia [52]. Reduced metabolism lowers PCO_2, whereas a reduced alveolar ventilation and increased solubility of CO_2 combine to increase the PCO_2. Thus, depending upon the prevalent factors, either a low PCO_2 [74, 79], or a respiratory acidosis can ensue [52]. If artificial ventilation is initiated, hypocapnia can readily develop and may be deleterious for hypothermia produces a leftward shift of the oxyhaemoglobin dissociation curve and this is further accentuated by hypocapnia. The resultant increased affinity of O_2 for haemoglobin threatens O_2 delivery. In addition, hypocapnia could theoretically increase peripheral vasoconstriction, and for clinical purposes, it is certainly important to pay attention to the PCO_2, especially in ventilated patients.

Finally, the need to correct PO_2 and PCO_2 remains questionable [51]. In a recent inquiry, carried out in 25 blood-gas laboratories, Hansen reported that 14 of them corrected both gas tensions and pH for the patient's temperature. He eventually concluded that for therapeutic purposes such correction is not necessary, whereas for physiological purposes the measured values should be corrected [29]. If it is considered that a correction must be made then the values can be derived from nomograms [2, 37, 80]; these decrease PCO_2 by some 4.4% and PO_2 by about 7% for each 1 deg. C of fall in body temperature.

Acid–base changes

Temperature also interferes with pH assessment. A fall of 1 deg. C in the temperature of sealed blood increases the pH by 0.0147 unit [75]. As pH is measured at electrode temperature (38°C), corrected values can be derived either from nomograms [37], or from Rosenthal's equation:

$$\text{blood pH} = \text{pH at } 38°C + 0.0147\,(38\text{-}t)$$

where t is the patient's temperature expressed in degrees centigrade.

Acidosis is frequent in hypothermic patients; it is commonly metabolic but sometimes both metabolic and respiratory acidosis coexist. Although inconstant [58], lactic and pyruvic acid levels are generally increased [22, 32, 62], presumably due to hypoxia, for many factors combine to reduce the tissue O_2 supply. These include an O_2 debt incurred either during cooling or rewarming, a low PO_2, and high affinity of O_2 for haemoglobin, hypocapnia, intense vasoconstriction, and increased blood viscosity. In addition, acidosis can readily develop during rewarming, due to the sudden return to the systemic circulation of large amounts of organic acids retained in tissue whilst the microcirculation was impaired, and by an increased muscle lactic acid production from shivering. The situation is aggravated by an impaired extraction of lactic acid by the liver [74] and a reduced renal capacity to excrete hydrogen ions [55, 78].

Renal changes

Cold exposure can quickly cause a diuresis, even before the central body temperature falls. It is generally agreed that skin vasoconstriction results in a shift of blood from superficial vascular beds to deep capacitance vessels; the so-called cold diuresis could be related to that mechanism, as could the loss of electrolytes and water that continues as the hypothermia progresses.

Hypothermia is commonly associated with renal failure, the incidence being related to the depth and duration of the hypothermia and resolves within the 24–48 h following rewarming; it is probably due to a reduced renal blood flow and defects in tubular transport.

Except during cardiac surgical bypass [25], the renal blood flow is constantly reduced [55, 74], by up to 60% at about 28°–30°C [46, p. 101]. Active tubular transfer is depressed, presumably due to the inhibition of enzymatic processes [7, 25, 55]. As a result, the urine gradually becomes dilute and nearly iso-osmotic to plasma; the tubules become insensitive to antidiuretic hormone. Finally, despite the low creatinine clearance, which accounts for the increased blood urea, diuresis is preserved, and polyuria may occur; natriuresis is also increased. By contrast oliguria has been reported in some instances, although no particular associated features have been found [52].

Although renal function commonly returns to normal, some patients with acute renal failure have been reported who required dialysis but who eventually recovered [24]. It is still not clear whether hypothermia alone can damage the kidney, and despite a reported case of chronic renal failure following hypothermia, it is difficult to rule out all the other factors that could affect the kidney [50].

Miscellaneous changes

Acute pancreatitis

The serum amylase is commonly elevated and many necropsies have shown oedematous, necrotizing, or haemorrhagic pancreatitis [17, 18, 45, 58, 67, 69, 70]. Nevertheless, the relation of pancreatitis to hypothermia is still unsolved.

It is a complication that is occasionally the cause of death after the patient has been rewarmed. Besides the amylasaemia, other enzymes are commonly found to be increased, such as creatine phosphokinase (CPK), aminotransferases (GOT and GPT), and hydroxybutyrate dehydrogenase (HBD) [47,92].

Gastric erosion

Acute gastroduodenal erosion and haemorrhage are sometimes mentioned [17, 24, 70], and are confirmed by the frequency of mucosal and submucosal erosions found at necropsy [8, 58]. Perforated duodenal ulcers have also been reported [48, 70], but it is not clear whether these lesions are directly related to the hypothermia. Obviously, in such critically ill patients there are many other well-known factors capable of producing acute gastric erosions.

Hyperglycaemia

A raised blood glucose level is common but it must be kept in mind that glycosuria may be noted without hyperglycaemia, for tubular transfer of glucose is impaired.

There are many metabolic changes that can affect the extent of the blood sugar change. It has been shown that in hypothermia glucose utilization by the tissues is inhibited either due to a resistance to the action of insulin on cell membrane transfer, or by an inactivation of hexokinase [32]. Similarly, initial liver glycogen breakdown, raised adrenocortical activity, and pancreatitis all influence the blood glucose level. Recently Stoner et al. stated that the apparent discrepancy between certain clinical reports could be accounted for by changing metabolic patterns as hypothermia deepens and is prolonged. Initially glucose is released from liver glycogen; and thereafter the utilization of glucose is first increased and finally depressed. These authors also demonstrated that plasma cortisol was high and probably contributed to the mobilization of body fuel stores; lipolysis and protein breakdown are associated. They finally concluded that no metabolic intervention is advisable [84]. For therapeutic purposes it must be emphasized that, unless hyperglycaemia is severe, insulin should not be used, because profound hypoglycaemia may follow during rewarming.

Coagulation

In man thrombocytopenia has been reported in hypothermia. Experimental studies have demonstrated a gradual fall in platelet count [46]. It has been experimentally suggested that in dogs, hepatic and splenic sequestration could account for this thrombocytopenia [64]. Neither thrombocytopenia nor miscellaneous coagulation changes [58], seem to be of particular clinical significance, however.

Cardiovascular changes

Overall

As already stressed, when man is exposed to a cold environment, the observed cardiovascular changes are due to thermoregulatory adjustments and the direct effects of the falling temperature on the heart, vessels, blood volume and viscosity. Figure 50.6 illustrates the circulatory changes in a man exposed to a cold and a hot temperature. When the ambient temperature is decreased from a neutral 28°C to 6°C, the systemic vascular resistances increase and there is a moderate elevation of diastolic arterial pressure and a slight decrease in both cardiac output and stroke volume, which may be a consequence of the increased afterload. Thereafter shivering occurs, with vasodilatation presumably in the muscles, and an increase in stroke volume, heart rate, and cardiac output to support the considerable increase in O_2 consumption [89].

Cold-induced

Thauer reviewed both experimental and clinical data correlating cardiac output and central body temperature (Fig. 50.7). Depending upon inhibition of thermoregulation by anaesthesia, two patterns of response have been observed. In unanaesthetized animals cardiac output initially increases to meet thermoregulatory requirements. Thereafter the suppression of thermoregulation by hypothermia accounts for a dramatic fall in cardiac output, similar to that observed in anaesthetized men and animals in whom body temperature closely parallels the decrease in cardiac output [88].

Brendel summarized the complete circulatory consequences of hypothermia in anaesthetized dogs [88]. As shown in Fig. 50.7, metabolic rate (expressed as O_2 consumption) and cardiac output gradually fall. The decrease in cardiac output results from bradycardia, whereas stroke volume remains constant and in spite of marked vasoconstriction, as documented by the increase in total peripheral resistance, mean arterial pressure decreases, with a marked drop below 25°C.

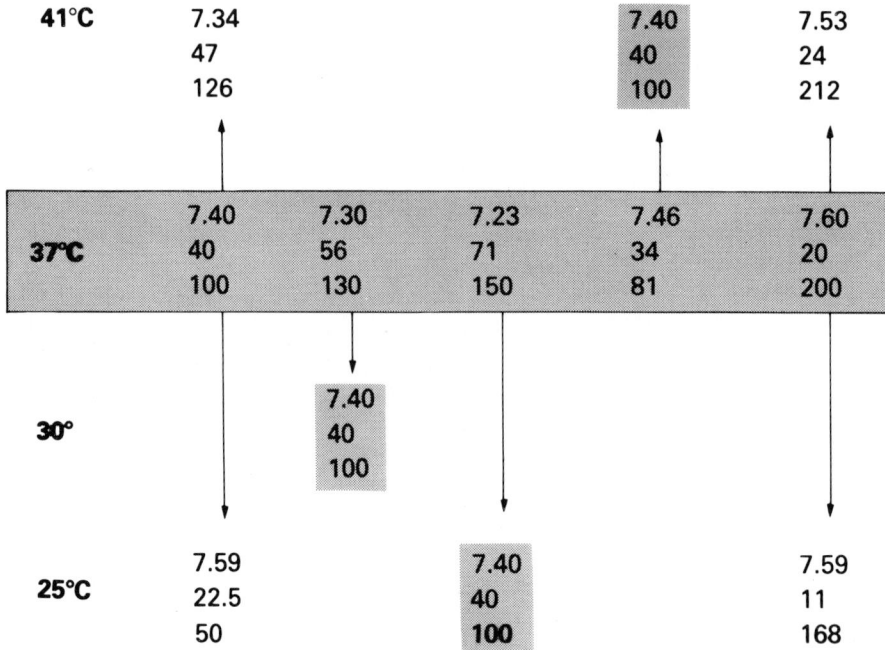

41°C	7.34			7.40	7.53
	47			40	24
	126			100	212

37°C	7.40	7.30	7.23	7.46	7.60
	40	56	71	34	20
	100	130	150	81	200

30°		7.40			
		40			
		100			

25°C	7.59		7.40		7.59
	22.5		40		11
	50		100		168

Fig. 50.5. *Gas tension and pH changes with temperature.* The *hatched area* represents the values measured at electrode temperature (37°–38°C). With standard formula or normograms, the corrected values are derived and indicated by *arrows*. The *shaded areas* indicate normal acid–base and gas tension values. It can be seen that normal pH and gas tensions at the patient's temperature indicate acidosis, hypercapnia, and hyperoxia when measured in the laboratory. Similarly, when measured pH is normal it means that an alkalosis exists in the hypothermic patient. If measured PO_2 and PCO_2 are within normal limits it signifies that the patient's values are low. The values obtained in a hyperthermic patient are also shown, to give a clearer illustration of the magnitude of the alterations.

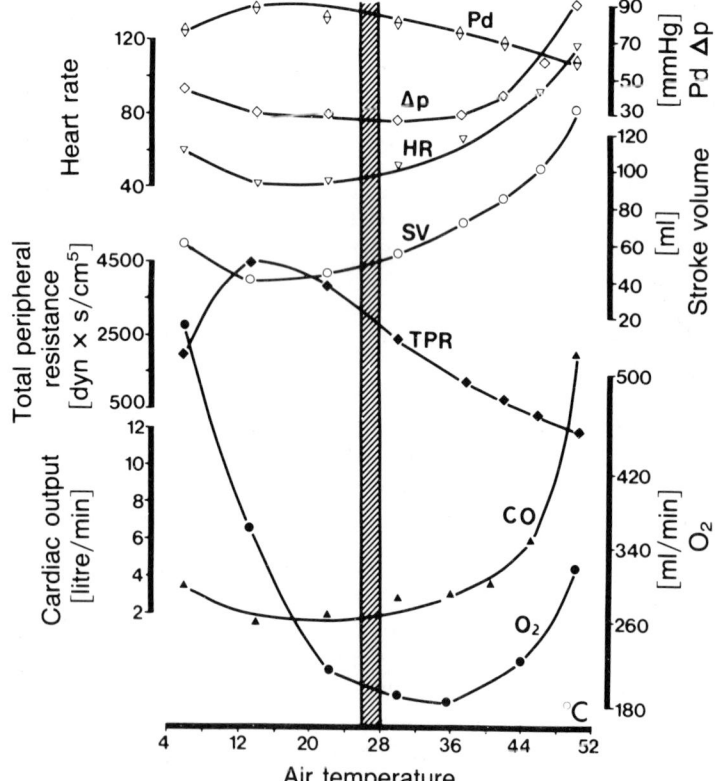

Fig. 50.6. *Cardiovascular changes related to environmental air temperature.* Changes in diastolic pressure (*Pd*), pulse pressure (*Δp*), heart rate (*HR*), stroke volume (*SV*), total peripheral resistance (*TPR*), cardiac output (*CO*), and O_2 consumption (*O_2*), in a naked resting, young man submitted to air temperatures ranging from +6° to +50°C (relative humidity 50%). From Thauer [89].

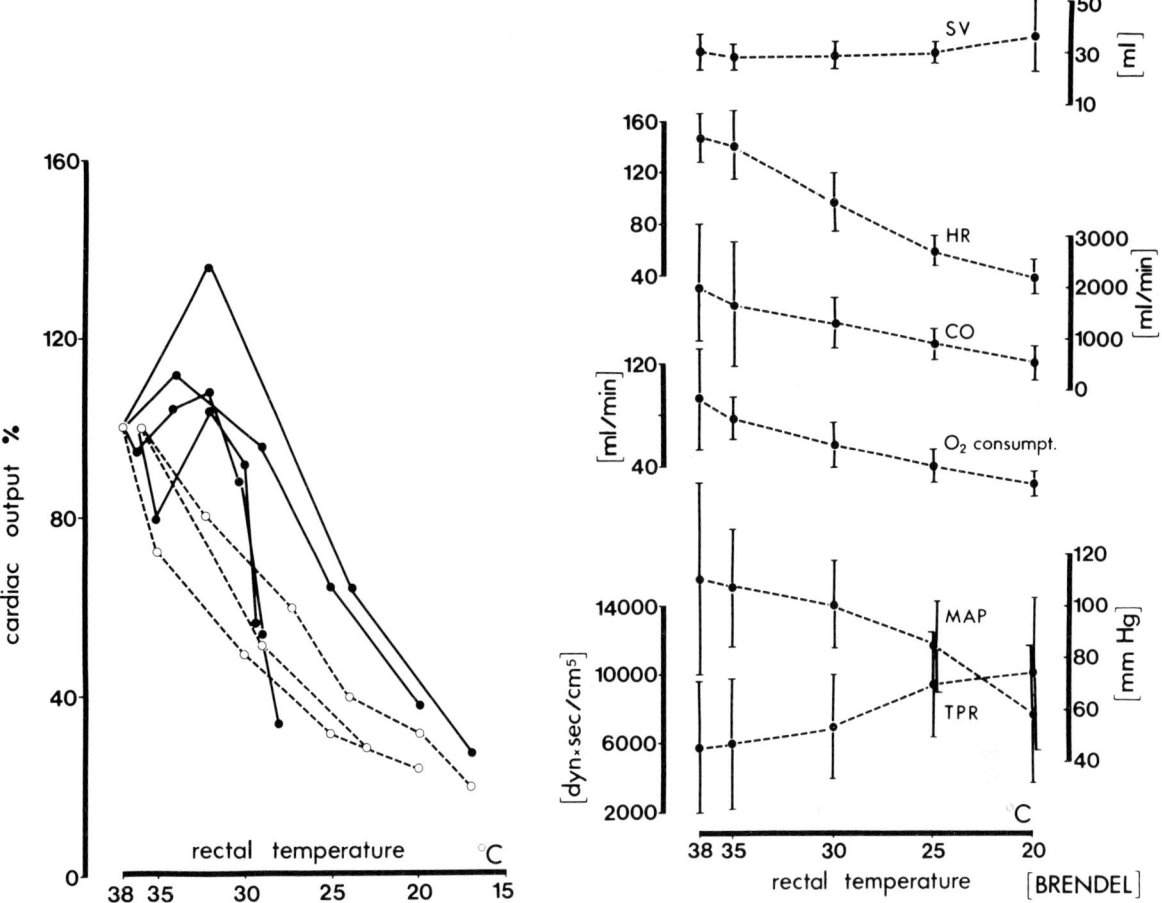

Fig. 50.7. *Cardiovascular changes in hypothermia.* On the *left*, data reviewed by Thauer [88] show clearly that in anaesthetized men and animals the cardiac output gradually falls with core temperature (*open circles, dotted lines*). By contrast, in unanaesthetized animals the drop in temperature is first associated with an increased cardiac output (*closed circles, solid lines*). At low temperatures, as thermoregulation is inhibited the cardiac output falls to the same level as that in anaesthetized animals. On the *right*, Brendel's summarized results the changes recorded in a surface-cooled dog. (*SV*, stroke volume; *HR*, heart rate; *CO*, cardiac output; O_2, oxygen consumption; *MAP*, mean arterial pressure; *TPR*, total peripheral resistances [88].

Clearly it could be that circulatory function is accurately adapted to metabolic rate. In deep hypothermia the cardiac index is commonly found to be as low as 1–1.5 litres/min per m² [30]. Accepting this interpretation, it is of interest to analyse the mechanisms that account for such a slowing of cardiovascular function. *Hypovolaemia.* In six patients with accidental hypothermia, whose central temperatures ranged from 26.3° to 28.2°C on admission, we found a haemodynamic pattern compatible with hypovolaemia [30]. Unfortunately, blood volume expansion had already been performed in three patients. In the three non-treated patients the cardiac index averaged 1.58 litres/min per m², whereas pulmonary artery wedge pressure

(PWP) was 1.6 mmHg and right atrial pressure (RAP) 1.25 mmHg. In the treated patients, despite fluid therapy with 1250–2600 ml colloid solutions, the cardiac index was 2.37 litres/min per m², and PWP and RAP were 10 and 5 mmHg respectively. Moreover, in these latter patients central venous pressure measured on admission was zero.

In the six patients, 500–2000 ml (mean = 1300) gelatin solution was infused over a mean period of 75 min. The cardiac index increased from 1.44 to 2.62 litres/min per m², mainly related to an increase in stroke volume (from 28.2 to 39.2 ml/beat per m²), whereas the heart rate accelerated only slightly, from 54 to 62 beats/min. Mean PWP and RAP rose from 1.6 to

13.5 mmHg and from 0.5 to 9.5 mmHg, respectively. Such an improvement in cardiac output associated with normal ventricular filling pressures strongly suggests hypovolaemia.

In five patients blood volume was measured with the Cr51-tagged red cell method. The total fluid volume and the red cell volume were found to be decreased to 70% and 60% of theoretical values, respectively [70]. Although under these conditions such measurements are controversial, our results are supported by other clinical observations [36, 57, 58], and experimental studies.

Data from several experimental works are summarized in Fig. 50.8. In anaesthetized dogs D'Amato found a 12% decrease in plasma volume at 20°C. As plasma specific gravity and the erythrocyte volume were not changed he concluded that there was a loss of whole plasma rather than of plasma water [13]. Later he demonstrated a 17% fall in thiocyanate space, which correlates with extracellular fluid, and therefore suggested that the plasma loss could be the result of trapping in peripherally vasoconstricted vessels from which erythocytes are excluded. In addition, the assessment of muscle

water and chloride (the latter being assumed to be extracellular) showed an intracellular space expansion [12]. Fedor further confirmed a decrease in plasma volume, while red cell volume remained constant. He also showed that following rewarming plasma volume increased substantially beyond control values [19]. Klussman confirmed these results but found that when the dogs were splenectomized hypothermia reduced both plasma and erythrocyte volumes [88].

It is therefore reasonable to acknowledge that there is a plasma volume reduction and a trend toward intracellular overhydration; the red cell volume can be affected by many other disorders which account for the wide scatter of haematocrit values reported in accidental hypothermia [17, 67, 90].

Vasomotor tone. The reported effects of hypothermia on arterial pressure vary. MacLean remarked that despite the decreased cardiac output, the arterial pressure remained constant because of intense vasoconstriction and a raised blood viscosity [46]. Blood viscosity increases by 3% for each centigrade degree fall in temperature [85], and the vasoconstriction is the result

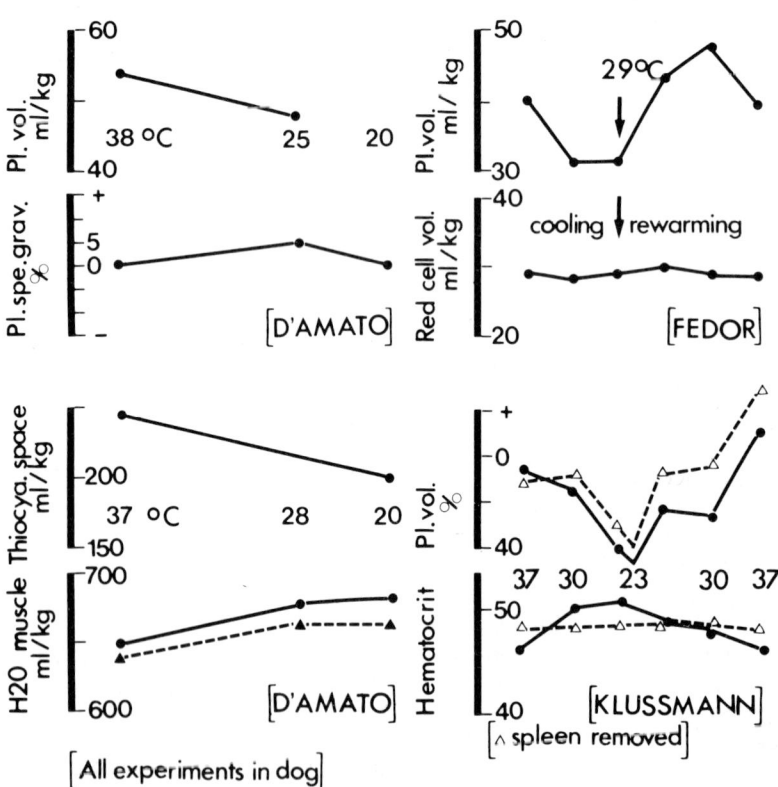

Fig. 50.8. *Mechanisms of hypovolaemia in hypothermic dogs.* Adapted from D'Amato [12, 13], Fedor [19], and Klussman [cited in 88].

of both a direct effect of cold on the vessels, and vasomotor control, which disappears below 23°–26°C [49].

In contrast to this, there are many published cases in which hypotension was present [36, 58, 62, 70], and it is likely that many factors have to be considered. For instance, the duration of hypothermia and the reduction in blood volume are probably more pronounced when this is prolonged. Arterial pressure is precariously maintained by vasoconstriction, so that moving the patient from a cold environment into a warm room can very readily lead to vasodilatation and significantly lower the arterial pressure. Similarly, therapeutic measures that affect viscosity, such as colloid infusion, or vasomotor tone, such as sedation, may all precipitate severe falls in arterial pressure.

Bradycardia and ECG. With hypovolaemia, bradycardia is the main factor contributing to the decreased cardiac output. In the six patients, whose admission temperatures were between 25.3° and 28.2°C, heart rate ranged between 32 and 60 beats/min [70]. Bradycardia is frequently noted in clinical reports, but occasionally tachycardia is found and usually implies a poor prognosis [46]. This is consistent with three of our cases, in whom the heart rate ranged from 70 to 120 beats/min despite central temperatures averaging 30°C. In all these patients severe complications, either neurological or cardiac, were associated, and shock quickly developed.

Kayser has clearly demonstrated the correlation between heart rate and temperature (Fig. 50.9) [35].

The ECG changes have been widely documented [18, 34] and are extensively reviewed by MacLean [46]. Sinus bradycardia is associated with hypothermia, the heart rate gradually slowing as the temperature falls. This bradycardia is not altered by atropine or vagotomy, suggesting that the cold directly affects the pacemaker. Progressively, sinus rhythm is followed by atrial flutter and fibrillation, occasionally accompanied by ventricular ectopic beats (VEBs). Thereafter an idioventricular rhythm occurs; at this point atrial activity may completely disappear.

It must be stressed that it is occasionally difficult to interpret an ECG, because of artefacts generally related to muscular activity [18, 58]. Myocardial conductivity is also gradually depressed, and this accounts for the prolonged PR, QRS, and QT intervals. The ST segment is generally depressed or concave, and sometimes elevated. The more specific change is the J deflection at the junction between the QRS and the ST segments (Fig. 50.10), and it is almost constant when the temperature falls to 31°C [59]. This deflection is upward in LV and downward in RV leads. It is thought that the deflection is the result of alterations in ionic fluxes across the myocardial sarcolemma [46]. None of the changes mentioned has any prognostic value.

Ventricular fibrillation is the most serious complication, and in most cases death in

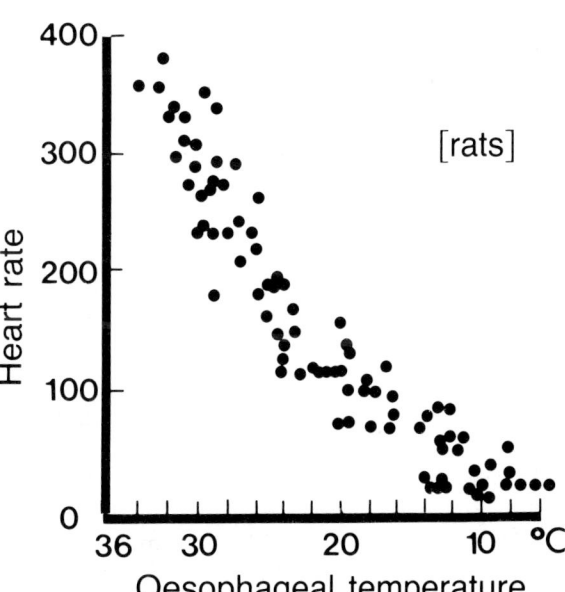

Fig. 50.9. *Changes in heart rate related to core temperature.* In an attempt to eliminate the proper effects of anaesthesia and shivering, the rats were curarized, then cooled in an ice-water bath [35].

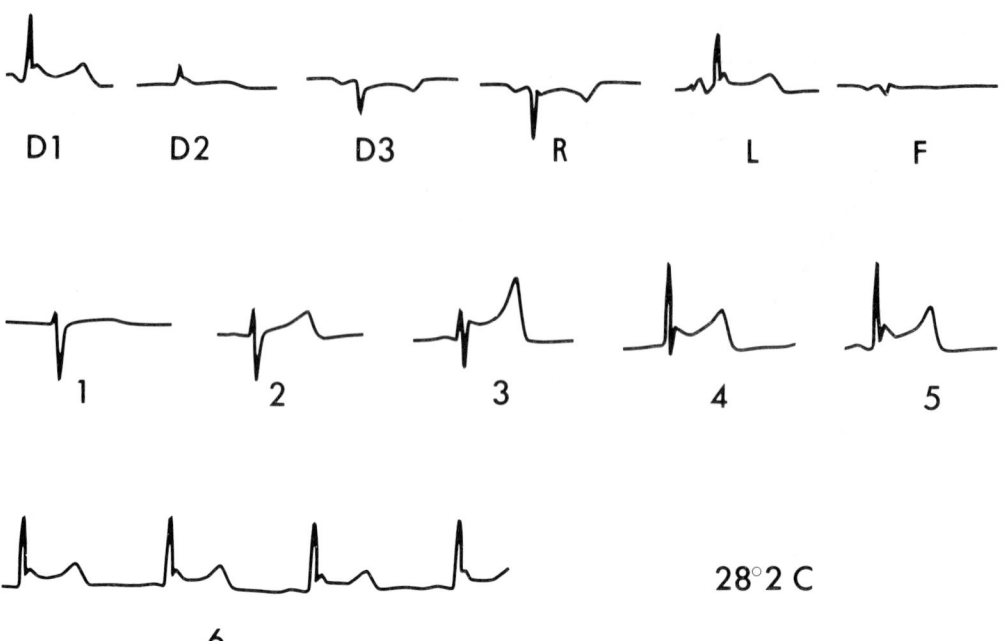

D1 D2 D3 R L F

1 2 3 4 5

6

28°2 C

Fig. 50.10. *ECG in accidental hypothermia (28.2°C).* The J deflections and the ST changes can be seen on D1, D2, and aVL, and from V3 to V6. There is a downward J deflection on D3 and aVR.

hypothermia is either initiated by or due to ventricular fibrillation or asystolic cardiac arrest [88]. The mechanism of ventricular fibrillation is still under discussion, but many contributory factors of practical importance have been recognized. They include heart catheterization, hypoxia, acceleration of heart rate, hypotension, endotracheal intubation, acidosis, and both hyper and hypocapnia [46, 88].

As shown in Fig. 50.11, the ECG changes are accounted for by alterations in the various phases of the action potential. For instance, delayed diastolic depolarization explains the bradycardia, and the changes in the intervals result from variable prolongation of each phase of the action potential [11].

Ventricular function. Low cardiac output in hypothermia is mainly related to bradycardia and hypovolaemia. Nevertheless, experimental data, and some clinical reports, suggest that ventricular performance might be impaired.

In the patients in whom haemodynamic patterns were recorded, we assessed ventricular function by plotting LV work against PWP as an index of LV filling pressure. Data were recorded before and after rapid blood volume expansion, and the assessment was repeated 48 h after the return to normothermia. Figure 50.12 shows that the LV power index (LVW) improved markedly after rewarming, but since this is an index of the work done in 1 min, the results

could merely signify that, as a result of increasing heart rate, LV work increased. Nevertheless when the LV work achieved for each systole (LVSWI) was plotted against PWP it appeared that some patients had decreased myocardial performance, which returned to normal on rewarming. It is also noteworthy that these patients had the longest periods of cold exposure, estimated to be more than 48 h [30].

In hypothermic dogs, Berne demonstrated a marked prolongation of the phases of isometric contraction, ejection, and isometric relaxation (Fig. 50.13) very similar in fact to the ventricular pressure curve we recorded in a patient at 28.2°C (Fig. 50.14) [4]. If, however, cardiac failure is characterized by a prolonged isometric contraction, then by contrast the ejection phase is abbreviated. He stated that in short periods of hypothermia the decline in arterial pressure and cardiac output do not result from myocardial failure. When the heart was electrically stimulated to give a rate of 57 beats/min, instead of 13, arterial pressure decreased further. This was interpreted as being due to a reduction in ventricular filling time leading to a decrease in stroke volume. He finally stressed that electrical acceleration of the heart is contraindicated [4]. In this context, Reissman demonstrated that if cardiac acceleration was obtained by epinephrine infusion, cardiac output increased markedly and was related to both an inotropic

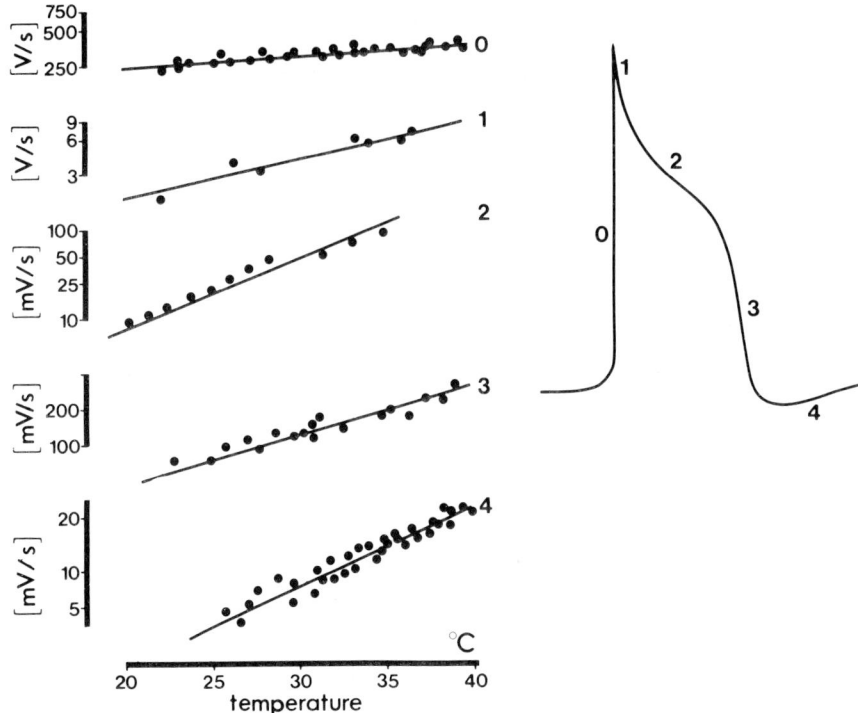

Fig. 50.11. *Effect of temperature on the rate of change of the potential difference in various phases of the action potential* [11]. It is apparent that the slow pacemaker depolarization and the falling phase of the action potential are much more influenced than the rising one.

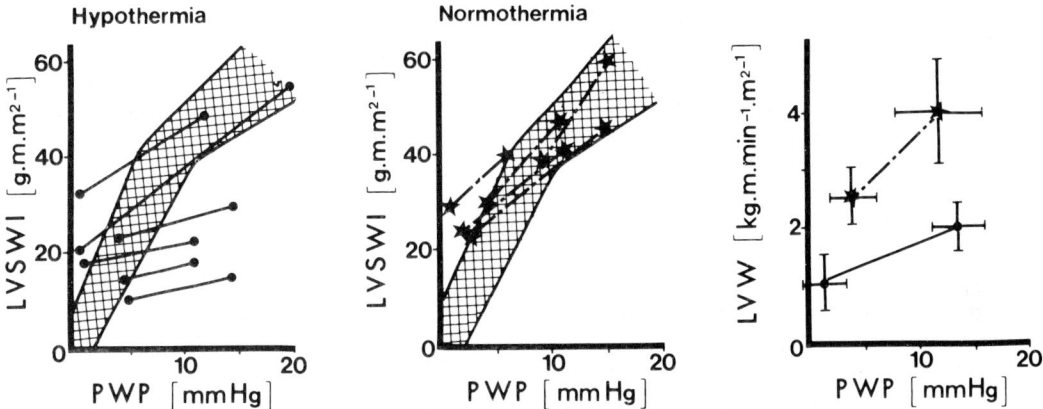

Fig. 50.12. *LV function in accidental hypothermia.* The *right hand diagram* shows the LVW plotted against the LV filling pressure. (pulmonary wedge pressure, PWP). Ventricular power is greatly increased after rewarming (*closed stars, dotted lines*), as compared with data recorded during hypothermia (*closed circles, solid lines*). This could be the result of an accelerated heart rate. Nevertheless, the *left-hand diagram* shows that the systolic work (expressed as the LVSWI) is depressed in four of six hypothermic patients; by contrast, after rewarming the five surviving patients exhibited normal L function. Thus, besides the lowered heart rate, depressed myocardial performance accounts for decreased cardiac activity.
(The *hatched areas* represent the accepted normal function in control euthermic patients).

effect and a rising heart rate. Cardiac acceleration was effective because epinephrine shortened both the contraction and relaxation phases but below 22°C it caused ectopic ventricular contractions [71]. In agreement with the experimental work several clinical studies have reported deleterious effects of cardiac pacing [30, 54, 57]. In a hypothermic patient whose heart was accelerated with either cardiac pacing or isoprenaline infusion, we found the stroke volume to be markedly decreased or slightly increased, respectively [30].

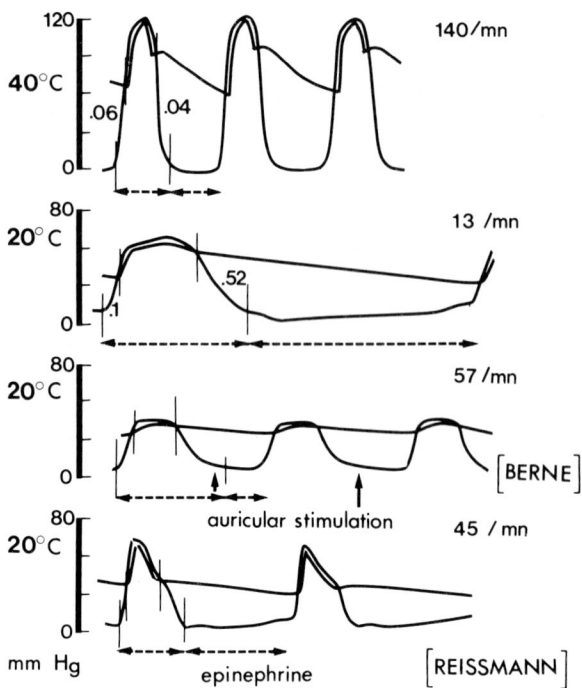

Fig. 50.13. *Myocardial function in hypothermia.* LV and arterial pressures were recorded in dogs at 40°C (*upper curve*), and then at 20°C. Heart rate decreased from 140 to 13 beats/min. The isometric contraction and relaxation phases, respectively, increased from 0.06 to 0.1 s, and from 0.04 to 0.52 s atrial electrical stimulation accelerated the heart rate to 57 beats/min. This led to a further decrease in arterial pressure. It must be noted that the ventricular filling time is markedly shortened, and furthermore that atrial stimulation occurs while the ventricle is not yet relaxed and the atrioventricular valves are still closed [4]. By contrast, the *lower curve* shows the effects of adrenaline infusion. Cardiac acceleration is associated with increased cardiac output because adrenaline markedly shortens the isometric contraction and relaxation phase, allowing the ventricular filling to be preserved period [71].

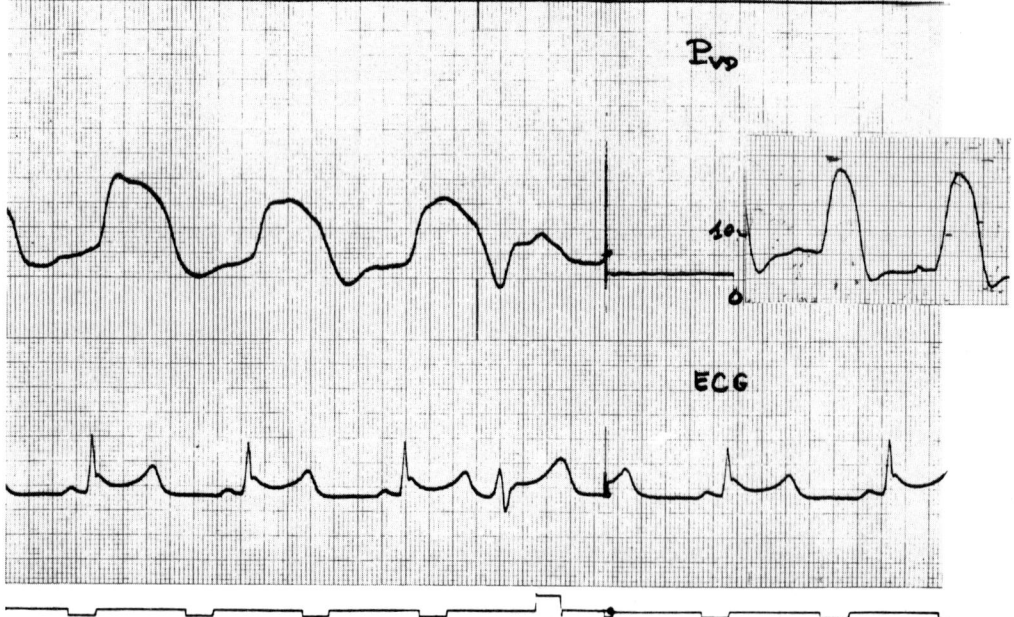

Fig. 50.14. *RV pressure curve.* Considerable slowing of contraction and relaxation are apparent on the pressure curve recorded in a patient at 28°C (heart rate = 45/min). At 34°C (on the *right*), the curve shows a shortening of both phases (heart rate = 60/min).

In four hypothermic patients, isoprenaline administration (10 μg/min) resulted in an increase in cardiac index from 2.4 to 4.6 litres/min per m^2, and in stroke volume from 41 to 46 ml/beats per min. Heart rate increased from 63 to 101 beats/min and both RAP and PWP decreased, respectively, from 5 to 2.5 mmHg and from 10 to 6 mmHg. The beneficial effects of isoprenaline on ventricular function are illustrated in Fig. 50.15.

Cardiac pacing can also compromise coronary blood flow [4, 88], and other factors such as decreased aortic pressure, increased coronary vascular resistance, high blood viscosity, and prolongation of systolic compression are associated. It should be emphasized that a satisfactory blood flow to cardiac muscle is guaranteed, provided the heart rate does not increase [88].

Finally, Templeton found a marked decrease in ventricular compliance in hypothermic dogs [87], and as a result of this elevated PWP does not necessarily signify that ventricular filling is adequate.

Circulation

In conclusion, in hypothermic patients, although there is a marked decrease in cardiac output, shock is not present because the metabolic requirements are proportionately reduced. Should rewarming, or an intercurrent complication, occur, this precarious equilibrium can be threatened and shock may develop. It is therefore necessary to remember that hypovolaemia, bradycardia, slowing of myocardial contraction and relaxation, and decreased myocardial compliance all combine to reduce cardiac output, and that because of vasoconstriction and increased blood viscosity, the microcirculation is considerably depressed.

Management

This involves the problems both of rewarming and of providing symptomatic treatment.

It has already been stressed that in hypothermia apparent death is ultimately compatible with survival, and Weyman has reinforced this: "Any hypothermic patient with evidence of cardiac or respiratory function, no matter how depressed, has the potential for full recovery" [92]. Moreover, survival following prolonged cardiac arrest or ventricular fibrillation has been reported. Thus every attempt should be made to resuscitate these patients, and those who are

seemingly dead, who are discovered after at least 12 h out of doors or in a cold room, and whose central temperature is less than 25°C but in whom no evidence of a rapidly fatal disease is found should be considered as profoundly hypothermic in the first instance.

Symptomatic treatment

Correction of hypoxaemia is essential and oxygenation is required, which becomes essential during rewarming. Mechanical ventilation is often needed. It is important to avoid severe hypocapnia, which accentuates vasoconstriction and may precipitate ventricular fibrillation.

Sodium bicarbonate should be given in whatever amounts are needed to maintain a normal pH. Initially 5% or 10% glucose is infused, and blood glucose must be carefully monitored. Initially, neither steroids nor antibiotics are indicated. Later, antibiotic treatment will depend upon relevant complications.

Apart from cardiac arrest or ventricular fibrillation, initial cardiovascular management is directed at ensuring correct filling of the heart. Hypovolaemia is constant [30], but filling pressures also depend upon ventricular functions and expansion of blood volume must be carried out continuously with monitoring of the central venous pressure (CVP) in all cases [58]. When the catheter is inserted for measurement of CVP, care must be taken to ensure that its tip does not enter the right atrium [72]; when the CVP is 5–10 cmH$_2$O the rate of perfusion should be reduced.

It is impossible to anticipate the fluid and electrolyte requirements because of the many factors that can influence fluid loss.

Age and the lung function obviously interfere with fluid therapy. Clinical and radiological evidence of pulmonary oedema calls for very cautious blood volume expansion. Nevertheless, we would like to stress that defects of ventilation are commonly associated with hypovolaemia, even in the elderly, and if the CVP is found to be low, such patients require both artificial ventilation, to re-open non-ventilated areas, and blood volume expansion.

There are two reasons for not advocating the insertion of a Swan–Ganz catheter. Firstly the published studies enable a prediction of what has happened to be made [30, 57]; and secondly, hypothermia alters RV and LV function in the same way and therefore CVP is a reliable predictor of LV filling pressure. Also, pulmonary artery catheterization may trigger off ventricular fibrillation.

Circulatory failure commonly supervenes during rewarming, and its diagnosis is not easy because hypotension and oliguria do not necessarily indicate circulatory impairment. Nonetheless, persistent hypotension, oliguria, metabolic acidosis, and a tachycardia are all suggestive of 'rewarming circulatory failure', which is closely related to the increasing peripheral vasodilatation. Blood volume expansion should be carefully continued [33], and we do not favour recooling or the use of vasopressors. In six patients, as rewarming progressed, blood volume expansion resulted in a gradual increase in cardiac output (Fig. 50.15) [70].

In rare instances CVP rises but circulatory failure persists. Isoprenaline has been shown to be effective in increasing cardiac output and lowering filling pressure with relief of pulmonary congestion [30, 54, 58]. However, because of the risk of ventricular fibrillation, it should be used cautiously; dopamine or dobutamine may be preferable, since these induce fewer rhythm abnormalities and do not provoke muscular vasodilatation.

Intracardiac pacing is generally ineffective and can be harmful [4, 30, 54, 57]. Despite some rare cases where it has been successfully used [54, 57], it seems reasonable to assume that in hypothermic sinus bradycardia pacing is not justified [46].

Ventricular fibrillation requires electrical defibrillation, and successful electrical shocks at temperatures as low as 24°C have been reported

[16, 82], but defibrillation is only likely to be efficient if the body temperature is 28°–30°C [43, 90, 91].

Rewarming

This is controversial, and a fundamental question is whether it is harmful to remain hypothermic for a long time? There is no definitive answer, but it can be argued that most of the complications that can arise are more likely to do so if the hypothermic state is prolonged [14, 52]. In the patients that we investigated, the most depressed ventricular function was associated with the more prolonged hypothermia [30], and reports of experimental studies suggest that the initial, apparently well-tolerated, phase of hypothermia is followed by a less safe period with circulatory and neurological complications particularly apparent [3, 22, 49, 65, 83]. We found that the spontaneous rate of rewarming was inversely related to the duration of hypothermia [70], and this is consistent with experimental findings [83]. A correlation between the rate of rewarming and the survival has also been suggested [92]. Finally, it is reasonable to assume that hypothermia for longer than 24 h is likely to be associated with both slow rewarming and problematic outcome.

Provided that correct insulation is ensured surgical patients at 26°–27°C can produce enough extra heat to rewarm themselves. Similarly, in accidental hypothermia some patients

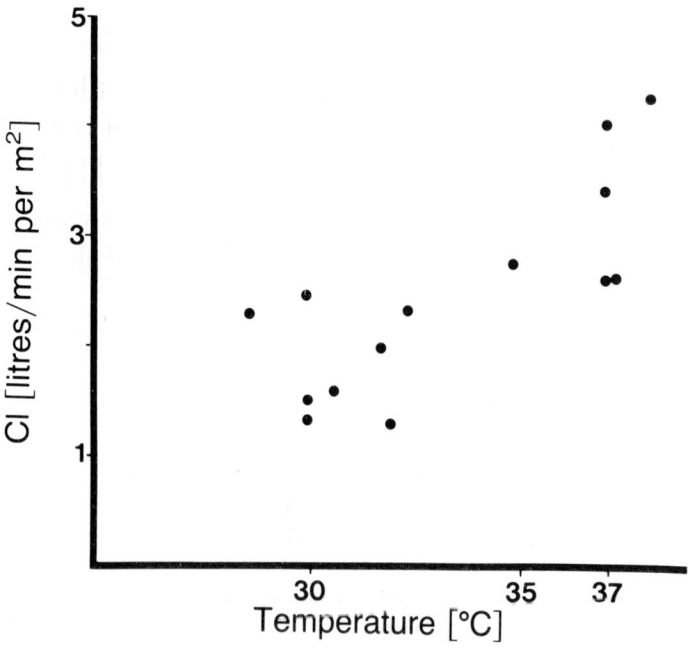

Fig. 50.15. *Cardiac index during rewarming.* In six hypothermic patients the rewarming was associated with increasing cardiac output. Blood volume expansion was performed to maintain central venous pressure between 5 and 10 cmH$_2$O during hypothermia as well as after rewarming.

are able to rewarm spontaneously, whereas in others, impairment of thermoregulation and an inability to shiver prevent a spontaneous rise of body temperature.

Thus it has been necessary to actively rewarm certain patients, by delivering heat through the skin, and such rapid and intensive surface rewarming has had opposing effects. The abrupt vasodilatation which it causes decreases both vascular resistances and venous return and accounts for 'rewarming shock'. Moreover, the cold blood from the superficial tissues is suddenly returned to the core, where it is sometimes responsible for a further fall in core temperature by some 3–4 deg. C, called the 'after-drop' [23, 26]. However, it can presumably be benefical, for profoundly hypothermic patients have been successfully treated in this fashion.

The complications of rapid surface rewarming, and the unsolved problem of cardiac arrest and ventricular fibrillation, however, suggest that it might be more appropriate to rewarm the core before the shell, which would also have the effect of warming the myocardium and improving cardiac performance.

It therefore is helpful to consider three techniques of rewarming: (1) slow spontaneous or passive rewarming; (2) rapid and active surface rewarming; and (3) rapid, active central rewarming. Table 50.1 gives the predicted rewarming rate achieved by each of the three methods.

Table 50.1. Rewarming rates

Technique	Rate of temperature rise
Slow spontaneous rewarming	0.1–0.7 deg. C/h
Rapid surface rewarming Heated blanket and mattress, cradles, etc.	1–4 deg. C/h
Hot baths	5–7 deg. C/h
Rapid central rewarming Peritoneal dialysis, warmed inhaled gases	1–1.5 deg. C/h
Extracorporeal blood rewarming	3–15 deg. C/h

Slow, passive spontaneous

The patient is removed from the cold environment, placed in a room at 25°–30°C, and insulated. His own heat production then achieves his own rewarming. Insulation is provided either by blankets supported by a bed cradle or by an insulating metallized plastic sheet

('space blanket') [46]. Rewarming rates average 0.1–0.7 deg. C per hour [17, 18, 24, 52, 58] and are related to heat production resulting from increasing metabolic rate and shivering, and from the circulatory adaption. The method reflects the capacity of the patient rather than the efficiency of the method. This fact accounts for the findings of Gregory, who showed that in a group of 201 patients the fatality rate was 60% in the actively rewarmed group, as against 44% in the passively rewarmed group [46, 72]. It is also consistent with the cases reported by Duguid [17], Weyman found a mean spontaneous rewarming rate of 3.7 deg. C per hour, whereas active rewarming commonly led to rates below 1 deg. C per hour. He stressed that no matter what method of rewarming was used, the rewarming rate was essentially correlated to the severity of underlying disease [92].

The spontaneous rate of rewarming therefore both has prognostic significance and is an indicator of the type of treatment to be used.

Rapid, active, surface

The techniques include hot water bottles, heat cradles, heated mattresses, heated sheets under an insulating blanket, electric blankets, and hot baths. It is therefore possible to vary the temperature of the apparatus and the surface of the body submitted to heat. In the literature the mean rewarming rate ranges from 5 to 7 deg. C per hour for hot baths, and from 1 to 4 deg. C for the other techniques [1, 21, 26, 33, 39, 53, 56, 62]. Nevertheless, depending upon the technique and the underlying disease, poor efficiency has been reported [92].

Two harmful effects should be noted. First, the danger of skin burns and second, the risk of provoking a fall in arterial pressure, accompanied occasionally by a temperature after-drop and a metabolic acidosis. Obviously the wider the temperature gradient across the skin and the larger the rewarmed surface the more severe are the haemodynamic changes. The intensity of rewarming should therefore be regulated according to the degree of cardiovascular tolerance. Hot baths should not be used in elderly patients, but are acceptable in the management of fit young adults [46].

In hypothermia following exposure, provided that intensive care is available, the patients can be quickly rewarmed by immersion in a bath at 40°–45°C: the trunk is fully immersed but the limbs are kept out to avoid the after-drop in temperature and to minimize the fall in arterial pressure. Should arterial pressure fall fluids are given IV and the legs are raised to increase venous return [36]. It is preferable to remove the patient from the bath as soon as the core temperature reaches 33°–34°C.

Rapid central rewarming

Rewarming the core before the shell should theoretically have several advantages. Since the heart is rewarmed first, it should be able to cope with the increased circulatory demand. Moreover, the hazardous changes of surface rewarming should not be encountered, and this is the only technique it is possible to apply in cases of ventricular fibrillation or cardiac arrest.

The central rewarming methods can be divided into two groups. First, extracorporeal blood rewarming, which allows the central temperature to rise by up to 15 deg. C per hour [14, 20, 90, 91]. Second, the methods that are designed to heat either via natural cavities (stomach, airways), or via less usual routes (peritoneum, pleural space, pericardium, vessels).

Extracorporeal rewarming by cannulation of the femoral artery and vein requires a blood heater and pump. Haemodialysis machines are also acceptable [42], and the blood may be heated to 40°C. Obviously such methods require specially trained personnel, and take a considerable time to set up; they also have complications of their own [92]. They should be strictly limited to the treatment of accidental hypothermia that is complicated by severe cardiac insufficiency.

Reported experience with peritoneal dialysis is slight, but in the few recorded cases rates of rewarming averaged 1–1.6 deg. C per hour. It is usually proposed in drug overdose and may facilitate elimination of excess drugs. The dialysis fluid is rewarmed to about 37°–43.5°C and exchanges should be as fast as possible [40, 63, 72]. More 'heroic' remedies, such as irrigation of the pericardium or pleural space after thoracotomy, have only been used in exceptional cases [43]. Gastro-intestinal irrigation, either intragastric or colonic, is easier but its efficiency remains unknown [72]. The IV administration of heated fluids at 40°C is inadequate when used alone.

More recently an attractive way of rewarming by inhalation of warmed humidified gases has been proposed [44, 81]. This method appears simple, is not invasive, and can be used outside the hospital [45]. Gas warmed to 60°C is given either via a specially designed apparatus, or via a conventional humidifier, and does not seem to involve any risk of damage to the airways. Lloyd, using this method, found an increase of 0.6–1 deg. C per hour in rectal temperature, but oesophageal temperature rose faster. He emphasized that this could be an appropriate way of rewarming the heart.

Which is the method of choice?

Deciding on a method of rewarming requires consideration of the depth, the duration and the aetiology of the hypothermia, and on the nature of the underlying disease, the age of the patient, and the availability of intensive care. Particular attention should be directed to cardiac rhythm disturbances and to the rate of spontaneous rewarming. Rapid rewarming has its dangers, but the prolongation of severe hypothermia is likely to cause more problems.

Figure 50.16 summarizes the principles of the management of rewarming [46, 54, 58]. Above 33°C patients are likely to rewarm spontaneously; and if they do not, a simple, non-aggressive means of surface rewarming is generally effective. Between 28° and 33°C the decision largely depends on the duration of the hypothermia and the age of the patient. Hypothermia from exposure of short duration (less than 12 h) in young patients should respond to active surface rewarming. By contrast, in the elderly patient with prolonged hypothermia and underlying diseases, passive rewarming should be used. If this is unsuccessful i.e., if the rate of rewarming is less than 0.75 deg. C per hour, active surface rewarming is indicated. In this case it would be appropriate to select a less aggressive surface technique and to regulate its potency according to cardiovascular, metabolic, and pulmonary tolerance. Below 28°C, cardiac arrest or ventricular fibrillation requires extracorporeal rewarming. In young patients following cold exposure or immersion, active surface rewarming is required and hot baths are appropriate. In debilitated patients after prolonged hypothermia, moderate active rewarming should be used first. If this does not ensure a minimal rewarming rate of 0.75°C per hour a more active method should be initiated.

In some cases it may be beneficial to combine methods of rewarming. For instance, moderate techniques of rewarming might be combined with warmed gas inhalation in patients with poor cardiovascular function.

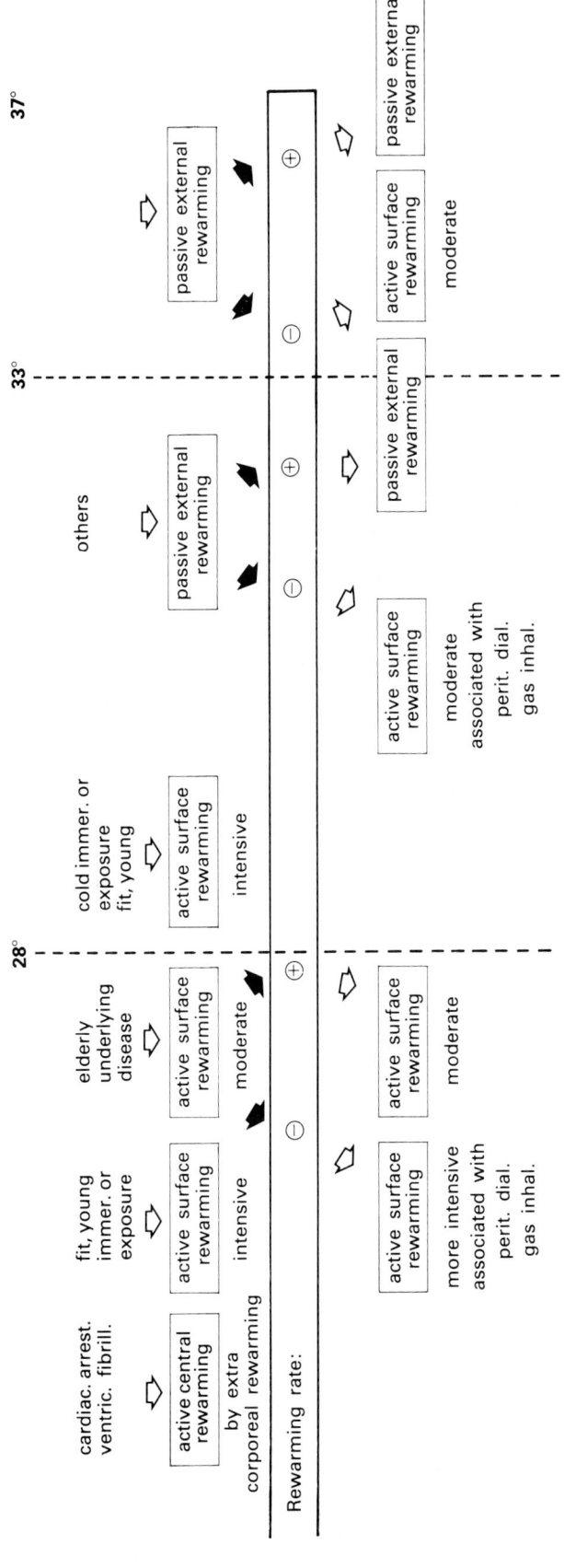

Fig. 50.16. Management of rewarming.

⊖ Rewarming rate less than 0.75 deg. C/h; ⊕ faster than 0.75 deg. C/h.

Prognosis

Accidental hypothermia is usually considered to have a poor prognosis. Weyman, reviewing the literature, found fatality rates ranging from 60% to 100% (Table 50.2). Nevertheless, in a group of patients he studied himself, he found a mortality rate of 75% in debilitated patients, which contrasted with a 6.25% fatality rate in young adults without underlying disease [92].

Besides age and associated disorders, aetiology plays a major role; for instance, the hypothermia accompanying drug intoxication carries a much better prognosis than other forms [48].

Table 50.2 also shows the correlation between depth of hypothermia and fatality, but apart from cold exposure or immersion, age is also correlated with the depth of hypothermia.

Table 50.2. Prognosis of accidental hypothermia, showing overall mortality (above)[a] and temperature-related mortality (below)[b]

		Cases (n)	Mortality (%)
Emslie-Smith	1958	8	100
Freuhan	1960	8	87
Duguid	1961	23	87
Prescott	1962	9	67
Rosin, Exton-Smith	1964	32	86
McNicol, Smith	1964	15	80
MacLean	1968	25	60
Coopwood, Kennedy	1970	11	82

Hypothermia (°C)	Cases (n)	Mortality (%)
32.2–34.3	31	26
26.7–31.7	122	52
26	41	66
31.8–35	22	40
26.1–31.7	43	46
26	5	80

[a]From Weyman et al. [92].
[b]From Gregory and Doolittle (cited in [46]; first three studies) and MacLean and Emslie-Smith [46] (last three studies).

References

1. Anderson S, Herbring BG, Widman B (1970) Accidental profound hypothermia: Case report. Br J Anaesth 42:653–655
2. Austin WH, Lacombe EH, Rand PW (1964) Correction of PCO$_2$ in hypothermia. J Appl Physiol 19:893–895
3. Azancot I, Dessange JF, Lemaigre D (1976) Evolution de la consommation d'oxygène et de la différence artérioveineuse au cours des hypothermies profondes expérimentales brèves et prolongées. CR Soc Biol (Paris) 170:1166–1172
4. Berne RM (1954) Myocardial function in severe hypothermia. Cir Res 2:90–95
5. Blair E, Esmond WG, Attar S, Cowley RA (1964) The effect of hypothermia on lung function. Ann Surg 160:814–823
6. Boutelier C, Timbal J, Colin J (1974) Echanges thermiques et réactions physiologiques à l'immersion en eau froide. Revue de Médecine Clinique 40:2631–2638
7. Boylan JW, Suk Ki Hong (1966) Regulation of renal function in hypothermia. Am J Physiol 211:1371–1378
8. British Medical Journal (1964) Dangers of cold immersion. Br Med J i:1202
9. British Medical Journal (1977) The old in the cold. Br Med J i:336
10. Collins KJ, Dore C, Exton-Smith AN, Fox RH, Mac Donald IC, Woodward PM (1977) Accidental hypothermia and impaired temperature homeostasis in the elderly. Br Med J i:353–356
11. Coraboeuf E, Weidmann S (1954) Temperature effects on the electrical activity of Purkinje fibres. Helv Physiol Pharmacol Acta 12:32–41
12. D'Amato HE (1954) Thiocyanate space and distribution of water in musculature of hypothermic dogs. Am J Physiol 178:143–147
13. D'Amato HE, Hegnauer AH (1953) Blood volume in hypothermic dogs. Am J Physiol 173:100–102
14. Davies DM, Millar EJ, Miller IA (1976) Accidental hypothermia treated by extra-corporeal blood rewarming. Lancet I:1036–1037
15. Deal CW, Warden JC, Monk I (1970) Effects of hypothermia on lung compliance. Thorax 25:105–109
16. Dominguez de Villota E, Barat G, Peral P, Juffe A, Fernandez de Miguel JM, Avello F (1973) Recovery from profound hypothermia with cardiac arrest after immersion. Br Med J iv:394–395
17. Duguid H, Simpson RG, Stowers JM (1961) Accidental hypothermia. Lancet II:1213–1219
18. Emslie-Smith D (1958) Accidental hypothermia. A common condition with a pathognomonic electrocardiogram. Lancet II:492–495
19. Fedor EJ, Fisher B (1959) Simultaneous determination of blood volume with 51 Cr and 1824 T during hypothermia and rewarming. Am J Physiol 196:703–705
20. Fell RH, Gunning AJ, Bardhan KD, Triger DR (1968) Severe hypothermia as a result of barbiturate overdose complicated by cardiac arrest. Lancet I:392–394
21. Fernandez JP, O'Rourke RA, Ewy GA (1970) Rapid active external rewarming in accidental hypothermia. JAMA 212:153–156
22. Fisher B, Fedor EJ, Lee SH (1958) Rewarming following hypothermia of two to twelve hours. Some metabolic effects. Ann Surg 148:32–36
23. Freeman J, Pugh LGCE (1969) Hypothermia in mountain accidents. Int Anesthesiol Clin 7:997–1007
24. Freuhan AE (1960) Accidental hypothermia. Arch Intern Med 106:218–229
25. Gil-Rodriguez JA, O'Gorman P (1970) Renal function during profound hypothermia. Br J Anaesth 42:557
26. Godeau P, Michaud A, Siguier F (1962) Hypothermie accidentelle réversible à 22°C. Mort subite 3 mois plus tard. Coeur Med Interne 1:497–504
27. Golden F, St C, Rivers JF (1975) The immersion incident. Anaesthesia 30:364–373
28. Gregory RT, Patton JF (1972) Treatment after exposure to cold. Lancet I:377

29. Hansen JE, Sue DY (1980) Should blood gas measurements be corrected for the patient's temperature? N Engl J Med 303:341

30. Harari A, Regnier B, Rapin M, Lemaire F, Legall JR (1975) Haemodynamic study of prolonged deep accidental hypothermia. Intensive Care Med 1:65–70

31. Hedley-Whyte J, Pontoppidan H, Lauer MB, Hallowell P, Bendixen HH (1965) Arterial oxygenation during hypothermia. Anaesthesiology 26:595–602

32. Henneman DH, Bunker JP, Brewster WR (1958) Immediate metabolic response to hypothermia in man. J Appl Physiol 12:164–168

33. Justin-Besançon L, Pequignot H, Etienne JP (1958a) Un cas de réfrigération à 23°5 suivi de guérison. Sem Hop Paris 34:63–69

34. Justin-Besançon L, Pequignot H, Etienne JP, Laurent D (1958b) Les modifications de l'électrocardiogramme au cours des hypothermies spontanées. Sem Hop Paris 34:84–96

35. Kayser C, Hiebel G (1953) La caractéristique de température ou l'incrément thermique critique de la fréquence cardiaque et de la vitesse de conduction intra-cardiaque au cours de l'hypothermie expérimentale profonde du rat blanc curarisé. CR Soc Biol (Paris) 147:1626–1633

36. Keatinge WR (1969) Survival in cold water. The physiology and treatment of immersion hypothermia and of drowning. Blackwell Scientific Publications, Oxford London Edinburgh Melbourne

37. Kelman GR, Nunn JF (1966) Nomograms for correction of blood PO_2, PCO_2, pH and base excess for time and temperature. J Appl Physiol 21:1484–1490

38. Kreger BE, Craven DE, McCabe WR (1980) Gram-negative bacteremia. IV. Re-evaluation of clinical features and treatment in 612 patients. Am J Med 68:344–355

39. Lancet (1972) Severe accidental hypothermia. (Leading article) Lancet I:237

40. Lash RF, Burdette JA, Ozoil T (1967) Accidental profound hypothermia and barbiturate intoxication. JAMA 210:269–270

41. Laufman H (1951) Profound accidental hypothermia. JAMA 147:1201–1212

42. Lee HA, Ames AC (1965) Haemodialysis in severe barbiturate poisoning. Br Med J i:1217–1219

43. Linton AL, Ledhingham I McA (1966) Severe hypothermia with barbiturate intoxication. Lancet I:24–26

44. Lloyd EL (1973) Accidental hypothermia treated by central rewarming through the airway. Br J Anaesth 45:41–48

45. Lloyd EL, Frankland JC (1974) Accidental hypothermia: Central rewarming in the field. Br Med J iv:717

46. MacLean D, Emslie-Smith D (1977) Accidental hypothermia, 1st edn. Blackwell Scientific Publications, Oxford London Edinburgh Melbourne

47. MacLean D, Griffiths PD, Emslie-Smith D (1968) Serum-enzymes in relation to electrocardiographic changes in accidental hypothermia. Lancet II:1266–1270

48. MacLean D, Murison J, Griffiths PO (1973) Acute pancreatitis and diabetic ketoacidosis in accidental hypothermia and hypothermic myxoedema. Br Med J 4:757–761

49. Malmejac J (1956) Incidences physiopathologiques cardiaques et nerveuses de l'hypothermie provoquée. CR Acad Sci [D] (Paris) 242:311

50. McKean WI, Dixon SR, Gwynne JF, Ivine ROH (1970) Renal failure after accidental hypothermia. Br Med J ii:463–464

51. McNicol MW (1967) Respiratory failure and acid–base status in hypothermia. Postgrad Med J 43:674–676

52. McNicol NW, Swith R (1964) Accidental hypothermia. Br Med J i:19–21

53. Meriwether WD, Goodman RM (1972) Severe accidental hypothermia with survival after rapid rewarming. Am J Med 53:505–510

54. Motin J, Bouletreau P, Petit P, Latarjet J (1973) L'hypothermie accidentelle au cours des intoxications par les neuroleptiques et les tranquillisants. Lyon Medical 230:53–62

55. Moyer JH, Morris GC, Debakey ME (1957) Effect of hypothermia on renal hemodynamics and on excretion of water and electrolytes in dog and man. Ann Surg 145:26–40

56. Niazi SA, Lewis FJ (1958) Profound hypothermia in man. Ann Surg 147:264–268

57. Nicolas G, Bounour JB, Heurtel A, Godin JF, Nicolas F (1971) Intérêt des données hémodynamiques dans la surveillance et la réanimation des hypothermies accidentelles. Rev Med Suisse Romande 91:707–720

58. Nicolas F, Nicolas G, Heurtel A, Baron D, Rodineau P, De Lajartre AY (1974) Vingt quatre observations d'hypothermies accidentelles. Anesth Anag (Paris) 31:485–538

59. Osborn JJ (1953) Experimental hypothermia. Respiratory and blood pH changes in relation to cardiac function. Am J Physiol 175:389–393

60. Otis AB, Jude J (1957) Effect of body temperature on pulmonary gas exchanges. Am J Physiol 188:355–359

61. Pagni CA, Courjon J (1964) Electroencephalographic modifications induced by moderate and deep hypothermia in man. Acta Neurochir [Suppl] (Wien) XIII:35–49

62. Phillipson EA, Herbert FA (1967) Accidental exposure to freezing. Clinical and laboratory observations during convalescence from near-fatal hypothermina. Can Med Assoc J 97:786–792

63. Pickering BG, Bristow GK, Craig DB (1977) Core rewarming by peritoneal irrigation in accidental hypothermia with cardiac arrest. Anesth Analg (Cleve) 56:574–577

64. Pina-Cabral JM, Amaral I, Pinto MM, Guerra E Paz LH (1973/1974) Haemostasis 2:235–244

65. Popovic VP, Kent KM (1965) Cardiovascular responses in prolonged hypothermia. Am J Physiol 209:1069–1074

66. Prakash O, Jonson B, Meij S, Hugenholtz PG, Hekman W (1978) Cardiorespiratory and metabolic effects of profound hypothermia. Crit Care Med 6:165–171

67. Prescott LF, Peard MC, Wallace IR (1962) Accidental hypothermia, a common condition. Br Med J 2:1367–1370

68. Pugh LGCE (1966) Accidental hypothermia in walkers, climbers and campers. (Report to the Medical Commission on accident prevention) Br Med J i:123–129

69. Read AE, Emslie-Smith D, Gough KR, Holmes R (1961) Pancreatitis and accidental hypothermia. Lancet II:1219–1221

70. Regnier B, Harari A, Azancot I (1973) Hypothermies accidentelles de l'adulte. In: Réanimation et médecine d'urgence. Expansion Scientifique, Paris, pp 5–23

71. Reissmann KR, Kapoor S (1956) Dynamics of hypothermic heart muscle. Am J Physiol 184:162–170

72. Reuler JB (1978) Hypothermia: Pathophysiology, clinical settings, and management. Ann Intern Med 89:519–527

73. Rolly G, Malcolm-Thomas B (1970) Measures de consommation d'oxygène au cours de l'hypothermie modérée. Anesth Analg Rean (Paris) 27:321–329

74. Rosenfeld JB (1963) Acid–base and electrolyte disturbances in hypothermia. Am J Cardiol 12:678–682

75. Rosenthal IB (1948) The effect of temperature on the pH of blood and plasma in vitro. J Biol Chem 173:25–30

76. Rosomoff HL (1964) Pathophysiology of the central

nervous system during hypothermia. Acta Neurochir [Suppl] (Wien) XIII:11–13

77. Sechzer PH (1958) Effect of hypothermia on compliance and resistance of the lung thorax system of anesthetized man. J Appl Physiol 13:53–56

78. Segar WE (1958) Effect of hypothermia on tubular transport mechanisms. Am J Physiol 195:91–96

79. Severinghaus JW (1950) Respiration and hypothermia. Ann NY Acad Sci 80:384–394

80. Severinghaus JW (1958) Oxyhaemoglobin dissociation curve correction for temperature and pH variation in human blood. J Appl Physiol 12:485–486

81. Shanks CA, Sara CA (1972) Temperature monitoring of the humidifier during treatment of hypothermia. Med J Aust 2:1351–1352

82. Siebke N, Brivik H, Rod T, Lind Djorn (1975) Survival after 40 minutes submersion without cerebral sequelae. Lancet I:1275–1277

83. Steen PA, Milde JH, Michenfelder JD (1980) The detrimental effects of prolonged hypothermia and rewarming in the dogs. Anesthesiology 52:224–230

84. Stoner HB, Frayn KN, Little RA, Threlfall CJ, Yates DW, Barton RN, Heath DF (1980) Metabolic aspects of hypothermia in the elderly. Clin Sci 59:19–27

85. Svanes K, Zweifach BW, Intaglietta M (1970) Effect of hypothermia on transcapillary fluid exchange. Am J Physiol 218:981–989

86. Swan H (1973) Clinical hypothermia: A lady with a past and some promise for the future. Surgery 73:736–758

87. Templeton GH, Wildenthal K, Willerson IT, Reardon WC (1974) Influence of temperature on the mechanical properties of cardiac muscle. Circ Res 34:624–634

88. Thauer R (1965a) The circulation in hypothermia of nonhibernating animals and men. In: Hamilton WF, Dow P (eds) Handbook of physiology. Circulation, vol III. American Physiological Society, Washington, Chapter 54, pp 1899–1920

89. Thauer R (1965b). Circulatory adjustments to climatic requirements. In: Hamilton WF, Dow P (eds) Handbook of physiology. Circulation, vol III. American Physiological Society, Washington, Chapter 55, pp 1921–1966

90. Towne WD, Geiss WP, Yanes HO, Rahimtoola SH (1972) Intractable ventricular fibrillation associated with profound accidental hypothermia. Successful treatment with partial cardiopulmonary bypass. N Eng J Med 287:1135–1136

91. Truscott DG, Firor WB, Clein LJ (1973) Accidental profound hypothermia. Successful ressuscitation by core rewarming and assisted circulation. Arch Surg 106:216–218

92. Weyman AE, Greenbaum DM, Grace WJ (1974) Accidental hypothermia in an alcoholic population. Am J Med 56:13–21

Chapter 51

Hyperthermia

Jean Marty and Kamran Samii

Hyperthermia denotes any elevation of core body temperature above normal. Such increases result from a disequilibrium in the overall heat balance, of such a kind that heat production exceeds heat loss. Hyperthermic states may be categorized according to the underlying impairments of thermoregulatory mechanisms. Factors governing the control of internal body temperature, the peripheral generation and dissipation of heat, and the heat-absorbing capacity of the environment may all play a role.

Fever

In physiological terms, fever is a type of hyperthermia. The pathophysiologic mechanism and the prognosis of fever are different from those of other hyperthermic conditions, however. Fever is a symptom, rather than a primary pathological state.

Pathophysiology

Fever is produced [1, 29] by the action of pyrogenic substances on the CNS. The site of action of the pyrogens is located in the pre-optic anterior hypothalamic area of the brain. Fever is independent of the ambient temperature. In a cold environment, fever is produced by a significant increase in heat production.

In a warm environment, fever may be primarily due to a decrease in heat loss without significant change in heat production.

Pyrogenic substances provoke a sudden upward shift in the thermal reference level. When this new set-point is reached, it is maintained by the normal thermoregulatory processes. Neither thermosensory nor thermo-effector mechanisms are impaired during fever. The hypermetabolic state associated with fever is rarely life-threatening in itself, although temperatures above 41°C may have direct deleterious effects on various physiological processes. Among the many causes of fever are infection, inflammatory processes, neoplasia, and malignant blood disorders.

Treatment

There are two main approaches to the treatment of fever [29]. Although it is a rather common practice, the treatment of fever by external cooling is in most instances an inappropriate manoeuvre. Such techniques are generally ineffective, because the body responds in such a way that the abnormally high temperature is maintained. Furthermore, cooling manoeuvres are uncomfortable for the patient. In contrast, pharmacological treatment is the more rational and potentially effective approach. The antipyretic action of aspirin and related compounds is thought to result from interference with the effect of circulating pyrogens on the CNS, shifting the set-point of temperature regulation toward normal.

In spite of its efficacy, however, the pharmacological treatment of fever may not always be advantageous. There is some question as to whether the presence of fever may enhance host defence mechanisms [17], impair the pathogenicity of invading organisms, or potentiate various forms of treatment. Therefore, it is advisable that antipyretic therapy be reserved for situations in which the presence of fever is thought to have marked deleterious physiological effects.

Heat stroke

Heat stroke is a pathophysiological condition characterized by circulatory and neurological dysfunction resulting from excessive body heat. It constitutes a medical emergency. Prompt recognition and treatment may prevent neurological sequelae and limit the mortality, which may range from 20% to 50% [4, 17, 22].

Pathogenesis

Heat stroke is induced when body heat production overwhelms the processes of heat dissipation [4, 5, 9, 15, 22, 23, 25, 27, 29]. Heat production may increase with muscular activity or generalized hypermetabolism.

Heat dissipation may be impeded by environmental conditions or by abnormalities of various physiologic functions. The rate of heat dissipation depends on several factors: (1) The temperature gradient between the body surface and the surrounding air; (2) the humidity of surrounding air, influencing evaporation of sweat; (3) the movement of air (breeze) across the skin surface, removing air of relatively higher temperature and humidity and allowing relatively cooler, dryer air to come in contact with the skin; (4) the rate of production of sweat; (5) the delivery of heat to the skin surface via the flow of blood; and (6) the presence of barriers to heat transfer, such as clothing and bedding. Changes in one or several of these factors can limit heat dissipation and contribute to hyperthermia.

In some cases, prolonged exposure to an ambient environment which is both humid and warmer than the body can itself lead to an elevated core body temperature with prolonged exercise, and the requirement of active muscle tissue for blood, together with the intravascular volume loss from prior sweating, limits the availability of blood flow to the skin. This limits both heat delivery to the skin and the rate of sweat formation, and thereby lowers the rate of heat dissipation [4, 23, 26].

These processes are responsible for the hyperthermia which may occur under normal climatic conditions during prolonged vigorous exercise, as is observed in sportsmen and military recruits [25]. Stimulant drugs may contribute to this by enhancing endurance to prolonged exercise [22]. In other circumstances, heat stroke may be observed in untrained and unacclimatized individuals who exhibit excessive sweating and volume loss [14, 22, 23, 29]. On the other hand, when people are subjected to heat stress they do not drink enough, and therefore suffer from 'voluntary dehydration', which predisposes to heat stroke [27].

Older patients are particularly predisposed to heat stroke [9]. Pre-existing hypovolaemia and cardiac insufficiency may limit the ability of the body to increase the cardiac output and peripheral blood flow, thus limiting heat dissipation. Conversely, the presence of hyperthermia may aggravate congestive failure [4]. Thus, heat stroke may be observed in sedentary elderly patients when exposed to a hot and humid environment over a long period.

Diagnosis

Heat stroke is characterized by an excessive elevation of body temperature, accompanied by a variety of neurological, circulatory, renal, coagulation, and hepatic abnormalities. The rectal temperature is generally higher than 41°C, and temperatures higher than 42°C involve a grave prognosis [18]. The skin is generally hot and dry [4, 18, 22]. Thus heat stroke represents a multiple-system disorder.

Neurological abnormalities

The initial neurological symptoms are headache, dizziness, weakness, mental confusion, and hyperventilation [4, 22, ,27]. Stupor and coma may supervene, with focal or generalized convulsions. Spinal fluid and EEG examinations are usually normal, but non-specific changes have been observed. The symptoms and signs of heat stroke generally resolve if treatment is instituted early. In some patients, however, recovery may be delayed, or permanent neurological deficit may result, in the form of cerebellar deficits, paresis, and mental or personality changes. This is more likely to occur if the heat stroke is prolonged and is accompanied by cardiovascular insufficiency. At autopsy, oedema, and petechial haemorrhages are found throughout the brain and meninges, with cellular abnormalities appearing particularly in the cerebellum.

Cardiovascular abnormalities

Increased core temperature is associated with increased cardiac output and heart rate [4, 5, 18, 21]. The ECG may show flattened or inverted T waves and depression of the S–T segment. Compensatory cutaneous vasodilatation occurs to enhance the efficiency of heat dissipation [23]. Haemodynamic monitoring during heat stroke generally reveals a hyperdynamic state with decreased peripheral resistance.

In some patients, however, initial or subsequent measurements reveal a hypodynamic state with decreased cardiac output and arterial pressure and increased or near normal peripheral resistance. This hypodynamic state may be due to hypovolaemia induced by sweating and by transudation of fluid into interstitial spaces [15]. Congestive heart failure with elevated ventricular pressures induced by the volume load may also be observed. Right ventricular failure has been observed, which may be due to pulmonary arterial hypertension of uncertain aetiology [8, 28]. A decrease in myocardial contractility has also been observed experimentally when body temperature exceeds 40°C [19]. In elderly patients, underlying ischaemic heart disease may contribute to the precipitation of congestive failure due to heat stroke.

Fluid electrolyte, and renal abnormalities

Heat stroke can cause fluid, electrolyte, and renal abnormalities [4, 14, 15, 18, 22, 25]. Prolonged sweating induces severe dehydration and sodium loss, particularly in unacclimatized patients. Compensatory sodium conservation is mediated by increased aldosterone secretion provoking a potassium deficit. The polyuria which is frequently observed in heat stroke is vasopressin resistant, and probably due to the potassium deficit. Such polyuria contributes to plasma hyperosmolality with hypernatraemia.

Metabolic acidosis may be observed, which is generally a lactic acidosis resulting from circulatory insufficiency.

Renal insufficiency is frequently seen. Prerenal azotaemia is generally reversible with the correction of hypovolaemia. However in 10%–35% of patients, acute tubular necrosis may ensue. This may result from severe diminution of renal blood flow, haemolysis, or rhabdomyolysis [30]. Rhabdomyolysis is indicated by myoglobinuria and elevated serum levels of skeletal muscle enzymes. Marked degrees of rhabdomyolysis can rapidly impair renal function, although modest degrees, as seen after intense muscular exercise, are compatible with normal renal function [18, 25].

Coagulation abnormalities

Petechiae or haemorrhages are observed in severe heat stroke, although the results of coagulation studies are generally within normal limits and disseminated intravascular coagulation is rare [3, 18, 27, 32].

Hepatic abnormalities

Mild hepatic dysfunction with elevation of bilirubin and transaminases is frequently noted [4, 16, 31]. More severe liver damage is observed in approximately 10% of patients. This may contribute to the overall mortality of heat stroke, although the precise role of hepatic failure in the death of patients with heat stroke is difficult to establish. The observed histologic changes include centrilobular necrosis and cholestasis. These may be due to hyperthermia or to the secondary circulatory insufficiency.

Treatment

The success of the treatment depends in large measure on the rapidity with which it is instituted. The main aims of treatment are cooling of body temperature and support of vital functions.

Cooling [18]

Central temperature should be measured frequently, preferably with a recording thermistor inserted in the oesophagus or rectum. If away from the hospital the clothing should be removed and the patient rapidly moved in a shaded and open vehicle. The patient should be placed in an iced bath as soon as possible. This is the most effective method of reducing the body temperature. During the bath, vigorous cutaneous massage helps prevent dermal circulatory stasis and enhances peripheral heat dissipation. Other methods of cooling have been proposed, including lavage of the stomach, bladder, and rectum with iced isotonic solutions. Peritoneal dialysis with iced solutions is a potential approach, but involves the risk of haemorrhage [11]. Ice bags and alcohol sponges, combined with ventilation or air conditioning, can also help the cooling. These measures should be continued until the central temperature has fallen below 39°C [16]. The use of neuroleptic drugs such as phenothiazines has been suggested, to decrease mental confusion and to reduce shivering [4, 22] by their suppressive influence on the thermoregulator centres. Shivering and metabolic heat production may also be decreased with curare if the patient has already been intubated and artificially ventilated [27]. Compared with immersion in iced water all the other forms of cooling therapy are relatively ineffective.

Haemodynamic management

A high cardiac output is necessary to supply the high surface blood flow required for effective heat dissipation. Haemodynamic management [4, 21] should include monitoring of arterial pressure, urine output, and central venous pressure. If predominantly LV heart failure seems probable a triple-lumen Swan–Ganz catheter should be inserted. This permits measurement of the right ventricular pressure, LV filling pressure and the cardiac output determined by the thermal dilution method. Hypovolaemia is the major cause of circulatory insufficiency, and must be treated by plasma volume expansion with iced Ringer's lactate solution with continuous monitoring of ventricular filling pressures. If heart failure supervenes, digitalis and/or adrenergic drugs such as isoprenaline, dopamine, or dobutamine may be called for. However, these measures may increase cardiac work and myocardial O_2 consumption, and may therefore have deleterious effects in the presence of underlying ischaemic heart disease. If ischaemic disease and potential heart failure are suspected, the use of vasodilator drugs (such as nitroprusside) with or without adrenergic drugs is a logical approach to decrease cardiac afterload and increase cardiac output once adequate plasma volume expansion has been accomplished. Nonetheless, it should be noted that vasodilator therapy during heat stroke has not yet been reported, and must be undertaken with caution and with careful haemodynamic monitoring.

Support of other vital functions

Rapid correction of circulatory insufficiency is the most important measure in prevention of renal failure. If urine output remains low despite the achievement of normal renal perfusion, frusemide may be used. The presence of intrinsic renal failure with a creatinine clearance below 10 ml/min is an indication for dialysis. When renal failure is due to rhabdomyolysis, severe hyperkalaemia may develop rapidly. This requires prompt recognition and management. Neurological deficits may impair respiratory function, and predispose to the retention of secretions and infectious complications. These may be prevented by chest physiotherapy or mechanical ventilation (MV). Barbiturates are recommended even if frank convulsions are not observed. If cerebral oedema supervenes, induction of some degree of fluid depletion is necessary. This may be dangerous, as it can further impair an already compromised circulation [4, 22]. If circulatory and renal functions are normal and neurological dysfunction occurs in the presence of hyponatraemia, suggesting CNS cellular hyperhydration, mannitol therapy may be used. Corticosteroids have not proved effective in the treatment of cerebral oedema. If a consumptive coagulopathy is demonstrated low-dose heparin therapy is logical, although its usefulness in this setting has not been studied [27].

Prevention

Heat stroke may be prevented in active individuals [4, 6, 8, 22, 23, 25, 26] by progressive muscular and cardiovascular training in anticipation of heavy exertion, avoidance of stimulant drugs to support exercise, progressive acclimatization to a hot and humid environment, and adequate water and salt intake. In sedentary and elderly individuals, avoidance of prolonged exposure to extreme environments and maintenance of water and salt intake are essential.

Malignant hyperthermia

Malignant hyperthermia is a drug-induced myopathy common to man and swine, and resulting from the use of inhalation anaesthetics and muscle relaxants [12].

Pathogenesis

It is generally accepted that the underlying cause of malignant hyperthermia is a defect in calcium transfer, which produces an elevation of intracellular calcium [2, 7, 24]. This activates phosphorylase, thereby increasing the catabolism of glycogen to lactic acid, CO_2, and heat. Higher concentration of calcium in the sarcoplasm activates myosin ATPase, which hydrolyses ATP to ADP and phosphate, with the release of heat and the induction of sustained muscular contraction. Elevation of the intramuscular temperature further activates these reactions, so that they become relatively self-sustaining and independent of the calcium concentration. In addition to the excessive heat generation, concomitant spasm of blood vessels tends to reduce peripheral blood flow and thereby impair heat loss. These two processes lead to the development of marked hyperthermia. This syndrome appears to result from an hereditary predisposition of muscle tissue to respond abnormally to drugs such as fluothane and succinylcholine [12].

Signs and symptoms

Tachycardia is a major sign of malignant hyperthermia. The observed heart rate is not appropriate for the patient's level of anaesthesia, and should not be attributed to the stage of light anaesthesia. Tachypnoea would be a frequent sign, were it not masked by the use of muscle relaxants. Bounding arterial pulses and cardiac arrythmias may also be observed. Frank fever has become rare because modern operating suites are usually kept cool. Therefore, temperature elevations of even 0.5 deg. C should be suspect in the setting of surgical anaesthesia. Muscular rigidity with trismus occurring immediately after administration of succinylcholine should also raise suspicion of this syndrome. The diagnosis is confirmed by findings of an elevated serum CPK, metabolic acidosis, and the presence of serum and urinary myoglobin [7, 8].

Treatment [7, 8]

Reversal of signs

Anaesthesia and surgery must be immediately interrupted. Once the anaesthetic appliance and tubing have been changed the patient is hyperventilated with 100% O_2. Sodium bicarbonate is administered to correct the metabolic acidosis and to decrease the hyperkalaemia. Cooling of the patient is achieved by lavage of the stomach, bladder, rectum, or peritoneal cavity with iced solutions and by the IV administration of iced saline. Ringer's lactate must be avoided to avoid contributing to a possibly high lactate level.

Surface cooling with ice baths or a hypothermia blanket or cold haemodialysis may also be used. A direct-acting skeletal muscle relaxant is useful, such as dantrolene 1 mg/kg IV up to a total dose of 10 mg/kg, or procainamide 15 mg/kg [10, 13, 20]. The administration of high-dose corticosteroids has also been proposed, but its usefulness has not been demonstrated.

Prevention

The relatives of any patient known to have reacted to anaesthetic agents or muscle relaxants with malignant hyperthermia should be evaluated for susceptibility. The following allow recognition of such a predisposition: (1) clinical muscular abnormalities, such as ptosis, kyphoscoliosis, and strabismus; (2) elevation of serum CPK; and (3) abnormal in vitro halothane and caffeine stimulation tests performed on muscle biopsy specimens. In susceptible individuals, a variety of agents should be avoided, including halothane and other volatile anaesthetics, succinylcholine, D-tubocurarine, adrenalin and atropine. If such agents are unavoidable, pretreatment with dantrolene seems logical [10].

Pathological and pharmacological hyperthermias [29]

Hypothalamic lesions

Cerebrovascular accident, tumor, infection, or surgical damage can cause hypothalamic lesions. The thermoregulatory responses are impaired and hyperthermia follows exposure to a hot environment in such circumstances.

Disturbances of central brain monoamine metabolism

Tricyclic antidepressants can induce such disturbances in a patient who is already receiving monoamine oxidase inhibitor therapy. Hyperthermia results from both increased heat production and suppressed heat dissipation mechanisms. A similar condition may occur during neuroleptic therapy.

Hypermetabolic states

Thyrotoxicosis and phaeochromocytoma are often accompanied by hyperthermia. In severe thyroid crisis, the body temperature can rapidly rise to dangerous levels, and measures to lower the temperature are vital.

Atropine

Atropine and similar drugs can block the production of sweat, thus impairing heat dissipation and possibly precipitating hyperthermia in individuals who undertake exercise in a hot environment.

References

1. Bernheim HA, Block LH, Atkins E (1979) Fever: pathogenesis, pathophysiology and purpose. Ann Intern Med 91:261–270
2. Britt BA (1979) Etiology and pathophysiology of malignant hyperthermia. Fed Proc 39:44–47
3. Britt BA, Locher WG, Kalow W (1969) Hereditary aspects of malignant hyperthermia Can Anaesth Soc J 16:89
4. Clowes GH, O'Donnel TF (1974) Heat stroke. N Engl J Med 291:564–567
5. Costrini AM, Pitt HA, Gustafson AB, Uddin DE (1979) Cardiovascular and metabolic manifestations of heat stroke and severe heat exhaustion. Am J Med 66:296–302
6. Dasler AP, Karas S, Bonman JS, et al (1973) Adverse effects of supplementary sodium chloride on heat adaptation. Fed Proc 32:336
7. Ellis FR (1980) Inherited muscular disease. Br J Anaesth 52:153–164
8. El Sherif NE, Shahwan L, Sorour AH (1970) The effect of acute thermal stress on general and pulmonary haemodynamics on the cardiac patient. Am Heart J 79:305–317
9. Fennell WH, Moore RE (1973) Responses of aged men to passive heating. J Physiol (Lond) 231:118–119
10. Flewellen EH, Nelson TE (1980) Dantrolene dose response on malignant hyperthermia susceptible (MHS) swine. Method to obtain prophylaxis and therapeusis. Anaesthesiology 52:303–308
11. Gjessing J, Barsa J, Tamlin PJ (1976) A possible means of rapid cooling in the treatment of MH. Br J Anaesth 48
12. Gronert GA, Theye RA (1976) Halothane-induced porcine malignant hyperthermia. Metabolic and haemodynamic changes. Anaesthesiology 44:36–43
13. Gronert GA, Milde JM, Theye RA (1976) Dantrolene in porcine malignant hyperthermia. Anaesthesiology 44:488–495
14. Harrison MH, Edwards RJ, Leitch DR (1975) Effect of exercise and thermal stress on plasma volume. J Appl Physiol 39:925–931
15. Kew M, Bersohn I, Seftel H, Kent G (1970) Liver damage in heat stroke. Am J Med 49:192–202
16. Klastersky J, Kass EH (1970) Is suppression of fever or hypothermia useful in experimental and clinical infectious diseases. J Infect Dis 121:81–86
17. Knochel JP, Beisel WR, Herndon EG, et al (1961) The renal, cardiovascular, haematologic and serum electrolyte abnormalities of heat stroke. Am J Med 30:299–309
18. Knochel JP, Dotlin LN, Hamburger RJ (1972) Pathophysiology of intense physical conditioning in a hot climate. Mechanisms of potassium depletion. J Clin Invest 51:242–255
19. Moore FT, Maroble SA, Ogden E (1966) Contractility of the heart in abnormal temperatures. Ann Thorac Surg 2:446–450
20. Nelson TE, Flewellen EH (1979) Rationale for dantrolene VS procainamide for treatment of malignant hyperthermia. Anaesthesiology 50:118–122
21. O'Donnell TF, Clowes GH (1972) The circulatory abnormalities of heat stroke. N Engl J Med 287:734–737
22. Radiguet de la Bastaie P, Poujol C (1979) L'hyperthermie maligne d'effort ou "coup de chaleur". Nouv Presse Med 27:2381–2385
23. Rowell LB, Marx MJ, Bruce RD, et al (1966) Reduction in cardiac output, central blood volume and stroke volume with thermal stress on normal men during exercise. J Clin Invest 45:1801–1816
24. Ryan J (1979) Physiology and pharmacology of malignant hyperthermia. Am Soc of Anaesth Annual meeting. Refr C Lect 103:1–4
25. Schrier RW, Hano J, Keller HI, Finkel RM, Gilliland PF, Cirksena WJ, Teschan PE (1970) Renal, metabolic and circulatory responses to heat and exercise. Ann Intern Med 73:213–223
26. Shapiro Y, Magazanik A, Udassin R, et al (1979) Heat intolerance in former heat stroke patients. Ann Intern Med 90:913–916
27. Shibolet S, Lancaster MC, Danon Y (1976) Heat stroke: A review. Aviat Space Environ Med 3:280–299
28. Sprung CL (1979) Haemodynamic alterations of heat stroke in the elderly. Chest 75:362–366
29. Stitt JT (1979) Fever versus hyperthermia. Fed Proc 38:39–43
30. Vertel RM, Knochel JP (1967) Acute renal failure due to heat injury. Am J Med 43:435–449
31. Vescia FG, Peck OC (1962) Liver disease from heat stroke. Gastroenterology 43:340
32. Weber MB, Blakely JA (1969) The haemorrhagic diathesis of heat stroke: A consumption coagulopathy successfully treated with heparin. Lancet I:1190–1192

Section J

Infection and Sepsis

Chapter 52

Hospital-Acquired Infections

J. C. Stoddart

The ICU is intended for the reception and treatment of patients who are suffering from failure of one or more major systems. Respiratory, cardiocirculatory, and renal failure are the most frequently encountered, but in terms of morbidity and mortality, failure of the complex system which provides defence against infection has the most frustrating and devastating results. Very few patients who remain in the ICU for more than 72 h can be shown to be entirely free from bacterial colonization, although only a small proportion of these require treatment [74].

From the outset it is important to distinguish between colonization and infection. The normal human being is colonized by bacteria from birth, and the skin and the respiratory and gastro-intestinal (GI) tracts have a bacterial population which is harmless and may be beneficial, provided it remains in its established place and is not activated by changes in its environment or in the host's defences. Colonization is defined as the identification of micro-organisms from any site; infection is the body's response to bacterial trespass and its effects depend upon a number of factors which are mentioned later.

When ICUs were first established it was widely believed that they would inevitably become sources of cross infection and of antibiotic resistance. Although in the properly designed and administered unit this should not occur it is an ever-present hazard. Many of the patients who are admitted are already suffering from some life-threatening illness in which infection plays a part, and the remainder are at risk because of either the nature of their presenting disease or its treatment. In this chapter the principal factors which cause infective illness in the ICU are outlined, together with some of the prophylactic and therapeutic measures which must be taken to minimize their effects. These observations are equally relevant in other specialized areas, such as those concerned with the treatment of patients who are suffering from burns, major trauma, and renal failure.

Causative Organisms

All known pathogenic organisms can cause infective illness in the ICU, but in this section only those which have been frequently incriminated will be listed (Table 52.1). Any discussion of this subject is dominated by Gram-negative organisms, because it has been realized for many years that these present a major problem in the ICU. There are many reasons for this, including the fact that most antibiotics are intrinsically more effective against Gram-positive than

Table 52.1. Micro-organisms which are responsible for infection in the ICU

E. coli	Proteus
Pseudomonas	Enterobacter
Klebsiella	Bacteroides
	Serratia

against Gram-negative organisms. The widespread use of antibiotics has encouraged the emergence of Gram-negative strains in the hospital population, which are resistant to all but a few antibiotics [32, 39, 45, 52, 70, 81]. The ability of such organisms to transfer R factors to other strains has compounded this problem [22, 54]. These and other points are discussed in more detail later. Viruses, mycoplasma, and Gram-positive organisms are also identified occasionally, but the diseases they cause are not peculiar to the hospital environment.

It is impossible to determine accurately the relative frequency with which Gram-negative infections occur, because this varies between hospitals and in different departments within the same hospital. Spink [93] reported that 23% of the organisms which he isolated from critically ill patients were *E. coli*. Other investigators have shown that *Pseudomonas* species, *Klebsiella*, *Proteus* and *Enterobacter* have been responsible for similar outbreaks, but hospital bacterial populations change unpredictably and in response to treatment [93, 95]. It was suggested above that the identification of an organism from a patient or a piece of equipment does not necessarily mean that a health hazard exists. The distinction between colonization and infection must constantly be borne in mind. For example, Burns [13] showed that in only 5 of 63 patients from whom *Pseudomonas* sp. were isolated was the organism acting as a pathogen. Many other authors have emphasized this distinction, with particular reference to the avoidance of unnecessary antibiotic therapy [32, 45, 52, 92].

Several methods have been used to determine whether or not such organisms are pathogenic, but none is universally accepted. The Limulus plasma assay has been used to demonstrate the presence of endotoxin in serum but it may be positive following aseptic tissue damage, in patients with fungal infections, and in infection with organisms which do not produce endotoxin [29, 59]. The nitroblue tetrazolium test (NBT) is said to make it possible to identify phagocytosis and to distinguish between bacterial and viral infections, but its reliability has not been generally acknowledged [30, 75]. Other methods based upon the establishment of leucocyte activation or of antibody response to systemic infection [1, 4, 36, 103, 104], while of interest, are either non-specific or take too long to perform to be of therapeutic value. In the final analysis the diagnosis and treatment of microbial infection are dependent upon clinical acumen. The relationship between the established signs of infective illness (pyrexia, leucocytosis, toxaemia, tachycardia), an infective source, and the identification of a pathogenic organism in pure culture are still the most useful guidelines to the institution of treatment.

Source of the infection

In the ICU infective illnesses arise from three sources: these are the patient himself [skin, respiratory tract, GI tract, and genito-urinary (GU) tract], from his environment, and from his attendants or fellow-patients. It will be realized from the subsequent sections that these are not mutually exclusive and in many cases the origin of the infection cannot be established with certainty. In particular, it must be recognized that micro-organisms require a vector for transmission, which is most frequently the patient's own hands or those of an attendant.

Autogenous

The natural habitat of the organisms listed in Table 52.1 is the GI tract, and it is widely believed that many of the patients who become infected do so from their resident bacteria [17, 24, 33, 57, 69, 90, 98].

Shooter and his colleagues [90] isolated *Pseudomonas aeruginosa* from 24% of patients on admission to a surgical ward, and found that 38% of patients were harbouring this organism at some time during their stay in hospital. By routinely taking rectal swabs from every patient admitted to the ICU, the present author showed that 11 of 21 patients who developed a *Pseudomonas* infection did so from their own GI tract [95].

Montgomerie and his co-workers [69] found that ten patients who had received renal transplants carried *Klebsiella* organisms in their GI tracts and that significant infection with this organism occurred in six of the patients.

Bacteroides is a normal inhabitant of the small intestine, where it is present in enormous numbers, and although isolation of this organism from human secretions and blood cultures is uncommon its incidence appears to be increasing [18, 31, 57, 79].

The potential importance of enteric organisms is referred to at several points later in this chapter, but awareness of their ubiquity permits precautions to be taken which may reduce their significance. There is some evidence that patients are at greater risk from acquired strains of enteric organisms than from their resident flora [39], but the work of Montgomerie et al. [69] indicates that autogenous infections are a real hazard.

The prevention of hospital infection is discussed later in this section, but it is appropriate to consider the problem of endogenous infection at this point. It is almost impossible to exclude this source completely. To do so would require all patients to undergo gut sterilization from the day of admission, to be fed with sterilized food, and to be isolated thereafter. Such treatment could not be guaranteed to be either effective or free from hazard. These techniques have been applied with some success to particularly vulnerable patients, for example, leukaemics who are undergoing bone marrow transplantation, but their adoption on a large scale is both impracticable and undesirable. Surgeons and others have become increasingly aware of the value of pre-operative bowel preparation and the selective use of pre-operative antibiotics in the prevention of infection, and it is possible that the effective use of these techniques could reduce the problem of infection in the ICU [8, 28, 35, 57, 74, 79, 99, 101]. However, patients who are admitted without prior warning following trauma or unexpected illness cannot be adequately prepared, and no pre-operative preparation can prevent infection from anastomotic leaks or perforation of the bowel [8, 28].

Environmental

Lowbury and Fox [60] isolated *Pseudomonas* from 94% of dust samples taken from a burns unit and from 86% of dust samples taken from a general ward. Most Gram-negative organisms do not readily survive in a dry environment and it is probable that these organisms originated from the patients rather than were the cause of the infection [24]. As will be emphasized later, this does not reduce the importance which is attached to maintaining a high level of social cleanliness in the ICU, and fungi and clostridia have no difficulty surviving in dust.

Alternative sources of Gram-negative organisms have been identified, and the more important of these are listed in Table 52.2. It is obvious from this list that the potential sources are almost limitless. It should also be noted that most of these have one thing in common, namely *moisture*. Since all types of breathing apparatus must be damp when in use and may be difficult to dry after use, it is not surprising

that ventilators, humidifiers, anaesthetic machines, and suction equipment are usually considered to be important potential sources of environmental infection and cross infection [14, 77, 82].

1) *Endotracheal and tracheostomy tubes* should be mentioned at this point. There is no doubt that the minor mucosal trauma which inevitably follows tracheal intubation increases the danger of local and systemic bacterial infection. The surgical procedure for insertion of tracheostomy tube causes still more damage. Any procedure which interrupts mucocutaneous continuity or requires the maintenance in situ of a foreign body will facilitate the growth and spread of micro-organisms [12, 38, 61]. The longer intubation is required, the greater the danger of mucosal damage and the hazard of infection. Intubation also reduces the efficiency of coughing and creates the need for tracheobronchial suction, both of which inevitably increase the risk of infection.

2) It is impossible to assess either the frequency with which infection from *foodstuffs* occurs or its significance, but it is considered by some investigators to be a major cause of hospital infection [23, 87, 91]. It has already been stated that patients' intestinal flora changes to the dominant hospital organism within 48 h of admission, and the hospital kitchen may be partly responsible for this. Patients who subsequently develop disease or dysfunction of any part of the GI tract, such as an anastomotic leak or fistula, are then at risk from the organisms they have acquired. It is widely believed that the stomach is sterile, but it has been repeatedly shown that in sick patients the stomach may be colonized by Gram-negative organisms [3, 71]. The possibilities of spread from this site through regurgitation and leakage are numerous. Nasogastric intubation reduces the efficiency of the cardiac sphincter and permits the passive regurgitation of gastric contents into the nasopharynx. Infective material can then readily enter the respiratory tract.

3) Of the causes of infection that are listed in Table 52.2, *intravenous catheters and contaminated infusion fluids* are frequently incriminated. There have been many examples quoted in which systemic infection has arisen from monitoring catheters and intravenous feeding lines [27, 34, 53, 80]. In addition to causing bacterial infections, parenteral nutrition has been specifically stated to be a cause of fungaemia [2, 39]. Intra-arterial monitoring devices have also been incriminated as a cause of bacterial infection [53].

Table 52.2. Sources of infection

Taps, sinks, overflows
Ventilators, humidifiers, nebulizers
Suction apparatus
Air-conditioning units
Tubes of lubricating jelly
Foodstuffs, food mixers, water jugs
Local anaesthetic solutions
Stock bottles, detergent, and antiseptic solutions
Baby baths, waste units, bedpan disposal units
Intravenous solutions, intravenous catheters
Urinary catheters, endotracheal and tracheostomy tubes

It is difficult to be certain how often the relationship is causal. If a patient develops septicaemia when an intravascular catheter is in situ the organism can usually be grown from the catheter tip, where a small plug of fibrin is often found. This does not necessarily mean that the catheter was the cause of the infection, but it is usual to remove and re-site intravenous lines if a patient develops the signs of septicaemia. If possible an interval of at least 24 h should be allowed to elapse before the re-introduction of long intravascular lines. Short peripheral infusion cannulae should be used in the interim. Three-way taps and Y-connectors should be used only if they are unavoidable, since all junction points increase the hazard of infection.

Various methods of reducing the risk of infection from intravascular catheters have been described, including channelled insertion and the use of low-dose heparin and of antiseptic dressings [5, 19]. All authors emphasize that intravenous catheters should not be used for routine injection of drugs. These should be administered through peripheral access points which are changed daily.

4) The association between *urinary catheters* and generalized sepsis has been known for many years. It is usually stated that within 3 days of catheterization the urine becomes contaminated, although with aseptic insertion and the use of closed-system drainage this should not be so [40, 49, 58, 98].

Cross infection

All infections other than those which are autogenous are the result of cross infection, but in this section cross infection is defined as the transfer of an organism directly or indirectly from one person to another. The preceding sections have given some other examples of cross infection, and overlap is inevitable.

Before cross infection can be diagnosed with confidence the source must be identified, and the patient must be known to have been initially free from the infection. Both these criteria are difficult to establish. Routine swabbing of all orifices and secretions, as described in the section on bacterial monitoring, is not certain to identify all pathogens [9], and the carrier may be an unsuspected member of the hospital staff or a transient [69]. It has been shown by all epidemiological studies that the hands of medical and nursing attendants are the most important vector of cross infection [11, 15, 40, 54].

Its prevention demands a high standard of nursing and medical care, with the emphasis being placed on adequate numbers and good teaching. Barrier nursing and other aspects of unit design are referred to later. It is unnecessary to emphasize that all equipment must be cleaned and sterilized after use, and that disposable items should be used whenever possible. In the final analysis the prevention of cross infection depends upon awareness of its potential hazards.

Systemic fungal infection

In general medical practice systemic fungal infections are very uncommon, but in the ICU infection with a variety of fungi may be encountered more frequently. *Candida albicans* is the usual causative organism, but other species of *Candida*, *Torulopsis glabrata*, and *Cryptococcus* may occasionally be identified. Fungi are frequently grown in cultures taken from the nose and throat, from tracheostomy sites, and from the skin. If treatment is indicated topical antifungal agents may be used. *Candida* may also be incriminated as the cause of diarrhoea in patients receiving antibiotic drugs, and its treatment is straightforward. However, when heavy growths of fungi are reported from urine or sputum specimens the problem becomes more difficult and blood cultures should be taken [51, 102].

Specific evidence of systemic fungal infections may occasionally be provided by the occurrence of endophthalmitis [102]. If he is conscious, the patient with endophthalmitis complains of visual disturbances, and on retinoscopy hard greyish-white exudates may be seen. Except in the case of aspergillosis, fungal pneumonitis has no specific radiographic appearances and the decision to institute antifungal treatment is based upon its probability and the presence of pneumonia that is resistant to standard methods of treatment. As with bacterial infection, the identification of *Candida* or other fungi from sputum is not automatically an indication for instituting treatment. However, if a heavy pure growth and the presence of pus cells is reported, consideration must be given to the possibility of significant infection.

The clinical picture of fungaemia is indistinguishable from that in septicaemia of bacterial origin, and a high index of suspicion is essential. The microbiological laboratory must be informed when fungaemia is suspected, since special culture methods must be employed. All the published series have certain features in common [2, 51, 86, 102]. Every patient has had at least one course of antibiotics and there is an equally high correlation with intravenous and urinary catheterization. Intravenous feeding and abdominal sepsis also predispose to the development of fungaemia, as does treatment with immunosuppressant and corticosteroid drugs. Homograft cardiac valves have been incriminated in one outbreak [100]. It will be realized that this list of associated factors differs in no way from those which predispose to bacterial sepsis.

The treatment of fungaemia includes, wherever possible, the removal of the provoking cause; for example, re-operation and replacement of infected prosthetic heart valves has been shown to aid eradication of the infection [56, 100]. A variety of effective antifungal agents is available [56, 67]. Amphotericin is the longest-established drug, but it may have undesirable side-effects. 5-Fluorocytosine is less dangerous and may be given together with amphotericin, so that a smaller dose of each can be used [84]. Miconazole has not been available long enough for its place to be defined, but it can be given safely to patients who are suffering from renal failure. Amphotericin and miconazole should not be given together because they may be chemically antagonistic [26].

The effectiveness of treatment is usually seen within a few days, but usually it must be continued for several weeks, and in some cases for months.

Predisposing causes

Many of the factors which predispose ICU patients to life-threatening infectious diseases have been listed or implied earlier in this sec-

Table 52.3. Factors associated with systemic fungal infection

Antibiotic therapy
Intravenous catheterization
Homograft valve replacement
Urinary catheterization
Intravenous feeding
Abdominal sepsis
Immunosuppressant and steroid therapy

tion. It has been shown that by the nature of their presenting disease ICU patients are particularly vulnerable to infection of all kinds. Invasive instrumentation and the use of antibiotics are common to most of them, and others are shown in Tables 52.3 and 52.4. The combination of abdominal sepsis of GI, biliary, or GU tract origin and the need for controlled ventilation and intravenous alimentation has the worst prognosis. However, other problems must be considered. These include the elements which interfere with the patient's resistance to infection (Table 52.4).

1) *Severe physical trauma* has been shown to depress the body's response to infection. This has been demonstrated in patients after surgery, burns and accidental injury [37, 64, 68, 72]. Antibody production is impaired [25, 103, 104] and there is evidence that patients with burns may produce a specific toxin from the burnt tissue which interferes with defence against infection [85].

2) *Leucocyte function, including motility and phagocytosis,* are reduced by many forms of trauma. This has been demonstrated by the techniques of granulocyte adherence assay and the observation of cell migration [1, 4, 36, 43]. Leukopenia in the presence of established infection is a bad prognostic sign [43, 55] and granulocyte transfusions have been used with some success in critically ill patients [41, 42].

Table 52.4. Factors which interfere with host defence

Extremes of age
Debilitating diseases (malignancy, renal failure, etc.)
Diabetes
Immunosuppressant and corticosteroid drugs
Major trauma, major surgery
Malnutrition
Complement depletion
Inhibition of antibody production
Failure of leucocyte activation
Leukopenia
Depression of the reticuloendothelial system

3) Several authors have presented results which suggest that *complement production is reduced* in patients who are suffering from acute infective illnesses, and the failure of treatment has been related to this mechanism [47, 65, 83]. The complement system serves mainly to potentiate the capability of granulocytes to kill bacteria.

4) Patients who are receiving *regular haemodialysis* may be particularly at risk of infection. The disease which has caused renal failure is, by definition, likely to increase the patients' vulnerability to infection. Vascular access in the form of an arteriovenous shunt or fistula, or peritoneal dialysis techniques, render the patient particularly vulnerable. A further factor which may be involved is the adverse effect that certain dialysis materials, particularly cellophanes, have upon granulocyte numbers and their function [21, 48]. All the organisms listed in Table 52.1 have been identified as causes of infectious illnesses in patients who are suffering from renal failure, and in addition *Listeria monocytogenes* and *Pneumocystis* may occasionally be isolated.

5) *Malnutrition* is now generally recognized as a major problem in the patient who is suffering from life-threatening disease, and it has been shown that this can increase the patient's vulnerability to infection [94].

Prevention

Recommendations for prevention can be discussed from the viewpoints of unit design; staff and their training and motivation; asepsis and antisepsis; bacterial monitoring; and antibiotic policy.

Unit design

Intensive care units differ widely, and the recommendations which follow refer to a unit of six to ten beds serving an acute general hospital.

1) The unit should be *situated* so that it cannot be used for access to other departments. It is difficult to prove that visitors and transients are causes of infection, but since they may be restrictions on entry are advisable. Quite apart from the bacteriological aspects of this recommendation, excessive traffic and noise create a nuisance. The access doors to the ICU should be clearly labelled so that all visitors are aware that they are entering an area which has special problems.

2) The second design consideration is *adequate space*. Overcrowding and difficulties with access and movement increase the risks of cross infection. Each bed should have approximately 16 m^2 of space [50] and the bed area should be so designed that the nurse and patient can be independent of the rest of the unit. The area allocated to each bed should be square so that the attendants can move freely all around the patient. The distribution of beds into open and closed areas is still debated, but it is probably advisable to have between one-third and one-half of the beds in cubicles. This distribution depends upon the usage of the unit. If many of the patients spend less than 48 h in the unit the need for cubicles is reduced, which reduces pressure upon the nursing staff.

3) If patients who have sustained *extensive burns* or *other major trauma* form a significant proportion of the total the number of enclosed beds must be increased. The increased vulnerability of severely traumatized patients has already been referred to. Because of the possibly adverse emotional effect that the general activity of the ICU may have upon them, children should be nursed in cubicles.

4) Full *barrier nursing facilities* should be provided in two of the cubicles, which should be larger (up to 20 m^2) than the others [20]. These facilities should include separation of the entry and exit points with adequate scrub, gowning, and divesting areas so that 'clean' and 'dirty' procedures can be separated. Two types of patient may be regarded as in need of barrier nursing, namely those who are particularly vulnerable to infection and those who present a hazard to the staff and other patients in the ICU. The first group includes patients who are maximally immunosuppressed or leukopenic or who are suffering from still uninfected burns. The second group includes patients with viral hepatitis, staphylococcal pneumonia and severe skin sepsis [10]. In some hospitals patients who have undergone major orthopaedic prosthetic surgery are barrier-nursed because it is felt that such patients are particularly at risk from secondary infection.

5) Barrier nursing cubicles should be equipped with *unidirectional plenum ventilation systems* with external exhaust pathways, both for the comfort of the patients and staff and for the protection of other patients. There is no hard evidence that bacterially filtered air-conditioning is of benefit for the patient in the open part of the unit, but air-conditioning is

essential for their comfort [7, 66, 68, 88]. It may be considered desirable to duct the expired gas from ventilators to the outside of the building to reduce the contamination of the atmosphere with airborne pathogens.

In addition to their other uses the cubicles can be used when extensive wound dressings or other surgical manoeuvres are carried out, unless the ICU has its own operating theatre.

6) Other aspects of design are considered elsewhere, but as much space as possible must be allocated to *storage* and to clean and dirty preparation and disposal areas. This facilitates the cleaning and storage of all types of equipment, bedding, and clinical materials.

7) It is appropriate at this point to re-emphasize that patients must be protected from *contamination by their own secretions.* Contaminated linen must be changed immediately soiling occurs, which may be as frequently as every hour. This creates a demand for a large linen storage area. The linen must be handled and disposed of in such a way as to prevent dissemination of infected material, and a dirty linen disposal point should be regarded as an essential feature of ICU design. Contaminated material must never be stored inside an ICU. Disposable and single-use items reduce the risk of cross infection and the need for resterilization, but they create a need for extensive storage facilities.

8) All parts of the ICU must be provided with facilities for *handwashing,* equipped with antiseptic surgical scrub solution. There must be at least as many handbasins as beds, situated so that all attendants and visitors can use them before approaching the patient. Hand towels and single-use scrubbing brushes are also required. Bar soap and some cleaning fluids may be good bacterial culture media and they should be monitored at regular intervals.

Handbasins have been identified as sources of infection [40, 96]. They should be of a streamlined design, without ledges or overflows, to facilitate daily cleaning. The outflow should be protected so that waste water cannot splash back onto the users' hands or garments while in use. Basins are available that can be maintained at a temperature above that at which pathogens grow, but they may emit an unpleasant smell. If taps and faucets are found to be persistently contaminated they can be sterilized by heating with a blow torch.

9) This emphasis on basic cleanliness also applies to the patient. Sick patients are frequently restless and may constantly be touching themselves and their surroundings. It is easy to picture the consequences of a patient touching his contaminated wound and then handling his tracheostomy tube or urethral catheter. This hazard can only be minimized by *good nursing.*

Shelves, cupboards, and ledges are potential dust traps and should be eliminated. An easily cleaned, freely mobile unit which combines the function of a screen with that of a working surface and supply unit is used in many ICUs. Other services should be provided on the 'wall rail' system, which is convenient, unobtrusive, and easily cleaned.

10) When a patient *leaves the unit,* the whole patient area should be stripped for cleaning and the equipment replaced. The bed should also be stripped and cleaned. In some units the bed and mattress are removed for autoclaving but this is probably unnecessary.

Most of the other aspects of design are covered elsewhere in this book, but in general the whole unit must be designed to facilitate cleaning and to eliminate regions where dust can accumulate and contaminated objects be lost or forgotten. Floors, walls, and ceilings should be smooth-surfaced; non-reflecting surfaces are more restful to the eye than are polished finishes.

Staff: Training and motivation

In any ICU the most important factor is the number, quality, and motivation of its medical, nursing, and ancillary staff. There should be enough nurses to remove the need for them to move between patients and they should not be constantly working under pressure, since otherwise basic aseptic routines may be neglected. These requirements are met by an establishment of four trained nurses per bed, i.e., an 8-bedded unit requires 32 trained nurses, together with supervisory and ancillary staff.

The ICU may be compared with the operating room, and a similar though more broadly based training is required for the ICU nurse. The patients in both situations are equally vulnerable and are undergoing procedures which are potentially equally hazardous. The importance of personal cleanliness and attention to aseptic procedures must be pointed out at every opportunity. At the same time unnecessarily rigid restrictions should be avoided.

The nursing and medical staff should wear simple, lightweight, comfortable but close-fitting garments, but except when open wounds are being dressed, caps and masks need not be worn.

Everyone who enters an ICU should be made to wear shoe covers and a clean gown over the outdoor clothing. This cannot be shown conclusively to reduce the incidence of infection, but it limits the number of casual visitors and therefore reduces the amount of contamination from skin bacteria.

Practical methods for the aseptic performance of such manoeuvres as tracheal suction, urinary drainage, drug administration, and the establishment and maintenance of intravenous fluid pathways should be laid down. These techniques may need to be a compromise between what is theoretically ideal but impossibly time-consuming, and what can be performed quickly and safely. However, no dangerous short-cuts must be allowed and carelessness must be discouraged. Medical staff of all grades of seniority are often haphazard in the observance of such rules but lax behaviour should be discouraged by personal example. In every instance the reasons for these practices should be explained.

Asepsis and antisepsis

This part of the programme of prevention is an extension of the above section. Self-discipline and awareness of the special problems which exist in the ICU are the most important aspects of asepsis. It is important to establish a regimen of aseptic maintenance so that all the precautionary measures are enacted routinely. Ventilator and oxygen lines, humidifiers, nebulizers, and suction tubing must be changed daily. Hypochlorite solution is a cheap and effective antiseptic for sinks and other surfaces, but all dirt and solid detritus must be removed by thorough cleaning before any antiseptic can be effective.

Many methods are available for sterilizing ventilators [62, 82]. Ethylene oxide gas, alcohol vapour, and formaldehyde have been shown to be satisfactory, although they are explosive, inflammable, malodorous, or time-consuming. They may also damage metallic and plastic components of the ventilators. Some ventilators may be autoclaved, which virtually guarantees sterility, at least for a time. The present author has sterilized ventilators with 20 vol% hydrogen peroxide vapour for many years and has found it to be completely satisfactory. It is odourless, non-explosive, and non-toxic, and the ventilator can be re-used within 4 h of the start of the cleaning procedure.

If a system of cleaning which involves liquids of any sort is used, the ventilator must be dried completely afterwards. The most practical way to do this is with compressed air. Any piece of apparatus which is stored damp will usually be found to be contaminated with bacteria after 24 h.

A sensible alternative method which is now widely used is to fit heated bacterial filters into the inspiratory and expiratory pathways of the ventilator [44, 62, 63]. Provided a record of the duration of ventilator usage is kept this should be an adequate safeguard against infection. Disposable, single-use bacterial filters are available. If it is difficult to establish a satisfactory cleaning and sterilizing regimen, these alternatives may be used. It is advisable when considering the purchase of new ventilators to determine whether they are easily cleaned and sterilized. Humidifiers, nebulizers, and suction apparatus which cannot be autoclaved or boiled are best sterilized with a solution of sodium hypochlorite. It should be possible to dismantle humidifiers and similar equipment so that the interior can be examined and cleaned. This should be done every 24 h, or more frequently if they are obviously contaminated. Ventilators must be sterilized every 3 days when in long-term use, and after every usage.

Stock solutions of antiseptics, saline, and distilled water which are used for topical and other purposes must be packaged in small-volume containers and any unused fluid discarded after opening. This also applies to sachets of lubricating jelly and topical anaesthetic cream and liquids, all of which are readily contaminated by handling or after contact with patients [6].

Intravenous infusion fluids and intravenous feeding materials easily become infected. Drugs and other additives must only be introduced into such fluids in a laminar flow chamber, and nothing should ever be added to blood products (whole blood, albumin solutions, coagulation factors) or to fat solutions, because of the risk of bacterial contamination and chemical incompatibility. The care of intravascular lines has been referred to earlier and all infusion sets must be renewed each 24 h. Ideally this would include the intravascular line, but this is usually not feasible.

The preceding section may suggest that the ICU must have an environment that is a combination of a bacteriological laboratory and a church. It is vital to realize that although many routine precautions need to be taken, the staff in the unit can be taught to perform them without in any way creating a restrictive working environment. This point is made elsewhere in this book, but an ICU which cannot combine self-discipline with relaxation is unlikely to function satisfactorily.

Bacterial monitoring policy

A bacterial monitoring policy is intended to facilitate the early recognition of colonization and infection. It acknowledges that however efficient cleaning and aseptic techniques are, their effects are short-lived and must be checked. It is applied to the patients in the unit and to their environment. Occasionally it may be necessary to exclude sources of infection amongst the ICU staff. With the support of the microbiological laboratory it can be simple and effective, and like many of the regimens in the ICU it should form part of the standard routine [89]. Again, as with other systems of observation and treatment it should not be inflexible, and should be modified when experience dictates that change is indicated.

On admission to the ICU every patient should have specimens taken for baseline microbiological data to be obtained. These should always include nose, throat, and sputum specimens, and when appropriate other secretions should be sampled. Urine, blood cultures, and specimens from abdominal drains and from venous and arterial cannulae should be included where indicated. If the patient requires controlled ventilation the ventilator and humidifier must be known not to be contaminated before being attached to the patient. In all cases, the results should be recorded so that the information obtained is immediately available.

These sites, and others which may become apparent during treatment, must be monitored at intervals after the initial samples have been taken. Ideally the monitoring would be performed daily, but a three-times-weekly routine is acceptable.

Area sampling should be performed at 3-monthly intervals as a routine. Agar plates should be exposed at known sites and samples taken from water taps, washhand basins, kitchen equipment, air-conditioning outlets, and any other appropriate position. A simple outline drawing of the ICU with the relevant features mentioned above marked upon it can be used to record the sites from which samples are taken. The results of such monitoring should be compared with those of previous tests, and any evidence which implies that dangerous colonization or failure of cleaning and antiseptic regimens has occurred should be discussed. The cleaning and technical staff should always be included in these discussions so that they can be made aware of the importance which is attached to their efforts.

The most important aspect of staff monitoring is concerned with the problem of serum hepatitis (HBA, Australian antigen-positive hepatitis). For medicolegal reasons it is advisable to ensure that all staff members are AA-negative when they join the unit. Thereafter HBA testing should be performed at intervals of approximately 6 months, and if serum-positive patients are nursed in the ICU, at an appropriate interval after they are discharged. All blood samples and other secretions from such patients should be clearly labelled and packed in tightly sealed containers, with great care being taken to avoid spillage. If the patient dies in the unit special precautions must be taken when handling the body. A double-layered plastic bag should be used and it is usually recommended that an autopsy is carried out only for the most exceptional reasons.

In most countries no policy decision has been taken with regard to the employment of medical and nursing staff who are antigen-positive.

Antibiotic policy

The problem of infection in the ICU must be considered in the context of the hospital as a whole. The widespread and often inappropriate use of antibiotics has contributed to the problem by encouraging the emergence of resistant strains of bacteria, and by devaluing many previously useful antibiotic and chemotherapeutic agents [16, 46, 79]. Failure to measure the blood antibiotic levels achieved during treatment has increased the dangers of undertreatment and the occurrence of toxic effects [73, 92].

Awareness of these difficulties has encouraged many hospitals to adopt an antibiotic policy [78]. This is established, reviewed, and monitored by an advisory committee, which is composed of clinical microbiologists, physicians, surgeons, and other interested personnel. Its purpose is to rationalize the use of antibiotics in the light of information which is obtained from general and local sources. It should also reduce the danger of undue influence on the part of the promoters of new antibiotics and the unwillingness of clinicians to change established and possibly outdated practices.

There is no doubt that if this type of policy was adopted throughout the hospital, all patients, not just those in the ICU, would benefit

[92]. It would limit the emergence of resistant strains of bacteria, discourage the use of useless antibiotics, and reserve others for the treatment of specific conditions inside and outside the ICU. It would probably also reduce the cost of treatment.

The antibiotic policy is based upon a number of factors. These are:

1) The laboratory identification of organisms, the frequency with which they occur in various sites, and their clinical significance
2) Changing patterns of antibiotic sensitivity
3) The effectiveness and toxicity of antibiotic treatment
4) The cost of such treatment.

This type of policy was originally necessitated by the emergence of the 'hospital *staphylococcus*' following the introduction of antibiotic and chemotherapeutic agents. The *staphylococcus* is not at present the major bacterial problem in hospitals, but the need for the advisory committee still exists. It should publish its findings at regular intervals. It should be sufficiently authoritative for its opinions to be respected by the hospital clinicians, but in the final analysis the decision with regard to treatment remains with the clinician who has direct responsibility for the care of patients.

In some circumstances the committee may suggest that certain antibiotics are no longer effective against the hospital's bacterial flora and may advise their total withdrawal. They may also give specific indications for the use of others. This type of advice has been shown to be of great value [16, 39, 78, 97].

A close relationship between the ICU and the hospital department of microbiology is essential. The routine monitoring policy referred to above is much more likely to be meaningful if the technicians who perform the isolation procedures understand their importance. The opinion of the clinical microbiologist should be obtained whenever a difficult problem arises and the department of microbiology staff should be encouraged to undertake epidemiological research in the ICU.

References

1. Alexander JW (1968) Neutrophil function in selected surgical disorders. Ann Surg 168:447–449
2. Ashcraft KW, Leape LL (1970) Candida sepsis complicating parenteral feeding. JAMA 212:454–456
3. Atherton ST, White DJ (1978) Stomach as source of bacteria colonizing respiratory tract during artificial ventilation. Lancet II:968–969
4. Atik M (1979) Granulocyte adherence assay in acute infection as a reflection of the host resistance. Surg Gynecol Obstet 149:879–883
5. Bailey MJ (1979) Reduction of catheter associated sepsis in parenteral nutrition using low-dose intravenous heparin. Br Med J i:1671–1673
6. Baird RM, Brown WRL, Shooter RA (1976) Pseudomonas aeruginosa in hospital pharmacies. Br Med J i:511–512
7. Barton FL, Branthwaite MA, English ICW, Prentis JJ (1973) Atmospheric contamination in intensive therapy units. Anaesthesia 28:160–163
8. Berger SA, Nagar H, Weitzman S (1978) Prophylactic antibiotics in surgical procedures. Surg Gynecol Obstet 146:469–475
9. Bettelheim KA, Faiers M, Shooter RA (1972) Serotypes of *Escherichia coli* in normal stools. Lancet II:1224–1226
10. Bridges K, Kidson A, Lowbury EJL, Wilkins MD (1979) Gentamicin- and silver-resistant Pseudomonas in a burns unit. Br Med J i:446–450
11. Bruun JN, Solberg CO (1973) Hand carriage of gram-negative bacilli and *Staphylococcus aureus*. Br Med J i:579–582
12. Bryant LR, Trinkle JK, Mobin-Uddin K (1972) Bacterial colonization profile with tracheal intubation and mechanical ventilation. Arch Surg 104:647–650
13. Burns MW (1973) Significance of *Pseudomonas aeruginosa* in sputum. Br Med J ii:382–383
14. Cartwright RY, Hargrave PR (1970) Pseudomonas in ventilators. Lancet I:40–42
15. Casewell M, Phillips I (1977) Hands as routes of transmission of *Klebsiella* sp. Br Med J ii:1315–1317
16. Castle M, Wilfert CM, Cate TR, Ousterhout S (1977) Antibiotic use at Duke University Medical Center. JAMA 237:2819–2823
17. Chow AW, Taylor PR, Yoshiwa TT, Guze LB (1979) A nosocomial outbreak of infections due to multiply resistant *Proteus mirabilis*: Role of intestinal colonization as a major reservoir. J Infect Dis 139:621–627
18. Clark LP, Marshall HA, Ackerman NB (1974) The role of Bacteroides as an infectious organism. Surg Gynecol Obstet 138:562–566
19. Colvin MP, Blogg CE, Savege TM, Jarvis JD, Strunin L (1972) A safe long-term infusion technique. Lancet II:317–320
20. Control of Infection Group (1974) Isolation system for general hospitals. Br Med J i:41–44
21. Craddock PR, Fehr J, Brigham KL, Kronenberg RS, Jacob HS (1977) Complement and leukocyte-mediated pulmonary dysfunction in hemodialysis. N Engl J Med 296 14:769–774
22. Craven DE, Bruins S, McCabe WR (1977) Sepsis due to gram negative bacilli: Epidemiology, pathogenesis and immunological aspects. In: Ledingham I McA (ed): Recent advances in intensive therapy, vol I. Churchill Livingstone, Edinburgh, p 177–190
23. Darell JH, Utley AHC (1976) Antibiotics in the perioperative period. Br J Anaesth 48:13–18
24. Darrell JH, Wahba AH (1964) Pyocine typing of hospital strains of *Pseudomonas pyocyanae*. J Clin Pathol 17:236–240
25. Diaz F, Mosovitch LL, Neter E (1970) Serogroups of *Pseudomonas aeruginosa* and the immune response of patients with cystic fibrosis. J Infect Dis 121:269–274
26. Duport B, Drouhet E (1979) In vitro synergy and antagonism of antifungal agents against yeast-like fungi. Postgrad Med J 55:683–686

27. Editorial (1974) Microbiological hazards of intravenous infusions. Lancet I:543–544

28. Eykin SJ, Jackson BT, Lockhart Mummery HE, Phillips I (1979) Prophylactic per-operative intravenous metronidazole in elective colo-rectal surgery. Lancet II:761–764

29. Fossard DP, Kakkar VV, Elsey PA (1974) Assessment of Limulus test for detecting endotoxaemia. Br Med J i:465–468

30. Freeman R, King B (1972) Infective complications of intravenous catheters and the monitoring of infection by the nitroblue tetrazolium test. Lancet I:992–993

31. Fry DE, Garrison RN, Polk HC (1979) Clinical implications in Bacteroides bacteremia. Surg Gynecol Obstet 149:189–192

32. Garrod LP (1972) Causes of failure of antibiotic therapy. Br Med J ii:473–475

33. Gaya H (1976) Infection control in intensive care. Br J Anaesth 48:9–12

34. Goldman DA, Martin WT, Workington JW (1973) Growth of bacteria and fungi in total parenteral nutritional solutions. Am J Surg 129:314–317

35. Goldring J, Sacott A, McNaught W, Gillespie G (1975) Prophylactic oral microbial agents in elective colonic surgery. Lancet II:997–999

36. Greco RS, Dick L, Duckenfield J (1978) Perioperative suppression of the leukocyte migration inhibition assay in patients undergoing elective operations. Surg Gynecol Obstet 147:717–720

37. Hamer-Hodges D, Woodruff P, Cuevas P, Kaufman A, Fine J (1974) Role of intra-intestinal gram negative bacterial flora in response to major injury. Surg Gynecol Obstet 138:599–603

38. Harris DM, Orwin JM, Colquhoun J, Schroeder HG (1969) Control of cross infection in an intensive care unit. J Hyg (Lond) 67:525–533

39. Haverkorn MJ, Michel MF (1979a) Nosocomial Klebsiellas: i. Colonization of hospital patients. J Hyg (Lond) 82:117–193

40. Haverkorn MJ, Michel MF (1979b) Nosocomial Klebsiellas: ii. Transfer in a hospital ward. J Hyg (Lond) 82:195–205

41. Herzig RH, Herzig GP, Graw RG, Bull MI, Ray KK (1977) Successful granulocyte transfusion therapy for gram-negative septicemia. N Engl J Med 296:701–705

42. Higby DJ (1977) Controlled prospective studies of granulocyte transfusion therapy. Exp Hematol [Suppl 1]:57–64

43. Hohn DC (1977) Leukocyte phagocytic function and dysfunction. Surg Gynecol Obstet 144:99–109

44. Holdcroft A, Lumley J, Gaya H (1973) Why disinfect ventilators? Lancet I:240–241

45. Hunt TK, Alexander JW, Burke JK, Maclean LD (1975) Antibiotics in surgery. Arch Surg 110:148–155

46. Jackson GG (1979) Antibiotic policies, practices and pressures. J Antimicrob Chemother 5:1–5

47. Jacobs HS (1978) Granulocyte–complement interaction. Arch Intern Med 138:461–463

48. Kaslow RA, Zellner SR (1972) Infection in patients on maintenance haemodialysis. Lancet II:117–119

49. Kass EH (1956) Asymptomatic infections of the urinary tract. Trans Assoc Am Physicians 69:56–60

50. Khanam T, Branthwaite MA, English ICW, Prentis JJ (1973) The control of pulmonary sepsis in intensive therapy units. Anaesthesia 28:17–28

51. Klein JJ, Watanakunakorn C (1979) Hospital acquired fungemia. Am J Med 67:51–58

52. Leading Article (1970) Prophylactic antibiotics. Lancet II:1231–1232

53. Leading Article (1979a) Monitoring devices and septicaemia. Br Med J i:1747–1748

54. Leading Article (1979b) Gut as a reservoir of resistant bacteria. Lancet II:945–946

55. Leading Article (1980a) Infection complicating severe granulocytopenia. Lancet I:25–26

56. Leading Article (1980b) Treating fungal infections. Br Med J i:668–669

57. Leigh DA (1974) Clinical importance of infection due to *Bacteroides fragilis* and role of antibiotic therapy. Br Med J i:225–228

58. Levin J (1964) The incidence and prevention of infection after urethral catherization. Ann Intern Med 60:914–922

59. Levin J, Poore TE, Zanbert NB, Oser L (1970) Detection of endotoxin in human blood. N Engl J Med 283:1313–1316

60. Lowbury EJL, Fox J (1954) The epidemiology of infection with *Pseudomonas pyocyanae* in a burns unit. J Hyg (Lond) 52:403–409

61. Lowbury EJL, Thorn BT, Lilly HA, Babb JR, Whitall K (1970) Sources of infection with *Pseudomonas aeruginosa* in patients with tracheostomy. J Med Microbiol 3:39–41

62. Lumley J (1976) Decontamination of anaesthetic equipment and ventilators. Br J Anaesth 48:3–8

63. Lumley J, Holdcroft A, Gaya H, Darlow HM, Adams DJ (1976) Expiratory bacterial filters. Lancet II:22–24

64. Maclean LD, Meakins JL, Taguchi K, Duignan JP, Dhillon KS, Gordon J (1975) Host resistance in sepsis and trauma. Ann Surg 182:207–212

65. McCabe WR (1973) Complement levels in gram-negative bacteremia. N Engl J Med 288:21–23

66. McLaughlan J, Logie JRC, Smylie HG, Singh G (1976) The role of clean air in wound infection acquired during operation. Surg Gynecol Obstet 143:6–8

67. Medoff G, Kobayashi GS (1980) Strategies in the treatment of systemic fungal infections. N Engl J Med 302:145–155

68. Miller RM, Polokavetz SH, Hornick RB, Cowley RA (1973) Analysis of infections acquired by the severely injured patient. Surg Gynecol Obstet 137:7–10

69. Montgomerie JZ, Doeck PB, Taylor DEM, North JDK, Martin WJ (1970) *Klebsiella* in faecal flora of transplant patients. Lancet II:787–792

70. Moody ML, Burke JP (1972) Infection and antibiotic use in a large private hospital. Comparisons among hospitals serving different populations. Arch Intern Med 130:261–265

71. Moore WEC, Cato EL, Holderman LV (1969) Anaerobic bacteria of the gastro-intestinal flora and their occurrence in clinical infection. J Infect Dis 120:641–650

72. Munster AM (1976) Post-traumatic immunosuppression is due to activation of suppressor T cells. Lancet I:1329–1330

73. Noone P, Parsons TMC, Pattison JR, Slack RCB, Garfield Davies D, Hughes K (1974) Experience in monitoring gentamicin therapy during treatment of serious gram-negative sepsis. Br Med J i:477–481

74. Northey D, Adess ML, Hartsuck JM, Rhoades ER (1974) Microbial surveillance in a surgical intensive care unit. Surg Gynecol Obstet 139:321–325

75. Park BN, Fikrig SM, Smith EM (1968) Infection and nitroblue–tetrazolium reduction by neutrophils. Lancet II:532–534

76. Parker TH, O'Leary JP (1978) Effect of preparation of the small intestine on microflora and postoperative wound infection. Surg Gynecol Obstet 146:379–382

77. Phillips I, Spencer G (1965) *Pseudomonas aeruginosa* cross infection. Lancet II:1325–1327

78. Phillips I (1979) Antibiotic policies. In: Reeves D, Geddes A (eds) Recent advances in infection, vol. I. Churchill Livingstone, Edinburgh and London, pp 151–163

79. Pollock AV, Arnott RS, Leaper DJ, Evans M (1978) The role of antibacterial preparation of the intestine in the reduction of primary wound sepsis after operations on the colon and rectum. Surg Gynecol Obstet 147:909–912

80. Prachar H, Dittel M, Jobst C, Kiss E, Machacek E, Nobis H, Spiel R (1978) Bacterial contamination of pulmonary artery catheters. Intensive Care Med 4:79–82

81. Price DJE, Sleigh JD (1970) Control of infection due to *Klebsiella aerogenes* in a neuro-surgical department by withdrawal of all antibiotics. Lancet II:1213–1216

82. Roberts RB (1970) The eradication of cross infection from anesthetic equipment. Anesth Analg (Cleve) 49:63–68

83. Robin M, Intrator L, Andre C, Lagrue G, Rapin M (1974) Anomalies du complement et choc infectieux. Nouv Presse Med 3:883–884

84. Saunders AM, Goolden AWG, Darrell JH (1978) Cryptococcosis: Survival attributed to combination antifungal treatment. Br Med J i:1930–1931

85. Schoenenberger GA, Burckhardt F, Kalberer F, Müller W, Städtler K, Vogt P, Allgöwer M (1975) Experimental evidence for a significant impairment of host defence for gram-negative organisms by a specific cutaneous toxin produced by severe burn injuries. Surg Gynecol Obstet 4:555–559

86. Seelig MS (1966) The role of antibiotics in the pathogenesis of Candida infections. Am J Med 40:887–890

87. Selden R, Lee S, Wang WLL, Bennett JV, Eickhoff TC (1971) Nosocomial colonization as a reservoir. Ann Intern Med 74:657–664

88. Shaw D, Doig CM, Douglas D (1973) Is airborne infection in operating theatres an important cause of wound infections in general surgery? Lancet I:17–20

89. Shield MJ, Hammill HJ, Neale DA (1979) Systemic bacterial monitoring of intensive care unit patients: The results of a twelve-month study. Intensive Care Med 5:171–181

90. Shooter RA, Walker KA, Williams VR, Horgan GM, Asheshar EA, Bullimore JF (1966) Faecal carriage of *Pseudomonas aeruginosa* in hospital patients. Lancet II:1331–1333

91. Shooter RA, Cooke EM, Gaya H, Kumar PJ, Parker MT, Thorn BT, Trace DB (1969) Foods and medicaments as possible sources of hospital strains of *Pseudomonas aeruginosa*. Lancet I:1227–1230

92. Speller DCE, Bint AJ, Stephens M (1977) Experience with amikacin and colistin in an outbreak of infection by resistant *Klebsiella aerogenes*. Antimicrob Chemother 3:483–491

93. Spink WW (1972) The ecology of human septic shock. In: Hershey SG, del Guercio LRM, McConn R (eds) Septic shock in man Little Brown, Boston, pp 3–14

94. Stinnett JD, Alexander JW (1978) Nutrition as related to host defence and infection. In: Richards JR, Kinney JM (eds) Nutritional aspects of care in the critically ill. Churchill Livingstone, Edinburgh, pp 557–569

95. Stoddart JC (1974) Gram-negative infections in the ICU. Crit Care Med 2:17–22

96. Teres D, Schweers P, Bushnell LS, Hedley Whyte J, Feingold DS (1973) Sources of *Pseudomonas aeruginosa* infection in a respiratory-surgical intensive therapy unit. Lancet I:415–417

97. Thadepalli H (1979) Principles and practice of antibiotic therapy for post-traumatic abdominal injuries. Surg Gynecol Obstet 148:937–951

98. Thornton GF, Andriole VT (1970) Bacteriuria during indwelling catheter drainage. JAMA 214:339–342

99. Vargish T, Crawford LC, Stallings RA, Wasilauskas BL, Myers RT (1978) A randomised prospective evaluation of orally administered antibiotics in operations on the colon. Surg Gynecol Obstet 146:193–198

100. Wain W, Ahmed M, Thompson R, Yacoub M (1979) The role of chemotherapy in the management of fungal endocarditis following homograft replacement. Postgrad Med J 55:629–631

101. Washington JA, Dearing WH, Judd IS, Elverback LR (1974) Effect of pre-operative antibiotic regimen on development of infection after intestinal surgery. Ann Surg 180:567–571

102. Weinstein AJ, Johnson EH, Moellering RC (1973) Candida endophthalmitis. A complication of Candidemia. Arch Intern Med 132:749–753

103. Young LS (1974) Role of antibody in infection due to Pseudomonas aeruginosa. J Infect Dis [Suppl] 130:5111–5118

104. Young LS, Yu BH, Armstrong D (1970) Agar-gel precipitating antibody in Pseudomonas infection. Infect Immun 2 4:495–503

Chapter 53

Management of Sepsis

Maurice Rapin and Claude George

The septic state is defined not only as the occurrence of an infection, but also as the general response of the body towards this infection.

In the critically ill, severe sepsis must be promptly recognized, though this is often difficult to achieve. For this reason the symptoms of severe sepsis are reviewed at the beginning of this chapter.

With the recognition of severe sepsis, three items of information should be sought: the location of infection; the causative organism; and the state of the host's immunity. Only with at least tentative answers to these questions can proper therapy be defined, a point which is developed in the final part of this chapter.

Recognition of severe sepsis

In the critically ill, recognition of sepsis is often difficult: the common symptoms due to sepsis may be absent whereas others, less commonly encountered, may be prominent. Furthermore, recent results [41] indicate that the clinical picture is not different whatever the micro-organism responsible.

Temperature

Fever is a frequent and early sign of infection and may be preceded by shivering. It is due to the passage of micro-organisms or their toxins into the bloodstream [13]. However, in the critically ill fever may be absent or even replaced by a fall in body temperature [3]. In these circumstances, hypothermia has the same diagnostic and bacteriological implications as a high fever. Furthermore, severe sepsis may be present despite a normal or only marginally raised temperature. This phenomenon is especially frequent in Gram-negative septicaemia and in patients with renal failure or hepatic cirrhosis. The reason for this is unclear but it may be due to a weakened inflammatory response. Since fever in the critically ill may be due to several non-bacterial causes (e.g., deep vein thrombosis, haematomas, drug intolerance), it is necessary to conclude that an abnormality in the temperature chart is a useful alarm signal but does not prove that an infection exists. On the other hand, normal temperature does not rule out severe infection.

Haemodynamic disturbances

Circulatory shock is frequently the first sign of severe sepsis. Septic shock is easily diagnosed when a low arterial pressure is found, but in fact this is a late sign. Tachycardia, cutaneous and neurological signs, and decreased urine output occur much earlier [14]. The clinical features of septic shock are analysed in Chap. 12.

Acute respiratory distress syndrome (ARDS)

As discussed previously, ARDS occurs frequently during severe sepsis and may be the most prominent feature. This syndrome is associated with non-haemodynamic pulmonary oedema and is usually accompanied by hypoxaemia and hypocapnia related to abnormalities in ventilation: perfusion ratios. Clinically, breathing is rapid and superficial, cough is nonproductive, and murmurs are rare.

Diaphragmatic excursion is decreased, especially with abdominal involvement in the infective process or after laparotomy. Chest x-ray examination reveals diffuse and extensive consolidation associated with micro-atelectasias. Pulmonary compliance is decreased, and in patients succumbing to this syndrome intra-alveolar hyaline membranes may be found on post-mortem examination. ARDS is an important prognostic factor in severe sepsis [23].

Acute renal failure

Acute renal failure occurs frequently during severe sepsis. It must be distinguished from simple nitrogen retention due to increased catabolism, in which the blood creatinine is normal. On urine analysis, it is possible to distinguish between functional and organic renal failure: in the former, urine is concentrated, urinary urea concentration is high (usually over 20 times the blood urea), and urinary sodium is low (less than 20 mMol/litre) and less concentrated than urinary potassium. Pathological examination in established renal failure has shown that the lesions involve both renal tubules and the intersitium, although in some cases there is also evidence of a glomerular lesion [5]. The mechanism of acute renal failure during severe sepsis is highly complex and probably several mechanisms can be implicated, including tubular obstruction, an increase in interstitial pressure from oedema, and alterations in renal blood flow associated with a decreased filtration pressure due to dilatation of afferent glomerular arterioles.

Abdominal symptoms and gastric bleeding

During severe sepsis, whatever its cause, abdominal symptoms are frequent. They usually start with meteorism and reflex ileus and may lead to acute necrotizing enterocolitis. Occasionally, one of the earliest signs of severe sepsis is gastro-intestinal (GI) haemorrhage. Prospective gastric fibroscopy during sepsis has demonstrated that gastro-duodenal lesions occur frequently. They begin as mucosal purpura, which is followed by superficial erosions, and the acute ulcers then become haemorrhagic if sepsis is not controlled [25]. Several factors account for these lesions, including mucosal ischaemia, rupture of the mucosal barrier, increased retrodiffusion of H^+ ions, and reflux of bile salts. They may appear rapidly after the onset of the infection but the bleeding stops abruptly when the infection has been overcome.

Jaundice

Jaundice occurs frequently during severe sepsis, and is related to hepatic dysfunction due to either infectious hepatitis or the hepatic complications of septic shock [30]. Intrahepatic cholestasis is associated with inflammatory infiltration of the portal tracts compressing biliary canaliculi. Septic shock causes hypoxia of hepatocytes by reducing portal blood flow, whereas hepatic arterial flow is usually preserved. The severity of jaundice is increased by acute renal failure, because excretion of conjugated bilirubin is reduced, and also by increased production of bilirubin consequent upon blood transfusions, resorption of haematomas, or haemolysis induced by bacteria. In the presence of clinically significant jaundice it is essential to exclude biliary tract infection.

Coagulation disorders

Occasionally in very severe acute sepsis, coagulation disorders are the hallmark of the disease; for example, purpura fulminans is mainly due to meningococcal infections but may also be observed with pneumococci in asplenic patients or even in very severe septicaemias due to Gram-negative bacilli. Sometimes, in vitro study of coagulation indicates the presence of true intravascular coagulation (IVC) thrombocytopenia associated with hypofibrinaemia, and a decrease in factor V and other co-factors. Experimentally, infusion of endotoxins has been shown to induce IVC in several species by an action on platelets, vascular endothelium, and the coagulation process. In man, however, intravascular thrombi are found far less frequently and IVC may be regarded as incidental [27]. More frequently, fibrin levels are increased and a decrease in partial thromboplastin time related to hepatic failure is observed, in which case the basic trouble is a thrombocytopenia, which may be profound (less than 30 000/mm^3), causing bleeding especially after surgical procedures. Recently the mechanisms of this thrombocytopenia have been studied and increased im-munoglobulin G associated with platelets has been found implicating the immune process [21].

Metabolic disturbances

During severe sepsis several metabolic disturb-ances occur which are characterized by low recovery of energy metabolism in spite of an increased demand [36]. Hyperglycaemia is due to secretion of cortisol, growth hormone, and glucagon, which increases hepatic gluco-neogenesis from amino acids. Hypersecretion of catecholamines causes glycogenolysis and inhibits insulin secretion. Nitrogen catabolism results from increased gluconeogenesis, which causes degradation of numerous important pro-teins, including those necessary for plasma transport, hepatic enzymes, and those involved in the immune response. Glucose becomes the main supply of energy, thereby increasing in-sulin secretion which may block fatty acid mobi-lization.

Encephalopathy

In the severely ill patient, consciousness is usually depressed as a result of diminished cerebral blood flow. In some patients, however this alteration may be pronounced and of long duration. Examination may reveal myoclonia and asterixis.

The white cell count

With most types of infection the white cell count (WCC) is elevated, especially when the sup-purative process is long-lasting. However, acute sepsis may be associated with the phenomenon of margination of leucocytes and the leucocyte count is consequently low. Similarly, in patients with depressed marrow function, as in folate deficiency, the WCC is reduced. As a conse-quence, a normal WCC cannot rule out severe sepsis.

Factors influencing the choice of treatment

Causative organisms

The identification of the micro-organisms re-sponsible for sepsis depends upon the conven-tional procedures for the isolation of bacteria, viruses, and protozoa. In the vast majority of cases, especially in countries where intensive care is well developed, severe sepsis is related to bacterial infections, and this section is de-voted primarily to these.

Knowledge of the site of infection enables a list of 'possible' causative organisms to be com-piled. Therefore, specific bacteriological prob-lems are considered for each site of infection.

In theory, bacteriological examination indi-cates the causative micro-organisms but in practice, except for direct examination of some biological fluids, the examination may take several days, and in some instances no bacteria grow. Whenever possible, all samples for bac-teriological study must be taken before antibio-tic therapy is started. All results have to be analysed critically; in some situations positive growth may represent contaminants.

Blood cultures

These should always be performed for it is of the utmost importance to know whether septi-caemia is really present, and bacteria isolated from several blood cultures have far greater significance than bacteria isolated from 'local' specimens.

A single blood culture only should never be performed, because of the risk of introducing contaminants from the patient's skin [34]. This is why only one positive culture of a Gram-negative bacterium is of doubtful significance, or conversely why several positive blood cul-tures are needed to incriminate *Staphylococcus epidermidis*.

Other examinations

Colonization of the patient by Gram-negative bacteria after admission to hospital explains why local examinations may have little value, especially sputum, urine, or wound swab ex-amination. The specific procedures for bacterial examination will be emphasized for each loca-tion of infection.

Location of infection

When blood cultures are performed the focus of infection is searched for methodically.

The investigation is based upon the symp-toms which have preceded the occurrence of severe sepsis, certain physical signs which may have a localizing value, and complementary examinations, especially x-ray and local bacteriological examinations.

Thereafter, surgical treatment of the septic foci should be considered in every case once it has localized.

Lungs and pleura

There are several types of agent that can cause pleuropulmonary infections, but with bacterial (especially anaerobes) and less frequently viral agents the clinical picture may be one of severe sepsis, sometimes dominating the symptoms of acute respiratory failure (ARF).

Clinical features. These are many, and include coryza, sore throat, cough with purulent, rust-coloured, or bloody sputum, pleuritic chest pain, and dyspnoea. The history should be checked for pharyngeal infection, alcoholism, or difficulty in swallowing, and the possibility of pleuropulmonary infection should always be considered after a general anaesthetic has been administered.

Symptoms of severe sepsis are associated with intense cyanosis, flaring of the ala nasi during inspiration, intense dyspnoea with tachypnea, inspiratory rales, and perhaps signs of consolidation and pleural friction rub or evidence of pleural fluid.

Investigations. Usually only an anteroposterior chest x-ray examination is possible at the bedside; it may reveal opacification of the lungs with a lobar or diffuse patchy distribution. Whereas the chest film is seldom diagnostic of a specific organism, it may be suggestive: lung abscesses are frequently multiple in the case of staphylococcal pneumonia, especially in children. Necrotizing pneumonia caused by aspiration of oral anaerobic organisms also causes abscesses.

Bacteriology. When pneumonia is suspected, a bacteriological examination of the sputum should be performed; this is helpful when the sputum is purulent or bloody but not particularly so when the cough is non-productive, when any isolates should be considered with caution. Very often in hospitalized patients growth of Gram-negative bacteria in the sputum is the result of oropharyngeal contamination. Direct aspiration of bronchial secretions may be more helpful in difficult cases, and samples can be obtained with transtracheal aspiration, or via an endotracheal tube or fiberoptic bronchoscope, although the last two techniques can introduce pharyngeal flora into the bronchial tree. Aspiration of a pleural effusion, if present,

may also yield valuable bacteriological information.

The diagnosis of viral infections is made by isolation of the virus in the sputum and by serologic assays. Mycotic or parasitic organisms infect predominantly immunosuppressed patients.

Surgery. Drainage of lung abscesses is helped by bronchial aspiration, physiotherapy, and an inclined position. Purulent pleural effusions should be evacuated as completely as possible by aspiration or surgical drainage.

Peritoneum

The clinical picture of an intraperitoneal infection varies according to whether the infection is initially generalized (peritonitis) or localized (intraperitoneal abscess).

Peritonitis. In secondary bacterial peritonitis, the numerous species of both aerobic and anaerobic micro-organisms that occur in the GI tract may all be found. In contrast, primary bacterial peritonitis is usually seen in patients with ascites and is often due to streptococci and *Enterobacteriaceae*.

Clinical features. These include abdominal pain, fever, and chills; abdominal distension, diffuse and/or localized tenderness with rigidity of the abdominal wall and absent bowel sounds are characteristic. The location of the pain and tenderness may suggest the nature of the underlying cause. Findings are usually less prominent at both extremes of age, in alcoholics, and in patients with ascites or receiving steroids.

Investigations. Supine and upright straight x-ray examination of the abdomen may show air in the peritoneal cavity, evidence of ileus or peritoneal fluid. In doubtful cases, peritoneal puncture or catheterization may be helpful in the diagnosis.

Bacteriology and surgery. After diagnosis, prompt surgery is indicated in most cases, the degree of urgency depending on the severity of the sepsis. Except in cases of primary peritonitis, bacteriologic examination of peritoneal pus is of little significance, since it always contains organisms from the GI tract. If no anaerobic strains are found it probably implies incorrect sampling.

Intraperitoneal abcess. After an intraperitoneal infection or any abdominal operation, subphrenic or pelvic abscesses may develop.

Clinical features. The onset of these is usually insidious, with low-grade fever, diarrhoea, abdominal distension, abdominal or thoracic pain, and finally the symptoms of severe sepsis. Localized tenderness of the abdomen, basal ileus (in the case of subphrenic abscess), or findings consistent with a pleural effusion may be present.

Investigations. The most consistent findings seen on chest and abdominal x-ray pictures are elevation of the diaphragm, basal atelectasis, pleural effusion, and gas-fluid levels. Localization of the abscess may be achieved by ultrasonic or CAT examination, possibly in association with a gallium scan [8]; sinograms may be possible in postoperative patients.

Surgery. After proper localization the abscess should be evacuated, care being taken to avoid seeding of the peritoneal cavity.

Female pelvis

As a complication of septic abortion or in association with pelvic thrombophlebitis, pelvic infection in the female can be life-threatening because of the presence of anaerobic organisms, particularly clostridial species.

Clinical features. A history of purulent and/or bloody vaginal discharge or of a preceding abortion is usually obtained.

Lower abdominal pain is a feature and serosanguineous material may be present in the vaginal vault. Following an abortion the uterus is enlarged and tender.

Investigations and treatment. After several blood cultures have been taken (cultures of the vaginal or uterine discharge are of no value) and antibiotics effective against anaerobes administered careful curettage of the uterus should be performed, even if most of the products appear to have been expelled spontaneously. If the patient's condition does not improve rapidly a hysterectomy must be considered.

Bile ducts

Infection of the bile ducts is usually associated with obstruction of the biliary tract.

Clinical features. Acute colicky pain in the right upper quadrant, rigor, and fever followed by jaundice are the typical symptoms. Sometimes the jaundice is more marked than the history of pain.

Examination may reveal right upper quadrant tenderness and guarding. Signs of a pleural effusion and pain on percussion of the liver are suggestive of an associated hepatic abscess, but this is extremely difficult to diagnose and can occur without biliary obstruction, for example in appendicitis, amoebic infection, or staphylococcal septicaemia.

Investigations. An ultrasound scan of the liver is the investigation of choice, or if this is not available abdominal angiography or radioisotope scanning may be used. Liver function tests show an elevation of conjugated bilirubin and moderate increases in alkaline phosphatase and the transaminases.

Surgery. When the infection of the bile ducts is associated with symptoms of severe sepsis immediate surgery is needed to relieve bile duct obstruction; this also makes it possible to perform a bacteriological examination of the bile, which very often grows *E. coli*. In some cases where a stone is at the lower end of the bile duct, endoscopic sphincterotomy may be possible.

Urinary tract

Numerous factors predispose to urinary tract infection, but the main one is obstruction to urinary flow of any origin. The common causative organisms are *E. coli, Proteus, Enterobacter,* group D *Streptococcus, Klebsiella,* and *Pseudomonas.*

Clinical features. A history of urgency and frequency of micturition, dysuria, haematuria, and nocturia may precede the onset of infection, which in turn will increase the intensity of these symptoms.

In the case of pyelonephritis or an intrarenal or perinephric abscess, pain and tenderness in the costovertebral angle is frequent, and this may be due to renal enlargement.

Investigations. Examination of the urine typically reveals mild proteinuria and haematuria. Quantification of organisms in the specimen discloses a number of organisms in excess of 100 000 and the number of white cells is frequently increased.

Urgent intravenous pyelography may identify a predisposing factor, but may not identify an intrarenal or perinephric abscess. Ultrasound and CAT are then the imaging techniques of choice [1, 32].

Treatment. When urinary retention or a major abscess is found appropriate surgical relief is mandatory.

Meninges

Clinical features. In a patient with severe sepsis the diagnosis of meningitis can be relatively easy, with headache, neck stiffness, and Kernig and Brudzinski signs all being present. However, the first signs are sometimes an altered level of consciousness and convulsions, without much in the way of localizing signs.

Investigations. In every case, lumbar puncture allows clinical and bacteriological diagnosis. Bacterial meningitis may be suspected when analysis of the cerebrospinal fluid (CSF) shows a low sugar level and a raised polymorphonuclear cell count. The organisms most frequently isolated in primary meningitis are meningococci, pneumococci, *Haemophilus influenzae* (especially in children), and *Listeria*; antibiotic treatment must be started immediately. A lymphocytic reaction in the CSF is most frequent in viral or tuberculous meningitis but may be found initialy with *Listeria* infection.

When focal neurological symptoms are present, encephalitis, thrombophlebitis or a cerebral abscess have to be looked for by means of CAT or other neuroradiological investigations.

Catheter-related

In patients in ICUs, infections related to intravascular catheters are frequent and serious. The main organisms responsible are *Staphylococcus aureus*, Gram-negative bacilli, and fungi, especially *Candida albicans*. Except when another site is clearly responsible for the infection, the catheter should be removed and its tip cultured. In many instances a complete recovery follows without antibiotics, but if the signs persist appropriate antibiotics should be given. Persisting positive blood cultures after removal of the catheter and antibiotics may be indicative of deep venous phlebitis or endocarditis.

Endocarditis

Cardiac valves may be involved by a wide variety of organisms, although *Streptococcus* and *Staphylococcus* are more likely than others to induce extensive damage.

Clinical features. Because of its widely variable clinical presentations, infective endocarditis is difficult to diagnose early, especially in a patient with severe sepsis. The sudden onset of congestive heart failure may be apparently related to septic shock and then a history of valvular heart disease is helpful but not essential.

The finding of a new heart murmur is of great value; however, murmurs may be absent in patients with right-sided endocarditis, which is especially frequent in drug addicts and after IV catheter infections. Finally, endocarditis should always be considered when the infection is disseminated to many organs, such as the CNS, spleen, kidneys, bones and joints. Cutaneous symptoms (Osler nodes, Janeway lesions) should be looked for on the palms of the hands and soles of the feet.

Investigations. Ultrasound is helpful because of its non-invasive nature, but when pulmonary oedema is extensive and cardiac surgery is contemplated, formal cardiac catheterization with angiography is necessary.

Soft tissues

Some soft tissue infections yield aerobic organisms, and less frequently anaerobic organisms, although there is good evidence to indicate that the latter are initially responsible. Gas gangrene is caused by several species of clostridii; aerobic and anaerobic streptococci are usually responsible for cellulitis.

Clinical features. Within several hours or days of injury or surgery of the GI tract, increased swelling and pain develop, with oozing of serous or serosanguineous material around the particular site.

On palpation the wound is very tender, and crepitations indicative of gas may be felt. Eventually bullae may cover the wound, beneath which the muscle tissue is pale and bleeds very little. If haemolysis occurs the patient rapidly becomes jaundiced and haemoglobinuria may occur.

Treatment. Immediate medical and surgical intervention is necessary. If possible hyperbaric O_2 should be given but this should not delay the surgical removal of dead tissue, which may require amputation of an extremity or extensive debridement.

Miscellaneous

Severe sepsis may be caused by a miscellany of organisms of the following types: bacterial (typhoid fever, leptospirosis), mycobacterial (tuberculosis), protozoal (malaria), and viral. The usual diagnostic procedures should be performed as in less severe cases.

Host defence mechanisms against infection

The management of the critically ill patient would not be complete without consideration of the state of the host defence mechanisms against infection. Many factors account for the increased susceptibility of critically ill patients to infection. Mechanical barriers against bacteria are weakened by instrumentation (endotracheal intubation, IV catheterization, urinary catheterization) and various surgical procedures. Defence mechanisms may be altered by drug therapy (steroids or cytotoxic drugs), surgery, and numerous underlying conditions (cirrhosis, malignancy, trauma, burns, diabetes, and renal failure). Furthermore, severe sepsis itself induces immunological disturbances. Thus the state of the host defence mechanisms against infection may be considered from the aspects of skin testing, cellular and humoral immunity, and the changes found in septic shock.

Skin testing as a means of assessing host defence mechanisms

Recent studies have indicated that the compromised host, who is highly susceptible to severe infection, may be recognized by delayed hypersensitivity to skin testing (DHST) [11]: in patients suffering from severe acute illness, a failure of the DHST response (anergy) is associated with high mortality, mainly from sepsis. In several studies carried out in ICUs, the mortality rate was 57%–58% in anergic patients, whereas when at least one response (e.g. induration greater than 5 mm) was recorded it was 16%–18% [11]. This relationship was initially shown in surgical patients, in whom the presence of anergy before surgery was associated with an increased incidence of postoperative septic complications [32]. The tests consist in intradermal injection of standard recall antigens, the most frequent being tuberculin, Candida, and streptokinase, which may be associated with skin tests with phytohaemagglutinin, dinitroclorobenzene or croton oil.

Old age and disseminated cancer apart, anergy may be due to several factors:

1) The effects of malnutrition have been studied extensively: either protein or calorie deprivation appears to alter the delayed hypersensitivity reactions, a defect which can be corrected by an appropriate diet.

2) It is firmly established that infections such as severe tuberculosis or measles are associated with a reduction of anergy. However, several other bacterial, viral, or parasitic infections have also been observed to produce the same effect [19]. The underlying process is rather complex, but antigenic stimulation and T cell depletion appear to be the most salient features.

3) Following surgery or trauma, both delayed hypersensitivity reactions and other immunological responses are depressed. There are decreased numbers of circulating lymphocytes and those that form E rosettes; leucocyte chemotaxis is reduced either under basal conditions or after stimulation with caseine: furthermore, immune depressant factors circulate in these patients [10].

Cellular and humoral immunity

Both circulating bacteria and endotoxin are cleared mainly by polymorphonuclear neutrophils and the hepatic reticuloendothelial system. This explains why serious infections frequently occur when leucocyte production is depressed or in the presence of portocaval anastomosis, as in hepatic cirrhosis. In contrast to the elimination of bacteria by the hepatic reticuloendothelial system, a non-specific phenomenon independent of the antibodies, phagocytic function of polymorphs appears to be dependent on its presence. Weinstein and Young [40] have shown that 40% of patients with septicaemia are infected by strains of bacteria that are resistant to phagocytosis by polymorphs. They found, however, that this defect was not related to an intrinsic white cell deficiency but to the absence of specific opsonizing antibodies; during recovery the capacity for phagocytosis is restored simultaneously with the rise in antibody titre.

From the time of colonization of the digestive tract by Gram-negative bacteria, antibodies will be formed against the serotypes of the bacteria present. These antibodies, principally of the IgM type, are known as natural antibodies, and in the presence of complement they confer on the serum a bactericidal power active against numerous strains of Gram-negative bacilli. The attachment of activated complement to the bacteria produces a lytic action causing bacterial death.

Thus a failure of the hepatic reticuloendothelial system, neutropenia, the presence of bacteria of an unknown serotype or the lack of opsonizing antibodies are conditions that may be found in the case of Gram-negative septicaemia. Similar factors account for infections due to cocci. Decreased humoral immunity raises the frequency and the severity of infections due to Streptococcus pneumoniae: fulminating infections due to this organism have also been described in asplenic patients.

Immunologic alterations due to septic shock

Several studies have shown that levels of complement components decrease during septic shock [11]. This decrease appears to be related to activation of complement via either classic or alternative pathways, and it has been found during infections due to Gram-negative bacilli, Gram-positive bacteria, and viruses. Serum immunoglobulins are decreased simultaneously and the two factors may be responsible for the major impairment in host defences. The presence of circulating immune complexes has been demonstrated during several infectious diseases, irrespective of the infecting organism. However, they cannot be detected during lethal septic shock [17]. The significance of this finding remains to be elucidated.

Treatment

Antimicrobial drug therapy

Several studies have shown that bacteria isolated from patients admitted to critical care units (CCUs) with severe sepsis were much more frequently multiresistant than those isolated from other parts of the hospital [38]. This is one reason why superinfections are more frequent and life-threatening in these patients [37]. The widespread and uncontrolled use of antibiotics has caused these phenomena and illustrates the need for a strict antibiotic policy [16].

Rules for antimicrobial drug therapy in CCU patients

Monotherapy. As often as possible, antimicrobial chemotherapy should be undertaken with only one drug. The combination of two antibiotics increases the risk of the emergence of multi-resistant strains and should be restricted to a limited number of infections, namely tuberculosis, mixed bacterial infection, bacterial endocarditis, and severe infection with Gram-negative rods in immunosuppressed patients.
Narrow-spectrum drug. When two drugs having an equal efficacy are considered, the one with the narrower spectrum should be preferred, because it is less likely to have a deleterious action on commensal bacteria and to increase the proliferation of those which have become resistant.
Restriction of antibiotic prophylaxis. The use of antibiotics enhances the emergence of bacterial resistance to useful antibiotic agents [24]. Therefore, antibiotic prophylaxis should be restricted

to clinical situations where controlled and prospective studies have clearly shown its efficacy in preventing the emergence of superinfections [7, 9, 20]. In critical care medicine, the circumstances in which it is most valuable are traumatology and surgery.

After surgical procedures, chemoprophylaxis appears to be beneficial in the case of operations in which endogenous bacterial contamination of the wound is unavoidable. It should also be considered for patients who require the insertion of foreign materials, e.g., prosthetic heart valves. In these cases, a simple dose of one antibiotic should be injected immediately before the start of the operation [39].

There is no definite evidence that prophylactic antibiotic therapy prevents superinfections following instrumental techniques for diagnosis or treatment, such as tracheostomy, bladder catheterization, and intravenous or intra-arterial catheterization.

Adherence to such rules for treatment and prophylaxis has considerably reduced the incidence of septicaemia due to superinfection from more than 10% to less than 5% of CCU patients [31].

Choice of antimicrobial drugs in CCU patients

Antimicrobial agents should be chosen with the following aims in mind:

● *The antibiotic must be active against the bacteria directly responsible for the sepsis that one has to treat or prevent.*

This means that bacteriological findings made in the laboratory must be critically examined. Providing that meticulous techniques are used, bacteria isolated by blood cultures, lumbar puncture, or bladder catheterization have an unequivocal value. On the other hand, in certain circumstances it is difficult to determine whether the identified strains are really responsible for the infection or result simply from colonization. Such dilemmas occur with the bacterial examination of specimens of sputum, tracheal aspirate, pus, wound dressings, etc. In such circumstances it is often possible to define the type that might be responsible by taking into account the locality of the sepsis and the usual epidemiological considerations, or by means of bacterial examinations that should be more specific, e.g., transtracheal aspiration of secretions.

● *The antibiotic used should have the appropriate pharmacological and pharmacokinetic properties to allow it to reach the infected focus in a sufficient concentration.*

• *The frequency and severity of adverse drug reactions should be weighed against the beneficial effects.*
• *The financial cost should be as low as possible without reduction of benefit.*

For these aims to be achieved, the different drugs may be separated into three groups. (Ball and Geddes [2] reviewed some new antibiotics in 1979.)

First group. The combined properties of these antibiotics are a narrow spectrum, a low incidence of adverse reactions, and a low risk of inducing proliferation of multiresistant Gram-negative rods. They should be chosen in every case in which bacteria susceptible to them are responsible for the infection.

Penicillin is the first drug of choice in infections due to streptococci, including *S. pneumoniae* (*Pneumococcus*) and anaerobic streptococci (*Peptostreptococcus* sp.), to *Neisseria meningitidis*, and to *Clostridia*.

The most frequent indications for the use of penicillin in critically ill patients are (1) Chemoprophylaxis of gas gangrene and other anaerobic infections in patients with a high risk of clostridial superinfection, i.e., post-partum or post-abortion infections, deep wounds, especially after road traffic accidents, open fractures, colonic and perineal surgery, especially in diabetics, and surgery for peripheral vascular disease; (2) acute pneumonia in patients with previously normal lungs, especially pneumococcal (primary pneumonia) or anaerobic (post-inhalation, foul odour, alcoholic patients with poor dental hygiene); and (3) acute meningitis due to *N. meningitidis*, *S. pneumoniae*, or *Listeria monocytogenes* needing combined therapy with an aminoglycoside (preferably gentamicin).

Besides allergy, the principal side-effects of penicillin are related to high blood levels which develop in the presence of renal insufficiency; they include metabolic encephalopathy (depressed consciousness, abnormal movements, and convulsions) [29] and bleeding due to functional platelet abnormalities [35]. These adverse effects disappear when the dosage is reduced.

Isoxazolyl-penicillins (methicillin, oxacillin, cloxacillin), which are resistant to beta-lactamases secreted by staphylococci, are the drugs of choice in infections due to staphylococci. Nevertheless, the sensitivity of staphylococci is very different from one strain to another and cannot be estimated from the bacteriostatic action in vitro alone. Therefore, the choice must be confirmed by, or modified in accordance with, the results of the in vitro bactericidal capacity of the antibiotic against the responsible strain.

When sepsis is severe, especially in septicaemia, combination with an aminoglycoside (gentamicin) is recommended because of its synergistic action with isoxazolyl-penicillins against staphylococci.

Macrolides (erythromycin) are the best alternative to penicillin in cases of streptococcal infections and of allergy to penicillin.

They are also efficient against other organisms, such as *Mycoplasma pneumoniae*, *Chlamydia trachomatis*, *Legionella pneumophila* and many anaerobic bacteria. For this reason, the macrolides are valuable antibiotics, highly recommended for use in acute, apparently primary, pneumonias.

Because of their good tissue penetration, their spectrum, and the low incidence of side-effects, they are the antibiotics of choice for the treatment of superinfections in chronic obstructive airways disease with acute respiratory insufficiency and encephalopathy [26].

Nitroimidazole compounds (metronidazole, ornidazole) are the drugs of choice against obligate anaeorobes, especially *Bacteroides fragilis*; aerobic and facultatively anaerobic bacteria are naturally resistant. Nitroimidazoles are highly effective in the treatment and prophylaxis of a wide variety of non-clostridial anaerobic infections and are compatible with many other antimicrobial agents [18].

Imperative indications include bacteraemia, endocarditis, meningitis, brain abscess, pneumonia, cellulitis, and necrotizing myositis or fasciitis due to obligate anaerobes. In addition, it is advisable to combine nitroimidazoles with surgical drainage from localized infections, which are known to include a high risk of anaerobic bacteraemia, such as intra-abdominal infections and pelvic sepsis originating from the female genital tract. In these cases, a useful preventative measure against aerobic Gram-negative bacteria is a combination of nitroimidazole compounds with gentamicin. Despite their lack of activity in vitro against aerobic organisms, nitroimidazoles have been shown to be effective both in surgical prophylaxis and in the treatment of mixed aerobic-anaerobic infections: aerobic and anaerobic bacteria disappear as the sepsis resolves in response to nitroimidazoles [15]. Their prophylactic use has been conspicuously successful in the prevention of postoperative sepsis in surgery of the GI and female genital tracts.

Quinolone compounds (nalidixic acid, pipemidic

acid) are mostly active against urinary infections caused by strains of *Escherichia coli* and *Proteus mirabilis*, when the sepsis has not invaded the kidney or related systems such as the prostate and when high tissue concentrations are not necessary. These compounds should be used preferably and initially in urinary infections due to long-standing bladder catheterization, when the infection has not been cured by removing the catheter and increasing the urinary output.
Second group. The joint property of this group is a wide spectrum inducing ecologic damage to commensal flora. On the other hand, some of these drugs have significant toxicity. However, these deleterious effects may be overlooked when these drugs are found to be effective against bacterial stains resistant to drugs of the first group.

For this reason, drugs in this group should be selected only when one is sure that drugs in the first group would be inactive.
Aminopenicillins (ampicillin, amoxycillin, metampicillin): the rising incidence of infections due to Gram-negative rods observed in surgical wards and CCUs since 1965 seems to be related to the wide use of aminopenicillins. Furthermore, these drugs are probably the ones most frequently implicated in the development of plasmidic resistance. They are also the antibiotics most frequently associated with pseudomembranous colitis due to *Clostridium difficile* toxin [4]. Therefore, the use of aminopenicillins should be restricted to those infections in which this group of antibiotics is irreplaceable.

Aminopenicillins are indicated in infections due to many strains of *E. coli*, *P. mirabilis* and *Klebsiella pneumoniae* for community-acquired infections. On the other hand, an increasing frequency of resistant hospital strains has been observed. Aminopenicillins have a special place in urinary tract infections due to these microbes, where widespread diffusion of the antibiotic is mandatory, i.e., in pyelonephritis.

The pharmacokinetics of aminopenicillins with their high biliary elimination support their preferential use in biliary tract infections, and IV metampicillin, has the highest biliary concentration.

Aminopenicillins are the most active antibiotics against *Haemophilus influenzae*. They should be used initially in infections where the bacterium has been isolated (pneumonia, meningitis) or before isolation when infection with *H. influenzae* is a possibility as in bacterial meningitis, especially in children.

Gentamicin remains the most frequently prescribed aminoglycoside antibiotic. The nephrotoxicity and ototoxicity of all aminoglycosides makes one cautious about their use in cases of renal insufficiency, or hypovolaemia or in association with the loop diuretics and other antibiotics such as the cephalosporins.

Their tissue distribution is poor, but because of their toxicity this disadvantage cannot be overcome by increasing dosage.

Aminoglycosides are potent against a great number of the bacteria responsible for some of the most serious infections seen in critically ill patients. But they do have a powerful tendency to induce resistant strains.

They are inactive against many strains of streptococci and against anaerobes, and are mainly used in association with compounds of other families when synergism is needed, as in severe sepsis due to staphylococci, *Enterobacteriaceae* and *Pseudomonas* Spp. However, in the last two instances, the new cephalosporins are tending to take their place.

Cotrimoxazole is potent against several bacterial species, especially streptococci and some *Enterobacteriaceae* such as *E. coli* and *P. mirabilis*; it has good tissue penetration [33]. In the cases of intolerance or resistance to the aminopenicillins, this drug might be used for serious or recurring infections of the urinary tract, especially in cases of pyelonephritis or prostatis. Its efficacy against *Pneumocystis carinii* makes it useful in opportunistic infections in immunodepressed patients.

Colistin is the main antibiotic of the polypeptidic group. In vitro, it is active against many strains of Enterobactericeae and Pseudomonas. It has a low tendency to induce plasmidic resistance but unfortunately, its in vivo efficacy is limited by its low diffusion, which cannot be overcome by increasing the dose because of its nephro and neurotoxicity. Its use in critical care medicine is therefore restricted.
Third-group. These drugs share either a high efficacy against several microbial strains or high financial cost. The emergence of bacterial resistance to each new antibiotic introduced into medical use is a phenomenon that has been repeatedly documented. Therefore these highly active new compounds should be reserved for specific cases to retain their efficacy for as long as possible.

They are indicated when in vitro testing shows that no drug of the preceding group is active and they should be reserved for serious life-threatening infections.
Carbenicillin and other semi-synthetic penicillins, such as ticarcillin, mezlocillin, and azlocillin,

have a broad spectrum of activity which includes 'problem' organisms such as *Pseudomonas aeruginosa* and the less common *Proteus* species (*P. vulgaris*, *P. morganii* and *P. rettgeri*). The potential of these antibiotics is limited by their susceptibility to beta-lactamases and by resistance to R-factors which may be acquired during treatment.

They may be useful in combination with an aminoglycoside in undiagnosed life-threatening infections in neutropenic patients.

Cephalosporins. Recently several new cephalosporins have been introduced. Some of these are highly insensitive to beta-lactamases: cefuroxime, cefamandole, cefoxitin (the first of a new family of antibiotics called cephamycins), cefotaxim, and cefsulodin; the last two are of special interest in critical care medicine.

Cefotaxim is the most potent antibiotic against *Enterobacteriaceae* and its resistance to inactivation by beta-lactamases is greater than that of other cephalosporins. Its minimum inhibitory concentration is the lowest of all known antibiotics active against Gram-negative bacteria, with the exception of *Pseudomonas aeruginosa* and obligate anaerobes (*Bacteroides fragilis*).

Cefotaxim is particularly useful in severe hospital-acquired infections due to multiresistant Gram-negative rods (*Escherichia coli*, *Klebsiella* sp., *Proteus* sp., *Serratia* sp.), especially during nosocomial bacteraemia and extensive pneumonia. Sufficient concentrations are achieved in CSF, and the successful treatment of meningitis by cefotaxim has been reported [6].

Cefsulodin has a very low minimum inhibitory concentration against *Pseudomonas aeruginosa* but poor efficacy against *Enterobacteriaceae*. Thus this compound may be considered as a narrow-spectrum antibiotic. It is now the first antibiotic of choice in serious infections due to *Pseudomonas aeruginosa*, especially in septicaemias and necrotizing pneumonias.

The *new aminoglycosides*, tobramycin, netilmicin, and amikacin, should be reserved for the management of serious infections caused by gentamicin-resistant organisms [28].

Extension of acquired resistance against one antibiotic (thus reducing the real spectrum of activity) is related to the duration of its use and therefore the oldest of the active drugs should be chosen.

Vancomycin is a nephrotoxic antibiotic that is highly active against staphylococci. It should be reserved for serious infections caused by that organism [12] and by *Clostridium difficile*.

Antibiotics of limited use in critical care. The following preparations have no or very few indications:

The *first and second-generation cephalosporins* (namely cephaloridin, cephalothin, cephalexin, cephacetril, cephanon, cephapirin, cefazolin and cefatricin) all have the disadvantages of the broad-spectrum antibiotics, and their widespread use has been recognized as being responsible for the development of nosocomial Gram-negative sepsis, especially that due to *Pseudomonas aeruginosa*. It is now possible to choose other drugs with fewer drawbacks in all cases.

Tetracyclines are bacteriostatic, broad-spectrum antibiotics, highly implicated in the development of bacterial resistance. The frequency with which resistance is found among streptococci, staphylococci, *Enterobacteriaceae*, *Clostridia*, and *Bacteroides* is so high that tetracyclines can no longer be advocated.

The *phenicol antibiotics* (chloraphenicol, thiamphenicol) have followed the same evolution as the tetracyclines, and furthermore their bone marrow toxicity makes them hazardous. However, because of the good CSF concentrations, they still have a definite advantage in treating meningitis due to beta-lactamase producing bacteria, and they are still the drugs of choice in enteric fever.

Lincomycin and *clindamycin* are active against streptococci, staphylococci, and *Bacteroides*, and their main advantage has been in their activity against *Bacteroides*. They have been proved to be the commonest cause of antibiotic-associated pseudomembranous colitis however, and therefore, since the introduction of nitroimidazoles there have been few, if any, indications for lincomycin and clindamycin in the prophylaxis or treatment of anaerobic infections.

Several active bactericidal compounds are now available for testing most of the severe infections found in CCUs.

The question that remains is how to adapt a strategy for their most effective use whilst keeping their unavoidable side-effects to a minimum. In this context it is worth remembering that many of the problems in severe sepsis are related more to a depressed host response or to difficulties in eliminating septic foci than to a lack of suitable antibiotics.

Treatment of the infected focus

Antibiotics are not the only weapon available for treating sepsis, and they are not even always the most effective one. Usually a septic condition is secondary to an infected focus, and the

Table 53.1. Efficacy of treatment of aerobic Gram-negative rod septicaemia in 77 patients

Treatment of the septic focus	Effective		Ineffective or ineradicable	
Antibiotic therapy	Appropriate		Appropriate	
	Yes	No	Yes	No
Mortality (%)	14	17	70	90

$P < 0.01$ NS   NS

discovery and eradication of this is the most important step in the treatment. For every case in which the infected focus can be treated with surgical drainage or removal of a foreign body, antibiotics are of secondary importance. Table 53.1 shows the results obtained in 77 personally treated patients with Gram-negative rod bacteraemia. The results clearly show that once the treatment of the primary lesion was effective, the prognosis did not differ significantly whether antibiotics were given or not. On the other hand, if the primary focus was not eradicated or if its treatment was ineffective, the prognosis was not significantly changed with the use of selected antibiotics. Nevertheless, in infections in which septic foci are diffuse and not amenable to surgical treatment, e.g., pneumonia, meningitis, or pyelonephritis, antibiotics are the most useful means of therapy.

Supportive therapy

In patients with impaired immune responses special treatment should be considered. In those with a reduced skin test response two main forms have proved useful: nutritional therapy and an aggressive approach to the infection.

The correction of established malnutrition or the prevention of its occurrence is an effective means of increasing host defence. This appears to be especially important in patients admitted to CCUs, where a high frequency of malnutrition has been shown [17]. Aggressive treatment of infection, especially when a septic focus is capable of being eradicated, is another procedure that has been shown to be effective [11].

In the future, forms of therapy acting directly on abnormalities in the immune response may be used, such as immunostimulation by drugs, infusion of non-specific immunoglobulins, and passive immunotherapy with serum containing antibodies against the toxic part of the LPS. At this time, only limited information is available and such therapy cannot yet be recommended.

References

1. Abbou C, Cordonnier C, Carlet J, Chopin D, Nebout T, Botto H (1981) Use of computerized tomography (CT) in the diagnosis of renal abscesses (RA). In: Shulman CC (ed) Advances in diagnostic urology. Springer, Berlin Heidelberg New York, pp 185–192
2. Ball AP, Geddes AM (1979) New antibiotics—a review. In: Reeves D and Geddes A (eds) Recent advances in infection, vol. 1. Churchill Livingstone, Edinburgh London New York, p 29
3. Barois A, Bourdain JL (1973) Les septicémies avec hypothermie. In: Goulon M, Rapin M (eds) Réanimation et médecine d'urgence. Expansion, Paris, pp 47–74
4. Barlett VG (1979) Antibiotic-associated pseudomembranous colitis. J Infect Dis 1:530–539
5. Beaufils M, Morel-Maroger L, Sraer JD, Kanfer A, Kourilsky O, Richet G (1976) Acute renal failure of glomerular origin during visceral abscesses. N Engl J Med 295:185–189
6. Belohradsky BH, Bruchk, Geiss D, Kafetzis D, Marget W, Peters G (1980) Intravenous cefotaxime in children with bacterial meningitis. Lancet I:61–63
7. Berger SA, Nagar H, Weitzman S (1978) Prophylactic antibiotics in surgical procedures. Surg Gynecol Obstet 146:469–475
8. Boelld DR, Levitt RG, Melson GL (1979) The role of gallium-67 scintigraphy, ultrasonography and computed tomography in the detection of abdominal abscesses. Semin Nucl Med 9:58–65
9. Chodak GW, Plant ME (1977) Use of systemic antibiotics for prophylaxis in surgery : A critical review. Arch Surg 112:326–334
10. Christou NV, Meakins JL (1979) Neutrophil function in surgical patients: Two inhibitors of granulocyte chemotaxis associated with sepsis. J Surg Res 26:355–363
11. Clumeck N, George C (1981) Immunological aspects of severe bacterial sepsis. Intensive Care Med 7:109–114
12. Cook FV, Farrar WE Jr (1978) Vancomycin revisited. Ann Intern Med 88:813–818
13. Dinarello CA, Wolff SM (1978) Pathogenesis of fever in man. N Engl J Med 298:607–612
14. Dussan J, Regnier B, Darragon T, Teisseire B, Le Gall JR, Lemaire F (1979) Hyperkinetic shock in viral and pneumococcal pneumonias. Intensive Care Med 5:59–64
15. Eykyn SJ, Phillips I (1978) Nitronidazole in surgical infections. J Antimicrob Chemother 4:75–81 [Suppl C]
16. Finland M (1970) Changing ecology of bacterial infections as related to antibacterial therapy. J Infect Dis 122:419–431
17. George C, Carlet J, Sobel A, Intrator L, Robin M, Sabatier C, Rapin M (1980) Circulating immune complexes in patients with Gram-negative septic shock. Intensive Care Med 6:123–127
18. Ingham HR, Sisson PR, Selkon JB (1980) Current concepts of the pathogenetic mechanisms of non sporing anaerobes: Chemotherapeutic implications. J Antimicrob Chemother 6:173–180
19. Kantor FS (1975) Infection, anergy and cell mediated immunity. N Engl J Med 292:629–634

20. Keighlet MRB, Burdon DW (1979) Antimicrobial prophylaxis in surgery. Pitman Medical, London
21. Kelton JG, Neame PB, Gauldie J, Hirsh J (1979) Elevated platelet associated IgG in the thrombocytopenia of septicemia. N Engl J Med 300:760–734
22. McLean LD, Meakins JL, Raguchi K, Ovignan JP, Omillon KS, Gordon J (1975) Host resistance in sepsis and trauma. Ann Surg 182:207–215
23. Ledingham I, McAedle CS (1978) Prospective study of the treatment of septic shock. Lancet I:1194–1196
24. Le Frock JL, Ellis CA, Weinstein L (1979) The relation between aerobic fecal and oropharyngeal microflora in hospitalized patients. Am J Med Sci 277:275–280
25. Le Gall JR, Mignon FC, Rapin M, Redjem M, Harari A, Bader JP, Soussy CJ (1976) Acute gastroduodenal lesions related to severe sepsis. Surg Gynecol Obstet 142:377–380
26. Lhoste F, Lemaire F, Tillement JP, Duval J, Rapin M (1980) Erythromycin lactobionate as a first choice parenteral antibiotic. In: Nelon JD, Grassi C (eds) Severe infective exacerbations of chronic bronchitis. Current chemotherapy and infectious disease. Nineteenth Interscience Conference on Antimicrobial agents and Chemotherapy, vol 2. American Society for Microbiology, Washington DC, pp 1018–1019
27. Mant MJ, King EG (1979) Severe acute disseminated intravascular coagulation. A reappraisal of its pathophysiology clinical significance and therapy based on 47 patients. Am J Med 67:557–563
28. Mouton RP (1980) Choice of an aminoglycoside. J Antimicrob Chemother 6:166–167
29. Nichols PJ (1980) Neurotoxic of Penicillin. J Antimicrob Chemother 6:161–165
30. Rangel DM, Dimbar A, Stewens GH, Cooper R, Fonkalsrud EW (1977) The hepatic response to endotoxin shock: Hemodynamic and enzymatic observations. Intensive Care Med 3:47–53
31. Rapin M, Duval J, Le Gall JR, Soussy CJ, Lemaire F, Harari A (1975) Les septicémies de surinfection en réanimation. Leur prévention par la restriction de l' antibiothérapie. Nouv Presse Med 4:483–486
32. Sagel SS, Staaley RJ, Levitt RG, Geisse (1977) Computed tomography of the kidney. Radiology 124:359–370
33. Schiffman DO (1975) Evaluation of an anti-infective combination. Trimethoprim-Sulfamethoxazole. JAMA 231:635–637
34. Semel JD, Trenholme GM, Harris AA, Jupa JE, Levin S (1978) Pseudomonas maltophilia pseudosepticemia. Am J Med 64:403–406
35. Shattil SJ, Bennett JS, McDonough M, Turnbull J (1980) Carbenicillin and penicillin G inhibit platelet function in vitro by impairing the interaction of agonists with the platelet surface. J Clin Invest 65:329–337
36. Siegel JM, Cerra FB, Coleman B, Giovannini I, Shetye M, Border JR, McMenamy RH (1979) Physiological and metabolic correlations in human sepsis. Surgery 86:163–193
37. Speller DCE (1980) Hospital infection by multiresistant Gram-negative bacilli. J Antimicrob Chemother 6:1970–1972
38. Stoddart JC (1974) Gram-negative infections in the ICU. Crit Care Med 2:17–22
39. Stone HH, Haney BB, Kolb LD, Geheber GE, Hooper CA (1979) Prophylactic and preventive antibiotic therapy—Timing, duration and economics. Ann Surg 189:691–699
40. Weinstein RJ, Young LS (1976) Neutrophil function in Gram negative rod bacteriema. J Clin Invest 58:190–198
41. Wiles JB, Cerra FB, Siegel JM, Border JR (1980) The systemic septic response: Does the organism matter? Crit Care Med 8:55–60

Chapter 54

Opportunistic Lung Infections in the Compromised Host

F. Cartier

In patients with altered immune defences, infection is a major cause of morbidity and mortality. Pulmonary infections, in particular, pose a special problem not only because of their frequent occurrence and severity but also because of the difficulties they invariably present in diagnosis and treatment. Pulmonary infections may be caused either by 'common' pathogens, which find a particularly easy prey in the immunocompromised patient, or by opportunistic micro-organisms.

The diagnostic work-up must take into account (1) the relative importance of unusual infections caused by opportunists; (2) the far-from-rare occurrence of mixed infections; (3) the extremely wide variety of possible infections, which casts doubt on the usefulness of broad-spectrum antibiotics and makes precise diagnosis essential; and (4) the need to formulate the diagnosis as quickly as possible in view of the severe course most of these infections run.

The compromised host

Immunological impairment concerns either specific or non-specific defences. Non-specific defences contribute to natural immunity against any invading organism. They consist of the skin–mucosal barrier, humoral defences involving the complement system, lysozyme, interferon, and cellular activity resulting in phagocytosis and destruction of the invading agent. Specific defences are initiated by recognition of the infective micro-organism. Their effect is to limit the spread of infection and bring about its resolution. They are subtended by lymphoid tissue. T lymphocytes retain the memory of and recognize foreign antigens, stimulate macrophage activity, and secrete leucotactic factors which attract macrophages to the site of infection. B lymphocytes are responsible for humoral antibody synthesis.

Immunodeficiency can be congenital. Defences can be altered by malignant diseases such as Hodgkin's disease and other lymphomas, leukaemia, and multiple myelomas and by cirrhosis, diabetes, and critical illness in general. Other factors can impair host defences, such as the administration of corticosteroids, cytotoxic agents, and antilymphocyte globulin, or venous or bladder catheterization, endotracheal intubation, and changes in microbial flora of the host through the use of broad-spectrum antibiotics.

Incidence of pulmonary infections

The reported incidence of pulmonary infection following renal transplantation ranges from 11% to 38% [31, 47, 60]. Onset of infection occurs within the first 3 months of transplantation in two out of three cases [31, 65], and the outcome is fatal in 21%–56% of cases [31, 47, 60]. In approximately half the cases, post-transplant mortality can be ascribed to pulmonary infection [47]. In a more recent study, however, Webb [65] reports only eight fatalities from pulmonary infection among 416 renal transplant recipients. He attributes this unprecedentedly low incidence to the use of low-dose prednisone.

Among patients with malignant disease, particularly haematological malignancy, pulmonary infection is often fatal, as was the case in 65% of the patients with acute leukaemia reported by Sickles [59] and in 60% of those, with diffuse interstitial pneumonia reported by Singer [62]. Pneumonia has been found post-mortem in 43% of patients with haematological malignancy [4].

In Hodgkin's disease and lymphosarcoma the risk of infection is low in the early stages of the disease and concerns particularly viruses, *Mycobacterium tuberculosis*, and fungi. In later stages, as a result of treatment-induced changes, infection by common bacterial pathogens is more frequent.

In acute leukaemia, bone-marrow aplasia makes the patient particularly vulnerable to common bacteria and to fungi. Even during non-critical periods, however, impairment of immune defences exposes the patient to virtually any infection, but more especially to that caused by opportunists and more commonly in patients with acute myeloblastic leukaemia than in those with acute lymphoblastic leukaemia.

In multiple myeloma the B cell deficiency increases the risk of infection from extracellular, particularly Gram-negative organisms. In patients with carcinoma the incidence of infection rises with the duration of the disease, local injury playing an important part in the onset of infection.

Clinical setting

Because of immunological impairment, the initial symptoms of pulmonary infection are often mild or atypical. A search for latent lesions in a standard chest film should be part of the routine diagnostic work-up in the immunocompromised patient. Fever, even when unaccompanied by other signs or symptoms, should immediately raise the suspicion of a pulmonary infection. Indeed, febrile episodes stem from infection in 70%–80% of adult leukaemia or lymphoma patients [40]. More commonplace symptoms, such as dyspnoea or a dry or productive cough, may also be due to infection.

Focal pneumonia may be bacterial, viral, mycotic, or tuberculous. The radiographic appearances show segmental or non-segmental opacities, which may be single or multiple, cavitary or homogeneous. These appearances can be seen on a simple routine chest film, which should be compared with earlier radiographs to check for less obvious abnormalities. Diffuse pneumonias may be due to bacterial or to fungal pathogens but are more commonly caused by viruses, particularly cytomegalovirus, or by *Pneumocystis carinii*. Radiographic evidence often lags behind the clinical signs.

A fall in PaO_2 is a useful diagnostic and prognostic pointer. The coexistence of neurological, hepatic, or cutaneous manifestations may direct suspicion to certain possible causative organisms.

Non-infectious pulmonary disease must be ruled out. Fluid accumulation in the lung may develop after renal transplantation as a result of renal failure induced by rejection. Malignant disease can also cause pulmonary lesions diagnosable on the strength of the clinical course and on cytological and histological examination. Sometimes pulmonary interstitial fibrosis is caused by chemotherapy, bleomycin being a known offender. The risk of phlebitis and pulmonary embolism should be kept in mind with bed-ridden patients, particularly those with malignant disease.

Diagnostic procedures

The slightest suspicion of a pulmonary infection, whether solitary or associated with another disease process, calls for a thorough search for the causative agent or agents. Once an organism is recovered, cytological and histological findings may clinch its aetiological responsibility. In deciding which diagnostic method to use, two main questions should be considered: How accurate is the information it provides? How hazardous is the procedure? An otherwise mild complication may, in these patients, have disastrous consequences, either immediate, as in the case of an exacerbated respiratory distress syndrome, or delayed, as in the case of superinfection. The conflicting nature of these contingencies accounts for the multiplicity of methods available.

Available methods

Sputum examination

Sputum production from the lower airways is not a constant feature of pulmonary infection in the immunocompromised host. Smear preparations are examined for predominant bacterial pathogens. During its passage through the upper airways, however, sputum is contaminated by bacteria or by *Candida*, thus clouding interpretation of the results, unless of course organisms normally absent from the respiratory tract, such as tubercle bacilli, are found. In fact sputum examination seldom provides a definitive diagnosis in these patients. In the absence of expectorated sputum, tracheal aspirates may be useful but again there is the risk of contamination from upper airways flora.

Transtracheal aspiration

Transtracheal aspiration via the cricothyroid membrane avoids oropharyngeal contamination. With a cooperative patient and in expert hands the risks of complications are minimal— one case of haemoptysis in 488 aspirations was reported by Bartlett in non-immunosuppressed patients [5]. In bacterial pneumonia false-negative results were exceptional in these patients provided no prior antibiotic therapy had been administered. False-positive results were seen in 5% of cases.

Bronchial brushing

Diagnostic material can be obtained from distal bronchial and alveolar sites by introducing nylon-bristle brushes through a fiberoptic bronchoscope under fluoroscopic guidance. The risk of complications is low: in 750 brush biopsies performed by Finley and Fenessy [23], mainly in immune-deficient patients, pneumothorax occurred in six, one of whom required chest tube placement, severe bleeding in two patients, and reversible respiratory arrest in one patient.

Brush biopsy has provided aetiological diagnosis in 28%–39% of immune-deficient patients [14, 23, 54]. Advocated mainly for detection of *P. carinii* and fungi, bronchial brushing is less useful in bacterial infections because of oropharyngeal contamination of the fiberoptic bronchoscope. This risk can be avoided if brushes are introduced through the cricothyroid membrane by way of a catheter. With this technique, however, the risk of complications is not negligible: in 38 brush biopsies, Aisner reports 7 significant although non-fatal complications, including five pneumothoraces requiring chest tube drainage, one case of severe bleeding, and one case of overt infection at the puncture site [2]. More recently Wimberley has proposed the use of a protected brush catheter [68].

Bronchioalveolar lavage

Bronchioalveolar lavage through a fiberoptic bronchoscope is an innocuous non-invasive technique. Washing in the middle lobe or lingula causes an average fall in PaO_2 of only 10 mm Hg [19] and secondary infection of this area occurs in only 0.5% of non-immunocompromised patients [63]. Interpretation of the bacteriological findings of bronchioalveolar lavage carries the same reservations as for 'unprotected' brush biopsy. In immunocompromised patients transtracheal aspiration has corroborated lavage findings in 57% of cases [18]. Lavage is at least as accurate as brush biopsy in diagnosing *P. carinii* and fungal pneumonias [18, 39].

Transbronchial lung biopsy

Transbronchial lung biopsy is usually effective in yielding lung tissue. In 2628 transbronchial lung biopsies, pneumothorax occurred in 5.5% of cases, bleeding in 1.3% of cases, and fatal complications, generally massive haemorrhage, in 0.2% of cases [30]. Pneumothorax was reported to occur in 10%–19% of immunodeficient patients [14, 21] and bleeding in 26% [14]. An aetiological diagnosis of pulmonary infection was established in 42%–76% of immunodeficient patients [14, 21].

Percutaneous transthoracic needle aspiration or biopsy

Transthoracic intrapulmonary sampling, obtained by simple needle aspiration or by needle biopsy, gives a diagnostic yield of 35%–76% for pulmonary infection, according to the different series reported [10, 27, 37]. The risks of complications, however, are fairly high—certainly higher than with endobronchial procedures. After needle aspiration, pneumothorax is reported to occur in 10%–37% of cases, with placement of a chest tube required in half the cases [10, 11, 27], pneumomediastinum in 3.5% of cases, and haemothorax in 1% of cases [11]. Percutaneous lung biopsy is associated with pneumothorax in 30% of cases and with bleeding in 15% [27].

Open lung biopsy

Open pulmonary biopsy through a limited thoracotomy generally provides sufficient tissue for histological and microbiological diagnosis. A common complication is pneumothorax. In a series of 416 immunodeficient patients Ray observed 6% who developed pneumothorax requiring placement of a chest tube [52]. Haemothorax occurred in 0.5% of cases and superficial wound infection in 0.7%. Mortality with this procedure was 0.4%. In immunocompromised patients with severe widespread pneumonia the main risk is respiratory failure. Several reports, however, testify to the rarity of pleural complications [27].

Choice of procedure

In the selection of a diagnostic procedure, the potential benefits must be weighed against the hazards. The benefits of a technique depend partly on the nature of the infective organism. Bacteriological findings are of doubtful significance if they have been obtained by the oropharyngeal route. Effectiveness also depends on the amount of diagnostic material produced. From this standpoint, open pulmonary biopsy tops the list. Next come transbronchial lung biopsy and percutaneous transthoracic needle biopsy, then bronchioalveolar lavage, brush biopsy, percutaneous transthoracic needle aspiration, and transtracheal aspiration. At the bottom of the list, although very useful in some cases, are tracheal aspirate and sputum examination.

The hazards associated with each diagnostic procedure are related to the patient's clinical status, the extent of patient cooperation, the degree of respiratory failure, and the presence and severity of coagulation disorders. Transtracheal aspiration, brush biopsy, and alveolar lavage carry low risks of complications. Other techniques, such as transbronchial lung biopsy, percutaneous transthoracic needle aspiration, and open lung biopsy, carry a low-to-moderate risk, depending on the patient's general condition. Open lung biopsy, of course, is already a surgical procedure performed under general anaesthesia. And quite a high risk is associated with percutaneous transthoracic needle biopsy.

Several biopsy methods may be used concurrently. For example, bronchioalveolar lavage, brush biopsy, and transbronchial lung biopsy can be performed during the same endoscopy session. Or again, several methods can be used in succession as needed and in accordance with the findings obtained at each stage of the workup. An important element in assessing the risk-to-benefit ratio of a method is the skill of the operator and the experience of the pathologist and microbiologist with the method in question.

Generally speaking, low-risk procedures can be justifiably used for routine investigation in even doubtful cases. Attempts to formulate an aetiological diagnosis, however, must be particularly 'aggressive' in immunocompromised patients, whose condition makes accurate early diagnosis imperative. Finally, diagnostic efforts should not cease when one organism has been isolated, since associated disease is common among immunocompromised patients.

Viruses

Cytomegalovirus

Incidence

Incidence figures for cytomegalovirus (CMV) pneumonias vary greatly with the type of underlying disease, with the diagnostic criteria used, and with the focus of the study undertaken. To considering retrospective studies first, among renal allograft recipients 1%–2% are reported to have pulmonary CMV disease and of those with pulmonary disease CMV is implicated in 6%–9% [31, 47, 65]; among marrow graft recipients, 53% of those with fatal pulmonary disease have CMV infection [45]; and among patients with malignant disease, CMV is causative in 4% of those with pulmonary disease [62]. In 'CMV-specific' prospective studies in renal allograft recipients, 3%–13% are reported to develop pulmonary CMV disease [3, 55, 61]. The wide variability in reported incidence clearly reflects the complexity of diagnosis.

CMV pneumonia is rare compared with active CMV infection, which is very common in the immunologically incompetent patient as a result either of reactivation of a latent CMV infection acquired in childhood or reinfection from transfused blood or a transplanted kidney [7]. Among renal transplant recipients, CMV infection is diagnosed by isolation of the virus either from urinary specimens (in 42%–73% of cases [3, 55, 61] or from tracheal aspirates. CMV has been isolated post-mortem from lung tissue in 17 of 159 patients with malignant disease [41], in 12 of 16 renal transplant recipients [13], and in 7 of 16 bone marrow transplant recipients [45]. In 46%–85% of renal allograft recipients, the frequency varying with assay technique, specific CMV antibodies show a rise over the first few weeks post-transplant [3, 7, 35, 61]. In the lungs, cytomegalic cells have been seen postmortem in 28%–52% of renal allograft recipients [3, 13, 46, 55] and in 53% of patients with interstitial pneumonitis following bone marrow transplantation [45].

Pathology

The pathologic findings are those of diffuse or focal interstitial pneumonia and include interstitial oedema associated with mononuclear cell infiltrates and obliteration of the alveolar spaces by protein accumulations and occasionally by hyaline membranes [13]. Inclusions are found both in pneumocytes and in macrophages. In certain cases, scattered inclusion-bearing macrophages are seen without an accompanying inflammatory reaction. Interstitial fibrosis may be present [1].

Clinical manifestations

Fever, dry cough and dyspnoea with hypoxaemia are the usual manifestations of CMV infection. Leucopenia with a WBC count of less than $5000/mm^3$ is common. Atypical lymphocytes in the blood and biochemical evidence of hepatitis are infrequently reported. Radiographic appearances show diffuse interstitial infiltrates beginning at the periphery of the lower lobes, and occasionally small nodular densities [1, 3, 45, 55, 61].

Diagnosis and treatment

In the immune-depressed patient isolation of CMV from the lower respiratory tract or lung

tissue and the occurrence of seroconversion are not enough to incriminate this organism in the causation of diffuse extensive pulmonary disease. Moreover, evidence of inclusion-bearing cells obtained by bronchial brushing [36] or bronchioalveolar lavage [6] is neither constant nor sufficient for aetiological diagnosis. Theoretically, before a firm diagnosis of pulmonary CMV disease can be made, sufficient amounts of lung biopsy specimens should be examined and virological and serological confirmation obtained. In practice, however, such exhaustive efforts to achieve diagnostic certainty seem unwarranted for a number of reasons. Some investigators, for example, consider solitary CMV pneumonia a non-fatal condition [3, 55, 61], albeit one which may predispose to other fatal infections. Secondly, the effectiveness of treatment of CMV infection with antiviral agents such as interferon, adenosine arabinoside, cytarabine, idoxuridine, and hyperimmune anti-CMV plasma is not established.

Herpes simplex

Herpes simplex virus (HSV) infection is a common clinical event in immune-deficient individuals. Virological and serological investigations confirm its relatively high frequency [35, 56]. Spread to the lower respiratory tract is sometimes seen. The picture is invariably one of tracheobronchial disease, rarely with associated pulmonary lesions. Exceptionally, pulmonary involvement by HSV infection is observed in the absence of tracheobronchitis [49].

Herpetic lesions of the lips or mouth so often accompany pneumonia in the immunodepressed patient that a diagnosis of pulmonary HSV infection is rarely considered at the outset.

Pulmonary lesions consist of necrosis of the alveolar walls and an intra-alveolar proteinaceous exudate, sometimes with haemorrhage. Intranuclear inclusions are found within alveolar lining cells.

Adenine arabinoside, used in the treatment of HSV encephalitis, has also been proposed for patients with herpetic pneumonia.

Varicella-zoster virus

The incidence of varicella-zoster infection has been estimated at 8.2% in renal transplant recipients, 25% in Hodgkin's disease patients, and 8.7% in patients with other lymphomas [58]. Varicella-zoster pneumonia developed in 3% of a series of children with herpes zoster and cancer [22]. Radiological signs consist of peribronchiolar bilateral nodular infiltrates. The infection is sometimes fatal.

Varicella-zoster rash accompanying pneumonitis may be suggestive. Isolation of the virus from sputum specimens and seroconversion are not enough to inculpate the virus in the pathogenesis of the pneumonia. The decision of undertake invasive biopsy techniques is based mainly on the possibility of another infection occuring singly or in association with the varicella-zoster infection. Proposed therapeutic agents include adenine arabinoside [66], which has given hopeful results, interferon, and acycloguanosine.

Other

Other viruses capable of causing pneumonia in immunologically incompetent individuals include adenovirus [70] and *Myxovirus influenzae* [9].

Pneumocystis carinii

Incidence

P. carinii pneumonia is common among infants with primary immunodeficiency disease, especially severe combined immunodeficiency [64]. In patients with acute lymphoblastic leukaemia, the incidence of *P. carinii* pneumonia is proportional to the intensity of chemotherapy [32]. Walzer reports an attack rate of 1.1% per year in patients with acute lymphoblastic leukaemia, 0.2% per year in those with acute myeloblastic leukaemia and 0.01%–0.05% per year in other haematological malignancies and lymphomas [64]. Lung biopsy or autopsy has disclosed the aetiological responsibility of *P. carinii* in 37.5%–83% of cases of diffuse interstitial pneumonia arising in the course of malignant disease [62]. *P. carinii* pneumonia has been reported to develop in 0.5%–9% of renal transplant patients [31, 60, 65], and 10% of cases of pulmonary infection are imputed to this organism [31, 65]. The figures are higher if only diffuse interstitial pneumonia is considered and if diagnosis is established from large quantities of biopsy material. They are lower among renal transplant patients who have received low doses of cortisone [65].

Pathology

The pulmonary lesions consist of a widening of the interstitial spaces, due mainly to hyper-plasia of the alveolar lining cells. Foamy eosinophilic material, made up of coalescent macrophages and clumps of microorganisms, fills the alveoli. The diagnostic form of *P. carinii* seen in light microscopic preparations is a cystic structure containing up to eight oval bodies. In patients responding to treatment interstitial fibrosis is sometimes observed [67].

Clinical manifestations

Dyspnoea, fever, and non-productive cough are the main symptoms of *P. carinii* pneumonia. Radiography most often initially shows interstitial and alveolar infiltration with bilateral perihilar distribution and sparing of peripheral lung fields and later, a more diffuse picture. Early infection, however, with fever, dyspnoea, and hypoxaemia may be present in the absence of abnormal chest radiographs. In the absence of specific treatment, *P. carinii* pneumonia in the immunologically incompetent child and adult has a fatal outcome. The more abrupt the onset of symptoms, the more rapidly fatal the course of the disease, death sometimes ensuing within a week.

Diagnosis

Diagnosis rests on demonstration of *P. carinii* in bronchial secretions or lung tissue. There are no helpful culture methods or serological techniques available. The organism is identified by microscopic examination of touch preparations or suspension smears stained by the Giemsa method, which rapidly produces evidence of the characteristic cyst contents; by the Grocott modification of the Gomori methenamine–silver nitrate method, which takes several hours and stains the cyst wall; or by the Gram–Weigert stain or the toluidine blue stain for demonstration of the intracystic bodies.

The organism is rarely demonstrated in sputum samples (in 6% of cases reported by Walzer [64]) or in transtracheal aspirates. Diagnosis is established by bronchial brushing in 62%–80% of cases [15, 23, 54]. The promising bronchioalveolar lavage method gave constant diagnostic information in series reported by Even et al. [18] and by Kelley et al. [39]. Demonstration of the organism was achieved by transbronchial lung biopsy in six cases described by Feldman, who noted no false-negative results. Percutaneous transthoracic needle aspiration has prompted diverse estimations of the hazards and benefits it involves: it was used by Johnson [37] to formulate diagnosis in 14 of 15 cases and by Chaudhary [11] in 87% of cases. Open lung biopsy, which enables rapid diagnosis to be made by examination of an imprint of the biopsied specimen, is the most reliable method.

Treatment

Until 1975 the preferred treatment for *P. carinii* pneumonia was pentamidine. This achieved cure in 75% of cases [33, 54], but adverse effects were numerous.

Hughes has used trimethoprim and sulphamethoxazole (TMP–SMX) in combination in an oral dose of 20 mg per kg daily for trimethoprim and 100 mg per kg daily for sulphamethoxazole over a 2-week period, resulting in cures in 12 of 14 cases [33]. Side-effects were mild and the treatment brought about clinical improvement within 3 days on average and normal chest films within an average of 8 days. In children with malignancies, Hughes also found TMP–SMX, in a daily dose of 150 mg (for trimethoprim) and 750 mg (for sulphamethoxazole), highly effective in the prevention of *P. carinii* pneumonitis [34].

Before chemotherapy takes effect, hypoxaemia should be treated by increasing the inspired O_2 concentration, associated if necessary with a positive airway pressure. If for any reason the patient needs tracheal intubation or if the arterial PO_2 cannot be maintained above 60 mmHg, MV may be necessary.

Fungi

Candida albicans

C. albicans is a normal saprophytic inhabitant of human mucosa, particularly of the GI tract. Candidal infection generally involves the superficial mucosa and its acquisition is favoured by spontaneous immunological impairment, diabetes, immunosuppressive therapy, and antibiotic therapy. Systemic candidal infection may occur with extensive lung involvement in leukaemia patients, renal transplant recipients, burn patients, and diabetics. Chest radiographs show disseminated infiltrative lesions tending to cavitation. Before a case of bronchopulmonary disease can be confidently ascribed to *C. albicans* it is necessary to demonstrate the presence in lung tissue of budding yeast-like cells and pseudohyphae within

nodular infiltrates, with blood vessel thrombi containing *Candida*. *C. albicans* is recovered from cultures of biopsy specimens. For ante-mortem aetiological diagnosis open lung biopsy is mandatory [67]. The recovery of *C. albicans* from specimens obtained by less invasive methods, including transtracheal aspiration, alveolar lavage, bronchial brush biopsy, and even percutaneous transthoracic needle aspiration, may be indicative of a mucosal infection but is not enough to inculpate this organism in the pathogenesis of the pulmonary disease. Nonetheless, the isolation of *C. albicans* from several sources—lower respiratory tract, blood culture, urine specimens—justifies suspicion of a systemic candidiasis and the possible involvement of *Candida* in the development of the extensive pulmonary lesions.

Precipitins directed against *Candida* have been found by immunodiffusion or more rapidly by counterimmunoelectrophoresis in the sera of patients with systemic candidiasis, but also in a certain number of healthy individuals. Among immune-deficient patients, precipitins may be absent or present in low amounts [17, 26]. Increased serum arabinitol levels may be associated with invasive candidiasis in high risk patients with neoplastic disease [25].

Pulmonary candidal infection, as a secondary focus of systemic infection from haematogenous spread, is life-threatening and calls for immediate treatment. Amphotericin B is given in a dose of 0.5 mg per kg on the first day and 0.75 mg per kg daily thereafter, with the dose adjusted to achieve a peak serum concentration of 2–2.5 μg per ml. An alternate-day regimen can then be instituted [26]. Addition of flucytosine to the regimen in a dose of 200 mg per kg daily may permit lower doses of amphotericin B to be used after determination of the MIC (minimal inhibitory concentration) for flucytosine [26]. Imidazole derivatives seem to be effective in patients with candidiasis. However, additional studies in immunosuppressed patients with systemic infection are needed.

Aspergillus

Invasive pulmonary aspergillosis is most often due to infection by *Aspergillus fumigatus* and has been found post-mortem in 16% of acute leukaemia patients and in 5% of lymphoma patients [44]. Among all renal transplant patients the incidence of pulmonary aspergillosis ranges from 0.7% to 2%, and of those with pulmonary disease 3%–15% are infected with this organism [31, 47, 65]. In immune-deficient patients the lung is nearly always the site of infection, although in 20%–50% of patients spread to other sites, particularly the brain, has been observed [67]. Pathologic features consist of necrotizing bronchopneumonia with invasion and occlusion of blood vessels by thrombi containing hyphae that grow through the vessel walls into lung parenchyma [44].

Clinical manifestations include fever, dyspnoea, non-productive cough, and occasionally pleuritic chest pain and haemoptysis [44]. Chest films may be normal in the early stages, and in some cases by the time the first radiographic signs appear the patient is already in critical condition. The picture is one of multiple infiltrates progressing to cavitation.

Sputum and transtracheal aspirate examination is often negative or sometimes false-positive [44], and serological tests are disappointing [67]. With brush biopsy or bronchial lavage, diagnosis can be formulated from direct examination and culture [18]. Transbronchial lung biopsy in addition may provide evidence of lung and vessel pathology. Where these methods prove fruitless and doubt still remains, recourse to open lung biopsy is still possible.

Untreated, invasive pulmonary aspergillosis is constantly fatal in the immune-deficient patient. In kidney and heart transplant patients amphotericin and flucytosine have resulted in cures [8, 28]. In patients with malignant disease these drugs are of little avail in stemming the infectious process [44].

Other

Pulmonary *Cryptococcus neoformans* is generally overshadowed by cryptococcal meningitis. *C. neoformans* may be found in sputum in the absence of infection. Transbronchial biopsy and open lung biopsy are of greater diagnostic help. Treatment consists of amphotericin B and flucytosine.

Disseminated pulmonary zygomycosis only occurs in the severely compromised host. Non-invasive diagnostic methods are often negative. Diagnosis requires the demonstration in lung tissue obtained by open biopsy of broad and non-septate hyphae in vessel thrombi and lung infarcts. Treatment with amphotericin may produce a cure [43].

Histoplasma capsulatum may, in endemic areas, produce a diffuse alveolar pulmonary disease in renal transplant recipients and patients with malignant disease [12]. Diagnosis can occa-

sionally be achieved by demonstration of the organism in sputum or bronchial biopsy specimens but more often on examination of open lung biopsy specimens [52]. Amphotericin B can result in cure [12].

Cases of pulmonary infection with *Coccidioides immitis* [16], *Blastomyces dermatitidis* [50], and *Torulopsis glabrata* [42] have also been reported.

Bacteria

Nocardia

Nocardia asteroides may cause pulmonary infection in the immuno-compromised patient [29, 55]. The disease may be asymptomatic and discovered on routine chest films showing infiltrates progressing to cavitation. Careful microscopic examination and culture of sputum specimens and tracheal aspirates may reveal the organism [29]. Alveolar lavage and bronchial brush biopsy are more helpful [18]. Sulphonamides or a combination of cefuroxime and amikacine can result in a cure [29].

Legionella pneumophila

L. pneumophila pneumonia occurs in local outbreaks [24]. Sporadic cases have been reported in immunosuppressed patients [57], among whom the disease tends to be more frequent and more severe. The clinical and radiographical signs are much the same as in the other bacterial pneumonias. In widespread forms severe respiratory failure is seen. Growing the organism in culture is difficult and diagnosis currently rests on direct fluorescent antibody staining of lung tissue, sputum specimens, and bronchial washings. Retrospective diagnosis can be established from evidence of raised serum immunofluorescent antibody titres. Erythromycin is effective in 2- to 4-g doses IV and the addition of rifampicin to the regimen has been proposed [57].

Pittsburgh pneumonia agent

Recently cases of pneumonia among immune-depressed patients have been attributed to a Gram-negative, weakly acid fast bacillus termed 'Pittsburgh pneumonia agent' (PPA). The disease is often fatal. The causative organism, often intracellular, has been observed in touch imprint smears of lung biopsy specimens. It does not grow on the usual culture mediums. PPA differs not only culturally but also tinctorially from *L. pneumophila*. The two diseases can also be distinguished serologically according to preliminary data. In vitro activity has been demonstrated with trimethoprim–sulphamethoxazole, rifampicin, and erythromycin [48].

Other

Common bacterial pneumonias are not strictly speaking opportunistic infections, since the causative organisms can produce pulmonary infection in the immunologically competent host. Nonetheless they are frequent among immune-deficient individuals, accounting for more than half the cases of lung infection in renal transplant patients [31, 47, 65], more than half in leukaemia patients [59], and for 41% of cases among patients with lowered resistance of diverse origin [18]. The causative organisms are for the most part Gram-negative bacilli: *Pseudomonas, Klebsiella, Escherichia coli, Haemophilus*, and less frequently, *Staphylococcus aureus, Streptococcus pneumoniae*, and anaerobic organisms.

Radiographic appearances generally consist of single or multiple foci of pneumonia and sometimes of diffuse extensive micronodular lesions. There is a general tendency to cavitation. Diagnosis rests on demonstration of the causative organisms in bronchial secretions uncontaminated by oropharyngeal flora. Transtracheal aspiration, protected bronchial brushing [68], and percutaneous transthoracic needle aspiration are therefore more reliable than examination of sputum or of bronchial secretions obtained by techniques employing the oropharyngeal route. In some cases examination of pleural fluid or blood culture discloses the causative bacterium. In general, strict criteria should be used in interpreting the bacteriological results of these methods and it should be borne in mind that several organisms may share pathogenic responsibility.

Other organisms

Toxoplasma gondii

T. gondii is an infrequent cause of diffuse interstitial pneumonia in immune-deficient individuals [53]. The disease is apparently due to reactivation of a latent infection. Diagnosis

rests on the demonstration of trophozoites of *T. gondii* in alveolar cells and pulmonary macrophages. A high IgM-fluorescent antibody titre is neither a constant finding in immunocompromised patients with pulmonary *T. gondii* infection [67] nor reason enough to incriminate this organism as the cause of the pulmonary disease. The combination of pyrimethamine and sulphonamides exerts an effective synergistic action [67].

Helminths

Extensive diffuse pulmonary disease due to *Strongyloides stercoralis* infection has been reported in the compromised host. Larvae have been found in sputum and bronchial washings [51]. Thiabendazole is the drug of choice.

Mycobacteria

Pulmonary mycobacterium tuberculosis infection is a significant problem in patients with Hodgkin's disease, lung carcinoma, lymphosarcoma, and reticulum cell sarcoma and after renal transplantation [38]. Reactivation of latent disease is an important factor, and isoniazid prophylaxis is apparently effective, in patients with tuberculous sequelae. Infection may be diffuse and fulminant. In some cases the first sign is an ulcerative nodular lesion seen on a routine chest film. Diagnosis calls for a careful search for the tuberculous bacillus on examination of sputum or tracheal aspirates. If this is negative, bronchial brush biopsy, bronchioalveolar lavage, or transbronchial biopsy is required.

Atypical mycobacterial infection may also occur in the compromised host [20]. The outcome is often unfavourable as a result of the variable effectiveness of tuberculosis therapy.

References

1. Abdallah PS, Mark JBD, Merigan TC (1976) Diagnosis of cytomegalovirus pneumonia in compromised hosts. Am J Med 61:326–332
2. Aisner J, Kvols LK, Sickles EA, Schimpff SC, Wiernik PH (1976) Transtracheal selective bronchial brushing for pulmonary infiltrates in patients with cancer. Chest 69:367–371
3. Andersen HK, Spencer ES (1969) Cytomegalovirus infection among renal allograft recipients. Acta Med Scand 186:7–19

4. Armstrong D, Young LS, Meyer RD, Blevins AH (1971) Infectious complications of neoplastic disease. Med Clin North Am 55:729

5. Bartlett JG (1977) Diagnostic accuracy of tracheal aspiration bacteriologic studies. Am Rev Respir Dis 115:777–782

6. Behrens HW, Quick CA (1974) Bronchoscopic diagnosis of cytomegalovirus infections. J Infect Dis 130:174

7. Betts RF, Freeman RB, Gordon Douglas R, Talley TE, Rundell B (1975) Transmission of cytomegalovirus infection with renal allograft. Kidney Int 8:387–394

8. Burton JR, Zacher JB, Bessin R, Rathbun HK, Greenough WB, Sterioff S, Wright JR, Salvin RE, Williams GM (1972) Aspergillosis in four renal transplant recipients: Diagnosis and effective treatment with amphotericin B. Ann Intern Med 77:383–388

9. Cartier F, Garré M, Thomas R, Fauconnier B (1977) Virus et pneumopathies des immunodéprimés. Rev Fr Mal Respir 5:543–552

10. Castellino RA, Blank N (1979) Etiologic diagnosis of focal pulmonary infection in immunocompromised patients by fluoroscopically guided percutaneous needle aspiration. Radiology 132:563–567

11. Chaudhary S, Hughes WT, Feldman S, Sanyal SK, Coburn T, Ossi M, Cox F (1977) Percutaneous transthoracic needle aspiration of the lung. Am J Dis Child 131:902–907

12. Cox F, Hughes WT (1974) Disseminated histoplasmosis and childhood leukemia. Cancer 33:1127

13. Craighead JE (1971) Pulmonary cytomegalovirus infection in the adult. Am J Pathol 63:487–504

14. Cunningham JH, Zavala DC, Corry RJ, Keim LW (1977) Trephine air drill, bronchial brush, and fiberoptic transbronchial lung biopsies in immunosuppressed patients. Am Rev Respir Dis 115:213–220

15. De Labarthe B, Kernec J, Kombila M, Garré M, Le Frèche JN, Doby JM, Danrigal A (1975) Diagnostic de la pneumonie á Pneumocystis carinii. Rev Fr Mal Respir 3:599–610

16. Deresinski SC, Stevens DA (1975) Coccidioidomycosis in compromised hosts: experience at Stanford University Hospital. Medicine 54:377–395

17. Drouhet E, Dupont B (1976) Infections mycosiques et parasitaires au cours des traitements immunosuppresseurs. Pathol Biol Paris 24:99–116

18. Even P, Caubarrère I, Sors H, Reynaud P, Hem B, Soulier A, Offredo C, Renault P (1979) Diagnostic des pneumopathies des sujets immunodéprimés par le lavage alvéolaire, In: Le lavage broncho-alvéolaire. Inserm 84:499–508

19. Fabre C, Gouget R, Dufat R, Dubois F, Ruff F, Chretien J (1979) Etude des gaz du sang au cours des fibroscopies bronchiques chez les malades normoxiques et hypoxiques et au cours de lavages bronchoalvéolaires. Rev Fr Mal Respir 7:602–607

20. Feld R, Bodey GP, Groschel D (1976) Mycobacteriosis in patients with malignant disease. Arch Intern Med 136:67–70

21. Feldman NT, Pennington JE, Ehrie MG (1977) Transbronchial lung biopsy in the compromised host. JAMA 238:1377–1379

22. Feldman S, Hughes WT, Kim HY (1973) Herpes zoster in children with cancer. Am J Dis Child 126:178–184

23. Finley R, Kieff E, Thomsen S, Fennessy J, Beem M, Lerner S, Morello J (1974) Bronchial brushing in the diagnosis of pulmonary disease in patients at risk for opportunistic infection. Am Rev Respir Dis 109:379–387

24. Frazer DW, Tsai TR, Orenstein W, Parkin WE, Beecham HJ, Sharrar RG, Harris J, Mallison GF, Martin SM,

McDade JE, Shepard CC, Brachman PS (1977) Legionnaires' disease: Description of an epidemic of pneumonia. N Engl J Med 297:1189–1197

25. Gold JWM, Carpentier F, Bernard EM, Kiehn TE, Wong B, Cook CA, Armstrong D (1980) Serum arabinitol antigen in patients with invasive candidiasis. In Symposium on infections in the immunocompromised host Eindhoven, June 1–5 1980. Abstracts book. Elsevier, North Holland Biomedical Press, Amsterdam, p. 97.

26. Goldstein E, Hoeprich PD (1977) Candidosis. In: Hoeprich PD (ed) Infections diseases, 2nd edn. Harper-Row, Hagerstown, pp 372–382

27. Greenman RL, Goodall PT, King D (1975) Lung biopsy in immunocompromised hosts. Am J Med 59:488–496

28. Gurwith MH, Stinson EB, Remington JS (1971) Aspergillus infection complicating cardiac transplantation: Report of five cases. Arch Intern Med 128:541–545

29. Hautefort B, Duboust A, Bedrossian J, El Etr M, Goldstein FW, Acar JF (1980) Three cases of Nocardia asteroides in the immunocompromised host. In Symposium on infections in the immunocompromised host. Eindhoven, June 1–5 1980. Abstracts book. Elsevier North-Holland Biomedical Press, Amsterdam, p. 59

30. Hert SM, Suratt PM (1978) Complications of transbronchial lung biopsies. Chest 73:759–760

31. Huertas VE, Port FK, Rozas VV, Niederhuber JE (1976) Pneumonia in recipients of renal allografts. Arch Surg 111:162–166

32. Hughes WT, Feldman S, Aur RJA, Verzosa MS, Hustu O, Simone JV (1975) Intensity of immunosuppressive therapy and the incidence of Pneumocystis carinii pneumonitis. Cancer 36:2004

33. Hughes WT, Feldman S, Sanyal SK (1975) Treatment of Pneumocystis carinii pneumonitis with trimethoprim-sulfamethoxazole. Can Med Assoc J 112:478

34. Hughes WT, Kuhn S, Chaudhary S, Feldman S, Verzosa M, Aur RJA, Pratt C, George SL (1977) Successful chemoprophylaxis for Pneumocystis carinii pneumonitis N Engl J Med 297:1419–1426

35. Huraux JM, Bricout F, Nicolas JC, Regnard J, Bogossian M, Descamps P, Grimfeld A, Gerbal A, Baptista-Lourenco MH (1975) Renal transplantation and viral infections. Results of follow-up studies. Biomedicine 22:311–319

36. Jain U, Mani K, Frable W (1973) Cytomegalic inclusion disease: Cytologic diagnosis from bronchial brushing material. Acta Cytol (Baltimore) 17:467–468

37. Johnson HD, Johnson WW (1970) Pneumonia in children with cancer: Diagnosis and treatment. JAMA 214:1067–1073

38. Kaplan MH, Armstrong D, Rosen P (1974) Tuberculosis complicating neoplastic disease. Cancer 33:850

39. Kelley J, Landis JN, Davis GS, Trainer TD, Jakab GJ, Green GM (1978) Diagnosis of pneumonia due to Pneumocystis by subsegmental pulmonary lavage via the fiberoptic bronchoscope. Chest 74:24–28

40. Levine AS, Graw RG, Young RC (1972) Management of infections in patients with leukemia and lymphoma: Current concepts and experimental approaches. Semin Hematol 9:141

41. Macasaet FF, Holley KE, Smith TF, Keys TF (1975) Cytomegalovirus studies of autopsy tissue. Incidence of inclusion bodies and related pathologic data. Am J Clin Pathol 63:859

42. Marks MI, Langston C, Eickhoff TC (1970) Torulopsis glabrata: An opportunistic pathogen in man. N Engl J Med 283:1131–1135

43. Medoff G, Kobayashi GS (1972) Pulmonary mucormycoses. N Engl J Med 286:86–87

44. Meyer RD, Young LS, Armstrong D, Yu B (1973) Asper-

gillosis complicating neoplastic disease. Am J Med 54:6–15

45. Meyers JD, Spencer HC, Watts JC, Gregg MB, Stewart JA, Troupin RH, Thomas ED (1975) Cytomegalovirus pneumonia after human marrow transplantation. Ann Intern Med 82:181–188

46. Milliard PR, Herbertson BM, Nagington J, Evans DB (1973) The morphological consequences and the significance of cytomegalovirus infection in renal transplant patients. Q J Med 152:585–596

47. Murphy JF, McDonald FD, Dawson M, Reite A, Turcotte J, Fekety R (1976) Factors affecting the frequency of infection in renal transplant recipients. Arch Intern Med 136:670–677

48. Myerowitz RL, Pasculle AW, Dowling JN, Pazin GJ, Puerzer M, Yee RB, Rinaldo CR, Hakala TR (1979) Opportunistic lung infections due to Pittsburgh pneumonia agent. N Engl J Med 301:953–958

49. Nash G, Foley FD (1970) Herpetic infection in the middle and lower respiratory tract. Am J Clin Pathol 54:857–863

50. Onal E, Lopata M, Lourenco RV (1976) Disseminated pulmonary blastomycosis in an immunosuppressed patient. Am Rev Respir Dis 113:83–86

51. Rassiga AL, Lowry JL, Forman WB (1974) Diffuse pulmonary infection due to Strongyloides stercoralis. JAMA 230:426–427

52. Ray JF, Lawton BR, Myers WO, Toyama WM, Reyes CN, Emanuel DA, Burns JL, Pederson DP, Dovenbarger WV, Wenzel FJ, Sautter RD (1976) Open pulmonary biopsy: Nineteen-year experience with 416 consecutive operations. Chest 69:43–47

53. Remington JS (1974) Toxoplasmosis in the adult. Bull NY Acad Med 50:211

54. Repsher LH, Schroter G, Hammond WS (1972) Diagnosis of Pneumocystis carinii pneumonitis by means of endobronchial brush biopsy. N Engl J Med 287:340–341

55. Rifkind D, Goodman N, Hill RB (1967) The clinical significance of cytomegalovirus infection in renal transplant recipients. Ann Intern Med 66:1116–1127

56. Ruffault A, Fauconnier B, Cartier F, Launois B (1975) Evolution des anticorps antiherpétiques chez 18 malades soumis aux immunodépresseurs aprés transplantation rénale. Pathol Biol (Paris) 23:371–374

57. Saravolatz LD, Burch KH, Fisher F, Madhavan T, Kiani D, Neblett T, Quinn EL (1979) The compromised host and legionnaires's disease. Ann Intern Med 90:538–542

58. Schimpff S, Serpick A, Stoler B, Rumack B, Mellin H, Joseph JM, Block J (1972) Varicella-zoster infection in patients with cancer. Ann Intern Med 76:241–254

59. Sickles EA, Young VM, Greene WH, Wiernik PH (1973) Pneumonia in acute leukemia. Ann Intern Med 79:528–534

60. Simmons RL, Uranga VM, Laplante ES, Buselmeier TJ,Kjellstrand CM, Najarian JS (1972) Pulmonary complications in transplant recipients. Arch Surg 105:260–261

61. Simmons RL, Lopez C, Balfour H, Kalis J, Rattazzi LC, Najarian JS (1974) Cytomegalovirus: Clinical virological correlations in renal transplant recipients. Ann Surg 180:623–634

62. Singer C, Armstrong D, Rosen PP, Walzer PD, Yu B (1979) Diffuse pulmonary infiltrates in immunosuppressed patients: Prospective study of 80 cases. Am J Med 66:110–120

63. Tonnel AB, Ramon Ph, Lafitte JJ (1979) Incidents et contre-indications du lavage broncho-alvéolaire. Rev Fr Mal Respir 7:651–656

64. Walzer PD, Perl DP, Krogstad DJ, Rawson PG, Schultz MG (1974) Pneumocystis carinii pneumonia in the united states: Epidemiologic, diagnostic, and clinical features. Ann Intern Med 80:83–93

65. Webb WR, Gamsu G, Rohlfing BM, Thorburn K, Kalifa LG, Amend WJC, Robertz M, Salvatierra O (1978) Pulmonary complications of renal transplantation: A survey of patients treated by low-dose immunosuppression. Radiology 126:1–8

66. Whitley RJ, Ch'ien LT, Dolin R, Galasso GJ, Alford CA (1976) Adenine arabinoside therapy of herpes zoster in the immunosuppressed. N Engl J Med 294:1193

67. Williams DM, Krick JA, Remington JS (1976) Pulmonary infection in the compromised host. Am Rev Respir Dis 114:359–394, 593–627

68. Wimberley N, Faling LJ, Bartlett JG (1979) A fiberoptic bronchoscopy technique to obtain uncontaminated lower airway secretions for bacterial culture. Am Rev Respir Dis 119:337–343

69. Wolff LJ, Bartlett MS, Baehner RL, Grosfeld JL, Smith JW (1977) The causes of interstitial pneumonitis in immunocompromised children: An aggressive systematic approach to diagnosis. Pediatrics 60:41–45

70. Zahradnik JM, Spencer MJ, Porter DD (1980) Adenovirus infection in the immunocompromised patient. Am J Med 68:725–732

Chapter 55

Tetanus

F. Vachon and F. Tremolières

Epidemiology

Tetanus has virtually disappeared in countries that have the benefit of good vaccination programmes. Since, to be effective, at least two successive injections of anatoxin are necessary, this vaccination is difficult to achieve in over-populated countries with poor social and medical backing. Therefore, the disease essentially affects neonates and infants in developing countries, where several hundred thousand die every year.

In Europe, only carelessness in maintaining the acquired immunity is responsible for the abnormally high occurrence of the disease in some countries such as Portugal and France (200–400 cases per year) [42]. It affects mostly women and the older age groups, two-thirds being over 65 years of age.

The sites of entry are often very minor wounds (punctures, cuts) that the patient does not think warrant medical attention, so that immunization is not sought. In 50% of cases, the site of entry is not due to trauma but is the result of varicose ulcers of the leg, arterial gangrene, especially in diabetic subjects, infected cancers, intramuscular injections (quinine and phenylbutazone), or bowel, pelvic, and obstetric surgery; in one case in ten the site of entry cannot be detected [54].

Preventative serum injections do not provide complete protection, whereas it is exceptional for tetanus to occur in vaccinated subjects who have received a booster of toxoid within the last 10 years.

Umbilical tetanus affects neonates born to unimmunized mothers undergoing unhygienic, sometimes ritual, customs.

Pathogenesis

Tetanus is due to the action of the exotoxin of Nicolaïer's bacillus, which is fixed on to the nervous tissues. The route of dissemination and sites of action have been studied by autoradiographic methods with iodine-labelled or tritiated toxin. After injection, the toxin (tetanospasmin) spreads by retrograde intra-axonal transport and accumulates particularly in the ventral root of the spinal cord, ipsilateral to the site of injection. It is distributed by both blood and nervous tissue to the different motor and sensory neurones. Preferential fixation of the toxin to nervous tissue may be the result of a particular affinity it has for certain cerebrosides. The rapidity of fixation depends on the length of the nerve and its electrical activity. The neurophysiological action of the toxin reveals itself only after it has passed across the synaptic cleft and reached the presynaptic terminals of inhibitory spinal interneurones where it interferes with the release of the inhibitory transmitter substance [26]. It produces a synaptic disinhibition of the gamma motor neurones, the interneurones, and the gamma segments of the medulla. The loss of this physiological inhibition renders some groups of neurones pathologically excitable, with the simultaneous contraction of agonist and antagonist muscles: the characteristic tetanospasm.

The effects of tetanus toxin on the autonomic nerve fibres are predominantly those of adrenergic stimulation [19].

Clinical aspects

Trismus

'Lockjaw' is the chief symptom: its occurrence alerts the patient and leads to the diagnosis. At first there is mild difficulty in opening the mouth, but as the trismus worsens the patient becomes completely unable to eat. Especially around the eyes, the face shows characteristic creasing because of the spasm of the superficial muscles of the face and neck.

Other possible causes of trismus are usually readily excluded. They are:

1) Local causes, such as a bad wisdom tooth or an inflamed tonsil, which give rise to unilateral signs and are often accompanied by fever, and traumatic causes, such as dislocation of the jaw; all these are easily recognized.

2) Temporo-maxillary arthritis often follows an injection of heterologous serum.

3) Spasm of the jaws and neck due to neuroleptic drugs (phenothiazine, butyrophenone, metoclopramide). These spasms are seen as a variable spasmodic torticollis and oculogyric crises. They disappear spontaneously in 24–48 h or under the influence of anti-Parkinson drugs.

4) Myalgic trismus, sometimes arising during a septicaemic state, may be misleading in that the disease may also be known to give rise to tetanus, for instance following a septic abortion.

5) Very occasionally, hysteria with neurological trismus (Gayet–Wernick disease) has to be considered.

If the trismus is the sole symptom and is not wholly characteristic the patient must be kept under medical observation in a special unit.

Feeding by mouth is not permitted and if the trismus is due to tetanus the remaining clinical symptoms will become manifest within a few days. There is no rise in temperature, and the consciousness remains normal. Constipation is usual and the reflexes become unusually brisk.

Spread of the spasms

Tetanus is considered to be generalized when it triggers off spasms of the neck and then of the trunk. These spasms essentially affect the trunk, and to a lesser extent, the limbs. At worst, the neck is rigid and hyperextended. Dysphagia is usual; oral feeding is impossible and swallowing of saliva is difficult. The contraction of paravertebral muscles produces such an intense lumbar lordosis that it is possible to pass one hand underneath the patient (opisthotonos). Board-like abdominal and thoracic rigidity impairs ventilation. The limbs remain relatively more supple, but spasm is present in the limb on which the site of entry is situated. The spasms are constant, but become greatly accentuated at times.

The paroxysms consist of tonic spasms with extension, or more rarely flexion, of the limbs, sometimes mimicking epilepsy. They provide further evidence, if needed, for the diagnosis, as does the bitten tongue.

Any spasm involves the risk of respiratory arrest, either because of a thoracic muscular spasm or, more frequently, because of severe glottic spasm which necessitates a tracheostomy. In addition to the respiratory problems, profuse sweating and paroxysmal hypertension with tachycardia may occur.

The diagnosis of tetanus is therefore a clinical concern. Investigations are of no help and should not delay transfer of the patient to a special ward.

Clinical forms

The cephalic tetanus of Rose occurs after a wound on the face. It includes peripheral facial paralysis on the same side as the wound, or bilateral paralysis if the wound is in the midline.

The ophthalmic tetanus of Worms follows injury to the orbit. It produces partial or complete ophthalmoplegia, and peripheral facial paralysis. This form is rare but is particularly severe.

Table 55.1. Scoring system for prognostic features of tetanus

No.	Prognostic feature	1 Score	0 Score
1	Incubation period[a]	<7 days	≥7 days or unknown
2	Period of onset[b]	<2 days (48 h)	8≥2 days or nil
3	Portal of entry	Umbilicus, uterus, open compound fractures; site of surgical incision or IM injection	All others + idiopathic cases
4	Spasms	Present	Absent
5	Fever (rectal temperature)	>38.4°C	≤38.4°C
6	Tachycardia		
	Adults	>120 beats/min	<120 beats/min
	Neonates	>150 beats/min	<150 beats/min

[a] Incubation period, time from wounding to first symptom (lockjaw).
[b] Period of onset, time from first symtom (lockjaw) to first spasm.

Prognosis

Following the suggestions adopted at the Fourth International Congress (1975), the prognostic features can be listed and scored as shown in Table 55.1. The prognosis is graded from 0 to VI according to the results of this scoring system (Table 55.2).

Table 55.2. Prognosis in tetanus, related to scores for different features

Grade	Score	Prognosis
0	0	Very good
I	1	Good
II	2	
↓	↓	↓
VI	6	Very poor

In addition to the signs and symptoms listed (Table 55.1), the survival rate is affected by age and by disease affecting other systems, e.g., hypertension, diabetes, and alcoholism.

Complications

In a few instances tetanus becomes generalized, with continuous spasms, high fever (42°C or over), hypertension, and tachycardia, in less than 24 h. The severe form of the condition requires high doses of sedative drugs and curarization from the outset. Major circulatory disorders occur, with hypotension, arrhythmias, and oliguria, and death generally then occurs in 24–48 h.

Cardiac arrest may occur during long periods of apnoea but is secondary to pulmonary embolism in most cases. Cardiovascular disorders with labile arterial pressures and profuse sweating are due to sympathetic hyperactivity of central origin. In some instances parasympathetic hyperactivity may also occur. These phenomena are generally transient, being seen during the first 2 weeks. The body weight often increases due to overhydration.

Infection and thrombo-embolic disease are the most frequent complications [41]. The infections seen as complications of tetanus are those that commonly affect recumbent patients receiving supportive treatment. Thrombo-embolism involves more serious risks, with confinement to bed, advanced age, and a history of poor venous circulation with varicose ulcers all favouring the occurrence of deep vein thrombosis and pulmonary embolism.

Recovery

Recovery is slow and rehabilitation with active and passive re-education of the muscles must be started early to avoid stiffness of the joints and muscles [58]. This type of disability is marked in 10%–15%, and 3% of people affected by tetanus develop ossification adjacent to the joints, especially the elbow.

The weight loss is very significant and interferes with recovery, especially in the elderly.

The acute phase of the disease lasts 3–4 weeks, whilst the recovery phase lasts a further 4 weeks. Sometimes, however, both these phases are substantially extended.

Treatment

The treatment now given for control of tetanus takes advantage of the most sophisticated techniques of intensive care, but it is still only symptomatic and demands a high degree of nursing and medical skill over the 2–6 week period of the illness. It is expensive and is generally felt to be badly out of date, especially since hospitals are now well suited to the delivery of complex treatments, and prophylactic action to eradicate the disease would theoretically be possible [7, 8, 16, 24, 26, 31, 46, 54, 57].

There are three aspects of treatment, but they are not of equal importance: (1) Eradication of the infection; (2) neutralization of the free toxin; and (3) intensive care.

Eradication of infection

A large dirty wound which does not heal easily must be washed, excised, and fully opened. Chronic wounds (e.g., varicose ulcers) are treated in a similar manner. Particular situations may warrant more specific treatment, such as curettage or hysterectomy in tetanus following abortion and limb amputation in the case of major and irreversible injuries of the limbs or of ulcerated tumours.

Wounds are often not explored because they seem too minor or because they have already healed (even though they may contain foreign material), or also because they are too apparently trivial to have attracted attention (e.g., ingrowing toenail). Such wounds should be opened and excised, however, since they may harbour proliferating tetanus bacilli. Indeed, ignoring them facilitates progression and exacerbation of the disease, with the possibility of relapse after the acute phase is over, because of the persisting release of free toxin from the wound.

In addition, penicillin G, 3–6 mU/day, is given, or larger doses in the case of extensive necrotic or dirty wounds. Any patient with penicillin intolerance should be treated with erythromycin or other appropriate antibiotics.

Neutralization of the toxin

This is the specific treatment for tetanus, but unfortunately once the disease has started the efficacy of the treatment is questionable.

The toxin can be neutralized by IM or IV injections of antitoxin if it is not already fixed on the nervous tissues [26]. Studies in ICUs have not shown any obviously significant advantages of high doses of antitoxin IM or IV [40, 56]. It is now rare for physicians to prescribe high doses of antitoxin, because of the side-effects of heterologous antitoxin and the cost of homologous serum. Many still recommend the use of small doses of antitoxin serum (500–1000 IU homologous serum and 1500–10 000 IU heterologous serum) [56], however, since the death rate has been found to increase in the absence of early serotherapy, particularly in countries with few intensive care facilities or none at all [11].

Serotherapy is of more benefit when administered by the intrathecal route. Animal experiments suggest that the antitoxin is able to combine with the fixed toxin in the intraneuronal areas when given intrathecally. Several studies have substantiated the beneficial effects of intrathecal antitoxin, especially where intensive care facilities are not available [4, 12, 18, 34, 36]. The various studies may have yielded different results because of differences in the experimental protocols: dose, type of antitoxin, and site of injection (lumbar or suboccipital) are only some of the variables that can affect outcome [23, 48, 55]. The precise protocol for correct intrathecal administration has still to be determined (route of injection, dose, type of antitoxin), and no specific antitoxin for this technique is yet commercially available. (The present antitoxin preparations are stabilized with phenol by-products and cannot be safely injected into the CSF.)

Intensive care

The main problem in the treatment of tetanus is the control of spasms. The drugs required to achieve this depress the ventilatory function, and the complications of the disease itself combine with this effect to make respiratory assistance necessary [30, 36, 37], which is only possible in a special unit with the facilities for managing all areas of treatment. Many of the problems that arise are in fact side-effects of the treatment, especially in elderly patients.

Pharmacological agents designed to restore cholinesterase levels to normal have been tried in tetanus but have not met with much acclaim.

Respiratory assistance

From the onset of generalized tetanus the overriding risk is that of asphyxia. In addition, food and/or saliva may be aspirated into the trachea. Treatment includes the administration of muscle relaxants and, if necessary, a tracheostomy, as the only technique that can make avoidance of glottic spasm possible while ensuring a free airway and allowing artificial ventilation as required. Tracheostomy should be performed as soon as the spasms start to spread, rather than waiting until respiration is already impaired. This course is recommended particularly in cases where the incubation period has been short [27, 54].

Some authors recommend prolonged intubation, but most consider that tracheostomy is safer for a disease whose course is expected to last 2–3 weeks.

Control of the spasms

Many drugs have been used for the control of tetanic spasms [14]. To date, the preparations detailed below merit attention:

Diazepam [10, 21, 50] has a remarkable muscle relaxant action, which has transformed the treatment of tetanus since 1965. Its haemodynamic side-effects are usually negligible even when high doses are used. An injection of 10 mg IV always depresses respiration, and respiratory assistance is often necessary when the total daily dose is as much as 120 mg.

The serum concentration of the drug reached after oral administration can vary some 20-fold in different patients. Diffusion is poor following injection IM and this mode of administration is not suitable for prolonged treatment. When an identical dose is given each day by mouth the serum concentration of the drug rises throughout the first week and then reaches a plateau. When the treatment is stopped a secondary release from the tissues, especially from the body fat, ensures a sufficient concentration of the drug for about a week. Therefore, it is better to use high doses at the start of treatment and to reduce them quickly afterwards. Smaller doses should be given in the case of hepatic insufficiency.

Clorazepate, which belongs to the same group of drugs, can be used as an alternative.

Carbamates are used in some countries (particularly meprobamate), but are of relatively little value.

Dantrolene has also been proposed for use in the treatment of tetanic spasm. Its action is good but it seems to have more side-effects than diazepam [2].

Barbiturates are used only in conjunction with diazepam, during severe tetanus or when curarization is necessary. Quick-acting barbiturates allow control of acute episodes but cause haemodynamic disorders. At the doses that are needed to treat tetanus they will all influence respiration, and consequently artificial ventilation is often required. They are widely stored in fatty tissue and doses must be modified in the presence of renal or hepatic failure.

Central analgesics have marked effects on spasms. From the haemodynamic point of view, phenoperidine and fentanyl are the best tolerated at present [44, 59]. When they are injected intermittently their action is short (30 min) and after a few days their effect is less pronounced.

Curare can also be used. Only non-depolarizing neuromuscular blocking agents are used for prolonged treatment of tetanus. Pancuronium bromide is particularly valuable because of its minimal cardiovascular effects and the lack of histamine release. It is excreted via the kidneys and does not accumulate; plasma concentrations rapidly fall below the activity threshold when administration is stopped, even after a 1- to 3-week course [15].

Guidelines

When trismus is isolated feeding by mouth is strictly forbidden. Intravenous infusions supply water and electrolytes, and IV feeding may be required later. Diazepam may be given in a continuous infusion, at a dose of 60–100 mg daily; close and constant surveillance is essential.

When signs of generalization are present tracheostomy must be performed. This is carried out under a local anaesthetic after premedication including atropine 0.25 mg and pethidine 1 mg/kg. Intravenous diazepam (5–10 mg/h) is started immediately, and the dose is increased as required up to a maximum of about 7–10 mg/kg per day. Over 2–5 days the enteral route, in the form of a naso-gastric tube, is gradually substituted for the parenteral route. The total dose is then distributed evenly every 2–3 h and adjusted daily for optimum control of the spasms. The mean daily dose for an adult is 250 mg.

Artificial ventilation is initiated according to the effects of diazepam on the level of consciousness and the respiratory status.

Treatment is eventually progressively reduced, depending on the evolution. The average duration of treatment is 2–3 weeks. In elderly and obese patients the drugs must be withdrawn sooner because they are metabolized differently in such patients.

Actual recovery does not really begin until 5–15 days after diazepam has been discontinued; the tracheostomy tube is not removed until the patient is able to swallow normally again.

Failure of the treatment is conceded when prolonged spasms persist despite a rapid increase of the dosage of diazepam to the maximum compatible with safety, and also when injections of diazepam 10 mg IV provide only very short periods of sedation (less than 5 min) or no sedation at all. Additional drugs are then prescribed, such as quick-acting *barbiturates* (thiopentone 2–4 g/day), which if effective may be followed by *phenobarbitone* (10 mg/kg per day in adults) for 2 or 3 days and *central analgesics*, particularly IV phenoperidine, as required.

If this treatment fails to improve the patient's condition intermittent injections of curare may prove useful and are usually the prelude to continuous curarization.

Paralysing the patient is a difficult decision to make because of the hazards that can be associated with prolonged curarization. It is not an alternative treatment for milder cases of tetanus, and most workers feel that it must be kept only for the severe forms that cannot be controlled by sedation.

The circulating blood volume must be adequate and sedation is continued. It is essential that curare be administered IV continuously by means of an infusion pump. Pancuronium has been the preferred preparation for curarization for the past 6–7 years; doses vary in adults and are determined individually for each patient within the range of 0.25–1.00 mg/kg per day. Serum concentrations, however, are less variable [15]; in eight of our patients they were between 0.27 and 0.48 μg/ml.

Curarized patients require absolutely constant surveillance since they cannot breathe without assistance. The balloon of the tracheostomy cannula must be inflated continuously and tracheal aspirations must be short to avoid hypoxia. When the clinical course allows curare is withdrawn and replaced by diazepam for a few days. The duration of treatment is 15–20 days on average; cardiac activity must be monitored for at least 10 days after curare has been stopped.

Other aspects

Careful attention to *fluid and electrolyte balance* is required. A high water intake is necessary usually between 3000 and 4000 ml per day to compensate for the large losses due to sweating [12, 25, 45]. Sweat also contains 60–100 mmol sodium/litre. Naso-gastric feeding can usually be started after 3–4 days; some authors advocate gastrostomy. A high calorie and protein intake is essential, at least 3000 calories and 120 g protein [49, 51, 52]. In curarized patients, paralytic ileus may prevent enteral feeding, and IV feeding should then be substituted.

Catheterization is usually needed to prevent urinary retention and to maintain a correct record of fluid balance. The importance of nursing and physiotherapy has already been stressed.

Pulmonary embolism used to be a frequent cause of death during tetanus, but preventative treatment with heparin SC has markedly reduced its incidence.

Hyperbaric O_2 therapy has been proposed by some authors [35] but does not seem to be of great use.

Circulatory disorders are not rare during tetanus and they vary in nature and severity. In the early stages of the disease they are generally related to hypovolaemia and often become manifest as hypotension after the administration of sedatives.

Disorders specific to tetanus are more severe; they are probably not frequent but their incidence is difficult to evaluate. In the last decade several studies have been devoted to the pathogenesis and treatment of these autonomic dysfunctions [3, 6, 9, 19, 33, 44, 53]. Signs of sympathetic hyperactivity appear a few days after the onset of the disease and consist in large and rapid variations in heart rate, arterial pressure, and (if they are measured) cardiac output and systemic vascular resistance. There appears to be a parallel increase in both alpha- and beta-adrenergic activities of either peripheral or central origin. Many types of drugs have been tried in such situations, with varying and sometimes contradictory results:

Beta blockers such as propranol or pindolol do not control the disorders fully.

Alpha blockers such as phenoxybenzamine or phentolamine, which controlled hypertension, have been abandoned in this condition because of the severe secondary hypotension that is likely to appear. Labetalol [13, 20, 39] was found to be effective in preliminary studies.

Central nervous system depressants, particularly chlorpromazine, which has also an alpha-adrenergic blocker action, can control the disorders with few side-effects [17, 28, 44, 59].

Neonatal tetanus

The treatment of neonatal tetanus is no different from that of the adult form, except that if barbiturates are used they must be prescribed at low doses because of a possible deleterious effect on cerebral development [54]. Only the techniques, particularly those for ventilation and feeding, are different, requiring specially trained medical staff for the management of the acute phase, which often lasts 4–6 weeks. In the best centres mortality should not be higher than 20% [1, 54]. Although neonatal tetanus has almost disappeared in western countries it remains a serious problem in countries with few or no technical resources [29, 43].

The main features of a simplified form of treatment are isolation of the neonate; early control of spasms with diazepam 0.3–1 mg/kg IV; passage of a naso-jejunal tube to allow administration of water, electrolytes, food, and drugs; and injections of antitoxin (10 000 IU IM, or 500–1000 IU intrathecally). Nonetheless, this treatment does not prevent a very high mortality of between 70% and 90%. Because of its geographical distribution this is the form of treatment that has most frequently to be adopted.

Similar sedative drugs are administered, but the doses are reduced to avoid undue respiratory depression. Because of the lack of intubation facilities it is not safe to insert a gastric tube.

This treatment protocol can be improved at little cost [11] by providing facilities for isolating the patient (which can be difficult in some societies) and for performing tracheostomy as required. Despite the lack of artificial ventilation, tracheostomy prevents the occurrence of severe apnoea due to glottic spasm and ensures a free airway. A naso-gastric tube could also then be inserted for parenteral feeding. This would entail the setting up of special care units and the mortality in this age group would be expected to fall to about 40%; the cost would be relatively low.

Prevention

Tetanus can occur when a person is wounded even if the wound is minor. Only active immunization (vaccination) before infection can provide actual protection.

Local treatment consists in washing, disinfection, and opening of the wound and removal of any foreign material.

The *immunoprophylaxis* to be given depends on the vaccination status of the patient and on the type of wound (Table 55.3).

Table 55.3. Indications for immunoprophylaxis

Immunization of the patient	Severity of the wound	
	Mild risks[a]	Severe risks[b]
Complete vaccination before the wound (at least two injections of toxoid and a booster dose) Last booster		
Up to 5 years earlier	Nothing	Nothing
5–10 years earlier	Nothing	Nothing
Over 10 years earlier	Booster dose	Booster dose + serum[c]
Incomplete vaccination before the wound (at least one injection of toxoid	Vaccination[d]	Vaccination[d] + serum[c]
No, or no known, vaccination	Vaccination[d] + serum[c]	Vaccination[d] + double dose of serum[c]

[a]Mild risks, minor wounds, not deep or dirty, with no foreign material, e.g., non-traumatic wounds (varicose ulcers) and some surgical incisions (on foot, gut, uterus, open recent or old fractures).
[b]Severe risks, large traumatic wounds, deep and dirty, with foreign material, left untreated for over 24 h (septic abortion, septic delivery, frostbite, necrotic ulcers, gangrene).
[c]Heterologous serum from animals (at least 1500 IU) or human antitetanus immunoglobulins (at least 250 U).
[d]Vaccination is completed later according to the simplified protocol recommended at present. If the injection is the first one received by the patient the second is given after 4–6 weeks and the booster dose 6 months later. If this is the second injection a booster dose 6 months later is sufficient.

References

1. Adams JM, Kenny JD, Rudolph AJ (1979) Modern management of tetanus neonatorum. Pediatrics 644:472–477
2. Ahmad MS, Mange MS, Kiblawi IS, Smith RC (1979) Treatment of tetanus with Dantrolene sodium. Proceedings of the Fifth International Conference on Tetanus, Sweden
3. Benedict CR, Kerr JH (1967) Assessment of sympathetic overactivity in tetanus. Br Med J iii:806
4. Bolot JF, Fournier G, Canton P, Cardinaud JP, Rey M, Stellman C, Triau R, Diop Mar I (1979) Intrathecal human specific antitenus. A multicentic controlled trial. Proceedings of the Fifth International Conference on Tetanus, Sweden
5. Boron P (1973) Inderal propanolol in the therapy of tetanus. Pol Tyg Lek 28/19:697–699
6. Buchanan N, Cane RD, Wolfson G, De Andrade M (1979) Autonomic dysfunction in tetanus: The effects of a variety of therapeutic agents with special reference to morphine. Intensive Care Med 5:65
7. Carrington Dacosta RB, Maul ER, Pimentel J, Cardoso D'Oliveira L, David Gomes J (1979) Is it possible to lower the lethality rate of tetanus? Proceedings of the Fifth International Conference on Tetanus, Sweden
8. Cole LB, Youngman HR (1969) Treatment of tetanus. Lancet I:1017
9. Corbett JL, Spalding JM, Harris PJ (1973) Hypotension in tetanus. Br Med J iii/5877:423–428
10. De Silva JA, Koechlin BA, Bader G (1966) Blood level distribution patterns of diazepam and its major metabolism in man. J Pharm Sci 55:692–702
11. Diop-Mar I, Sow A (1975) Traitement simplifié du tétanos en l'absence de soins intensifs. Proceeding of the 4th International Conference on Tetanus. Dakar, Mérieux I:583–605
12. Diop-Mar I, Badiane S, Sow A, Ba A, (1979) Treatment of tetanus by intrathecal heterologous antitoxin. Proceedings of the Fifth International Conference on Tetanus, Sweden
13. Dundee JW, Morrow WF (1979) Labetalol in severe tetanus. Br Med J i:1121
14. Duvaldestin P, Desmont JM (1976) Pharmacocinétique des médicaments utilisés dans le traitement symptomatique du tétanos. In: L'année en réanimation médicale 1975/76. Flammarion, Paris, p 151–162
15. Duvaldestin P, Gibert C, Henzel D, Guy P, Desmont JM (1979) Pancuronium blood level monitoring in patients with tetanus. Intens Care Med. 5:111–114
16. Emondson RS, Flowers MW (1979) Intensive care in tetanus: Management, complications and mortality in 100 cases. Br Med J i:1401–1404
17. Fraisse F, Amoudry C, Tremolieres F, Comoy E, Gibert C, Vachon F (1979) Interest of Chlorpromazine versus Pindolol in the treatment of hemodynamic dysfunction in severe tetanus. Proceedings of the Fifth International Conference on Tetanus, Sweden
18. Gallais H, Moreau J, Cornet C, Odehouri K, Abisse A, Echimane A (1979) Therapeutic evaluation of 404 cases of tetanus: Advantages of intrathecal serotherapy. Proceedings of the Fifth International Conference on Tetanus, Sweden
19. Gustafson I, Carlsson C, Nilsson E (1979) Sympathetic hyperactivity in tetanus. Proceedings of the Fifth International Conference on Tetanus, Sweden
20. Hanna W, Grell GA (1978) Labetalol in hypertensive emergencies. Br Med J iii:772
21. Hendrickse RG, Shermann PM (1965) Therapeutic trial of diazepam in tetanus. Lancet I:737–738
22. Holloway R (1970) Fluid and electrolyte status in tetanus. Lancet II:1978–1279
23. Ildirim I (1974) Intrathecal serotherapy of tetanus. Turk J Pediatr 16:103
24. Kerr JH (1977) Problems in severe tetanus. In: Hill ED, Peregrinus P (eds) Management of the acutely ill. p 92
25. Kerr JH (1979a) Insensible fluid losses in tetanus. Proceedings of the Fifth International Conference on Tetanus, Sweden
26. Kerr JH (1979b) Current topics in tetanus. Intensive Care Med 5:105–110
27. Kerr JH, Spalding JM, Crampton-Smith A (1970) Experience with tracheostomies in Oxford. Int Anesthesiol Clin 8:875
28. Kryshanovsky GN (1973) The effect of several substances of phenothiazine series and alpha-adrenoblockers on spinal cord activity with inhibitory mechanisms disrupted by tetanus toxin. Farmakol Toksikol 3:276–280
29. Kurosu Y, Tamura K, Yamamoto Y, Inami K (1979) Airway management in neonatal tetanus. Proceedings of the Fifth International Conference on Tetanus, Sweden
30. Lassen HC, Bjornerboe M, Ibsen B, Neukirch F (1954) Treatment of tetanus wirh curarization, general anaesthesia and intra-tracheal positive pressure ventilation. Lancet II:1040–1044
31. Lazar M, Pikelj F, Vidmar L (1979) Modern views on the pathogenesis and therapy of tetanus. Proceedings of the Fifth International Conference on Tetanus, Sweden
32. Leonardi G, Nair KG, Dastur FD, Kamat JS, Desai BT (1973) Evaluation of cholinesterase agents restoring in the treatment of tetanus in man. J Infect Dis 128:652–657
33. Levell MJ (1970) Adrenal cortical function in patients with tetanus. Br J Anaesth 42:531
34. List WF (1979) Tetanus treatment with high doses of tetanus antitoxin. Proceedings of the Fifth International Conference on Tetanus, Sweden
35. Milledge JS (1968) Hyperbaric oxygen therapy in tetanus. JAMA 203:875–876
36. Mollaret P, Bastin R, Damoiseau B, Goulon M, Pocidalo JJ (1955) Le traitement héroïque du tetanos gravissime (curarisation maxima sous anesthésie mais avec trachéotomie et respiration artificielle par controle volumétrique interne des modifications de pression). Nouv Presse Med 63:1413–1416
37. Mollaret P, Vic Dupont V, Cartier F, Margairaz A, Monsallier JF, Pocidalo JJ, Grosblas A (1965) Traitement du tétanos à la Clinique de Réanimation Médicale de l'hopital Claude Bernard. Enseignement tiré des 150 derniers cas d'une statistique de 1000 sujets. Nouv Presse Med 73:2153–2156
38. Nilsson E (1979) Experience of tetanus treatment in an ICU. Proceedings of the Fifth International Conference on Tetanus, Sweden
39. Omar MA, Wesley AG, Pather M (1979) Labetalol in severe tetanus. Br Med J ii:274
40. Patel JC, Mehta BC (1979) Homologus tetanus immune globulin in the treatment of tetanus. A preliminary report. Proceedings of the Fifth International Conference on Tetanus, Sweden
41. Poisot D, Benissan CG, Castaing Y, Gabinski C, Cardinaud JP (1979) Causes of death in tetanus. Importance of complications of intensive care. Proceedings of the Fifth International Conference on Tetanus, Sweden
42. Rey M (1979) Le tétanos en question. Rev Fr Transfus Immuno Hématol XXII/4:415–426

43. Rhea JW (1975) New approaches to simple neonatal tetanus treatment. Proceedings of the 4th International Conference on Tetanus, Dakar, vol I. Mérieux, Lyon, pp 607–610

44. Rie MA, Wilson RS (1978) Morphine therapy controls autonomic hyperactivity in tetanus. Ann Intern Med 88:653

45. Ruzic A, Pavlovic J, Jorgacevic D (1970) Troubles de l'équilibre hydro-électrolytique transcutané au cours du tétanos grave. Vème Congrès International de Maladies Infectieuses, A 2n, 5, vol 56 pp 229–234

46. Sanders RK (1979) Treatment of tetanus. Br Med J ii:49

47. Sanders RK, Joseph R, Martyn B, Peacock ML (1977) Intrathecal antitetanus serum (horse) in the treatment of tetanus. Lancet I:974

48. Sedaghatian MR (1979) Intrathecal serotherapy in neonatal tetanus: A controlled trial. Arch Dis Child 54:623–625

49. Shelestink PI (1966) Changes in basal metabolism in patients with tetanus. Urachebroe Delo (Kiev) 11:99–102

50. Takano K (1979) Tetanus toxin and gamma motor system: A theoretical background of a good use of diazepam in tetanus therapy. Proceedings of the Fifth International Conference on Tetanus, Sweden

51. Tremolières F, Gibert C, Henzel D, Vachon F (1974a) Dépenses énergétiques et azotées au cours du tétanos. Adaptation des apports nutritionnels aux besoins. Nouv Presse Med 3:943–946

52. Tremolieres F, Gibert C, Vachon F, Pocidalo JJ (1974b) Effect of curarization on energy and nitrogen balances in acute tetanus treated by prolonged administration of d-tubocurarine. Biomedicine [Express] 4/21:186–189

53. Tseuda K, Oliver PB, Richter RW (1974) Cardiovascular manifestations of tetanus. Anesthesiology 40:588

54. Vachon F, Gibert C, Tremolieres F, Manuel C, Huault G, Vic Dupont V (1975) Traitement intensif du tétanos aigu géneralise. Proceedings of the Fourth International Conference on Tetanus, Dakar, vol I. Mérieux, Lyon, pp 497–526

55. Vakil BJ, Armittage P, Rosemary E, Clifford E, Laurence DR (1979) Therapeutic trials of intrathecal (intracisternal) administration of human tetanus immunoglobulin in severe tetanus. Proceedings of the Fifth International Conference on Tetanus, Sweden

56. Vic Dupont V, Vachon F, Gaudebout C, Manuel C, Tremolieres F, Gibert C (1975) Essai en double aveugle de gammaglobulines humaines antitétaniques hyperimmunes par voie intraveineuse dans le traitement du tétanos généralisé. Proceedings of the Fourth International Conference on Tetanus, Dakar, vol I. Mérieux, Lyon, pp 401–408

57. Vic Dupont V, Vachon F, Gibert C, Tremolieres F, Manuel C, Goursot G (1976) Traitement intensif du tétanos généralisé de l'adulte. Nouv Presse Med 5/1:31–34; 5/2:83–86

58. Warter K, Mantz JM, Otteni JC, Kempf F (1965) L'ossification paraarticulaire, complication fréquente du tétanos. Nouv Presse Med 73:1203

59. Woods KL (1978) Hypotensive effect of propanolol and phenoperidine in tetanus. Br Med J ii:1164

Section K

Methods of Investigation

Chapter 56

Monitoring Equipment and Unit Design

D. W. Hill

Design considerations

Size

An estimate of the proportion of the patients admitted to an acute hospital who will need intensive therapy at some time is between 1% and 2% [9]. Units of less than six beds are uneconomical in terms of staffing, accommodation, essential services and equipment, while one with more than ten beds becomes unwieldy. In a general hospital it is usually possible for the ICU to accept all types of emergency, but the coronary care unit (CCU) should be adjacent to the ICU if this is feasible.

Siting

The ICU should preferably be located close to the operating and recovery rooms and on the same floor, and also to the accident and emergency and diagnostic radiology departments. This arrangement allows a sharing of air conditioning plant and switchgear rooms, eases communications, and may allow staff and ancillary accommodation to be shared with the recovery room. Consideration must be given when selecting the site to allow for adequate stores accommodation, offices, rest room, and relatives' room, plus some flexibility to allow for a small laboratory area, for example.

The Department of Health and Social Security Building Note [9] makes the point that there are advantages in having natural daylight and, if possible, an attractive view from the windows in the bed areas and staff rooms so that the occupants do not feel aware of a psychological barrier between them and the outside world.

Rooms

The basic design of an ICU encompasses a fully observable bed area with sufficient space to position the beds with regard to the nursing procedures and associated equipment. The base for the duty staff should be close to the beds and designed to keep the movement both of staff and of clean and dirty articles to a minimum.

Patient area

This is usually arranged as one large area with at least two single rooms. The single rooms should each have a minimum area of 26 m^2 and be approximately square in shape; and each should be fitted with an airlock to allow for the nursing of infectious and susceptible patients. Beds in multi-bed areas should be spaced at at least 3.3 m, centre to centre. Glare from windows or direct sunlight must be controlled by blinds. Partition walls between the single rooms and the multi-bed area should be partly glazed, preferably with double glazing and a Venetian blind between the glass panes. Thus privacy can be preserved in the cubicles, but observation of the beds can be arranged from the staff base. Glare from lights and brightly coloured walls must also be avoided.

Furnishings

The siting of fixtures and fittings is important and provision must be made for ample electrical outlets (8 per bed has been found to be insufficient in practice) and piped suction, compressed air, oxygen, and nitrous oxide if these are available in the operating room suite. Commercial trunking systems are made to house these outlets and rail systems are also available for holding such items as an automatic lung ventilator, sphygmomanometer, and adjustable lamp. Bed curtaining is not recommended because it would interfere with the overall view of the bed area and restrict the possible positions for beds. Low mobile screens (0.95–1 m high) can be used to screen patients from each other when they are lying down, but do not obstruct observation by the staff. The low screens can be supplemented by mobile screens about 1.8 m high or these may be preferred. A shelf behind can be used for a patient's personal belongings, such as glasses and toilet articles, with the patient's clothing being stored in a locker not at the bedside. Comfortable stacking chairs will be needed for staff and visitors at the bedside, and these are removed to the equipment store when not in use.

Staff base

This is the focal point of the ICU and should be an open area to allow for both audible and visual communication with the patients. The base should have a desk of adequate size to allow for two people working simultaneously, at least two chairs, a telephone, space for patients' records, a central patient monitoring console, and an x-ray viewing box.

Washbasins

There should be a washbasin with elbow-operated taps in each single-bed area and at least two similar basins in the multi-bed area, sited so as not to restrict the positioning of the beds.

Clean utility area

The staff base should be close to a clean utility area equipped with a sink with elbow-operated taps, drinking water, a lockable drug cupboard, space for medicine trolleys, space for any mobile equipment which is in regular use, and cupboards/shelves for medicines, lotions, disposable items such as syringes, catheters, cannulas, and packs of general clean supplies. This stock will normally be supplied from the hospital's central sterile supply department. If transport difficulties are foreseen a small, portable, electrically heated pressure steam sterilizer may be needed.

Office

Office accommodation is required for the sister, for interviewing staff and preparing reports. It may also be used by visiting medical staff or a separate office may be provided for the 'intensivist' if such a person is in charge of the ICU. Furniture will include a desk, chairs, table, lockable storage cupboard, shelves, and a filing cabinet. The office(s) should be within the ICU and near to the entrance.

Staff rest room

Work in an ICU is arduous and a rest-room should be available close to the bed area. In addition to easy chairs and a table, facilities should be available for the preparation of beverages and snacks only, e.g., a small refrigerator, electric kettle, hot plate, crockery cupboard, and food/drink cupboard.

Equipment store

This room must be large enough to hold all the reserve or specialist apparatus such as automatic lung ventilators, patient monitors, suckers, and defibrillators. It should be within the ICU and kept tidy.

Dirty utility/sluice room

Here dirty and used articles can be cleaned, if necessary, and stored temporarily pending disposal or transfer to the central sterile supply department, laundry, or incinerator. It should have a worktop sink with elbow-operated taps, draining board, disposal bins, and stands for soiled linen bags. There should be a bed-pan washer and disinfector or bed-pan disposal unit, a flushing sink and slab, and a heated bed-pan cabinet if required. Shelving and a ventilated storage cabinet cater for stool specimens and for 24-h urine specimens. The room will be used for urine testing and for the emptying, cleaning, and storage of bed-pans and urine bottles.

Doctor's room/overnight stay

The ICU should contain a room which the doctor on duty can use as a bedroom when he is on call at night, and it can also double as an office. Equipment should include a desk or table, chairs, bookcase or shelves, a twin x-ray viewing box, a convertible settee or divan, a hanging cupboard for clothes, and a washbasin.

Linen store

Storage cupboards are required to hold the ICU's working stock of linen, with high-level shelving for items such as pillows. One or two cupboards each with an area of approximately 2.5 m^2 will suffice, and these can contain the linen trolleys if these are used to bring over the linen from a central supply.

Lavatory and changing accommodation

A cloakroom should be located at the entrance to the ICU so that nurses can don gowns and leave their ordinary uniform or outdoor clothes. Full-length lockers are needed for each nurse and a changing and locker space of at least 0.75 m^2 per person. A toilet, washbasin, and shower should be available next to the nurses' cloakroom. Doctors can change in the office(s).

Space may need to be provided at the entrance to the ICU for visiting staff and relatives to don protective clothing. Accommodation will be necessary for outdoor clothes, clean garments, and containers for used garments. A bench seat assists with the donning of overshoes. Entrance to the gowning area should be via a lobby fitted with double doors to provide some control of the air-flow within the ICU. It must be borne in mind that protective clothing for visitors is not insisted on in all ICUs.

Relatives' room

A room for relatives of patients in the ICU should be available outside the unit and should be fitted with comfortable chairs, a divan, and a hanging cupboard for clothes. Toilet, washing, and telephone facilities should be available nearby.

Cleaners' room

Located inside the ICU, it should contain a bucket sink with hot and cold water, drainer, and space for cleaning equipment and utensils.

Laboratory

In some ICUs, such as those for post-cardiac surgery patients, space may be provided for a blood gas laboratory, and occasionally this may also house 'Stat' instrumentation such as that required to measure electrolytes. Apart from automated blood gas analysis, it is now generally considered that other biochemical tests should be performed in a proper hospital laboratory by professional biochemistry staff.

The 'laboratory' should be fitted with a laboratory sink and benches, storage cupboards, and engineering service outlets. A refrigerator may also be needed.

Workshop

A case can sometimes be made for a small workshop for handling minor repairs and maintenance to items such as patient monitors, defibrillators, suckers, ventilators, and infusion pumps. However, the technical staff will also work with operating room and cardiology equipment, and it may be better to think in terms of a central clinical workshop for the hospital but with staff having a priority for the needs of the ICU.

Engineering services

The plant room for the engineering services may often be shared with other departments, e.g., the operating rooms. The noise and vibration carrying to the ICU must be minimal.

Heating

The heating system should be designed for continuous operation and should be available at all times of the year for use in the patient areas on cold days. With an outside ambient temperature of 1°C it should be possible to maintain the patient areas at 21°C and provide 15 changes of air per hour. A conventional hot water heating system with flush-fitting radiators is generally satisfactory for an ICU.

Ventilation

The main bed area should be provided with supply and extract ventilation and the introduction of 15 air changes per hour of fresh air at the end of the ICU furthest from the door and the extraction of 30 air changes per hour close to the door should provide a sufficient current of air through the open doorway to prevent air from flowing in.

Monitoring equipment

General requirements

Intensive therapy must involve close and regular observation of the patients by the nursing staff. At such times not only can numerical information be obtained, such as the patient's temperature from a clinical thermometer, but important clinical observations can be made, for example whether the patient is restless or sweating. Thus in many ICUs, the only electronic monitoring equipment may be cardioscopes, supplemented with direct observation of the blood pressure, temperature, and respiration. In ICUs associated with major surgery, e.g., cardiac surgery, it is normal to use pressure transducers for monitoring systemic arterial, left atrial, and pulmonary artery pressures. In some ICUs of this type a large range of instrumentation will be encountered, including cardiac output measurements and equipment for measuring fluid loss and infusion.

Haemodynamic measurements

Undoubtedly the most commonly encountered signal in ICUs is the electrocardiogram (ECG). It is non-invasive and contains a wealth of diagnostic information on the rhythmicity of the heart and the state of the myocardium. However, the ECG by itself does not give any quantitative information on the pumping ability of the heart and needs to be supplemented with pressure and flow data when a detailed knowledge of a patient's haemodynamics is required.

For a diagnosis, a conventional 12-lead ECG is normally taken, with a standard heated stylus, ink jet, or pressure-sensitive electrocardiograph with conventional plate and suction electrodes. Since limb leads are prone to severe motion artefacts in a restless patient, longer-term routine ECG monitoring is usually performed with disposable self-adhesive chest electrodes in a simulated lead 2 arrangement [20]. The electrodes now used are of the fluid column type with a silver–silver chloride electrode recessed in a plastic cup containing a foam impregnated with conductive gel. The skin should be cleaned with an ether–methylated spirit mixture and rubbed but not heavily abraded.

The resulting ECG is displayed on a digital storage-type oscilloscope so that it is possible to 'freeze' the tracing when it is desired to inspect it at leisure. The older type of 'bouncing ball' displays with a long-persistence screen, are being rapidly replaced with storage displays. A heart-rate meter is often provided, driven from the R waves of the ECG. The latest approach is to employ a microcomputer so that the R waves are selected on the basis of a software algorithm rather than by hardware circuitry. This provides for a more flexible approach in terms of a matching filter to selectively amplify the QRS complex, an adjustable inhibitory period to prevent R wave detection during the T wave of the ECG, and automatic adjustment of the QRS detection threshold so that it is raised when R waves are unlikely and lowered when they are likely. In this way a substantial degree of immunity against noise on the waveform is possible.

The simpler types of R wave detector based upon filtering and peak detection are prone to high-frequency artefacts and thus false alarms can be a problem. The microprocessor approach reduces false alarms by averaging the R–R intervals to derive the heart rate. If too much noise is found on the ECG waveform the previous heart rate is stored and continues to be displayed. If the noise persists for a significant period of time a 'noisy signal' message is displayed and an alarm raised.

Significant advances have also occurred in the design of blood pressure transducers such as the quartz diaphragm model 1290A by Hewlett Packard, which operates on the capacitance manometer principle. The rugged diaphragm can withstand a high overload pressure of +6000 mmHg and can also be gas-sterilized and scrubbed with a brush and detergent. The transducer is light in weight (105 g including cable), and its flat shape enables it to be taped directly to the patient's wrist. The pressure range is −30 to +400 mmHg and the sensitivity is 40 mV per volt per mmHg with an excitation voltage of 3.5–5 V r.m.s. at 2400 Hz. The volume displacement is 0.2 mm^3 per 100 mmHg and the operating temperature range is 10–40°C. The body of the transducer is made of a glass-filled polyester material and can be either liquid or gas-sterilized. Disposable domes (cuvettes) made from a polycarbonate for the dome and polyvinyl chloride for the dome membrane can be attached to the transducer's body with a simple 'twist-and-lock' action. The disposable dome provides protection against cross infection since it is presterilized, and also minimizes electrical leakage currents. The electrical insulation of the model 1290A is quoted in terms of a leakage current to earth of less than 5 μA at 120 V r.m.s. via the fluid column, and each transducer is tested to withstand 10 000 Vdc defibrillator pulses.

Both the quartz diaphragm transducer and differential transformer type blood pressure transducers require energizing with ac at some 2.4 kHz 5 V r.m.s. and the use of a carrier amplifier, whereas bonded and unbonded strain gauge pressure transducers can be energized from a stable amplitude source of either ac or dc. Compact displays are readily available with a storage-type display of the ECG and one or more blood pressures (Fig. 56.1), with numerical indications of the heart rate, systolic and diastolic pressures, mean pressures, and temperature information. Sandman and Hill [33] and Klevenhagen and Storey [16] describe circuitry for the separation of the systolic, diastolic and mean pressures from an arterial pressure wave form.

Care needs to be exercised to ensure that clots do not dampen the blood pressure waveform and arouse suspicions concerning the patient's cardiovascular status. One way to guard against clotting is to continuously flush the catheter system with a small flow (e.g. 4 ml/h)

with heparinized saline from a pressurized reservoir. Shinebourne and Pfitzner [35] give details of such an arrangement, while Weinstein [37] deals with the problems of cross-infection between patients arising from the use of the same transducer on successive occasions. Gram-negative bacteria from a contaminated transducer cuvette can grow through several feet of tubing over a period of 3 days.

The development of flow-directed Swan–Ganz catheters, which are radio-opaque, have gauges for adults of 6 or 7 French, a pressure-measuring lumen opening at the distal tip, a natural latex balloon mounted just proximal to the tip, and a second lumen which opens 30 cm proximal to the tip for the injection of cool saline, has encouraged catheterization of the right heart and pulmonary artery and the use of the thermal dilution technique for the measurement of cardiac output (Chap. 1). The catheter carries a small thermistor located 4 cm from the tip, which senses the passage of the cool saline. The proximal end of the catheter is fitted with a stopcock for inflation of the balloon, two insulated jack plugs for connecting the thermistor to the associated cardiac output computer, and Luer-Lok fittings for attachment to the pressure transducer and for the injectate.

Once the cardiac output has been determined

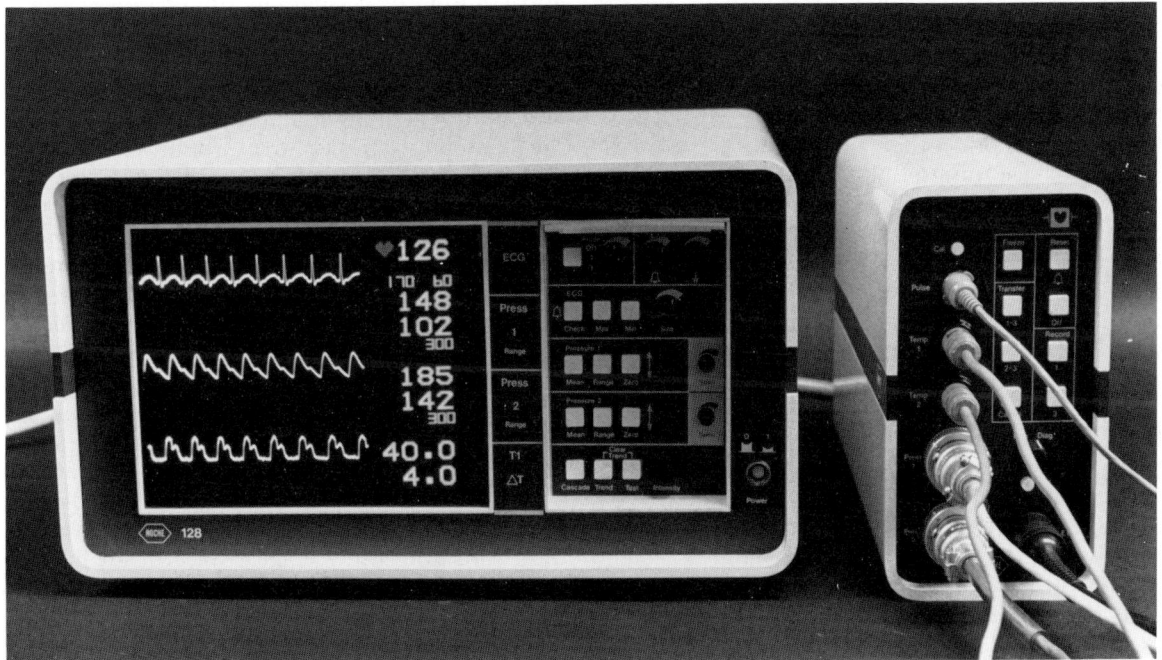

Fig. 56.1. Digital storage–type monitor for the display of the ECG and one or more blood pressure wave forms, with numerical indications of the heart rate, systolic and diastolic pressures, mean pressures, and temperature information. Courtesy of Roche Ltd.

the average stroke volume can be found from: cardiac output = stoke volume × heart rate.

An index of changes in myocardial contractility is also of value in the management of patients developing cardiac failure, and non-invasive techniques for doing this are the electrical impedance approach of Welham et al. [38] or the Doppler shift ultrasound method of Light [18, 19], known as transaortic velography. This effectively monitors the velocity of ejection of the stroke volume into the aorta and the use of the technique in the ICU has been evaluated by Buchtal et al. [6].

Apart from the monitoring of central blood flow, there is also a requirement in some critically ill patients for monitoring of limb blood flow and the volume flow into a segment of a limb can conveniently be monitored by means of venous occlusion plethysmography.

Arenson and Mohapatra [2] compared 119 pairs of simultaneous calf blood flow values obtained by the mercury-in-rubber strain gauge and impedance plethysmogram methods with manual inflation of the cuff; and in 20 conscious volunteers and 20 anaesthetized patients who had no clinical evidence of cardiovascular disease, the correlation coefficient was 0.88.

Body temperature

While the conventional mercury-in-glass clinical thermometer is still widely used in ICUs, electronic thermometers are normally available on most modular patient monitoring systems and differential temperature modules are used for recording the difference between the core temperature and the temperature at the periphery. Henning et al. [11] showed that for patients with acute myocardial infarction, bacteraemia, or blood and fluid loss the difference (great toe temperature minus ambient temperature) is a reliable indicator for assessing tissue perfusion. Joly and Weil [15] showed that the great toe temperature follows changes in the patient's cardiac output.

Thermistors are almost universally used as the temperature-sensitive element in patient monitors. A thermistor consists of a bead of semiconductor material with a marked negative coefficient of resistance with temperature. The bead is mounted in a plastic or stainless steel probe so that it is mechanically robust and can be chemically sterilized. After ageing treatment to stabilize its characteristics, the thermistor is mounted in its housing together with shunt and series resistors chosen to linearize the resistance temperature change and to equalize this

for individual probes so that more than one probe can be used with the same calibrated meter. The thermistor forms one arm of a Wheatstone bridge circuit. A typical temperature range would be 32–42°C with a probe time constant of 10 s for a skin probe and 90 s for a rectal probe. It is important to be sure that the temperature range is adequate if hypothermic patients are to be monitored.

Respiration

For adult patients, most modular patient monitoring systems provide facilities for monitoring the respiratory rate, often by sensing the rhythmic changes of resistance of a thermistor bead mounted in the tidal air stream. The thermistor can be located in a facemask if O_2 therapy is in use or taped beneath a nostril, but care may be required to obtain reproducible signals over extended periods of time. A length of strapping around the patient's chest can be used to actuate a switch, or the ends of the strapping may be connected to the closed ends of a short length of corrugated rubber tubing which in turn is joined to a pressure transducer. The expansion of the chest during inspiration stretches the tubing and raises the pressure, and the increase in the signal from the transducer is used to trigger the respiratory rate meter. Alternatively, if a pneumotachograph is employed for flow rate and volume measurements the respiratory rate can be derived from its output signal.

For spontaneously breathing patients, the rate may be continously monitored and the tidal and minute volume monitored as required by means of a facemask and a turbine-type volume meter such as the well-known Wright respirometer [40].

A continuous indication of tidal and minute volume is possible from an integrating pneumotachograph. The pneumotachograph essentially consists of a linear pneumatic resistance to gas flow such as a 400 mesh gauze screen or a number of narrow tubes in parallel. The pressure drop across the head is only a few millimetres of water and is linearly proportional over a stated range to the volume flow rate of gas passing through the head. The calibration should be the same in the forward and reverse directions and some types are electrically heated to prevent a condensation of breath moisture from affecting the calibration. The calibration against known flow rates depends on the composition of the gas mixture and calibration techniques have been described by Hobbes [12] and Turney and Blumenfeld [36].

A rectifier arrangement can be used to select the signals from the pneumotachograph's pressure transducer corresponding to either the inspiratory or the expiratory flow rates and these can be integrated on an individual basis to give the inspiratory or expiratory tidal volumes. The tidal volumes can be summed over a period of 1 min to yield the minute volume on a minute-by-minute basis.

The monitoring of the high-frequency electrical thoracic electrical impedance changes with respiration is used as a respiratory rate monitor in some patient monitoring systems. A simple two-terminal arrangement operating at a frequency such as 25 kHz is convenient. The same pair of electrodes serves to pass a constant current across the chest and to detect the resulting voltage changes with respiration. The electrodes can be placed bilaterally along the midaxillary line. The standing impedance across the chest would be of the order of 200 ohms and the change with each breath of the order of a few ohms per litre. An ac-coupled amplifier detects only the changes in impedance and feeds these via a shaping network to the respiratory rate meter.

Neonates are prone to periods of apnoea and much thought has been devoted to the development of apnoea detectors for babies (Chap. 64).

The continuous breath-by-breath monitoring of respiratory gases in the ITU has been greatly helped by the availability of compact quadripole mass spectrometers. These function as a mass filter for the gas molecules in the breath. The tuning of the filter can be swept electronically over a mass range of typically 1 to 150 in a time interval of less than 100 ms [25]. The output for specific gases, such as O_2, CO_2, and N_2, can be displayed on a set of digital displays and pen recorder channels. Once evacuated, the mass spectrometer head is maintained at a high vacuum by means of a silent ion pump, while a separate rotary pump draws a sample of the respired gases down a heated metal capillary tube to a molecular leak through which a small portion diffuses through into the head where it becomes ionized and split up by the mass filter into selected components.

McAslan [21] has described the use of a mass spectrometer for the automatic hourly sampling of airway gases on a 24-h basis in a 12-bed ICU. Riker and Haberman [31] found the availability of a mass spectrometer of value in a community hospital for weaning patients from ventilators and determining the optimum ventilator settings. This was also reported by Potter [29], who also used the device to guide the differential

ventilation of the lungs when their mechanical properties differ. Yakulis et al. [41] found that monitoring by mass spectrometer of the end-tidal CO_2 concentration could detect changes in blood gas variables caused by alterations in cardiopulmonary function which might otherwise have remained undetected until they were potentially life-threatening.

Blood gas analysis

It is usual for an ICU to have its own blood gas analyser for the measurement of blood pH, PO_2 and PCO_2 on blood samples of the order of 500 μl. A glass electrode is used for pH, a polarographic electrode for the PO_2, and a CO_2 electrode for PCO_2. The CO_2 electrode consists of a pH electrode having a thin film of sodium bicarbonate solution held in contact with it by a membrane through which CO_2 from the blood sample can diffuse. All three electrodes are in a common cuvette which is maintained at 37°C by either a water bath or a heated metal block.

The current tendency is to build a microcomputer into the blood gas analyser and this makes possible automatic calibrations and checking for the end-point of the electrode responses, the presence of an adequate amount of buffer solutions, and the need to empty the waste bottle. The microcomputer also provides a sophisticated system of diagnostics to check for instrumentation malfunction and the calculation of derived variables such as the percentage O_2 saturation, actual bicarbonate, total CO_2, and standard base excess. Once the operator presses the start button, the sample is automatically drawn from the syringe or capillary and measured; then the system is rinsed out and the results calculated. The analyser may have its own electronic barometer and may use calibrated gas mixtures contained in cylinders or prepare its own mixtures from cylinders of O_2 and CO_2 via a gas mixing device. Modern analysers are now available 24-h per day and can be used by junior medical staff or nursing staff without the need for a skilled technician. A microsampling mode is normally available for O_2 measurements only with fetal scalp samples of 125 μl [13]. There are numerous references to the use of modern blood gas analysers in the literature [4, 23, 32, 34]. A thin-film tonometer is an invaluable device for checking on the accuracy of blood gas and pH measurements [7].

The analysers so far mentioned all record in vitro measurements on discrete samples preferably of the patient's arterial blood. A new development has been the design of heated electrodes for the transcutaneous monitoring of PO_2 and PCO_2, particularly in neonates, where there is a good agreement with the arterial values (Chap 65) [1, 3, 14, 28, 39].

A heated sampling probe may be used for transcutaneous blood gas measurements in conjunction with a mass spectrometer. The inlet capillary tube of the mass spectrometer is connected to a membrane-covered heated inlet chamber which is attached to the skin by means of a double-sided adhesive ring [8, 22].

In neonates a polarographic or fuel cell type of O_2 sensor can be mounted at the tip of an umbilical artery catheter to provide a continuous recording of the PaO_2 [10] and catheters are available for measurement of both PO_2 and PCO_2 measurements [26].

Safety aspects

In choosing monitoring equipment consideration must be given to the physical aspects of safety—mechanical and electrical, chemical—and sterility where appropriate.

Items such as transducers, catheters, cannulas, or conductive creams used in or on patients must be chemically safe, i.e., non-toxic and non-irritant, and when used in the blood stream they must not lead to any more than a minimal formation of thrombus. Brantigan et al. [5] designed a membrane-covered Teflon sampling catheter for the direct measurement by mass spectrometer of arterial blood gas tensions; this was thrombo-resistant during in vivo use for 7 days. ECG monitoring electrodes may have to be left in place for 24 h or more and should be disposable to minimize cross infection. To ensure stable electrical characteristics, such electrodes are of the fluid column type mounted in a plastic housing with a silver–silver chloride electrode and a conducting gel [17, 27]. Both the gel and the adhesive used to attach the electrode assembly to the skin should be non-irritant, and if adhesive plaster is employed this should be of the micropore type, which will allow the passage of moisture evolved from the skin. Only minimal abrasion of the skin should be used in preparing the skin site for the electrode, to minimize irritation and possible infection. The electrode assembly should be light in weight with a relatively large skin contact area to ensure a stable fixation to the skin.

It goes without saying that a good mechanical construction must be employed for items such as catheter-tip pressure transducers and Swan–Ganz catheters so that pieces do not became detached within the patient's body.

Wherever possible, steam sterilization of apparatus should be employed for items intended for in vivo use, but for electronic and optical equipment this is generally not possible and recourse to chemical or gas sterilizing is necessary. The makers' instructions on sterilizing expensive items such as pressure transducers and fibre-optic catheters should be followed carefully or damage may arise. The problems of cross infection arising from the use of pressure transducers with a succession of patients have been discussed by Weinstein [37]. Modern automatic lung ventilators are designed so that all the porting in contact with the patient's breath can be removed for autoclaving if necessary and bacterial filters are commonly fitted to the gas exhaust port in cases of infection [24]. Humidifiers used with ventilators and incubators represent a particular source of infection and need to be kept in a sterile condition.

Much has been written about the electrical safety requirements for patient monitoring equipment, particularly for apparatus which has a direct connection to the heart, such as external cardiac pacemakers or arterial pressure transducers. The electrical risk to a patient depends on a number of factors, including the patient's condition, the route taken by the current, the nature of the current, and its magnitude.

The present specifications for the safety of medical electrical equipment are contained in the International Electrotechnical Commission's Document IEC 601.1 *Safety of Medical Electrical Equipment*, Part 1: *General requirements*. IEC class 1 equipment does not rely for protection against electric shock on basic insulation only; its accessible conductive parts are connected to a protective (earth) conductor in the fixed wiring of the installation so that they cannot become live in the event of a failure of the basic insulation. Class 2 equipment also does not only rely on basic insulation, but has additional safety precautions such as double insulation or reinforced insulation, there being now no provision for protective earthing or reliance upon installation conditions. In class 3 equipment, protection against electric shock relies on the use of a safety extra-low voltage (SELV) and voltages higher than SELV are not generated in the equipment. In the case of class 3 medical equipment the supply is limited to a medical SELV, i.e., MSELV.

In IEC terms, if an item of equipment is directly connected to a patient, the applied part consists of all those parts of the equipment, including the patient leads, which come into contact with the patient.

Equipment without an applied part, i.e., not directly connected to the patient, can be class 1, 2, or 3 as regards protection, and has an internal electric power source. Type BF equipment is type B equipment but with an isolated floating applied part for connection to the patient. Type CF equipment is class 1 or 2 equipment with an internal electric power source and an isolated (floating) applied part for connection to the patient.

Equipment or equipment parts specifically designed for application where a conductive connection is established directly to the heart must be of type CF. Such equipment may be mains-operated, in which case its protection must be of class 1 or 2, or it may derive its power supply from an internal electrical power source, e.g., a battery.

Leakage current is defined as non-functional current through or across an insulation. Of particular interest is the patient leakage current, which is defined as the current flowing from the applied part via the patient to earth (excluding any functional current), or flowing from the patient via a floating applied part to earth, originating from the unintended appearance of a voltage from an external source on the patient. The magnitude of the patient leakage current has to be measured under a number of specified single fault conditions: With one supply conductor interrupted at a time; with the interruption of a single protective earth conductor; the short-circuiting of each of the constituent parts of a double insulation in turn; a voltage equal to 110% of the highest rated mains voltage applied between the floating applied part and earth. The following are the maximum permitted values:

Current path	Type B		Type BF		Type CF	
	NC	SFC	NC	SFC	NC	SFC
Patient leakage current	0.1	0.5	0.1	0.5	0.01	0.05 mA

NC normal condition; SFC single fault condition.

For 50–60 Hz ac applied through the skin via either the upper or the lower limbs the threshold of sensation is approximately 1 mA r.m.s., and muscular paralysis commences between 10 and 15 mA. It must be remembered that seriously enfeebled patients or those who are anaesthetized and paralysed will be much more at risk from electrical shock than fit, conscious, subjects!

The heart is at maximum risk from ventricular fibrillation for 50–60 Hz currents and whereas currents greater than 3 mA r.m.s. are required to pass into an atrium to produce rhythm disturbances, in man currents as low as 80 μA at 50 or 60 Hz into the right ventricle have been known to cause ventricular fibrillation [30].

In contrast, dc currents are approximately four times less effective than 50–60 Hz ac currents. However, low-voltage electrolytic burns can be the cause of inconvenience and even disfigurement when these occur beneath metal electrodes through which a dc current passes, and the IEC regulations limit the dc current which may pass between electrodes to 10 μA.

A full system of equipment management for ICUs should be in operation. This commences with the choice of reliable equipment which will perform the required clinical function and fulfil the relevant national safety standards. During its working life the equipment should be regularly checked and maintained and due provision made for its ultimate replacement. Type CF amplifiers and isolated pressure transducers are readily available for direct connection to the heart and can withstand the discharge of a dc defibrillator.

References

1. Al-Diady W, Skeates SJ, Hill DW, Tinker J (1977) The use of transcutaneous oxygen electrodes in intensive therapy. Intensive Care Med 3:33–39
2. Arenson Helena M, Mohapatra SN (1976) Evaluation of electrical impedance plethysmography for the non-invasive measurement of blood flow. Br J Anaesth 49:105
3. Beran AV, Sigezawa GY, Young HN, Huxtable RF (1978) An improved sensor and a method for transcutaneous CO_2 monitoring. Acta Anaesthesiol Scand, 22 [Suppl 68]:110–117
4. Blackburn JP (1978) What is new in blood-gas analysis? Br J Anaesth 50:51–62
5. Brantigan JW, Dann DL, Albo D (1976) Clinical catheter for continuous blood gas measurement by mass spectrometry. J Appl Physiol 40:443–446
6. Buchtal Anna, Hanson Gillian C, Peisach AR (1976) Transcutaneous aortovelography: Potentially useful technique in management of critically ill patients. Br Heart J 38:451

7. Chalmers C, Bird BD, Whitwam JG (1976) Evaluation of a new thin film tonometer. Br J Anaesth 46:253
8. Delpy D, Parker D (1979) The application of mass spectrometry to transcutaneous blood-gas analysis. In: Payne JP, Bushman JA, Hill DW (eds) Medical and biological applications of mass spectrometry. Academic Press, London, pp 179–191
9. Department of Health and Social Security (1974) Hospital Building Note No 27, Intensive therapy unit. HM Stationery Office, London
10. Goddard PJ, Keith I, Marcovitch H, Rolfe P, Scopes JW (1972) A catheter-tip oxygen electrode: Experience in newborn infants with respiratory distress. Arch Dis Child 47:675
11. Henning RJ, Wiener F, Valdes S, Weill MH (1979) Measurement of toe temperature for assessing the severity of acute circulatory failure. Surg Gynecol Obstet 149:1–7
12. Hobbes AFT (1967) A comparison of methods of calibrating the pneumotachograph. Br J Anaesth 39:899
13. Hochberg HM (1978) New instrument developments for fetal pH monitoring. Arch Gynecol 226:79–84
14. Huch R, Huch A, Lubbers DW (1973) Transcutaneous measurement of blood PO_2 (tcPO$_2$): Method and application in perinatal medicine. Perinatal Med 1:183
15. Joly HR, Weil MN (1963) Temperature of the great toe as an indication of the severity of shock. Circulation 39:131–138
16. Klevenhagen SC, Storey P (1978) Display stabilising circuit for systolic-diastolic blood pressure monitors. Med Biol Eng Comput 16:65–67
17. Klingler DR, Schoenberg AA, Worth NP, Egleston CF, Burkart JA (1979) A comparison of gel-to-gel measurements of electrode impedance. Med Instrum 13:266–268
18. Light LH (1970) A recording spectrograph for analysing Doppler blood velocity signals (particularly aortic flow) in real time. J Physiol (Lond) 207:42–44
19. Light LH (1976) Transcutaneous aortovelography. A new window on the circulation? Br Heart J 38:443
20. Marriott HJL, Fogg E (1970) Constant monitoring for cardiac dysrhythmias and blocks. Modern Concepts of Cardiovascular Disease 39
21. McAslan TV (1976) Automated respiratory gas monitoring of critically injured patients. Crit Care Med 4:255–260
22. McIlroy MB, Simbruner G, Sonoda Y (1978) Transcutaneous blood gas measurement using a mass spectrometer. Acta Anaesthesiol Scand 22 [Suppl 68]:128–130
23. Minty BD, Barrett AM (1978) Accuracy of automated blood-gas analyser operated by untrained staff. Br J Anaesth 50:1031–1039
24. Mitchell NJ, Gamble DR (1973) Evaluation of the new Williams anaesthetic filter. Br Med J ii:653–654
25. Mosharaffa M (1970) Mass spectrometry in clinical and medical research. Research Development 21:24
26. Parker D, Delpy D, Lewis M (1978) Catheter-tip electrode for continuous measurement of PO_2 and PCO_2. Med Biol Eng Comput 16:599–600
27. Patterson RP (1978) The electrical characteristics of some commercial ECG electrodes. J Electrocardiol 11:23–26
28. Peabody JL, Willis MN, Gregory GA (1978) Clinical limitations and advantages of transcutaneous oxygen electrodes. Acta Anaesthesiol Scand 22 [Suppl 68]:76–82
29. Potter WA (1976) Mass spectrometry for innovative techniques of respirator care, ventilator weaning and differential ventilation in an intensive care unit. Crit Care Med 4:235–238
30. Raftery EB, Green NL, Gregory LC (1975) Disturbances of heart rhythm produced by 50 Hz leakage current in human subjects. Cardiovasc Res 9:256–262
31. Riker JB, Haberman B (1976) Expired gas monitoring by mass spectrometry in a respiratory intensive care unit. Crit Care Med 4:223–229
32. Rubin P, Bradbury S, Prowse K (1979) Comparative study of automatic blood-gas analysers and their use in analysing arterial and capillary samples. Br Med J 1:156–158
33. Sandman AM, Hill DW (1974) An analogue preprocessor for the analysis of arterial blood pressure waveforms. Med Biol Eng Comput 12:360–363
34. Selmers RJ, Tait AR (1976) Towards blood-gas autoanalysis: An evaluation of the Radiometer ABL1. Br J Anaesth 48:487
35. Shinebourne EA, Pfitzner J (1973) Continuous flushing device for indwelling arterial and venous cannulae. Br J Hosp Med Equip [Suppl] 9:64
36. Turney SZ, Blumenfeld W (1973) On-line respiratory waveform analysis using a digital desk calculator. Med Biol Eng Comput 11:275–285
37. Weinstein RA (1976) The design of pressure monitoring devices: Infection control considerations. Med Instrum 10:287–290
38. Welham KC, Mohapatra SN, Hill DW, Stevenson L (1978) The first derivative of the transthoracic electrical impedance as an index of changes in the myocardial contractility in the intact anaesthetised dog. Intensive Care Med 4:43–50
39. Willard D, Messer J, Eberhard P (1980) Non-invasive cutaneous PCO_2 monitoring. Intensive Care Med 6:137
40. Wright BM (1955) A respiratory anemometer. J Physiol (Lond) 127:25P
41. Yakulis R, Snyder JV, Powner D, Fusco D, Grenvik A (1978) Mass spectrometry monitoring of respiratory variables in an intensive care unit. Respiratory Care 23:671–679

Chapter 57

Techniques for Investigating Cardiovascular Function

H. J. C. Swan and William Ganz

This section describes the purpose of measurement of significant cardiovascular variables in the critically ill patient, the instrumentation required, the procedures used, the indications for measurement, and the commonly associated complications. The techniques reviewed including monitoring of (1) heart rate and rhythm, (2) arterial blood pressure, (3) central venous pressure, (4) intracardiac (right heart) pressure, and (5) cardiac output.

The uses of noninvasive procedures, including nuclear scintigraphy, M-mode and two-dimensional echocardiography, and applications of the Doppler technique, are currently less well-defined in clinical practice. Present noninvasive instrumentation is not well-suited for critical care application because of the size of instrumentation, the complexity of the associated processing equipment, the high level of operator skills and experience required, and the need in critical care medicine for multiple and repetitive measurements. With miniaturization of transducer systems and application of modern computer processing techniques, noninvasive procedures may have broad application for the future. However, for the reasons stated above, they will not be considered further in this chapter.

Heart rate and rhythm

Purpose

The regulation of heart rate and the management of cardiac arrhythmias play a major role in the care of the critically ill. Since a significant number of such patients suffer also from serious intrinsic cardiac diseases, the presence of heart rates that are too fast or too slow, or even of minor cardiac arrhythmias, may have serious negative hemodynamic consequences. The purpose of monitoring includes the identification of (1) the presence of an optimal ventricular rate, (2) the presence of coordinated atrioventricular activity, (3) the occurrence of potentially fatal arrhythmias, and (4) the presence of other abnormalities of cardiac rhythm of less immediate adverse significance.

In the presence of intrinsic myocardial or coronary artery disease, maintenance of an optimal heart rate, preferably with an atrioventricular mechanism, may prevent the development of the other accompaniments of low-output states, such as electrolyte disorders, catecholamine excess, and alterations in acid–base balance, which in themselves further depress cardiac output. The addition of an alarm function in the case of ventricular fibrillation or flutter, cardiac arrest, or complete heart block, warns the appropriate critical care personnel to obtain immediate confirmation of the apparent disturbance of rhythm and to promptly correct it and, if possible, the underlying cause. Techniques for such correction include cardioversion, cardiac pacing, and the use of rapidly acting drugs such as atropine or vasopressors. Less serious abnormalities of cardiac rate or rhythm may respond to appropriate medication, or require placement of a cardiac pacemaker. Evaluation of the significance of an arrhythmia must include not only the presence and identity of a specific disturbance of cardiac rhythm, but also some appraisal, even subjective, of the underlying state of the myocardium and the circulation. Many abnormalities of cardiac rhythm are well tolerated in the presence of healthy and appropriately perfused myocardium.

Techniques and procedures

The ECG may be monitored by direct 'hard wire' connection between the patient and the display oscilloscope or recorder, or by means of telemetry in which the ECG signal is transmitted to appropriate receiving antennas connected to display, recording, or computing devices. Computerized monitors are available to identify and to tabulate the numbers and varieties of ectopic cardiac impulses that fall during pre-identified observation periods. Telemetry is particularly useful in the patient with primary cardiac arrhythmias and in patients receiving specific anti-arrhythmic therapy. The majority of automated data processing devices provide an adequate identification and computation of ventricular ectopy, but appear deficient in the analysis of supraventricular ectopy and atrial fibrillation or when an intracardiac pacemaker is being used. The telemetry signal is of particular value in that the patient may be mobile and not restricted to his bed or room during monitoring. Such equipment is, in general, more acceptable to less critically ill patients than a permanent 'hard wire' monitored system. However, telemeterized and computerized systems do not appear to have a substantively lower incidence of false alarms and the other artifactual interferences that have substantively reduced the warning value of cardiac monitors.

Monitoring leads may consist of a standard bipolar lead system in which electrodes are placed below the right clavicle, below the left clavicle, and at the seventh intercostal space in the mid-clavicular line. By means of an appropriate lead selector, the complex which provides the most suitable ECG complex is selected. Alternatively, the Marriott lead (MCL-1) offers several advantages. Electrodes are placed in the right and left intraclavicular regions and also in the fourth intercostal space just to the right of the sternum. This has the specific advantage of improved P-wave definition, improved diagnosis of right and left bundle-branch block, and improved differential diagnosis of supraventricular ectopy.

In all instances, care must be taken to minimize the skin resistance so as to provide the optimal ECG signal. After careful skin preparation, appropriate electrodes must be carefully moistened with a conducting gel and, in general the electrodes should be changed at approximately 60–72 h. The electrodes are also positioned in locations of minimal muscle artifact and away from the hairy areas of the body whenever possible.

Complications

Monitoring of the surface ECG offers no significant complications apart from irritating skin rashes associated with allergic reactions to the applied electrode gels or adhesives. When intracardiac monitoring is carried out for purposes of identification and dignosis of complex arrhythmias, the possibility of significant current leakage with generation of ectopy or of ventricular fibrillation must always be considered.

Arterial pressure

Purpose

Systemic arterial blood pressure is one of the most fundamental variables related to cardiac performance and is a mainstay of decision-making in treatment of the critically ill. Arterial pressure may be measured by the traditional indirect methods or by direct recording of the intra-arterial blood pressure. This measurement provides numerical values describing the phasic and mean levels of pressure in the systemic arterial bed, so as allowing a judgement on the overall performance of the cardiovascular system and the adequacy of blood flow to the tissues and the organs of the body. The arterial blood pressure is a function not only of cardiac output but also of the resistance or impedance offered by the small arterial vessels to the outflow of blood from the central arterial tree. In the critically ill patient, large swings in vasomotor tone may occur with constriction of systemic arterioles to a fraction of their normal average diameter. Vasoconstriction differs between body organs: may be maximal in skin and muscle arterioles and only partial in cerebral, hepatic, and coronary vessels, thus favoring redistribution of cardiac output both in absolute and in proportionate terms.

The phasic characteristics of the arterial pressure are also determined by the behaviour of the arterial tree. These changes may be particularly significant in conditions of substantiable alteration in the resistive or capacitive characteristics of the arterial tree secondary to disease processes, pathophysiological responses, or the use of pharmacological agents. Thus, while mean arterial pressure falls progressively from the central arterial bed to the peripheral arteries, phasic peak systolic pressure normally increases and diastolic pressure falls in comparison to the central aorta [25]. This increase is a function of the vessel in which the arterial pressure is measured. Thus, pressures measured in the tibial arteries or the radial arteries demonstrate higher systolic and lower diastolic pressures than values simultaneously obtained at the aortic root. The magnitude of systolic amplification is enhanced when regional vasodilation is present. Severe constriction of the peripheral large arteries that frequently characterizes patients in shock can distort and damp arterial pressures measured peripherally.

There is a general relationship between the average pressures obtained indirectly by the sphygmomanometer method with the average systolic and diastolic pressures recorded directly in the arterial tree. In patients with profound shock, the indirect method of determining arterial blood pressure may be misleading [12], with values for systolic and average pressures as low as one-half actual pressure levels within the central arterial tree. The phasic recording of arterial blood pressure is also important for effective synchronization of diastolic augmentation with the intra-aortic balloon assist device.

Techniques and procedures

Arterial blood pressure may be measured by the traditional sphygmomanometer compressive technique with detection of the blood flow by the generation of turbulance as blood passes the partially occluded vessel, or by partially automated systems such as the Arteriosonde or various applications of the Doppler technique. These methods are, by their very nature, discontinuous and have the disadvantage of not providing a phasic tracing of the arterial pressure. They have the advantage, of course, of being noninvasive and not associated with significant discomfort.

In the management of the critically ill, continuous and direct monitoring of intra-arterial pressure is widely accepted. Phasic intra-arterial pressure can be displayed as a continuous function on an appropriate oscilloscope with calibration; magnitudes can be quantified; and alterations in the levels of arterial blood pressure, heart rate, and other phasic phenomena can be recognized nearly instantaneously and accurately quantified by the means of digital read-out devices. A strip chart device allows for a permanent record. Techniques for the measurement of intra-arterial pressure frequently utilize a peripheral arterial site, commonly the radial artery [9]. Less commonly, the brachial or axillary artery are selected while the femoral artery is a useful location for short-term arterial pressure monitoring (e.g., in the cardiac catheterization laboratory). In general, femoral insertion is less desirable in patients in whom arterial pressure monitoring extends over several days. In certain patients, critical care physicians and surgeons will approach the radial artery by way of a small skin incision with direct cannulation of the vessel. In all probability, the greatest information content of pressure pulses is obtained if a catheter is advanced into the aortic root, the ascending aorta, or its proximal branches. In the majority of instances, however, percutaneous placement of a needle or catheter is practiced in a relatively peripheral portion of the arterial system. This has the advantage of avoiding the risk of central emboli, which might have serious consequences.

The site commonly selected is the radial artery. After application of Allen's test for adequacy of ulnar arterial flow, the selected wrist is prepared, with sterile technique and appropriate draping. Under local anesthesia, a Longdwell cannula is inserted and advanced 1–2 in. into the artery according to the exact technique preferred [21]. The presence of adequate backflow of arterial blood is confirmed and the cannula attached by means of a non-compliant connecting catheter, preferably less than 30 cm in length, through a stopcock to an appropriate pressure transducer. The arm is mounted on a supporting board and secured appropriately. In some instances, physicians will place a small suture at the point of insertion of the cannula into the vessel to insure stability.

Calibration of the pressure transducer is achieved by adjusting the gauge itself to ambient atmospheric pressure. Small errors in the exactness of establishment of zero reference are of less significance than in the case of the (low) right heart pressure in which zero reference errors may have a profound effect on the measured values. The arterial pressure should be displayed on an oscilloscope and a permanent recording of the observed pressure levels should be obtained. The levels of pressure should be documented hourly. While it is also possible to automatically identify alarm situations based on maximal/minimal or average arterial blood pressures, these criteria are not commonly used in ICUs at the present time. Blood samples may be obtained intermittently from the intra-arterial cannula for measurement of arterial blood gases and electrolytes. Such blood samples are not suitable for coagulation studies—small quantities of heparin may result in major errors in these values.

The monitoring and maintenance of intra-arterial cannulae and associate equipment is the responsibility of specially trained personnel, including critical care nurses.

Patency of the lumen of the intra-arterial cannula is maintained by use of a high-pressure forward flush system to intermittently expel blood elements from the cannula and to maintain a small continuous 'forward flow'. A Sorenson intra-flow is frequently used to maintain a fluid infusion rate of 3–6 ml per hour. Usually the solution contains heparin 10–20 mg in 500 ml physiological solution or 5% dextrose in water.

Complications

Complications of intra-arterial cannulation include local hematoma, infection, or vaso-spasm. Severe arterial trauma resulting in local or distal thrombosis may result in loss of the local arterial pulse. However, the development of gangrene in the distribution of arterial occlusion is rare. Many surgeons and anesthetists believe that if percutaneous puncture of the radial artery is not promptly achieved, direct exposure of the vessel and direct cannulation is perferable to further arterial damage.

Central venous pressure

Purpose

This measurement provides an index of the filing levels (preload) of the right ventricle, since the overall function of the right ventricle in relation to its afterload (PAP) is the principal determinant of central venous pressure. In addition, central venous pressure is a secondary reflection of venous tone and the relative venous volume. Changes in intrathoracic pressure, including the effects of IPPV, also alter the level of central venous pressure. The phasic central venous pressure is seldom used in critical care patients.

It is important to recognize that central venous (right atrial) pressure does not necessarily give guidance about the LV pressure dynamics [8, 38]. RV function is itself highly dependent upon pulmonary vascular resistance and left-sided preload (pulmonary artery wedge pressure). Hence, RV competence is affected by RV afterload. The presence of disease of the right ventricle may cause dramatic alterations in the central venous pressure. If disease is dominantly right-sided and if LV function is reasonably normal, then high central venous pressures may be found in the presence of normal or even reduced left atrial pressures [19]. RV infarction is characterized by profound depression of cardiac output because of severe generalized destruction of the right, as opposed to the left ventricle, whereas LV dynamics may approximate normal [14]. Pericardial disease, pericardial effusion, and mediastinal malignancies may also affect the central venous pressure significantly.

Techniques and procedures

Central venous pressure was regarded as one of the mainstays of clinical hemodynamic monitoring up to the time of the introduction of balloon-flotation (Swan–Ganz) catheters. Placement of central venous pressure lines (polyvinylchloride tubing 1.5 mm outer diameter, 1.0 mm inner diameter) has been achieved by open venostomy, usually in antecubital fascia, or by the percutaneous technique. The percutaneous techniques are considered in greater detail in the section on balloon-flotation catheters. Mean central venous pressure is usually estimated by use of a water-filled manometer. Phasic pressures are infrequently measured. Careful calibration to establish a zero reference at the level of the mid-right atrium is necessary. The central venous pressure catheter is usually disconnected from the water manometer between readings and is irrigated intermittently to ensure patency. The catheter is usually advanced until its tip lies just in the high portion of the right atrium and fluctuations of the level of the manometer, coincidental with respiration, can be identified.

Complications

Complications may be associated with insertion, including hematoma, and in the case of percutaneous puncture of the internal jugular vein, trauma of the common carotid artery. A particular and perhaps overlooked complication of central venous pressure measurements include the development of atrial or ventricular arrhythmias. The latter can be occasioned by the unrecognized migration of the central venous catheter into the low right atrium with intermittent stimulation of the right ventricle. Right atrial ectopy (PAC) is not uncommon, and atrial fibrillation has been reported. A further complication specific to central venous pressure measurement is the insertion of the cannula into mediastinal tissues or perforation of great veins. Withdrawal of blood after the catheter has been positioned in the central circulation is essential to avoid this rare complication.

A final 'complication' is an erroneous interpretation of the significance of values for central venous pressure. Its useful role in the management of the critically ill is of particular value in previously healthy or young patients who have been involved in serious trauma, have experienced hemorrhage or burns, and in whom substantive alterations in fluid balance have occurred without changes in the pulmonary vascular bed or with imbalances between the functions of the right and left ventricle. In the absence of these complicating factors, continuous measurement of central venous pressure is a valuable adjunct to fluid management in such instances.

Intracardiac right heart pressures and cardiac output

Purpose

The importance of ventricular input pressure (pre-load), and ventricular outflow resistances (afterload) are now recognized as critical variables in the overall control of cardiac function [5, 6]. The levels of these values and the direction of their changes may not be readily identifiable from clinical examination in general, but in particular, in the critically ill. Balloon-flotation (Swan-Ganz) catheters [41] were developed to allow application of the basic principles of diagnostic cardiac catheterization to specific clinical settings in which data initially observed in the laboratory setting is vitally required. These include the medical, respiratory, and cardiac ICUs; shock, burn and trauma management facilities and the anesthesia suite, operating rooms and recovery areas [1, 3, 4, 5, 7]; and the cardiac catheterization laboratory itself. The flow-directed balloon-tipped catheter allows measurement of the pulmonary artery systolic, diastolic and mean pressures; PCWP, right atrial pressure, and cardiac output. Mean PCWP is a relatively precise correlate of mean left atrial pressure and, in the presence of a normal mitral valve, of the mean LV diastolic pressure. In important disorders of ventricular function, the relationship between end-diastolic ventricular pressure and mean LV diastolic end-mean wedge pressures deviate considerably [33]. In conditions which importantly increase ventricular stiffness, the LV end-diastolic pressure may exceed mean LV diastolic and mean wedge pressure by 15–20 mmHg. However, this deviation is only seen at the higher levels of mean LV diastolic pressure (30–35 mmHg) and is not a serious practical limitation of the wedge technique. Diastolic PAP agrees closely with mean PCWP in the majority of patients, but in those who have primary pulmonary vascular disease, pulmonary embolus, or cor pulmonale, this relationship no longer holds. Diastolic pulmonary pressure and PCWP show a much poorer correlation with left atrial pressure in patients receiving ventilatory support.

Specifications of balloon-flotation (Swan–Ganz) catheters

Modification of catheter specifications allows for the basic catheterization technique to be applied in the absence of facilities for fluoroscopic manipulation of catheters, and with a minimum of significant complications. Collection of those data elements that are critical to the understanding of the underlying patyhophysiologic processes is a prime objective of monitoring in critical care. The balloon-flotation catheter, so utilized, allows definition of pre-load conditions for both right and left ventricles (right atrial and mean PCWP, respectively), quantification of blood flow to the body (cardiac output), and outflow resistance or afterload (PAP and resistance, systemic arterial resistance). In addition, balloon-flotation catheters and associated instrumentation possess qualities of simplicity, practicality, and ready applicability in the appropriate clinical environment.

Technique and instrumentation

Effective and safe application of balloon-flotation catheterization is best achieved if all aspects of the techniques employed in a given institution are as uniform and as consistent as is practically possible. Variations between units or between individual physicians' practices favors error and the development of needless complications. The uniformity should extend to the equipment, data display and recording, and procedures. A wide range of catheter sizes is available for a variety of monitoring (and cardiac pacing) purposes from several established manufacturers. A manual of procedures and practices for all personnel, including physicians, must be maintained and be consistent among different departments of a given institution.

Balloon-flotation catheters have several important physical characteristics. First, they are intrinsically less stiff than the conventional instruments used in routine catheterization procedures. This is to facilitate flotation of the catheter tip by the flowing bloodstream into the central circulation. Second, they carry a balloon so located that, when inflated, it not only acts as a flotation or directional device but, in addition, protects the endocardium of the right atrium and right ventricle from stimulation occasioned by the passage of an unprotected tip across the subendocardial myocardium. Double-lumen catheters are available for the measurement of pressure at the catheter tip, the second lumen being used for the inflation and deflation of the guiding balloon [41]. Additional, larger catheters allow for the presence of three and four lumens for the simultaneous measurement of tip (pulmonary artery) and side hole (right atrial) pressures and for the passage of leads from a thermistor located just proximal to the balloon (cardiac output) [17]. A further catheter addition includes electrodes for sensing of electrograms from the right ventricle and right atrium, and for pacing either in the atrial or ventricular mode or in atrioventricular sequence [11].

Procedure

Introduction of catheters into the vascular system may be achieved (1) by venous cutdown in the antecubital fossa, (2) percutaneously in a central venous site via a large-bore introducer, and (3) percutaneously by means of a dilator set and modified Seldinger technique [36, 44]. The latter is currently the insertion procedure of choice.

It is also necessary to have appropriate transducers and an oscilloscopic display and, preferably, a device for the recording of selected pressure wave forms during the passage of the catheter through the right side of the heart. The preferred method of insertion of balloon-flotation catheters is the right internal jugular vein [23], since potential applications include measurement during surgery and this method has the advantages of speed of insertion and a high success rate. With this technique, it has been reported that 72% of catheters have been in place in the pulmonary artery in under 2 min. However, the exact selection of insertion site will depend upon prior skills and on assessment of the individual patient. The right or left subclavian vein is also suitable [31], but the femoral veins are less desirable, although appropriate for patients undergoing short-term diagnostic catheterization procedures. With the preferred technique, the exact point of venous insertion should be accurately predetermined by a probing no. 22 needle, followed by strict adherence to one of the established techniques including the guidewire sheath insertion procedures. Supervised performance is required before an individual should undertake these techniques alone, since complications may be serious and are, in general, associated with inexperience. Placement by direct antecubital fossa venostomy, widely practiced by cardiologists, is less satisfactory, since the time for insertion is considerably longer, the absolute failure rate is increased, the procedure immobilizes the arm of introduction, and it is associated with a higher frequency of catheter displacement and migration. Irrespective of the site of insertion, the procedure is carried out under strict aseptic conditions, particularly in those instances in which longer-term hemodynamic monitoring may be contemplated.

The anatomy of the region is defined and appropriate draping and aseptic preparation of the area are performed. The procedure is carried out with the operator gowned and gloved as for a formal surgical procedure. After identification of the desired vein by a probing needle and syringe, an 18-gauge thin-walled $2\frac{1}{2}$ in. Teflon catheter is placed into the vein and threaded down the vessel. It is important that blood be freely aspirated through the introducer. The guidewire is then inserted and it should be possible to advance the wire without significant resistance. After enlargement of the insertion location, the dilator introducer set, consisting of an internal vascular dilator, is passed into the selected vein over the guidewire until the catheter sheath lies well into the internal jugular vein, or into the subclavian vein and advanced centrally. The wire is then removed and the catheter, filled with fluid and attached to a transducer, is advanced through the introducer to the region of the right atrium, where its position may be recognized by intravascular pressure fluctuations concordant with the respiratory cycle. The catheter is then advanced 3–5 cm and the guidance balloon inflated to the volume recommended. Volumes differ for different catheter sizes, from 0.8 to 1.5 ml. With the guidance balloon inflated, the catheter is then slowly, but consistently, advanced and the balloon is deflected medially through the tricuspid valve to the mid- or outflow portions of the right ventricle by the flowing bloodstream. The propulsive effects of RV contraction will then drive the balloon catheter into the pulmonary artery, its progress continuing until it impacts in a vessel slightly smaller than the distended balloon diameter. A permanent recording of cardiac rhythms and pressures within the right atrium, right ventricle, pulmonary artery, and pulmonary wedge positions is desirable. Pressure recordings over at least one complete respiratory cycle should be obtained in each of the locations. The balloon is then deflated and, provided advancement has not been too rapid, the catheter will recoil 2–4 cm into the main pulmonary artery or one of the principal (right or left) branches. A final recording of PAP through at least two respiratory cycles is then obtained. The catheter should not be advanced too rapidly during its traversal of the right ventricle, since redundant loops may form in the right atrium. If, following deflation of the guidance balloon, the pressure trace on inspiration suggests ventricularization or the presence of cardiac arrhythmias, the balloon should be re-inflated slowly and allowed to advance into the main pulmonary artery, with insertion of 1–2 cm of additional catheter shaft. The final position of the catheter with the balloon deflated should lie in a central pulmonary artery and not in a distal branch. An x-ray picture

should be obtained when possible to define the location of a monitoring catheter.

Comparison of the mean pulmonary artery wedge pressure and the pulmonary diastolic pressure should be undertaken promptly, together with diagnostic interpretation of the pressure contours obtained from the right atrial, right ventricular, pulmonary artery, and the pulmonary wedge positions. If the pulmonary diastolic pressure is within 1–3 mmHg of the mean wedge pressure, then the values of diastolic pulmonary pressure are adequate to monitor mean wedge pressure under most circumstances for clinical purposes. The catheter shaft should then be securely anchored at the site of insertion, with due attention to appropriate sterile techniques. Under no circumstance should advancement of a catheter be anticipated, once the sterile component of the procedure is completed. When the catheter is properly located, cardiac output, usually in triplicate, is determined by injection of thermal indicator into the proximal orifice of the flotation catheter, which should rest in the mid-right atrium or superior vena cava [17].

Data collection

Great vessel and intracardiac pressures

Pressures measured by flotation catheters must be referenced to an appropriate zero, usually related to the level of the tricuspid valve orifice, the point of lowest potential energy in the circulation. With careful establishment and maintenance of this zero reference point, and appropriate calibrations, pressures in the right heart may be measured with an accuracy of ±2 mmHg under clinical circumstances. Appropriate corrections for the influences of respiration, particularly under conditions of positive pressure ventilation, are essential [24, 26]. If large fluctuations in intrathoracic pressures are occurring, then some quantitative correction must be made for the extravascular intrathoracic pressure changes.

The dynamic response characteristics and inertial artifacts seen with balloon-flotation catheters are similar to those associated with conventional (stiff) right heart catheters [45]. The ideal dynamic response for catheter systems employed in human physiology include a flat frequency response to approximately 7 Hz, depending upon heart rate and vascular characteristics of the individual patient, and a rapid cutoff to frequencies in excess of 10–12 Hz. The lower frequencies contain the great majority of valuable hemodynamic information, although important data, such as heart sound tracings, can only be obtained with higher-frequency systems. Unfortunately, the natural frequency of artifacts commonly characterizing fluid-filled catheter systems occurs between 12 and 24 Hz in most instances and may render the reading of pulmonary capillary wedge and pulmonary diastolic phase of pressures difficult.

Cardiac output measured by the dilution principle [47]

Thermodilution is the now most frequently used technique for the measurement of cardiac output in critical care circumstances in the human, because of the simplicity of application and inherent precision. To obtain a useful level of precision the technique of measurement must be standardized, and attention to detail is essential. The injectate temperature and volume and the speed of injection must be carefully controlled and replicated.

Certain models of the balloon-flotation catheter incorporate a thermistor embedded in the catheter wall just proximal to the balloon, connected with the exterior by means of two insulated wires [17]. The electrical resistance of the thermistor is inversely related to its ambient temperature and therefore, when incorporated as the variable resistor in a wheatstone bridge circuit, allows definition of the transient change in pulmonary artery temperature consequent upon injection of cold solution into the right atrium. Mixing is believed to be complete and adequate, provided the bolus of blood and injected thermal indicator passes through a system consisting of at least two valves and one contracting chamber. A number of small, dedicated, and relatively inexpensive computer devices are available from a range of manufacturers for the incorporation of the calculation of the transient change in pulmonary artery blood temperature into cardiac output.

The injection of cold fluid into the right atrium is harmless and detection of a change in blood temperature in the pulmonary artery is readily accomplished without withdrawal of blood from the body as for the determination of concentration of indicator dyes. The procedure can be carried out at the bedside by a single individual and relevant data, including the calculated cardiac output and the form of the thermodilution curve, displayed immediately for acceptance or rejection. The thermodilution technique satisfies the assumptions underlying Fick's principles, although there is a minimal heat transfer to the walls of the catheter during injection. This is corrected by a constant introduced into the calculation. Also, a minimal heat transfer to the walls of the cardiac chamber occurs during the initial passage of the cold fluid through these chambers. This temperature flux is promptly returned to the flowing bloodstream and recognized by the detecting thermistor on the tail of the dilution curve. The use of automated and calibrated computer devices allows for uniformity in the recognition and calculation of cardiac output [33].

Precision—the variability between repeated measurements of the same phenomenon—determines the significance of directional alterations in cardiac output. Precision in such determinations is highly dependent upon the attention to the performance of thermodilution technique. In a series of triplicate determinations obtained from patients in a steady state, the sum of methodologic and biologic variances was 3.9% [17]. This is the lowest variance obtained by any of the techniques commonly used for the measurement of cardiac output in man. Thus, changes from a previous value of ±10% almost certainly have directional significance. Therefore, important prognostic information and therapeutic direction can be derived. In the non-steady state, and if details of the procedure are not followed precisely, methodologic variations may be expected; changes of 15% above and below an initial value do not truly establish directional validity.

Other methods commonly in use for the measurement of cardiac output include the standard Fick procedure based upon O_2-consumption and A–V O_2 difference. This technique is complex and cumbersome and is unsuitable for routine application in a clinical care setting. The indicator-dilution method using Indocyanine Green has been regarded as an established and precise measurement of cardiac output. However, this technique requires sampling of arterial blood with withdrawal through a sampling densitometer external to the vascular system. More importantly, however, the blood which has been withdrawn from the arterial system (usual sampling volume, 20–40 ml) has to be re-infused into the vascular system, a procedure which has proved to be cumbersome and consuming of personnel in a clinical care setting. Also, Indocyanine Green recirculates and must be corrected for in the estimation of flow. Hence, the applications of Fick's principle on the basis of O_2 exchange and on the basis of indicator dye dilution are infrequently used in clinical practice in the management of the critically ill.

Indications

Application of this technique is indicated in those situations in which the therapeutic decision-making will be substantively improved by the availability of critical hemodynamic data [1, 7, 10, 39, 42]. The technique also appears to be of value in the application of advance pacing concepts by optimization of the heart rate and atrial contraction by use of the multipurpose flow-directed electrode catheter system [11]. For appropriate application of these techniques, certain intrinsic human aptitudes also must be identified. Individuals using these procedures must have the ability to carefully apply the technique with a minimum of complication and an ability to identify and assess the relevant data in the light of the underlying pathophysiology and clinical problem, and most importantly, a successful therapeutic plan, based on the derived data, must be possible. Under other conditions and in those institutions in which programs of potentially beneficial interventions are absent or uncertain, invasive hemodynamic monitoring is contraindicated [15].

Surgical patients [21, 46]

Flotation catheters are used throughout anesthesia and into the early phases of recovery [29, 32]. Patients who may benefit include those in whom either the surgical procedure contemplated carries a higher risk than usual or who, because of intrinsic cardiac disease, are faced with a greater than average hazard for a non-cardiac surgical procedure. The indications for hemodynamic monitoring during non-cardiac surgery are listed in Table 57.1, and those for its application in cardiac surgery, in Table 57.2. The objective of monitoring is to minimize cardiovascular stress during the induction and maintenance of anesthesia [29, 32] during the critical phases of the surgical procedure; and in particular when surgery is associated with large fluid shifts and in early postoperative recovery. The purpose is to reduce mortality and, perhaps as important, postoperative morbidity. In practice, hemodynamic monitoring appears to allow the inclusion of patients otherwise unsuitable by reason

Table 57.1. Indications for hemodynamic monitoring in surgical setting

---

I. Cardiac surgery
    Valve replacement (multiple, elderly)
    Severe associated pulmonary disease (mitral stenosis)
    Coronary artery bypass grafting
    Resection of ventricular aneurysm
    Pre-operative congestive heart failure
II. Vascular procedures
    Dissecting aneurysm
    Resection of thoracic aneurysm
III. Prostatic resection
IV. Extensive bowel resection (tumor)
V. Prolonged orthopedic procedures (elderly)
VI. Severe burns
VII. Multiple injuries

---

of age or pre-existing disease for significant surgical procedures [37]. Although it is difficult, if not impossible, to document the scope and variety of surgical procedures attempted in high-risk patients, they appear to be increasing.

Medical patients [2, 19, 39, 41, 43]

In medical ICUs, including specialized cardiac and respiratory care facilities, hemodynamic

Table 57.2. Indications for hemodynamic monitoring in a medical setting

---

I. Acute cardiac conditions
    Acute myocardial infarction—complicated
    Right ventricular infarction
    Perforated ventricular septum, mitral regurgitation
    Postinfarction angina
    Acute bacterial endocarditis
    Acute cardiac tamponade

II. Chronic cardiac insufficiency
    Congestive cardiomyopathy
    End-stage cardiac failure (therapy)
    Constrictive pericarditis, tamponade

III. Acute respiratory disorders
    Acute pulmonary edema (non-infarct)
    Pulmonary embolus
    Cor pulmonale with pneumonia
    Fat embolism (trauma)
    Ventilator function

IV. Miscellaneous indications
    Severe non-cardiac hypotension
    Extensive multisystem infections
    Dialysis
    Overdose
    Intra-aortic balloon support
    Acute vasodilator therapy

V. Research
    Development of physiologic subsets
    Therapeutic responses

---

monitoring is currently confined to the management of the critically ill and, particularly, of the near-moribund patient (Table 57.3). In some of these instances, the essential nature of the cardiovascular component of the illness can be clearly identified and, at times, reversed. While hemodynamic monitoring is generally not believed to be helpful in the management of patients with acute, but uncomplicated, myocardial infarction [15], a more aggressive approach may be possible in the future [2, 13, 14, 19, 42]. It is now recognized that effective interventions in the patient suffering from acute myocardial infarction (AMI) must be instituted within a very short time (1–2 h) of the onset of the symptoms of an actual infarctive process. This also applies to acute ischemic events occurring in the course of AMI (postinfarction angina, ventricular septal rupture, and acute mitral regurgitation). Such patients may be candidates for early operative intervention, intra-aortic balloon counterpulsation, coronary dilatation (Grunzig procedure), or dissolution of intracoronary thrombi [20, 35]. In respiratory ICUs, confusion as to the presence or absence of significant degrees of right or left heart failure may complicate the clinical picture and questions as to the role of pulmonary emboli, and the state of fluid loading may be rapidly and precisely determined by hemodynamic monitoring [26]. In the majority of instances, these

Table 57.3. Complications associated with hemodynamic monitoring (balloon-flotation catheters)

I. Associated with insertion
   Vascular damage, venous, arterial
   Hematoma
   Infection
   Local thrombosis

II. Associated with advancement
   PACs, PVCs
   Ventricular tachycardia
   Ventricular fibrillation
   Complete heart block
   Right bundle-branch block

III. Associated with maintenance
   Venous thrombosis, pulmonary embolus
   Bacteremia, endocarditis, valve rupture
   Pulmonary infarction
   Pulmonary hemorrhage (arterial rupture)
   Catheter knotting
   Balloon rupture

IV. Complications associated with data collection and
    management
   Faulty calibration
   Interpretative error (clotting, etc.)
   Inappropriate decision-making
   Failure to use data in a timely fashion

procedures are still believed to be in the 'investigative' category, but greater practical utilization in patient care is a consequence of a clearer understanding of the complex pathophysiologic problems facing the critical care clinician, combined with the perceived errors related to current clinical methods of evaluation [18, 39].

Complications associated with bedside catheterization [29, 30, 40]

Those associated with insertion include vascular damage, venous or arterial hematoma, localized infection, and thrombosis. Inexperience in vascular puncture procedures and poor attention to sterile techniques favor such complications. Difficulty in the cannulation of an internal jugular vein may be encountered in patients with diseases of the cervical spine or with a tortuous carotid arterial system. Pneumothorax is a particular complication (occurring in 1%–4%) when the subclavian vein is to be catheterized. The occurrence of this complication is inversely related to the experience of the physician. Complications associated with the advancement of the catheter include atrial (rare) and ventricular (uncommon) ectopy. The inflated balloon serves to minimize the forces which may initiate arrhythmias by stimulation of the subendocardial myocardium. Careful, continuous advancement of the catheter ensures that the locus of the ectopic impulses changes continuously and sustained ectopy is not generated. Nevertheless, reports of ventricular tachycardia (usually brief and self-limited) and of at least four episodes of fatal ventricular fibrillation have been published. Cases of persistent supraventricular tachycardia and heart block have been reported. Complete heart block has occurred during catheterization (with conventional and balloon guided catheters) in patients with pre-existing right bundle-branch block.

Pulmonary infarction is probably a frequent complication of balloon-flotation catheterization. It may be associated with wedging of a catheter, as has been reported in catheterization with standard catheters. Infusion of a hypersomotic solution or prolonged wedging and distortion of the nutrient blood supply may cause localized infarction. This may occur in an as many as 10% of subjects and is rarely productive of symptoms. However, if careful roentgenograms of the chest are taken, localized areas of infarction concordant with the position of the catheter tip may be identified.

Significant pulmonary vascular damage is uncommon, and the most serious complication, pulmonary artery rupture, is rare. However, this complication appears to be specific to the use of balloon-flotation catheters [15, 30] and has not been reported in conjunction with the use of semi-stiff (non-balloon-tipped) catheters. Twenty-one cases of pulmonary artery rupture have now been identified in the world literature. The majority of these were fatal, due to intractable pulmonary hemorrhage. These complications appear to be more common in elderly patients and particularly in those with evidence of pulmonary hypertension. Experimentally, it is difficult to rupture a pulmonary artery in animal models or in small human pulmonary vessels obtained in autopsy. The mechanism of pulmonary arterial rupture and the consequent pulmonary hemorrhage appear to be either due to erosion of a pulmonary arterial branch by continuous impaction and leverage of the tip of the catheter, or by physical rupture by inflation of the balloon when lying in a peripheral pulmonary radical. In either case, migration of the catheter, deliberate positioning of the catheter tip in the periphery, or rapid balloon inflation in a distal pulmonary branch appear to be operator-related, and probably largely preventable, in the majority of cases. Pulmonary artery rupture has been reported in the setting of the cardiac catheterization laboratory, under conditions of anesthesia and open-heart surgery, and (uncommonly) in ICU application. It is somewhat surprising that few, if any, reports of such complications have occurred in the large experience obtained in balloon-flotation catheterization of patients undergoing rehabilitation, particularly in the Federal Republic of Germany.

Other late complications include thrombosis, particularly in patients in whom a thrombotic tendency exists. Such thrombi are possible sources of pulmonary emboli. Ventricular ectopy due to migration of the catheter tip from the pulmonary artery into the outflow tract of the right ventricle can occur, and may be recognized by continuous oscilloscopic recording of the catheter tip pressure. Prolonged maintenance of intravascular catheterization favors the development of bacteremia and possibly endocarditis. This is particularly true in critical care patients in whom ventilators are utilized as part of the therapy. Therefore, it is strongly recommended that flotation catheters used for hemodynamic monitoring be re-moved as soon as stability has been attained and cardiac compensation achieved. Failure of catheter performance due to balloon rupture, luminal occlusion, or fractured thermistor or sensing electrode leads may also occur, and is probably more often due to misuse and mishandling by the user than to manufacturing deficiencies.

Although the variety of complications of balloon-flotation catheters is wide, nevertheless, the incidence of serious complications appears to remain small. Recognition of the possibility of complications and attention to specific details, as well as restrictions of the applications of these techniques to a limited number of trained, skilled, and well-informed professional personnel, will maximize the effective application of balloon-flotation catheter systems and appropriate levels of safety in hemodynamic monitoring.

References

1. Allardyce DB (1978) Symposium on intensive care—monitoring of the critically ill surgical patient. Can J Surg 21:75–78
2. Amsterdam EA, DeMaria AN, et al (1978) Hemodynamic evaluation in acute myocardial infarction. Adv Cardiol 23:132–141
3. Barash TG, Chen Y, et al (1980) The hemodynamic tracking system: A method of data management and guide for cardiovascular therapy. Anesth Analg (Cleve) 59:169–174
4. Benis AM, Fitzkee HL, et al (1980) Improved detection of adverse cardiovascular trends with use of a two-variable computer alarm. Crit Care Med 8:341–344
5. Bland R, Shoemaker WC, et al (1978) Physiologic monitoring goals for the critically ill patient. Surg Gynecol Obstet 145:833–841
6. Bloch A, Scheidegger D (1980) Hemodynamic monitoring: Correlation of clinical and invasive methods. Schweiz Med Wochenschr 110:52–55
7. Bourdois M, Freysz M, et al 1979 Swan–Ganz catheters during surgical intensive care. Anesth Analg (Paris) 36:127–150
8. Brisman R, Parks LC, et al (1967) Pitfalls in the clinical use of central venous pressure. Arch Surg 95:902
9. Brown AE, Sweeney DB, et al (1969)Percutaneous radial artery cannulation. Anesthesiology 24:532 (1969)
10. Buchbinder N, Ganz W (1976) Hemodynamic monitoring. Anesthesiology 45:146
11. Chatterjee K, Swan HJC, et al (1975) Use of a balloon-tipped flotation electrode catheter for cardiac monitoring. Am J Cardiol 36:56
12. Cohn JN (1967) Blood pressure reassessment in shock. JAMA 19:972
13. Cohn JN, Franciosa JA (1977) Vasodilator therapy of cardiac failure. N Engl J Med 297:27
14. Cohn JN, Guiha NH, et al (1976) Right ventricular infarction. Am J Cardiol 33:209–216

15. Dalen JE (1979) Bedside hemodynamic monitoring. N Engl J Med 301:1176–1178
16. Forrester JS, Diamond G, et al (1971) Filling pressures in the right and left sides of the heart in acute myocardial infarction N Engl J Med 285:190–193
17. Forrester JS, Ganz W, et al (1972) Thermodilution cardiac output determination with a single flow directed catheter. Am Heart J 83:306
18. Forrester JS, Diamond G, et al (1976) Medical therapy of acute myocardial infarction by application of hemodynamic subsets (Parts I and II). N Engl J Med 295:1356–1362; 1404–1413
19. Forrester JS, Diamond GA, et al (1977) A correlative classification for clinical and hemodynamic abnormalities associated with acute myocardial infarction. Am J Cardiol 39:144
20. Ganz W, Buchbinder N, et al (1981) Intracoronary thrombolisis in evolving myocardial infarction. Am Heart J 101:4–13
21. Gardner RN, Schwartz R, et al (1974) Percutaneous in-dwelling radial artery catheters for monitoring cardiovascular function. N Engl J Med 290:1227
22. Holliday RL, Doris PJ (1979) Monitoring the critically ill surgical patient. Can Med Assoc J 121:931–935
23. Kaplan JA, Miller ED (1976) Insertion of the Swan–Ganz catheter. Anesth Rev, Nov., 22–25
24. King EG (1979) Influence of mechanical ventilation on pulmonary disease and pulmonary artery pressure monitoring. Can Med Assoc J 121:901–904 (1979)
25. Kroeker EJ, Wood EH (1955) Comparison of simultaneously recorded central and peripheral pressure pulses during rest, exercise and tilted position in man. Circ Res 3:623–632
26. Kubler A, Arohnski A (1978) Monitoring pulmonary artery pressures in critically ill patients. Resuscitation 6:43–46
27. Lauwers P, Ferdinande T, et al (1978) Computer-assisted monitoring in intensive medicine. Acta Anesthiol Belg 29:287–304
28. Moore CH, Lombardo TR, et al (1978) Left main coronary artery stenosis. Hemodynamic monitoring to reduce mortality. Ann Thorac Surg 26:445–451
29. Pace NL (1977) A critique of flow-directed pulmonary arterial catheterization. Anesthesiology 45:455 (1977)
30. Pape LA, Haffajee Cl, et al (1979) Fatal pulmonary hemorrhage after use of the flow-directed balloon-tipped catheter. Ann Intern Med 90:344–347
31. Pego RF, Luria MH (1979) Left subclavian vein puncture for insertion of Swan–Ganz catheter. Heart & Lung 8:507–510
32. Pietak SP, Teasdale SJ (1979) Hemodynamic monitoring and care of the patient of high risk for anesthesia. Can Med Assoc J 121:922–928
33. Powner DJ, Snyder JB (1978) In vitro comparison of six commercially available thermodilution cardiac output systems. Med Instrum 12:122–127
34. Rahimtoola SH, Loeb HS, et al (1972) Relation of pulmonary artery to left ventricular diastolic pressures in acute myocardial infarction. Circulation 46:283–290
35. Rentrop P, Blanke H, et al (1979) Acute myocardial infarction: Intracoronary application of nitroglycerin and streptokinase in combination with transluminal recannulazation. Clin Cardiol 5:354
36. Seldinger SI (1953) Catheter replacement of the needle in percutaneous arteriography. Acta Radiol 39:368
37. Sorenson MB, Bille-Brahe NE, et al (1978) Hemodynamic observation in relation to extensive surgical treatment of patients with increased operative risk. Acta Anesth Scand 22:287–302
38. Swan HJC (1974) Central venous pressure monitoring is an outmoded procedure of limited practical value. *In* Controversies in internal Inglefinger FJ, Ebert, RV, Finland M, Relman AS (eds) medicine, vol 2. WB Saunders, Philadelphia, pp 185–194
39. Swan HJC (1975) The role of hemodynamic monitoring in the management of the critically ill. Crit Care Med 3:86
40. Swan HJC, Ganz W (1975) Use of balloon-flotation catheters in critically ill patients. Surg Clin North Am 55:501
41. Swan HJC, Ganz W, et al (1970) Catheterization of the heart in man with use of a flow-directed balloon-tipped catheter. N Engl J Med 283:447
42. Theroux P, Waters DD, et al (1978) The value and limits of hemodynamic monitoring in acute myocardial infarction. Ann Cardiol Angeiol (Paris) 27:439–442
43. Todres ID, Crome RK, et al (1979) Swan–Ganz catheterization in the critically ill newborn. Crit Care Med 7:330–334
44. Turnbull AD, Carlong, et al (1979) Multipurpose central venous access using the Cordis sheath introducer system. Crit Care Med 7:30–32
45. Wood EH, Leusen IR, et al (1954) Measurement of pressures in man by cardiac catheters. Circ Res 2:294–303
46. Wynands JE (1978) The high-risk cardiac patient undergoing general surgery. Can J Surg 21:475
47. Zierler KL, Meier P (1954) On the theory of the indicator dilution method for measurement of blood flow and volume. J Appl Phys 6:731

Chapter 58

Techniques for Assessing Respiratory Function

W. J. Russell

The development of greater understanding of lung physiology and the improvement in measuring techniques have given the clinician great scope in evaluating respiratory disease. This has enabled thoracic physicians to make useful analyses of small and large airway conduction disorders, to assess respiratory drive, and to examine gas distribution within the lungs. For evaluation of many of the common chronic problems in respiratory medicine, the simple (three-part) model [55] is inadequate, but in the critically ill patient this model is helpful as bulk gas transport is the significant respiratory problem and few of the sophisticated techniques now common in respiratory medicine are used. Generally there is either an acute failure of ventilation from a gross mechanical cause or a failure of gas exchange within the lung. The recognition that intensive care patients in respiratory trouble have critical problems with gas transport means a different emphasis on monitoring respiratory function. Continuous or frequent estimates of CO_2 and O_2 status are essential. Thus devices with a high reliability and accuracy are most desirable, preferably requiring no invasion of the patient. The standard for respiratory assessment is the arterial blood gas analysis, which unfortunately is both intermittent and invasive.

Although arterial PCO_2 and PO_2 tensions are the final arbiters in the critically ill patient, other approaches in assessment are used because they are continuous or because they are simpler and less invasive than arterial sampling. If lung parameters, particularly compliance, flow resistance, and shunt, are stable or slowly changing, simple observation of lung mechanics may suffice for long periods. However, rapid changes in gas exchange can only be managed by observing O_2 and CO_2 levels. These may be monitored indirectly, by the expired gas, transcutaneously, or for O_2 by haemoglobin saturation. With some of these measurements, additional information can be derived to assist in patient management.

Lung mechanics

The most-used measurement in this group is the expired volume. Other measurements, such as the vital capacity, peak flow, and inspiratory force, assume importance in the weaning of a patient from the ventilator after the acute illness [40, 51, 54] but during respiratory support the inspired O_2 and expired volume are paramount.

Lung volumes

Probably the most widely used instrument is the Wright's respirometer. This inferential volume meter or anemometer is popular because of its light weight and reliability. However, in routine clinical use there may be errors as large as 15% of the measured value [38]. It has a very low flow resistance; even at 30 litres/min back pressure is less than 2 mmH₂O [9].

The Wright's respirometer tends to under-read by more than 10% at flows below about 0.1 litre/s and may not move at all with flows less than 0.06 litre/s [7]. It tends to over-read at flows above 1.0 litre/s. However, the intermittent nature of respiration with various flows during each surge results in good accuracy between 4 and 8 litres/min [7]. In most situations expired minute volumes of 4–24 litres/min will be accurate within 5% (Fig. 58.1). It is important that no 'jetting' occurs

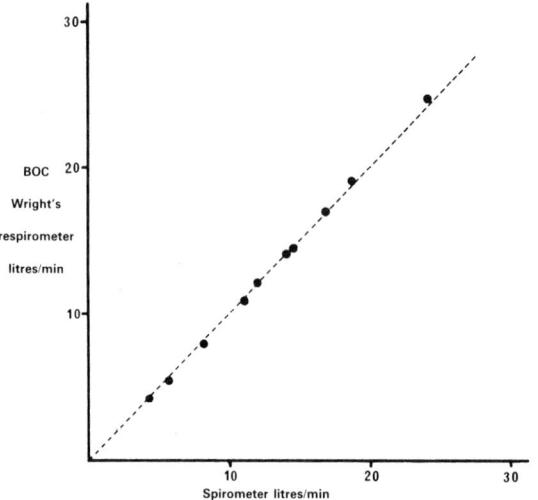

Fig. 58.1. Accuracy of Wright's respirometer over flows from 4 to 24 litres/min in spontaneously breathing subjects. The *line of identity* is shown. Reference values were derived from volume timed into a volume spirometer and corrected to BTPS. Low flows under-read slightly and high flows over-read. No flow was in error by more than 5%.

against the anemometer slots, as this will create an unpredictable over-read [46]. Thus the respirometer should not be used close to a flow constriction such as a catheter mount. Readings are also affected by gas density, but if 50% nitrous oxide in O₂ is used, the additional error is unlikely to exceed 5%. In most clinical situation these errors are of little consequence as the respirometer is used to check the constancy of a set minute or tidal volume and the appropriateness of this ventilation is independently determined by blood gas analysis.

An alternative device for measuring minute or tidal volume is Bourn's ventilation monitor LS75. This operates by creating turbulence within the gas stream by a cross bar. The vortex

downstream of the cross bar oscillates with a set volume flow, nominally 1 ml. Oscillations are detected by an ultrasonic beam. The device has no moving parts and appears to be robust. Examination of one unit showed it to have reasonable linearity over the full scale from 5 to 40 litres per minute volume (Fig. 58.2). The respiratory rate is also counted and displayed.

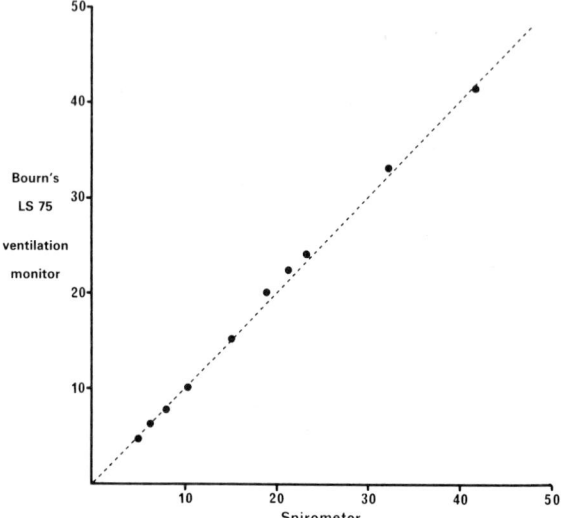

Fig. 58.2. Accuracy of Bourn's LS75 ventilation monitor over flows from 4 to 40 litres/min in spontaneously breathing subjects. The *line of identity* is shown. Reference values were derived from a volume timed into a volume spirometer and corrected to BTPS. No flow was in error by more than 6%.

The dry gas meter is the most accurate of all simple devices and records volumes greater than 50 litres with accuracy of at least 1% [3]. It cannot be connected in reciprocating flows, however, and therefore can only be used with systems in which the expired gas is uncontaminated by driving gas.

Other techniques

Although pneumotachographs have been available for many years, they have not become established in ICUs. The Fleisch pneumotachograph [22] has been most commonly employed for research and in the pulmonary function laboratory. The small tubes which make up its parallel resistive network are easily blocked by moisture or mucus. Although heating and mucus traps have been used to reduce these problems, generally the device has not been found sufficiently robust to withstand continuous clinical use. The development of microelectronics has made the use of pressure drop across turbulent flow devices attractive, as the electronics can provide a linear output if necessary [20, 48, 58]. Because these devices operate with turbulent flow, they are relatively insensitive to temperature changes but are slightly altered by the density of the measured gas. Switching from air (nominal mol. wt. 29) to O_2 (mol. wt 32) is likely to cause over-read by only a few percent. However, devices of this type may still be subject to errors which have been found to result from asymmetries in the differential pressure transducers with the older pneumotachographs [1, 12]. A recent evaluation of spirometers found flow-measuring devices less effective than direct volume measurement, so that some caution is necessary in accepting flow devices for respiratory measurement [24].

Special techniques are of uncertain value. High-frequency resistance seems altered by conditions such as pulmonary water [35], and may eventually prove of prognostic value. However, its place remains to be determined. Similarly pulmonary occlusion pressure seems to be a logical index of central drive [72] but is unlikely to be of interest in critically ill patients. Compliance measurements have been claimed to be a guide to the optimal end-expiratory pressure [69]. But in practice, most centres seem content to rely on trial and error to find the minimum pressure to achieve a PaO_2 above 60 mmHg (8 kPa) with, if possible, an FIO_2 0.4 [23].

Gas monitoring

Apart from volume measurement, the commonest method of respiratory monitoring is associated with gas composition. Usually, inspired gas is monitored only for O_2 level but expired gas may be monitored for both CO_2 and O_2.

Inspired oxygen

Three methods of measurement are used commonly. They are the paramagnetic, polarographic, and fuel cell methods. Instruments based on any of these methods give an acceptable accuracy, but require that calibration is done immediately before use. The degree of accuracy required determines how much care should be taken in calibration. If the expected reading is within 20%–50% O_2 calibration on air alone will give accuracy within 5% of the read-

ing. However, for accuracy within 1%, calibration with at least air (20.95%) and medical O_2 (99.5%) is necessary. Paramagnetic devices are most accurate [21, 47] but generally cannot be connected into the circuit. They are usually used only for intermittent O_2 analysis. For practical use, they are totally specific for O_2.

The polarographic method is suitable for continuous O_2 assessment but has a response time of 60 s or more [6], which makes it unsuitable for breath-by-breath analysis unless special electronics are used. It is, however, not completely specific. Most polarographic systems are affected by nitrous oxide. Generally this corresponds to about a 2%–4% O_2 reading for 100% nitrous oxide, but the percent reading should be checked for each machine [68].

Fuel cell methods are generally robust and reliable, although they are not usually very accurate. A common value is about ±3% of the reading. Mostly calibration is performed only on air if values less than 50% are anticipated, or 100% O_2 if values above 50% are to be measured. The readings are little affected by nitrous oxide. Fuel cell O_2 analysers depend on the consumption of a small quantity of O_2 to generate a voltage proportional to the O_2 tension [70]. The continued exposure to O_2 at any tension eventually depletes the cell, which must be replaced. Most medical devices with fuel cell analysers have a life of at least 1 000 000 mmHg O_2 hours, which is about $8\frac{1}{2}$ months in air. If exposed to O_2, fuel cell sensors continue to deteriorate even if no measurements are being taken. Generally the response time of fuel cell analysers is between 10 and 60 s which makes them unsuitable for expired gas analysis.

Expired gas

Apart from volume measurement of the ventilated patient, which should always be done on expired gas, expiratory measurements of CO_2 and O_2 can give useful information on the patient. For any satisfactory measurements on a breath-by-breath basis, measuring devices should have response times in the 100 ms range or less, require small sampling flows (preferably less than 100 ml/min), and be resistant to disturbance of zero or linearity by water vapour. In practice, compromises are often made.

Carbon dioxide

The most commonly used method of measurement is by non-dispersive infra-red analysis

(NDIR). This depends on the absorption of infra-red radiation in the 4.25-μm region of the spectrum [30]. The presence of CO_2 within the sample cell decreases the infra-red transmission. Unfortunately other diatomic gases, such as nitrous oxide, also have this effect. The use of microphonic differential detectors in these analysers means they are sensitive to heat and vibration. Careful warm-up and calibration are essential. The detector gives an alinear output and special linearizing electronic circuits are usually designed for a specific flow sampling, commonly 100 ml or 500 ml; a several-point calibration is required if another flow is used. If gas is sampled close to the patient, water condensation and mucus can be a problem. Water or mucus may be aspirated into the sample cell and block infra-red transmission. This makes the analyser impossible to zero. Non-dispersive infra-red analysers require careful handling and close attention to operate satisfactorily in the intensive care environment.

Other detectors exploiting infra-red absorption with a direct optical pathway are available (Datex, Finland). Although they suffer from similar problems with moisture and mucus and nitrous oxide cross interference, they are more robust optically and more compact. Detectors of this type are currently used in at least one ventilator system (Servo 900 series, Siemens), although not as a control parameter for ventilation. Infra red absorption has also been used for transcutaneous CO_2 monitoring [19].

A recent suggestion for CO_2 detection in expired gas was made by Bushman [8]. The ionization of water by CO_2 is used to measure FI CO_2. The water is de-ionized by a resin bed and recirculated. This ionization of water reduces the electrical resistance, which is sensed as a change in current and displayed on an ammeter as percent CO_2.

Although still being developed, CO_2 electrodes for transcutaneous PCO_2 may in future find a place in respiratory gas measurement. However, at present their response time is too long to be useful in this context [76]. An alternative approach to CO_2 estimates can be by the estimate of mixed venous PCO_2 [31, 52]. This is a well-established, non-invasive technique which can give useful information, and when combined with $PaCO_2$ it can be a guide to the cardiac output [41, 42]. It does, however, require hand ventilation of the patient with a closed circuit containing an equilibration CO_2/O_2 mixture. Mixed expired and rebreathing CO_2 levels can be measured conveniently and cheaply by chemical means with caustic absorption as no fast response time is required. One simple device with good accuracy is the Lloyd Haldane volumetric analyser [10].

Oxygen

The rapid response times required limit the type of sensor which is suitable for breath by breath analysis. Paramagnetic systems cannot respond rapidly, because of their high volumes. They are also sensitive to error when sampling at a fast flow, which tends to cause instability of the N_2 dumbell in the cell [47]. Polarographic methods are normally too slow, but electronic enhancement of the tracking can achieve a sufficiently rapid response to be effective on a breath-by-breath basis. This system is used in the Beckman OM-11.

Many systems now use mass spectrometry, which gives a good zero stability and linearity and an excellent response time for breath-by-breath analysis.

Mass spectrometry

Mass spectrometers use the different masses of gases and vapours to identify constituents of a mixture. The molecules in a sample are charged in a high vacuum and accelerated onto a detector plate. To reach the detector the charged particles must traverse a sieving system. This was a magnetic field in the first spectrometers. Lighter mass particles being deflected more within the magnetic field arrive at a different point in the detector system [16]. A further development has been the quadripole mass spectrometer, in which the sieving is done by tuning the charged quadripole stack through which the charged particles pass. Rapid frequency oscillations of the field exclude all but one mass/charge ratio from penetrating the field to reach the detector. Shifting the frequency allows successive masses to be detected. Quadripole systems are more compact than magnetic mass spectrometers but generally do not have the ability to select masses above 100 atomic mass units. They are also limited slightly in that only one mass can be detected at any one time. In practice, however, neither of these limitations is a problem in respiratory medicine.

Mass spectrometry allows rapid, virtually continuous detection of O_2, CO_2, and H_2O vapour. Generally zero stability and linearity are well maintained and a continous read-out of inspired and expired O_2, humidity, and CO_2 can be obtained. If lung function is reasonable, estimates of end-tidal CO_2 and O_2 can be obtained. If these are combined with volume measurements, O_2 consumption and CO_2 production can be calculated [53]. With arterial measurements, A-a gradients and effective shunt also can be calculated [39, 74].

Mass spectrometry uses a high vacuum and consumes considerable power. In a closed room heating can be a significant problem with some devices. The need for a steady entrainment into the high vacuum also means that care must be taken to avoid plugging with mucus. This can be a particular problem when good end-tidal sampling is sought and the catheter is placed in or very near to the patient's trachea. Mass spectrometers are only suitable for units with a high level of technical support, as sophisticated electronics and high-vacuum technology need regular servicing and maintenance.

Blood gas measurement

The disadvantages associated with arterial blood PO_2 and PCO_2 make alternative methods attractive. The need for repeated arterial sampling means the technique is intermittent, involves a delay of at least several minutes, and is possibly painful. The invasiveness also carries a risk of infection and arterial thrombosis. Any alternative must offer more continuous readings or less invasion to be acceptable. However it is important to appreciate that even though arterial measurement is the standard for judging current blood gas status, the current measurement techniques involve some degree of error, which will increase unless careful quality control is maintained.

Automatic blood gas analysis

Many ICUs are equipped with automatic or semi-automatic machines for blood gas analysis. Although the errors and difficulties associated with the early manual machines have been well documented [2, 45] it is often not appreciated that automatic machines suffer from similar difficulties [36]. An uncritical approach to the results from an automated analyser may result in clinical errors.

Most machines have a controlled input of capillary samples, but allow larger syringe samples to be injected. Larger samples, usually about 0.5 ml, enter a block in which are set the PO_2, PCO_2, and pH electrodes [61]. Small

channels lead the blood past each electrode and equilibration is allowed for 0.5–3 min. Many machines accept very small samples typically, 150 μl. If not specially treated as microsamples they can become contaminated by residual washing solution, which may markedly decrease the PCO_2 but usually has little effect on the PO_2 and pH. Errors can also arise in PO_2, PCO_2, and pH if the final temperature differs by more than 0.2°C from the set temperature [2, 29, 63] (conventionally 37°C). For each centigrade degree, PO_2 increases by about 7% and PCO_2 by about 8% overall; the blood pH rises by 0.0147 per centigrade degree decrease. With pH however, the change with temperature is altered slightly by the pH level itself, the temperature coefficient being lower with a low pH. Temperature errors arise most commonly because too large a cold sample has been injected, which seriously delays the return of the temperature of the electrodes to within 0.2°C of their specification (Fig. 58.3).

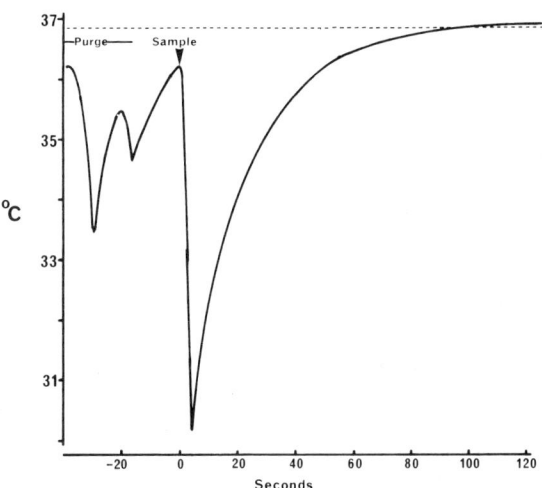

Fig. 58.3. Temperature effect of injection of a 2-ml arterial sample previously stored in ice for 20 min. The automatic blood gas analyser had been standing for some time prior to the injection and so a purge cycle occurred when the sample button was pushed. On injection, the block temperature fell to 30.3°C and did not recover to 36.8°C, the bottom of the specified range, for 100 s. A similar temperature dip occurred with a 1-ml sample, but the minimum was 34°C and the block returned to 36.8°C in 60 s.

Also of concern is the general practice of calibration with reference gases, which are humidified and passed across the PO_2 and PCO_2 electrodes. Often very small volumes of gas are used and the gas actually used may have been standing for some hours in the tubing between the cylinders and the machine. Permeability of the tubing may result in loss of CO_2 or accumulation of O_2. Usually two gases are used: one with zero O_2 and about 10% CO_2 and a second, commonly with 12% O_2 and 5% CO_2. Generally, however, a better clinical accuracy can be obtained with a second gas of 17% O_2 and 3% CO_2, which spans the common clinical range for intensive care work better. It is important that the gases are calibrated on site by multiple analyses as most workers find that mixtures supplied commercially are not reliable to the accuracy required (preferably better than one part in 1000 for each gas) [37, 63]. The use of the standard chemical methods of gas analysis by Haldane or Schölander can now be minimized by use of rapid accurate physical methods such as mass spectrometry [27].

Even with careful service and maintenance, quality control checks are essential. There are several commercially available checking solutions, but none have the characteristics of whole blood. Good quality control can only be maintained by regular tonometry of whole blood. However, great care must be taken in gas and temperature control of the tonometer. Generally a film tonometer with temperature control is used [11]. Tonometry should be done with two gases, 60 mmHg O_2 (8 kPa) with 60 mmHg (8 kPa) CO_2 and 100 mm (13.3 kPa) O_2 with 30 mmHg CO_2 (4 kPa), which span the most important clinical range. Tonometry can only assess PO_2 and PCO_2 accuracy and not pH, but tonometered standards may be the only means of quality control. For example, errors can arise in all three measurements owing to gradual protein build-up within the analyser. Generally this results in under-reading. Protein build-up causes a low reading with the pH electrode and instability with the PO_2 and PCO_2 electrodes. The build-up slows diffusion of CO_2 and O_2 which results in slower equilibration and low gas tension values if the automatic machine fails to detect the slow change and stop the analysis (assuming complete equilibrium).

Poor technique may also contribute to errors. Operators of automatic blood gas analysers must still take care to handle samples correctly [45]. Errors commonly occur because red cell mixing is incomplete in cold-stored samples, if too much blood is injected, or if blood is not properly stored at 0°C and handled aerobically before analysis. Even with optimal quality control by tonometry and careful operations, a ±4% reading for PO_2 and ±3% reading for PCO_2 and ±0.01 units pH must be expected (Fig. 58.4).

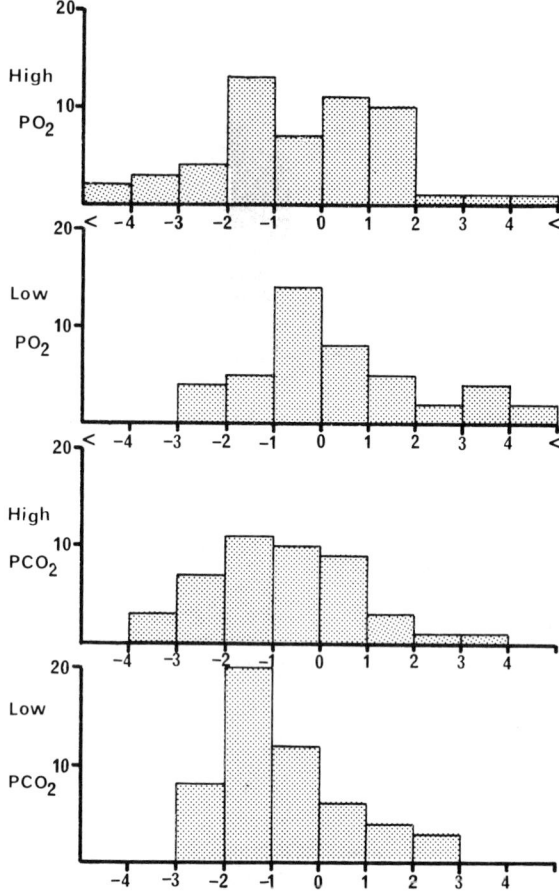

Fig. 58.4. Percentage deviation of quality control checks with film-tonometered blood (IL 237) over a 2-month period. *Bins* are percent points. *Bars* are the number of samples with each error. No systematic errors occurred. Normal maintenance and membrane changes were done as appropriate. Errors are approximately distributed about zero. For the low PO_2 90% of values are within −2% and +4%. For the high PO_2, 90% are within ± 3%. For the low and high PCO_2, 90% are within −3% to 2%.

Other measurement on arterial blood

Few measurements are done other than PO_2, PCO_2, and pH. Most other blood gas values are calculated, usually from standard curves or formulae. Values commonly calculated are standard bicarbonate, base excess, haemoglobin saturation, O_2 content.

Oxygen saturation may be calculated or more accurately measured by optical devices, such as the Co-oximeter, with absorbance at 548, 568 and 578 mm [16]. If O_2 content is to be calculated from these measurements, it is important that carboxyhaemoglobin, which may be over 10%, be taken into account [15]. Oxygen content may be measured by traditional chemical methods or by Lexi-O_2-Con analysis. Calculated values may differ by several percent from values obtained directly. The Lexi-O_2-Con has a close correspondence with value by Van Slyke within 1 ml/100 ml to 95% confidence. However, the estimate is sensitive to the rate of carrier flow [62].

Oxygen saturation

The physiologically important levels are between about 100 mmHg (13.3 kPa) and 50 mmHg PO_2 (6.6 kPa), which is also the level at which significant haemoglobin desaturation begins in normal blood. Below a saturation of 90%, which corresponds to a PO_2 of about 60 mmHg desaturation increases sharply (Fig. 58.5). If

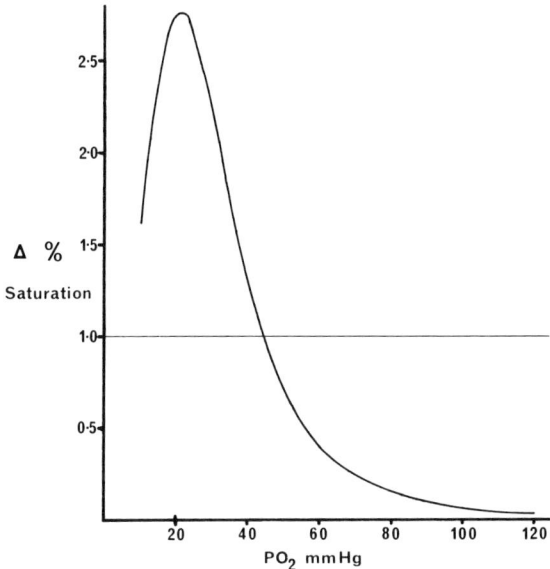

Fig. 58.5. Graph showing percent change in saturation for each 1 mmHg change in PO_2 for normal blood (pH 7.4, PCO_2 40, P 50, 27.2 mmHg). Below 60 mmHg the rate of change is rapid. The 1:1 point occurs at 45 mmHg. The maximum saturation change occurs at 22 mmHg.

blood gas machines read to 1 mmHg and oximeters to 1 percentage point, below 45 mmHg (80% saturation) the oximeter is more sensitive to desaturation than blood gas estimation. Thus O_2 saturation is equally useful as a clinical guide to oxygenation. Oximetry offers a continuous assessment of O_2 saturation.

Fibre-optic catheters can provide an intravascular assessment of O_2 saturation in the central venous system [4] or, in neonates, arterial saturation can be monitored through the umbilical artery by reflective oximetry [73]. These techniques are, however, invasive. An alternative approach is to estimate saturation by transmission oximetry through the skin.

Although several skin oximeters [59, 60, 75] are available, usually for the ear, most require a null and standardization on 100% O_2 to cope with differences in skin pigmentation and haemoglobin which is inactive, e.g., carboxyhaemoglobin.

The most suitable instrument currently available is the Hewlett Packard oximeter 47201A. This can resolve skin pigment and carboxyhaemoglobin by measuring eight wavelengths in rapid succession (Fig. 58.6) and averaging

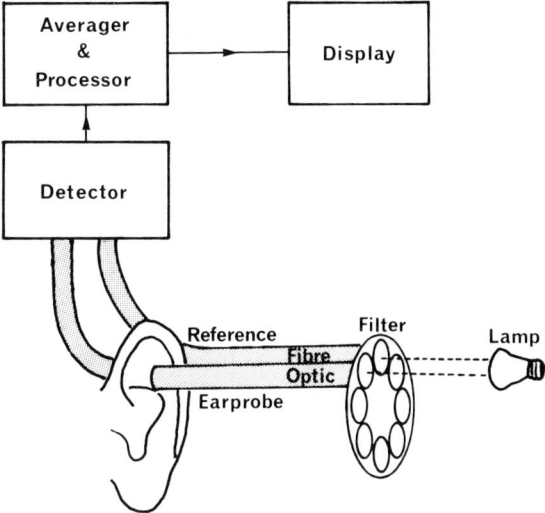

Fig. 58.6. Functional diagram of the Hewlett Packard 47201A. Eight paired narrow band filters compare the ear transmission with a reference transmission. Transmission values are each averaged and the logarithmic transmittance ratios of the eight pairs with 18 empirical coefficients are then used to calculate a true percentage O_2 saturation of haemoglobin excluding carboxyhaemoglobin and other inactive pigments.

samples to reduce noise [43]. Calculated estimates of saturation are then made and presented about every 0.5 s. For ear oximetry, good ear perfusion is essential. Some indication of the oximeter error can be obtained if perfusion is first assessed with the Hewlett Packard 47205A perfusion indicator. This indicates the level of perfusion and gives an estimate of the potential error of oximeter readings. Local low perfusion can be partly corrected by persistent rubbing and warming. However, in patients with a poor general output state, ear oximetry is unsuitable. Usually a very low reading is found or the 'off ear' alarm occurs. Calibration of the oximeter is by an automatic internal standardization procedure which takes less than 1 min before the oximeter is applied to the ear. Thus this oximeter can give a reliable saturation measurement even in subjects whose haemoglobin cannot be fully saturated for instrument calibration.

In addition to low perfusion states, oximetry with this device is affected by jaundice. A bilirubin level of 25 mg/100 ml (N < 0.8 mg/100 ml) can be expected to reduce the saturation reading by about 4%. In one patient with a PaO_2 of 150 mmHg (20 kPa) and a bilirubin of 390 mg/100 ml, the oximeter saturation reading was consistently about 75%. However, the saturation reading continued to follow his PaO_2 with a 20% offset.

Usually ear oximetry with the H-P47201A will give a correct or slightly low reading and therefore is a useful guide to the respiratory state of a severely ill patient whose cardiovascular system is stable. This is particularly helpful in patients who are likely to develop adult respiratory distress syndrome, as monitoring for several days is feasible. Generally, the unit should be checked and repositioned on the ear about every 4 h, although longer periods have occurred in our ICU without problems. It is also useful in patients during weaning, as a safety measure. However, as a criterion for successful weaning the unit is not useful, as weaning is normally done with a high FIO_2 and the adequacy of ventilation is assessed by the arterial PCO_2.

The unit is not suitable for restless patients and patients with severe facial or ear damage, such as burns. However in cooperative or paralysed patients it can be tolerated for long periods with no discomfort.

Transcutaneous gas measurement

Skin is not completely impervious to O_2 and CO_2. This property can be exploited to obtain transcutaneous estimates of body O_2 and CO_2 levels [18, 65].

Oxygen

Transcutaneous O_2 is usually measured by a polarographic technique [17] or by mass spectrometry [49] as an O_2 tension (tcPO_2). The electrode is generally heated to 43–45°C and firmly applied to skin on the trunk. The transcutaneous O_2 concentration depends upon the level of tissue O_2, the permeability of the skin, and the O_2 consumption of the skin and of the sensing electrode [18]. The measurement is usually done at about 44°C, which increases O_2 tension and capillary flow to 'arterialize' the skin O_2 level. However, skin O_2 consumption is

increased by about 40% [66]. Usually these conflicting factors cancel and transcutaneous tcPO_2 closely reflects PaO_2 [18]. In neonates, the relationship is close, the transcutaneous O_2 being almost identical with PaO_2 with little offset [17, 44, 50, 57]. In adults with thicker skin, tcPO_2 is generally about 19.5 mmHg (2.6 kPa) below the arterial tension [25] at 43°C. Some compensation for the longer diffusion pathway can be achieved by heating to 45°C [57] but the skin must be observed closely. In both adults and neonates, changes in arterial O_2 tension are closely followed by the transcutaneous O_2 measurements.

Some factors may make tcPO_2 diverge from the PaO_2. Electrode temperature is important: at 37°C tcPO_2 bears almost no relation to PaO_2. Anything which adversely affects the 'luxury' capillary blood flow will reduce tcPO_2. Thus hypotension reduces tcPO_2 both in neonates [50, 71] and in adults [26]. If circulation is stable other O_2 transport factors, such as haematocrit and blood volume, appear to have little impact. Some drugs may upset tcPO_2. Tolazoline in neonates appears to diminish tcPO_2 [50], possibly because of subdermal shunting, and a similar effect may occur with sodium nitroprusside [26]. Halothane appears to affect measurements: The magnitude of the effect appears to depend on the polarization. This may also occur with nitrous oxide, although most systems appear to be unaffected.

In use, the electrode is first calibrated. A zero O_2 environment is used first. It may be N_2 or sometimes a sulphite solution, although some electrodes are not suitable for immersion in sulphite. A second calibration point should be close to the expected upper value of measurement. Ethylene glycol, room air, and air in a temperature-controlled chamber have all been used. Ethylene glycol 50% approximates the same 'stirring' effect as for skin. The stirring effect is related to diffusion of O_2 into the electrode as it is consumed [64]. In practice, air can be bubbled through the warmed solution to give a reference of 145 mmHg (19.3 kPa) O_2. For most situations, air calibration alone provides reasonable accuracy, particularly when arterial sampling is available to establish the initial tcPO_2: PaO_2 relationship. Transcutaneous O_2 monitoring has found a ready place in neonatal intensive care [13, 56] for monitoring oxygenation. It also has a useful place in other situations, such as judging the efficiency of therapeutic manoeuvres where changes can be expected within hours [28].

Although calibration of this method is more

cumbersome than oximetry, a chest electrode is probably more acceptable in a restless patient. Transcutaneous methods can also measure well above 150 mmHg (20 kPa) O_2, which is impractical by oximetry. This probably has little clinical importance.

The transcutaneous Clark PO_2 electrode has some disadvantages. The electrode must be handled with care and the membrane needs to be changed at least every week. The electrode may also be susceptible to other gases, particularly nitrous oxide [49] and halothane [26], which penetrate the skin. It is also necessary to heat the skin to 43°C or over, which may sometimes cause mild skin blistering.

Transcutaneous measurements by mass spectrometry would probably involve less difficulty with calibration but most not exceed the available O_2 consumption of about 10^{-5} ml.cm^{-2}.s^{-1} [49]; a transcutaneous CO_2 probe would also seem practical with mass spectrometry.

Carbon dioxide

Theoretically, CO_2 has some advantages which make transcutaneous measurement less difficult than that for O_2. Carbon dioxide is a much more permeable gas, diffusing readily through intact skin [5]. The measurement of PCO_2 by a buffered pH electrode does not consume CO_2, and so any stirring effect is avoided. Skin warming increases tcPCO_2, however, both because temperature increases the gas tension and because metabolism increases [65]. An alternative approach has been to measure CO_2 by an infrared microchamber [19]. This does not require heating but does require stripping of the stratum corneum, the tcPCO_2 being about 0.7 kPa above the $PaCO_2$.

Transcutaneous pCO_2 seems particularly attractive when patients are being weaned from a ventilator [19] or when mechanical respiratory difficulties such as flail chests or asthma, where failure can be an insidious progression, are assessed.

Derived values

The ready availability of hand-held programmable calculators and powerful computers has resulted in the use of values derived from the measurements of gases and volumes. These values may be calculated by use of small hand-held computers or directly, by an integrated system [34, 67].

While it is usually appreciated that the assumption of a fixed value such as 5 vol % for the arteriovenous O_2 difference can result in large errors of derived parameters, such as cardiac output, it is important to remember that measurements also have a potential error. Even with care, most respiratory measurements will not be more accurate than ±2%. Derived values must therefore have this degree of potential error or greater. The more measurements used to calculate a value, the greater the potential error (roughly at least the sum of the errors of the individual measurements). Derived values such as O_2 transport from at least three measured values may be substantially inaccurate by 10% or more from the additive effects of errors. Only large fluctuations in the derived values should be considered significant.

It is not usually noted that errors of only a few percent may have a very large effect when the calculations use differences between measurements. This is seen most commonly in calculations of dead space:tidal volume ratio and physiological shunt. A 2% random variation in the arterial and venous O_2 contents can result in a true value of Qs/Qt of 20% being spread from 0% to 35% [33].

The future

Although derived values are subject to potentially wide errors, this can be reduced by integration and averaging. The use of integrated respiratory measurements with ventilation and gas delivery systems allows a feedback control to optimize body values. Experimental designs for adjusting O_2 in relation to PaO_2 [14] and adjusting ventilation in response to CO_2 production [32] have been published.

As more integration of the separate measurement is achieved the information supplied may also influence the decision-making of the clinician. For example, the easier availability of values for CO_2 production (from end-tidal CO_2 and flow measurement) may allow an assessment of the state of paralysis in ventilated afebrile patients by this measurement alone. We may also see a resurgence of non-invasive Fick estimates of cardiac output to help in deciding when a closer monitoring of cardiac function is necessary. The wider availability of mass spectrometry in intensive care may allow intensivists to utilize information in expired nitrogen or argon to evaluate lung performance and ventilation. Although the concepts of nitrogen fluctuation have been used for assessment in respiratory medicine this is not yet widespread in ICUs.

References

1. Abrahams N, Fisk GC, Churches AE, Loughman J, Vonwiller JB, Agzarian J, Harrison GA (1975) Errors in pneumotachography with intermittent positive pressure ventilation. Anaesth Intensive Care 3:284–294

2. Adams AP, Morgan-Hughes JO, Sykes MK (1967, 1968) pH and blood-gas analysis: Methods of measurement and sources of error using electrode systems. Part 1 and 2. Anaesthesia 22:575–597, 23:47–64

3. Adams AP, Vickers MDA, Munroe JP, Parker CW (1967) Dry displacement gas meters. Br J Anaesth 39:174–183

4. Armstrong RF, Walker JS, Andrew DS, Cobbe SM, Cohen SL, Lincoln JCR (1978) Continuous monitoring of mixed venous oxygen tension (Pv O_2) in cardiorespiratory disorders. Lancet I: 632–634

5. Beran AV, Shigezawa GY, Yeung HN, Huxtable RF (1978) An improved sensor and method for transcutaneous CO_2 monitoring. Acta Anaesthesiol Scand [Suppl] 68:111–117

6. Blackburn JP (1978) What is new in blood gas analysis? Br J Anaesth 50:51–62

7. Bushman JA (1979) Effect of different flow patterns on the Wright respirometer. Br J Anaesth 51:895–898

8. Bushman JA, Askill S, Serafinowicz H and James B (1975) A new method for the measurement of carbon dioxide in the expired air. Br J Anaesth 47:439–442

9. Byles PH (1960) Observations on some continuously-acting spirometers. Br J Anaesth 32:470–475

10. Campbell EJM (1960) Simplification of Haldane's apparatus for measuring CO_2 concentration in respired gas in clinical practice. Br Med J i:457–458

11. Chalmers C, Bird BD, Whitwram JG (1974) Evaluation of a new thin-film tonometer. Br J Anaesth 46:253

12. Churches AE, Loughman J, Fisk GC, Abrahams N, Vonwiller JB (1977) Measurement errors in pneumotachography due to pressure transducer design. Anaesth Intensive Care 5:19–29

13. Clarke T, Manning F, Baird K and Gluck L (1978) Experience and problems in the first six months of transcutaneous PO_2 (tc PO_2) monitoring in routine neonatal intensive care. Acta Anaesthesiol Scand [Suppl] 68:83–86

14. Collins P, Levy NM, Beddis IR, Godfrey S, Silverman M (1979) Apparatus for the servo-control of arterial oxygen tension in preterm infants. Med Biol Eng Comput 17:449–452

15. DeVillota ED, Carmona MTG, Estada J, Avello F (1976) The influence of carboxy haemoglobin on the oxygen-binding capacity of blood; a comparison of Manometric (Van Slyke) and optical (Co-Oximeter) measurements. Br J Anaesth 48:111–117

16. Donovan DJ, Johnston RP, MacDonnell KF (1977) Respiratory monitoring: Systems and devices. In: MacDonnel KF, Segal MS (eds) Current respiratory care. Little Brown, Boston, Ch 2

17. Eberhard P and Mindt W (1978) Reliability of cutaneous oxygen measurement by skin sensors with large size cathodes. Acta Anaesthesiol Scand [Suppl] 68:20–27

18. Eberhard P, Severinghaus JW (1978) Measurement of

heated skin O_2 diffusion conductance and PO_2 sensor induced O_2 gradient. Acta Anaesthesiol Scand [Suppl] 68:1–3

19. Eletr S, Jimison H, Ream AK, Dolan WM, Rosenthal MJ (1978) Cutaneous monitoring of systemic PCO_2 on patients in the respiratory intensive care unit being weaned from the ventilator. Acta Anaesthesiol Scand [Suppl] 68:123–127

20. Elliott SE, Shore JH (1977) Turbulent airflow meter for long term monitoring in patient-ventilator circuits. J Appl Physiol 42:456

21. Ellis FR, Nunn JF (1968) The measurement of gaseous oxygen tension utilizing paramagnetism: An elevation of the Servomex OA150 analyzer. Br J Anaesth 40:569–578

22. Fleisch A (1925) Der Pneumotachograph–ein Apparat zur Geschwindigkeitsregistrierung der Atemluft. Pfluegers Arch 209:713–722

23. Gallagher TJ, Civetta JM, Kirby RR (1978) Terminology update: Optimal PEEP. Crit Care Med 6:323–326

24. Gardner RM, Hankinson JL, West BJ (1980) Evaluating commercially available spirometers. Am Rev Respir Dis 121:73–82

25. Gothgen I and Jacobsen E (1978a) Transcutaneous oxygen tension management I. Age variation and reproducibility. Acta Anaesthesiol Scand [Suppl] 67:66–70

26. Gothgen I, Jacobsen E (1978b), Transcutaneous oxygen tension measurement II. The influence of halothane and hypotension. Acta Anaesthesiol Scand [Suppl] 67:71–75

27. Hallback I, Karlsson E, Ekblom B (1978) Comparison between mass spectrometry and Haldane technique in analysing O_2 and CO_2 concentrations in air gas mixture. Scand J Clin Lab Invest 38:285–288

28. Hedstrand U, Liw M, Roth G, Ögren CH (1978) Effect of respiratory physiotherapy on arterial oxygen tension. Acta Anaesthesiol Scand 22:349–352

29. Hill DW, Dolan AM (1976) Intensive Care Instrumentation. London Academic Press

30. Hill DW, Powell T (1965) Non-dispersive infra-red gas analysers in science, medicine, and industry. Hilger & Watts, London

31. Howell JBL (1962) Rebreathing methods for measurement of blood CO_2 tension. Br J Anaesth 34:617–620

32. Jordan WS, Westenskow DR (1979) Microprocessor control of ventilation using carbon dioxide production. Anesthesiology 51:S380

33. Kelman GR (1972) Errors in Riley Analysis. Br J Anaesth 44:433–435

34. Kenny GNC (1979) Programmable calculator: A program for use in the intensive care unit. Br J Anaesth 51:793–796

35. Kirk BW (1980) Pulmonary function following acute myocardial infarction: Abstract. Combined meeting RACS, RACP and RC Phys and Surg. Canada Sydney, Feb

36. Ladegaard-Pedersen HJ (1978) Accuracy and reproducibility of arterial blood-gas and pH measurements. Acta Anaesthesiol Scand [Suppl] 67:63–65

37. Lewis DG, Burn N (1972) Homogeneity of carbon dioxide/oxygen mixture. Br J Anaesth 44:473–476

38. Lunn JN, Hillard EK (1970) The effect of repairs on the performance of the Wrights respirometer. Br J Anaesth 42:1127–1130

39. McAslan TC (1976) Automated respiratory gas monitoring of critically ill patients. Crit Care Med 4:255–260

40. MacDonnell KF (1977) Weaning: Criteria: Intermittent mandatory ventilation. In: MacDonnell KF, Segal MS (eds) Current respiratory care. Little Brown, Boston, chap 12

41. McHardy GJR (1967) The relationship between the

differences in pressure and content of carbon dioxide in arterial and venous blood. Clin Sci 32:299

42. McHardy GJR, Jones NL, Campbell EJM (1967) Graphical analysis of carbon dioxide transport during exercise. Clin Sci 32:289–298

43. Merrick EB, Hayes TJ (1976) Continuous, non-invasive measurements of arterial blood oxygen levels. Hewlett Packard Journal, October:2–9

44. Messner JT, Lous PC, Grossman LB (1979) Intraoperative transcutaneous pO_2 monitoring in infants. Anesthesiology 51:S319

45. Nunn JF (1962) Measurement of blood oxygen tension: Handling of samples. Br J Anaesth 34:621–630

46. Nunn JF, Ezi-Ashi TI (1962) The accuracy of the respirometer and ventilator. Br J Anaesth 34:422–432

47. Nunn JF, Bergman NA, Coleman AJ, Casselle DC (1964) Evaluation of the servomex paramognetic analyzer. Br J Anaesth 36:666–673

48. Osborn JJ (1978) A flow meter for respiratory monitoring. Crit Care Med 6:349–351

49. Parker D, Delpy D, Reynolds EOR (1978) Transcutaneous blood gas measurement by mass spectrometry. Acta Anaesthesiol Scand [Suppl] 68:131–136

50. Peabody JL, Willis MM, Gregory GA, Tooley WH, Lucey JF (1978) Clinical limitations and advantages of transcutaneous oxygen electrode. Acta Anaesthesiol Scand [Suppl] 68:76–82

51. Pontoppidan H, Browne DRG (1978) Weaning from mechanical ventilation. In: Weil MH, Da Luz PL (eds) Critical care medicine manual. Springer-Verlag, New York

52. Powles ACP, Campbell EJM (1978) An improved rebreathing method for measuring mixed venous carbon dioxide tension and its clinical application. Can Med Assoc J 118:501–504

53. Prakash O, Meij S (1977) Use of mass spectrometry and infrared CO_2 analyzer for bedside measurement of cardio-pulmonary function during anaesthesia and intensive care. Crit Care Med 5:180–184

54. Prakash O, Meij S, Bos E, Frederiksz PA, Hekman W, Jonson B (1978) Lung mechanics in patients undergoing mitral valve replacement. Crit Care Med 6:370–372

55. Riley RL, Cournand A (1949) Ideal alveolar air and the analysis of ventilation–perfusion relationship in the lungs. J Appl Physiol 1:825–847

56. Roaf ER, Slavin R, Epstein M, Cohen A (1979) Applications of the transcutaneous oxygen electrode in neonatal intensive care. Anesthesiology 51:S296

57. Rooth G (1978) Continuous transcutaneous monitoring of PO_2 and PCO_2. Acta Anaesthesiol Scand. [Suppl] 70:175–179

58. Saklad M, Sullivan M, Paliotta J, Lipsky M (1979) Pneumotachography: A new, low-dead-space humidity-independent device. Anesthesiology 51:149–153

59. Saunders NA, Powles ACP, Rebuck AS (1976) Ear oximetry: Accuracy and practicability in the assessment of arterial oxygenation. Am Rev Respir Dis 113:745–749

60. Scoggin C, Nett L, Petty TL (1977) Clinical evaluation of a new ear oximeter. Heart Lung 6:121–126

61. Selman BJ, Tait AR (1976) Towards blood-gas autoanalysis: An evaluation of the Radiometer ABL1. Br J Anaesth 48:487–494

62. Selman BJ, White YS, Tait AR (1975) An evaluation of the Lex-O_2-Con oxygen content analyzer. Anaesthesia 30:206–211

63. Severinghaus JW, Bradley AF (1971) Blood gas electrodes or what the instructions didn't say. Copenhagen Radiometer publication ST 59

64. Severinghaus JW, Thunstrom A (1978) Problems of calibration and stabilization of tcPO$_2$ electrodes. Acta Anaesthesiol Scand [Suppl] 68:68–72

65. Severinghaus JW, Stafford M, Bradley AF (1978a) tcPCO$_2$ electrode design, calibration and temperature gradient problems. Acta Anaesthesiol Scand [Suppl] 68:118–122

66. Severinghaus JW, Stafford M, Thunstrom AM (1978b) Estimation of skin metabolism and blood flow with tcPO$_2$ and tcPCO$_2$ electrodes by cuff occlusion of the circulation. Acta Anaesthesiol Scand [Suppl] 68:9–15

67. Shabot MM, Shoemaker WC, State D (1977) Rapid bedside computation of cardiorespiratory variables with a programmable calculator. Crit Care Med 5:105–111

68. Smith NT, Rader CD (1975) Oxygen monitoring and end-tidal gas analysis in anaesthesia. RSA Miniworkshop on monitoring, October

69. Suter PM, Fairley HB, Isenberg MD (1975) Optimum end-expiratory airway pressure in patients with acute pulmonary failure. N Engl J Med 292:284–289

70. Torda TA, Grant GC (1972) Test of a fuel cell oxygen analyser. Br J Anaesth 44:1108–1112

71. Versmold HT, Linderkamp O, Holzmann M, Strohhaker I, Riegel KP (1978) Limits of tcPO$_2$ monitoring in sick neonates: Relations to blood pressure, blood volume, peripheral blood flow and acid base status. Acta Anaesthesiol Scand [Suppl] 68:88–90

72. Whitelaw WA, Derenne J, Milic-Emilic J (1975) Occlusion pressure as a measure of respiratory centre output in conscious man. Respir Physiol 23:181–199

73. Wilkinson RR, Phibbs RH, Gregory GA (1979) Continuous vivo oxygen saturation in newborn infants with pulmonary disease. Crit Care Med 7:232–236

74. Yakulis R, Snyder JV, Powner D, Fusco D, Grenwik A (1978) Mass spectrometry monitoring of respiratory variables in an intensive care unit. Respiratory Care 23:671–679

75. Yoshiya I, Shimada Y, Tanaka K (1980) Spectrophotometric monitoring of arterial oxygen saturation in the finger-tip. Med Biol Eng Comput 18:27–32

76. Yeung HN, Beran AV, Huxtable RF (1978) Low impedance pH sensitive electrochemical devices that are potentially applicable to transcutaneous PCO$_2$ measurements. Acta Anaesthesiol Scand [Suppl] 68:137–141

Chapter 59

Assessment of Renal Function

A. M. Joekes and C. A. Lawrence

The assessment of renal function and of homeostatic abnormalities occupies a central place in the management of critically ill patients. The kidney plays an essential role in maintaining the volume and composition of the body fluids. Although gross changes in concentration of certain constituents, of which urea and creatinine are the most obvious, it is possible that alteration in the *ratio* of physiologically active plasma constituents may be more likely to interfere with cell function acting as the primary abnormality, triggering off a series of changes which may ultimately prove fatal.

Renal function may be compromised with almost any major insult, complicating trauma in road traffic accidents or battle and following major surgery as well as with loss of body fluids and electrolytes due to gastro-intestinal upsets. The acute renal failure that may complicate major cardiovascular surgery is a particularly important instance where advances in monitoring could salvage many lives. The acute renal failure complicating so many insults is in the great majority of cases totally reversible if the patient can be kept alive until renal function is re-established. When elective surgery is undertaken renal functional assessment should be carried out before surgical intervention. Should this not be done the assessment of renal functional status following operation can be misleading.

A major factor in the relatively high fatality rate of acute *reversible* renal failure, which has shown very little improvement over the last two decades, is due to the failure to recognise the *onset* of the kidney functional impairment allowing major homeostatic disturbances to develop before strict metabolic management is started.

In this chapter the approach to the management of patients with acute renal failure (ARF), which must be assumed to be reversible, falls into three main parts:

1. a Recognition of the onset of acute renal functional impairment
   b Reversal of the renal functional abnormality
2. Metabolic management during the renal failure
3. Recognition of primary and secondary changes in homeostasis that may progress to a fatal outcome.

Recognition of onset

During the first 24–48 h after the onset of acute renal damage the renal functional abnormality *cannot* be recognized from changes in blood biochemistry. When relative oliguria is associated with acute renal failure (ARF) the character of the urine, in particular the urine: plasma ratio of urea or creatinine, can establish the functional abnormality from the moment that it occurs. In the less common situation where a maintained urine volume is present the presence of ARF can only be recognized in the early

Table 59.1. Procedure to be followed with urine specimens from bladder catheter in suspected oliguric renal failure

i	Urine sample	Specific gravity Laboratory: Culture Urea, Na, K
ii	*Timed* urine collection (30 ml is adequate)	Specific gravity Laboratory: Urea, Na, K
iii	If oliguric renal failure	Mannitol 20%, 200 ml IV in 10 min
iv	If no response	Ethacrynic acid 50 mg IV
v	If no response	Acute insufficiency established

stages by measuring the *rate* of urea or creatinine excretion. As a rough guide an adult will excrete about 1 mg (11 μmol) creatinine per minute. This can, however, vary greatly from one individual to another, depending on their muscle mass, and further emphasizes the importance of establishing renal functional status before any elective surgery.

It has been shown [7] that the excretion of urea, sodium, and potassium are not significantly affected during the first 48–72 h after cessation of protein or electrolyte intake. In the absence of trauma the summated osmolar excretion of urea and sodium and potassium and their anions will not be less than 720 mmol/24 h during the first 48 h after intake is limited to water and glucose. Following major trauma or surgery, tissue catabolism would in fact lead to a considerably increased excretion of urea. With a urine volume of 720 ml/24 h or 0.5 ml/min the osmolar excretion with normal renal function must be in the order of 1000 mmol/litre, with a specific gravity exceeding 1020.

If oliguric renal failure is suspected the following steps detailed in Table 59.1 should be taken.

If the initial untimed specimen of urine has a high specific gravity or osmolar concentration the presence of oliguric renal failure is excluded. It should be remembered that very high urinary specific gravities may follow intravenous urography (IVU) because of the presence of the contrast medium in the urine. Glycosuria also increases the specific gravity.

Once a timed urine volume has been sent to the laboratory three main settings of urine composition may be found, as shown in Table 59.2. The first setting shows a physiological oliguria and renal function is not compromised. The second setting shows a situation in which there is a major sodium retention by the kidney and not infrequently some minor impairment of renal function is present. If this metabolic situation is allowed to continue for several days the typical reversible ARF can result. The management of this sodium-retaining phase requires careful analysis of the patient's condition, including the measurement of plasma or whole-blood volume and a consideration of hormonal settings. Merely to fill a patient up with some sodium salt may be extremely dangerous. In the third setting acute renal tubular functional damage is established, showing the characteristic inability to concentrate either urea or creatinine. The electrolyte content may vary considerably depending on the aetiology of the renal damage.

Ancillary investigations

Although urine characteristics during oliguria are reliable and quick further diagnostic help may be required in the presence of oliguric failure to determine whether the type II oliguria is developing into fully established ARF or to exclude obstructive uropathy. Other investigations that may prove helpful are: (1) High-dose IVU; (2) radioactive renography; and (3) gamma-camera scintigraphy.

High-dose IVU with acute parenchymal renal failure will show the characteristic long-persisting nephrographic phase without opacification of the urinary tract. In obstructive uropathy late films will show the collecting systems filled with contrast medium [3, 14].

Radioactive renography with radioactive hippuran is a rapid and reliable method of de-

Table 59.2. Urine composition in oliguria (<0.5 ml/min)

Setting	Specific gravity	osmol/litre	÷ Urine: plasma ratio		mmol/litre	
			Urea	Creatinine	Na	K
I	>1020	>800	>50	>100	>100	>40
II	<1016	<600	>50	>100	<20	?
III	<1014	<450	<15	<25	?	?

tecting and roughly assessing the degree of functional damage [11]. This can be of particular importance in monitoring a gradual change from type II to type III oliguria and in obtaining evidence of 'potential' renal function despite prolonged oliguria or anuria. Gradual recovery of renal function may be demonstrated by repeated renography despite the absence of any improvement in convential renal function tests.

Gamma-camera scintigraphy is a sophiscated method of obtaining evidence of potential renal function. It is of particular importance when renography shows no significant function, when scintigraphy can demonstrate vascular perfusion of the kidneys and potential function not detectable by renography. Scintigraphy can also differentiate between parenchymal and obstructive uropathy [5].

A detailed description of nuclear medicine techniques for elucidation of renal function and diagnosis is not possible in this chapter.

If renal damage (type III urine) is recognized in the first 48 h after the onset, reversal of the renal functional impairment can be achieved in a minority of patients. As in the second setting, the cardiodynamic situation of the patient must be carefully assessed, and where necessary or possible, corrected. While various claims have been made that ARF can be *prevented* this is extremely difficult in a clinical situation although in animal experiments there is, for example, conflicting evidence that beta blockade with propranolol prevents or reduces the incidence or severity of ischaemic renal damage. In the clinical situation, once ARF is established the rapid infusion of 40–50 g of mannitol as a 20% or 25% solution is the only generally accepted manoeuvre that may reverse the renal functional impairment. In our hands this has never succeeded later than 48 h after the proven onset. If a mannitol infusion is effective this will be immediately apparent, with a dramatic increase in urine flow during or within minutes of the mannitol infusion. It must be emphasized that the mannitol should be infused as rapidly as possible and that the solution should be warmed to body temperature to be sure that none of the mannitol remains as crystals at the bottom of the bottle. If such a rapid return of urine flow occurs this appears to result in a complete reversal of the renal abnormality and the ability of the tubules to concentrate the urine is re-established.

Despite many claims, there is no documented evidence that frusemide can reverse the renal tubular damage, although it may succeed in increasing urine flow. An IV infusion of 1 mg frusemide/min can be useful in maintaining a urine flow of approximately 2 litres for 48 h, diminishing the dangers of water overload and hyperkalaemia, whilst arrangements are made for transfer of the patient to a specialized unit with necessary back-up facilities to handle acute reversible renal failure. The frusemide infusion should not be continued beyond 48 h as there is suggestive evidence that myocardial damage may occur if it is continued beyond this time.

In our own hands we have seen five patients, all with a background of severe cardiac lesions, in whom IV administration of 50 mg ethacrynic acid has resulted in a reversal of ARF. Possibly these were patients who had slipped from the type II oliguria and it was a fortuitous moment at which to have given this diuretic. We have never seen this occur with frusemide.

Metabolic management during renal failure

The common course of ARF, acute tubular dysfunction, is a period of oliguria with volumes between 200 and 700 ml/24 h, followed by a step-wise increase of urine volume to over 2000 ml/24 h. For a period approximately the length of the oliguric phase an 'early diuretic phase' still shows an inability of the nephron to concentrate or significantly modify the urine composition. This early diuretic phase is functionally similar to ARF with maintained urine volume.

During oliguria the patient is virtually a 'closed system'. The most important potentially dangerous factors are water, potassium and hydrogen ion, or acid–base balance. The aetiology of the ARF can have a profound bearing on clinical management. When it is a complication of non-septicaemic abortion the patient is anabolic and can frequently be treated conservatively on the simple principle of not putting in what does not come out, i.e., no more than the basic 500 ml water requirement plus any urine output or gastro-intestinal (GI) loss and no potassium, sodium or protein other than measured as lost from the body. However, with haemodialysis or peritoneal dialysis available it is no longer acceptable to manage patients purely conservatively unless careful monitoring can be undertaken. In the mid-1940s and early 1950s abortion was by far the commonest cause of ARF but it now accounts for only a small minority of cases; major surgery, in particular open-heart surgery with bypass, trauma, and septicaemia are the main causes, with a rather ill-defined group possibly related to antibiotic sensitivity. In many cases there is significant or even intense catabolism and conservative management is impossible.

In the non-catabolic patient management during the oliguric phase is basically very simple: (1) Fluid administration is restricted to maintaining a daily weight loss of 0.5 kg. Requirements may increase dramatically in hot climates; (2) The calorie intake is kept moderate, avoiding potassium, protein, and salt; (3) Soluble vitamins are given; (4) Mouth hygiene should be maintained by stimulating salivation, achieved by sucking lemon or chewing gum; (5) Proven infection must be treated promptly; (6) Plasma K should be measured daily and when necessary ECG monitoring should be instituted.

With peritoneal dialysis the non-catabolic patient can be safely managed, allowing both increased fluid and calorie and nutritional intake and maintenance of a steady body weight with normal plasma potassium and bicarbonate concentrations. Experience suggests that 'continuous' peritoneal dialysis with dwell times of about 6 h with 2 litres dialysate avoids unnecessary swings in homeostasis. This procedure should not be started until overhydration and/or hyperkalaemia have been corrected by more frequent cycles, if necessary with hypertonic dialysate.

If hyperkalaemia with ECG changes is present and there is delay in instituting dialysis, glucose and insulin (25 g glucose, 8 U insulin) should be given IV as a bolus, if necessary followed by oral calcium.

Once the early diuretic phase is achieved, with urine volumes in excess of 2 litres/24 h, the electrolyte losses in the urine *must* be replaced and fluid intake increased to maintain constant body weight. Sodium and potassium loss in the early diuretic phase varies greatly from patient to patient, but remains fairly constant irrespective of urine volume. In general terms severe trauma is associated with a higher potassium and a low sodium (possibly less than 5 mmol/litre) urine concentration. Non-traumatic cases tend to have a sodium concentration of about 60 mmol/litre and potassium 30 mmol/litre. Unless measured in each patient major homeostatic disturbances can be induced by guessing the required replacement of urinary losses. If replacement is not undertaken prerenal disturbances can result in a further episode of ARF with oliguria.

Whether dialysis needs to be continued during the early diuretic phase is a decision particular to each patient. The inability of the tubules to concentrate the urine during this phase results in the plasma concentrations of urea and creatinine either continuing to rise or remaining unchanged. Overhydration and hyperkalaemia should no longer be a major danger, but in hypercatabolic patients acidosis may require correction by sodium replacement as bicarbonate.

In the hypercatabolic patient following trauma, major surgery, or infection, the nutritional state of the patient is of paramount impeding diaphragmatic movement if the pa-intake is only possible with frequent haemodialysis, which should whenever possible be commenced within 48 h of the onset of the renal failure, virtually always at the time of the trauma. Peritoneal dialysis is rarely sufficiently effective, quite apart from the disadvantage of impeding diaphragmatic movement if the patient has cardiac or pulmonary involvement. The nutritional requirements in hypercatabolic ARF have recently been reviewed [10].

In the severely catabolic patient plasma electrolyte concentrations may alter very rapidly, which can cause cardiac arrhythmias or arrest, and with delay in starting haemodialysis the rapid correction of such electrolyte disturbance is extremely likely to induce cardiac arrhythmias that would make it impossible to continue dialysis and thereby almost certainly have a fatal outcome. The critical monitoring of electrolyte disturbance is discussed in the next section.

Recognition of potentially fatal primary and secondary changes in homeostasis

For effective monitoring of any major abnormality affecting the body that may result in a fatal outcome, it is first necessary to ask what is the likely immediate cause of death, and secondly the physiological disturbances that may lead up to the critical point must be sought. With isolated renal failure, when other systems are normal at the outset, death is virtually always from either cardiac arrest due to hyperkalaemia or cardiac failure due to water overload. With the daily measurement of plasma potassium and body weight both these potentially fatal factors should be avoided, and isolated ARF with a reversible renal lesion should have zero mortality if proper metabolic management with dialysis facilities is available.

Acute renal failure occurring as a complication of open-heart bypass surgery presents a very difficult challenge with respect to monitoring. Again the two main immediate causes of death are cardiac arrest and pulmonary oedema, but the myocardium is already damaged and may prove to be extremely 'brittle' as regards arrhythmias, thus being likely to be in 'failure' overtly or by physiological definition. The mortality in renal failure complicating open-heart surgery is depressingly high although the renal lesion is potentially reversible, and is far higher than would occur with the cardiac lesion and surgery alone. Is it possible to define the factors occurring with the renal failure that are primarily responsible for the high mortality?

In our approach to patients with ARF and primary cardiopulmonary problems we have selected what may be 'primary' metabolic factors and 'secondary' functional changes. The importance both of calcium and potassium plasma concentrations individually and of the K:Ca ratio has long been known to be of vital importance to myocardial function. In the presence of oliguric renal failure plasma potassium is likely to increase, more particularly in the presence of hypercatabolism, and plasma calcium to decrease. With these two ions moving in opposite directions the K:Ca may change rapidly and dramatically. If haemodialysis is delayed beyond the first 48 h a major reversal of the K:Ca is likely to result early in dialysis. It is a common experience to find that cardiac arrhythmias, cardiac arrest, or worsening myocardial function frequently occur soon after delayed haemodialysis is started. With the careful control of intravascular and extravascular circulatory volumes with modern dialysis techniques the asumption must be that the cardiac deterioration is dependent on some metabolic change. Apart from a rapid fall in the K:Ca ratio the two other ion concentrations that may show major changes are phosphate and bicarbonate or hydrogen ion. A change in both phosphate concentration and, more particularly, the plasma pH can be expected to affect the ionized calcium fraction, which is presumably the physiologically active component, as opposed to that which is protein-bound or complexed.

If it may be argued that a rapid change in K: ionized Ca is the primary reason for inducing cardiac arrhythmia or arrest or reduced efficiency of myocardial concentration, then on-line continuous monitoring of potassium and ionized calcium could provide the most important information likely to improve the survival rate in patients with ARF complicating open-heart surgery.

The most closely related secondary effect would be myocardial 'contractibility' or ejection efficiency (inevitably altered by arrhythmias) and cardiopulmonary efficiency reflected in blood PO_2 and PCO_2. A fall in blood pressure or peripheral circulation and skin: core temperature ratio are at best late indications of possibly impending disaster. In a prospective study to monitor critically ill patients with renal failure we are developing continuous monitoring of: (1) Plasma potassium and ionized calcium; (2) cardiac efficiency, by non-invasive methods; and (3) PO_2 and PCO_2.

Continuous plasma potassium and ionized calcium measurement

Intravascular electrode probes for potassium have been tried [1], but the problem of interference due to protein deposition, the difficulty of sterilization, and the impossibility of recalibration in situ have frustrated most clinical attempts. On-line potassium monitoring with a continuous extracorporeal blood flow can overcome the problem of recalibration [6, 13]. Usually, however, multiple blood samples are measured by flame photometry or bench electrodes. Calcium electrodes can similarly be used, but how frequently should samples be taken? It is extremely unlikely that any predictable pattern of the rate of change in K:Ca ratio can be established for individual patients.

Over the last few years we have developed on-line continuous monitoring of potassium and ionized calcium, for which we use a very small-capacity dialysis unit, the protein-free dialysate passing over the electrodes with the blood returning to the patient [8]. This technique has allowed continuous monitoring for up to 48 h.

Cardiac contractility or myocardial efficiency

Electrical thoracic impedance has given very valuable information on myocardial function [4, 9, 8, 15]. It is totally non-invasive and cardiac contraction can be followed from beat to beat. This has proved extremely valuable in assessment of the effect of therapeutic manoeuvres in cardiac function.

Echocardiography, equally non-invasive, may give valuable although slightly different information, but is less well adapted to continuous monitoring.

Continuous blood gas analysis

Many different approaches to this have been undertaken [2, 12, 16], and we have not yet developed any advance which would allow this to be incorporated into a single monitoring read-out unit, including ion electrode and cardiac measurements.

It is our contention that unless it is possible to establish 'prime movers' in the metabolic abnormalities cascading to an ultimately fatal outcome, the mortality rate resulting from ARF complicating open-heart surgery, severe trauma, or severe infection is unlikely to be improved. Whether K:Ca ratio will prove to be the, or one of the, 'prime movers' is not established. The techniques outlined, in particular the on-line potassium and calcium monitoring can be adapted for other ions or substances that may be thought to be of importance.

References

1. Band DM, Treasure T (1976) Continuous monitoring of blood potassium demonstrated in an animal. J Physiol 266:12–13
2. Brantigan JW (1976) Catheters for continuous in vivo blood and tissue monitoring. Crit Care Med 4:239–244
3. Fry IK, Cattell WR (1972) The nephrographic pattern during excretion urography. Br Med Bull 28:227–232
4. Girling Margery (1978) Thesis, London University
5. Hilson AJW, Maisey MN, Brown CB, Ogg CS, Bewick MS (1978) Dynamic renal transplant imaging with Tc-99m DTPA (Sn) supplemented by transplant perfusion index in the management of renal transplant. J Nucl Med 19:994
6. Jank K, Mosoglu E, Hicquet J, Demeester M (1977) A multi-sensor support for in vivo monitoring of blood parameters with in situ sensor calibration. Pfluegers Arch 371:175–178
7. Joekes AM, Mowbray JF, Dormandy K (1957) Oliguria with urine of 'fixed' specific gravity. Lancet II:864
8. Joekes AM, Lawrence CA, Simpson RJ (1980) Demonstration of continuous bedside potassium and ionised calcium measurement using a combined haemofiltration and flow-through electrode system. J Physiol 307:1–2P
9. Kubicek WG, Kottke FJ, Ramos MU, Patterson RG, Witsoe DA, Labree JW, Remole W, Layman TE, Schoening H, Garamela T (1974) Minnesota Impedance cardiograph–cleaning and applications. Biomed Eng 9:410–416
10. Lee HA (1980) Acute renal failure. In: Chapman A (ed). Churchill Livingstone, Edinburgh, pp 106–122
11. O'Reilly PH, Shields RA, Testa HJ (1979) Nuclear medicine in urography and renography. Butterworths, London
12. Parker D, Key A, Davies RS (1971) Catheter-tip transducer for continuous in vivo measurement of oxygen tension. Lancet II:952–953
13. Schindler JG, Dennhardt R, Simon W (1977) Kontinuierlicher ionselektive und elektrochemishe enzymatische Direktmessung an Menschen. Chimia 31:404–407
14. Sherwood T, Doyle FH, Boulton-Jones M, Joekes AM, Peters KD, Sissons P (1974) The intravenous urogram in acute renal failure. Br J Radiol 47:368–372
15. Thompson FD, Joekes AM (1981) Thoracic impedance. Cardiodynamic assessment: validation and clinical use. Ciba-Geigy, London
16. Vurek GG, Kolobow T, Clem TR (1978) Blood gas monitor for extended extracorporeal procedures. Ann Biomed Eng 6:544–554

Chapter 60

Radiology

John M. Stevens, William R. Lees,
and Richard R. Mason

Modern radiology offers an expansive range of imaging modalities and techniques which have become virtually indispensable in the management of many life-threatening diseases. This section reviews some aspects of modern radiological and ultrasonographic interpretation and procedure which it is hoped will be found useful by non-radiologists responsible for the care of the acutely ill.

General observations

Mobile x-ray equipment

Much of the radiography in critically ill patients is performed with portable equipment. Mobile generators cannot deliver the high tube currents available from the large fixed generators of most x-ray departments, and to achieve adequate exposures in some situations the tube voltage must be raised, the exposure time lengthened, or the object-tube distance shortened. These are all manoeuvres which significantly degrade the radiographic image. Because the chest requires relatively low exposures, films of reasonable quality can be expected from modern mobile machines. However, in thick regions of the body, such as the abdomen, ward mobile films are less satisfactory for demonstrating anything

but large gas accumulations and dense bone; contrast studies such as intravenous urography (IVU) may be inadequately performed. Some ICUs have their fixed generator and x-ray tube [98], but a well-chosen modern mobile machine should meet most requirements.

Silhouettes and the silhouette sign

The obliteration of the borders created by differences in radiographic density between normal soft-tissue structures and aerated lung is an extremely useful sign for localizing abnormal shadows in frontal radiographs of the chest. Felson ascribed this phenomenon to contact between the abnormal area and that part of the soft-tissue surface profiled by the tangential x-ray beam [35]. Others have recognized that a positive silhouette sign requires only that the abnormal area be of comparable radiographic density to the border, which it may overlap rather than contact [81]. Nevertheless, Felson's original concept remains a very useful one: heart borders are obliterated by anteriorly located lesions and are seen distinctly through posteriorly located ones.

Mach's bands

These are purely visual effects, which result in enhanced contrast at borders. The Mach band is a thin line, usually of low density, visible along a border defined by only slight differences in radiographic density. It is a phenomenon produced in the retina of the observer and not on the film [75]. The effect has caused confusion in certain situations. A longitudinal skin fold may be raised by the film cassette pressing against a patient's back, and result in perception of a lucent line passing downward across a lung field easily misdiagnosed as a pneumothorax; lines produced across bone by soft-tissue folds or thinner overlying bone have been erroneously called fractures [21] (Fig. 60.1).

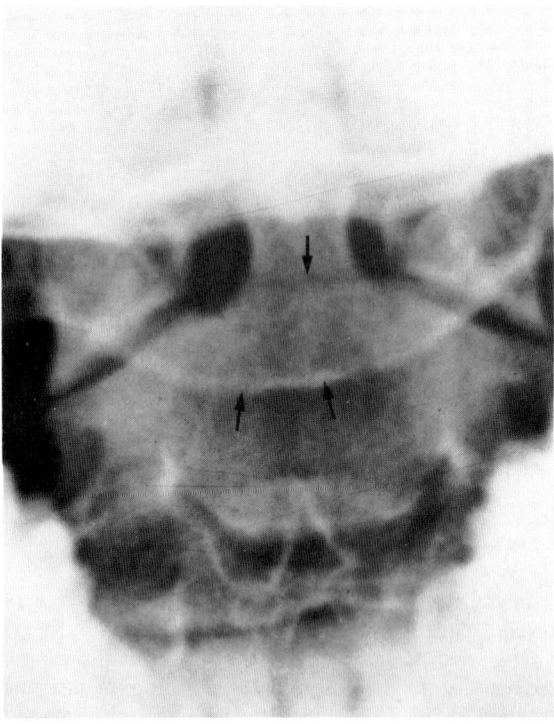

Fig. 60.1. Pseudo-fracture of the dens. A lucent line (*arrow*) crosses the base of the dens. It runs parallel to the lower margin of the posterior arch of the atlas (*arrows*), and is produced by slight differences in density caused by the thin bone of the posterior arch. It is a phenomenon generated in the retina of the observer, due to lateral inhibition, and does not exist physically on the film.

Co-operation

Positioning of the patient prior to the radiographic exposure is crucial to the interpretability of the result. Lordotic positions produce misleading density at the lung bases; rotation of the patient or lateral off-centering of the x-ray tube suggest unilateral transradiancy of a lung [65].

That radiographers using ward mobiles should receive every assistance from ward staff

to achieve optimum positioning is a point which cannot be overemphasized. Close liaison between clinician, radiographer, and radiologist is essential if errors are to be avoided.

Chest x-ray

Anatomical considerations

Pleura and mediastinum

Figures 60.2–60.4 illustrate the lateral mediastinum, the normal right hilum, and the interlobar fissures. Some unusual locations of central venous pressure lines are illustrated in Fig. 60.5. If a catheter is difficult to see, it can be filled with 1 or 2 ml contrast medium (e.g., Urograffin 76%) prior to another radiographic exposure. If the vessel in which it is located requires identification, 20 or 30 ml contrast can be injected down the catheter and a film taken. Such procedures are rarely necessary, however [98].

Pulmonary parenchyma

Modern radiology defines two compartments in which abnormal lung opacity may be recognized: alveolae and interstitium.

Alveolar filling processes (pulmonary oedema, consolidation, pulmonary haemorrhage). The smallest radiologically recognizable unit of lung tissue is the acinus, which is defined as the air spaces distal to a terminal bronchiole [43]. A fluid-filled acinus is 7.4 mm in mean size, round when fully filled and rosette-shaped when incompletely filled [45]. Because acini communicate freely, alveolar filling diseases involve large aggregates of acini in which the individual units usually cannot be recognized. Occasionally, however, a nodular pattern is seen, comprising a profusion of discrete acinar shadows (Fig. 60.6).

A larger radiologically identifiable unit of lung tissue is the pulmonary lobule, which comprises several acini [58]. These may be up to 2.5 cm in size, and are demarcated by substantial connective tissue septa. They are best-developed in the outer zones where they define

Fig. 60.2. A and **B** Lateral view of the normal hila. *LPA*, left ▷ pulmonary artery; *RPA*, right pulmonary artery; *PV*, pulmonary veins. The *arrow* points to the posterior wall of the bronchus intermedius, which is defined posteriorly by aerated lung in the azygo-oesophageal pleural recesses; it is usually easy to identify. The right middle lobe bronchus is seen below the RPA.

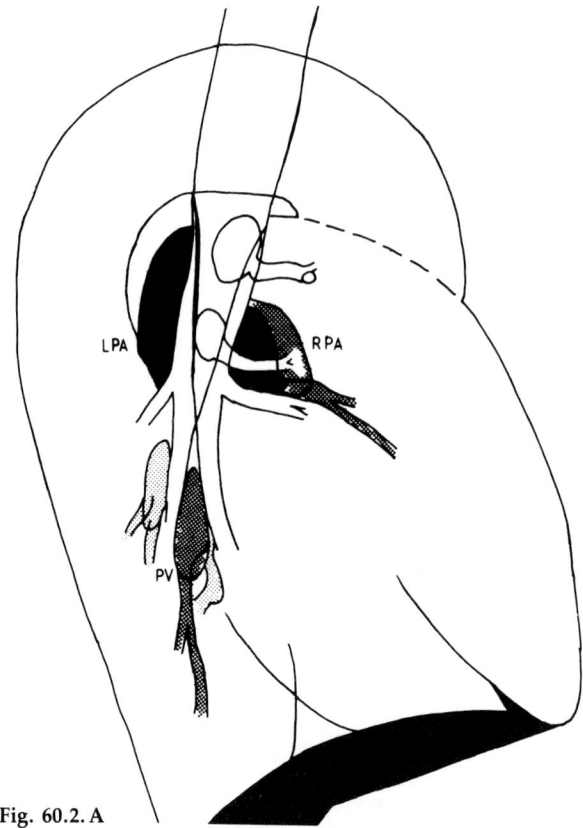

Fig. 60.2. A

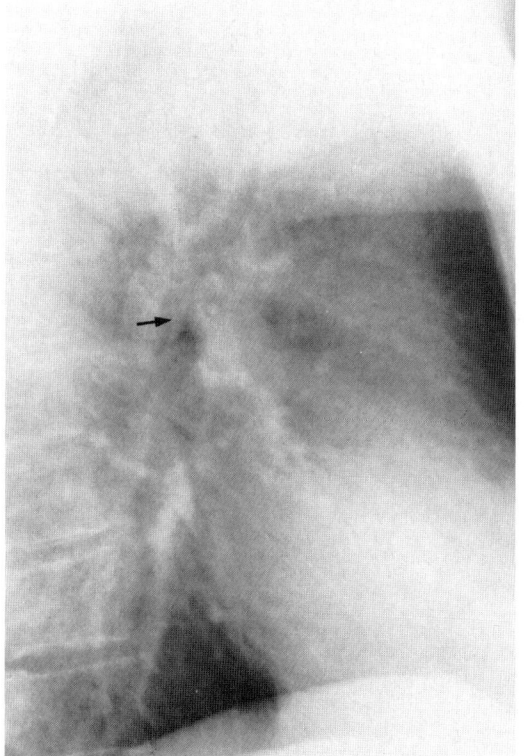

Fig. 60.2. B

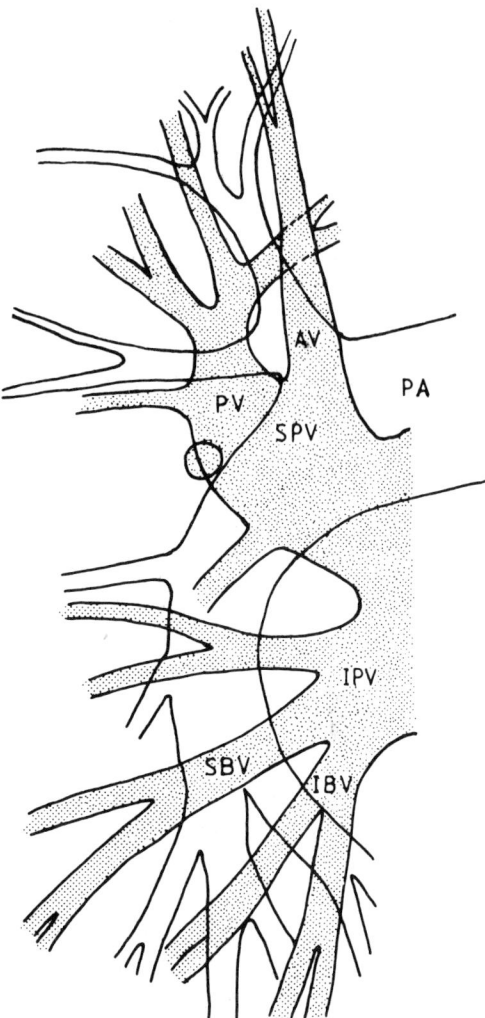

Fig. 60.3. Frontal view of the right hilum, to show the relationship between pulmonary arteries and veins. These structures are usually easier to identify in patients with pulmonary venous hypertension than in normal subjects. *AV*, apical vein; *IBV*, inferor basal vein; *IPV*, inferior pulmonary vein; *PA*, pulmonary artery; *PV*, posterior vein; *SBV*, superior basal vein; *SPV*, superior plumary vein.

a region often designated the cortex of the lung (Fig. 60.7). Lobular boundaries form the margins of consolidating and oedematous processes, and individual lobules are frequently spared within involved areas, imparting inhomogeneity to the radiographic opacity.

That alveolar filling processes seldom produce homogeneous shadows is a most helpful differential observation: the other features of these processes, namely air bronchogram and obliteration of vascular markings, are helpful signs only if film quality permits. Finally, nodular patterns in alveolar diseases are more commonly seen in patients with chronic lung

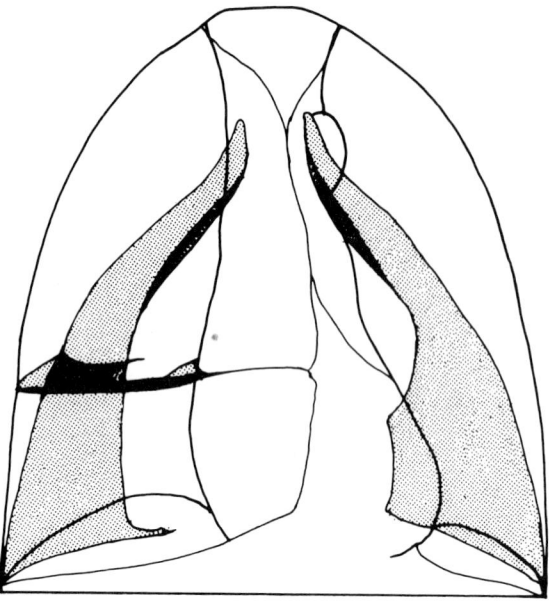

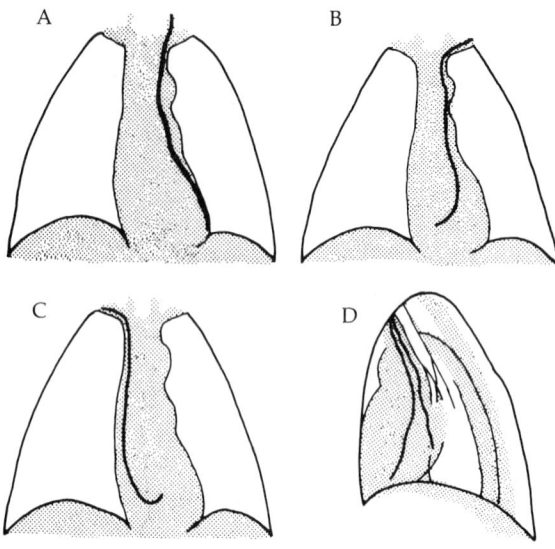

Fig. 60.5. Some unsatisfactory positions of central venous pressure catheters: **A** Left cardiaco-phrenic vein. **B** left superior vena cava. **C** Coronary sinus. **D** Lateral view showing the pericardiaco-phrenic vein (anterior) and the left superior vena cava (posterior).

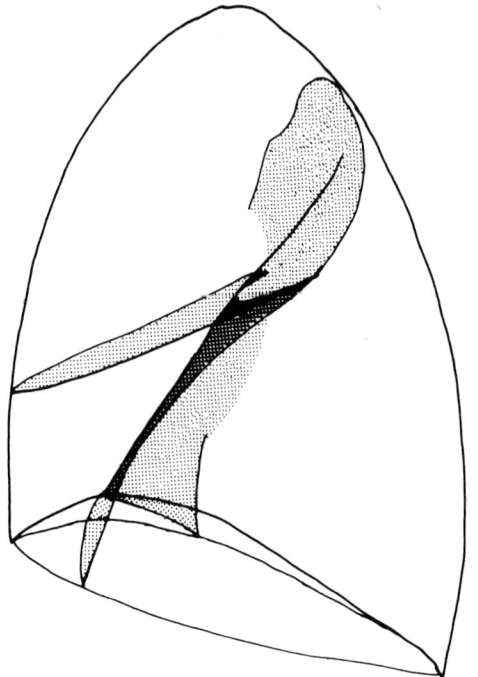

Fig. 60.4. The interlobar fissures, drawn in perspective to illustrate the orientation to the frontally and laterally directed x-ray beam. The fissures are incomplete and their undulations slightly exaggerated. Note the portions of each fissure, which tend to be aligned tangentially to the beam and hence appear on the radiograph, and what meagre information about the position of the fissure as a whole this provides.

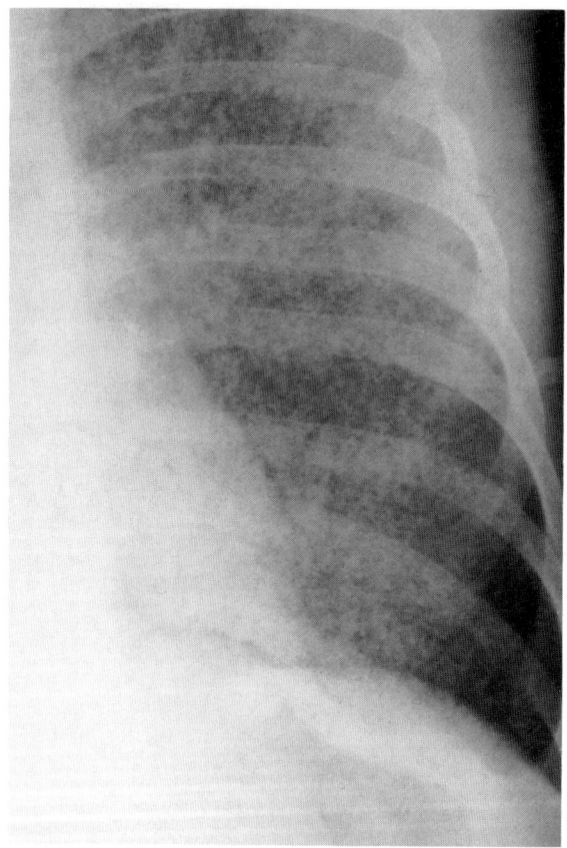

Fig. 60.6. Intra-alveolar haemorrhage. Acinar shadows and indistinct rosette forms can be seen in the left lung field. A similar appearance may be produced by pulmonary oedema or pneumonitis.

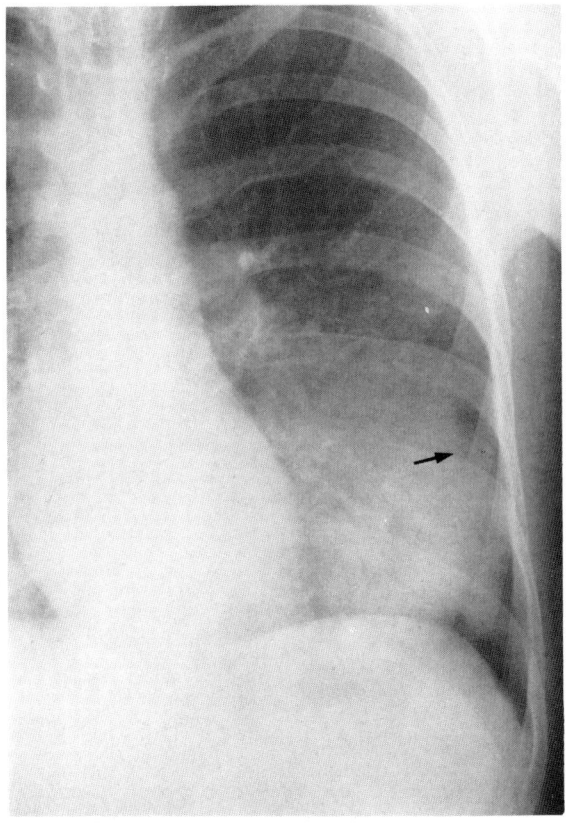

◁ **Fig. 60.7.** Intra-alveolar oedema confined to the central portion of the lower zone of the left lung field. The cortical region of the uninvolved pulmonary lobules is sharply demarcated (*arrow*).

disease, and are due to discrete non-confluent opacification of acini or lobules (see section: *Pulmonary oedema*).

Interstitium. It is now firmly established [59] that Kerley's lines represent thickened connective tissue septa between lobules in the cortex of the lung and less well-defined interstitial planes within the medulla of each lung. The following definitions of Kerley's lines may be helpful: *B-lines* are horizontal, pleurally based, 1 mm thick, 1–2.5 cm in length, and are seen best laterally near the lung bases; *A-lines* are straight or angulated, 1 mm thick, 3–5 cm in length, and are best seen in the upper zones of each lung field directed towards the hilum; *C-lines* are a fine reticular network only occasionally seen around the hila or at the right lung base. However, in addition to these are numerous other interstitial lines, which have recently been designated *D-lines* [72]. The commonest of these are 2–3 mm thick, 5–10 cm in length, straight or angulated, and are best seen anteriorly in the lateral chest film (Fig. 60.8).

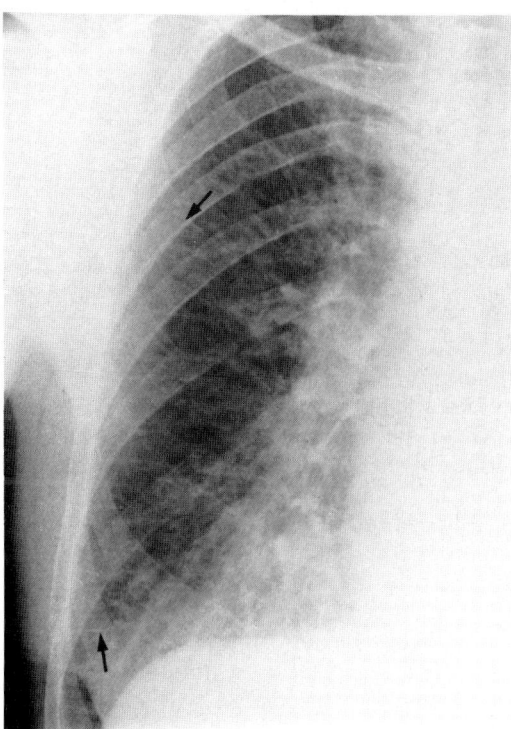

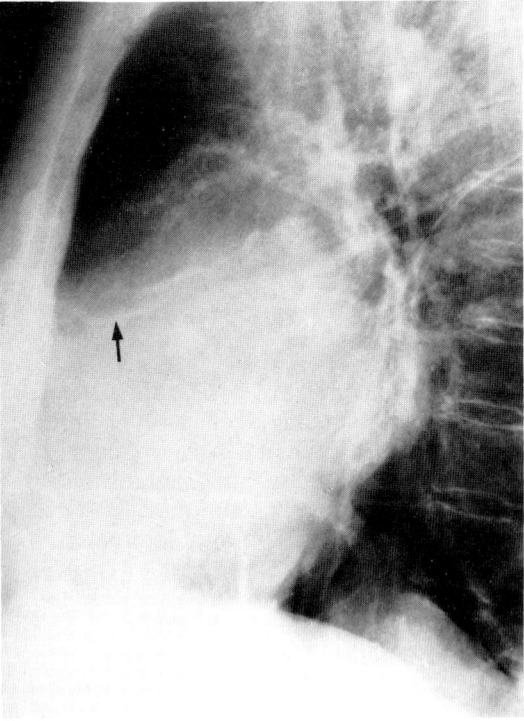

A   B

Fig. 60.8. Kerley's lines. **A** Frontal view: *upper arrow*, A-line; *lower arrow*, B-line. **B** lateral view. *arrow*, D-lines. Two patients with interstitial oedema due to left heart failure.

Physiological considerations and pulmonary oedema

The demonstration of regional differences in pulmonary blood flow and the early detection of increases in extravascular lung water are potentially among the most valuable contributions plain chest radiography can make in the intensive therapy situation. However, much of the experimental work on which this statement is based derives from animal models [89] or otherwise idealized radiographic situations [105]. In everyday practice it is frustrating how frequently the signs cannot be applied with confidence, a failure which is usually ascribable to poor film quality when it matters most, in the sickest patients.

Pulmonary blood flow and volume

Regional differences in blood flow are seen as areas where the vascular shadows are reduced in size and number compared to those elsewhere [89, 90]. The effect of gravity is usually visible, causing lower zone vessels to be larger than those in the upper zones in erect chest films. Reversal of this apex to base gradation frequently accompanies elevated left heart pressures [63, 77, 89]. However, this sign is most easily seen in chronic pressure elevation such as mitral valve disease, and may be unreliable in acute states such as myocardial infarction [90]. A *generalized* increase in pulmonary blood volume and flow may obliterate the normal gravitational effect and result in distension of upper and lower zone vessels to an equal degree [90]. This sign is helpful in identifying patients whose major problem is overhydration, or salt retention and renal failure.

Pulmonary oedema

Careful studies correlating the radiological assessment of interstitial oedema with accurate estimation of extravascular lung water have established the plain chest radiograph as a sensitive indicator of early pulmonary oedema [105]. However, many of the radiological signs of interstitial oedema are seen best in chronic rather than acute oedema states. The most frequent are blurring of the hilar shadows and peribronchial oedema. The latter is of particular help in acute oedema (Fig. 60.9), and presumably arises from the bronchial artery circulation where these vessels drain into pulmonary veins from a systemic arterial pressure [24]. Endo-

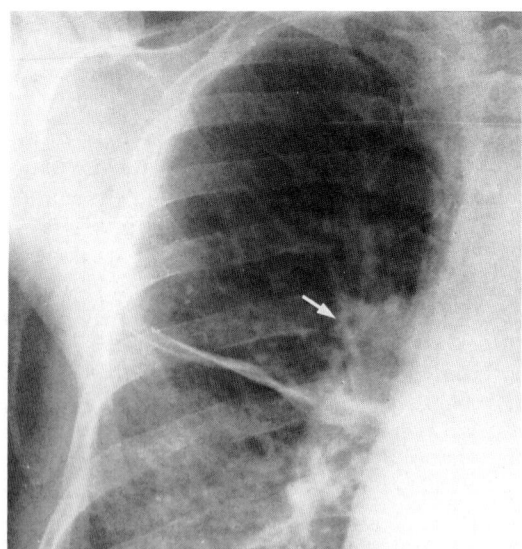

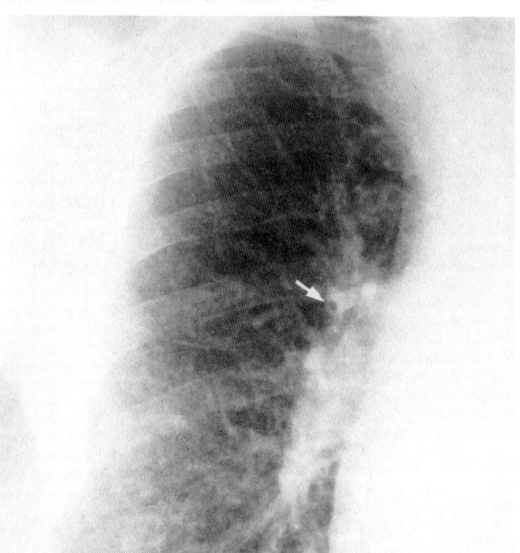

Fig. 60.9. Peribronchial oedema. Two PA chest films in the same patient taken 24 h apart. Note the difference between the two films in the appearance of the anterior segmental bronchus of the right upper lobe (*arrow*).

bronchial thickening due to mucosal oedema also occurs, which may explain why air trapping can dominate the appearance of early pulmonary oedema, especially in children [51]. Of Kerley's lines, B-lines are the most commonly seen overall, whereas the less frequent A-lines have been noted slightly more often in acute than in chronic oedema states [105]. D-lines were observed in 25 of 64 premortem chest x-rays in patients with autopsy-proven interstitial oedema and were usually associated with B-lines [72]. Other signs include thickening of interlobar fissures, micronodular mottling, and a diffuse increase in lung density [98, 105].

It is common to see atypical patterns of pulmonary oedema in patients with chronic lung disease. The subject was reviewed by Hublitz et al. [61], who found lobar or segmental alveolar oedema indistinguishable from pneumonia to be the commonest atypical pattern. Significantly, the oedema tended to affect normal rather than bullous regions of the lung. In other patients they observed merely an accentuation of the pre-existing interstitial reticular and linear markings; the increased incidence of nodular patterns in these patients has already been mentioned (section: *Pulmonary parenchyma*).

Gravitational dependence of intra-alveolar oedema is frequently demonstrable. In one group of patients receiving assisted ventilation [78] gravity-dependent asymmetry was observed in 68%, and major shifts in the opacity could be induced by a position change of 2 h. Occasionally purely unilateral alveolar oedema is seen which is not related to a lateral recumbent position or the other established causes. It is usually right-sided and remains unexplained [147]; an association with the LV failure accompanying arrhythmias has been observed.

Respiratory distress syndrome

Chest radiographs made during a latent phase prior to clinical deterioration are frequently normal. Although specific but subtle abnormalities have been described shortly after the onset of the clinical features [97], the coalescing parenchymal opacities which typify the radiological appearances of the syndrome [64, 97] develop 12–24 h later [34]. Spreading opacities appear rapidly, but once present they tend to persist unchanging from day to day, unlike the shadows of pulmonary oedema or haemorrhage, which come and go within hours. Cavitation and pleural effusion indicate complicating secondary infection or infarction and do not occur until the end of the first week [64].

The application of positive end-expiratory pressure (PEEP) ventilation often produces an immediate radiological improvement, which is not necessarily due to re-aeration of atelectatic alveoli. It may indicate overdistension of the smaller conducting airways [127], or if associated with marked clinical deterioration, pulmonary interstitial emphysema (see section: *Complications of assisted ventilation*).

Aspiration syndromes

Aspiration is usefully grouped into four clinico-radiological patterns.

Pulmonary oedema

This is usually due to aspiration of gastric juice, in which case the alveolar injury is related to the pH of the aspirate [6, 13]. The immediate chest radiograph is usually abnormal, but the extent of the opacities at this time does not predict the outcome. The shadows clear within 5 days in survivors, but secondary infection can be expected in 25% of patients [13]. Similar patterns are seen in drowning [108] and several other inhalation situations [6].

Pleuropneumonia

This pattern is due to aspiration of infected oropharyngeal contents. It is frequently due to anaerobic organisms [13], and the radiological features of pleuropneumonia from this cause have been reviewed recently [73]. Consolidations appear, which progress slowly over 5–7 days despite appropriate treatment, and may take weeks to clear. Cavitation and empyema formation are common, and may develop rapidly; infected pleural exudates are consistently unilateral.

Granulomas

This group includes reticular patterns, nodules, and large solid masses, which frequently need to be distinguished from carcinoma. They are the result of fibrosis around the aspirated vegetable fibre [11], chronic aspiration in oesophageal diseases [6], and aspiration of exogenous lipid [80].

Major atelectasis or air trapping

These are the patterns seen with aspiration of food particles, broken teeth, or dentures.

Pulmonary embolism

Focal redistribution of blood flow has been reported as one of the commonest radiographic signs of pulmonary embolism. However, the sign is usually misleading, being subtle when present and often requiring tomography for its demonstration; whereas obvious areas of focal

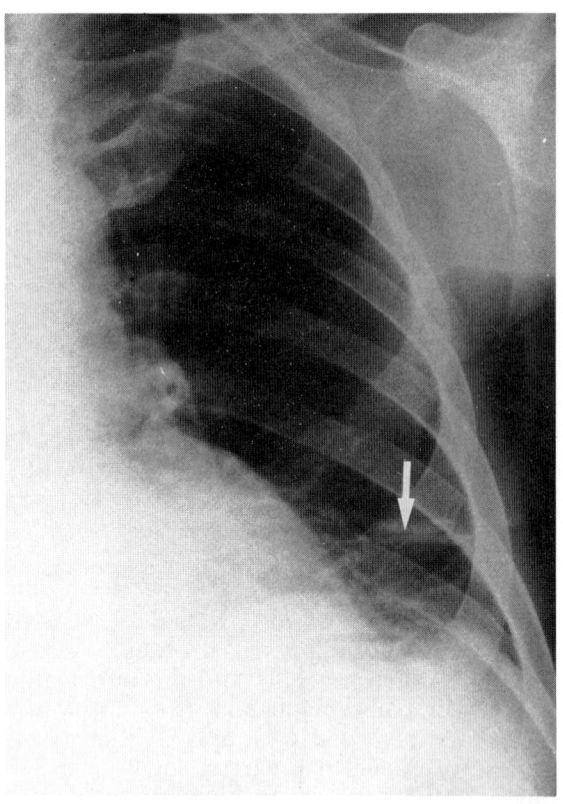

◁ **Fig. 60.10.** Fleischner lines. The patient suffered left-sided pleuritic chest pain and showed multiple perfusion defects in a perfusion lung scan, presumed to be due to pulmonary emboli.

diminution in blood flow are almost invariably due to emphysema, not pulmonary emboli [44].

The most useful radiological signs of embolism in the chest x-ray are homogeneous lung shadows, pleural effusion, and perhaps reduced lung volume. In a review of 155 patients with angiographically proven emboli, 88% exhibited one or more of these signs [14]. *Lung shadows* characteristically have no air bronchogram, which can be useful in distinguishing infarction from pneumonia [4]. Many of these shadows clear completely within 5 days without scarring [44]. *Pleural effusions* are usually unilateral, small in size, diminish after three days, and in as many as 18% of cases are the only abnormal finding [14]. *Loss of lung volume* may be accompanied by the basal shadows often referred to as Fleischner's lines. These are horizontal sheets of atelactatic lung and infolded pleura 2 or 3 mm thick [5], but are a very non-specific finding (Fig. 60.10).

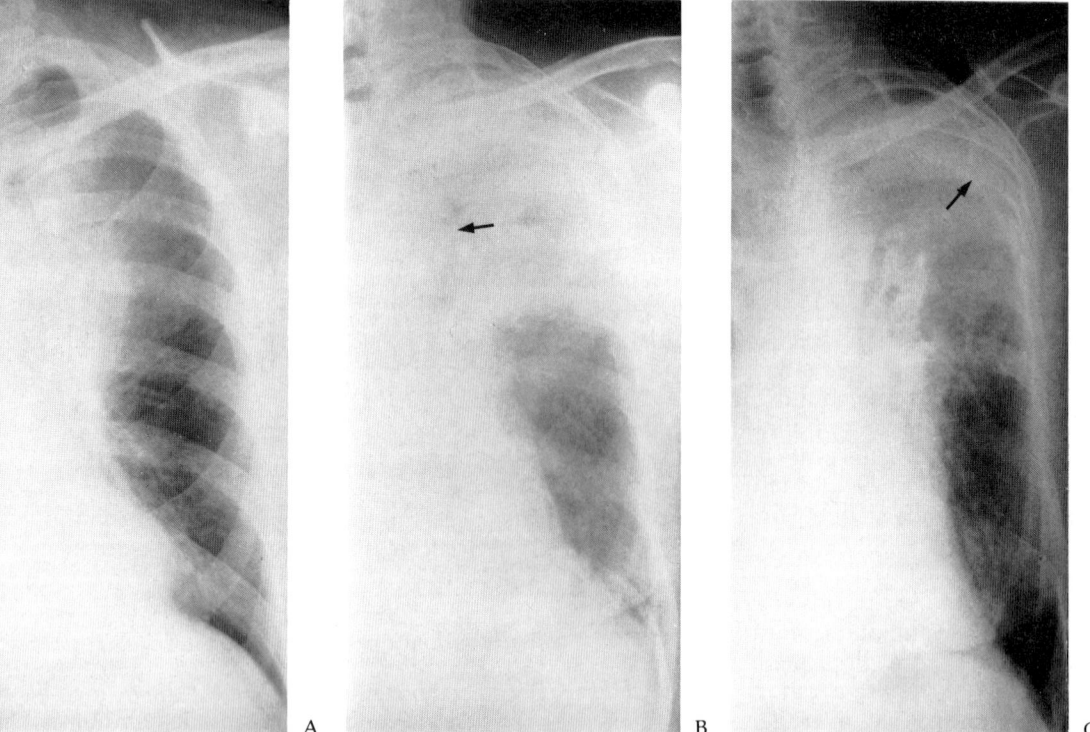

        A   B   C

Fig. 60.11. Two patients with left upper lobe collapse. **A** Typical pattern of central collapse, the bulk of the collapse shadow lying anteriorly and medially. The hilar wedge crosses and obscures the aortic arch. **B** Peripheral collapse, the central parts of the left lung remaining aerated. The aortic arch can be seen (*arrow*). **C** One day later, and at greater radiographic exposure, the lateral portion of the collapse shadow is clearly seen (*arrow*). This could be misinterpreted as an apical effusion.

Septic embolism tends to produce multiple shadows which characteristically cavitate [50]. Multiple pneumatoceles have recently been described [147], and cavitating lesions of similar aetiology have occurred with peripheral migration of Swan-Ganz catheters [119].

Pulmonary collapse

Patterns of lobar collapse have been recently reviewed [106] and new signs of major atelactasis relating to mediastinal [66] and diaphragmatic [67] alterations described. Peripheral forms of lobar collapse may be mistaken for atypical pleural effusions (Fig. 60.11); and during the resolution of large pleural exudates, a ball-like area of atelactasis may arise and be misdiagnosed as an underlying tumour mass [53, 116].

Pleural

Effusion

The distinction between a pleural and a parenchymal location is often all that can be concluded about a shadow on a single portable chest film. Pleural shadows tend to veil lung markings, whereas those in the parenchyma obliterate them. The effect of incomplete interlobar fissures on the appearance of the fluid extending into them [22] is illustrated in (Fig. 60.12). Subpulmonary effusions show their most characteristic appearance (Fig. 60.13) in expiratory films [10].

Pneumothorax

In the supine patient an anteriorly located pneumothorax may be impossible to detect without a lateral film. In infants, such collections may bulge anteriorly across the mediastinum in a characteristic way [41]. Basal pneumothoraces usually displace the lateral margin of the lung from the chest wall and are not difficult to detect (Fig. 60.14), but occasional subpulmonary pneumothoraces do not and can easily be overlooked [15].

Mediastinum

Post-cardiac surgery

Mediastinal widening seen in the immediate postoperative period should begin to reduce within 2 or 3 days [98]. Clinical deterioration in

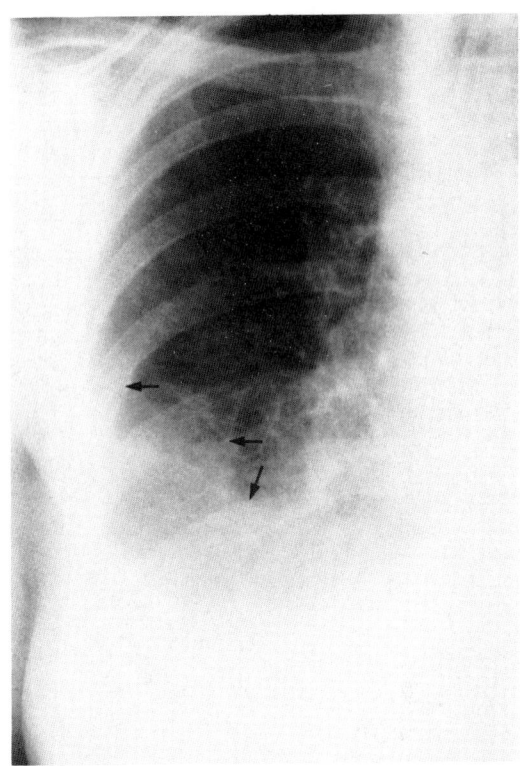

Fig. 60.12. Right pleural effusion. Fluid extends into a very incomplete oblique fissure (*horizontal arrow*). The curved margin (*arrows*) probably defines the central extent of an incomplete fissure. (The lateral view showed considerable fluid in the horizontal fissure.)

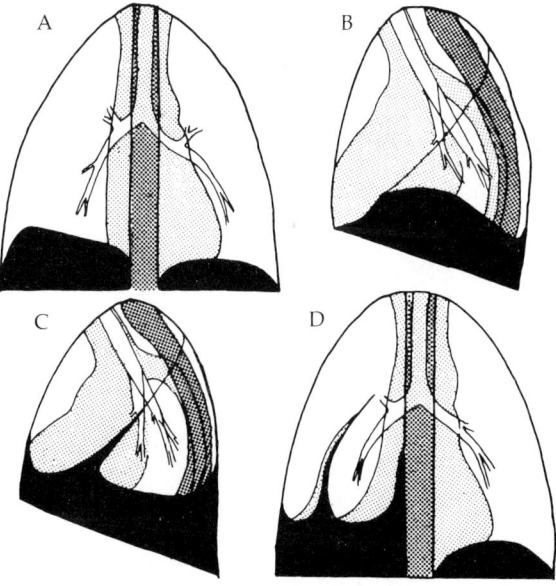

Fig. 60.13. Basal pleural effusions. **A** Right subpulmonary effusion. **B** Lateral view; the subpulmonary fluid is demarcated anteriorly by the oblique fissure. **C** More typical appearance of a larger effusion on which the right lung is floating. Fluid extends into the oblique fissure. **D** Frontal view of **C**.

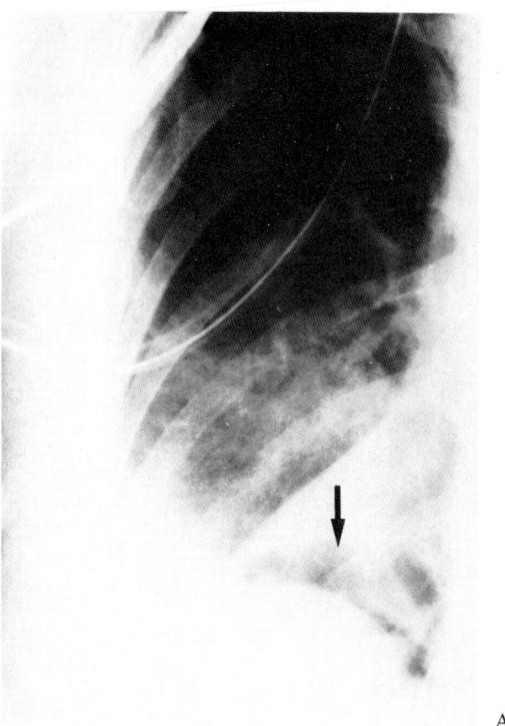
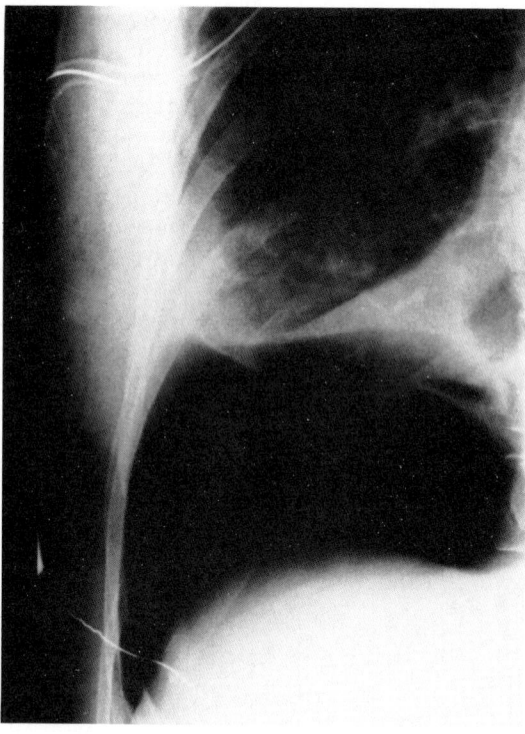

Fig. 60.14. Basal pneumothorax, right middle and lower lobe collapse. The small basal pneumothorax (*arrow*) (**A**) rapidly enlarged over 24 h, as can be seen in the film on the *right* (**B**).

the face of normal lung fields may be due to anterior loculation of mediastinal fluid causing tamponade, or to sternal dehiscence. The former is seen as widening of the cardiopericardial shadow, especially anteriorly in the lateral view [32], and the latter as alterations in the alignment of sternal wire sutures, or a verticle lucent line in the sternal area [150].

Acute mediastinal widening

Major arterial trauma. The wide superior mediastinum in a severely traumatized patient is a frequent diagnostic problem. One solution is to take serial chest radiographs at hourly or even more frequent intervals to demonstrate progressive widening [40]; subtle changes may be progressive drift of the trachea or a nasogastric tube to the right [132]. Suggestive findings on a single film however are thick apical pleural 'caps', due to extrapleural haematoma dissecting over the apex of the lung from the mediastinum, widening of the paraspinal lines [42], especially the left [109], and the appearance of a large pleural effusion (Fig. 60.15). Urgent aortography provides the difinitive answer and in experienced hands holds no special hazard in this group of patients.

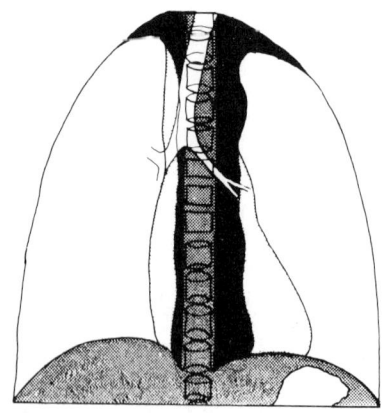

Fig. 60.15. The mediastinal haematoma in acute rupture of the aorta, parietal pleura intact. Note extrapleural extension of blood over the apex of each lung, depression of the left principal bronchus, and displacement of the trachea to the right.

Other mediastinal catastrophes. The signs of acute aortic dissection both on plain films and at aortography have been reviewed by Itzchak et al. [62]; the plain film findings are similar to aortic rupture. Mediastinal air is the cardinal sign of ruptured oesophagus, for which water-soluble contrast examination of the oesophagus is the definitive investigation (see section: *Emergency contrast studies*).

Complications of assisted ventilation

The endotracheal tube

The position of the tube is precisely revealed on chest radiographs. Intubation of the right principal bronchus is associated with increased mortality [151]. We have reviewed a small series of patients with tubes less than 2.5 cm above the carina, and have noticed an increased incidence of consolidation in the left lung even when only the tip of the bevel entered the right bronchus, and that significant reduction of left lung volume always accompanied descent of the entire tube orifice into the right bronchus. Movement of the tube with flexion and extension of the head can be considerable, especially in neonates [133], and head position should be taken into account when the tube level is assessed radiologically. Other abnormalities of the tube such as kinks are usually identifiable.

Extra-alveolar air

Radiological signs of pulmonary barotrauma frequently occur before the clinical ones [98, 112]. Pulmonary interstitial emphysema has been described by Swischuk [127] as a pattern of wormy, tortuous bubbles which radiate from the hila and do not change in size with the phases of respiration. The bubbles are best seen against consolidated lung and usually progress rapidly to produce large subpleural blebs. However in one group of 108 patients with extra-alveolar air reviewed by Rohlfing [112] only five were recognized as having pulmonary interstitial emphysema. Pneumothorax was the commonest abnormality in this group; they were usually under tension, and 50% were associated with pneumomediastinum. Abdominal air was present in 37%. The air was usually retroperitoneal and characteristically formed a lucent crescent over the right lobe of the liver extending down into the right flank. Moreover, free intraperitoneal gas was present in 12% of patients, and only half of these showed air in the retroperitoneal tissues as well: nevertheless, if a pneumoperitoneum is seen in a patient receiving assisted ventilation, a perforated abdominal viscus should still be suspected, especially if mediastinal or subcutaneous emphysema are not present. Finally, pulmonary venous air embolism can be induced by barotrauma and gas in the cardiac chambers and abdominal vessels has been seen on plain radiographs [120].

Positive end-expiratory pressure ventilation

The application of this form of ventilation therapy often produces a dramatic change in the chest radiograph: lungs become overinflated, airways measurably enlarge, and parenchymal infiltrates often clear rapidly (see section: *Respiratory distress syndrome*). Compression of areas of persistent atelectasis by surrounding hyperinflated lung can suggest deterioration, however, and if one lung happens to inflate more than another an erroneous suspicion of diaphragmatic paralysis on the unexpanded size may arise [94]. In a group of patients studied by McLoud [86] pulmonary barotrauma occurred in as many as 25%; all pneumothoraces were under tension, and 50% were bilateral. Finally, when ventilation is withdrawn parenchymal shadowing may reappear without clinical deterioration.

Abdomen

Detection of pneumoperitoneum

In the critically ill patient a large pneumoperitoneum may be clinically silent. Air loculating anteriorly in the supine position is detectable if of sufficient volume to separate loops of bowel (Fig. 60.16). Unusual gas shadows within the abdomen are frequently problematical. If free gas is suspected it is useful to lie the patient on the left side for ten minutes prior to making an

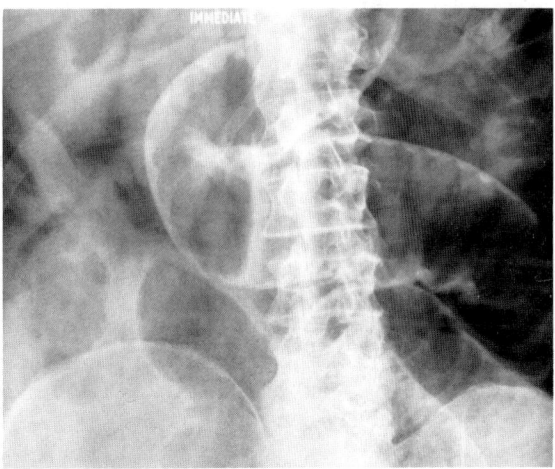

Fig. 60.16. Massive pneumoperitoneum in a moribund uraemic patient, noted on the preliminary film of an urgent IVU. The cause was a perforated diverticulum of the sigmoid colon. Air can be clearly seen both inside and outside the walls of several jejunal loops.

erect radiograph. This encourages the gas to move over the right lobe of the liver where its nature may be more easily recognised; but failure of the gas to move in this way does not of course prove it to be intraluminal. The observation has been made that small amounts of free peritoneal gas are better detected on the erect abdominal film exposed in full expiration when the diaphragms are held as high as possible [93].

Diagnosis of bowel obstruction

Fluid levels within the abdomen less than 3 cm in length and less than three in number are unlikely to be significant. The *step-ladder* pattern is due to multiple fluid levels of varying heights, and the *string-of-beads* sign is due to a chain of small gas bubbles which have collected between the plicae semicirculares of the upper wall of an otherwise fluid-filled loop of jejunum. Both signs are seen more frequently in mechanical obstruction than in adynamic ileus. The diagnosability of certain types of closed loop obstruction on plain radiographs has been recently emphasized; these are caecal volvulus [144], sigmoid volvulus [145], small-bowel closed loops [137], and ileosigmoid knot [146].

Emergency contrast studies

Water-soluble contrast agents in the gastro-intestinal tract

Barium sulphate suspensions provide better anatomical detail than water-soluble media and should be used wherever possible. The disadvantages of barium in some emergency applications are its relatively slow transit time through the small bowel; its tendency to inspissate in the large bowel may convert a partial into a complete obstruction; and leakage into the peritoneal cavity or soft tissues may cause adhesions or granulomas. On the other hand, water-soluble agents (of which Gastrografin is the most palatable) transit rapidly through the small bowel because they are hygroscopic and act as cathartics; they are quickly absorbed across the peritoneum and from soft tissues. Their use is confined by Margulis [85] to the identification of perforations of the GI tract, including leaking anastomoses, and the delineation of mechanical obstruction. *Perforations* are usually outlined by contrast leaking from the lumen, and because these agents are rapidly absorbed across the

peritoneum urinary tract opacification occurs. Indeed, if the urinary tract is well opacified, especially if calyces are seen, a perforation can be presumed to be present even if the actual leak has not been delineated. *Intestinal obstruction* is rapidly revealed, as Gastrografin normally transits the small bowel in less than 30 min and opacifies the colon within about 1 h even in the presence of ileus; it may opacify an obstructed closed loop [137].

There are two dangers in the use of water-soluble media. The first is the very real possibility of inducing dehydration or electrolyte imbalance, especially if injudiciously large quantities are given; and the second is that entering on the respiratory tract in concentrations exceeding 20% they cause pulmonary oedema [110]. If there is a suspicion that ingested contrast medium may enter the respiratory tract, other media should be used.

Intravenous urography

For investigation of patients with deteriorating renal function the administration of 40 or 50 g iodine may be required. At these doses anuria has occasionally occurred. Diabetics with cardiac and renal dysfunction and patients with paraproteinaemia are at the greatest risk [30, 91]; it is important to have patients well hydrated prior to the administration of high doses of contrast medium [30].

Computed axial tomography (CT)

Cranial

This imaging modality is firmly established as the first-line investigation in suspected intracranial disease and can easily be performed on critically ill patients. It should be realized that contrast enhancement is often utilized during the examination, involving the IV administration of 30 or 40 g iodine, as in high-dose urography

Head injury

There have been several general reviews illustrating the types of abnormality shown by CT with discussion of their clinical significance [134].
Parenchymal injury. Focal areas of low attenuation sometimes enhance after contrast, and focal

haematomas (Fig. 60.17) are associated with cerebral contusion, including shearing injuries of the white matter [149]. Intraventricular haematoma is quite common; it clears within 5 days or so, usually without sequelae, contrary to what was thought prior to CT.

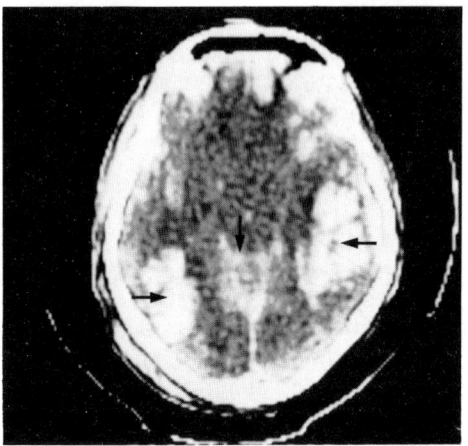

Fig. 60.17. Head injury, showing large bilateral intracerebral haematomas in the temporal lobes (*horizontal arrows*), and also subarachnoid blood in the quadrigeminal cistern (*vertical arrow*).

Extracerebral collections. These acute surgical emergencies are well shown, and the distinction between subdural, epidural, or subarachnoid location can usually be made. An occasional problem is presented by isodense subdural haematomas, which cannot be differentiated from normal brain and are seen only by their mass effect (Fig. 60.18). Techniques for enhancing the attenuation of normal brain have been devised to assist recognition of these collections [55, 70]. In a recent review of the findings in non-accidental head injury in children [148] acute subdural haematomas were the commonest abnormality and were frequently found alongside the falx cerebri.

Stroke

Cerebral infarction is detected within 12–24 h of onset [29], and is usually diagnosed with confidence [71, 141]. *Intracerebral haemorrhage* is easy to see even if only a few millimetres in size. Haematomas become very dense 3–4 h after extravasation and gradually shrink from the periphery over a few days. *Pressure cones* produced by mass effect from any cause can be recognised on CT at the tentorial hiatus (Fig. 60.19) and sometimes foramen magnum

levels [96]. *Spontaneous subarachnoid haemorrhage* is demonstrable by the recognition of subarachnoid haematoma in 90% of cases, provided they are scanned within 5 days of bleeding [118].

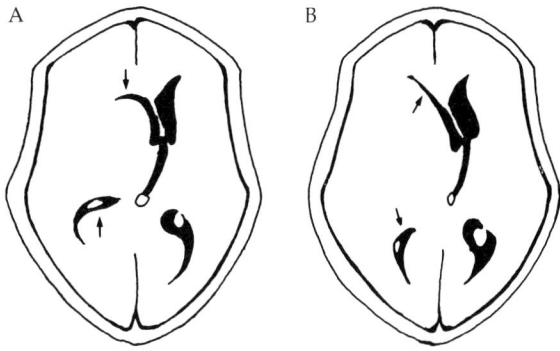

Fig. 60.18. A Isodense subdural haematoma. **B** Isodense deep cerebral tumour of the left hemisphere. Note how the diffuse mass effect in **A** produces posterior displacement of the trigone region as well as dislocation of midline structures to the right. This is characteristic of subfalcine herniation of the cingulate gyrus and suggests the presence of an extracerebral convexity collection, whereas the ventricular distortion shown in **B** does not.

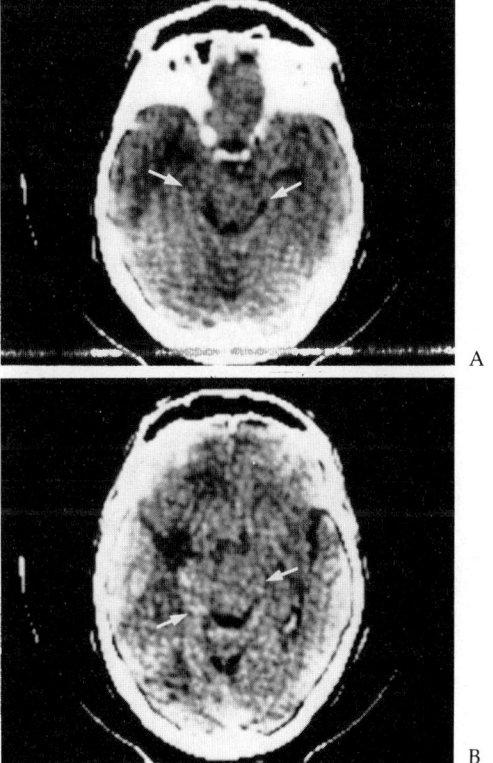

Fig. 60.19. The uncus (**A**, *arrow*) and parahippocampal and lingual gyri (**B**, *arrow*) presenting at the tentorial hiatus and compressing and rotating the brain stem (**A** and **B**, *right arrows*).

Encephalitis

Scans are usually normal, or show very non-specific abnormalities, such as altered white matter attenuation or a little patchy enhancement after IV contrast. *Herpes simplex* encephalitis, however, may have a characteristic pattern of low attenuation in a temporal lobe with occasional pathological enhancement occurring in the opercular gyri [23].

Body

This modality lacks a well-defined place in the investigation of acutely ill patients. Some areas have been explored [20, 57, 84, 104, 107, 121] but serious problems are created by ECG wires, endotracheal tubes, central venous pressure lines, etc., which induce disturbing artefacts in the reconstructed images.

Diagnostic ultrasonography

Technical considerations

The last year has seen the general availability of ultrasound instruments which are portable and produce dynamic images (real-time) but which have image quality comparable to conventional static B-scanners. Virtually all the diagnostic capabilities of ultrasonography can now be realised at the bedside.

Diagnostic aspects

Fluid spaces are imaged preferentially, so that ultrasonography is most effective in demonstrating anatomical abnormalies of vessels, ducts, and fluid-filled viscera.

Vascular imaging

Abdominal aortic aneurysms are detected in over 90% of cases. The extent and size of the true lumen, and of intramural thrombi are more readily assessed than by any other imaging modality [33]. A clinical diagnosis of acute dissection can be confirmed by careful study of the walls of the aneurysm [9] (Fig. 60.20). Vascular thrombosis of small vessels is difficult to assess, but is apparent in major vessels, such as the inferior vena cava, portal vein, and renal veins [88, 128]. Measurements of the calibre of veins correlate well with venous pressure, particularly in portal venous hypertension. Renal vein thrombosis is diagnosed by changes in renal

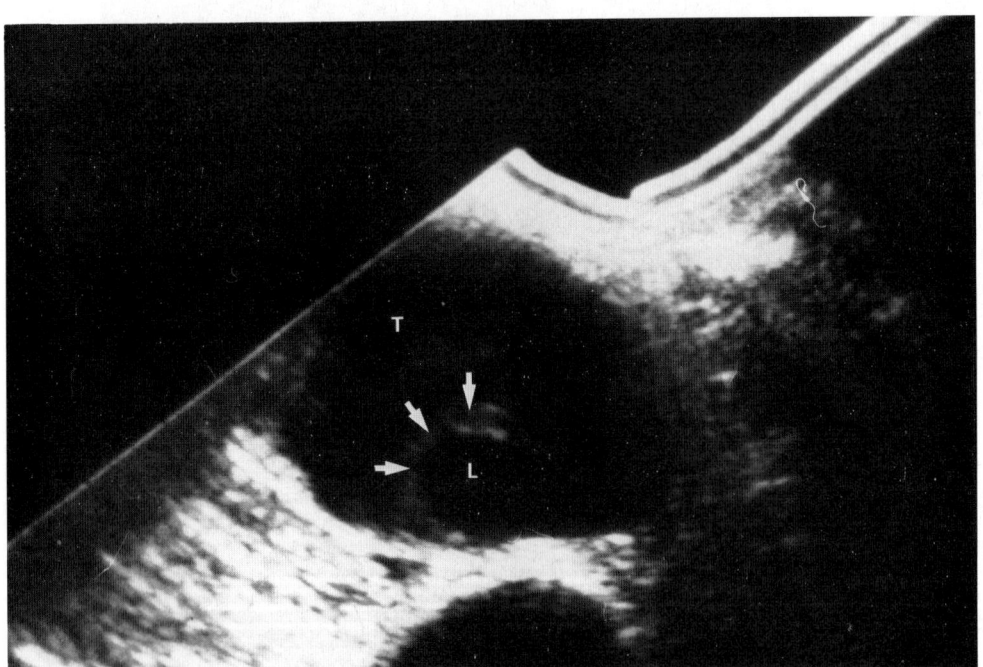

Fig. 60.20. Aortic aneurysm: A horizontal section 4 cm below the origin of the renal arteries, showing a posteriorly placed fluid lumen with an echogenic rim; surrounding this is the poorly reflective, thrombus-filled aortic wall. *L*, lumen; *T*, thrombus; *arrows*, intima.

size and parenchymal appearance, and also by a failure to demonstrate renal vein patency or pulsation when the renal hilus has been well visualized [39].

Trauma

Trauma to the kidney, spleen or liver is assessed by studying the integrity of the organ capsule and by seeking both intra- and extra-organ haematoma formation [2, 68]. Retroperitoneal haematomas appear as poorly reflective masses.

Renal failure

A hydronephrosis is readily recognized by distension of the pelvicalyceal system and ureter, and the obstructing lesion is often demonstrated. Sensitivity is as high as 98%, which is similar to that of IVU [142] (Fig. 60.21). Other recognizable causes of renal failure include renal and perirenal abscesses [117], polycystic kidneys, end-stage nephritides and acute tubular or cortical necrosis. It is becoming accepted that ultrasonography is the first-choice imaging investigation in newly discovered renal failure [115].

Biliary system and pancreas

The capabilities of ultrasonography in the diagnosis of gallbladder stones [19], jaundice [114, 135], and chronic pancreatic disease [79, 95] are well known. Of greater relevance to this discussion are the effects of trauma [136], infection, or acute pancreatitis. Fluid leaks from the biliary tree [139], pancreatic pseudocysts, or abscesses [27] can be detected in virtually all cases.

Liver

Cystic spaces within the liver as small as 2–3 mm are readily detected and can be separated on ultrasonographic criteria alone into simple or hydatid cysts and amoebic or pyogenic abscesses, or necrotic tumours [8, 87, 131] (Fig. 60.22).

Extravisceral fluid collections

Thorax. Bone and gas block the transmission of the ultrasound beam. Thus thoracic ultrasonography is limited to the study of masses, fluid collections, and abscesses in continuity with the diaphragm or intercostal spaces, such as pericardial and pleural effusions, cysts, and mediastinal abscesses.

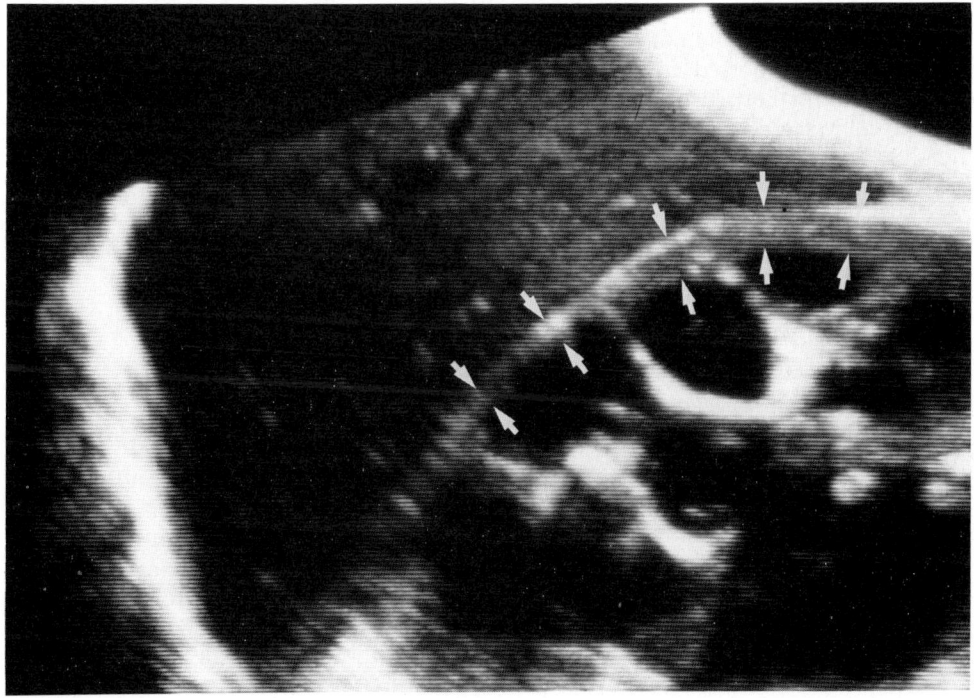

Fig. 60.21. Right hydronephrosis: A parasagittal section through the right lobe of the liver and long axis of the right kidney. The kidney contains multiple large fluid spaces grouped around a central large fluid space. These are the distended calyces and renal pelvis. Significant thinning of the cortex is noted between liver and distended calyx (*arrows*).

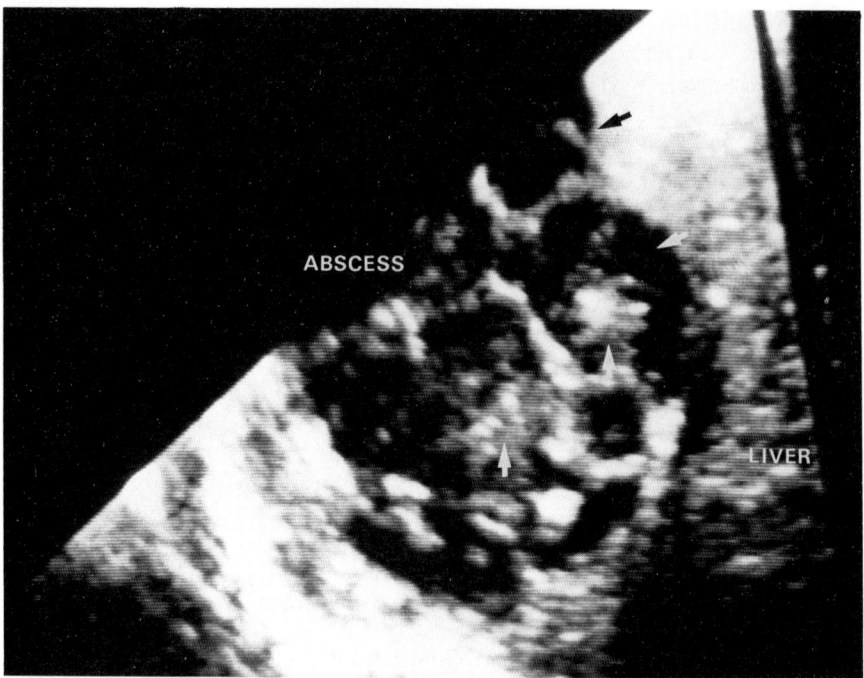

Fig. 60.22. Liver abscess: A small-angle sector scan through the intercostal spaces, demonstrating an intrahepatic abscess. The abscess is part solid, part cystic (*open* and *closed arrows*) and septation is seen. There is a sharp border between the abscess and surrounding normal liver parenchyma.

Intra-abdominal fluid collections. Detection and recognition of pus in the abdomen can be very reliable. In a recent series 70 of 75 intra-abdominal abscesses were detected [130]. Abscesses were correctly excluded in 143 of 145 cases and similar results are reported for all common sites of intra-abdominal abscesses [74, 83]. Study of associated viscera and of the acoustic properties of the fluid will usually indicate the nature and origin of the pus, blood, or ascitic fluid [28, 31, 143].

Monitoring the progress of disease

Two decades of experience in obstetric ultra-sonography have proven the technique to be ideal for measurement. The calibre of vessels, the size of organs, fluid collections, tumours, haematomas, or pseudocysts measured serially allows documentation of the response to treatment.

Ultrasonographic guidance of biopsy needles and drainage catheters

Echoes returning from a needle or catheter are clearly seen and allow guidance to a target to be controlled by 'direct vision' with great accuracy [46].

Malignant disease can be diagnosed by fine-needle aspiration biopsy [38]. Drainage catheters can be placed into pleural or pericardial effusions, into abscesses, pseudocysts [52], or extrabiliary collections [124]. Percutaneous nephrostomy [125, 126] is similarly performed to relieve an obstructive uropathy and multifocal liver abscesses have been treated by a combination of aspiration and direct injection of antibiotic into the cavities (W.R. Lees, 1980, unpublished work).

Contrast radiology and therapeutic implications

In addition to the role of contrast radiology in diagnosis, an increasing number of radiologically guided therapeutic procedures are being reported. These therapeutic manoeuvres in most cases follow on logically from diagnostic procedures. They may be considered as alternatives to conventional surgical procedures but have the advantages that they are less traumatic and do not require general anaesthesia. In some cases they constitute definitive management, in others they are temporising, improving the patient's condition for later surgery. There is considerable scope for further innovation in interventional radiology.

Pulmonary embolism

The diagnosis of acute massive pulmonary embolism may be confirmed by pulmonary arteriography. A technique of transvenous basket extraction of emboli through a femoral or internal jugular venotomy under local anaesthesia has been described by Greenfield and Zocco [49], but the indications are not yet clearly established. The likelihood of further embolism may be reduced by interruption of inferior vena caval flow with a filter introduced through the venotomy and sited accurately under radiological control [48]. Berland et al. [7] have critically compared the two designs of filter in common use.

Oesophageal varices

A percutaneous transhepatic catheter may be introduced under local anaesthesia into a branch of the portal vein and directed retrogradely into the portal branches supplying varices. A variety of agents has been injected to sclerose or occlude these portosystemic shunts [82, 101], and the indications and results have been critically discussed by Passariello et al. [100].

Biliary tract

The diagnosis of obstructive jaundice is usually confirmed by ultrasound. For a precise demonstration of the site of obstruction and the cause cholangiography is required, and in the presence of jaundice contrast must be introduced into the biliary tree direct. This may be accomplished by the percutaneous transhepatic method or by endoscopic retrograde cannulation.

The obstructed biliary system may be drained externally through a catheter introduced transhepatically under local anaesthesia [25, 37, 92]. Drainage avoids the need for urgent surgery, which can be performed electively when the patient's liver function and general condition have improved. This may be of particular value in the hepatorenal syndrome and when multiple liver abscesses complicate obstructive cholangitis; such abscesses rapidly resolve with adequate drainage [87]. Percutaneous biliary diversion may also be useful in the management of postoperative biliary leaks.

Burhenne [12] has described a technique for the extraction of retained biliary stones through the T-tube track. His steerable catheter can be used under radiological control to resite a biliary drain, e.g., above an obstruction when there is complicating sepsis; dislodged or blocked drainage tubes can be replaced in the bile duct or other sites.

Alternatively, drainage catheters may be positioned on gallstones removed endoscopically under radiological guidance [17, 18, 76].

Urinary tract

Supravesical obstruction accompanied by uraemia or infection has traditionally been managed by retrograde ureteric catheterization, or by surgical nephrostomy when catheterization fails. However, an alternative method of management is to introduce a drainage catheter directly into the renal pelvis under local anaesthesia with radiological or ultrasound guidance. The technique is reviewed by Stables [126] and is applicable also to the transplanted kidney [102]. After the uraemia and infection have been brought under control definitive surgery may be performed or stones extracted percutaneously [36, 99]. If surgery is contraindicated a catheter can be placed through a ureteric stricture as an internal splint, a manoeuvre performed over a guide wire introduced through the percutaneous nephrostomy [47, 103].

Angiography

Acute GI haemorrhage

Provided the patient is actively bleeding at the time, angiography usually shows the site [1], and selective infusion of vasopressin or embolization with various agents usually arrests the haemorrhage. Bleeding lesions in the stomach, duodenum [138], colon [3, 122], rectosigmoid [16], and liver have been successfully managed in this way.

Renal

Haemorrhage in polycystic disease [54] and following renal biopsy [113] has been arrested by embolization. Life-threatening massive proteinuria in a dialysis patient unfit for surgical nephrectomy has been stopped by 'embolization nephrectomy' [26] and severe hypertension in a renal transplant patient relieved by percutaneous dilatation of a stricture at the site of arterial anastomosis [123].

Unusual indications

Emergency hepatic embolisation resulted in immediate relief of severe hypercalcaemia secondary to hepatoma [111] relieving intractable cardiac arrhythmia and illustrating the versatility of the technique. Epistaxis [69], puerperal pelvic haemorrhage [56], bleeding from carcinoma of the cervix and other tumours, haemoptysis (bronchial artery embolization), bleeding from pelvic fracture [140] and several other critical situations [60] have all been successfully managed by arterial embolization.

References

1. Allison DJ (1980) Gastrointestinal bleeding. Radiological diagnosis Br J Hosp Med 23:358–365
2. Asher WM, Parvin S, Virgilio RW, Harber K (1980) Echographic evaluation of splenic injury after blunt trauma. Radiology 118:411–415
3. Athanasoulis CA, Baum S, Rösch J et al. (1975) Mesenteric arterial infusions of vasopressin for haemorrhage from colonic diverticulosis. Am J Surg 129:212–216
4. Bachynski JE (1971) Absence of the air bronchogram sign. A reliable finding in pulmonary embolism with infarction or haemorrhage. Radiology 100:547–552
5. Baron NG (1972) Fleischner lines and pulmonary emboli. Circulation 45:171–178
6. Berkman YM (1980) Aspiration and inhalation pneumonias. Semin Roentgenol 15:73–84
7. Berland LL, Maddison FE, Bernhard VM (1980) Radiological follow-up of vena cava filter devices. AJR 134:1047–1052
8. Boultbee JE, Simjee AE, Rooknoodeen F, Engelbrecht HE (1979) Experience with Grey-scale ultrasonography in hepatic amoebiasis. Clin Radiol 30:683–689
9. Bresnihan R, Keates PG (1980) Ultrasound and dissection of the abdominal aorta. Clin Radiol 31:105–108
10. Bryk D (1976) Infrapulmonary effusion. Radiology 120:33–36
11. Bulmer SR, Lamb D, McCormack RJM, Walbaum PR (1978) The aetiology of unresolved pneumonia. Thorax 33:307–314
12. Burhenne HJ (1974) The technique of biliary stone extraction. Radiology 113:567–572
13. Bynum LJ, Pierce AK (1976) Pulmonary aspiration of gastric contents. Am Rev Respir Dis 114:1129–1136
14. Bynum LJ, Wilson JE (1978) Pleural effusions in pulmonary embolism. Am Rev Respir Dis 117:829–834
15. Christensen EE, Dietz GW (1976) Subpulmonary pneumothorax in patients with chronic obstructive pulmonary disease. Radiology 121:33–37
16. Chuang VP, Wallace S, Zornoza J, Davis LJ (1979) Transcatheter arterial occlusion in the management of rectosigmoidal bleeding. Radiology 133:605–609
17. Cotton PB (1980) Non-operative removal of bile duct stones by duodenoscopic sphincterotomy. Br J Surg 67:1–5
18. Cotton PB, Burney PG, Mason RR (1979) Trans-nasal bile duct catheterisation after endoscopic sphincterotomy. Gut 20:285–287
19. Crade M (1980) Comparison of ultrasound and oral cholecystogram in the diagnosis of gallstones. In: Taylor KJW (ed) Diagnostic ultrasound in gastrointestinal disease. Churchill Livingstone, London, pp 123–136
20. Crowe JK, Brown LR, Buhm JR (1978) CT of the mediastinum. Radiology 128:75–87
21. Daffner RH (1977) Pseudofracture of the dens: Mach bands. AJR 128:607–612
22. Dandy WE (1978) Incomplete pulmonary interlobar fissure sign. Radiology 128:21–25
23. Davis JM, Davis KR, Kleinman GM, Kirschner HS, Taveras JM (1978) CT of herpes simplex encephalitis with clinico-pathological correlation. Radiology 129:409–417
24. Don C, Johnson R (1977) The nature and significance of peribronchial cuffing in pulmonary oedema. Radiology 125:577–582
25. Dooey JS, Dick R, Olney J, Sherlock S (1979) Nonsurgical treatment of biliary obstruction. Lancet II:1040–1043
26. Dotter CT, Goldman ML, Rösch J (1975) Instant selective arterial occlusion with isobutyl 2-cyanoacrylate. Radiology 114:227–230
27. Doust BD, Pearce JA (1976) Grey-scale ultrasonic properties of the normal and inflamed pancreas. Radiology 120:653–657
28. Doust BD, Thompson R (1978) Ultrasonography of abdominal fluid collections. Gastrointest Radiol 3:273–279
29. Drayer BP, Dujouny M, Boehnke M, Wolfson SK (1977) The capacity for computed tomographic diagnosis of cerebral infarction. Radiology 125:393–402
30. Dure-Smith P (1976) Opinion: Fluid restriction before excretory urography. Radiology 118:487–489
31. Edell SL, Gefter WB (1979) Ultrasonic differentiation of types of ascitic fluid. AJR 133:111–114
32. Ellison LH, Kirsh MM (1974) Delayed mediastinal tamponade after open heart surgery. Chest 65:64–66
33. Eriksson I, Hemmingsson A, Lindgren PG (1980) Diagnosis of abdominal aortic aneurysm by aortography, computer tomography and ultrasound. Acta Radiol [Diagn] (Stockh) 21:209–214
34. Feldman F, Ellis K, Green WM (1975) Fat embolism syndrome. Radiology 114:535–542
35. Felson B, Felson H (1950) Localisation of intrathoracic lesions by means of the PA roentgenogram. The silhouette sign. Radiology 55:363–374
36. Fernström I, Johansson B (1976) Percutaneous pyelolithotomy. A new extraction technique. Scand J Urol Nephrol 10:257–259
37. Ferrucci JT, Mueller PR, Harbin WP (1980a) Percutaneous transhepatic biliary drainage. Radiology 135:1–13
38. Ferrucci JT, Withenberg J, Mueller PR, et al. (1980b) Diagnosis of abdominal malignancy by radiologic fine needle aspiration biopsy. AJR 134:323–330
39. Finberg HJ, Hillman B, Smith EH (1980) Ultrasound in the evaluation of the non-functioning kidney: In Rosenfield AT (ed) Genitourinary ultrasonography. Churchill Livingstone, London, pp 105–123
40. Fishbone G, Robbins DI, Osborn DJ, Grinja V (1973) Trauma to the thoracic aorta and greater vessels. Radiol Clin North Am 11:543–554
41. Fletcher BD (1978) Mediastinal herniation of parietal pleura: A useful sign of pneumothorax in supine neonates. AJR 130:469–472
42. Forrest JV, Shackelford GD, Bramson RT, Anderson LS (1973) Acute mediastinal widening. AJR 117:881–885
43. Fraser RG, Paré JAP (1977a) The Acinar shadow. In:

Diagnosis of diseases of the chest, 2nd edn, vol 1. Saunders, Philadelphia, pp 344–345

44. Fraser RG, Paré JAP (1977b) Embolic and thrombotic diseases of the lungs. In: Diagnosis of diseases of the chest, 2nd edn, vol 2. Saunders, Philadelphia, pp 1135–1175

45. Gamsa G, Thurlbeck WM, Macklem PT, Fraser RG (1971) Roentgenographic appearance of the human pulmonary acinus. Invest Radiol 6:171

46. Goldberg BB, Cole-Beuglet C, Kurtz AB (1980) Real-time aspiration biopsy transducer. J Clin Ultrasound 8:107–112

47. Goldin AR (1977) Percutaneous ureteral splinting. Urology 10:165–168

48. Greenfield LJ (1979) Technical considerations for insertion of vena caval filters. Surg Gynecol Obstet 148:422–426

49. Greenfield LJ, Zocco JJ (1979) Intraluminal management of acute massive pulmonary thromboembolism. J Thorac Cardiovasc Surg 77:402–410

50. Griffith GL, Maull KI, Sachatello CR (1977) Septic pulmonary embolisation. Surg Gynecol Obstet 144:105–108

51. Griscom NT, Wohl MEB, Kirkpatrick JA (1978) Lower respiratory tract infection: How infants differ from adults. Radiol Clin North Am 16:367–387

52. Hancke S, Pedersen JF (1976) Pseudocyst needle drainage. Surg Gynecol Obstet 42:551

53. Hanke R, Kretzschmer R (1980) Round atelectasis. Semin Roentgenol 15:174–182

54. Harley JD, Shen FH, Carter SJ (1980) Transcatheter infarction of a polycystic kidney for control of recurrent haemorrhage. AJR 134:818–820

55. Hayman LA, Evans RA, Hinck VC (1979) Rapid high dose contrast CT of isodense subdural haematoma and cerebral swelling. Radiology 131:381–383

56. Heaston DK, Mineau DE, Brown BJ, Miller FJ (1979) Transcatheter arterial embolization for control of persistent massive puerperal haemorrhage after bilateral surgical hypogastric artery ligation. AJR 133:152–154

57. Heitzman ER, Goldwin RL, Proto AV (1977a) Radiological analysis of the mediastinum utilizing computed tomography. Radiol Clin North Am 15:309–329

58. Heitzman ER, Markarian B, Berger I, Daily E (1969) The secondary pulmonary lobule: A practical concept for interpretation of chest radiographs. I. Roentgen anatomy of the normal secondary lobule. II. Application of the anatomic concept to an understanding of the roentgen pattern in disease states. Radiology 93:507–512

59. Heitzman ER, Ziter FM, Markarian B, McClennan B, Sherry H (1977b) Kerley's interlobular septal lines: Roentgen pathological correlation. AJR 100:578–582

60. Higgins CB, Siemers PT, Bookstein JJ, Utley JR (1979) Control of haemorrhage from a common carotid arterio-cutaneous fistula by temporary implantation of a balloon catheter. Radiology 132:224–226

61. Hublitz VF, Shapiro JH (1969) A typical pulmonary patterns of congestive failure in chronic lung disease. The influence of pre-existing diseases on the appearance and distribution of pulmonary oedema. Radiology 93:995–1006

62. Itzchak Y, Rosenthal T, Adar R, Rubinstein ZJ, Leiberman Y, Deutsch V (1975) Dissecting aneurysm of the thoracic aorta: Reapprasal of the radiographic diagnosis. AJR 125:559–570

63. Jefferson K, Rees S (1973) Pulmonary venous hypertension. In: Clinical cardiac radiology. Butterworths, London, pp 84–94

64. Joffe N (1974) Adult respiratory distress syndrome. AJR 112:719–732

65. Joseph AEA, de Lacey GJ, Bryant THE, Stoker DJ, Ayr G (1978) The hypertransradiant hemithorax. The importance of lateral decentering, and the explanation for its appearance due to rotation. Clin Radiol 29:125–131

66. Kattan KR (1980) Upper mediastinal changes in lower lobe collapse. Semin Roentgenol 15:183–186

67. Kattan KR, Eyler WR, Felson B (1980) The juxtaphrenic peak in upper lobe collapse. Semin Roentgenol 15:187–193

68. Kay CJ, Rosenfield AT, Armm M (1980) Grey-scale ultrasonography in the evaluation of renal trauma. Radiology 134:461–466

69. Kendall BE, Zilkha E, Loh L, Hayward R, Radue EW, Ingram GS (1978) Diagnosis of subdural haematoma by computed axial tomography: Use of xenon inhalation for contrast enhancement. J Neurol Neurosurg Psychiatry 41:370–373

70. Kendall BE, Joyner M, Grant H (1977) Hereditary haemorrhagic telangiectasia—microembolization in the management of epistaxis. Clin Otolaryngol 2:249–261

71. Kinkel WR, Jacobs L (1976) CAT in cerebral vascular disease. Neurology 26:924–930

72. Kreel L, Slavin G, Herbert A, Sandin B (1975) Intralobular septal oedema. D-Lines. Clin Radiol 26:209–221

73. Landay MJ, Christensen EE, Bynum LJ, Goodman C (1980) Anaerobic pleural and pulmonary infections. AJR 134:233–240

74. Landay MJ, Harless W (1977) Ultrasonic differentiation of right pleural effusion from sub-phrenic fluid on longitudinal scans of the right upper quadrant. Radiology 123:155–8

75. Lane EJ, Proto AV, Phillips TW (1976) Mach Bands and density perception. Radiology 121:9–17

76. Laurence BH, Cotton PB (1980) Decompression of malignant biliary obstruction by duodenoscopic intubation of bile duct. Br Med J 280:522–523

77. Lavender JP, Doppman J (1963) The hilum in pulmonary venous hypertension. Br J Radiol 35:303–313

78. Leeming BWA (1973) Gravitational oedema of the lungs observed during assisted respiration. Chest 64:719–722

79. Lees WR, Vallon AG, Denyer ME, Vahl SP, Cotton PB (1979) Prospective study of ultrasonography in chronic pancreatic disease. Br Med J i:162–4

80. Lipinski JK, Weisbrod GL, Sanders DE (1980) Exogenous lipoid pneumonitis. J Can Assoc Radiol 31:92–98

81. Longuet R, Phelan J, Tanous H, Buskong S (1977) Criteria of the silhouette sign. Radiology 122:581–585

82. Lunderquist A, Börjesson B, Owman T, Bengmark S (1978) Isobutyl 2-cyanoacrylate (Bucrylate) in obliteration of gastric coronary vein and oesophageal varices. AJR 130:1–6

83. Maklad NF, Doust BD, Baum JK (1974) Ultrasonic diagnosis of post-operative intra-abdominal abscesses. Radiology 113:417–422

84. Mall JC, Kaiser JA (1980) CT diagnosis of splenic laceration. AJR 134:265–269

85. Margulis AR (1973) The use of iodinated water-soluble contrast agents in acute gastrointestinal diseases. In: Margulis AR, Burhenne JH (eds) Alimentary tract roentgenogology, vol 1, 2nd edn. Mosby, St Louis, pp 271–280

86. McLoud T, Barash PG, Ravin C (1977) PEEP: Radiographic features and associated complications. AJR 129:209–213

87. Meire HB, Husband J (1979) Demonstration of focal

liver disease by ultrasound and computed tomography. In: Taylor KJW (ed) Diagnostic ultrasound in gastrointestinal disease: Churchill Livingstone New York, London pp 35–38

88. Merritt CRB (1979) Ultrasonographic demonstration of portal vein thrombosis. Radiology 133:425–427

89. Milne ENC (1973) Correlation of physiological findings and chest roentgenology. Radiol Clin North Am 11:17–48

90. Milne ENC (1978) Some new concepts of pulmonary blood flow and volume. Radiol Clin North Am 16:515–536

91. Myers GH, Witten DM (1971) Acute renal failure after excretory urography in multiple myeloma. (Editorial) AJR 113:583–588

92. Nakayama T, Ikeda A, Okuda K (1978) Percutaneous transhepatic drainage of the biliary tract. Gastroenterology 74:554–559

93. Oestreich AE (1977) Pneumoperitoneum: A technical remark concerning detection (Abstract) Radiology 125:567

94. Oh KS, Stitik FP, Galvis AG, Mearman SB, Heller RM, Dorst JP (1974) Radiological manifestation in patients on continuous positive pressure breathing. Radiology 110:627–630

95. Ohto M, Saotome N, Saisho H (1980) Real-time sonography of the pancreatic duct. Application to percutaneous pancreatic ductography. AJR 134:647–652

96. Osborn A (1977) Diagnosis of descending transtentorial herniation by cranial CT. Radiology 123:93–96

97. Ostendorf P, Birzle H, Vogel W, Mittermayer C (1975) Pulmonary radiographic abnormalities in shock: Roentgen–clinical–pathological correlation. Radiology 115:257–263

98. Ovenfors CO, Hedgcock MW (1978) Intensive care unit radiology: Problems of interpretation. Radiol Clin North Am 16:407–439

99. Palestrant AM, Rad FF, Sacks BA, Klein LA (1980) Post-operative percutaneous kidney stone extraction. Radiology 134:778–779

100. Passariello R, Rossi P, Simonetti G, Ciolina A, Rovight L (1979) Emergency transhepatic obliteration of bleeding varices. Cardiovasc Radiol 2:97–106

101. Pereiras R, Viamonte M, Russell E, Le Page J, White P, Hutson D (1977) New techniques for interruption of gastro-oesophageal venous blood flow. Radiology 124:313–323

102. Petrek J, Tilney NL, Smith EH, Williams JS, Vineyard GC (1977) Ultrasound in renal transplantation. Ann Surg 185:441–447

103. Pingoud EG, Bagley DH, Zeman RK, Glancy KE, Pais AS (1980) Percutaneous antegrade bilateral ureteral dilatation and stent placement for internal drainage. Radiology 134:780

104. Pistolesi GF, Marzoli GP, Colasso PO, Pederzoli P, Procoicci C (1978) Computed tomography in surgical pancreatic emergencies. J Comput Assist Tomogr 2:165–169

105. Pistolesi M, Giuntini C (1978) Assessment of extravascular lung water. Radiol Clin North Am 16:551–574

106. Proto AV, Tocino I (1980) Lobar collapse. Semin Roentgenol 15:117–173

107. Pugatch RD, Faling LJ, Robbins AH, Snider GL (1978) Differentiation of pleural and pulmonary lesions using CT. J Comput Assist Tomogr 2:601–606

108. Putman CE, Tummillo DA, Myerson DA, Myerson PJ (1975) Drowning: Another plunge. AJR 125:543–548

109. Raphael MJ (1963) Mediastinal haematoma, description

of some radiological appearances. Br J Radiol 36:921–924

110. Reich SB (1969) Production of pulmonary oedema by aspiration of water-soluble; non absorbable contrast media. Radiology 92:367–370

111. Roche A, Franco D, Dhumeaux D, Bismuth H, Doyon D (1979) Emergency hepatic arterial embolization for secondary hypercalcaemia in hepatocellular carcinoma. Radiology 133:315–316

112. Rohlfing BM, Webb WR, Schlobohm RM (1976) Ventilator-related extra-alveolar air in adults. Radiology 121:25–31

113. Rosen RJ, Feldman L, Wilson AR (1978) Embolization for post-biopsy arteriovenous fistula: Effective occlusion using homologous clot AJR 131:1072–1073

114. Sample WF, Sarti DA, Goldstein LI, Winer M, Kadell BM (1978) Grey-scale ultrasonography of the jaundiced patient. Radiology 128:719–725

115. Sanders RC, Bearman S (1976) B-scan ultrasound in the evaluation of renal failure. Radiology 119:199–202

116. Schneider HJ, Felson B, Gonzalez LL (1980) Round atelectasis. AJR 134:225–232

117. Schneider M, Becher JA, Staiano S (1976) Sonographic correlation of renal and peri-renal infections. AJR 127:1007–1004

118. Scotti G, Ethier R, Melancon D, Terbrugge K, Tchang S (1977) CT in the evaluation of intracranial aneuryms and subarachnoid haemorrhage. Radiology 123:85–90

119. Shin MS, Ho K (1979) Cavitatory pulmonary lesions complicating use of flow directed balloon tipped catheters in two cases. AJR 132:650–1652

120. Shook DR, Cram KB, Williams AJ (1975) Pulmonary venous air embolism in hyaline membrane disease. AJR 125:538–542

121. Sinner WN (1978) Computed tomographic patterns of pulmonary thromboembolism and infarction. J Comput Assist Tomogr 2:395–399

122. Sniderman FW, Franklin J, Sos TA (1978) Successful transcatheter Gelfoam embolization of a bleeding cecal vascular ectasia. AJR 131:157–159

123. Sniderman KW, Sos TA, Sprayregen S, Saddekni S, Cheigh JS, Tapia L, Tellis V, Veith FJ (1980) Percutaneous transluminal angioplasty in renal transplant arterial stenosis for relief of hypertension. Radiology 135:23–26

124. Smith EH, Bartrum RJ (1974) Ultrasonically guided percutaneous aspiration of abscesses. AJR 122:308

125. Stables DP, Ginsberg NJ, Johnson ML (1978) Percutaneous nephrostomy: A series and review of the literature AJR 130:75–82

126. Stables DP, Johnson ML (1980) Percutaneous nephrostomy. The role of ultrasound. In: Rosenfield AT (ed) Genitourinary ultrasonography. Churchill Livingstone, New York, pp 73–87

127. Swischuk LE (1977) Bubbles in hyaline membrane disease. Differentiation of three types. Radiology 122:417–426

128. Taylor KJW (1975) Ultrasonic investigation of inferior vena-caval obstruction. Br J Radiol 48:1024–1026

129. Taylor KJW, McCready VR (1976) A clinical evaluation of Grey-scale ultrasonography. Br J Radiol 49:244–252

130. Taylor KJW, Sullivan DC, Wasson JFM, Rosenfield ART (1978a) Ultrasound and gallium for the diagnosis of abdominal and pelvic abscesses. Gastrointest Radiol 3:281–286

131. Taylor KJW, Wasson JF, De Graaf C, Rosenfield AT, Andriole VT (1978b) Accuracy of Grey-scale ultrasound diagnosis of abdominal and pelvic abscesses in 220 patients. Lancet i:83–86

132. Tisnado J, Tsai FY, Als A, Roach JF (1977) A new sign

of acute traumatic rupture of the thoracic aorta: Displacement of the nasogastric tube to the right. Radiology 125:603–608

133. Todres D, de Bois F, Kramer SS, Moylan FMB, Shannon DC (1976) Endotracheal tube displacement in the newborn infant. J Paediatr 89:126–127

134. Tsai FY, Huprich JE, Gardner FC, Segall HD, Teal TS (1978) Diagnostic and prognostic implication of CT of head trauma. J Comput Assist Tomogr 2:323–331

135. Vallon AG, Lees WR, Cotton PB (1979a) Grey-scale ultrasonography in cholestatic jaundice. Gut 20:51–54

136. Vallon AG, Lees WR, Cotton PB (1979b) Grey-scale ultrasonography and endoscopic pancreatography after pancreatic trauma. Br J Surg 66:169–172

137. Vest B (1962) Roentgenographic diagnosis of strangulated closed loop obstruction of the small intestine. Surg Gynecol Obstet 115:561–567

138. Waltman AC, Greenfield AJ, Novelline RA, Athanasoulis CA (1979) Pyloroduodenal bleeding and intra-arterial vasopressin: Clinical results. AJR 133:643–646

139. Weissman HS, Chun KJ, Frank M (1979) Demonstration of traumatic bile leakage with cholescintingraphy and ultrasonography. AJR 133:843–847

140. White RI, Kaufman SL, Barth KH, DeCaprio V, Strandbert JD (1979) Emblotherapy with detachable balloon catheters. Radiology 131:619–627

141. Wing SD, Norman D, Pollock JA, Newton TH (1975) Contrast enhancement of cerebral infarcts in CT. Radiology 121:89–92

142. Winston M, Pritchard J, Paulin P (1978) Ultrasonography in the management of unexplained renal failure. J Clin Ultrasound 6:23–27

143. Yeh HC, Wolf BS (1977) Ultrasonography in ascites. Radiology 124:783–790

144. Young WS (1980) Further observations in caecal volvulus. Clin Radiol 31:479–483

145. Young WS, Englebrecht HE, Stoker A (1978) Plain film analysis in sigmoid volvulus. Clin Radiol 29:553–560

146. Young WS, White A, Grave F (1978) The radiology of ileo-sigmoid knot. Clin Radiol 29:211–216

147. Youngberg AS (1977) Unilateral diffuse lung opacity. Radiology 123:277–281

148. Zelefsky MN, Lutzker LG (1977) The target sign: New radiological sign of septic pulmonary embolism. AJR 129:453–455

149. Zimmerman RA, Balaniuk LT, Bruce D, Schut L, Uzzell B, Goldberg H (1979) CT of cranio-cerebral injury in the abused child. Radiology 130:687–690

150. Zimmerman RA, Balaniuk LT, Gennerall LT (1978) CT of shearing injuries of cerebral white matter. Radiology 127:393–396

151. Ziter FMH (1977) Major thoracic dehiscence: Radiographic considerations. Radiology 122:587–590

152. Zwillich CW, Pierson DJ, Creagh CE, Sutton FD, Shatz E, Petty TL (1974) Complications of assisted ventilation. A prospective study of 354 consecutive cases. Am J Med 57:161–170

Chapter 61

Nuclear Imaging

Robert M. Donaldson

The applications of radionuclide techniques to the diagnosis and management of critically ill patients are developing so quickly that the average clinician needs guidance on what is likely to be useful in particular circumstances. In the majority of these nuclear studies, a radioactive tracer is administered to evaluate a particular function: no more than an intravenous injection is required, the studies can be performed swiftly with minimal manipulation to the patient, and the radiation dose is often far lower than in equivalent radiological investigations.

Increased interest in nuclear techniques has been linked to the introduction of new radionuclides and the development of detection devices interfaced with advanced data loggers and computers which provide continuously expanding data-processing capabilities and improved detector performance. In addition, mobile (and in the future, portable) instrumentation allows non-invasive studies to be performed at the bedside of the acutely ill patient unable to leave the ICU [43].

This section will outline some aspects of these investigations, which can contribute greatly to successful management and treatment, emphasizing recent progress in the respiratory and cardiovascular area. No attempt will be made to cover the field completely, and it should be borne in mind that in many circumstances the results obtained by nuclear techniques only complement those obtained by other methods, in particular ultrasound and transmission computerized tomography (CT).

Radionuclides

The biological property of the radiopharmaceutical must be matched to the physiology under investigation and the instrument employed to make the measurement [5]. The radioisotope to be used should not emit any nuclear particles (i.e. α or β particles), since these have very limited ranges and are absorbed by tissues, contributing significantly to radiation exposure and aiding very little in detection and diagnosis. Thus, gamma-emitting radionuclides which do not emit nuclear particles are preferred. Some commonly used radiotracers, applications, and mechanisms of localization are summarized in Table 61.1. There are other groups of isotopes that decay by positron (β^+) emission (positron emitting radionuclides). The positrons undergo annihilation reaction, emitting two gamma rays at 180° to each other, which can be measured by annihilation coincidence detection (ACD) with very good spatial resolution. Developments in emission computerized tomography (ECT) with positrons have encouraged the introduction of new radiopharmaceuticals with positron-emitting isotopes. The very short half-life of these agents enables sequential studies to be performed with reduced radiation exposure to the patient, and they have been used, for example, to produce three-dimensional images of tissues, for nuclear angiography in cyanotic neonates (^{191m}iridium), pulmonary ventilation imaging (^{81m}krypton and ^{15}oxygen) in the study of metabolic pathways

Table 61.1. Commonly used radiotracers

Radiopharmaceutical	Use	Mechanism of localization
Radioiodinated fibinogen (fibrinogen uptake test)		Detection of fresh thrombi (active fibrin deposition)
Radioiodinated plasminogen fibrinolytic agents	Thrombus detection (venous thrombosis)	Detection of pre-existing thrombi
99mTc-MAA or pertechnetate (TcO4⁻) (Radionuclide venography)		Blockade (demonstrates mechanical obstruction)
99mTc-Albumin macro-aggregates (MAA) or microspheres	Lung perfusion	Blockade of capillaries
Xenon–133 Xenon–127 Krypton-81 m	Lung ventilation	Diffusion
Thallium ions (2o1 TL)	Myocardial perfusion imaging	Diffusion and exchange
99mTc-Pyrophosphate 99mTc-Imidodiphosphate	Detection of acutely damaged myocardium	Controversial. ? Calcium salt precipitates
99mTc-Albumin or red blood cells	LV function, multiple-gated studies	Intravascular substance
99mTc Pertechnetate or DPTA	LV function (first pass)	First passage through the central circulation
99mTc-Diethylene-triamine-pentacetic acid (DTPA)	Dynamic renal imaging	In compartmental space; excretion by glomerular filtration
99mTc-Dimercapto-succinic acid (DMSA)	Static renal imaging	Fixed in the parenchyma
131-I-Hippuran	Isotope renography	Renal excretion
99mTc-Sulphur colloid	Hepatosplenic imaging	Phagocytosis by reticuloendothelial cells
N-Substituted iminodiacetic acid derivatives (99mTc-HIDA, diethyl IDA); I-131 Rose Bengal	Radionuclide hepatobiliary procedures	Accumulate in hepatocyctes, later excreted into bowel through bile ducts
Gallium 67	Intra-abdominal sepsis and malignancy	Leucocyte labelling and migration to inflamed areas (? Bound to lactoferrin)
99mTc-TcO4⁻, DTPA, or glucoheptonate	Brain imaging and cerebrovascular flow studies	Diffusion.? Increased binding to abnormal tissue.? Alteration in blood-brain barrier

(labelled fatty acids), for pancreatic imaging (^{11}C-labelled amino acids), in bone scanning ([18]fluorine) to assess myocardial perfusion and necrosis ([82]rubidium and [13]ammonia), etc. The limiting factor in the use of positrons is that they are produced by nuclear reactions in a cyclotron, which has to be close to the place of use.

Most clinically useful radiopharmaceuticals are 'substrate-non-specific' and do not participate in a specific chemical reaction. For example, regional perfusion can be measured by capillary blockade, but the agent need not be a specific substance, as a number of different radiolabelled particles of the appropriate size can be used. Substrate-specific radiotracers participate in a chemical reaction or take part in a ligand–substrate interaction; as they are changed according to highly specific biochemical and pharmacologic processes, they provide precise diagnostic information of the particular pathway studied.

Commercially available generator systems are utilized to provide isotopes for medical and research purposes. These are systems by which a longer-lived 'parent' radionuclide decays continuously to shorter-lived radiotracers.

Instrumentation

All detectors use one or more sodium iodide scintillation crystals attached to one or more photomultiplier tubes. The function of this assembly is to detect and amplify the interaction of a gamma-ray within the scintillation crystal. Since its output is proportional to the energy of the incident gamma-ray, by pulse-height analysis it is possible to separate interactions from photons of differing energies, permitting dual isotope studies. The inclusion of a lead collimator in front of this detector assembly allows only those gamma photons which are emitted parallel to the axis of collimator holes to be detected, enabling a one-to-one correspondence between point of emission from the patient and the detected image. There are a wide variety of detection devices [24], each with different properties.

Non–imaging techniques

A probe system is an external radiation detector consisting of a single photomultiplier/scintillation crystal which can be applied to monitor the passage of an injected bolus isotope through the kidneys, heart, lungs, vessels, and other organs.

Imaging techniques

Gamma cameras (Anger cameras)

These consist of a large single sodium iodide crystal and an array of photomultiplier tubes. Photons are emitted in all directions from the point of disintegration; those that travel perpendicular to the crystal pass through the holes in the lead collimator and interact with the sodium iodide crystal. The position of the interaction within the crystal is detected by a bank of photomultiplier tubes that convert the electromagnetic energy to electrical current and determine the position of the disintegration within the crystal. The resultant image is a map of the radioactive distribution within the patient. If sequential images are obtained, the regional change in radioactivity as a function of time can be measured. The advantages of this system are: (1) The ease with which it can be interfaced with the computer, making measurement possible; (2) the speed with which investigations can be performed; (3) the ability to do dynamic studies where rapid time sequence images are required; and (4) the relative ease of positioning the patient.

Rectilinear scanners

These have two crystals that localize the origin of photons by viewing one point in space at a time, using a focused collimator and mechanically moving the detector in a rectilinear fashion over the object. They are useful for evaluating static spatial distribution of tracers and have some advantages in imaging high-energy photons, but are for the most part cumbersome and not ideally suited for imaging the acutely ill patient.

Multicrystal gamma cameras

The multicrystal camera consists of an array of scintillation crystals connected to an array of photomultiplier tubes. Localization of the incident gamma photon is achieved by identification of the crystal in which the interaction took place; a collimator is again used to give spatial resolution. Although the best resolution that can be achieved in dynamic mode is 1 cm full-width half maximum (compared with the conventional gamma camera, which has resolution capabilities of 5 mm FWHM), this device has increased sensitivity ($\times 10$) over the Anger camera, and high count-rate capabilities. It is therefore the instrument of choice for 'first pass' dynamic cardiac studies, giving statistically significant images with 20–50 ms frame acquisition times for the passage of a bolus through the central circulation. A computerized on-line data processor is adapted to the camera.

Tomographic methods

Tomographic imaging techniques overcome the geometric limitations of the standard two-dimensional scintigraphy. Both transmission (CT) and emission (ECT) tomography techniques use a computer for image reconstruction. In CT, a beam of x-rays shines through the body and absorption coefficients are used for image reconstruction [67]; in the ECT, the radiation emitted from the organ and recorded by scintillation detectors is used for image processing. The ECT technique has been described as 'in vivo autoradiography' [103], and the images contain a combination of morphological and functional information.

ECT may be carried out with either single-photon nuclides (^{99m}Tc-labelled radiopharmaceuticals and other commercially available radionuclides [26, 75, 76] or positron-emitting isotopes (^{13}ammonia, ^{15}oxygen, ^{11}carbon, ^{82}rubidium etc.) [105]. An advantage in the use of single-photon emitters is that a cyclotron does not need to be located within the institution. However, positron emitters have higher and more uniform sensitivity and attenuation correction is easier [104].

These two approaches are being vigorously pursued at present, and it is likely that both will develop into areas of significant clinical application, primarily because of the technique's unique potential for improvement in the contrast of structures compared with that of conventional planar views [23]. An important contribution of ECT is also its capability to section an organ tomographically into a map of quantitative tracer concentration with high resolution and accuracy; positron-emitting radiopharmaceuticals can be used to examine a wide variety of function indicators (perfusion, metabolism, necrosis, substrate transport, etc.)[36]. Although most ECT devices are not portable, clinically useful images have been obtained with a seven-pinhole collimator and a commercially available mobile gamma camera [142].

Miniaturization and portability

Although several manufacturers have produced mobile scintillation cameras (Fig. 61.1), the ideal light-weight portable system designed strictly for data collection is not yet available. The development of a reliable floppy disc system and microprocessors and the appearance of high-density bubble memories on the semiconductor market make such a machine now technologically feasible. No doubt the expanding market and the need to perform radionuclide studies on the critically ill patient will stimulate the development of such equipment in the very near future.

Data processors

Scintigraphic data processing devices incorporating on-line computer systems and interfaced to the gamma camera are generally provided by the manufacturers options to their systems. Data is recorded by the gamma camera as signals of certain intensity and in certain positions on the crystal, changed to digital form and stored within the computer memory (discs or

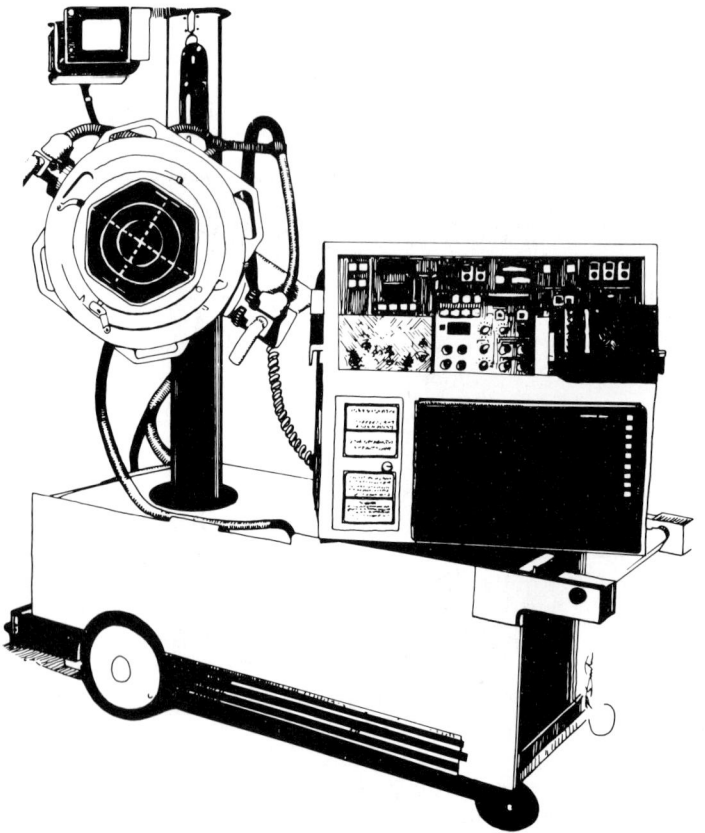

Fig. 61.1. Mobile gamma camera.

tapes) which can be replayed for later analysis. These processors are essential for data acquisition and imaging (including background subtraction smoothing) [107] and for analysing dynamic function data.

Clinical applications

Thrombus detection

Early detection of venous thrombosis with a view to prevention of embolization is difficult to achieve; the clinical diagnosis in acutely ill patients is unreliable, and often late when definite. Prevention of embolization in the lung is important, as it carries a mortality rate of 8%–9% in those patients surviving for more than 1 h [33]. A number of radionuclide agents have been used to locate thrombi in the veins; these include radioiodinated fibrinogen (fibrinogen uptake tests, FUT) [14, 28, 29, 72], which is useful in localizing fresh thrombi, labelled plasminogen and fibrinolytic agents [63, 114] that detect pre-existing thrombi and radionuclide venography [45, 120, 131, 141]. They have their limitations: several conditions, such as oedema, cellulitis, and superficial thrombophlebitis, may lead to false-positive FUT and their overall accuracy is around 50%, with a 75% correlation with contrast venography [61]. FUT are more sensitive than venography in detecting small thrombi in muscular veins in the calf, but cannot be used for diagnosing common femoral or pelvic vein thrombosis because of the high background count in surrounding structures. Radionuclide venography (RNV) (Fig. 61.2) with labelled macro-aggregated albumin or pertechnetate injected through the foot veins bilaterally depends upon the demonstration of mechanical obstruction: it appears to be simple, safe and highly accurate [46] and is the study of choice for detecting pelvic venous abnormalities. With portable imaging facilities, thromboembolism can be fully assessed in intensive care patients, and RNV can ensure more appropriate selection of patients for contrast studies. Initial experience with [111]indium-labelled human platelets [59] is encouraging and permits the study of platelet kinetics and distribution; venous and arterial accumulation of platelets has been visualized in thrombophlebitis, arterial trauma, in intracardiac thrombus, arterial embolization, and recent pulmonary embolism. It is likely that the emergence of other radionuclide techniques will contribute significantly to the early detection of thromboembolism.

Ventilation–perfusion lung scanning

One of the most frequent clinical problems in intensive care management is the differential diagnosis of pulmonary embolism in patients with tachypnoea, chest discomfort, left ventricular failure, uncontrolled arrhythmias, or 'intractable' congestive cardiac failure. The clinical picture is frequently non-specific and

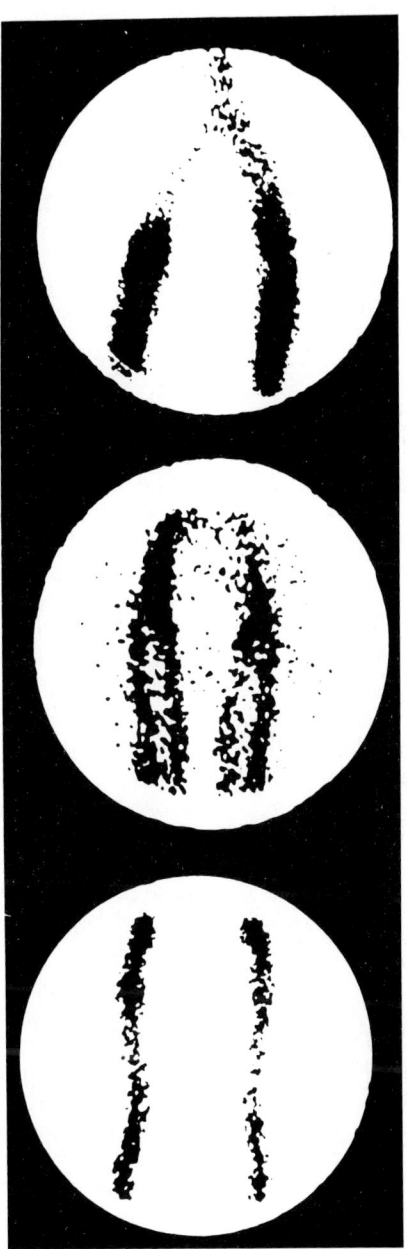

Fig. 61.2. Normal radionuclide venography (RNV) following the administration of technetium into the veins in the dorsum of the feet. The course of the radioactive tracer through the popliteal, superficial femoral, great saphenous, femoral, and common iliac veins to the inferior vena cava is visualized.

hence underdiagnosed. Radionuclide perfusion and ventilation (P/V) studies of the lung are widely used to screen patients with suspected pulmonary embolism and select those requiring angiography; their accuracy has beeen extensively documented [35, 94, 95, 140, 143].

For perfusion scanning, [99m]technetium-labelled albumin particles of different sizes (macro-aggregates or microspheres) are injected IV and as these are scattered through the pulmonary circulation they become obstructed temporarily in the terminal arterioles and capillaries in proportion to regional perfusion; the distribution of gamma ray emission from these microparticles is therefore proportional to regional perfusion. It is important to obtain anatomical information about regional perfusion, in particular the lobar and segmental nature of perfusion defects, and a number of views of the lung taken from the different surfaces of the thorax should be obtained.

For ventilation imaging, 133 and 127 xenon and [81m]krypton are used. Radioactive xenon [6] is most widely used, but its solubility in interstitial fluid and fat is a disadvantage when measurements of regional ventilation are to be made from the 'washout' curves. [127]Xenon is probably preferable to [133]xenon because of higher count rates, a lower patient radiation dose and longer shelf-life. Studies of regional ventilation are usually performed by inhaling radioactive xenon to total lung capacity and measuring its distribution during this initial 'wash-in' breath, proceeding to equilibrium during a rebreathing phase [56] and finishing with the dynamic washout phase while breathing air [92].

[81m]Krypton offers a new approach to ventilation imaging: it has a very short half-life (13 s), remains in continuing wash-in phase (during which regional ventilation is assessed) [50], and is currently the radionuclide of choice. The ventilation scan obtained with [81m]krypton is comparable to the perfusion image obtained with the labelled microparticles, in that both are obtained with the patient at rest and breathing quietly. These radionuclides have gamma ray emissions which are suitable for high-resolution images with a gamma camera [51]. Furthermore, when the 'energy window' of the gamma camera is used, the emissions from each may be imaged separately without changing the position of the patient to obtain successively an image of regional perfusion and of regional ventilation. This is of particular value when assessing the 'matching' between ventilation and perfusion, as pulmonary embolism results

in defects in regional (usually segmental) perfusion without comparable change in ventilation [7, 91] (Fig. 61.3) and airways disease usually produces matching ventilation–perfusion abnormalities.

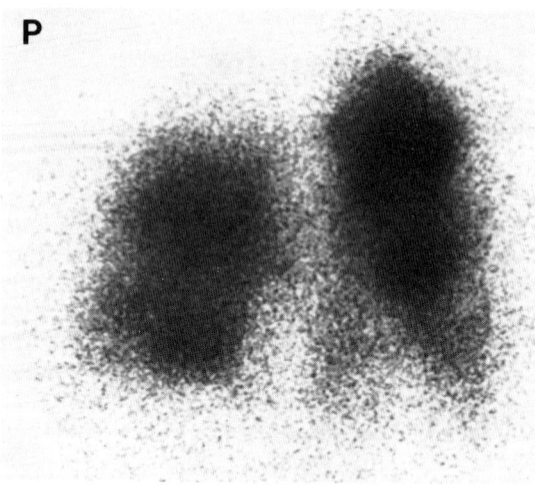

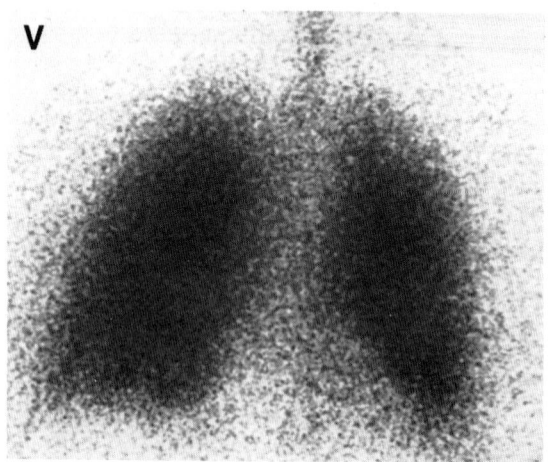

Fig. 61.3. Perfusion (*P*) and ventilation (*V*) mismatch (anterior views). The perfusion lung scan displays a large defect involving the right upper lobe; the corresponding [81m]krypton ventilation scan shows normal homogeneous ventilation of both lungs. This P/V mismatch is very suggestive of pulmonary emboli. Courtesy of Dr. J. P. Lavender, Hammersmith Hospital, London

One current strategy for the diagnosis of pulmonary embolism [90] recommends that if the perfusion study is normal or has certain minor abnormalities, the patient should be assumed not to have pulmonary embolism; if there are major perfusion abnormalities (segmental or larger) without associated ventilatory abnormalities, the patient is assumed to have pulmonary embolism and is so treated. Other abnormal patterns ('indeterminate scans') are not diagnostic and such patients (about 10%– 25%) should undergo pulmonary angiography, as other clinical and laboratory studies offer little aid in further defining the probability of embolism [52]. Conversely, if P/V studies demonstrate perfusion defects which correspond in size and location to zones of decreased ventilation (Fig. 61.4) (P/V match) embolism is

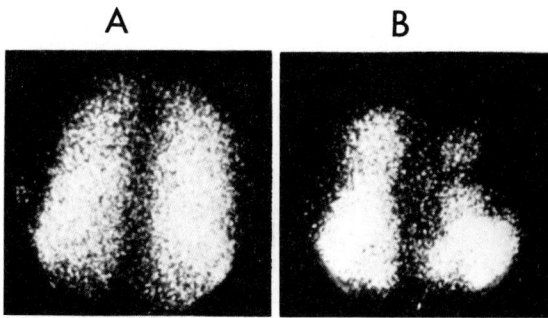

Fig. 61.4. Posterior Xe–133 (single-breath) ventilation studies: **A** Normal homogenous ventilation of both lung fields; **B** abnormal scan demonstrating area of decreased ventilation in right upper lobe due to obstructive airways disease.

unlikely. This approach, involving the combination of scintigraphic perfusion–ventilation studies and selected pulmonary angiography, has been reported as having a true-positive rate greater than 95% and a false-positive rate of 2% in a large general patient population [90]. There are some limitations to this strategy (e.g., ventilation abnormalities can be infrequently present in embolic sites) but it is ideally suited to the management of the acutely ill patient [43].

The diagnosis of pulmonary emboli is more difficult in patients with congestive cardiac failure or chronic obstructive pulmonary disease, because of multiple perfusion and ventilation defects which are common in these disorders [4, 126]. The delayed washout phase of the ventilation scan, however, is usually quite sensitive in detecting regional airways disease, showing uneven retention of the radioactivity [8]. Locally delayed clearance from the lungs reflects impaired exchange of air, and this can be due to small airways disease or to a more proximal partial or complete obstruction; widespread irregularly delayed clearance is usually due to generalized obstructive airway disease.

A new method for the detection of pulmonary embolism is based on the rate of washout of H_2 $^{15}O_2$ from regions of the lung [96]. The $^{15}O_2$ is introduced by inhalation of radioactive CO_2 ($^{15}CO_2$), which is then converted by carbonic anhydrase in pulmonary erythrocytes to O_2-

labelled water; embolized zones have slower washout than normal ones and appear as areas of increased radioactivity ('hot spot') on positron imaging. The principal applications of this technique may be determination of the resolution rates of pulmonary emboli during anticoagulant or thrombolytic therapy and detection of pulmonary emboli among patients with chronic pulmonary disease or congestive heart failure. However, this method requires a positron camera and the production of $^{15}O_2$ necessitates the availability of a cyclotron.

In the therapeutic approach to a patient in an intensive care environment, it is foreseeable that more rapid indices of lung function will be required in the evaluation of the respiratory status. In this context, the availability of an ^{81m}krypton generator seems of particular importance. The very short half-life of this radioactive gas allows rapid changes in regional ventilation to be studied (because equilibrium is reached within a minute or so of the change) without undue stress to the patient and permits moment-to-moment assessment of the respiratory status and its modification with therapy. Radionuclide lung function tests measure aspects that are different from the regular pulmonary function tests and probably reflect more accurately the usual exchange of air in the alveoli. The new information available may require a revision of the approach to emergency therapy and drug evaluation.

Cardiac studies

Profound advances have been made in the use of isotope emission scanning in the study of the heart. With the development of high-resolution scintillation cameras and highly sophisticated minicomputers, radionuclide techniques have taken their place alongside electrophysiologic and biochemical methodologies for the routine day-to-day assessment of patients with known and suspected cardiac disease. Myocardial perfusion can be evaluated, acutely damaged cardiac tissue detected, and non-invasive physiological data obtained for studies of cardiac performance. The extension of these methods with three-dimensional reconstruction techniques and longitudinal tomography has remarkable potential for further developments. The function measured with a radioactive tracer procedure will depend on the type of radiopharmaceutical administered, the time of observation and the sensitivity of the instrument used to make the measurement.

Myocardial perfusion imaging (MPI)

Radionuclide techniques provide information that is useful for the detection and evaluation of coronary artery disease and in the assessment of therapies aimed at limiting the degree of ischaemia and the extent of tissue necrosis. Myocardial perfusion is studied with radionuclides which accumulate maximally in normal myocardium, through diffusion and exchange with potassium, the chief intracellular cation. The regional distribution of ^{201}thallium in the myocardium reflects perfusion at tissue level [106]. Studies are performed following thallium administration at the time of maximal exercise stress testing (exercise scintigraphy) (Fig. 61.5); a zone of abnormality is detected as an area of decreased radionuclide accumulation ('cold spot'). By re-imaging with the patient at rest 3–4 h later (redistribution scans), it is possible in most cases to differentiate regions of severe ischaemia (reversible uptake defects) from infarcted tissue (which shows persistent reduction of regional activity) [108]. Perfusion scintigraphy cannot, however, differentiate between old and new infarction; ancillary clinical information and the use of ^{99m}Tc-labelled phosphates aid in this distinction. As characteristic patterns of regional tracer distribution are seen with specific coronary lesions, this technique is a highly sensitive and useful adjunct to conventional exercise testing in the detection and localization of myocardial ischaemia [20].

Pharmacologic coronary vasodilation with IV dipyridamole [3] appears to be as effective as maximal treadmill exercise in creating regional myocardial perfusion abnormalities detectable with thallium imaging, and this method is useful for those patients who are unable to undergo exercise testing. Visualization of the right ventricle in MPI at rest is suggestive of RV hypertrophy or enlargement secondary to pulmonary hypertension or other causes; perfusion imaging has also been employed in the evaluation of patients who have undergone coronary bypass grafting [60].

Abnormal resting scintigrams have been reported in unstable angina pectoris and in coronary spasm [87]. Interpretation of the scintigrams is quite subjective; the high cost of thallium and the problem of overlying myocardial structures, liver and lung (which can obscure areas of mildly decreased perfusion) are limitations in myocardial imaging. In addition, determination of the extent of damaged myocardium cannot be made accurately and correlations between estimates of infarct size determined at post-mortem examination and from two dimensional scintigraphy have been only fair.

Myocardial imaging with non-ionic gamma-emitting tracers (i.e., labelled fatty acids) is being developed and this reflects regional myocardial metabolism as opposed to the uptake patterns based primarily on perfusion. It should be possible in future to provide hot spot demonstration of stress-induced ischaemia by injecting the tracer with the patient at rest and determining which areas differentially retain radioactivity when the heart is subjected to stress [139]. With recent developments in emission computerized tomography (ECT), transaxial cross-sectional imaging of the heart has become possible. These tomographic imagers overcome the geometric limitations of standard scintigraphy and, as they reflect quantitatively the distribution of radioactive indicator concentrations in myocardium, provide a potential

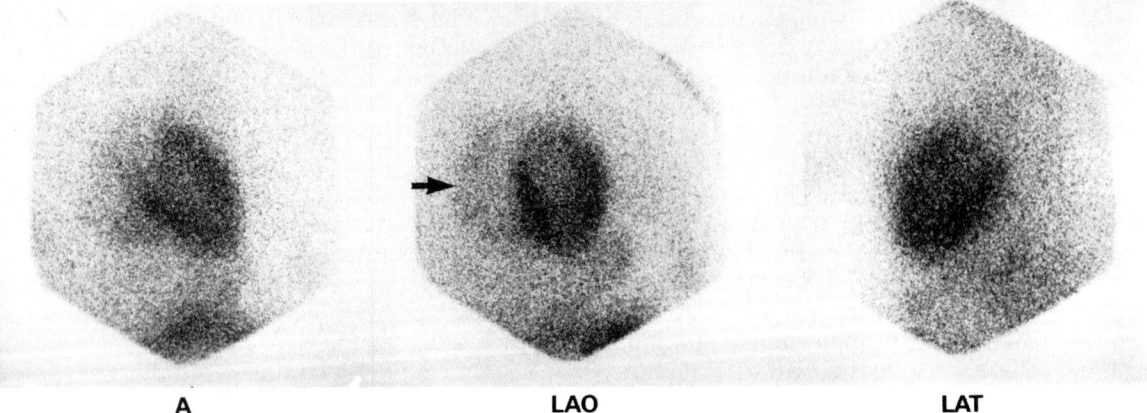

A   **LAO**   **LAT**

Fig. 61.5. Normal myocardial perfusion imaging (MPI) with 201T1 following exercise. The normal 'horseshoe'-shaped homogeneous pattern of the LV myocardium is seen; the cavity is visualized as a central area of decreased activity. A hint of RV uptake is visible (*arrowed*). *A*, anterior; *LAO*, left anterior oblique; *LAT*, left lateral projections.

means of accurately estimating altered regional perfusion and infarct size [103, 125].

Detection of acutely damaged myocardium

Bone-seeking agents (^{99m}Tc-labelled phosphates) define infarcted myocardial tissue as a zone of increased radioactivity (hot spot); although the exact mechanism of uptake of these labelled phosphates is still unclear, it is a highly sensitive technique for detecting infarction within 24 h after the onset of pain [71]. This approach is especially useful in a number of selected clinical situations in which the presence or absence of recent infarction cannot be accurately determined by applying conventional clinical criteria (equivocal ECGs, re-infarction, peri-operative infarction). Although a single positive (discrete) scintigram may not be diagnostic of infarction in all patients, evolving scintigraphic abnormalities provide strong support for the diagnosis in most instances (Fig. 61.6). False-positive scintigrams have been documented, particularly if a diffuse uptake pattern is present (calcified valves, post-cardioversion, ventricular aneurysm, unstable angina, old infarction, etc.) [85]. As discrete uptake occurs in only a minority of patients with subendocardial infarction, infarct scintigraphy is relatively insensitive in this condition [88]. The technique can document infarct extension and may be of value in attempting to estimate infarct size, although quantification is difficult because of the inherent limitations leading to disparity between injured tissue and its two-dimensional display. Except in the subgroup of patients with RV dysfunction as a cause of low cardiac output in acute inferior infarction [127], myocardial scintigraphy does not yet provide information which is essential for management. However, the 'doughnut' uptake pattern in acute infarction appears to identify a subgroup of patients with a very poor long-term prognosis [2].

Emission computerized tomography contributes further to the accurate assessment of the extent and location of myocardial damage [66]. The multiple-level images obtained permit quantification of infarct size; in addition, the difficult diagnosis of subendocardial infarction appears to benefit from the improved contrast in the ECT sections (Fig. 61.7).

Other causes of myocardial necrosis

Radionuclide techniques identify myocardial necrosis resulting from other causes, such as myocarditis, myocardial abscess, hypoxic or acidotic injury, cardioversion, and metabolic infiltration. Scintigraphy is extremely useful in the diagnosis of myocardial injury secondary to blunt trauma and penetrating wounds [57]. The scans can be obtained with mobile equipment in seriously injured patients, in most of whom myocardial contusion cannot be diagnosed without a positive scan, which thus provides information essential to management [132].

Evaluation of ventricular function

Ventricular performance is a prime factor in determining appropriate medical and surgical management in patients with coronary heart disease. Left ventricular ejection fraction and regional wall motion are directly related to the clinical prognosis in chronic coronary heart disease and after myocardial infarction. Invasive techniques provide reliable measurements of ejection fraction and regional wall motion [73]. However, they have limited applicability in clinical situations requiring serial assessments of ventricular function and in the evaluation of critically ill patients. Nuclear techniques are safe and repeatable, and they do not induce measurable haemodynamic alterations. Critically ill patients too sick to be transported to the clinical nuclear medicine unit can be studied at the

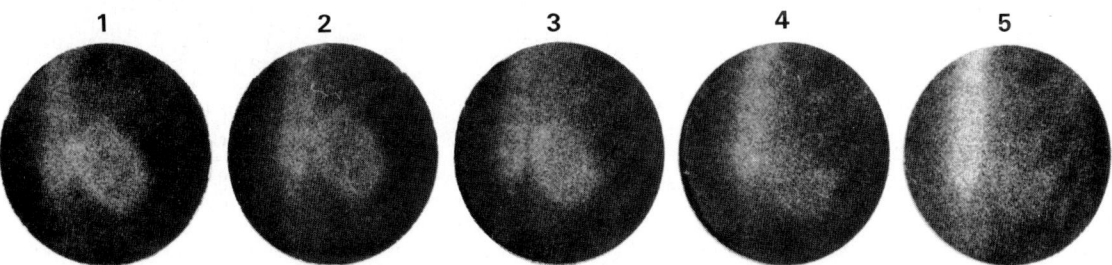

Fig. 61.6. Detection of acutely damaged myocardium. Serial scans (left anterior oblique projection) obtained over 5 days in a patient with anterior infarction using ^{99m}Tc-labelled phosphate. The infarcted tissue is seen as an evolving zone of increased radioactivity (hot spot); there is progressive diminished uptake by day 5. The bone-seeking agent clearly defines the sternum and ribs: quantification of cardiac uptake is based upon a comparison with the bone uptake.

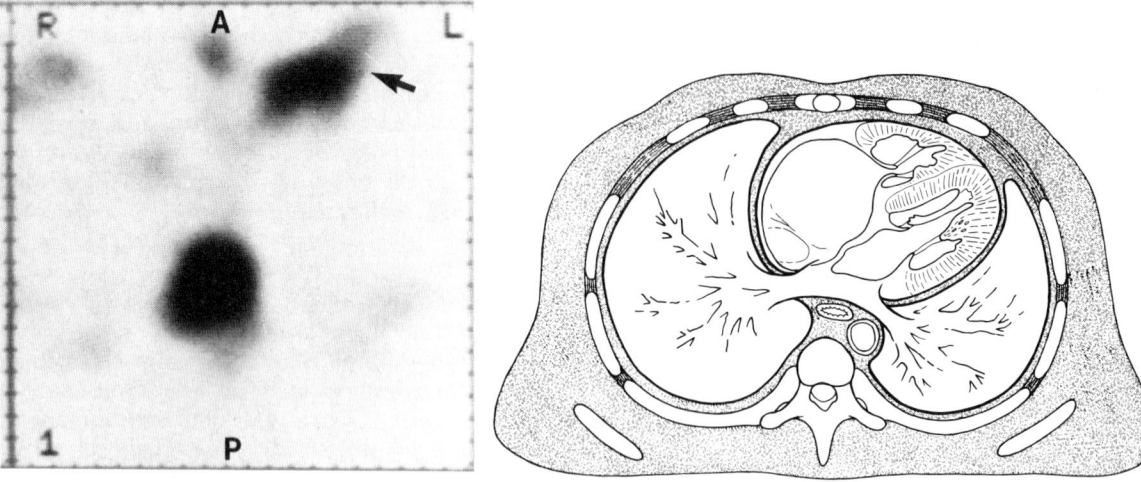

Fig. 61.7. Emission tomography study with ^{99m}Tc-labelled phosphate in a patient with a large anterior myocardial infarction (*arrowed*). Numerous slices are obtained, orientated as though the viewer is looking from below, with anterior surface up. The uptake of the radionuclide into the sternum, ribs and spine is seen. Slice 1 corresponds to the base of the heart. *A*, anterior; *P*, posterior.

bedside with mobile scintillation cameras and probe detectors [13], and haemodynamic measurements can thus be obtained at any location throughout the hospital.

There are two general types of radionuclide techniques for studying ventricular performance: (1) First-pass techniques, which provide indices of cardiac performance from the initial transit of the radiotracer through the heart; and (2) equilibrium studies, which measure ventricular function by means of radiotracers that have reached equilibrium in the intravascular space.

First-pass method (dynamic imaging). A bolus of a ^{99m}technetium-labelled pharmaceutical is administered IV and data are recorded during the initial passage of the tracer through the heart. The study of the derived time–activity curves allows quantitative analysis of ejection fraction for either ventricle [11], which correlates well with data obtained from ventriculography [53] and is independent of geometric assumptions inherent in volume determinations made from cavity outlines. A high count-rate, background corrected "representative" cycle (which is usually the summation of equivalent phases of several cycles), is recorded. Regional wall motion is evaluated from end-diastolic and endsystolic images obtained from this cycle (Fig. 61.8); the frames can also be displayed as a cine-film format. Sequential images also provide information concerning the anatomical relationship of the intracardiac chambers and great vessels.

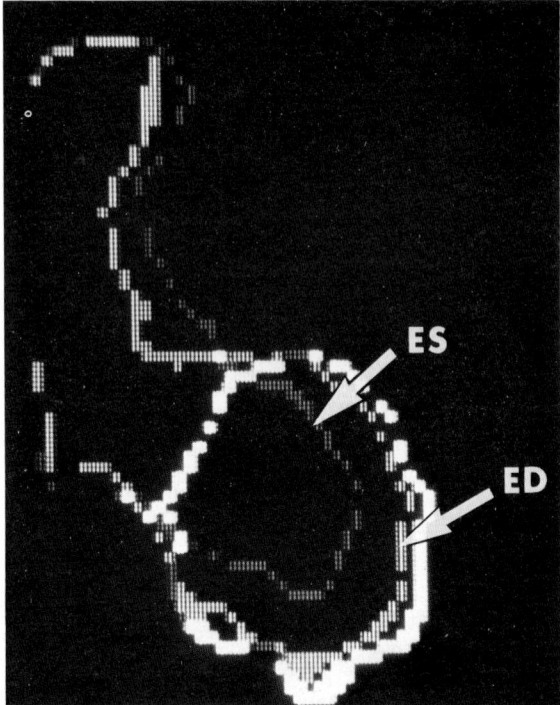

Fig. 61.8. Evaluation of ventricular function. Regional wall motion studies obtained from the first pass of radionuclide through the left ventricle (right anterior oblique view) in a patient with normal ventricular function. Each image represents a composite consisting of a computer generated end-diastolic (*ED*) ring superimposed upon the end-systolic image (*ES*). A region of interest is drawn through the level of the aortic valve and encompasses the perimeter of the left ventricle.

The advantages of the method include the short time (20–30 s) required for data acquisition (and this is crucial in critically ill patients), and the fact that studies can be performed in any projection (particularly the right anterior oblique projection, which is the best view for assessing LV wall motion). It also permits measurement of the relative regional ejection fraction during maximal exercise, as imaging may be performed at peak stress (because of the short data acquisition time), which may be of value in the detection of ischaemic heart disease. The multicrystal detection system, coupled with its computer capabilities, is capable of performing virtually all nuclear cardiology studies. The disadvantages of the method are: (1) Only one view is recorded with each injection; (2) haemodynamic changes following various therapeutic interventions are difficult to evaluate; and (3) energy resolution is poor (this is particularly so with low-energy isotopes).

Multiple-gated acquisition images (MUGA). Ventricular function can also be studied with a tracer that equilibrates in the blood pool vasculature (equilibrium technique). Multiple, high-spatial resolution images of consecutive cycles are recorded with a computer-assisted scintillation camera at selected points with an electronic switch (gate) synchronized to the patient's ECG. The mean representative cardiac cycle is then divided into numerous frames (20–30) displayed in a real-time cine format as an endless loop. The number of cycles recorded can be controlled by the operator (usually 800–1000 cycles). From the end-diastolic and end-systolic gated images, the ejection fraction can be determined (Fig. 61.9). Since the biological half-life of the radiopharmaceutical (^{99m}technetium-labelled albumin or red blood cells) is approximately 40 h, serial measurements of ventricular function can be made over extended periods of time (up to 4 h) and multiple views recorded. From the time-activity curve, ventricular filling and emptying rates are analysed and defined; this has been found to correlate well with angiographic volumes [27, 53]. The advantages of the method include: (1) Additional instrumentation required is minimal for those workers already possessing a gamma camera; (2) the safety and ease of performing repetitive studies allows the evaluation of therapeutic interventions; (3) mobile instrumentation permits studies to be performed at the bedside of the acutely ill patient; and (4) statistically reliable data are easier to obtain, as the radioactivity is analysed over numerous beats.

Disadvantages of the multiple-gated technique are: (1) the lengthy acquisition time required, (5–15 min); (2) the difficulty in determining the background contribution; (3) views are limited to the LAO and AP projections (some areas of LV wall motion are suboptimally seen in these views); and (4) inaccuracy in patients with irregular rhythm.

In addition to the non-invasive measurement

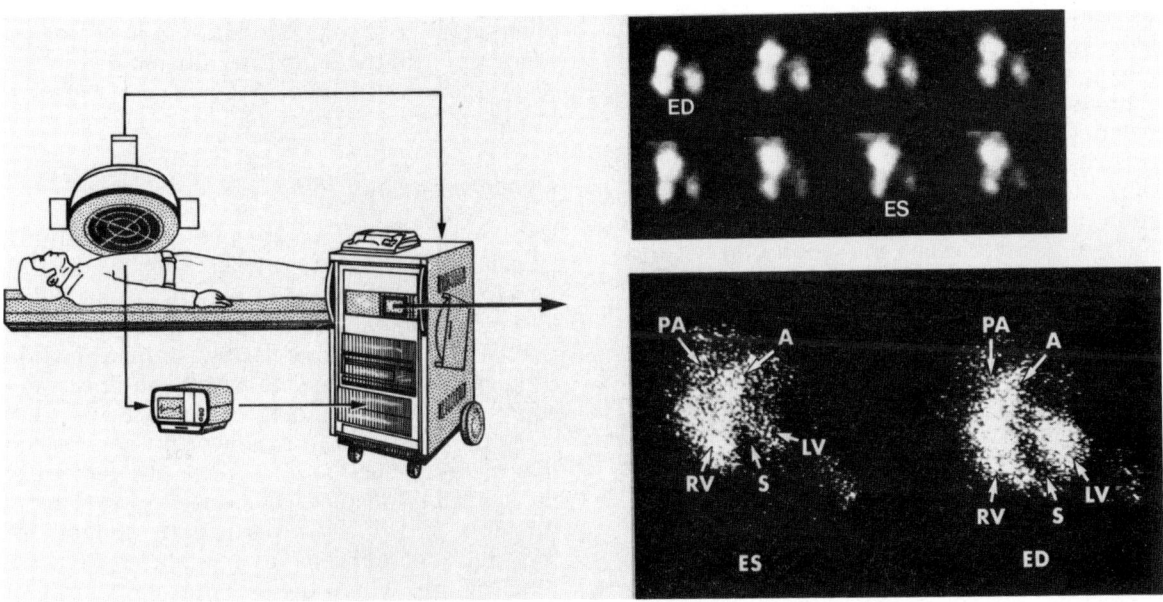

Fig. 61.9. Normal multiple-gated studies. Images recorded using a mobile scintillation camera and a computer system; the counts are synchronized to the ECG to obtain end-diastolic (*ED*) and end-systolic (*ES*) frames. Selected left anterior oblique frames shown. *LV*, left ventricle; *RV*, right ventricle; *S*, septum; *PA*, pulmonary artery; *A*, aorta.

of haemodynamic parameters and assessment of ventricular size and regional wall motion abnormalities [147] first-pass and gated studies are of value in the evaluation of biventricular contraction patterns after acute infarction [112, 116], in congestive heart failure [97] and hypertrophic cardiomyopathy [109], and in the detection of ventricular aneurysm and

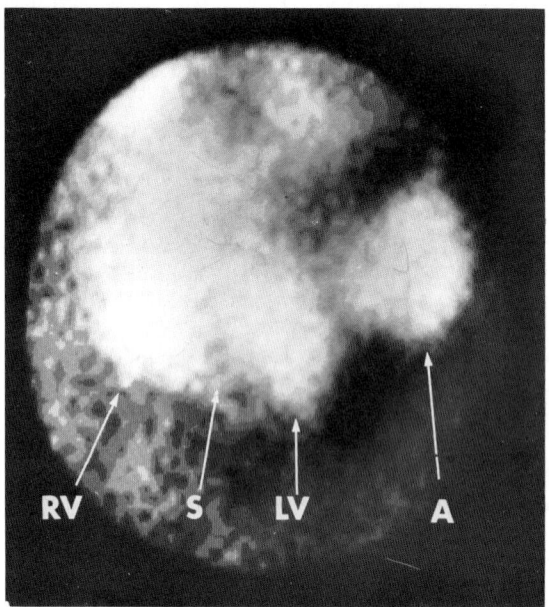

Fig. 61.10. Gated scan (left anterior oblique, systolic frame) demonstrating an LV aneurysm (*A*).

pseudoaneurysm [39, 115] (Fig. 61.10). Particularly useful clinical applications are: (1) the initial diagnostic screening prior to cardiac catheterization; (2) determination of serial haemodynamic changes following drug therapy or surgical intervention; (3) prospective evaluation of cardiotoxic drugs; (4) prognostication from the severity of ventricular dysfunction following myocardial infarction; (5) to document non-invasively the efficacy or adverse effects of drugs on ventricular function; and (6) studies performed after stress may be helpful in visualizing regional asynergy or relative ejection fraction changes which provide evidence of regional myocardial ischaemia [18, 19], and this is of value in the detection and localization of ischaemic heart disease.

Pericardial effusion

The use of radioactive tracers in the diagnosis of pericardial effusion is less versatile and less sensitive than echocardiography [30]. However,

the correct echocardiographic diagnosis requires technically good recording of all components of the LV posterior wall, and a satisfactory study may be extremely difficult in ill, ventilated patients and in those with an emphysematous chest. It is this technical problem that causes most false-positive and false-negative results [78, 133]. Radioisotopes provide an alternative bedside technique for the confirmation of a pericardial effusion and, if used together with myocardial scintigraphy, may offer an insight into associated cardiac necrosis (i.e. haemopericardium following non-penetrating chest trauma with its attendant risk of cardiac rupture and tamponade) [133]. The imaging procedure is usually performed with ^{99m}technetium-labelled human serum albumin or red cells.

Renal scanning

Probe system

The uptake and excretion of tracers handled by the kidneys can be measured by means of external radiation detectors or probes. This 'isotope renography' with ^{131}I-hippuran or ^{99m}Tc-glucoheptonate is used as a screening test for possible renal disease and gives an assessment of divided renal function. Combined with rapid-sequence urography, it is useful in those patients for whom a high clinical suspicion of renovascular disease exists [49], the early rapid rise of radioactivity on the curve being greatly attenuated on the side affected by functional obstruction. The complementary role of isotope renography to the Saralasin infusion test in the diagnosis of angiotensinogenic hypertension has been recently reviewed [89].

Dynamic renal imaging

Dynamic renal imaging with technetium-labelled radiopharmaceuticals such as DTPA, which is handled by glomerular filtration, allows comprehensive evaluation of renal function, while quantitative analysis of the excretion of the agent (by means of an on-line mini-computer generating activity–time curves from a region of interest) improves the accuracy of this method. Such studies allow assessment of the contribution of each kidney to total renal function, and they are particularly suitable for the study of critically ill patients with acute renal failure, where the size and vascularity of the kidneys can readily be evaluated with a mobile gamma camera. In acute tabular necrosis, the scan shows the kidneys to be relatively well perfused in the early stages (2–3 min); they are then seen progressively less well. In obstruction, perfusion is normal in the early stages (in prolonged obstruction it may be altered); in acute nephritis, there is usually some impairment of perfusion. In acute-on-chronic renal failure, the small kidneys are poorly seen. Serial dynamic studies permit measurement of changes in the perfusion of transplanted kidneys and this is known to be one of the earliest indicators of rejection [10, 34, 111]. Renal imaging can also be used for observing changes in function as a result of urinary tract obstruction and hydronephrosis, but ultrasound is more accurate in demonstrating the anatomy and pathology of obstruction [44].

Static renal imaging

Static renal imaging with Technetium-labelled dimercaptosuccinic acid (^{99m}Tc-DMSA) (which is fixed in the parenchyma) also allows visualization of the distribution of function between and within the kidneys, as well as its quantification. Summation of the activity in each kidney provides information on divided renal function that could previously only be obtained by invasive and often unreliable techniques involving ureteric catheterization. Knowledge of the distribution of function within a kidney is particularly useful when planning operations for staghorn calculi and in distinguishing islands of hypertrophied parenchyma from tumours of cysts.

There is at present no investigation of choice for the localization of space-occupying lesions in the kidney. A combination of radionuclide static imaging and ultrasound may serve as a primary imaging procedure [110]; the value of ultrasonography derives from its ability to separate cystic from solid masses [58]. In other cases, computerized tomography (CT) affords an accurate method of obtaining a definitive delineation of a renal or perirenal abnormality, including differentiation of cysts from tumours [123].

Hepatosplenic imaging

Liver scanning

The radionuclide scan with ^{99m}Tc-labelled sulphur colloid (which is taken up by the reticuloendothelial cells), in combination with ultrasound and CT has refined the investigation of lesions within the liver and spleen [22, 124, 136].

Space-occupying lesions appear as areas devoid of radioactive material (cold spots), and at present radionuclide scanning is the preferred technique for the initial hepatic screening because of its high sensitivity and easy performance [41, 82]. The weakness of hepatic scanning resides in its high [up to 20%] false-positive or equivocal rate; ultrasonography is an effective complementary technique to confirm or characterize equivocal scan defects further [130, 137]. Computerized tomography has yielded comparable although not clearly superior results for detection of focal or diffuse liver disease. Newer imaging modalities, such as emission computerized tomography (ECT), have been used to give better definition of scan abnormalities, either deep in the liver or in the porta hepatis [124]. Multinuclide and multiple non-invasive imaging techniques are indicated when there is a high degree of suspicion concerning a mass lesion on the colloid liver scan.

A diminished uptake of sulphur colloid is seen in the scan of diffuse parenchymal liver disease; more is therefore available for other reticuloendothelial sites such as the spleen and bone marrow. The CT scan, although unable to show parenchymal abnormalities, can provide a specific diagnosis of fatty infiltration.

Sepsis

Acute pyogenic and chronic abscesses can also be clearly defined; intra-abdominal sepsis, inflammatory lesions, and malignancy may be localized by the abnormal accumulation of ^{67}gallium (^{67}Ga), an element closely akin to aluminium, which has an affinity for these lesions [64]. In problem cases with suspected intra-abdominal abscesses, the combination of gallium scan with ultrasound and CT is the recommended approach [68, 77, 138]. A combined liver/lung scan can be performed to define the extent of a subphrenic abscess, an entity that is difficult to diagnose and can be fatal [101].

Obstructive jaundice

Radionuclide hepatobiliary procedures are performed with ^{131}I-Rose Bengal or technetium-labelled iminodiacetic acid derivatives (HIDA, IDA), which accumulate in the hepatocytes and are later excreted into the bowel through the bile ducts. These techniques are useful for the diagnosis of biliary obstruction [48, 121, 122, 144]: prompt appearance of activity within the small bowel indicates that the biliary tree is patent; persistent activity within the gall bladder and delayed entry into the gut suggests common duct obstruction. However, the excretion of these agents is diminished in the presence of hepatocellular failure and marked hyperbilirubinaemia [62], and this limits the use of these procedures in the diagnosis of partial hepatic obstruction. Ultrasound [135] and CT scanning [81], generally followed by percutaneous transhepatic cholangiography or endoscopic retro-grade cholangiopancreatography, can demonstrate the distended biliary tree and are the investigations of choice for distinguishing between hepatocellular and obstructive jaundice.

Cystic duct obstruction

Cystic duct obstruction can be evaluated by cholescintigraphy. Cystic duct obstruction initiates acute cholecystitis, so that detection of obstruction is diagnostic during the acute phase of the disease. An accurate radionuclide assessment of cystic duct patency is performed by IV administration of cholecystokinin, followed by a hepatobiliary radiopharmaceutical [42]. Subsequent accumulation of radioactivity in the gallbladder indicates that the cystic duct is patent. Failure to visualize the gallbladder is highly specific and sensitive for cystic duct obstruction if hepatic excretory function is adequate to produce detectable tracer in the bowel.

The rapid evolution of ultrasound in the diagnosis of cholelithiasis [17] will undoubtedly overshadow some of these nuclear techniques which, however, appear to be useful in the differential diagnosis of any state of jaundice and may also be used to assess the patency of surgically devised drainage pathways of the biliary system, particularly after liver transplantation and surgery for biliary atresia [102, 119].

Liver injury

Early diagnosis of hepatic trauma is essential for the correct management of this condition and this is sometimes difficult, particularly in cases of blunt abdominal injuries. Simultaneous liver/spleen scanning with mobile gamma cameras is a rapid screening method which provides valuable information for the assessment of these patients [47], and follow-up data can be obtained from repeat scans.

Splenic imaging

A liver/spleen scan is useful for the investigation of splenomegaly and space-occupying lesions, and of particular relevance to suspected splenic trauma. In this respect, the diagnosis of post-traumatic subcapsular haematomas is clinically important, as there is a significant probability of delayed rupture. The high (90%) sensitivity of scintigraphy in detecting splenic rupture [47, 55, 69, 83, 100] makes radionuclide scanning (Fig. 61.11) and splenic ultrasound [12] the screening tests of choice following blunt

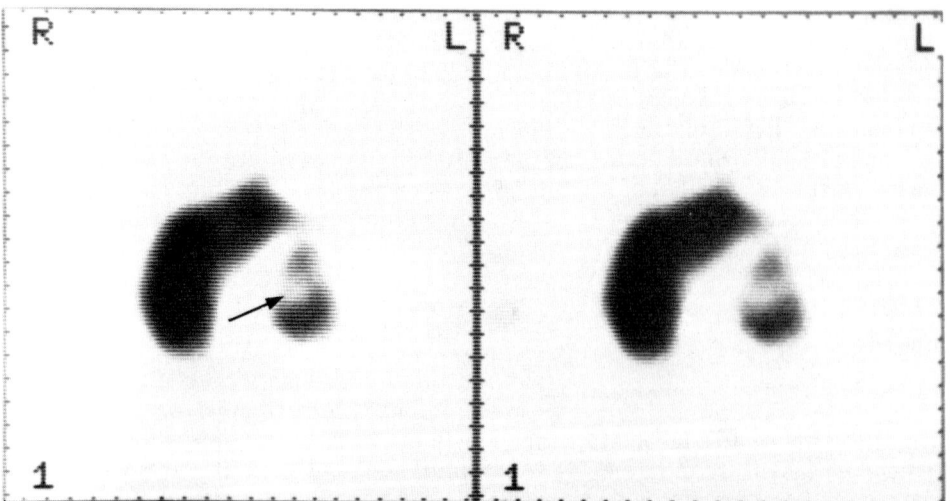

Fig. 61.11. Splenic trauma. Emission tomographic transverse section scans (ECT) through the liver and spleen. Within the spleen there is a round area of impaired tracer uptake (*arrow*) compatible with a haematoma. This followed blunt abdominal trauma. Courtesy of Dr. O. Khan, Middlesex Hospital, London.

abdominal trauma. Continued scintigraphic follow-up is mandatory if pain develops or a mass becomes palpable in the left upper quadrant. Sequential renovascular imaging may demonstrate an associated peri-renal haematoma.

Gastro-intestinal studies

Pancreas

When an abdominal tumour is suspected or when the aetiology of gastro-intestinal (GI) symptoms cannot be readily established, a normal pancreatic scan with selenomethione (^{75}Se) (which is taken up by most tumours) is helpful in ruling out the presence of pancreatic carcinoma. Nuclear imaging has also been moderately successful in distinguishing tumours of the head of the pancreas from other entities [1] but is infrequently used because of its high false-positive rate and its inability to differentiate a benign from a malignant lesion [9]. Sonography is the study of choice in acute pancreatitis, pseudocyst, and carcinoma of the head of the pancreas [40], and CT when chronic pancreatitis, abscess, or carcinoma of the body and tail of the pancreas is suspected [15, 37, 128, 129]. Recent developments in imaging with positron tomography (ECT) by means of ^{11}C-labelled amino acids [25], which permits selective pancreatic function analysis, should overcome the present limitations of pancreatic scanning.

Acute GI bleeding

Contrast radiography, angiography, endoscopy, and laparotomy may fail to localize GI bleeding. Preliminary results with an isotopic method based on ^{99m}Tc-human albumin [93] for detecting the site of bleeding are promising, and this technique has the advantage of being non-invasive and easy to perform. Further clinical experience is necessary to establish its role in the management of the acutely ill patient.

Neurological investigations

Radionuclide and CT scanning are the primary investigations for intracranial space-occupying lesions [31, 118]; the ability of the mobile gamma camera to go to the bedside in the ICU makes the nuclear technique more easily applicable to acutely ill patients. When focal intracranial space-occupying lesions, such as a tumour, abscess, or infarct, are present there is a localized uptake o the isotope (^{99m}Tc-labelled per-technetate, DTPA, or glucoheptonate) relative to the surrounding brain, producing a positive scan. The actual mechanism of localization has not been completely defined, but uptake is probably due to an alteration in the blood–brain barrier, which allows the agent to penetrate in and around the lesion. Nuclide brain scanning of intracranial inflammation is extremely sensitive and will detect nearly all abscesses over 1 cm in diameter (Fig. 61.12); the enhanced CT scan is especially suited for following the evolution of focal cerebritis into an encapsulated abscess. Static studies should preferably be associated with dynamic studies that estimate the regional distribution of blood flow through the brain [16, 134] and are the most effective screening test for arteriovenous malformations [54]. Dynamic imaging is great value in the timing of the surgical management of subarachnoid haemorrhage, as those patients with markedly impaired cerebral circulation on imaging are at increased risk of cerebral infarction after aneurysm clipping [74, 98] and operation should be deferred until the normalization of scan. Isotopic static and dynamic brain scans are also highly sensitive for the recognition of post-traumatic chronic subdural haematoma [21, 32]; CT (particularly with contrast enhancement) is, however, more reliable in the diagnosis of this condition and is the imaging procedure of choice when the clinical problem is acute. It is also of value in differentiating structural lesions of a chronic nature (such as brain atrophy or hydrocephalus) that will not take up isotope. Nuclear techniques are used particularly in subacute problems, but in many cases the two methods are complementary. Section scanning [146] and emission tomographs (ECT scans) [65, 70, 79] appear to increase the sensitivity of detection of the space-occupying lesions, and positron ECT studies permit the measurement of blood flow and metabolic activity in small defined parts of the brain [80, 113].

Nuclear techniques can accurately detect the presence of cerebrospinal fluid (CSF) rhinorrhoea. This is usually secondary to severe head trauma, and is complicated by pyogenic meningitis in up to 25% of the cases. The nuclear methods consist in measurements of gastric or nasal pledget radioactivity following the intrathecal injection of a radiopharmaceutical or visualization of nasal, pharyngeal or middle ear radioactivity on radionuclide cisternography [38, 84, 99]. Quantitative radionuclide pledget tests are probably the most accurate method available for both the diagnosis and localization of the CSF fistula.

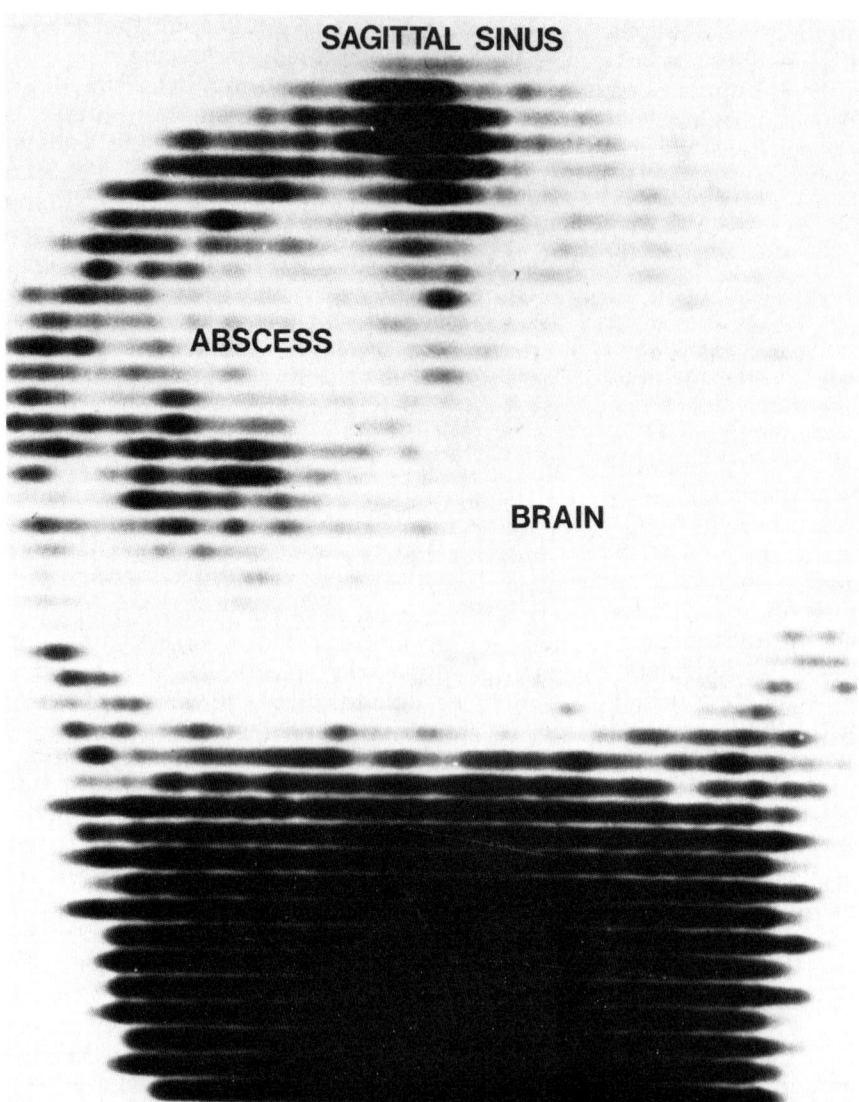

Fig. 61.12. Brain scan (posterior view) showing an intracranial abscess with the characteristic 'doughnut' appearance (ring of activity with no tracer in the centre due to central necrosis).

Probable advances in brain imaging will continue along the lines of transmission scanning for analysis of structure and dynamic studies of function; their future contributions to the investigation and management of the acutely ill patient will undoubtedly be significant.

Future prospects

The expected developments in technology, such as improved detector speed and efficiency, fast reliable labelling methods, availability of desk-top isotope generators, and cyclotrons,

single-photon transverse devises etc., will undoubtedly influence nuclear investigations. The rapid progress in computer-based quantitative techniques emphasizes the value of cross-sectional and three-dimensional images produced by various forms of radiant energy (ultrasound, x-rays, positrons, gamma rays, etc.) for clinical and biochemical research. A dynamic, three-dimensional spatial reconstructor (DSR) in which multiple x-ray sources and computer-based spatial reconstruction techniques are to be used is being developed [117, 145] and will allow the study of structural functional relationships of moving organ systems such as the heart, lungs and the circulation.

Emission transaxial tomography systems (ECT) in which short-lived positrons and biologically active radiopharmaceuticals are used should overcome the present limitations of conventional imaging, permitting measurements of metabolic activity and blood flow to small defined parts of the body [103, 105]. Quantitative dynamic scanning of the sequential organ distribution of specific ionic and non-ionic substrates is a new approach into the metabolic consequences of disease and the introduction of radiopharmaceuticals based on specific antibodies points to the possibility of their use in both the diagnosis and treatment.

References

1. Agnew JE, Maze M, Mitchell CJ (1976) Pancreatic scanning. Br J Radiol 49:979–995
2. Ahmad M, Logan KW, Martin RH (1979) Doughnut pattern of technetium^{-99m} pyrophosphate myocardial uptake in patients with acute myocardial infarction: A sign of poor long-term prognosis. Am J Cardiol 44:13–17
3. Albro PC, Gould KL, Westcott RJ, Hamilton GW, Ritchie JL, Williams DL (1978) Non-invasive assessment of coronary stenosis by myocardial imaging during pharmocologic coronary vasodilation. III. Clinical trial. Am J Cardiol 42:751–760
4. Alderson PO, Secker-Walker RH, Forrest JV (1974) Detection of obstructive pulmonary disease: Relative sensitivity of ventilation-perfusion studies and chest radiography. Radiology 112:643–648
5. Alderson PO, Krohn KA, Welch MJ (1976a) Radiopharmaceuticals. In: Gottschalk A, Potchen EJ (eds), Diagnostic nuclear medicine. Williams & Wilkins, Baltimore, pp 24–46
6. Alderson PO, Rujanavech N, Secker-Walker RH, Knight MC (1976b) The role of ^{133}Xe ventilation studies in the scintigraphic detection of pulmonary embolism. Radiology 120:633–640
7. Alderson PO, Doppman JL, Diamond SS, Mendenhall KG, Baron EL, Girton M (1978) Ventilation-perfusion lung imaging and selective pulmonary angiography in animals with experimental pulmonary embolism. J Nucl Med 19:164–171
8. Alderson PO, Lee H, Summer W, Motazedi A, Wagner HN (1979) Comparison of Xe^{133} washout and single breath imaging for the detection of ventilation abnormalities. J Nucl Med 20:917–922
9. Andrews JT, Kidd G, Steven IW, McKay WJ, Lichtenstein M (1977) Interpretation of radionuclide substraction scan in pancreatic carcinoma. Australas Radiol 21:53–59
10. Aquino HC, Preston DF, Luke RG (1971) ^{99m}Pertechnetate uptake in the transplanted kidney. Proceedings of the Dialysis and Transplantation Forum, pp 83–88
11. Ashburn WL, Schelbert HR, Verba JW (1978) Left ventricular ejection fraction: A review of several radionuclide angiographic approaches using the scintillation camera. Prog Cardiovasc Dis 20:267–284
12. Asher WM, Parvin S, Virgilio RW, Haber K (1976) Echographic evaluation of splenic injury after blunt trauma. Radiology 118:411–415
13. Bacharach SL, Green MV, Borer JS, Ostrow HG, Redwood DR, Johnston GS (1977) ECG-gated scintillation probe measurement of left ventricular function. J Nucl Med 18:1176–1183
14. Back N, Ambrus JL, Mink IB (1961) Distribution and fate of I-131-labeled componentes of the fibrinolysis system. Circ Res 9:1208–1216
15. Barkin J, Vining D, Miale A Jr, Gottlieb S, Redlhammer D, Kalser MH, (1977) Computerized tomography, diagnostic ultrasound, and radionuclide scanning: Comparison of efficacy in diagnosis of pancreatic carcinoma. JAMA 238:2040–2042
16. Barnes BD, Finklestein S, Winestock DP (1978) Radionuclide angiography: A sensitive diagnostic test for anterior circulation ischaemia. Neurology (Minneap) 28:775–781
17. Bartrum RJ Jr, Crow HC, Foote SR (1977) Ultrasonic and radiographic cholecystography. N Engl J Med 296:538–541
18. Bodenheimer MM, Banka VS, Fooshee CM, Gillespie JA, Helfant RH (1978) Detection of coronary heart disease using radionuclide-determined regional ejection fraction at rest and during handgrip exercise: Correlation with coronary arteriography. Circulation 58:640–648
19. Borer JS, Bacharach SL, Green MV, Kent KM, Epstein SE, Johnston GS (1977) Real-time radionuclide cineangiography in the non-invasive evaluation of global and regional left ventricular function at rest and during exercise in patients with coronary artery disease. N Engl J Med 296:839–844
20. Botvinick EH, Taradash MR, Shames DM, Parmley WW (1978) Thallium-201 myocardial perfusion scintigraphy for the clinical clarification of normal, abnormal and equivocal electrocardiographic stress tests. Am J Cardiol 41:43–51
21. Brown R, Weber PM, Dos Remedios LV, (1975) Dynamic/static brain scintigraphy: An effective scanning test for subdural hematoma. Radiology 117:355–360
22. Bryan PJ, Dinn WM, Grossman ZD, Wistow BW, McAfee JG, Kieffer SA (1977) Correlation of computed tomography, gray scale ultrasonography and radionuclide imaging of the liver in detecting space-occupying processes. Radiology 124:387–393
23. Budinger TF, Gullberg GT (1977) Transverse section reconstruction of gamma-ray emitting radionuclides in patients. In: Ter-Pogossian MM, Phelps ME, Brownell G, Cox JR, Davis DO, Evens RG (eds) Reconstruction tomography in diagnostic radiology and nuclear medicine. University Park Press, Baltimore, pp 315–342
24. Budinger TF, Rollo FD (1977) Physics and instrumentation. Prog Cardiovasc Dis 20:19–53
25. Buonocore E, Hübner KF (1979) Positron-emission computed tomography of the pancreas. A preliminary study. Radiology 133:195–201
26. Burdine JA, Murphy PH, DePuey EC (1979) Radionuclide computed tomography of the body using routine radiopharmaceuticals. II. Clinical applications. J Nucl Med 20:108–114
27. Burow RD, Strauss HW, Singleton R, Pond M, Rehn T, Bailey IK, Griffith LC, Nickoloff E, Pitt B (1977) analysis of left ventricular function from multiple gated acquisition cardiac blood pool imaging. Circulation 56:1024–1028
28. Carretta RF, DeNardo SJ, DeNardo GL, Jansholt A-L, Rose AW (1977) Early Diagnosis of venous thrombosis using ^{125}I-fibrinogen. J Nucl Med 18:5–10

29. Charkes ND, Dugan MA, Maier WP, Soulen R, Escovitz E, Learner N, Dubin R, Kozar J (1974) Scintigraphic detection of deep-vein thrombosis with ^{131}I-fibrinogen. J Nucl Med 15:1163–1166

30. Christensen EE, Bonte FJ (1968) The relative accuracy of echocardiography, intravenous CO_2 studies and blood-pool scanning in detecting pericardial effusions in dogs. Radiology 91:265–270

31. Claveria LE, Du Boulay GH, Moseley IF (1976) Intracranial infections: investigation by computerized axial tomography. Neuroradiology 12:59–71

32. Cowan RI, Maynard CD (1974) Trauma to the brain and extracranial structures. Semin Nucl Med 4:319–338

33. Dalen JE, Alpert JS (1975) Natural history of pulmonary embolism. Prog Cardiovasc Dis 17:259–270

34. Delmonico FL, McKusick KA, Cosimi AB, Russell PS (1977) Differentiation between renal allograft rejection and acute tubular necrosis by renal scan. AJR 128:625–628

35. DeNardo GL, Goodwin DA, Ravasini R, Dietrich PA (1970) The ventilatory lung scan in the diagnosis of pulmonary embolism. N Engl J Med 282:1334–1336

36. Depresseux JC (1977) Positron emission tomography and its applications. J Belge Radiol 60:483–500

37. DiMagno EP, Malagelada J-R, Taylor WF, Go VLW (1977) A prospective comparison of current diagnostic tests for pancreatic cancer. N Engl J Med 297:737–742

38. Doge H, Johannsen BA (1977) Radioactivity in gastric juice: A simple adjunct to the Yb-169 DTPA cisternographic diagnosis of rhinorrhea. J Nucl Med 19:1202–1204

39. Donaldson RM, Jarrit PH, Liversedge S, Ell PJ (1979) Ventricular pseudoaneurysm demonstrated by multiple gated cardiac imaging. Nuklearmedizin 18:283–285

40. Doust BD (1978) Ultrasonic examination of the pancreas. Radiol Clin North Am 13:467–478

41. Drum DE, Christacopoulos JS (1972) Hepatic scintigraphy in clinical decision making. J Nucl Med 13:908–915

42. Eikman EA, Cameron JL, Colman M, Natarajan TK, Dugal P, Wagner HN (1975) A test for patency of the cystic duct in acute cholecystitis. Ann Intern Med 82:318–322

43. Ell PJ, Donaldson RM (1978) Cardiovascular nuclear medicine and intensive care. Intensive Care Med 4:119–122

44. Ellenbogen PH, Scheible FW, Talner LB, Leopold GR (1978) Sensitivity of gray scale ultrasound in detecting urinary tract obstruction. AJR 130:731–733

45. Ennis JT, Elmes RJ (1977) Radionuclide venography in diagnosis of deep vein thrombosis. Radiology 125:441–449

46. Ennis JT, Elmes RJ (1978) Radionuclide venography in the diagnosis of deep vein thrombosis. Clin Nucl Med 3:276–277

47. Evans GW, Curtin FG, McCarthy HF, Kieran JH (1972) Scintigraphy in traumatic lesions of liver and spleen. JAMA 222:665–667

48. Eyler WR, Schuman BM, DuSault LA, Hinson RE (1965) The radioiodinated rose bengal liverscan as an aid in the differential diagnosis of jaundice. AJR 94:469–476

49. Fair WR (1975) Renal perfusion/excretion determination renogram: A new tool in the diagnostic evaluation of renovascular hypertension. J Urol 113:595–600

50. Fazio F, Jones T (1975) Assessment of regional ventilation by continuous inhalation of radioactive Krypton-81m. Br Med J iii:673–676

51. Fazio F, Lavender JP, Steiner RE (1978) Krypton-81m ventilation and ^{99m}Tc perfusion scans in chest disease: Comparison with standard radiographs. AJR 130:421–428

52. Fischer KC, McNeil BJ (1979) The indeterminate lung scan; its characteristics and its association with pulmonary embolism. Eur J Nucl Med 4:49–53

53. Folland ED, Hamilton GW, Larson SM, Kennedy JW, Williams DL, Ritchie JL (1977) The radionuclide ejection fraction: A comparison of three radionuclide techniques with contrast angiography. J Nucl Med 18:1159–1166

54. Gates GF, Fishman LS, Segall HD (1978) Scintigraphic detection of congenital intracranial vascular malformations. J Nucl Med 19:235–244

55. Gilday DL, Alderson PO (1974) Scintigraphic evaluation of liver and splenic injury. Semin Nucl Med 4:357–370

56. Glazier JB, DeNardo GL (1966) Pulmonary function studied with the xenon[133] scanning technique. Normal values and a postural study. Am Rev Respir Dis 94:188–194

57. Go RT, Doty DB, Chui CL, Christie JH (1975) A new method of diagnosing myocardial contusion in man by radionuclide imaging. Radiology 116:107–110

58. Goldberg BB, Ostrum BJ, Isard HJ (1968) Nephrosonography: Ultrasound differentiation of renal masses. Radiology 90:1113–1118

59. Goodwin DA, Bushberg JT, Doherty PW, Lipton MJ, Conley FK, Diamanti CI, Meares CF (1978) Indium-111-labelled autologous platelets for location of vascular thrombi in humans. J Nucl Med 19:626–634

60. Greenberg B, Hart R, Werner J, Brundage B, Botvinick E, Chatterjee K, Parmley W (1977) Thallium-201 stress imaging in the followup evaluation of coronary bypass patients. Circulation 56: [Suppl III] 111–230

61. Harris WH, Salzman EW, Athanasoulis C, Waltman A, Baum S, DeSanctis RW, Potsaid MS, Sise H (1975) Comparison of ^{125}I fibrinogen count scanning with phlebography for detection of venous thrombi after hip surgery. N Engl J Med 292:665–667

62. Harvey E, Loberg M, Ryan J, Sikorski S, Faith W, Cooper M (1979) Hepatic clearance mechanisms of ^{99m}Tc-HIDA and its effect on quantitation of hepatobiliary function. J Nucl Med 20:310–313

63. Harwig SS, Harwig JF, Sherman LA, Coleman RE, Welch MJ (1977) Radioiodinated plasminogen: An imaging agent for pre-existing thrombi. J Nucl Med 18:42–45

64. Hayes RL (1977) The tissue distribution of gallium radionuclides. J Nucl Med 18:740–742

65. Hill TC, Costello P, Gramm HF, Lovett R, McNeil BJ, Treves S (1978) Early clinical experience with a radioisotope computerized emission tomographic brain imager system. Radiology 128:803–806

66. Holman BL, Hill TC, Wynne J, Lovett RD, Zimmerman RE, Smith EM (1979) Single photon emission computed tomography of the heart in normal subjects and in patients with infarction. J Nucl Med 20:736–748

67. Hounsfield GN (1973) Computerized transverse axial scanning (tomography) 1 Description of system. Br J Radiol 46:1016–1022

68. Houser MF, Alderson PO (1978) Gallium 67 imaging in abdominal disease. Semin Nucl Med 8:251–270

69. Jackson GL, Albright D (1968) Splenic rupture: Application of radioisotopic techniques in diagnosis. JAMA 204:930–931

70. Jaszczak RJ, Murphy PH, Huard D, Burdine JA (1977) Radionuclide emission computed tomography of the head with ^{99m}Tc and a scintillation camera. J Nucl Med 18:373–380

71. Joseph SP, Pereira-Prestes AV, Ell PJ, Donaldson R,

Somerville W, Emanuel RW (1979) Value of positive myocardial infarction imaging in coronary care units. Br Med J i:372–374

72. Kakkar VV (1977) Fibrinogen uptake tests for detection of deep vein thrombosis. Semin Nucl Med 7:229–244

73. Karliner JS, Gault MD, Eckberg D, Mullins CB, Ross J Jr (1971) Mean velocity of fiber shortening: A simplified measure of left ventricular myocardial contractility. Circulation 44:323–333

74. Kelly PJ, Gorten RJ, Grossman RG, Eisenberg HM (1977) Cerebral perfusion, vascular spasm and outcome in patients with ruptured intracranial aneurysm. J Neurosurg 47:44–49

75. Keyes JW, Leonard PF, Svethoff DJ, Brody SI, Rogers WL, Lucchesi BR (1978) Myocardial imaging using emission computed tomography. Radiology 127:809–812

76. Kircos LT, Leonard PF, Keyes JW (1978) Optimized collimator for single-photon computed tomography with a scintillation camera. J Nucl Med 19:322–323

77. Korobkin M, Callen PW, Filly RA, Hoff PB, Shimshak RR, Kressel HY (1978) Comparison of computed tomography, ultrasonography, and gallium-67 scanning in the evaluation of suspected abdominal abscess. Radiology 129:89–93

78. Kotler MN, Segal BL, Mintz G, Parry WR (1977) Pitfalls and limitations of M-mode echocardiography. Am Heart J 94:227–249

79. Kuhd DF, Edwards RQ, Ricci AR, Yacob RJ, Mich TJ, Alavia A (1976) The MARK IV system for radionuclide computed tomography of the brain. Radiology 121:405–413

80. Lassen NA, Obrist W, Risberg J (1979) Cerebral blood flow by Xe 133 inhalation and single photon emission tomography. Contributon to the International Symposium of Cerebral Circulation, Toulouse

81. Levitt RG, Sagel SS, Stanley RJ, Jost RG (1977) Accuracy of computed tomography of the liver and biliary tract. Radiology 124:123–128

82. Lunia S, Parthasarathy KL, Bakshi S, Bender MA (1975) An evaluation of ^{99m}Tc-sulfur colloid liver scintiscans and their usefulness in metastatic workup: A review of 1,424 studies. J Nucl Med 16:62–65

83. Lutzker L, Koenigsberg M, Meng C, Freeman LM (1974) The role of radionuclide imaging in spleen trauma. Radiology 110:419–425

84. Magmaes B, Solheim D (1977) Controlled overpressure cisternography to localize cerebrospinal fluid rhinorrhea. J Nucl Med 8:109–111

85. Marcus ML, Kerber RE (1977) Present status of the ^{99m}technetium pyrophosphate infarct scintigram. Circulation 56:335–339

86. Marshall RC, Berger HJ, Costin JD, Freedman GS, Wolberg J, Cohen LS, Gottschalk A, Zaret BS (1977) Assessment of cardiac performance with quantitative angiocardiography. Circulation 56:820–829

87. Maseri A, Parodi O, Severi S, Pesola A (1976) Transient transmural reduction of myocardial blood flow, demonstrated by thallium-201 scintigraphy, as a cause of variant angina. Circulation 54:280–288

88. Massie BM, Botvinick EH, Werner JA, Chaterjee K, Parmley WW (1979) Myocardial scintigraphy with technetium-99m stannous pyrophosphate: An insensitive test for non-transmural myocardial infarction. Am J Cardiol 43:186–199

89. McAfee JG, Thomas FD, Grossman DHP, Streeten E, Dailey E, Gagne G (1977) Diagnosis of angiotensinogenic hypertension: Complementary roles of renal scintigraphy and saralasin infusion test. J Nucl Med 18:664–675

90. McNeil BJ (1976) A diagnostic strategy using ventilation-perfusion studies in patients suspect for pulmonary embolism. J Nucl Med 17:613–616

91. McNeil BJ, Holman BL, Adelstein SJ (1974) The scintigraphic definition of pulmonary embolism. JAMA 227:753–756

92. Miller JM, Ali MK, Howe CD (1970) Clinical determination of regional pulmonary function during normal breathing using xenon 133. Am Rev Respir Dis 101:218–229

93. Miskowiak J, Nielsen SL, Munck O, Andersen B (1977) Abdominal scintiphotography with technetium-99m labelled albumin in acute gastro-intestinal bleeding: Experimental study and case report. Lancet II:852–854

94. Moser KM (1977) Pulmonary embolism. Am Rev Respir Dis 115:829–852

95. Moses DC, Silver TM, Bookstein JJ (1974) The complementary roles of chest radiography, lung scanning and selective pulmonary angiography in the diagnosis of pulmonary embolism. Circulation 49:179–188

96. Nichols AB, Cochavi S, Hales CA, Strauss W, McCusick KA, Wastman AC, Beller GA (1978) Scintigraphic detection of pulmonary emboli by serial positron imaging of inhaled ^{15}O-labelled carbon dioxide. N Engl J Med 299:279–284

97. Nichols AB, McKusick KA, Strauss HW, Dinsmore RE, Block PC, Pohost GM (1978) Clinical utility of gated cardiac blood pool imaging in congestive left heart failure. Am J Med 65:785–793

98. Nilsson BW (1977) Cerebral blood flow in patients with subarachnoid haemorrhage studied with an intravenous isotope technique: Its clinical significance in the timing of surgery of cerebral arterial aneurysms. Acta Neurochir (Wien) 37:33–38

99. Oberson R (1972) Radioisotopic diagnosis of rhinorrhea. Radiol Clin Biol 41:28–35

100. O'Mara RE, Hall RC, Dombroski DL (1970) Scintigraphic scanning in the diagnosis of rupture of the spleen. Surg Gynecol Obstet 131:1077–1079

101. Passalaqua AM, Oster ZH, Chandra R, Braunstein P (1978) Liverpleural cavity scan for diagnosis of subphrenic abscess. Clin Nucl Med 3:209–211

102. Pauwels S, Steel SM, Piret L, Beckers C (1978) Clinical evaluation of ^{99m}Tc-diethyl-ida in hepatobiliary disorders. J Nucl Med 19:783–788

103. Phelps ME (1977) What is the purpose of emission computed tomography in nuclear medicine. J Nucl Med 18:399–402

104. Phelps ME, Hoffman EJ, Mullani NA, Ter-Pogossian MM (1975) Application of annihilation coincidence detection to trans-axial reconstruction tomography. J Nucl Med 16:635–647

105. Phelps ME, Hoffman EJ, Huang SC, Kuhl DE (1978) ECAT: A new computerized tomographic imaging system for positron-emitting radiopharmaceuticals. J Nucl Med 19:635–647

106. Pitt B, Strauss HW (1976) Myocardial perfusion imaging and gated cardiac blood pool scanning: Clinical application. Am J Cardiol 38:739–746

107. Pizer SM, Todd-Pokropek AE (1978) Improvement of scintigrams by computer processing. Semin Nucl Med 8:125–146

108. Pohost GM, Zir LM, Moore RH, McKusick DA, Guiney TE, Beller GA (1977a) Differentiation of transiently ischemic from infarcted myocardium by serial imaging after a single dose of thallium-201. Circulation 55:294–302

109. Pohost GM, Vignola PA, McKusick KA, Block PC, Myers GS, Walker HJ, Copen DL, Dinsmore RE (1977)

110. Pollack HM, Goldberg BB, Morales JO, Bogash M
Hypertropic cardiomyopathy. Evaluation by gated cardiac blood pool scanning. Circulation 55:92–99
(1974) A systematized approach to the differential
diagnosis of renal masses. Radiology 113:653–659

111. Preston DF, Luke RG (1979) Radionuclide evaluation of
renal transplants. J Nucl Med 20:1095–1097

112. Reduto LA, Berger HJ, Cohen LS, Gottschalk A, Zaret
AL (1978) Sequential radionuclide assessment of left
and right ventricular performance after acute transmural myocardial infarction. Ann Intern Med 89:441–447

113. Reivich M, Kuhl D, Wolf A, Greenberg J, Phelps M,
Ido T, Casella V, Fowler J, Gallagher B, Hoffman E,
Alavi A, Sokoloff L (1977) Measurement of local cerebral glucose metabolism in man with 18F-2fluoro-2-
deoxy-D-glucose. Acta Neurol Scand 56 [Suppl 64]:
190–191

114. Rhodes BA, Bell WR, Malmud LS (1975) Labeling and
testing of urokinase and streptokinase: New tracers for
the detection of thromboemboli. In: Radiopharmaceuticals and labeled compounds, vol 2. IAEA,
Viena, pp 163–169

115. Rigo P, Murray M, Strauss HW, Bitt B (1974a) Scintiphotographic evaluation of patients with suspected
left ventricular aneurysm. Circulation 50:985–991

116. Rigo P, Murray M, Strauss HW, Taylor D, Kelly D,
Weisfeldt M, Pitt B (1974b) Left ventricular function in
acute myocardial infarction evaluated by gated scintiphotography. Circulation 50:678–684

117. Ritman EL, Robb RA, Johnson SA, Chevalier PA,
Gilbert BK, Greenleaf JF, Sturm RE, Wood EH (1978)
Quantitative imaging of the structure and function
of the heart, lungs and circulation. Mayo Clin Proc
53:3–11

118. Rollo FD, Cavalieri RR, Born M, Blei L, Chew M (1977)
Accuracy of brain scanning in paediatric craniocerebral
neoplasms. Radiology 123:379–383

119. Ronai PM (1977) Hepatobiliary radiopharmaceuticals:
Defining their clinical role will be a galling experience. J
Nucl Med 18:488–490

120. Rosenthall L (1966) Radionuclide venography using
99mTc pertechnetate and the gamma-ray scintillation
camera. Semin Roentgenol 97:874–879

121. Rosenthall L, Shaffer EA, Lisboka R, Pare P (1978)
Diagnosis of Hepatobiliary Disease by 99mTc-HIDA
cholescintigraphy. Radiology 126:467–474

122. Ryan J, Cooper M, Loberg B, Harvey E, Sixorski S
(1977) Technetium-99m-labelled [N-(2, 6-dimethyl-
phenylcarbamoylmethyl)] iminodiacetic acid (Tc-99m
HIDA): A new radiopharmaceutical for hepatobiliary
imaging studies. J Nucl Med 18:997–1004

123. Sagel SS, Stanley RJ, Levitt RG, Geisse G (1977)
Computed tomography of the kidney. Radiology
124:359–370

124. Sample WF, Gray RK, Poe ND, Graham LS, Bennett
LR (1977) Nuclear imaging, tomographic nuclear imaging, and gray scale ultrasound in the evaluation of the
porta hepatis. Radiology 122:773–779

125. Schelbert HR, Phelps HE, Hoffman EJ, Huang SC,
Selin CE, Kuhl DE (1979) Regional myocardial perfusion assessed with N13 labelled ammonia and position
emission computerized tomography. Am J Cardiol
43:209–218

126. Secker-Walker RH (1978) Pulmonary physiology,
pathology and ventilation-perfusion studies. J Nucl
Med 19:961–968

127. Sharpe DN, Botvinick EM, Shames DM, Schiller NB,
Massie BM, Chatterjee K, Parmley WW (1978) The
non-invasive diagnosis of right ventricular infarction.
Circulation 57:483–490

128. Sheedy PF II, Stephens DH, Hattery RR, Macarty RL
(1977) Computed tomography in the evaluation of
patients with suspected carcinoma of the pancreas.
Radiology 124:731–737

129. Stanley RJ, Sagel SS, Levitt RG (1977) Computed
tomographic evaluation of the pancreas. Radiology
124:715–722

130. Sullivan DC, Taylor KJW, Gottschalk A (1978) The use
of ultrasound to enhance the diagnostic utility of the
equivocal liver scintigraph. Radiology 128:727–732

131. Sy WH, Lao RS, Bay R, Nash M (1978) Technetium 99m
pertechnetate radionuclide venography: Large volume
injection without tourniquet. J Nucl Med 19:1001–1006

132. Symbas PN (1978) Trauma to the heart and great
vessels, 2nd edn Grune & Stratton, New York, pp 55–
65

133. Tajik AJ (1977) Echocardiography in pericardial effusion. Am J Med 63:29–40

134. Tanasescu DE, Wolfstein RS, Waxman AD (1977) Critical evaluation of Tc99m glucoheptonate as brain scanning agent (Abstract) J Nucl Med 18:630

135. Taylor KJW, Carpenter DA, McCready VR (1974) Ultrasound and scintigraphy in the differential diagnosis of
obstructive jaundice. J Clin Ultrasound 2:105–116

136. Taylor KJW, Sullivan D, Simeone J, Rosenfield AT
(1977a) Scintigraphy, ultrasound and CT scanning of
the liver. Yale J Biol Med 50:437–455

137. Taylor KJW, Sullivan D, Rosenfield AT (1977b) Gray
scale ultrasound and isotope scanning: Complementary techniques for imaging the liver. AJR
128:277–281

138. Taylor KJW, Sullivan DC, Wasson JFM, McI JF,
Rosenfield AT (1978) Ultrasound and gallium for the
diagnosis of abdominal and pelvic abscesses. Gastrointest Radiol 3:281–286

139. Thrall JH, Swanson DP, Wieland DM (1978) Development of non-ionic gamma-emitting radiopharmaceuticals for myocardial imaging. J Nucl Med 19:969

140. Tow DE, Simon AL (1975) Comparison of lung scanning and pulmonary angiography in the detection and
follow-up of pulmonary embolism: The Urokinase-
Pulmonary Embolism Trial Experience. Prog Cardiovasc Dis 17:239–245

141. Tow DE, Wagner HN, North WA (1967) Detection of
venous obstruction in the legs with Tc99m albumin. J
Nucl Med 8:277

142. Vogel RA, Kirch D, Le Free M, Steele P (1978) A new
method of multiplanar emission tomography using a
seven pinhole collimeter and an anger scintillation
camera. J Nucl Med 19:648–654

143. Wagner HN Jr, Strauss HW (1975) Radioactive tracers
in the differential diagnosis of pulmonary embolism.
Prog Cardiovasc Dis 17:271–282

144. Winston MA, Blahd WH (1972) I-131 Rose Bengal
imaging techniques in differential diagnosis of jaundiced patients. Semin Nucl Med 2:167–175

145. Wood EH (1976) Cardiovascular and pulmonary dynamics by quantitative imaging. Circ Res 38:131–139

146. Woolley JL, Williams B, Venkatesh S (1977) Cranial
isotopic section scanning. Clin Radiol 28:517–528

147. Zaret BL, Strauss HW, Hurley PJ, Natarajan TK, Pitt B
(1971) A non-invasive scintiphotographic method for
detecting regional ventricular dysfunction in man. N
Engl J Med 284:1165–1170

Chapter 62

Blood Gas Analysis

B. Teisseire

This chapter focuses on four problems confronting the staff of an intensive care laboratory.

The first is that of quality control of blood gas analysers. These machines, which function 24 h a day, are not always installed within the specialized laboratory; we have tried, therefore, to give the overall outlines of realistic quality control that will ensure constantly reliable results.

The second problem, a direct result of quality control, is the use of tonometered total blood and control solutions, aqueous solutions or reconstituted blood, in the analysers. The user has, in effect, a wide choice of control solutions available, and in addition to a thorough knowledge of the blood gas equipment employed their use requires familiarity with the properties of the various solutions and with the advantages and disadvantages of each.

The third problem is that of correction of the PO$_2$ in accordance with the patient's temperature. Depending upon the apparatus used, a given PO$_2$, measured at 37°C, will give different values after correction for the patient's temperature. Variations obtained with the different blood gas analysers raise the problem of the validity of such a correction, given that it varies according to the apparatus and that such variations in values for PO$_2$ far exceed the accuracy of the measurement.

Finally, with the advent of the possibility of rapid determination of blood lactic acid concentrations (within 1 min), we have cited our own experience of combining this measurement with the measurement of acid–base equilibrium and oxymetry.

Quality control

Until 1960, determination of the parameters of acid–base equilibrium was the exclusive domain of specialized laboratories whose personnel were thoroughly trained in measurement of these, with the Van Slyke manometric apparatus, Natelson's microgasometer, and the Schölander machine. In 1960, the advent of the first machines capable of direct measurement of the partial pressures of O$_2$ and CO$_2$ together with measurements of pH at 37°C allowed a certain level of standardization. These so-called manual devices were extremely simple, consisting of three electrodes and a measurement chamber immersed in a waterbath at 37°C. The quality of the measurement depended to a great extent on the operator, for he or she was responsible for carrying out calibrations on gases and pH, for introducing the specimen to be measured into the machine, and for performing the necessary rinses. In 1970, with the arrival of the electronic era, the machines became semi-automatic and automatic. By 1980, the simple manual apparatus of 1960 had given way to a highly sophisticated and complex push-button machine with a multiplicity of predetermined cycles and logic circuits capable of commanding these, and much internal tubing but because of the more complicated and unpredictable breakdowns that occur in such apparatus, trained and specialized personnel are needed to keep it in perfect functioning order.

A blood gas analysis is usually requested only

in an emergency, and the results of such an examination will lead to therapeutic decisions which could have grave consequences if the original results are incorrect. Unfortunately, there are many possible sources of error, and the built-in security of an automatic apparatus cannot in itself reduce their number.

Errors due to calibration

Standard gas mixtures used for the calibration of PO_2 and PCO_2 electrodes are generally precisely constituted. It is wise, however, to verify this composition by the method of Schölander, for although errors are very rare, they do happen. The calibration gas bottles should be kept in a horizontal position to avoid stratification and should be attached to the blood gas analyser by means of thick Neoprene tubing. Some automatic machines are equipped with a gas mixer which, using air and pure CO_2, can produce two standard gases. An obvious precaution is to place this machine in a well-ventilated room, remote from any source of O_2. The presence of a gas mixer in the automated apparatus does not preclude the use of the Schölander machine, for ageing or clogging of the gas mixer membranes can modify the gaseous mixture. If the calibration is performed during a liquid phase after tonometry of the pH buffer solutions, not only PCO_2 and PO_2 will be affected, but also the pH value. Deficiencies in the smooth functioning of the gas mixer are very difficult to detect, for they tend to build up very gradually. Thus, it is essential to verify the performance of the gas mixer by using a Schölander machine every 6 months. Isolated calibration of pH by means of ampoules containing standard buffer solution does not pose any problem providing they have not been exposed to air for more than 2 h.

Errors due to faulty sampling

To minimize the probability of such errors we have very strict rules, viz.:

1) An *arterial blood sample* of 3 ml taken into an American luer-lock glass syringe, free of bubbles should be used.

2) The person taking the blood sample should *carry it personally* to the laboratory, together with a *request form* giving the *ventilatory conditions* (FIO$_2$, current volume, frequency, PEEP, etc.) *and the patient's temperature.*

3) *No more than 20 min* should elapse between sampling and analysis.

4) Heparin must only remain in the syringe's 'dead' space; too small a volume of blood (less than 1 ml) when diluted with a similar volume of heparin will lead to a decrease in pH, PCO_2, and total CO_2.

Three other points merit discussion, however:

1) Conservation of the sample in ice should only be envisaged for blood samples with high numbers of leucocytes ($>30\ 000/mm^3$; i.e., in leukemia and septicaemia cases, etc.). Routine storage of blood samples in ice has two disadvantages in our opinion: the notion of emergency is lost; and there is a certain instability in the measurement of PO_2 on some machines whose heating system is not adequate to ensure thermal equilibrium at 37°C.

2) Capillary sampling: If exact values for arterial pH, PCO_2, and PO_2 are desired, then capillary sampling is not a satisfactory alternative.

3) Plastic syringes must not be used to take samples with high values of PO_2 [>200 mmHg (26.7 kPa)] and PCO_2.

Errors due to poor condition of the apparatus

The analysers must be kept impeccably clean. Errors can be caused by polluted electrolyte solutions, a faulty KCl bridge, coating of the electrode membranes with protein, bacteria in the measurement chamber, and other factors.

During measurement

Oxygen saturation (sat HbO$_2$) must be determined simultaneously with the measurements of PO_2 and pH. It will then be possible to compare the measured sat HbO$_2$ and the calculated sat HbO$_2$ by means of a standard curve for O$_2$–Hb dissociation and the Bohr effect. Except where there is a large modification in the intra-erythrocyte 2,3-DPG concentration, these two values are within 1%–2% of each other. This supplementary measurement, besides giving a very good approximation of the O$_2$ content, helps to avoid large errors in PO_2 and pH measurements. Any discrepancy between measured and calculated sat HbO$_2$ should be followed up by a repeat measurement of the preceding parameters on another machine. This comparison between measured and calculated sat HbO$_2$ cannot be carried out in the presence of abnormally structured haemoglobin (this is extremely rare) or fetal (newborn) haemoglobin specimen.

It is essential to have two blood gas analysers constantly functioning in the same laboratory. Achievement of identical results with passage of the same blood specimen on each of these two machines is perhaps the best method of checking the accuracy of measurement [10].

All blood gas results should be catalogued for each patient; the record must include the date and time of sampling, precise ventilatory conditions, and the temperature of the patient.

Monitoring of apparatus function

Use of tonometered blood

This method, which appears simple and involves equilibration of a blood sample with a gaseous mixture of known composition, is in fact complex and difficult. It can only give reliable results if the following requirements are carefully adhered to:

In the gaseous phase, the gas mixtures employed should be analyzed according to Schö-lander and the gas mixture should be preheated to 37°C and saturated in water vapour.

Pressure should not be excessive when equilibration takes place in the tonometer, and the tonometry chamber must be perfectly clean. The duration of tonometry will depend on the blood volume and gas debit ratio: the lower the liquid volume, the higher the gas debit, and the shorter the time necessary for achieving equilibrium [18].

Heparinized human blood samples without high white cell counts should be used, to preserve the haemoglobin characteristics. The tonometered blood sample must be transferred to the measurement cell without any gaseous contamination or change in pressure or temperature with respect to the tonometry conditions, and determinations must be carried out immediately on tonometered blood.

For thermal equilibration, the temperature of the equipment used for tonometry must be identical with that of the measurement cell–electrode unit. The temperature of tonometry must be conserved during transfer by means of preheated syringes, and preheated solutions should be used to rinse the tonometer [22].

Only if all these rules are adhered to will it be possible to obtain perfectly tonometered blood for monitoring of the blood gas measurement apparatus. This procedure, cumbersome as it

may be, is the only one that is entirely satisfactory [7, 12].

Aqueous control solutions

These are standard aqueous buffer solutions equilibrated with gas mixtures of O_2 and CO_2 at 37°C. These liquids are now commercially stabilized and stored in ampoules. The addition of 30% glycerol makes it possible to obtain solutions whose viscosity and diffusion current are similar to those of total blood with the same partial pressures of O_2 and CO_2. When produced, these solutions are very carefully equilibrated with gaseous mixtures of known composition, but their target value and range in the final ampoule are determined on a blood gas analyser. Behavioural differences between such solutions and blood, as well as differences in the physical characteristics of blood gas analysers, explain why target values for the same check are not identical. Several different models, all produced by the same manufacturer, may show variations in target values and notable differences in PO_2, depending on the O_2 concentration of the gas used for tonometry of the aqueous buffer solution [10, 21].

The aqueous buffer solutions contained in ampoules are acceptable for checking the pH electrode. They are available in three grades (acid, normal, and alkaline), with ranges of around ±0.02 pH units. They should not under any circumstances be confused with commercially available pH calibration solutions.

As a control for the PCO_2 electrode, a liquid in the more general sense of the word is preferable to a gaseous mixture, since it detects electrical wastage at the level of the electrode, tears in the membrane, variations in measurement temperature, and anomalies due to introduction of the specimen [19].

In quality control of the PO_2 electrode, aqueous buffer solutions in ampoules do not give satisfactory results, as O_2 is present in such liquids only in a dissolved form. This has been documented in two analysers (the BMS 3 manual and the ABL II automatic, both from Radiometer). Tonometry was performed with fresh blood and with commercially available aqueous buffer solutions, and with a gaseous mixture whose composition had been determined according to Schölander's method. The tonometer was equipped with a PO_2 verification electrode. The results are shown in Fig. 62.1. The two machines were in perfect functioning order, since the values for PO_2 obtained from tonometered blood are in perfect agreement

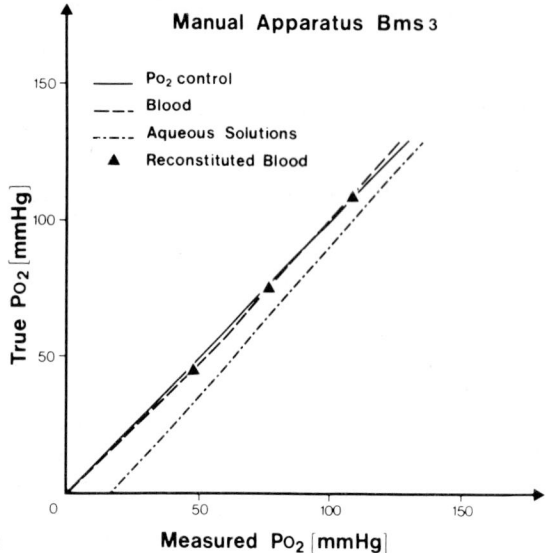

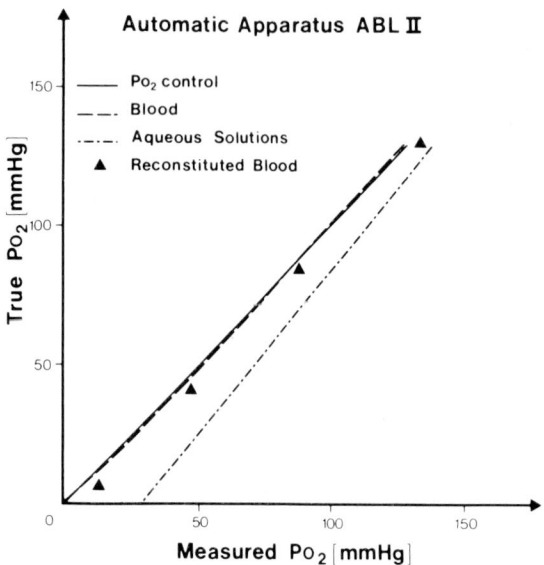

Fig. 62.1. a Effects of contamination by humidity or gas on the PO_2 measured by a manual blood gas analyser. Total blood, aqueous buffer solutions, and reconstituted blood are compared;

b Effects of contamination by humidity or gas on the PO_2 measured by an automatic blood gas apparatus. Total blood, aqueous buffer solutions, and reconstituted blood are compared.

with the calculated values. Significant differences were observed for tonometered aqueous buffer solutions, however. Three factors combined to make results with aqueous buffer solutions unreliable:

Contamination of the aqueous control solution by calibration gas left over in the measurement chamber before the sample was

introduced, or by traces of humidity in the measurement chamber;

Contamination by O_2 from the air of the aqueous buffer solution when the ampoule was opened or when it was decanted into the syringe. (This factor was not present in our study);

The existence of the blood/gas factor, i.e., a difference in the response of a PO_2 electrode in the gaseous or the aqueous and blood phases [1].

To set target values for these aqueous buffer solutions, manufacturers must base them not on the tonometry values at the time of manufacture, but on the overall values these solutions register on many new apparatuses of the same type. It is normal for calibration gas or traces of humidity to remain inside the measurement chamber without necessarily changing the PO_2 measured on the blood specimens.

'Control' blood

This is a suspension of human blood cells stabilized in a buffer medium. It does not appear to have any advantages over tonometered aqueous solutions for measuring pH and PCO_2. Despite a curve of O_2–Hb dissociation which is non-sigmoid and strongly displaced toward the left (P_{50}: 5 mmHg at pH 7.40 and 37°C), it nonetheless retains some buffer strength, giving excellent results (Fig. 62.1) [9].

Correction of PO_2 for the patient's temperature

Automated blood gas apparatuses are equipped with computers permitting correction of values for pH, PCO_2, and PO_2 (measured at 37°C) for the patient's temperature. While formulae for correction of pH and PCO_2 are nearly identical on the different analysers [2, 3, 11, 13], this is not the case for correction of the PO_2, according to the results in the literature [5, 6, 11, 16, 17, 20]. We find, in fact, some formulae which use a saturation value calculated from pH and PO_2 measurements for the AVL 940, BG II, and Corning 175 machines, and other formulae which only take into account the value of the measured PO_2. Table 62.1 raises the problem of the validity of these corrections. It gives values, calculated at 25°C, of 100 mmHg for PO_2

Table 62.1. Correction at 25°C of a PO₂: 100 mmHg measurement with three acid-base statuses at 37°C by means of various automatic blood gas analysers

Apparatus \ pH:37°C	6.90	7.40	7.60
AVL, BG II, CORNING 175	46.1	58.8	62.5
IL 813	42.5	53.5	59.1
ABL II	51.5	51.5	51.5
ABL III	47.0	47.0	47.0
IL 1303	48.8	48.8	48.0

measured at 37°C on the different automatic blood gas analysers. Those whose formulae include saturation show results that are modified as a function of the pH value measured at 37°C, thus differing from those that calculate corrected PO₂ starting from the level of the PO₂ measured at 37°C. This variation is significant (from 46 mmHg to 62.5 mmHg) and is far greater than the measurement error. The problem of correction of PO₂ is complicated due to the action of different haemoglobin ligands, depending on the temperature level, the interactions of these different ligands, and especially on the change in the effect of H^+, CO_2, 2, 3-DPG, and temperature as a function of the oxygenation level of the haemoglobin molecule [8, 14, 15].

In the light of these scattered results obtained for correction of PO₂ for the patient's temperature, it would be wise for manufacturers to try and create uniformity in their correction formulas (R. Herigault et al., 1981, unpublished work).

Rapid assay of blood lactic acid

The arrival on the market of semi-automatic apparatuses for L-lactate assays has meant that it is now possible to obtain the lactic acid concentration of a blood specimen very rapidly (in 1 min for 50 μl blood). We felt it would be of interest to study both acid–base equilibrium and oxymetry values, and lacticaemia values of blood samples from resuscitation centres or cardio-vascular surgery wards simultaneously [4]. We were unable to show any relationship

between the lactic acid concentration value and the values of pH and bicarbonate. We should, nonetheless, emphasize two points: (1) The possible co-existence of a high level of lacticaemia and normal parameters for acid–base equilibrium; and (2) a progressive increase of lacticaemia with time while acid–base equilibrium remains nearly normal because of the resuscitation procedure. This dissociation has always signified a bad prognosis.

Figure 62.2 shows the evolution of lacticaemia in the course of extracorporeal circulation in a child. Hypothermia systematically leads to an increase in lactic acid concentration, which should not exceed 2–3 mM/litre. Lacticaemia with values higher than 5 mM/litre are a cause for alarm, and there seems to be a critical threshold at 10 mM/litre. Above such a value for lacticaemia, one can expect problems with the decline in extracorporeal circulation. Another important factor to take into consideration is the return to normal of postoperative lactic acid levels.

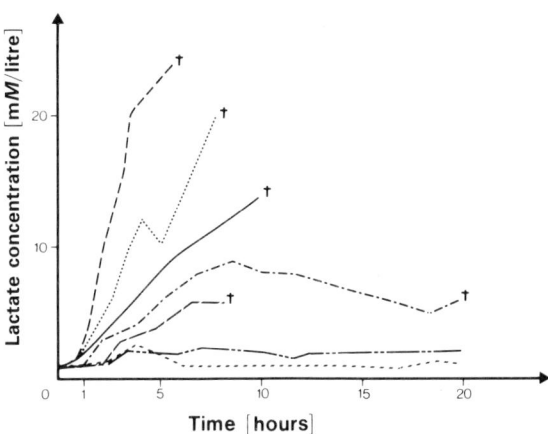

Fig. 62.2. Evolution of the blood lactate concentration (mM/litre) versus time during and after extracorporeal circulation in open-chest surgery.
†, death of the patient.

References

1. Adams AP, Morgan-Hughes JO (1967) Determination of the blood gas factor of the oxygen electrode using a new tonometer. Br J Anaesth 39:107–110
2. Adamson K, Daniel SS, Gandy G, James LS (1964) Influence of temperature on blood pH of the human adult and newborn. J Appl Physiol 19:897–900
3. Astrup P, Engel K, Severinghaus JW, Munson E (1965) The influence of temperature and pH on the dissociation curve of oxyhemoglobin of human blood. J Clin Lab Invest 17:515–523

4. Bossart H, Perret C (1979) Lactate in acute conditions. S. Karger, Basel New York
5. Bradley AF, Stupfel M, Severinghaus JW (1956) Effect of temperature on PCO_2 and PO_2 of blood in vitro. J Appl Physiol 9:201–204
6. Burnett RW (1978) Erroneous temperature corrections for blood pH and gas measurements. Clin Chem 24:1850–1859
7. Farhi LE (1965) Continuous duty tonometer system. J Appl Physiol 20:1098–1101
8. Hlastala MP, Woodson RD, Wranne B (1977) Influence of temperature on hemoglobin ligand interaction in whole blood. J Appl Physiol 43:545–550
9. Matthews H, Schneider A (1976) Quality control materials for pH and PCO_2 determinations. Clin Chem 22:1821–1824
10. Noonan DC, Burnett RW (1974) Quality control system for blood pH and gas measurements, with the use of a tonometered bicarbonate-chloride solution and duplicate samples of whole blood. Clin Chem 20:660–665
11. Nunn JF, Bergman NA, Bunatyan A, Coleman AJ (1965) Temperature coefficients for PCO_2 and PO_2 of blood in vitro. J Appl Physiol 20:23–26
12. Ravin MB, Briscoe WA (1964) Blood gas transfer, hemolysis, and diffusing capacity in a bubble tonometer. J Appl Physiol 19:784–790
13. Rosenthal TB (1948) The effect of temperature on the pH of blood and plasma in vitro. J Biol Chem 173:25–30
14. Severinghaus JW (1966) Blood gas calculator. J Appl Physiol 21:1108–1116
15. Severinghaus JW, Stupfel M, Bradley AF (1956) Accuracy of blood pH and PCO_2 determination. J Appl Physiol 9:189–196
16. Siggard-Andersen O (1974) The acid–base status of the blood, 4th edn. Munksgaard, Copenhagen
17. Siggard-Andersen O (1976) Blood gases. In: Tietz N (ed) Fundamentals of clinical chemestry. Saunders, Philadelphia, p 854
18. Steiner MC, Shapiro BA, Kavanaugh J, Walton JR, Johnson W (1978) A stable blood product for pH-blood gas quality control. Clin Chem 24:793–795
19. Teng Leary E, Delaney CJ, Kenny MA (1977) Use of equilibrated blood for internal blood gas quality control. Clin Chem 23:493–503
20. Thomas LJ Jr (1972) Algorithms for selected blood acid-base and blood gas calculations. J Appl Physiol 33:154–158
21. Veefkind AH, Van der Camp RAM, Mass AHJ (1975) Use of carbon dioxide and oxygen tonometered phosphate-bicarbonate-chloride-glycerol-water mixtures for calibration and control of pH, PCO_2 and PO_2. Clin Chem 21:685–693
22. Weisbrot JM, Kambli VB, Gorton L (1974) An evaluation of clinical laboratory performance of pH-blood gas analyses using whole-blood tonometer specimens. Am J Clin Pathol 61:923–929

Section L

Paediatric Problems

Chapter 63

Temperature Regulation in Sick Infants

Edmund Hey

Homoeothermy is achieved in the baby in very much the same way as it is in adult life, and its maintenance is probably just as important in later life as it is in the neonatal period. Such differences as there are are quantitative rather than qualitative.

Surroundings that provide reasonable comfort for a growing child or adult may, nevertheless, impose a severe cold stress on an ill baby in the first 3 months of life. Differences in basal metabolism per unit surface area are the main reason for this disparity. The problem is aggravated by a limited behavioural response to cold stress and by an inability to communicate. No nurse would ever respond to an adult patient who complained of feeling cold by just taking their temperature and then saying, 'Nonsense, you cannot be cold; your temperature is quite normal'; but this, I fear, is how we often approach small babies. We tend to confuse feeling cold and being cold. And we do this despite all we now know about the way in which thermal stress can affect the body long before homoeothermic temperature regulation starts to break down. Comfort and warmth are at least as important to the patient receiving intensive care as they are to the wellbeing and recovery of every other patient requiring nursing care. We ignore these needs at the patient's peril.

There is nothing unique about the mechanisms underlying homoeothermy in the neonatal period. The principles of neonatal management are almost certainly just as relevant to the care of older children and adults. While, therefore, this chapter will concentrate on the needs of babies in the first few months of life, attention will be drawn to parallel issues affecting the care of older patients where appropriate.

Factors affecting thermal exchange

Resting heat production

Resting heat production on a weight-for-weight basis is often twice as high in babies a few weeks old as it is in adult life. Heat loss is proportional to surface area (or that fraction of total area sufficiently exposed to participate in heat exchange), however, and resting heat production per unit surface area in a 1-kg baby shortly after birth may be only one-third that in adult life [60]. On this count alone, these babies need an environment three times as warm as that required by their attendants to experience comparable warmth, since ambient warmth is inversely proportional to the difference between environmental temperature and deep body temperature. Thus where a clothed adult with a deep body temperature of 37°C might be comfortably warm in a room at 22°C, a comparably dressed 1-kg baby might only feel warm in a room at 32°C.

Resting heat production rises fairly rapidly in healthy babies during the first week or so of life, [55], and then more slowly until heat production per unit surface area approaches a value similar to that found in adult life 3–5 months after birth [72]. Thereafter heat production per unit surface area remains almost constant throughout childhood [77] and through most of adult life. In consequence, while it is generally safe to assume that any environment that seems reasonably warm to an adult will be equally appropriate for a comparably clothed child more than 3 months old, assessment is very much more difficult in the neonatal period.

Starvation can cause a fall in resting heat production in the neonatal period [117], as in later childhood [1], while specific dynamic action and the high calorie intake associated with rapid growth [21, 22] can cause a rise. Drugs can also have an effect on resting metabolism in the neonatal period [48]. More importantly, basal heat production is quite markedly reduced in babies with severe cyanosis and a low cardiac output, and even more markedly elevated in others with a left-to-right shunt and congestive heart failure [73]. There is evidence that heat production is also greatly increased in babies recovering from the acute stages of respiratory distress in the neonatal period [79]. Little is known about the way in which laboured breathing increases heat production in babies and young children with other respiratory disorders.

Response to cold stress

Healthy babies can more than double their heat production in response to acute cold stress. Naked babies usually become restless in cold surroundings, but shivering is not seen and muscular activity is often poorly sustained [55]. Clothed babies show even less overt muscular activity in response to cold stress [65], and much of the increase in heat production is thought to be due to oxidation of fat within strategically situated areas of brown adipose tissue around the heart, kidneys, and great vessels in the neck, chest, and abdomen [68].

Despite this response, there is usually some fall in rectal temperature and this cannot be ascribed to an inability to respond, since it often occurs when heat production is well below the maximum that can be achieved [55]. A similar 'heterothermic' response is seen in many neonatal mammals and has been considered to be an adaptive response influencing survival. The response to cold stress is further reduced by severe chronic hypoxia [25] and abolished by acute hypoxia when arterial PO_2 falls below about 46 mm Hg (6 kPa) [103]. Severe asphyxia also disturbs temperature regulation for a variable time after birth [24]. Sedative drugs also mute the metabolic response to cold stress, making small babies vulnerable to hypothermia [30].

Thermal insulation

Tissue insulation is marginally lower in infancy than it is in adult life, and is significantly reduced in babies of less than 1.5 kg [67, 101], probably as a result of the reduced amount of subcutaneous fat. Even very immature babies have almost as much control over skin blood flow and tissue insulation as adults [23, 61], but the importance of this variation in tissue insulation is dwarfed by the extent to which total thermal insulation varies in response to external factors.

Considerable heat can be lost by conduction when an unclothed baby lies on an unwarmed plastic or metal surface of high thermal conductivity [67], but conductive loss is negligible in most clinical settings. Convective and radiant loss account for the remaining bulk loss of sensible heat, with the boundary layer of still air over the body surface, which is nearly 1 cm thick, playing a much larger part in controlling heat loss than is generally appreciated. The overall resistance to heat loss caused by this layer of still air is almost as high in infancy as it is in adult life, any small difference being largely due to the body's lower average radius of curvature [67].

Radiant loss is responsible for rather more than half of all sensible heat loss in a draught-free environment when the radiant surfaces are the same temperature as the air, and radiant loss increases still further when environmental radiant temperature is lower than the air temperature. Transparent single-walled incubators pose problems in this regard because their surfaces are only heated indirectly, with the result that wall temperature is influenced almost as much by room temperature as it is by internal air temperature [64]. Radiant loss can, in consequence, more than double when a baby in a single-walled incubator is moved from a warm hospital ward into an unheated transport vehicle at 10°C, even if the incubator air temperature remains completely unaffected.

Convective loss accounts for slightly less than half of all sensible heat loss in draught-free surroundings, but air movement causes a rapid increase in this loss. The baby's own movements can cause a measurable increase in convective loss by decreasing the depth of the boundary layer of still air [67], and small increases in the speed with which air circulates within an enclosed incubator can also cause a significant increase in heat loss [29]. Major draughts could easily double convective heat loss, although this factor has never been subjected to direct study.

Changes in posture are the only way a small infant can exert any personal control over these major sources of heat loss. There is some evidence that a prone baby can exert some postural control over these losses when naked, but less evidence that a supine baby has this ability. Clothes and bedding offer the most effective way of decreasing these losses: a single light sheet or drape greatly reduces the loss, and a vest, nightdress, and napkin more than halve the loss [65]. Relatively little heat is lost from the extremities in the clothed or unclothed baby, but the head is a major source of heat loss, partly on account of its relatively large size in early infancy, partly because of the brain's continuous metabolic activity, and partly because skin blood flow over the head appears to vary relatively little in response to changes in the thermal environment [61].

There is no reliable way of judging cold stress merely from a child's appearance. Shivering may be absent and muscular activity minimal. Posture may provide a clue but is far from reliable. Vasomotor tone is equally hard to assess visually, but the cold hands and feet of the vasoconstricted infant are a useful sign of probable cold stress in the absence of hypovolaemia or generalized shock.

Insensible water loss

Throughout childhood and adult life insensible water loss from the skin and respiratory tract normally accounts for a quarter of all heat loss at rest [59, 78], with respiratory loss responsible for about a quarter of this total. However, babies born more than about 9 weeks before term lose quite excessive amounts of water through the skin [41, 91, 98].

Respiratory water loss is always directly proportional to the difference between ambient water vapour pressure and the vapour pressure of fully humidified air at deep body temperature [86]. Skin water loss in the absence of active sweat production bears a similar [53] (but probably non-linear) relation to ambient humidity. Total loss at rest in an environment of moderate humidity [ambient vapour pressure ~15 mm Hg (~2 kPa)] amounts to a little over 1 g/kg per hour throughout infancy (compared to a basal value of 0.5 g/kg in adult life), but insensible water loss may be 3 or even 6 times as high as this in babies of less than 28 weeks' gestation during the first day of life (Fig. 63.1). The loss

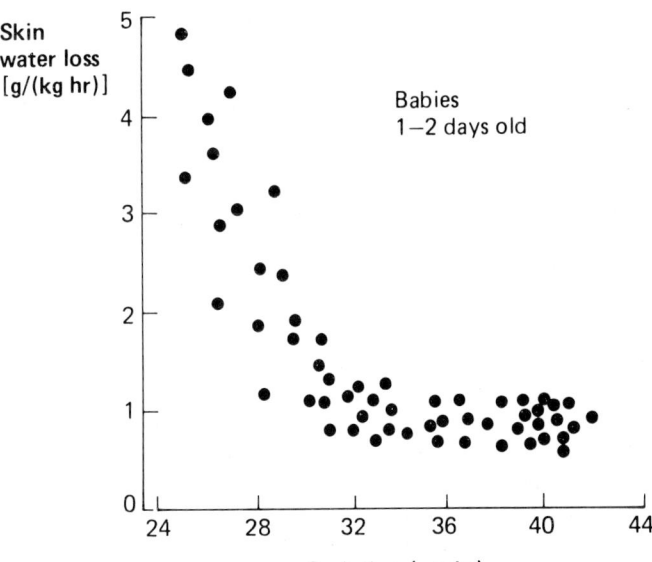

Fig. 63.1. Skin water loss in naked babies 1–2 days old in a moderately humid draught-free environment (P H_2O = 2kPa). Note that a preterm 1-kg baby can easily lose 100 ml water over 24 h through the skin (10% of the initial body weight). Comparable losses in an older patient with third-degree burns would quickly prove fatal.

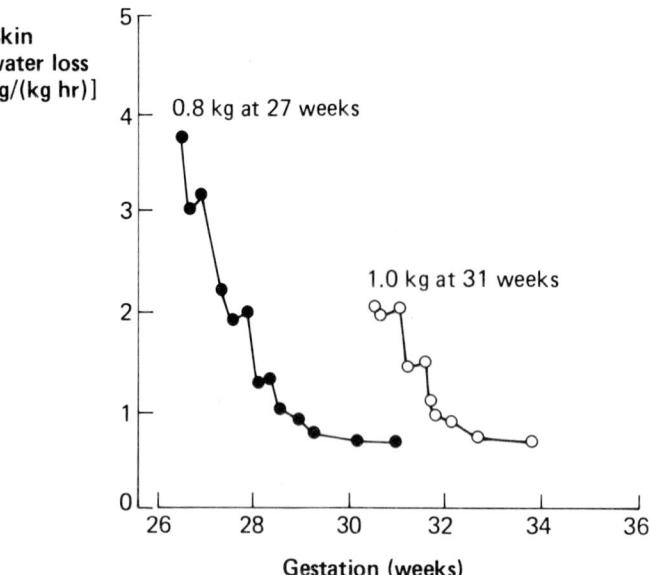

Fig. 63.2. Skin water loss falls rapidly in the first 2 weeks after birth as the skin becomes better keratinized. Enhanced skin maturation in response to premature delivery results in a month-old baby born at 26 weeks' gestation having a much more 'waterproof' skin (and sweat glands that are more functionally mature) than a 1-day-old baby of 30 weeks' gestation.

falls rapidly over the first 2 or 3 weeks of life [98] as the thin and easily traumatized skin becomes more fully keratinized (Fig. 63.2), but it often exceeds the baby's fluid intake during the first 2 or 3 days of life, and may cause so much heat loss during the first 24 h that deep body temperature can only be maintained if convective and radiant heat loss is effectively eliminated by increasing environmental temperature to the point where it equals mean skin temperature.

Sweat production

Few infants seem able to more than quadruple their evaporative loss by sweating in the first 2 weeks of life before rectal temperature exceeds 38°C [59]. As a result, the ability to maintain a constant body temperature in unduly warm surroundings at birth is even more limited than the ability to withstand cold stress. Sweat function is more limited still in babies born 3 weeks before term, and babies born more than 8 weeks before term seem unable to sweat at all [59]. Glandular immaturity appears to limit sweat function in babies of short gestation [44, 52], but what limits sweat function in the full-term baby is less certain, because the skin appears to contain 6 times as many active sweat glands as the same area in an average adult, and the peak response of each gland to direct chemical stimulation is about one-third that found in most adults. On this basis the baby's response to thermal stress would be expected to exceed that of the average adult: in fact the reverse appears to be the case and there is therefore a

very real risk of hyperthermia. How long this increased risk lasts is uncertain because few tests of sweat function have been conducted in later infancy. There is some evidence to suggest that the risk may continue for several months after birth [45].

Sweating is usually most copious and most noticeable, both in babies and in later life, over the temples, forehead and upper trunk [97], but evaporative loss can rise markedly before it becomes visible, especially at low ambient humidity.

Optimal warmth

Homeothermic animals utilize O_2, increase their metabolism, and generate extra heat to defend their deep body temperature when faced with an unfavourably cold environment. Similarly, in hot surroundings, body temperature eventually begins to rise and, as a result, metabolic rate also rises above basal levels. Between these two extremes lies a relatively narrow environmental zone in which the thermal conditions can be considered 'neutral'. Many factors affect the position of this neutral zone. An environment that suits one animal species is often quite intolerable for another, and an environment that provides neutral conditions for a grown adult may be lethally cold for its unprotected offspring.

Whether every environment that is consistent with minimum heat production is necessarily neutral in all its effects is questionable, however. Certainly an animal that is only maintaining a normal deep body temperature by panting or sweating cannot really be considered to be in a neutral environment, and it is now generally agreed that the term should only be used to describe an environment in which resting metabolism and thermoregulatory water loss are both at a minimum [57]. The true thermoneutral range in man, defined in this way, is narrow. The degree of control that can be achieved by adjusting skin blood flow is small, and evaporative water loss increases before maximum vasodilatation occurs. In consequence, the thermoneutral range tends to shrink from a zone to a point [57].

Thermal balance

Evidence has accumulated over the past 25 years to suggest that a thermoneutral environment may provide the optimum environment in which to care for small preterm babies in the first week of life. Survival data from six separate controlled trials are summarized in Table 63.1. No comparable data exist relating the thermal environment to survival in later life, but there is no reason to suppose that thermal stress only affects survival in the neonatal period. Animal evidence certainly points to the relation being of more general significance. What caused the excess mortality in the studies listed in Table 63.1 is uncertain: one major factor seems to be an increase in the number of deaths from respiratory distress due to hyaline membrane disease and surfactant deficiency [94]. Minimizing O_2 consumption may be equally important to survival in other cardiorespiratory conditions where adequate tissue oxygenation is critical.

Warmth can be overdone, however, and one study (Table 63.1, study 5) produced evidence to suggest that neonatal mortality increases in babies of less than 2 kg if incubator air temperature is kept at 34°C instead of 32°C without regard to age or weight even when steps are taken to prevent rectal temperature exceeding 37.8°C [123]. That such a small rise in deep body temperature should also be associated with increased mortality is surprising, because the fetus grows at just such a temperature in utero.

Because of this evidence concerning the narrowness of the optimum temperature range, many hospitals now use servo-controlled heaters to regulate incubator air temperature with a sensing thermistor taped to the child's abdomen, although no controlled study has ever been done to establish the wisdom of such an arrangement. Servo-control devices can certainly cause overheating if the skin sensor comes loose, obscure the signs of early septicaemia and, theoretically at least, subject an infected infant with a raised thermoregulatory 'set-point' to marked cold stress. Temperature receptors in the hypothalamus probably play a part in the diurnal variation of body temperature in later life. A change of about half a degree centigrade in the set-point of this central thermostat is almost certainly responsible for the abrupt fall in body temperature that occurs with

Table 63.1. Factors shown to affect survival in small newborn babies enclosed and nursed naked in an incubator

Authors and study population	Humidity (% RH)	Environmental conditions under test	Birth weight (kg)	Change in mortality
Silverman et al. 1958 154 babies [106]	80–90	Air temperature maintained at 31.7° *instead of* 28.9°C for the first 5 days after birth.	1.0–1.5 > 1.5	37% fall 67% fall
Jolly et al. 1962 148 babies [70]	≤ 100	Air temperature "high enough to keep rectal temperature at 35.6–37.2" *instead of* a fixed air temperature of 29.4°C.	1.0–1.5 1.5–2.0	21% fall 26% fall
Day et al. 1964 93 babies [39]	60–90	Supplementary radiant heat "to keep abdominal skin temperature at 36°C" *in addition to* an air temperature of 31.5°C.	1.0–1.4 1.4–1.8	60% fall 48% fall
Buetow & Klein 1964 158 babies [27]	50–65	As in the study by Day et al. for the first 4 days after birth.	1.0–1.5	22% fall
Yashiro et al. 1973 72 babies [123]	50	Air temperature maintained at 34° *instead of* 32°C.	1.0–2.0	100% rise
Perlstein et al. 1976 182 babies [94]	60–70	Computer-assisted servo-control used to minimise temperature fluctuation in the incubator.	0.8–2.2	56% fall

the onset of sleep from quite an early age [38]. We know little about the speed with which these rhythms become established after birth, and even less about their significance. Neither do we know what happens if these rhythms are ignored or overridden.

Small differences in enviromental warmth not only have a major impact on survival in the first 2 weeks of life, but also have an impact on subsequent growth [49, 50]. It is a pity, therefore, that many manually controlled incubators still have a safety thermostat adjusted so that air temperature cannot be set to more than 35°C, and still have an unlockable temperature-control knob that is all too easily altered when touched or leant on. Fluctuations in environmental temperature can easily precipitate apnoea [93], and may even have an effect on overall mortality (Table 63.1, study 6). Such fluctuations are readily minimized by light clothing or deflected by a suitable perspex baffle [7]. They are only a serious problem in incubators in which air temperature is controlled by an 'on/off' thermostat rather than a proportional heat-control unit.

Several studies show that there is more to defining an optimum incubator environment than merely prescribing conditions of thermoneutrality. Some thermoneutral conditions (as currently defined) are far from neutral in their effects on the baby and there is still no incontrovertible proof that any strictly thermoneutral environment necessarily provides optimal conditions for the smallest preterm babies [57]. Adults often profess to find maximum comfort in an environment slightly below the neutral range [46], and even young animals often display a similar preference [88]. School children even think better in classrooms kept slightly below the thermal comfort zone [4–6]! Nurses left to use their own judgement in selecting incubator temperature tend to make a similar choice [100], and thermoneutral conditions are not the best environment in which to develop thermoregulatory ability after birth [49]. Apnoeic attacks are also said to be less frequent when babies are nursed at the lower end of the thermoneutral range [34].

Many of the smallest babies in the various controlled trials already referred to had deep body temperatures of rather less than 36°C for several days after birth even in the warmest conditions under test, and other data suggest that very small babies actually adapt to such low body temperatures within 1 or 2 days of birth [26]. Nevertheless, such adaptations almost certainly have strict limits. There is, for example,

indirect evidence that the more primitive of the two biochemical pathways involved in surfactant production (and the only pathway active in most preterm babies at birth) is disrupted if deep body temperature falls below 35°C [51]. There is as yet no incontrovertible evidence that it is essential to keep deep body temperature permanently above .36°C in babies less than 1.5 kg in the first week of life, however.

Certain facts are clear. Prolonged hypothermia (<35.5°C) usually carries a high mortality in the neonatal period. Fluctuating environmental conditions are hazardous for small babies, especially in the period immediately after birth. The optimum temperature range is small and a stable nursing environment close to the lower end of the thermoneutral temperature zone probably provides optimum conditions for survival in the neonatal period. Whether these factors are applicable to nursing care outside the neonatal period is anyone's guess. They probably are.

Fluid balance

Environmental humidity only has a modest effect on thermal balance in babies with a reasonably well-keratinized skin. The increase in evaporative heat loss that occurs when relative humidity fall 50% in a sub-thermoneutral environment can be counterbalanced by increasing the operative environmental temperature by something over 0.5°C, while in warmer surroundings spontaneous changes in skin blood flow and increased sweating serve to maintain thermal equilibrium without any net change in heat balance [62].

Much more consideration has to be given to evaporative water loss from the skin in babies of less than 31 weeks' gestation, especially in the first week of life when water loss is often the single most important channel of obligatory heat loss from the skin. Halving this loss by increasing ambient humidity 50% (Fig. 63.3) [53] may have as potent an effect as increasing environmental temperature by nearly 1.5°C in these small babies (as Silverman [105] showed in the first of his classical clinical trials of incubator management). Placing a clear plastic drape [82], or a perspex radiant-heat shield with closed ends [41], over the baby works in much the same way by decreasing air movement and increasing the humidity of the microenvironment around the baby. Paraffin wax on the skin can also be used to nearly halve the evaporative loss [99].

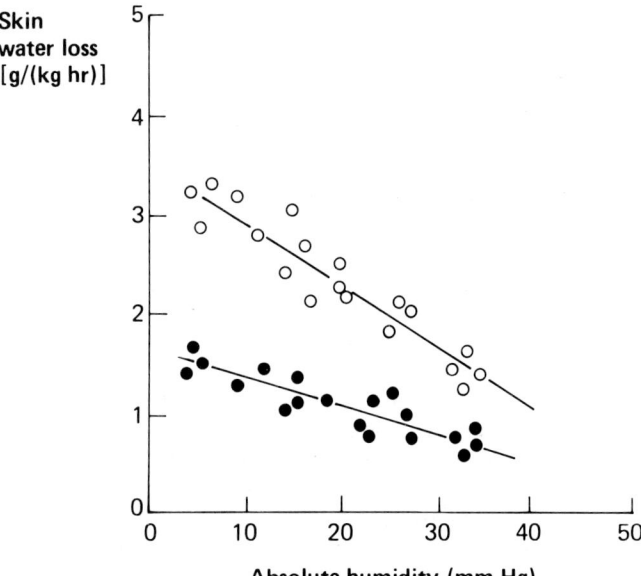

Fig. 63.3. The relation between skin water loss and ambient humidity in a 1-week-old baby of 1.7 kg at 32 weeks' gestation (○) and in a 1-week-old baby of 1.1 kg at 28 weeks' gestation (●) nursed naked in a thermoneutral environment.

Insensible water loss is particularly variable in small babies, and the factors influencing this loss are still not fully understood. Total insensible water loss increases when air speed increases [116] and when the baby becomes active [59] (partly, no doubt, because of increased respiratory loss [114]) and skin water loss rises if abrasions traumatize the delicate and only half-keratinized skin. Significant heat loss will also occur if water or urine evaporate from the skin. Phototherapy causes an increase in skin blood flow [90, 122] and in water loss from the skin [89] (even when steps are taken to compensate for the change in the radiant environment) that is only partly due to increased fluid loss in the stool [121]. Overhead radiant heaters appear to have a similar effect [119, 120] (although some of the reported difference may have been due to differences in the air speed and in the absolute humidity of the two environments under test). The combination of phototherapy and direct radiant heat may be additive [12]. The reason for this increased loss is not known. Focal radiant heat could conceivably cause local sweating over the trunk, even in surroundings that left the majority of the body still very cool. Clinicians (and research workers) should be warned that many devices for measuring ambient humidity and changes in body weight are not as accurate and reliable as they seem, and that small changes in air speed influence evaporative loss more than was previously appreciated when skin permeability is high.

Important as it is to allow for evaporative heat loss when trying to optimize the thermal en-vironment, recent studies show that it may be even more important to control fluid balance accurately in these babies. Evidence has recently been presented to suggest that differences of as little as 2 ml/kg an hour in net fluid intake can significantly increase the risk of congestive failure due to patent ductus arteriosus [14], and necrotizing enterocolitis [13], in babies of less than 1.5 kg with respiratory distress. The indications are that it may be hazardous to increase daily fluid intake more than 80 ml/kg above insensible water loss until such time as respiratory problems have settled, particularly if there is reason to believe that the ductus arteriosus is still not fully closed.

Whether there is such a thing as an optimal ambient humidity is more doubtful [107] although Blackfan and Yaglou's early study [18] certainly suggested that a low ambient humidity was associated with an increased incidence of gastro-intestinal (GI) symptoms and temperature instability. Humidifying devices are easily contaminated with *Pseudomonas* and other hygrophylic bacteria, but ventilators, sinks, and suction bottles seem, in practice, to be much more hazardous than incubator humidity tanks in this regard. Very high ambient humidity will cause troublesome condensation and limit visibility into the incubator unless room temperature is also kept high [9], but a relatively high ambient humidity certainly serves to reduce insensible water loss in the smallest preterm babies, making it easier to assess overall fluid balance with slightly greater accuracy in the first 2 weeks of life. The disadvantages of running the incubators 'dry' outweigh the advantages when nursing babies of less than 30 weeks' gestation under 1 week old.

Heat loss from the respiratory tract is not usually a major problem unless the inspired air is unusually dry, but dry air can certainly make tracheal secretions more viscid, especially when inspired air bypasses the nose. Small babies have a relatively weak and ineffective cough reflex anyway [43], and the smaller the baby, the greater the potential problem with retained secretions. Babies with an artificial airway almost always have moisture added to the air they breathe, but little attention has been paid in the past to the form this humidification should take. Recent animal data suggests that nebulized droplets of water may eventually have a traumatizing effect on the smaller airways, which is avoided when all inspired water is vaporized at delivery (as with most warm air humidifiers) [69]. In the light of these findings, the habit of injecting boluses of sterile water or saline down the airway at regular intervals over any period of time appears due for reappraisal.

Delivery room care

Countless papers attest to the fact that preterm babies who become cold immediately after delivery are much more likely to die [109]. Hyaline membrane disease appears to be the greatest hazard [110], and there is evidence that hypothermia and acidosis both inhibit surfactant production by the only metabolic pathway functional in the preterm baby at birth [51]. Many babies probably become cold because they are already ill, but the importance of not allowing any baby to become ill as a result of becoming cold cannot be overemphasized. Even healthy babies subjected to cold stress at this time become hypoxic [112] and acidotic [47]. The normal metabolic response to cold stress is muted at birth [55], and heat production is particularly limited in babies who have been sedated [28, 30, 55] or asphyxiated [24] during delivery.

Evaporative heat loss alone exceeds resting heat production at birth by a factor of 4, and only decreases exponentially over a period of 2 h [54] if active steps are not taken to dry the wet skin. Net heat loss from convection and radiation is equally high if the baby is left unclothed even in a room at 26°C, and draughts will further increase this loss. With heat loss

exceeding heat production by a factor of 8 it is not surprising that deep body temperature frequently falls more than a degree within 10 min of delivery even in a big, healthy, full-term baby. Drying the skin with a soft, absorbent towel rapidly reduces the evaporative loss, however, while a 400 watt overhead radiant heat source ($\lambda > 1.5\ \mu$) some 60 cm above the baby can be used to counterbalance most of the sensible heat loss [33]. Heat conservation is probably particularly important in the ill baby, and no baby is ever too ill for these two steps to be omitted in the rush to start resuscitation after birth.

Obsessional concern with minimizing heat loss, on the other hand, is all too common in the management of healthy full-term infants. The mother is at least as effective a source of physical warmth as of emotional warmth, and her arms at least as effective as blankets in checking sensible heat loss [54] (though it is still wise to dry the baby gently before the mother holds her unclothed child for any length of time). It is also wise to cover both mother and baby with a light blanket or drape to reduce convective loss unless the room is unusually warm. Any extensive form of examination or toilet only increases heat loss. Bathing, like circumcision, should be considered an unnecessary ritual undertaken only at the express wish of the parents. The rush to clothe and swaddle the baby before allowing the parents any extended period of contact is misplaced because there is, in fact, no evidence that this reduces the risk of hypothermia.

Delivery rooms should be draught-free and some trouble taken to try and keep room temperature from falling below 24°C. Unfortunately many units are currently run at a much lower temperature than this. A temperature of 26°C would be more consistent with the baby's need at this time, and would reduce the perceived need to separate mother and child at a time when there are many important reasons for allowing extended contact [40, 74].

Subsequent clinical management

Incubator care

There is no such thing as a completely safe incubator. Any device capable of providing enough warmth to protect a frail 1-kg baby from hypothermia is necessarily capable of rendering a larger and more mature baby hyperthermic

[60], and there are few good reasons for nursing babies of more than 1.5 kg in an incubator unless they have to be nursed naked or given increased O_2 or humidity.

Indirect estimates of the conditions most likely to produce thermal neutrality for a baby being nursed in a closed warm-air incubator were first made on the basis of laboratory studies [56] between 1966 and 1970 (Table 63.2). The predictions have stood the test of time remarkably well, and have now been vindicated by more direct measures of heat production and evaporative loss in the nursery itself [15]. Nevertheless, it has to be remembered that published data relate to mean findings, and cannot, therefore, be relied upon to predict optimum conditions for any individual baby largely because the basal metabolism is so variable [100] (see section: *Resting heat production*).

The effect of radiant heat loss to the cold incubator walls is another important variable that has to be taken into account [64]. One approach is to minimize the problem by keeping the incubator in a very warm room. An alternative approach is to shield the baby from the loss by placing a second perspex surface the same temperature as the air in the incubator between the baby and the outer incubator wall [63]. Moveable radiant shields have been widely used for nearly 15 years, and specially constructed double-walled incubators are now becoming fashionable [125]. The excess radiant loss can also be counterbalanced more simply, however, by increasing incubator air temperature 1°C for every 7°C by which incubator air temperature exceeds room temperature. The only limitation to this approach is that many incubators still have their safety thermostat set to cut out if air temperature in the incubator exceeds 35°C.

Each of these procedures has been validated in clinical practice, and there is nothing to suggest that the more cumbersome and expensive alternatives confer any special advantage [16]. Such reports as have appeared suggesting that one technique is better than another [125] are as yet unconfirmed [83]. It is clear, however, that there are important theoretical advantages in using a double wall for transport incubators, because external air temperature is then both variable and unpredictable. It must be also be said that an incubator does not necessarily provide optimal conditions merely because it normalizes body temperature and minimizes O_2 consumption [57]. The incubators in use today bear little resemblance to the equipment used in the trials that finally established the importance of environmental warmth on neonatal survival in 1964 (Table 63.1) [92]. Some modern incubators have very indifferent humidity controls and many clinicians, worried by the risk of *Pseudomonas* infection, have stopped providing supplemental humidification altogether. While a slight increase in air temperature serves to offset the result of the increase in evaporative heat loss without affecting O_2 consumption [36], we know nothing about the effect of such a change in management on survival. There also seem to be important advantages in using proportional heat control units rather than on/off thermostats to minimize incubator air temperature fluctuation [94].

Radiant heat

Similar considerations apply to the recent increase in the use of servo-controlled radiant heat cradles. Early studies produced conflicting data, but there is now reasonably good (if somewhat belated) evidence that babies nursed under these cradles consume some 10% more oxygen than babies nursed in warm-air incubators [16, 84, 118]. Furthermore, it is still not

Table 63.2. The mean temperature needed to provide thermal neutrality for a healthy baby nursed naked in draught-free surroundings of uniform temperature and moderate humidity (50%–70% RH) after birth

Birth weight (kg)	Operative environmental temperature[a]			
	35°C	34°C	33°C	32°C
1.0	For 10 days[b] →	After 10 days →	After 20 days →	After 5 weeks
1.5	—	For 10 days →	After 10 days →	After 4 weeks
2.0	—	For 2 days →	After 2 days →	After 3 weeks
2.5	—	—	For 2 days →	After 2 days

[a]To estimate operative temperature in a single-walled incubator subtract 1°C from incubator *air* temperature for every 7°C by which this exceeds room temperature.
[b]A temperature of 36° may be necessary in many babies of less than 1 kg in the first 2–3 days because of high evaporative heat loss through the skin.

known whether survival is as good. Some babies certainly have rather cool extremities when nursed under a radiant heater [80] even though core temperature is normal and peripheral skin blood flow sometimes high.

Convenience has been a major factor in their increased use. They certainly make handling easier (which is sometimes a mixed blessing). Parents also find them less daunting (which is an unmixed blessing). There is no evidence that their use increases the risk of cross infection [87], but it certainly doubles evaporative water loss, rendering very small babies vulnerable to dehydration and hypernatraemia if fluid loss is not compensated [71] (Fig. 63.4). Perspex heat shields have been used to try and reduce this loss [16, 124], but are not very satisfactory: the perspex also blocks the direct transfer of radiant heat between the canopy and the baby. A transparent tented plastic drape is more satisfactory [42]. Even regular skin treatment with paraffin oil significantly reduces evaporative heat loss. A light plastic sheet can also be used to swaddle the baby loosely. Ordinary clothes have less effect in reducing evaporative loss [65], but do not interfere with the efficiency of the heat cradle or the operation of the servo-control sensor, and some babies seem to be less restless if lightly clothed.

Radiant heat cradles should not be used to provide long-term nursing care unless heat output is controlled by a thermocouple or thermistor. Some of the advantages and disadvantages associated with servo-control have already been reviewed (section: *Thermal balance*). The cali-bration of some early probes was seriously inadequate, and errors of up to 1°C are still encountered now. It is conventional to monitor abdominal skin temperature, although it has recently been argued that the upper arm might be a more representative site to monitor. Air currents, evaporative losses, direct radiant heat, and the technique of attachment all influence the temperature recorded by such a skin sensor, and these sometimes cause potentially dangerous fluctuations in environmental temperature in warm-air incubators with an on/off heater. Such considerations are of lesser significance in units provided with proportional heat control. Even the rectum can now be used for monitoring with these units, despite earlier experience suggesting that this produced dangerous 'hunting' of the servo-control mechanism [2].

For many years it was conventional to keep the abdominal skin at 36°C [27, 39], and this is probably ideal for any child more than a few weeks old. More recently many neonatal units have favoured 36.5° or even 36.8°C for younger babies [16]. The latter may be appropriate when rectal temperature is monitored, but is almost certainly too high for skin temperature in any baby over 1.5 kg. In very small babies with a high evaporative heat loss, however, abdominal skin temperature may actually exceed rectal temperature when environmental humidity is low [11], partly because taping the thermistor to the skin produces a falsely high indication of true skin temperature. A temperature of 36.8°C may, therefore, be appropriate in these babies in the first few days of life. There is as yet no

HEAT LOSS IN A ONE DAY OLD BABY OF 0.75 Kg
(watts/m^2)

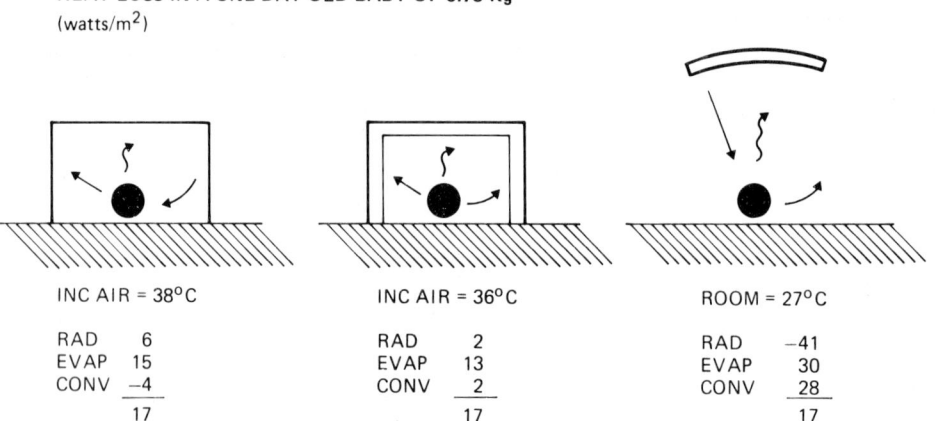

INC AIR = 38°C		INC AIR = 36°C		ROOM = 27°C	
RAD	6	RAD	2	RAD	−41
EVAP	15	EVAP	13	EVAP	30
CONV	−4	CONV	2	CONV	28
	17		17		17

Fig. 63.4. Three different ways of achieving thermoneutrality for a 1-day-old baby weighing 0.75 kg at 27 weeks' gestation. Evaporative heat loss is high even when the baby is nursed in a fully humidified incubator (75% RH), and doubles when the baby is exposed under a radiant cradle in an unhumidified room (25% RH) at 27°C. Uniform surroundings at 36°C provide thermoneutral conditions as long as the walls are the same temperature as the air in the incubator, but air temperature needs to exceed the baby's own deep body temperature in a single-walled incubator (room temperature 24°C [75°F]) to compensate for the continued radiant and evaporative loss.

evidence that survival is improved by further increasing body temperature once rectal temperature exceeds 36°C, and there are many potential hazards associated with overheating.

Phototherapy is now frequently given to any small baby with a direct bilirubin of more than 170 μmol/litre to minimize the risk of kernicterus. Blue light with a wavelength of 460 nm is thought to be most effective, but a light source with a spectrum more similar to that of natural sunlight makes it easier to judge the child's colour and condition. Phototherapy is extremely effective when a 150- or 200-watt bank of fluorescent lamps with high irradiance at the relevant wavelength is placed less than 45 cm from the baby (as is possible with most incubators). Unfortunately, it is often difficult to get such a bank within 90 cm of a baby when a radiant cradle is in use, and this renders treatment almost totally ineffective because irradiance varies with the square of the distance between the light source and the subject.

Radiant heaters are also of limited use during major surgery. They also get in the way of bulky x-ray equipment during cardiac catheterization, angiography, and other radiological investigations. A heated air bed or thermostatically controlled warm water mattress is capable of providing a certain amount of warmth, and this may be all that is necessary if room temperature is also high, but very ill babies benefit from the supplementary warmth provided by the servo-controlled radiotranslucent heat canopy first described in 1965 [97].

This piece of equipment was first designed for use during exchange transfusion and other minor operative procedures. In this connection it is sometimes forgotten that the infusion of a large quantity of cold blood or other fluid also imposes a significant heat debt on a small baby [67]. Any fluid rapidly equilibrates to within a few degrees of room temperature as it passes down the donor tubing if the rate of infusion is reasonably low. Heat exchange coils are therefore relatively ineffective unless placed within 60 cm of the baby. A 2-volume exchange of blood (180 ml/kg) for donor blood at 26°C will cause the body temperature of an infant in a neutral environment to fall by 1.7°C unless heat production rises. Oxygen consumption would have to increase by 50% for more than 1.5 h to balance such a heat debt [67].

Clothes and bedding

A short woollen vest, a napkin, and a long cotton nightdress with sleeves provide as much thermal insulation as the clothing worn by an average adult indoors. Nevertheless, because of differences in basal heat production, a baby of 2–4 kg so dressed will only be tolerably warm in an environment of about 28°C, whereas an adult would find 20°C quite acceptable [65]. For much the same reason a healthy full-term baby lying fully clothed under three or four blankets in a cot starts to become hypothermic if the environmental temperature falls below about 10°C even though the mother, asleep in the same bedroom, fails to sense any undue cold stress.

Healthy babies over 2 kg in weight merely need to be clothed and well wrapped up in a cot. A draught-free room of moderate humidity at 26°C will normally offer thermoneutral conditions in the first 24 h, and a room at 24°C provides appropriate warmth for a cot-nursed baby more than 2 days old. Swaddling an unclothed child in a large flannelette sheet provides considerable insulation against heat loss, but not as much as the insulation offered by clothes. Even a single thin sheet decreases heat loss considerably by trapping a micro-environment of warm air round the body. Two blankets and a sheet are enough to increase the insulation round a clothed baby by half [65]. Further blankets have little measurable effect, but some additional benefit can be gained by covering the head [113] (Table 63.3). A small waterproof electric heating pad placed immediately above the mattress can also be used to provide useful supplementary warmth, but it is essential for any such device to contain a separately wired safety thermocouple to stop surface temperature exceeding 41°C.

Babies of 1.5–2 kg can also be nursed very adequately in cots, as long as the room is kept at 28°C or more for the first few days of life, and cot nursing makes the baby more accessible to the parents as well as providing protection from fluctuations in environmental temperature. A naked baby can only accommodate a 2°C fall in environmental temperature if energy and O_2 consumption increase by more than a quarter (unless deep body temperature falls), but a cot-nursed infant can accommodate a 6°C fall in environmental temperature before experiencing comparable cold stress [66]. For more than 50 years most babies in incubators were nursed fully clothed [104]. The tradition has largely been lost, but this is a pity. Lack of clothes can help to minimize handling and reduce the skin trauma caused by moisture and abrasion in some of the very smallest babies, but observation is not significantly impeded by covering the

Table 63.3 Resistance to heat loss (in clo units[a]) in a 2.5-kg baby laying supine on a thick foam mattress in a cool draught-free room

Resistance due to	Completely naked	Wearing bonnet and wrapped in one sheet	Fully clothed under blankets in a clot
One flannelette sheet and two blankets round a clothed baby	—	—	0.61
One flannelette swaddling sheet round an unclothed baby	—	0.81	—
Thick gauze bonnet over head	—	0.22	0.22
Vest, napkin, and long nightdress	—	—	1.25
Boundary layer of still air round skin	0.78	0.78	0.78
Body tissues (when vaso-constricted)	0.29	0.29	0.29
Total resistance	1.07	2.10	3.15

[a]1 clo unit = $0.155°C.m^2.W^{-1}$ or $0.18°C.m^2h.kcal^{-1}$

trunk, and many babies seem to be less restless when lightly covered or clothed.

A number of plastic swaddling devices have been described. The silver swaddler uses the same principle as the emergency 'exposure blanket' used by mountaineers [10]. When used as originally described to protect a baby from cold stress immediately after birth it works primarily by preventing (or, more probably, postponing) evaporative water loss. When used in older babies, however, where evaporative loss is less substantial, it works largely by reducing convective and radiant heat loss. In this respect it provides slightly more insulation than a single flannelette swaddling sheet (Table 63.3), but no more insulation than a thick cellular cotton blanket and slightly less insulation than conventional clothes. The non-abrasive aluminium coating makes the baby less easy to see, and is only responsible for a fifth of the overall thermal insulation. An alternative approach [17] in which bags of 'bubble wrap' packaging material (Saran) are used also reduces evaporative heat loss. It probably provides marginally more insulation than the silver swaddler and does not limit visibility to quite the same extent, but it is much more bulky. Both devices are designed to cover the head as well as the body.

The use of these devices to further reduce heat loss from a baby already in an incubator or under a radiant cradle is largely misconceived, and the child's appearance is certainly distressing to some parents. The devices function in this situation mainly by reducing evaporative heat loss, and this can easily be achieved with a clear plastic drape. The most obvious use for such a drape is in the care of a baby with a gastroscheisis or ruptured exomphalos immediately after birth.

Phototherapy cannot be given to a clothed child, but this does not mean that every baby requiring phototherapy has to be nursed in an incubator. Even relatively large babies will suffer cold stress if left naked under a bank of lights in a room at 24–26°C, but a perspex cover over the top of the cot is usually enough to minimize heat loss in most healthy babies weighing more than 2 kg [108].

Disturbed thermoregulation

Hyperthermia

Body temperatures in excess of 41°C are at least as hazardous in the neonatal period as they are in later life: homeothermy soon breaks down and heat stroke, brain damage, and death are only prevented by rapid external cooling [75]. Small babies are at increased risk of heat stroke because of their limited ability to sweat, and there is some circumstantial evidence that this risk may persist throughout the first year of life. There is no published information (and very little unpublished information) on the effect of hyperpyrexia in the neonatal period, but several babies have been found dead with temperatures in excess of 41°C in incubators that had overheated as a result of an electrical fault. Closed warm-air incubators now always contain a safety thermostat to prevent any such mishap, but it is difficult to devise a similar device for use with overhead radiant heaters. In the few unpublished neonatal deaths known to the author, death was remarkably rapid, there were no abnormal features prior to collapse (other than restlessness), and no abnormal findings at autopsy. Older children, in whom death is less rapid, may show all the clinical and postmortem features classically associated with heat stroke [8, 111]. Even when sweat function is reasonably adequate, there remains the hazard of heat prostration in any infant fed entirely on unmodified cow's milk, because of the high solute load such a diet imposes on the kidney [35, 37].

Lesser degrees of fever are common [76] even in the neonatal period, and are sometimes a source of unnecessary anxiety [102]. Even small infants can develop a raised thermoregulatory set-point in response to fever [85], although deep body temperature more often falls when a small baby is ill. Most increases in body temperature, however, are due to environmental changes, or to restlessness. Where this is the case the extremities are often as hot as the trunk, and there may be some small beads of sweat on the back, forehead, or temples. Babies with pyrexia due to infection and 'disease-related fever', in contrast, are generally vasoconstricted with cold extremities [95], but this distinction cannot always be relied upon. Direct sunlight rapidly turns an incubator into a greenhouse [64], and this can be a particularly potent cause of otherwise unexplained pyrexia.

The brain is such a metabolically active organ, even in the neonatal period [32], that any sudden fall in deep body temperature must suggest seriously reduced cerebral blood flow and brain death, especially where the head is significantly cooler than the trunk. Babies with spina bifida may have thermoregulatory problems [45] because of their paraplegia, while those with extensive congenital damage to the mid-brain, (cf. some babies with hydranencephaly and severe occipital encephalocele) may be poikilothermic [31]. Severe intrapartum asphyxia can also derange thermoregulation for a variable number of days after birth [24]: these babies nearly always prove to have permanent brain damage at follow-up.

Hypothermia

Hypothermia is, nevertheless, still probably the commonest problem in the neonatal period [81], and at least as common in the tropics as it is elsewhere (although it often goes unrecognized because a low-reading rectal thermometer is not routinely used). Accidental hypothermia due to overwhelming cold stress can easily occur at birth, but in many cases also occurs later, in the first 2 weeks of life [19]. A small baby left in an unheated room is at particular risk of cold injury if the weather turns unexpectedly cold in the night, while older infants are sometimes rendered vulnerable to cold injury by infection or marasmus [3, 20].

Babies are probably best rewarmed in a warm-air incubator with the air temperature so adjusted that the deep body temperature rises between 1° and 2°C per hour [115]. More complex procedures may be preferable in older patients. It is important to warm the trunk before the limbs. There is some limited anecdotal evidence to suggest that patients who have been cold a long time should be rewarmed more slowly than usual.

Hypoglycaemia is not particularly common at the time of diagnosis, but may occur during rewarming, and a slow infusion of glucose IV should probably be started once the circulation starts to improve and deep body temperature reaches about 32°C. Electrolyte and hydrogen ion abnormalities (after correction for low body temperature) are uncommon in the absence of some secondary underlying illness. Acute haemorrhagic pulmonary oedema is the greatest hazard during recovery, while necrotizing enterocolitis may occur if oral feeding is re-introduced too quickly. Babies appear to become poikilothermic once body temperature falls below about 32°C, and thermoregulatory ability only returns on recovery over a period of 1 or 2 days. Hypothermia usually appears to be caused by the metabolism being overwhelmed, but cases have been described in a number of very small babies where exhaustion of the brown adipose tissue's energy reserves appeared to be a factor [58]. Although this tissue preferentially utilizes its own adipose store for heat production during cold stress, it is also capable of using fatty acids derived from other body tissues, rendering hypothermia due to 'fuel starvation' unlikely except in severe marasmus.

A rather more unusual form of adaptive hypothermia has been found in a number of preterm babies weighing less than 1.5 kg in the first 2 weeks of life [24], after prolonged nursing at what would now be considered an undesirably low environmental temperature. In these babies, a rectal temperature of 33°–36°C is associated with reduced O_2 consumption, but any further lowering of environmental temperature triggers an immediate rise in heat production. Vasodilatation and sweating are only clearly demonstrable when body temperature rises to normal, suggesting that the baby's homeothermic mechanisms are now allowing deep body temperature to range over a band of temperature instead of regulating it around a closely defined set-point. Such adaptation is rare, however, and there is little documentary evidence that large babies ever lower their metabolism under similar conditions, even when treated with drugs such as chlorpromazine and promethazine. There is, therefore, at the moment, no proven use for therapeutic hypothermia in the neonatal period, although it remains possible that there may be some value in its use under carefully controlled conditions in the intensive care management of severe intrapartum cerebral anoxia.

Bibliography

Documentary evidence for the vast majority of the statements made in this chapter can be found in the following books and review articles:

Editorial (1979) Heat disorders. Lancet I:910–911
Editorial (1980) Incubating babies. Br Med J 281:1443–1444
Hey EN (1971) The care of babies in incubators. In: Gairdner D, Hull D (eds) Recent advances in paediatrics, 4th edn. Churchill, London, pp 171–215
Hey EN (1975) Thermal neutrality. Br Med Bull 31:69–74
Maclean D, Emslie-Smith D (1977) Accidental hypothermia. Blackwells, Oxford
Sinclair JC (1978) Temperature regulation and energy metabolism in the newborn. Grune Stratton, New York

References

1. Ablett JG, McCance RA (1971) Energy expenditure of children with kwaschiorkor. Lancet II:517–519
2. Agate FJ, Silverman WA (1963) The control of body temperature in the small newborn infant by low-energy infra-red radiation. Pediatrics 31:725–733
3. Arneil GC, Kerr MN (1963) Severe hypothermia in Glasgow infants in winter. Lancet II:756–759
4. Auliciems A (1969) Thermal requirements of secondary school children in winter. J Hyg (Camb) 67:59–65
5. Auliciems A (1972a) Classroom performance as a function of thermal comfort. Int J Biometeorol 16:233–246
6. Auliciems A (1972b) Some observed relationships between the atmospheric environment and mental work. Environ Res 5:217–240
7. Aynsley-Green A, Roberton NRC, Rolfe P (1975) Air temperature recordings in infant incubators. Arch Dis Child 50:215–219
8. Bacon C, Scott D, Jones P (1979) Heat stroke in well-wrapped infants. Lancet I:422–425
9. Bardell E, Freeman J, Hey EN (1968) Relative humidity in incubators. Arch Dis Child 43:172–177
10. Baum JD, Scopes JW (1968) The silver swaddler: device for preventing hypothermia in the newborn. Lancet I:672–673
11. Belgaunkar TK, Scott KE (1975) Effects of low humidity on small premature infants in servo controlled incubators. 1. Decrease in rectal temperature. Biol Neonate 26:337–347
12. Bell EF, Neidich GA, Cashore WJ, Oh W (1979a) Combined effect of radiant warmer and phototherapy on insensible water loss in low birth weight infants. J Pediatr 94:810–813
13. Bell EF, Warburton D, Stonestreet BS, Oh W (1979b) High-volume fluid intake predisposes premature infants to necrotising enterocolitis. Lancet II:90
14. Bell EF, Warburton D, Stonestreet BS, Oh W (1980a) Effect of fluid administration on the development of symptomatic patent ductus arteriosus and congestive heart failure in premature infants. N Engl J Med 302:598–604
15. Bell EF, Gray JC, Weinstein MR, Oh W (1980b) The effects of thermal environment on heat balance and insensible water loss in low-birth weight infants. J Pediatr 96:452–459
16. Bell FE, Weinstein MR, Oh W (1980c) Heat balance in premature infants: comparative effect of convectively incubated and radiant warmer, with and without plastic heat shield. J Pediatr 96:460–465
17. Besch NJ, Perlstein PH, Edwards NK, Keenan WJ, Sutherland JM (1971) The transparent baby bag. A shield against heat loss. N Engl J Med 284:121–124
18. Bladkfan KD, Yaglou CP (1933) The premature infant. Am J Dis Child 46:1175–1236
19. Bower BD, Jones LF, Weeks MN (1960) Cold injury in the newborn. Br Med J i:303–309
20. Brooke OG (1972) Hypothermia in malnourished Jamaican children. Arch Dis Child 47:525–530
21. Brooke OG (1980) Energy balance and metabolic rate in preterm infants fed with standard and high-energy formulas. Br J Nutr 44:13–23
22. Brooke OG, Ashworth A (1972) The influence of malnutrition on the postprandial metabolic rate and respiratory quotient. Br J Nutr 27:407–415
23. Brück K (1961) Temperature regulation in the newborn infant. Biol Neonat 3:65–119
24. Brück K, Brück M, Lemtis H (1960) Die Temperaturregelung Neugeborener und Frühgeborener nach spontaner und pathologisher Geburt. Geburtshilfe Frauenheilk 20:461–472
25. Brück K, Adams FH, Brück M (1962) Temperature regulation in infants with chronic hypoxemia. Pediatrics 30:350–360
26. Brück K, Parmelee AH, Brück M (1962) Neutral temperature range and range of "thermal comfort" in premature infants. Biol Neonat 4:32–51
27. Buetow KC, Klein SW (1964) Effects of maintenance of "normal" skin temperature of survival of infants of low birth weight. Pediatrics 34:163–170
28. Burnard ED, Cross KW (1958) Rectal temperature in the new-born asphyxia. Br Med J ii:1197–1199
29. Clarke PP, Cross KW, Goff MR, Mullen BJ, Stothers JK, Warner RM (1978) Neonatal natural and forced convection. J Physiol (Lond) 284:22–25P
30. Cree JE, Meyer J, Hailey DM (1973) Diazepam in

labour: its metabolism and effect on the clinical condition and thermogenesis of the new-born. Br Med J iv:251–255

31. Cross KW, Hey EN, Kennaird DL, Lewis SR, Urich H (1971) Lack of temperature control in infants with abnormalities of the central nervous system. Arch Dis Child 46:437–443

32. Cross KW, Dear PRF, Hawthorn MKS, Hyams A, Kerslake DM, Milligan DW, Rahilly PM, Stothers JK (1979) An estimation of intracranial blood flow in the newborn infant. J Physiol (Lond) 289:329–345

33. Dahm LS, James LS (1972) New-born temperature and calculated heat losses in the delivery room. Pediatrics 49:504–513

34. Daily WJR, Klaus M, Meyer HBP (1969) Apnoea in premature infants: monitoring, incidence, heat rate changes and an effect of environmental temperature. Pediatrics 43:510–518

35. Danks DM, Webb DW, Allen J (1962) Heat illness in infants and young children. A study of 47 cases. Br Med J ii:287–293

36. Darnall RA, Ariagno RL (1979) Resting oxygen consumption in premature infants covered with a plastic thermal blanket. Pediatrics 63:547–551

37. Darrow DC, Cooke RE, Segar WE (1954) Water and electrolyte metabolism in infants fed on cow's milk mixture during heat stress. Pediatrics 14:602–617

38. Day RL (1941) Regulation of body temperature during sleep. Am J Dis Child 61:734–746

39. Day RL, Caliguiri L, Kamenski C, Ehrlich F (1964) Body temperature and survival of premature infants. Pediatrics 34:171–181

40. De Chateau P, Wyberg B (1977) Long-term effects on mother-infant behaviour of extra contact during the first hour post-partum. Acta Paediatr Scand 66:137–141, 145–151

41. Fanaroff AA, Wald M, Gruber HS, Klaus MH (1972) Insensible water loss in low birth weight infants. Pediatrics 50:236–245

42. Fitch CW, Corones SB, Wade JE (1980) Measured reduction of radiant energy requirements in special heat shield. Pediatr Res 14:597

43. Fleming PJ, Bryan AC, Bryan MH (1978) Functional immaturity of the pulmonary irritant receptors and apnea in new-born preterm infants. Pediatrics 61:515–518

44. Foster KG, Hey EN, Katz G (1969) The response of the sweat glands of the new-born baby to thermal stimuli and to intradermal acetylcholine. J Physiol (Lond) 203:13–29

45. Foster KG, Hey EN, O'Connell B (1971) Sweat function in babies with defects of the central nervous system. Arch Dis Child 46:444–451

46. Gagge AP, Hardy JD, Rapp GM (1965) Experimental study on comfort for high temperature sources of radiant heat. Trans Am Soc Heat Refrig Air-Cond Eng 71:19–26

47. Gandy GM, Adamsons K, Cunningham N, Silverman WA, James LS (1964) Thermal environment and acid–base homeostasis in human infants during the first few hours of life. J Clin Invest 43:751–758

48. Gerhardt T, McCarthy J, Bancalari E (1979) Effect of aminophylline on respiratory centre activity and metabolic rate in premature infants with idiopathic apnoea. Pediatrics 63:537–542

49. Glass L, Silverman WA, Sinclair JC (1968) Effect of the thermal environment on cold resistance and growth of small infants after the first week of life. Pediatrics 41:1033–1046

50. Glass L, Silverman WA, Sinclair JC (1969) Relationship of thermal environment and calorie intake to growth and resting metabolism in the late neonatal period. Biol Neonate 14:324–340

51. Gluck L, Kulovich MV, Eidelman Al, Cordero L, Kahzin AF (1972) Biochemical development of surface activity in mammalian lung. IV. Pulmonary lecithin synthesis in the human fetus and new-born and etiology of the respiratory distress syndrome. Pediatr Res 6:81–99

52. Green M, Behrendt H (1970) Drug-induced localised sweating in neonates. Am J Dis Child 120:434–438

53. Hammarlund K, Sedin G (1979) Transepidermal water loss in new-born infants. III. Relation to gestational age. Acta Paediatr Scand 68:795–801

54. Hammarlund K, Nilsson GE, Öberg PA, Sedin G (1980) Transepidermal water loss in new-born infants. V. Evaporation from the skin and heat exchange during the first hours of life. Acta Paediatr Scand 69:385–392

55. Hey EN (1969) The relation between environmental temperature and oxygen consumption in the new-born baby. J Physiol (Lond) 200:589–603

56. Hey E (1971) The care of babies in incubators. In: Gairdner D, Hull D (eds). Recent advances in paediatrics, 4th ed. Churchill, London, pp 171–184

57. Hey EN (1975) Thermal neutrality. Br Med Bull 31:69–74

58. Hey EN, Katz G (1969a) Temporary loss of metabolic response to cold stress in infants of low birth weight. Arch Dis Child 44:323–330

59. Hey EN, Katz G (1969b) Evaporative water loss in the new-born baby. J Physiol (Lond) 200:605–619

60. Hey EN, Katz G (1970a) The optimum thermal environment for naked babies. Arch Dis Child 45:328–334

61. Hey EN, Katz G (1970b) The range of thermal insulation in the tissues of the new-born baby. J Physiol (Lond) 207:667–681

62. Hey EN, Maurice NP (1968) Effect of humidity on production and loss of heat in the new-born baby. Arch Dis Child 43:166–171

63. Hey EN, Mount LE (1966) Temperature control in incubators. Lancet II:202–203

64. Hey EN, Mount LE (1967) Heat losses from babies in incubators. Arch Dis Child 42:75–84

65. Hey EN, O'Connell B (1970) Oxygen consumption and heat balance in the cot-nursed baby. Arch Dis Child 45:335–343

66. Hey EN, Kohlinsky S, O'Connell B (1969) Heat losses from babies during exchanged transfusion. Lancet I:335–338

67. Hey EN, Katz G, O'Connell B (1970) The total thermal insulation of the new-born baby. J Physiol (Lond) 207:683–698

68. Hull D (1966) The structure and function of brown adipose tissue. Br Med Bull 22:92–96

69. John E, Ermosilla R, Golden J, Cash R, McDevitt M, Cassady G (1980) Effects of gas temperature and particulate water on rabbit lungs during ventilation. Pediatr Res 14:1186–1191

70. Jolly H, Molyneaux P, Newell DJ (1962) A controlled study of the effect of temperature on premature babies. J Pediatr 60:889–894

71. Jones RWA, Roshefort MJ, Baum JD (1976) Increased insensible water loss in new-born infants nursed under radiant heaters. Br Med J ii:1347–1350

72. Karlberg P (1952) Determination of standard enery metabolism (basal metabolism in normal infants. Acta Paediatr Scand 41:Suppl 89

73. Kennaird DL (1976) Oxygen consumption and evaporation water loss in infants with congenital heart

disease. Arch Dis Child 51:34–41

74. Kennell JH, Jerauld R, Wolfe H, Chesler D, Creager NC, McAlpine W, Steffin M, Claus MH (1974) Maternal behaviour one year after early and extended post-partum contact. Dev Med Child Neurol 16:172–179

75. Khogali M, Weiner JS (1980) Heat stroke: Report on 18 cases. Lancet II:276–278

76. Kluger MJ (1980) Fever. Pediatrics 66:720–724

77. Lee VA, lliff A (1956) The energy metabolism of infants and young children during postprandial sleep. Pediatrics 18:739–749

78. Levine SZ, Marples E (1930) The insensible perspiration in infancy and in childhood. III. Basal metabolism and basal insensible perspiration of the normal infant: A statistical study of reliability and of correlation. Am J Dis Child 40:269–284

79. Levison H, Delivoria-Papadopoulos M, Swyer PR (1964) Oxygen consumption in new-born infants with the respiratory distress syndrome. Biol Neonate 7:255–269

80. Levison H, Linsao L, Swyer PR (1966) A comparison of infra-red and convective heating for new-born infants. Lancet II:1346–1348

81. Mann TP, Elliott RIK (1957) Neonatal cold injury due to accidental exposure to cold. Lancet I:229–234

82. Marks KH, Friedman Z, Maisels MJ (1977) A simple device for reducing insensible water loss in low-birth weight babies. Pediatrics 60:223–226

83. Marks KH, Bolan CD, Maisels MJ (1980a) The double-walled effect of oxygen consumption and mean skin temperature in premature infants in a forced convection incubator. Pediatr Res 14:605

84. Marks HK, Gunther RC, Rossi JA, Maisels MJ (1980b) Oxygen consumption and insensible water loss in premature infants under radiant heaters. Pediatrics 66:228–232

85. Matsaniotis N, Pastelis V, Agathopoulos A, Constantsas N (1971) Fever and biochemical thermogenesis. Pediatrics 47:571–576

86. McCutchan JW, Taylor CL (1950) Respiratory heat exchange and varying temperature and humidity of inspired air. J Appl Physiol 4:121–124

87. Merenstein GB, Cozial DF, Brown CL, Weisman LE (1979) Radiant warmers vs incubators for neonatal care. Am J Dis Child 133:857–858

88. Mount LE (1963) Environmental temperature preferred by the young pig. Nature 199:1212–1213

89. Oh W, Karecki H (1972) Phototherapy and insensible water loss in the new-born infant. Am J Dis Child 124:230–232

90. Oh W, Yao AC, Hansen JS, Lind J (1973) Peripheral circulatory response to phototherapy in new-born infants. Acta Paediatr Scand 62:49–54

91. Okken A, Jonxis JHP, Rispens P, Zijlstra WG (1979) Insensible water loss and metabolic growth rate in low birth weight new-born babies. Pediatr Res 13:1072–1075

92. Perlstein PH (1978) Games with children. Pediatrics 61:666–669

93. Perlstein PH, Edwards NK, Sutherland JM (1970) Apnoea in premature infants and incubator-air-temperature changes. N Engl J Med 282:461–466

94. Perlstein PH, Edwards NK, Atherton HD, Sutherland JM (1976) Computer-assisted new-born intensive care. Pediatrics 57:494–501

95. Pomerance JJ Brand RJ, Meredith JL (1981) Differentiating environmental from disease-related fevers in the term new-born. Pediatrics 67:485–487

96. Rodaway KA, Oliver TK (1965) Incubator accessory for exchanged transfusion. Lancet I:1220

97. Rutter N, Hull D (1979a) Response of term babies to a warm environment. Arch Dis Child 54:178–183

98. Rutter N, Hull D (1979b) Water loss from the skin of term and preterm babies. Arch Dis Child 54:858–868

99. Rutter N, Hull D (1981) Reduction in skin water loss in the newborn. I. Effect of applying topical agents. Arch Dis Child 56:669–672

100. Rutter N, Brown SM, Hull D (1978) Variation in the resting oxygen consumption of small babies. Arch Dis Child 51:34–41

101. Ryser G, Jéquier E (1972) Study by direct calorimetry of thermal balance on the first day of life. Eur J Clin Invest 2:176–187

102. Schmitt BD (1980) Fever phobia. Am J Dis Child 134:176–181

103. Scopes JW, Ahmed I (1966) Indirect assessment of oxygen requirements in new-born babies by monitoring deep body temperature. Arch Dis Child 41:25–29

104. Silverman WA (1979) Incubator-baby sideshows. Pediatrics 64:127–141

105. Silverman WA, Blanc WA (1957) The effect of humidity on survival of newly born premature babies. Pediatrics 20:477–487

106. Silverman WA, Fertig JW, Berger AP (1958) The influence of the thermal environment upon the survival of newly born premature infants. Pediatrics 22:876–885

107. Silverman WA, Agate FJ Jr, Fertig JM (1963) A sequential trial of the non-thermal effect of atmospheric humidity on survival of infants of low birth weight. Pediatrics 31:719–724

108. Smales ORC (1978) Effect of phototherapy on thermal environment of the newborn. Arch Dis Child 53:172–174

109. Stanley FJ, Alberman ED (1978a) Infants of very low birth weight. I. Perinatal factors affecting survival. Dev Med Child Neurol 20:300–312

110. Stanley FJ, Alberman ED (1978b) Infants of very low birth weight. II. Perinatal factors in conditions associated with respiratory distress syndrome. Dev Med Child Neurol 20:313–322

111. Stanton AN, Scott DJ, Downham MAPS (1980) Is overheating a factor in some unexpected infant deaths? Lancet I:1054–1057

112. Stephenson JM, Du JN, Oliver TK (1970) The effect of cooling on blood gas tension in new-born infants. J Pediatr 76:848–852

113. Stothers JK (1981) Head insulation and heat loss in the new-born. Arch Dis Child 56:530–534

114. Sulyok E, Jequier E, Prod'hom LS (1973) Respiratory contribution to the thermal balance of new-born infants under various ambiant conditions. Pediatrics 51:641–650

115. Tafari N, Gentz J (1974) Aspects on rewarming new-born infants with severe accidental hypothermia. Acta Paediatr Scand 63:595–600

116. Thomson MH, Stothers JK (1981) The effect of forced convection on neonatal water loss. Paper to the Neonatal Society, July 1981

117. Varga F (1959) The respective effect of starvation and changed body composition on energy metabolism in malnourished infants. Pediatrics 23:1085–1090

118. Weldon AE, Rutter N (1982) The heat balance of small babies nursed in incubators and under radiant warmers. Early Hum Dev (to be published)

119. Williams PR, Oh W (1974) Effects of radiant warmer on insensible water loss in new-born infants. Am J Dis Child 128:511–514

120. Wu PYK, Hodgman JE (1974) Insensible water loss in preterm infants: changes with postnatal development and non-ionizing radiant energy. Pediatrics 54:504–512

121. Wu PYK, Moosa A (1978) Effect of phototherapy on nitrogen and electrolyte levels and water balance in jaundice preterm infants. Pediatrics 61:193–198

122. Wu PYK, Wong WH, Hodgman JE, Levan N (1974) Changes in blood flow in the skin and muscle with phototherapy. Pediatr Res 8:257–262

123. Yashiro K, Adams FH, Emmanoulides GC, Mickey MR (1973) Preliminary studies on the thermal environment of low-birth-weight infants. J Pediatr 82:991–994

124. Yeh TF, Amma P, Lilien LD, Baccaro MM, Matwynschyn J, Pyati S, Pildes RS (1979) Reduction of insensible water loss in premature infants under the radiant warmer. J Pediatr 94:651–653

125. Yeh TF, Voora S, Lilien LD, Matwynshyn J, Srinivasan G, Pildes RS (1980) Oxygen consumption and insensible water loss in premature infants in single-space vs double-walled incubators. J Pediatr 97:967–971

Chapter 64

Monitoring the Sick Infant

A. D. Milner and G. Smith

Modern neonatal intensive care has had a dramatic effect on mortality, so that well-equipped and staffed units are achieving 50%–70% survival rates in babies with a birth weight of 750–1000 g, compared with 10%–20% only 5–10 years ago, the improvement having been made possible only through the development and introduction of monitoring techniques. For the very small baby to survive intact the environmental challenge must be kept to a minimum, since in utero the baby would be growing in a protected fluid environment maintained at 37°C, with all its nutritional requirements supplied in a readily utilizable form.

In some respects the preterm baby is quite tolerant to adverse challenge, coping with periods of hypoxia which would prove fatal to the older child, and apparently being unharmed by relatively low blood glucose levels. In contrast, the neonate is much more likely to develop severe hypothermia if the environmental temperature is low [30] and has particular problems relating to its immaturity, including hyperoxic retinal artery sensitivity, retrolental fibroplasia, and an incompetent blood–brain barrier predisposing to kernicterus when the serum concentration of unconjugated bilirubin becomes grossly elevated. Once critical metabolic conditions are exceeded, the rapidly developing brain may be severely damaged,

leading to various degrees of cerebral palsy and mental subnormality. The skilful use of monitoring allows us to identify the onset of potentially damaging processes and enables us to initiate the appropriate remedial steps.

Monitoring devices have a major role in reducing the need to handle the baby, all involved in neonatal care agreeing that the more the baby is left undisturbed in an appropriate environment, the less will be the need for intensive cardiorespiratory support and the lower the associated morbidity.

Temperature

After provision of adequate resuscitation facilities, maintenance of an appropriate thermal environment is probably the most important single aspect of neonatal care. Body core temperature is most easily estimated with a rectal thermometer. This is not without its problems. The child has to be handled and the incubator door opened. Occasionally the bulb bursts, leading to local injury. In fact, all methods have their problems.

Body core temperature

Rectal

Rectal temperature can be monitored continuously with a suitably mounted thermistor head having a response time of 1–2 min. The main practical disadvantage is the tendency for this to be expelled regularly and frequently. In 1948 Bazett et al. [1] demonstrated that the rectal temperature tended to underestimate the true core temperature, due to local cooling by blood returning from the legs via the iliac veins. In addition faeces in the rectum may effectively insulate the probe. Rectal probes must never be used to control incubator or radiant heater output since the time taken for core temperature to respond to ambient temperature changes is too long, and large swings in environmental temperature will result. Marked changes in ambient temperature have been shown to induce potentially dangerous apnoea in preterm neonates [25].

Aural

An alternative method of core temperature estimation, with the zero gradient aural thermometer, was devised in 1974 by Cross and Stratton [34]; it involves the use of paired thermistor probes and a servo-controlled heating pad attached to the pinna, and the results correlate well with those of oesophageal temperature monitoring, but this again should not be used to control environmental heating.

Skin temperature

Devices consisting of a thermistor mounted in a disc are available for monitoring skin temperature; these measure accurately to within 0.5°C and remain stable over long intervals. Periodic checking of calibration is required, usually by immersion in warm water in a Dewar flask and comparison with a mercury-in-glass thermometer. The devices often become detached and may be affected either by environmental temperature or by heat loss due to evaporation of liquids in contact with the probe [22]. Additionally, they do not measure core temperature, but provided the probe is placed over the upper abdomen the recording is likely to be within 1.0°C, assuming a stable temperature state. Peripheral circulatory failure may cause gradients as high as 1.5°C to develop.

The temperature difference between peripheral and core or abdominal skin temperature has been used to help identify poor peripheral perfusion or low environmental temperature [4]. Abdominal skin temperature can undoubtedly be used to control the heat output of an incubator, and when used carefully can provide a sensitive reliable system [29]. Although radiant heater output may be similarly controlled, this constitutes a far greater hazard to the child. There is a major need for a system to be developed which will alarm when the probe becomes detached, avoiding the exposure of the baby to excessive radiant heat, although to date no commercial system is available.

Respiration

Apnoea is a common and major problem in preterm and in sick full-term babies. Many attacks are self-limiting but others are potentially fatal. Prolonged attacks are accompanied by progressive hypoxia and acidosis. Termination of apnoea is relatively easily achieved by simple stimulation if the metabolic changes are not too severe. Because of their tendency to apnoeic attacks, all preterm or sick babies admitted to a neonatal unit require respiratory monitoring, which can be discontinued when the child's condition permits and no longer proves to be a practical problem.

Respiratory rate is variable in the neonatal period, depending on sleep state as well as underlying cardiorespiratory, neurological, and metabolic derangement, thus making it more important to utilize a system which will reliably identify apnoea rather than accurately record respiratory rate. Many preterm infants have periodic respiration for several weeks, and to avoid frequent alarm signals the apnoea device should be activated after a variable delay of 10–20 s.

Since no commercially available apnoea monitor is ideal, systems have proliferated and there are now at least eight different techniques in use.

The apnoea alarm mattress

This is one of the cheapest and most widely used devices, consisting of a compartmented inflatable mattress with tubes leading from each compartment to a central manifold containing a heated thermistor head (Fig. 64.1). Redistribution of the infant's weight with respiration

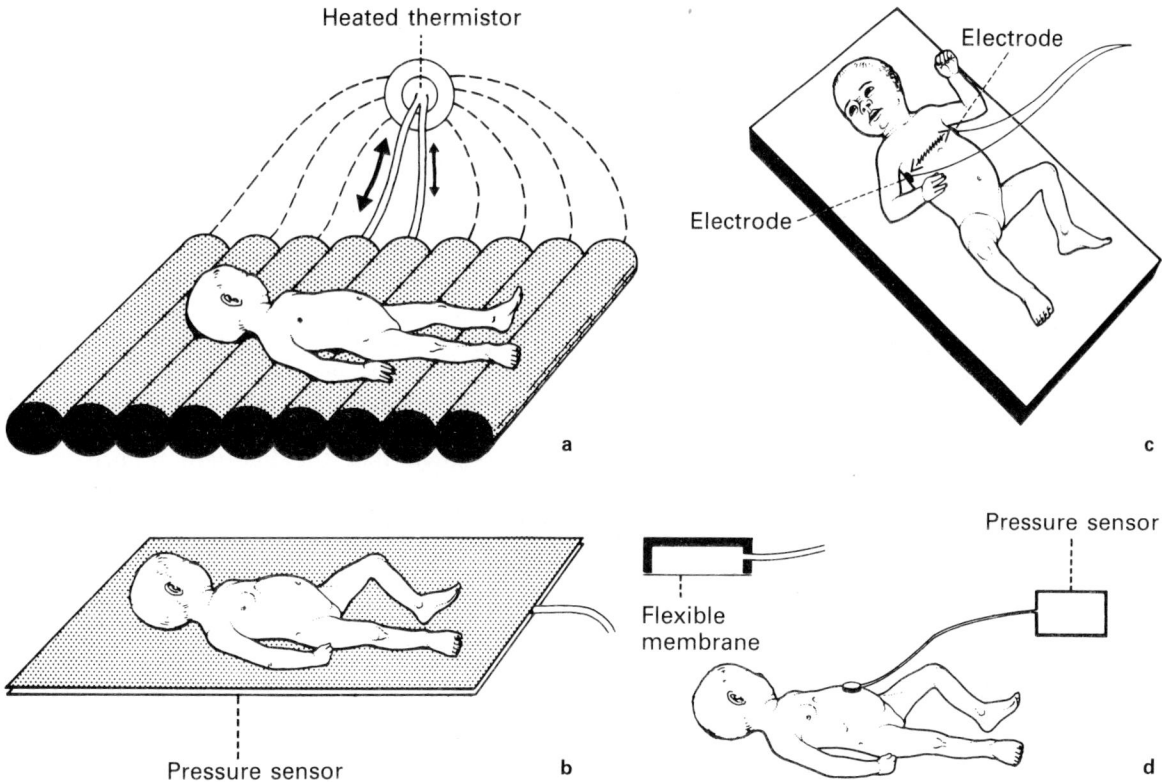

Fig. 64.1. Diagrams of systems for detecting apnoea: **a** Apnoea mattress; **b** mattress transducer; **c** impedance system; and **d** Wright respiration monitor.

causes a net airflow through the manifold and across the thermistor [16]. The principal advantages of the system are its relative cheapness and the absence of any electrical contact to the baby. The disadvantages are the need to maintain a critical level of inflation and sensitivity. False-negative alarms are common, due to too low a sensitivity setting, overinflation of the mattress, or simply because the baby has rolled off [28]. False-positive alarm failures are more worrying, and occur if the baby is in obstructive apnoea and making respiratory efforts although no tidal flow is occurring, or is fitting. Alarm failures also occur if the sensitivity is set too high, as the thermistor will respond to cardiac oscillations which become accentuated with the progression of apnoea [32]. The mattress is also vulnerable to puncture.

The mattress pressure transducer

This device also depends on the baby's weight redistribution during respiration, as sensed by a piezoresistive transducer, and has similar advantages and disadvantages to the apnoea mattress, with the exception of lack of susceptibility to puncture [31].

Impedance systems

This is probably the most popular technique, although electrodes are required, one attached to each side of the chest. In this system, the subject is coupled to an oscillator so that respiration will cause amplitude and/or frequency modulation of the oscillator signal [4, 26]. This device is usually combined with an ECG monitor, sharing two of the three electrodes; it provides a read-out of respiratory rate as well as indicating apnoea. False-negative alarms are less frequent than with the previously described systems, but nevertheless it will not detect obstructive apnoea when respiratory movements are present, and is prone to movement artefact. This device may also fail to alarm on apnoea because of accentuation of the cardiac artefact [21].

Magnetometers

The principle used by the monitor is that of distance measurement performed magnetically. The distance variations between two points on the chest produced by respiration are used to identify respiratory movement [27]. Although used extensively in research projects, their introduction into routine clinical use has been restricted due to practical problems with positioning and calibration.

The Wright apnoea device

Respiration is detected by measuring changes in the curvature of the abdominal wall by means of a flat cylindrical capsule with a diaphragm attached. A transducer system converts pressure changes due to distortion of the diaphragm into electrical signals and an electronic display is provided [42]. The capsule in contact with the baby inevitably makes nursing care a little more difficult, but otherwise this device shows similar advantages and disadvantages to the mattress devices.

Nasal thermistors

Nasal thermistors were introduced in an attempt to develop a system detecting obstructive as well as central apnoea. With tidal flow, the thermistor temperature and therefore its resistance will vary, lack of resistance change indicating apnoea [7]. While not affected by cardiac artefact, the system has the disadvantage that it lacks a reliable fixation system which will not occlude the nares.

Microphone system

An alternative to the nasal thermistor technique has been the use of a small microphone placed over the trachea, recording and amplifying the noise produced by non-laminar air flow in the airway. This promising device is still in the developmental stage, a reliable attachment system again proving problematic [40].

Radar/Doppler system

A radar beam is directed from an overhead transmitter receiver module at the infant, and chest wall movement detected by shifting of the standing wave pattern on the recorder [3]. The system has the advantage that it is not attached to the baby and is not influenced by cardiac oscillation. It is prone to movement artefact and is considerably more expensive than mattress devices, and so is no longer commercially available.

Heart rate

The main function of heart monitoring in the neonatal period is to identify bradycardia and tachycardia. Although arrhythmias do occur, these are relatively rare and so a continuous reading of heart rate is more important than a high-quality ECG display. The heart rate meter is also of considerable value if used in conjunction with respiration monitors, since clinically significant apnoea is usually associated with bradycardia. It is also very useful in identifying attacks of obstructive apnoea when bradycardia occurs early and rapidly [32]. Recent studies have shown that the frequent occurrence of bradycardia in preterm babies in situations where the apnoea alarm is not triggered are usually due to bradycardia brought on by respiratory effort against a closed airway, presumably via a Valsalva manoeuvre [38].

Any ECG-based monitor is satisfactory for neonatal use, providing the meter scale extends to at least 250/min, and preferably up to 300/min, as rates in excess of 200/min are frequently seen. Of greater importance is the need for suitably small lightweight electrodes which do not damage the very thin skin of the preterm baby.

Blood pressure

It is essential that all neonatal units have the facilities for blood pressure monitoring as it is not always easy to identify the existence of shock in the sick neonate. There may also be difficulty in diagnosing coarctation of the aorta in babies who are in cardiac failure, with a rapid low volume pulse. As blood pressure can rarely be measured with the occlusive cuff and stethoscope combination, other systems, including continuous blood pressure monitoring, are needed. Although the pattern varies widely, most well-equipped units use their systems only intermittently, despite the potentially valuable information to be gained.

Ultrasound system—Doppler shift principle

There are now many inexpensive units available which can detect minimal arterial flow in small vessels, and used in conjunction with a suitable cuff and pressure manometer can measure blood pressure in either the upper or the lower limb. The Doppler principle has been touched upon earlier, in connection with apnoea monitors. It is essential to ensure that the occlusive cuff is soft and extends over at least two-thirds of the upper or lower portion of the limb if accurate results are to be achieved [33, 35]. If upper and lower limb pressures are needed to exclude coarctation the calf region should be used, as these results compare more accurately with upper limb measurements [8].

Automatic sphygmomanometry

Devices are available which will record systolic and diastolic pressure automatically at preset time intervals by detecting infrasonic arterial wall oscillations associated with the Korotkoff sounds [36]. The real advantage of the system is that a record of blood pressure may be obtained non-invasively and may be updated every 1–10 min [15]. The pressure readings correlate well with direct intra-arterial measurements and the devices are not excessively expensive.

Continuous intra-arterial pressure monitoring

Accurate measurement of blood pressure is best achieved by linking an indwelling cannula in umbilical, radial, posterior tibial, dorsalis pedis, or superficial temporal arteries to a pressure transducer by a suitable manometer line. As the majority of babies with severe respiratory problems have an arterial line in situ primarily for sampling purposes, the addition of an arterial pressure-monitoring facility need not be dismissed on the grounds of being an unnecessarily invasive technique. Satisfactory pressure wave recordings can be achieved with even 3.5 fg lines although inevitably there will be a damping effect if a catheter of less than 5 fg is used [10]. A syringe pump is essential to provide a low-volume continuous flush through the cannula, other infusion systems tending to produce a large recording artefact and an excessively high fluid input.

It should be remembered that the recorded pressure will depend on the vertical height between the top of the cannula and the transducer. Baseline drift is common, and the oscilloscope or recorder display must be re-zeroed at least every 12 h by obstructing the arterial line and opening the pressure transducer to air.

The inherent technical problems have discouraged many from routinely using available systems, but information on impending cardiovascular collapse can often be gained by observing trends in the arterial pressure, allowing appropriate therapy to be instituted to prevent dangerous decompensation.

An extremely simple hydrostatic method of measuring mean aortic pressure in sick neonates already undergoing umbilical arterial perfusion has been described recently by Ogata and Hewing [20], basically using the infusion line as a passive manometer and the infusion burette chamber as gravity reservoir.

EEG and cerebral function

Systems have been developed which will continuously monitor voltage variations of filtered cerebral electrical activity [23], possibly proving useful in determining whether apnoeic episodes are a manifestation of fits, or due to a failure of respiratory drive. More information is needed on patterns in normal infants before these devices can be routinely used in the neonatal unit.

Oxygen

The dangers of hypoxia or hyperoxia are always present in the neonatal period so that it is no longer acceptable to estimate O_2 concentrations in incubators or headboxes simply by calculation from fresh gas flow rates, or to accept concentrations preset on ventilator control panels. It is essential that the F_IO_2 be measured whenever an O_2-enriched environment is selected. There are currently three O_2-monitoring systems in widespread clinical use, one being the paramagnetic O_2 analyser and the other two respectively polarographic Clark electrode devices and fuel cells (Fig. 64.2).

Paramagnetic O_2 analysers

Oxygen is a strongly paramagnetic gas (i.e., attracted into a magnetic field) and paramagnetic O_2 analysers utilize this property in such a way that the scale deflection produced on the meter is proportional to the number of O_2 molecules attracted into the magnetic field, and synonymous with O_2 concentration. The system has the advantages of very high sensitivity,

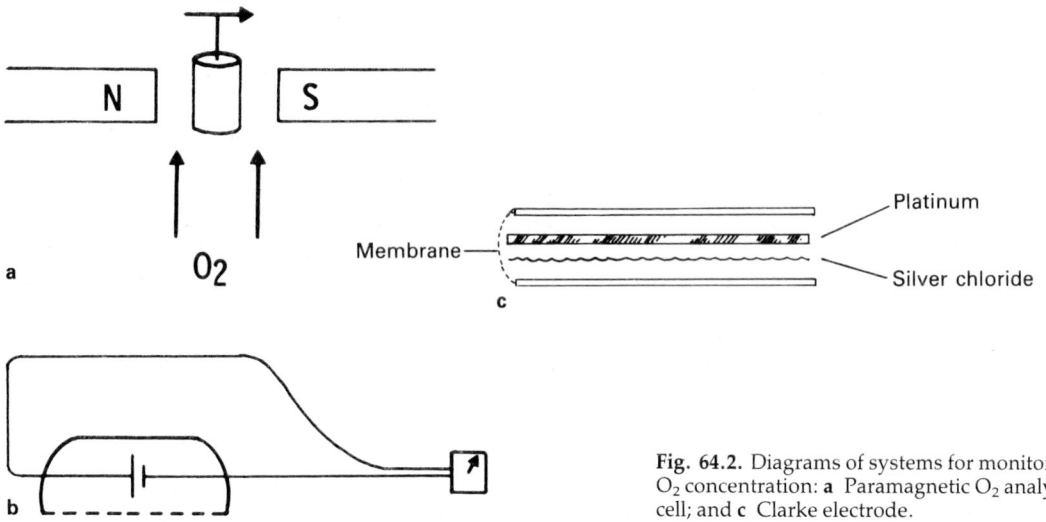

Fig. 64.2. Diagrams of systems for monitoring ambient O_2 concentration: **a** Paramagnetic O_2 analyser; **b** fuel cell; and **c** Clarke electrode.

linearity, and stability over prolonged periods, and minimal running costs. The main disadvantage is that they may be destroyed by humidity, necessitating the incorporation of reusable silica gel drying chamber in the sampling line. They are also pressure-sensitive, necessitating the inclusion of a needle valve proximal to the sampling chamber if continuous sampling is required in a pressure fluctuating circuit.

Fuel cells

A fuel cell is a device which converts the potential chemical energy of a fuel, in this case O_2, directly into electrical energy, by-passing intermediate energy states such as thermal and kinetic.

In view of their precision and potential capability of continuous O_2 analysis combined with relatively rapid response times, they are undoubtedly the most popular devices available for measuring inspired O_2 concentrations [38]. Despite good stability, as the cells age so their sensitivity decreases. However, they remain virtually insensitive to water vapour or anaesthetic gases, and may be included in any circuit. Relatively high cost and short life after exposure to O_2 limits their usefulness.

Clark polarographic O_2 electrode device

This system, introduced in 1960, consists of a platinum cathode and silver anode dipping into buffered electrolyte solution, the cathode tip being separated from the blood sample by a gas-permeable plastic membrane. For O_2 analysis, an electrode potential of 0.6 V is maintained, and at the cathode the process of electroreduction of O_2 occurs, the higher the O_2 tension in the sample the greater the current produced. The main advantage of the system is its relative cheapness, while poor stability combined with the necessity for daily calibration have detracted from their widespread use.

End-tidal CO_2

Until relatively recently it has not been possible to monitor end-tidal CO_2 in newborn infants, as the commercially available CO_2 analysers all had minimum flow requirements that were too high. Now infrared CO_2 analysers are available which will function with reasonable response times (90–100 ms) at flow rates down to 50 ml/min. Their place in the management of babies with respiratory failure, whether spontaneously breathing or artificially ventilated, has yet to be determined.

Blood gas analysis

The facility which above all other monitoring systems determines whether a unit can provide intensive care or should transfer babies in established or predictable respiratory failure elsewhere, is that of blood gas analysis. By choice, the analyser should be either in or immediately adjacent to the unit, thus making sampling logistically easier for the staff and reducing errors due to inefficient cold storage prior to analysis. Warm blood has a metabolic rate such that at 37°C the O_2 tension will fall and CO_2 tension rise by approximately 0.75 mmHg (0.1 kPa)/min [12]. To prevent these errors, blood samples which cannot be immediately analysed should be immersed in ice and analysed as soon as possible. Any conveniently sited artery may be used for sampling, with a heparinized 2 ml syringe and a fine gauge needle (21–25). The femoral artery is less preferable, due to the relative ease with which femoral venous blood may be accidentally aspirated and in the sick hypoxic neonate differentiation between arterial and venous blood gas results may not be easy. Blood sample volume should be minimized as repeated sampling may significantly affect the child's blood volume, which is only in the region of 80 ml/kg body weight. The main disadvantage of intermittent sampling, apart from the technical problems, is that the procedure is almost always associated with a dramatic fall in arterial O_2 tension [5]. The alternative is to insert an indwelling arterial cannula.

Umbilical arterial catheterization

The main advantage of the umbilical arteries is their accessibility so that catheters can be passed up to the descending aorta with a reasonably high success rate with a minimum of experience. Blood samples can be withdrawn over periods of up to 2 weeks without disturbing the child. The disadvantages of this route are that the arteries are only available for catheterization in the first 24 h of life and even within that period spasm sometimes prevents passage; it is relatively easy to produce a false passage in the wall of the artery, and peritoneal perforation has been experienced [37]. Post-mortem studies have shown that thrombi frequently form on the tip of the catheter, although clinically obvious emboli are rare. In view of potential embolic damage to the kidney, the practice has developed of advancing the catheter until the tip lies at the radiological level of the 2nd or 3rd lumbar vertebra. Recent studies [18] indicating that emboli are less common if the catheter tip is higher have resulted in a policy of advancing the catheter tip till it comes to lie above the diaphragm. Passage of the catheter may occasionally obstruct branches of the descending

aorta or cause spasm, producing blanching of the leg progressing to severe tissue damage unless the catheter is withdrawn within a few minutes [13]. Blood samples from umbilical artery catheters are post-ductal, and it is well known that hypoxia or metabolic acidosis in the neonate may lead to pulmonary hypertension and a right-to-left shunt through the ductus arteriosus [24], thus making the blood in the descending aorta considerably desaturated compared with carotid and retinal arteries. The tension difference is unlikely to exceed 30 mmHg (4 kPa).

Percutaneous arterial catheterization

With skill and luck, it is possible to insert a cannula into any superficially sited artery. Radial artery cannulation is facilitated by transillumination of the wrist with a fibre-optic light source. A catheter of up to 4 fg can be introduced into peripheral arteries of babies over 1500 g in weight, but below this a maximum of 3 fg should be used. Temporal artery cannulation may lead to superficial necrosis of areas of the scalp, and radial or posterior tibial catheterization to the loss of digits. The problems of maintaining cannula patency have already been mentioned.

Because retrolental fibroplasia has been observed in severely preterm babies breathing only air no degree of hyperoxia may be considered entirely safe, and most authorities would recommend that preductal arterial O_2 tension should be between 60 and 120 mmHg (8 and 16 kPa) and postductal blood between 50 and 90 mmHg (6.7 and 12 kPa) [24].

Continuous blood gas monitoring

Although the time constant for CO_2 in the blood is relatively slow, rising by 3.8–7.6 mmHg (0.5–1 kPa)/min during apnoea [19], the O_2 tension is far more labile and 4-hourly sampling can be misleading and lead to inappropriate changes in therapy. For this reason, methods have been developed for continuously monitoring arterial O_2 tension.

Catheter tip polarographic O_2 electrode

Presterilized 4 and 5 fg catheters have been produced that incorporate a small Clark electrode at the tip. The cell is activated by immersing the tip in saline for approximately 30 min [11]. Because of the idiosyncratic output from the electrode, the catheter has a lumen for blood sampling, so that in vivo calibration can be carried out. The catheter is only suitable for insertion via the umbilical artery and 5%–15% fail to work once introduced, due either to a manufacturing fault or to damage during insertion. The electrode life is variable and unpredictable, from less than 1 to more than 20 days, and during this period drift and sensitivity changes necessitate direct arterial sampling at least every 6 h. The response time to a change in arterial concentration is approximately 15 s. Although the lumen is small, it is possible to monitor blood pressure by connecting a transducer to the sample line.

The continuous O_2 electrode records the dramatic fall in O_2 tension on handling the neonate, and so acts as a useful reminder to nursing and medical staff to avoid unnecessary or prolonged techniques.

Sampling probe with mass spectrometer

By by-passing the critical collecting chamber in the mass spectrometer, it is possible to measure the blood gas constituents at a sampling gas flow rate of 10^{-5} ml/s, comparable with the rates of diffusion of O_2 and CO_2 across a gas-permeable membrane mounted at the tip of the sampling catheter [6]. These systems are under further development, and will allow continuous monitoring of any gas within the mass range of the spectrometer. As with all sampling catheters utilizing semi-permeable membranes, a limiting factor has been the tendency for fibrin and blood clot to accumulate, decreasing sensitivity and slowing system response times.

Sampling probe with gas chromatograph

An ingenious system has been recently developed whereby arterial O_2 and CO_2 diffused across a membrane on the catheter tip and were allowed to reach equilibrium, using helium as a carrier gas (2). At short intervals, the helium and blood gas mixture was sampled by the gas chromatograph and the contents analysed. Although attractive in concept, this proved too expensive for routine clinical use and in addition problems were experienced maintaining membrane continuity.

In vivo oximetry

As an alternative to O_2 tension monitoring, haemoglobin O_2 saturation can also be con-

tinuously monitored with a flexible fibre-optic catheter placed in the umbilical artery [9]. This allows spectral analysis of the light reflected from arterial blood and calculation of the percentage of oxidized haemoglobin to within ±1%. The system is calibrated in vitro, is unlikely to be damaged during insertion, and proves to be remarkably stable, often not needing a change in calibration over 1–2 weeks. Disadvantages are that the catheter tip may impinge over a vessel wall, although systems for detecting this are built in, and that staff are often not used to dealing with percentage saturation readings. It is necessary to keep the maximum saturation below 96%, as the arterial O_2 tension can rise dramatically with only small subsequent changes in saturation due to the shape of the O_2–Hb dissociation curve. An additional disadvantage is the relatively high cost of these disposable catheters.

Since the continuous monitoring systems mentioned above all require insertion of an arterial line, new equipment has been developed for transcutaneous estimation of arterial blood gases. The transcutaneous systems depend on producing local vasodilatation in the skin by heating to 42–44°C, thereby increasing transcutaneous gas diffusion and also a right shift of the O_2–Hb dissociation curve, providing an increased diffusion gradient for O_2.

Transcutaneous O_2 analysers

There is now a variety of commercially available systems on the market that utilize a modified Clark polarographic O_2 electrode and a servo-controlled heater in the probe [14]. Calibration of the transcutaneous electrode is usually carried out in air, and once it is correctly placed on the skin reasonably accurate results are obtained within a few minutes. As the heater produces local burns, the probe must be removed, recalibrated, and repositioned every 2–6 h, depending on the individual system and its probe heater temperature. The response time is usually between 30 and 60 s. Major problems arise with membrane decay, which tends to be quite rapid in the clinical situation, necessitating membrane changes occasionally after a few days but usually after 1–3 weeks. Accurate monitoring depends on good local perfusion, and the onset of peripheral circulatory failure with decreased tissue perfusion will produce an underestimate of the arterial PO_2. Many systems include a probe heater power input display, since it is hoped that when hypoperfusion occurs this will be recorded by an increase in the power input. Unfortunately, under some circumstances the flow through the skin capillaries may fall before the deeper vessels are affected, a condition not picked up by the equipment, which is heating the tissues down to a depth of at least 0.5 cm [17].

Sometimes grossly inaccurate recordings of PO_2 are obtained for no obvious reason, and there is a small group of preterm babies in whom the system is totally inaccurate, presumably reflecting a variation in their skin structure. Although these devices are undoubtedly very useful in the management of neonates with severe respiratory problems, they cannot at present be considered a viable alternative to regular arterial blood gas analysis, their main use being as trend monitors. Tragedies are likely to occur if they are used in any other way.

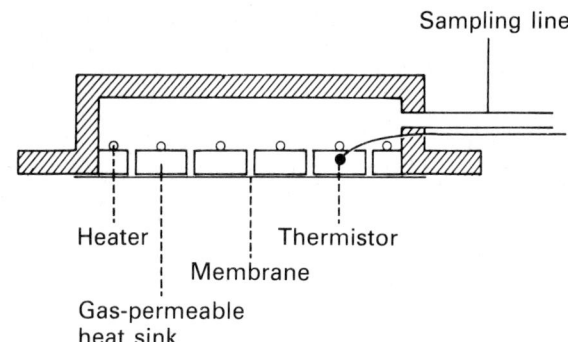

Fig. 64.3. Diagram of probe for measuring transcutaneous gases by mass spectrometry.

Transcutaneous CO_2 electrodes

Transcutaneous CO_2 electrodes are now becoming clinically available, either as single probes or combined with a transcutaneous oxygen device [41]. Further information is still required on their reliability and indeed on their most appropriate probe heater temperature setting, although the devices appear most accurate when the heater is set at 37°C. At this temperature the response time is slow, about 4–6 min, but if the skin temperature is raised to 44°C the response time drops to 30–60 s while the device consistently over-records by 30%–40%.

Transcutaneous arterial gas analysis with skin probe and mass spectrometer

The rate of diffusion of CO_2 and O_2 across skin heated to 43–44°C is sufficient to match the minimum flow requirements of the mass spectrometer [42] commercially available, which makes it possible to measure these gases by means of a membrane-covered probe with a heater included, feeding via a fine-bore gas-impermeable tube to a mass spectrometer (Fig. 64.3). This is an expensive system, sharing the limitation of the electro-chemical transcutaneous devices. In addition it is bulky, generates a high heat output, and has proved time-consuming and temperamental to set up for initial use.

We are now reaching a point at which more and more sophisticated and inevitably expensive monitoring equipment is available. The cost of the equipment has, in these days, to be matched against the possible benefit and must

be looked at against other facilities. When buying new equipment the ability of the staff to use and carry out day-to-day maintenance must be considered, and nursing staff should always be involved in selection. It is also very important to take into account the servicing record of the supplying company in your own area and to assess the running costs, which can be considerable and may lead to the rapid rejection of a system.

A centralized display of monitoring devices has largely been rejected in the neonatal unit, as there is no substitute for having nurses around the babies. Despite these problems there is no doubt that appropriate and sensible use of monitoring devices saves lives and limits long-term damage in newborn babies.

References

1. Bazett HC, Love L, Newton M, Eisenberg L, Day R, Foster R (1948) Temperature changes in blood flowing in arteries and veins in man. J Appl Physiol 1:3–19
2. Behrens-Tepper JC, Messaro TA (1977) New continuous monitoring of arterial gas tension by gas chromatography: Animal and initial clinical evaluations. In: The association for the advancement for medical instrumentation. Arpington, Virginia–Proceedings: AAMI 12th Annual Meeting, March, p 234
3. Caro CG, Bloice JA (1971) Contactless apnoea detector based on radar. Lancet II:959–961
4. Daily WJR, Klaus M, Meyer HBP (1969) Apnoea in premature infants: Monitoring, incidence, heart rate changes and an effect of environmental temperature. Adv Pediatr 43:510–518
5. Dangman BC, Hegyi T, Hiatt M, Indyk L, James LS (1976) The variability of PO_2 in newborn infants in response to routine care. Pediatr Res 10:422 (Abstract 728)
6. Delpy DT, Parker D (1979) In vivo and transcutaneous blood gas measurement by mass spectrometry. In: Payne JP, Bushman JA, Hill DW (eds) The medical and

biological applications of mass spectrometry. Academic Press, London, p 179–191

7. Dransfield DA, Lewis J, Fox WW (1980) Efficacy of airflow measurements by nasal determinations without oral measurements in neonatal apnoea. Pediatr Res 14:595

8. Elseed AM, Shinebourne EA, Joseph MC (1973) Assessment of techniques for measurement of blood pressure in infants and children. Arch Dis Child 48:932–936

9. Enson Y, Briscoe WA, Polangi ML, Cournand A (1962) In vivo studies with an intravascular and intracardiac reflection oximeter. J Appl Physiol 17:552–558

10. Geddes LA (1970) The direct and indirect measurement of blood pressure. Year Book Medical Publishers, Chicago

11. Goddard P, Keith I, Marcovitch H, Roberton NRC, Rolfe P, Scopes JW (1974) Use of a continuously recording intravascular oxygen electrode in the newborn. Arch Dis Child 49:853–860

12. Greenbaum R, Nunn JF, Prys-Roberts C, Kelman GR (1967) Metabolic changes in whole human blood in vitro at 37°C. Respir Physiol 2:274–282

13. Gupta JM, Roberton NRC, Wigglesworth JS (1968) Umbilical artery catheterisation in the newborn. Arch Dis Child 43:382

14. Huch R, Lubbers DW, Huch A (1974) Reliability of transcutaneous monitoring of arterial oxygen tension in newborn infants. Arch Dis Child 49:213–218

15. Kwong M, Mehta J, Goldberg AD (1980) Evaluation of an automatic sphygmomanometer in the neonatal intensive care unit. Pediatr Res 14:603 Abst 1063

16. Lewin JE (1969) An apnoea alarm mattress. Lancet II:667–668

17. Matsen FA, Wyss CR, King RV, Summons CW (1980) Effect of acute haemorrhage on transcutaneous, subcutaneous, intramuscular and arterial oxygen tension. Pediatrics 65:881–883

18. Mokrohisky ST, Levine RL, Blumhagen JS (1978) Low positioning of umbilical-artery catheters increases associated complications in newborn infants. N Engl J Med 299:561–564

19. Nunn JF (1969) Applied respiratory physiology, 1st edn. Butterworths, London, p 308

20. Ogata CS, Herring GR (1980) Rapid measurement of blood pressure in the sick neonate. Intensive Care Med 6:7–8

21. Pacela AF (1966) Impedance pneumograph: A survey of instrumentation techniques. Med Biol Eng Comput 4:1–15

22. Perlstein PH, Edwards NK, Sutherland JM (1970) Apnoea in premature infants and incubator air temperature changes. N Engl J Med 282:461–466

23. Prior P (1980) Non invasive monitoring of cerebral function. Br J Clin Equip 5:54–63

24. Roberton NRC (1968) Oxygen therapy in the newborn. Lancet I:1323–9

25. Roberton NRC (1976) Respiratory disease in early life. In: Stretton T (ed) Recent advances in respiratory medicine, vol 1. Churchill Livingstone, Edinburgh, p 241

26. Robins KE, Marko AR (1962) An improved method of registering respiration rate. In: Paper 5, Session V, Digest of the 15th Annual Conference on Engineering in Medicine and Biology, Chicago, Illinois, p 18

27. Rolfe P (1971) A magnetometer respiration monitor for use in premature babies. Biochem Eng 6:402–404

28. Rolfe P (1975) Monitoring in newborn intensive care. Med Biol Eng Comput 10/11:399–404

29. Scopes JS (1970) Control of body temperature in newborn babies. Scientific basis of medicine series, Athlone Press, London

30. Silverman WA, Fertig JW, Berger AP (1958) The influence of the thermal environment upon the survival of newly born premature infants. J Appl Physiol 22:876–885

31. Smith JE, Scopes JN (1972) A new apnoea alarm for babies. Lancet II:545–546

32. Smith ML, Milner AD (1981) Bradycardia and associated respiratory changes in the neonate. Arch Dis Child 56:645–648

33. Stegall HF, Kardon MB, Kemmeren WT (1968) Indirect measurement of arterial blood pressure by ultrasonic sphygmomanometry. J Appl Physiol 25:793–798

34. Stratton D (1977) Aural temperature of the newborn infant. Arch Dis Child 52:865–9

35. Swiet M de, Fayers P, Shinebourne EA (1980) Systolic blood pressure in a population of infants in the first year of life. The Brompton Study. Pediatrics 65:1028–1035

36. Ur A, Gordon M (1970) Origin of Korotkoff sounds. Am J Physiol 218/2:524–529

37. Van Leenwen G, Patney M (1969) Complications of umbilical vessel catheterisation: Peritoneal perforation. Pediatrics 44:1028

38. Vyas H, Milner AD, Hopkin IE (1981) Relationship between apnoea and bradycardia in preterm infants. Acta Paed Scand 70:785–790

39. Weil JV, Sodal IE, Speck RP (1967) A modified fuel cell for the analysis of oxygen concentration of gases. J Appl Physiol 23:419–422

40. Westhammer J, Stark A, Krasner J, Dibenedetto J (1980) Apnoea monitoring by accoustic detection of airflow. Pediatr Res 14:653

41. Whitehead MD, Pollitzer MJ, Parker D, Halsall D, Delpy DT, Reynolds EOR (1980) Transcutaneous estimation of arterial PO_2 and pCO_2 in newborn infants with a single electrochemical sensor. Lancet I:1111–1114

42. Wright BM (1977) An abdominal respiratory detector. J Physiol 271:11–12

Chapter 65

Principles of Neonatal Intensive Care

F. Beaufils, Y. Aujard, and Y. Bompard

The neonatal period extends from birth to the 27th day of postnatal age. This definition is important because during 4 weeks the newborn is in transition in all the aspects of his life. The suppression of placental circulation requires an acute adaptation of almost all the organs, particularly the cardiopulmonary system, kidneys, and liver. Profound adjustments are necessary for all the vital processes, such as carbohydrate metabolism, endocrine systems, neurological development, and coagulation. The newborn passes suddenly from a pathogen-free environment to an environment rich in a great variety of pathogens and is not always able to protect himself against these pathogens. Although very complicated, the adjustments are generally successful. But any of them may fail and raise important problems.

Knowledge concerning the pathology of the newborn has increased dramatically in the last 15 years, and the subject of neonatal intensive care is very extensive. We have therefore not attempted to be comprehensive, but have chosen to illustrate the importance of this pathology and how it relates to neonatal intensive care, taking account of the fact that the newborn is *in constant development*. This chapter is directed at physicians who are not familiar with this particular age group but have occasionally to deal with neonates. Neonatologists and physicians who require a more extensive account of neonatal intensive care are referred to other publications [16, 46, 52, 68, 69, 72].

Technological problems involved in the emergency treatment of this particular age are given in the Technical Appendix.

Cardiopulmonary adaptation [11, 12]

In utero the gaseous environment of the fetus is maintained by the placenta and the fetal lung does not function as an organ of gas exchange. At birth it has suddenly to assume this role. In a few seconds the fetus changes from an aquatic state dependent on the mother to an air-breathing state where he is independent and has to 'breathe by himself'. This change requires major adjustments in the circulatory and respiratory systems. For most babies, these adjustments are successfully made and cardio-respiratory functions are normal within a few hours. But for some these mechanisms fail, which results in a vital state of distress. Our aim is to present the main steps of cardiopulmonary adaptation and then to show how each of them may be a cause of distress if they don't perfectly succeed.

Normal cardiopulmonary adaptation
[16, 27, 43, 66, 68, 72]

Fetal lung and the first breath

Alveolar capillary units are formed between the 27th and 29th weeks of gestation and proliferate from this time until term. It is generally considered that sustained ventilation is impossible before 28 weeks of gestational age. In utero, the alveoli are liquid-filled with lung fluid, which arises from both blood and alveolar lining cells. Alveolar type II cells produce surfactant on which depends the ability of the neonate to maintain a normal functional residual capacity (FRC) at birth. The main component of surfactant is the surface active lecithin and its secretion can be evaluated in utero by the L:S (lecithin-to-sphingomyelin) ratio [32]. The L:S ratio is low until approximately 32 weeks gestation, which means that a premature baby of less than 32 weeks gestational age has a maximum risk of respiratory distress due to the inability of the lung to maintain an adequate FRC. At 35 weeks the L:S ratio increases suddenly, and from then on gestation increases steadily until term.

'At birth, the action of taking the first breath is the key event in the transfer from placental to pulmonary gas exchange' [72]. This is achieved by the following sequence of events.

1) During the birth process, the thorax is compressed by pressures which may reach up to 100 cmH$_2$O. Such pressure removes an important volume of the pulmonary liquid and the residue is rapidly removed by absorption into the lymphatics and the pulmonary vascular bed.

2) With delivery, the extrathoracic positive pressure decreases and a sudden increase in chest volume occurs, which sucks air into the upper airways.

3) After 10–20 s the first breath occurs, which requires a negative intrathoracic pressure of −20 cmH$_2$O to −40 cmH$_2$O and sometimes as great as −75 cmH$_2$O [43].

4) The first expiration occurs with a partially closed glottis and a positive pressure (recorded in the oesophagus) of 20–30 cmH$_2$O. This distributes air throughout the lung and establishes the FRC.

5) Following the first respiratory movement, each successive breath requires less and less inspiratory force.

Several stimuli contribute to the initiation of breathing but their relative importance has not yet been defined. A fall in PaO$_2$ and arterial pH and a rise in PaCO$_2$ (which are common during delivery) may stimulate respiration but if they are pronounced they can depress it. Clamping the umbilical cord seems to initiate breathing in experimental animals, but in man it is known that the first breath may occur before the cord has been clamped. Other stimuli are physical [16, 68, 72]: lowering of environmental temperature, change of the environment from liquid to air, and exposure to tactile stimuli.

Table 65.1. Blood gas equilibrium at birth

	Fetal scalp (during labour)	Neonate H1
pH	7.30	7.30
Bicarbonate	19 mmol/litre	19 mmol/litre
PaCO$_2$	44 mmHg (5.9 kPa)	37 mmHg (4.9 kPa)
PO$_2$	20–25 mmHg (2.7–3.3 kPa)	60–65 mmHg (8–8.7 kPa)

Adequate respiratory function is rapidly established in normal newborns, as can be shown by clinical examination, chest x-rays and assessment of blood gases (Table 65.1).

Pulmonary circulation and adaptation at birth

The pulmonary circulation in utero is characterized by a high resistance and a low flow. Only about 3%–7% of the combined outputs of the two ventricles goes to the lung [69] and this plays no significant role in gas exchange. Most of the inferior vena cava blood flow is diverted from the right atrium to the left through the foramen ovale, and most of the superior vena caval flow is diverted from the right atrium and right ventricle to the aorta via the ductus arteriosus. Blood from the left atrium is ejected by the left ventricle into the ascending aorta and cephalad portion of the body which receives well-oxygenated blood (62% saturation). Blood flowing from the ascending aorta and from the ductus arteriosus is mixed in the descending aorta and the residual saturation is 58%. Half of the flow is to the systemic circulation of the fetus and half to the placenta via the umbilical arteries, which have a low resistance.

The high resistance in the pulmonary arteries is probably due to several factors. The medial smooth muscle in the walls of the smallest arteries is thick, averaging 14%–17% of the external diameter [53, 68]. Hypoxia maintains constriction of the vessels and hydrostatic pressure produced by the pulmonary fluid and intrapleural pressure are additional forces that augment vascular resistance.

At birth, as soon as air breathing begins, *pulmonary vascular resistance falls* and the pulmonary blood flow abruptly increases [12]. Venous return to the left atrium increases and flow to the right heart from the placenta decreases so that the atrial pressure gradient is reversed and the foramen ovale can be functionally closed. The arterial O_2 saturation rapidly increases so that the ductus arteriosus constricts. With the fall in pulmonary vascular resistance, the two vascular shunts existing during fetal life disappear. Vascular resistances in umbilical arteries increase and umbilical flow decreases and eventually ceases. The umbilical cord occlusion has two consequences: (1) to reduce venous return and reduce the pressure in the right heart; and (2) to increase left heart and systemic resistances by removing blood flow from the placental circulation [3].

At birth the main modification for circulatory adaptation is *the abrupt fall of pulmonary vascular resistance*. Several factors may contribute to this: removal of pulmonary fluid, decrease of the positive intrapleural pressure existing in utero, lung inflation, increase of O_2 concentration particularly in the muscle of the pulmonary arteries. Acetylcholine, histamine, and bradykinin have vasodilator effects but their exact role has not been defined. The fall in vascular resistance continues during the next month with involution of the medial smooth muscle [53].

Though abrupt and essential for normal breathing, the vascular modifications occuring at birth are not immediately definitive. During the early postnatal period, the foramen ovale and ductus arteriosus are not permanently closed and right-to-left or left-to-right shunting through them is possible. The direction of flow depends on the level of vascular, pulmonary, and systemic resistances. Hypoxia and acidosis may increase pulmonary vascular resistance. The foramen ovale and ductus arteriosus are functionally but not yet anatomically closed, and may reopen in pathological situations. In fact, approximately the first week of life is characterized by a *transitional state*, which must be taken into account in every abnormal situation of respiratory function that may develop at this time.

Disorders of cardiopulmonary adaptation

Every cause of neonatal respiratory distress (Table 65.2) giving rise to hypoxia and acidosis may disturb the cardiopulmonary adaptation to extra-uterine life. Some diseases can be con-

Table 65.2. Causes of respiratory distress in the newborn

I. Obstruction of the upper airways
  Choanal atresia
  Pierre-Robin syndrome
  Congenital laryngeal stridor
  Laryngeal webs
  Laryngeal stenosis and tracheal stenosis
  Cysts of larynx
  Vocal cord paralysis

II. Lung parenchymal diseases
  Aspiration syndrome
  Transient tachypnoea of the newborn
  Respiratory distress syndrome
  Pneumonia
  Pneumothorax, pneumo-mediastinum. Interstitial emphysema

III. Non-direct pulmonary causes
  Oesophageal atresia tracheo-oesophageal fistula
  Diaphragmatic hernia
  Diaphragmatic paralysis
  Heart failure
  Apnoeic spells

sidered as direct disturbances of cardiopulmonary adaptation, namely neonatal asphyxia at birth, aspiration syndrome, retained lung liquid, and hyaline membrane disease. They may induce hypoxia, acidosis, elevated pulmonary arterial resistances, pulmonary hypoperfusion, and right-to-left shunting through a patent ductus arteriosus and foramen ovale. Actually, all this means *a return to a fetal circulation* but without the placenta. Such a situation leads to a vicious circle (Fig. 65.1) in which hypoxia and acidosis induce pulmonary arterial vasoconstriction, which further increases the hypoxia and acidosis. The aim of the treatment is to break this vicious circle as quickly as possible, by correction of hypoxia and acidosis. Persistent fetal circulation (PFC) is also observed in some cases of diaphragmatic hernia after operation. Finally, primary PFC, i.e., PFC without appa-

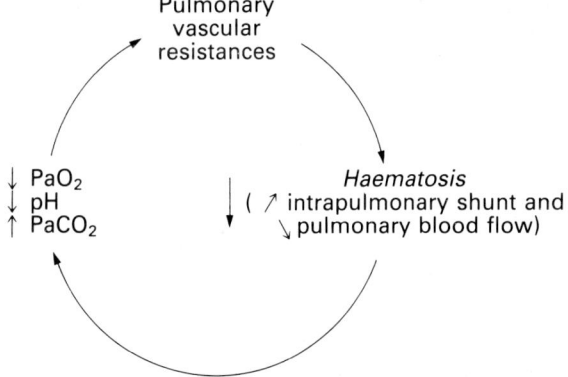

Fig. 65.1. Vicious circle of hypoxia in neonates.

rent pulmonary parenchymal disease, may be observed and this raises some problems of understanding and therapy.

Asphyxia at birth [16, 20, 34, 46]

Asphyxia at birth may be responsible for death or permanent and severe brain damage, with fitting and secondary, profound, developmental retardation. The major effort must be directed at identifying those pregnant women who are more likely than others to have an infant at risk of asphyxia. This is possible by continuous monitoring of fetal heart rate and intra-uterine pressure, and by measuring blood pH from the fetal scalp when the membranes are ruptured and the cervix dilated. Adequate monitoring is particularly important for the fetus at risk. When a fetus is suspected of being in distress, the paediatrician on call must be alerted and the equipment for resuscitation of the newborn must be prepared and checked.

Circulatory adjustments protecting vital organs from hypoxia have been described, but these protective effects are quickly overwhelmed after short periods of asphyxia. It is therefore important to detect significant abnormalities at a time when operative intervention has the greatest chance of promoting the delivery of a potiential normal baby. For the baby born asphyxiated, resuscitative measures must be started at once. The longer the delay in initiating these, the greater are the risks of death or neurological sequelae.

The classic and most practical guidelines for such emergencies are based on the Apgar score (Table 65.3) evaluated at 1, 5, and 10 min after birth. Two abnormal situations may be observed.

1) *When the Apgar score is under 3*, in fact *when the heart rate* (detected by heart sounds or beats of the umbilical arteries) *is under 100*, resuscitation is directed at providing O_2 and removing

CO_2 by positive pressure ventilation, maintaining the circulation by external cardiac massage, and then providing alkali for buffering the excess acid produced during anaerobic metabolism. After brief suction to clear the airway, the patient is intubated and ventilated with O_2 at a rate of 40–50 times per minute. External cardiac massage is done at a rate of 120 compressions per minute.

The infusion of alkali has been mentioned. In fact, during total experimental asphyxia in rhesus monkeys delivered by caesarean section, Dawes [16] has shown that dramatic changes occurred in acid base parameters with a fall of pH from 7.3 just prior to asphyxia to 6.8 at 10 min, and a rise of $PaCO_2$ from 45 mmHg (6 kPa) prior to asphyxia to 150 mmHg (20 kPa) at 10 min. So it is necessary to ensure adequate ventilation before any sodium bicarbonate is given. If after adequate ventilation and external cardiac massage the infant does not improve, then the slow administration (over 2–3 min) of $NaHCO_3$ 2–3 mmol/kg via an umbilical vein is indicated and may exert a beneficial effect. Although hypoglycaemia is unusual in infants being resuscitated, the administration of 10% glucose (5–10 ml/kg) may be of value because a decrease in the content of glucose in brain cells has been reported in experimental anoxia. Even if they fail, resuscitative measures must be continued for at least 20 min and sodium bicarbonate infusions repeated. If despite adequate techniques, the heart rate remains low or is absent, 1 or 2 ml calcium chloride may be infused, and if this fails to increase the heart rate, adrenaline (1–2 ml 1:10 000) may be tried but even when everything has been tried, resuscitative measures do not always succeed and cannot always prevent the consequences of prolonged prenatal anoxia.

2) *When the initial heart rate is over 100 beats per minute* (Apgar score between 3 and 6), brief

Table 65.3. Apgar score

Sign	Score		
	0	1	2
Heart rate	Absent	100/min	100/min
Respiratory effort	Absent	Weak, poor cry	Strong, good cry
Muscle tone	Limp	Some flexion of extremities	Active motion
Reflex irritability	No response	Weak response	Cough or sneeze
Colour	Blue, pale	Body pink, limbs blue	Completely pink

suctioning of the airway may be immediately followed by rapid improvement. If this is not the case, positive pressure ventilation with an O_2 mask and bag will often result in improvement. Before starting any ventilation with a mask, it is necessary to confirm the site of the heart sounds in the chest. If they are heard to the right side, a left diaphragmatic hernia must be suspected and the patient immediately intubated. Indeed in case of a diaphragmatic hernia, respiratory distress would be made worse by ventilation with a mask. If suctioning and ventilation with a mask do not improve the state of the infant within 3 min, management should proceed as for severe asphyxia.

The consequences of asphyxia on the brain are well known and all the states between neuronal destruction and cerebral edema can exist [8]. For the latter, intravenous phenobarbitone associated with fluid restriction, frusemide, or mannitol seem to have a good protective effect [34].

Asphyxia may affect other organs, especially the heart, sometimes giving rise to frank myocardial ischaemia [10, 19, 27].

Some cases, prolonged prenatal asphyxia, very low birth weight infants (<1000 g) or infants with apparent severe congenital malformation may raise the question of the advisability of resuscitation. In all such situations, resuscitative measures must be started immediately to avoid any loss of time and the risk of causing severe anomalies secondary to anoxia. The difficult ethical problem of proceeding with the intensive care can be decided upon later.

Whatever the problem, heat losses are very important during resuscitation and the infant needs to be kept warm. Overhead radiant heat sources placed over the resuscitation table can be adapted to maintain the neonate's temperature at over 36° C.

Congenital malformations and respiratory distress

Some major congenital malformations may induce respiratory distress. They should be detected immediately at birth:

Choanal atresia is detected by catheterization of the nostrils and oesophageal atresia by oesophageal catheterization and the 'syringe test': injection of a 5-ml bolus of air normally produces a noise which is heard on auscultation of the epigastrium. If an obstruction is encountered 9–13 cm from the anterior nares and/or if auscultation of the epigastrium is silent, an AP x-ray of the chest with the oesophageal catheter in place will confirm the diagnosis. Immediate transfer to a neonatal surgical unit is mandatory in such cases.

Left diaphragmatic hernia should be suspected, with or without severe respiratory distress, when heart sounds are heard in the right part of the chest. An AP chest x-ray rapidly confirms the diagnosis by showing displacement of the mediastinum to the right and typical gas-filled intestinal loops on the left. Emergency surgical treatment is required. A right diaphragmatic hernia is more rare and is not usually apparent at birth.

Pierre-Robin syndrome is easily recognized by the observation of three major anomalies in an infant with respiratory distress: mandibular retrognathia, cleft palate, and glossoptosis.

Other anomalies at birth

Secondary apnoea may be observed with a birth by caesarean section. Transient positive pressure ventilation with a mask will usually rapidly improve the situation.

Severe anaemia may be recognized at birth by the appearance of the infant and inferred from the obstetric history. Blood replacement at a rate of 2–3 ml/kg/min should be carried out after determination of the infant's and the mother's blood type. Measurement of the haematocrit is a guide to the quantity of blood to be infused. In severe bleeding, emergency transfusion should be done with non-dangerous group O rhesus negative blood or, as proposed by Fisher [46], with placental blood drawn aseptically from the umbilical vein.

Severe anaemia secondary to erythroblastosis fetalis should be treated by an exchange transfusion. In severe cases, anaemia is accompanied by respiratory distress secondary to cardiac failure and pulmonary oedema. Such cases require resuscitative measures; this means simultaneous exchange transfusion and assisted ventilation with intermittent positive pressure and sometimes a positive end-expiratory pressure. In fact, the proper management of severe erythroblastosis fetalis means transfer of the mother to a special centre for prenatal care and delivery. The same may be said for other high-risk pregnancies such as those complicated by toxaemia or occurring in diabetic mothers.

Lung parenchymal diseases

Meconium aspiration [16, 17, 28, 69, 72]. In cases of intra-uterine asphyxia, amniotic fluid may enter the lungs. In this instance, the liquid may contain meconium so that when air-breathing is started aspiration pneumonia occurs.

If signs of fetal distress are detected, and especially if meconium is found in the amniotic fluid during labour, meconium aspiration must be suspected. Immediately after birth, the mouth and the pharynx should be suctioned and the larynx visualized directly with a laryngoscope; suction of the trachea either directly or through an endotracheal tube then removes the meconium. If this is done before any positive pressure ventilation, meconium will not be pushed into small bronchi and alveoli and a good prognosis may be anticipated.

If positive pressure ventilation is performed before suction there is an increased risk of meconium aspiration and severe respiratory distress will be observed with tachypnoea, enlargement of the chest along the AP axis, hypoxia, and respiratory and metabolic acidosis. Chest x-ray shows coarse, irregular shadows and over-inflation of the lungs. Even at this stage suction of meconium through an endotracheal tube is necessary and usually productive. If possible, positive pressure ventilation should be avoided but in some cases respiratory distress is so severe that even with positive pressure ventilation there is a profound hypoxia [16]. Some of these cases may be dramatically improved by infusion of a pulmonary vaso dilatator such as tolazoline (cf. persistent fetal circulation). Other complications of meconium aspiration with intermittent positive pressure ventilation are pneumomediastinum, pneumothorax, and subcutaneous emphysema.

The diagnosis of meconium aspiration is obvious when endotracheal suction is productive, however it may be more frequent than usually admitted, as reported by Dehan et al. who have described a urinary meconium index [17].

Transient tachypnea of the newborn. Mild respiratory distress of a usually full-term infant may be due to delayed clearance of fetal lung liquid in the first few hours of life. The most important clinical sign is a high respiratory rate, sometimes with grunting and moderate cyanosis. The pH and $PaCO_2$ are within normal limits. PaO_2, often low initially, usually increases quickly. The chest x-ray shows well-expanded lungs with widened interlobular lines, pleural fluid, widened interlobular fissures and, sometimes, Kerley's lines [69]. Most cases need moderate oxygenation and improve over a few hours. Nevertheless in some cases the O_2 requirement increases to an FiO_2 of 60%, and in rare instances intubation and ventilation with a low PEEP (+3–4 cmH_2O) are required.

This syndrome is more frequent after caesarean section and breech delivery.

Respiratory distress syndrome (hyaline membrane disease). Respiratory distress syndrome (RDS) is the most common cause of respiratory distress in the premature infant. It is the most typical anomaly of respiratory adaptation. In preterm infants of less than 37 weeks of gestation, the absence or reduction of surface-active lecithin may be responsible for RDS. An extensive description of the condition and its management can be found in Chap. 66.

Persistent fetal circulation (PFC) [5, 31, 33, 60, 61]

The PFC syndrome is characterized by severe hypoxia which indicates a right-to-left shunt through the ductus arteriosus and the foramen ovale. This disorder is secondary to pulmonary hypertension and may occur in isolation (idiopathic PFC) or as a complication of parenchymal lung disease in the absence of structural malformations of the heart (Table 65.4).

Table 65.4. Principal causes of persistent fetal circulation

Idiopathic
Meconium aspiration
Diaphragmatic hernia
Miscellaneous lung disorders (RDS, infection)
Metabolic: hypoglycemia
Polycythemia

Idiopathic. Idiopathic PFC usually occurs in full-term infants and the pulmonary hypertension can be explained on the basis of pulmonary vasospasm complicating an increased medial smooth muscle in the small pulmonary arteries [53]. This disorder is seen particularly in fetuses who have been exposed to chronic hypoxia in utero. It presents as severe respiratory distress with cyanosis that is unresponsive to O_2 and artificial ventilation; PaO_2 is less than 60 mmHg (8 kPa) when pure O_2 is breathed. The chest x-ray is usually normal, apart from mild cardiac enlargement in some cases. Cardiac catheterization will confirm the pulmonary hypertension and normal cardiac status.

Echocardiography is very helpful for the exclusion of cardiac malformation and for indication of pulmonary hypertension from elevation of the ratio of right ventricular pre-ejection period to the right ventricular ejection time (RPEP/RVET). Tolazoline (Priscoline) has proved to be very useful in the treatment; 1–2 mg/kg is infused over 10 min and followed by a continuous IV infusion of 1–2 mg/kg/h [33]. It is generally given via a scalp or upper limb vein, and if this is not possible, via an umbilical vein or umbilical artery. An increase in PaO_2 of at least 30 mmHg (4 kPa) is considered to be a positive response. The dosages of tolazoline are gradually decreased when the PaO_2 reaches 60–80 mmHg (8–10.7 kPa) with an $FiO_2 < 0.60$. Monitoring of arterial blood pressure, central venous pressure, and urine output is recommended. Systemic hypotension may occur necessitating a decrease of the tolazoline and some times expansion of the blood volume. Other complications that have been described are abdominal distension, gastrointestinal haemorrage, seizures, thrombocytopenia and, rarely hypertension.

Secondary Secondary PFC [28, 49] must be suspected if hypoxia is lower than may be expected from the radiological signs or if there is severe hypoxia unresponsive to adequate ventilation without gross changes of pulmonary disease, particularly in the absence of pneumothorax. An elevated RPEP/RVET ratio indicates pulmonary hypertension and may predict a positive response to tolazoline [42] but this treatment must be stopped in the absence of a rapid increase of PaO_2. It is seen particularly with meconium aspiration and in diaphragmatic hernia severe hypoxia may occur after the 'honeymoon' period following operation. If *AaDO2* is greater than 600 mmHg (80 kPa) postoperatively, it has been proposed that tolazoline should be started before refractory hypoxia occurs.

Patent ductus arteriosus (PDA)
[6, 14, 29, 50]

Congestive heart failure may develop in small preterm infants due to PDA. Closure of the ductus arteriosus is delayed in premature infants and the left-to-right shunt through it increases cardiac output and gives rise to pulmonary hypertension. Clinically a systolic or continuous murmur is associated with accentuated peripheral pulses, tachypnoea and tachycardia. If the left-to-right shunt is large, congestive heart failure occurs, with pulmonary oedema, hepatomegaly, cardiomegaly, and excessive weight. An elevated ratio of the diameter of left atrial and aorta on echocardiography to above 0.9 indicates a left-to-right shunt. Study of left ventricle LPEP/LVET is also necessary when the first ratio is subnormal and the clinical signs are present [6, 38].

Closure of the ductus arteriosus can be achieved either by surgery or with drugs. Conservative management with diuretics, digitalis, and fluid restriction may control the heart failure meanwhile. If the infant is less than 34 weeks old and there are no contra-indications, indomethacin [14, 29, 30], which is an inhibitor of prostaglandin E1 (PGE1) that dilates the ductus arteriosus, is often used. Doses are 0.3 mg/kg by mouth or rectally, or 0.1 mg/kg IV, administered 8- to 12- hourly. One to three doses are usually necessary, and a decrease in the ratio of the left atrial to the aortic diameter will confirm the reduction of the shunt [6]. During indomethacin medication renal digestive, and haematological functions should be carefully monitored. Renal failure is common but usually transient; thrombocytopenia is not rare and may accentuate GI bleeding. Hence a blood urea level above 0.50 g/litre, thrombopenia of less than 100 000, bleeding problems, jaundice with a bilirubin level higher than 100 mg/litre, and digestive problems are contra-indications to the use of indomethacin. If conservative management or indomethacin is not successful or if drugs are contra-indicated surgical closure is indicated [50]. PDA can be the only disorder present but it may also complicate RDS. For the very small preterm infant of birth weight less than 1200 g, quick closure of the DA seems to improve the prognosis of the disease [41].

Miscellaneous

There are special circumstances during pregnancy or delivery that may produce problems with cardiopulmonary adaptation at birth. Three of them merit some comment, because of the special effect on the heart. These are encountered in neonates of diabetic mothers, rhesus haemolytic disease, and birth asphyxia.

Respiratory distress syndrome

RDS is more frequent in neonates of *diabetic mothers* [62]. Maybe there is an inhibiting interaction with insulin abolishing the effect of cortisol in stimulating phosphatidylcholine synthesis.

Neonates with Rh haemolytic disease often have RDS, which can be due either to lung oedema or to surfactant deficiency aggravated by oedema. Both conditions are treated by artificial ventilation with PEEP. Hypoglycaemia and hypocalcaemia are common metabolic complications of the two diseases.

Fetal asphyxia may produce RDS secondary to lung oedema, without meconium aspiration. The pathogenesis is not yet clear.

Myocardial dysfunction

In these three conditions alteration of myocardial contractility plays a role [7, 9, 10, 19, 27, 36, 48, 78]. Myocardial dysfunction has been suspected for many years, because of the cardiomegaly observed in these cases. Echocardiographic studies have now established its presence and attempts have been made to distinguish between alterations of myocardial contractility and myocardial distensibility. The therapeutic consequences are important, for a disturbance of distensibility requires a reduction of fluid intake whereas impaired contractility requires inotropic drugs. Cardiogenic shock, if present, may be due to myocardial ischaemia [27, 60, 64] or to an ischaemic papillary necrosis [19].

Fluid and electrolyte requirements

Factors regulating fluid balance

Three important factors are involved in fluid balance in the newborn: changes in the distribution of body water in the first days of life, *particularly* pronounced extrarenal water losses, and the postnatal adaptation of renal function.

Changes in the distribution of body water

At birth total body water represents approximately 75% of the body weight of the full-term infant, 30%–35% as intracellular fluid (ICF), and 40%–45% as extracellular fluid (ECF). In the first 3 days of life, there is a mean weight loss of 5%–8% of body weight, together with a redistribution of body fluids. The volume of ECF decreases and there is a relative increase in the volume of ICF. These changes are most marked in premature babies and in both full-term and preterm they continue during the first months

of life. By 12 months of age, the ECF is approximately 20%–25% and the ICF 40% of total body weight.

Extrarenal water losses

The variation of water losses from the respiratory tract and skin are important and are affected by many factors, including the nature of the skin, its blood flow, the degree of sweating, postnatal age, and environmental conditions. The skin of the newborn infant is thinner than that of the adult, and in premature infants there are numerous blood vessels beneath the skin, which increase the convective transfer of internal body heat to the surface. This may increase the amount of water lost from the skin. Environmental influences greatly affect insensible water loss; at 30%–60% relative humidity the average full-term infant loses 24 ml water/ kg per day, 60% from the lungs and 40% from the skin [56]. Infants of low birth weight are vulnerable to excess fluid losses in the early neonatal period, but loss of water can be reduced by using a heat shield [21]. Radiant heat warmers greatly increase insensible water losses, by some 50%–100% for infants under 1500 g and by 80%–190% for infants greater than 1500 g [80]. Phototherapy for the treatment of jaundice increases the insensible water loss by 1.7–2.4 ml/kg per hour [57]. Sweating may be increased by high ambient temperatures but is not marked in infants of less than 2000 g body weight.

Gastrointestinal losses are generally not important except in babies receiving phototherapy and with diarrhoea, who may lose up to 19 ml water/kg per day [65].

Postnatal development of renal function [63, 70]

At birth, suppression of the placental circulation requires an acute adaptation of the kidney to extra-uterine life. The kidney of the neonate, compared with the kidney of the adult, seems to be functionally immature, but it is sufficiently developed to regulate the functional adjustments. In fact, "contrary to earlier notions, it may well be that it is not the functional limitations which dictate growth rate but in fact normal growth with its increasing metabolic requirements which stimulates appropriate functional development" [54]. Furthermore, the level of function is influenced by the duration of postnatal existence, being for instance better in a premature baby at an age equivalent to term than for a full-term infant.

Glomerular filtration rate (GFR) The GFR at birth is approximately 20–30 ml/min per 1.73 m² for a premature baby and 35–40 ml/min per 1.73 m² for a newborn at term. It doubles in the first 2 postnatal weeks [35] and this rapid increase has been attributed to several factors, the most important of which may be haemodynamic changes [35] such as have been observed in puppies. Aschinberg et al. [4, 58], using a xenon washout technique, showed a linear increase of mean renal blood flow of almost 10-fold, from 0.23 to 2.06± 0.12 ml/g/min; the increase was greatest for the outer cortical flow, which reached adult values after 6–10 weeks. The rapidity of this change is suggestive of a change in renal vascular resistance in the outer cortex.

Renal concentrating capacity [22, 23, 76] A relatively low capacity of urinary concentration has been demonstrated by water deprivation and with the DDAVP test. There is a postnatal increase of mean concentrating capacity from 385 mosmol/kg at 1–3 weeks to 565 mosmol/kg at 4–6 weeks in full-term infants and from 359 mosmol/kg at 1–3 weeks to 524 mosmol/kg at 4–6 weeks in preterm infants. This low urine osmolarity is related in part to a low concentration of urea in the glomerular filtrate and is increased in infants fed with a high-protein diet [22].

Renal control of sodium balance Urinary sodium excretion is increased in immature infants and can produce a negative sodium balance in very premature infants. For instance, Engelke et al. [25] reported a negative sodium balance of 9.25 mmol/kg/day in infants of less than 30 weeks gestational age. Sulyok [75] demonstrated that the rate of urinary sodium excretion and fractional sodium excretion were higher in premature than in full-term infants at 1 week. This natriuresis is related to a decreased reabsorption of sodium in the proximal tubule and unresponsiveness of the distal tubule to aldosterone [75]. Both proximal and distal tubular sodium reabsorption improves with increasing postnatal age. In premature babies the increased sodium excretion causes a tendency to hyponatraemia, which disappears after 4–6 weeks.

The renal response to a salt load is reduced in full-term infants, particularly in those with a high haematocrit, as was shown by Aperia [1]. Even full-term babies with abnormal haematocrits may retain abnormal amounts of sodium if given more than 12 mmol/kg/day. In preterm

infants the basal sodium excretion is at a higher level than in full-term infants [2].

Clinical implications

Water and electrolyte requirements

These are indicated in Table 65.5. As shown the needs differ according to gestational and postnatal age. On the first day, the fluid requirement is approximately 60–80 ml per kg; it then gradually increases by 20 ml per day, up to 150–200 ml/kg per day. This is calculated for oral intake; parenteral intake must not exceed 120–150 ml/kg per day.

Table 65.5. Daily fluid and electrolyte requirements

Water	130–200 ml/kg
	(First day 60–80 ml/kg)
Sodium	2–4 mmol/kg
Chloride	1–2 mmol/kg
Potassium	1–2 mmol/kg

The sodium needs of premature babies are significant: 3–4 mmol/kg per day and then decrease progressively after 4–6 weeks of age, to 1–2 mmol/kg per day.

Urine output and body weight are important guides for prescribing water and sodium. An absence of growth in a premature infant receiving adequate calories may be due to insufficient sodium. Conversely, Hornych and Amiel-Tison [39] reported infants of low birth weight, preterm or small for their dates, who had a sudden increase in weight and head circumference at approximately 40 weeks corrected gestational age. This abnormal pattern may have been due to an excess sodium intake at a time when the proximal tubular reabsorption of sodium increased and became normal. Stopping sodium supplementation and, in some cases, giving frusemide 1 mg/kg promptly restored the situation to normal.

The risks of giving too much sodium also need to be considered. Intracranial haemorrhages in premature infants have been attributed to rapid infusions of sodium bicarbonate [71].

Management of water and sodium intake in some abnormal states

Intestinal obstruction Fluid and electrolyte requirements may be increased *in intestinal obstruction* because of vomiting, gastric suction, or loss from an ileostomy, as in necrotizing enterocolitis. Ideally these abnormal fluid and electrolyte losses should be measured and replaced but in many cases it is difficult to evaluate accurately the exact volume of fluid that has been lost and consequently the exact rate of electrolyte loss. Blood concentrations of protein, electrolytes and urea may be helpful, but in some cases these are normal or subnormal although the total content of electrolytes has decreased. Weight, daily urine output, and electrolyte concentration are the best indicators of the state of hydration and electrolyte balance. For example, a high urinary osmolality together with a low concentration of sodium in the urine implies that intake of both water and sodium is inadequate and needs to be increased. For a proper control of sodium chloride and potassium balance it is important to measure the total daily urine output rather than calculating the requirements, from a single sample of urine.

Acute dehydration Acute dehydration (AD) in the neonate is similar in many ways to dehydration of older infants. Nevertheless, some aspects need highlighting, namely severity and causation. AD of the newborn infant may be very severe [59]; Pillion reported 46 cases, of whom 16 died, 26 developed renal complications, mainly renal vein thrombosis, and 34 neurological complications. Hypernatraemia (Na > 160 mmol/litre) is frequently seen and may be due either to a disproportionate loss of water and salt or to an excessive intake of solute that is followed by dehydration due, for instance, to an error in preparing proprietary feed. Such states are often complicated by fitting and coma, which are related to cerebral water content [9]; only rarely are they due to haemorrhage. The risk is particularly high when the rate of fluid infusion is too rapid, and Finberg recommends gradual replacement over 48 h at an infusion rate of 100 ml/kg per day with approximately 75–100 mmol sodium/litre solution. (For the complete management of hypernatraemic dehydration the reader is referred to the work of Finberg [26].)

The main cause of AD is gastro-enteritis, but it may be due to congenital diseases, particularly congenital malformations of the kidney and congenital adrenal hyperplasia with a sodium-losing state. Congenital malformations of the kidney, principally obstructive uropathy, are a likely cause when the dehydration is accompanied by renal failure with polyuria and low urinary osmolality (<400 mosmol/kg).

Adrenal hyperplasia with a sodium-losing state (Debré–Fibiger syndrome) is suggested by dehydration with vomiting, severe hypo-natraemia with increased urinary sodium losses and hyperkalaemia [15, 40]. The hyperkalaemia is sometimes very pronounced (>10 mmol/litre) and may therefore be life threatening. Emergency treatment requires an ion exhange resin (1 g/kg) for the hyperkalaemia, prompt and rapid infusion of sodium (10 mmol/kg/day or more), hydrocortisone (20–25 mg/m^2) and 9 α fluorohydrocortisone (100 mg per day on the first day).

Acid–base balance

Acid–base homeostasis

Almost all diseases of the newborn may disturb acid–base homeostasis, a tendency that is facilitated by the kidney's limited ability to excrete hydrogen ions at this age, [44, 73, 74, 77], particularly in preterm infants. Sulyok and his group [73, 74] in infants of 1650–1900 g birth weight, found a maximal urinary hydrogen ion output of 30 μmol/min per 1.73 m^2 in the 1st week and 60 μmol/min per 1.73 m^2 in the 6th week of life. This decrease of acidifying capacity is due in part to a decrease of NH_4^+ and titrable acidity and in part to a low bicarbonate threshold. In the same infants, these authors found a renal bicarbonate threshold of 12 mmol/litre, which rose to 17–18 mmol/litre at the end of the 4th week of postnatal age and 20–21 mmol/litre in children of 1 year [24]. It is probably related to a decrease in proximal tubular reabsorption of sodium [51]. Excretion in the distal tubule is normal, so that in cases of acidosis the urine pH can decrease to 5.5 or less, as in children and adults.

Clinical implications

Acid–base homeostasis is generally normal in full-term infants but in preterm infants, a late metabolic acidosis has been described developing in the 2nd and 3rd weeks of postnatal life by Kildeberg [45]. It occurred in approximately 20% of premature babies and 5% of full-term infants [77]. The incidence may be increased by a high protein diet. Generally infants with this condition do not show any symptoms, since the pH and bicarbonate are only moderately decreased (7.30 and 17 mmol/litre). In fact, hydrogen ion excretion by the kidney is adapted to the metabolic needs of healthy newborns, but may be insufficient for sick newborns. For this reason, in both neonates and premature infants, the blood acid–base status should be monitored closely.

Pathology of acid–base disturbances

Acidosis

Severe acidosis produces a number of effects that are observed at all ages, such as arrhythmias, neurological complications and haemostatic disorders such as disseminated intravascular coagulation [13]. More important in the present context are two anomalies it produces in the neonatal period, namely the displacement of bilirubin from plasma albumin and pulmonary vasoconstriction.

The displacement of bilirubin from albumin may be quite deleterious in premature and even in full-term infants, increasing the risk of kernicterus and severe neurological damage.

Severe acidosis and hypoxaemia [67] both induce pulmonary vasoconstriction with elevation of pulmonary arterial pressure, reduction of pulmonary capillary blood flow, and right-to-left shunt of blood through the foramen ovale and ductus arteriosus. This results in a vicious circle which can be reversed only by correction of hypoxaemia and acidosis.

The important causes of acidosis are shown in Table 65.6 and in all these circumstances it must be evaluated and corrected. This implies artificial ventilation in respiratory acidosis and bicarbonate infusion in metabolic acidosis. The quantity of bicarbonate to be administered can be calculated from the base excess (BE): Q. mmol = BE × body wt (kg)/3. The infusion must always be given slowly (over 1 h) because rapid infusions increase the risk of intracranial haemorrhage, particularly in premature infants. In mixed disturbances, bicarbonate should not be given unless the infant is ventilated, because without ventilation it will augment the $PaCO_2$ [18, 37]. In fact, at any elevation of $PaCO_2$, some bicarbonate will leak in interstitial fluid, and the concept of 'base deficit' should not be used for calculation of bicarbonate dosage.

Alkalosis

Alkalosis is less frequent than acidosis. A respiratory alkalosis may be produced by artificial ventilation and is easily corrected by adjustment of the ventilation.

The main mechanism by which metabolic alkalosis is produced in the newborn is loss of hydrochloric acid from vomiting or prolonged gastric suction. The most common cause is pyloric stenosis [79], where the metabolic alkalosis is accompanied by low plasma chloride and potassium concentrations and by marked dehydration. All these anomalies must be corrected by infusion of large amounts of sodium chloride and potassium chloride, up to 10–15 mmol/kg per day for NaCl and up to 5 mmol/kg per day for KCl [79].

Table 65.6. Principal causes of acidosis in neonates

Mechanism	Causes	
Increased H^+ ions production	Tissue hypoxia	Cardiorespiratory arrest
		Respiratory distress
		Cardiac failure
		Cyanotic heart malformations
		Neonatal infections
		Necrotizing enterocolitis
		Acute dehydration
		Hypothermia
	Inborn errors	Amino acid metabolism
		Organic acids
	Parenteral feeding	
Decreased H^+ ion excretion by the kidney		Renal agenesis
		Bilateral vein thrombosis
		Cortical necrosis
		Distal tubular acidosis
		Proximal tubular acidosis
Decreased CO_2 excretion by the lung	All causes of respiratory distress	

A metabolic alkalosis due to an exogenous gain of bicarbonate is quite rare. We have observed it in some cases of severe fetal erythroblastosis after several exchange transfusions.

Some principles of neonatal pharmacology [52, 55]

A full treatment of this field is beyond the scope of this chapter. The points made here emphasize some of the difficult problems that are encountered in prescribing drugs for neonates. For a more detailed description the reader is referred to the work of Neims et al. [55]. Table 65.7 gives therapeutic schedules for some of the drugs must often used in neonates.

The binding of many drugs to plasma protein is diminished, and for this reason the drugs may cause a more marked response.

The absorption of many orally administered drugs is slow but complete.

The capacity to oxidize drugs is diminished, with wide individual variations depending on the nature of the drug, the gestational age, and the postnatal age; the capacity matures at birth. Certain pathologies, such as hypoxia and malnutrition, may cause a reduction in oxidative capacity.

Glycuronidation is deficient.

Some drugs compete with bilirubin for binding to plasma protein. This may be increased by prematurity, low serum albumin concentrations, and acidosis.

The excretion of drugs is affected by the relative renal immaturity at birth, especially the low GFR and reduced tubular function; both influence the dose and rate of administration of antibiotics in the first 7 days of life.

A number of general recommendations can be made on the basis of these points:

1) Use a loading dose in the order of that used in children
2) Use a maintenance dose that is substantially lower than that given to children
3) Remember that fixed-dosage regimens cannot be defined
4) Be aware of possible clinical consequences and abnormal symptoms after drug administration
5) Monitor drug levels whenever possible.

Technical appendix

Endotracheal intubation

Body weight of the infant	2500 g	≥2500 g
Laryngoscope blades	Guedel no. 1	
	Miller no. 0	Miller no. 1
	Oxford	
Endotracheal tube { Oral/Nasal	Portex no. 2.5	no. 3
{ Oral	Cole no. 12	no. 14

Basic principles

1) All resuscitation efforts should be carried out under a radiant heat unit.
2) Except in emergencies use naso-tracheal intubation with the help of MacGill forceps to guide the tip of the tube into the glottis.
3) The tip of the tube should be placed midway between the carina and the glottis. This position should always be checked radiologically and the tube well secured with adhesive tape.
4) Oxygen should be provided (a) before intubation by normal ventilation with a positive pressure mask and bag; and (b) during intubation by a catheter connected to the tracheal tube and to the ventilator.

Closed-chest cardiac message

Closed-chest cardiac massage should be done:

1) When the heart rate is <100/min
2) With the fingertips over the middle third of the sternum (the infant resting on a firm surface for the massage to be effective)
3) With adequate force to depress the sternum the desired 1–1.5 cm
4) At a rate of 120 compressions per min
5) With one lung inflation to every four compressions
6) For as long as the heart rate remains low.

Table 65.7. Therapeutic schedule for drugs commonly used in neonatal period

Drugs	Route	Total daily dose mg/kg/day	No. of divided doses	Remarks
Ampicillin	IV, IM	50–100 75–200	2 < J7 3 > J7	High doses in case of mening-itis
Carbenicillin	IV (1 h)	200 300–400	2 < J7 3–4 > J7	
Oxacillin	IV, IM	50–75 75–100	2 < J7 3–4 > J7	
Penicillin	IV, IM	50 000 Units 75 000 Units	2 < J7 3 > J7	
Colistin	IM, IV	50 000–75 000 Units	2 < J7 3 > J7	Blood level monitoring necessary
Gentamicin	IM, IV (1 h)	3–5	2 < J7 3 > J7	Blood level monitoring necessary
Tobramycin	IM, IV (1 h)	3–5	2 < J7 3 > J7	
Amikacin	IM, IV (1 h)	10–15	2 < J7 3 > J7	
Metronidazole	IV (1 h)	30	3	
Diazepam	IV, PR, IM	0.1–0.8	6	
Phenobarbitone	IM, PO, IV	Loading dose 20 mg/kg; maintenance dose 1 mg/kg per day after 48 h	1	Use only glass syringe Blood level monitoring necessary
Diphenylhydantoin	IM, IV	Loading dose 20 mg/kg; maintenance dose 1 mg/kg per day after 48 h	1	Blood level monitoring necessary
Digoxin	PO	PO loading dose 15 μg/kg; maintenance dose after 8 h:	3	Blood level monitoring neces-sary
	IV	15 μg/kg/24 h IV 75% of the loading and maintenance dose PO	3	
Dopamine	IV	2.5–7.5 μg/kg per min	Continuous infusion	
Dobutamine	IV	5–10 μg/kg per min		
Isoprenaline	IV	0.1–1 μg/kg per min		
Frusemide	IM, IV, PO	2 5	6 4	
Indomethacin	PO or IM IV	0.3 0.1	1–3 1–3	IV = Route ++
Tolazoline	IV	Loading dose 1–2 mg/kg per 10 min; maintenance dose 1–2 mg/kg/h		Gradual decrease when FiO2 $\leq$ 0.6

IV, intravenous; IM, intramuscular; PO, by mouth; PR, per rectum.

Emergency relief of a tension pneumothorax

1) Insert a scalp needle (no. 23) attached to a three-way stopcock and a 20-ml syringe into the third intercostal space at the mid-clavicular line
2) Remove air until the condition improves
3) If the x-ray examination-reveals persistent trapped air, insert a chest drain (Vygon no. 12), either via the previous route or by the 4th intercostal space in the midaxillary line, and have another x-ray examination per-formed
4) Place a continuous suction of 10–20 cmH$_2$O on the chest tube.

Umbilical vessel catheterization[a]

The use of umbilical catheterization requires careful consideration of the risks involved. We can expect that the number of indications will be reduced due to the development of noninvasive technique of monitoring

	Indications	Complications
Arterial catheter (safest location: body of the 3rd lumbar vertebra)	Sampling for arterial blood gas and acid–base status Monitoring blood pressure	Sepsis Renal artery thrombosis, infarction Haemorrhage from loose connection Microemboli iliac arteries; limb ischaemia mesenteric arteries Enterocolitis (if displaced upwards) medullary arteries; paraplegia Trauma to the vessel wall activation of the intrinsic coagulation; aortic thrombosis
Venous catheter (safest location: inferior vena cava through the ductus venosus.)	Unexpected emergency (delivery room); not to be left in place for over 24 h	Liver necrosis (if in a portal branch) Portal vein thrombosis Perforation of the colon

[a]Technique: Use a 3.5 (French size) argyle umbilical catheter. Identify the umbilical vein, a thin-walled wide-open oval lumen located at 12 o'clock in the cord stump, and the two umbilical arteries. These are thick-walled and tightly constricted located at 5 and 7 o'clock on the cord stump. Insert the catheter to a length of 12 cm in the artery or to over 8 cm in the vein. Identify the position of the catheter immediately and withdraw if it has been inserted too far. If it is not far enough in it must be removed and another catheter inserted. If it is in a safe position, tie with silk suture. Both arterial and venous catheters should be removed as soon as possible: 24 h is the maximum for a venous catheter and 5 days for an arterial catheter.

Rules for blood transfusion in neonates and infants under 3 months of age

Laboratory tests before any transfusion
　　Mother: Blood type
　　Infant:　Blood type
　　　　　　Direct Coomb's test

Choice of donor blood type

Mother's blood type	Infant's blood type	Donor blood type
OAB	O	O
O	AB	Non-dangerous O = without irregular agglutinin anti-A and anti-B
A	B	
B	A	
A	A–AB	A
B	B–AB	B
Rh+	Rh+	Rh+
	Rh−	Rh−
Rh−	Rh+	Rh−
	Rh−	Rh−

Volume to transfuse

Whole fresh blood: 6 ml/weight (kg/g Hb)
Red packed cells:　3 ml/weight (kg/g Hb)

If mother's blood type is not known, use non-dangerous O blood type (without irregular agglutinin anti-A and anti-B).

References

1. Aperia A, Broberger O, Thodenius K, Zetterstrom R (1972) Renal response to an oral sodium load in newborn full-term infants. Acta Paediatr Scand 61:670
2. Aperia A, Broberger O, Thodenius K, Zetterstrom R (1974) Developmental study of the renal response to an oral salt load in preterm infants. Acta Paediatr Scand 63:517
3. Arcilla RA, Coll OHW, Lind J, Gessner IH (1966) Pulmonary arterial pressures of the newborn infants born with early clamping of the cord. Acta Paediatr Scand 35:305
4. Aschinberg LC, Goldsmith DI, Olbing H, Spitzer A, Edelmann CM Jr, Blaufox MD (1975) Neonatal changes

in renal blood flow distribution in puppies. Am J Physiol 228:1453

5. Aujard Y, Beaufils F, Bourrillon A (1978) La persistance de la circulation foetale. Arch Fr Pediatr 35:681

6. Baylen BG, Meyer RA, Kaplan S, et al (1975) The critically ill premature infant with patent ductus arteriosus and pulmonary disease—an echocardiographic assessment. J Pediatr 86:423

7. Breitweiser JA, Meyer RA, Sperling MA, Tsang RC, Kaplan S (1980) Cardioseptal hypertrophy in hyperinsulinemic infants. J Pediatr 96:535

8. Brown JK, Habel AH (1975) Toxic encephalopathy and acute brain swelling in children. Dev Med Child Neurol 17:659

9. Bucciarelli RL, Nelson RM, Egan EA II, Eitzman DV, Gessner IH (1977) Transient tricuspid insufficiency of the newborn: A form of myocardial dysfunction in stressed newborns. Pediatrics 59:330

10. Cabal LA, De Voskar U, Siassi B, Hodgman JE, Emmanouilides G (1980) Cardiogenic shock associated with perinatal asphyxia. J Pediatr 96:705

11. Cassin S, Dawes GS, Ross BB (1964a) Pulmonary blood flow and vascular resistance in immature fetal lambs. J Physiol (Lond) 171:80

12. Cassin S, Dawes GS, Mott JC, Ross BB, Strang LB (1964b) The vascular resistance of the fetal and newly ventilated lung of the lamb. J Physiol (Lond) 171:61

13. Chessels JM, Wigglesworth JS (1971) Coagulation studies in severe birth asphyxia. Arch Dis Child 46:253

14. Cotton RB, Stahlman MT, Kovar I, Katterton WZ (1978) Medical management of small preterm infants with symptomatic patent ductus arteriosus. J Pediatr 92:467

15. David M, Ghali P, Gillet P, Bertrand J, Francois R, Jeune M (1977) Management of congenital adrenal hyperplasia by determinations of plasma testosterone, 17-OH-progesterone, and ACTH levels and plasma renin activity. In: Lee PA, Plotnick LP, Kowarski AA, Migeon CJ (eds) Congenital adrenal hyperplasia. University Park Press, Baltimore, p 183

16. Dawes G (1968) Fetal and neonatal physiology. Year Book Medical Publishers, Chicago

17. Dehan M, Ropert JC, Francoual C et al. (1979) Diagnostic biologique de la maladie des membranes hyalines et de l'inhalatation amniotique—Une étude de 100 nouveaux-nés en détresse respiratoire. Arch Fr Pediatr 36:886

18. Dell RB, Winters RW (1972) Acid-base effects of hypertonic sodium bicarbonate solutions. (Commentary) J Pediatr 80:681

19. Donnelly WH, Bucciarelli RL, Nelson RA (1980) Ischemic papillary muscle necrosis in stressed newborn infant. J Pediatr 96:295

20. Dorand RD (1977) Neonatal asphyxia—An approach to physiology and management. Pediatr Clin North Am 24:455

21. Dreszer M (1977) Fluid and electrolytes requirements in the newborn. Pediatr Clin North Am 24:537

22. Edelmann CM Jr, Wolfish NM (1968) Dietary influence on renal maturation in premature infants. Pediatr Res 2:421

23. Edelmann CM Jr, Barnett HL, Troupkou V (1960) Renal concentrating mechanisms in newborn infants. Effect of dietary protein and water content, role of urea and responsiveness to anti-diuretic hormone. J Clin Invest 39:1062

24. Edelmann CM, Soriano JR, Bolchis H, Gruskin AB, Acosta MI (1967) Renal bicarbonate reabsorption and hydrogen ion excretion in normal infants. J Clin Invest 46:1309

25. Engelke SC, Shah BL, Vasan U, Raye JR (1978) Sodium balance in very low birth weight infants. J Pediatr 93:837

26. Finberg L (1973) Diarrheal dehydration. In Winters RW (ed) The body fluids in pediatrics. Little Brown, Boston, 349

27. Finley JP, Howman-Giles RB, Gilday DL, Bloom KR, Rowe RD (1979) Transient myocardial ischemia of the newborn infant demonstrated by Thallium myocardial imaging. J Pediatr 94:263

28. Fox WW, Gewitz MH, Dinwiddie R, Drummont WH, Peckham GJ (1977) Pulmonary hypertension in the perinatal aspiration syndromes. Pediatrics 59:205

29. Friedman WF, Hirschklan MS, Printz M, Pitlich PT, Kirkpatrick SE (1976) Pharmacological closure of P.D.A. in the premature infant. N Engl J Med 295:526

30. Friedman WF, Heymann MA, Rudolph AM (1977) New thoughts on an old problem: patent ductus arteriosus in the premature. (Commentary) J Pediatr 90:338

31. Gersony WM (1973) Persistence of the fetal circulation. Commentary J Pediatr 82:1103

32. Gluck L, Kulovich MV (1973) L/S ratios in amniotic fluid in normal and abnormal pregnancies. Am J Obstet Gynecol 120:524

33. Goetzam BW, Sunshine P, Johnson JO et al. (1976) Persistence of fetal circulation. Hypoxia and pulmonary spasm: Response to tolazoline. J Pediatr 89:617

34. Gold F, Bourin M, Granry JC, Breteau M, Laugier J, (1979) Intérêt de la voie intra-veineuse pour l'utilisation du phénobarbital chez le nouveau-né à terme asphyxié. Arch Fr Pediatr 36:610

35. Guignard JP, Torrado A, Da Cunha O, Gautier E (1975) Glomerular filtration rate in the first three weeks of life. J Pediatr 87:268

36. Gutgesell HT, Speer M, Rosenberg HS (1978) Further characterization of the hypertrophic cardiomyopathy of infants of diabetics mothers. Am J Cardiol 41:406

37. Haworth SG, Sarcia SR, Daniel SS, James LS (1968) Dangers of rapid correction of pH following asphyxia. Pediatr Res 2:395

38. Hirschfeld S, Meyer R, Schwartz DC, Korfhagens J, Kaplan S (1975) Measurement of right and left ventricular systolic time intervals by echocardiography. Circulation 51:304

39. Hornyck H, Amiel-Tison C (1977) Rétention hydrosaline chez les enfants de faible poids de naissance. Arch Fr Pediatr 34:206

40. Huseman CA, Varma MM, Blizzard RM, Johanson A (1977) Treatment of congenital virilizing adrenal hyperplasia with multiple and single daily doses of prednisone. J Pediatr 90:538

41. Jacob J, Gluck L, Di Sessa T, et al (1980) The contribution of P.D.A. in the neonate with severe R.D.S. J Pediatr 96:79

42. Johnson GL, Douglas Cunningham M, Desai NS, Cottril CM, Noonan JA (1980) Echocardiography in hypoxemic neonatal pulmonary disease. J Pediatr 96:716

43. Karlberg P (1960) The adaptative changes in the immediate post natal period wih particular reference to respiration. J Pediatr 56:560

44. Kerpel-Fronius E, Hein T, Sulyok E (1970) The development of the renal acidifying processes and their relation to acidosis in low-birth-weight infants. Biol Neonat 15:156

45. Kildeberg P (1964) Disturbances of hydrogen ion homeostasis. II. Late metabolic acidosis. Acta Paediatr Scand 53:517

46. Klaus MH, Fanaroff AA (1979) Care of the high-risk neonote, 2nd edn. Saunders, Philadelphia, p 34

47. Koch G, Lind J (1973) La circulation foetale et l'adaptation cardio-respiratoire néonatale. Bull Physiopathol Respir 9:1389

48. Mace S, Hirschfeld SS, Riggs T, Fanaroff AA, Markatz IR, Franklin W (1979) Echocardiographic abnormalities in infants of diabetic mothers. J Pediatr 95:1013

49. McIntosh N, Walters RD (1979) Effect of tolazoline in severe hyaline membrane disease. Arch Dis Child 54:105

50. Meurit TA, Di Sessa TG, Feldman BH, Kirkpatrick SE, Gluck L, Friedman WF (1979) Closure of the patent ductus arteriosus with ligation and indometocin. A consecutive experience. J Pediatr 95:639

51. Moore ES, Fine BP, Satrasook SF, Vergel ZM, Edelmann CM (1972) Renal reabsorption of bicarbonate in puppies: Effect of extracellular volume contraction on the renal threshold for bicarbonate. Pediatr Res 6:859

52. Morselli PL, Garattini S, Sereni F (1975) Basic and therapeutic aspects of perinatal pharmacology. Raven Press, New York

53. Naeyve RL, Letts HW (1962) The effect of prolonged neonatal hypoxemia on the pulmonary vasculary bed and heart. Pediatrics 30:902

54. Nash MA, Edelmann CM Jr (1973) The developing kidney. Immature function or inappropriate standard? Nephron 11:71

55. Neims AH, Aranda JV, Laughnan PM (1977) Principles of neonatal pharmacology. In: Schaffer AJ, Avery ME (eds) Diseases of the newborn, 4th edn. Saunders, Philadelphia London Toronto, p 1020

56. O'Brien D, Hansen JDL, Smith CA (1954) Effect of supersaturated atmospheres an insensible water loss in the newborn infant. Pediatrics 13:126

57. Oh W, Karecki H (1972) Phototherapy and insensible water loss in the newborn infant. Am J Dis Child 124:230

58. Olbing H, Blaufox MD, Aschinberg LC et al. (1973) Postnatal changes in renal glomerular blood flow distribution in puppies. J Clin Invest 52:2885

59. Pillion G, Beaufils F (1978) Etude de 46 cas de déshydratation grave du nouveau-né. Facteurs de gravité prévention. In: Journées Parisiennes de Pédiatrie. Paris Flammarion Médecine-Sciences, 481

60. Rienmenschneider TA, Nielsen HC, Ruttenberg HD, Jaffe RB (1976) Pulmonary hypertension and myocardial dysfunction. J Pediatr 89:622

61. Riggs T, Hirschfeld S, Fanaroff AA, Liebman J, Meyer R (1977) Persistence of fetal circulation syndrome-an echocardiographic study. J Pediatr 91:626

62. Robert MF, Neff RK, Hubbell JP, Talusch HW, Avery ME (1976) Association between maternal diabetes and respiratory distress syndrome in the newborn. N Engl J Med 294:357

63. Ross B, Cowett RM, Oh W (1977) Renal functions of low

birth weight infants during the first two months of life. Pediatr Res 11:1662

64. Rowe RD, Hoffman T (1961) Transient myocardial ischemia of the newborn infant: A form of severe cardiorespiratory distress syndrome. Pediatrics 27:551

65. Rubaltelli FF, Larga Jolli G (1973) Effect of light exposure on just transit time in jaundiced newborns. Acta Paediatr Scand 62:146

66. Rudolph AM, Heymann MA (1970) Circulation changes during growth in fetal lamb. Circ Res 26:289

67. Rudolph AM, Yuan S (1966) Response of the pulmonary vasculature to hypoxia and H+ concentration changes. J Clin Invest 45:399

68. Scarpelli EM (1975) Pulmonary physiology of the fetus, newborn and child. Lee & Febiger, Philadelphia, p 117

69. Schaffer AS, Avery ME (1977) Diseases of the newborn, 4th edn, Saunders, Philadelphia, p 34

70. Siegel SR, Oh W (1976) Renal function as a marker of human fetal maturation. Acta Paediatr Scand 65:481

71. Simmons MA, Adcok EW, Bard H, Battaglia FC (1974) Hypernatremia intracranial hemorrhage and $NaHCO_3$ administration in neonates. N Engl J Med 291:6

72. Strang LB (1977) Neonatal respiration-physiological and clinical studies. Blackwell Scientific, Oxford London Edinburgh, Melbourne

73. Sulyok E, Heim T (1971) Assessment of maximal urinary acidification in premature infants. Biol Neonat 19:200

74. Sulyok E, Heim T, Soltesz G, Jaszai V (1972) The influence of maturity on renal control of acidosis in newborn infants. Biol Neonat 21:418

75. Sulyok E, Varga F, Györy E, Jobst K, Csaba IF (1980) On the mechanism of renal sodium handling in newborn infants. Biol Neonate 37:75

76. Svenningsen NW, Aronson AS (1974) Post natal development of renal concentration capacity as estimated by DDAVP-test in normal and asphyxiated neonates. Biol Neonate 25:230

77. Svenningsen NW, Lindquist B (1973) Incidence of metabolic acidosis in term, preterm, and small for gestational age infants in relation to dietary protein intake. Acta Paediatr Scand 62:1

78. Way GL, Walfe RR, Estregpour E, Bender RL, Jaffe RB, Ruttenberg HD (1979) The natural history of hypertrophic cardiomyopathy in infants of diabetic mothers. J Pediatr 95:1020

79. Winters RW (1973) Metabolic alkalosis of pyloric stenosis. In: Winters RW (ed) The body fluids in pediatrics. Little Brown, Boston, p 402

80. WU PYK, Hodgman JE (1974) Insensible water loss in preterm infants: Changes with post natal development and non ionizing radiant energy. Pediatrics 54:704

Chapter 66

The Newborn Respiratory Distress Syndrome

Mary Ellen Leder Skalina, Richard J. Martin, and Avroy A. Fanaroff

Respiratory distress syndrome (RDS), also known as hyaline membrane disease (HMD), continues to be one of the most important causes of mortality and morbidity in newborn babies; however, lack of a precise definition necessitates cautious interpretation of any statistics regarding incidence, mortality, and results of treatment [13, 31, 40, 43, 44, 55, 60]. The diagnosis can be clearly established if hyaline membranes are present at autopsy or a deficiency of pulmonary surfactant is documented after delivery; but most series will rely on differing combinations of clinical features, biochemical derangements, and radiologic abnormalities to establish the diagnosis. This chapter will be concerned with various aspects of hyaline membrane disease, with particular emphasis on respiratory support.

Incidence

Approximately 10%–15% of babies weighing less than 2.5 kg at birth will manifest RDS, the highest incidence being observed among the lowest-birth-weight groups. The disease occurs throughout the world, with a slight male predominance. Although the overall mortality has declined during the past decade, raw mortality figures are of little use unless accompanied by a detailed description of the infants, including birth weight, gestational age, and sex, as well as the indications for and modes of therapy.

The greatest risk factor appears to be gestational age, while other risk factors include maternal diabetes and cesarean section. As RDS or its associated complications still account for 50% of neonatal deaths in the United States, or approximately 12 000 infants annually, major efforts must be directed at the prevention of RDS, especially through prevention of prematurity. This is achieved in part through uniform screening of all pregnant women, identification of risk, and optimal prepartum management. Pharmacologic inhibition of premature labor is successful in suitably selected pregnancies. Furthermore, where premature delivery is inevitable, consideration must be given to accelerating pulmonary surfactant maturation pharmacologically. Avoidance of iatrogenic prematurity is mandatory.

Pathophysiology

The pathogenesis of RDS is outlined schematically in Fig 66.1. A deficiency of pulmonary surfactant at the linings of the alveoli is a key factor. Although some of the components of surfactant are produced by the type II alveolar cells in the lung as early as at 20 weeks of gestation, the ratio of the various components differs markedly from that in mature surfactant, which appears at approximately 35–36 weeks of gestation (see below). In addition, these substances are not released onto the surface of the alveolus until well after surfactant production is under way. The lack of surfactant at the alveolar surface in turn produces extremely high surface tension with resultant alveolar collapse. This leads to decreased lung compliance and alveolar hypoventilation with ventilation/perfusion (V/Q) imbalance. Hypoxemia, and in more severely affected infants hypercarbia, result.

In uncomplicated cases surfactant production and release improves by 2–3 days of life with a concomitant decrease in clinical symptoms. However, surfactant synthesis is a process that is adversely affected by acidosis, cold stress, hypoxemia, and hypovolemia, frequent occur-

rences in these infants. In addition, exposure to high concentrations of O_2 and mechanical ventilation (MV) may further injure the alveolar and bronchial tissues and delay surfactant production. Thus, multiple factors associated with the disease itself, its complications, and its treatment contribute to a cascade of events which may increase the severity of the course and delay recovery.

Assessment of pulmonary maturity

After 36 weeks of intrauterine life, nearly all infants will have mature lungs. However, dating according to the mother's last menstrual period may be quite inaccurate. Estimation of fetal size and hence age according to uterine fundal height in single pregnancies is also an inexact method, especially in the last trimester when normal variation in the amount of amniotic fluid and the possibility of intrauterine growth retardation confuse the issue. An ultrasound scan may be performed to measure fetal biparietal diameter; however, after 30 weeks this method also becomes less accurate.

The goal of accurate estimation of gestational age is, of course, to predict which infants are at risk for the complications of prematurity, including RDS. However, a more specific method of determining pulmonary maturity is clearly

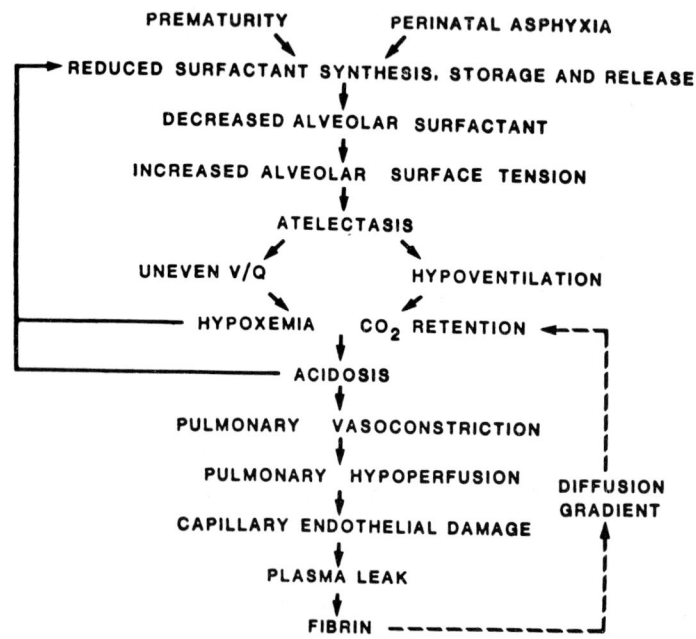

Fig. 66.1. Schematic representation of the pathogenesis of RDS [19].

needed, since gestational age alone is an extremely inaccurate predictor of the likelihood of RDS. Thus, where the clinical setting allows, amniocentesis should be performed [24]; both qualitative and quantitative measures of the amount of surface active material (surfactant) present in the amniotic fluid, and by inference in the pulmonary effluent, may then be determined.

The understanding of the biochemical nature of lung surfactant, which is responsible for decreasing alveolar surface tension and hence maintaining alveolar patency, was greatly expanded by the work of Gluck in the early 1970s [23, 25]. It is now known that surfactant has several phospholipid components. Phosphatidylcholine (lecithin) is the major component, present in low concentrations until approximately 26 weeks, after which it rises steadily. This phospholipid is found in most mammalian cells; however, that which is found in pulmonary surfactant is unique in that a high percentage contains palmitic acid esterified at both the α and the β positions of the glycerol backbone. This difference allows separation of the disaturated from the non-surface-active monosaturated compound. Phosphatidylinositol is found in minute concentrations until 26–30 weeks. It then rises steadily until 36 weeks, after which it decreases to one-half the peak value by term. Phosphatidylglycerol is first detected at 35–36

weeks gestation, and by term has become the second most abundant phospholipid. Its presence in the amniotic fluid assures pulmonary maturity. Sphingomyelin remains relatively constant in concentration over gestation, and it is this aspect of surfactant composition which lends the lecithin:sphingomyelin (L:S) ratio its significance. As the concentration of lecithin rises, the value of this ratio rises and pulmonary maturity is usually present when it exceeds 2:1. Lower values serve to identify the population of babies at risk for RDS.

The shake test, a simple bedside procedure, involves mixing the amniotic fluid with ethanol, diluting with saline, shaking in a prescribed manner, and gauging the stability of the resulting bubbles [11]. (A modification of this test, useful as an aid in differential diagnosis once the infant has already been delivered, may be performed on a gastric aspirate obtained from the infant immediately after delivery.) Positive results (stable bubbles) reflect the amount of mature surfactant present and thus indicate fetal lung maturity.

Fetal pulmonary maturity as determined by an L:S ratio of >2.0 occurs at a mean gestational age of 35 ± 2 weeks in normal pregnancies. However, certain fetomaternal conditions are known to be associated with acceleration or delay of maturation (Fig. 66.2). Accelerated maturity has been described in the presence of

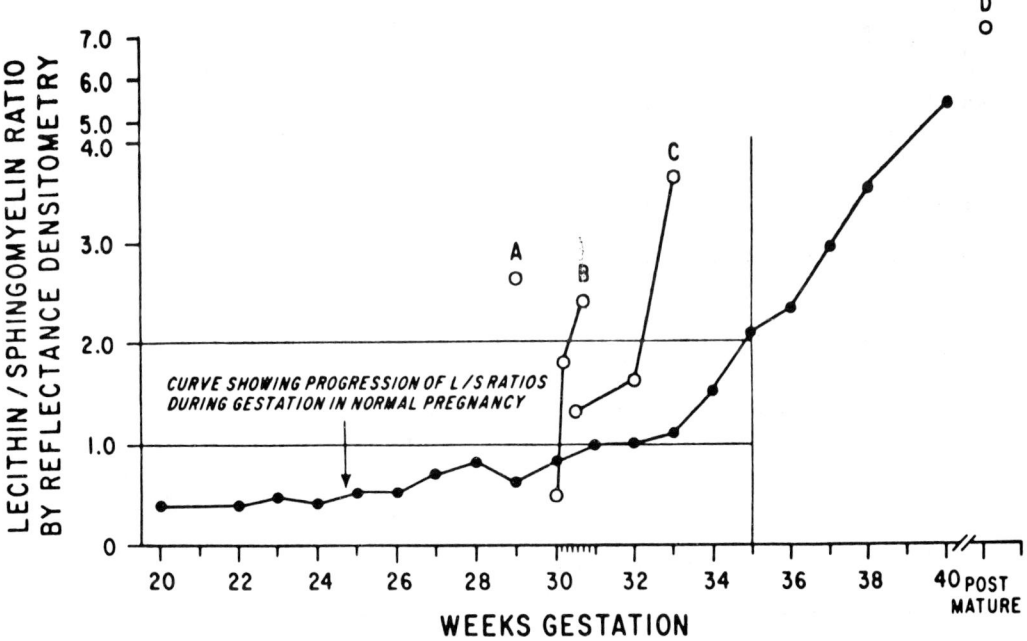

Fig. 66.2. Abnormal elevations of L:S ratio as compared with the L:S ratio curve for normal pregnancy [23]. *A*, chronic stress (retroplacental bleeding); *B*, acute stress (membranes ruptured 72–96 h); *C*, acute stress (placental infarction); *D*, chronic stress (postmaturity).

maternal hypertensive disease of multiple etiologies, placental insufficiency syndromes (including placental infarct and chronic abruptio placenta with retroplacental bleeding), maternal diabetes mellitus of advanced stage with vascular disease, and narcotic addiction. In addition, prolonged rupture of membranes may be associated with decreased risk of RDS. Delayed fetal pulmonary maturity is seen with several conditions, by far the most common of which is maternal diabetes mellitus, classes A, B and C [49]. It has been shown that infants of diabetic mothers are at greater risk for RDS at any given gestational age than infants of non-diabetic mothers. The situation is further complicated by the fact that mature L:S ratios in these infants do not always indicate mature lungs, i.e., there is a possibility of obtaining false-positive results, especially before 38 weeks gestation. Decisions regarding management may thus be difficult when early delivery is being contemplated for other reasons.

Pharmacologic acceleration

If premature delivery of any infant appears probable or necessary, lung maturation can now be accelerated. In recent years much attention has been focused on hormonal and other pharmacologic agents which achieve this result. The effects of various catecholamines and of aminophylline have been studied. However, the most promising method of this time appears to be prepartum glucocorticoid administration. Although conflicting evidence has appeared in the literature, it appears that these agents, when administered to the mother at least 24–48 h prior to delivery, decrease both the incidence and the severity of RDS (Table 66.1). Note that corticosteroids appear to be only effective before 34 weeks gestation and when administered at least 24 h and no longer than 7 days

before delivery [39]. To date, there are no proven complications of this treatment, but concern has been expressed about the possibility of increased infection in both mother and infant, as well as possible effects on the infant's later growth and development. Also, the administration of beta-mimetic drugs to inhibit uterine activity together with corticosteroids to accelerate pulmonary maturation have produced fulminant pulmonary edema in some mothers.

Prevention of prematurity

Factors known to predispose to premature delivery include lower socioeconomic class, poor antenatal care, multiple pregnancy, infection, uterine malformations, and cervical incompetence. However, the majority of premature deliveries are not associated with any specific risk factor. Adequate prenatal care for all pregnant mothers is thus required to prevent prematurity.

Several classes of pharmacologic agents have been studied for their ability to stop premature labor. Ethanol IV [6] has been widely used with moderate success, but the side-effects are marked and continued oral therapy, once labor has been arrested, is difficult to regulate. More recently, several beta-mimetic adrenergic agents have been tested for their ability to inhibit uterine contractions. Beta agonists with maximal inhibition of uterine contraction and minimal cardiovascular side-effects and fetal toxicity are being actively sought. Among those most commonly used are ritodrine, isoxuprine, salbutamol, fenoterol, and metaproterenol (Table 66.2). To date, the incidence of side effects of the beta-mimetic agents on both mother and fetus have been minimal although hypoglycemia and

Table 66.1 Occurrence of RDS related to entry-delivery interval in liveborn infants delivered after unplanned premature labor [39]

Entry-delivery interval	Betamethasone-treated group			Control group			P^a
	No.	RDS	%RDS	No.	RDS	%RDS	
Under 24 hrs.	55	14	25.5	56	15	26.8	NS^b
1 and under 7 days	115	10	8.7	99	26	26.3	0.005
More than 7 days	109	7	6.4	98	5	5.1	NS
All liveborn infants	279	31	11.1	253	46	18.2	0.04

[a]P values were derived by using the x^2-test with Yates' correction.
[b]NS, not significant ($P > 0.1$).

Table 66.2. Prolongation of pregnancy: mean time gained (days) [38]

	Singletons (120)	Twins (15)	Combined[a] (135)
Ethanol	26.6 ± 3.4	30.7 ± 9.2	27.6 ± 3.1
Ritodrine	46.2 ± 4.1	22.0 ± 6.0	44.0 ± 3.9

[a] $P < 0.001$

alterations in heart rate and rhythm have been encountered. No adverse long-term side-effects have been documented. Inhibitors of prostaglandin synthesis act to relax the pregnant uterus and indomethacin has been used with some success to arrest premature labor. However, investigations in both animals and humans have revealed instances of premature closure of the ductus arteriosus in utero and pulmonary artery hypertension after birth, severely limiting the attractiveness of this agent. Other drugs which have been noted to arrest premature labor include magnesium sulfate and diazoxide, but extensive studies have not yet been performed to determine their overall usefulness.

In summary then, there exist a number of pharmacologic agents capable of inhibiting premature labor, but further experience is necessary to delineate fully their relative advantages and disadvantages. Despite the fact that only approximately 25% of patients delivering prematurely will be candidates for pharmacologic inhibition of labor if appropriate indications and contraindications are followed, these agents offer promise for the future in this select group of patients.

Iatrogenic RDS

It is a disturbing reality that as many as 10%–12% of the total number of cases of RDS seen at major referral centers are iatrogenic, i.e., infants delivered electively without adequate prenatal assessment of gestational age or pulmonary maturity [28]. When elective delivery is planned (as for repeat cesarean sections), all efforts should be made to ascertain fetal pulmonary maturity or wait for the spontaneous onset of labor. In this way a significant amount of RDS can be prevented. The precise role of cesarean section in the incidence of RDS has been carefully evaluated and it is now felt that it is the timing of the delivery relative to pulmonary maturity rather than the method of delivery which is important.

Diagnosis and clinical course

The diagnosis of RDS is based on both x-ray and clinical criteria. Clinically, the affected infant will exhibit tachypnea, expiratory grunting, flaring of the nasal alae, and chest wall retractions of the sub-and intercostal and suprasternal areas. These symptoms are frequently apparent within the first minutes of life, but in less severe cases may take longer to become fully manifest. The infant will show evidence of hypoxia in room air, but the severity varies from duskiness of the nail beds and oral mucosa to overall frank cyanosis. Apneic episodes are indicative of severe hypoxia, respiratory failure, or infection. Auscultation of the chest is frequently not a useful tool in newborns, because there is excellent transmission of all breath sounds throughout the thorax. Auscultation may reveal decreased or harsh tubular breath sounds but may also be entirely within normal limits. The differential diagnosis of RDS in the neonatal period is extensive. Some conditions to be considered are shown in Table 66.3.

Table 66.3. Some causes of respiratory distress in the newborn

Respiratory disorders (common)
Hyaline membrane disease
Transient tachypnea of the newborn (retained pulmonary fluid)
Aspiration meconium
Pneumonia: bacterial, viral
Pneumothorax
Pulmonary hemorrhage or edema

Extra pulmonary causes (less common)
1. Neuromuscular disorders
   Brain: asphyxia, hemorrhage, edema, drugs, infection
   Spinal cord: trauma, Werdnig–Hoffman disease
   Peripheral nerves: phrenic or recurrent laryngeal nerve injury
   Myasthenia gravis
   Muscular dystrophies
2. Mechanical obstruction/restriction
   Airway obstruction: e.g., choanal atresia, tracheomalacia
   Rib cage abnormalities: thoracic dystrophies, bone disease
   Diaphragmatic disorders: congenital eventration or hernia, abdominal distention
3. Cardiovascular
   Congenital heart disease with cyanosis and/or pulmonary edema
   Hypovolemia and/or hypotension
   Primary pulmonary artery hypertension (PFC)
4. Hematologic disorders: e.g., anemia, polycythemia
5. Metabolic abnormalities: e.g., acidosis, hypothermia

The *chest radiograph* typically reveals a reticulogranular pattern to the lung fields, which has also been described as a 'ground glass' appearance. There is decreased lung volume as well. The presence of air bronchograms is a variable finding. In less severe cases, they may be evident only centrally and behind the cardiac silhouette; however, the most severe radiographic evidence of disease will include air bronchograms visible to the periphery throughout all lung fields. This degree of disease is frequently accompanied by 'white out' lung fields, i.e., the density of the pulmonary parenchyma is so great as to obliterate all other lung markings as well as the cardiothymic silhouette. The findings described above are all caused by diffuse alveolar atelectasis, the result of the underlying surfactant deficiency, which leads to non-aerated parenchyma outlining air-filled bronchi. It is important to recognize that x-rays taken in the first minutes or hours of life may appear normal despite obvious symptoms of respiratory distress, and only later is there a typical radiographic appearance (Fig. 66.3). Although evidence of the disease is usually uniform throughout the lung fields, this is not always the case. This may be especially true when pulmonary edema (of any etiology) is a complicating factor. (It is imperative to recognize that pneumonia due to group B β-hemolytic streptococcus may mimic some or even all of the above findings; therefore, antibiotics are included in the initial treatment regimen of any infant with respiratory distress.) The cardiac silhouette is frequently normal early in the course of the disease, but may be enlarged if the infant has suffered severe asphyxia or has been fluid-overloaded iatrogenically. Patency of the ductus arteriosus, a frequent complication of RDS, if associated with significant left-to-right shunting, may also cause cardiomegaly and pulmonary edema. The thymus is usually prominent in the initial radiographs.

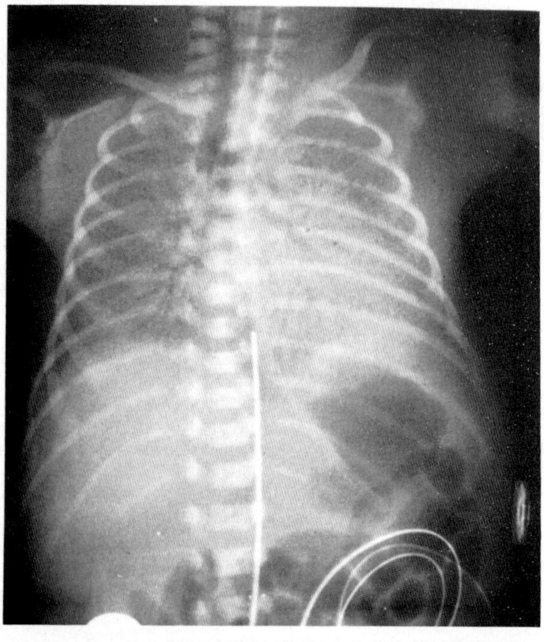

The severity of the disease process progressively increases through the first 48–72 h of life, and then, in uncomplicated cases, resolves over the ensuing days. However, this time course may be altered by various confounding developments, specifically those associated with assisted ventilation. Mechanical ventilation with high rates, pressures, and O_2 concentrations may further damage the lungs, producing interstitial emphysema, pneumothoraces, and subsequently bronchopulmonary dysplasia. The requirement for supplemental O_2 may be prolonged by days, weeks, or even months. Development of a patent ductus arteriosus frequently causes congestive heart failure with pulmonary edema severe enough to increase requirements for O_2 and ventilatory support. Recovery from RDS is characterized by a gradual decrease in the FiO_2 and ventilator settings needed by the infant. In the mild or moderate cases that do not require MV recovery may be complete by 1 week of life.

Fig. 66.3. The typical radiographic appearance of RDS, with prominent air bronchograms. Note the presence of an endotracheal tube and umbilical arterial catheter.

General management

Supportive measures for infants with RDS include those important in the care of all premature infants. They should be maintained in a neutral thermal environment, i.e., that ambient temperature which will maintain normal core temperature with minimal O_2 expenditure. This can be achieved by means of either an incubator or a radiant warmer, although the latter may be associated with higher convective and evaporative heat losses. We have found it useful to place the smallest infants under plastic heat shields within the incubator, thereby reducing radiant losses [37]. In addition, the air within the incubator should be humidified to approximately 50%–60%.

Heart rate and respirations must be monitored constantly by electrical monitors with audio alarms to alert staff members early to a baby with apnea or bradycardia. In addition, intra-arterial catheters may be attached to transducers to provide constant display of blood pressure. Alternatively, blood pressure should be monitored at specific intervals with a Doppler device. (Palpation, auscultation, and the flush method of determining blood pressure have all been shown to give measurements which differ significantly from those obtained via intra-arterial determination and are therefore inadequate.)

Blood pressure must be supported as necessary. Although the graphs of 'normal' blood pressures for infants of various birth weights based on the work of Kitterman et al. [35] are useful as general guidelines, they are only that. Clinical signs of pallor, poor peripheral perfusion, and tachycardia, as well as persistent metabolic acidosis, may indicate intravascular depletion in spite of an apparently normal blood pressure. In such cases, volume expansion may be accomplished with whole blood, plasma, or crystalloid solutions (normal saline or lactated Ringer's). The hematocrit should be maintained above 45% with transfusions to maximize oxygen-carrying capacity. Exchange transfusions were advocated in the treatment of RDS at one time, for the purpose of replacing circulating fetal hemoglobin with adult hemoglobin, and thus increasing O_2 release to the tissues. However, it has been suggested that this form of therapy is associated with an increased incidence of retrolental fibroplasia and it is therefore no longer advocated [16].

Frequent evaluations of arterial blood gas status are imperative in all infants with RDS; arterial catheters are therefore routinely placed in such infants upon admission. The umbilical arteries are by far the most accessible and therefore the most frequently used sites, although the radial and dorsalis pedis arteries may also be used. The complications of such catheters are many, and include spasm of the artery, thromboembolic phenomena (which have been linked to renovascular hypertension, necrotizing enterocolitis, and vascular compromise of portions of the lower extremities), hemorrhage secondary to dislodgement or disconnection of the catheter, and introduction of infection. Arteriolized capillary blood samples obtained from a warmed heel of the infant are useful indicators of pH and $PaCO_2$, but their correlation with PaO_2 is poor. The complications of arterial catheters noted above are thus overcome, but maceration of the heel and infection

of the soft tissues and even bone are well described problems with this technique.

In the past few years, transcutaneous (Tc) monitoring techniques have been developed for use in neonates, and the small warmed sensors which are placed on the infant's skin provide accurate, continuous, non-invasive assessments of PaO_2 and $PaCO_2$ [33, 42]. The in vivo response time of the O_2 electrode is only 5–10 s. The sensor must be warmed to 44 °C to obtain accurate readings, but may underestimate PaO_2 when the infant is suffering from hypotension with tissue hypoperfusion, when the postnatal age is greater than 2 months, and when the PaO_2 is extremely high (greater than 100 mmHg). Despite these limitations the $TcPO_2$ monitor has proved a valuable adjunct in the management of infants with HMD (Fig 66.4). It obviates the need for intermittent arterial puncture in infants without indwelling catheters, specifically those who have only mild disease with low O_2 requirements and those whose catheters have already been removed. It decreases the total number of blood gases and therefore the total amount of blood drawn in some infants, and facilitates rapid weaning in infants who are over-oxygenated. In addition it has made possible the accumulation of a body of information on the effects of various forms of intervention by physicians and nurses on PaO_2, e.g., suctioning, bagging, and positioning, as well as data regarding the fluctuations in PaO_2 these infants suffer even without intervention. More recently $TcPCO_2$ monitors have become available for use in newborns. Although their response time is slightly greater than that of the O_2 monitors (60–90 s), they are proving a useful adjunct to these in the noninvasive management and study of newborns of all gestational ages.

Fluid and electrolyte balance must be maintained. Maintenance fluid requirements increase from 60–80 cm^3/kg per day to approximately 120 cm^3/kg per day by day 5 of life. However, fluid needs may be modified by several factors (Table 66.4). Many of these infants suffer some degree of asphyxia at birth and develop acute tubular necrosis, which also modifies their fluid needs.

Most premature neonates will be able to tolerate a solution containing 10% dextrose. The goal is to provide at least 4–6 mg glucose/kg per min, which is sufficient to meet glucose requirements and prevent hypoglycemia. Maintenance of sodium balance is usually achieved with administration of 3–4 mmol/kg per day. However, renal inability to

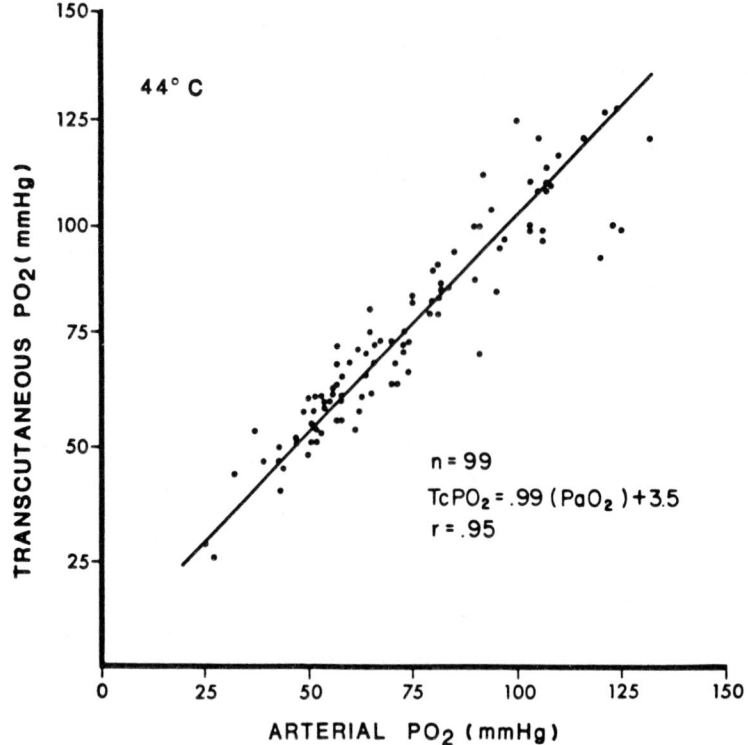

Fig. 66.4. Correlation between transcutaneous and arterial O_2 tension measurements in 25 preterm infants with RDS [36].

Table 66.4 Factors that increase fluid requirements [18]

1. Increased insensible water loss in immature infants
2. Phototherapy
3. Radiant warmers
4. Labile body temperature, labile ambient temperature
5. Increased urinary volume associated with glycosuria and acute tubular necrosis
6. Abnormal fluid losses—post surgery, e.g., colostomy chest tube drainage
7. Third space losses
8. Diarrhea or vomiting, etc.

conserve sodium, particularly in the presence of glucosuria or with the use of diuretics, may increase these requirements. Overzealous sodium administration, on the other hand, may result in hypernatremia as well as peripheral edema. Potassium requirements are approximately 1–2 mmol/kg per day. Calcium is supplied as one of several salts and 20 mg elemental calcium/kg per day usually suffices to maintain serum calcium levels.

Management of acid–base disturbances may present significant difficulty. Metabolic acidosis is frequently encountered subsequent to hypoxia and hypovolemia. This may require IV sodium bicarbonate therapy, which commences with 1–2 mmol/kg and is repeated until the acidosis has been corrected, provided that the total dose does not exceed 8 mmol/kg in 12 h

[52]. Although untreated acidosis may result in an increased risk of intracranial hemorrhage, decreased myocardial contractility, and metabolic dysfunction at the cellular level, the treatment is also not without hazards. Fluid overload and hypernatremia are well-described complications of repeated administration of bicarbonate; an association has also been suggested between intracranial hemorrhage and rapid infusion of hypertonic materials such as bicarbonate.

Abdominal decompression with an orogastric or nasogastric tube should be maintained in all infants with respiratory distress, to prevent compromise of diaphragmatic excursion. This is especially important in infants being treated with nasal or pharyngeal CPAP (continuous positive airway pressure), as extensive swallowing of air with abdominal distension may result.

Providing adequate nutrition for these infants is frequently quite difficult. In our nursery enteral feedings are not begun until the infant is well on the road to recovery, generally not until he or she is stable in supplemental O_2 alone without other assistance to ventilation. Until that time parenteral nutrition is administered. Protein, carbohydrate, and fats are all supplied IV, with trace elements, vitamins, and electrolytes added. Although this is far from the ideal method to supply calories, it does prevent catabolism of the body's tissues and at a higher level provides enough calories for growth. There are, unfortunately, a number of side-effects to this aspect of treatment, some of them serious, and therefore the goal should be full enteral nutrition as early as possible [18].

Continuous positive airway pressure

Prior to 1970 MV was utilized in the treatment of RDS only when severe respiratory failure supervened despite administration of increased O_2 concentrations. Consequently, the results were extremely discouraging, with only 65% survival expected for infants weighing greater than 2 kg, approximately 33% at 2 kg, and 20% if they were smaller. In 1970, Gregory et al. introduced a new approach with the application of CPAP via headbox or endotracheal tube to infants who were breathing spontaneously [27]. Their initial results were encouraging, for they not only demonstrated a significant increase in PaO_2 with a resultant decrease in O_2 requirements; their outcome data also suggested improved survival. Soon thereafter multiple reports describing different techniques of application appeared. These included a pressurized face chamber, face mask, plastic bags, and nasal prongs [1, 34, 48]. Other investigators chose to produce positive transpulmonary pressure by exerting continuous negative pressure around the chest wall with either a modified negative pressure ventilator or a chamber within the incubator to which a vacuum was applied [10, 20]. The purpose of all these different modes of therapy is to achieve continuous distending pressure (CDP) throughout the respiratory cycle. It should be apparent that this may be accomplished either by exerting a CPAP or by exerting negative pressure around the thorax (CNP). Debate continues as to the most efficacious method by which to deliver CDP as well as the optimal time to initiate therapy; there is, however, no argument as to its benefit, despite the limited number of controlled studies.

The physiologic basis for the use of continuous distending airway pressure was first suggested by Harrison, who investigated the role of grunting in RDS [30]. He concluded that grunting (exhaling against a partially closed glottis with active contraction of the abdominal muscles) represented an attempt by the infant to overcome atelectasis. When grunting was eliminated with endotracheal intubation, a fall in PaO_2 ensued. The grunting resumed after extubation, and PaO_2 rose promptly. Although it has been widely accepted that CPAP increases PaO_2, thereby allowing a reduction in FiO_2, it is not entirely clear what physiologic factors account for these effects. It has been postulated that recruitment of previously collapsed alveoli results in better oxygenation by improving ventilation–perfusion relationships within the lungs. After application of CPAP there is an increase in functional residual capacity (FRC), [2], which presumably decreases intrapulmonary right-to-left shunting, lending credence to this idea. However, there is a variable effect on lung compliance [2, 61]. This suggests that in addition to recruitment of some alveoli, there may also be overdistention of others. The breathing pattern becomes slower and more regular [61], and grunting generally ceases after CDP has been applied. Because of the rapidity with which these changes occur, it has been postulated that they result from modification of the Hering-Breuer reflex with the change in FRC [41].

There is conflicting evidence regarding the effect of CDP on $PaCO_2$. Several studies have shown no consistent changes in $PaCO_2$ [2, 61] with increasing levels of CDP while others have demonstrated significant increases. Even when $PaCO_2$ remains unchanged, however, minute ventilation tends to decrease [2, 61], suggesting a reduction in physiologic dead space.

The optimal level of CDP may be defined as that airway pressure at which arterial O_2 tension is maximal with minimal effect on cardiovascular function. If the pressure is increased above this level, PaO_2 decreases slightly and $PaCO_2$ rises [4]. There is a sharp rise in esophageal pressure when the optimal CDP is achieved, suggesting recruitment of alveoli, improved compliance, and enhanced transmission of airway pressure to the intrapleural space. The optimal CDP is not static in any given patient.

The initial report by Gregory described the use of either a pressurized headbox or an endotracheal tube. However, an alternative to endotracheal CPAP was vigorously sought to avoid intubation and its attendant risks. The head chamber presented many difficulties: it was not easy to construct, in addition to which it limited access to the infant and at times produced constriction about the neck, with subsequent skin breakdown. It also required an extremely high air flow and thus produced an unacceptable noise level for the infant. Various modifications were suggested to overcome some of these problems, including development of the face chamber and modification of a pneumask, essentially a large plastic bag, to fit over the infant's head. A mask which would cover only the nose and mouth was tried, but an adequate seal was difficult to achieve without exerting great pressure on the head and face. Various devices for CNP were also developed. However, an obvious drawback to these is that therapy must be interrupted for procedures to be performed on the infant; in addition, with any leak in the chamber, thermoregulation becomes a problem as a result of the torrential air flow. In summary then, the positive pressure hood, plastic head bag, or CNP body chamber all tend to isolate the infant and prevent access without temporary interruption of therapy. The potentially harmful effects of positive pressure to the eyes, cooling of the face, high sound levels, and fluctuation of O_2 concentration were other problems encountered when these systems were employed.

In 1973 Kattwinkel [34] reported a modification of Agostino's method with the development of the now widely used nasal prongs for delivering CDP (Fig. 66.5). There are several advantages to this technique: it is relatively atraumatic, causes lower airway resistance than an endotracheal tube, allows constant access to the baby, is simple to set up and care for, and requires lower flow rates than head or face chambers. Furthermore, there are no problems with thermoregulation. An alternative method to the short nasal prongs is nasopharyngeal delivery by way of modified endotracheal tubes placed in one or both nares. However, a recent study by Goldman [26] has demonstrated a considerably higher work of breathing with nasal prongs than with the face mask, thought to be due to the resistance of the tubing. The systems for delivery of continuous distending airway pressure, therefore, continued to be modified.

Indications and outcome

Increases in the fractional concentration of inspired O_2 represent the minimum level of respiratory support which an infant with RDS may require. However, such support is frequently not sufficient, as evidenced by falling

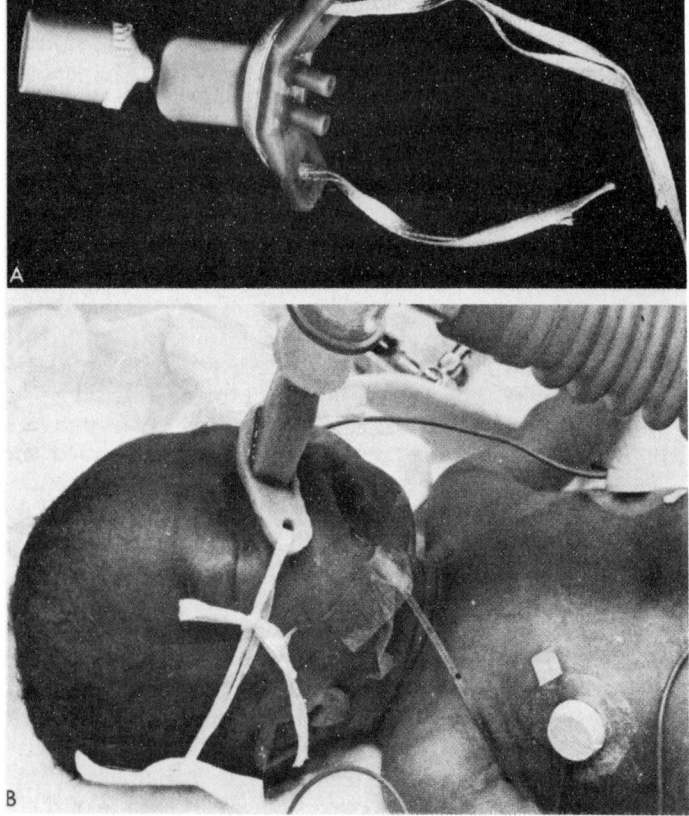

Fig. 66.5. A Silastic device for the administration of nasal CPAP; **B** nasal CPAP unit in place on an infant.

PaO_2 and rising $PaCO_2$, and further assistance is required. Because the only consistently documented effect of CPAP on respiratory status is to raise PaO_2, hypoxia remains the only universally accepted rationale for institution of this therapy. Specific guidelines, however, are more variable. In our nursery the inability of the infant to maintain PaO_2 at or above 60 mmHg with FiO_2 of approximately 0.7 constitutes adequate indication for beginning CPAP in most infants. CPAP is applied earlier under certain circumstances, particularly in small infants with clearcut RDS. Because CPAP has a variable effect on $PaCO_2$, one must monitor the blood gases closely and if respiratory failure ensues [i.e., $PaCO_2$ greater than 65 mmHg (8.7 kPa), pH less than 7.20] endotracheal intubation with MV should be instituted instead. Recently, Tanswell et al. [59] studied the effects of application of CPAP in the first hours of life in infants with RDS, without awaiting the conventional indication of high FiO_2 requirements. Their results showed that early CPAP was associated with lower O_2 and pressure requirements, as well as improved pH, $PaCO_2$, and A-aDO_2. Although such data must be considered somewhat preliminary at this point, in view of the low complication rate many neonatal units are following this approach.

In summary, CDP has proven an extremely effective tool for the management of hyaline membrane disease. The level and duration of high O_2 concentrations required by these infants are both reduced, and the need for MV appears to be decreased [7, 20]. In addition, CPAP is extremely useful as an intermediate step in weaning infants from mechanical ventilation, and there is evidence that the duration of intubation is decreased. Several studies have shown an improved outcome as well, with decreases in both the mortality rate [7, 48] and the incidence of bronchopulmonary dysplasia (BPD) among the survivors. If the need for and duration of endotracheal intubation are truly decreased, these could lead to a decline in the incidence of the long-term upper airway problems that sometimes follow this procedure. Despite almost a decade of experience the indications for elective intervention with CDP remain controversial.

Mechanical ventilation

In 1929 Drinker introduced the negative pressure ventilator for adults [17], and positive pressure ventilators followed thereafter. Although sporadic reports on the use of MV in infants appeared as early as the 1940s, it was to be many years before ventilators appropriate for use in small infants were available. By the late 1960s the use of ventilators in newborns became more common, and in the past decade MV appears to have contributed significantly to the drastic reduction of perinatal mortality.

Despite several reports attesting to the efficacy of intermittent assisted ventilation with mask and bag, it became apparent that for many infants with hyaline membrane disease and respiratory failure the only chance for survival was continuous ventilatory support. Early uncontrolled trials described the use of both intermittent negative pressure ventilation (INPV) [55, 56] and intermittent positive pressure ventilation (IPPV) [14, 31, 43]. Intermittent negative pressure ventilation was delivered initially with a ventilator–incubator combination which enclosed the infant's entire body from the neck down. The smallest babies were tossed about by the relatively large flows and changes in pressure, became bruised, developed skin breakdown beneath the seals at the neck, and also experienced significant thermal stress. Later modifications attempted to stabilize the infant's body by limiting the negative pressure chamber to extend only from the neck to the hips. Stahlman et al. reported a series of 80 patients treated with INPV [55]. Although these patients were severely ill, exhibiting PaO_2 less than 30–40 mmHg with an FiO_2 of 1.0, prolonged apnea, gasping respirations or bradycardia, the derangements of pH, $PaCO_2$, and PaO_2 were corrected in many and 39% survived. Stern's group from Montreal reported a similar success rate [56]. Previously only 10% of these infants would have been expected to survive.

Intermittent positive pressure ventilation was simultaneously undergoing trials at other centers. In controlled and uncontrolled studies employing both pressure- and volume-cycled ventilators, the efficacy of this mode of therapy in correcting derangements of ventilation and oxygenation was demonstrated. Although controlled studies revealed statistically significant decreases in mortality, the results at this time were still very disappointing (Table 66.5). Proponents of INPV were quick to point out that it eliminated the morbidity of endotracheal intubation and was associated with a reduced incidence of air leak syndromes and chronic lung disease as well. Access to the infant, however, was considerably more restricted and

Table 66.5. Survival by birth weight following assisted ventilation for hyaline membrane disease[a]

Year		Birth weight (g)			
		<1500	1500–2000	>2000	Overall
CPAP	1970–74	52% (n = 153)	←————— 95% combined —————→ (n = 219)		77% (n = 372)
	1975–79	63% (n = 175)	89% (n = 35)	90% (n = 48)	71% (n = 258)
MV	Before 1965	←—————	30% combined (n = 222)	—————→	30% (n = 222)
	1965–74	19% (n = 213)	39% (n = 201)	57% (n = 218)	39% (n = 632)
	1975–79	29% (n = 125)	47% (n = 32)	70% (n = 54)	42% (n = 211)

[a]Combined data from references 1, 6, 7, 9, 10, 13, 14, 20, 27, 31, 34, 40, 43, 44, 48, 55, 56, 58, 60, 61.

necessitated interruption of MV, thereby limiting its usefulness. Thus, because of their greater versatility, positive-pressure ventilators are used almost exclusively at most major centers today; few units continue to employ negative pressure ventilation. The remainder of this section will therefore be confined to IPPV.

With the original positive pressure ventilators, gas flow to the patient occurred only during the inspiratory phase of the cycle. The expiratory phase was characterized by passive emptying of the lungs. Attempts at spontaneous ventilation during periods without gas flow would have entailed a markedly increased work of breathing for the patient as well as inhalation of recently exhaled, and therefore CO_2-enriched, gas. It was thus necessary to abolish spontaneous ventilation either by increasing alveolar ventilation to the point that respiratory drive was overcome, or by neuromuscular blockade. The concept of intermittent mandatory ventilation (IMV), during which a fresh flow of gas is delivered to the patient throughout the respiratory cycle, represented a major step forward in MV of neonates. This mode permits both spontaneous and artificial ventilation concurrently.

Gregory and co-workers demonstrated the efficacy of CPAP in spontaneously breathing infants. The application of distending airway pressure throughout the respiratory cycle combined with IPPV and known as positive end-expiratory pressure (PEEP) followed naturally [13]. The addition of positive pressure throughout the cycle prevents recurrent collapse of alveoli and improves oxygenation by improving the ventilation/perfusion (V/Q) relationships within the lungs.

Despite much experience and significant success with MV there is still considerable difference of opinion regarding the optimal method of ventilating infants, particularly those with persistent derangement of blood gases. Both volume- and pressure-cycled ventilators have been used [6, 40], with the latter gaining more favor as attempts are made to adequately ventilate infants with low pressures. With a volume-cycled machine, one presets the tidal volume (generally 7–10 cm³/kg) to be delivered to the patient and adjusts the flow rate to determine the time over which it is delivered, and hence, the ratio of inspiratory to expiratory phase (I:E ratio). It must be recognized, however, that such ventilators will deliver these volumes irrespective of the pressure generated. This assumes increasing importance in infants with severe RDS, in whom compliance is so markedly diminished that delivery of a 'normal' tidal volume requires a tremendous peak inspiratory pressure (PIP). Furthermore, the high flow rates of these machines limit the adjustment of the I:E ratio. The alternative is the use of a pressure-cycled ventilator, wherein flow is delivered to the patient until the predetermined PIP is reached. At this point the pressure may be immediately allowed to return to end-expiratory levels, producing a saw-tooth pressure curve, or it may be maintained at peak levels for some period of time before the expiratory phase begins, producing a pressure curve with plateaus (Fig. 66.6). Within this framework the I:E ratio may be widely manipulated. Prolonged I:E ratios to the extent of reversal of the ratio (that is, inspiratory time greater than expiratory time) often produce an increased PaO_2 [32, 47] but may cause CO_2 retention if alveolar ventilation

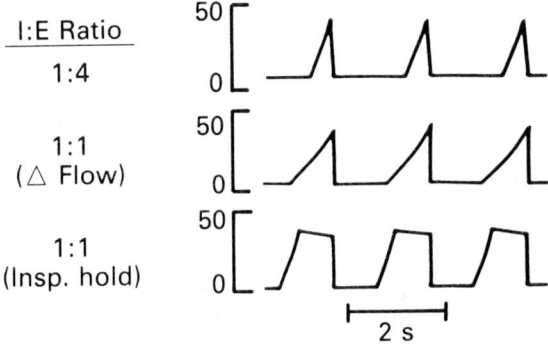

Fig. 66.6. The different airway pressure waves produced while the I:E ratio is increased either by decreasing inspiratory flow rate or by employing the inspiratory time hold mechanism [5].

is impaired. In contrast to adults, compromise of cardiac function with decreased venous return secondary to prolonged high intrathoracic pressures has not been a significant clinical problem in neonates with decreased lung compliance.

Increases in peak inspiratory pressure will generally decrease $PaCO_2$ [54] but may also result in increased incidence of serious air leaks and chronic lung disease. It has been suggested that lower peak inspiratory pressures combined with higher I:E ratios may result in decreased morbidity and even mortality. Increases in the level of PEEP tend to improve PaO_2 [32], but one is limited in this aspect of therapy by the increased risk of air leaks as well as decreased alveolar ventilation and possibly cardiac output. Indeed, some studies suggest that mean airway pressure (MAP) is the most important determinant of changes in blood gases as well as complications such as air leaks and bronchopulmonary dysplasia [5, 8, 32].

There remains much confusion regarding the optimal rate at which to ventilate these infants. Although it is clear that an increased rate results in improved alveolar ventilation and decreased $PaCO_2$ [54], the effect on arterial O_2 tension may be none or detrimental. In fact, some studies suggest that slower rates in combination with an increased I:E ratio are associated with decreased morbidity and mortality [40], while other reports describe high survival rates with rapid ventilation at low pressures [3]. Recent studies have demonstrated adequate oxygenation and ventilation of infants with RDS when oscillation at frequencies as high as 1800/min was used [22]. Perhaps this is the direction of the future.

At our own institution the indications for ventilator therapy are deterioration of blood gases or clinical condition. The infant may be unable to maintain adequate oxygenation [PaO_2 more than 50 mmHg (6.7 kPa)] or adequate ventilation [$PaCO_2$ less than 55–60 mmHg (7.3–8 kPa) with pH greater than 7.20] on an FiO_2 of 1.0 with a nasal CPAP of 10 cmH$_2$O, or may exhibit increasing periods of apnea and/or bradycardia requiring vigorous stimulation or positive-pressure bagging. We prefer to perform endotracheal intubation with tubes of at least 3 mm internal diameter, as it is exceedingly difficult to accomplish effective pulmonary toilet with smaller tubes. However, as a greater number of smaller babies are being ventilated, 2.5 mm tubes are increasingly used. Pressure-cycled ventilators are employed for most infants with RDS.

Weaning the infant from ventilatory support is frequently as difficult a problem as the initial management. In milder cases it may be easily accomplished, but with severe disease, the superimposition of iatrogenic lung disease may make the processs difficult or even impossible. The approach is usually to decrease peak inspiratory pressure as tolerated until it reaches 20–25 cmH$_2$O, and then to direct one's attention to O_2 concentration and rate. It has been suggested that treatment with aminophylline to stimulate the respiratory drive will facilitate the weaning process, but the evidence for this is scanty. When low IMV of approximately 10 breaths/min is tolerated a short trial of endotracheal CPAP is in order. Prolonged periods of endotracheal CPAP in small infants with resolving lung disease are usually unsuccessful. This is because the infant may be incapable of sustaining the additional work of breathing associated with the increased airway resistance and the added dead space of the endotracheal tube. Endotracheal CPAP should not be decreased to less than 2 cmH$_2$O as this represents the normal end-expiratory pressure and is the optimal CPAP for weaning. The infant is then extubated, but may benefit from nasal CPAP in the post-extubation period.

Complications

Complications associated with hyaline membrane disease include entities which are directly related to its respiratory management, as well as those whose relationship is less clear, may involve other organ systems, and may occur in premature infants without HMD. Major factors which have been linked with the morbidity of this disease include O_2 administration, MV, endotracheal intubation, and placement of arterial catheters. In addition to the various sites of injury along the respiratory tract, the cardiovascular and central nervous systems may be affected by the course of the disease or its treatment.

Air leaks

Among the most common complications of RDS are the various air leak syndromes which may occur, including pneumothorax, pneumomediastinum, pneumopericardium, and even pneumoperitoneum. Recent data have shown little if any increase in the risk of air leak when patients with RDS treated with CPAP are compared with those who are treated only with supplemental O_2, both being less than 5%. However, there is no question that the addition of MV with PEEP to the treatment regimen increases this risk, with reported incidences of 14%–33% in this group. However, it is not clear what individual aspects of ventilator management are most important in increasing the risk of this complication. Pneumothorax and pneumopericardium usually result in a sudden deterioration of the baby's condition, with development of cyanosis, mottling, and bradycardia. Although the most severely affected infants who require high ventilatory pressures early in their course may suffer this complication in the first few hours of life, many infants will develop an air leak after several days. Presumably, as their disease resolves and lung compliance increases, airway pressures are not decreased quickly enough and normal alveoli rupture. Clinical criteria of an asymmetric chest wall configuration with decreased breath sounds on the affected side may or may not be present. A radiograph of the chest obtained at this time may show air outlining the lung tissue, with mediastinal structures shifted to the contralateral side (Fig. 66.7). However, because of the remarkable stiffness of lungs severely affected with RDS, collapse is frequently incomplete and the pneumothorax may be visible only anteriorly on a lateral view of the chest. Increased lucency of one hemithorax compared with the other on an AP view may suggest the diagnosis of anterior pneumothorax. Although the definitive diagnosis is made by chest x-ray, the patient's condition may not allow time for this procedure. Transillumination of the chest has proven a useful bedside aid in this situation. Evacuation of the air may be accomplished with

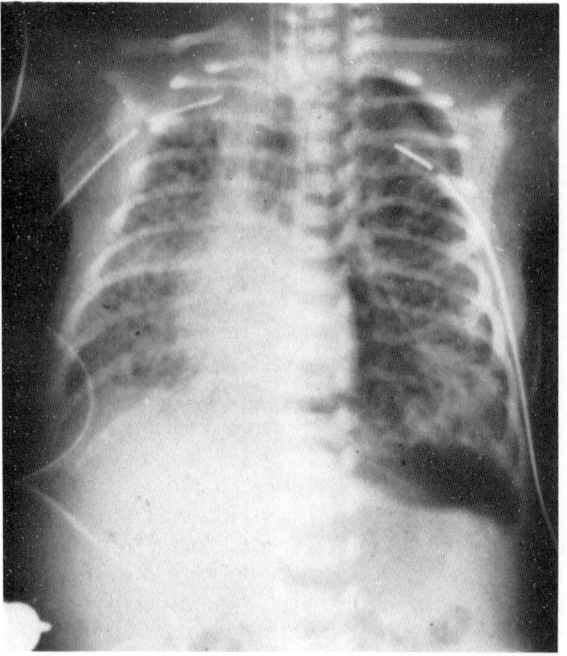

Fig. 66.7. A tension pneumothorax in an infant with RDS. Note the incomplete collapse of the lung on the affected side, despite mediastinal shift and depression of the diaphragm.

needle and syringe if the proper equipment is not available for tube thoracotomy.

Bronchopulmonary dysplasia

Pulmonary interstitial air (Fig. 66.8), though related to major air leaks as discussed above, is equally important as a harbinger of BPD, the chronic lung disease which often follows inten-

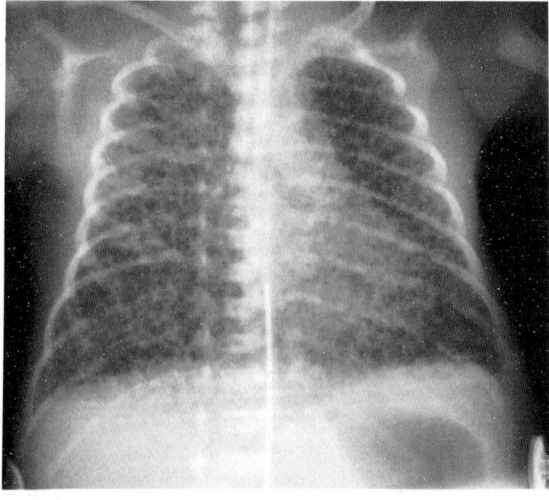

Fig. 66.8. Severe pulmonary interstitial emphysema which developed in the first 24 h of life in an infant receiving MV for RDS.

sive respiratory therapy with high O_2 concentrations and MV [45]. Individual small areas of emphysema may become progressively more distended until they compromise the expansion of the remaining lung tissue, and surgical removal of the affected lobe may be necessary. In less severe cases, selective intubation of the mainstem bronchus of the less affected side has been suggested as an alternative manner in which to manage this problem. In the majority of babies who survive with BPD, however, the interstitial emphysema recedes as the infant is weaned from ventilatory support. Nonetheless, their lungs remain severely damaged with marked interstitial fibrosis, microscopic emphysema, and mucosal destruction. Indeed, there is evidence that even infants treated with positive pressure ventilation who have normal pulmonary function prior to discharge from the hospital may develop increased airway resistance later during their first year [57]. It is clear that infants who suffer from BPD have an increased incidence of serious lower respiratory tract illness during the first 2–3 years of life, and that many require readmission to the hospital during this period [21]. However, it is fortunate that the lungs have such tremendous regenerative capacity. Widespread experience has revealed that the natural history of this disease is one of gradual improvement over the first few years. Most affected children will have clinically normal pulmonary function by the time they reach school age. While it is true that cor pulmonale compromises the cardiorespiratory function in some of these infants, especially those most severely affected, it is unclear what prognostic implications this sequela carries in and of itself. What are the most important aspects of ventilatory support in the pathogenesis of this disease? Unfortunately, this remains a subject of great controversy, but O_2 concentration and various aspects of pressure have been implicated, and probably all play some role.

Upper airway obstruction

Complications of endotracheal intubation itself are a direct result of mechanical trauma. Laryngeal edema may cause upper airway obstruction after extubation severe enough to result in marked CO_2 retention and reintubation. Steroids are not routinely used prior to extubation, but if stridor thought to be due to laryngeal edema develops, racemic epinephrine aerosols may be administered. Subglottic stenosis of varying degrees may develop. Milder cases may be characterized by croup-like symptoms or stridor observed only during intercurrent infections once the child has been discharged. However, there are unfortunately a number of children in whom the stenosis is so severe that tracheostomy becomes necessary. This procedure is associated with a very high morbidity and mortality through infancy, even in the most experienced hands, and therefore should not be undertaken lightly. Evidence of stenosis extending as far as the carina or even into the mainstem bronchi has been documented in some cases, presumably secondary to movement of the tube and suction catheters. Orotracheal intubation may result in gingival and dental complications which become apparent as the infant's teeth erupt. Nasotracheal intubation, although felt by some to afford greater stability of the tube, may be technically more difficult. In addition, necrosis of the skin of the nostril, erosion of the nasal septum, and strictures of the nasal vestibule have been reported. Furthermore, increased rates of colonization and subsequent infection have been suggested with this technique.

Atelectasis

Atelectasis is a frequent problem in the post-extubation period, the result of increased secretions in infants recovering from RDS and decreased pulmonary toilet once the tube is removed. Chest x-rays may show a wide spectrum of involvement from small areas of atelectasis found locally or diffusely, to collapse of an entire lobe or even lung. The right upper lobe is the most frequently affected. Clinically the infants exhibit increased respiratory distress with nasal flaring and chest wall retractions. Oxygen requirements increase, and frequently hypercarbia ensues. Respiratory failure may be severe enough to require reintubation and reinstitution of MV. However, the recent development of a flexible fiberoptic bronchoscope which is small enough for use in premature neonates and which provides O_2 to the infant during the procedure, has made it possible to perform endotracheal suction under direct vision, remove mucus plugs, and thus re-expand the atelectatic areas without prolonged reintubation. There is evidence that vigorous chest physiotherapy begun prior to extubation and continued into the post-extubation period will decrease the incidence of this complication markedly.

Pneumonia

Pneumonia, especially that secondary to infection with group B β-hemolytic streptococcus, may coexist with RDS, but it may also mimic RDS clinically and radiographically in an infant with mature lungs. Risk factors for infection, such as prolonged rupture of membranes and maternal fever, are not always present. Because of the frequently fulminant course of neonatal sepsis and the difficulty distinguishing it from RDS, all infants with symptoms of respiratory distress should be treated with antibiotics after appropriate cultures are obtained. A penicillin combined with an aminoglycoside is the usual choice. Furthermore, infants who require prolonged intubation appear to be at greater risk for colonization and subsequent infection of their respiratory tract. *Staphylococcus aureus* and *Candida* are more frequent pathogens under these circumstances.

Persistent fetal circulation

Persistence of the fetal circulation (PFC), a syndrome characterized by pulmonary artery hypertension and right-to-left shunting at the level of the foramen ovale and/or the ductus arteriosus has classically been associated with larger asphyxiated infants with or without meconium aspiration pneumonia. However, it has become increasingly clear over recent years that immature infants are also capable of developing elevated pulmonary artery pressures, and this may complicate the treatment of some infants with RDS. The diagnosis is suggested by hypoxia out of proportion to the degree of lung disease noted radiographically, and may be confirmed by the echocardiographic finding of an elevated RVPEP:RVET (right ventricular pre-ejection period to right ventricular ejection time) ratio, which is indicative of the increased afterload caused by the pulmonary artery hypertension. In such cases the pulmonary artery also tends to be hyperreactive, and these infants may suddenly become deeply cyanotic after the smallest change in ventilator settings or minimal tactile stimulation. For this reason an attempt should be made to achieve minimal handling of any infant suspected of having a component of persistent fetal circulation.

Hyperventilation may be beneficial for these infants. Neuromuscular blockade with pancuronium should be considered in any infant whose blood gas derangements are refractory to the usual levels of respiratory support, or who continues to breathe out of phase with the ventilator. However, preliminary evidence has linked use of this drug with an increased incidence of intracranial hemorrhage, and its use should not be undertaken lightly. Tolazoline has been advocated by some investigators for use in cases of PFC or severe RDS. However, there are no controlled trials which support its efficacy. Furthermore, its side-effects, especially systemic hypotension and gastrointestinal bleeding, may be life-threatening, and it should therefore be used only when other therapeutic measures have been exhausted.

Patent ductus arteriosus

Patency of the ductus arteriosus (PDA) is a frequent complication of prematurity and is especially common in those premature infants with RDS [50]. Although tissue hypoxia, acidosis, and fluid overload, among other things, have been implicated in the genesis of this problem, it is clearly a multifactorial condition. The opening of a previously functionally closed ductus may be heralded by an acute deterioration in the infant's status, with the onset of periods of apnea, bradycardia, or sudden worsening of the blood gas status (i.e., hypoxia, hypercarbia, and acidosis). However, its onset may also be more insidious, with hyperactivity of the precordium, bounding pulses, the typical continuous murmur, and varying degrees of right- and left-sided congestive heart failure becoming evident. Failure of the infant with RDS to improve clinically after 2–3 days should alert the physician to the possibility of a PDA. The diagnosis may be confirmed radiographically or by echocardiogram [51]. Echocardiographic features include the presence of an increased ratio of the left atrial:aortic root size of greater than 1.2 or evidence of increased left atrial or ventricular end-diastolic dimensions. Initial medical management centers on fluid restriction and vigorous diuresis, and in some infants with RDS this will suffice to control failure and close the ductus. Commonly though, additional measures are necessary. Digitalis has been used but its efficacy is unproven and there is evidence of marked toxicity in premature infants. Indomethacin, an inhibitor of prostaglandin synthesis, has been studied extensively for its ability to constrict the patent ductus, but its use remains somewhat controversial. The definitive treatment continues to be surgical ligation, a procedure which, in experienced hands, carries minimal intraoperative risk [12].

Cardiovascular effects of assisted ventilation

The effects of increased airway pressures due to CPAP or MV with PEEP on cardiac function have been well demonstrated in adults. The increase in intrathoracic pressure transmitted from the airways to the right side of the heart impedes venous return and thus compromises cardiac output. However, because of the marked decrease in lung compliance in infants with RDS, transmission of this pressure is greatly impaired. Although direct monitoring of cardiac output and central venous pressure is difficult in such small infants, and therefore infrequently performed, clinically apparent changes in cardiac function have not been noted [32, 40, 61].

Intracranial hemorrhage

Intracranial hemorrhage, especially in the subependymal, periventricular, and intraventricular regions [46], is a frequent complication of RDS [29]. Many factors have been linked to its occurrence, including asphyxia neonatorum, rapid volume expansion, rapid changes in serum osmolarity due to administration of hypertonic materials such as sodium bicarbonate, coagulation disorders, and hypoxia and acidosis. The use of CPAP and MV, especially with high inflating pressures, has been implicated in the pathogenesis as well [15]. It has been suggested that transmission of increased intrathoracic pressures to the right atrium and then to the intracranial veins results in increases in both the volume and the pressure of these vessels. When this is complicated by the fragility of the structural supports of the cerebral vasculature in the premature neonate, especially in the subependymal and periventricular areas, hemorrhage may result. However, this remains a controversial issue, since many of the other risk factors mentioned above are also associated with severe RDS. In addition, when CPAP is administered via a face mask, the tightness with which the mask must be fastened about the infant's head to maintain an adequate seal has been implicated in the pathogenesis of cerebellar hemorrhage. Further study is necessary to delineate the most important causes of intracranial hemorrhage.

Retrolental fibroplasia

Although the relationship of oxygen administration to retrolental fibroplasia (RLF) was noted decades ago, eradication of this disease from the nursery remains incomplete. Factors associated with its development include degree of prematurity, length of oxygen exposure, and duration of hyperoxia. It appears, however, that other factors must play some role as well, since the disease has been described in term infants after minimal oxygen exposure. Nonetheless, it remains most common in premature infants with RDS, despite newer techniques which allow closer monitoring of arterial oxygen tension. Luckily, the majority of cases are mild and resolve spontaneously over the first months of life. However, we continue to see infants with retinal detachment and blindness as a result of RLF.

References

1. Ahlstrom H, Jonson B, Svenningsen NW (1976) Continuous positive airways pressure treatment by a face chamber in idiopathic respiratory distress syndrome. Arch Dis Child 51:13
2. Bancalari E, Garcia OL, Jesse MJ (1973) Effects of continuous negative pressure on lung mechanics in idiopathic respiratory distress syndrome. Pediatrics 51:485
3. Bland RD, Kim MH, Light MJ et al (1980) High frequency mechanical ventilation in severe hyaline membrane disease: An alternative treatment. Crit Care Med 8:275
4. Bonta BW, Uauy R, Warshaw JB et al (1977) Determination of optimal continuous positive airway pressure for the treatment of RDS by measurement of esophageal pressure. J Pediatr 91:449
5. Boros SJ (1979) Variations in inspiratory: Expiratory ratio and airway pressure wave form during mechanical ventilation: The significance of mean airway pressure. J Pediatr 94:114
6. Boros SJ, Orgill AA (1978) Mortality and morbidity associated with pressure, and volume, limited infant ventilators. Am J Dis Child 132:865
7. Boros SJ, Reynolds JW (1975) Hyaline membrane disease treated with early end-expiratory pressure: One year's experience. Pediatrics 56:218
8. Boros SJ, Matalou SV, Ewald R, et al (1977) The effect of independent variations in inspiratory-expiratory ratio and end-expiratory pressure during mechanical ventilation in hyaline membrane disease: The significance of mean airway pressure. J Pediatr 91:794
9. Brady JP, Gregory GA (1979) Assisted ventilation. In: Klaus MH, Fanaroff AA (eds) Care of the high-risk neonate. Saunders, Philadelphia
10. Chernick V, Vidyasagar D (1972) Continuous negative chest wall pressure in hyaline membrane disease: One year experience. Pediatrics 49:753
11. Clements JA, Platzker ACG, Tierney DF et al (1972) Assessment of the risk of the respiratory distress syndrome by a rapid test for surfactant in amniotic fluid. N Engl J Med 286:1077
12. Cotton RB, Stahlman MT, Bender HW et al (1978) Randomized trial of early closure of symptomatic patent

ductus arteriosus in small preterm infants. J Pediatr 93:647

13. Cumarasamy N, Nussli R, Vischer D et al (1973) Artificial ventilation in hyaline membrane disease: The use of positive end-expiratory pressure and continuous positive airway pressure. Pediatrics 51:629

14. Daily WJR, Sunshine P, Smith PC (1971) Mechanical ventilation of newborn infants. V. Five years' experience. Anesthesiology 34:132

15. de Lemos RA, Tomasovic JJ (1978) Effects of positive pressure ventilation on cerebral blood flow in the newborn infant. Clin Perinatol 5:395

16. Delivoria-Papadopoulos M, Miller LD, Foster RD et al (1976) The role of exchange transfusion in the management of low-birth-weight infants with and without severe respiratory distress syndrome. J Pediatr 89:273

17. Drinker P, Shaw LA (1929) An apparatus for the prolonged administration of artificial respiration. J Clin Invest 7:229

18. Fanaroff AA, Klaus M (1979) The gastrointestinal tract-feeding and selected disorders. In: Klaus MH, Fanaroff AA (eds) Care of the high-risk neonate. Saunders, Philadelphia

19. Fanaroff AA, Martin RJ (1982) Respiratory disorders. In: Fanaroff AA, Martin RJ (eds): Behrman's neonatal perinatal medicine, to be published

20. Fanaroff AA, Cha CC, Sosa R et al (1973) Controlled trial of continuous negative external pressure in the treatment of severe respiratory distress syndrome. J Pediatr 82:921

21. Fitzhardinge PM (1978) Follow-up studies in infants treated by mechanical ventilation. Clin Perinatol 5:451

22. Frantz ID, Stark AR, Dorkin HL (1980) Ventilation of infants at frequencies up to 1800/min. Pediatr Res 14:642

23. Gluck L, Kulovich MV (1973) Lecithin/sphingomyelin ratios in amniotic fluid in normal and abnormal pregnancy. Am J Obstet Gynecol 115:539

24. Gluck L, Kulovich M, Borer R et al (1971) Diagnosis of the respiratory distress syndrome by amniocentesis. Am J Obstet Gynecol 109:440

25. Gluck L, Kulovich MV, Eidelman AI et al (1972) Biochemical development of surfactant activity in mammalian lung. IV. Pulmonary lecithin synthesis in the human fetus and newborn and etiology of the respiratory distress syndrome. Pediatr Res 6:81

26. Goldman SL, Brady JP, Dumpit FM (1979) Increased work of breathing associated with nasal prongs. Pediatrics 64:160

27. Gregory GA, Kitterman JA, Phibbs RH et al (1971) Treatment of the idiopathic respiratory-distress syndrome with continuous positive airway pressure. N Engl J Med 284:1333

28. Hack M, Fanaroff AA, Klaus MH et al (1976) Neonatal respiratory distress following elective delivery. A preventable disease? Am J Obstet Gynecol 126:43

29. Harrison VC, de V Heese H, Klein M (1968a) Intracranial haemorrhage associated with hyaline membrane disease Arch Dis Child 43:116

30. Harrison VC, de V Heese H, Klein M (1968b) The significance of grunting in hyaline membrane disease. Pediatrics 41:549

31. Heese H de V, Harrison VC, Klein M et al (1970) Intermittent positive pressure ventilation in hyaline membrane disease. J Pediatr 76:183

32. Herman S, Reynolds EOR (1973) Methods for improving oxygenation in infants mechanically ventilated for severe hyaline membrane disease. Arch Dis Child 48:612

33. Herrell N, Martin RJ, Pultusker M et al (1980) Optimal temperature for the measurement of transcutaneous

carbon dioxide tension in the neonate J Pediatr 97:114

34. Kattwinkel J, Fleming D, Cha CC et al (1973) A device for administration of continuous positive airway pressure by the nasal route. Pediatrics 52:131

35. Kitterman JA, Phibbs RH, Tooley WH (1969) Aortic blood pressure in normal newborn infants during the first 12 hours of life. Pediatrics 44:959

36. Klaus M, Fanaroff A, Martin R (1979a) Respiratory problems. In: Klaus M and Fanaroff AA (eds) Care of the high risk Neonate. Saunders, Philadelphia

37. Klaus M, Fanaroff A and Martin RJ (1979b) The physical environment. In: Klaus MH and Fanaroff AA (eds) Care of the high risk neonate. Saunders, Philadelphia

38. Lauersen N, Merkatz I, Tejani N et al (1977) Inhibition of premature labor: A multicenter comparison of retodrine and ethanol. Am J Obstet Gynecol 127:837

39. Liggins GC, Howie RN (1974) The prevention of RDS by maternal steroid therapy. In: Gluck L (ed) Modern perinatal medicine. Year Book Medical Publishers, Chicago

40. Manginello FP, Grassi AE, Schechner S et al (1978) Evaluation of methods of assisted ventilation in hyaline membrane disease. Arch Dis Child 53:878

41. Martin RJ, Nearman HS, Katona PG et al (1977) The effect of a low continuous positive airway pressure on the reflex control of respiration in the preterm infant. J Pediatr 90:976

42. Martin R, Okken A, Rubin D (1979) Arterial oxygen tension during active and quiet sleep in the normal neonate. J Pediatr 94:271

43. Martin-Bonyer G, Monset-Couchard M, Bomsel F et al (1970) Artificial ventilation in hyaline membrane disease. Biol Neonate 16:164

44. Murdock AI, Linsao L, Reid M et al (1970) Mechanical ventilation in respiratory distress syndrome: A controlled trial. Arch Dis Child 45:524

45. Northway WH, Rosan RC, Parker DY (1967) Pulmonary disease following respirator therapy of hyaline membrane disease. N Engl J Med 276:357

46. Papile L, Burstein J, Burstein R et al (1978) Incidence and evolution of subependymal and intraventricular hemorrhage: A study of infants with birth weights less than 1,500 gm. J Pediatr 92:529

47. Reynolds EOR (1971) Effect of alterations in mechanical ventilator settings on pulmonary gas exchange in hyaline membrane disease. Arch Dis Child 46:152

48. Rhodes PG, Hall RT (1973) Continuous positive airway pressure delivered by face mask in infants with the idiopathic respiratory distress syndrome: A controlled study. Pediatrics 52:1

49. Robert MF, Neff RK, Hubbell JP et al (1976) The association between maternal diabetes and the respiratory distress syndrome in the newborn. N Engl J Med 294:357

50. Siassi B, Blanco C, Cabal LA et al (1976) Incidence and clinical features of patent ductus arteriosus in low-birth-weight infants: A prospective analysis of 150 consecutively born infants. Pediatrics 57:347

51. Silverman NH, Lewis AB, Heymann MA et al (1974) Echocardiographic assessment of ductus arteriosus shunt in premature infants. Circulation 50:821

52. Simmons MA, Adcock EW, Bard H et al (1974) Hypernatremia and intracranial hemorrhage in neonates. N Engl J Med 291:6

53. Smith PC, Daily WJR, Fletcher G et al (1969) Mechanical ventilation of newborn infants. I. The effect of rate and pressure on arterial oxygenation of infants with respiratory distress syndrome. Pediatr Res 3:244

54. Smith PC, Schach E, Daily WJR (1972) Mechanical ventilation of newborn infants: II. Effects of independ-

ent variation of rate and pressure on arterial oxygenation of infants with respiratory distress syndrome. Anesthesiology 37:498

55. Stahlman MT, Malan AF, Shepard FM et al (1970) Negative pressure assisted ventilation in infants with hyaline membrane disease J Pediatr 76:174

56. Stern L, Ramos AD, Outerbridge EW et al (1970) Negative pressure artificial respiration: Use in treatment of respiratory failure in the newborn. Can Med Assoc J 102:595

57. Stocks J, Godfrey S (1976) The role of artificial ventilation, oxygen and CPAP in the pathogenesis of lung damage in neonates: Assessment by serial measurements of lung function. Pediatrics 57:352

58. Swyer PR (1969) An assessment of artificial respiration in the newborn. In: Lucey JF (ed) Problems of neonatal intensive care. Report of the Fifty-Ninth Ross Conference on Pediatric Research, Ross Laboratories, Columbus, Ohio

59. Tanswell AK, Clubb RA, Smith BT et al (1980) Individualized continuous distending pressure applied within 6 hours of delivery in infants with respiratory distress syndrome. Arch Dis Child 55:33

60. Thompson T, Reynolds J (1977) The results of intensive care therapy for neonates with respiratory distress syndrome: I. Neonatal mortality rates for neonates with RDS. II. Long-term prognosis for survivors with RDS. J Perinat Med 5:149

61. Weinstein L, Hack M, Gordon D et al (1980) RDS in VLBW infants—Outcome 1975–1977. Pediatr Res 14:615

62. Yu VYH, Rolfe P (1977) Effect of continuous positive airway pressure breathing on cardiorespiratory function in infants with respiratory distress syndrome. Acta Paediatr Scand 66:59

Chapter 67

Acute Renal Failure in Infancy and Childhood

G. B. Haycock

Acute renal failure (ARF), defined as an episode of potentially reversible loss or impairment of renal function, may affect children of all ages and as a result of many different diseases and injurious events. There is much overlap with the adult patient as regards specific causes, but the relative importance of particular disorders varies greatly with age, and certain types of ARF are unique to, or greatly over-represented within, particular age groups. Of particular importance in this respect is the newborn period, when ARF is relatively common and may be unusually difficult to recognize. Successful management requires, firstly, familiarity with the natural history of the specific disorders likely to be involved, and secondly, an understanding of the physiology of the developing individual and its implications with respect to fluid and electrolyte balance and nutrition. Detailed accounts of these subjects may be found in standard textbooks [7, 17].

Water and electrolyte balance

Metabolic rate is approximately proportional to body surface area (BSA). The ratio between BSA and body mass is inversely related to body size, so that the requirement for calories, water, and other nutrients is much higher in relation to weight in small individuals than in large ones.

Thus, whereas an adult man normally ingests each day a quantity of water equivalent to 2%–3% of his weight, the corresponding figure for a healthy infant of 3–5 kg is 15%. It follows that serious derangements of hydration and extracellular fluid (ECF) chemistry may occur with extreme rapidity in infants deprived of renal function, and monitoring of these parameters must be extremely sensitive if homeostasis is to be maintained.

The resting water intake of a child is approximately 1500 ml/min per m^2 BSA, of which some 400 ml/m^2 is insensible; the latter may therefore be taken as the basal water requirement of the anuric patient. An alternative formulation for total daily water intake, avoiding the necessity for BSA calculations, is as follows: for each of the first 10 kg body weight, 100 ml/kg; for the second 10 kg, 50 ml/kg; and for each additional 1 kg (21 kg+), 20 ml/kg. Insensible loss may be taken as 25% of the resulting total. The latter formula is not applicable to small infants, in whom it leads to an underestimation of needs. Babies in the weight range 5–10 kg need 120 ml/kg daily, while those of 2.5–5 kg require 150 ml/kg daily. Low-birthweight (less than 2.5 kg) infants may need even more, sometimes in excess of 200 ml/kg per day; however, it is entirely inappropriate to consider managing such infants anywhere other than a competent intensive care baby unit, where such considerations are part of daily routine. The above formulae are summarized and contrasted in Fig. 67.1. It should be noted that however the water requirement is arrived at, it increases by about 12% for every 1 deg. C *body* temperature above 37°C, and by 30 ml/kg for every 1 deg. C *ambient* temperature above 30°C, the temperature at which thermal sweating normally begins under resting conditions.

The normal requirement for sodium and potassium is 1–3 mmol/kg/day, with chloride making up most of the attendant anion. However, since most of this is replacement of urinary output, in the oliguric patient intake should be based on measured urinary, gastrointestinal (GI) and other losses, and measured plasma concentrations.

Energy needs are directly proportional to BSA, and therefore to normal water requirement. The importance of meeting the nutritional demands of the child in ARF cannot be exaggerated, and will be discussed below.

Causes of acute renal failure

It is customary, and useful, to assign the oliguric patient with raised blood urea concentration to one of three major categories:

1) *'Pre-renal failure'*: oliguria resulting from reduced renal perfusion. Strictly speaking, this is not renal failure at all, but an entirely appropriate attempt by the kidney to conserve as much water (and salt) as possible. Urine flow returns promptly on restoration of renal perfusion, which is normally achieved by filling the vascular compartment to the appropriate degree. Pre-renal failure, perhaps more appropriately called *physiological oliguria*, may be found in association with dehydration, blood loss, hypotension due to trauma or severe infection, and other similar disorders. Differentiation of physiological oliguria from true renal failure is discussed below.

2) *'Post-renal failure'*: i.e., obstruction of the lower urinary tract. Provided that secondary renal damage has not occurred, relief of the obtruction is followed by diuresis and the return of normal function. Obstruction in the childhood years is most often the result of congenital anomalies, especially posterior urethral valves in boys, which may present as oliguric ARF immediately after birth. Incomplete obstruction is often missed, only to present unsuspected chronic renal insufficiency months or years later, the kidneys having been irrecoverably damaged.

3) *True renal failure*: intrinsic disease of, or injury to, the kidney itself. Rehydration will *not* be followed by diuresis; recovery of renal function will only occur after resolution or healing of the underlying cause. The term 'acute renal failure' (ARF) as used subsequently in this chapter refers solely to this class of disease. The principal causes of true acute renal failure are listed in Table 67.1. Inspection of Table 67.1 reveals that the causes of acute tubular necrosis

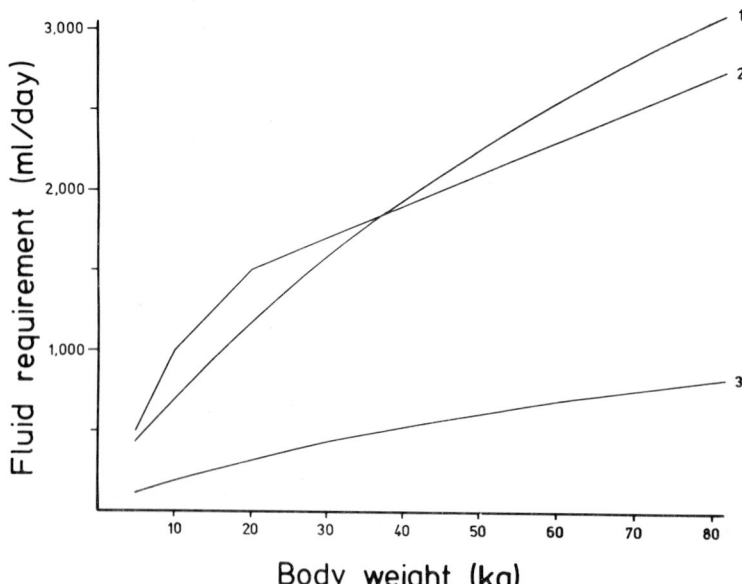

Fig. 67.1. *Lines 1 and 2* indicate normal daily water requirements according to the two formulae given in the text, assuming average body proportions. *Line 3* shows insensible loss, estimated as 400 ml/m² per day, based on the same assumption.

Table 67.1. Causes of ARF

1. Primary glomerular disease (glomerulonephritis)
   Acute post-streptococcal glomerulonephritis
   Nephritis of Henoch–Schönlein purpura
   Systemic lupus erythematosus
   Others

2. Interstitial nephritis
   Drug-induced (methicillin, frusemide)
   Post-viral
   Idiopathic

3. Acute tubular necrosis:[a] Renal damage due to:
   Anoxia/ischaemia/hypovolaemia/hypotension
   Septicaemia (especially Gram-negative organisms)
   Nephrotoxins, e.g., mercury, myoglobin
   Combination of above (burns, crush injuries, surgery)

4. Vascular disorders
   Haemolytic–uraemic syndrome
   Renal vein thrombosis

5. Crystalluria
   Uric acid (following antileukaemia therapy)
   Sulphadiazine
   Oxalic acid (ingestion of polyethylene glycol)

6. Miscellaneous (rare) causes

[a]The diagnostic term 'acute tubular necrosis' is disliked by many nephrologists as histologically inaccurate. However, it is the label most commonly applied to this form of renal failure.

(ATN) are similar to those responsible for physiological oliguria. This reflects the fact that if severe hypotension, anoxia, or dehydration is allowed to persist untreated, especially in the presence of sepsis, pre-renal failure may progress to ATN, thus seriously compromising the patient's chance of survival. The categories listed in Table 67.1 are not always as clear-cut as is often thought: thus, ATN and renal vein thrombosis may represent parts of the same spectrum or response to renal injury, while glomerulonephritis and interstitial nephritis may co-exist in a patient with post-streptococcal disease.

Pathophysiology

The pathophysiology of ARF is complex and beyond the scope of this Chapter. A number of excellent recent reviews are available to the interested reader [11, 15, 16].

Clinical features

These will to some extent depend on the cause. Where because of primary renal disease (e.g.,

glomerulonephritis, haemolytic uraemic syndrome) the oliguria and uraemia previously referred to are usually associated with oedema and hypertension secondary to salt and water retention. The urine contains blood and protein as well as casts. The fluid retention may be severe enough to cause congestive cardiac failure or convulsions, which may be the presenting feature. Specific details of history and physical findings may indicate a particular cause (previous respiratory infection or GI disturbance, rashes, etc.); descriptions of the individual diseases will be found in standard textbooks [5, 10].

In ATN the patient's condition will reflect the causative disorder. Typically he will be dehydrated, ill, and possibly shocked; the contributing causes will often be obvious from the history. Acidotic respiration, tetany, and other consequences of the complex metabolic disturbance which is likely to be present may be seen. Sometimes, particularly when ATN has occurred unrecognized in a hospital setting, overenthusiastic rehydration therapy will have led to fluid overload, but with a high index of suspicion the condition should be recognized before this has occurred.

The natural history of ATN is distinctive, and may be divided into four main phases:

1. Inciting cause or insult (see above)
2. Oliguric (occasionally anuric) phase
3. Polyuric (diuretic) phase
4. Recovery.

In a minority of cases, for reasons which are not well understood, the oliguric phase is omitted and urine output is high from the outset (polyuric or high-output ATN). This variant may be commoner than is generally realized, particularly if milder episodes of ATN are considered, perhaps accounting for as many as 25% of the total. This represents failure of tubular reabsorption of filtrate out of proportion to the fall in GFR; in such cases the urine, though abundant in quantity, is abnormal in quality (see below).

Diagnosis

The usual starting point in the investigation of ARF is a patient who, either in the context of a pre-existing illness or without prior warning, becomes oliguric (occasionally polyuric) and is found to have disordered ECF chemistry, including a high blood urea concentration. The diagnostic process may then be divided into two phases: (1) Establishing whether the uraemia is of pre-renal, renal, or obstructive origin (see above); and (2) identifying the underlying cause.

The first step is of extreme urgency, since it dictates the immediate management of the patient. Unless the cause of the condition is clear at the outset, obstruction must be excluded without delay. It is the practice at Guy's Hospital to perform, as soon as possible after admission, (1) abdominal ultrasound examination, (2) plain abdominal x-ray and micturating cysto-urethrogram, and (3) dynamic renal scan with ^{99m}Tc DTPA. Taken together, these provide the following information: The size and general shape of the kidneys, the presence or absence of dilatation of pelvicalyceal systems, ureters and bladder, the presence or absence of radio-opaque calculi, whether or not the urethra is obstructed, and some indication of the perfusion and functional state of the kidneys. In particular, by these means obstruction may be excluded with confidence.

The distinctive functional characteristics of ARF proper are reduced GFR and impaired tubular reabsorption of sodium. In contrast, GFR is well maintained and sodium reabsorption avid in physiological oliguria. These facts allow a clear distinction to be made between the two on biochemical grounds. Formal demonstration of low GFR by clearance or other techniques, although diagnostic, does not provide a result quickly enough to be helpful in the management of the acute situation, and a number of simpler (and much quicker) tests are available.

The plasma urea concentration has almost no value in this context; simple dehydration alone will produce levels similar to those seen in renal failure due to enhanced tubular reabsorption of urea under conditions of low urine flow rate. The plasma creatinine concentration, on the other hand, is a reliable guide to GFR [4, 12] and if grossly elevated confirms the presence of intrinsic renal insufficiency; a concentration greater than 4–5 times the upper limit of normal for age [13] is diagnostic in itself and requires no confirmation from other tests. Frequently, however, the patient will be investigated very early in the course of the disease, before the creatinine has had time to rise to diagnostic levels; thus, while a very high creatinine confirms the presence of renal failure, a lower one does not exclude it. Examination of the urine is then helpful. The urine in ARF (ATN) has the following characteristics: high sodium and low nitrogen (urea and creatinine) concentration and approximate isosmolality with plasma (250–400 mosmol/kg water; specific gravity about 1010). The oliguric patient with good renal function produces urine with exactly opposite composition: high urea, creatinine, and osmolality and very low sodium concentration.

Various permutations of these urinary and plasma values have been explored in an attempt to add precision to the biochemical diagnosis of ARF. Of these, the calculated fractional sodium excretion has been shown to be clearly the most effective, i.e., the proportion of filtered sodium which is excreted in the urine. This is obtained by dividing sodium clearance by creatinine clearance, and reduces to the simple formula:

$$FENa\ (\%) = \frac{U_{Na} \times P_{cr}}{P_{Na} \times U_{cr}} \times 100$$

where FENa is fractional sodium excretion and the other terms represent the urine and plasma concentrations of sodium and creatinine, respectively. Note that timed urinary collections are not required, a 'spot' blood and urine sent immediately the presence of ATN is suspected is sufficient. The value of this calculation has been documented in adults, children, and the newborn [6, 8]. The tests which may be used the diagnosis of ATN are listed in Table 67.2.

Table 67.2. Biochemical differentiation of pre-renal and renal failure.

	Pre-renal failure	Renal failure
Plasma urea	Raised	Raised
Plasma creatinine	Normal	Raised
Urine urea	High	Low
Urine creatinine	High	Low
Urine osmolality	High (>500)	Low (200–400)
Urine specific gravity	High (>1025)	Low (1008–1012)
U:P[a] urea	High (>10)	Low
U:P[a] creatinine	High (>40)	Low
U:P[a] osmolality	High (>2)	Low (~1)
FENa[b]	Low (<1%)	High (>3%)

[a] U:P, urine:plasma ratio.
[b] FENa, fractional sodium excretion.

The child who, when first seen, has no recent history of a disease or event likely to predispose to ATN, and who is normally hydrated or overloaded at presentation, presents a somewhat different diagnostic problem. Assuming obstruction has been excluded and ultrasound examination shows the kidneys to be of normal size, the likely diagnoses are: (1) some form of glomerulonephritis; (2) acute interstitial nephritis; (3) haemolytic uraemic syndrome, or (4) a drug-induced or toxic form of ATN. If there is no clinical or serological clue to help discriminate among these, urgent renal biopsy is indicated, since early specific therapy of some of these possibilities may influence the eventual outcome. If the kidneys are not well visualize on IV urography (as is probable in this setting) the procedure should be performed either under ultrasound control or as a formal open biopsy; in either case it is essential that an experienced operator obtain the tissue and that clotting defects be corrected first.

In addition to tests designed to establish the presence and *cause* of ARF, the patient should be assessed to evaluate the *effects* of the condition on the general condition and in particular on the composition of his ECF. This is discussed further in the next section.

Metabolic consequences

Acute loss of renal function leads to predictable disturbances of body chemistry. The prime function of the kidney is regulation of the volume and composition of the ECF; the changes typical of renal failure are listed in Table 67.3.

Table 67.3. Typical changes in plasma composition in ARF

Increased	Creatinine
	Urea
	Uric acid
	Potassium
	Hydrogen ion (acid)
	Phosphate
Decreased	Bicarbonate (metabolic acidosis)
	Calcium
Variable	Sodium
	Chloride

The alterations in salt and water balance are variable, and depend largely on the patient's intake during the interval between *onset* of ARF and its clinical *recognition*. By the time the diagnosis is made, continuing intake in the face of diminished output has often led to overload of salt and water, usually with water predominating. Thus, the patient is frequently oedematous, hypertensive, and hyponatraemic. Since patients with ARF are usually ill as a result of the precipitating cause of the failure, they are likely to be catabolic; this leads to increased production of urea and other nitrogenous products, hydrogen ion, potassium, and phosphate, exaggerating the increase in plasma concentration of these substances. In consequence, the *conservative* management of ARF is largely aimed at reducing the effective input of these substances into the system, while management by *dialysis* is directed towards removing them by artificial means.

Conservative management

This consists in adjusting the input of various dietary components in response to the damaged kidneys' limited capacity to excrete and regulate them. In addition, specific treatment may need to be given for the underlying disease, and attention must be directed to the general care and maintainance of the child, especially to his nutrition.

Circulating blood volume, if depleted, must be restored as a matter of urgency. This is best done with blood plasma in the first instance, and the circulation should be monitored by means of measurement of central venous pressure and the central–peripheral temperature gap. If peripheral perfusion is poor in the face of high venous pressure the judicious use of vasodilator drugs is often helpful, as described elsewhere in this book. If circulatory insufficiency is allowed to persist the effects may be very damaging; not only may further damage be sustained by the kidneys, but acidosis and hyperkalaemia may become uncontrollable due to release of hydrogen ion and potassium from hypoxic tissues. The alternative problem of *circulatory overload* can, if mild, be reversed by reducing input below normal requirements, but if more than mild is an indication for dialysis without delay.

When the circulation is secure, external balance for *water* is achieved by restricting input to insensible loss (see above) plus a volume equivalent to measured urinary and other output. In the oliguric or anuric patient whose general condition is stable, fluid intake may be calculated on a daily basis according to the previous day's output, but the polyuric patient must be reassessed at much more frequent intervals; it may even be necessary to adjust the rate of infusion hourly or half-hourly to 'chase' an obligate diuresis. This is *not* a task which can safely be delegated to a nurse; close medical supervision is mandatory. The patient who is well enough to drink presents a particular problem in approximately inverse proportion to his age, in that it is often extremely difficult or impossible to prevent a thirsty child from drinking. In a busy ward the only person who can be relied upon to exercise the necessary continuous control may well be the mother, who should be actively recruited into the treatment team whenever possible.

Sodium input is adjusted according to plasma concentration and measured output. If output is considerable, the sodium concentration should be measured whenever possible. If this information is lacking, the assumption should be made that insensible losses are sodium-free, while urine is 'half-normal' (70–80 mmol sodium/litre) and all other losses (GI, wound drainage, etc.) are isotonic. When interpreting plasma concentrations of electrolytes as a measure of ECF chemistry, ECF volume should be taken as one-third of body weight (30%–35%) in infants below 1 year, and 20%–25% in older children. Thus, for example, if a sodium concentration of 135 mmol/litre is desired and the measured value is 128 (assuming the patient is not water overloaded), the deficit is 7 times the body weight (kg) × 0.3 mmol for a 2-year-old. It is extremely important to avoid hypernatraemia, which acts as an irrestible stimulus to thirst; a hyperosmolar child will, if permitted to do so, happily drink his way into pulmonary oedema.

Alkali (usually sodium bicarbonate) is given in amounts sufficient to correct acidosis, the dose being calculated on the basis of estimated ECF volume as for sodium. Frequently the amount of alkali required exceeds that which can be given without endangering the patient's sodium status, in which case dialysis should be instituted.

Potassium is severely restricted unless (unusually) the plasma concentration is low. If dangerously high levels are present (6 mmol/litre or more) emergency measures must be taken to prevent cardiac arrhythmias; these are listed in Table 67.4. These measures will normally be followed immediately by dialysis; a cardiac monitor (showing wave form as well as

Table 67.4. Treatment of acute hyperkalaemia

---

1. IV sodium bicarbonate (1 mmol/kg)
2. IV calcium gluconate (0.1–0.2 ml 10% solution/kg)
3. Oral and/or rectal calcium resonium (1 g/kg)
4. IV glucose and insulin
5. Dialysis

---

rate) should be employed until the emergency is contained.

Phosphate absorption from the gut is reduced by giving aluminium hydroxide gel by mouth, forming insoluble aluminium phosphate in the lumen. This is worth doing in the hyperphosphataemic patient, even if he is not eating, since a significant amount of phosphate is present in GI secretions, particularly saliva. The low-protein diet which the patient will be receiving (see below) will already be low in phosphate, and little further can be achieved in this respect by dietary manipulation.

Calcium may need to be given to correct severe hypocalcaemia, which should not be allowed to persist, particularly in the presence of hyperkalaemia. A combination of hypocalcaemia and marked hyperphosphataemia will not be corrected by the administration of calcium alone, and is another indication for dialysis.

Detailed attention to *nutritional* requirements forms an essential part of the management of any sick child, and the child with renal failure is no exception. The exact policy to be adopted will vary somewhat according to the cause and duration of the renal failure; energy requirements must be met as fully as possible in all cases, while protein, vitamin, and trace element intake becomes progressively more important as time passes. If renal failure persists for more than a few days, modern practice requires that dialysis is routinely instituted, so that the need to provide *full* nutrition in the context of *conservative* management is rarely encountered.

If the child is well enough he should be fed orally if at all possible. If he cannot (or will not) eat, intragastric or jejunal tube feeding should be attempted, with IV feeding reserved for failure of enteral feeding. The usual limiting factor in the oliguric patient is *volume*. It is not easy to pack sufficient energy into a volume not much more than 400 ml/m²daily, but a good approach to this ideal can be made with modern highly concentrated energy supplements. Table 67.5 shows the composition of a 'renal feed' based on glucose polymer as a carbohydrate source and arachis oil emulsion as fat. Mixed in these proportions it provides 1385 calories in a total water volume of 465 ml (65 ml water being contained in 130 ml Prosparol). The mixture may be flavoured with chocolate or milk shake flavouring for oral consumption, or given unflavoured down a tube. The aqueous phase of the feed is hyperosmolar with respect to plasma, and it is therefore wise to start with a quarter- or half-strength preparation, working

Table 67.5. Composition of 'renal feed'

Caloreen[b]	200 g
Prosparol[c]	130 ml
Water	400 ml

[a]This provide 1385 calories in a total water content of 465 ml (see text). Protein may be added e.g., in the form of Clinifeed (Laboratoires Sopharga, Puteaux, France), which contains 4 g protein in 100 ml.
[b]Roussel Laboratories, London, England.
[c]Duncan, Flockhart & Co. Ltd, London, England.

up to the full concentration over 3 or 4 days. Small amounts of protein can be added as required, with either milk-based protein (e.g. 'Clinifeed') or amino acid preparations; the latter are very expensive and offer no theoretical or actual advantage over protein unless digestive function is impaired.

The object of intensive nutritional therapy in ARF is threefold: (1) To support the child's general condition and prevent cachexia; (2) to minimize catabolism and thus limit the rate of rise of urea, potassium, hydrogen ion and phosphate concentrations in the ECF; and (3) theoretically, to accelerate healing of the renal lesion. There is no experimental evidence in support of the third named objective, but the importance of the first two is well established.

Once the cause of the renal failure is known, there may be an indication for specific treatment of the underlying disease, such as steroids [3] or 'cocktail' therapy [2] for glomerulonephritis, plasma infusions for the haemolytic uraemic syndrome [9] or antibiotics for septicaemia associated with ATN. If antibiotics or other drugs are to be used, special attention must be directed to the metabolism and excretion of the drug in question. If excretion is wholly or partly via the kidney, appropriate modifications must be made to dosage and blood levels, where relevant, should be obtained. A very valuable review of the effects of renal failure on drug metabolism and dosage has been published [1].

The use of powerful loop *diuretics*, particularly frusemide, has been advocated as a means of accelerating the resolution of ATN. There is in fact no convincing evidence of benefit in man, and very little in animals, resulting from the administration of frusemide (or mannitol) after the onset of ARF. A variable protective effect has been demonstrated when the drug is given *before* renal failure is induced, but not more so than can be achieved by simple saline diuresis, and this is probably a consequence of high urine flow rate preventing occlusion of the tubular lumina by cell debris. Frusemide is

known to potentiate the toxic effects of aminoglycosides and other nephrotoxic drugs, and therefore has no place in the routine management of ARF in childhood.

Treatment by dialysis

The general principles governing the use of dialysis techniques in ARF are discussed elsewhere in this book (Chap. 24). The same methods which are used in the adult patient can be applied to children, but various adaptations must be made in respect of the smaller size and different metabolism of the child if good results are to be obtained.

Indications for dialysis are summarised in Table 67.6. Frequently multiple indications will

Table 67.6. Indications[a] for acute dialysis

1. Hyperkalaemia
2. Severe acidosis
3. Salt and/or water overload (manifest as hypertension, generalized or pulmonary oedema)
4. Hyperphosphataemia/hypocalcaemia
5. Failure of early improvement with conservative management
6. Impairment of other systems in a very sick patient

[a]The presence of two or more of these indications at the time of presentation suggests that dialysis should probably be instituted immediately, without prior attempts at conservative management.

be present, and the need for dialysis will then be obvious from the outset. On other occasions the choice between conservative management and dialysis may be difficult, but certain generalizations may be made as a result of experience. Firstly, the child who is ill and catabolic and in renal failure should be dialysed early, since the probability of succeeding with conservative management alone in such patients is remote; further, if dialysis is delayed until the last possible moment the risks are greatly increased. Secondly, very small infants and children are less readily controlled conservatively than larger individuals and should be dialysed for lesser indications than might be required in the latter, i.e., the threshold for dialysis is relatively low. Thirdly, once the decision has been taken that dialysis is going to be required for a particular patient, it should be commenced immediately—delay can only increase risk. Fourthly, if you are in doubt as to whether dialysis is indicated, it probably is. Provided that the staff concerned are properly trained in the techniques, both peritoneal and extra-corporeal dialysis are relatively low-risk pro-cedures and patients are much more often lost through failure to begin dialysis in time than through dialysing someone who might have survived without it.

The choice of methods lies between peritoneal dialysis (PD) and haemodialysis (HD). Both are highly effective as a means of managing ARF, and local practice will to some extent determine which is selected in a particular case. In general, the smaller the child the more difficult it is to establish access to the circulation; thus PD is almost universally used as the treatment of choice in babies. Very small patients aside, HD is advantageous in (1) very prolonged ARF, since the time spent on dialysis is much less and a much greater degree of mobility and activity is possible; (2) in hypercatabolic patients, in whom even continuous PD may not be efficient enough to keep pace with the rate of accumula-tion of urea and other metabolic products; and (3) arguably, in the haemolytic uraemic syn-drome, since the same shunt as is used for dialysis can be used for the administration of the large volumes of plasma which have re-cently been advocated as active treatment for the disease [9].

The basic technique of PD in infants and children is much the same as for adults. Special cannulae are available for paediatric use, being essentially miniature versions of the adult ones. If these are not available, the perforated end of an adult cannula can be shortened with a pair of scissors, the ideal length being the maximum which can be accommodated within the abdo-men with all the side holes contained inside the peritoneal cavity. The cut end should be flamed with a match to remove sharp edges, and the cannula should be mounted on its trochar in the usual way but with the short length which has been cut off *behind* it; thus the total length of tubing on the introducer remains the same (Fig. 67.2). The conventional sub-umbilical placement of the cannula is not satis-factory in infants and small children, allowing insufficient length of intra-abdominal tubing for efficient dialysis. The preferred sites are in the mid-line *above* the umbilicus and in either flank above the anterior superior iliac spine (Fig. 67.3). Great care must be taken to avoid injury to the liver, the spleen, and the great vessels when using these high insertion sites; the most skilled operator available should place the cannula, and the technique should be learnt at first hand from an expert by beginners (not from a book, even this one!).

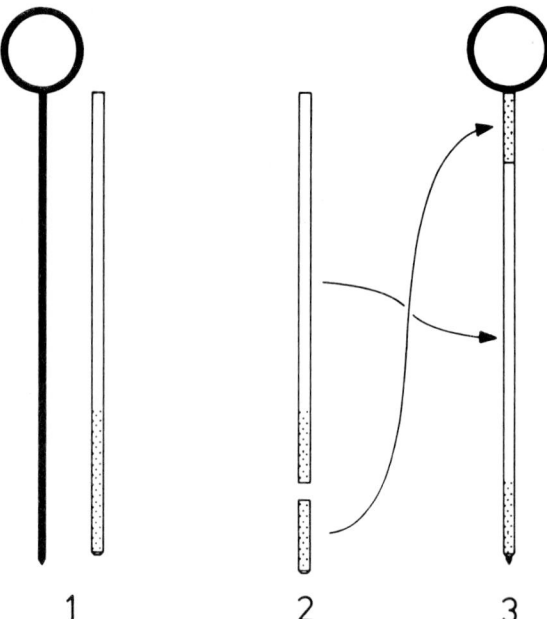

Fig. 67.2. Method for shortening a peritoneal dialysis cath-eter for use in small patients.

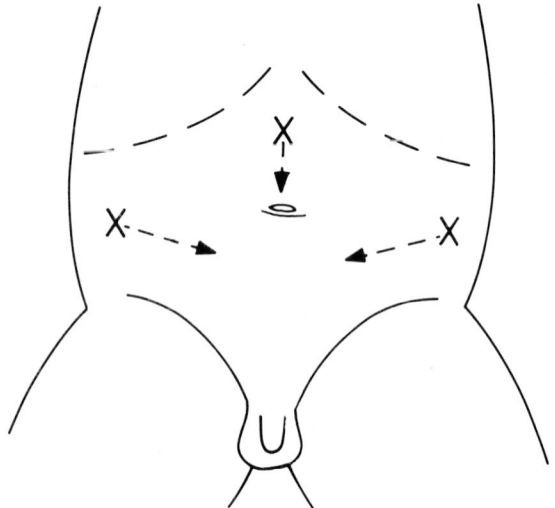

Fig. 67.3. Alternative sites for placement of peritoneal catheters in infants. The *arrows* indicate the direction in which the catheter should be advanced.

The cycle volume must of course be reduced in proportion to the size of the patient. Effective dialysis usually requires 20–50 ml/kg per cycle, or approximately 1 litre/m^2 BSA. The most efficient volume is the maximum which can comfortably be tolerated without abdominal pain, respiratory embarrassment, or interfer-ence with venous return from the lower half of the body. Rapid exchanges, up to three to four per hour, increase the efficiency of dialysis but are more uncomfortable for the patient; one to two per hour is usually adequate. A mechanical dialyser is an immense help in relieving nursing staff of much of the burden of supervision of the procedure, and a number of satisfactory models are available. That manufactured by LKB Instruments Ltd (South Croydon, England) has been found to be safe and reliable, and can be adapted to instil volumes as small as 125 ml per cycle.

The duration and frequency of dialysis must be determined on a day-to-day basis according to the patient's condition. If renal failure is prolonged, a routine of about 12 h treatment in every 24 h is usually satisfactory, the procedure being performed overnight for convenience if adequate nursing supervision is available. This schedule may not be sufficient for ill patients, and continuous dialysis for days or weeks may be required. If treatment is likely to be needed for a prolonged period a soft Tenckhof catheter, surgically placed, is better tolerated than the more rigid 'acute' type; alternatively, a change to HD may be considered.

Larger children may be haemodialysed via shunts placed as in the adult patient, or by the Shaldon technique, in which intermittent femoral venous catheterization is used [14]. The smaller the child, however, the greater the problem of circulatory access, and it is this which limits the use of the technique in infancy. If there is no alternative to HD, access is nearly always possible by way of the femoral vessels, but since this involves the eventual sacrifice of the femoral artery this is generally regarded as an expedient of last resort. Fortunately the capacity to develop adequate collateral blood supply to the affected limb is inversely related to age, and ischaemia to the limb does not appear to be a problem in practice in young children.

The choice of equipment for the extracorporeal circulation can be difficult in smaller children, and is constrained by two considerations. Firstly, not more than 8%–10% of the calculated blood volume should be outside the body at one time. Assuming a blood volume of 85 ml/kg, the smallest commercially available equipment is unsatisfactory for infants smaller than 8 kg, since the priming volume of the circuit is about 70 ml. This can be reduced by improvising a set of tubing lines on an ad hoc basis, but this is difficult and time-consuming. Work currently in progress in several centres should result in the general availability of a smaller set in the near future, which will greatly simplify the problem of HD in infants.

Secondly, because metabolic rate is more closely related to BSA than to weight, the smaller the patient the greater the excretory and homeostatic load on the kidney per unit weight; this is clearly reflected in the development of the normal kidney, GFR being closely related to BSA. The logical solution to this problem in the child with renal failure is to use a proportionately larger dialyser (considered per unit body weight) the smaller the patient. In practice, this approach is limited by the size of the extracorporeal circuit, as discussed above. The only alternative is to increase the time spent on dialysis, and experience shows that infants and small children require either longer periods on the machine or, preferably, shorter interdialytic intervals than larger subjects. Daily dialysis is therefore the optimal regimen in such patients and should be employed electively if resources (i.e., the availability of skilled staff) permit. A further reason for daily dialysis is the need to remove fluid to make room for the provision of adequate nutrition which, as discussed above, may be critically important in supporting the patient's general condition. Usually a daily dialysis of 3–4 h is sufficient, but it is not possible to lay down such hard and fast rules as is the case for chronic dialysis; adequacy of treatment must be assessed on an individual basis according to the degree of control of extracellular fluid volume and chemistry.

Providing proper account is taken of the differences in metabolism and physiology that exist between individuals at different stages of development, application of the above principles should allow children in ARF to be managed with results at least as good as can be obtained in adult practice, perhaps better in view of the child's superior ability to heal damaged tissues and the lower incidence of unrelated disease in other systems. It must be recognized, however, that the appropriate place for sick children to be treated is a paediatric unit equipped with all the specialized expertise relevant to the child's condition. In the particular case of ARF this means a paediatric ICU with more than occasional experience of management of renal failure, especially PD and HD of paediatric patients. The optimal treatment is therefore to transfer the child to such a centre as soon as ARF is diagnosed, unless his condition makes this impossible.

References

1. Bennett WM, Singer I, Coggins CJ (1974) A guide to drug therapy in renal failure. JAMA 230:1544–1553

2. Brown CB, Wilson D, Turner D, Cameron JS, Ogg CS, Chantler C, Gill D (1974) Combined immunosuppression and anticoagulation in rapidly progressive glomerulonephritis. Lancet II:1166–1172

3. Cole BR, Brocklebank JT, Kienstra RA, Kissane JM, Robson AM (1976) "Pulse" methylprednisolone therapy in the treatment of severe glomerulonephritis. J Pediatr 88:307–314

4. Counahan R, Chantler C, Ghazali S, Kirkwood B, Rose F, Barratt TM (1976) Estimation of glomerular filtration rate from plasma creatinine concentration in children. Arch Dis Child 51:875–878

5. Edelmann CM Jr (ed) (1978) Pediatric kidney disease. Little, Brown, Boston.

6. Mathew OP, Jones AS, James E, Bland H, Groshong E (1980) Neonatal renal failure: Usefulness of diagnostic indices. Pediatrics 65:57–60

7. McLaren DS, Burman D (eds) (1981) Textbook of paediatric nutrition, 2nd ed. Churchill Livingstone, Edinburgh

8. Miller TR, Anderson RJ, Linas SL, Henrich WL, Berus AS, Gabow PA, Schrier RW (1978) Urinary diagnostic indices in acute renal failure: A prospective study. Ann Intern Med 89:47–50

9. Remuzzi G, Misiani R, Marchesi D, Livio M, Mecca G, de Gaetano G, Donati MB (1979) Treatment of the haemolytic uremic syndrome with plasma. Clin Nephrol 12:279–284

10. Rubin MI, Barratt TM (1975) Pediatric nephrology. Williams & Wilkins, Baltimore

11. Schrier RW (1979) Acute renal failure. Kidney Int 15:205–216

12. Schwartz GJ, Haycock GB, Edelmann CM Jr, Spitzer A (1976a) A simple estimate of glomerular filtration rate in children derived from body length and plasma creatinine. Pediatrics 58:259–263

13. Schwartz GJ, Haycock GB, Spitzer A (1976b) Plasma creatinine and urea concentration in children: Normal values for age and sex. J Pediatr 88:828–830

14. Shaldon S, Silva H, Pomeroy J, Rae AI, Rosen SM (1964) Percutaneous femoral venous catheterisation and reusable dialyzers in the treatment of acute renal failure. Trans Am Soc Artif Intern Organs 10:133–135

15. Stein JH, Lifschitz MD, Barnes LD (1978) Current concepts on the pathophysiology of acute renal failure. Am J Physiol 234:F171–F181

16. Thurau K, Boylan JW (1976) Acute renal success: The unexpected logic of oliguria in acute renal failure. Am J Med 61:308–315

17. Winter RW (ed) (1973) The body fluids in pediatrics. Little, Brown, Boston

Nutritional Problems

C. Ricour and J.– F. Duhamel

The metabolic stresses induced by severe infection, trauma, or major surgery may create a protein energy deficit within a few days, adding the risk of malnutrition to the already high risks inherent in the primary disease. In septic patients, malnutrition occurs almost immediately. A vicious circle is formed with serious consequences, particularly for children with a severe malnutrition syndrome [11, 88].

Risk factors in childhood malnutrition

The hazards of malnutrition have been attributed to three factors: metabolic dysfunction, depression of defence mechanisms, and malfunction of the gastrointestinal (GI) system. An understanding of these three interrelated factors should help to prevent or limit the risks.

Metabolic dysfunction

This is related to water and electrolyte abnormalities, protein deficiency, decreased energy reserves, and a diminished endocrine adaptation to stress.

Abnormalities of body fluids and electrolytes

Total body water, whether measured by isotope dilution or tissue analyses, has been found to be greater in most studies, particularly in the presence of oedema [3]; increases of some 20%–25% have been reported [40], with total body water levels reaching 89% of body weight in some cases, whereas water accounts for only 60%–67% of body weight in normal children [128]. Some of the excess water is found in the intracellular space, but most is found extracellularly [3, 43].

In the cell compartments sodium and water accumulation is probably due to dysfunction of the glycolytic pathway and citric acid cycle, both of which contribute to ATP depletion [71].

Extracellular water accumulates, for the most part, in the interstitial spaces as the result of hypoalbuminaemia and a fall in plasma-osmotic pressure; intravascular volumes may be reduced by nearly 50% because of decreased plasma and red cell volumes [122]. The ensuing reduction in renal plasma flow, hyperaldosteronism, and increased levels of antidiuretic hormone prolong and aggravate the fluid retention [3]. The haemodynamic consequences of this abnormal distribution of extracellular fluid are an elevation of pulmonary and systemic vascular resistance, a fall in ventricular pressure, and a prolongation of circulation time, which explains the hypotension and bradycardia with risk of hypovolaemic shock [122].

Total body sodium is increased [3], being 8 times higher than normal in the cells [72]; like body water, sodium accumulates in the interstitial spaces and plasma sodium is normal or low. The effects of a calorie deficiency on cellular function together with hyperaldosteronism probably explain these abnormalities.

Total body potassium is reduced, in certain cases by as much as 50% [40], attaining levels of 25–30 mmol/kg (normal 45–50 mmol/kg) [2];

the depletion is both intra- and extracellular, and is related to a reduction in total body protein as well as to a true potassium deficiency. Both factors should be taken into account during recovery, particularly the incorporation of potassium during protein synthesis.

Magnesium is diminished by 20%–30% in muscle [3]; plasma magnesium levels, however, are variable, and because of the close correlation between potassium and magnesium simultaneous correction of both levels is necessary [102].

Phosphorus is always decreased. A fall in its urinary excretion with hypercalciuria and hypophosphataemia signals the phosphorus depletion, which may only become apparent when the anabolic process begins [92].

Iron deficiency is frequent [37] and is partly responsible for alterations in immune defence mechanisms. It also has an anti-infectious role by inhibition of bacterial growth [29].

Deficiencies of copper, chromium, selenium, and zinc are usual [102], especially when there are GI losses. Because of their importance in protein synthesis, glucose utilization, haematopoiesis, and polyunsaturated fatty acid metabolism, it is essential that deficits be corrected [95, 102].

Levels of most vitamins are usually lower, as evidenced by reduced plasma and leucocyte levels and in urinary excretion [31, 68, 78]. Because of the many metabolic processes which vitamins govern, it is important to correct deficiency not only of fat-soluble vitamins but also of ascorbic acid and most of the B vitamins, especially at the onset of anabolism [31]. Requirements should be adjusted to protein intake, and particularly energy needs.

Protein deficiency

Total body protein decreases by 20%–30% [40], and by 50% in muscle [87].

The rates of albumin synthesis and breakdown fall by 50%, and total reserve is reduced by 50%, especially in the extravascular pool, because the albumin is shifted into the plasma [127]. Despite this adaptive process, hypoalbuminemia is one of the most reliable indices of malnutrition. Transferrin, caeruloplasmin, and retinol-binding protein are lowered to varying degrees [81], as are fibrinogen and other coagulation proteins, such as factors II, VII, X, V; because of their short half-life the rapid variations in their plasma levels serve as indicators of the nutritional status [74, 81].

The plasma concentration of essential amino acids decreases by 50%, which explains the fall in the essential:non-essential amino acid ratio. The decrease in plasma concentration is greatest for the branched-chain amino acids; valine levels may be decreased eightfold [3]. High cortisol and growth hormone levels and a fall in insulin have been cited as possible causes of this phenomenon. It is also probable that an increase in their muscle catabolism, as indicated by increased transaminase activity, contributes to the decrease [125]. On the other hand, this mechanism may initially raise plasma alanine levels and lysine and histidine levels remain normal because of their decreased catabolism. The same is true for phenylalanine, although the phenylalanine:tyrosine ratio falls as a result of a reduction in tyrosine concentration [3].

There are a number of mechanisms of adaptation to low nitrogen intake. In rats, rates of protein synthesis are maintained by the reutilization of 90%–95% of amino acids (normal 75%) [125]. In the liver the enzymes activating amino acids are greater, but the activity of the enzymes of the urea cycle is reduced, urea production is decreased, and its excretion in the urine falls from 65% to 37%, so conserving nitrogen. Ammonia excretion, however, increases, because of potassium depletion and the acidosis that is induced by protein and fatty acid catabolism [3].

In muscle, unlike liver, protein synthesis rapidly decreases; synthetase activity decreases, whereas transaminase activity increases, as shown by the urinary excretion of creatinine, hydroxyproline, and 3-methylhistidine [3].

Adaptation to low nitrogen intake involves (1) utilization of muscle protein reserves to maintain the plasma and liver amino acid pool and to assure the production of alanine as a glycogenic liver substrate by transamination of branched-chain amino acids, and (2) the utilization of liver amino acids for protein synthesis rather than urea production. Liver protein synthesis is thus spared in comparison with that of muscle protein.

Energy depletion

Glycogen stores are reduced by 50% [3]. Blood glucose levels are maintained by increased hepatic glucose-6-phosphatase activity and particularly by increased gluconeogenesis, which is dependent on cortisol and growth hormone secretion and utilizes glycerol, glucogenic amino acids, lactate, pyruvate, and alanine [59]. Reduction of glucose utilization also contributes to the adaptation, and if the stress persists the abnormalities in response to a carbohydrate load show the metabolic disturbance, which may be due to a reduction in insulin synthesis and secretion [120], but in many cases blood levels of insulin are high, indicating 'peripheral insulin resistance'. This resistance is the result of several factors, such as chromium and potassium depletion and increased secretion of growth hormone, cortisol, catecholamines, and free fatty acids.

A marked decrease in adipose tissue, indeed its almost complete disappearance, has been observed [120]. Plasma triglyceride, cholesterol, phospholipid, and linoleic acid concentration levels fall; very low-density lipoproteins (VLDL) are undetectable and low-density lipoprotein (LDL) levels are diminished [120]. By contrast, under the stress of an acute infection most of these values increase [63]. On the other hand, an increase in liver triglycerides may account for 40% of the hepatic volume [120], and several factors may account for this overload, namely deficiencies of VLDL, more specifically a decrease in apoprotein VLDL synthesis, and the lack of lysine-carnitine [14], choline, and essential fatty acids [120]. As a result of these, the liver function and clearance and synthesis of triglycerides are critically impaired. Moreover, peripheral triglyceride utilization is reduced, due in particular to decreased lipoprotein lipase activity, and the use of IV fat emulsions in such cases is dangerous and inappropriate [93].

As already noted, impaired cellular ATP production and utilization partly account for sodium and water retention as well as potassium, phosphorus, and magnesium depletion, which may be corrected by administering glucose [71]. Adaptation to energy deficiency is characterized by a relative reduction of energy expenditure; the changes in basal metabolic rate are difficult to interpret, but may fall from 230 to 221 kJ/g per day [3, 13]; maintenance energy requirements may fall from 335 to 250 kJ/g per day if the child is not fed orally [89]. If the energy intake does not supply these minimum requirements then the endogenous stores—free fatty acids, amino acids, and ketone bodies—are used immediately. Any infections, surgical stress, or GI losses accelerate the process. With a lack of energy stores thermoregulation is impaired and hypothermia is a constant threat and can be fatal [3].

Endocrine adaptation

Endocrine adaptation to stress is characterized by an increase in growth hormone secretion during fasting and after stimulation, with reduced somatomedine activity; levels return to normal 24–72 h after elimination of the stress factors. Cortisol levels, particularly the free fraction of plasma cortisol, increase as the plasma albumin falls. Plasma glucagon levels are normal or elevated; insulin is either low or high and shows little response to stimulation [47]. This endocrine profile explains some of the problems encountered when nutrition is restarted.

Depression of the immune system

The large number of studies devoted to this subject is an indication of the frequency of infections in malnourished infants. Progress in techniques of studying the defence mechanisms has provided a better understanding of the causes of superinfection and the malnutrition–infection synergy appears to be due to abnormalities affecting specific, non-specific, and nutritional immunity [19, 29, 53, 67, 105, 108, 113, 129]. More specifically it may be a result of protein energy, vitamin, and mineral deficiencies, acting separately or in association, directly or indirectly, on each of the immune response systems [18, 21, 26, 46, 66].

Cellular immunity and T lymphocytes

Impairment of cell immunity has been known for some time. Delayed hypersensitivity reactions to various antigens, candida, trichophyton, streptococcus, mumps, dinitrochlorobenzine, dinitrofluorobenzine, or tuberculin, are constantly present, as are abnormalities of the lymphoblastic transformation tests [19, 46, 66, 105, 114]. Studies of lymphocyte distribution based on rosette formation have also shown that the number of T lymphocytes is reduced both proportionately and absolutely; while the number of B lymphocytes remains constant and the number of null cells increases proportionately [20]. T lymphocytes with an IgM surface marker (Tu) are the most affected, while the number of T cells with IgG receptors (Ty) is increased [20].

The mechanism and the significance of these various abnormal responses are complex, probably multifactorial, and are probably related to thymic atrophy, with degeneration of Hassal's corpuscles, lymphoid depletion, and involution of the thymus-dependent peripheral areas accompanied by reduction of cell proliferation and protein synthesis [114]. All these features are reversible when the malnutrition is treated. They are due primarily to protein energy deficiency, but isolated or associated vitamin or trace element deficiencies of iron [18, 66, 129], folate [46], pyridoxine [19], and zinc [26] are also involved.

Humoral immunity and B lymphocytes

Plasma levels of the various classes of immunoglobulins are generally normal, which compares with the normal number of B lymphocytes but does not exclude the possibility of a defective humoral response; additional infection may lead to an increase of immunoglobin levels [113]. Isohaemagglutinin titres are normal, but antibody responses to viral, bacterial, or parasitic infections may be abnormally low in malnourished children [50, 113]. The production of secretory IgA 11S in nasopharyngeal secretions, tears, and saliva may be normal [66] but is usually reduced [19, 21, 53, 113], and this may account for the entry of organisms responsible for infections of the respiratory and GI tracts. There may be a correlation between this disorder and the reduced synthesis of IgA by the fewer IgA plasma cells in the submucosae, and/or decreased synthesis of the secretory component in the atrophied epithelia. These abnormalities, which have also been observed in cases of iron deficiency [21], are reversible with nutritional therapy, but deficiencies of some of the B vitamins, pyridoxine, riboflavin, and pantothenic acid, appear to limit antibody production [26].

Non-specific immunity

Total haemolytic complementary activity is frequently reduced, the more so if there have been repeated infections; the same is true of the serum levels of almost all the components: C_{19}, C_{15}, C_3, C_5, C_6, C_8, C_9, $C_{3P.A.}$. Only C_4 remains within normal limits [113]. This may be due to decreased synthesis, increased consumption during infection, and greater anticomplement serum activity. However, with the exception of C_9, these abnormalities are usually corrected after a few weeks of nutritional therapy [113]. Opsonin activity is only reduced at lower concentrations and may then limit bacterial phagocytocis by neutrophils [19]; furthermore,

the bactericidal activities are always disturbed but are also reversible when feeding is restarted [19, 108]. The same is true when iron alone is deficient [21]. Serum chemotaxis is decreased and is corrected after 2–3 weeks of feeding [4]. The significance of alterations of lysozyme and interferon in such cases has not yet been determined [19].

Nutritional immunity

This immune system is related to the presence of ligands with a strong affinity for substrate indispensable to bacterial growth. They limit their biological availability and thus have bacteriostatic properties. This is the case of transferrin in relation to iron [29]. The reduced synthesis of these proteins, especially transferrin, can therefore facilitate bacterial proliferation [29, 67]. However, when the plasma transferrin level is low, correction for iron deficiency may be dangerous [7].

These results clearly show the essential role of malnutrition in promoting infection because of disturbances in cellular immunity, IgA secretion, neutrophilic bactericidal effects, serum chemotacticity and transferrin levels. In addition, infection aggravates malnutrition by mobilizing muscle amino acids, so increasing urinary nitrogen excretion [57]. These catabolic events also release minerals and vitamins, and produce a vicious circle in which each component adds to the deleterious effects of the others [26, 57].

Gastrointestinal dysfunction

Dysfunction of the GI tract in the malnourished child includes varying degrees of abnormal bacterial proliferation, and both morphological and functional intestinal disturbances. These aggravate the malnutrition, and explain the difficulties of restarting GI nutrition.

The presence of an abnormal intestinal bacterial flora, in either qualitative or quantitative terms, is indicative of the changes in the gastric and intestinal defence systems. The gastric bactericidal barrier is modified because of mucosal atrophy and a decrease in hydrogen ion secretion [42, 123]. In the intestine, apart from oral gastric contamination, other factors that combine to explain the abnormal bacterial proliferation are a decrease in intestinal motility, a reduction of biliary and pancreatic secretions [123], an excess of residual intraluminal unabsorbed nutrients, a reduction in IgA secretion [86], and adherence to the mucosa of bacteria such as *E. coli*. Changes in the mucosal barrier also allow endotoxin absorption and transfer of bacterial and alimentary antigens conducive to Gram-negative sepsis, and perhaps to an immuno-allergic process [124]. Morphological changes are variable and may be characterized by mucosal atrophy with the disappearance of the villous structure, a reduction in the mitotic index, and cellular infiltration of the lamina propria [118]. On the other hand, there may only be structural changes of the enterocyte, visible only with electron microscopy at the brush border and in the endoplasmic reticulum [15, 62].

The reduction in most of the enzyme activity is virtually constant [118]. Specific disturbances in the ileum for vitamin B_{12} and conjugated bile acid absorption [4, 123], and that in the colon for sodium–potassium exchange and water absorption [118], are also frequent. Conditions for defective digestion and malabsorption of nutrients, water, and electrolytes are therefore present.

Appropriate nutrition

Principles

The infective, metabolic, and GI problems that have been outlined must be constantly taken account of during treatment. The risk of infection, an expression of both specific and non-specific depression in immunity, may jeopardize the prognosis and aggravate nutritional problems at any time. Clinical and paraclinical investigations must be performed repeatedly, to look for widening foci of infection (respiratory, GI, skeletal, and urinary) and for their systemic spread. When a localized or systemic infection is identified, specific treatment is urgently required. The routine use of antibiotics in the absence of bacteriologic evidence in a malnourished child is inadvisable, antibiotics should be given if sufficient indirect evidence points to the likelihood of an infection [3]. Active intestinal parasitosis should of course be vigorously treated. The evidence or suspicion of an infection is an essential factor in modifying water, electrolyte, and nutrient intake and also of the choice of the feeding technique.

The metabolic risk requires changes in therapeutic decisions to avoid serious iatrogenic accidents both at the beginning and later.

The first 72 h are governed by the following emergency measures: the risk of water and sodium intoxication because of their excessive retention, accentuated by an abnormal secretion of vasopressin and aldosterone, requires a reduction in their intake except in cases of acute dehydration. This reduction aims to compensate for insensible and possible GI losses, but it should be emphasized that losses into a third sector, intraperitoneal or intestinal, can be very difficult to recognize.

Correction of potassium depletion is essential but should be achieved gradually with careful diuresis and cardiac monitoring. It can be dangerous to correct the deficit completely at the stage at which the capacity for fixing potassium is especially low, because the protein mass is reduced; excessive intake leads to the risk of hyperkalaemia [89].

Haemodynamic problems may require infusions of albumin, plasma, or blood depending on the haematocrit and CVP recording, and if the cardiorespiratory response is poor, MV may be required.

Oral or parenteral carbohydrates are necessary for blood glucose homeostasis, but the risk of hyperglycaemia with osmotic diuresis and hyperosmolar coma must be avoided [91]. Energy intake at this stage can only cover maintenance needs, and has to be in the form of carbohydrate because of the limited clearance of plasma triglycerides [93].

It is illusory and dangerous to attempt to suppress protein catabolism under these conditions of stress and a relative lack of energy. Excessive protein intake may lead to hyperammonaemia and/or acidosis by exceeding renal clearance capacity for H^+ ions and for phosphate. An intake of 0.5–1 g parenteral amino acids or oral peptides per kilogram combines to maintain the plasma amino acid pool by compensating for their digestive losses.

Maintenance of a stable body temperature between 36.5 °C and 37 °C by appropriate warming techniques, and the prevention of cutaneous lesions and musculotendinous contractions by careful nursing are all essential.

On subsequent days, following the initial period of stress, it is important to correct the protein energy deficiency and the other related disorders. This type of correction has to be made carefully and gradually since the deficits are profound and of long standing. An excessive or imbalanced intake, especially if given too rapidly, will jeopardize the prognosis [89]. It is essential to provide both nitrogen and calories simultaneously and in the correct ratio [89]. Excess nitrogen must be avoided, especially branched-chain amino acids because of the risk or hyperazotaemia, acidosis, and hyperammo-naemia [74]. Thus a ratio of 3–4 g protein/kg to 500–625 kJ/kg is adequate [89]. A higher energy intake may sometimes be necessary but should never be excessive especially if given parenterally at a constant rate over a 24-h period. The continuous stimulation of insulin secretion thus results in an overload of trig-lyceride and glycogen in the liver and in an alteration of the pattern of nitrogen anabolism by preferentially facilitating muscle protein synthesis. This metabolic imbalance can be prevented by avoiding excessive carbohydrate and lipid intake and by establishing a regimen of alternating periods of feeding and fasting which stimulates insulin and glucagon secretion alternately [60, 99]. The increase in energy intake, if progressive (41.6 kJ/kg to 332 kJ/kg per day) avoids acute episodes of sodium and water retention accompanied by oliguria and a fall in urinary sodium and potassium output. It is likely that these changes are related to the carbohydrates, for it has been shown that their occurrence and equally rapid reversal develop with changes in glucose intake [89]. This anti-natriuretic effect of glucose appears to be similar to the antinatriuresis observed during feeding after a phase of experimental fasting [103]. The insulin secreted induces sodium tubular reab-sorption [25] and the alkalosis that develops might be explained by the increased tubular absorption of bicarbonate [115].

Compensation for the energy deficit initiates an anabolic response which requires an under-standing of the nutritional relationships be-tween nutrients, electrolytes, vitamins, and trace elements. If their intake is not initially correct, it is during this phase that a deficit will become apparent, either clinically or in biologi-cal terms. The prevention of these deficits is usually assured by giving them in the following proportions: 1045 kJ, nitrogen 1 g, calcium 1.8 mmol, phosphorus 2.9 mmol, magnesium 1.0 mmol, potassium 10 mmol, sodium and chloride 7 mmol, zinc 1.2 mg. Similarly, it is essential to adapt the intake of copper, man-ganese, chromium, iron, iodine, cobalt, and fluoride, and the vitamins, especially group B. Also, the intakes of essential fatty acids, tocopherol, and selenium in the ratio: 100 mg/0.6 mg/3 μg are also closely correlated.

The degree of GI tolerance during the first attempts at feeding is of great importance in planning. Oral feeding, sophisticated if neces-sary, despite its technical difficulties, should be attempted if there is no contra-indication to the use of the GI tract. If this cannot be done

immediately then IV feeding is necessary with the introduction of oral feeding over succeed-ing days. Digestive autonomy should return within 10 days, but if it does not long-term parenteral nutrition may become necessary.

Constant-rate enteral nutrition (CREN)

The facility to provide water, electrolytes, and nutrients at a constant rate by gastric, duodenal or jejunal routes represents an important advance of the last decade. Whether started immediately or during the later phase of paren-teral feeding, this technique can correct electro-lyte and nutritional imbalance. It is widely used in neonates as well as in infants and children when oral nutrition is not possible or is contra-indicated. The method we have developed and used in over 500 children is described below.

Infusion material

The tube is made of radio-opaque polyvinyl-chloride or silicon; its diameter (size 4–10) varying as a function of the child's weight and age. It is inserted nasogastrically without dif-ficulty by using the nose–umbilicus distance as a point of reference. Its position is routinely checked by epigastric auscultation during the injection of air and the aspiration of liquid with a pH less than 3. Duodenal or jejunal feeding, only used in oesophageal or gastric pathology, is more difficult, and requires a weighted tube, with the patient placed in the right lateral position, and if necessary, an IM injection of metoclopramide (0.5 mg/kg). The position of the distal end of the tube is then checked radiographically. Careful nasal fixation of the tube is used to avoid displacement, and it is stuck to the upper lip, the ipsilateral cheek, and the external ear. Depending on the child's age and the indications for the CREN, the tube may also be introduced through the mouth [8] or via a gastrostomy or jejunostomy. It is changed every 3 days when placed in the stomach and every 8 days when in the duodeno-jejunal area. Only silicone tubes can be maintained for sev-eral weeks and they are preferentially used in transpyloric feeding. If vomiting occurs the tube is immediately moved.

A constant infusion pump is essential, and in some models the rate of flow can be read directly. Miniaturized and battery-powered pumps have been used for ambulatory feeding. During infusion the solution may be kept stirred and refrigerated.

Composition of the solutions

The choice of nutrients varies according to the state of digestion and absorption.

For non-GI conditions it is possible to use breast or humanized milk in newborns and young infants, and ordinary liquid feeds for children over 1 year of age. In other cases, the preparation of the solution must take into account not only the child's age and nutritional status but also the aetiology of the digestive pathology. The presence of anatomical and functional changes in the intestine, whether due to an extensive reduction of the absorptive surface or to an enteropathy, makes artificial feeding necessary. The limiting factors in these cases are impairment of gastric, biliary, and pancreatic secretions, disturbances of the intestinal flora, and malabsorption. The preparation of the solutions should be based on an absence of fibre; the maintenance of an osmolality below 320 mosmol/kg; the use of substrates with a rapid, intestinal transfer and no intraluminal residue, with exclusion of those that require intraluminal hydrolysis (proteins, starch, long-chain triglycerides); the elimination of cow milk proteins, gluten and soya, which are potentially highly antigenic; the use of sterile solution, because of the high risk posed by bacterial antigens and rupture of intestinal barriers; the exclusion of elements that can facilitate bacterial proliferation, such as iron. For all these reasons, to begin enteral feeding it is appropriate to have recourse to an elemental diet, in which each constituent can be independently modified.

Carbohydrates: Lactase activity is nearly always diminished and lactose should therefore be excluded. The same is true initially for the other disaccharides whose enzymatic activities in the brush border are reduced. During the first days, carbohydrate intake is exclusively glucose but its high osmolality (5.5 mosmol) limits the rate and amount that can be given. The later addition of fructose may provoke an increase of disaccharidase activity and so make it easier to substitute maltose and sucrose for glucose. Subsequently the introduction of low-osmolality oligosaccharides may allow the intake to reach 20 or indeed 24 g/kg per day, especially in infants.

Nitrogen: Because of the very rapid absorption of amino acids in the form of peptides, the initial use of a solution of polypeptides with a lower osmolality than that of a mixture of amino acids, such as a casein hydrolysate, is preferable. Nitrogen needs vary depending on toler-ance, and range from 350 to 500 mg/kg per day, or even more in some highly catabolic situations. In premature infants protein intake should represent 10% of the energy intake [106].

Fats: Medium-chain triglycerides whose absorption does not require lipase hydrolysis or previous micellar solubilization are preferable at the beginning, especially in premature infants [107]; intake varies from 0.5 to 4 g/kg per day. The poor tolerance to long-chain triglycerides at this stage is due to a number of factors: long-chain fatty acids stimulate biliary and pancreatic secretions, which promote increased intestinal motility; an excess of them in the intestinal lumen, especially if they are hydroxylated by bacteria, reverses the rate of water and electrolyte absorption and aggravates the malabsorption. In these conditions the addition of cholestyramine may be appropriate and supplementation with essential fatty acids either IV or percutaneously (100 mg/kg per day) is then essential.

Water, electrolyte, and energy intake: Recommendations are shown in Table 68.1. In the older child the energy intake varies from 350 to 450 kJ/kg per day, and water rarely exceeds 80 ml/kg per day. The recommendations for average intake of vitamins and trace elements are shown in the Tables 68.2 and 68.3; competition between trace elements such as copper and zinc has been taken into account in these recommendations; a daily supplement higher in premature than in full-term infants is suggested, especially in vitamins D, E, C and folates [75, 76] as well as in iron and in zinc [110, 111].

Table 68.1. Recommended intake of energy, water and electrolytes in premature babies[a] and full-term infants

	Premature babies	Infants
Energy (kJ/kg per day)	500–550	500–600
Water (ml/kg per day)	150–250	120–200
Electrolytes (mmol/kg per day)		
Calcium	1.0	0.75
Phosphorus	1.0	1.3
Magnesium	0.3	0.4
Sodium	3.0	2.0
Chloride	3.0	2.0
Potassium	3.0	3.0–4.0

[a]Adapted from Senterre [106].

Table 68.2. Vitamin requirements in premature babies and full term infants[a]

	Daily requirements (/100 kcal)	
	Premature babies	Infants
A IU	250–500	250–500
E mg	3	0.7/g EFA
D IU	200–300	40–80
K μg	5–40	4–40
B$_1$ μg	100	100
B$_2$ μg	150	100
B$_5$ μg	400	400
B$_6$ μg	80	80
PP μg	500	250–500
B$_{12}$ μg	0.3	0.15
Folic acid (μg)	20	10
Biotine μg	5	5
C mg	20	10

[a]Adapted from Moran [75, 76] and Navarro [78].

Table 68.3. Trace element requirements in premature babies and full-term infants[a]

	Daily requirements (μg/100 kcal)			
	Parenteral		Enteral	
	Premature babies	Infants	Premature babies	Infants
Iodine	—	5	—	10
Copper	30–50	20	90	70
Zinc	300	100	1000	500
Manganese	2–10	5–10	—	40
Fluoride	—	30	—	50
Iron	100–200	50	2000–5000	1000
Selenium	—	3	—	6
Chrome	5	0.2–2	—	2

[a]Modified from Greene et al. [45], James and McMahon [51] and Shaw [110, 111].

Practical procedures

A suitable environment is necessary if these techniques are to be used effectively and safely. The daily preparation of feed requires strict asepsis, dieticians, and an appropriate work area. In cases of high risk where a sterile elemental diet is essential, sterile nutrients and a laminar flux process are necessary.

To limit the risk of bacterial contamination, rigorous aseptic measures must be used when bottles and connections are changed. To prevent bacterial growth, the feed should be continously refrigerated at 4 °C during its pre-servation and infusion, and it may be necessary for the solution to be stirred continuously to ensure perfect homogenization, especially after the addition of triglycerides and when there are no oligosaccharides. To have a constant rate of infusion a pump is necessary.

Regulation of intake

Whether used after a prolonged period of parenteral nutrition or simply after a brief phase of peripheral venous infusion CREN can be considered in three successive stages of varying complexity depending on the child's nutritional state and the indications for its use.

Initial phase of mixed nutrition: This first step includes the progressive reduction of the parenteral intake and a stepwise increase in the enteral feed according to tolerance.

Water and electrolytes: The progressive replacement of IV hypertonic solutions by isotonic solutions in the intestine initially leads to an increase in the water intake. Its intake should be increased to compensate for the intestinal losses generally induced by this kind of feeding and its tolerance is estimated from the weight of the child, the volume and osmolality of urine samples taken at 6-h intervals and from the plasma osmolality. Sodium intake is also increased and the tolerance and needs are estimated from 24-h urine analyses, whilst attempting to maintain a natriuresis of 2–3 mmol/kg per day. At the same time, potassium intake is determined by urinary excretion and calcium, phosphorus, and magnesium intake are adjusted as a function of the nitrogen and energy intake, after consideration of their plasma concentrations.

Nutrients and calories: Glucose is used at first and the amount is increased progressively and controlled according to the stool volume pH and absence of reductory bodies. In the first days of feeding at least a molar ratio of glucose and sodium is maintained. The introduction of casein hydrolysate usually occurs 48 to 72 h later, that of lipids 5–7 days later and their increase is also gradual and linked to digestive tolerance. During the course of this initial phase, caloric enteral intake usually increases from 50 to 300 kJ/kg per day over a week.

The second phase of exclusive CREN: The following qualitative and quantitative changes are now gradually carried out: fructose is added to the glucose, in proportions of 1/3 and 2/3; disaccharides are then introduced, starting with maltose. Simultaneously, nitrogen and lipids are increased, usually allowing 500–600 kJ/kg per day to be reached in the infant in 10–18 days. During this period the introduction of oligosaccharides precedes that of such synthetic preparations as Nutramigen and Pregestimil or even breast milk, all of which replace the basic solutes in 10–15 days.

The weaning period: The duration of this stage varies from 8 days to several weeks. It is facilitated by the maintenance of the suckling and swallowing functions during the period of CREN, which is usually simple if the duration of CREN does not exceed 4 months. It includes a period of continuous night-time feeding supplemented by five or six meals in the daytime until the volume of the latter reaches 50% of the total intake.

Results and prevention of complications

In our experience, of 500 children treated in this way, 10% died because of the serious nature of their initial pathology; in all other cases, the results were positive. Infants under 1 year of age gained 25 g per day on average, grew 2–3 cm per month, and had cranial circumference increases of 1.5 cm per month. All the children were able to return to fractionated oral feeding after 3 weeks to 36 months of CREN, this lengthy course being due either to the initial shortness of the small intestine or to a chronic disturbance of metabolism.

Technical complications in CREN are rare but serious. Strict adherence to the techniques indicated and careful supervision are essential. The presence of the tube may predispose to local nasal, pharyngeal, and ear infections. The tube may also be responsible for causing a haemorragic oesophagitis with subsequent stenosis, because of gastro-oesophageal reflux which it can induce. Prevention rests on the use of silicone tubes, the oral administration of a suitable lubricant, and at times the insertion of a second tube for the aspiration of gastric contents during duodenal feeding. Finally, whenever possible, the child should be nursed in an upright position.

Malposition of the tube or its displacement may result in oesophageal infusion with the risk of bronchial aspiration; passage beyond the pylorus will provoke diarrhoea with dehydration and/or carbohydrate imbalance similar to the dumping syndrome. Careful supervision and fixation of the tube limit such risks. The risk is greatest with duodenojejunal tubes in low-birth-weight infants. Pyloric stenosis has been reported after prolonged duodenal feeding in premature babies; this is probably due both to the presence of the transpyloric tube and to spasm of the pylorus secondary to the direct infusion of lipid into the duodenum. GI haemorrhage, perforation and intestinal intussuception have been described [22, 82] with polyvinylchloride tubes that have been left in place for 8 days. These tubes lose their flexibility after 36 h and their relative rigidity predisposes to such complications. Vascular enteropathy [8] may occur in premature babies and neonates suffering from hypoxia and infections, and the abdomen must therefore be observed very carefully. Factors that may be responsible for this are bacterial proliferation induced by the tube [104], and the use of hyperosmolar solutions with an excess of carbohydrate and protein. The use of suitable solutions together with silicon tubes, which must never be pushed back when displaced, should reduce the incidence of these complications, but the risk of perforation cannot be totally eliminated [82]. There are some who prefer parenteral nutrition rather than this technique in premature babies weighing less than 1500 g who require respiratory assistance [8]. We think that one of the best ways of preventing complications is to use gastric infusions as much as possible, strictly limiting duodenal infusions.

Because of the risks of vomiting and, especially, of diarrhoea, resulting from the irregularity of the flow, the technique always requires constant regulation of the infusion rate by means of a pump. Finally, the preparation of the feed, and the manipulations of the line and bottles can be the source of severe bacterial GI infection in high-risk children; and bacteriological control of samples of the solute is mandatory [104].

Metabolic problems. The tolerance of this constant-rate enteral infusion is satisfactory if the supervision is rigorous. No overloading or water and electrolyte depletion should occur and the regularity of the infusion maintains a stable blood sugar level, which is also characterized by low and stable insulin and glucagon levels throughout 24 h [97]. However, hypo- or hyperglycaemia may occur and a high level of suspicion must be maintained.

At the intestinal level, there is reduction of the anatomical or functional absorptive surface. Constant infusion of elemental diets increases the intestinal utilization of nitrogen, calcium, phosphorus, sodium, and potassium above that with discontinuous feeding; the stool volume is markedly reduced [97]. Its effectiveness is probably due to a reduction in gastric acid and peptic secretion with a decrease in vagal response and induced hypergastrinaemia and a reduction of exocrine pancreatic and biliary secretions [61, 97]. Although the absorptive functions of the proximal small intestine are preserved, in the distal small intestine and colon there is a preservation of histologic structure but a reduction of enzyme hydrolysis and transfer activities; in animals a concentration of DNA and proteins in the mucosa is reduced [77]. A decrease in luminal flora has been noted [130] and there is reduced muscle activity with a slowing of gastric emptying [17]. Under these conditions, especially if CREN is prolonged, it is necessary gradually to re-induce secretory function, motility, and intestinal function by using polymeric and fractionated feeds.

Indications

CREN, whether used as a follow-up to parenteral nutrition or the first step in renutrition, or simply to provide support when oral feeding has become impossible, can be considered in two different contexts, namely in digestive and extradigestive pathology.

During digestive disturbances, gastric CREN is preferred in most instances. The effect on severe, protracted diarrhoeas is particularly favourable if the technique is instituted sufficiently early. A number of serious cholera-like syndromes in older children, which occur in association with travel, respond, to CREN when it is instituted early [30, 97]. Certain types of particularly serious coeliac disease, intolerance to cow milk proteins, or specific malabsorption, such as Anderson's disease or saccharose intolerance, may also benefit.

In oncology, serious enteropathies caused by abdominal radiation or chemotherapy are also strong indications, and the complications of abdominal radiation have been greatly reduced [27]. Inflammatory bowel disease, ulcerative colitis, and Crohn's disease are also important indications. The CREN allows correction or maintenance of the nutritional state especially during a relapse; the use of a hypoallergenic low-residue diet avoids irritation of affected areas. It is a good preparation for surgical interventions and may be useful during recovery, especially after intestinal resections or enterostomies.

The development of ambulatory and domiciliary techniques has also broadened the indications for its use [90]. Some forms of chronic pancreatitis, recurrent gastroduodenal ulcera-

tive diseases, and intestinal tuberculosis may sometimes benefit.

In neonatal abdominal surgery for congenital or acquired disease, CREN, usually combined with parenteral nutrition, offers a programme of prolonged nutritional support which has transformed the prognosis in many illnesses and is particularly important in the following situations: (1) Reduction in the absorptive surface [97], enterocutaneous fistulae [79]; and extensive intestinal resection [97]. (2) Functional anomalies of transit, such as malfunctions of duodenojejunal anastomosis, 'plastic' peritonitis after repeated interventions, laparoschisis [32]; and omphalocele and adynamic small bowel [33].

In the treatment of oesophageal fistulas, atresias, and perforations, and in some cases of malposition of the cardia and some exceptional instances of congenital microgastria [97], as after any surgical intervention in a child with cystic fibrosis, the tube is placed via a gastrotomy. Duodenojejunal feeding is then required.

Extra-GI indications have broadened in recent years and can be listed in four groups.

For many it is the method of choice in premature babies and sick neonates. It offers a better prognosis and fresh mother's milk is given, preferably transpylorically rather than into the stomach when birth weight is less than 1000 g [73, 121]. Extreme care of all the factors previously mentioned is mandatory in this high-risk group. Some clinicians prefer to stop continuous feeding if respiratory difficulties are encountered, and to institute total parenteral nutrition [8].

Certain metabolic disorders provide rare indications for its use: amino-acidopathies (leucinosis, methylmalonic proprionic acidaemia); glycogenosis [35], resistant hypoglycaemia [56]; marked hypercholesterolaemia, cystinosis, and congenital nephrotic syndrome, in all of which it improves the management.

More frequent are cases where oral feeding is difficult, or dangerous, such as coma or cardiorespiratory distress; and when protein energy intake can only be tolerated when given by continuous infusion over a 24-h period; and in the presence of multiple injuries, extensive burns and certain congenital cardiopathies.

Domiciliary indications for CREN are increasing with improvements in technology and the elimination of problems of management outside hospital [90]. It should now be considered in each case when the initial pathology is well controlled and does not necessarily justify continued hospitalization, e.g. in cases of subtotal small bowel resection, of primary or secondary problems of intestinal peristalsis, and in certain cases of inborn errors of metabolism.

Parenteral nutrition

Recent developments have opened a new era of parenteral nutrition therapy in children, and it is now possible to maintain nutrition for several weeks or months when enteral nutrition is impossible or contra-indicated. Our experience with more than 700 children has demonstrated its potential for changing the course of both medical and surgical patients. The topics which will be considered below are:

The vascular approach;
The water and electrolyte and nutrient intake;
The prevention of technical and metabolic complications;
The selection of cases for its use.

Vascular approach

The vascular approach can be accomplished in three possible ways. Perfusion of superficial veins [12, 48, 52, 85] is certainly the simplest method and the least hazardous. It demands rigorous asepsis in the malnourished child and to avoid superficial phlebitis, only iso-osmolar solutes should be used, so that the energy intake has to be provided in part by a lipid emulsion [52]. Two factors limiting this approach are the degree of malnutrition or of the infection which contra-indicates the use of an artificial emulsion [93]; and also restriction or even the absence of superficial venous access.

Infusion into the superior vena cava offers the only vascular access in many instances. Considering the risks of this method, we believe that it should only be attempted in specialized neonatal units or GI ICUs. Only silicon catheters should be used, of a size adapted to the weight and age of the child. Their insertion can be achieved percutaneously through an epicranial vein or through a superficial vein in one of the upper limbs [109]. In older children it is more often necessary to use a jugular, subclavian or humeral vein [36, 91]. The cutaneous and venous entry sites should be spaced apart by a 5–10-cm SC tunnel and the cutaneous exit should be protected by an occlusive dressing and the extracutaneous portion of the catheter fixed by a sheath. An antibacterial filter (Millipore, 0.22 μm) should be inserted between the infusion bottle and the catheter and an infusion

pump will assure a constant flow of the solution. The solution to be used must be prepared with strict asepsis after Millipore filtration under laminar flux [83].

Perfusion into a rapid flow venous area is an alternative reserved for prolonged nutritional intervention; the arterialized venous axis below an arterial–venous fistula may be used, but there is a risk that thrombosis may be caused by blocking of the fistula, especially in infants [99]. Perfusion of the cannula of an arterio-venous shunt has also been suggested [112], and whilst such vascular approaches have undoubted advantages, they should be strictly reserved for discontinuous parenteral nutrition in children or adolescents [99].

Intakes

It is essential that the composition of the IV feeding solution be adjusted at least daily according to the clinical and biochemical criteria and according to some a transition between parenteral and enteral feeding. It is suggested, with the reservations noted above that the following procedures be introduced from the 8th to the 12th day.

Nitrogen intake obviously depends on the age and degree of malnutrition. In premature babies, the intake varies, according to the literature, from 400 mg [100], 500 mg [69] to 650 mg/kg per day [109]. In infants the intake varies from 400 mg [12, 91] to 800 mg/kg per day when GI losses are great [52]. In older children 300 mg/kg per day is usually sufficient. Such intakes, which are higher than the needs for growth, cover the demands of catabolism and nitrogen debt. More than this is unsuitable, because with a constant caloric intake there is a negative correlation between nitrogen intake and the amount retained [92], and in premature babies there may be a danger of hyperaminoacidaemia [41], metabolic acidosis [49], and iso-osmolar coma. Such intakes may also be responsible for some of the anomalies in phosphorus and calcium metabolism that have been observed [92]. Qualitatively, only mixtures of crystalline L-amino acids, with a composition close to reference proteins (egg and breast milk), are now used. They assure an intake of 18 amino acids, 12 of which are essential or semi-essential. Because of malfunction of certain enzyme systems in the malnourished infant or because of their immaturity in premature babies, solutions intended for use in these two high-risk groups may require modification of their profile. Threonine, phenylalanine, and methionine are reduced and cystine, taurine, histidine, proline, and lysine are increased [91]. It is also suggested that the ratio of essential amino acids to total amino acids is of the order of 0.45 to 0.53 [100].

Energy intake is closely correlated with that of nitrogen. In premature babies intake varies from 418 kJ/kg per day [69] to 527 kJ/kg per day [106]; the same is true in infants, but in older children the intake is reduced to 325 kJ/kg per day [91].

Glucose is the principal carbohydrate but it is not possible when using superficial veins to exceed 15 g/kg per day because of its osmolality. However, with central catheters, intakes 1.5–2 times higher are possible if tolerance is satisfactory [58, 94] and as long as the carbohydrate osmotic load is increased stepwise without exceeding 100 mosmol/100 ml. It is essential that the infusion rate be kept constant at 1 g or 1.5 g/kg per hour. Under these conditions the appearance of a glucosuria indicates a technical problem with the infusion or some stress, particularly an infection.

The use of other carbohydrates is not advised in children; fructose has been recommended, but it induces a severe lactic acidosis when its intake exceeds 0.3 g/kg per hour [48].

The use of a lipid emulsion, for which Intralipid seems to be the preparation of choice, offers undoubted advantages. The raised energy intake and reduced osmolality make peripheral parenteral nutrition possible. Furthermore, the emulsion covers the essential fatty acid needs. It is preferably continuously infused over 24 h/ 2–4 g lipid/kg per day [5, 12, 16, 48, 49] in association with a continuous inflow of glucose and amino acids [49], especially to avoid the risk of hypoglycaemia. The addition of 25–50 IU heparin/kg is advised by some workers, according to the total lipid concentration and the turbidity index [23]. On the other hand lipid emulsions are not recommended in certain conditions, such as septicaemia and thrombocytopenia, particularly when there is a reduction of the post-heparin lipoprotein lipase (PHLL) activity. Also a reduction in antibody production, a concentration of fat in the reticuloendothelial cells, and a decrease in polynuclear chemotaxis have been observed when lipid emulsions have been used [80]. The onset of infection and/or a depressed immune response are therefore contra-indications to their use, especially in malnourished children in whom the risk of a decreased PHLL activity adds to the other risks [1, 93]. The possibility of displacing non-conjugated bilirubin from albumin by free fatty acids implies that intralipid should not be infused during neonatal jaundice [6] and hepatic dysfunction. It is also contra-indicated in cases of cardiac or respiratory distress because alveolar capillary diffusion problems may arise if lipid particles overload the alveolar macrophages and the capillaries [39]. Phospholipid metabolism, which promotes the stability of the lipid emulsion, produces hydrogen ions (37 mmol 10% Intralipid/litre) [34], and this makes its use hazardous in metabolic acidosis, particularly in renal insufficiency, when again PHLL activity is reduced. Finally, the contraindications include all the disorders of lipid metabolism, hyperlipoproteinaemia types I, II, III, and V; nephrotic syndrome; acute pancreatitis, etc.

If energy intake in the form of lipids is contraindicated then only glucose–amino acid solutions should be used and their osmolality requires that they be infused via a central vein. The prevention of essential fatty acid deficiencies can then be achieved by the cutaneous application of sunflower-seed oil [38] and parenteral injection of selenium and tocopherol [78, 95].

Water and electrolyte intake must be varied according to the age and condition of the child, needing adjustment, for example, if there are intestinal losses. Premature babies need 150–200 ml water/kg body weight daily to maintain equilibrium [100, 107]; infants require 120–140 ml/kg and older children 80–100 ml/kg [91], and all normal babies and children need 3–5 mmol chloride, sodium, and potassium/kg daily. When there are losses due to vomiting or gastric aspiration 8 mmol sodium, 1 mmol potassium, 6 mmol H^+ ions, and 12 mmol chloride should be added to each 100 ml water. In the case of an enterostomy, sodium 14 mmol, potassium 1 mmol, chloride 10 mmol and bicarbonate 5 mmol should be added for each 100 ml water. Severe colitis requires 5 mmol sodium, 10 mmol potassium, and 12 mmol chloride per 100 ml water.

With a nitrogen intake of 400 mg/kg per day and a calcium intake of 1.68 mmol/kg per day, the daily requirement of phosphorus is 2.3 mmol/kg for bone growth and nitrogen anabolism; if the phosphorus intake is lower or the intake of nitrogen and/or calcium is higher severe phosphorus depletion results. This involves neurological problems, hypophosphataemia, hypercalciuria [91] and osteoporosis, an increase in the affinity of haemoglobin for O_2 [119], acidosis due to reduced renal H^+ excretion [54], and phagocyte malfunction [24]. These metabolic conditions aggravate the imbalance caused by malnutrition, thus worsening the prognosis. Magnesium requirements are usually satisfied by 1 mmol/kg daily.

Vitamin and trace element intakes are provided as a function of the intake of the respective nutrients and their anabolism; in infants and older children observance of the recommendations in Tables 68.2 and 68.3 helps to prevent depletion or excess. It is necessary to adjust them in cases of catabolic stress, however, such as an infection or intestinal losses [78, 95]. The needs for vitamins and trace elements may be different in premature babies [45, 51, 110, 111].

Prevention of complications

Technical considerations: Infection is the overriding problem with IV feeding. Its prevention demands careful attention during insertion and the use of superficial veins whenever possible. The introduction of a central venous catheter undoubtedly increases the risk of infection. In our experience it has arisen in 5%–10% of catheterizations. Its prevention demands strict, continuous asepsis during insertion of the catheter, and when filters and infusion sets are changed. The solution should be prepared in sterile air and should be filtered at 0.22 μm. The work areas should be as aseptic as possible.

The care of the child should be assigned to personnel highly trained in this technique. Fever or clinical signs suggestive of infection should lead to a detailed search for a source, together with a white cell count and coagulation studies. Blood cultures via the catheter are essential and the tubing and filter must be replaced after the catheter has been washed out with a heparinized solution (1 mg/ml). Removal of the catheter is not considered unless the parenteral nutrition program is close to completion and in other cases it can only be considered if the patient continues to deteriorate even when appropriate antibiotic therapy had been started. Prophylactic antibiotics present more disadvantages than benefits and are contra-indicated [91]. On the other hand the presence of suppurating foci and/or septicemia in a severely malnourished child is not a contra-indication to parenteral nutrition but an additional reason for its use in combination with appropriate antibiotic therapy.

With good technique, displacement or obstruction of the catheter, or thrombosis of the superior vena cave are rare. Careful technique should also help prevent superficial venous thrombophlebitis and the risk of dissemination of septic emboli.

Metabolic considerations: Most complications can be prevented by careful supervision and the provision of appropriate intakes. It is essential that the infusion rate, body temperature, cardiac and respiratory function, urinary volume and digestive output are continuously monitored. During the first 5 days and also when the osmotic load is increased, urine should be checked for osmolality, pH, glucose, and protein. The plasma and urinary ion controls with the calcium, phosphorus, magnesium, glucose and haematocrits should be obtained twice during the first week, and then once weekly; plasma proteins, albumin, bilirubin, alkaline phosphatase and transaminases, bimonthly. With these data available, and knowledge of the patient's state and age, it should be possible to progressively regulate and control the intake and avoid problems of overload or depletion. In practice the criteria of appropriate nutrition are:

Regular and non-excessive weight gain;
Regular increase in morphometric indices (triceps and subscapular skinfold, midarm circumference etc.);
Retention of 50%–70% of the infused nitrogen;
Normal plasma levels of albumin, transferrin, coagulation proteins and haemoglobin;
Absence of protein and glucose in the urine;
Balanced sodium and potassium excretion;
Calciuria not exceeding 5 mg/kg per day with persistence of a "safety" phosphaturia [92].

Hepatobiliary complications such as cholestasis and/or steatosis during parenteral nutrition [9, 84, 101, 131] are difficult to control because of the numerous factors which may be involved. The first signs are an increase in bilirubin, the transaminases, and alkaline phosphatase; they serve as an alarm signal and point to the need for certain measures. It is important to watch for: a deficiency in essential fatty acids [60], an excess energy intake, especially of glucose [70], and toxic derivatives of tryptophane, which result from the action of sodium hyposulfite that is used as an antioxidizing agent [44]. On the other hand the stimulation of the enterobiliary axis is advisable when possible by the periodic ingestion of a mixture of peptides and long-chain triglycerides, or by the injection of cholecystokinin or cerulein [88]; cyclic nutrition may also induce normal liver function [60].

Functional suppression of the intestinal tract during parenteral nutrition may be the cause of vomiting and diarrhoea when reinstituting enter al nutrition. Again several factors are involved:

Reduction in gastric and biliopancreatic secretions

Decrease in enzyme activities at the brush border, and changes in the luminal flora

Slowing of intestinal motility and gastric emptying [55, 97].

In this situation, prevention of poor intraluminar digestion and intestinal malabsorption is based on a progressive decrease in parenteral intake with substitution of elemental enteral diets, administered at a constant rate over a 24-h period, so encouraging a regulated reintroduction of secretory and enzyme activities.

Indications

Parenteral nutrition has to be considered in all malnourished children, whatever the cause of the malnutrition when it is impossible to feed via the GI tract. The indications for its use have widened during the last decade. But because of the iatrogenic and technical risks involved with the method if it has to be used for several weeks, it should only be used in centres with special experience.

Quantitative or qualitative reductions of the intestinal surface, responsible for severe malabsorption, are obvious indications. Indeed it is the final therapeutic recourse after failure of CREN in numerous cases of intractable diarrhoea in the infant and in cases of the choleralike syndromes in the older child, whatever aetiologic factors may be responsible [98]. Extensive intestinal resections, enterocutaneous fistulae [79], and high enterostomies are elective indications for IV feeding combined with, whenever possible, elemental CREN, so as to provide the residual intestinal surface with the best conditions for adaptation. This is also true of some neonatal intestinal abnormalities where parenteral nutrition allows a successful transition over several critical weeks, e.g. in laparoschisis, ruptured omphalocele, and certain cases of adynamic bowel, congenital or secondary to adhesive peritonitis [32].

In other circumstances, parenteral nutrition not only provides relief from symptoms by correcting the protein energy deficit but may constitute specific therapy:

By inhibiting the secretion of gut hormones which aid gastric and biliopancreatic stimulation and also intestinal motility;

By reducing the abnormal growth of intestinal flora;

By suppressing most of the luminal proteins of high antigenic potential;

By modifying the haemolymphodynamic conditions in intestinal circulation.

The interplay of these different parameters apparently explains the remarkable results obtained by parenteral nutrition in: (a) Inflammatory bowel diseases—Crohn's disease, ulcerative colitis, and some cases of unidentified colitis [117]. (b) Acute hemorrhagic pancreatitis [28] and fulminating gastric ulcerogenic hypersecretion. (c) Radiation enteritis— intestinal obstruction; fistulae, etc. [27]. (d) Vascular enteropathies such as necrotizing enterocolitis of premature babies and infants, idiopathic or complicating Hirschsprung's disease, or the severe arteriolitis seen in some forms of rheumatoid purpura and periarteritis nodosa.

In extradigestive pathology, some metabolic disturbances, congenital or acquired, such as hepatic insufficiency, may benefit from appropriate amino acid solutions [116]. In other circumstances, hypercatabolism and losses of nitrogen and energy are indications for providing them parenterally when the GI tract cannot be used or when the intake required exceeds the absorptive capability. This may be the case in large premature babies, in children with multiple injuries or with extensive burns, and in certain cases of nephropathies complicated by total gastric intolerance or intractable diarrhoea.

References

1. Agbedana EO, Johnson AO, Taylor GO (1979) Studies on hepatic and extrahepatic lipoprotein lipases in protein-calorie malnutrition. Am J Clin Nutr 32:292–298
2. Alleyne GAO (1975) Mineral metabolism in protein-calorie malnutrition. In: Olson RE (ed) Protein-calorie malnutrition. Academic Press, New York San Francisco London, pp 201–212
3. Alleyne GAO, Hay RW, Picou DI, Stanfield JP, Whitehead RG (1977) Protein-energy malnutrition, 1st edn. Edward Arnold, London, p. 54
4. Alvarado J, Vargas W, Diaz N, Viteri FE (1973) Vitamin B_{12} absorption in protein-calorie malnourished children and during recovery: Influence of protein depletion and of diarrhea. Am J Clin Nutr 26:595–599
5. Andrew G, Chan G, Schiff D (1976a) Lipid metabolism in the neonate: I The effects of intralipid infusion on plasma triglyceride and free fatty acid concentration in the neonate. J Pediatr 88:273–278
6. Andrew G, Chan G, Schiff D (1976b) Lipid metabolism in the neonate. J Pediatr 88:279–284

7. Barry DMJ, Reeve AW (1977) Increased incidence of gram-negative neonatal sepsis with intramuscular iron administration. Pediatrics 60:908–912

8. Beddis I, McKenzie S (1979) Transpyloric feeding in very low birth weight infant. One year's experience in an intensive care neonatal unit. Arch Dis Child 54:213–217

9. Bernstein J, Chang CH, Bough AJ, Heidelberger KP (1977) Conjugated hyperbilirubinemia in infancy associated with parenteral alimentation. J Pediatr 90:361–367

10. Blackburn GL (1977a) Lipid metabolism in infection. Am J Clin Nutr 30:1321–332

11. Blackburn GL (1977b) Nutritional assessment and support during infection. Am J Clin Nutr 30:1493–1497

12. Borresen HC (1972) Balanced intravenous nutrition in pediatric surgery. Nutr Metab 14:114–117

13. Brooke OG, Cocks T, March Y (1974) Resting metabolic rate in malnourished babies in relation to total body potassium. Acta Paediatr Scand 63:817–825

14. Broquist HP, Horne DW, Tanphaichitr V (1975) Lysine metabolism in protein-calorie malnutrition with attention to the synthesis of carnitine. In: Olson RE (ed) Protein-calorie malnutrition. Academic Press, New York San Franscisco London pp 49–60

15. Brunser O, Castillo C, Araya M (1976) Fine structure of the small intestinal mucosa in infantile marasmic malnutrition. Gastroenterology 70:495–507

16. Bryan H, Shennan A, Griffin E, Angel A (1976) Intralipid, its rational use in parenteral nutrition of the newborn. Pediatrics 58:787

17. Bury KD, Jambunathan G (1974) Effects of elemental diets on gastric emptying and gastric secretion in man. Am J Surg 127:59–64

18. Chandra RK (1973) Reduced bactericidal capacity of polymorphs in iron deficiency. Arch Dis Child 48:863–866

19. Chandra RK (1979a) Interactions of nutrition, infection and immune response. Immuno-competence in nutritional deficiency, methodological considerations and intervention strategies. Acta Paediatr Scand 68:137–144

20. Chandra RK (1979b) T and B lymphocyte subpopulations and leucocyte terminal deoxynucleotidyl-transferase in energy-protein undernutrition. Acta Paediatr Scand 68:841–845

21. Chandra RK, Au B, Woodford G, Hyam P (1977) Iron status, immune response and susceptibility to infection. In: CIBA Foundation Symposium 51. Symposium on iron metabolism. London, December 1976. Amsterdam, Elsevier Excerpta Medica, pp 249–268

22. Chen JW, Wonk PKK (1974) Intestinal complication of nasojejunal feeding in low birth weight infants. J Pediatr 85:109–110

23. Coran AG (1975) Intravenous use of fat for the total parenteral nutrition of the infant. In: Winters RW, Hasselmeyer EG (ed) Intravenous nutrition in the high risk infant. John Wiley, New York London Sidney Toronto, pp 343–67

24. Craddock PR, Yamata Y, Vansauten L, Gilberstadt S, Silvis S, Jacob HS (1974) Acquired phagocyte dysfunction. A complication of the hypophosphatemia of parenteral hyperalimentation. N Engl J Med 290:1403–1407

25. DeFronzo RA, Cooke CR, Andres R, Faloona GR, Davis PJ (1975) The effect of insulin on renal handling of sodium, potassium, calcium and phosphate in man. J Clin Invest 55:845–855

26. Dionigi R, Gnes F, Bonera A, Dominioni L (1979) Nutrition and infection. JPEN 3:62–68

27. Donaldson SS, Jundt S, Ricour C, Sarrazin D, Lemerle J, Schweisguth O (1975) Radiation enteritis in children. Cancer 35:1167–1178

28. Duhamel JF, Ricour C (1978) Les pancréatites aigues graves. In: Journées Parisiennes de Pédiatrie. Flammarion, Paris, pp 184–192

29. Duhamel JF, Rey J (1980) L'immunité nutritionnelle. Arch Fr Pediatr 37:289–291

30. Duhamel JF, Royer P (1980) Les diarrhées du retour. In: Journées Parisiennes de Pédiatrie. Flammarion, Paris, pp 203–210

31. Duhamel JF, Ricour C, Dufier JL, Saurat JH, Drillon P, Navarro J (1979 a) Deficit en vitamine B_2 et nutrition parentérale exclusive. Arch Fr Pediatr 36: 342–346

32. Duhamel JF, Coupris L, Revillon Y et al (1979 b) Laparoschisis: Etude d'une série de 50 cas de 1960 à 1976. Arch Fr Pediatr 36: 40–48

33. Duhamel JF, Ricour C, Dupont C et al (1980) L'adynamie intestinale chronique primitive à révélation néonatale (à propos de 3 observations). Arch Fr Pediatr 37:293–297

34. Erny Ph, Laval M, Bourdalle C, Gardien P, Didelot F, Cabanne A (1977) Métabolisme des ions H^+ et alimentation parentérale. Ann Anestesiol Fr 18:1043–1049

35. Fernandes J, Jansen H, Jansen TC (1979) Nocturnal gastric feeding in glucose-6-phosphatase deficient children. Pediatr Res 13:225–229

36. Filler RM, Eraklis AJ, Rubin VG, Das JB (1969) Long term parenteral nutrition in infants. N Engl J Med 281:589–594

37. Finch CA (1975) Erythropoiesis in protein-calorie malnutrition. In: Olson RE (ed) Protein-calorie malnutrition. Academic Press, New York San Francisco London, pp 247–256

38. Friedman Z, Shochat SJ, Maisels MJ, Marks KH, Lamberth EL (1976) Correction of essential fatty acid deficiency in newborn infants by cutaneous application of sunflower-seed oil. Pediatrics 58:650–654

39. Friedman Z, Marks KH, Maisels MJ, Thorson R, Naeye R (1978) Effect of parenteral fat emulsion on the pulmonary and reticulo endothelial systems in the newborn infant. Pediatrics 61:694–698

40. Garrow JS, Fletcher K, Halliday D (1965) Body composition in severe infantile malnutrition. J Clin Invest 44:417–425

41. Ghadimi H, Abaci F, Kumar S, Rathi M (1971) Biochemical aspects of intravenous alimentation. Pediatrics 48:955–965

42. Gracey M, Stone DE, Suharjono MD (1974) Isolation of candida species from the gastrointestinal tract in malnourished children. Am J Clin Nutr 27:345–349

43. Graham GG, Cordano A, Blizzard RM, Cheek DB (1969) Infantile malnutrition: Changes in body composition during rehabilitation. Pediatr Res 3:579–589

44. Grant JP, Cox CE, Kleinman LH et al (1977) Serum hepatic enzyme and bilirubin elevations during parenteral nutrition. Surg Gynecol Obstet 145:573–580

45. Greene HL, Vandervorm D, Helinek GL, Nicholalds G (1979) Trace elements in parenteral feeding of infants. In: Visser HKA (ed) Nutrition and metabolism of the fetus and infant. Martinus Nijhoff, The Hague Boston London, pp 377–389

46. Gross RL, Reid JVO, Newberne PM, Burgess B, Marston R, Hift W (1975) Depressed cellmediated immunity in megaloblastic anemia due to folic acid deficiency. Am J Clin Nutr 28:225–232

47. Hansen JDL (1975) Endocrines and malnutrition. In: Olson RE (ed) Protein-calorie malnutrition. Academic Press, New York San Francisco London, pp 229–241

48. Harris JT (1971) Intravenous feeding in infants. Arch Dis Child 46:855–63

49. Heird WC, Winders RW (1975) Total parenteral nutrition. J Pediatr 86:2–16

50. Ifekwunigwe AE, Grasset N, Glass R, Foster S (1980) Immune response to measles and smallpox vacinations in malnourished children. Am J Clin Nutr 33:621–624

51. James BE, McMahon RA (1976) Balance studies of nine elements during complete intravenous feeding of small premature infants. Aust Paediatr J 12:154–162

52. Jean R, Rieu D, Montoya F, Castel J, Alquier J (1973) Conduite pratique de l'alimentation parentérale. Rev Pediatr 9:409–18

53. Katz M, Stiehm ER (1977) Host defense in malnutrition. Pediatrics 59:490–495

54. Kohant EC, Klish WJ, Beachler CW, Hill LL (1977) Reduced renal acid excretion in malnutrition: A result of phosphate depletion. Am J Clin Nutr 30:861–867

55. Koretz RL, Meyer JH (1980) Elemental diets. Facts and fantasies. Gastroenterology 78:393–410

56. Lejeune C, Bouille C, Paillerets F (1976) Prevention et traitement de l'hypoglycémie neonatale par l'alimentation entérale continue. Ann Pediatr 23:699–704

57. Lindblad BS (1978) Free amino acid diets in the vicious circle of diarrhoea-malnutrition-malabsorption during infancy. Acta Paediatr Scand 67:393–396

58. Lindblad BS, Sehergren G, Feychting H, Persson B (1977) Total parenteral nutrition in infants. Acta Paediatr Scand 66:409–419

59. Long CL (1977) Energy balance and carbohydrate metabolism in infection and sepsis. Am J Clin Nutr 30:1301–1310

60. Maini B, Blackburn GL, Bistrain BR et al (1976) Cyclic hyperalimentation an optional technique for preservation of visceral protein. J Surg Res 20:515–525

61. Malagelada JR, Go VLW, Summerskill WHJ (1979) Different gastric, pancreatic and biliary responses to solid-liquid or homogenized meals. Dig Dis Sci 24:101–110

62. Martins Campos JV, Neto VF, Patricio FRS, Wehba J, Carvalho AA, Shiner M (1979) Jejunal mucosa is marasmic children. Clinical, Pathological, and fine structural evaluation of the effects of protein-energy malnutrition and environmental contamination. Am J Clin Nutr 32:1575–1591

63. Masoro EJ (1977) Fat Metabolism in normal and abnormal states. Am J Clin Nutr 30:1311–1320

64. Maurage C, Duhamel JF, Tardieu M, Pham HT, Ricour C (1979) Correction of immunodeficiency syndrome in severe protein-calorie malnutrition by total parenteral nutrition in children. (Abstract) JPEN 3:307

65. McDonald AT, Philipps J, Jeejeebhoy KN (1973) Reversal of fatty liver by intralipid in patients on total parenteral alimentation. (Abstract) Gastroenterology 64:885

66. McDougall LG, Anderson R, McNab GM, Katz J (1975) The immune response in iron-deficient children: Impaired cellular defense mechanisms with altered humoral components. J Pediatr 86:833–843

67. McFarlane H, Reddy S, Adcock KJ, Adeshina H, Cooke AR, Akene J (1970) Immunity, transferrin and survival in kwashiorkor. Br Med J iv:268–270

68. McLaren DS (1975) The fat-soluble vitamins and protein-calorie (energy) malnutrition. In: Olson RE (ed) Protein-calorie malnutrition. Academic Press, New York San Francisco London, pp 181–194

69. Meng HC, Stahlman MT, Otten A, Dolanski EA, Caldwel MD, O'Neill JA (1977) The use of a crystalline amino acid mixture for parenteral nutrition in low-birth weight infants. Pediatrics 59:699–709

70. Messing B, Bittoun A, Galian A, Mary JY, Grell A, Bernier JJ (1977) La steatose hépatique au cours de la nutrition parentérale dépend-elle de l'apport calorique glucidique? Gastroenterol Clin Biol 1:1015–1025

71. Metcoff J (1975) Cellular energy metabolism in protein-calorie malnutrition. In: Olson RE (ed) Protein-calorie malnutrition. Academic Press, New York San Francisco London pp 65–85

72. Metcoff J, Frenk S, Yoshida T, Pinedo RT, Kaiser E, Hansen J (1966) Cell composition and metabolism in Kwashiorkor. Medecine 45:365–390

73. Minoli I, More G, Ovadia MF (1978) Nasoduodenal feeding in high risk newborns. Acta Paediatr Scand 67:161–168

74. Morali A, Ricour C, Duhamel JF, Parvy P, Kamoun P (1979) Total parenteral nutrition in severe protein-calorie malnutrition in children: Effects of branched chain aminoacid supplementation. (Abstract) JPEN 3:308

75. Moran RJ, Greene HL (1979a) The B vitamins and vitamin C in human nutrition: I General considerations and obligatory B vitamins. Am J Dis Child 133:192–199

76. Moran RJ, Greene HL (1979b) The B vitamins and vitamin C in human nutrition:II Conditional B vitamins and vitamin C. Am J Dis Child 133:308–314

77. Morin CL, Ling V, Bourassa D (1980) Small intestinal and colonic changes induced by a chemically defined diet. Dig Dis Sci 25:123–128

78. Navarro J, Ricour C, Duhamel JF, Desquiibet N (1979) Apports en vitamines A, E, C, B_{12} et folates pendant la renutrition parentérale exclusive en pédiatrie. Arch Fr Pediatr 36:121–133

79. Nihoul-Fekete C, Ricour C, Duhamel JF, Lecoultre C, Pellerin D (1978) Enterocutaneous fistulas of the small bowel in children (25 cases). J Pediatr Surg 13:1–4

80. Nordenstrom J, Jarstrand C, Wiernik A (1979) Decreased chemotactic and random migration of leucocytes during intralipid infusion. Am J Clin Nutr 32:2416–2422

81. Olson RE (1975) The effect of variations in protein and calorie-intake on the rate of recovery and selected physiological responses in Thai children with protein-calorie malnutrition. In: Olson RE (ed) Protein-calorie malnutrition. Academic Press, New York San Francisco London pp 275–297

82. Perez-Rodrigues J, Quero J, Frias EG, Omenaca F (1978) Duodenorenal perforation in a neonate by a tube of silicone rubber during transpyloric feeding. J Pediatr 92:113–114

83. Porquet D, Beaune P, Pellerin P, Regnat A, Goris A, Ricour C (1978) Nutrition parentérale prolongée par cathéter cave chez l'enfant. Realisation pratique des solutés. Ann Pharm Fr 36:329–336

84. Postuma R, Trevenen C (1979) Liver disease in infants receiving total parenteral nutrition. Pediatrics 63:110–115

85. Puri P, Guiney EJ, O'Donnall B (1975) Total parenteral feeding in infants using peripheral veins. Arch Dis Child 50:133–136

86. Reddy V, Raghuramulu N, Bhaskaramc (1976) Secretory IgA in protein-calorie malnutrition. Arch Dis Child 51:871–874

87. Reeds PJ, Jackson AA, Picou D, Poulter N (1978) Muscle mass and composition in malnourished infants and children and changes seen after recovery. Pediatr Res 12:613–618

88. Ricour C (1979) Problèmes métaboliques et indications de la nutrition parentérale exclusive et prolongée chez l'enfant. Int J Vitam Nutr Res 18:61–66

89. Ricour C, Duhamel JF (1977) Marasme extrême de

l'enfant. Traitement par nutrition parentérale exclusive. In: Journées Parisiennes de Pédiatrie. Flammarion, Paris, pp 257–270

90. Ricour C, Duhamel JF (1979) La nutrition entérale á débit constant à domicile chez l'enfant. In: Journées Parisiennes de Pédiatrie. Flammarion, Paris, pp 124–130

91. Ricour C, Nihoul-Fekete C (1973) Nutrition parentérale prolongée chez l'enfant. Arch Fr Pediatr 30:469–490

92. Ricour C, Millot M, Balsan S (1975) Phosphorus depletion in children on long term total parenteral nutrition. Acta Paediatr Scand 64:385–329

93. Ricour C, Hatemi N, Etienne J, Polonovski J (1976) Plasma post heparin lipolytic activity before and during total parenteral nutrition in children. Acta Chir Scand 466:114–115

94. Ricour C, Hatemi N, Assan R, Czernichow P, Rappaport R (1976) Hormonal adaptation in infants on total parenteral nutrition. Acta Chir Scand [Suppl] 466/1:112–113

95. Ricour C, Duhamel JF, Gros J, Maziere B, Comar D (1977a) Oligo-elements chez l'enfant en nutrition parentérale exclusive: estimation des besoins. Arch Fr Pediatr 34:92–99

96. Ricour C, Duhamel JF, Nihoul-Fekete C (1977a) Utilisation de la nutrition parentérale et entérale élémentaire dans le traitement de la maladie de Crohn et de la colite ulcéreuse de l'enfant. Arch Fr Pediatr 34:505–513

97. Ricour C, Duhamel JF, Nihoul-Fekete C (1977b) Nutrition entérale à débit constant chez l'enfant. Arch Fr Pediatr 34:154–170

98. Ricour C, Navarro J, Frederich A, Ghisolfi J, Rieu D, Duhamel JF (1977) La diarrhée grave rebelle du nourrisson. Arch Fr Pediatr 34:844–859

99. Ricour C, Duhamel JF, Revillon Y (1980) Metabolic response to cyclic total parenteral nutrition. (Abstract) JPEN 4:420

100. Rigo J (1980) Contribution à l'étude de l'apport optimal en acides aminés chez le prématuré alimenté par voie orale ou parentérale. Mémoire de Docteur en Sciences Cliniques, Liège

101. Rodgers BM, Hollenbeck JI, Donnelly WH (1976) Intrahepatic cholestasis and parenteral alimentation. Am J Surg 131:149–155

102. Sandstead HH (1975) Mineral metabolism in protein malnutrition. In: Olson RE (ed) Protein-calorie malnutrition. Academic Press, New York San Francisco London, pp 213–220

103. Saudek CD, Felig P (1976) The metabolic events of starvation. Am J Med 60:117–126

104. Schreiner RL, Eitzen H, Gfell MA et al (1979) Environmental contamination of continuous drip feedings. Paediatrics 63:232–237

105. Scrimshaw NS (1975) Interactions of malnutrition and infection:Advances in understanding. In: Olson RE (ed) Protein-calorie malnutrition. Academic Press, New York San Francisco London, pp 353–367

106. Senterre J (1979) Nitrogen balance and protein requirements. In: Visser HKA (ed) Nutrition and metabolism of the fetus and infants. Martinus Nijhoff, The Hague Boston London, p 195

107. Senterre J, Rigo J (1974) Les besoins nutritionnels du prematuré et son alimentation orale ou parentérale. In: Minkowski A (ed) Rapport des journees nationales de néonatalogie. J. Gaulier, Paris, pp 55–73

108. Seth V, Chandra RK (1972) Opsonic activity, phagocytosis, and bactericidal capacity of polymorphs in undernutrition. Arch Dis Child 47:282–284

109. Shaw JCL (1973) Parenteral nutrition in low birth weight babies. In:Jonxis JHP (ed) Therapeutic aspects of nutrition. Stenfert HE Kroese BV, Leiden p 258–271

110. Shaw JCL (1979) Trace elements in the fetus and young infant (I). Am J Dis Child 133:1260–1268

111. Shaw JCL (1980) Trace elements in the fetus and young infant (II). Am J Dis Child 134:74–81

112. Shils ME, Wright WL, Turnbull A, Brescia F (1970) Longterm parenteral nutrition through an external arteriovenous shunt. N Engl J Med 283:341–344

113. Sirisinha S (1975) Immunoglobulins and complement in protein-caloric malnutrition. In:Olson RE (ed) Protein-calorie malnutrition. Academic Press, New York San Francisco London, pp 369–375

114. Smyth PM et al (1971) Thymolymphatic deficiency and depression of cell mediated immunity protein-calorie malnutrition. Lancet II:939–943

115. Stinebaugh BJ, Schloeder FX (1972) Glucose-induced alkalosis in fasting subjects. J Clin Invest 51:1326–1336

116. Striebel JP, Holm E, Lutz H, Storz LW (1979) Parenteral nutrition and coma therapy with aminoacids in hepatic failure. JPEN 3:240–246

117. Strobel CT, Byrne WJ, Ament ME (1979) Home parenteral nutrition in children with Crohn's disease:An effective management alternative. Gastroenterology 77:272–279

118. Suskind RM (1975) Gastrointestinal changes in the malnourished child. Pediatr. Clin North Am 22:873–883

119. Travis SF, Sugerman HJ, Ruberg RL et al (1971) Alterations of red-cell glycolytic intermediates and oxygen transport as a consequence of hypophosphatemia in patients receiving intravenuous hyperalimentation. N Engl J Med 285:763–768

120. Truswell AS (1977) Carbohydrate and lipid metabolism in protein-calorie malnutrition. In:Olson RE (ed) Protein-calorie malnutrition. Academic Press, New York San Francisco London, pp 119–141

121. Van Caillie M, Powel GK (1975) Nasoduodenal versus nasogastric feeding in the very low birth weight infant. Pediatrics 56:1065–1072

122. Viart P (1977) Hemodynamic findings in severe protein-calorie malnutrition. Am J Clin Nutr 30:334–348

123. Viteri FE, Schneider RE (1974) Gastrointestinal alterations of protein-calorie malnutrition. Med Clin North Am 58:1487–1505

124. Walker WA, Isselbacher KJ (1977). Intestinal antibodies. N Engl J Med 297:767–773

125. Wannemacker RW (1977) Key role of various individual aminoacids in host response to infection. Am J Clin Nutr 30:1269–1280

126. Waterlow JC (1975) Adaptation to low-protein intakes. In:Olson RE (ed) Protein-calorie malnutrition. Academic Press, New York San Francisco London, pp 23–35

127. Waterlow JC, Golden M, Picou D (1977) The measurements of rates of protein turnover, synthesis, and breakdown in man and the effects of nutritional status and surgical injury. Am J Clin Nutr 30:1333–1339

128. Weil WB, Bailie MD (1977) Fluid and electrolyte metabolism in infants and children. Grune-Stratton, New York San Francisco London, pp 5

129. Weinberg ED (1974) Iron and susceptibility to infectious disease. Science 184:952–956

130. Winitz M, Adams RF, Seedman DA, Davis PN, Jayro LG. Hamilton JA (1970) Studies in metabolic nutrition employing chemically defined diets. II. Effect on gut microflora populations. Am J Clin Nutr 23:546–559

131. Zarif MA, Pildes RS, Szanto PB, Vidyasagar D (1976) Cholestasis associated with administration of aminoacids and dextrose solutions. Biol Neonate 29:66–76

Appendix

List of Abbreviations

AA	Australia antigen
AaDO$_2$	alveolar-arterial O$_2$ tension difference
AC	acetylcholine
ac	alternating current
ACCR	amylase:creatinine clearance ratio
ACCT	acute cervical cord trauma
ACD	acid citrate dextrose; annihilation coincidence detection
AD	acute dehydration
ADH	anti-diuretic hormone
ADP	adenosine-5-diphosphate
AI	anatomic index
AIP	acute intermittent porphyria
AMI	acute myocardial infarction
AMP	adenosine monophosphate
ARDS	adult respiratory distress syndrome
ARF	acute renal failure; acute respiratory failure
AST	aspartate transaminase
ATG	antithymocyte globulin
ATN	acute tubular necrosis
ATP	adenosine triphosphate
AUC	area under the curve
A-V	arteriovenous
AV	artificial ventilation; atrioventricular
BAT	brown adipose tissue
BBB	blood–brain barrier
BCM	body cell mass
BCNU	bacterially controlled nursing unit
BE	base excess
BF	body fat
BMR	basal metabolic rate
BP	blood pressure
BPD	bronchopulmonary dysplasia
BSA	body surface area
BTPS	body temperature and pressure, saturated with water vapour
BW	body weight
CABG	coronary artery bypass grafting
CABS	coronary artery bypass surgery
CAD	coronary artery disease
(Ca)i	intercellular calcium
cAMP	cyclic 3'5'-adenosine monophosphate
CAP	cardiac action potential
CAT	computerized axial tomography

CBF	cerebral blood flow
CBV	cerebral blood volume
CCU	coronary care unit
CDP	continuous distending pressure
CFM	cerebral function monitor
cGMP	cyclic 3'5'-guanyl monophosphate
CHR	chronic hypercapnic respiratory failure
CI	cardiac index
CIVD	cold-induced vasodilation
CL$_{ss}$	total systemic clearance
CMS	cytomegalovirus
CN	cyanide
CNP	continuous negative pressure
CNS	central nervous system
CO	carbon monoxide
C.O.	cardiac output
COAD	chronic obstructive airways disease
COMT	catechol-O-methyl transferase
COP	colloid oncotic pressure
COPD	chronic obstructive pulmonary disease
CPAP	continuous positive airways pressure
CPC	cerebral performance category
CPCR	cardiopulmonary–cerebral resuscitation
CPD	citrate phosphate dextrose; continuous peritoneal dialysis
CPK	creatinine phosphokinase
CPP	cerebral perfusion pressure
CPPV	continuous positive pressure ventilation
CPR	cardiopulmonary resuscitation
Cr	renal clearance
CREN	constant rate enteral nutrition
CRF	chronic (hypercapnic) respiratory failure
CSF	cerebrospinal fluid
CSMI	cardiogenic shock following acute myocardial infarction
CT	transmission computerized tomography
CVP	central venous pressure
CVS	cardiovascular system
DA	ductus arteriosus
dc	direct current
DDAVP	desamino-D-8-arginine-vasopressin
2,3 DPG	2,3 diphosphoglycerate
DHST	delayed hypersensitivity to skin testing
DIAR	dextran-induced anaphylactoid reactions
DIC	disseminated intravascular coagulation

DIT	diet-induced thermogenesis		HFPPV	high-frequency positive-pressure ventilation
$D_L CO$	diffusing capacity of the lung for CO		HFV	high-frequency ventilation
D_M	diffusing capacity of the alveolar–capillary membrane		HMD	hyaline membrane disease
DOCA	deoxycorticosterone acetate		HONK	hyperosmotic non-ketotic (coma)
DOPA	dihydroxyphenylalanine		HP	haemoperfusion
DPTI	diastolic pressure time index		HPA	hypothalamo-pituitary-adrenal (axis)
DRA	dextran-reactive antibodies		HR	heart rate
DSR	dynamic three-dimensional spatial reconstructor		HSA	human serum albumin
			HSV	herpes simplex virus
DTC	d-Tubocurarine (curare)		5-HT	5-hydroxytryptamine
DVT	deep vein thrombosis		HUS	haemolytic-uraemic syndromes

EACA	epsilon aminocaproic acid		IABCP	intra-aortic balloon counterpulsation
ECF	extracellular fluid		IAPB	intra-aortic balloon pumping
ECG	electrocardiogram		ICDA	international classification of disease-adapted (code)
ECM	extracellular mass			
ECMO	extracorporeal membrane oxygenation		ICF	intracellular fluid
ECS	extracellular space		ICP	intracranial pressure
ECT	emission computerized tomography		ICU	intensive care/therapy unit
ECW	extracellular water		IDA	iminodiacetic acid derivatives
EDTA	calcium disodium edetate		I:E	inspiration: expiration time ratio
EEG	electroencephalogram		IFP	interstitial fluid pressure
EFA	essential fatty acids		IM	intramuscular
EPAP	expiratory positive airway pressure		IMV	intermittent mandatory ventilation
ERCP	endoscopic retrograde cholangio-pancreatogram		INPV	intermittent negative pressure ventilation
ESR	erythrocyte sedimentation rate		IP	intraperitoneal
EVLW	extravascular lung water		IPPV	intermittent positive pressure ventilation
EVR	endocardial viability ratio			
			IRV	inverse ratio ventilation
			IS	incentive spirometer
FDP	fibrinogen degradation product		ISDN	isosorbide dinitrate
FENa	fractional sodium excretion		ISS	injury severity score
FET	forced expiratory technique		IV	intravenous
FEV_1	forced expiratory volume in one second		IVC	intravascular coagulation
FFA	free fatty acids		IVP	intravenous pyelography
FFP	fresh frozen plasma		IVU	intravenous urography
$F_I O_2$	fraction of inspired oxygen			
FRC	functional residual capacity		K_e	total exchangeable potassium
FUT	fibrinogen uptake tests		K_m	Michaelis constant
FWHM	full-width half maximum			

GAG	glycosaminoglycan		LAD	left anterior descending
GFR	glomerular filtration rate		LAO	left anterior oblique
GI	gastro-intestinal		LBM	lean body mass
GOT	glutamic-oxaloacetic transaminase		LDL	low-density lipoproteins
G6P	glucose-6-phosphate		LFPPV-ECCO$_2$R	low-frequency positive-pressure ventilation with extracorporeal CO_2 removal
GPT	glutamic-pyruvic transaminase			
GU	genito-urinary		LMCA	left main coronary artery
GX	glycinexylidide		LPEP/LVET	left ventricular pre-ejection period/left ventricular ejection time
			L:S	lecithin: sphingomyelin
HAFOE	high air flow with O_2 enrichment		LVEDP	left ventricular end-diastolic pressure
Hb	haemoglobin			
HBA	Australia antigen positive hepatitis			
HBD	hydroxybutyrate dehydrogenase		MAO	monoamine oxidase
HD	haemodialysis		MAP	mean airway pressure
HES	hydroxyethyl starch		MAST	military anti-shock trousers
HFO	high-frequency oscillation		MDF	myocardial depressant factor

MEGX	monoethyl glycinexylidide
MHP	microvascular hydrostatic pressure
MMV	mandatory minute volume
$\bar{M}_n$	average molecular number
MPI	myocardial perfusion imaging
MSOF	multiple system organ failure
MUGA	multiple gated acquisition images
MV	mechanical ventilation
$\bar{M}_w$	average molecular weight
Na_e	total exchangeable sodium
NAPA	n-acetyl procainamide
NBT	nitroblue tetrazolium
NDIR	non-dispersive infra-red analysis
NST	non-shivering thermogenesis
O_2	oxygen
ODC	O_2 dissociation curve
OPC	overall performance category
PAC	premature atrial contraction
$PaCO_2$	arterial carbon dioxide tension
PAEDP	pulmonary artery end-diastolic pressure
PAF	platelet activating factor
PAH	pulmonary artery hypertension
PAO_2	arterial oxygen tension
PAP	pulmonary artery pressure
PBF	pulmonary blood flow
PCO_2	carbon dioxide tension
PCP	pulmonary capillary pressure
PCWP	pulmonary capillary wedge pressure
PD	peritoneal dialysis
PDA	patent ductus arteriosus
PDE	phosphodiesterase
PE	pulmonary edema
PEEP	positive end-expiratory pressure
PFC	persistent fetal circulation
PGE1	prostaglandin E1
PGI_2	prostacyclin
PHILL	post-heparin lipoprotein lipase
PIP	peak inspiratory pressure
PMN	polymorphonuclear leucocyte
PNMT	phosphoethanolamine-N-methyl transferase
PO	per os
PO_2	oxygen tension
POAH	pre-optic region of anterior part of hypothalamus
POB	phenoxybenzamine
PPC	postoperative pulmonary complications
PPF	plasma protein fraction
$P_{50}PO_2$	oxygen tension necessary to produce 50% saturation of Hb
PPS	pasteurized protein solution
P_{ss}	plasma steady-state concentration
PTH	parathyroid hormone
PTLF	passive transferable lethal factor
PTT	prothrombin time

PV	plasma volume
P/V	perfusion/ventilation
$P_{\bar{v}}O_2$	mixed venous oxygen tension
PVR	pulmonary vascular resistance
$\dot{Q}$	distribution (perfusion)
$\dot{Q}_S$	physiological shunt
$\dot{Q}_S/\dot{Q}_T$	intrapulmonary shunt fraction
$\dot{Q}_{VA}/\dot{Q}_T$	venous admixture
$\dot{Q}_T$	cardiac output
R	relaxed (Hb)
RAP	right atrial pressure
RAST	radio-allergo-solvent test
RBF	renal blood flow
RDS	respiratory distress syndrome
REM	rapid eye movement
RISA	^{125}I-labelled human serum albumin
RLF	retrolental fibroplasia
RNV	radionuclide venography
RPEP/ RVET	right ventricular pre-ejection period/ right ventricular ejection time
RPGN	rapidly progressive glomerulonephritis
RVT	renal vein thrombosis
S.A.I.M.R.	South African Institute for Medical Research
SAP	systemic arterial pressure
$satHbO_2$	oxygen saturation
SBP	systolic blood pressure
SC	subcutaneous
SCI	spinal cord injury
SCN	thiocyanate
SE	status epilepticus
SER	somatosensory cortically evoked responses
SGOT	serum glutamic oxalo-acetic transaminase
SIMV	synchronized IMV (qv.)
SMA	superior mesenteric artery
SNP	sodium nitroprusside
SRS-A	slow-reacting substance of anaphylaxis
STPD	standard temperature and pressure, dry
T	tense (Hb)
T_3	tri-iodothyronine
T_4	thyroxine
TA	titratable acid
TBW	total body water
$tcPCO_2$	transcutaneous CO_2 tension
$tcPO_2$	transcutaneous O_2 tension
THAM	tris-(hydroxymethyl) aminomethane
T_h	temperature of hypothalamus
TMP-SMX	trimethoprim and sulphamethoxazole
TNG	trinitroglycerin
TNZ	thermoneutral zone
TPN	total parenteral nutrition
T_s	set-point temperature

TSH	thyroid-stimulating hormone	$\dot{V}_E$	expired minimum volume
TTI	tension time index	VEB	ventricular ectopic beats
TRH	thyrotrophin-releasing hormone	VEDP	ventricular end-diastolic pressure
		VF	ventricular fibrillation
		VFP	ventricular filling pressure
U/P	urine/plasma	VIP	vaso-active intestinal peptide
$\dot{V}$	ventilation	VLDL	very low-density lipoproteins
V_A	alveolar volume	VMA	vanilmandelic acid
$\dot{V}_A$	alveolar ventilation	VMC	vasomotor centre
$\dot{V}_A/\dot{Q}$	ventilation: perfusion ratio	$\dot{V}O_2$	oxygen consumption
V_C	blood volume of the capillary bed	V_T	tidal volume
V_D	anatomical dead space		
$\dot{V}_D$	dead space ventilation		
VD	volume of distribution	WBC	white blood cell
V_D/V_T	dead space to tidal volume ratio	WCC	white cell count

Subject Index